FOURTH EDITION

Moore | Linscott

Vattoth | Koch | Jhaveri | Nagaraj | Ross

Diagnostic Imaging
Pediatric Neuroradiology

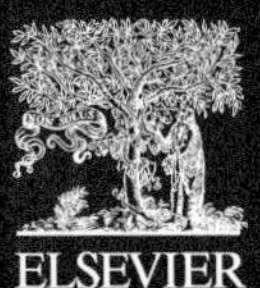

ELSEVIER

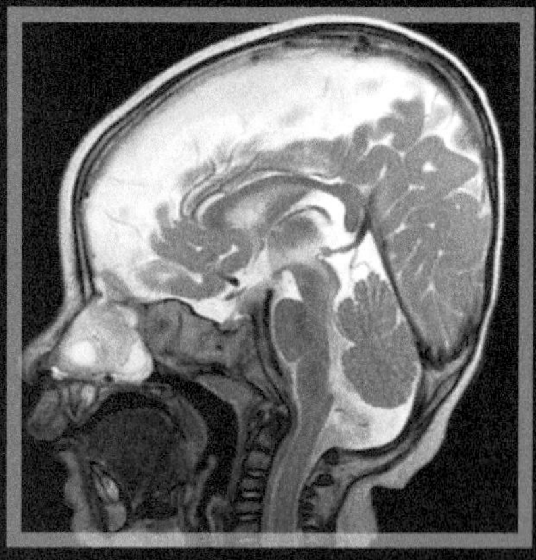

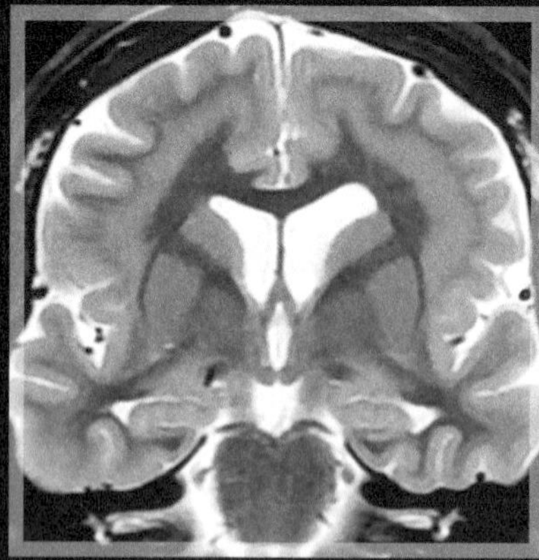

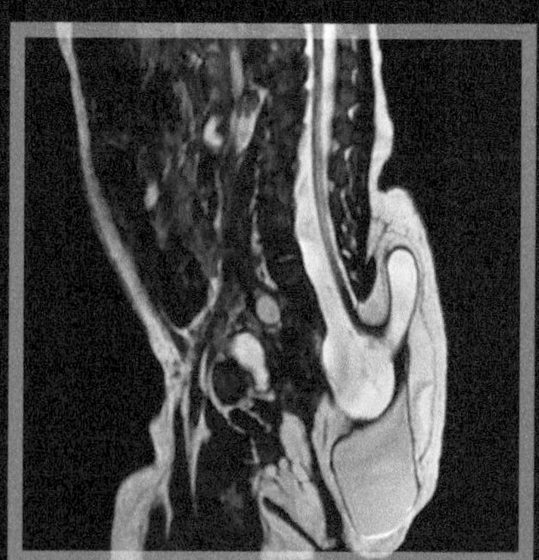

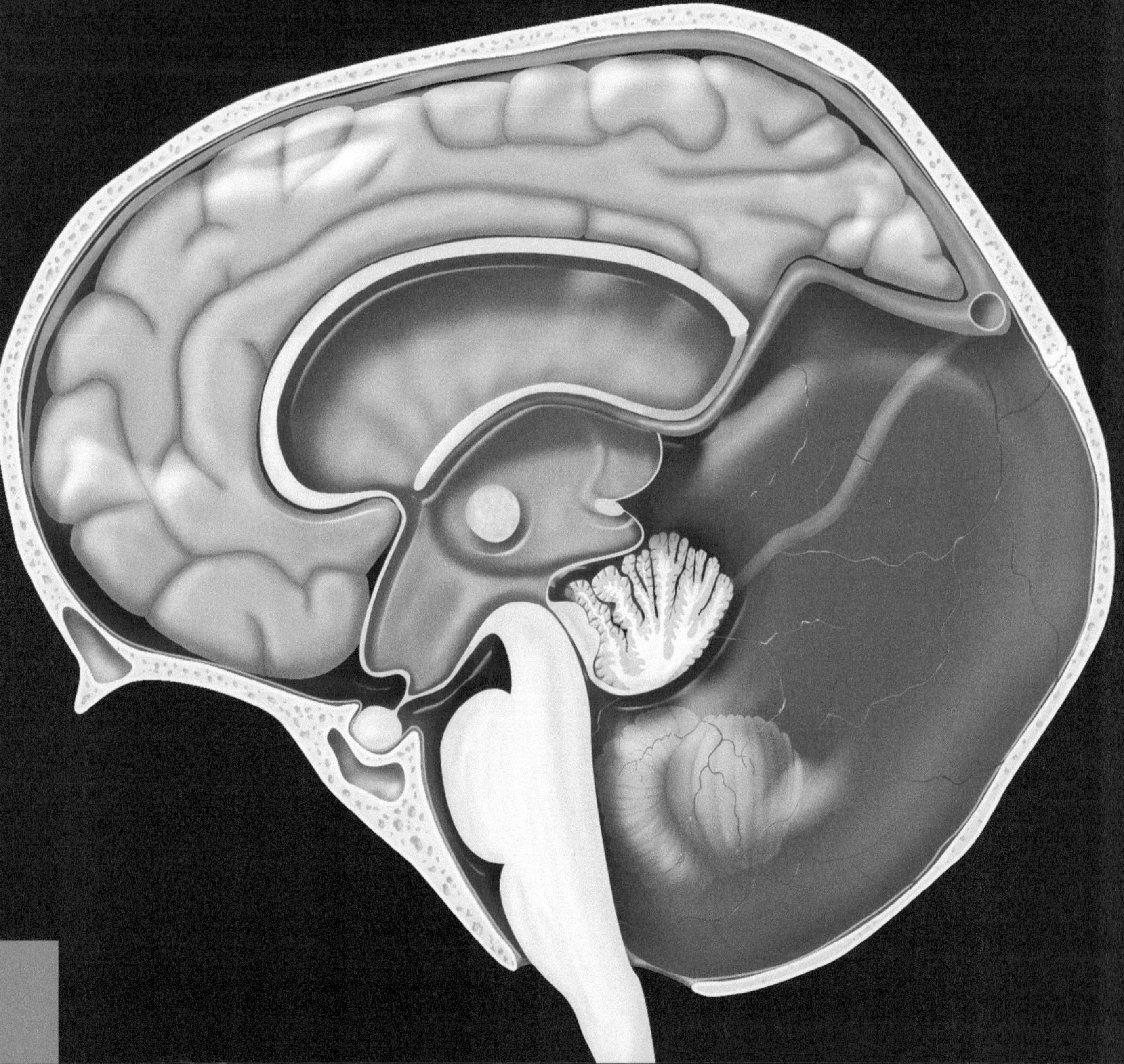

Diagnostic Imaging

Pediatric Neuroradiology

FOURTH EDITION

Kevin R. Moore, MD

Pediatric Radiologist and Neuroradiologist
Intermountain Pediatric Imaging
Primary Children's Hospital
Adjunct Professor of Radiology
University of Utah School of Medicine
Salt Lake City, Utah

Luke L. Linscott, MD

Pediatric Radiologist and Neuroradiologist
Chair, Department of Medical Imaging
Primary Children's Hospital
Adjunct Associate Professor of Radiology
University of Utah School of Medicine
Salt Lake City, Utah

Elsevier
1600 John F. Kennedy Blvd.
Ste 1800
Philadelphia, PA 19103-2899

DIAGNOSTIC IMAGING: PEDIATRIC NEURORADIOLOGY, FOURTH EDITION ISBN: 978-0-443-23492-7

Notices

Practitioners and researchers must always rely on their own experience and knowledge in evaluating and using any information, methods, compounds or experiments described herein. Because of rapid advances in the medical sciences, in particular, independent verification of diagnoses and drug dosages should be made. To the fullest extent of the law, no responsibility is assumed by Elsevier, authors, editors or contributors for any injury and/or damage to persons or property as a matter of products liability, negligence or otherwise, or from any use or operation of any methods, products, instructions, or ideas contained in the material herein.

Previous edition copyrighted 2020.

Library of Congress Control Number: 2024931135

Printed in Great Britain

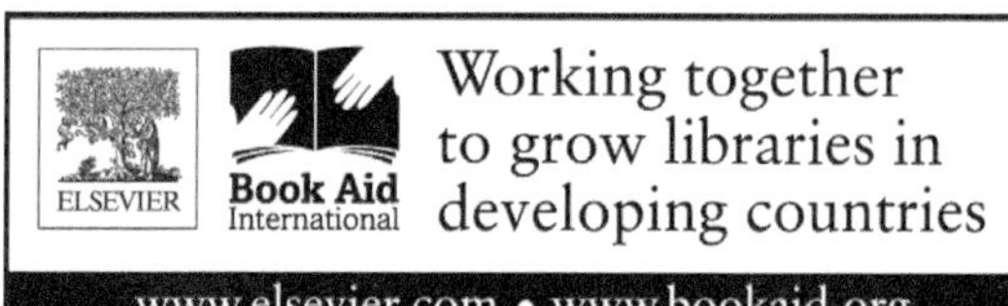

Last digit is the print number: 9 8 7 6 5 4 3 2

Dedications

You hold the fourth edition of Diagnostic Imaging: Pediatric Neuroradiology, *successor to the three highly successful editions that preceded it. Building on past editions of these excellent books, our author team has focused our attention toward both refining and updating the previously written chapters, as well as adding new introductory and diagnosis chapters to introduce important, but previously unknown (or misunderstood), disorders. Many new images have been added to reflect advances in imaging quality and techniques as well as to expand the portrayal of disease variants.*

I have been fortunate to work again with an outstanding group of coauthors for this edition. I am delighted to work with the entire author team from the third edition. In addition to their outstanding experience and depth of knowledge on all topics in pediatric neuroradiology, they bring deep experience with authorship within the Elsevier Diagnostic Imaging *series ecosystem.*

For this edition, Luke Linscott, MD, has joined me as colead author for this edition. I am greatly indebted to Luke for his excellent ideas and sharing of the many tasks involved in bringing a comprehensive textbook to publication.

I would also like to shine light on the many individuals within the editorial and production staff, who spend countless hours in the background attending to the many tiny details that distinguish an excellent book. Although they frequently work in anonymity, the importance of these team members is difficult to overstate. We are deeply indebted to them. In particular, it would not have been possible to bring this edition to fruition without the excellent assistance of Nina Bennett, our outstanding lead editor.

Finally, the authors would like to acknowledge (and thank!) their spouses and significant others, children, and colleagues who directly or indirectly support our devotion of many hours' time committed to completing this project. In my case, I wish to acknowledge my wife of 35 years, Margaret, for her selfless and complete support for my time spent working on this project.

We sincerely hope that you find this book useful in your daily practice.

KRM

I am grateful to my friend, mentor, and colleague, Dr. Kevin Moore, for his willingness to bring me on as a coeditor on this amazing project! Kevin has been a great role model, a huge advocate, and a true friend to me for many years.

Many thanks to my wife, Carrie, for her constant love and support!

Thanks to my kids, Abby, Katie, Alex, and Sarah, who often take sincere interest in my book writing and are understanding when it takes away from our "fun time."

Many thanks to my parents, who built my foundation for learning and set me on the road to success.

LLL

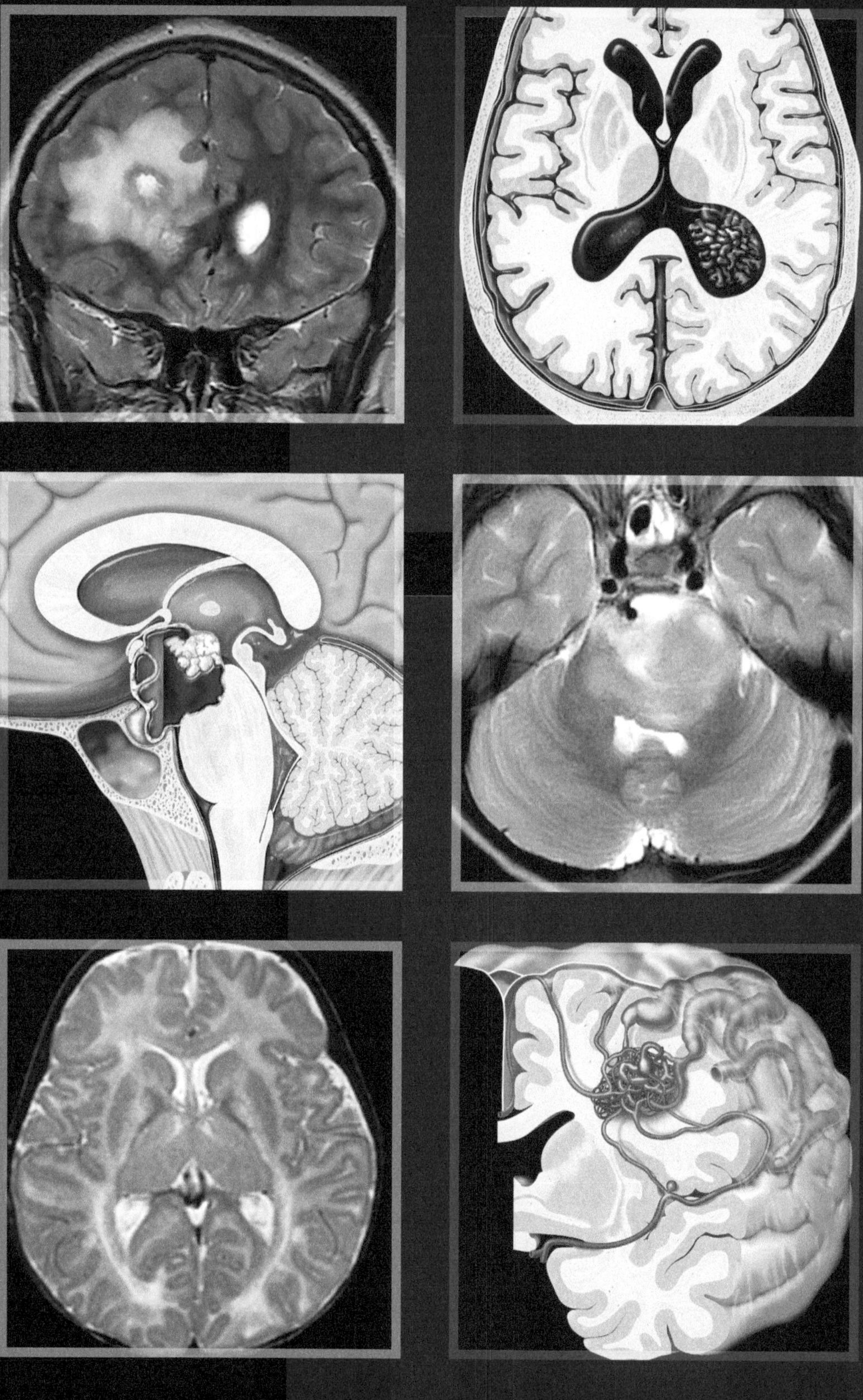

Contributing Authors

Blaise V. Jones, MD
Division Director, Neuroradiology
Cincinnati Children's Hospital Medical Center
Professor, Radiology and Pediatrics
University of Cincinnati College of Medicine
Cincinnati, Ohio

Bernadette L. Koch, MD
Associate Chief, Radiology
Cincinnati Children's Hospital Medical Center
Professor, Radiology and Pediatrics
University of Cincinnati College of Medicine
Cincinnati, Ohio

Usha D. Nagaraj, MD
Faculty Radiologist
Cincinnati Children's Hospital Medical Center
Associate Professor of Radiology
University of Cincinnati College of Medicine
Cincinnati, Ohio

Surjith Vattoth, MD, FRCR
Professor
Department of Diagnostic Radiology & Nuclear Medicine
Division of Neuroradiology
Rush University Medical Center
Chicago, Illinois

Additional Contributors

Susan I. Blaser, MD, FRCPC
Philip R. Chapman, MD
Bronwyn E. Hamilton, MD
H. Ric Harnsberger, MD
Miral D. Jhaveri, MD, MBA
Nicholas A. Koontz, MD
Daniel E. Meltzer, MD
Anne G. Osborn, MD, FACR
Jeffrey S. Ross, MD
Karen L. Salzman, MD, FACR

Preface

Welcome to the fourth edition of *Diagnostic Imaging: Pediatric Neuroradiology.* Time flies, and we are delighted that users continue to find this book useful for their daily practice! I am personally grateful and excited that we have returned the entire outstanding author group from the prior edition for this new edition, and the authors have carefully reviewed the third edition to identify areas that have experienced advances in pathophysiology knowledge or genetic characterization. Not surprisingly, our concepts of many disorders described in the prior edition have significantly changed thanks to advances in molecular genetics of pediatric brain tumors and WHO brain tumor updated criteria, as well as more granularity and better imaging markers for pediatric demyelinating diseases. As a direct result, the previous book has undergone extensive revision in an attempt to reflect the most current understanding of these as well as many other disorders. We have introduced entirely new chapters covering important but previously undiscussed pediatric brain and spine neoplasms and have updated terminology that is no longer in use. We have also updated and expanded our coverage of pediatric demyelinating disorders, including a new introductory prose chapter covering these important and very different entities.

Despite these changes, we have endeavored to retain many popular features of prior editions. We continue to utilize bulleted, succinct text for fast and easy comprehension of essential information, including terminology, imaging findings, key facts, differential diagnoses, pathology, clinical issues, diagnostic checklist, and selected references. Introductory chapters before major book sections are written to provide pertinent embryologic, anatomic, and physiologic background to help readers understand fundamental concepts of the disorders described in the sections that follow. The authors have scrutinized color graphics from prior editions, updating many older graphics to improve accuracy as well as developing entirely new graphics to more helpfully demonstrate key diagnosis features and findings. The print and digital image galleries have also been extensively revised to cull older images, and many new images have been added to reflect evolving knowledge and improvements in imaging technology.

As was the case in the previous editions, this book reflects the contributions of many colleagues (too numerous to name individually) who helped us write (and rewrite) the many chapters. We would be remiss, however, in not mentioning by name our outstanding lead editor, Nina Bennett, without whom this project would have been very difficult to complete on time and at as high a quality level. We are indebted to one another for sharing our valuable (and finite) time and expertise to ensure that the completed project meets the high standards of the authors and the publisher. We are particularly indebted to the dedicated editorial and production staff at Elsevier for their many hours of largely anonymous work attending to the many small details that result in a quality book. We believe that the end result is a comprehensive but accessible textbook that describes a large number of important pediatric disorders, both common and uncommon, that affect the brains, heads, necks, and spines of children. In disorders that affect both adults and children, the diagnoses are written and figures selected to emphasize the pediatric aspects of these disorders.

The authors and publisher hope that you, the reader, will find this fourth edition of *Diagnostic Imaging: Pediatric Neuroradiology* to be a handy and useful resource at the workstation or clinic within your daily practice.

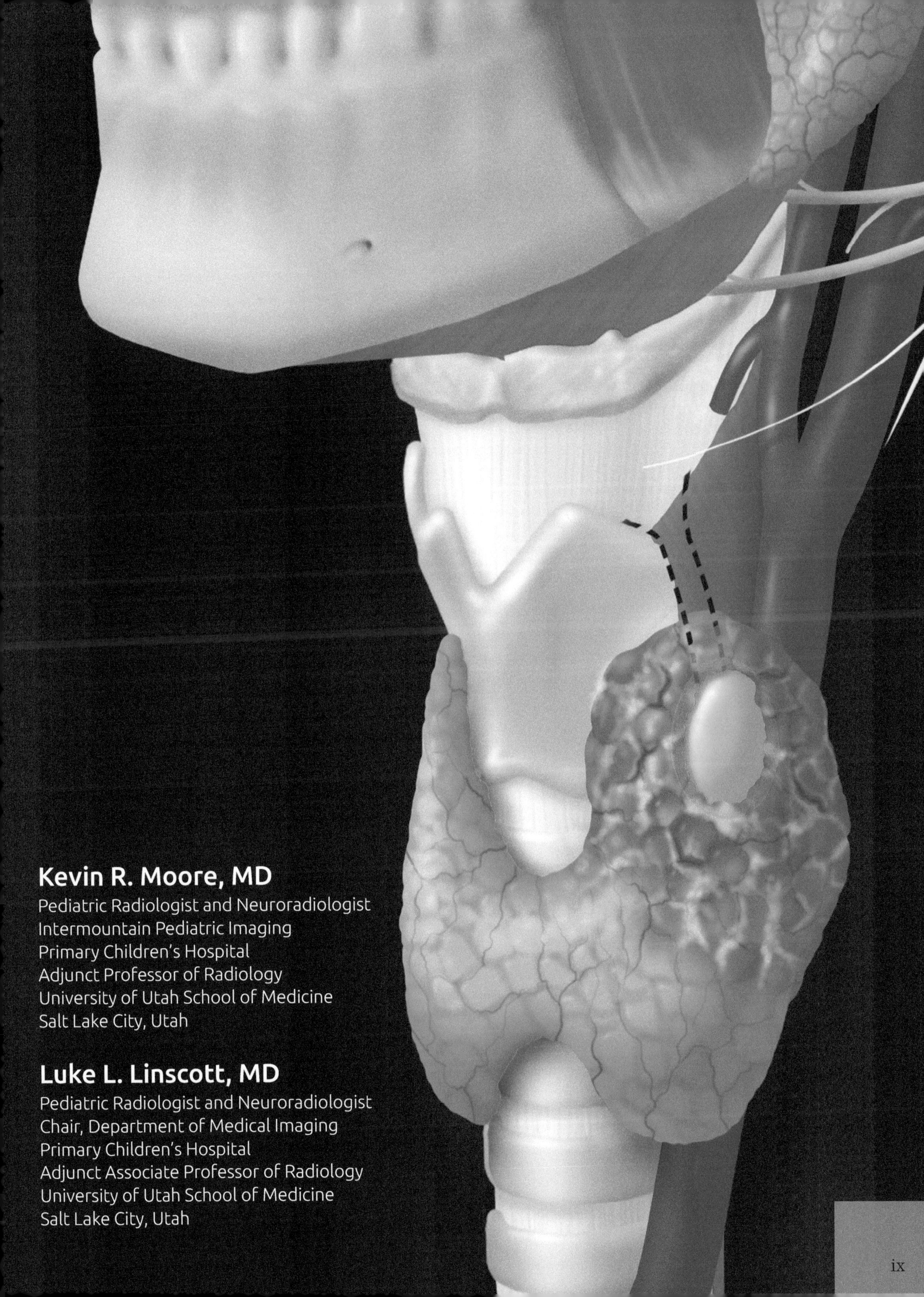

Kevin R. Moore, MD
Pediatric Radiologist and Neuroradiologist
Intermountain Pediatric Imaging
Primary Children's Hospital
Adjunct Professor of Radiology
University of Utah School of Medicine
Salt Lake City, Utah

Luke L. Linscott, MD
Pediatric Radiologist and Neuroradiologist
Chair, Department of Medical Imaging
Primary Children's Hospital
Adjunct Associate Professor of Radiology
University of Utah School of Medicine
Salt Lake City, Utah

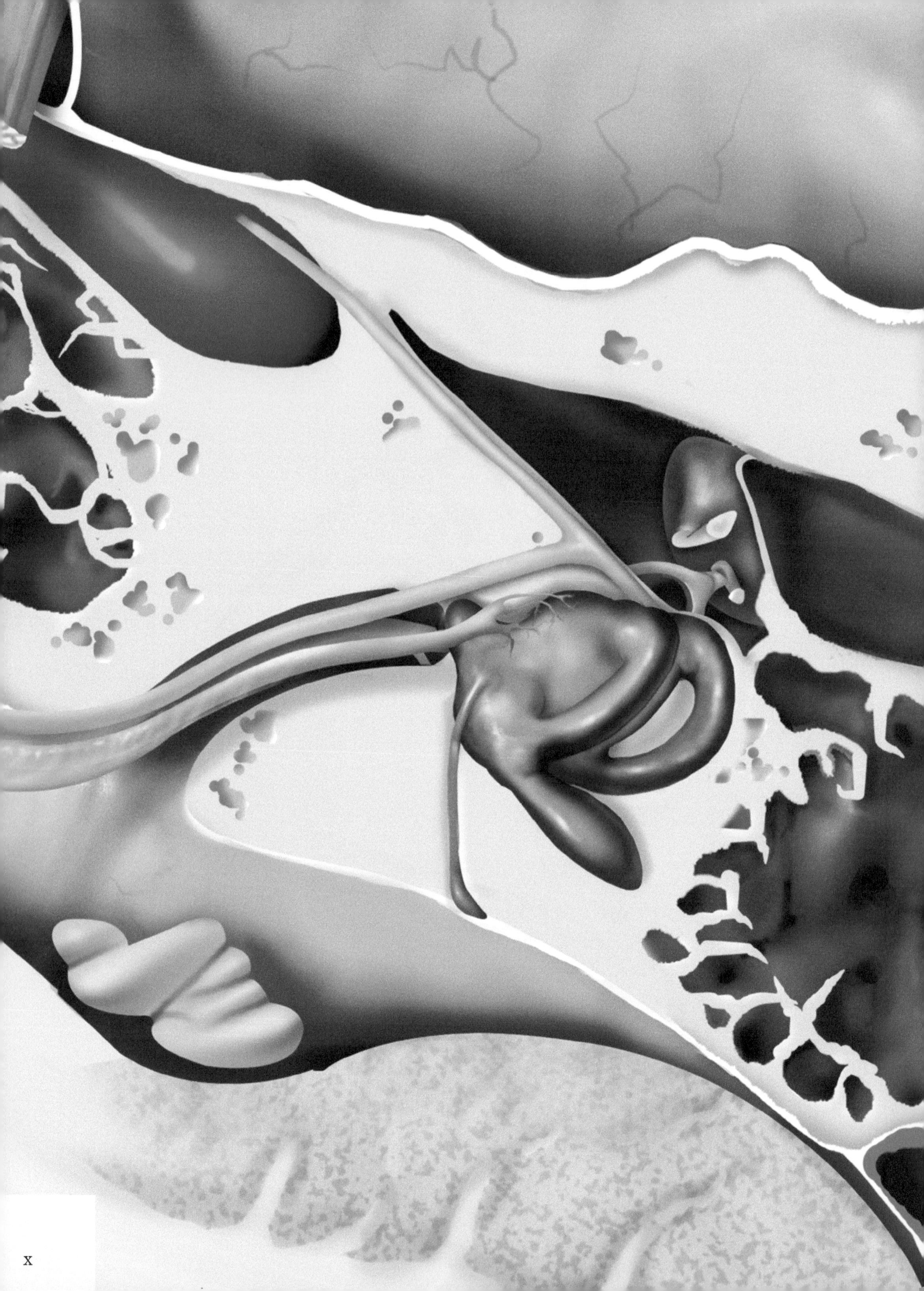

Acknowledgments

LEAD EDITOR
Nina Themann, BA

LEAD ILLUSTRATOR
Lane R. Bennion, MS

TEXT EDITORS
Arthur G. Gelsinger, MA
Rebecca L. Bluth, BA
Terry W. Ferrell, MS
Megg Morin, BA
Kathryn Watkins, BA
Shannon Kelly, MA

ILLUSTRATIONS
Richard Coombs, MS
Laura C. Wissler, MA

IMAGE EDITORS
Jeffrey J. Marmorstone, BS
Lisa A. M. Steadman, BS

ART DIRECTION AND DESIGN
Cindy Lin, BFA

PRODUCTION EDITORS
Emily C. Fassett, BA
John Pecorelli, BS

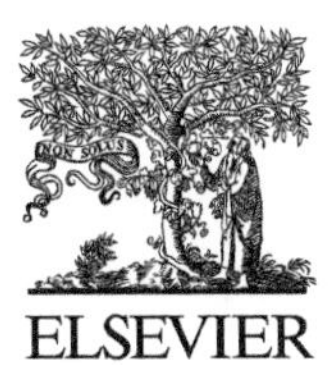

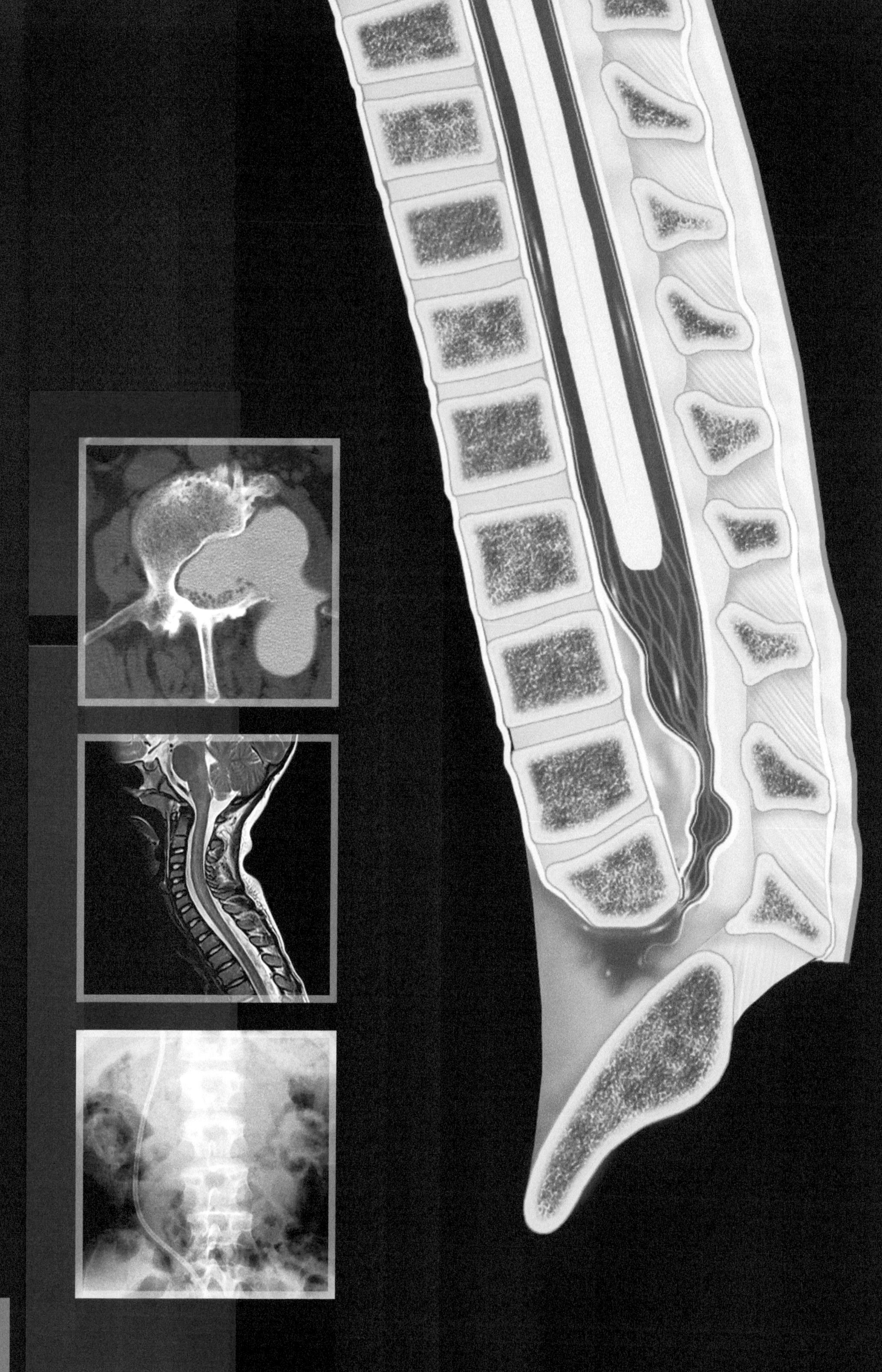

Sections

TABLE OF CONTENTS

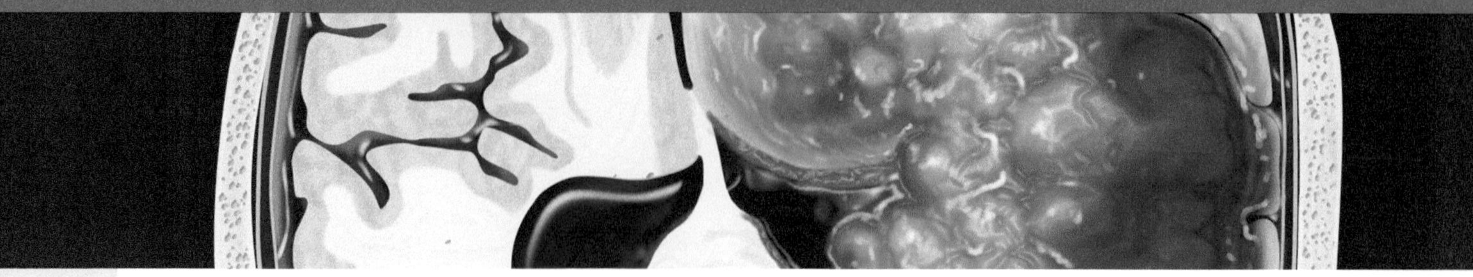

Part I: Brain

SECTION 1: PATHOLOGY-BASED DIAGNOSES

TABLE OF CONTENTS

TABLE OF CONTENTS

TABLE OF CONTENTS

SECTION 2: ANATOMY-BASED DIAGNOSES

VENTRICLES AND CISTERNS

SELLA AND PITUITARY

SKULL, SCALP, AND MENINGES

CONGENITAL

TRAUMA

NONNEOPLASTIC AND TUMOR-LIKE DISORDERS

Part II: Head and Neck

SECTION 1: TEMPORAL BONE AND SKULL BASE

SECTION 2: ORBIT, NOSE, AND SINUSES

TABLE OF CONTENTS

TABLE OF CONTENTS

TABLE OF CONTENTS

FOURTH EDITION

Moore | Linscott

Diagnostic Imaging
Pediatric Neuroradiology

PART I
SECTION 1
Pathology-Based Diagnoses

Congenital Malformations

Trauma

Stroke

Vascular Malformations

Neoplasms

General Imaging Approach to Brain Malformations

Whenever an infant or child is referred for imaging because of either seizures or delayed development, the possibility of a brain malformation should be carefully investigated. If the child appears dysmorphic in any way (low-set ears, abnormal facies, hypotelorism), the likelihood of an underlying brain malformation is even higher, but a normal appearance is no guarantee of a normal brain. In all such cases, imaging should be geared toward showing a structural abnormality. The imaging sequences should maximize contrast between gray matter and white matter, have high spatial resolution, and be acquired as volumetric data whenever possible so that images can be reformatted in any plane or as a surface rendering. The high resolution and ability to reformat will aid in the diagnosis of subtle abnormalities. High-resolution T1-weighted volumetric images are essential for this purpose. High-resolution 2D coronal T2 images remain a workhorse for evaluation of midline structures, hippocampi, and optic nerves. High-resolution 3D FLAIR images may be particularly helpful in evaluating for focal cortical dysplasia (FCD). The use of diffusion tensor imaging (DTI) to acquire color fractional anisotropy (FA) maps and perform tractography is useful to better understand the connectivity of the malformed brain, particularly in the brainstem, and may become clinically useful in the near future.

After acquisition of appropriate images, image analysis must take place in an orderly manner. The midline structures (including cerebral commissures, septum pellucidum, nose and rhinencephalon, pituitary gland, optic chiasm, and hypothalamus), the cerebral cortex (cortical thickness, gyral pattern, and cortical gray matter-white matter junction), the cerebral white matter (myelination, presence of nodules or clefts), the basal ganglia, the ventricular system (all ventricles completely present and of normal size and shape), the interhemispheric fissure (IHF), and the midbrain and hindbrain structures (brainstem and cerebellum) should all be scrutinized in every patient.

Evaluate the midline structures first, as many disease processes of children take place in the midline, including anomalies of the cerebral commissures (corpus callosum, anterior commissure, and hippocampal commissure), midline tumors (suprasellar, pineal, brainstem, and 4th ventricle), anomalies of the cerebellar vermis, and anomalies of the craniocervical junction. Anomalies of the cerebral commissures are the most common brain malformations; > 130 syndromes involving them have been described. Many of these malformations are associated with anomalies of the hypothalamus, so always look at the hypothalamus and pituitary gland to ensure that the posterior pituitary lobe is in the sella turcica and not in the median eminence of the hypothalamus. The midline leptomeninges are important in commissural development, so be sure to look for other anomalies associated with abnormal midline leptomeninges, such as interhemispheric lipomas and interhemispheric cysts, when the commissures are absent or dysmorphic. Remember that large CSF spaces in the posterior fossa may be a sign of associated anomalies of the cerebellum. The reason for this has only recently been discovered. Several cerebellar growth factors derive from the overlying leptomeninges. Therefore, abnormalities of the cerebellar leptomeninges may result in anomalies of the cerebellum itself, as well as abnormalities of the surrounding CSF spaces. This is the basis for development of the Dandy-Walker malformation; it requires abnormal development of the cerebellum itself and of the overlying leptomeninges. Looking at the midline image also gives an idea of the relative head size through assessment of the craniofacial ratio. In the normal neonate, the ratio of the cranial vault: face on midline images is 5:1 or 6:1. By 2 years, it should be 2.5:1, and by 10 years, it should be ~1.5:1.

After looking at the midline, evaluate the brain from outside to inside. Start with the cerebral cortex. Is the thickness normal (2-3 mm)? If it is too thick, think of pachygyria or polymicrogyria. Is the cortical white matter junction smooth or irregular? If it is irregular, think of polymicrogyria or cobblestone cortex. Polymicrogyria is seen in many underlying disorders, including congenital cytomegalovirus (CMV) and genetic syndromes, among others. Cobblestone cortex may be associated with congenital muscular dystrophies, such as muscle-eye-brain disease. Pachygyria that is more severe in the parietal and occipital lobes suggests a mutation of *PAFAH1B1* (LIS1) or *TUBA1A* (*TUBA1A* is also associated with microcephaly), whereas pachygyria that is worst in the frontal lobes suggests a mutation of *DCX*. Similarly, there are many different polymicrogyria syndromes that depend upon the location of the polymicrogyria. Bilateral frontal polymicrogyria is a different entity than bilateral perisylvian polymicrogyria or bilateral parasagittal parietooccipital polymicrogyria; it is important to be specific in reporting the location of the abnormality. If the cortex is abnormally thin and associated with diminished underlying white matter, one should think of a prenatal injury (infectious or ischemic), particularly if the thinning is focal or multifocal.

After the cortex, look at the cerebral white matter. Make sure myelination is appropriate for age (there are many sources of normal myelination charts, including journal articles and textbooks). Then, look for areas of abnormal myelination within the deep white matter. Diffuse layers of hypomyelination or amyelination associated with overlying polymicrogyria should raise suspicion for congenital CMV infection. Generalized ipsilateral ↑ T1 and ↓ T2 signal in the white matter of a neonate with overlying cortical malformation should prompt one to think of hemimegalencephaly, which is often accompanied by ipsilateral hemisphere and ventricular enlargement. FCDs are often most conspicuous at birth with ↑ T1 and ↓ T2 in the subcortical white matter. After myelination, FCDs are typically most conspicuous on FLAIR, where one may see a curvilinear cone-shaped abnormality coursing from the cortex to the superolateral margin of a lateral ventricle (known as the transmantle sign). Narrowing the window on FLAIR images ↑ conspicuity of FCD. Also, look for nodules of heterotopic gray matter in the periventricular or deep white matter. Transmantle gray matter heterotopia typically extends from the cortex all the way to the lateral ventricular wall, whereas periventricular nodular heterotopia is more localized to the immediate subependymal/periventricular region. Heterotopia might be difficult to differentiate from unmyelinated or injured white matter on T1-weighted images, so be sure to look at T2-weighted images or FLAIR images to ensure that the lesion is isointense to gray matter on all sequences.

The basal ganglia are sometimes abnormal in neuronal migration disorders, as they are formed from neurons generated in the medial and lateral ganglionic eminences, the same germinal zones that produce GABAergic neurons that migrate to the cerebral cortex. In particular, the basal ganglia

Brain Anomaly Imaging Checklist

Anomaly	Findings
Anomalies of Cerebral Cortex	
Agyria/pachygyria	Thick cortex, smooth inner margin, few shallow sulci
PMG	Nodular cortex & gray matter-white matter junction
Cobblestone cortex	Thick cortex, irregular inner margin, abnormal myelin
Focal cortical dysplasia	Thick cortex, blurred gray-white junction, ± deep sulcus
White Matter Abnormalities With Cortical Malformation	
Hemimegalencephaly	↑ T1, ↓ T2 in neonatal white matter; dysplastic neurons
Cobblestone cortex	Delayed myelination, patchy hypomyelination
Congenital cytomegalovirus	Deep layers of hypomyelination/gliosis
Focal cortical dysplasia	"Tail" of signal abnormality extending toward ventricle
Malformations Associated With Absent Septum Pellucidum	
Septo-optic dysplasia	ON hypoplasia, pituitary anomaly, ± PMG/schizencephaly
Holoprosencephaly	Varying degrees of incomplete hemispheric separation
Malformations with severe prolonged hydrocephalus	Absent septum typically thought to be destructive

ON = optic nerve; PMG = polymicrogyria.

tend to be dysmorphic in appearance in patients with subcortical heterotopia. In addition, the hippocampi are often abnormal in cortical development malformations. In patients with lissencephaly, in particular, the hippocampi are incompletely folded. Sometimes, the only structural abnormalities in children with developmental delay are hippocampal; always ensure that they are fully folded and not too round. In the case of longstanding seizures, carefully inspect the hippocampi for asymmetric atrophy and ↑ signal to suggest hippocampal sclerosis.

Always look at the entire IHF; if the cerebral hemispheres are continuous across the midline, holoprosencephaly should be diagnosed. In severe holoprosencephalies, the IHF is completely absent, whereas, in milder forms of holoprosencephaly, certain areas of the IHF will be absent (anterior IHF in semilobar holoprosencephaly, central IHF in syntelencephaly). Look at the septum pellucidum; absence of the septum is seen in corpus callosum dysgenesis/agenesis and septo-optic dysplasia. When septo-optic dysplasia is identified, look carefully for pituitary abnormalities, most commonly an ectopic posterior pituitary. Additionally, whenever septo-optic dysplasia is suspected, a careful search for associated schizencephaly or polymicrogyria is warranted. If present, a diagnosis of septo-optic dysplasia **plus** is established. While checking the septum, look at the lateral ventricles to ensure they are normal in size and shape. Abnormally enlarged trigones and temporal horns are often associated with callosal anomalies and pachygyria. Enlarged frontal horns are often seen in bilateral frontal polymicrogyria.

Remember to look carefully at the posterior fossa; anomalies of the brainstem and cerebellum are commonly overlooked. Make sure that the 4th ventricle and cerebellar vermis are normally sized. In newborns, the vermis should extend from the inferior colliculi to the obex, whereas infants and older children should have a vermis that extends from the intercollicular sulcus to the obex. Also, make sure the vermian fissures are normal. If the fissuration of the vermis looks abnormal, refer to an axial or coronal image to make sure the vermis is present; if the cerebellar hemispheres are continuous without a vermis between them, make a diagnosis of rhombencephalosynapsis. Whenever aqueductal stenosis is encountered, look carefully for rhombencephalosynapsis. If the 4th ventricle has an abnormal rectangular shape (with a horizontal superior margin) with a narrow isthmus and small vermis, consider a molar tooth malformation. To confirm this diagnosis, look on axial images for the molar tooth sign of the lower midbrain, consisting of large, horizontal superior cerebellar peduncles extending posteriorly toward the cerebellum, and a longitudinal cleft in the superior vermis. Make sure that the brainstem components are of normal size; in a child, the height of the pons should be double that of the midbrain on the midline sagittal image. Looking at the size of the pons compared to that of the cerebellar vermis can provide an important clue. Because much of the anterior pons is composed of the decussation of the middle cerebellar peduncles, development hypoplasia of the cerebellum is nearly always associated with hypoplasia of the ventral pons. If the pons is normal in the setting of a small cerebellum, it is most likely that the cerebellum lost volume near the end of gestation or after birth. Remember that in a small posterior fossa, intracranial **hypo**tension, **or** intracranial **hyper**tension can result in descent of the cerebellum below the foramen magnum. Look for causes of a small posterior fossa (clival anomaly, anomaly of the craniovertebral junction), intracranial hypertension (space-occupying mass, hydrocephalus), or evidence of intracranial hypotension (large dural venous sinuses, large pituitary gland, "slumping" brainstem) before making a diagnosis of Chiari 1. Finally, remember to look at the size of the CSF spaces in the posterior fossa, enlargement of which may be a sign of abnormal leptomeningeal development.

Selected References

1. Chaudhari BP et al: Congenital brain malformations: an integrated diagnostic approach. Semin Pediatr Neurol. 42:100973, 2022
2. Fenton LZ: Imaging of congenital malformations of the brain. Clin Perinatol. 49(3):587-601, 2022

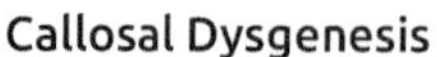

Callosal Dysgenesis

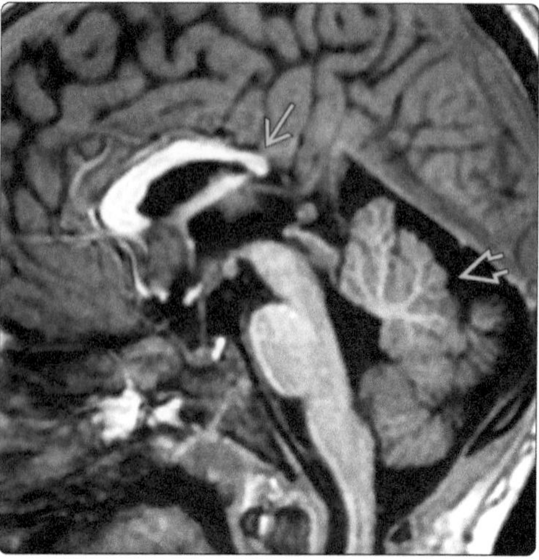

Callosal Dysgenesis With Pericallosal Lipoma

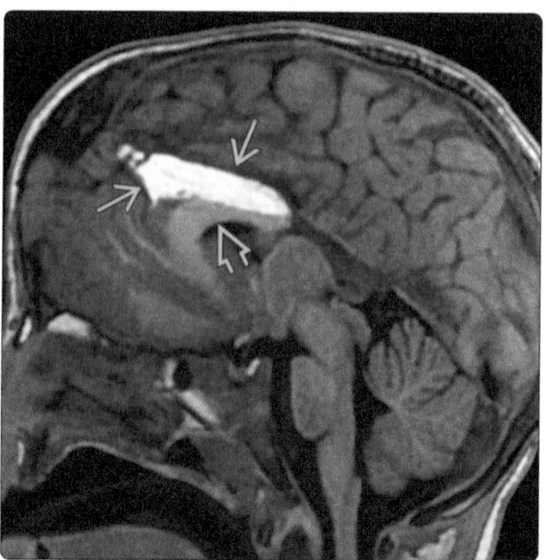

(Left) *Sagittal T1 MR in a 10-year-old with callosal dysgenesis shows a short and dysmorphic corpus callosum (CC) with small splenium ⇨. This patient had other associated anomalies, including cerebellar dysplasia ⇨.* **(Right)** *Sagittal T1 MR in a 5-year-old with a large tubulonodular pericallosal lipoma ⇨ and callosal dysgenesis ⇨ is shown. Pericallosal lipomas are associated with varying degrees of callosal dysgenesis. Typically, the larger the lipoma, the more dysgenetic the CC.*

Pachygyria

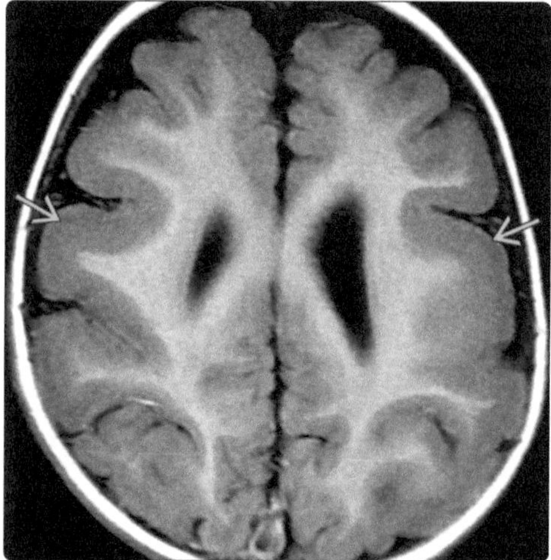

Polymicrogyria

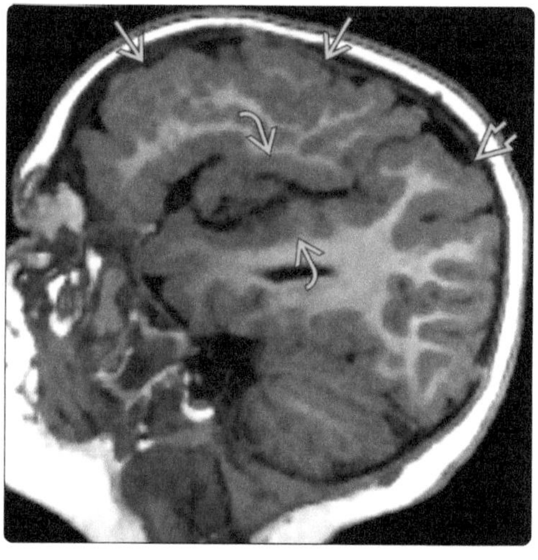

(Left) *Axial T1 MR in a 1-year-old shows bilateral symmetric areas of smooth, ↓ sulcation with cortical thickening ⇨, typical of pachygyria. In contrast to polymicrogyria (PMG), pachygyria has a smooth cortical surface and gray matter-white matter junction.* **(Right)** *Sagittal T1 MR in a 2-year-old with new-onset seizures shows PMG predominantly in perisylvian area ⇨ and frontal lobe ⇨. Note the continuation of the sylvian fissure into the superior parietal lobule ⇨, a characteristic appearance for PMG.*

Focal Cortical Dysplasia

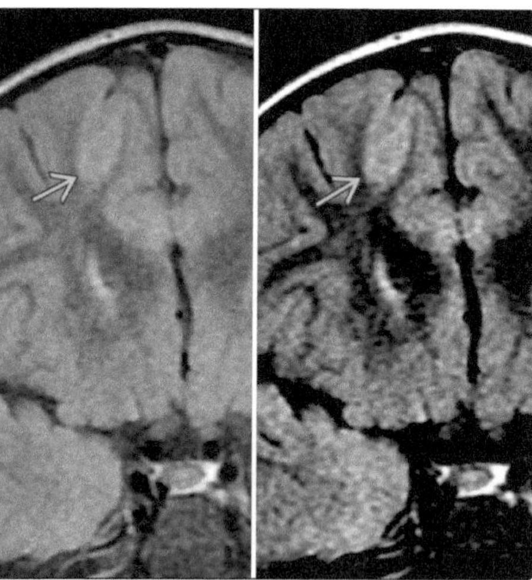

Subependymal Gray Matter Heterotopia

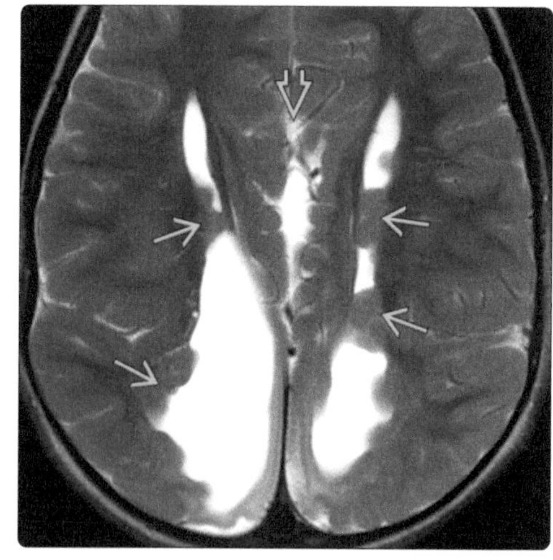

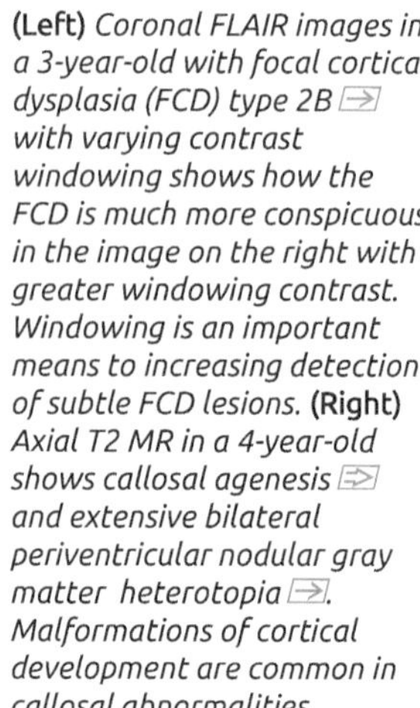

(Left) *Coronal FLAIR images in a 3-year-old with focal cortical dysplasia (FCD) type 2B ⇨ with varying contrast windowing shows how the FCD is much more conspicuous in the image on the right with greater windowing contrast. Windowing is an important means to increasing detection of subtle FCD lesions.* **(Right)** *Axial T2 MR in a 4-year-old shows callosal agenesis ⇨ and extensive bilateral periventricular nodular gray matter heterotopia ⇨. Malformations of cortical development are common in callosal abnormalities.*

Septo-Optic Dysplasia

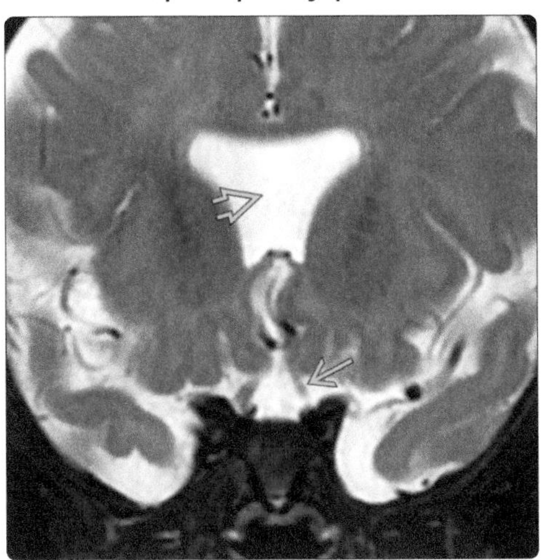

Septo-Optic Dysplasia Plus

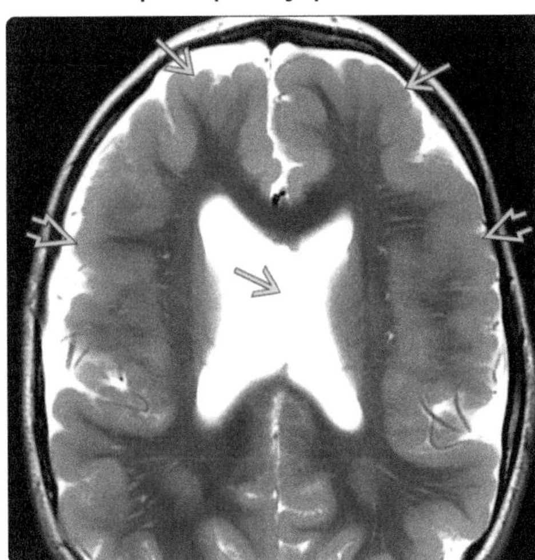

(Left) *Coronal T2 MR in a 5-year-old with septo-optic dysplasia (SOD) shows absence of septum pellucidum and a very small left optic nerve. Right optic nerve looks grossly normal in size. Asymmetric optic nerve hypoplasia is very common in this diagnosis.* **(Right)** *Axial T2 MR in a 6-year-old shows absent septum pellucidum and bilateral frontal PMG. Findings of SOD with associated cortical malformation is termed SOD plus.*

Semilobar Holoprosencephaly

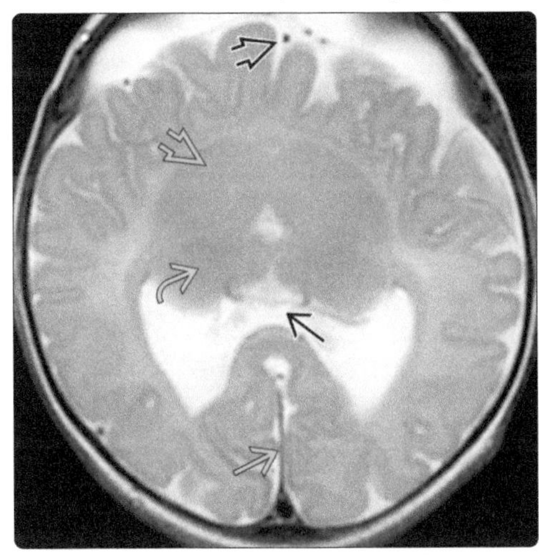

Rhombencephalosynapsis

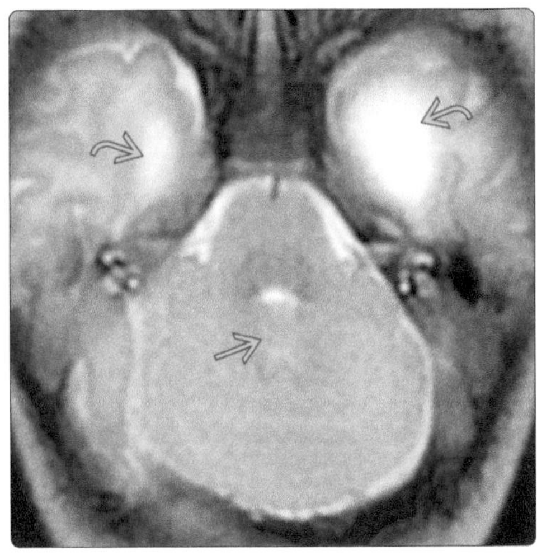

(Left) *Axial T2 MR in a 3-day-old with semilobar HPE shows absence of the anterior interhemispheric fissure, frontal horns, and septum pellucidum, fused basal ganglia and thalami. Note the normal posterior interhemispheric fissure and the azygos anterior cerebral artery.* **(Right)** *Axial T2 MR in a 2-month-old with RES shows absence of the cerebellar vermis and fusion of the dentate nuclei. Note the enlarged temporal horns due to congenital hydrocephalus secondary to aqueductal stenosis.*

Joubert Syndrome

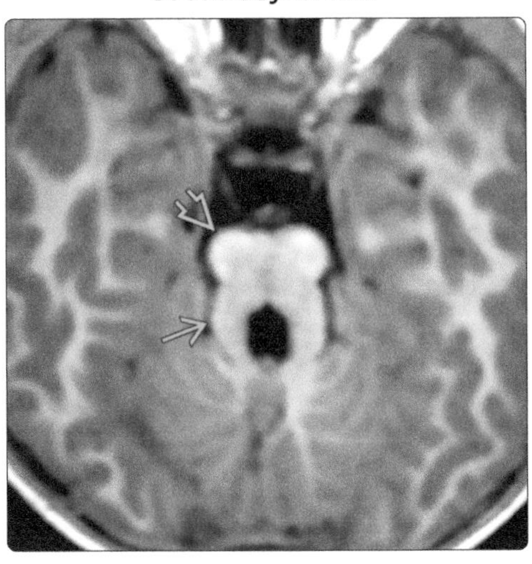

Dandy-Walker Malformation

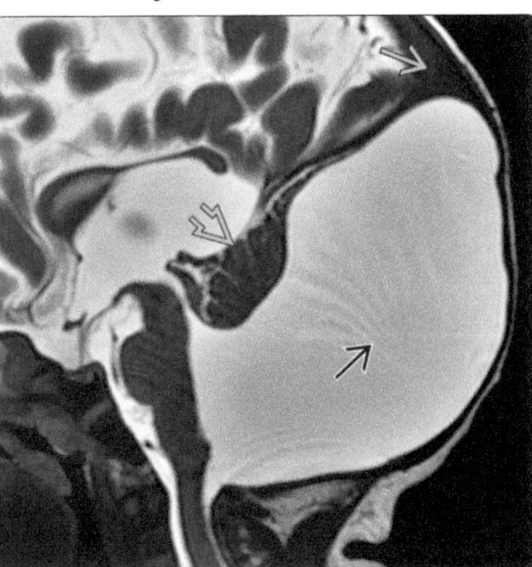

(Left) *Axial T1 MR in a 4-month-old with molar tooth sign shows the prominent thickening of the superior cerebellar peduncles that form the "roots" of the molar tooth while the pons forms the "crown" of the molar tooth.* **(Right)** *Sagittal T2 MR in an infant with classic Dandy-Walker malformation shows marked cystic enlargement of the posterior fossa in continuity with the 4th ventricle, hypogenetic cerebellar vermis, and elevation of the torcula Herophili.*

Dandy-Walker Continuum

KEY FACTS

TERMINOLOGY

- Dandy-Walker continuum is clinically & radiologically heterogeneous group of posterior fossa (PF) malformations
  - Classic Dandy-Walker malformation (DWM)
  - Vermian hypoplasia (VH)
  - Blake pouch (BP) remnant/cyst
  - Mega cisterna magna (MCM)

IMAGING

- Most severe to mildest: Classic DWM → VH → BP → MCM
- Classic DWM
  - Triad of vermian agenesis/hypogenesis, 4th ventricle cystic dilation, & enlarged PF with elevation of torcular Herophili (torcular-lambdoid inversion)
  - ± hydrocephalus
- VH
  - Variable VH ± rotation of vermis (coexisting BP)
  - No upward sloping of tentorium or torcular-lambdoid inversion
- BP remnant
  - Elevated tegmentovermian angle
  - Normal size & morphology of vermis
- MCM
  - Enlarged retrocerebellar CSF cistern (≥ 10 mm)

TOP DIFFERENTIAL DIAGNOSES

- PF arachnoid cyst
- Joubert syndrome & related disorders
- Dystroglycanopathies
- Cerebellar hypoplasia

CLINICAL ISSUES

- Conflicting terminology, not universally agreed upon
- Wide range of clinical severity
- Classic DWM & VH may be difficult to distinguish; anatomic descriptions may be most useful clinically

(Left) *Graphic of the classic Dandy-Walker malformation (DWM) shows an enlarged posterior fossa, elevated torcular Herophili ➡ (above the lambdoid suture ➡), superior rotation of a hypoplastic cerebellar vermis ➡, & posterior cystic expansion of the 4th ventricle.* **(Right)** *Sagittal T2WI MR in a 2-day-old girl with prenatally diagnosed classic DWM shows the hypoplastic rotated vermis ➡, upward slanting tentorium with elevated torcular Herophili ➡, & obstructive hydrocephalus.*

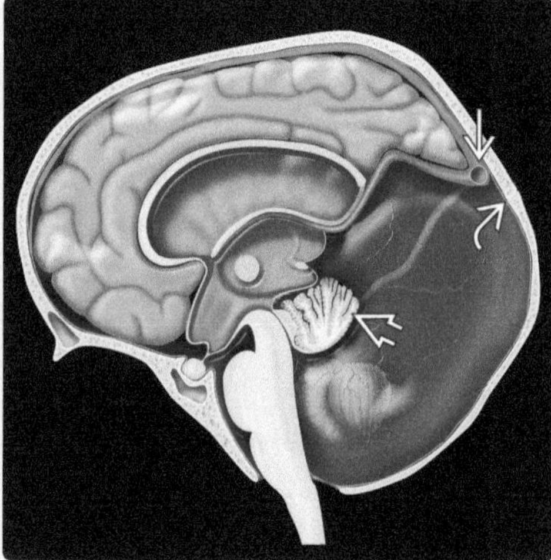

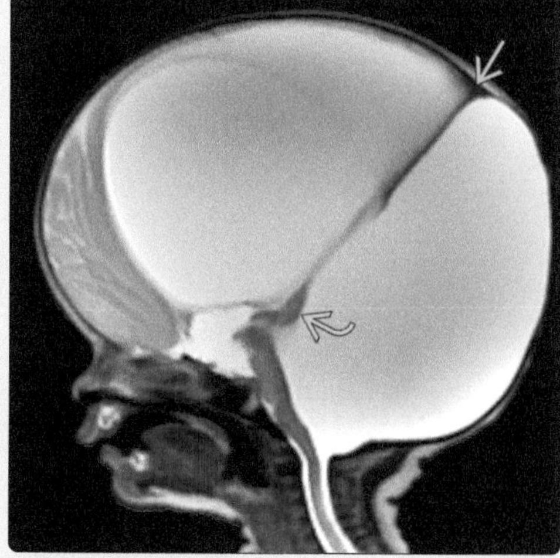

(Left) *Axial T2WI MR in the same patient shows lateral displacement of the cerebellar hemispheres ➡ & obstructive hydrocephalus with dilated lateral ventricular temporal horns ➡. The presence of hydrocephalus & other associated brain malformations are critical in helping to establish prognosis.* **(Right)** *Sagittal 3D FIESTA MR of the craniocervical junction in the same patient demonstrates the abnormal persistence of Blake pouch (BP) remnant ➡ obstructing the 4th ventricular outflow tracts.*

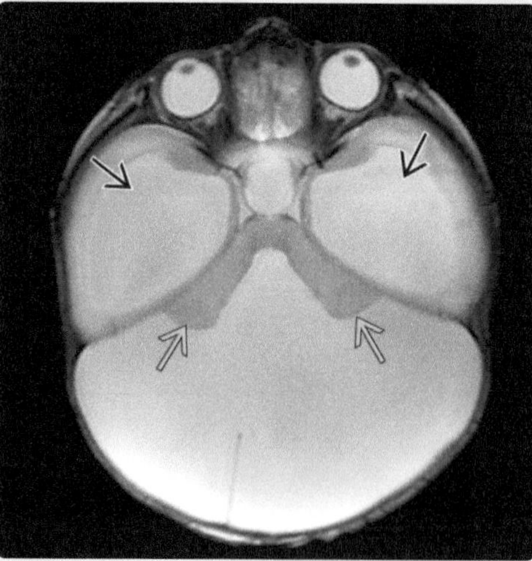

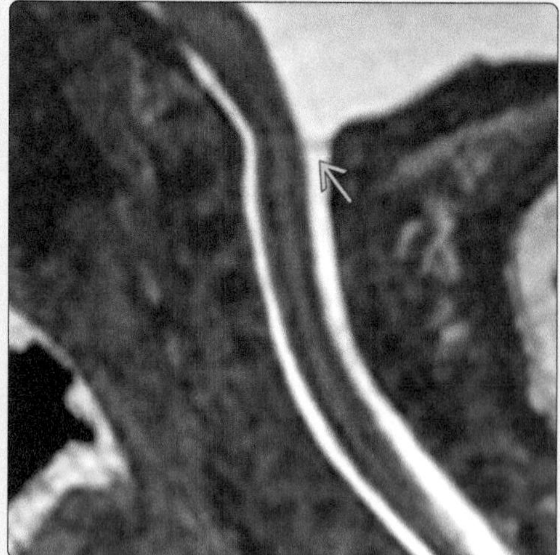

TERMINOLOGY

Abbreviations

- Dandy-Walker malformation (DWM)

Synonyms

- Terms DW spectrum, DW variant, & DW complex have complicated clinical & imaging implications in literature

Definitions

- DW continuum: Clinically & radiologically heterogeneous group of posterior fossa (PF) malformations
- Referred to as continuum by some based on belief that DWM, vermian hypoplasia (VH), Blake pouch (BP) remnant/cyst, & mega cisterna magna (MCM) are spectrum of developmental anomalies of rhombencephalic vesicle roof
  - Terminology is controversial & not uniformly accepted
  - Consortium recommends term DW **phenotype instead**
  - Clinical severity ranges widely in this group

IMAGING

General Features

- Best diagnostic clue
  - Classic DWM triad: Vermian agenesis/hypogenesis, 4th ventricle cystic dilation, & enlarged PF with elevation of torcular Herophili (torcular-lambdoid inversion)
  - VH: Vermis is small & usually rotated (coexisting BP), may be dysplastic; no torcular-lambdoid inversion
  - BP: Vermis is normal in size & morphology with rotation marked by elevated tegmentovermian angle (≥ 18°)
  - MCM: Enlarged retrocerebellar CSF space (≥ 10 mm) with normal size & orientation of vermis (normal tegmentovermian angle)
- Morphology
  - DW continuum (from most to least severe)
    - DWM classic triad
      - □ Complete or partial agenesis of vermis
      - □ Cystic dilation of 4th ventricle → rotation of hypoplastic vermis
      - □ Enlarged PF with upward displacement of tentorium & torcular Herophili (torcular-lambdoid inversion)
      - □ Obstructive hydrocephalus: 70-90%; callosal anomalies: 20%; polymicrogyria or gray matter heterotopia: 5-10%
    - VH
      - □ Variable degree of VH ± rotation/BP remnant
      - □ ± abnormal vermian foliation/dysplasia
      - □ No upward slanting tentorium, no torcular-lambdoid inversion
      - □ May be difficult to distinguish from DWM
    - BP remnant (a.k.a. BP "cyst")
      - □ Elevated tegmentovermian angle (a.k.a. "open" 4th ventricle)
      - □ Normal size & morphology of vermis
    - MCM
      - □ Enlarged retrocerebellar cistern (≥ 10 mm) without mass effect on hindbrain
      - □ Normal vermis, 4th ventricle, & tegmentovermian angle
      - □ Incidental finding in isolation

CT Findings

- NECT
  - DWM: Large PF
    - Torcular-lambdoid inversion (torcular above lambdoid sutures)
  - Scalloped occipital bone, remodeled in all types of DW continuum

MR Findings

- T1, T2, FLAIR
  - DWM
    - Vermian agenesis/hypogenesis, hypoplastic vermis with superior rotation/elevation
    - Variable cerebellar hemisphere & brainstem hypoplasia &/or compression
    - Enlarged 4th ventricle communicating with retrocerebellar cystic space
    - Elevated torcular Herophili with upward-slanting tentorium
    - Hydrocephalus is common
  - VH
    - Varying degrees of vermian tissue are present
    - Vertical height of vermis does not reach level of obex
    - ± rotation of vermis
      - □ Normal tegmentovermian angle is usually close to 0°; however, < 18° has been reported as normal
      - □ Angle as large as 30° may be normal before 20-weeks gestation on fetal MR
    - ± abnormal foliation/dysplasia
    - May be difficult to distinguish from DWM, particularly in fetus in which there are no reliable landmarks to identify lambdoid sutures
  - BP remnant
    - Rotated but normal-appearing vermis
    - 4th ventricle communicates inferiorly with retrocerebellar CSF cystic space
    - Cyst wall is variably present, often imperceptible on MR
    - Choroid plexus may be seen along inferior surface of vermis (superior margin of cyst wall)
  - MCM
    - Enlarged retrocerebellar CSF space
    - Normal vermis (not rotated, dysplastic, or hypoplastic)
  - ± callosal anomalies, polymicrogyria, gray matter heterotopia, occipital cephalocele, decreased myelination
  - Other described imaging signs in DWM
    - Tail sign: Presence of vermian tail has been described as characteristic of DWM; however, not it is always present & can be seen with other PF pathologies
    - Taenia-tela choroidea complex: Position of this complex has been described as way to differentiate DWM from BP but not consistently seen

Imaging Recommendations

- Protocol advice
  - Routine MR with thin-section sagittal 3D true FISP/FIESTA to look for cyst wall

DIFFERENTIAL DIAGNOSIS

Posterior Fossa Arachnoid Cyst

- True cyst that does not communicate with 4th ventricle

Joubert Syndrome & Related Disorders

- Hypoplastic/dysplastic vermis, "bat wing" 4th ventricle on axial images, thickened & horizontal superior cerebellar peduncles with midbrain cleft → molar tooth appearance on axial images

Dystroglycanopathies

- VH with cobblestone cortex & Z-shaped brainstem (Walker-Warburg phenotype)

Cerebellar Hypoplasia

- ± brainstem hypoplasia (pontocerebellar hypoplasia)

PATHOLOGY

General Features

- Etiology
  - DW continuum is result of abnormal development of PF mesenchyme
  - Rhombencephalic vesicle roof divides into cranial [anterior membranous area (AMA)] & caudal [posterior membranous area (PMA)] segments
    - AMA invaded by neural cells → cerebellum
    - PMA expands then disappears to form outlet foramina of 4th ventricle
  - Hindbrain development arrest
    - Defective AMA & PMA → DWM & VH
    - Defective PMA only → BP (incomplete/nonperforation of foramen of Magendie) & MCM (delayed perforation)
- Genetics
  - Multiple causative genes identified
    - *FOXC1* (chromosome 6p25.3)
    - Deletion of 3q24 (includes *ZIC1* & *ZIC4* genes)
    - *FGF17*, *LAMC1*, *NID1*
  - DWM can be in isolation or in well-defined syndrome
    - Ritscher-Schinzel syndrome
    - Cranio-cerebello-cardiac syndrome
- Associated abnormalities
  - 2/3 of DWM & related disorders have associated CNS &/or extracranial anomalies
    - Midline anomalies, neurocutaneous melanosis, PHACE(S) syndrome
    - Craniofacial, cardiac, urinary tract, & orthopedic anomalies
    - Trisomy 18 > other trisomies
- Embryology
  - Common association of DWM/VH with facial & cardiovascular anomalies suggests onset between formation & migration of neural crest cells

CLINICAL ISSUES

Presentation

- Most common signs/symptoms
  - DWM: Macrocephaly, bulging fontanelle (obstructive hydrocephalus)
  - MCM: Incidental finding
- Clinical profile
  - Motor developmental delay, spastic paraplegia, seizures, variable intellectual disability
    - Marked heterogeneity in clinical findings, even in families with same genetic mutations

Demographics

- Age
  - DWM: 80% diagnosed by 1 year of age
    - Age of diagnosis depends on degree of hydrocephalus, supratentorial anomalies, & cerebellar dysfunction
- Epidemiology
  - 1:25,000-30,000 births

Natural History & Prognosis

- Cognitive outcome depends on associated syndromes, supratentorial anomalies, & hydrocephalus
- Classic DWM: Poor prognosis overall
  - Though developmental delay was previously reported in 40 60%, recent literature suggests much higher incidence in true DWM
  - 70-90% with hydrocephalus
  - Seizures, hearing &/or visual difficulties, systemic abnormalities
- VH: Highly variable
  - Cognitive abnormalities in 40-50%, but normal neurodevelopment has been reported in isolated VH
  - Strong association with genetic conditions & congenital heart disease
- BP: Favorable outcome in isolation; however, significant proportion are associated with other anomalies
  - When identified prenatally, postnatal follow-up recommended to excluded developing hydrocephalus
- MCM: Normal neurodevelopmental outcome in isolation

Treatment

- CSF diversion for hydrocephalus: Ventriculoperitoneal shunt ± cyst shunt or marsupialization

DIAGNOSTIC CHECKLIST

Reporting Tips

- Terms, such as DW spectrum, variant, & continuum, can be confusing
  - Use clear description & best categorization of abnormal PF findings when possible (may not always be clear cut)
  - Note hydrocephalus & supratentorial anomalies

SELECTED REFERENCES

1. Whitehead MT et al: Refining the neuroimaging definition of the Dandy-Walker phenotype. AJNR Am J Neuroradiol. 43(10):1488-93, 2022
2. Nagaraj UD et al: evaluation of posterior fossa biometric measurements on fetal MRI in the evaluation of Dandy-Walker continuum. AJNR Am J Neuroradiol. 42(9):1716-21, 2021
3. Venkatesan C et al: Short- and long-term outcomes of prenatally diagnosed Dandy-Walker malformation, vermian hypoplasia, and blake pouch cyst. J Child Neurol. 36(12):1111-9, 2021
4. Aldinger KA et al: Redefining the etiologic landscape of cerebellar malformations. Am J Hum Genet. 105(3):606-15, 2019
5. Robinson AJ: Inferior vermian hypoplasia–preconception, misconception. Ultrasound Obstet Gynecol. 43(2):123-36, 2014

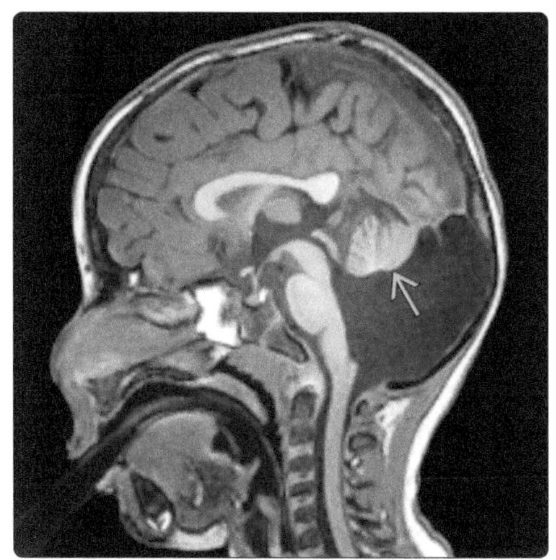

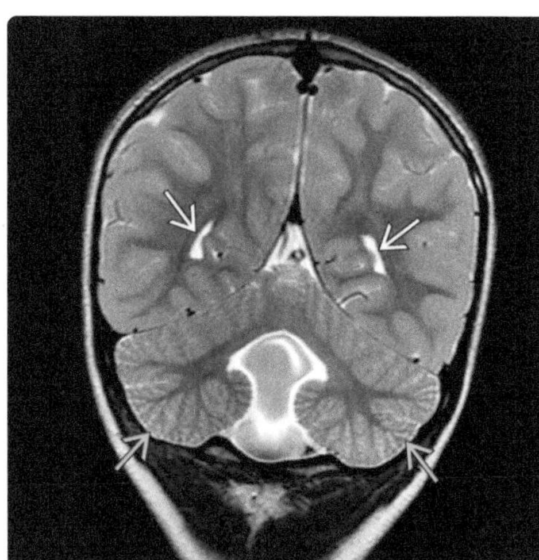

(Left) *Sagittal T1WI MR in a 4-year-old with vermian hypoplasia with associated BP remnant shows a small & rotated vermis → with no significant torcular-lambdoid inversion (though the lambdoid suture is difficult to see on this image).* **(Right)** *Coronal T2WI MR in the same patient demonstrates mild separation of the cerebellar hemispheres →. The supratentorial ventricles are normal in size ➔, & there is no evidence of ventricular obstruction.*

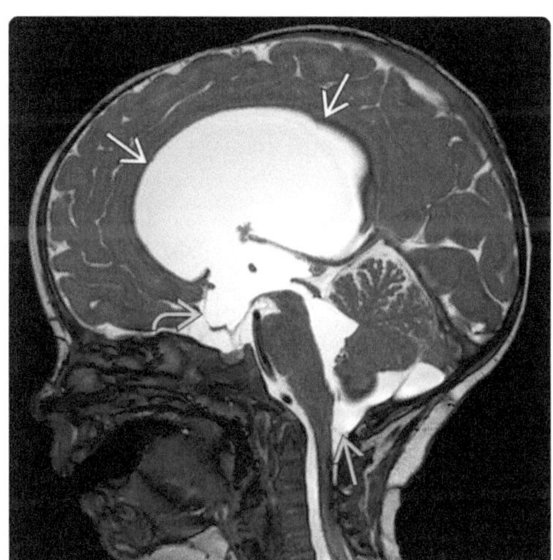

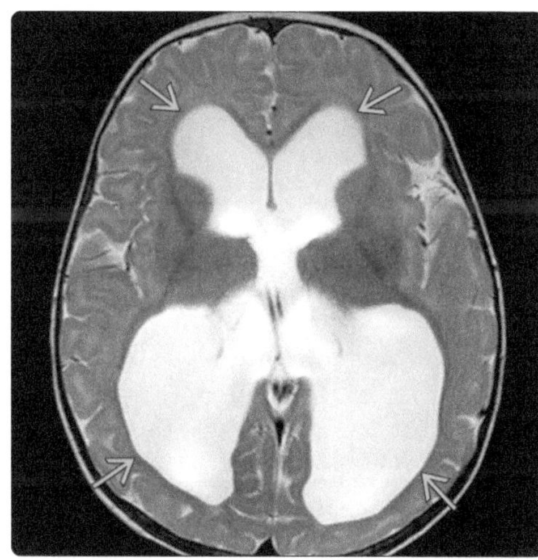

(Left) *Sagittal 3D FIESTA MR in a 9-month-old with a BP remnant → shows ventricular obstruction with upward stretching of the corpus callosum ➔ & anterior bowing of the lamina terminalis ↷. The vermis is normal in size.* **(Right)** *Axial T2WI MR in the same patient demonstrates ventriculomegaly of the lateral → & 3rd ventricles. However, there is evidence of chronic compensation, as there is no periventricular edema or sulcal effacement.*

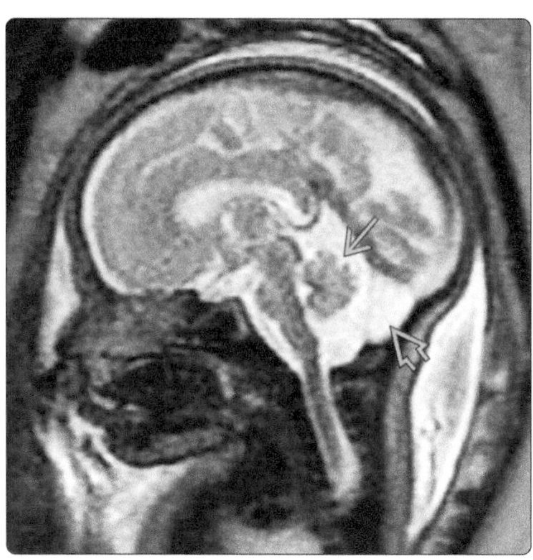

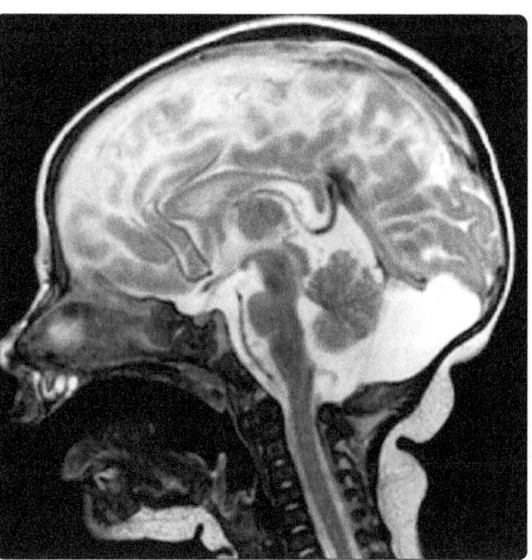

(Left) *Sagittal T2 SSFSE fetal MR at 33-weeks gestation shows a mega cisterna magna. In this patient, the cisterna magna ⇨ is enlarged, measuring 15 mm in the AP dimension. The vermis → is normal in size, morphology, & orientation.* **(Right)** *Postnatal sagittal T2 MR in the same patient at 6 weeks of age shows that the cisterna magna remains enlarged with a normal vermis. Note the lack of mass effect on the cerebellum & brainstem. In isolation, this is an incidental finding.*

Rhombencephalosynapsis

KEY FACTS

TERMINOLOGY

- Rhombencephalosynapsis (RES): Congenital continuity (lack of division) of cerebellar hemispheres
  - Complete or partial absence of vermis
  - Varying degrees of midline fusion of cerebellar hemispheres, dentate nuclei
  - May be partial; any portions of hemispheres may be affected

IMAGING

- Small, single hemisphere cerebellum
  - Continuous white matter (WM) tracts crossing midline
  - Absent primary fissure
  - Fused dentate nuclei
  - Small, diamond- or keyhole-shaped 4th ventricle
  - ± aqueductal stenosis → hydrocephalus
  - ± corpus callosum dysgenesis (especially posterior)

TOP DIFFERENTIAL DIAGNOSES

- Molar tooth malformations
- Lhermitte-Duclos syndrome
- Vermian hypoplasia
- Diffuse cerebellar cortical dysplasia

PATHOLOGY

- Failure of vermian differentiation
  - Differentiation of vermis required to separate cerebellar hemispheres

DIAGNOSTIC CHECKLIST

- Seen in ~ 50% of patients with aqueductal stenosis
- Remember to define associated supratentorial anomalies
- Can be mimicked by mechanically induced cerebellar deformation in chronically shunted patients
- Look closely for RES in setting of aqueductal stenosis

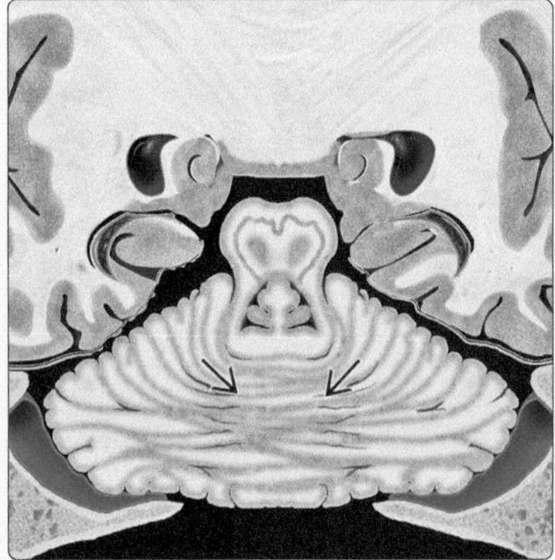

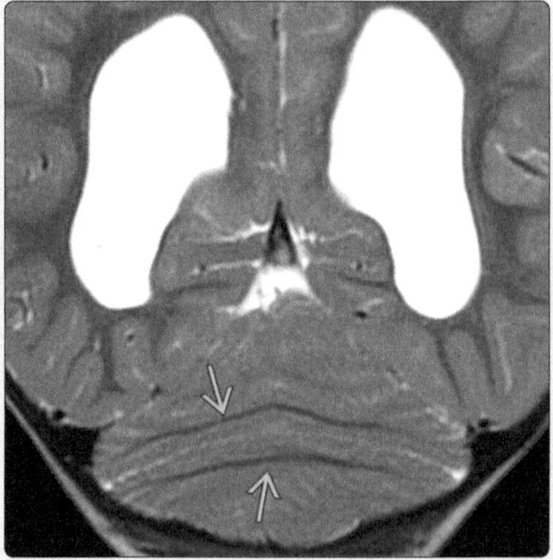

(Left) *Coronal graphic of rhombencephalosynapsis (RES) shows that no vermis is present in the midline of the cerebellum. Instead, the folia, interfoliate sulci, and cerebellar white matter ⇒ are continuous across the cerebellar midline.* **(Right)** *Coronal T2 MR in a syndromic (karyotype 47,XYY) patient with RES shows absence of the vermis and continuous bands of white matter ⇒ coursing uninterrupted across the midline cerebellum.*

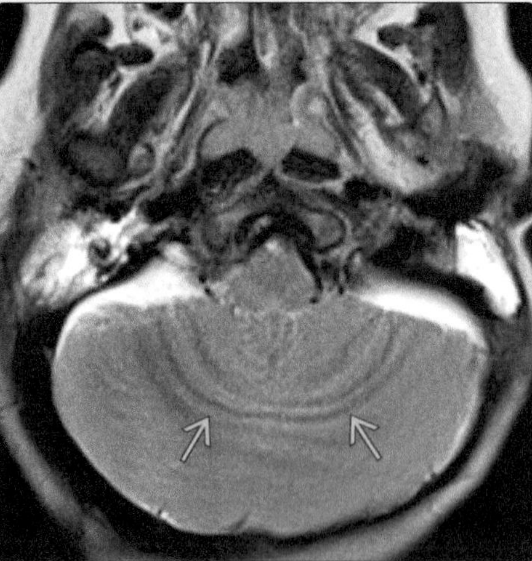

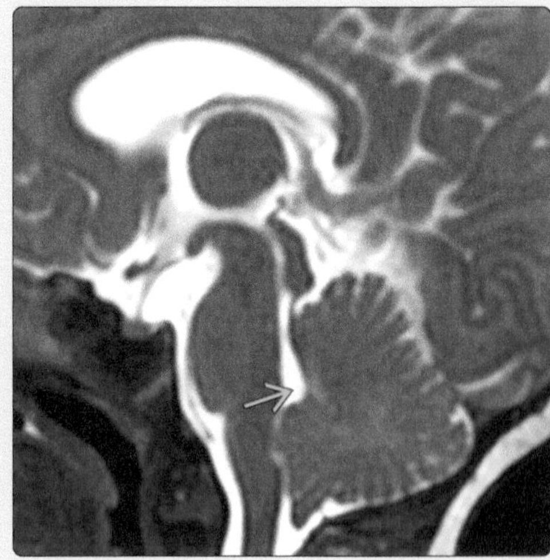

(Left) *Axial T2 MR in a 4-year-old shows absence of the cerebellar vermis and uninterrupted bands of white matter ⇒ coursing across the midline cerebellum, consistent with RES.* **(Right)** *Midline sagittal T2 MR in a newborn with isolated RES shows absence of the normal vermian landmarks (e.g., primary and prepyramidal fissures). In RES, the cerebellar folia are continuous across the midline. This also results in blunting or rounding of the normally sharp 4th ventricular fastigium ⇒.*

TERMINOLOGY

Abbreviations

- Rhombencephalosynapsis (RES)

Definitions

- Congenital continuity (lack of division) of cerebellar hemispheres
  - Complete or partial absence of vermis
  - Varying degrees of midline fusion of cerebellar hemispheres, dentate nuclei
    - Hemispheres usually continuous across midline
    - May be partial, affect any part(s) of hemispheres
  - Best classified as abnormal induction of dorsal cerebellar midline

IMAGING

General Features

- Best diagnostic clue
  - Single (often small) hemisphere cerebellum with continuous white matter (WM) tracts crossing midline
    - Small, diamond- or keyhole-shaped 4th ventricle
    - Fused dentate nuclei
- Location
  - Midline posterior fossa
- Size
  - Posterior fossa typically smaller than usual
- Morphology
  - Round or oval solitary cerebellar hemisphere

CT Findings

- NECT
  - Cerebellar hemispheric fusion
  - Diamond- or keyhole-shaped 4th ventricle
  - Narrowed transverse diameter of cerebellum
  - Often hydrocephalus with absent septum

MR Findings

- T1WI
  - Sagittal
    - Absent primary fissure of vermis
    - ± upwardly rounded fastigial recess of 4th ventricle
      - Nodulus preserved if fastigial recess present
    - ± aqueductal stenosis → hydrocephalus
    - ± corpus callosum dysgenesis (especially posterior)
  - Axial
    - ± collicular fusion
    - ± supratentorial cortical dysplasias
- T2WI
  - Coronal
    - Fused cerebellar hemispheres → total or partial
      - Continuous WM tracts across midline
      - Midline superior "tenting" of WM
    - Absent or severely hypoplastic vermis
    - Transverse folia
    - ± absent septum pellucidum
    - ± fused thalami and fornices
  - Fetal
    - Can be identified on fetal MR
      - Typically performed to investigate hydrocephalus seen on US
    - Abnormal shape of 4th ventricle and absence of vermis most reliable signs

Ultrasonographic Findings

- Grayscale ultrasound
  - Occasionally identified on fetal sonography

Imaging Recommendations

- Best imaging tool
  - MR
- Protocol advice
  - High-resolution FSE T2WI in multiple imaging planes
    - T2WI more clearly defines posterior fossa structures in neonate and infant

DIFFERENTIAL DIAGNOSIS

Molar Tooth Malformations

- Joubert syndrome
  - Vermian dysplasia with prominent superior cerebellar peduncles
  - 4th ventricle has bat wing shape

Lhermitte-Duclos Disease

- Dysplastic cerebellar gangliocytoma
- Striated cerebellar hemisphere
- Associated with Cowden syndrome

Vermian Hypoplasia

- Small vermis without hemispheric fusion
- Vermis develops enough to separate hemispheres, then arrests

Single Hemisphere Cerebellar Hypoplasia

- Often secondary to in utero insult

Diffuse Cerebellar Cortical Dysplasia

- May be associated with congenital muscular dystrophies
- Type 2 lissencephaly

PATHOLOGY

General Features

- Etiology
  - Unknown; 2 major theories
    - Failure of vermian differentiation
      - Based on evidence that hemispheres develop as unpaired structure from cerebellar primordium
      - Differentiation of vermis required to separate cerebellar hemispheres
      - Better explains cases of partial RES
    - Vermian agenesis allowing hemisphere continuity
      - Based on theory that hemispheres form separately from rhombic lips
      - Absence of vermian development allows hemispheres to become apposed and then fuse in midline
- Genetics
  - *FGF8* and *LMX1A* genes may influence expression of isthmic organizer
    - Isthmic organizer

- ▫ Controls/influences patterning of midbrain and anterior hindbrain
- ▫ Located within neuroepithelium of isthmic constriction at midbrain-hindbrain boundary
- o No genetic mutations have been found in RES
- o Syndromes associated with RES
  - – Gomez-Lopez-Hernandez syndrome
- Associated abnormalities
  - o Aqueductal stenosis: ~ 50% have associated RES
  - o Frequently occurs with other midline anomalies
    - – Absent septum pellucidum, holoprosencephalies
    - – Callosal and anterior commissure dysgenesis
    - – Thalamic fusion with 3rd ventricle atresia (diencephalosynapsis)
    - – Collicular fusion ± aqueductal stenosis/atresia, hydrocephalus
  - o Prosencephalic and midline facial anomalies
  - o Occasional associated extracranial anomalies
    - – Segmentation and fusion anomalies in spine
    - – Cardiovascular (conotruncal) anomalies reported
    - – Variable respiratory, GU anomalies reported
    - – Musculoskeletal anomalies common: Phalangeal and radial ray

Staging, Grading, & Classification

- Partial fusion
  - o Fusion may be in any part of cerebellum
- Presence or absence of supratentorial anomalies

Gross Pathologic & Surgical Features

- Typical
  - o Fused cerebellar hemispheres
  - o Fused cerebellar WM → large corpus medullare
  - o Absent posterior cerebellar incisura, vallecula
  - o Horseshoe-shaped dentate nuclei
  - o Agenesis or hypogenesis of anterior vermis, velum medullare anterior, and nuclei fastigii
  - o Hypoplastic posterior vermis
    - – Nodulus may form
- Rare
  - o Aventriculy (a.k.a. synencephaly or telencephalosynapsis)
  - o Encysted 4th ventricle

CLINICAL ISSUES

Presentation

- Most common signs/symptoms
  - o Variable neurologic signs
    - – Ataxia, gait abnormalities, seizures
    - – Developmental delay
    - – RES discovered in near-normal patients at autopsy
  - o Most common associated congenital syndrome is Gomez-Lopez-Hernandez syndrome
    - – Cerebello-trigeminal-dermal dysplasia
      - ▫ RES with scalp alopecia, abnormal head shape
      - ▫ Trigeminal anesthesia
      - ▫ Craniofacial dysmorphisms, short stature common

Demographics

- Age
  - o Usually found during early infancy or childhood
  - o Rarely incidental finding
- Epidemiology
  - o Rare but increasingly recognized on MR

Natural History & Prognosis

- Developmental delay
- Psychiatric disorders (self-injurious, bipolar, hyperactive)
- Additional midline supratentorial anomalies and hydrocephalus → worse prognosis

Treatment

- Treat related hydrocephalus, monitor hypothalamic-pituitary axis

DIAGNOSTIC CHECKLIST

Consider

- Look closely for RES in setting of aqueductal stenosis
- Isolated RES is less common than with supratentorial anomalies

Image Interpretation Pearls

- Can be mimicked by mechanically induced cerebellar deformation in chronically shunted patients

Reporting Tips

- Remember to define associated supratentorial anomalies

SELECTED REFERENCES

1. Fouda MA et al: Rhomboencephalosynapsis: review of the literature. World Neurosurg. 159:48-53, 2022
2. Moosavi A et al: Congenital malformations of cerebellum. Clin Perinatol. 49(3):603-21, 2022
3. Choudhary N et al: Gomez-López-Hernandez syndrome: the triad of cerebello-trigemino-dermal dysplasia. BMJ Case Rep. 14(10):e246189, 2021
4. Haratz KK et al: Prenatal diagnosis of rhombencephalosynapsis: neuroimaging features and severity of vermian anomaly. Ultrasound Obstet Gynecol. 58(6):864-74, 2021
5. Aldinger KA et al: Rhombencephalosynapsis: fused cerebellum, confused geneticists. Am J Med Genet C Semin Med Genet. 178(4):432-9, 2018
6. Kline-Fath BM et al: Prenatal aqueduct stenosis: association with rhombencephalosynapsis and neonatal outcome. Prenat Diagn. 38(13):1028-34, 2018
7. Chapman T et al: Diagnostic imaging of posterior fossa anomalies in the fetus and neonate: part 2, posterior fossa disorders. Clin Imaging. 39(2):167-75, 2015
8. Passi GR et al: Rhombencephalosynapsis. Pediatr Neurol. 52(6):651-2, 2015
9. Poretti A et al: Fetal diagnosis of rhombencephalosynapsis. Neuropediatrics. 46(6):357-8, 2015
10. Poretti A et al: Cerebellar hypoplasia: differential diagnosis and diagnostic approach. Am J Med Genet C Semin Med Genet. 166(2):211-26, 2014
11. Whitehead MT et al: Rhombencephalosynapsis as a cause of aqueductal stenosis: an under-recognized association in hydrocephalic children. Pediatr Radiol. 44(7):849-56, 2014
12. Weaver J et al: Rhombencephalosynapsis: embryopathology and management strategies of associated neurosurgical conditions with a review of the literature. J Neurosurg Pediatr. 11(3):320-6, 2013
13. Ishak GE et al: Rhombencephalosynapsis: a hindbrain malformation associated with incomplete separation of midbrain and forebrain, hydrocephalus and a broad spectrum of severity. Brain. 135(Pt 5):1370-86, 2012
14. Barkovich AJ et al: A developmental and genetic classification for midbrain-hindbrain malformations. Brain. 132(Pt 12):3199-230, 2009
15. Dill P et al: Fetal magnetic resonance imaging in midline malformations of the central nervous system and review of the literature. J Neuroradiol. 36(3):138-46, 2009
16. Jellinger KA: Rhombencephalosynapsis with and without associated malformations. Acta Neuropathol. 117(2):219, 2009
17. Pasquier L et al: Rhombencephalosynapsis and related anomalies: a neuropathological study of 40 fetal cases. Acta Neuropathol. 117(2):185-200, 2009

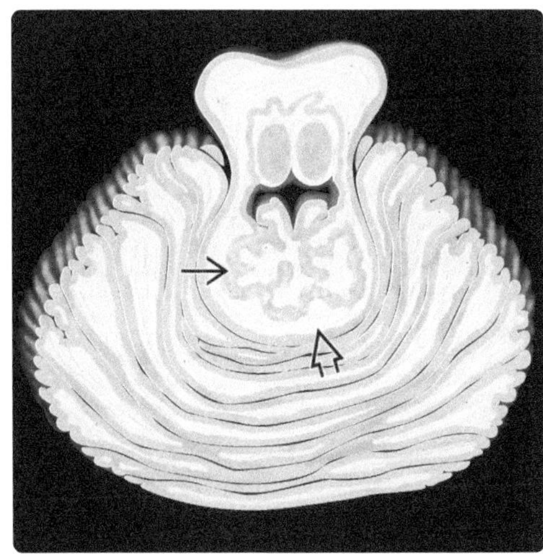

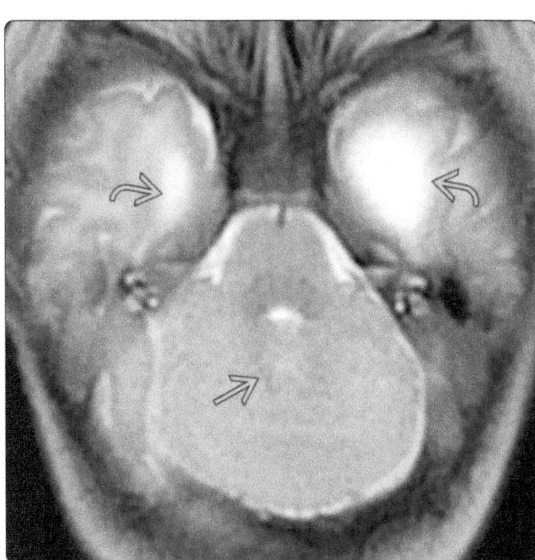

(Left) *Axial graphic of RES shows absence of the vermis. There is fusion of the folia, interfoliate sulci, dentate nuclei ➔, and cerebellar white matter ➔ across the midline.* **(Right)** *Axial T2 MR in a 2-month-old with aqueductal stenosis and RES shows absence of the cerebellar vermis and fusion of the dentate nuclei ➔. Also note the enlarged temporal horns ➔ in this patient with congenital hydrocephalus secondary to aqueductal stenosis.*

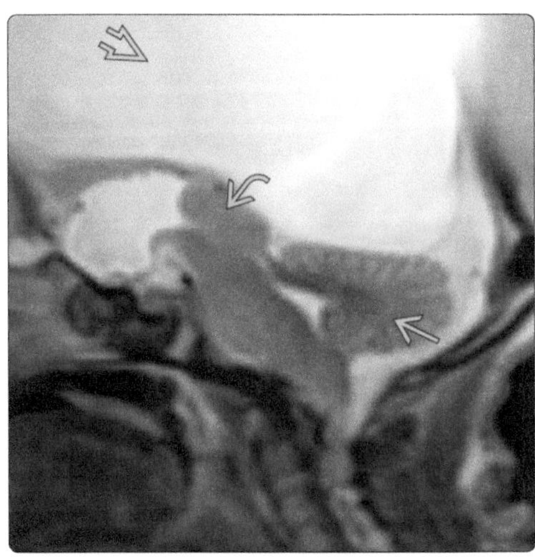

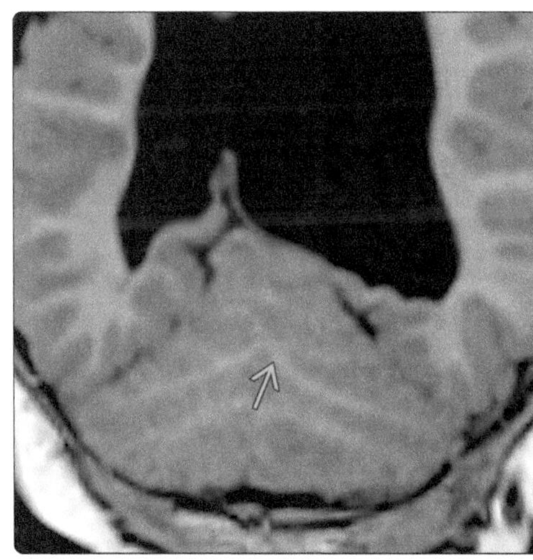

(Left) *Midline sagittal T2 MR in the same neonate shows absence of the normal vermian fissures ➔. Also note the thickened tectum ➔ with absence of the cerebral aqueduct and ventricular enlargement ➔. Aqueductal stenosis and RES are highly associated with one another.* **(Right)** *Coronal T1 MR in the same patient shows the myelinated white matter ➔ crossing the midline, consistent with RES in this patient with ventriculomegaly from aqueductal stenosis.*

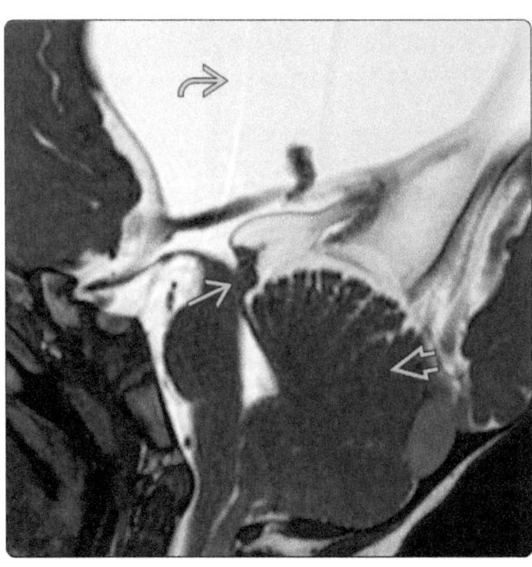

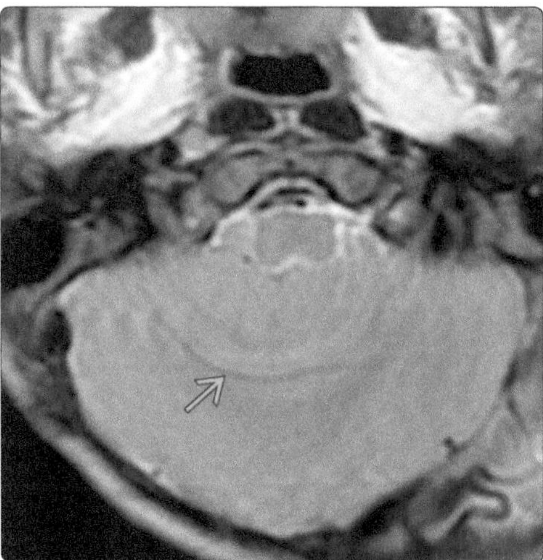

(Left) *Midline sagittal FIESTA MR in a 12-month-old with aqueductal stenosis and RES shows absence of normal vermian morphology (e.g., no primary fissure) ➔, absence of the distal cerebral aqueduct ➔, and ventriculomegaly ➔. There is a high association between aqueductal stenosis and RES.* **(Right)** *Axial T2 MR in the same patient shows white matter crossing the midline ➔ with absence of the vermis, pathognomonic findings for RES.*

Unclassified Cerebellar Dysplasias

KEY FACTS

TERMINOLOGY

- Focal or diffuse dysplasias of cerebellar hemispheres or vermis not associated with other known malformations or syndromes

IMAGING

- Asymmetry or focal disruption of cerebellar folial and sulcal morphology
    - Sometimes frank cleft is present
- Bumpy gray matter-white matter (GM-WM) interface in cerebellum
- Lack of normal arborization of WM
- Abnormal hyperintense signal in subcortical WM → cyst-like foci
- Cerebellar GM heterotopia
- Enlarged and vertically oriented fissures
- Disordered foliation

PATHOLOGY

- Most likely result of in utero insult with somatic mutations thought to be less likely cause

CLINICAL ISSUES

- In isolation, usually asymptomatic or mildly symptomatic, though more severe neurologic deficits have been described
- Milder clinical features include autism spectrum disorder, speech delay, oculomotor apraxia

DIAGNOSTIC CHECKLIST

- When considering diagnosis of isolated cerebellar dysplasia, check clinical presentation and available genetic studies
- Look for and document associated posterior fossa and supratentorial anomalies

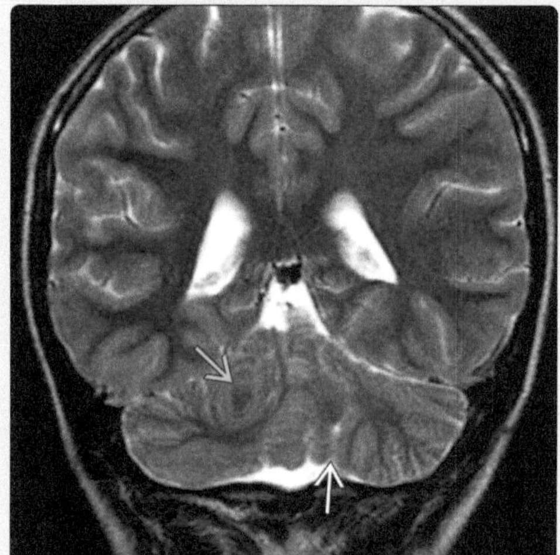

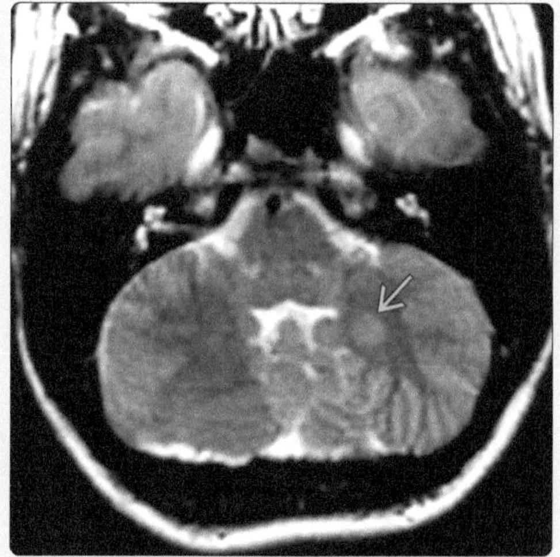

(Left) *Coronal T2WI MR in a 12-year-old girl with headaches demonstrates focal abnormal foliation of the right cerebellar hemisphere ⇨ and abnormal vertical cleft ➡ in the left cerebellar hemisphere compatible with cerebellar dysplasia. There is no other past medical history, and this is likely unrelated to clinical presentation.* **(Right)** *Axial T2WI MR in the same patient demonstrates left cerebellar gray matter heterotopia ⇨. While these are uncommon in the cerebellum, they are associated with cerebellar dysplasia.*

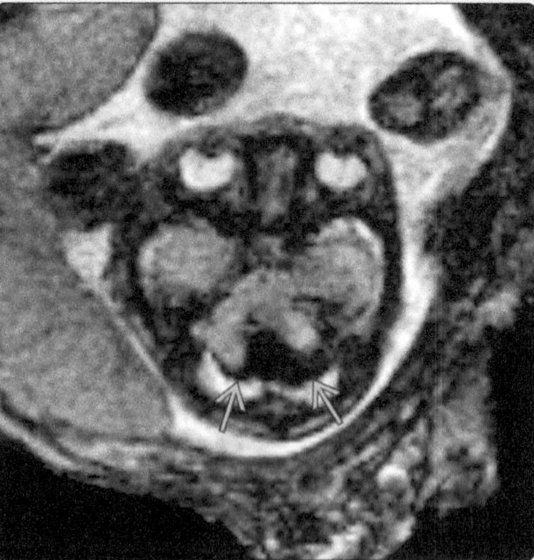

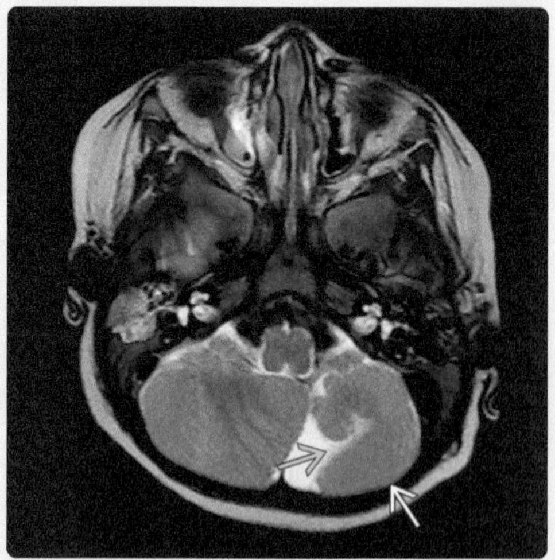

(Left) *Axial echo planar image from a fetal MR in a 25-weeks-gestation fetus referred for absence of normal cerebellar landmarks on fetal US shows a hemorrhage in the L > R cerebellar hemispheres ⇨. TORCH and neonatal alloimmune thrombocytopenia (NAIT) work-up were negative.* **(Right)** *Axial T2WI MR in the same patient at 12 months of age referred to ophthalmology for an esotropia work-up demonstrates hypoplasia ➡ and clefting ⇨ of the left cerebellar hemisphere as a result of prenatal injury.*

TERMINOLOGY

Synonyms

- Cerebellar polymicrogyria, cerebellar heterotopia, cerebellar dysgenesis

Definitions

- Descriptive term referring to abnormal morphology of cerebellum not associated with other known posterior fossa malformations, syndromes, or pathologic spectrums
  - Excludes Dandy-Walker continuum, Lhermitte-Duclos, rhombencephalosynapsis, Joubert syndrome and related disorders (JSRD/molar tooth malformations), dystroglycanopathies, other described genetic or nongenetic syndromes involving cerebellum and brainstem [e.g., PHACE(S), tubulinopathies, pontocerebellar hypoplasia]

IMAGING

General Features

- Best diagnostic clue
  - Abnormal orientation of cerebellar folia and sulcal morphology, usually with associated decreased volume
  - ± underlying heterotopic gray matter (GM) in cerebellar white matter (WM)
- Location
  - Variable: Can be uni- or bilateral; ± varying degrees of vermian involvement
- Morphology
  - Focal or global
  - Abnormal foliation, fissuration, WM arborization, loss of normal GM-WM differentiation

MR Findings

- T1WI, T2WI, FLAIR
  - Cerebellar clefting
  - Lack of normal arborization of WM
  - Cyst-like foci in subcortical WM
  - GM heterotopias, usually with abnormal foliation of overlying cortex
  - Abnormal sulcation and fissure orientation
  - Typically with decreased volume of affected area

Imaging Recommendations

- Best imaging tool: MR
- Protocol advice: Use thin-slice profile T2WI in axial and coronal planes to define cerebellar morphology

DIFFERENTIAL DIAGNOSIS

Rhombencephalosynapsis

- Incomplete separation of cerebellar hemispheres with associated partial or complete absence of vermis

Joubert Syndrome and Related Disorders (Molar Tooth Malformations)

- Thickened, elongated superior cerebellar peduncles in molar tooth configuration

Cerebellar Dysplasia Associated With Dystroglycanopathies

- Congenital muscular dystrophies

Dysplastic Cerebellar Gangliocytoma (Lhermitte-Duclos)

- Focal enlargement of cerebellar folia

Dandy-Walker Continuum

- Look for elevation of tegmentovermian angle/counter-clockwise rotation of vermis

PHACE(S) Syndrome

- **P**osterior fossa malformation, **h**emangioma, **a**rterial abnormalities, **c**ardiac abnormalities, **e**ye abnormalities, **s**ternal cleft

PATHOLOGY

General Features

- Cerebellar cortex does not assume adult-like histology prior to 1 year of age
- In one study of 147 normal infants, minor cerebellar dysplasias were identified in close to 85%
  - Some minor dysplasias involute after 9 months of age

Associated Findings

- Supratentorial cortical dysplasia or other malformation of cortical development
- Macro-/microscopic heterotopia in cerebellar WM

Causes

- Most likely secondary to in utero disruptive event
- Disruption of cerebellar cortical development by mosaic genetic abnormality possible but less likely
- Potential etiologies: *COL4A1* mutation, TORCH infection, hypoxic-ischemic encephalopathy (HIE), in utero toxins

CLINICAL ISSUES

Presentation

- Most common signs/symptoms
  - Highly variable, ranging from incidental to severe neurologic impairment
  - In absence of supratentorial anomalies, patients either mildly affected or asymptomatic
- Other signs/symptoms
  - Ataxia, facial malformations, abnormal eye movements, motor delay

DIAGNOSTIC CHECKLIST

Consider

- When considering diagnosis of isolated cerebellar dysplasia, check clinical presentation and available genetic studies
- In isolation, focal cerebellar dysplasia is usually incidental and result of some type of in utero insult

Reporting Tips

- Look for and document associated posterior fossa and supratentorial anomalies

SELECTED REFERENCES

1. Barkovich AJ et al: Pediatric Neuroimaging. 6th ed. Wolters Kluwer: 545-8, 2019
2. Bosemani T et al: Congenital abnormalities of the posterior fossa. Radiographics. 35(1):200-20, 2015
3. Barkovich AJ et al: A developmental and genetic classification for midbrain-hindbrain malformations. Brain. 132(Pt 12):3199-230, 2009

KEY FACTS

TERMINOLOGY

- Joubert syndrome and related disorders (JSRD)
  - Hindbrain anomaly characterized by dysmorphic vermis, lack of decussation of superior cerebellar peduncle, central pontine tracts, corticospinal tracts
- Also sometimes called molar tooth malformation (MTM)

IMAGING

- Molar tooth appearance of midbrain on axial images
- Midline vermian clefting
- Thick, horizontal (perpendicular to brainstem) superior cerebellar peduncles
- Midline depression of 4th ventricular floor at isthmus (thin isthmus on midline)
- High-definition T2 (CISS/FIESTA) provides exquisite structural analysis

TOP DIFFERENTIAL DIAGNOSES

- Dandy-Walker continuum
- Vermian and pontocerebellar hypoplasia
- Cerebellar vermian hypoplasia
- Cerebellar vermian atrophy

PATHOLOGY

- > 20 causative genes have been discovered so far
  - All encode for proteins expressed in primary cilium/its apparatus
- Absence of decussation of superior cerebellar peduncles
- Near-total absence of pyramidal decussation

CLINICAL ISSUES

- Ataxia, developmental delay, oculomotor and respiratory abnormalities

DIAGNOSTIC CHECKLIST

- Look for MTM whenever scanning infants/children with severe hypotonia and ocular anomalies

(Left) *Axial graphic depicts Joubert malformation. Thickened superior cerebellar peduncles ➔ around the elongated 4th ventricle form the classic "molar tooth" seen in this anomaly. Note the sagittal cleft within the small dysplastic cerebellar vermis ➔.* **(Right)** *Axial T1WI MR in a 4-month-old with molar tooth sign shows the prominent thickening of the superior cerebellar peduncles ➔ that forms the "roots" of the molar tooth while the pons ➔ forms the "crown" of the molar tooth.*

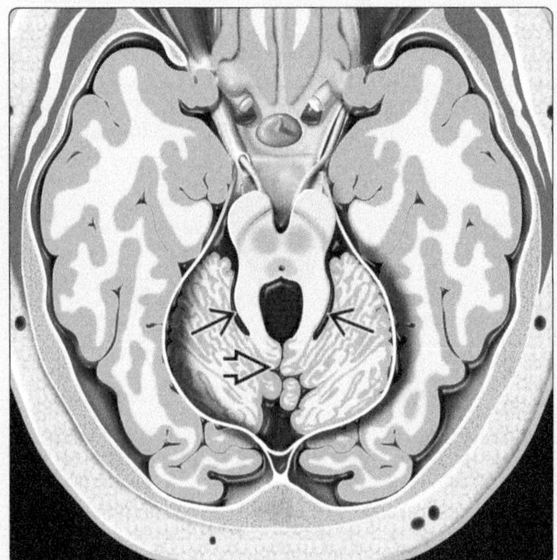

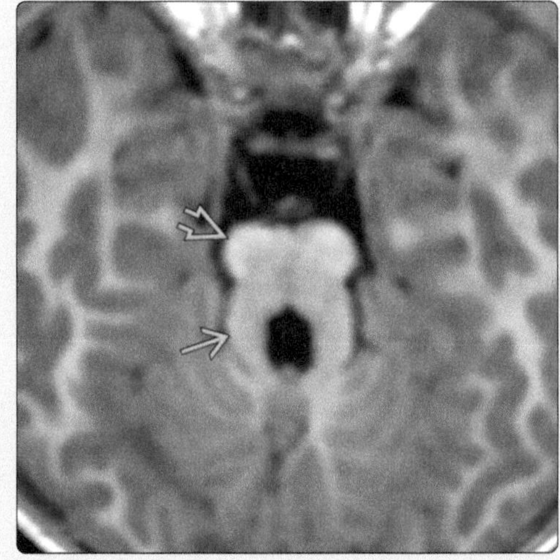

(Left) *Axial T1WI MR in a 2-day-old with nystagmus and molar tooth sign shows the prominent thickening of the superior cerebellar peduncles ➔. Note how they are myelinated structures in this neonate.* **(Right)** *Sagittal T2WI MR in the same patient shows the abnormal small vermis ➔ in this patient with molar tooth sign and Joubert syndrome. Note the dysplastic roof of the 4th ventricle with loss of the normal fastigial point. These are typical findings in Joubert syndrome.*

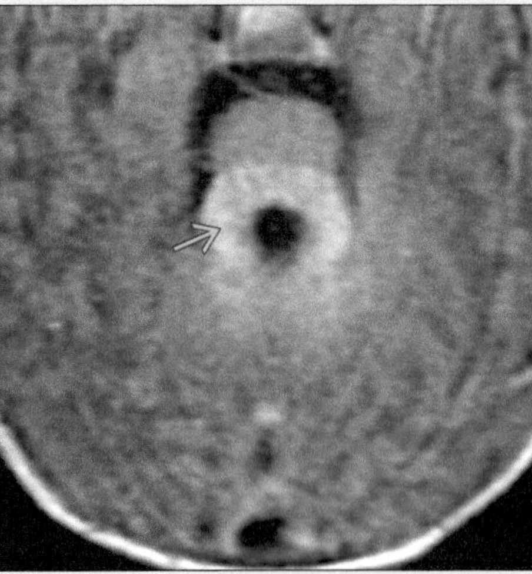

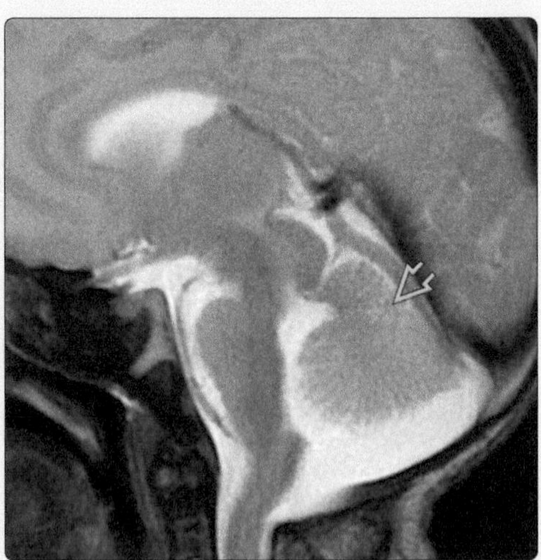

TERMINOLOGY

Abbreviations

- Molar tooth malformation (MTM)

Definitions

- Joubert syndrome and related disorders (JSRD)
  - Include Joubert, Dekaban-Arima, COACH (**c**erebellar vermis hypo-/aplasia, **o**ligophrenia, congenital **a**taxia, ocular **c**oloboma, **h**epatic fibrosis), Senior-Loken, Varadi-Papp, Joubert-polymicrogyria syndromes, oral-digital-facial syndrome
  - New genes/syndromes with MTM continue to be described
  - JSRD considered as ciliopathy
- Hindbrain anomaly characterized by dysmorphic vermis, thick horizontal superior cerebellar peduncles (SCPs)
  - Sagittal clefting of cerebellar vermis
  - Abnormal brainstem nuclei
  - SCPs, central pontine tracts, corticospinal tracts do not decussate

IMAGING

General Features

- Best diagnostic clue
  - Molar tooth appearance of midbrain on axial images
  - Small vermis with midline clefting
- Location
  - Brainstem isthmus (pontomesencephalic)
  - Vermis and superior (efferent) cerebellar peduncle
- Morphology
  - Hard to identify vermis with midline sagittal cleft
    - Dorsal 4th ventricle has dysmorphic, irregular fastigium
  - Thick, horizontal (perpendicular to brainstem), SCPs
  - Midline depression of 4th ventricular floor at isthmus (thin isthmus on midline)
  - Frequently associated with other brain malformations (e.g., polymicrogyria)

CT Findings

- NECT
  - Vermis clefting
  - 4th ventricle has bat wing configuration

MR Findings

- T1WI
  - Sagittal
    - Normal midline appearance of vermis lost
    - Dysmorphic roof of 4th ventricle with fastigial point lost
    - Large CSF spaces, but tentorium is in normal location
  - Coronal
    - Vermian clefting above apposed hemispheres (cleft lined with cortex)
  - Axial: Vermian clefting, molar tooth appearance
    - Anteriorly pointed ventricular floor at pons-midbrain junction (thin isthmus)
    - Prominent, in-plane, parallel SCPs (molar roots)
    - Bat wing appearance of 4th ventricle
- T2WI
  - Same findings as T1WI
    - Better contrast than T1WI
    - Prominent CSF spaces common
    - Abnormal myelination sometimes
  - High-definition T2 (CISS/FIESTA) provides exquisite structural analysis
  - HASTE allows clear identification of molar tooth sign in fetuses
- Diffusion tensor imaging (DTI)
  - SCPs fail to decussate in mesencephalon
  - ± thinning of middle cerebral peduncle, ventral pontocerebellar tracts

Ultrasonographic Findings

- Prenatal ultrasound shows small vermis, large cisterna magna
  - May show supernumerary digits, heart disease, kidney disease, etc.

Imaging Recommendations

- Best imaging tool
  - MR
- Protocol advice
  - Use high definition; posterior fossa structures are small
  - DTI is useful complementary technique

DIFFERENTIAL DIAGNOSIS

Dandy-Walker Continuum

- Hypo-/agenetic vermis (not clefting)
- Cerebellar hemispheres often small
- Elevated tentorium

Vermian and Pontocerebellar Hypoplasia

- Vermis is small, no clefting
- Variable abnormalities of pons, medulla, midbrain

Rhombencephalosynapsis

- Cerebellar hemispheres/dentates are fused without differentiated midline vermis

Cerebellar Vermian Atrophy

- Midbrain, cerebellar peduncles normal; normal vermian foliation with enlarged fissures
- Causal context (prematurity, metabolic, etc.)

PATHOLOGY

General Features

- Etiology
  - Thought to result from mutations of ciliary/centrosomal proteins that can affect cell migration, axonal pathway, other still unknown mechanisms
    - Referred to as ciliopathy
    - Seen in many syndromes [Meckel-Gruber, orofacial-digital syndrome type VI (OFD VI), Bardet-Biedl, Senior-Loken, others]
- Genetics
  - Predominately autosomal recessive
  - > 20 causative genes discovered so far
    - All encoding proteins expressed in primary cilia and its apparatus

- Associated CNS findings include ocular anomalies, polymicrogyria, cephaloceles, hamartomas
- Mutations in *CSPP1* → classic Joubert syndrome
- Malformation complexes probably result from disruption of several different processes involving cilia
- Associated abnormalities
  - Polymicrogyria; renal, retinal, hepatic abnormalities
    - Prominent CSF spaces and ventriculomegaly
    - Rarely: Meningoencephaloceles, microcephaly, lissencephaly, agenesis of corpus callosum
    - Hypothalamic hamartomas
  - Juvenile nephronophthisis or multicystic dysplastic kidney
  - Ocular anomalies (retinal dysplasias and colobomata)
  - Hepatic fibrosis and cysts, heart disease, polydactyly

Gross Pathologic & Surgical Features

- Midbrain-hindbrain malformation characterized by
  - Dysmorphic vermis with midline cleft
  - Thick, horizontal SCPs
  - Ocular colobomas, polymicrogyria can be found

Microscopic Features

- Absence of decussation of SCPs
- Near-total absence of pyramidal decussation
- Dysplasias and heterotopia of cerebellar nuclei
- Structural anomalies in multiple locations
  - Inferior olivary nuclei, descending trigeminal tract, solitary fascicle, dorsal column nuclei

CLINICAL ISSUES

Presentation

- Most common signs/symptoms
  - Core features: Hypotonia, ataxia, intellectual disability
  - Other: Variable involvement of retina, kidneys, liver
- Other signs/symptoms
  - Neonate: Nystagmus, alternating apnea, hyperpnea (Joubert syndrome), seizures
  - Characteristic facial features
    - Large head
    - Prominent forehead
    - High, rounded eyebrows
    - Epicanthal folds
    - Upturned nose with evident nostrils
    - Tongue protrusion and rhythmic tongue motions
    - In OFD VI, teratomas of tongue
  - Retinal anomalies
    - Congenital retinal dystrophy
    - Pigmentary retinopathy
    - Chorioretinal colobomata
    - Fundus flavus

Demographics

- Age
  - Infancy and childhood; isolated oculomotor apraxia may present later
- Sex
  - M = F

Natural History & Prognosis

- Early death in affected infants
- Older children → problems with temperament, hyperactivity, aggressiveness, and dependency
  - Most affected children are severely impaired

Treatment

- Genetic counseling, physical therapy, occupational therapy

DIAGNOSTIC CHECKLIST

Consider

- MTM whenever scanning infants/children with severe hypotonia and ocular anomalies

Image Interpretation Pearls

- If vermis not recognized or looks small and dysmorphic on sagittal image
- Sometimes vermis looks nearly normal
  - Look for vermian cleft and molar tooth sign on axials

SELECTED REFERENCES

1. Dong Y et al: Clinical and genetic characteristics of 36 children with Joubert syndrome. Front Pediatr. 11:1102639, 2023
2. Liao DW et al: Analysis of CT and MRI manifestations of Joubert syndrome. J Belg Soc Radiol. 107(1):78, 2023
3. Moosavi A et al: Congenital malformations of cerebellum. Clin Perinatol. 49(3):603-21, 2022
4. Surisetti BK et al: Clinical and imaging profile of patients with Joubert syndrome. J Mov Disord. 14(3):231-5, 2021
5. Aljeaid D et al: A novel pathogenic variant in OFD1 results in X-linked Joubert syndrome with orofaciodigital features and pituitary aplasia. Am J Med Genet A. 179(6):1010-4, 2019
6. Hardee I et al: Defective ciliogenesis in INPP5E-related Joubert syndrome. Am J Med Genet A. 173(12):3231-7, 2017
7. Poretti A et al: Joubert syndrome: neuroimaging findings in 110 patients in correlation with cognitive function and genetic cause. J Med Genet. 54(8):521-9, 2017
8. Vilboux T et al: Molecular genetic findings and clinical correlations in 100 patients with Joubert syndrome and related disorders prospectively evaluated at a single center. Genet Med. 19(8):875-82, 2017
9. Quarello E: Enlarged intracranial translucency and molar tooth sign in the first trimester as features of Joubert syndrome and related disorders. Ultrasound Obstet Gynecol. 48(4):532-4, 2016
10. Chapman T et al: Diagnostic imaging of posterior fossa anomalies in the fetus and neonate: part 2, posterior fossa disorders. Clin Imaging. 39(2):167-75, 2015
11. Hsu CC et al: High-resolution diffusion tensor imaging and tractography in Joubert syndrome: Beyond molar tooth sign. Pediatr Neurol. 53(1):47-52, 2015
12. Huppke P et al: Tectonic gene mutations in patients with Joubert syndrome. Eur J Hum Genet. 23(5):616-20, 2015
13. Van Battum EY et al: Axon guidance proteins in neurological disorders. Lancet Neurol. 14(5):532-46, 2015
14. Akizu N et al: Mutations in CSPP1 lead to classical Joubert syndrome. Am J Hum Genet. 94(1):80-6, 2014
15. Poretti A et al: The molar tooth sign is pathognomonic for Joubert syndrome! Pediatr Neurol. 50(6):e15-6, 2014
16. Romani M et al: Joubert syndrome: congenital cerebellar ataxia with the molar tooth. Lancet Neurol. 12(9):894-905, 2013
17. Simms RJ et al: Modelling a ciliopathy: Ahi1 knockdown in model systems reveals an essential role in brain, retinal, and renal development. Cell Mol Life Sci. 69(6):993-1009, 2012
18. Lee JE et al: Cilia in the nervous system: linking cilia function and neurodevelopmental disorders. Curr Opin Neurol. 24(2):98-105, 2011
19. Poretti A et al: Joubert syndrome and related disorders: spectrum of neuroimaging findings in 75 patients. AJNR Am J Neuroradiol. 32(8):1459-63, 2011
20. Saleem SN et al: Prenatal magnetic resonance imaging diagnosis of molar tooth sign at 17 to 18 weeks of gestation in two fetuses at risk for Joubert syndrome and related cerebellar disorders. Neuropediatrics. 42(1):35-8, 2011
21. Sattar S et al: The ciliopathies in neuronal development: a clinical approach to investigation of Joubert syndrome and Joubert syndrome-related disorders. Dev Med Child Neurol. 53(9):793-8, 2011

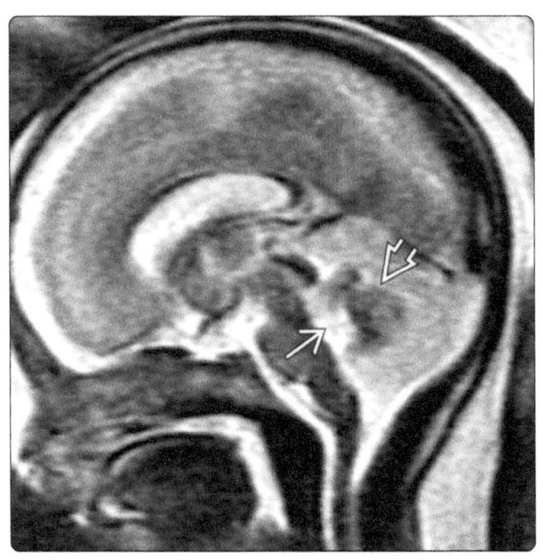

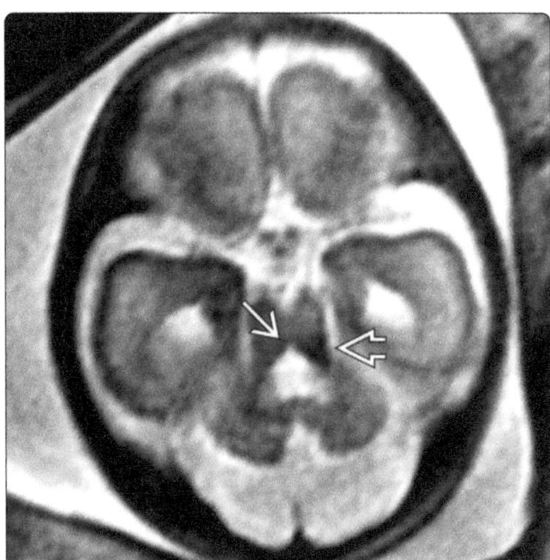

(Left) *Sagittal T2WI HASTE MR in a 27-week fetus shows a dysmorphic 4th ventricle ➡ with a hardly recognizable vermis ➡ (abnormal shape, no normal fissures identified). The posterior fossa cisterns are markedly enlarged. Supratentorial structures are normal.* **(Right)** *Axial T2WI HASTE MR in the same patient demonstrates an anteriorly pointed 4th ventricle ➡ and thick superior cerebellar peduncles ➡, giving the appearance of a molar tooth.*

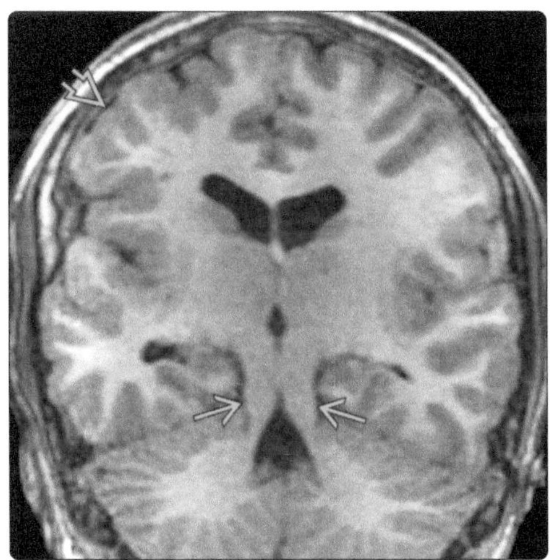

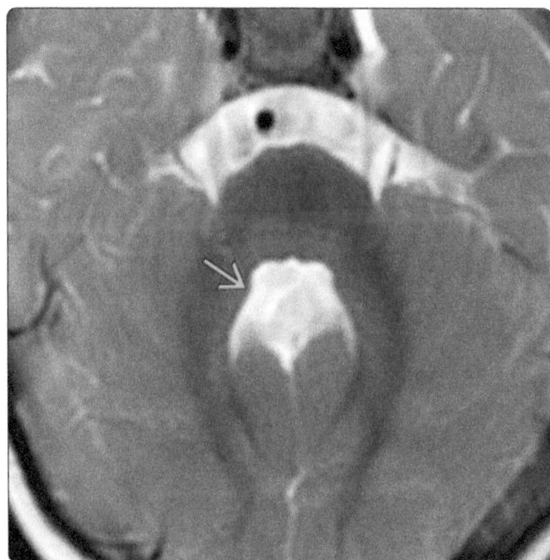

(Left) *Oblique coronal T1WI MR in a 14-year-old boy with Joubert syndrome shows elongation of the superior cerebellar peduncles → and associated right frontal operculum polymicrogyria ⇒. Associated brain malformations are common in JSRD.* **(Right)** *Axial T2WI MR in a 1-year-old with Joubert syndrome shows absence of the inferior vermis, which often results in a bat wing appearance of the 4th ventricle →. Sometimes, the inferior 4th ventricle appears effaced due to absence of the inferior 4th ventricle.*

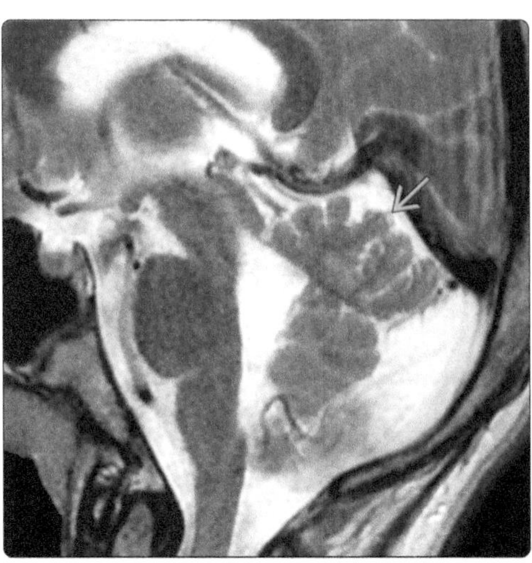

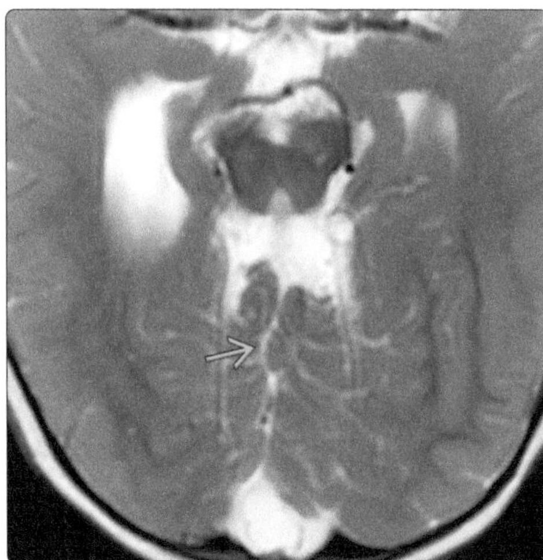

(Left) *Midline sagittal T2WI MR in a 14-year-old boy with Joubert syndrome shows a small dysplastic vermis → that is located superiorly, a characteristic finding in JSRD. In the axial plane, the superior vermis typically has an irregular clefted appearance.* **(Right)** *Axial T2WI MR in a 1-year-old with Joubert syndrome shows a sagittal cleft → in the small dysmorphic vermis, a common finding in JSRD.*

Cerebellar Hypoplasia

KEY FACTS

TERMINOLOGY

- Microcerebellum, cerebellar hypogenesis
- Inherited or acquired condition, isolated or syndromic/malformative
- Characterized by ↓ or disorganized cerebellar growth, injury, or ↑ apoptosis

IMAGING

- Morphology
  - Global cerebellar hypoplasia
  - Cerebellar with brainstem hypoplasia (includes pontocerebellar hypoplasia)
  - Vermian predominant cerebellar hypoplasia (Dandy-Walker continuum)
  - Unilateral cerebellar hypoplasia usually (not always) acquired from prenatal insult
- MR is study of choice
  - Small cerebellum ± pontine hypoplasia or clefting
  - May see vermian hypogenesis, anomalous fissuration, cortical dysplasias, supra-/infratentorial malformations
- Thin-section 3D MR acquisition of entire brain with multiplanar reformats

TOP DIFFERENTIAL DIAGNOSES

- Cerebellar atrophy
  - Loss of cerebellar tissue after formation: Many causes, and there can be overlap
  - Metabolic/neurodegenerative disorders, posttraumatic, paraneoplastic, epilepsy, radiation therapy, toxic

CLINICAL ISSUES

- Wide variety of clinical presentations due to heterogeneous pathologies and numerous genetic associations
- Poor correlation with degree of cerebellar deformity and clinical outcome
  - Additional imaging findings, prenatal history/exposures, and genetic profile are extremely important

(Left) *Sagittal T1 MR in a child with microcephaly, colobomas, choreoathetosis, and strabismus shows severe hypoplasia of cerebellum and pons. The posterior fossa is small with downward-sloping tentorium. No mutations for known types of pontocerebellar hypoplasia were found.* **(Right)** *Sagittal T2 MR in a preterm infant after a complicated NICU course shows hydrocephalus and hypoplasia of the cerebellum and pons. Intraventricular hemorrhage in preterm neonates is associated with cerebellar hemorrhage.*

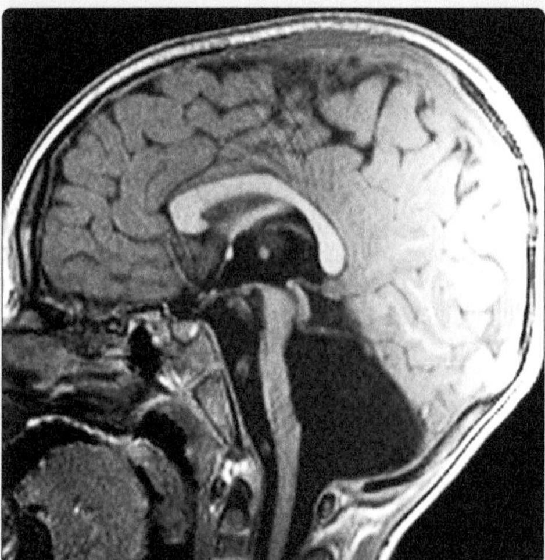

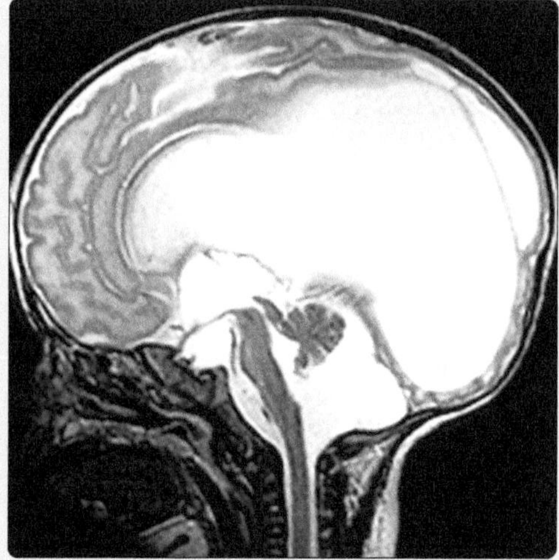

(Left) *Sagittal T1 MR in a 7-year-old with pontocerebellar hypoplasia from an EXOSC3 mutation demonstrates a very small cerebellar vermis with disproportionate hypoplasia of the inferior vermis ⇨. Note mild flattening of the ventral pons ⇨.* **(Right)** *Coronal T2 MR in the same patient demonstrates severe cerebellar hypoplasia of the cerebellar hemispheres ⇨ with marked enlargement of the cerebellar sulci. Also note mild ventriculomegaly of the lateral ventricles ➡.*

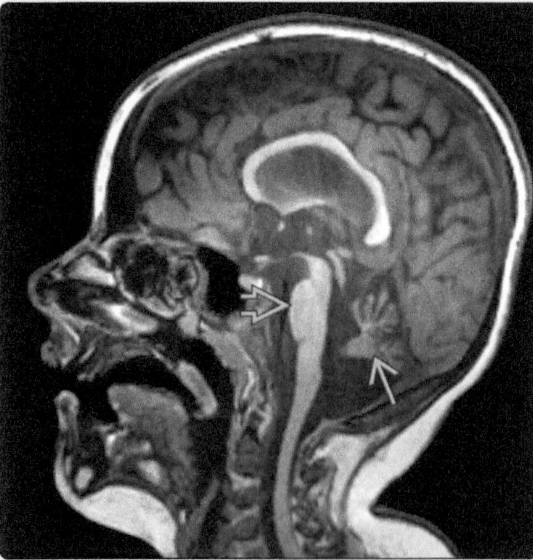

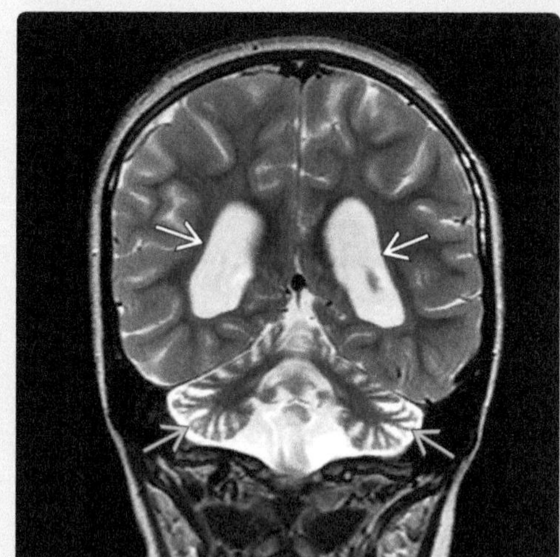

TERMINOLOGY

Synonyms

- Microcerebellum, cerebellar hypogenesis

Definitions

- Spectrum of malformative or disruptive conditions
  - There can be overlap
- Characterized by ↓ or disorganized growth, injury, or ↑ apoptosis

IMAGING

General Features

- Best diagnostic clue
  - ↓ cerebellar volume ± cerebellar dysplasia
- Location
  - May be isolated to posterior fossa structures or may include supratentorial brain malformation
  - Can be primarily vermian, global, unilateral, ± brainstem involvement
- Size
  - Variable
- Morphology
  - Global cerebellar hypoplasia
    - Numerous genetic abnormalities and syndromes
    - Congenital infection (CMV most common), prenatal drug exposure, prematurity
  - Cerebellar and brainstem involvement
    - Pontocerebellar hypoplasia (PCH), Joubert syndrome and related disorders (JSRD), dystroglycanopathies (a.k.a. congenial muscular dystrophies), other genetic disorders
  - Unilateral hypoplasia is often (not always) secondary to prenatal injury
    - PHACE(S), *COL4A1* mutation, cerebellar cleft
  - Vermian hypoplasia/aplasia
    - Dandy-Walker continuum
    - Rhombencephalosynapsis

CT Findings

- NECT
  - Bony posterior fossa variable in size
    - Enlarged with classic Dandy-Walker malformation, small with Chiari 2

MR Findings

- T1WI
  - Small cerebellum
    - ± pontine hypoplasia or clefting
    - ± vermian hypogenesis, anomalous fissuration, cortical dysplasias, infra-/supratentorial malformations
- T2WI
  - ± hypomyelination
- FLAIR
  - Hyperintense gliosis may suggest atrophy rather than hypogenesis

Imaging Recommendations

- Best imaging tool
  - Volumetric MR for entire brain with multiplanar reformats
- Protocol advice
  - Consider thin-section TruFISP/FIESTA images through posterior fossa for Dandy-Walker spectrum to look for coexisting Blake pouch remnant or arachnoid cyst for surgical planning

DIFFERENTIAL DIAGNOSIS

Cerebellar Atrophy

- Loss of cerebellar tissue after formation: Many causes, and there can be overlap
  - ± gliosis, focal volume loss, enlarged cerebellar fissures/interfoliate sulci
- Progressive inborn errors of metabolism or neurodegenerative
  - Partial list: Zellweger, Smith-Lemli-Opitz, GM2, congenital disorders of glycosylation type 1, ataxia-telangiectasia (ATM), infantile neuraxonal dystrophy, coenzyme Q deficiency, spinocerebellar atrophy, olivopontocerebellar atrophy
- Posttraumatic brain injury, posterior fossa surgery
- Paraneoplastic syndromes
  - Hodgkin disease, Langerhans cell histiocytosis, opsoclonus myoclonus syndrome
- Chronic epilepsy
- Radiation therapy
- Malnutrition
  - Vitamin B12 deficiency
- Toxic
  - Antiepileptics, such as phenytoin, tacrolimus, EtOH, solvents, heavy metals

PATHOLOGY

General Features

- Etiology
  - Genetic mutations or acquired prenatal insults
  - Acquired insults
    - Cerebellum susceptible to prenatal hemorrhages; may be germinal matrix in origin
    - Congenital infection: Rubella, parvovirus, and CMV in particular have all been implicated in cases of cerebellar or pontocerebellar "arrest"
- Genetics
  - Nonprogressive cerebellar hypoplasias: Many
    - Familial neocerebellar hypoplasias: X-linked (*OPHN1, DKC1*) and autosomal recessive forms
    - Aneuploidy: Trisomies 13, 18, 21; Cornelia de Lange, etc.
  - PCH
    - Has become descriptive term rather than diagnosis comprising heterogeneous group of disorders
    - > 20 described types/genetic anomalies; list is growing
    - Pons is often small in patients with cerebellar hypoplasia due to diminished associated axonal pathways and is not diagnostic of genetic diagnosis
  - Neuronal migrational anomalies
    - Reelin pathway: *RELN, VLDLR*
    - Tubulin genes: *TUBA1A, TUBB2B, TUBB3*
  - Vermian malformations and hypoplasias
    - Dandy-Walker continuum (*ZIC1/ZIC4, FOXC1*), JSRD (*NPHP1, AHI1*); rhombencephalosynapsis

- Dystroglycanopathies (a.k.a. congenital muscular dystrophies)
  - Walker-Warburg syndrome, Fukuyama congenital muscular dystrophy, muscle-eye-brain disease
- Associated abnormalities
  - Clinical associations
    - PHACE syndrome: **P**osterior fossa malformations, **h**emangiomas, **a**rterial anomalies, **c**oarctation of aorta and cardiac anomalies, **e**ye anomalies
    - Ciliopathies (± renal, digital, ocular anomalies): JSRD
    - CHARGE: **C**oloboma, **h**eart defects, **a**tresia choanae, **r**estricted growth and development, **g**enital hypoplasia, **e**ar anomalies
    - Velocardiofacial syndrome (DiGeorge syndrome): 22q11.2 deletion, inner ear anomalies, choanal atresia, congenital heart disease, facial anomalies
- Embryology anatomy
  - Abnormal expression of superior rhombic lip progenitors may cause diffuse granule cell hypoplasia → severe diffuse cerebellar hypoplasia
    - *ATOH1, ZIC1, ZIC3, MEIS1, PAX6*
  - Abnormal development of cerebellar ventricular zone causes cerebellar hypoplasia or agenesis
    - *PTF1A, FOXC1, CXCL12*
  - Unilateral cerebellar hypoplasia likely secondary to early fetal injury or genetic mutations with somatic mosaicism
    - Prenatal hemorrhage leading cause

Staging, Grading, & Classification

- Cerebellar agenesis: Near-complete absence of cerebellar tissue
- Global cerebellar hypoplasia
- Unilateral cerebellar hypoplasia
- Vermian hypoplasia
- Refine grading by assessing additional features: ± cerebellar dysplasia, brainstem involvement, supratentorial malformation, hypomyelination, extra-CNS anomalies

Gross Pathologic & Surgical Features

- Neocerebellar, ± pontine hypoplasia, ± fissuration anomalies

Microscopic Features

- ↓ number of cerebellar cortical neurons
- ± dentate nucleus disorganized
- ± nuclear gray matter of brainstem hypoplastic or absent
- ± heterotopic islands within white matter or cortical heterotopias

CLINICAL ISSUES

Presentation

- Most common signs/symptoms
  - Wide range of symptomatology
    - Poor correlation between severity of cerebellar deformity and clinical symptoms
  - Cerebellar hypoplasia must be assessed in context of other anomalies, genetic profile, and clinical history/prior exposures
- Other signs/symptoms
  - Renal, ocular, hepatic, or cardiac malformations may be clue to specific diagnosis
- Clinical profile
  - Variable hypotonia, ataxia (may be mild or severe), tremor or titubation, strabismus, nystagmus, cognitive and speech delays

Demographics

- Age
  - Infancy and early childhood
- Ethnicity
  - Population isolates: Hutterite variant, Cayman Island variant
- Epidemiology
  - Extremely heterogeneous

Natural History & Prognosis

- Isolated cerebellar hypoplasia: Nonprogressive congenital ataxia, cognitive impairment in up to 85%
- Nonisolated cerebellar hypoplasia has highly variable prognosis depending on other contributing factors

Treatment

- Supportive

DIAGNOSTIC CHECKLIST

Consider

- Terms cerebellar hypoplasia and cerebellar atrophy are often used interchangeably and can overlap/coexist along spectrum

Image Interpretation Pearls

- Pattern descriptions and identification of additional anomalies important
  - Allows for more accurate genotype-phenotype correlations
- Correlation between severity of cerebellar deformity and clinical symptoms is poor
  - Coexisting supratentorial abnormalities ↑ incidence of neurodevelopmental disabilities

SELECTED REFERENCES

1. Accogli A et al: Diagnostic approach to cerebellar hypoplasia. Cerebellum. 20(4):631-58, 2021
2. Rüsch CT et al: Pontocerebellar hypoplasia: a pattern recognition approach. Cerebellum. 19(4):569-82, 2020
3. Barkovich et al: Pediatric Neuroimaging. 6th ed. Wolters Kluwer, 2019
4. Bosemani T et al: Congenital abnormalities of the posterior fossa. Radiographics. 35(1):200-20, 2015
5. Poretti A et al: Differential diagnosis of cerebellar atrophy in childhood: an update. Neuropediatrics. 46(6):359-70, 2015
6. Adachi Y et al: Posterior fossa in primary microcephaly: relationships between forebrain and mid-hindbrain size in 110 patients. Neuropediatrics. 45(2):93-101, 2014
7. Bahi-Buisson N et al: The wide spectrum of tubulinopathies: what are the key features for the diagnosis? Brain. 137(Pt 6):1676-700, 2014
8. Massoud M et al: Prenatal unilateral cerebellar hypoplasia in a series of 26 cases: significance and implications for prenatal diagnosis. Ultrasound Obstet Gynecol. 44(4):447-54, 2014
9. Poretti A et al: Cerebellar hypoplasia: differential diagnosis and diagnostic approach. Am J Med Genet C Semin Med Genet. 166(2):211-26, 2014
10. Doherty D et al: Midbrain and hindbrain malformations: advances in clinical diagnosis, imaging, and genetics. Lancet Neurol. 12(4):381-93, 2013
11. González G et al: Location of periventricular nodular heterotopia is related to the malformation phenotype on MRI. AJNR Am J Neuroradiol. 34(4):877-83, 2013
12. Tam EW: Potential mechanisms of cerebellar hypoplasia in prematurity. Neuroradiology. 55 Suppl 2:41-6, 2013
13. Pisano T et al: Peritrigonal and temporo-occipital heterotopia with corpus callosum and cerebellar dysgenesis. Neurology. 79(12):1244-51, 2012

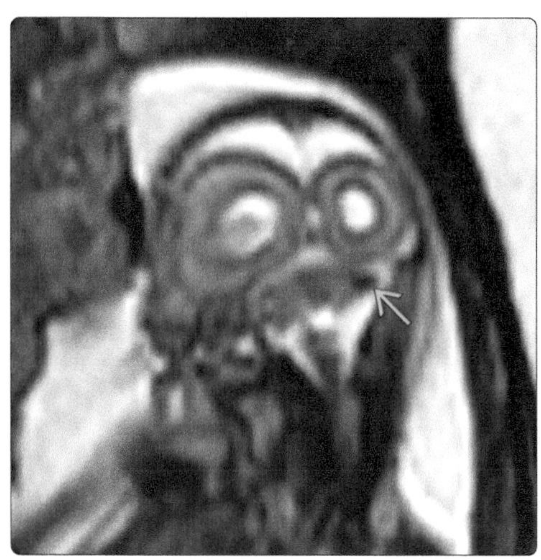

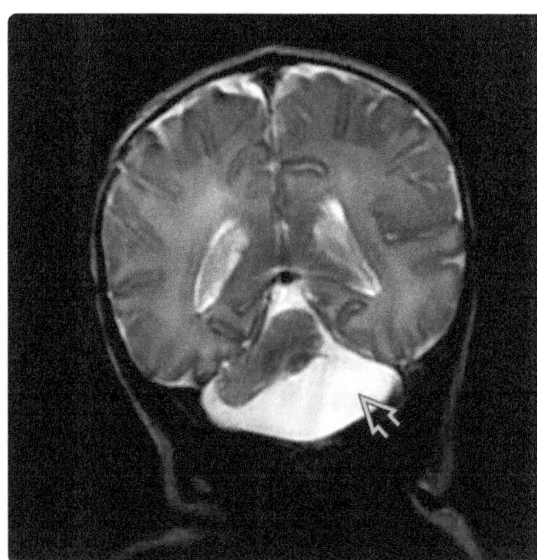

(Left) *Coronal T2 MR from a fetal MR performed at 20-weeks, 6-days gestational age demonstrates T2-hypointense hemorrhage and volume loss in the left cerebellar hemisphere* ➔. **(Right)** *Coronal T2 MR in the same patient on day 1 of life demonstrates near-complete absence of the left cerebellar hemisphere/unilateral cerebellar hypoplasia* ➔ *as a result of in utero cerebellar hemorrhage.*

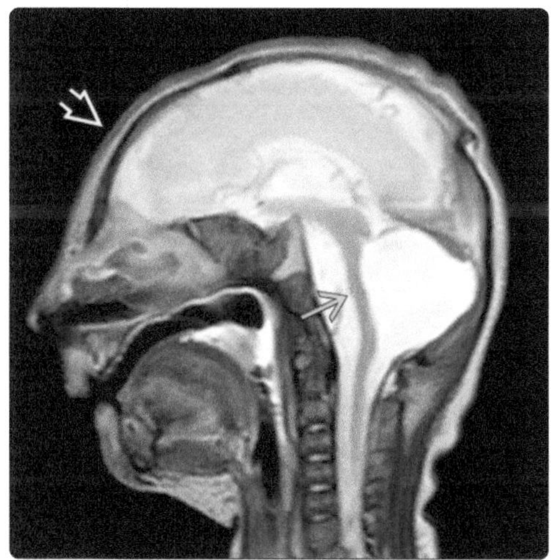

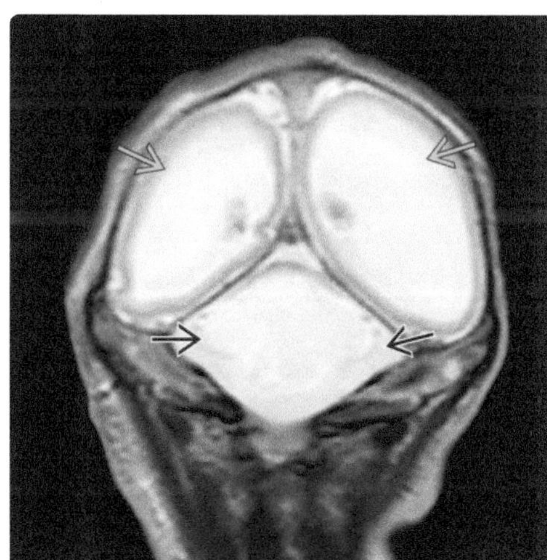

(Left) *Sagittal T2 MR in a 4-day-old boy shows severe cerebellar hypoplasia marked by near-complete absence of cerebellar tissue. There is also marked brainstem hypoplasia* ➔ *and microcephaly marked by a decreased craniofacial ratio* ➔. **(Right)** *Coronal T2 MR in the same patient shows near-complete absence of the cerebellum* ➔ *with severe ventriculomegaly* ➔ *and thinning of the cerebral mantle. WES showed homozygosity at an 11.8 Mb region of chromosome 19, uncertain significance. Care was withdrawn on 7th DOL.*

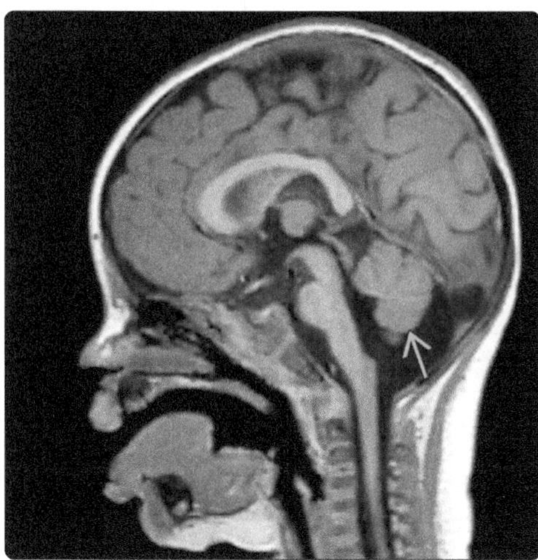

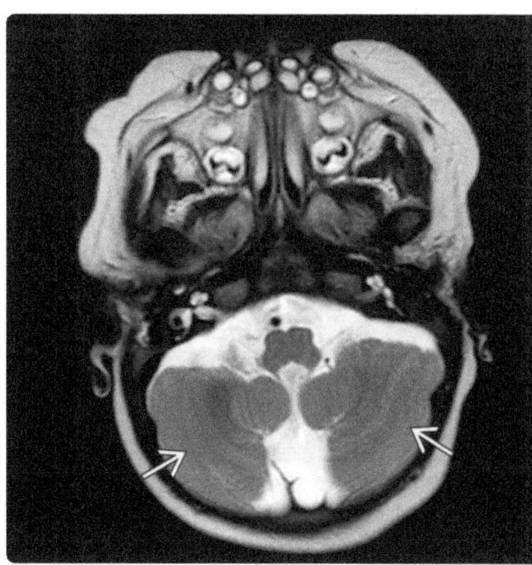

(Left) *Sagittal T1 MR in a 1-year-old girl with trisomy 21 demonstrates mild vermian hypoplasia as the bottom edge of the vermis* ➔ *is above the location of the obex. Better seen on other images is mild simplification of the cerebral gyral sulcal pattern.* **(Right)** *Axial T2 MR in the same patient shows mild hypoplasia of the cerebellar hemispheres* ➔ *marked by enlargement of the surrounding subarachnoid fluid spaces in the posterior cranial fossa.*

Holoprosencephaly

KEY FACTS

TERMINOLOGY

- Incomplete separation of cerebral hemispheres

IMAGING

- Anomaly and severity defined by degree of forebrain cleavage
  - Spectrum; no clear division between types
- Alobar holoprosencephaly (HPE)
  - Single "ball," "cup," or "pancake" brain around primitive monoventricle
  - ± dorsal cyst, dysmorphic facies
- Semilobar HPE
  - Frontal lobes > 50% fused
  - Thalami, hypothalamus "fused"
  - Posterior interhemispheric fissure (IHF), falx may be present
  - ± dorsal cyst, mild/absent facial malformations
- Lobar HPE
  - IHF present along most of midline
  - Only most inferior frontal lobes fused
  - Thalami almost/completely separated
  - Septum pellucidum always absent
  - Rudimentary frontal horns, ± 3rd ventricle, corpus callosum normal or incomplete

TOP DIFFERENTIAL DIAGNOSES

- Maximal obstructive hydrocephalus
- Hydranencephaly
- Syntelencephaly or middle interhemispheric variant (MIH) of HPE
- Septo-optic dysplasia
- Schizencephaly

PATHOLOGY

- Multifactorial; at least 13 HPE-associated genes but no strict genotype-phenotype correlation

DIAGNOSTIC CHECKLIST

- Evaluate basal forebrain for cleavage failure to detect HPE

(Left) *Coronal US in a neonate with alobar HPE shows absence of an interhemispheric fissure with continuous mantle of cerebrum crossing the midline & dysmorphic monoventricle.* **(Right)** *Axial T2 MR in a neonate with alobar HPE shows continuous mantle of cerebrum extending across the midline with a large monoventricle in communication with a large dorsal cyst. Alobar HPE patients are often microcephalic at birth but often develop hydrocephalus, requiring shunting.*

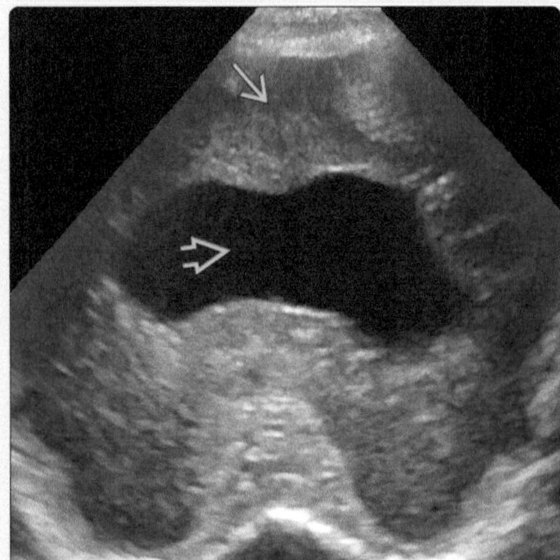

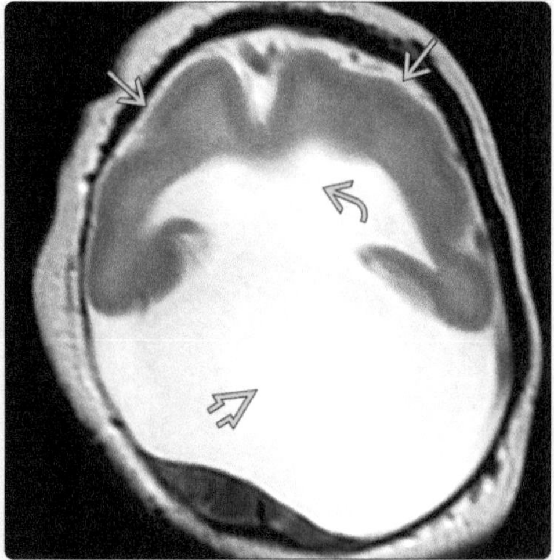

(Left) *Midline sagittal T1 MR in a 2-year-old with semilobar HPE shows absence of the cingulate gyrus & normal corpus callosum with gray matter (GM) extending across the entire midline from anterior to posterior.* **(Right)** *Axial T2 MR in a 3-day-old girl with semilobar HPE shows absence of the anterior interhemispheric fissure, frontal horns, & septum pellucidum, fused basal ganglia & thalami. Note the normal posterior interhemispheric fissure & the azygos anterior cerebral artery.*

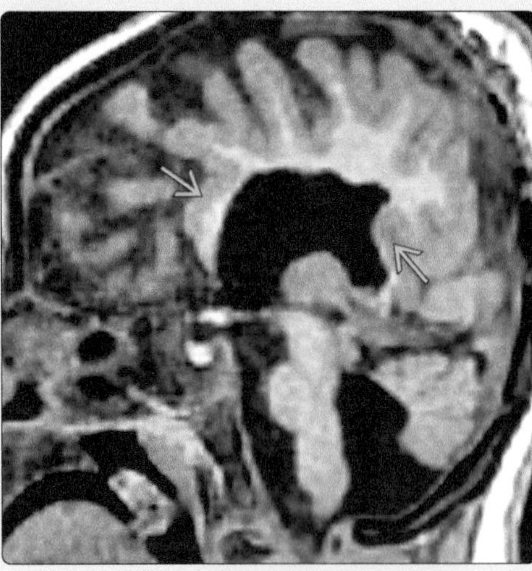

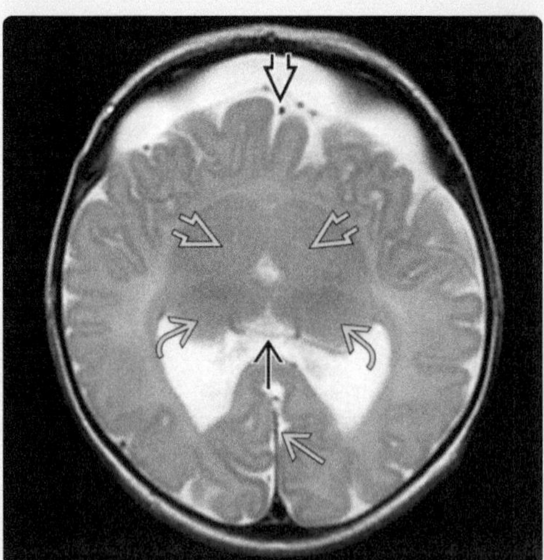

TERMINOLOGY

Abbreviations

- Holoprosencephaly (HPE)

Synonyms

- Formerly called arrhinencephaly

Definitions

- Incomplete separation of prosencephalon (hemispheres + deep gray nuclei)

IMAGING

General Features

- Best diagnostic clue
  - Single ventricle
  - Absent or partial hemispheric and basal cleavage with absent/incomplete interhemispheric fissure (IHF)/falx
  - Azygous anterior cerebral artery (ACA)
  - ± associated midline facial defects
- Location
  - Forebrain ± midface
- Morphology
  - Anomaly and severity defined by degree of forebrain cleavage
    - Spectrum; no clear division between types
  - Alobar HPE
    - Single "ball," "cup," or "pancake" brain around primitive monoventricle
      - ± dorsal cyst, dysmorphic facies
  - Semilobar HPE
    - Frontal lobes > 50% fused
    - Posterior IHF, falx may be present
    - Thalami, hypothalamus "fused"
    - ± dorsal cyst, mild/absent facial malformations
  - Lobar HPE
    - IHF present along most of midline
    - Only most inferior frontal lobes fused
    - Thalami almost/completely separated
    - Septum pellucidum always absent
    - Rudimentary frontal horns, ± 3rd ventricle, corpus callosum normal or incomplete

CT Findings

- NECT
  - Single ventricle without septum pellucidum
  - Uncleaved deep gray nuclei
  - Variable extent of posterior IHF
  - Variable degree of aplasia of midface, nasal cavity, and paranasal sinuses (all derived from neural crest)

MR Findings

- T1WI
  - Evaluates severity: Alobar, semilobar, or lobar HPE
    - Degree of differentiation of single ventricular cavity, presence of dorsal cyst
      - 3rd ventricle identified when thalami are separated
    - Hemispheric cleavage (extent of IHF), falx defines anatomic severity
      - Alobar: No fissure
      - Semilobar: Divided temporal lobes around midbrain
      - Lobar: Fissure extends anteriorly to frontal lobes, posterior callosum present
      - All intermediate degrees can be encountered
    - Gyration variably developed, from agyria to well convoluted
    - Variable extent of basal cleavage: Thalami, striatum, hypothalamus
  - Sylvian angle (SA) reflects frontal development, hence severity of HPE as well
    - Superiorly tilted sylvian fissures (↑ SA) = less developed frontal lobes, more severe HPE
- T2WI
  - Same as T1WI
  - In addition, evaluates myelin maturation, optic nerves/globes, olfactory nerves, pituitary
- DWI
  - DTI helps in identifying white matter (WM) tracts
- MRA
  - ACA
    - May present with early fan-like array of branching arteries over surface of single frontal lobe
- MRV
  - Absent venous sinuses correlate falx/tentorium malformations

Ultrasonographic Findings

- Grayscale ultrasound
  - HPE diagnosable on fetal US and MR

Angiographic Findings

- Azygous ACA

Imaging Recommendations

- Best imaging tool
  - MR without contrast
- Protocol advice
  - 3D fast GE sequence (e.g., FSPGR, MP-RAGE) with multiplanar reconstructions allows for optimal evaluation of midline structures

DIFFERENTIAL DIAGNOSIS

Severe Obstructive Hydrocephalus

- May have massively enlarged ventricles, thin rim of cortex
- Falx present; basal ganglia (BG) separated

Hydranencephaly

- Water bag brain appearance; little or no cortex; falx present
- Typically with complete absence of brain supplied by internal carotid artery with preservation of posterior cerebral artery (PCA) distribution

Syntelencephaly or Middle Interhemispheric Variant of Holoprosencephaly

- Single ventricular cavity: No septum pellucidum, no fornix, no 3rd ventricular roof
- Azygous ACA
- Noncleavage of anterior-inferior BG
- Interhemispheric cortical continuity usually in posterior frontal-parietal area
- Anterior &/or posterior corpus callosum found

Absent Septum Pellucidum

- False single ventricular cavity and paired ACA
- Septo-optic dysplasia (fornices fused but present)
- Schizencephaly (hemispheric clefts, fornices present)

Torn Septum Pellucidum

- Severe, usually congenital hydrocephalus
- Typically macrocephalic (HPE usually microcephalic), fornices present

PATHOLOGY

General Features

- Etiology
  - Primary defect of ventral induction, patterning
    - Results in total or partial failure of separation of prosencephalon into 2 separate hemispheres
  - Multifactorial; at least 13 HPE-associated genes but no strict genotype-phenotype correlation
    - Other: Environmental/maternal factors: Diabetes (1% HPE in diabetic mothers), alcohol, retinoid acid, plant alkaloids (*Veratrum californicum*)
- Genetics
  - Cytogenetic abnormalities in 25-50%: Trisomy 13, 18q-, 18p-, 3p, 7-, trisomy 9, 1q15q, 11q12-q13 (*DHCR7* gene mutation = Smith-Lemli-Opitz)
  - Sonic hedgehog (*SHH*) (7q36), *ZIC2* (13q13.2), *SIX3* (2p21), *TGIF1* (18p11.3), *GLI2* (2q14.2) → ventrodorsal gradient → noncleavage anterobasal midline, disorganized neocortex (anterior)
    - *SHH* also controls neural crest (midface) and oligodendrocytic (myelination) development
  - Patterns of genotype-phenotype correlation
    - *ZIC2* and *SIX3* → severe phenotype (alobar and semilobar)
    - *SHH* → less severe phenotype (lobar)
- Associated abnormalities
  - HPE mostly sporadic, sometimes familial, 25% syndromic
  - 80% of facial anomalies; correlate with severity of HPE
    - Cyclopia, proboscis; single nare; single nasal bone/absent internasal suture
    - Midline cleft lip or palate; premaxillary agenesis
    - Single maxillary central incisor (SMCI); absent superior lingual frenulum

Staging, Grading, & Classification

- Class 1 HPE spectrum: All ranges of decreasing severity may be found in same pedigree
  - Includes alobar, semilobar, lobar
  - Midfacial abnormalities without overt brain malformation
    - Flat face, maxillary hypoplasia, midline cleft lip/palate, hypotelorism
  - Isolated SMCI
    - Often associated with, but not always indicator of, HPE
- Class 2 syntelencephaly, or MIH variant of HPE
  - Posterior frontal-parietal cortical continuity across midline; both callosal genu and splenium often present

Gross Pathologic & Surgical Features

- Variable hypoplasia of cortex, variable gyral development
- Variable degree of separation of diencephalon and BG with incorporation into upper brainstem
- Dorsal cyst represents posteriorly located tela choroidea of single ventricle

CLINICAL ISSUES

Presentation

- Most common signs/symptoms
  - Facial malformation with hypotelorism
  - Seizures (50%) and developmental delays
  - Hypothalamic/pituitary malfunction (75%, mostly diabetes insipidus), poor body temperature regulation
  - Dystonia and hypotonia: Severity correlates with degree of BG nonseparation
  - Microcephaly (macrocephaly may occur with alobar HPE)
- Clinical profile
  - Intellectually disabled microcephalic infant with hypotelorism

Demographics

- Age
  - Presentation in infancy or early childhood
    - Can be diagnosed with fetal US or MR
- Sex
  - M:F = 1.4:1
- Epidemiology
  - Most common malformation of brain and face in humans
  - 1.3/10,000 live births, but 1 in 250 conceptuses

Natural History & Prognosis

- Overrepresented in fetal demise, stillbirths
- Clinical severity and life expectancy relate to degree of hemispheric and deep gray nuclei nonseparation (alobar HPE = worst)

Treatment

- Treat seizures and endocrine dysfunction
- Alobar HPE may develop hydrocephalus and require shunting

DIAGNOSTIC CHECKLIST

Consider

- Whenever HPE in doubt, look at basal forebrain for cleavage failure

Image Interpretation Pearls

- Not all cases of missing septum pellucidum are single ventricles

SELECTED REFERENCES

1. Malta M et al: Holoprosencephaly: review of embryology, clinical phenotypes, etiology and management. Children (Basel). 10(4):647, 2023
2. Chaudhari BP et al: Congenital brain malformations: an integrated diagnostic approach. Semin Pediatr Neurol. 42:100973, 2022
3. Fenton LZ: Imaging of congenital malformations of the brain. Clin Perinatol. 49(3):587-601, 2022
4. Montaguti E et al: Sonography of fetal holoprosencephaly: a guide to recognize the lesser varieties. J Matern Fetal Neonatal Med. 35(25):9717-23, 2022
5. Yang E et al: A practical approach to supratentorial brain malformations: what radiologists should know. Radiol Clin North Am. 55(4):609-27, 2017
6. Winter TC et al: Holoprosencephaly: a survey of the entity, with embryology and fetal imaging. Radiographics. 35(1):275-90, 2015

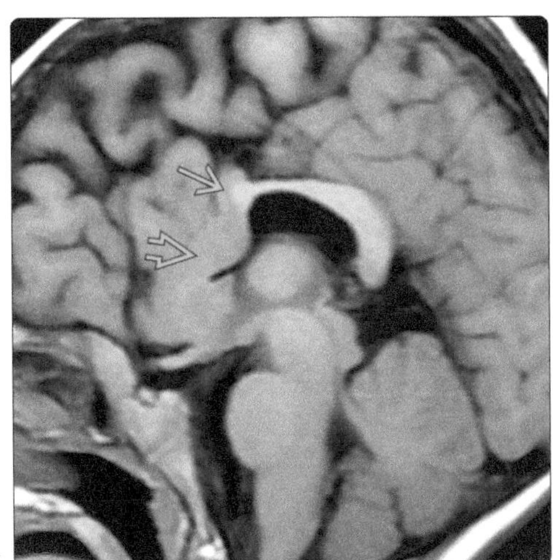

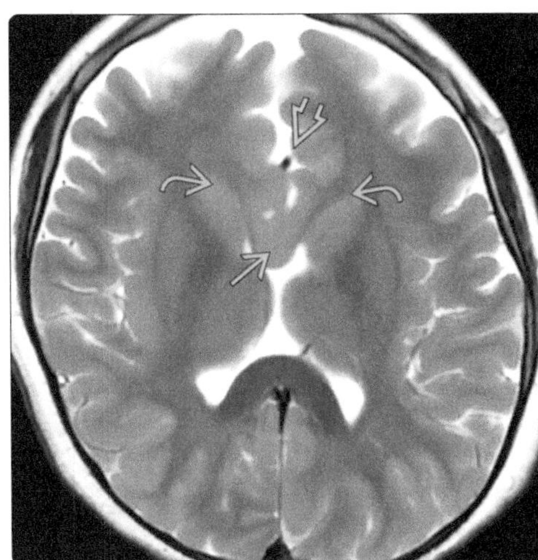

(Left) *Sagittal T1 MR in a 3-year-old with lobar HPE shows absence of the anterior genu & rostrum of the corpus callosum → with GM crossing the midline →. The posterior ~ 3/4 of the corpus callosum is normal in morphology.* **(Right)** *Axial T2 MR in the same patient 10 years later shows failure of midline cleavage of the anterior cerebrum. There is cortical GM → crossing the midline anteriorly with absence of the frontal horns →. Also note the single azygous anterior cerebral artery →.*

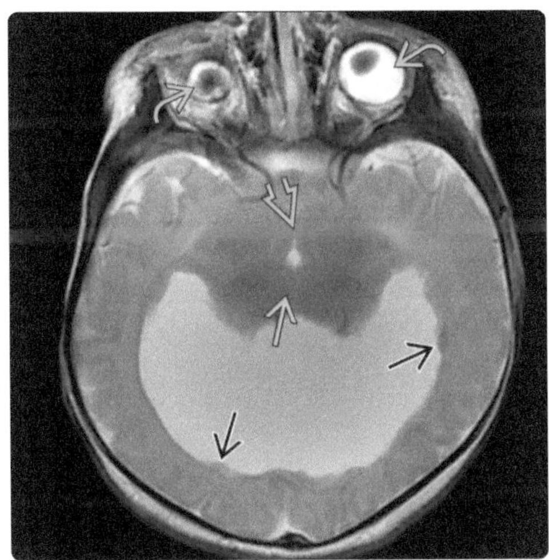

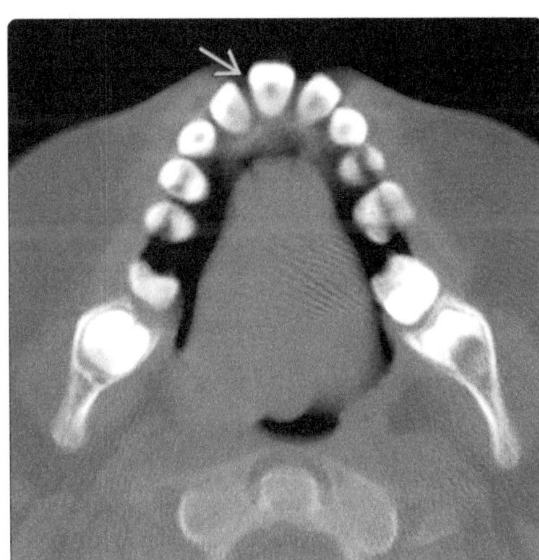

(Left) *Axial T2 MR in a patient with alobar HPE shows fusion of the thalami → & basal ganglia → & complete lack of midline cleavage of the cerebral hemispheres. Also note the associated dysplastic globes → & GM heterotopia →.* **(Right)** *Axial NECT in a 10-year-old with HPE shows a solitary midline incisor →, another associated midline abnormality seen in HPE. The severity of the midline facial anomalies does not always correlate with severity of brain anomalies but may depend more on the genotype.*

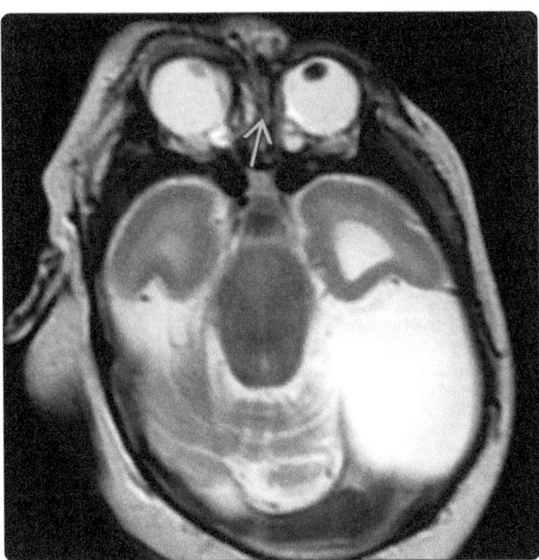

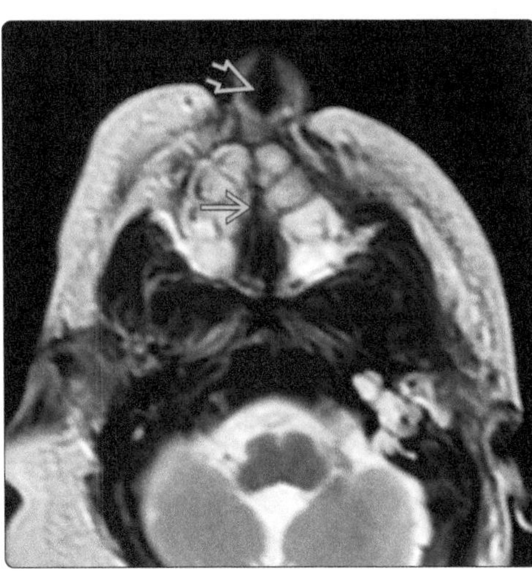

(Left) *Axial T2 MR in a neonate with alobar HPE shows decreased intraocular spacing →, consistent with hypotelorism, a common facial dysmorphism in HPE.* **(Right)** *Axial T2 MR in the same patient with alobar HPE shows hypoplastic maxilla → with crowding of the teeth & absence of the midline nasal septum → with a single nasal cavity. Look carefully for midline facial anomalies when intracranial HPE is evident & vice versa.*

Syntelencephaly (Middle Interhemispheric Variant)

KEY FACTS

TERMINOLOGY

- Syntelencephaly; middle interhemispheric (MIH) variant of holoprosencephaly (HPE)

IMAGING

- Single ventricular cavity (100%)
- Fused dorsal mid- or posterior hemispheric cortex (100%) (by definition)
- Azygous anterior cerebral artery (ACA) (100%)
- Abnormal sylvian fissure (SF) spans both hemispheres (86%)
- Heterotopia, cortical malformations (86%)
- Dysgenetic corpus callosum (CC)
- Hypertelorism (most HPEs have hypotelorism)

TOP DIFFERENTIAL DIAGNOSES

- Classic HPE
- Septo-optic dysplasia
- Bilateral schizencephaly
- Bilateral perisylvian polymicrogyria (PMG)

PATHOLOGY

- High occurrence of syntelencephaly (as well as other forms of HPE) has been observed in babies born from diabetic mothers
- *ZIC2* mutation at 13q32 is observed in 5-6% of patients

CLINICAL ISSUES

- Spasticity (86%), hypotonia (57%), dystonia (50%), seizures (40%), developmental delay (common)
- Facial dysmorphisms (less common than classic HPE): Hypertelorism, cleft lip/palate

DIAGNOSTIC CHECKLIST

- Always look for interhemispheric fissure, septum pellucidum
- Look at bridging cortex lining upper surface of pseudo-CC
- Distortion of anterior interhemispheric fissure on prenatal imaging: Look for cerebral midline anomalies

(Left) *Axial graphic depicts classic findings of syntelencephaly with an anomalous coronal fissure ⇒ and both gray matter (GM) and white matter (WM) bridges ⇒ crossing the interhemispheric fissure in several locations. The GM in the cortical bridges appears thickened and dysplastic.* **(Right)** *Axial T2WI MR in a 14-year-old with severe microcephaly shows a coronally oriented cleft ⇒ with columns of WM ⇒ coursing uninterrupted across the midline both anterior and posterior to the cleft.*

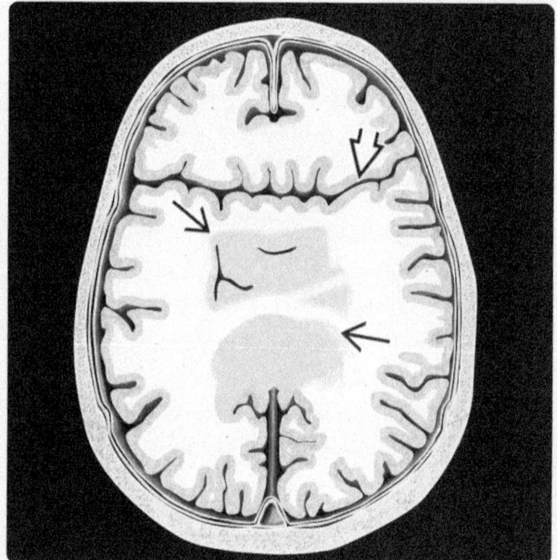

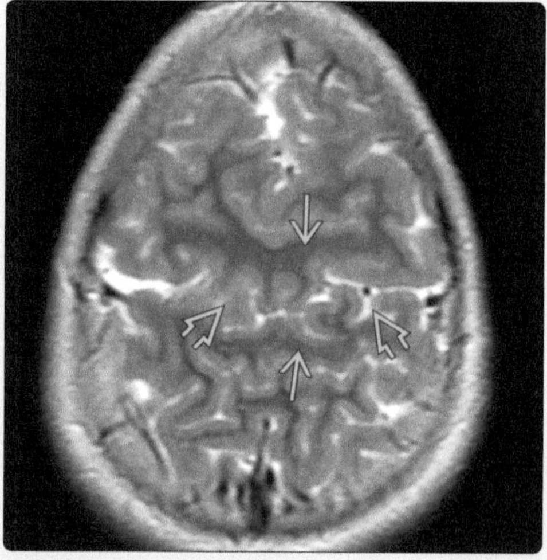

(Left) *Midline sagittal T1WI MR in a 13-year-old with syntelencephaly shows an undulating and irregular body of corpus callosum (CC) ⇒ with GM ⇒ along the dorsal aspect of the CC. Such an appearance on midline sagittal is typical for syntelencephaly.* **(Right)** *Coronal T2WI MR in a 13-year-old with middle hemispheric variant of holoprosencephaly (HPE) shows absence of the septum pellucidum ⇒ and continuation of GM ⇒ across the midline within the central or middle portion of the hemispheres.*

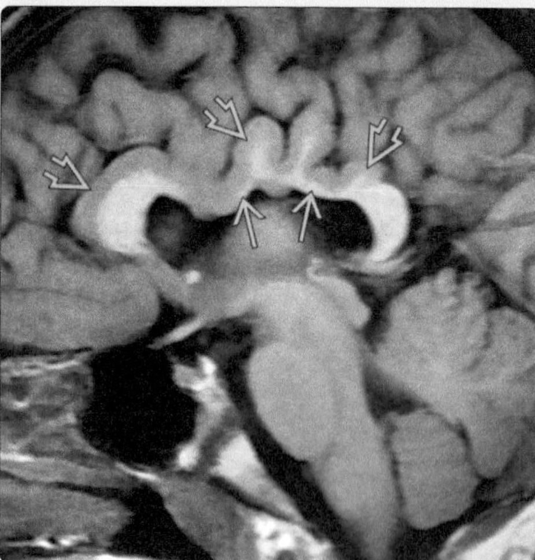

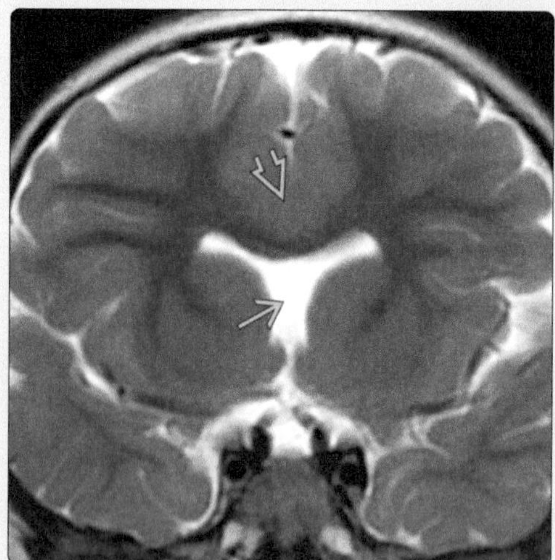

TERMINOLOGY

Synonyms

- Syntelencephaly
- Middle interhemispheric variant (MIH) of holoprosencephaly (HPE)

Definitions

- Variant of HPE characterized by lack of separation of midportion of hemispheres

IMAGING

General Features

- Best diagnostic clue
  - Midline continuity of posterior frontal/parietal cortex with normal separation of frontal pole
  - Single ventricular cavity
- Location
  - Midline
- Size
  - Typically normocephalic
- Morphology
  - Noncleavage of dorsal aspect of cerebral hemispheres, usually posterior frontal lobes
  - Single ventricular cavity
  - Single (azygous) anterior cerebral artery (ACA)
  - Mostly normal ventral hemispheres, basal ganglia, and hypothalamus

CT Findings

- Axial view: Absent septum pellucidum
- Sagittal reformats: Segmented corpus callosum (CC) (typically, only genu and splenium present)
- Coronal reformats: Cortical bridge between midportion of hemispheres, convex upper border of lateral ventricles
- Bone algorithms of facial bones: Cleft lip, cleft palate, hypertelorism
  - Never hypotelorism (unlike true HPE)

MR Findings

- T1WI
  - Hemispheres
    - Unseparated ("fused") dorsal midhemispheric cortex (100%) (by definition)
    - Single ventricular cavity (100%)
    - Single abnormal sylvian fissure (SF) spans both hemispheres dorsally (86%)
    - Heterotopia, cortical malformations (86%)
      - Thick cortex lining anterior interhemispheric fissure (IHF)
      - Heterotopic gray matter nodules often situated on top of lateral ventricle bodies
    - Dysgenetic CC
      - Genu and splenium only (61%)
      - Genu or splenium (22%)
      - Genu, splenium, and some of body (20%)
    - Olfactory sulci normal (57%), olfactory bulbs (64%)
    - Hippocampi poorly developed
  - Deep gray matter
    - Lentiform nuclei normal, anterobasal caudate fused (11%)
    - Hypothalamus usually normal
    - Thalami fused (33%)
  - Midbrain
    - Incomplete segmentation of diencephalon-mesencephalon (18%)
  - Posterior fossa
    - Chiari, cerebellar hypoplasia possible
  - Meninges
    - Dorsal cyst (25%); may require CSF diversion
    - Rarely, cephaloceles overlying unseparated portion of hemispheres
  - Others
    - No endocrinopathy (unlike HPE)
    - Normal thermoregulation (unlike HPE)
- T2WI
  - Brain morphology
    - Similar to T1WI
  - Brain maturation
    - Myelination is normal in keeping with patient age (unlike in classic HPE)
- MRA
  - Azygous ACA (100%)

Imaging Recommendations

- Best imaging tool
  - MR
- Protocol advice
  - Multisequence triplanar
  - T1-weighted IR, MP-RAGE/SPGR provide exquisite gray-white contrast
  - DTI may help in understanding white matter organization

Ultrasonographic Findings

- Grayscale ultrasound
  - Absent septum pellucidum
  - Absence of middle portion of IHF
- Color Doppler
  - Azygous ACA

DIFFERENTIAL DIAGNOSIS

Classic Holoprosencephaly

- Single hemisphere and ventricle
- Failure of cleavage
  - Hypothalamus
  - Basal ganglia
  - Prefrontal cerebrum
- Midline facial anomalies much more common

Septo-Optic Dysplasia

- Absent/incomplete septum pellucidum
- Well-separated cerebral hemispheres
- Well-separated basal ganglia and thalami
- Normal CC
- Bilateral ACA

Bilateral Schizencephaly

- Clefts communicate with ventricles
- Well-separated cerebral hemispheres
- Bilateral ACA

Bilateral Perisylvian Polymicrogyria

- Well-divided hemispheres and ventricles
- Bilateral ACA

PATHOLOGY

General Features

- Etiology
  - Mitosis/apoptosis of embryonic roof plate form IHF after neural tube closure (fetal weeks 3-4)
    - Impaired expression of roof plate properties alters mitosis and apoptosis → faulty dorsal IHF formation, poor cleavage of cerebral hemispheres
  - High occurrence of syntelencephaly (as well as other forms of HPE) has been observed in babies born from diabetic mothers
- Genetics
  - Presumably linked to dorsal induction genes
    - Genes linked to classic HPE [e.g., sonic hedgehog (*SHH*)] mostly affect ventral induction
      - May explain importance of facial defects in classic HPE
    - By contrast, dorsal induction disorder is predominant in syntelencephaly
      - May explain lack of severe midline facial dysmorphisms
      - Presumably, induction of neural crest that forms midfacial skeleton proceeds normally
    - *ZIC2* mutation at 13q32 is observed in 5-6% of patients
      - Involved in differentiation of embryonic roof plate
- Associated abnormalities
  - Hypertelorism
  - Cleft lips, palate
  - Cystic vestibulocochlear anomalies

Staging, Grading, & Classification

- Classic spectrum of HPEs from alobar to lobar
- Syntelencephaly considered milder end of spectrum
  - Clinically severe, although less than complete HPE

Gross Pathologic & Surgical Features

- IHF present at frontal, occipital poles
  - Hemispheric fusion posterior frontal and parietal lobes
- Lentiform nuclei normal, caudate fused
- Thalami fused in 1/3
- Hypothalamus not fused

CLINICAL ISSUES

Presentation

- Most common signs/symptoms
  - Developmental disorders
    - Spasticity (86%)
    - Hypotonia (57%)
    - Dystonia (50%)
    - Seizures (40%)
    - Developmental delay (speech, etc.) (100%)
    - Absence of choreoathetosis (common in classic HPE)
- Other signs/symptoms
  - Mild facial dysmorphisms less common than with classic HPE
    - Hypertelorism
    - Cleft lip/palate
- Clinical profile
  - Developmental delay
  - Spasticity
  - Seizures

Demographics

- Age
  - Presents in infancy

Natural History & Prognosis

- Static course

Treatment

- Rehabilitation

DIAGNOSTIC CHECKLIST

Consider

- Always look for normal IHF, septum pellucidum in fetuses, developmentally delayed children

Image Interpretation Pearls

- Distortion of anterior IHF on prenatal imaging: Look for cerebral midline anomalies
- Look at ventricle
- Look at bridging cortex lining upper surface of pseudo-CC

SELECTED REFERENCES

1. Malta M et al: Holoprosencephaly: review of embryology, clinical phenotypes, etiology and management. Children (Basel). 10(4):647, 2023
2. Tavano I et al: Prenatal diagnosis of middle interhemispheric variant of holoprosencephaly: review of literature and prenatal case series. J Matern Fetal Neonatal Med. 35(25):4976-84, 2022
3. Zantow E et al: Prenatal diagnosis of middle interhemispheric variant of holoprosencephaly: report of two cases. J Clin Ultrasound. 49(7):765-9, 2021
4. Calloni SF et al: Disorders of ventral induction/spectrum of holoprosencephaly. Neuroimaging Clin N Am. 29(3):411-21, 2019
5. Dubourg C et al: Recent advances in understanding inheritance of holoprosencephaly. Am J Med Genet C Semin Med Genet. 178(2):258-69, 2018
6. Fallet-Bianco C: Neuropathology of holoprosencephaly. Am J Med Genet C Semin Med Genet. 178(2):214-28, 2018
7. Kousa YA et al: Prenatal diagnosis of holoprosencephaly. Am J Med Genet C Semin Med Genet. 178(2):206-13, 2018
8. Yang E et al: A practical approach to supratentorial brain malformations: what radiologists should know. Radiol Clin North Am. 55(4):609-27, 2017
9. Akyol Y et al: Syntelencephaly associated with cystic cochleovestibular malformations. Neurology. 86(2):198-9, 2016
10. Bulakbasi N et al: The middle interhemispheric variant of holoprosencephaly: magnetic resonance and diffusion tensor imaging findings. Br J Radiol. 89(1063):20160115, 2016
11. Griffiths PD et al: In utero MR imaging of fetal holoprosencephaly: a structured approach to diagnosis and classification. AJNR Am J Neuroradiol. 37(3):536-43, 2016
12. Winter TC et al: Holoprosencephaly: a survey of the entity, with embryology and fetal imaging. Radiographics. 35(1):275-90, 2015
13. Simon EM et al: The middle interhemispheric variant of holoprosencephaly. AJNR Am J Neuroradiol. 23(1): 151-6, 2002
14. Barkovich AJ et al: Middle interhemispheric fusion: an unusual variant of holoprosencephaly. AJNR Am J Neuroradiol. 14(2):431-40, 1993

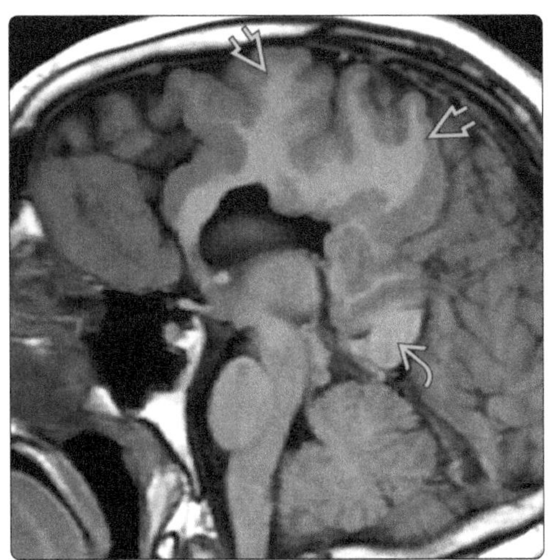

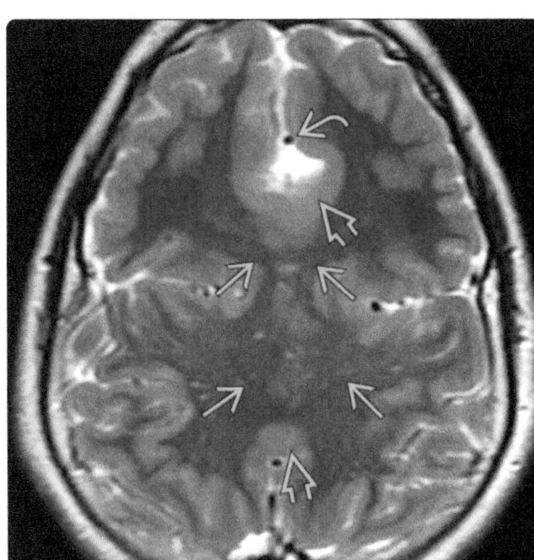

(Left) *Sagittal T1WI MR in a 14-year-old with severe microcephaly shows absence of the normal CC with bizarre-appearing gyri* ➲ *connecting the cerebral hemispheres. Note the small residual splenium* ➲ *of the CC.* **(Right)** *Axial T2WI MR in the same patient shows WM* ➲ *and cortical GM* ➲ *coursing across the midline with a lack of the interhemispheric fissure. The location and size of WM tracts and cortical GM crossing the midline varies greatly. Also note the azygous anterior cerebral artery (ACA)* ➲.

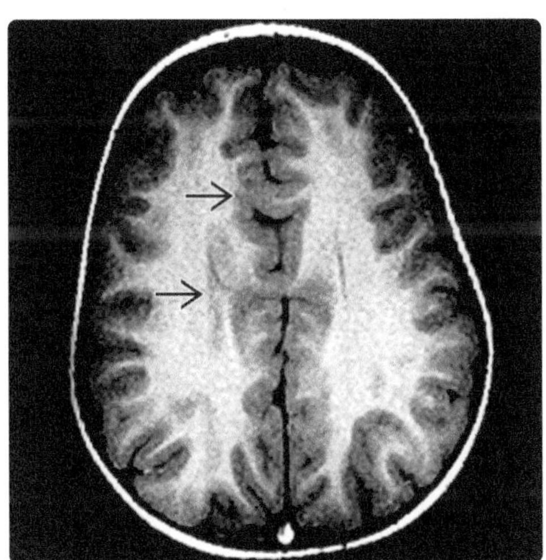

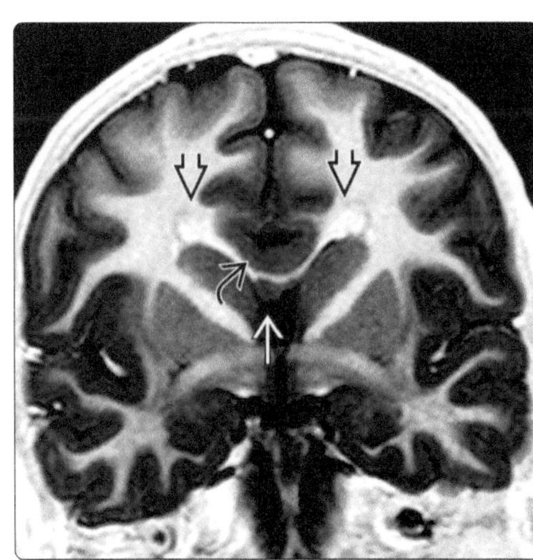

(Left) *Axial T1WI MR shows WM and GM crossing the interhemispheric fissure in the midline* ➲*, creating several interhemispheric cortical bridges.* **(Right)** *Coronal T1WI MR in the same patient shows a thick layer of cortex* ➲ *crossing the interhemispheric fissure; some GM* ➲ *protrudes into the ventricular lumen. Note the parasagittal bright T1 signal bundle of WM* ➲ *on each side, which may represent misdirected callosal fibers.*

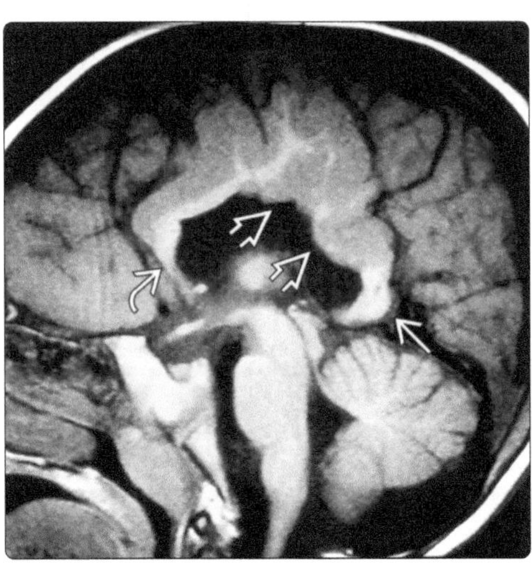

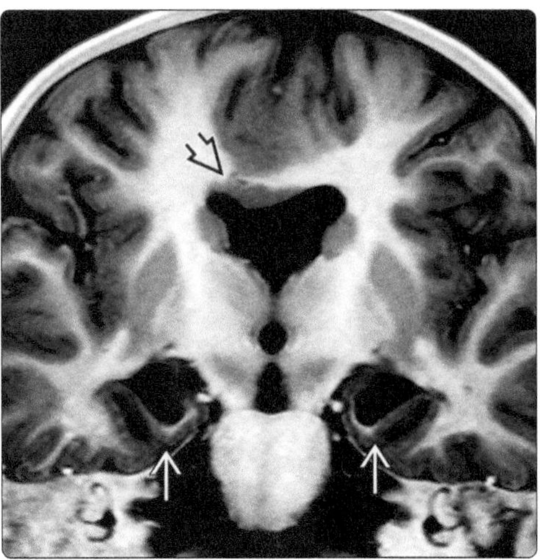

(Left) *Sagittal T1WI MR shows middle hemispheric fusion. The splenium* ➲ *and rostrum* ➲ *are well delineated. In the area of interhemispheric continuity, GM encroaches on the ventricular lumen* ➲*. Interhemispheric fissure was normal in the anterior frontal and the parietooccipital areas.* **(Right)** *Coronal T1WI MR shows a single ventricular cavity and interhemispheric cortical continuity. Note the heterotopic GM on the ventricular roof* ➲ *and the poorly developed hippocampi* ➲.

KEY FACTS

TERMINOLOGY

- Septo-optic dysplasia (SOD)
- De Morsier syndrome

IMAGING

- Optimal imaging: MR with 3D acquisitions and MPRs
  - 3D GRE-based T1 → optic nerves (ONs) and ectopic neurohypophysis
  - 3D-balanced SS-GRE → ONs and pituitary infundibulum
- ON hypoplasia (ONH) (often asymmetric)
- ± absent septum pellucidum (sometimes partial)
  - Flat-roofed ventricles, inferiorly pointed frontal horns
- ± pituitary abnormalities (often ectopic neurohypophysis)
- Look for associated polymicrogyria &/or schizencephaly
  - SOD plus

CLINICAL ISSUES

- Child with short stature, endocrine dysfunction
- ONH: Normal or color blindness, visual loss, nystagmus, strabismus
- Pituitary dysfunction in majority of patients
  - Abnormal pituitary anatomy ↑ risk for endocrine dysfunction; however, normal pituitary on imaging can have endocrine dysfunction, and abnormal pituitary on imaging can have normal endocrine function
- SOD plus: Seizures, cognitive and motor dysfunction
- ± intellectual disability, spasticity, microcephaly, anosmia

DIAGNOSTIC CHECKLIST

- SOD in small-stature pediatric patient with absent septum pellucidum
- Look closely for associated midline anomalies and cortical malformations

SCANNING TIPS

- Perform high-resolution 3D imaging with MPRs for optimal evaluation

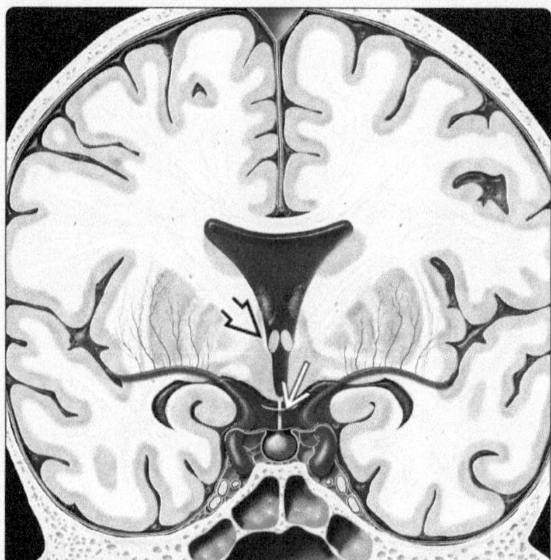

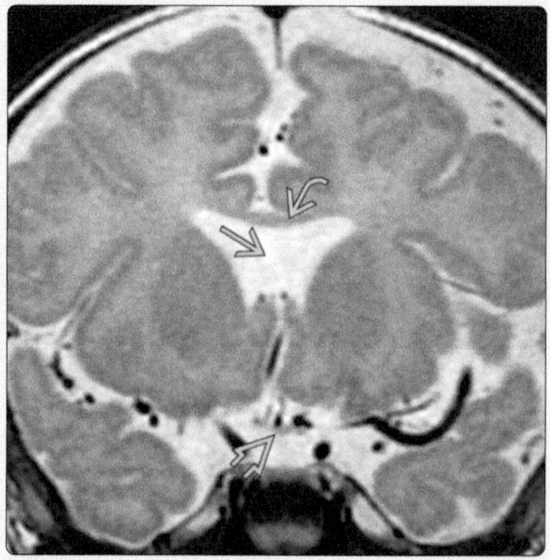

(Left) *Coronal graphic depicts flat-roofed anterior horns and the absence of a midline septum pellucidum (SP) in septo-optic dysplasia (SOD). The anterior horns are draped inferiorly around the fornices ⇨, and the optic chiasm ➡ is small.* **(Right)** *Coronal T2WI MR in an 11-week-old with SOD shows absence of the SP ⇨, flat-roofed lateral ventricles ⇨, and a very small optic chiasm ⇨. When such findings are encountered, the search for additional midline and cortical malformations should ensue.*

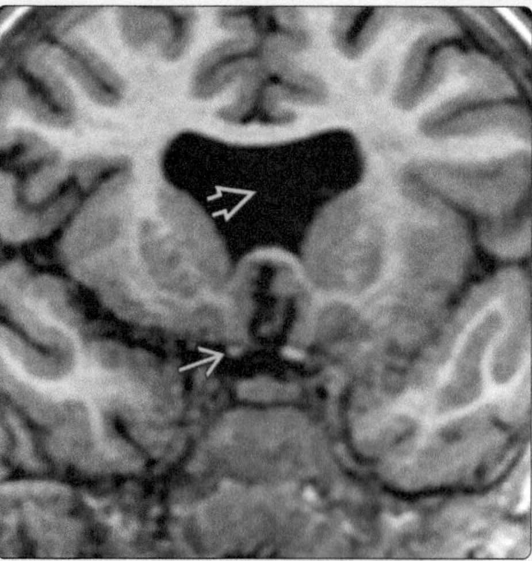

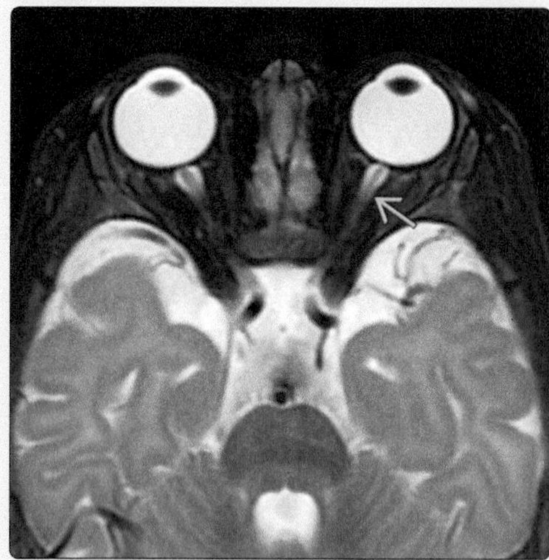

(Left) *Coronal T1WI MR in a 10-year-old boy with poor vision in the right eye shows absence of the SP ⇨ and right prechiasmatic optic nerve hypoplasia (ONH) ⇨, a typical appearance for SOD. SOD may involve 1 or both optic nerves, sometimes including the optic chiasm.* **(Right)** *Axial T2WI MR in a 5-year-old with poor vision in the left eye shows decreased size of the left optic nerve ⇨ throughout its course, including the intraorbital segment. Thin-slice imaging of the orbits is helpful in establishing ONH.*

TERMINOLOGY

Abbreviations

- Septo-optic dysplasia (SOD)

Synonyms

- De Morsier syndrome
- Kaplan-Grumbach-Hoyt syndrome
- Suprasellar dysgenesis
- Septo-optic-pituitary dysgenesis

Definitions

- Heterogeneous association characterized by optic nerve hypoplasia (ONH), absent septum pellucidum, hypothalamic-pituitary dysfunction
  - De Morsier (1956): Described 7 patients with SOD
  - Hoyt (1978): Described association of SOD with hypopituitarism
- SOD plus: SOD + polymicrogyria &/or schizencephaly

IMAGING

General Features

- Best diagnostic clue
  - Absent septum pellucidum, small optic chiasm
- Location
  - Optic nerves (ONs), pituitary gland, septum pellucidum
- Size
  - Small ONs (often asymmetric)
  - Small pituitary gland with ectopic posterior lobe
  - Absent septum pellucidum
- Morphology
  - Coronal imaging shows
    - Flat-roofed ventricles
    - Downward-pointing anterior horns

CT Findings

- NECT
  - Absent septum pellucidum
  - Large lateral ventricles
  - Small bony optic foramina on axial and coronal imaging

MR Findings

- T1WI
  - 3D GRE-based T1WI with MPRs is ideal
    - ± thin pituitary stalk, small anterior lobe of pituitary
    - ± posterior pituitary ectopia
    - ± thin corpus callosum
    - ± vertical hippocampi
    - ± polymicrogyria &/or schizencephaly
    - ± midbrain-hindbrain abnormalities (short midbrain, small pons, thick quadrigeminal plate, vermian dysplasia) significant but underrecognized component of SOD spectrum
- T2WI
  - Thin coronal plane is most helpful in SOD
    - Small ONs best seen on thin coronal T2WI
    - Absent septum pellucidum (remnants may be present)
    - Flat roof of frontal horns, pointed inferior frontal horns
    - Callosal-forniceal continuation or fused midline fornices
    - ± hypoplastic/absent olfactory nerves
    - Deficient falx (especially anteriorly) ± hypomyelination
- FLAIR
  - Axial FLAIR is helpful for identifying pituitary infundibulum
- Balanced SS-GRE (e.g., FIESTA, CISS, b-FFE)
  - High spatial resolution with elimination of CSF flow artifact
  - Sagittal plane is excellent for identification of ON/chiasm hypoplasia and pituitary infundibulum abnormalities

Imaging Recommendations

- Best imaging tool
  - MR with 3D acquisitions and MPRs
- Protocol advice
  - Coronal, sagittal thin sections through sella/orbits
  - Balanced SS-GRE (e.g., FIESTA, CISS, b-FFE) to optimally identify midline anomalies

DIFFERENTIAL DIAGNOSIS

Syndromes Overlapping With Septo-Optic Dysplasia

- Optic-infundibular dysplasia, normal septum pellucidum
- Schizencephaly with absent septum

Kallmann Syndrome

- Absent olfactory nerves
- ± visual, septal, pituitary abnormalities

Holoprosencephaly

- Shares absence of septum pellucidum; otherwise, different constellation of findings
- Requires gray matter to cross midline, which is not finding of SOD

Isolated Ectopic Posterior Pituitary Lobe

- Normal chiasm/nerves, septum pellucidum

PATHOLOGY

General Features

- Etiology
  - Theories
    - Midline heritable defect (mild holoprosencephaly variant)
    - Damage to cerebral and ON ~ 6-weeks gestation
      - Secondary degeneration of ON fibers
    - Vascular disruption (field defect) during brain development
    - Teratogens: CMV, antiepileptic drugs, alcohol, maternal diabetes
- Genetics
  - Majority are sporadic
  - Some are autosomal dominant or recessive
  - Some cases have mutations in *HESX1* gene
    - Homozygous mutations = full syndrome
    - Heterozygous mutations = milder pituitary phenotypes
  - Inactivation of *HESX1* (3p21.2-3p21.2) by Arg53Cys substitution leads to deficient anterior pituitary lobe (does not occur in sporadic SOD)

- Mutations of *FGFR1*, *PROKR2* also described
- Associated abnormalities
  - Frequently associated with other cerebral anomalies
    - Most common: Polymicrogyria &/or schizencephaly
    - Midline malformations (callosal dysgenesis, etc.)
    - Ocular anomalies (coloboma, anophthalmia, microphthalmia)
    - Olfactory tract/bulb hypoplasia
    - Incomplete hippocampal rotation
  - Overlapping syndromes with optic, septal, frontal lobe, midline, olfactory deficiencies

Staging, Grading, & Classification

- Isolated ONH: Visual defect only; intelligence normal; at risk for pituitary dysfunction
- ONH and septal deficiency: Same as isolated
- ONH and septal and pituitary abnormality: At ↑ risk for pituitary dysfunction
- SOD plus: Most severe form with neurocognitive dysfunction likely

Gross Pathologic & Surgical Features

- Small optic chiasm/nerves
- Small or absent geniculate nucleus
- Deficient/absent septum pellucidum
- Forniceal columns (± fused) → run along roof of 3rd ventricle
- ± pituitary anomalies
- ± absent olfactory bulbs

Microscopic Features

- ONs, chiasm have sparse or absent myelinated fibers
- Geniculate nucleus (if found): Disorganized layering of small neurons

CLINICAL ISSUES

Presentation

- Most common signs/symptoms
  - Newborns: Hypoglycemic seizures, apnea, cyanosis, hypotonia, prolonged conjugated jaundice, and (in boys) microphallus
  - Pituitary dysfunction
    - Imperfect correlation between anatomic abnormalities on MR and clinical pituitary dysfunction
      - Normal pituitary: Still at risk for development of endocrine dysfunction
      - Abnormal pituitary: At ↑ risk for endocrine dysfunction, but some have normal hormone status
    - Regardless of imaging findings, patients are screened annually for development of pituitary dysfunction
  - SOD plus: Seizures, cognitive dysfunction, motor dysfunction
- Clinical profile
  - Child with short stature, endocrine dysfunction
  - Normal or color blindness, visual loss, nystagmus, strabismus
  - ± intellectual disability, spasticity, microcephaly, anosmia

Demographics

- Age
  - Generally detected in infants
  - More common among younger mothers and 1st-born children
- Sex
  - M = F
- Epidemiology
  - 1 in 50,000 worldwide
  - ONH
    - 60% have brain abnormalities; 62-88% have pituitary insufficiency
      - 30% have both
    - 25-50% have absent septum pellucidum
  - SOD
    - 75-90% have brain abnormalities; 45% have pituitary insufficiency
    - Bilateral ONH (70%)

Natural History & Prognosis

- Hypothalamic and pituitary crises; sudden death (hypocortisolism)
- Depends upon severity of associated brain and pituitary malformations

Treatment

- Hormonal replacement therapy

DIAGNOSTIC CHECKLIST

Consider

- SOD in small-stature pediatric patient with absent septum pellucidum

Image Interpretation Pearls

- Small ONs, ± absent septum pellucidum, ± ectopic posterior pituitary lobe
- Look for associated cortical malformation (SOD plus)

SELECTED REFERENCES

1. Fenton LZ: Imaging of congenital malformations of the brain. Clin Perinatol. 49(3):587-601, 2022
2. Pickup EES et al: Isolated absent septum pellucidum: a retrospective study of fetal diagnosis and postnatal outcomes. Pediatr Neurol. 136:8-14, 2022
3. Ward DJ et al: Review of the MRI brain findings of septo-optic dysplasia. Clin Radiol. 76(2):160.e1-14, 2021
4. Wang CY et al: Neuroimaging of septo-optic dysplasia-plus with midbrain hypoplasia and ophthalmoplegia. eNeurologicalSci. 19:100235, 2020
5. Benson JC et al: Septo-optic dysplasia: assessment of associated findings with special attention to the olfactory sulci and tracts. Clin Neuroradiol. 29(3):505-13, 2019
6. Dahl S et al: High prevalence of pituitary hormone deficiency in both unilateral and bilateral optic nerve hypoplasia. Acta Paediatr. 108(9):1677-85, 2019
7. Qian X et al: Neuroimaging and endocrine disorders in paediatric optic nerve hypoplasia. Br J Ophthalmol. 102(7):906-10, 2018
8. Alt C et al: Clinical and radiologic spectrum of septo-optic dysplasia: review of 17 cases. J Child Neurol. 32(9):797-803, 2017
9. Cemeroglu AP et al: Spectrum of clinical presentations and endocrinological findings of patients with septo-optic dysplasia: a retrospective study. J Pediatr Endocrinol Metab. 28(9-10):1057-63, 2015
10. Lenhart PD et al: The role of magnetic resonance imaging in diagnosing optic nerve hypoplasia. Am J Ophthalmol. 158(6):1164-71.e2, 2014
11. Severino M et al: Midbrain-hindbrain involvement in septo-optic dysplasia. AJNR Am J Neuroradiol. 35(8):1586-92, 2014
12. Garcia-Filion P et al: Optic nerve hypoplasia syndrome: a review of the epidemiology and clinical associations. Curr Treat Options Neurol. 15(1):78-89, 2013

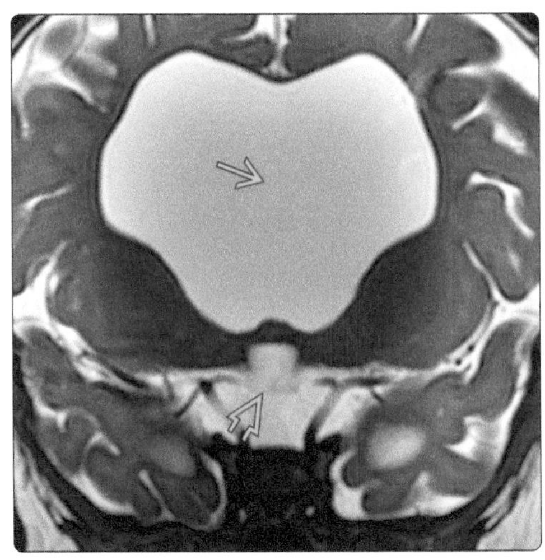

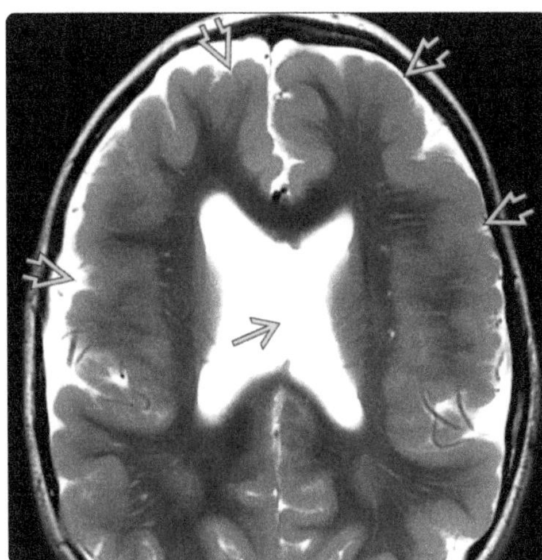

(Left) *Coronal FIESTA in a 4-month-old with SOD shows absence of the SP ⇨ and ventriculomegaly. There is near-complete absence of the optic chiasm ⇨. High-resolution balanced SS-GRE sequences (e.g., FIESTA, CISS, b-FFE) are helpful to evaluate the optic nerves and pituitary infundibulum.* **(Right)** *Axial T2WI MR in a 6-year-old shows absent SP ⇨ and bilateral frontal polymicrogyria (PMG) ⇨. Findings of SOD with associated cortical malformation are termed SOD plus.*

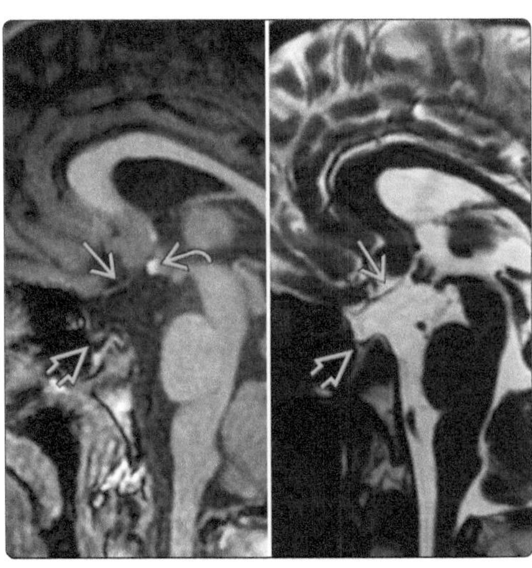

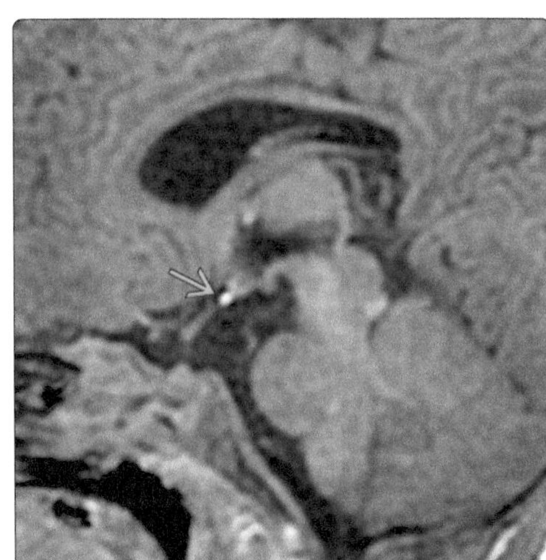

(Left) *Midline sagittal T1WI (left) and FIESTA (right) MR images in a 15-year-old show a very small optic chiasm ⇨, ectopic posterior pituitary ⇨, small anterior pituitary ⇨, and absence of the pituitary infundibulum. The spectrum of pituitary malformations associated with SOD are broad.* **(Right)** *Sagittal T1WI MR in an 11-week-old with SOD and ectopic neurohypophysis shows the posterior pituitary bright spot ⇨ at the base of the hypothalamus near the expected origin of the pituitary infundibulum.*

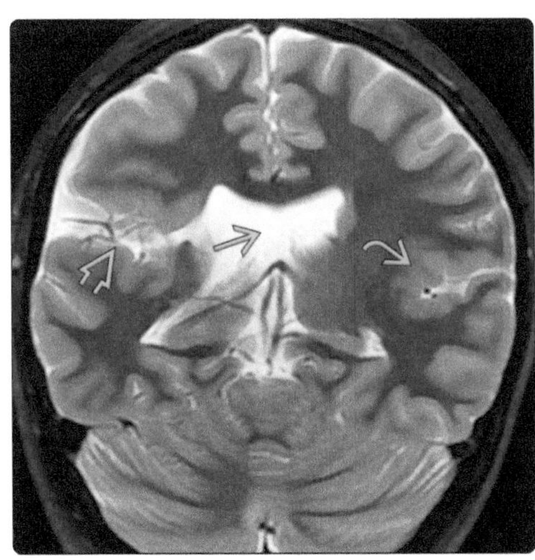

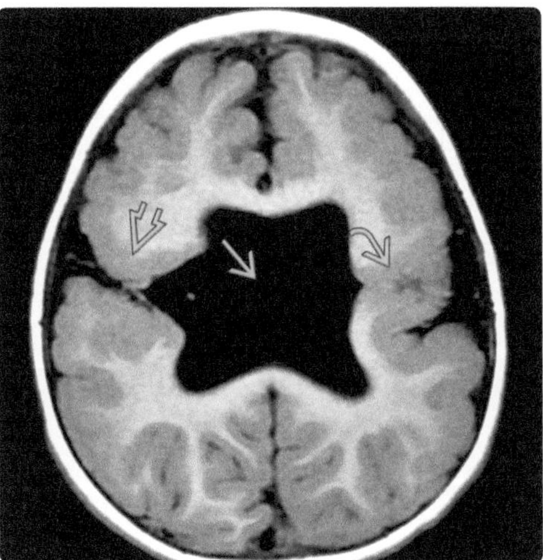

(Left) *Coronal T2WI MR in a 12-year-old with absent SP ⇨, ONH (not shown), right closed-lip schizencephaly ⇨, and left PMG ⇨ is shown. Both schizencephaly and PMG are often associated with SOD and should be carefully evaluated for.* **(Right)** *Axial T1WI MR in an 11-month-old with SOD shows absence of the SP ⇨, bilateral schizencephaly, open-lip schizencephaly ⇨ on the right, and closed-lip schizencephaly ⇨ on the left. Findings are consistent with SOD plus.*

KEY FACTS

TERMINOLOGY

- Partial or complete absence of corpus callosum and hippocampal commissure

IMAGING

- MR: Absent corpus callosum on sagittal, coronal views
  - Axial: Atrium/occipital horns dilated ("colpocephaly"); parallel ventricles
  - Sagittal: Absent cingulate gyrus
  - Coronal: Separate, vertically oriented frontal horns
  - DTI: Callosal fiber tracts form Probst bundles instead of crossing, where corpus callosum is absent
  - MRA: Vertical/posterior course of anterior cerebral artery (no genu to sweep around)
- CT: Multiplanar reconstructions key to diagnosis

PATHOLOGY

- Most common feature seen in CNS malformations
  - > 130 syndromes
- May be complete or variably partial
- May have interhemispheric dysplasia: Meningeal cysts, lipomas

CLINICAL ISSUES

- Any age; classically identified in early childhood; most common malformation found in fetuses
- Seizures, developmental delay, cranial deformity/hypertelorism
- Sporadic/isolated agenesis/dysgenesis of corpus callosum: Normal/near normal at 3 years (75%), but subtle cognitive defects apparent with increasing complexity of school tasks
- Agenesis/dysgenesis of corpus callosum with associated/syndromic anomalies = worst outcome

DIAGNOSTIC CHECKLIST

- Look for both direct signs (e.g., absent/incomplete corpus callosum) and indirect signs (e.g., absent cingulate gyrus, colpocephaly)
- Fully assess for associated lesions

(Left) *Coronal graphic shows a lack of transverse corpus callosum (CC) and separated lateral ventricles. The interhemispheric fissure extends to the 3rd ventricle. The bundles of Probst ➡ contain the rerouted callosal fibers.* **(Right)** *Coronal ultrasound in a newborn shows absence of the septum pellucidum ⇨, the widely spaced Viking helmet appearance of the frontal horns ⇨, and a high-riding 3rd ventricle ⇨. The frontal horns are located lateral to the Probst bundles ➡.*

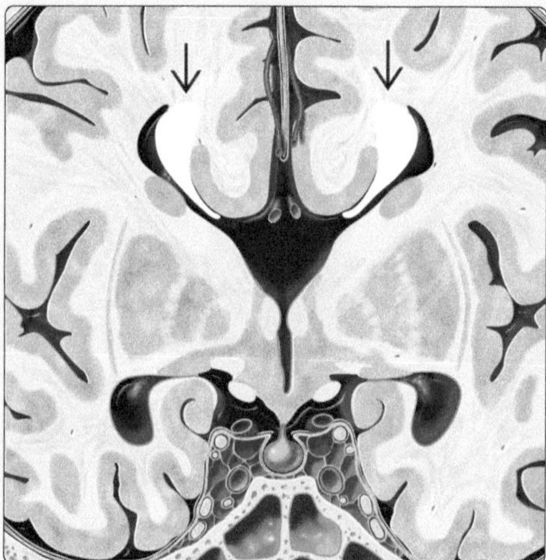

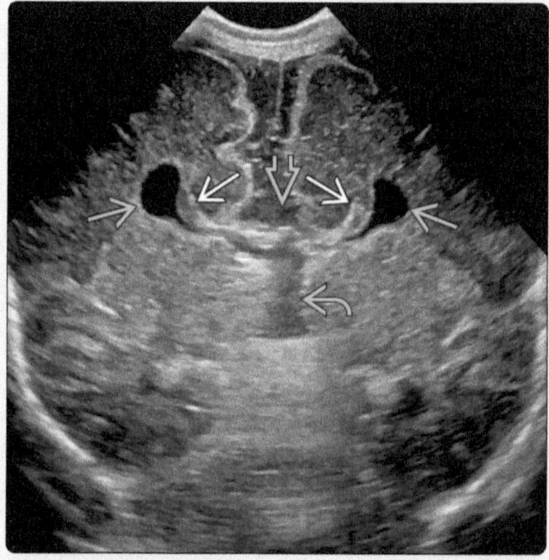

(Left) *Sagittal T2 MR in a 2-year-old shows absence of the CC with gyri and sulci ⇨ radiating vertically from the roof of the 3rd ventricle and internal cerebral vein ⇨. The cingulate sulcus is conspicuously absent in callosal agenesis.* **(Right)** *Axial T2 MR in the same patient shows a parallel configuration of the lateral ventricles with focal expansion of the atria and occipital horns ⇨ of the lateral ventricles, consistent with colpocephaly. Note the more posterior location of the anterior cerebral arteries ⇨ in the absence of the CC.*

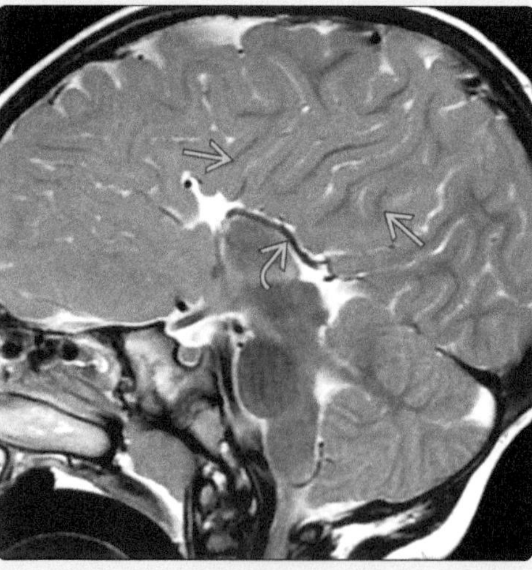

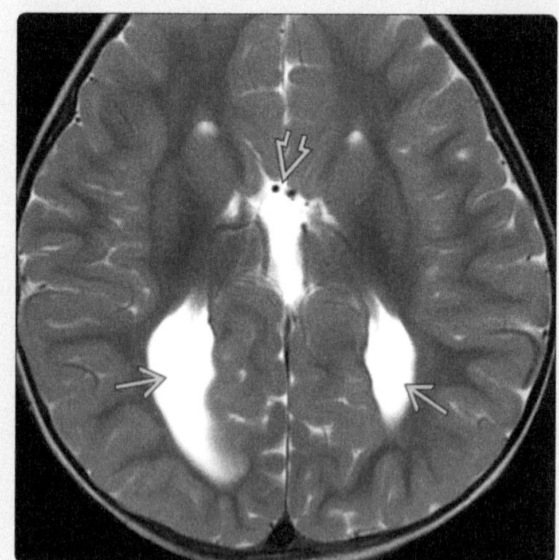

TERMINOLOGY

Abbreviations

- Agenesis/dysgenesis of corpus callosum (ACC)

Synonyms

- Callosal agenesis/dysgenesis, commissural agenesis/dysgenesis

Definitions

- Partial or complete absence of corpus callosum (CC), hippocampal commissure (HC), or anterior commissure (AC)

IMAGING

General Features

- Best diagnostic clue
  - Partially or completely absent CC on midline sagittal and coronal planes
  - Lateral ventricles separate and parallel (axial), bull's-head, trident, Viking helmet, or moose head appearances (coronal)
- Size
  - When present, CC remnants vary in size, extent, shape
    - Prior to myelin maturation, may be difficult to define (T2WI is better)
- Morphology
  - Commissural plate, clockwise
    - AC
    - Lamina rostralis and rostrum
    - Genu, body and isthmus, splenium
    - HC below CC, largest posterior to septum pellucidum

CT Findings

- NECT
  - On axial CT, lateral ventricles key to diagnosis
    - Parallel and separate
    - Atrium/occipital horns dilated ("colpocephaly")
- CTA
  - Anterior cerebral arteries (ACAs) course directly upward in interhemispheric fissure

MR Findings

- T1WI
  - Sagittal
    - Absent or incomplete commissures, expanded 3rd ventricular roof
    - Absent cingulate gyrus: Radiating sulcal pattern
    - AC may be absent, small, or normal
    - ± lipomas: Tubulonodular, curvilinear
  - Coronal
    - Interhemispheric fissure extends down to 3rd ventricular roof
    - Probst bundles: Medial parasagittal white matter tracts, brighter than other myelin on T1WI, indent lateral ventricles ("bull's head," etc.)
    - Bifid temporal horns and rounded hippocampi
  - Axial
    - Parallel separate lateral ventricles, colpocephaly
- T2WI
  - Same morphology as on T1WI
    - Probst bundles darker than rest of white matter
  - Separate and vertically oriented frontal horns, bull's-head, trident, Viking helmet, or moose head appearances
  - Variants and associated malformations
    - High-riding 3rd ventricle
    - Partial agenesis usually affects posterior CC and HC
    - Multiple interhemispheric cysts (meningeal dysplasia)
    - Malformations of cortical development (MCD): Polymicrogyria-like cortical malformation (often along midline cysts), subcortical or periventricular nodular heterotopia
    - Malformation of eyes, hindbrain (Dandy-Walker), hypothalamus-pituitary, cord, heart
- DWI
  - DTI: Callosal fiber tracts form Probst bundles instead of crossing, where CC is absent
  - Callosal remnants may contain axons from any part of cerebrum
- MRA
  - Vertical/posterior course of ACA (no genu to sweep around), ± azygous ACA
- MRV
  - Occasional midline venous anomalies, persistent falcine sinus

Ultrasonographic Findings

- Grayscale ultrasound
  - Coronal
    - Absent CC, "bull's-head" lateral ventricles, separated lateral ventricles, colpocephaly
  - Sagittal
    - Radially arranged gyri "point to" 3rd ventricle
- Color Doppler
  - Abnormal posterior ACA course

Imaging Recommendations

- Best imaging tool
  - MR
- Protocol advice
  - Multiplanar MR (look for associated malformations)
  - If MR unavailable, multiplanar CT will diagnose ACC
  - In fetuses, use ultrafast single-shot T2WI in 3 planes

DIFFERENTIAL DIAGNOSIS

Destruction of Corpus Callosum

- Surgery (callosotomy), trauma
- Hypoxic-ischemic encephalopathy, infarcts, hemorrhages
- Metabolic (Marchiafava-Bignami) with necrosis, longitudinal splitting of CC

Stretched Corpus Callosum

- Thinned CC (e.g., hydrocephalus), but all parts present

Hypoplastic Corpus Callosum

- CC thin, but all parts present

Immature Corpus Callosum

- Premyelinated CC may be difficult to confirm; look for cingulate gyrus

PATHOLOGY

General Features

- Etiology
  - Axons fail to form
    - Rare: CRASH syndrome/*L1CAM* gene defect, "cobblestone" lissencephaly
  - Axons not guided to midline (mutations in adhesion molecules)
  - Axons reach midline but fail to cross (absence or malfunction of midsagittal guiding substrate)
    - Turn and form large, aberrant, parasagittal Probst bundles
  - Miscellaneous
    - Toxic: Fetal alcohol exposure may affect *L1CAM*
    - Infection: In utero CMV
    - Inborn errors of metabolism: Nonketotic hyperglycinemia, pyruvate dehydrogenase deficiency, maternal phenylketonuria (PKU), Zellweger
- Genetics
  - Genetics of associated/syndromic CC anomalies
    - Most common abnormality seen as part of CNS malformations: > 130 syndromes
    - Chiari 2, frontonasal dysplasia, syndromic craniosynostoses, MCD, tubulin mutations, etc.
    - Aicardi syndrome: X-linked ACC, polymicrogyria and heterotopia, infantile spasms, retinal lacunae, developmental delay
- Associated abnormalities
  - MCD: Heterotopia, polymicrogyria, etc.
  - Ocular/hypothalamic-pituitary/cord/facial anomalies
  - Heart, limbs

Staging, Grading, & Classification

- May be complete or partial
- May be isolated anomaly or part of syndrome (> 130)
- May have interhemispheric dysplasia: Meningeal cysts, lipomas

Gross Pathologic & Surgical Features

- Leaves of septum pellucidum laterally displaced, contain Probst bundles
- Probst bundles contain parasagittal callosal bundle
  - Only form if callosal neurons present
  - Variable-sized bundles smaller than normal CC
- Associated dysgenetic brain lesions

CLINICAL ISSUES

Presentation

- Most common signs/symptoms
  - Seizures, developmental delay, cranial deformity-hypertelorism
  - Hypopituitarism-hypothalamic malfunction
  - Autism spectrum disorders
- Clinical profile
  - None specific

Demographics

- Age
  - Any; classically identified in early childhood; most common malformation found in fetuses
- Sex
  - M > F, if isolated finding
- Epidemiology
  - 0.5-70 per 10,000 live births
  - 4% of CNS malformations
  - Can be isolated (often male patients) or part of other CNS malformations

Natural History & Prognosis

- Sporadic/isolated ACC: Normal/near normal at 3 years (75%), but subtle cognitive defects apparent with increasing complexity of school tasks
- ACC with associated/syndromic anomalies = worst outcome

DIAGNOSTIC CHECKLIST

Consider

- Syndromic associations common

Image Interpretation Pearls

- Look for absent/incomplete CC rather than indirect signs
- Fully assess for associated brain lesions

SELECTED REFERENCES

1. Nguyen T et al: Abnormalities of the corpus callosum. Can prenatal imaging predict the genetic status? Correlations between imaging phenotype and genotype. Prenat Diagn. 43(6):746-55, 2023
2. Fenton LZ: Imaging of congenital malformations of the brain. Clin Perinatol. 49(3):587-601, 2022
3. Severino M et al: Imaging characteristics and neurosurgical outcome in subjects with agenesis of the corpus callosum and interhemispheric cysts. Neuroradiology. 64(11):2163-77, 2022
4. Shwe WH et al: Outcome of agenesis of the corpus callosum diagnosed by fetal MRI. Pediatr Neurol. 135:44-51, 2022
5. Manor C et al: Magnetic resonance imaging findings in fetal corpus callosal developmental abnormalities: a pictorial essay. J Pediatr Neurosci. 15(4):352-7, 2020
6. Raile V et al: Clinical outcome of children with corpus callosum agenesis. Pediatr Neurol. 112:47-52, 2020
7. des Portes V et al: Outcome of isolated agenesis of the corpus callosum: a population-based prospective study. Eur J Paediatr Neurol. 22(1):82-92, 2018
8. Leombroni M et al: Fetal midline anomalies: diagnosis and counselling part 1: corpus callosum anomalies. Eur J Paediatr Neurol. 22(6):951-62, 2018
9. Jarre A et al: Value of brain MRI when sonography raises suspicion of agenesis of the corpus callosum in fetuses. Radiologia. 59(3):226-31, 2017
10. Yang E et al: A practical approach to supratentorial brain malformations: what radiologists should know. Radiol Clin North Am. 55(4):609-27, 2017
11. Edwards TJ et al: Clinical, genetic and imaging findings identify new causes for corpus callosum development syndromes. Brain. 137(Pt 6):1579-613, 2014
12. Lau YC et al: Autism traits in individuals with agenesis of the corpus callosum. J Autism Dev Disord. 43(5):1106-18, 2013
13. Owen JP et al: The structural connectome of the human brain in agenesis of the corpus callosum. Neuroimage. 70:340-55, 2013
14. Santo S et al: Counseling in fetal medicine: agenesis of the corpus callosum. Ultrasound Obstet Gynecol. 40(5):513-21, 2012
15. Vasudevan C et al: Long-term outcome of antenatally diagnosed agenesis of corpus callosum and cerebellar malformations. Semin Fetal Neonatal Med. 17(5):295-300, 2012
16. Hopkins B et al: Neuroimaging aspects of Aicardi syndrome. Am J Med Genet A. 146A(22):2871-8, 2008
17. Miller E et al: The old and the new: supratentorial MR findings in Chiari II malformation. Childs Nerv Syst. 24(5):563-75, 2008
18. Lee SK et al: Diffusion tensor MR imaging visualizes the altered hemispheric fiber connection in callosal dysgenesis. AJNR Am J Neuroradiol. 25(1):25-8, 2004
19. Küker W et al: Malformations of the midline commissures: MRI findings in different forms of callosal dysgenesis. Eur Radiol. 13(3):598-604, 2003
20. Moutard ML et al: Agenesis of corpus callosum: prenatal diagnosis and prognosis. Childs Nerv Syst. 19(7-8):471-6, 2003
21. Sato N et al: MR evaluation of the hippocampus in patients with congenital malformations of the brain. AJNR Am J Neuroradiol. 22(2):389-93, 2001

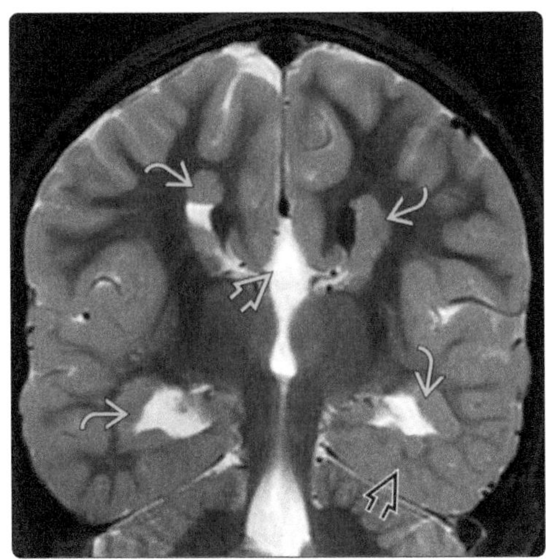

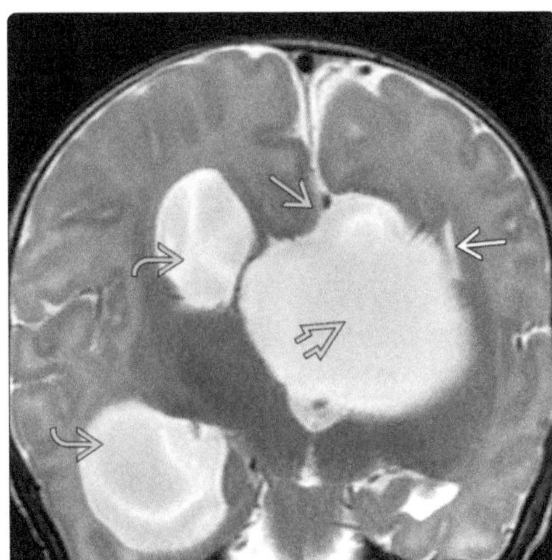

(Left) *Coronal T2 MR in a 4-year-old with callosal agenesis → shows associated malformations of cortical development: Bilateral subependymal gray matter heterotopia → and left temporal dysplasia → with too many gyri/sulci and abnormal white matter signal.* **(Right)** *Coronal T2 MR in a 5-week-old with callosal agenesis and associated interhemispheric cyst → shows absence of the CC → and the dilated right lateral ventricle →. The left frontal horn → is widely separated and effaced.*

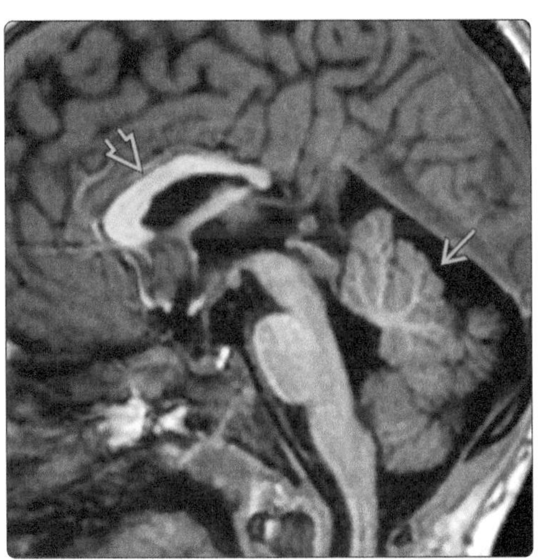

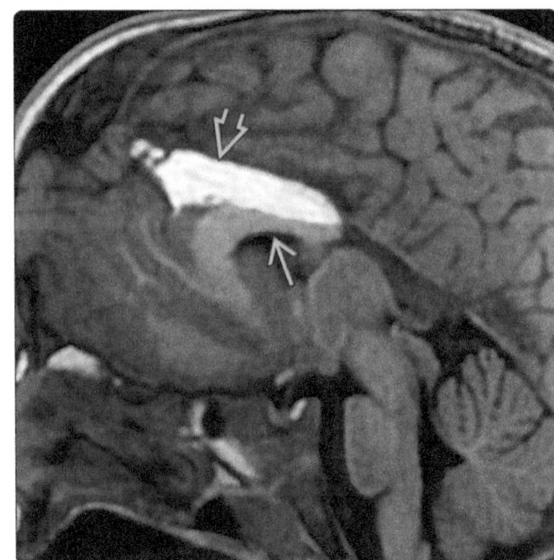

(Left) *Sagittal T1 MR in a 10-year-old with callosal dysgenesis shows a short and dysmorphic CC with small splenium →. This patient had other associated anomalies, including cerebellar dysplasia →.* **(Right)** *Sagittal T1 MR in a 5-year-old with a large tubulonodular pericallosal lipoma → and callosal dysgenesis → is shown. Pericallosal lipomas are associated with varying degrees of callosal dysgenesis. Typically, the larger the lipoma, the more dysgenetic the CC.*

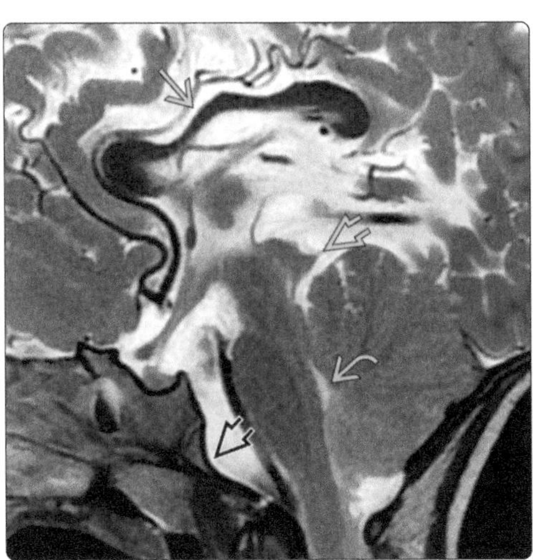

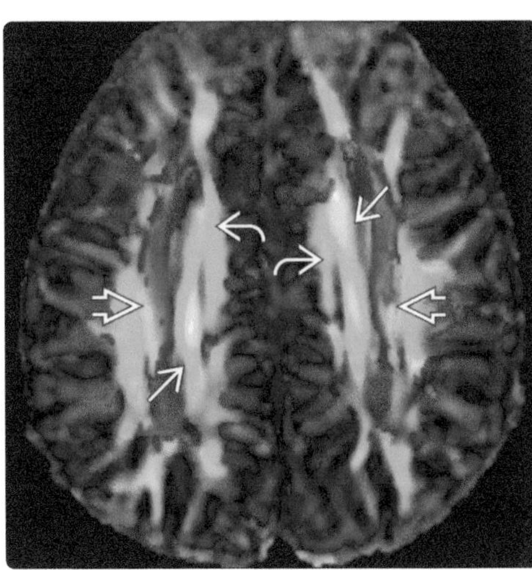

(Left) *Midline sagittal T2 MR in a child with repaired myelomeningocele and Chiari 2 malformation (beaked tectum →, small 4th ventricle →, and scalloped clivus →) shows a thinned dysmorphic CC →.* **(Right)** *Axial DTI of a child with complete callosal agenesis is shown. Transverse is shown by red, dorsoventral by green, and craniocaudal by blue. Probst bundles (uncrossed callosal fibers →) form a thick, dorsoventral bundle on each side of the midline, medial to the corona radiata → and lateral to the cingulum →.*

Congenital Microcephaly

KEY FACTS

TERMINOLOGY

- Microcephaly: Abnormally small head size
- Microencephaly: Abnormally small brain size

IMAGING

- Lateral radiograph, CT, or sagittal MR: ↓ craniofacial proportions
  - Normal craniofacial ratios: Preterm (5:1), term (4:1), 2 years (3:1), 3 years (2.5:1.0), 12 years (2:1), adult (1.5:1.0)
  - Microcephaly: ↓ craniofacial ratio, slanted forehead, closely apposed or overlapping calvarial sutures
- Imaging findings dictated by cause of primary microcephaly (MCPH)

TOP DIFFERENTIAL DIAGNOSES

- **Secondary microcephaly**
  - Perinatal: Hypoxic-ischemic encephalopathy (HIE), infection
  - Postnatal: Prolonged status epilepticus, HIE, hypoglycemia, meningoencephalitis, neurodegenerative, abusive head injury

PATHOLOGY

- Reduced growth of brain, ↓ proliferation of glia and neurons (all causes)

CLINICAL ISSUES

- Sloping forehead, flattened cranial vault, prominent ears, ± upslanting palpebral fissures
- Cognitive function ranges normal to developmental delay, intellectual disability, ± seizures

DIAGNOSTIC CHECKLIST

- Microcephaly may be first indication of underlying congenital, genetic, or acquired problem
  - Many genetic conditions are associated with abnormal head growth pattern

(Left) *Sagittal T1WI MR in a patient with familial primary microcephaly (MCPH) (autosomal recessive) shows a diminished craniofacial ratio but otherwise normal-appearing brain.* **(Right)** *Sagittal T1WI MR in an 11-month-old infant shows severe microcephaly with normal posterior fossa structures. Notice the very low craniofacial ratio, which is < 1. The cerebellum and brainstem are disproportionately large.*

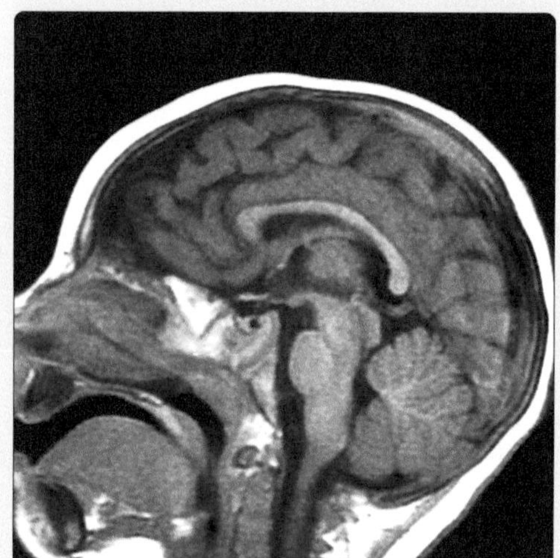

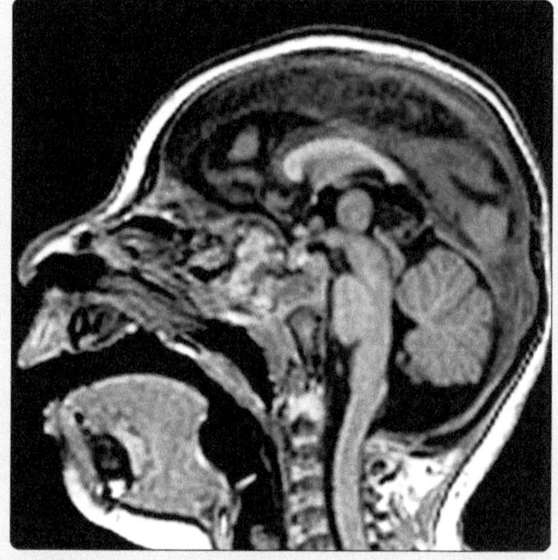

(Left) *Coronal T2WI MR in a severely microcephalic young adult with profound cognitive deficits reveals a smooth, thin cortex with minimal sulcation and gyration typical of microlissencephaly. Ventriculomegaly is attributed to passive expansion related to brain volume loss.* **(Right)** *Axial T2WI MR in a 12-month-old boy with moderate microcephaly and profound cognitive delay reveals smooth brain surface with aberrant cortical migration resulting in absence of sulcation and gyration. Findings are typical of classic lissencephaly.*

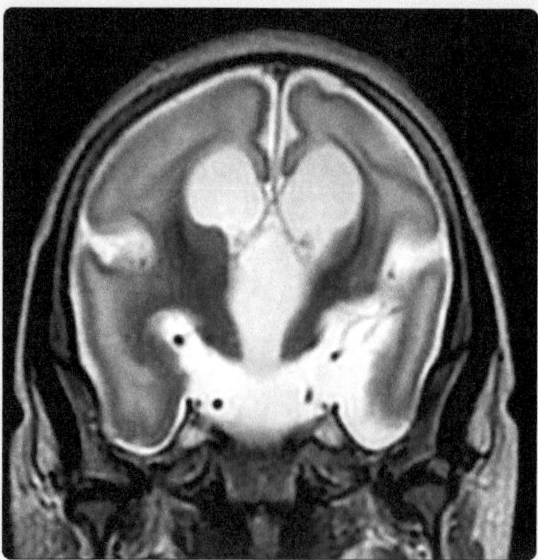

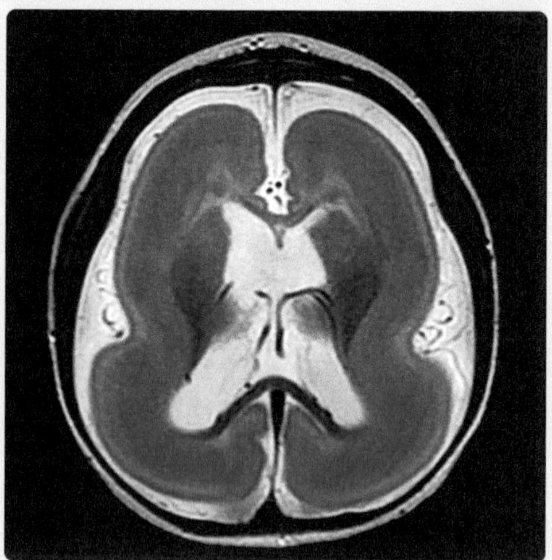

TERMINOLOGY

Definitions

- Microcephaly: Abnormally small head size
- Microencephaly: Abnormally small brain size
  - Because head growth is driven by brain growth, microcephaly usually implies microencephaly, but microencephaly does not always indicate microcephaly
- Microcephaly is sign, not diagnosis, so is defined with qualifying terms
  - Borderline microcephaly: Occipitofrontal circumference (OFC) 2-3 standard deviations (SD) below mean for age, sex, and gestation
  - Moderate microcephaly: OFC 3-5 SD below mean for age, sex, and gestation
  - Severe microcephaly: OFC ≥ 5 SD below mean for age, sex, and gestation

IMAGING

General Features

- Best diagnostic clue
  - Lateral radiograph, CT, or sagittal MR: ↓ craniofacial proportions
    - Normal craniofacial ratios: Preterm (5:1), term (4:1), 2 years (3:1), 3 years (2.5:1.0), 12 years (2:1), adult (1.5:1.0)
    - Microcephaly: ↓ craniofacial ratio, slanted forehead, closely apposed or overlapping calvarial sutures
    - Small cranial vault: Sutures closely apposed, overlapping ± secondary craniosynostosis
- Morphology
  - Imaging findings dictated by cause of microcephaly
    - More severe associated with gyral pattern simplification
    - Look for ↓ craniofacial proportions, suture overlap, simplified gyri, shallow sulci
  - Primary microcephaly (MCPH): Autosomal recessive sporadic neurodevelopmental ailment with head size ≤ 3-4 SD of normal
    - Group of autosomal recessive developmental disorders with microcephaly present at birth and intellectual disability
    - Smaller version of architecturally normal brain with significant size ↓ in cerebral cortex
    - Presentation at birth with nonprogressive intellectual disability
  - Gyral simplification
    - Small, grossly normal brain → oligogyria, mildly shallow sulci
    - Corpus callosum may be thick, lacks isthmus
    - Mild presentation sometimes described as small but perfect brain
  - Cortical dysplasia
    - Focal or diffuse gray matter malformation
    - More severe → pachygyria, lissencephaly
  - Microlissencephaly
    - Very small brain, smooth surface
    - Z-shaped brainstem
    - Callosal agenesis
  - Midline anomalies
    - Holoprosencephaly
      - Ranges lobar → alobar in order of severity
      - Most severe → smallest head
    - Callosal dysgenesis/agenesis
      - Consider fetal alcohol syndrome (FAS) in proper clinical context
    - Cerebellar hypoplasia
      - Pontocerebellar hypoplasia, spinocerebellar ataxia, carbohydrate-deficient glycoprotein syndrome type 1a, microlissencephaly
      - *TUBA1A* mutations: Lissencephaly + cerebellar hypoplasia
  - Hypomyelination (may be clue to rare disorders)
    - Early-onset West syndrome with cerebral hypomyelination, ↓ white matter
    - 3-phosphoglycerate dehydrogenase deficiency
    - Progressive encephalopathy, edema, hypsarrhythmia, optic atrophy (PEHO)
  - Pseudo-TORCH (Aicardi-Goutières)
    - CMV-like findings: Ca^{++}, hypomyelination, atrophy
    - Autosomal recessive (early-onset *TREX1*, late-onset *RNASEH2B* mutations)
  - Progeroid syndromes (Cockayne syndrome)
    - Disorder of DNA repair → cachectic dwarfism with intellectual disability
    - Basal ganglia/dentate Ca^{++}, demyelination, atrophy
    - Characteristic facies, progressive neuroimaging findings

DIFFERENTIAL DIAGNOSIS

Secondary Microcephaly

- Perinatal
  - Hypoxic-ischemic encephalopathy (HIE): Cortical atrophy (boundary zone vs. total) &/or basal ganglia/thalamus encephalomalacia
    - Look for classic patterns of involvement
  - Infection [particularly group B strep (GBS), HSV]: Asymmetric encephalomalacia ± hemosiderin, Ca^{++}
    - Late pregnancy TORCH infection (especially CMV) may produce white matter scarring and cysts without cortical dysplasia
- Postnatal
  - Prolonged status epilepticus, HIE
  - Hypoglycemia (occipital lobe predilection)
  - Meningoencephalitis: Asymmetric encephalomalacia ± hemosiderin, Ca^{++}
  - Neurodegenerative/metabolic: ± thickened calvariae, subdurals from shrinking brain (consider glutaric - acidemia, Menkes kinky hair)
  - Sturge-Weber syndrome: Cortical Ca^{++} + volume loss, leptomeningeal enhancement
  - Abusive head injury: Encephalomalacia, chronic subdurals, ± parenchymal lacerations
  - Multiple sutural craniosynostosis: Characteristic skull deformity
- Secondary microcephaly usually results from injury within first 2 years of life
- Cerebellum often spared → normal size compared to abnormal small cerebrum

PATHOLOGY

General Features

- Classify by gene mutation, if known; also assess
  - Relative size of supratentorial/infratentorial structures
  - Supratentorial anomalies (polymicrogyria, heterotopia, callosal anomalies)
  - Association with extra-CNS anomalies
- Etiology
  - From any cause, there is reduced growth of brain, ↓ proliferation of glia and neurons
  - Genetic: Mendelian inheritance **or** associated with genetic syndrome
    - Genetic or presumably genetic (e.g., numeric chromosome aberrations, microdeletions/duplications, monogenic disorders, genetic syndromes): 29%
    - Most MCPH mutations affect mitosis of neurons/glia (tubulins, microtubule-associated proteins)
  - Nongenetic
    - Noxious chemical or infectious agent (teratogenic exposure)
      - Maternal ingestion of anticonvulsants, alcohol, cocaine, excessive vitamin A affects fetal brain growth
    - Fetal vascular injury (in utero, preeclampsia)
      - Hydranencephaly most severe manifestation
    - Consequence of maternal systemic disease (rheumatologic, diabetes, etc.)
    - Congenital infection: TORCH (including Zika)
    - Early pregnancy injury mechanism may produce gray matter disorders of migration and organization
  - Unknown etiology: 41% (likely that many of these patients have genetic etiology)
- Genetics
  - Primary (genetic) MCPH is typically autosomal recessive (e.g., familial form → 1/40,000 births)
    - 18 MCPH loci (MCPH1-MCPH18) mapped to date (as of 2018)
  - Syndrome associations
    - Down (trisomy 21), Edward (trisomy 18), Cri-du-chat (5p-), Cornelia de Lange, Rubinstein-Taybi
    - Rare: DOOR, PEHO, Menkes, Seckel, X-linked FG syndrome, Cockayne, and pseudo-TORCH syndromes
- Associated abnormalities
  - Extra-CNS anomalies: Musculoskeletal, cardiac, gastrointestinal, etc.

Gross Pathologic & Surgical Features

- Skull capacity < 1,300 mL, brain weight < 900 g
  - Extreme microcephaly, as low as 300 g; head circumference = 5-10 SD below mean
- Simple gyral pattern (oligogyria), short central sulcus, enlarged sulcus parietooccipitalis (simian fissure), incomplete operculization
- ± lissencephaly, oligogyria, heterotopias, holoprosencephaly, cortical dysgenesis, cerebellar hypoplasia

CLINICAL ISSUES

Presentation

- Most common signs/symptoms
  - Small head (OFC > 3 SDs below mean for age, sex)
  - Severe intellectual disability, ± seizures, developmental delay
- Clinical profile
  - Receding forehead, flat occiput, conical head, ± overlapping sutures

Demographics

- Age
  - Congenital microcephaly often detected in utero or shortly after birth
- Sex
  - Variable based on etiology, genetic vs. nongenetic
- Ethnicity
  - Common genetic forms approximately panethnic
  - Certain syndromic causes may show ethnic preference
- Epidemiology
  - Incidence of MCPH in general population: 0.06-0.16%
  - Incidence of genetically determined microcephaly: Familial: 1/40,000; Down syndrome: 1/800

Natural History & Prognosis

- Dictated by cause: Variable seizures, intellectual disability, motor handicap

Treatment

- Supportive; genetic testing available for some microcephalic disorders

DIAGNOSTIC CHECKLIST

Consider

- Microcephaly is important neurologic finding
  - Deviations from normal head growth may be first indication of underlying congenital, genetic, or acquired problem
  - Many genetic conditions are associated with abnormal head growth pattern
  - Important to determine if head circumference was ever normal
- Cerebellar hypoplasia more common in genetic causes of microcephaly
- Consider FAS if midline anomalies accompany microcephaly

Image Interpretation Pearls

- Reduced craniofacial proportions on sagittal MR helpful but may be erroneous if brachycephalic: Tape measure best

SELECTED REFERENCES

1. Farcy S et al: Genetic primary microcephalies: when centrosome dysfunction dictates brain and body size. Cells. 12:1807, 2023
2. Gomes JA et al: Molecular mechanisms of ZIKV-induced teratogenesis: a systematic review of studies in animal models. Mol Neurobiol. 60(1):68-83, 2023
3. Naveed M et al: Comprehensive review on the molecular genetics of autosomal recessive primary microcephaly (MCPH). Genet Res (Camb). 100:e7, 2018
4. Zaqout S et al: Autosomal recessive primary microcephaly (MCPH): an update. Neuropediatrics. 48(3):135-42, 2017

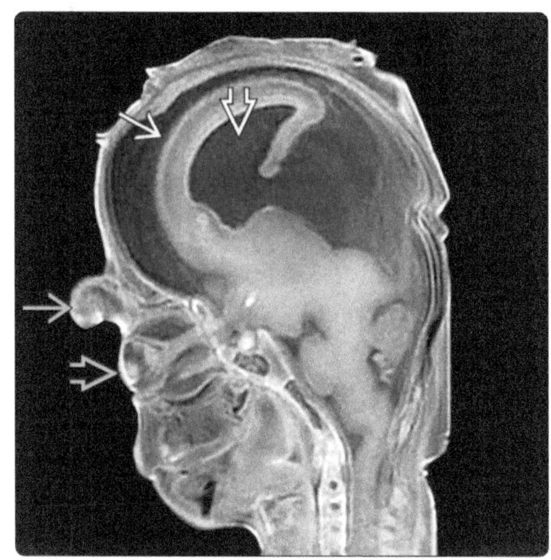

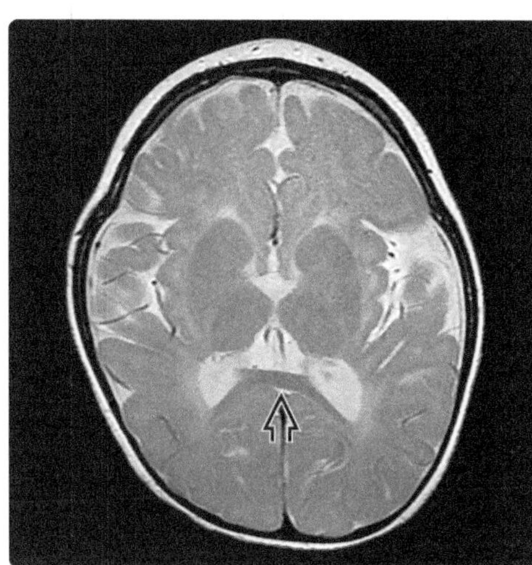

(Left) *Sagittal postnatal T1WI MR in a deceased 18-month fetus with alobar holoprosencephaly reveals marked microcephaly with small anterior "fused" cortical mantle ➡ and large central monoventricle ➡. Note also midline proboscis ➡ and phthisis bulbi ➡.* **(Right)** *Axial T2WI MR in a 22-month-old boy with abnormal facies and microcephaly (Cockayne syndrome) reveals profound hypomyelination with the most conspicuous myelination detected within the corpus callosum splenium ➡.*

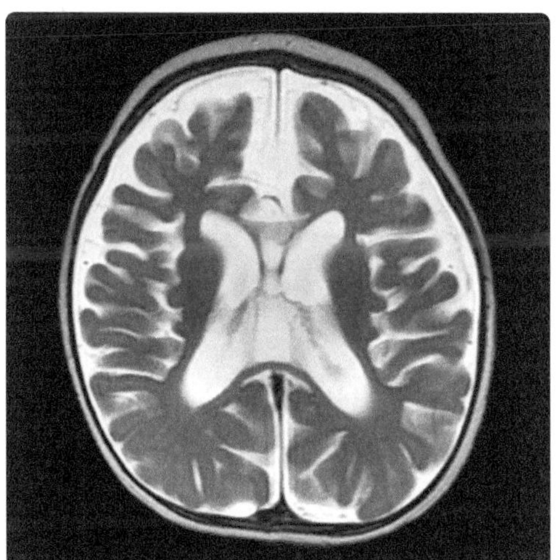

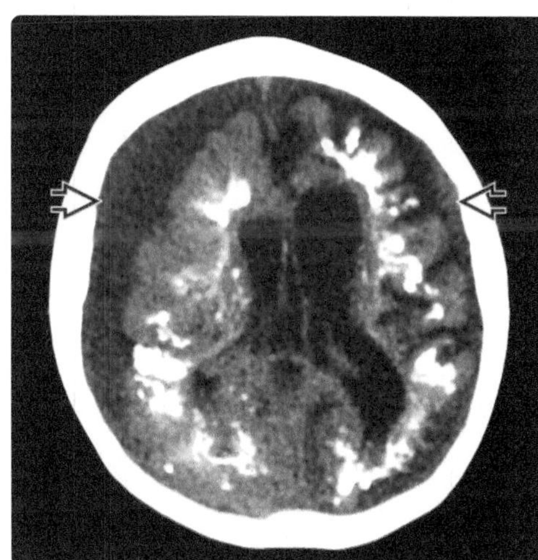

(Left) *Axial T2WI MR in a boy with Aicardi-Goutières syndrome and microcephaly reveals prominent sulci and ventricles compatible with diffuse brain volume loss.* **(Right)** *Axial NECT in the same patient when older shows progressive brain volume loss with extensive parenchymal calcifications. Bilateral subdural hematomata ➡ have developed as well due to brain shrinkage.*

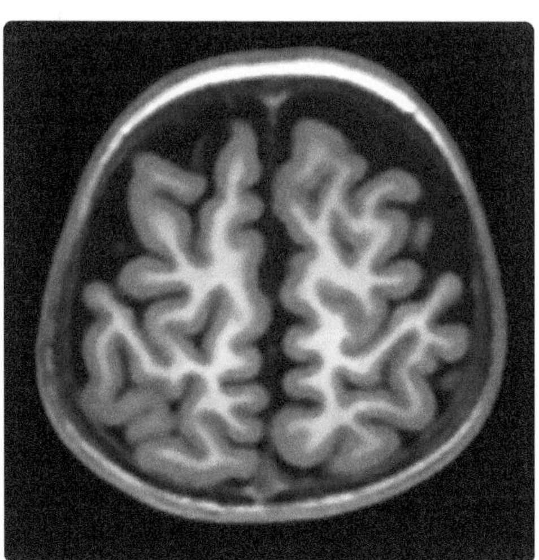

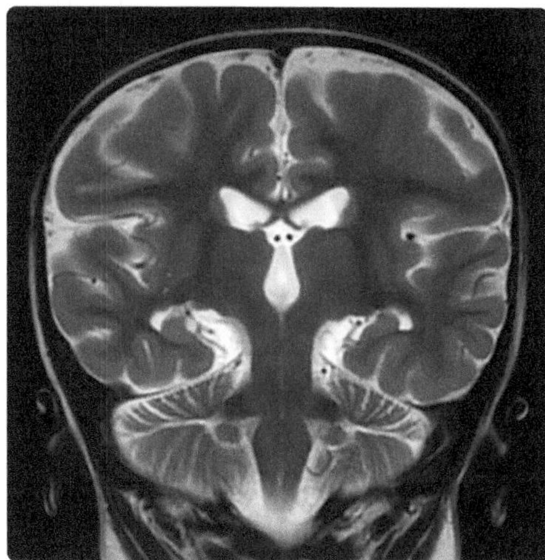

(Left) *Axial T1WI MR in a 2-year-old patient with Cornelia De Lange syndrome and microcephaly reveals a mild simplified gyral pattern.* **(Right)** *Coronal T2WI MR in the same patient confirms the simplified gyral pattern, particularly in the frontal and parietal lobes, with comparatively more advanced gyral development in the temporal lobes.*

Congenital Muscular Dystrophy

KEY FACTS

TERMINOLOGY

- Congenital muscular dystrophies (CMDs): Heterogeneous group of autosomal recessive myopathies presenting at birth with hypotonia
- Cobblestone malformations: CMDs with wide spectrum of brain imaging abnormalities

IMAGING

- Cobblestone malformation: Thick cortex with undersulcated surface and abnormal striated gray matter-white matter (WM) junction
- Hypoplastic brainstem, characteristically Z-shaped in Walker-Warburg phenotype (WWP)
- Dysplastic cerebellum: Polymicrogyria and cysts
- Polymicrogyria, hypomyelination
- Eye abnormalities: Retinal detachments, colobomas, persistent hyperplastic primary vitreous, microphthalmia, buphthalmos

PATHOLOGY

- Cobblestone malformations: 5 main phenotypes
  - WWP: Most severe phenotype, death in early infancy
  - Fukuyama CMD (FCMD)
  - Muscle-eye-brain phenotype (MEB)
  - *ADGRG1*-related cobblestone malformation [a.k.a. bilateral frontoparietal "polymicrogyria" (BFPP)]
  - Occipital cobblestone malformations
- Muscle biopsy: Necrosis, regenerating fibers, fiber size variability, increased perimysial and endomysial connective tissue

CLINICAL ISSUES

- Hypotonia, "floppy" newborn
- Cobblestone malformations: Developmental delay, poor vision, seizures

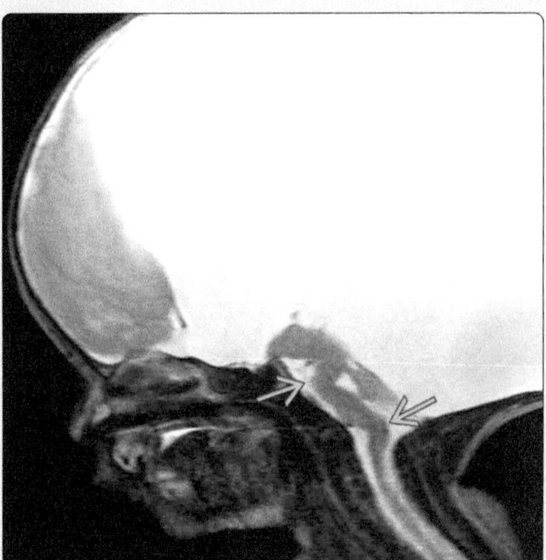

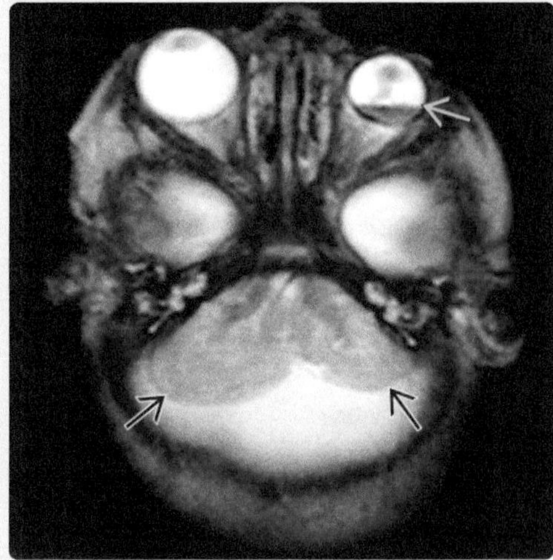

(Left) *Sagittal T2WI MR from a 7-day-old with hypotonia and elevated serum creatine kinase with intracranial findings of Walker-Warburg phenotype (WWP) shows a Z-shaped brainstem with ventral and dorsal apex angulation of the pontomesencephalic and cervicomedullary junctions, respectively ➡.* **(Right)** *Axial T2WI MR from the same patient is shown with additional findings of WWP, including left microphthalmia with retinal dysplasia and fluid-fluid level ➡ and asymmetric cerebellar dysplasia ➡.*

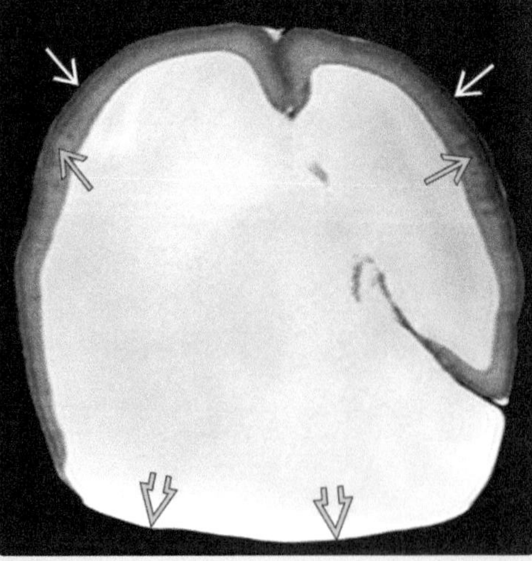

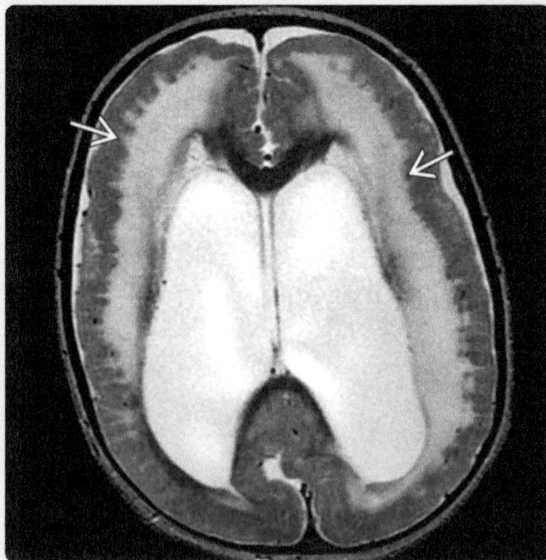

(Left) *Axial T2WI MR of the same patient with findings of cobblestone malformation with undersulcated outer cortical surface ➡ and finely serrated gray matter-white matter junction ➡ is shown. Also present is secondary aqueductal stenosis with ventriculomegaly and right ventricular dehiscence ➡.* **(Right)** *Axial T2WI MR shows classic serrated gray matter-white matter junction of cobblestone cortex ➡. Ventriculomegaly and white matter hypomyelination are also present.*

TERMINOLOGY

Abbreviations

- Congenital muscular dystrophy (CMD)

Definitions

- CMDs: Heterogeneous group of genetic disorders primarily characterized by onset of hypotonia within first 2 years of life
- Cobblestone malformations: Congenital muscular dystrophies with brain abnormalities primarily characterized by cobblestone malformation, commonly described phenotypes include
  - Walker-Warburg phenotype (WWP)
  - Fukuyama CMD (FCMD)
  - Muscle-eye-brain phenotype (MEB)
  - *ADGRG1*-related cobblestone malformation [a.k.a. bilateral frontoparietal "polymicrogyria" (BFPP)]
  - Occipital cobblestone malformations

IMAGING

General Features

- Best diagnostic clue
  - Cobblestone cortex and Z-shaped brainstem in hypotonic infant for WWP
  - Cobblestone malformation: Abnormality of neuronal migration characterized by protrusion of neurons beyond 1st cortical layer at pial surface of brain
    - Abnormal undersulcation of cerebral surface, thick cortex and characteristic striated cat's comb appearance of gray matter-white matter (WM) junction
    - Can sometimes be difficult to differentiate from true polymicrogyria and may fall along same pathologic spectrum
    - Formerly called "type II lissencephaly," though this term has been discarded
- Morphology
  - Cobblestone malformations
    - WWP (most severe phenotype)
      - Diffuse cobblestone cortex
      - Z-shaped brainstem: Enlarged rounded tectum, pontine hypoplasia with ventral apex kink at pontomesencephalic junction, 2nd dorsal apex kink, and cervicomedullary junction
      - Small dysplastic vermis and cerebellum
      - Obstructive hydrocephalus
      - Ocular abnormalities: Colobomas, microphthalmia, retinal dysplasias/detachments
      - Occipital cephalocele (10%)
    - FCMD
      - Polymicrogyria (frontal predominance) > cobblestone cortex (occipital predominance)
      - Delayed myelination
      - Dysmorphic cerebellum with subcortical cysts
      - Variable pontine hypoplasia, ± rounded tectum
      - Ocular abnormalities (retinal dysplasias)
    - MEB
      - Cobblestone cortex, polymicrogyria
      - Delayed myelination, patchy T2-hyperintense WM even after myelination complete
      - Brainstem: Large rounded tectum, hypoplastic pons with vertical midline cleft
      - Hypoplastic/dysmorphic cerebellum with subcortical cysts
      - Ocular abnormalities: Retinal dysplasia/detachments, hypoplastic optic nerve
      - Severity of findings intermediate between WWP and FCMD
    - *ADGRG1*-related cobblestone malformation (BFPP)
      - Phenotype similar to MEB but milder
    - Occipital cobblestone malformation
      - ± cerebellar dysplasia
      - Abnormal, diffuse, symmetric, T2-hyperintense WM signal
      - ± mild pontine hypoplasia
      - No ocular anomalies
      - Cortical abnormalities may be subtle and often not seen by imaging

MR Findings

- T1WI
  - Cobblestone malformations
    - Abnormal cortex: Cobblestone cortex, polymicrogyria
    - Cerebellar and vermian hypoplasia and dysplasia
    - Brainstem hypoplasia: Rounded tectum, Z-shaped if WWP
    - Varying degrees of WM hypointensity
- T2WI
  - Cobblestone malformations: Polymicrogyria or pebbled cortex, abnormal myelin, cysts in cerebellum
    - FCMD, MEB: WM abnormalities in 50%
    - WWP: Severe WM hypomyelination

Imaging Recommendations

- Best imaging tool
  - Multiplanar MR
- Protocol advice
  - Multiplanar, multisequence for WM, brainstem, and cerebellar changes

DIFFERENTIAL DIAGNOSIS

Joubert Syndrome and Related Disorders

- Look for molar tooth appearance of brainstem on axial images

Aqueductal Stenosis

- Can be difficult to differentiate from WWP prenatal and perinatal
- Brainstem can appear falsely kinked secondary to supratentorial mass effect
- Cortex difficult to evaluate in setting of severe obstructive hydrocephalus

Isolated Polymicrogyria

- Can be isolated or diffuse, though most commonly seen in perisylvian distribution

Leukodystrophies

- Some can appear similar to laminopathies; need to correlate clinically

PATHOLOGY

General Features

- Etiology
  - Dystroglycanopathies
    - Includes WWP, FCMD, MEB
    - Gene mutations cause underglycosylation of α-dystroglycan with O-linked carbohydrates
      - Results in anomalies of brain, eyes, and muscles
    - Inhibits binding of extracellular matrix proteins
    - Cortical malformations result from abnormal neuronal migration through gaps in basement membrane
  - *ADGRG1*-related diseases
    - *ADGRG1* is present in radial glial endfeet; when deficient, results in defective pial basement membrane
  - Laminopathies a.k.a. merosin-deficient CMD
    - Includes occipital cobblestone malformation
    - Absence of laminin α-2 chain (formerly known as merosin)
    - Inhibits cellular attachment and stability of skeletal muscle fibers and Schwann cells in peripheral nerves
- Genetics
  - Usually autosomal recessive
    - Some autosomal dominant, spontaneous mutations or mosaicism
    - Though clinical genetic testing available for nearly all associated genes, some affected patients do not have genetic diagnosis; there are still genes that have not been identified

Gross Pathologic & Surgical Features

- Supratentorial: Coarse gyri, agyric regions, ± ventriculomegaly and focal interhemispheric fusion
- Brainstem: Variable degrees of pontine hypoplasia and fused colliculi; flat, cleft, or Z-shaped brainstem
- Cerebellum: Cerebellar hypoplasia, polymicrogyria, and cysts ± encephalocele
- Ocular: Retinal/optic nerve dysplasias, retinal detachments, microphthalmia, buphthalmos, glaucoma, anterior chamber dysplasias, cataracts, persistent hyperplastic primary vitreous, myopia

Microscopic Features

- Muscle biopsy
  - Necrosis, regenerating fibers, fiber size variability, increased perimysial and endomysial connective tissue
  - Immunohistochemical staining
    - Cobblestone malformation/dystroglycanopathy: Deficiency of α-dystroglycan
    - Merosin-deficient CMD: Deficiency of laminin α-2 (merosin)
- Cobblestone cortex
  - Disruption of pial surface basement membrane with gliosis
  - Areas of fusion across intervening sulci
  - Abnormal clustering of neurons in upper levels of cortex
  - One hypothesis is that, depending on size of pial membrane defects, resulting cortex may present as polymicrogyria (small gaps) or cobblestone malformation (large gaps)

CLINICAL ISSUES

Presentation

- Most common signs/symptoms
  - Hypotonia, developmental delay, poor vision, seizures
  - Elevated serum creatine kinase

Demographics

- Age
  - Clinical presentation within first 2 years of life
  - Diagnosis of WWP can be suggested on fetal MR
- Sex
  - M = F usually (some M > F or M < F variants)
- Ethnicity
  - WWP has worldwide distribution
  - FCMD most common in Japan (carrier state 1:88)
  - MEB more prevalent in Finland

Natural History & Prognosis

- WWP: Lethal in infancy
- FCMD: Early contractures, rarely learn to walk; death < 20 years
- MEB: May survive to 20 years but with spasticity and contractures

Treatment

- No treatment other than supportive

DIAGNOSTIC CHECKLIST

Consider

- Typical brainstem and cerebellar findings should prompt diagnosis in hypotonic infant even if eyes and supratentorial cortex radiographically normal
- Polymicrogyria-like cortex with myelination defects: Look for brainstem, cerebellar, and ocular findings
- Clinical features are key; consider diagnosis in hypotonic newborn with abnormal brainstem morphology

Image Interpretation Pearls

- Not all Z-shaped brainstems are WWP
- Cobblestone malformation and polymicrogyria can be hard to differentiate by imaging and may fall along same pathologic spectrum

SELECTED REFERENCES

1. Camelo CG et al: Brain MRI abnormalities, epilepsy and intellectual disability in LAMA2 related dystrophy - a genotype/phenotype correlation. J Neuromuscul Dis. 10(4):483-92, 2023
2. Severino M et al: Definitions and classification of malformations of cortical development: practical guidelines. Brain. 143(10):2874-94, 2020
3. Barkovich AJ et al: Pediatric Neuroimaging. 6th ed. Wolters Kluwer, 2019
4. Kang PB et al: Evidence-based guideline summary: evaluation, diagnosis, and management of congenital muscular dystrophy: report of the Guideline Development Subcommittee of the American Academy of Neurology and the Practice Issues Review Panel of the American Association of Neuromuscular & Electrodiagnostic Medicine. Neurology. 84(13):1369-78, 2015

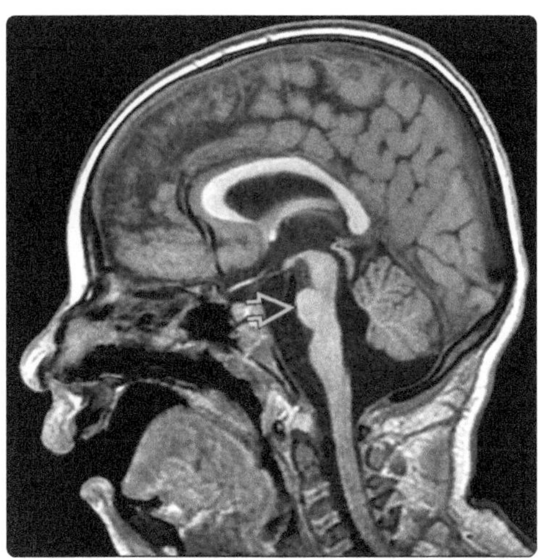

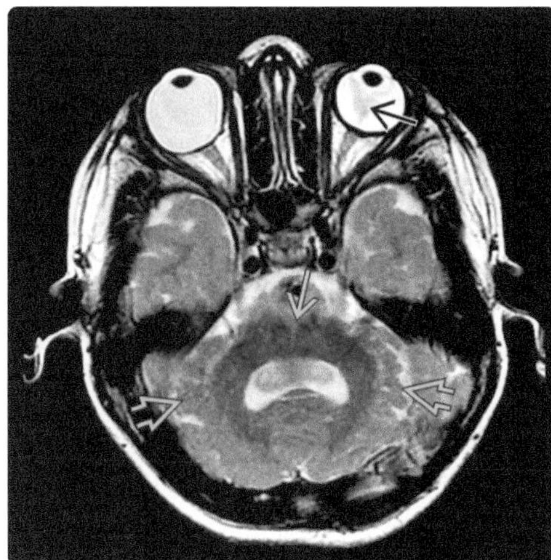

(Left) *Sagittal T1WI MR of a 5-year-old with a history of hypotonia, developmental delay, and abnormal vision with FKRP mutation, consistent with muscle-eye-brain disease, shows marked hypoplasia of the pons ⇒.* **(Right)** *Axial T2WI MR in the same patient shows a central pontine cleft →, cerebellar polymicrogyria ⇒, and eye abnormalities, including right buphthalmos and left microphthalmia with the retrolental linear signal abnormality consistent with persistent hyperplastic primary vitreous ⇒.*

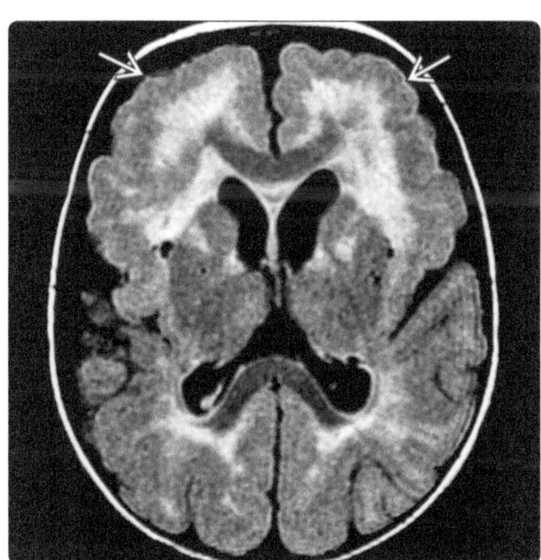

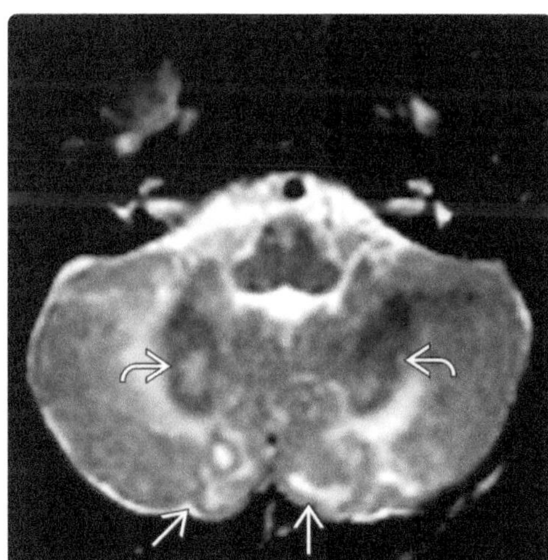

(Left) *Axial FLAIR MR in a 1-year-old with Fukuyama CMD shows characteristic bilateral frontal polymicrogyria ➡. There are large pericerebral spaces, mild ventriculomegaly, and abnormal myelination sparing the corpus callosum.* **(Right)** *Axial T2WI MR in the same patient shows blurred cerebellar cortex due to polymicrogyria. Note the poor myelination of arbor vitae with prominence of dentate nuclei ➡. Multiple high T2 signal cortical microcysts ➡ are typical of cobblestone malformations, such as Fukuyama CMD.*

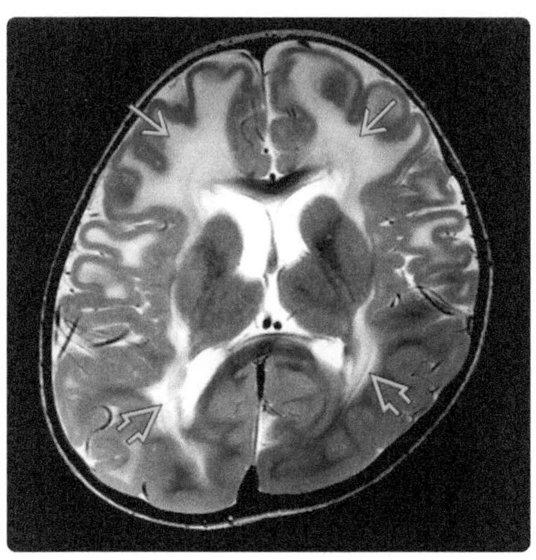

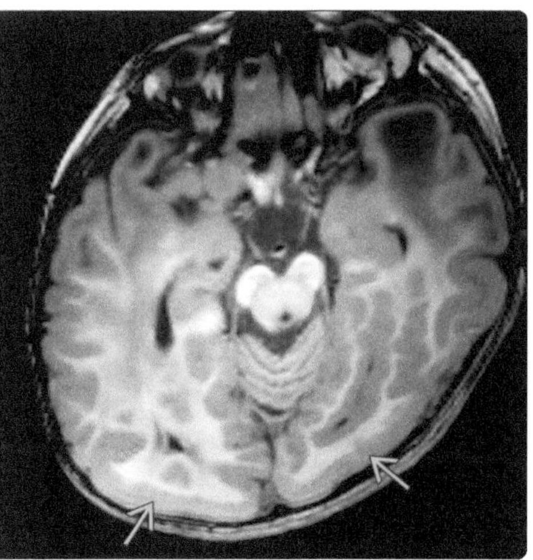

(Left) *Axial T2WI MR in a 5-year-old boy with LAMA2 mutation is shown. There is diffuse abnormal T2-hyperintense signal in the bilateral frontal lobes → and R > L occipital lobes ⇒.* **(Right)** *Axial T1WI MR in the same patient demonstrates subtle cobblestone malformation involving the bilateral occipital cortices →. Imaging findings are consistent with occipital cobblestone malformation phenotype of CMD.*

KEY FACTS

TERMINOLOGY

- Heterotopia (HTP): Abnormally located gray matter (GM) due to foreshortened or prolonged neuronal migration
  - Anywhere from periventricular germinal zone (GZ) to pia

IMAGING

- Ectopic nodular or ribbon-like foci following GM signal intensity on every MR sequence
- Locations: Periventricular, subcortical, pial
  - Periventricular nodular HTP (most common)
  - Synonyms: Band HTP, laminar HTP, double cortex
  - Subcortical nodular HTP (focal or multinodular)
  - Pial: "Cobblestone" cortex
- Best MR sequences (with multiplanar reformats)
  - Myelinated brain: 3D T1 spoiled-GRE (e.g., SPGR)
  - Unmyelinated brain: 3D T2 FSE (e.g., Cube/VISTA/SPACE)

TOP DIFFERENTIAL DIAGNOSES

- Tuberous sclerosis
- Closed-lip schizencephaly
- Ependymal spread of tumor
- Congenital CMV

PATHOLOGY

- Genetic and acquired etiologies cause disturbed neuronal migration, resulting in ectopic rests of GM
  - At GZ → periventricular HTP
  - Before reaching cortex → subcortical and band HTP
  - At pia → "cobblestone" brain

CLINICAL ISSUES

- Symptoms: Developmental delay, motor dysfunction, seizures (40% of intractable epilepsy cases)
- Palliative surgery reserved for intractable seizures

DIAGNOSTIC CHECKLIST

- Look closely for associated anomalies of adjacent cortex

(Left) *Axial T2WI MR in an 18-month-old girl with Aicardi syndrome and seizures shows extensive bifrontal periventricular and subcortical gray matter heterotopia ➡. Note the thin, irregular cortex ⇨ overlying the heterotopia. The corpus callosum is absent ⮳.* **(Right)** *Axial T1WI MR in a 2-month-old with seizures shows extensive, symmetric heterotopic gray matter ➡ with a brain-in-brain appearance. The more superficial cortex is thinner than usual with poor sulcation.*

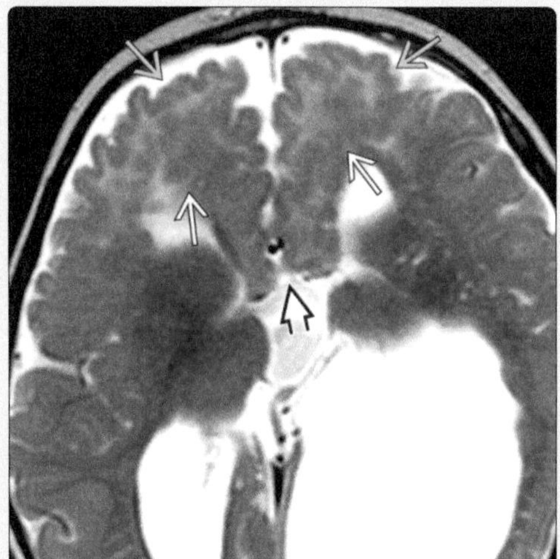

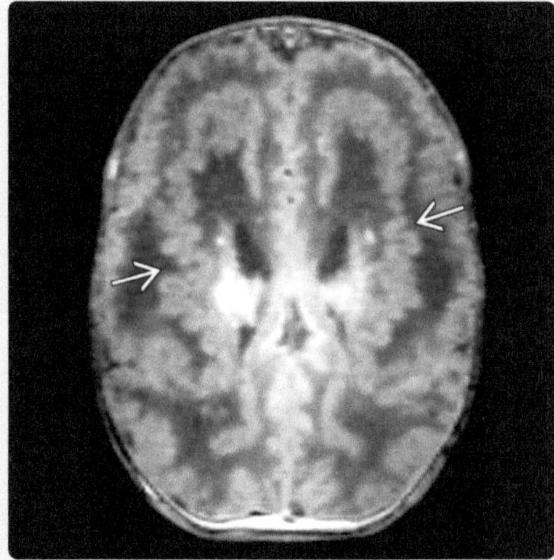

(Left) *Coronal T2WI MR in a 15-year-old with epilepsy shows a heterotopic band of gray matter of variable thickness ➡ within the deep and subcortical white matter, consistent with band heterotopia. Note the thin layer of intervening white matter ⇨ between the band of heterotopic gray matter and cortex.* **(Right)** *Axial T1WI MR in a 9-year-old boy with epilepsy shows the diffuse form of periventricular nodular heterotopia ➡. Note the abnormal overlying cortex ⇨ in multiple areas.*

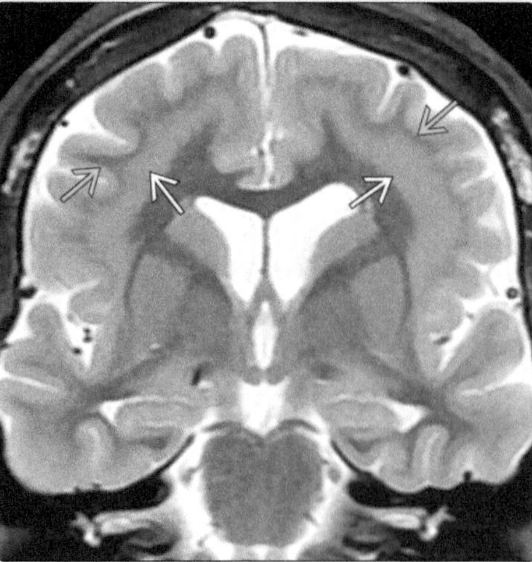

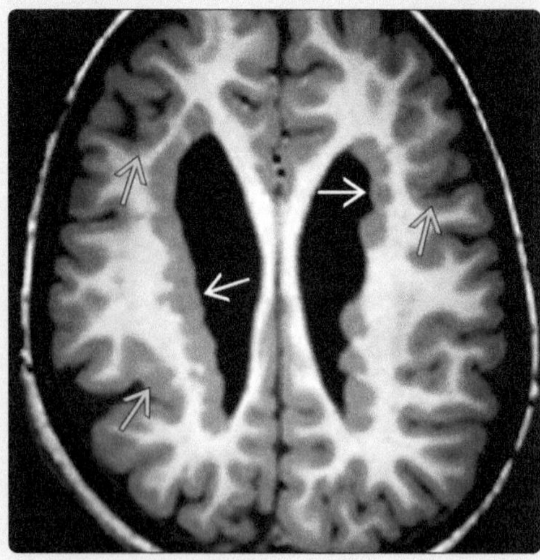

Heterotopic Gray Matter

TERMINOLOGY

Synonyms

- Gray matter (GM) heterotopia (HTP)
- Band HTP, double cortex

Definitions

- Abnormally located GM due to foreshortened or prolonged migration of neuronal groups
  - Occurs anywhere from periventricular germinal zone (GZ) to pia

IMAGING

General Features

- Best diagnostic clue
  - Nodules or ribbons of ectopic tissue that follow GM on all MR sequences
- Location
  - Periventricular, subcortical/transcerebral, pial

CT Findings

- **NECT**: Isodense with GM; rare dysplastic Ca^{++}

MR Findings

- T1WI: Isointense to GM; well marginated
- T2WI: Isointense to GM
- FLAIR: Isointense to minimally hyperintense to GM
- DWI: Isointense to GM
- T1 C+: No enhancement
- Fetal MR: Nodular, irregular ventricular lining ± abnormal sulcation

Ultrasonographic Findings

- Nodular periventricular HTP may be evident as irregular/lobulated ventricular margin

Imaging Recommendations

- Protocol advice
  - Multiplanar reconstructions of
    - 3D T1 spoiled-GRE MR (e.g., SPGR) in myelinated brain
    - 3D T2 FSE MR (e.g., Cube/VISTA/SPACE) in unmyelinated brain
  - Look closely for subtle dysplasia of overlying cortex

DIFFERENTIAL DIAGNOSIS

Tuberous Sclerosis

- Subependymal nodules in regions of fetal germinal matrix
- Often calcify; may enhance
- Associated with cortical/subcortical tubers

Closed-Lip Schizencephaly

- Polymicrogyric GM lines apposed walls of pial-ependymal cleft with funnel-shaped outpouching of ventricular wall

Ependymal Spread of Tumor

- Nodular or crescentic foci along ventricular lining
- Usually enhance, may restrict diffusion

Congenital CMV

- Periventricular Ca^{++} without protrusion into ventricle
- ± white matter injury, polymicrogyria, schizencephaly, cerebellar hypoplasia, microcephaly

PATHOLOGY

General Features

- Etiology
  - Genetic: Mutations alter molecular interactions at multiple migration points → migration arrest → HTP
  - Acquired: Fetal insult (ischemia, infection, etc.) → disturbed neuronal migration/cortical positioning
- Genetics
  - Diffuse periventricular nodular HTP often genetic
    - *FLNA* (Xq28), *ARFGEF2* (20q13.13), 5p15
  - Band HTP: Mild form of classic lissencephaly (agyria/pachygyria/double cortex)
    - *PAFAH1B1*/LIS1 (17p13.3), *DCX* (Xq22.3-q23), tubulin genes
- Associated abnormalities
  - Focal periventricular nodular HTP in 30% of Chiari 2
- Embryology
  - Abnormal neuronal migration
    - At GZ → periventricular HTP
    - Before reaching cortex → subcortical and band HTP
    - At pia → "cobblestone" brain

Microscopic Features

- Multiple types of immature/dysplastic cells
  - Excitatory exceed inhibitory

CLINICAL ISSUES

Presentation

- Most common signs/symptoms
  - Developmental delay, seizures, motor dysfunction
  - Age of onset and severity of symptoms depend on location and extent of abnormalities

Demographics

- Epidemiology
  - Found in up to 40% of patients with intractable epilepsy

Natural History & Prognosis

- Prognosis depends on location and extent of HTP, associated malformations, and seizure severity
- Focal HTP can be incidental on imaging/autopsy

Treatment

- Palliative surgery reserved for intractable seizures
- New radiofrequency or laser ablation of focal epileptogenic HTP

DIAGNOSTIC CHECKLIST

Image Interpretation Pearls

- HTP commonly associated with other anomalies
  - Look closely for overlying cortical abnormalities
- GM HTP does not enhance

SELECTED REFERENCES

1. Di Nora A et al: Gray matter heterotopia: clinical and neuroimaging report on 22 children. Acta Neurol Belg. 122(1):153-62, 2022
2. Zampeli A et al: Structural association between heterotopia and cortical lesions visualised with 7 T MRI in patients with focal epilepsy. Seizure. 101:177-83, 2022
3. Neuhaus E et al: Heterotopia in individuals with 22q11.2 deletion syndrome. AJNR Am J Neuroradiol. 42(11):2070-6, 2021

Polymicrogyria

KEY FACTS

TERMINOLOGY

- Traditionally considered malformation of late neuronal migration & cortical organization, resulting in abnormal distribution of neurons; disputed by some literature

IMAGING

- Excessively small & disorganized gyral convolutions with shallow sulci, creating appearance of nodular cortex
- Commonly perisylvian; may be unilateral or bilateral
- Imaging findings depend on patient age
  - Fetal: Premature appearance of sulci
  - 1-2 years: Abnormal sulcation pattern
  - > 2 years: Abnormally thick, irregular cortex
- NECT may detect Ca^{++} in CMV
- Polymicrogyria (PMG) lines clefts of schizencephaly
- Optimal imaging sequence depends on brain maturation
  - Incomplete myelination (< 1 year): Thin-section T2WI MR
  - Complete myelination (> 1-2 years): 3D SPGR T1WI MR

TOP DIFFERENTIAL DIAGNOSES

- Microcephaly with simplified gyral pattern
- Hemimegalencephaly
- Pachygyria
- Cobblestone malformations

PATHOLOGY

- Causes: Fetal infection, ischemia, or genetic/syndromic
- Associated syndromes: Aicardi, Zellweger, DiGeorge, Warburg microsyndromes

CLINICAL ISSUES

- Most common symptoms: Seizures, developmental delay, spasticity; varies with extent/location of PMG
- Age: Neonatal (in severe) vs. adolescence (in mild, focal)

DIAGNOSTIC CHECKLIST

- Look for secondary findings to suggest underlying CMV or metabolic or syndromic diagnosis

(Left) *Coronal oblique graphic shows thickened "pebbly" or nodular gyri of polymicrogyria (PMG) involving the frontal ⇒ & temporal ⇒ opercula. Note the abnormal sulcation & irregular gray matter-white matter (WM) junctions ⇒ in the affected regions.* **(Right)** *Sagittal T1WI MR in a 2-year-old with new-onset seizures shows PMG predominantly in the perisylvian area ⇒ & frontal lobe ⇒. Note the continuation of the sylvian fissure into the superior parietal lobule ⇒, a characteristic appearance for PMG.*

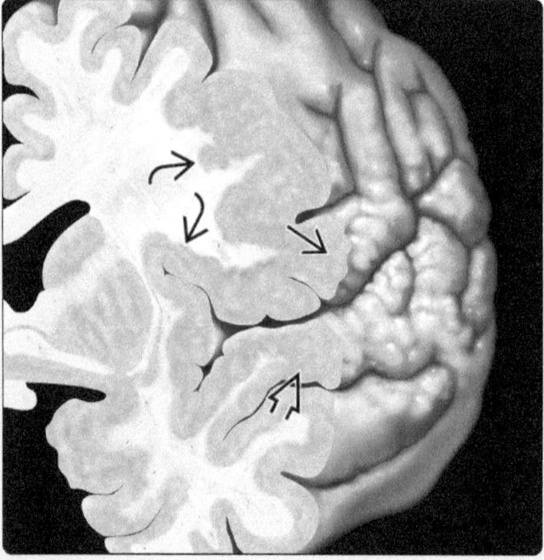

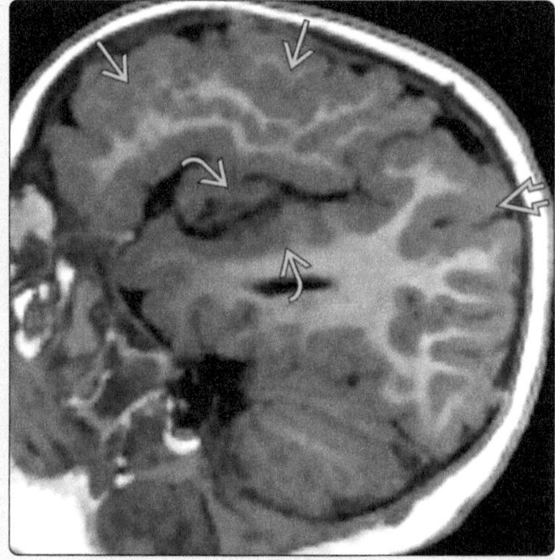

(Left) *Axial T2WI MR in the same 2-year-old shows extensive left frontoparietal PMG. Note the characteristic shallow sulci ⇒ & thickened, irregular cortex ⇒. The brain surface & the gray-white junction have an irregular nodular appearance. Contrast this to the normal right cerebral hemisphere.* **(Right)** *Coronal SSFSE MR in a 25-week-gestation fetus shows bilateral foci of irregular cortex ⇒, consistent with extensive PMG. The cortex in these regions should appear smooth at this time in gestation.*

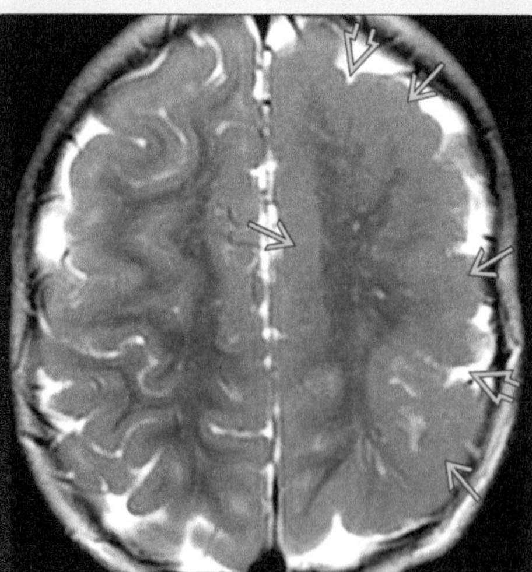

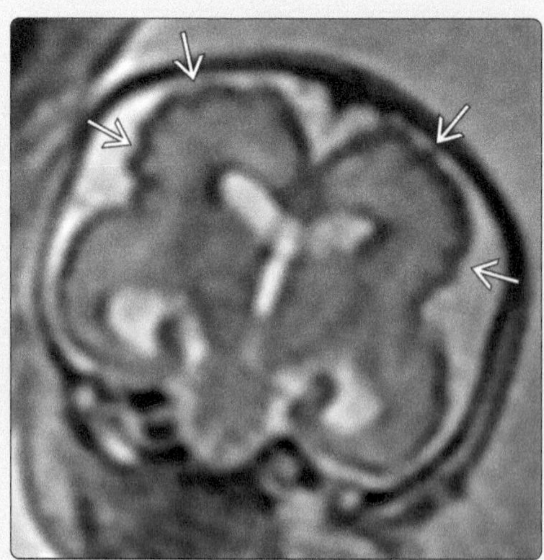

TERMINOLOGY

Abbreviations

- Polymicrogyria (PMG)

Definitions

- Traditionally considered malformation of late neuronal migration & cortical organization, resulting in abnormal distribution of neurons; disputed by some literature
  - Regardless, macroscopic result is nodular cortex with disorganized small undulating gyri & shallow sulci
    - May give false impression of several large, thick gyri

IMAGING

General Features

- Best diagnostic clue
  - Excessively small & numerous gyri
- Location
  - Can be unilateral, bilateral, multifocal
    - When bilateral, often symmetric
  - Most common in perisylvian regions (60-70%)
- Size
  - Ranges from single gyrus to entire cerebrum
- Morphology
  - Small irregular gyri
    - Irregular gyri best seen on thin-section (1- to 2-mm) imaging
    - Appearance of cortical thickening more common with thick-section (3- to 5-mm) imaging
  - Thick nodular cortex with irregular gray matter-white matter junctions
  - May appear as deep infolding of thick cortex
  - Schizencephalic clefts lined by PMG
  - Sylvian fissure may extend into parietal lobe

CT Findings

- Look for altered sulcation pattern (suggests PMG)
- Periventricular Ca^{++} in CMV
- Excessive small convolutions difficult to detect on CT due to poor contrast resolution

MR Findings

- **T1WI**: Irregular cortical surface; thick-appearing cortex; deep infolding of irregular cortex
  - Irregular cortical surface, often seen best on thin parasagittal images
  - May appear as arc of thick (5- to 7-mm) cortex with irregular gray matter-white matter junction without normal sulci
  - May appear as deep infolding of irregular thick cortex
  - Less sensitive for diagnosis before myelination (< 1 year)
- **T2WI**: 2 imaging patterns depending on patient age
  - < 12 months: Undulating cortex of normal thickness
  - > 18 months: Thick, bumpy cortex (6-8 mm)
  - Most sensitive sequence for PMG detection before myelination (< 1 year)
- **FLAIR**: May be difficult to see microgyri because of poor contrast between cortex & white matter
  - Allows differentiation between dilated perivascular spaces (common in PMG) & abnormal myelination (suggests cobblestone malformation or prenatal infection, such as CMV)
- **SWI/T2* GRE**: Hypointense periventricular foci → Ca^{++} in CMV
- **T1WI C+**: Amplifies dysplastic leptomeningeal veins (when present) overlying regions of PGM
- **MRS**: ↓ NAA at seizure-precipitating, atrophic, &/or hypomyelinated sites
- **MRV**: Demonstrates large leptomeningeal veins overlying abnormal cortex

Angiographic Findings

- May see large veins in clefts of PMG

Nuclear Medicine Findings

- **PET**: Ictal hypermetabolism & interictal hypometabolism

Other Modality Findings

- **Fetal MR & US**
  - Irregular cortex or premature appearance of sulci
  - Important to know expected sulcation pattern for gestational age to detect PMG on fetal MR
  - Can detect PMG & other anomalies of cortical development as early as 22 weeks

Imaging Recommendations

- Best imaging tool
  - MR comprehensively assesses malformation
  - NECT for suspected Ca^{++} (CMV)
- Protocol advice
  - Volumetric 3D SPGR (T1WI) MR in mature brain
  - Thin-section T2WI MR if unmyelinated

DIFFERENTIAL DIAGNOSIS

Polymicrogyria Secondary to Inborn Errors of Metabolism

- Mitochondrial & pyruvate metabolism disorders
- Zellweger syndrome: Severe hypomyelination, PMG

Microcephaly With Simplified Gyral Pattern

- Disorder of stem cell proliferation; head circumference < 3 standard deviations below mean
- Normal cortex with primary & secondary sulci but absent tertiary sulci

Hemimegalencephaly

- Disorder of neuronal proliferation, migration, & differentiation
- ↑ size of involved hemisphere (vs. ↓ in PMG)
- Abnormal T1/T2 signal in white matter of involved hemisphere

Pachygyria

- Thick cortex (8-10 mm), smooth gray matter-white matter junction
- Simplified gyral pattern

Cobblestone Malformations

- Hypomyelination, cerebellar dysgenesis, pontine hypoplasia
- Often associated with congenital muscular dystrophy (e.g., Walker-Warburg)

PATHOLOGY

General Features

- Etiology
  - Intrauterine infection, ischemia, or gene mutations
    - Timing: 2nd half of 2nd trimester
  - Recent research suggests that abnormalities in overlying pia & leptomeninges contribute significantly to abnormal cortical development
- Genetics
  - Mutations in following genetic pathways: mTORopathies, tubulinopathies, laminopathies, & glycosylation disorders
  - Most common: 1p36.3 & 22q11.2 microdeletions
  - Mutations of Xq28, Xq21.33-q23 (*SRPX2*),16q12.2-21, 1p36, & 22q11.2, & genetic loci on chromosomes 1p36.3, 2p16.1-p23, 4q21.21-q22.1, 6q26-q27, & 21q21.3-22.1 have been identified
- Associated abnormalities
  - CMV: Periventricular Ca^{++}, white matter signal abnormality, anterior temporal cysts, & hearing loss
  - Aicardi, Zellweger, Warburg microsyndromes
  - Congenital bilateral perisylvian syndrome (Foix-Chavany-Marie)
  - Corpus callosum dysgenesis, periventricular nodular heterotopia, & subcortical heterotopia
  - Microcephaly (~ 50%); more common in generalized forms of PMG
  - Schizencephaly thought to be more severe outcome of similar etiologies (fetal CMV, ischemia, etc.), as evidenced by frequent contralateral PMG
  - Septo-optic dysplasia (SOD) plus syndrome: SOD with associated PMG &/or schizencephaly

Gross Pathologic & Surgical Features

- Multiple small gyri lie in haphazard orientation
- Multiple appearances & locations
  - Unilateral: Focal, perisylvian, or hemispheric
  - Bilateral symmetrical: Perisylvian, frontal, frontoparietal, lateral parietal, medial parasagittal parietooccipital
  - Bilateral asymmetrical

Microscopic Features

- Derangements of normal 6-layered cortex
  - Reduced numbers of neurons
  - Areas of 2-, 4-, & 6-layered cortex described, even in different regions of same brain
    - Normal vs. abnormal laminar arrangement disputed
  - Leptomeningeal embryonic vasculature overlies malformation
  - Myelination within subcortical or intracortical fibers changes cortical appearance on T2WI

CLINICAL ISSUES

Presentation

- Most common signs/symptoms
  - Seizures, developmental delay, spasticity
    - Congenital bilateral perisylvian syndrome: Bilateral perisylvian PMG + oromotor dysfunction & seizure disorder
    - Unilateral PMG often leads to hemiparesis/seizures
    - Onset & severity of seizures, neurologic deficits relate to location & extent of malformation
  - Associated sensorineural hearing loss suggests CMV

Demographics

- Age
  - Symptom onset varies with extent/location of malformation
    - Neonatal manifestations in severely affected vs. 2nd decade of life for focal unilateral PMG
- Sex
  - No preference
- Ethnicity
  - Found in all populations
- Epidemiology
  - Malformations of cortical development found in ~ 40% of children with intractable epilepsy

Natural History & Prognosis

- Variable based on severity of genetic mutation, resultant malformation, associated anomalies
- Many patients with isolated unilateral PMG highly functional
  - Often otherwise healthy until presenting in 1st or 2nd decade with seizures

Treatment

- Surgical options with medically refractory seizures
  - Focal PMG may be resected
  - Corpus callosotomy if bilateral or unresectable lesions

DIAGNOSTIC CHECKLIST

Image Interpretation Pearls

- Look for PMG in congenital hemiplegia with epilepsy
  - Schizencephaly always lined by PMG
  - Open sylvian fissures with thick cortex suggest PMG
- Look for secondary findings of CMV or syndrome
  - With macrocephaly, think of MPPH (**m**acrocephaly, **P**MG, **p**olydactyly, **h**ydrocephalus)

SELECTED REFERENCES

1. Kolbjer S et al: Polymicrogyria: epidemiology, imaging, and clinical aspects in a population-based cohort. Brain Commun. 5(4):fcad213, 2023
2. Khandelwal A et al: Magnetic resonance imaging of malformations of cortical development-a comprehensive review. World Neurosurg. 159:70-9, 2022
3. Arrigoni F et al: Characterizing white matter tract organization in polymicrogyria and lissencephaly: a multifiber diffusion MRI modeling and tractography study. AJNR Am J Neuroradiol. 41(8):1495-502, 2020
4. Guimaraes CVA et al: Imaging phenotype correlation with molecular and molecular pathway defects in malformations of cortical development. Pediatr Radiol. 50(13):1974-87, 2020
5. Jalloh I et al: The role of surgery in refractory epilepsy secondary to polymicrogyria in the pediatric population. Epilepsia. 59(10):1982-96, 2018
6. Jansen AC et al: The histopathology of polymicrogyria: a series of 71 brain autopsy studies. Dev Med Child Neurol. 58(1):39-48, 2016
7. De Ciantis A et al: Ultra-high-field MR imaging in polymicrogyria and epilepsy. AJNR Am J Neuroradiol. 36(2):309-16, 2015
8. Stutterd CA et al: Polymicrogyria: a common and heterogeneous malformation of cortical development. Am J Med Genet C Semin Med Genet. 166C(2):227-39, 2014
9. Barkovich AJ et al: A developmental and genetic classification for malformations of cortical development: update 2012. Brain. 135(Pt 5):1348-69, 2012
10. Mavili E et al: Polymicrogyria: correlation of magnetic resonance imaging and clinical findings. Childs Nerv Syst. 28(6):905-9, 2012

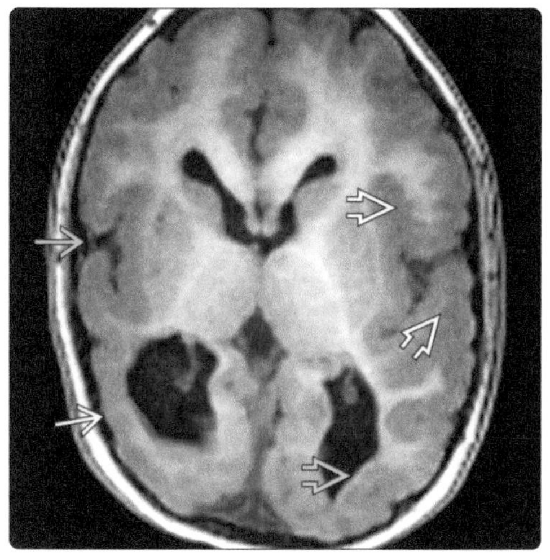

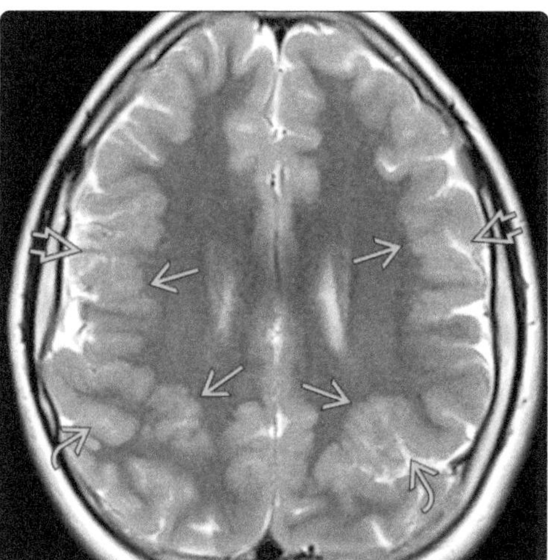

(Left) *Axial T1WI MR in a 2-year-old girl shows a lack of normal sulci ➔ with thickened nodular cortex ➔ & an "open" sylvian fissure on the right ➔, characteristic of PMG. Note the WM thinning ➔ (with ex vacuo ventricular dilation) from congenital CMV.* **(Right)** *Axial T2WI MR in a 9-year-old shows bilateral PMG in the perisylvian region, including the frontal operculum ➔ & the superior parietal lobule ➔. Note the irregular junction of the cortical gray matter and subcortical WM ➔.*

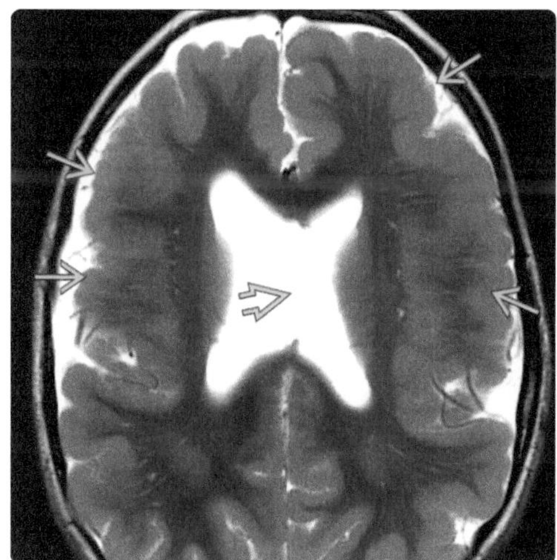

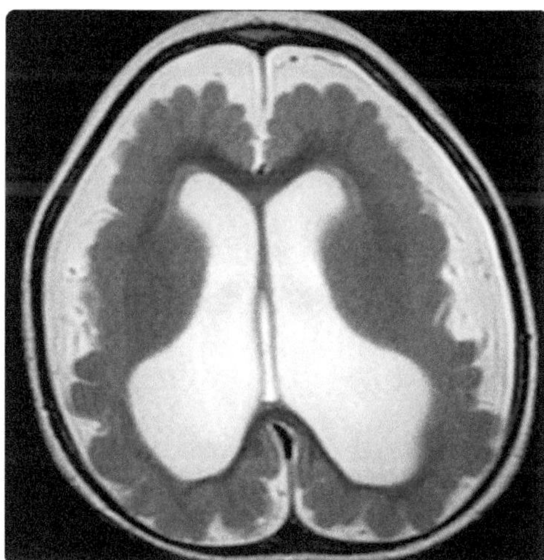

(Left) *Axial T2WI MR in a 6-year-old with septo-optic dysplasia (SOD) plus with extensive bilateral PMG ➔ is shown. Note the lack of the septum pellucidum ➔. When you see signs of SOD, look closely for associated PMG, which would suggest SOD plus.* **(Right)** *Axial T2WI MR shows a 21-month-old with bilateral holohemispheric PMG & a mutation in 17p13.1. This severe PMG is associated with significant brain parenchymal volume loss with very little WM & prominent ventricles & extraaxial CSF spaces.*

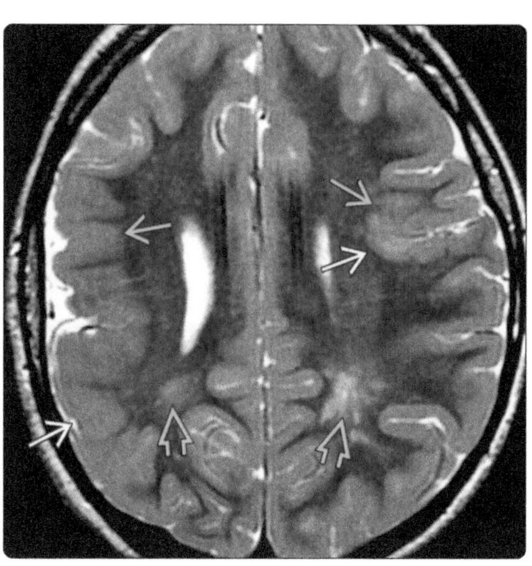

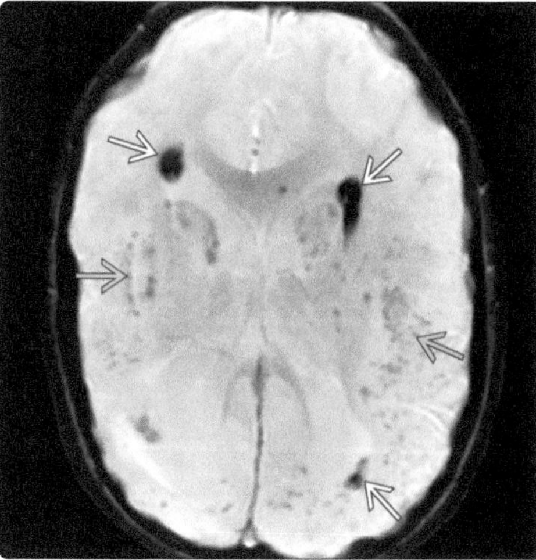

(Left) *Axial T2WI MR in a 4-year-old boy with hearing loss shows abnormal sulcation ➔ & nodular cortical thickening ➔ bilaterally (R > L), consistent with PMG. Also note the periatrial WM injury ➔. The combination of hearing loss, PMG, & WM injury suggests congenital CMV infection.* **(Right)** *Axial SWI in a 2-year-old girl shows multiple periventricular ➔ & parenchymal ➔ Ca^{++} along with extensive WM volume loss. PMG, Ca^{++}, & WM volume loss are a typical constellation of findings seen in congenital CMV.*

KEY FACTS

TERMINOLOGY

- Cortical disorganization & abnormal laminar architecture

IMAGING

- Focal cortical dysplasia (FCD) type 1
    - MR imaging findings present in 22-64%; may be lower in children
        - White matter (WM) volume loss
        - Ill-defined WM increased signal
        - Blurring of gray matter (GM)-WM junction
        - Cortical signal change
        - Abnormal sulcal & gyral pattern
- FCD type 2
    - MR imaging findings more commonly present (60-100%)
        - Focal signal abnormality in subcortical WM
        - Blurring of GM-WM junction
        - Cortical thickening & signal change
        - Abnormal sulcal & gyral pattern

PATHOLOGY

- FCD type 1
    - Abnormal lamination of cortex **without** dysmorphic neurons
- FCD type 2
    - Abnormal lamination of cortex **with** dysmorphic neurons, ± balloon cells
- FCD type 3
    - FCD associated with other structural lesions

CLINICAL ISSUES

- FCD is most common pathology seen in pediatric patients with surgically treated epilepsy
    - Type 1 dysplasias more commonly seen in adults
- Epilepsy surgery effectiveness dependent on type of underlying pathology
    - FCD type 1: 13-21% seizure free
    - FCD type 2: 52-91% seizure free

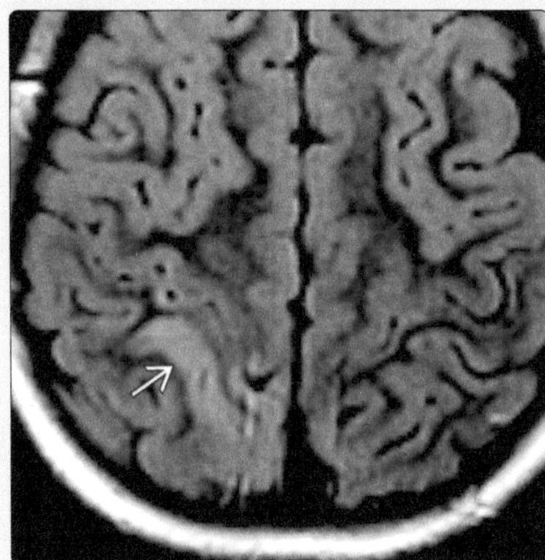

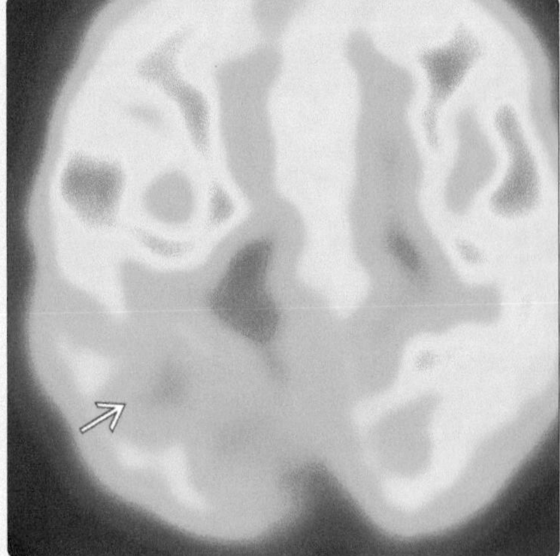

(Left) *Axial FLAIR MR in an 8-year-old girl shows hyperintense signal ➡ in the right parietal cortex, a common finding in focal cortical dysplasia (FCD). Pathology demonstrated FCD type 2B.* **(Right)** *Axial color-coded FDG PET in the same patient shows focally decreased metabolism ➡ in the area of MR signal abnormality. FDG PET is particularly helpful in identifying FCD lesions that are not visible or very subtle on conventional MR imaging.*

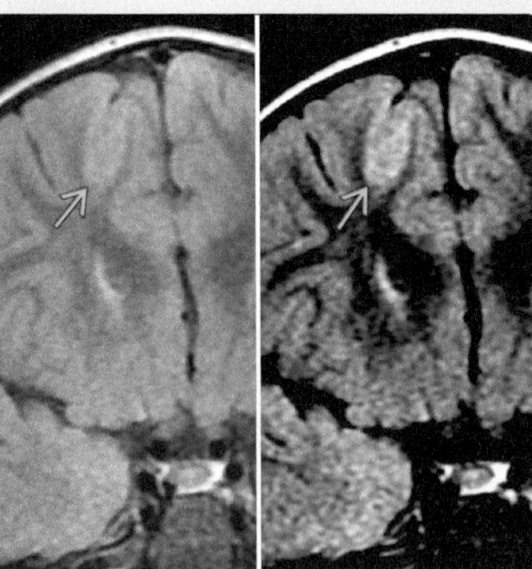

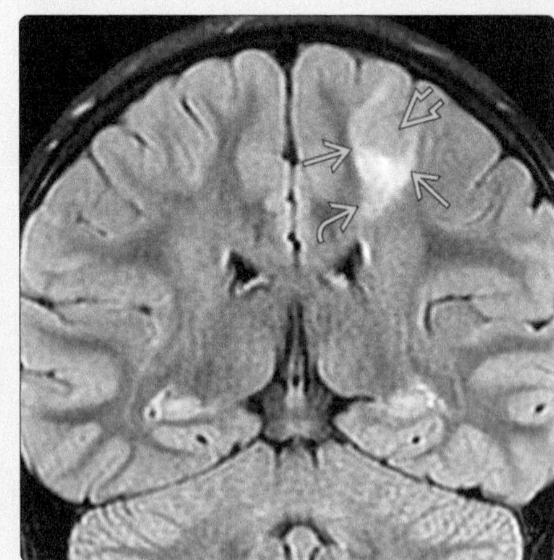

(Left) *Coronal FLAIR images in a 3-year-old with FCD type 2B show varying contrast windowing ➡. Note how FCD is much more conspicuous in the image on the right with greater contrast windowing. Windowing allows for improved detection of subtle FCD.* **(Right)** *Coronal FLAIR MR in a 10-year-old with epilepsy shows hyperintense thick cortex ➡ & subcortical white matter ➡ focused at the depth of the sulcus. Note the characteristic tapering ↗ of signal abnormality toward the ventricle, typical of FCD type 2B.*

TERMINOLOGY

Definitions

- Focal cortical dysplasia (FCD)
  - Cortical disorganization & abnormal laminar architecture

IMAGING

General Features

- FCD type 1
  - Only 22-64% have imaging findings; may be lower in children (12%)
  - When present, MR findings are often subtle
    - White matter (WM) volume loss
    - Ill-defined WM increased signal
    - Blurring of gray matter (GM)-WM junction
    - Cortical signal change
    - Abnormal gyral & sulcal pattern
- FCD type 2
  - 60-100% have identifiable abnormalities on MR
    - Focal signal abnormality in subcortical WM
    - Blurring of GM-WM junction
    - Increased cortical thickness
    - Cortical signal change
    - Abnormal gyral & sulcal pattern
  - MR findings highly suggestive of type 2
    - Transmantle sign: WM signal tapering from subcortical region to ventricular margin
    - Depth of sulcus morphology: Increased signal at depth of abnormal sulcus ± transmantle sign

Nuclear Medicine Findings

- PET
  - Decreased interictal vs. increased ictal metabolic activity
- Perfusion SPECT
  - Comparative ictal & interictal scans with Tc-99m HMPAO or Tc-99m ECD
    - Increased ictal vs. decreased interictal perfusion

Imaging Recommendations

- Protocol advice
  - Higher field strength (3T) preferred
  - 3D isotropic MR techniques (T1 & FLAIR) allow multiplanar reconstruction, PET/SPECT/MEG fusion, & intraoperative guidance
  - DTI may better detect FCD & discriminate FCD subtypes

DIFFERENTIAL DIAGNOSIS

Tuberous Sclerosis

- Radial migration lines & cortical tubers share many imaging features with FCD, especially FCD type 2B
- Tubers & FCD type 2B share similar histopathology

Cortical Neoplasm

- Especially dysembryoplastic neuroepithelial tumor (DNET), ganglioglioma, or other low-grade glioma
- Abnormal enhancement excludes FCD

Incomplete or Delayed Myelination

- Focal incomplete myelination may mimic FCD
- Follow-up imaging after myelin maturation helpful

PATHOLOGY

General Features

- Etiology
  - FCD type 1: Disturbance of cortical organization
  - FCD type 2: Disturbance of cellular proliferation

Staging, Grading, & Classification

- FCD type 1
  - Isolated alterations in cortical organization & lamination
    - 1A: Abnormal radial cortical lamination
    - 1B: Abnormal tangential cortical lamination
    - 1C: Abnormal radial & tangential cortical lamination
- FCD type 2
  - Isolated alterations in cortical organization & lamination **with dysmorphic neurons**
    - 2A: Presence of dysmorphic neurons
    - 2B: Dysmorphic neurons **& balloon cells**
- FCD type 3
  - FCD associated with another principal (non-FCD) lesion
    - 3A: FCD associated with **hippocampal sclerosis**
    - 3B: FCD associated with **glial or glioneuronal tumor**
    - 3C: FCD associated with **vascular malformation**
    - 3D: FCD associated with early-acquired **encephaloclastic lesion**

CLINICAL ISSUES

Presentation

- 10% of all epilepsy patients
- 50% of children undergoing surgery for intractable epilepsy

Natural History & Prognosis

- Seizure-free outcome following surgery much better in FCD type 2 (52-91%) compared to FCD type 1 (21%)

Treatment

- Focal resection ± preceding subdural EEG grid localization

DIAGNOSTIC CHECKLIST

Consider

- Review localizing EEG findings during image interpretation if available

Image Interpretation Pearls

- Consideration of seizure semiology, localizing EEG findings, & nuclear medicine imaging help localize MR abnormalities
- ~ 1/3 of cases are initially missed because findings are subtle
- Proper MR imaging technique improves lesion detection
- Windowing to increase contrast on T2 & FLAIR imaging is helpful to improve subtle FCD detection

SELECTED REFERENCES

1. Gennari AG et al: Diffusion tensor imaging discriminates focal cortical dysplasia from normal brain parenchyma and differentiates between focal cortical dysplasia types. Insights Imaging. 14(1):36, 2023
2. Tahta A et al: Focal cortical dysplasia: etiology, epileptogenesis, classification, clinical presentation, imaging, and management. Childs Nerv Syst. 36(12):2939-47, 2020
3. Jayalakshmi S et al: Focal cortical dysplasia and refractory epilepsy: role of multimodality imaging and outcome of surgery. AJNR Am J Neuroradiol. 40(5):892-8, 2019

Lissencephaly

KEY FACTS

TERMINOLOGY

- Extensive cortical malformation caused by ↓ transmantle neuronal migration
  - Results in thick cortex & ↓ sulcation
- Spectrum of agyria, pachygyria, & band heterotopia

IMAGING

- Spectrum of ↓ number & depth of sulci + broad gyri
  - Graded based on extent, anteroposterior predominance ± band heterotopia
- Thick cortex
  - May see 3-layer pattern on MR with thinner outer molecular layer, cell-sparse zone, & thicker inner neuronal layer
- Hourglass or figure 8 cerebral hemispheres in agyria or near agyria
- Additional anomalies: Marked callosal dysgenesis, dysmorphic basal ganglia, cerebellar hypoplasia
- Deep white matter: Volume loss, ↓ arborization
- Ventriculomegaly
- Normocephalic or microcephalic

TOP DIFFERENTIAL DIAGNOSES

- Microcephaly with simplified gyral pattern
- Congenital muscular dystrophies: Dystroglycanopathies
- Expected immature sulcation pattern of prematurity
- Polymicrogyria

PATHOLOGY

- Result of arrested migration or undermigration of neurons, which is highly dependent on microtubule activity
- Many genetic mutations → spectrum of phenotypes
- *PAFAH1B1* (LIS1), *DCX*, & *TUBA1A* mutations account for majority of cases

DIAGNOSTIC CHECKLIST

- Imaging classification now based on severity, gradients/location, cortical thickness, & presence of associated brain malformations

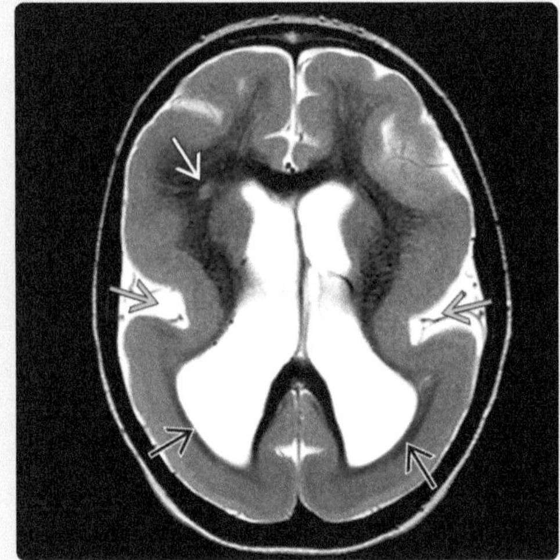
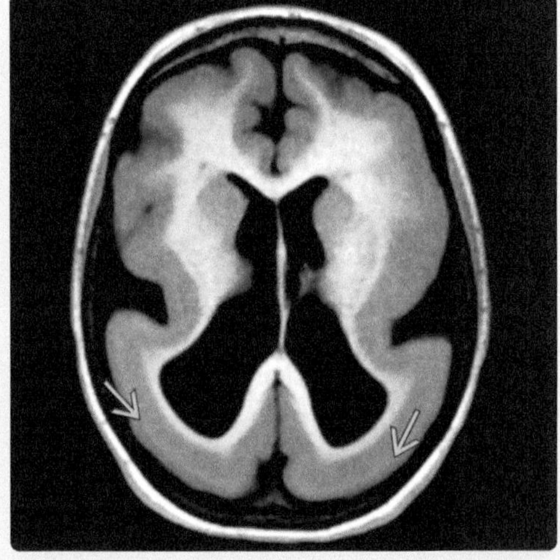

(Left) *Axial T2WI MR in a 10-year-old girl with a PAFAH1B1 (LIS1) gene mutation shows posterior predominant agyria & bifrontal pachygyria. There is diffuse cortical thickening & vertically oriented sylvian fissures ➾, consistent with classic lissencephaly. Posterior predominant ventriculomegaly ➾ is seen as well as right frontal periventricular gray matter heterotopia ➡.* **(Right)** *Axial T1WI MR in the same patient shows similar findings. The T1-hyperintense cell-sparse zone ➾ can be faintly seen posteriorly.*

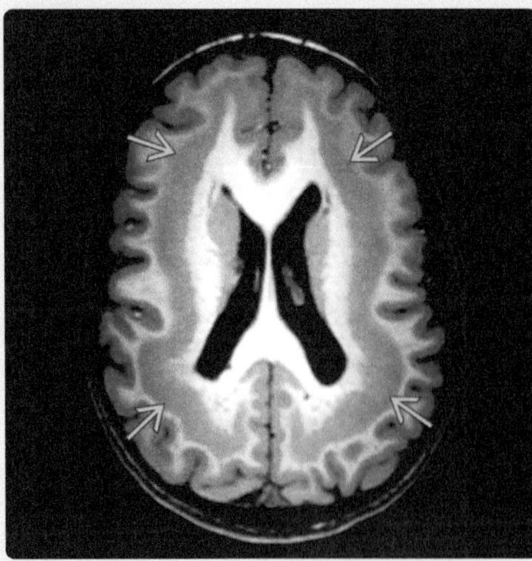
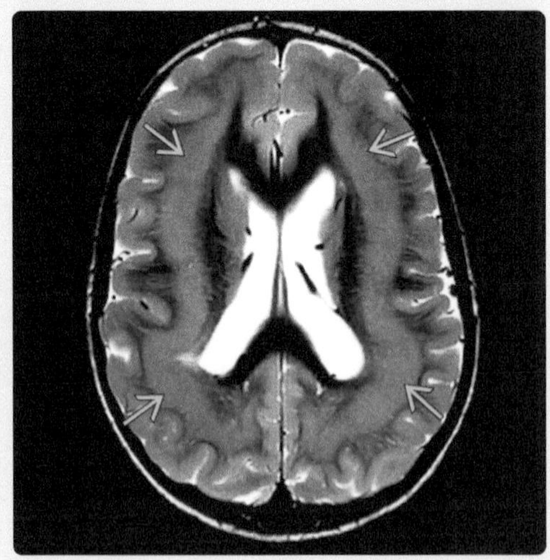

(Left) *Axial T1WI MR in an 8-year-old girl with a DCX mutation & generalized seizures shows diffuse subcortical band heterotopia ➾, which is in the lissencephaly spectrum.* **(Right)** *Axial T2WI MR in the same patient shows bilateral hemispheric band heterotopia ➾. The overlying gyral-sulcal pattern is normal with normal cortical thickness. Band heterotopia can be diffuse (as in this case) but, in some cases, may only involve the frontal or parietooccipital regions.*

TERMINOLOGY

Synonyms

- Agyria-pachygyria complex

Definitions

- Spectrum of cortical malformation caused by arrested or ↓ transmantle neuronal migration
  - Agyria, pachygyria, & subcortical band heterotopia (BH)
- Advances in genetic testing have made previously described classification systems less useful clinically
- Abnormalities of neuronal proliferation (microlissencephaly, microcephaly with simplified gyral pattern, megalencephalies) & dystroglycanopathies (cobblestone malformations) are described in separate categories
  - However, there is phenotypic & genetic overlap with congenital microcephaly & tubulinopathies

IMAGING

General Features

- Best diagnostic clue
  - Thick cortex with absence (agyria) or ↓ (pachygyria) number of sulci
  - Hourglass or figure 8 shape of cerebral hemispheres on axial images
- Location
  - Gradients of anterior vs. posterior cerebral hemispheric involvement are described in some of most commonly encountered genetic etiologies

MR Findings

- Smooth cortical surface
  - Spectrum of ↓ number & depth of sulci with large, broad gyri
- Thick cortex with ↓ gyri/sulci
  - MR can potentially resolve 3-layer pattern with cell-sparse zone (T1 & T2 prolongation) deep to thin outer molecular layer & superficial to thick deeper neuronal layer
    - Not always seen on MR; can be difficult to distinguish from BH in certain cases
- Deep white matter abnormalities
  - ↓ volume with ↓ arborization
- Enlarged lateral ventricles
- Common associated findings
  - Callosal dysgenesis/agenesis
  - Pontocerebellar hypoplasia
  - Hippocampal anomalies

DIFFERENTIAL DIAGNOSIS

Microcephaly With Simplified Gyral Pattern

- Head circumference ≥ 3 standard deviations below normal
- Broad gyri, ↓ number of sulci without cortical thickening

Congenital Muscular Dystrophies: Dystroglycanopathies

- Cobblestone cortex
- Z-shaped hypoplastic brainstem on sagittal images

Delayed Gyral-Sulcal Pattern

- Seen in preterm infants, infants with prenatal/neonatal systemic stressors, or genetic abnormalities/syndromes

PATHOLOGY

General Features

- Genetics
  - Many identified mutations → spectrum of phenotypes
  - Tubulinopathies
    - Most lissencephalies fall under this category, most caused by MAP mutations [50% *PAFAH1B1* (LIS1), 10% *DCX*], but up to 7% are from tubulin mutations
    - *DCX* mutations: Classic lissencephaly in male patients, BH in female patients
    - Microtubules are essential in neuronal proliferation, migration, & axonal pathfinding
    - Mutations of genes encoding microtubule-associated proteins [(MAPs): *PAFAH1B1*, *DCX*, *KIF5C*, *NDE1*, *KIF2A*, & *DYNC1H1*], α-tubulin (TUBA genes, mainly *TUBA1A*), & β-tubulin (TUBB genes, mainly *TUBB2B* & *TUBB3*)
    - MAP mutations: Milder brain growth impairment (normal or near-normal head circumference) but can have mild callosal dysgenesis & vermian hypoplasia
    - Tubulin mutations (*TUBA1A*): Microcephaly, callosal dysgenesis, basal ganglia abnormalities, cerebellar hypoplasia
  - Miller-Dieker syndrome
    - LIS1 (a.k.a. *PAFAH1B1*) mutation with additional *YWHAE* (14-3-3ε) gene mutation
    - Dysmorphic facies ± congenital heart disease, omphalocele, cleft palate, genital anomalies in male patients
  - Baraitser-Winter Syndrome
    - Mutation of actin genes *ACTB* & *ACTG1*
    - Microcephaly, ocular anomalies, ptosis, intellectual disabilities, dysmorphic features, short stature

CLINICAL ISSUES

Presentation

- Clinical profile depends on severity of malformation & associated anomalies
  - Complete/near-complete agyric lissencephaly: Neonatal hypotonia, gradual spasticity, severe epilepsy
  - Isolated BH: Intellectual disability, seizures, may be asymptomatic

DIAGNOSTIC CHECKLIST

Reporting Tips

- Describe severity & regions of involvement ± associated abnormalities to help in classification

SELECTED REFERENCES

1. Kolbjer S et al: Lissencephaly in an epilepsy cohort: molecular, radiological and clinical aspects. Eur J Paediatr Neurol. 30:71-81, 2021
2. Lerman-Sagie T et al: A practical approach to prenatal diagnosis of malformations of cortical development. Eur J Paediatr Neurol. 34:50-61, 2021
3. Severino M et al: Definitions and classification of malformations of cortical development: practical guidelines. Brain. 143(10):2874-94, 2020

KEY FACTS

IMAGING

- Transmantle cleft of brain parenchyma extending from cortical surface to ventricle
  - Cleft lined by dysplastic gray matter (GM)
    - Polymicrogyria (PMG), heterotopia
  - Closed-lip defect: Cleft walls closely apposed/fused
    - Dimple of lateral ventricle laterally at cleft
  - Open-lip defect: Cleft walls separated by CSF; widths & shapes of clefts variable
- Bilateral in up to 1/2 of patients
  - Unilateral, often shows contralateral PMG
- ± hemosiderin staining of cleft, ventricles
- ± Ca^{++} if due to in utero infection (e.g., CMV)
- Associated with absence of cavum septum pellucidum ± optic nerve hypoplasia (septo-optic dysplasia)
  - Anomalies of hypothalamic-pituitary axis
  - Callosal hypogenesis, other midline anomalies
- MR protocol advice
  - Multiplanar sequences ± volumetric acquisition, particularly important for closed-lip type
  - Prior to myelination, GM-lined cleft best seen on T2WI

TOP DIFFERENTIAL DIAGNOSES

- Encephaloclastic porencephaly
- Hydranencephaly
- Alobar holoprosencephaly

PATHOLOGY

- In utero insult affecting neuronal migration
- Etiologies include: Vascular insult, infection (CMV, HSV), maternal trauma, toxins; possible genetic etiologies

CLINICAL ISSUES

- Seizures, motor abnormalities, developmental delay
- Type & severity of clinical impairment determined by
  - Number, size, & location of clefts
  - Presence of associated malformations
- 1 in 3 children have non-CNS abnormalities

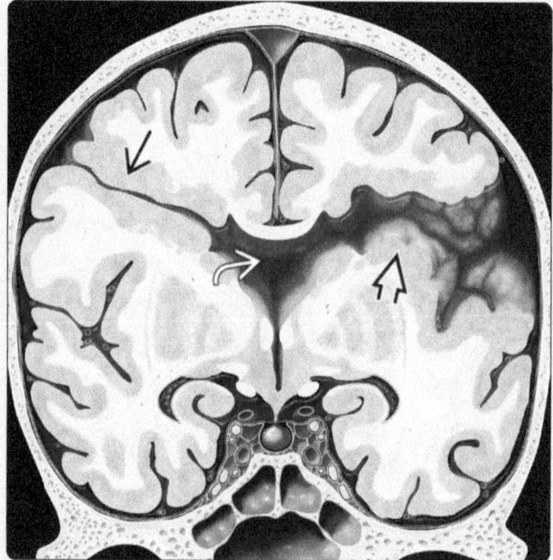

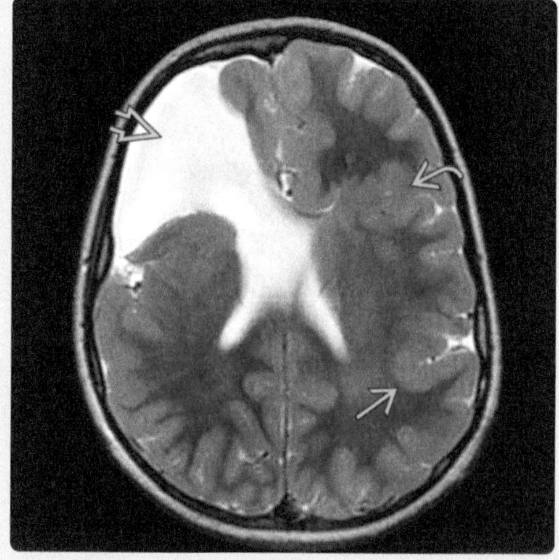

(Left) *Coronal graphic shows bilateral schizencephalic clefts, closed lip on the right ➡ & open lip on the left ➡. Both clefts are lined by dysplastic gray matter. Note the absence of the septum pellucidum ➡.* **(Right)** *Axial T2WI MR of a 7-year-old patient with schizencephaly shows bifrontal clefts, open lip on the right ➡ & closed lip on the left ➡. Both clefts are lined by abnormal gray matter. Note the polymicrogyria (PMG) ➡ affecting the left perisylvian region. PMG is a common association.*

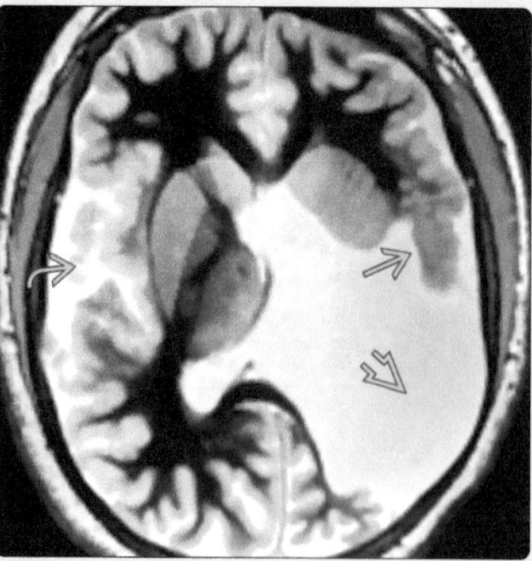

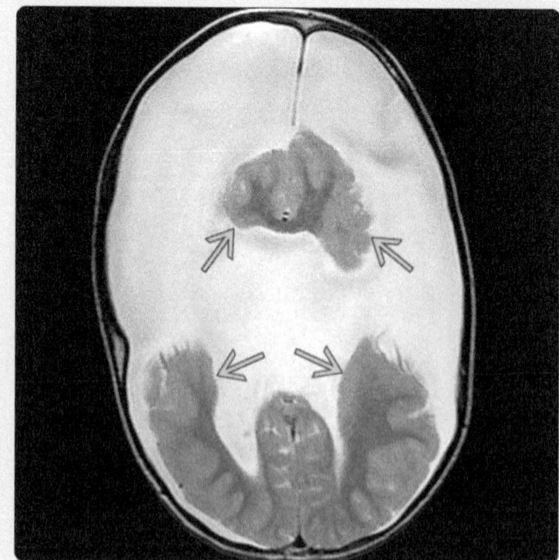

(Left) *Axial BRAVO white matter-null MR in a teen with seizures shows a large left open-lip schizencephaly ➡. Note the dysplastic gray matter lining the margins of the cleft ➡, especially anteriorly. Also note the extensive right insular and perisylvian PMG ➡.* **(Right)** *Axial T2WI MR in an 8-year-old with bilateral, large, open-lip schizencephalic clefts in the midportions of the cerebral hemispheres, mimicking hydranencephaly. The key feature of schizencephaly is the dysplastic gray matter ➡ that lines the clefts.*

TERMINOLOGY

Synonyms

- Agenetic porencephaly

Definitions

- Transmantle cleft in brain parenchyma extending from cortical surface to ventricle (i.e., pia to ependyma)
  - Lined by dysplastic gray matter (GM)
- Types I (closed-lip) & II (open-lip) defects
- Most consider schizencephaly to be severe form of polymicrogyria (PMG), given their common association with one another

IMAGING

General Features

- Best diagnostic clue
  - Full-thickness transmantle GM-lined cleft extending from pial to ependymal surfaces
    - Closed lip (type I): Walls of cleft in direct contact
    - Open lip (type II): CSF throughout cleft
      - Variable cleft widths
      - Wider clefts result in smaller volume of normal brain
- Location
  - Most common location: Frontal & parietal lobes near central sulcus
    - Can involve any region
  - Up to 50% bilateral
- Size
  - Open-lip schizencephaly may result in large cystic cavity often mistaken for cyst
  - Closed-lip schizencephaly may be very small & subtle, mimicking transmantle GM heterotopia

CT Findings

- NECT
  - Cerebral cleft of CSF density (in open-lip type)
  - GM lining clefts may appear hyperdense
  - Dimple on lateral wall of lateral ventricle indicates ependymal margin of closed-lip cleft
  - Periventricular Ca^{++} if due to infection (CMV)
  - Thinned, expanded calvarium with large open-lip clefts
- CECT
  - Large, primitive-appearing veins near cleft

MR Findings

- T1WI, T2WI, FLAIR
  - Closed-lip type may appear as irregular tract of GM from cortical surface to ventricle (fused cleft)
    - Look for dimple in wall of lateral ventricle
    - Transmantle heterotopia may be considered mild spectrum of closed-lip schizencephaly
  - Open-lip type can be wide & wedge-shaped or have nearly parallel walls
    - CSF-filled cleft connects lateral ventricle with subarachnoid space
  - Abnormal GM lining cleft: PMG or heterotopia
  - ± thin overlying membrane of pia or ependyma
    - More common on prenatal MR
  - GM heterotopia often seen adjacent to cleft
  - Contralateral PMG common
  - Look for associated optic nerve hypoplasia
    - ± absent septum pellucidum
  - Associated arachnoid cysts common
- T2* GRE
  - ± hemosiderin staining of ventricles &/or cleft from prenatal insult
  - May show Ca^{++} when associated with CMV
- MRV
  - Abnormal veins overlying cleft
- fMRI: Functional reorganization of undamaged hemisphere reported

Ultrasonographic Findings

- May be visualized with pre- & postnatal imaging
- Sensitive for type II (open lip), less sensitive for type I (closed lip)

Nuclear Medicine Findings

- Normal or ↑ glucose metabolism (PET) & perfusion (SPECT) of cleft wall (by GM)

Imaging Recommendations

- Best imaging tool
  - MR with 3D acquisitions
- Protocol advice
  - Multiplanar sequences (± volumetric acquisition) particularly important for closed-lip type
  - Ultrafast GRE T1-weighted 3D acquisitions allow for exceptional GM-white matter (WM) contrast
  - Prior to myelination, T2WI provides best GM-WM differentiation

DIFFERENTIAL DIAGNOSIS

Encephaloclastic Porencephaly

- Parenchymal cavity due to insult after migration complete
- Lined by gliotic WM, not dysplastic GM

Hydranencephaly

- Destruction of middle & anterior cerebral artery territories
  - Residual tissue supplied by posterior circulation
    - Posterior fossa, occipital poles, medial temporal lobes

Alobar Holoprosencephaly

- Anterior monoventricle with large dorsal cyst

Bilateral Arachnoid Cysts

- No communication with underlying ventricles
- No true cerebral cleft, only displaced parenchyma

PATHOLOGY

General Features

- Etiology
  - In utero insult to germinal zone prior to neuronal migration
  - Etiologies may be hypoxic-ischemic, vascular, teratogenic (alcohol, warfarin, & cocaine), infectious (CMV, HSV)
- Genetics
  - Many potential genetic etiologies
    - Aneuploidy
    - Single-gene mutations

- Mutations of *COL4A1* associated
- Previously hypothesized roles of *EMX2*, *LHX2*, *HESX1*, & *SOX2* without definitive association in larger cohorts
- Syndromes: Adams-Oliver, septo-optic dysplasia (SOD)

- Associated abnormalities
  - SOD plus
    - SOD is seen in ~ 70% of all cases of schizencephaly
    - Heterogeneous disorder with 2 or more features of classic triad
      - Agenesis of septum pellucidum &/or corpus callosum
      - Optic nerve hypoplasia
      - Pituitary abnormalities
    - Septum pellucidum absent in large percentage of schizencephaly cases, especially bilateral clefts
      - Complete absence more common in frontal clefts
      - Partial posterior absence more common in parietal clefts
  - GM heterotopia often seen adjacent to cleft
  - Contralateral PMG common
  - Hippocampal & callosal anomalies

Gross Pathologic & Surgical Features

- Transmantle clefts with separated or apposed GM lining
- Thalami, corticospinal tracts may be atrophied or not formed

Microscopic Features

- Little, if any, glial scarring
- Loss of normal laminar architecture
- Pachygyria, PMG, or heterotopic GM

CLINICAL ISSUES

Presentation

- Most common signs/symptoms
  - Seizures, hemiparesis, developmental delay
  - Bilateral clefts: Tetraparesis, blindness, more severe cognitive impairment
- Other signs/symptoms
  - Psychiatric disorders, perisylvian syndrome

Demographics

- Epidemiology
  - Incidence: 1.5/100,000 births
  - 1 in 3 children have non-CNS abnormalities
    - > 50% likely due to vascular disruption
      - Gastroschisis, bowel atresias, & amniotic band disruption sequence
  - Associated with ↓ maternal age, lack of prenatal care

Natural History & Prognosis

- Type & severity of clinical impairment determined by
  - Number, size, & location of clefts
    - Bilateral & open defects have worse prognosis than unilateral & closed types
      - May change from open-lip to closed-lip forms between pre- & postnatal imaging, which could alter prognosis & prenatal counseling
      - Malformation stable postnatally
  - Presence of associated malformations
    - Bilateral clefts, motor impairment, microcephaly, & callosal agenesis are strongly associated with neurocognitive impairment

Treatment

- Surgery for medically intractable epilepsy
  - Lesionectomy, lobectomy
  - Corpus callosotomy, functional hemispherotomy

DIAGNOSTIC CHECKLIST

Consider

- Look for evidence of SOD when schizencephaly is encountered & vice versa

Image Interpretation Pearls

- Multiplanar imaging (± volumetric acquisition) to avoid in-plane oversight of closed-lip clefts
  - If plane of imaging same as plane of cleft, abnormality may be overlooked
- Contours of lateral ventricular walls should be smooth
  - Dimple may indicate subtle closed-lip schizencephaly
- Bilateral clefts may by asymmetric in size
  - Look closely for small contralateral cleft
- Absence of septum pellucidum should raise suspicion for SOD & be correlated with ophthalmologic exam
  - Search for associated midline anomalies, including corpus callosum & hypothalamic-pituitary axis

SELECTED REFERENCES

1. Fenton LZ: Imaging of congenital malformations of the brain. Clin Perinatol. 49(3):587-601, 2022
2. Khandelwal A et al: Magnetic resonance imaging of malformations of cortical development-a comprehensive review. World Neurosurg. 159:70-9, 2022
3. Severino M et al: Definitions and classification of malformations of cortical development: practical guidelines. Brain. 143(10):2874-94, 2020
4. Braga VL et al: Schizencephaly: a review of 734 patients. Pediatr Neurol. 87:23-9, 2018
5. Griffiths PD: Schizencephaly revisited. Neuroradiology. 60(9):945-60, 2018
6. Hung PC et al: Schizencephaly in children: a single medical center retrospective study. Pediatr Neonatol. 59(6):573-80, 2018
7. Halabuda A et al: Schizencephaly-diagnostics and clinical dilemmas. Childs Nerv Syst. 31(4):551-6, 2015
8. Kutuk MS et al: Prenatal diagnosis and postnatal outcome of schizencephaly. J Child Neurol. 30(10):1388-94, 2014
9. Nabavizadeh SA et al: Correlation of prenatal and postnatal MRI findings in schizencephaly. AJNR Am JNeuroradiol. 35(7):1418-24, 2014
10. Cui Z et al: Resection or multi-lobe disconnection for intractable epilepsy with open-lip schizencephaly. J Clin Neurosci. 20(12):1780-2, 2013
11. Dies KA et al: Schizencephaly: association with young maternal age, alcohol use, and lack of prenatal care. J Child Neurol. 28(2):198-203, 2013
12. Rios LT et al: Prenatal and postnatal schizencephaly findings by 2D and 3D ultrasound: pictorial essay. J Clin Imaging Sci. 2:30, 2012

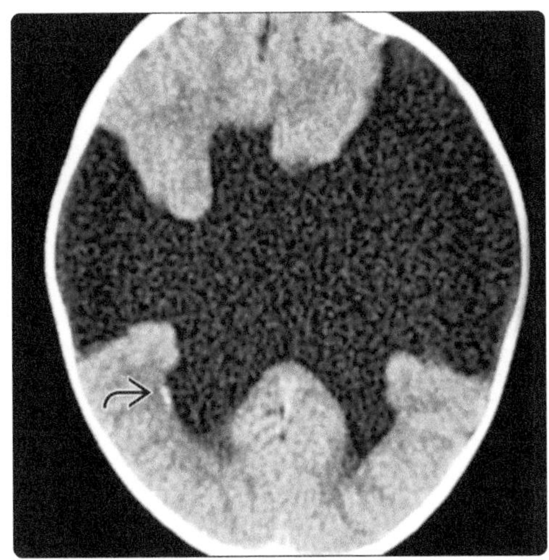

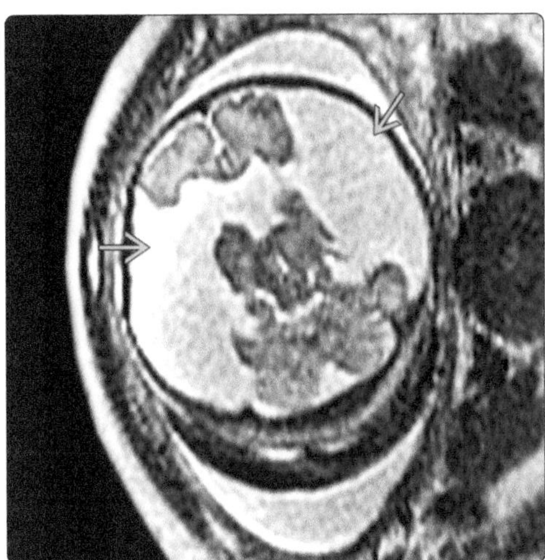

(Left) *Axial NECT shows a bat wing configuration of the lateral ventricles due to bilateral, large open-lipped schizencephaly. Note the dystrophic* Ca^{++} *bordering the right lateral ventricle wall ⮫, suggesting a history of intrauterine CMV infection as the source of this child's migrational abnormality.* **(Right)** *Axial T2WI MR in a fetus shows huge, bilateral open-lip schizencephalic clefts ⇨. Fetal MR is a complementary evaluation to fetal US for characterization of schizencephaly.*

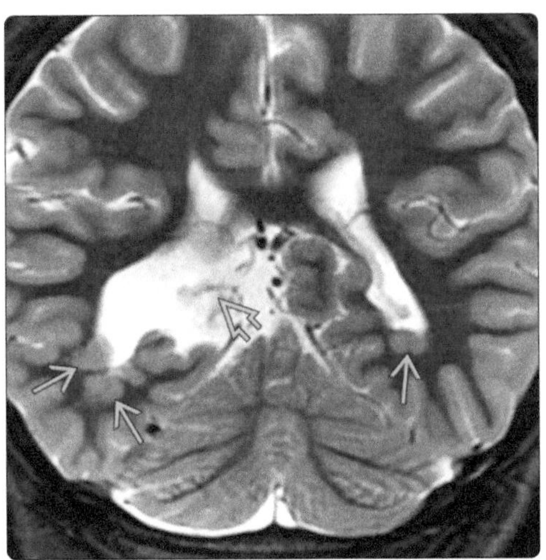

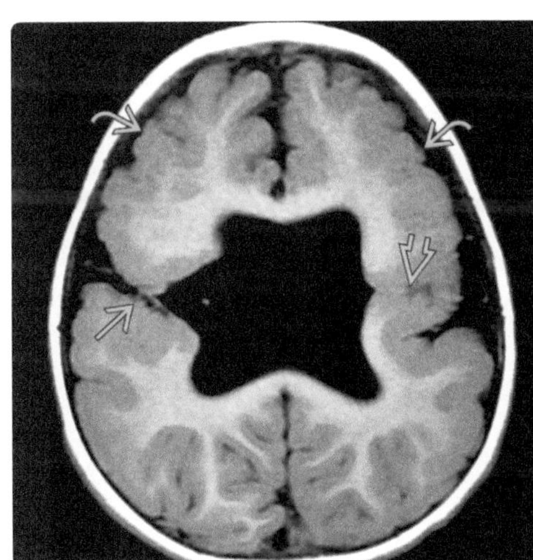

(Left) *Coronal T2WI MR in a 15-year-old with right medial temporal schizencephaly ⇨ shows associated bilateral subependymal gray matter heterotopia ⇨. Schizencephaly is usually associated with other cortical malformations, often involving the contralateral brain.* **(Right)** *Axial T1WI MR in the same patient shows the bilateral schizencephaly lined by PMG. The right side is open lip ⇨, & the left side is closed lip ⇨. Again, note the PMG ⮫ involving the bilateral frontal lobes.*

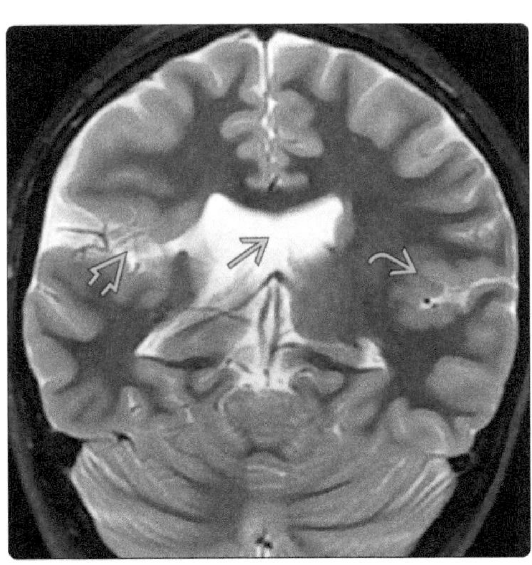

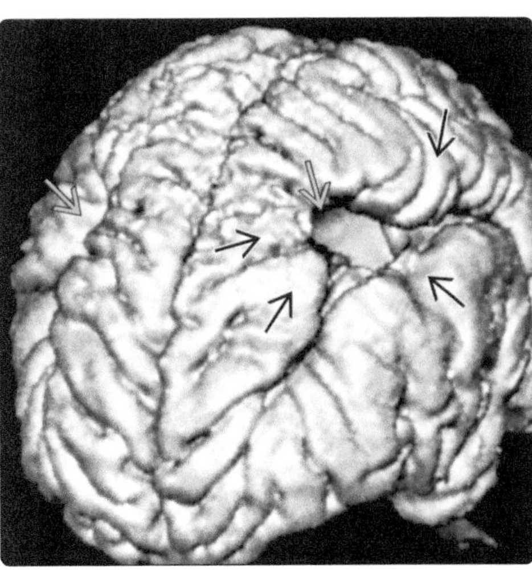

(Left) *Coronal T2WI MR in a 12-year-old with absent septum pellucidum ⇨, optic nerve hypoplasia (not shown), right closed-lip schizencephaly ⇨, and left perisylvian PMG ⮫ is shown. This constellation of findings is consistent with septo-optic dysplasia (SOD) plus.* **(Right)** *Coronal oblique 3D CT surface rendering shows bilateral open-lip schizencephaly ⇨. Note the gyri radially arranged ➔ around the left cleft, giving the appearance of diving into the cleft.*

Hemimegalencephaly

KEY FACTS

TERMINOLOGY

- Hemimegalencephaly (HMEG): Overgrowth & malformation of part vs. entire hemisphere
- Due to defects in neuronal proliferation, migration, & organization

IMAGING

- Large cerebral hemisphere & hemicranium
  - Displaced posterior falx & occipital pole extending to contralateral side
  - Enlarged ipsilateral ventricle with abnormally shaped frontal horn (often pointed)
- Associated cortical malformations include pachygyria, polymicrogyria, & heterotopias
- White matter (WM) abnormalities
  - ↑ volume, abnormal T2 signal intensity
    - Often dark prior to typical myelination time frame
  - Poor gray matter (GM)-WM differentiation
- Size & signal intensity of HMEG can change over time
  - May atrophy with chronic seizure activity

PATHOLOGY

- Classified as cortical dysgenesis with abnormal cell proliferation but without neoplasia
- Same pathologic & genetic spectrum as focal cortical dysplasia type II & tuberous sclerosis complex

CLINICAL ISSUES

- Most common presentations: Seizures, hemiparesis, developmental delay
  - 50% have associated skin lesions, truncal/extremity overgrowth, &/or vascular malformations
    - Seen in *PIK3CA*-related overgrowth spectrum (PROS)
- Functional hemispherectomy is used for seizure control (as anticonvulsants are usually ineffective)

DIAGNOSTIC CHECKLIST

- Evaluation for contralateral abnormalities important for surgical prognostication

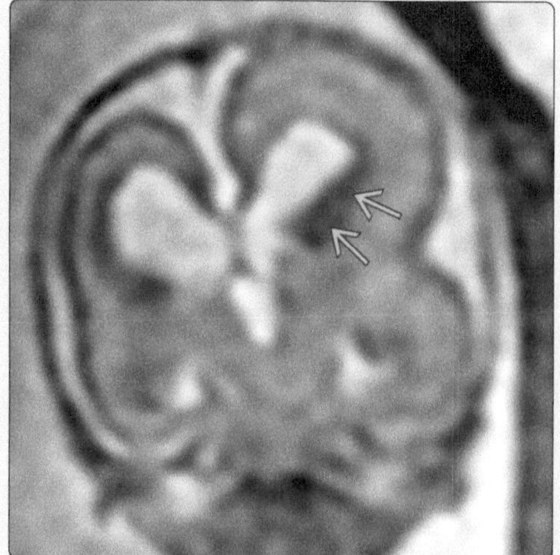

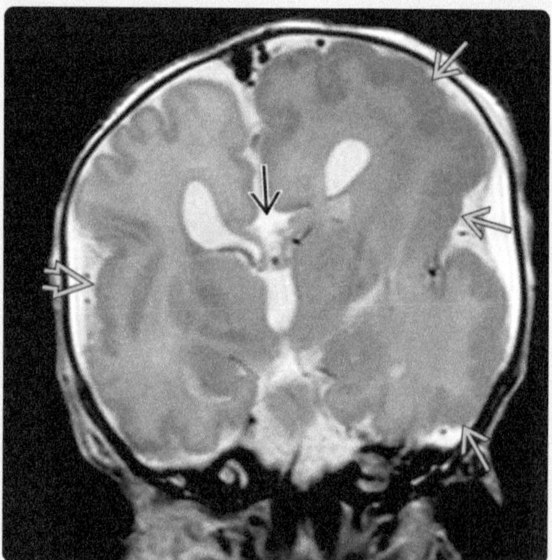

(Left) *Coronal SSFSE T2 fetal MR at 20-weeks gestational age shows left hemimegalencephaly (HMEG). The left germinal matrix ⇨ is asymmetrically larger than the right, compatible with ↑ neuronal proliferation.* **(Right)** *Coronal T2 MR in the same patient after delivery shows extensive associated left polymicrogyria ⇨, consistent with abnormal neuronal organization. There is also callosal hypogenesis ➡ & right perisylvian polymicrogyria ⇨, which is important in predicting the success of surgery.*

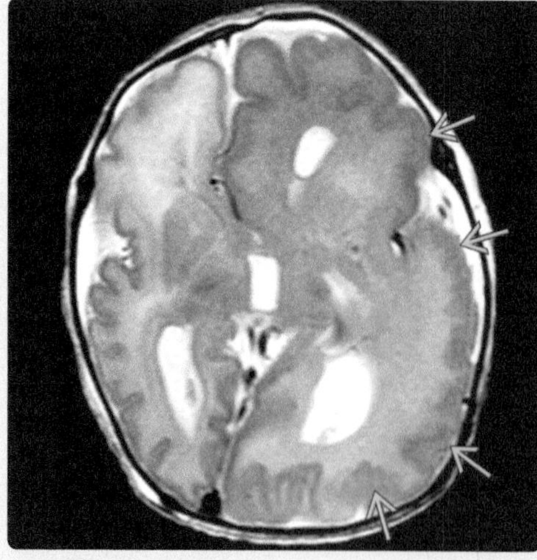

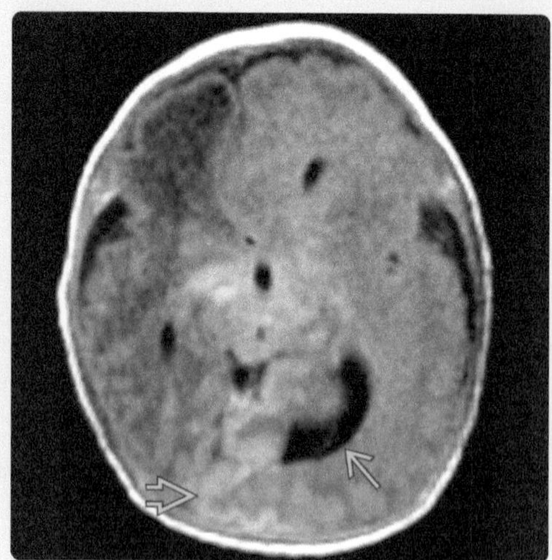

(Left) *Axial T2 MR in the same patient with left HMEG shows asymmetric relative T2 hypointensity of the white matter in the left cerebral hemisphere, compatible with abnormal neuronal migration. Extensive left polymicrogyria ⇨ is again seen.* **(Right)** *Axial T1 MR in the same patient shows characteristic asymmetric enlargement of the lateral ventricle on the affected side ⇨ with the occipital lobe crossing midline posteriorly ⇨. Note the abnormal gray matter-white matter differentiation on the left.*

TERMINOLOGY

Definitions

- Megalencephaly is spectrum of brain overgrowth disorders
  - Can be bilateral or unilateral with involvement of all or portion of cerebral hemisphere
  - Most caused by somatic mosaic mutations
- Hemimegalencephaly (HMEG): Nonneoplastic overgrowth of part or entire hemisphere
  - Classic HMEG (unilateral megalencephaly): Holohemispheric or near-holohemispheric involvement
  - Partial HMEG (focal megalencephaly): Portion of hemisphere involved
- Dysplastic megalencephaly (DMEG): Macrocephaly with significant portions of both hemispheres involved
- Same pathologic & genetic spectrum as focal cortical dysplasia type II & tuberous sclerosis complex (TSC)

IMAGING

General Features

- Best diagnostic clue
  - Enlarged dysplastic cerebral hemisphere (or portion of hemisphere) with enlarged ipsilateral lateral ventricle
    - Abnormal gray matter (GM) & white matter (WM)
  - Displaced posterior falx with enlarged occipital lobe crossing midline

MR Findings

- T1, T2, FLAIR
  - Abnormal GM: Pachygyria, polymicrogyria, heterotopia
  - Abnormal WM: ↑ volume, ↓ T2 signal intensity prior to expected myelination time frame, variable T2 signal intensity after myelination is complete
  - Blurring of GM-WM junction
  - Enlarged ipsilateral ventricle, pointed frontal horn
  - ± cerebellar, brainstem ipsilateral overgrowth
- T2* GRE
  - Signal loss from dystrophic Ca^{++}
- Fetal MR
  - Disruption of normal cerebral mantle lamination (described on SSFSE T2) secondary to abnormal neuronal migration & proliferation
  - Mass-like low T2 signal proliferation of germinal matrix/ventricular zone mimics hemorrhage

DIFFERENTIAL DIAGNOSIS

Rasmussen Encephalitis

- Unilateral encephalitis with progressive atrophy

Gliomatosis Cerebri

- Diffusely infiltrating glioma effaces ipsilateral ventricle (rather than enlarging it)

Unilateral Cerebral Edema

- May be seen with trauma, infarction, or infection

PATHOLOGY

General Features

- Etiology
  - Defect in neuronal proliferation, migration, & organization
- Genetics
  - Currently believed to be result of gene mutations coding PI3K-AKT-mTOR pathway proteins
    - TSC
  - *PIK3CA*-related overgrowth spectrum (PROS)

CLINICAL ISSUES

Presentation

- Most common signs/symptoms
  - Macrocephaly
  - Seizures, hemiparesis, developmental delay
- Other signs/symptoms
  - 50% of patients have associated abnormalities
    - Cutaneous lesions, hemihypertrophy

Demographics

- Usually diagnosed during 1st year of life

Natural History & Prognosis

- Intractable seizures with progressive hemiparesis
- Best seizure control is offered by functional hemispherectomy, though motor deficits/hemiparesis frequently persist
- Some infants develop obstructive hydrocephalus requiring CSF diversion

Treatment

- Anticonvulsants are usually ineffective
- Functional hemispherectomy or hemispherotomy
  - Earlier surgical intervention yields better outcomes
  - Confirming normal or abnormal contralateral hemisphere can help with prognostication
- Endovascular embolic hemispherectomy
  - Transarterial embolization of affected cerebral hemisphere is relatively new technique

DIAGNOSTIC CHECKLIST

Consider

- HMEG in setting of PI3K-AKT-mTOR pathway anomalies

Image Interpretation Pearls

- Unlike other pathologies, unilateral ventriculomegaly in classic HMEG is seen in involved cerebral hemisphere

Reporting Tips

- Identification of contralateral abnormalities is important in presurgical evaluation & prognostication

SELECTED REFERENCES

1. Pearl MS et al: Definitive treatment of seizures due to hemimegalencephaly in neonates and young infants by transarterial embolization: technical considerations for 'endovascular embolic hemispherectomy'. J Neurointerv Surg. 16(1):81-7, 2023
2. Severino M et al: Definitions and classification of malformations of cortical development: practical guidelines. Brain. 143(10):2874-94, 2020
3. Barkovich AJ et al: Pediatric Neuroimaging. 6th ed. Wolters Kluwer. 448-51, 2019
4. Keppler-Noreuil KM et al: PIK3CA-related overgrowth spectrum (PROS): diagnostic and testing eligibility criteria, differential diagnosis, and evaluation. Am J Med Genet A. 167A(2):287-95, 2015

Neurofibromatosis Type 1, Brain

KEY FACTS

IMAGING

- Nonenhancing, T2-/FLAIR MR hyperintense lesions
  - 60-85% of children with neurofibromatosis type 1 (NF1)
  - Characteristic sites: Globus pallidus, cerebellar WM
  - Little/no mass effect, no enhancement
  - Higher lesion burden may ↓ cognitive functioning
  - ↓ with puberty, gone by adulthood
- Optic pathway gliomas (OPGs)
  - 15-20% of children with NF1
  - From optic nerve (ON) through optic radiations
  - Fusiform to lobular in shape, ± ON tortuosity
  - ± contrast enhancement
- Plexiform neurofibromas (PNFs)
  - Lobular infiltrating soft tissue masses
  - Target appearance in cross section on T2WI MR
  - Orbital PNFs associated with sphenoid wing defects
- Vascular dysplasia (moyamoya arteriopathy)
  - 3-7% of children with NF1
  - Vessel narrowing (especially distal ICA) with collaterals

PATHOLOGY

- *NF1* gene locus → long arm of chromosome 17
- Autosomal dominant; 50% new mutations
- Variable expression, virtually 100% penetrance

CLINICAL ISSUES

- 1:3,000-5,000 people have NF1
- NF1-related learning disability in 30-60%
- OPGs & brainstem gliomas have more indolent behavior in NF1 compared to non-NF1 patients
  - OPGs typically not progressive; treatment in ~ 15%
- Phenotype quite variable: Can be dominated by peripheral, paraspinal, or intracranial lesions

DIAGNOSTIC CHECKLIST

- Include dedicated imaging of orbits with all brain MRs
- Look closely for vascular dysplasia

(Left) *Axial graphic of the orbits shows an infiltrating plexiform neurofibroma (PNF) extending from the cavernous sinus through the orbit into the temporal fossa with associated "dysplasia" of the sphenoid wing* ➡. **(Right)** *Axial T2 FS MR in a 12-year-old girl with NF1 shows a large hyperintense lesion* ➡ *in the right orbit, consistent with a PFN. Note the absence of the greater sphenoid wing* ⇨, *consistent with sphenoid wing dysplasia. Such osseous changes in the sphenoid occur almost exclusively in the setting of a PFN.*

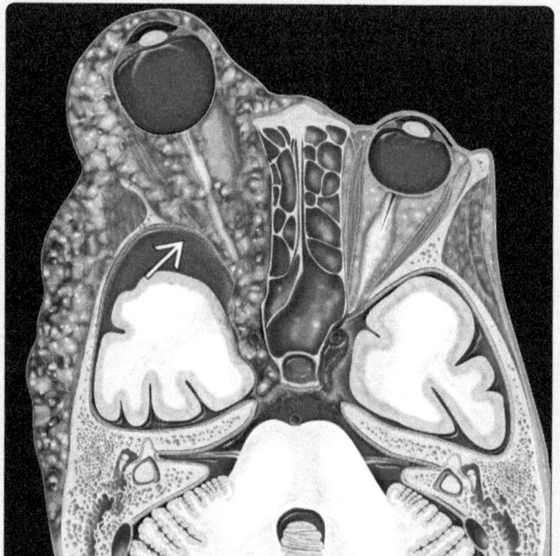

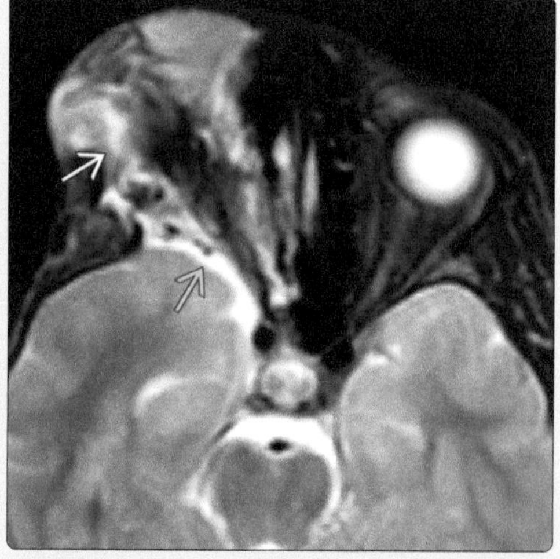

(Left) *Axial MIP of a CISS MR in a 3-year-old girl with NF1 shows enlargement and tortuosity of the orbital* ➡ *and prechiasmatic optic nerves* ⇨, *optic chiasm* ⇨, *and optic tracts* ➡, *consistent with an OPG.* **(Right)** *Axial T1 C+ FS MRs in a patient with NF1 at 3 years (top) & 6 years (bottom) are shown. The initial image shows mild enlargement and marked enhancement of the left orbital optic nerve* ⇨, *consistent with an OPG. Without any therapy, the lesion has resolved spontaneously over a 3-year period* ⇨.

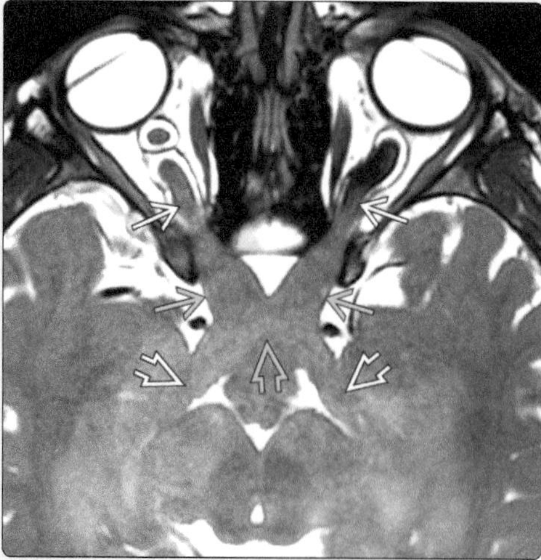

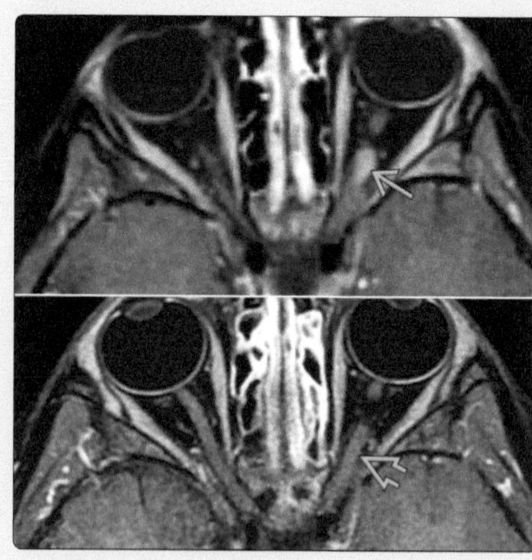

TERMINOLOGY

Abbreviations

- Neurofibromatosis type 1 (NF1)

Synonyms

- von Recklinghausen disease

Definitions

- Neurocutaneous disorder (phakomatosis) characterized by
  - Nonenhancing, T2-/FLAIR MR signal abnormalities at characteristic brain locations
    - Unidentified bright objects (UBOs) or focal abnormal signal intensities (FASIs)
  - Plexiform neurofibromas (PNFs) of soft tissues
    - Differ from diffuse & localized NFs
  - Astrocytomas, primarily optic pathway gliomas (OPGs)
  - Vascular dysplasias (moyamoya arteriopathy)
  - Skeletal dysplastic lesions
  - Café au lait spots of skin

IMAGING

General Features

- Best diagnostic clue
  - Nonenhancing, T2-/FLAIR hyperintense foci
    - a.k.a. UBOs, FASIs
  - OPGs
  - PNFs
- **Nonenhancing, hyperintense T2-/FLAIR MR lesions**
  - 60-85% of children with NF1
  - Commonly found in deep gray matter (especially globus pallidus & thalamus), hippocampus, brainstem, cerebellar white matter (WM)
  - Hyperintense on T2/FLAIR, little/no mass effect
  - Often inapparent on T1WI & CT
  - No enhancement
  - Characteristic time course
    - Not present in first 1-2 years of life
    - ↑ in number/size in young children; peak at ~ 7 years
    - ↓ in teenage years with resolution in late teen years
- **Increased WM volume**
  - Macrocephaly &/or thickened corpus callosum
- **OPGs**
  - Occur in ~ 15-20% of children with NF1
  - Anywhere from ONs through optic radiations
  - Fusiform enlargement ± enhancement
    - Tortuosity in orbit: Dotted i sign on axial images
- **PNFs**
  - Infiltrating soft tissue lobules along peripheral nerves
  - Hyperintense on T2/STIR MR
    - Target sign in cross section (central hypointensity)
  - Variable enhancement, classically central
- **Sphenoid wing dysplasia**
  - Almost always associated with orbital PNF
  - Distortion/absence of lateral orbital wall with anterior expansion of middle cranial fossa
- **Vascular dysplasia (moyamoya arteriopathy)**
  - Occurs in 3-7% of children with NF1
  - Vessel narrowing (especially distal internal carotid artery) with collateral formation

CT Findings

- NECT
  - Bone defects of sphenoid wing & lambdoid suture
  - Enlargement of ON, chiasm, superior orbital fissure
- CECT
  - ± enhancement in OPG
  - PNFs typically have little enhancement
- CTA
  - May be best test to determine degree of stenosis in moyamoya arteriopathy

MR Findings

- T1WI
  - Thick corpus callosum on sagittal images
  - OPG: Enlargement of ON, chiasm
  - PNF: Isointense to brain/cord
  - May see hyperintense globus pallidus & dentate nuclei in older patients who have had multiple gadolinium administrations from prior screening MRs
    - Pathologically proven to represent gadolinium deposition
- T2WI
  - Poorly defined, round, or ovoid hyperintense WM lesions in characteristic locations
- T2WI FS
  - OPGs may have hyperintense signal
- STIR
  - Helpful to identify soft tissue PNFs
- FLAIR
  - Best sequence to identify nonenhancing parenchymal signal abnormalities
- DWI
  - ↑ ADC values in nonenhancing signal abnormalities
- T1WI C+
  - PNFs & OPGs have variable enhancement patterns that often change over time
  - Parenchymal signal abnormalities should not enhance (which would suggest gliomatous degeneration)
- MRA
  - Major cerebral artery narrowing (especially carotid terminus) in moyamoya arteriopathy
- MRS
  - Can help distinguish nonenhancing signal abnormalities from glioma
    - Nonenhancing signal abnormalities → elevation of myoinositol (mI), preserved NAA
    - Glioma → elevation of choline, ↓ NAA

Angiographic Findings

- Conventional
  - Typically reserved for cases of moyamoya arteriopathy where revascularization is contemplated

Imaging Recommendations

- Best imaging tool
  - Brain/orbits MR C+
- Protocol advice
  - Dedicated orbital protocol T1 C+ FS MR for optimal detection of OPG & orbital PNF
  - Thin-section T2WI or MRA for vascular dysplasia

DIFFERENTIAL DIAGNOSIS

Neurocutaneous Syndromes: Phakomatoses

- **Tuberous sclerosis complex (TSC)**
  - Multiple hamartomas
- **Sturge-Weber syndrome (SWS)**
  - Retinal & pial angiomatosis with focal/lobar cerebral atrophy due to abnormal cerebral venous drainage
- **NF2**
  - Multiple meningiomas, schwannomas, & ependymomas
- **PHACES**
  - **P**osterior fossa malformations, infantile **h**emangiomas, **a**rterial anomalies, **c**ardiac anomalies, **e**ye anomalies, & **s**ternal clefting
- **von Hippel-Lindau (VHL) disease**
  - Hemangioblastomas, retinal angiomas, renal cysts & carcinomas
- Multiple others, including ataxia telangiectasia, neurocutaneous melanosis, incontinentia pigmenti, basal cell nevus syndrome

PATHOLOGY

General Features

- Etiology
  - Inactivation of neurofibromin allows cell proliferation & tumor development
  - Oligodendrocyte myelin glycoprotein within *NF1* gene
    - May cause myelin dysplasia → UBOs & FASIs
- Genetics
  - *NF1* gene locus → long arm of chromosome 17
    - Gene product → neurofibromin, inactivated in NF1
    - Neurofibromin: RAS GTPase-activating protein responsible for tumor suppression
  - Autosomal dominant; 50% new mutations
  - Variable expression; virtually 100% penetrance
- Associated abnormalities
  - Pheochromocytomas, malignant peripheral nerve sheath tumors (MPNSTs)

Staging, Grading, & Classification

- NF1 if ≥ 2 of following
  - ≥ 6 skin café au lait spots, > 5 mm
  - ≥ 2 NFs or 1 PNF
  - Axillary/inguinal freckling
  - ON glioma
  - Distinctive bone lesion
  - 1° relative with NF1

Gross Pathologic & Surgical Features

- Visual pathway glioma, usually low grade
  - Can extend to geniculate bodies & optic radiations
  - Perichiasmatic infiltration → more likely to be aggressive, ↑ frequency of precocious puberty
- Lisch nodules (iris hamartomas) in 85% > 10 years old
- Buphthalmos (globe)

Microscopic Features

- Nonenhancing, T2-/FLAIR MR hyperintense lesions: Foci of "myelin vacuolization"; no inflammation/demyelination
- PNFs: Schwann cells, perineural fibroblasts, growth along nerve fascicles

CLINICAL ISSUES

Presentation

- Most common signs/symptoms
  - > 95% have skin lesions
  - > 95% have Lisch nodules (adults)
  - ~ 50% have macrocephaly → ↑ WM volume
  - > 30% have learning disabilities
  - ~ 15% have scoliosis
  - ~ 15% have OPGs
- Phenotype quite variable: Can be dominated by peripheral, paraspinal, or intracranial lesions

Demographics

- Age
  - Café au lait spots appear in 1st year of life
  - OPGs usually occur in 1st few years
    - Median age at diagnosis: 3 years
    - If OPGs not identified before 15 months, patient unlikely to develop symptomatic OPGs
- Sex
  - M = F
- Epidemiology
  - Most common autosomal dominant disorder
  - 1:3,000-5,000 people have NF1

Natural History & Prognosis

- NF1-related learning disability in 30-60%
  - May be associated with ↑ number of characteristic T2/FLAIR MR parenchymal lesions
- 1-3% risk of other CNS glial tumors
  - Typically low grade in children, higher grade in adults
- 8-13% lifetime risk of MPNST
- Vascular dysplasia: If progressive, may cause ischemic injury
- OPGs typically have indolent course with observation sufficient in most cases
  - Chiasmatic & postchiasmatic more likely to progress than prechiasmatic
  - Small percentage resolve spontaneously

Treatment

- Observation/surveillance sufficient unless symptoms arise
- PNF: Debulking surgery if symptomatic
  - MEK inhibitors (e.g., selumetinib) for inoperable lesions
- OPG: ~ 15% require chemotherapy for progression
  - Decision to treat based on combination of clinical & radiologic findings
- Moyamoya arteriopathy: Surgical revascularization

DIAGNOSTIC CHECKLIST

Image Interpretation Pearls

- Remember to look for vascular lesions
- Signal abnormalities with mass effect, enhancement, or atypical location should be viewed with suspicion

SELECTED REFERENCES

1. Wang MX et al: Neurofibromatosis from head to toe: what the radiologist needs to know. Radiographics. 42(4):1123-44, 2022
2. Calvez S et al: Focal areas of high signal intensity in children with neurofibromatosis type 1: expected evolution on MRI. AJNR Am J Neuroradiol. 41(9):1733-9, 2020

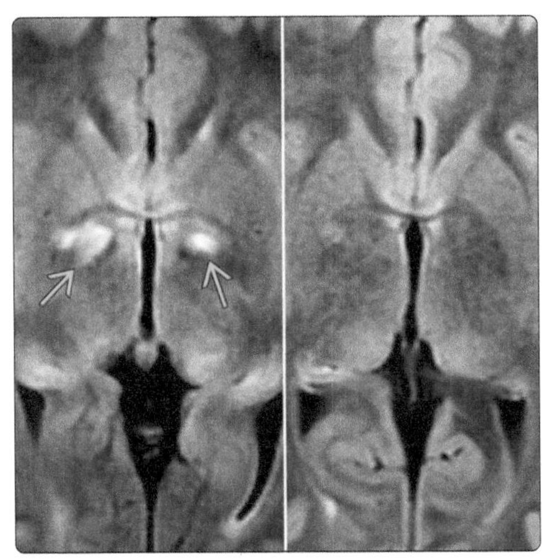

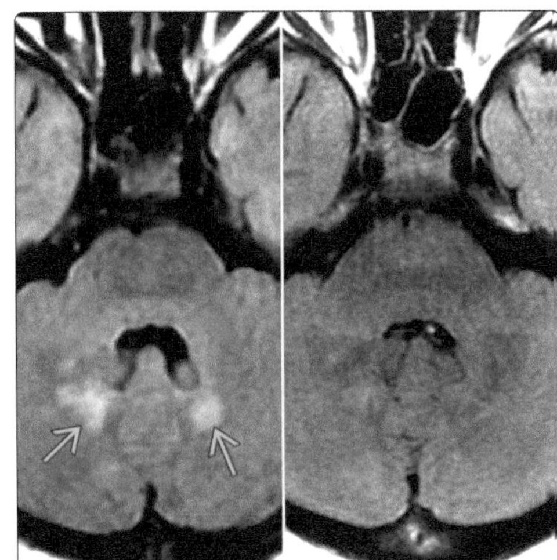

(Left) *Axial FLAIR MR images in a patient with NF1 at 10 years (left) & 15 years of age (right) show near-complete resolution of the characteristic nonenhancing signal abnormalities → within the globus pallidus nuclei.* **(Right)** *Axial FLAIR MR images in a patient with NF1 at 10 years (left) & 15 years of age (right) show near-complete interval resolution of the nonenhancing signal abnormalities → within the cerebellar white matter and dentate nuclei. These signal abnormalities typically resolve in the late teenage years.*

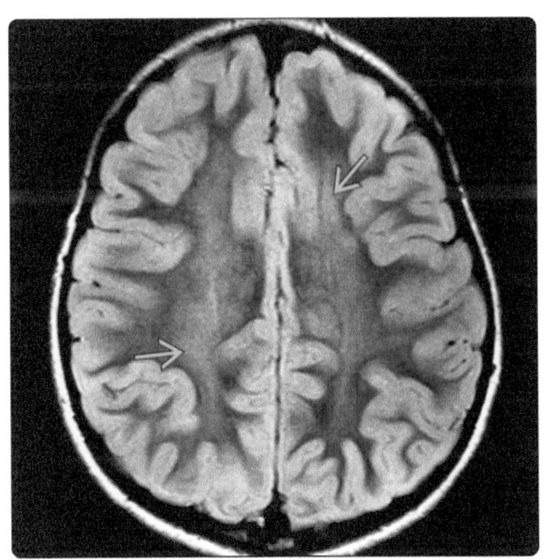

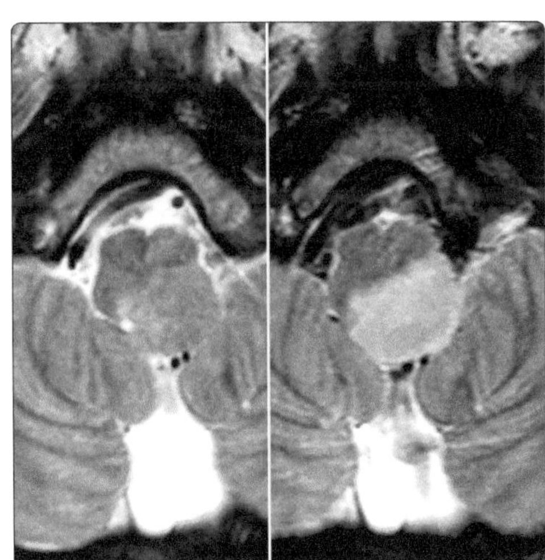

(Left) *Axial FLAIR MR in an 8-year-old boy with NF1 shows nearly symmetric increased signal within the centrum semiovale → without volume loss. This degree of delayed/abnormal myelination is uncommon, but mildly delayed myelination in younger patients is frequently seen in NF1.* **(Right)** *Axial T2WI MRs in a patient with NF1 at 6 years (left) & 9 years (right) show minimal change in the lesion over time. Brainstem masses in NF1 typically have a more indolent behavior than brainstem masses seen in otherwise healthy individuals.*

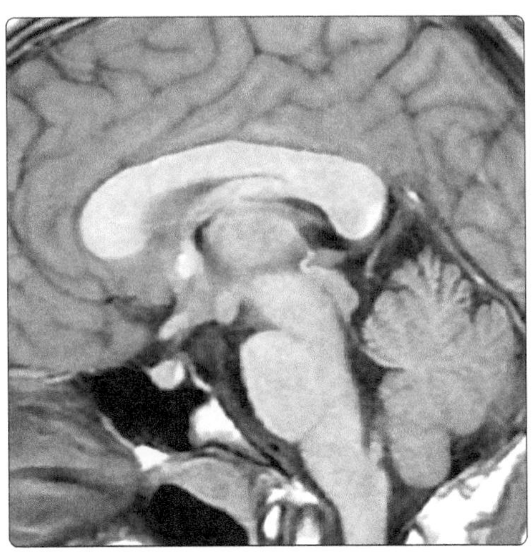

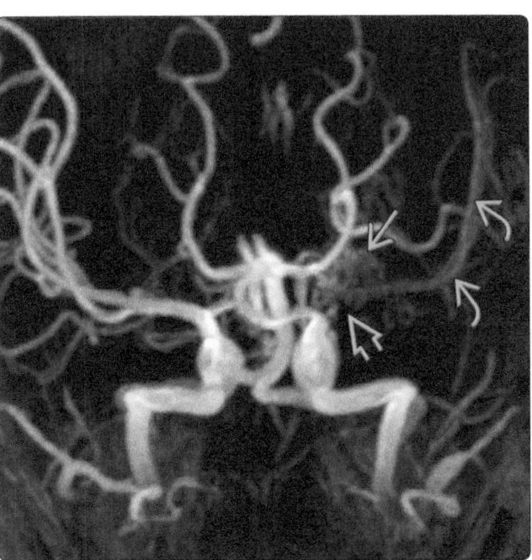

(Left) *Sagittal T1WI MR in a 15-year-old with NF1 shows a diffusely thickened corpus callosum with normal signal. On average, NF1 patients have higher corpus callosum volumes compared to normal subjects.* **(Right)** *3D surface rendering MRA in a 5-year-old boy with NF1 shows absent flow in the region of the M1 segment → of the left middle cerebral artery (MCA), tangle of collateral vessels →, and diminished flow in the more distal left MCA branches →. These findings are consistent with NF1-associated moyamoya arteriopathy.*

KEY FACTS

TERMINOLOGY

- Familial cancer syndrome
  - Multiple cranial nerve (CN) schwannomas, meningiomas, & spinal tumors

IMAGING

- Best diagnostic clue: Bilateral vestibular schwannomas (VSs)
- Multiple extraaxial tumors
  - Schwannomas of CNs & spinal nerve roots
  - Meningiomas on dural surfaces (up to 50%)
- Intraaxial tumors
  - Ependymomas in spinal cord & brainstem (6%)
- Recommendation: Use high-resolution T1 C+ FS & FIESTA MR through basal cisterns to evaluate CNs

TOP DIFFERENTIAL DIAGNOSES

- Schwannomatosis
- Multiple meningiomas
- Metastases

PATHOLOGY

- All neurofibromatosis type 2 (NF2) families have chromosome 22q12 abnormalities
- *NF2* gene encodes for merlin protein

CLINICAL ISSUES

- Usually presents between 2nd & 4th decades with hearing loss, ± vertigo
- Incidence: 1:25,000-30,000
- Life span substantially shortened by presence of meningiomas & by complications related to lower cranial neuropathies (i.e., aspiration)

DIAGNOSTIC CHECKLIST

- Carefully evaluate other CNs in any new diagnosis of schwannoma or meningioma in child/adolescent/young adult
- Look for commonly associated cerebral & cerebellar subcortical lesions (likely dysplasias)

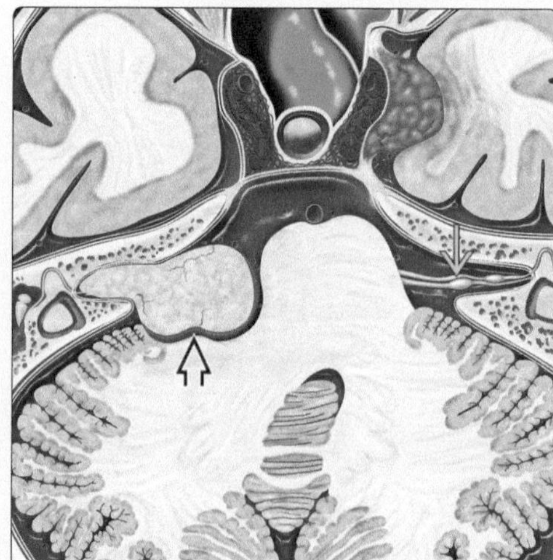

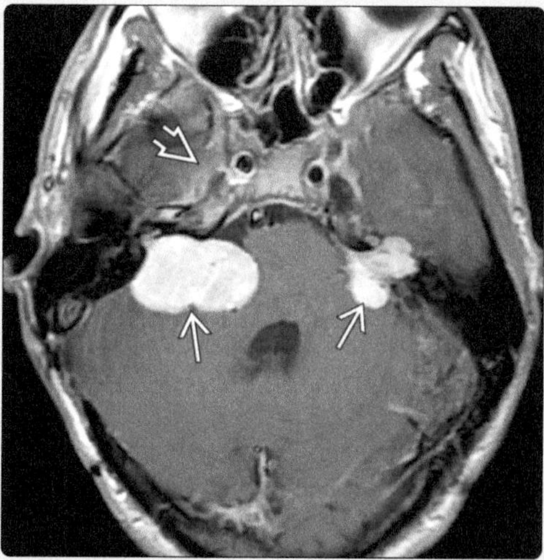

(Left) *Axial graphic shows bilateral cerebellopontine angle (CPA) schwannomas pathognomonic in children with neurofibromatosis type 2 (NF2). The tumor ⇨ on the right is large, and several small schwannomas ⇨ are seen on the left vestibulocochlear nerves.* **(Right)** *Axial T1 C+ MR in typical NF2 shows bilateral vestibular schwannomas (VSs) ➡ and a right cavernous sinus meningioma ➡. Look carefully for lesions throughout the skull base when there is clinical suspicion of NF2.*

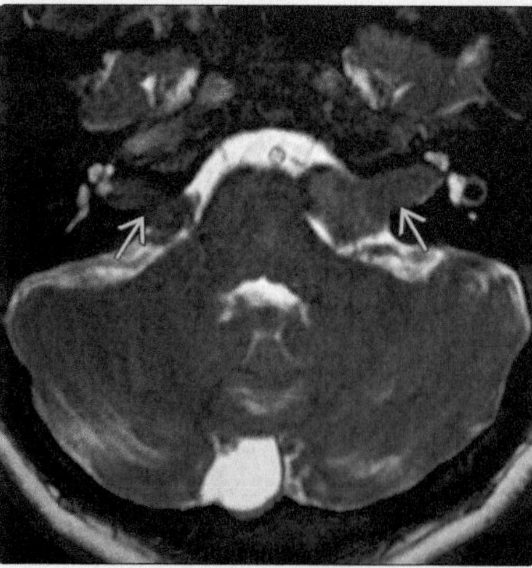

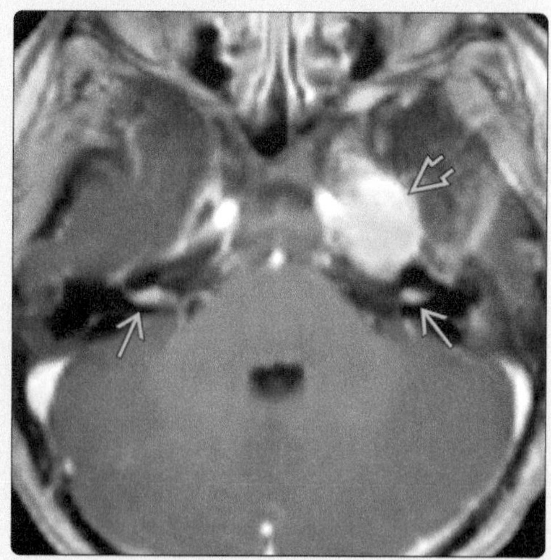

(Left) *Axial FIESTA MR in a teenager with NF2 shows expansion of the bilateral internal auditory canals (IACs) with soft tissue filling the IACs ⇨ and extending into the CPA cisterns. FIESTA is a great sequence to evaluate the cisternal segments of the cranial nerves (CNs) for detection of small schwannomas.* **(Right)** *Axial T1 C+ MR in a 10-year-old with NF2 shows a large schwannoma ⇨ in the left cavernous sinus as well as small bilateral enhancing VSs ⇨.*

TERMINOLOGY

Abbreviations

- Neurofibromatosis type 2 (NF2)

Synonyms

- Acoustic neurofibromatosis, central neurofibromatosis
- Multiple intracranial schwannomas, meningiomas, & ependymomas (MISME)

Definitions

- Familial cancer syndrome causing multiple cranial nerve (CN) schwannomas, meningiomas, & spinal ependymomas

IMAGING

General Features

- Best diagnostic clue
  - Bilateral vestibular schwannomas (VSs)
- Location
  - Multiple extraaxial tumors
    - Schwannomas of CNs & spinal nerve roots
    - Meningiomas on dural surfaces (up to 50%)
  - Intraaxial tumors
    - Ependymomas in spinal cord & brainstem (6%)
- Size
  - CN tumors typically symptomatic while still small but can achieve great size
- Morphology
  - Tumors grow spherically but accommodate to bony canals [e.g., internal auditory canal (IAC)]
- Multiplicity of lesions
  - Schwannomas of other CNs in 50%
    - CNV most common; CNIII, CNXII also common
  - Schwannoma of spinal nerves (up to 90%)
  - Meningiomas (often multiple)
  - Intramedullary ependymomas (spinal cord)
- Associated abnormalities
  - Wedge-shaped T2/FLAIR signal abnormalities in subcortical white matter (~ 65%)
    - Similar abnormalities in cerebellum (~ 15-20%)
    - Pathology is uncertain, suspected dysplastic lesions
  - Meningioangiomatosis
  - Posterior lens opacities (juveniles, in 60-80%)

CT Findings

- NECT
  - Schwannoma
    - Cerebellopontine angle (CPA) mass ± widened IAC
    - Isodense to hyperdense
    - Rarely cystic/necrotic
  - Meningioma
    - High-density, dural-based mass(es)
  - Nonneoplastic cerebral Ca^{++} (uncommon)
    - Extensive choroid plexus Ca^{++}
    - Cortical surface
    - Ventricular lining
- CECT
  - CN tumor enhancement
  - Meningioma enhancement

MR Findings

- T1WI
  - Schwannoma
    - Hypointense to isointense
    - Rare cystic change
  - Meningioma
    - Isointense to hypointense
    - Occasional hyperintense foci from Ca^{++}
- T2WI
  - Schwannoma
    - Small intracanalicular lesions can be shown on high-resolution T2WI
  - Meningioma
    - May incite significant adjacent edema
  - Look for associated subcortical cerebral (~ 65%) & cerebellar (~ 17%) wedge-shaped signal abnormalities
- T2* GRE
  - Shows nonneoplastic Ca^{++} to best advantage
- DWI
  - Some meningiomas have restricted diffusion
    - Characteristic of atypical or malignant meningioma
  - May be helpful to distinguish sporadic from NF2-related schwannomas
- T1WI C+
  - Schwannoma
    - Diffuse enhancement
    - Usually homogeneous
    - T1 C+ with fat saturation & thin-slice profile essential for identification of small CN tumors
    - VSs typically "bulge" into CPA cistern from IAC
  - Meningioma
    - Diffuse enhancement of tumor; may be plaque-like
- MRS
  - Schwannoma
    - Absent NAA peak, ↑ myoinositol, usually no lactate
  - Meningioma
    - Absent NAA peak, ↑ alanine, ± lactate

Nonvascular Interventions

- Myelography
  - Will demonstrate multiple spinal tumorlets
    - Replaced by contrast-enhanced MR

Imaging Recommendations

- Best imaging tool
  - Contrast-enhanced MR
- Protocol advice
  - Use high-resolution T1 C+ FS MR through basal cisterns to evaluate CNs
  - Evaluation for spinal disease is critical

DIFFERENTIAL DIAGNOSIS

Schwannomatosis

- Multiple schwannomas without vestibular tumors
- No cutaneous stigmata or meningiomas

Cerebellopontine Angle Masses

- Arachnoid cyst: Follows CSF on all sequences
- Epidermoid: DWI easily distinguishes from arachnoid cyst
- Aneurysm

- Posterior inferior cerebellar artery (PICA)/anterior inferior cerebellar artery (AICA)/vertebral artery (VA) aneurysms may project into CPA
- Pulsation artifact in phase-encoding direction
- Ependymoma: Extends into CPA from 4th ventricle

Multiple Meningiomas

- Recurrent or metastatic
- Secondary to radiation therapy

Metastases

- CNS primary: Glioblastoma, medulloblastoma, germinoma, ependymoma
- Non-CNS primary

Inflammatory Disease

- Granulomatous disease: Sarcoidosis, tuberculosis
- Neuritis: Bell palsy, Lyme disease

PATHOLOGY

General Features

- Etiology
  - 50% with known family history of NF2; 50% new mutations
  - Mutations cause truncated, inactivated merlin protein (**m**eosin-**e**rzin-**r**axidin-**li**ke protein)
  - Tumor cells are usually hemizygous or homozygous for *NF2* mutations
- Genetics
  - Autosomal dominant
  - All NF2 families have chromosome 22q12 abnormalities
  - Germline, somatic *NF2* gene mutations
    - *NF2* gene encodes for merlin protein
    - *NF2* gene functions: Links cytoskeleton & cell membranes; also tumor suppressor gene
    - Molecular pathway mTORC1 is affected; inhibitors may inhibit tumor growth
- Multiple schwannomas, meningiomas, ependymomas

Staging, Grading, & Classification

- NF2-associated schwannomas are WHO grade 1
- Diagnostic criteria
  - Bilateral VS, or
  - 1st-degree relative with NF2 & 1 VS, or
  - 1st-degree relative with NF2 & 2 of following
    - Neurofibroma
    - Meningioma
    - Glioma
    - Schwannoma
    - Posterior subcapsular lenticular opacity

Gross Pathologic & Surgical Features

- Schwannomas are round-ovoid, encapsulated masses
- Meningiomas are unencapsulated but sharply circumscribed

Microscopic Features

- NF2-related schwannomas have higher proliferative activity than sporadic tumors but not necessarily more aggressive course

CLINICAL ISSUES

Presentation

- Most common signs/symptoms
  - Usually presents between 2nd & 4th decades with hearing loss, ± vertigo
  - 1/3 of children with NF2 present with hearing loss, 1/3 present with other CN symptoms
  - May present with meningioma before VSs develop
    - Children presenting with meningioma should have testing for NF2
- Other signs/symptoms
  - Scoliosis, paraplegia, or neck pain from spinal lesions
- Clinical profile
  - Wishart type: Early onset, rapid progression before adulthood, more severe presentation
  - Gardner type: Later onset, less severe manifestations

Demographics

- Epidemiology
  - 1:25,000-30,000

Natural History & Prognosis

- Life span substantially shortened by presence of meningiomas & by complications related to lower cranial neuropathies (i.e., aspiration)

Treatment

- Schwannoma
  - Bevacizumab (Avastin) has been shown to reduce tumor size, slow growth, & improve auditory symptoms
  - Complete microsurgical resection of CNVIII schwannoma, if feasible
    - Can be difficult as schwannomas tend to splay/envelop CNs instead of displace them
    - Stereotactic radiosurgery is also option
  - Subtotal microsurgical resection with functional cochlear nerve preservation in last hearing ear
- Meningioma
  - Surgical resection, if accessible
  - Stereotactic radiosurgery also option

DIAGNOSTIC CHECKLIST

Consider

- Carefully evaluate other CNs in any new diagnosis of VS or meningioma in child/adolescent
- Study entire neuraxis in suspected cases (multiple small, asymptomatic schwannomas on cauda equina common)
- Look for associated cerebral & cerebellar dysplastic lesions

Image Interpretation Pearls

- Coronal thin-slice T1 C+ FS & FIESTA MR to assess CNs

SELECTED REFERENCES

1. Ishi Y et al: Variations and natural history of primary intraparenchymal lesions associated with neurofibromatosis type 2. Neuroradiology. 64(2):393-6, 2022
2. Ota Y et al: Neurofibromatosis type 2 versus sporadic vestibular schwannoma: the utility of MR diffusion and dynamic contrast-enhanced imaging. J Neuroimaging. 32(3):554-60, 2022
3. Wang MX et al: Neurofibromatosis from head to toe: what the radiologist needs to know. Radiographics. 42(4):1123-44, 2022

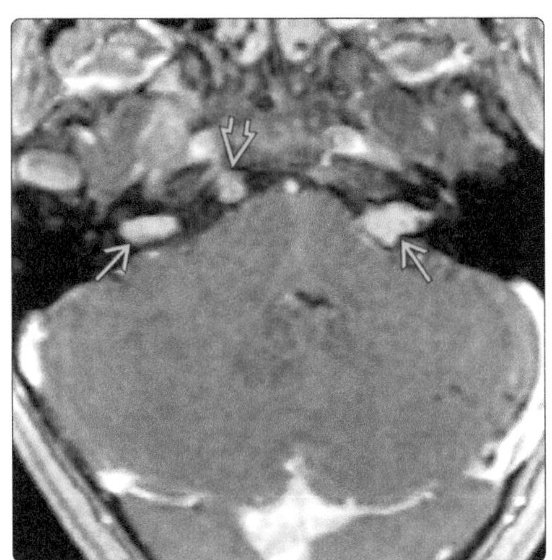

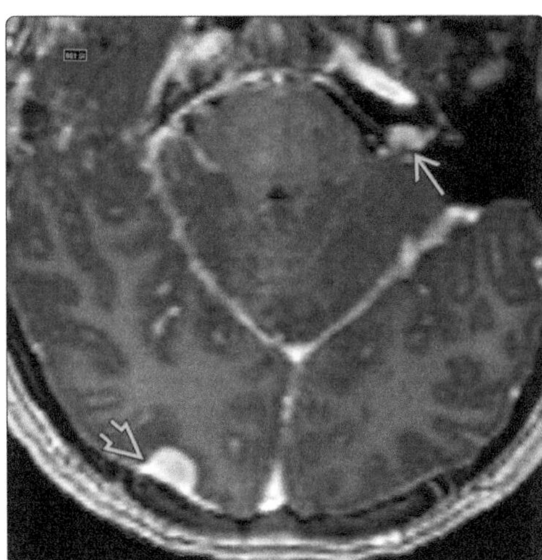

(Left) *Axial T1 C+ MR in a 10-year-old with NF1 shows enhancing lesions within the bilateral IACs ➡, consistent with VS. If one looks carefully, they will also note a schwannoma involving the right CNV ➡.* **(Right)** *Axial T1 C+ MR in a 17-year-old with NF2 shows a VS ➡ in the left IAC as well as a dural-based lesion ➡ in the right occipital region, consistent with meningioma. The combination of a VS and meningiomas qualifies a patient for a diagnosis of NF2.*

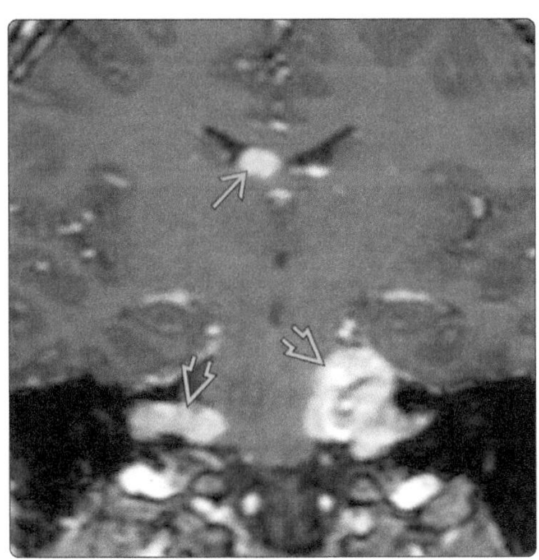

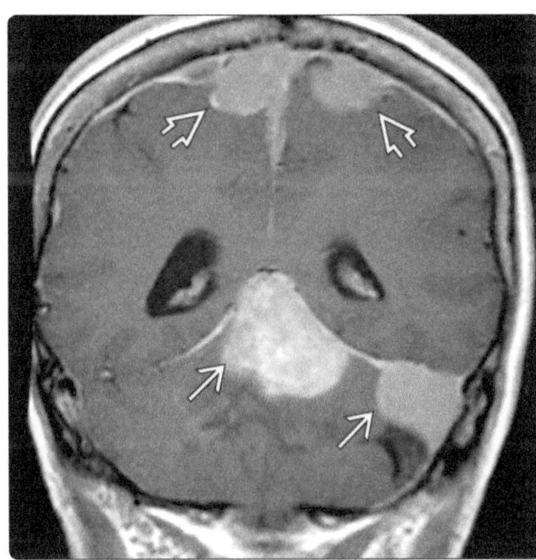

(Left) *Coronal T1 C+ MR in a 17-year-old with NF2 shows a large, bilateral VS ➡ as well as an enhancing lesion in the right lateral ventricle associated with the choroid plexus, consistent with a choroid plexus meningioma ➡.* **(Right)** *Coronal T1 C+ MR in an older adult shows dural-based meningiomas in the posterior fossa ➡ and along the falx and convexities ➡. In this patient, the meningiomatosis predominates over the schwannomas.*

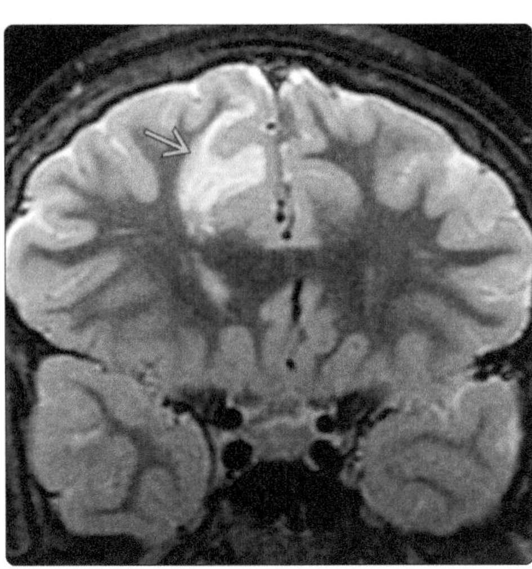

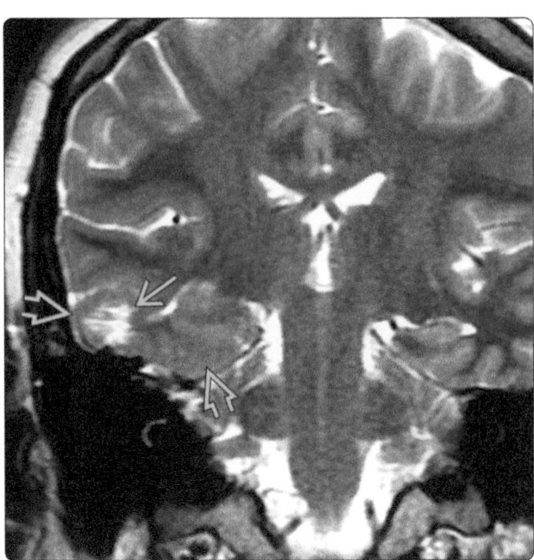

(Left) *Coronal T2 FS MR in an 18-year-old with NF2 shows a wedge-shaped area of hyperintense signal ➡ in the right frontal subcortical white matter. When such abnormalities are searched for in NF2, they are seen in a significant proportion of cases.* **(Right)** *Coronal T2 MR in the same patient shows another subcortical lesion ➡ within the right temporal lobe with adjacent cortical malformation ➡. The etiology of these abnormalities is uncertain, but they are suspected to represent congenital dysplastic lesions.*

von Hippel-Lindau Syndrome

KEY FACTS

TERMINOLOGY

- Autosomal dominant familial syndrome with hemangioblastomas (HGBLs), clear cell renal cell carcinoma (RCC), cystadenomas, pheochromocytomas

IMAGING

- 2 or more CNS HGBLs or 1 HGBL + visceral lesion or retinal hemorrhage
- HGBL: Vary from tiny enhancing mass to large cystic mass with enhancing mural nodule
- HGBL: Marked ↑ CBV & ↑ CBF; endolymphatic sac tumor: Enhancing destructive lesion in petrous bone

TOP DIFFERENTIAL DIAGNOSES

- Vascular metastasis; solitary hemangioblastoma
- Pilocytic astrocytoma
- Hemispheric medulloblastoma in teenager or young adult
- Multiple arteriovenous malformations in vascular neurocutaneous syndrome

PATHOLOGY

- von Hippel-Lindau phenotypes, subtypes based on absence or presence of pheochromocytoma
  - Type 1: Low risk of pheochromocytoma
  - Type 2: High risk of pheochromocytoma
    - Type 2A: Low risk of RCC
    - Type 2B: High risk of RCC
    - Type 2C: Familial pheochromocytoma without either HGBL or RCC

CLINICAL ISSUES

- Earliest symptom in VHL often visual
  - Retinal HGBL, peak in teenage
- HGBLs → multiple periods of tumor growth (usually associated with increasing cyst size) separated by periods of arrested growth

DIAGNOSTIC CHECKLIST

- Follow NIH screening guidelines

(Left) *Sagittal graphic shows 2 hemangioblastomas (HGBLs) in von Hippel-Lindau (VHL). In this patient, the spinal cord tumor has an associated cyst ➢ and would cause myelopathy. The small cerebellar HGBL ➢ would be asymptomatic.* **(Right)** *Sagittal T1 C+ MR in a 17-year-old with VHL shows a large cystic lesion → in the medulla with an avidly enhancing mural nodule ➢. Also note the additional enhancing lesions ↪ lower in the cervical cord. Multiplicity of HGBLs is essentially diagnostic of VHL, especially in children.*

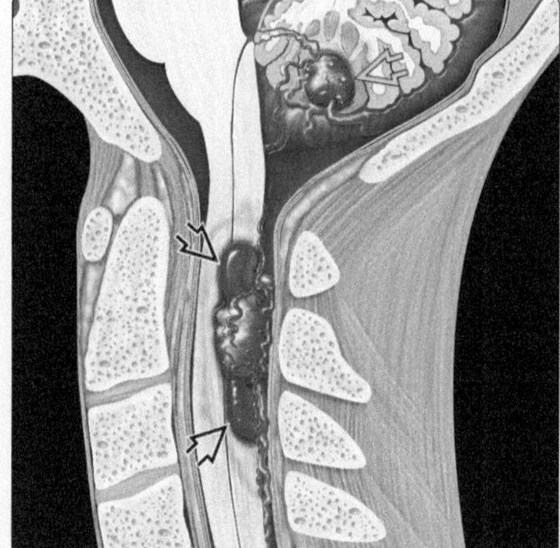

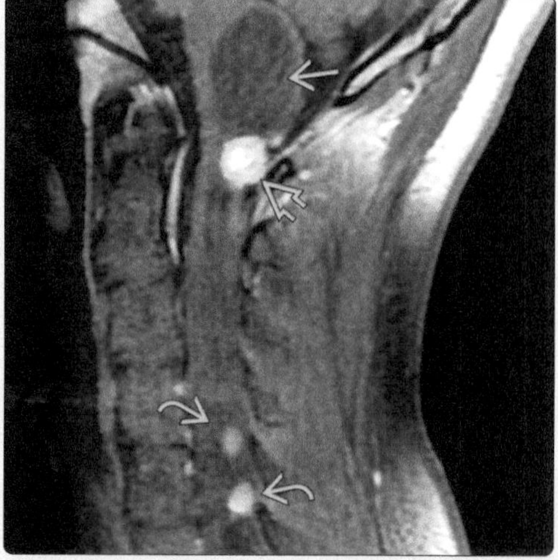

(Left) *Coronal T1 C+ FS MR in an asymptomatic 26-year-old man with pancreatic cysts and a family history of VHL shows 2 solid ➡ and 1 cystic HGBL with a mural nodule ➢.* **(Right)** *Sagittal T1 C+ FS MR in a 17-year-old with VHL shows an avidly enhancing spinal lesion ➢ with multiple hypointense central flow voids →, consistent with tumor vessels. The identification of flow voids is very helpful in establishing a diagnosis of HGBL.*

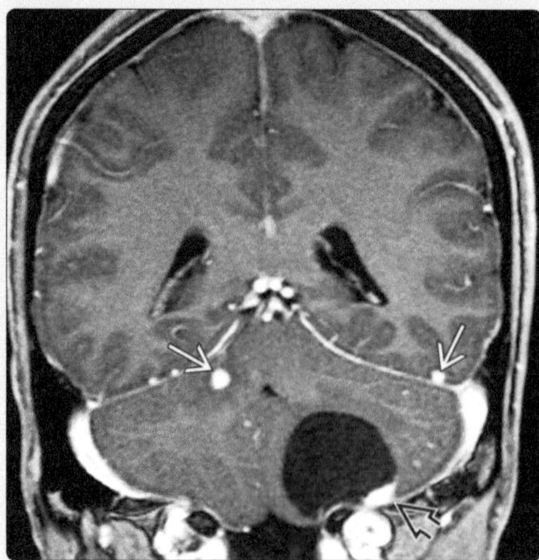

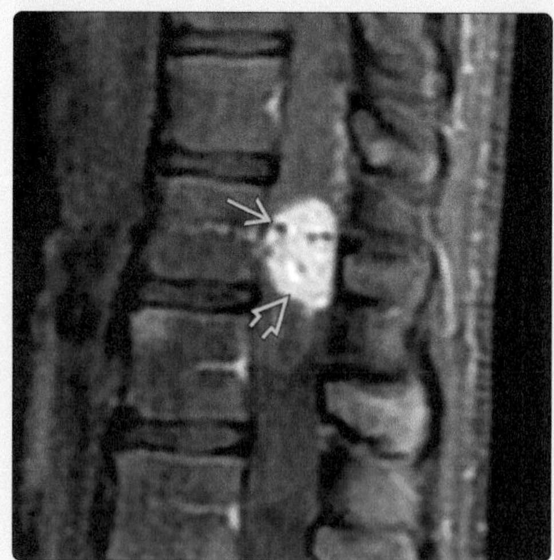

TERMINOLOGY

Abbreviations

- von Hippel-Lindau (VHL) syndrome

Definitions

- Autosomal dominant familial syndrome with hemangioblastomas (HGBLs), clear cell renal cell carcinoma (RCC), cystadenomas, pheochromocytomas
  - Affects 6 different organ systems, including eye, ear, and CNS
  - Involved tissues often have multiple lesions
  - Lesions → benign cysts, vascular tumors, carcinomas

IMAGING

General Features

- Best diagnostic clue
  - 2 or more CNS HGBLs, or 1 HGBL + visceral lesion or retinal hemorrhage
- Location
  - HGBLs in VHL in 60-80% of patients
    - Typically multiple
    - 40-50% in spinal cord (posterior 1/2)
    - 44-72% cerebellum (posterior > anterior 1/2)
    - 10-25% brainstem (posterior medulla)
    - HGBLs arise from pia; if lesion is in deep white matter or in center of cord, it is not HGBL
  - Ocular angiomas
    - Found in 25-60% of *VHL* gene carriers
    - Cause retinal detachment, hemorrhage
  - Endolymphatic sac tumors (ELSTs)
    - Large temporal bone mass; located posterior to internal auditory canal near vestibular aqueduct
- Size
  - HGBLs vary from tiny mass to very large with even larger associated cysts
- Morphology
  - HGBL may be solid, solid with central necrosis, or cystic with enhancing mural nodule

CT Findings

- NECT
  - HGBL: 2/3 → well-delineated cerebellar cyst with nodule
    - Nodule typically abuts pial surface
    - 1/3 solid, without cyst
  - ELST → permeative, destructive changes in petrous bone
- CECT
  - Intense enhancement of tumor nodule

MR Findings

- T1WI
  - HGBL: Mixed iso- to hypointense nodule, ± flow voids
  - Associated cyst iso- to slightly hyperintense to CSF
  - Cystadenoma of endolymphatic sac (ELS): Heterogeneous hyper-/hypointense
- T2WI
  - HGBL: Hyperintense nodule, cyst
  - HGBL: Look for adjacent or intratumoral flow voids
  - Cystadenoma of ELS: Hyperintense mass
- FLAIR
  - HGBL: Hyperintense cyst with variable edema
  - Cystadenoma of ELS: Hyperintense mass
- T2* GRE
  - HGBL: Blooms if hemorrhage present
- PWI
  - HGBL: Marked ↑ cerebral blood volume (CBV) & ↑ cerebral blood flow (CBF)
  - Perfusion very helpful in distinguishing HGBL from other posterior fossa tumors
- T1WI C+
  - HGBL: Tumor nodule enhances strongly; cyst wall does not enhance
  - Tiny, asymptomatic enhancing nodules commonly found
  - Cystadenoma of ELS: Heterogeneous enhancement

Angiographic Findings

- Conventional
  - HGBL: DSA shows intensely vascular mass, prolonged stain
  - Arteriovenous shunting (early draining vein) common

Imaging Recommendations

- Best imaging tool
  - Brain: MR ± contrast
- Protocol advice
  - Scan entire brain and spine
- NIH recommendations
  - Contrast-enhanced MR of brain/spinal cord every 2 years from age 11 years
  - US of abdomen from 11 years, yearly
  - Abdominal CT from 20 years, yearly/every other year
  - MR of temporal bone if hearing loss/tinnitus/vertigo

DIFFERENTIAL DIAGNOSIS

Vascular Metastasis

- Usually solid, not cyst with nodule
- Some tumors (e.g., clear cell RCC) can resemble HGBL histopathologically

Solitary Hemangioblastoma

- 25-40% of HGBLs occur in VHL
- No *VHL* mutations, family history, other tumors or cysts

Pilocytic Astrocytoma

- Usually younger than VHL patients
- Tumor nodule lacks vascular flow voids (more characteristic of HGBL)
- Tumor nodule often does not abut pial or ependymal surface

Hemispheric Medulloblastoma in Teenager or Young Adult

- Rare; occur in peripheral cerebellar hemisphere
- May appear extraparenchymal
- Solid, gray matter intensity on T2WI

Multiple Arteriovenous Malformations in Vascular Neurocutaneous Syndrome

- Osler-Weber-Rendu, Wyburn-Mason, etc.
- Small arteriovenous malformations may resemble HGBL at angiography

PATHOLOGY

General Features

- Genetics
  - Autosomal dominant inheritance with high penetrance, variable expression
    - 20% of cases due to new mutation
  - Germline mutations of *VHL* tumor suppressor gene
    - Chromosome 3p25-26
    - Gene product: pVHL; inactivation of pVHL results in overexpression of hypoxia-inducible mRNAs, including vascular endothelial growth factor (VEGF)
    - Involved in cell cycle regulation, angiogenesis
    - Disease features vary depending on specific *VHL* mutations
    - Posterior distribution of HGBLs = result of tumor development during embryogenesis
      - Tumors are derived from embryonic multipotent cells

Staging, Grading, & Classification

- Capillary hemangioblastoma: WHO grade 1

Gross Pathologic & Surgical Features

- HGBL seen as well-circumscribed, very vascular, reddish nodule
  - 75% at least partially cystic; fluid is amber colored

Microscopic Features

- 2 components in HGBL
  - Rich capillary network
  - Large, vacuolated stromal cells with clear cytoplasm

CLINICAL ISSUES

Presentation

- Most common signs/symptoms
  - VHL is clinically very heterogeneous; phenotypic penetrance: 97% at 65 years
    - Rate of new tumor development not constant, varies with age (peak at 30-34 years)
  - Retinal angiomas
    - Earliest symptom in VHL often visual; peak in teenage years
    - Retinal detachment, vitreous hemorrhages
  - Cerebellar HGBLs
    - Headache (obstructive hydrocephalus)
    - Peak 4th decade
    - Nearly 75% of symptom-producing tumors have associated cyst, peritumoral edema
  - Spinal cord HGBLs
    - Progressive myelopathy
    - 95% associated syrinx
  - ELSTs
    - Prevalence in VHL patients is 3.6%
    - Can be 1st presentation of VHL, so molecular testing is needed
- Clinical profile
  - Diagnosis of VHL: Capillary hemangioblastoma in CNS/retina and 1 of typical VHL-associated tumors or previous family history
  - VHL phenotypes, subtypes based on absence or presence of pheochromocytoma
    - Type 1: Low risk of pheochromocytoma
    - Type 2: High risk of pheochromocytoma
      - Type 2A (low risk of RCC)
      - Type 2B high risk of RCC
      - Type 2C (familial pheochromocytoma without either HGBL or RCC)

Demographics

- Age
  - VHL presents in young adults: Mean age of presentation
    - Retinal angioma: 25 years
    - Cerebellar HGBL, pheochromocytoma: 30 years
    - Endolymphatic sac tumor: 31 years
    - RCC: 33 years
- Epidemiology
  - 1:35,000-50,000

Natural History & Prognosis

- RCC proximal cause of death in 15-50%
- HGBLs → multiple periods of tumor growth (usually associated with increasing cyst size) separated by periods of arrested growth
- On average, new lesion develops every 2 years in VHL

Treatment

- Ophthalmoscopy yearly from infancy
- Physical/neurologic examination yearly
- Surgical resection of symptomatic cerebellar/spinal HGBL
  - Presurgical tumor embolization commonly performed
- Stereotactic radiosurgery provides tumor control in 70-90%
- Laser treatment of retinal angiomas

DIAGNOSTIC CHECKLIST

Consider

- Follow NIH screening guidelines
- Look for ELS tumors in VHL patients with dysequilibrium, hearing loss, or aural fullness

Image Interpretation Pearls

- Solitary HGBL in young patient may indicate VHL
- Perform perfusion imaging to distinguish HGBL from pilocytic astrocytoma

SELECTED REFERENCES

1. Daniels AB et al: Guidelines for surveillance of patients with von Hippel-Lindau disease: consensus statement of the International VHL Surveillance Guidelines Consortium and VHL Alliance. Cancer. 129(19):2927-40, 2023
2. Mazzapicchi E et al: Sporadic and von Hippel-Lindau related hemangioblastomas of brain and spinal cord: multimodal imaging for intraoperative strategy. Cancers (Basel). 14(22), 2022
3. Mehta GU et al: Endolymphatic sac tumor screening and diagnosis in von Hippel-Lindau disease: a consensus statement. J Neurol Surg B Skull Base. 83(Suppl 2):e225-31, 2022
4. Takami H et al: Presentation, imaging, patterns of care, growth, and outcome in sporadic and von Hippel-Lindau-associated central nervous system hemangioblastomas. J Neurooncol. 159(2):221-31, 2022
5. Huntoon K et al: Hemangioblastoma diagnosis and surveillance in von Hippel-Lindau disease: a consensus statement. J Neurosurg. 1-6, 2021
6. Schweizer L et al: Molecular characterisation of sporadic endolymphatic sac tumours and comparison to von Hippel-Lindau disease-related tumours. Neuropathol Appl Neurobiol. 47(6):756-67, 2021
7. Dornbos D 3rd et al: Review of the neurological implications of von Hippel-Lindau disease. JAMA Neurol. 75(5):620-7, 2018

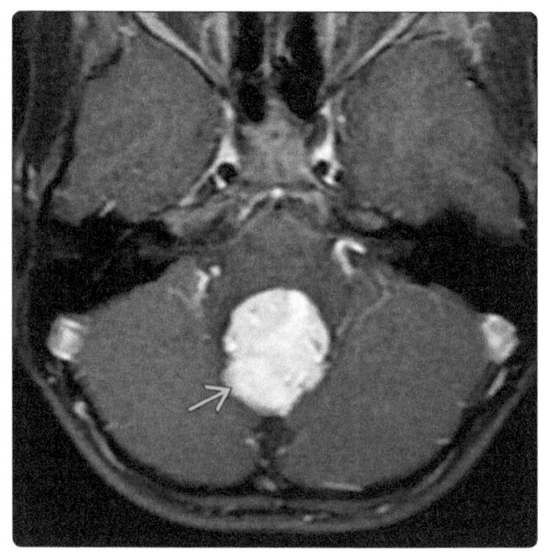

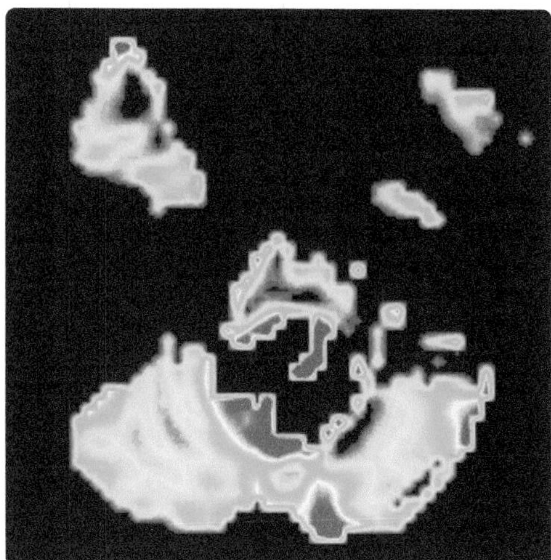

(Left) *Axial T1 C+ FS MR in a 7-year-old with VHL and an HGBL shows an avidly enhancing midline posterior fossa mass* ➡ *with enhancement equal to blood pool.* **(Right)** *Axial dynamic MR perfusion in a 7-year-old with VHL and an HGBL shows marked ↑ perfusion. The black areas are from aliasing (perfusion above the threshold). Markedly ↑ perfusion is a distinguishing characteristic of an HGBL. This markedly ↑ perfusion helps to distinguish HGBL from mimics, such as pilocytic astrocytoma.*

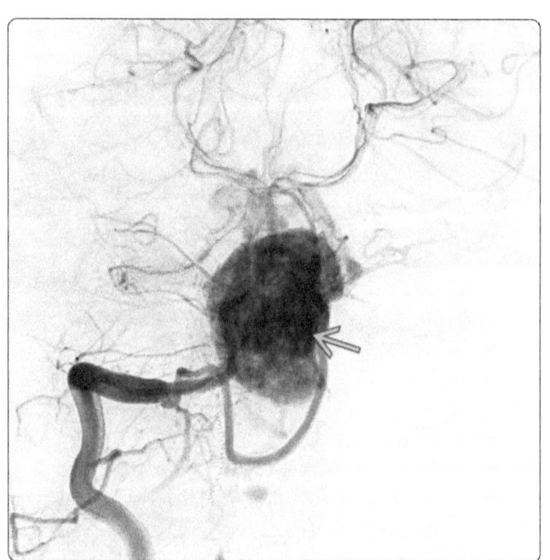

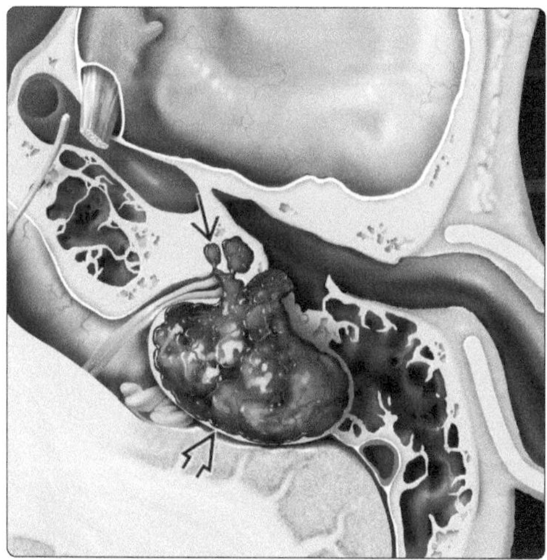

(Left) *Frontal projection DSA in the same patient shows the extensive enhancement* ➡ *during arterial phase, reflecting the very high perfusion in HGBLs. This patient went on to have preoperative embolization of the tumor to minimize blood loss during resection.* **(Right)** *Axial graphic depicts an endolymphatic sac tumor in a patient with VHL. The lesion is a lytic, vascular, hemorrhagic mass* ➡ *that lies between the internal auditory canal and sigmoid sinus. Note the tendency to fistulize the inner ear* ➡*.*

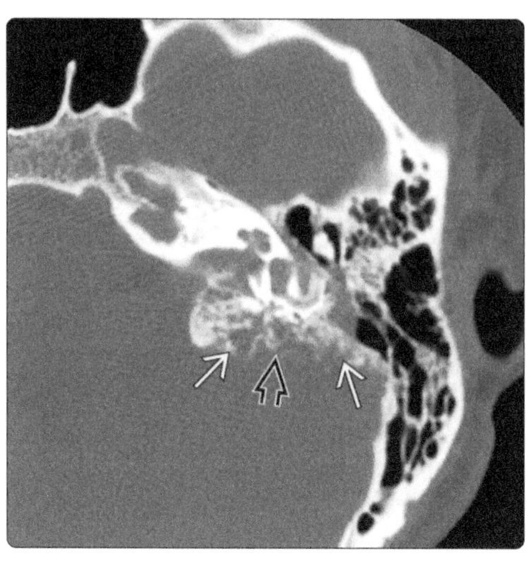

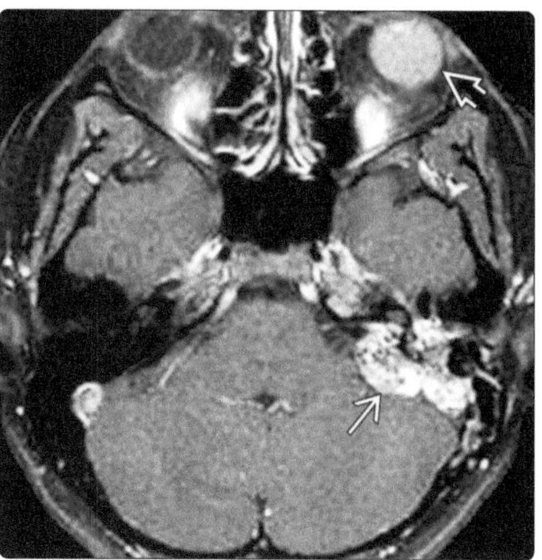

(Left) *Axial temporal bone CT in the same patient shows a lytic, infiltrative lesion* ➡ *along the left posterior petrous temporal bone. Note the preserved spicules of bone* ➡ *within the lesion. The location and appearance are characteristic for endolymphatic sac tumors (ELSTs).* **(Right)** *Axial T1 C+ FS MR in the same patient shows that the lesion* ➡ *enhances intensely but heterogeneously. The retinal hemorrhage* ➡ *is hyperintense on T1. (Courtesy D. Shatzkes, MD.)*

KEY FACTS

TERMINOLOGY

- Hamartomas of multiple organs → CNS, skin, kidney, bone

IMAGING

- Cerebral tubers
  - Cortical/subcortical lesion expanding overlying gyri
  - T2/FLAIR hyperintense, T1 hypointense after myelination
  - T1 hyperintense prior to myelination
- Cerebellar tubers
  - Wedge-shaped foci of volume loss
  - Often enhance & calcify
- Subependymal nodules (SENs)
  - Elongated nodules in locations of fetal germinal matrix
  - Increasing Ca^{++} over time
  - 30-80% enhance
- Subependymal giant cell astrocytoma (SEGA)
  - Growing nodule at caudothalamic groove
  - WHO grade 1 neoplasm

TOP DIFFERENTIAL DIAGNOSES

- Focal cortical dysplasia
- Dysembryoplastic neuroepithelial tumor
- Ganglioglioma
- TORCH infections that cause periventricular Ca^{++}
- X-linked subependymal heterotopia

PATHOLOGY

- 2 distinct gene loci
  - *TSC1* (9q34) encodes **hamartin**
  - *TSC2* (16p13) encodes **tuberin** → more severe

CLINICAL ISSUES

- Medical antiseizure therapy, resection of seizure focus
- mTOR inhibitors now 1st-line therapy for SEGA

DIAGNOSTIC CHECKLIST

- Tubers + SEN pathognomonic for TSC
- Surveillance imaging is performed to detect SEGA

(Left) *Axial FLAIR MR in a 6-year-old boy with tuberous sclerosis complex (TSC) shows a moderate to severe burden of cerebral tubers and right subependymal giant cell astrocytoma (SEGA) ⇨. Cystic change is seen in a left parietal lobe tuber ⇨. Tubers are dysplastic lesions that are present in nearly all patients with TSC.* **(Right)** *Axial T1 C+ MR in a 9-year-old girl with TSC shows a lobular, homogeneously enhancing mass ⇨ in the left caudothalamic groove, consistent with a SEGA. Note the subependymal nodule ⇨.*

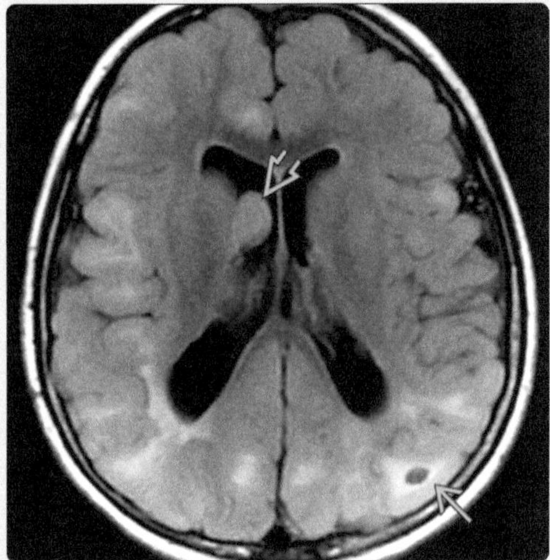

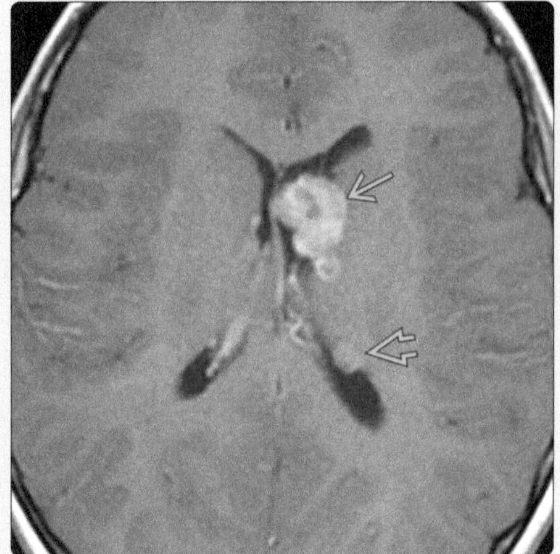

(Left) *Axial T1 C+ MR in a 4-year-old boy shows a wedge-shaped, enhancing left cerebellar tuber ⇨. The majority of cerebellar tubers enhance, in contrast to the supratentorial cerebral hemisphere tubers, which rarely enhance.* **(Right)** *Axial NECT in a 23-month-old girl with TSC shows multiple calcified subependymal nodules ➡. Note that the location of the nodules adheres to the distribution of fetal germinal matrix with a preponderance in the caudothalamic grooves.*

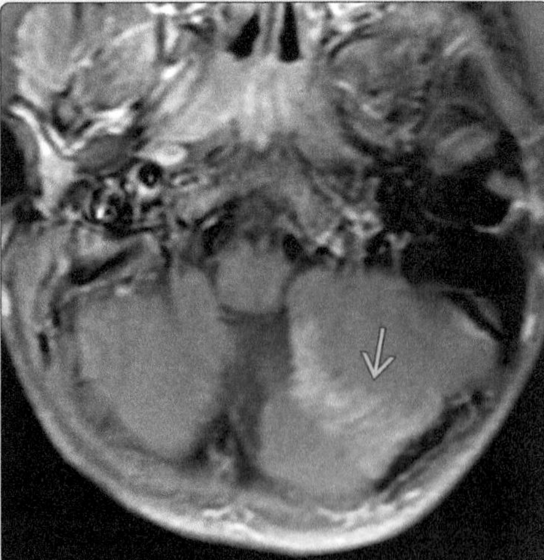

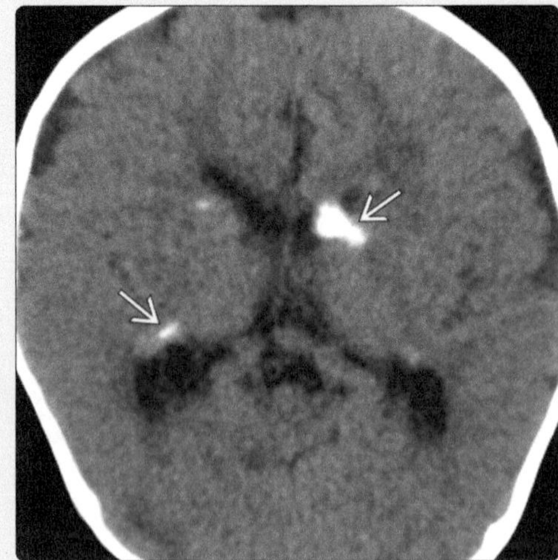

TERMINOLOGY

Abbreviations

- Tuberous sclerosis complex (TSC)

Synonyms

- Bourneville syndrome, Pringle disease, epiloia

Definitions

- Neurocutaneous syndrome: Hamartomatosis
  - Hamartomas of multiple organs → CNS, skin, kidney, bone

IMAGING

General Features

- Best diagnostic clue
  - Cerebral & cerebellar "tubers"
    - Tubers = potato-like texture observed at surgery
    - Dysplastic lesions present from birth
  - Subependymal nodules (SENs)
  - Subependymal giant cell astrocytoma (SEGA)
- Location
  - Tubers → cerebrum (90%) > cerebellum (24-36%)
  - SEN → anatomic distribution is same as fetal germinal matrix with preponderance in caudothalamic grooves
    - Caudothalamic groove > body/atrium > temp horn
  - SEGA → enlarging mass at foramen of Monro
- Morphology
  - Tubers
    - Cerebral
      - Cortical/subcortical tubers expand overlying gyri
      - Cystic tuber degeneration → "empty gyri"
      - Often associated with radial migration lines extending toward lateral ventricles
    - Cerebellar
      - Typically wedge-shaped foci with volume loss & folia distortion
  - SENs
    - Usually small, nodular foci along ventricle margin
    - Majority calcify (↑ Ca^{++} with ↑ age)
  - SEGAs become more spherical with ↑ size

CT Findings

- NECT
  - SENs → Ca^{++} ↑ with time
  - Tubers → low-attenuation subcortical lesion expanding overlying gyri
    - Cerebral tubers usually noncalcified (↑ Ca^{++} with ↑ age)
    - Cerebellar tubers often calcified (~ 30%)
  - Hamartomatous lobe → Ca^{++} in dysplasia/hamartoma of entire lobe (frontal) or hemisphere
  - Giant optic drusen → Ca^{++} in retinal hamartoma
- CECT
  - Most SENs enhance → may be masked by Ca^{++}
  - Some tubers faintly enhance
- CTA
  - Aneurysms occur infrequently (0.74%)

MR Findings

- T1WI
  - SENs → typically slightly hyperintense
    - Best shown on sagittal & coronal images
  - Tubers & radial migration lines are T1 hyperintense in very young patients prior to myelination
  - Tubers & radial migration lines become T1 hypointense after myelination
  - Magnetization transfer ↑ detection of cortical tubers & radial migration lines in children
- T2WI
  - Tubers/radial migration lines typically inconspicuous in very young patients prior to myelination
    - More apparent (hyperintense) with maturation of normal myelin (hypointense)
- FLAIR
  - Tubers → hyperintense
    - "Empty gyri" & periventricular cysts suppress completely
  - Best sequence for detection of tubers & radial migration lines
- T2* GRE
  - Helpful to show Ca^{++} in tubers & SENs
- DWI
  - ↑ ADC values reported in epileptogenic tubers
  - ↑ diffusivity & ↓ fractional anisotropy (FA) values in normal-appearing white matter (WM)
- T1WI C+
  - Best sequence for showing SEN enhancement
  - 3-4% of cortical tubers enhance
  - 33-92% of cerebellar tubers enhance
- MRA
  - Aneurysms (0.74%) & ectasias occasionally encountered
- MRS
  - ↑ myo-inositol (mI) in central & peripheral lesions
  - ↓ NAA with ↑ mI in SEN at foramen of Monro = SEGA

Nuclear Medicine Findings

- PET
  - Tubers are hypometabolic

Other Lesions

- Cerebral aneurysms (0.78%) & dolichoectasia
- Retinal hamartoma
- Renal angiomyolipoma (RAM)
- Lymphangioleiomyomatosis (LAM)
- Cardiac rhabdomyoma
- Sclerotic bone islands & cysts

Imaging Recommendations

- Best imaging tool
  - MR ± contrast
- Protocol advice
  - Use DWI to assess epileptogenic foci
  - ↑ MR field strength may improve tuber detection

DIFFERENTIAL DIAGNOSIS

Infection

- TORCH infections that cause periventricular Ca^{++}
  - CMV, toxoplasmosis
  - May be distinguished by location outside distribution of fetal germinal matrix

- Periventricular, not subependymal
- Hematogenous spread of infections that cause subcortical lesions
  - Fungus
  - Neurocysticercosis

Neoplasms

- Superficial tumors that can resemble tubers
  - Dysembryoplastic neuroepithelial tumor (DNET)
  - Ganglioglioma
  - Angiocentric glioma
- Intraventricular tumors
  - Choroid plexus tumors
  - Subependymoma
  - Central neurocytoma

Focal Cortical Dysplasia

- Especially type II

X-Linked Subependymal Heterotopia

- Gray matter heterotopia along lateral ventricle margins
- No Ca^{++} or enhancement

Subcortical Ischemia, Infarction

- Regions of hyperintense subcortical signal on T2WI & FLAIR
- Restricted diffusion, gyral swelling

PATHOLOGY

General Features

- Etiology
  - Tuberin & hamartin combine to form complex in vivo
    - Act together to regulate mTOR pathway
      - **M**ammalian **t**arget **o**f **r**apamycin
    - Normally inhibit part of mTOR activity
    - Regulate cell growth & proliferation
  - Mutations prevent them from downregulating mTOR
  - Affects germinal matrix → disordered neuronal migration & growth
- Genetics
  - 2 distinct gene loci
    - *TSC1* (9q34) encodes **hamartin**
    - *TSC2* (16p13) encodes **tuberin**
    - *TSC2* most common with severe phenotype
      - More likely to have complex partial seizures, infantile spasms, SEGAs, & intellectual disability
  - 1/3 familial
    - Autosomal dominant, high penetrance
- Associated abnormalities
  - RAM → 40-80% incidence, amenable to embolization
  - Cardiac rhabdomyomas → majority involute spontaneously

Staging, Grading, & Classification

- SEGA = WHO grade 1 neoplasm
- Diagnostic criteria: 2 major (definite) or 1 major + 1 minor (probable)
  - Major: Tubers &/or radial migration lines, SEN, SEGA, cardiac rhabdomyoma, RAM, LAM, adenoma sebaceum, sub-/periungual fibroma, hypomelanotic macules, shagreen patch, retinal hamartoma
  - Minor: WM lesions, dental pits, gingival fibromas, rectal polyps, bone cysts, nonrenal hamartoma, retinal achromic patch, confetti skin lesions, multiple renal cysts
- Genetic testing detects mutations in 60-80% of affected individuals

Gross Pathologic & Surgical Features

- Firm cortical masses with umbilication

Microscopic Features

- Tubers: Balloon cells, giant cells, ectopic neurons
  - Tubers share many histopathologic features with focal cortical dysplasia (FCD) type 2B
- Myelin loss, vacuolation, & gliosis

CLINICAL ISSUES

Presentation

- Classic clinical triad: Adenoma sebaceum, seizures, intellectual disability
  - Seen in only 30-40%
- Infantile spasms → poorer outcome
- Autism

Demographics

- Age
  - Rhabdomyomas present prenatally & in infancy
  - CNS lesions present in infancy & childhood
  - Skin lesions present in childhood
  - Renal, lung, & bone lesions present in adolescence & adulthood
- Epidemiology
  - 1:10,000 incidence

Natural History & Prognosis

- Prognosis dependent upon severity of symptoms (seizures, arrhythmias, renal insufficiency) & success of treatment

Treatment

- Medical antiseizure therapy, resection of seizure focus
- mTOR inhibitors now 1st-line therapy for SEGA
  - Have been shown to be highly effective at reducing seizure frequency

DIAGNOSTIC CHECKLIST

Consider

- ↑ incidence of non-CNS lesions as patients age

Image Interpretation Pearls

- Do not forget to look for vascular lesions

SELECTED REFERENCES

1. Goergen SK et al: Prenatal MR imaging phenotype of fetuses with tuberous sclerosis: an institutional case series and literature review. AJNR Am J Neuroradiol. 43(4):633-8, 2022
2. Northrup H et al: Updated international tuberous sclerosis complex diagnostic criteria and surveillance and management recommendations. Pediatr Neurol. 123:50-66, 2021
3. Wang MX et al: Tuberous sclerosis: current update. Radiographics. 41(7):1992-2010, 2021
4. Russo C et al: Neuroimaging in tuberous sclerosis complex. Childs Nerv Syst. 36(10):2497-509, 2020
5. Gül Mert G et al: Factors affecting epilepsy prognosis in patients with tuberous sclerosis. Childs Nerv Syst. 35(3):463-8, 2019

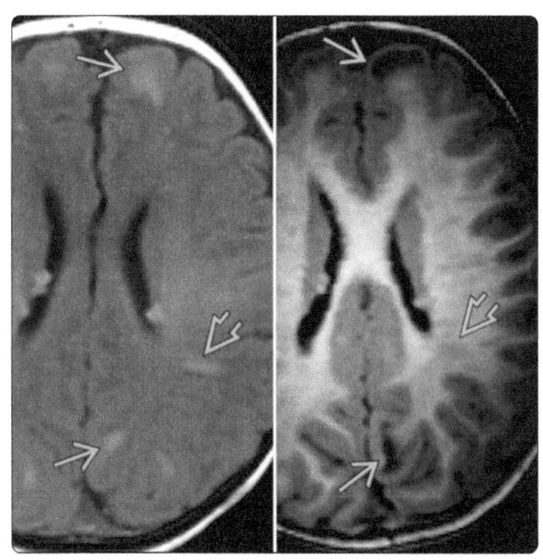

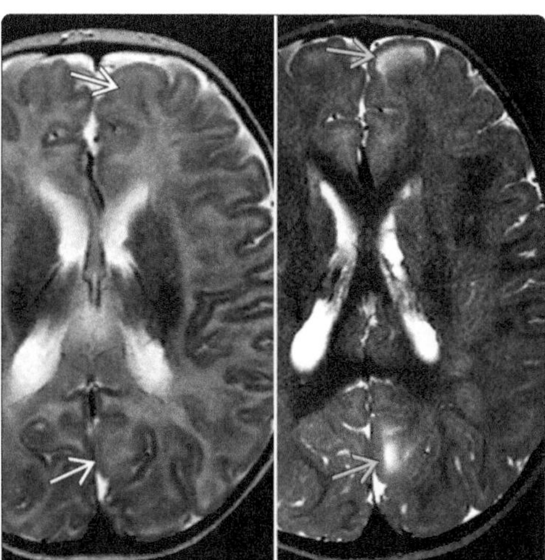

(Left) *Axial T1 MR in a female infant with TSC at 3 months (left) & 10 months (right) of age shows how the cerebral tubers ➡ & radial migration lines ⇨ are relatively hyperintense before myelination (left) & relatively hypointense after myelination (right).* **(Right)** *Axial T2 MR in the same patient at 3 months (left) & 10 months (right) of age shows how the cerebral tubers are inconspicuous prior to myelination ➡ (left) but become conspicuous after myelination ➡ (right).*

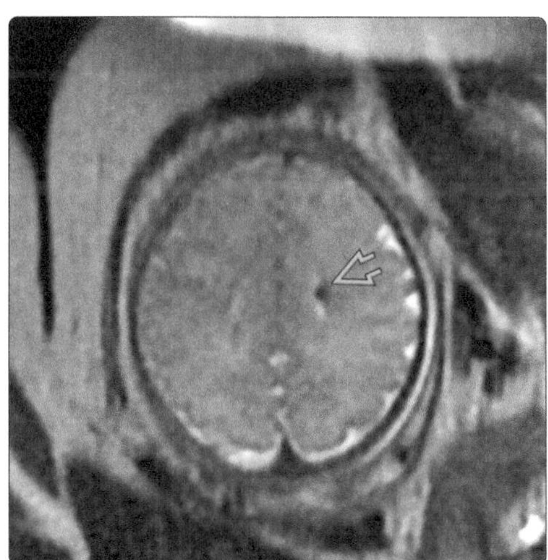

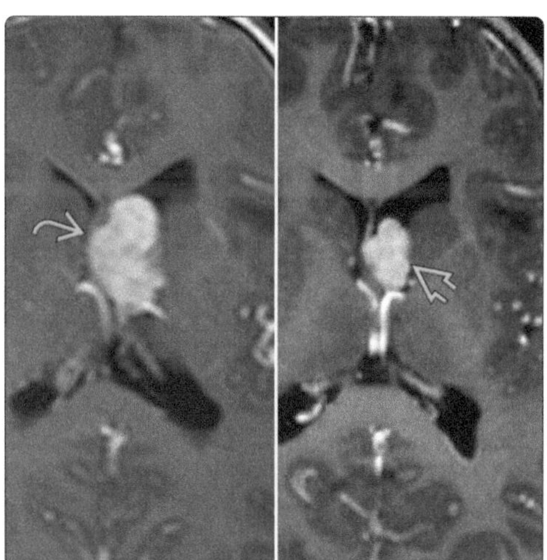

(Left) *Axial T2 MR SSFSE of a 36-weeks gestation fetus shows a hypointense subependymal nodule ⇨. Other non-CNS features confirmed a diagnosis of TSC.* **(Right)** *Axial T1 C+ MR in a 4-year-old girl shows a large SEGA ↷ in the left caudothalamic groove (left). Three months after initiation of an mTOR inhibitor (right), the SEGA ⇨ has substantially decreased in size. mTOR inhibitors are often used as 1st-line therapy for symptomatic SEGAs & have secondary benefits of decreased seizure frequency.*

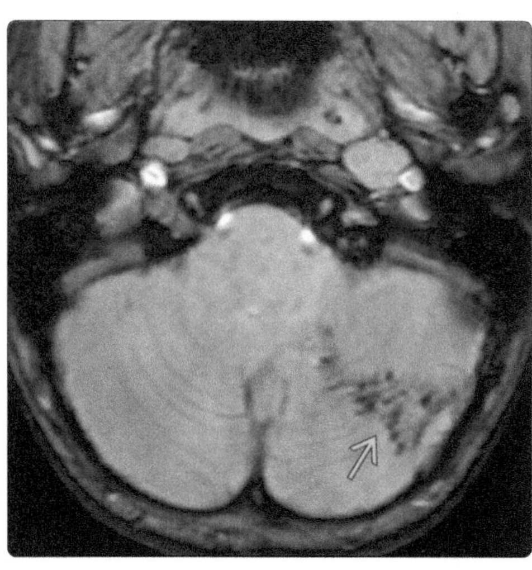

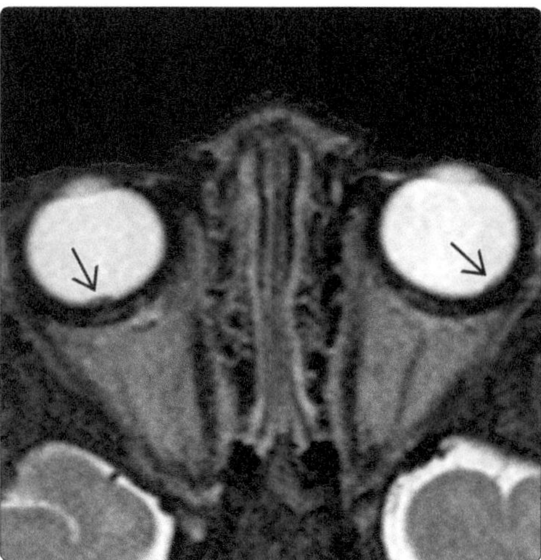

(Left) *Axial SWI MR in a 4-year-old boy with TSC shows signal loss within a calcified, wedge-shaped cerebellar tuber ➡. Approximately 1/3 of all cerebellar tubers are calcified. In contrast to cerebral tubers, which show gyral expansion, cerebellar tubers typically show volume loss.* **(Right)** *High-resolution axial T2 TSE MR in a 10-month-old girl with TSC shows small, bilateral retinal contour abnormalities ➡, consistent with retinal hamartomas.*

Sturge-Weber Syndrome

KEY FACTS

TERMINOLOGY

- Syndrome of abnormal cortical venous development
- Imaging features result from progressive venous occlusion, recruitment of alternate drainage pathways, & chronic venous ischemia

IMAGING

- **CT**: Gyral/subcortical Ca^{++} (may be tram-track appearance)
  - ± calvarial thickening & sinus hyperpneumatization
- **MR**: Regions of atrophy ± abnormal myelination
  - **T2WI**: Flow voids in enlarged deep/transcerebral veins
  - **FLAIR**: Atrophied lobe(s) ± bright sulcal signal of leptomeningeal angiomatosis
  - **SWI/T2* GRE**: ↓ cortical/subcortical signal from Ca^{++}
  - **T1WI C+**: Enhancing leptomeningeal angiomatosis
    - Abundant medullary & deep-draining veins
    - Choroidal globe enhancement of angioma
  - **MRV**: Absent normal cortical veins in affected region
  - **PWI**: ↑ perfusion early, ↓ perfusion late
- **FDG PET**: Progressive ↓ metabolism in affected brain

TOP DIFFERENTIAL DIAGNOSES

- Acquired meningeal processes; PHACES syndrome
- Blue rubber bleb nevus syndrome
- Meningioangiomatosis

CLINICAL ISSUES

- Seizures (75-90%), hemiparesis (30-66%)
  - Holohemispheric/bilateral angiomatosis (10-20%) worse than focal involvement
- Forehead cutaneous capillary malformation (port-wine stain) in ~ 95%
- Choroidal angioma in 70% → glaucoma
- Treatment: Aggressive seizure control, resection/hemispherectomy for intractable epilepsy

DIAGNOSTIC CHECKLIST

- MR in early infancy may be normal: Recommend follow-up if patient at risk for Sturge-Weber syndrome clinically

(Left) *Axial NECT in an 11-year-old girl with intractable epilepsy shows bilateral (right > left) subcortical Ca^{++} ➡, characteristic of Sturge-Weber syndrome (SWS).* **(Right)** *Axial T1 C+ FS MR in the same patient shows bilateral leptomeningeal enhancement ➡ & enlargement of the right choroid plexus ➡. Note the low signal within the subcortical white matter at the depth of sulci ➡, consistent with Ca^{++}. There is mildly increased right calvarial thickness ➡ secondary to underlying brain parenchymal volume loss.*

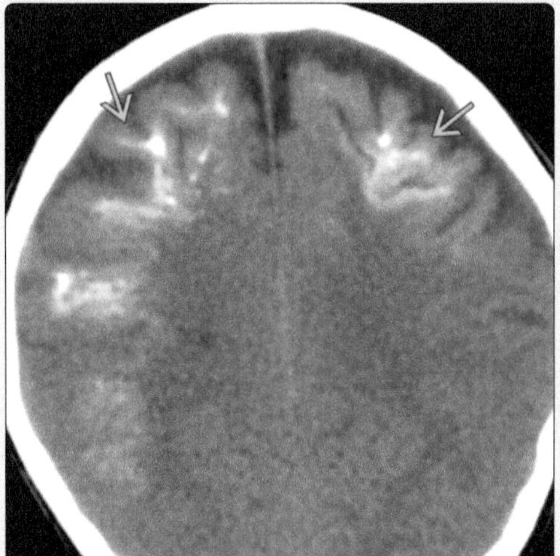

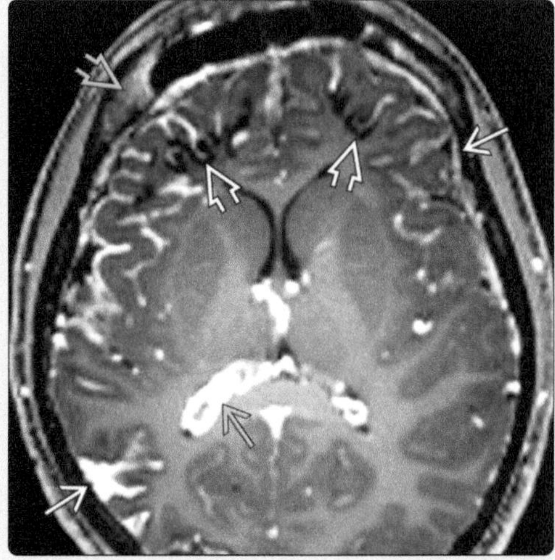

(Left) *Axial T2 MR in a 10-year-old boy with right-sided hemiplegia & seizures shows marked parenchymal volume loss & low signal ➡ corresponding to an area of cortical/subcortical Ca^{++} seen on CT. Also note the ipsilateral, enlarged, deep-draining vein ➡.* **(Right)** *Axial T1 C+ MR in the same patient shows extensive left cerebral leptomeningeal enhancement ➡ with multiple prominent medullary veins ➡ & a large, subependymal-draining vein ➡. Enlargement of the left lateral ventricle is secondary to left cerebral volume loss.*

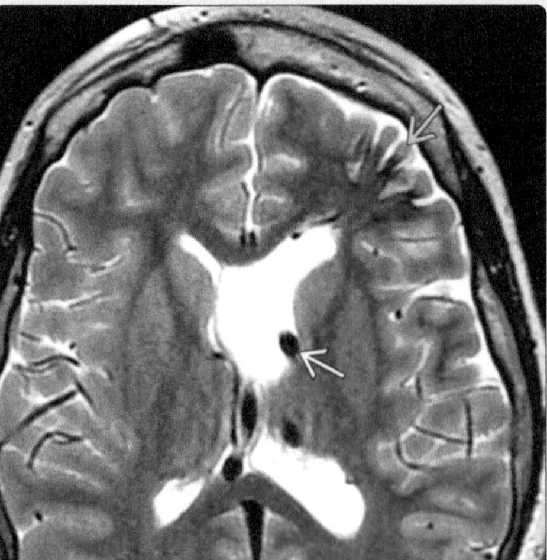

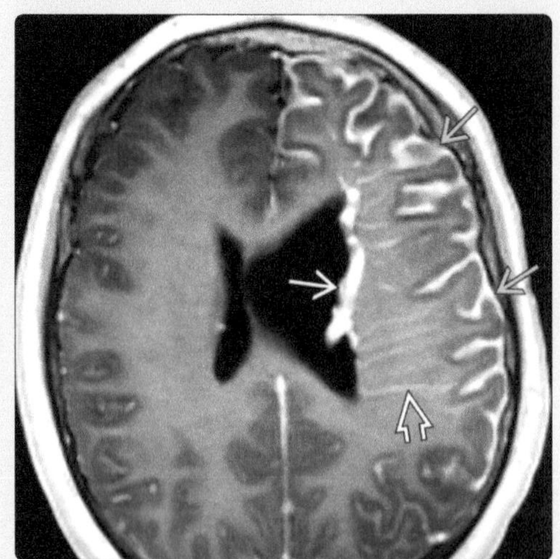

TERMINOLOGY

Abbreviations

- Sturge-Weber syndrome (SWS)

Synonyms

- Sturge-Weber-Dimitri, encephalotrigeminal angiomatosis

Definitions

- Congenital (but not inherited) syndrome in which cortical veins fail to develop normally, leading to numerous long-term intracranial manifestations of chronic ischemia & expanded alternate routes of venous drainage

IMAGING

General Features

- Best diagnostic clue
  - Cerebral lobar atrophy with cortical/subcortical Ca^{++}, leptomeningeal enhancement, & enlarged ipsilateral choroid plexus
- Location
  - Leptomeningeal angiomatosis unilateral in 80-90%, bilateral in 10-20%

Radiographic Findings

- May see cortical/subcortical Ca^{++} &/or calvarial thickening

CT Findings

- NECT
  - Gyral/subcortical Ca^{++} (may be tram-track appearance)
    - Progressive process, usually not present in very young
  - Calvarial thickening & hyperpneumatization of sinuses
    - Secondary to brain parenchymal volume loss
- CECT
  - Leptomeningeal enhancement of angiomatosis
  - Ipsilateral choroid plexus enlargement

MR Findings

- T1WI
  - Altered ("accelerated") white matter (WM) myelination in young patients
- T2WI
  - Hypointense subcortical signal of Ca^{++} at depth of sulci
  - ↓ WM signal of accelerated myelination &/or low oxygen tension
  - Enlarged deep medullary vein flow voids
- FLAIR
  - Gliosis often seen late in affected regions
- T2* GRE
  - ↓ cortical/subcortical signal (Ca^{++})
  - SWI: Most sensitive to transcerebral medullary collaterals
- DWI
  - Typically qualitatively normal, but subtle ↑ in ADC values of involved brain
- PWI
  - Early: Variable, but usually ↓ cerebral blood flow (CBF)
  - Late: ↓ perfusion in affected regions
    - ↓ perfusion associated with frequent seizures, ↑ duration of epilepsy, & brain atrophy
- T1WI C+
  - Leptomeningeal enhancement (angiomatosis)
  - Late stage: ↓ leptomeningeal enhancement, atrophy
  - Choroidal globe enhancement (choroidal angioma)
    - Best seen on T1 C+ FS
- MRA
  - Normal early, but ↓ artery size in affected areas later
- MRV
  - Absent cortical veins in affected region
  - ↑ size of medullary & deep-draining veins
- MRS
  - ↓ NAA, ↑ choline in affected areas

Ultrasonographic Findings

- Pulsed Doppler
  - ↓ middle cerebral artery velocity in late disease

Angiographic Findings

- Conventional
  - Pial blush, but findings mostly venous: Paucity of normal cortical veins, extensive medullary & deep collateral veins

Nuclear Medicine Findings

- **FDG PET**: Progressive hypometabolism in affected regions
  - Hypermetabolism may be seen in very young before or shortly after developing seizures
  - Areas of hypometabolism often extend beyond extent of brain Ca^{++}
- **SPECT**: Hyperperfusion (early), hypoperfusion (late) on interictal scans
  - Pattern inconsistent; may be smaller or larger than abnormality detected on CT/MR
- Note that ictal scans (which may be intentional on SPECT or unintentional on FDG PET) will show ↑ activity

Imaging Recommendations

- Best imaging tool
  - MR with contrast
- Protocol advice
  - MR C+: May be normal at early age; consider follow-up
    - FLAIR C+ improves detection of leptomeningeal angiomatosis
    - Perfusion may predict progression

DIFFERENTIAL DIAGNOSIS

Acquired Meningeal Processes

- Meningitis, tumor spread, hemorrhage, high inspired oxygen content of CSF (usually with anesthesia)

PHACES Syndrome

- **P**osterior fossa malformations, infantile **h**emangiomas, **a**rterial anomalies, **c**oarctation of aorta, **c**ardiac, **e**ye, & **s**ternal anomalies
- Segmental hemangioma of face not fully present at birth

Blue Rubber Bleb Nevus Syndrome

- Multiple small soft tissue venous malformations + intracranial developmental venous anomalies

Klippel-Trenaunay Syndrome

- Extremity overgrowth with extensive capillary-venolymphatic malformations & abnormal deep venous system

Wyburn-Mason Syndrome

- Facial vascular nevus; high-flow visual pathway &/or brain arteriovenous malformation

Meningioangiomatosis

- Rare, meningovascular, hamartomatous, plaque-like mass ± Ca^{++} & cyst formation
  - Ca^{++} common; variable leptomeningeal enhancement; atrophy usually absent
  - May invade brain through Virchow-Robin perivascular spaces

PATHOLOGY

General Features

- Etiology
  - Congenital (but not inherited) syndrome in which cortical veins fail to develop normally
    - Secondary recruitment of alternate venous drainage pathways
    - Imaging features result from progressive venous occlusion & chronic venous ischemia
- Embryology
  - 4-8 weeks: Embryonic cortical veins fail to coalesce & develop → persistent primordial vessels
  - Visual cortex & upper fetal face adjacent in developing embryo
- Sporadic: Mosaic somatic mutation in gene *GNAQ* (9q21) most common
  - Somatic mutations in *GNA11* and *GNB2* genes also uncommonly implicated
  - Timing of somatic mutation may determine severity of clinical phenotype
  - Fibronectin (found in SWS port-wine-derived fibroblasts & SWS surgical brain samples) regulates angiogenesis & vasculogenesis

Staging, Grading, & Classification

- Roach scale
  - Type 1: Facial stain, leptomeningeal angiomatosis ± glaucoma
  - Type 2: Facial stain only, ± glaucoma
  - Type 3: Leptomeningeal angiomatosis only (5% of all)

Microscopic Features

- Leptomeningeal angioma = multiple thin-walled vessels in enlarged sulci
- Cortical atrophy, Ca^{++}
- May have underlying cortical dysplasia

CLINICAL ISSUES

Presentation

- Most common signs/symptoms
  - Seizures (75-90%), hemiparesis (30-66%)
  - Stroke-like episodes, neurologic deficit, headaches, & intellectual disability
  - Facial capillary malformation (port-wine stain) in ~ 95%
    - V1 distribution classic
  - Choroidal angioma (70%), especially with eyelid stain
    - ↑ intraocular pressure/congenital glaucoma → buphthalmos
    - Retinal telangiectatic vessels, scleral angioma, iris heterochromia
- Clinical profile
  - Triad of port-wine stain, seizures, hemiparesis
    - 50% have extracranial port-wine stains (torso or extremities)

Demographics

- Rare: 1:20,000-50,000
- Facial lesion visible at birth
  - Leptomeningeal angiomatosis may be occult if no facial lesion & no seizures to prompt imaging
- Seizures typically develop in 1st year of life

Natural History & Prognosis

- Progression of lobar involvement & atrophy → ↑ likelihood of seizures
- Seizures exacerbate vascular compromise to affected brain → progressive brain injury
- Holohemispheric &/or bilateral involvement worse compared with focal involvement
- Progressive hemiparesis (30%), homonymous hemianopsia (2%)

Treatment

- Presymptomatic: Some recommend low-dose aspirin ± anticonvulsant
- Symptomatic: Aggressive medical management of seizures
- Symptomatic & medically refractory: Consider surgical resection/hemispherectomy

DIAGNOSTIC CHECKLIST

Consider

- Child with facial capillary stain who reaches 2 years of age with normal neurologic & MR exams probably does not have brain involvement

Image Interpretation Pearls

- FLAIR C+ most sensitive sequence to detect leptomeningeal angioma, especially in infancy
- MR in infancy may be normal; recommend follow-up if patient at risk for SWS clinically
  - ASL may increase sensitivity in young patients

SELECTED REFERENCES

1. Sánchez-Espino LF et al: Sturge-Weber syndrome: a review of pathophysiology, genetics, clinical features, and current management Approache. Appl Clin Genet. 16:63-81, 2023
2. Pouliquen G et al: Arterial spin-labeling perfusion imaging in the early stage of Sturge-Weber syndrome. AJNR Am J Neuroradiol. 43(10):1516-22, 2022
3. Yeom S et al: Updates on Sturge-Weber syndrome. Stroke. 53(12):3769-79, 2022
4. Sabeti S et al: Consensus statement for the management and treatment of Sturge-Weber syndrome: neurology, neuroimaging, and ophthalmology Recommendations. Pediatr Neurol. 121:59-66, 2021
5. Bar C et al: Early magnetic resonance imaging to detect presymptomatic leptomeningeal angioma in children with suspected Sturge-Weber syndrome. Dev Med Child Neurol. 62(2):227-33, 2020
6. Warne RR et al: The bone does not predict the brain in Sturge-Weber syndrome. AJNR Am J Neuroradiol. 39(8):1543-9, 2018
7. Zallmann M et al: Retrospective review of screening for Sturge-Weber syndrome with brain magnetic resonance imaging and electroencephalography in infants with high-risk port-wine stains. Pediatr Dermatol. 35(5):575-81, 2018
8. Zallmann M et al: Screening for Sturge-Weber syndrome: a state-of-the-art review. Pediatr Dermatol. 35(1):30-42, 2018

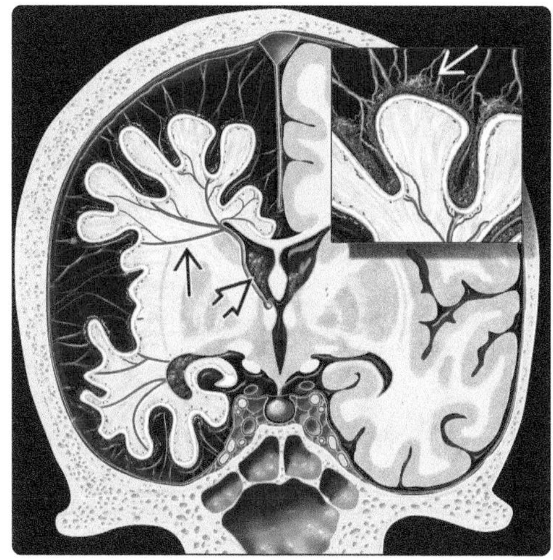

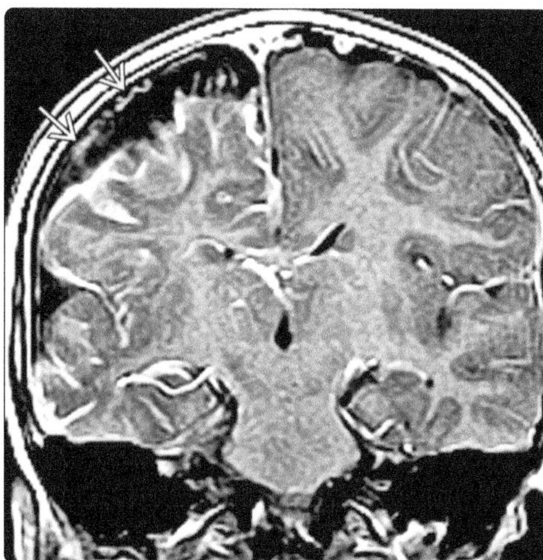

(Left) *Coronal graphic shows extensive pial angiomatosis ➔ surrounding affected gyri. There are prominent medullary venous collaterals ➔ shunting venous blood to the deep system. The ipsilateral choroid plexus is enlarged ➔, & there is atrophy of the right cerebral hemisphere. These findings are all characteristic of SWS.* **(Right)** *Coronal T1 C+ MR shows right frontal atrophy, extensive pial enhancement, & involvement of the prominent overlying subarachnoid space by pial angiomatosis ➔.*

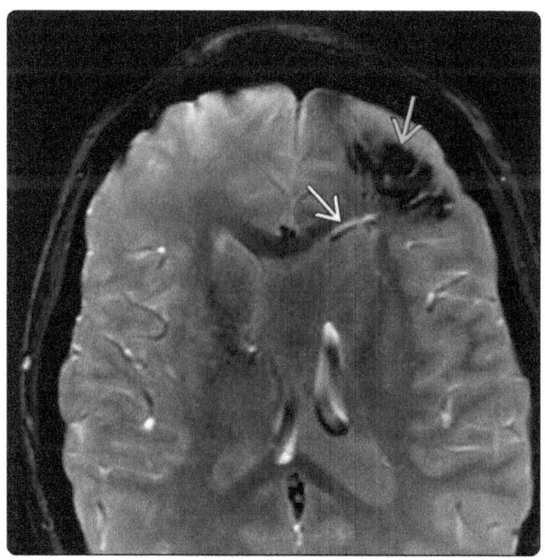

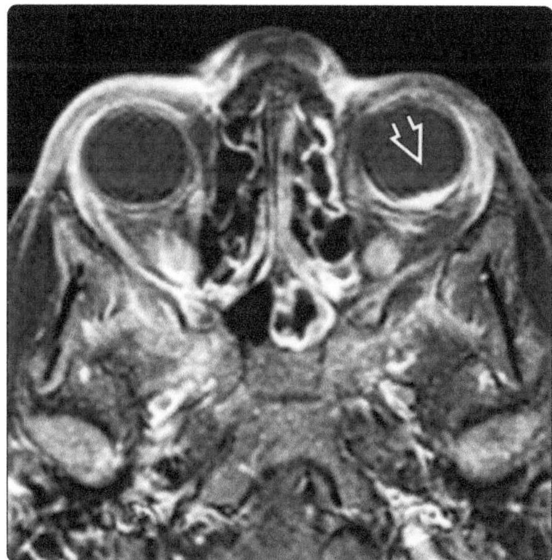

(Left) *Axial SWI MR in a 10-year-old boy with right-sided hemiplegia & seizures shows contiguous loss of signal ➔ within the subcortical white matter of the left frontal lobe, suggesting Ca^{++}. Also note the enlarged subependymal vein ➔ in the left frontal horn.* **(Right)** *Axial T1 C+ FS MR in a 10-year-old with SWS shows orbital involvement by choroidal angioma, revealed as crescentic enhancement ➔ of the posterior left choroid. One should look for orbital enhancement, as it indicates ↑ risk of intraocular pressure & glaucoma.*

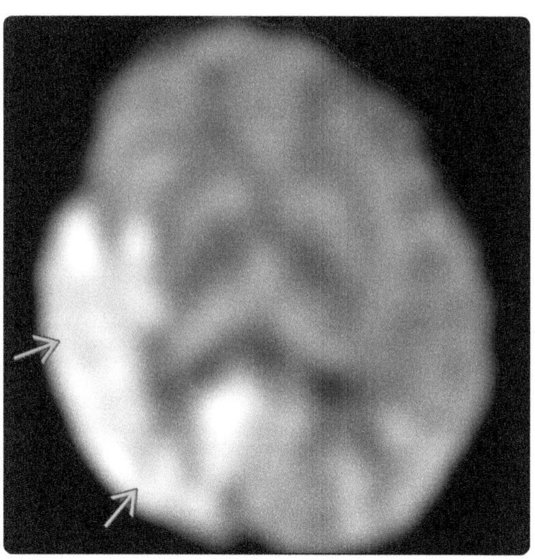

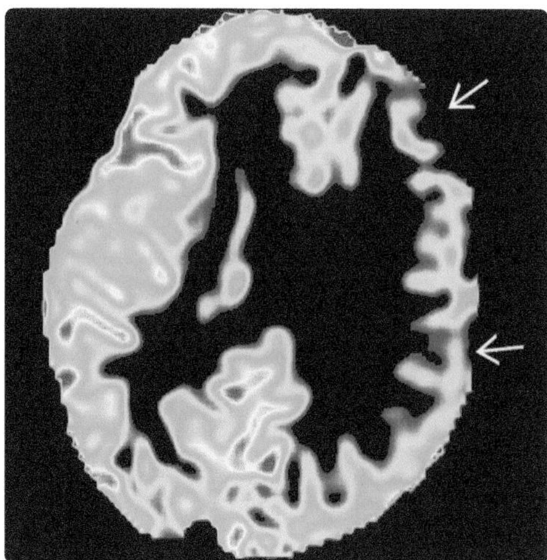

(Left) *Axial ASL perfusion MR in a 10-month-old with SWS and extensive right temporal and occipital leptomeningeal angiomatosis ➔ shows a geographic area of ↑ cerebral blood flow (CBF) in the affected areas. This is an atypical appearance. Most SWS patients have ↓ CBF in affected regions even early in the disease.* **(Right)** *Axial ASL MR perfusion MR in the same patient with right-sided hemiplegia & seizures shows substantially ↓ perfusion ➔ in the left frontal lobe that is affected by leptomeningeal angiomatosis.*

KEY FACTS

TERMINOLOGY

- Benign hamartomatous cortical, subcortical white matter (WM) lesion with leptomeningeal vascular malformation

IMAGING

- Cortical/subcortical WM mass characterized by Ca^{++}, enhancing meningovascular proliferation
- NECT: Linear, gyriform, or nodular Ca^{++}
- MR
  - T1WI: Cortex isointense, WM hypointense
  - T2/FLAIR: Cortex hypointense, WM hyperintense
  - T1 C+: Slight gyriform + meningeal enhancement

TOP DIFFERENTIAL DIAGNOSES

- Meningioma
- Oligodendroglioma
- Sturge-Weber disease
- Other: Dysembryoplastic neuroepithelial tumor (DNET), granuloma, parasites, ganglioglioma

PATHOLOGY

- Uncertain etiology: Hamartoma, meningioma invading brain, or vascular malformation
- Association with neurofibromatosis (NF), particularly NF2
- Gross appearance
  - Vascular-appearing gyriform mass in cortex, subcortical WM
- Microscopic
  - Proliferation of meningothelial cells, irregularly branched blood in both cortex, subcortical WM
  - No malignant degeneration

CLINICAL ISSUES

- Gross total resection for treatment of seizure disorder; excellent prognosis with excision

DIAGNOSTIC CHECKLIST

- Consider meningioangiomatosis for calcified cortical/subcortical WM mass ± gyriform enhancement

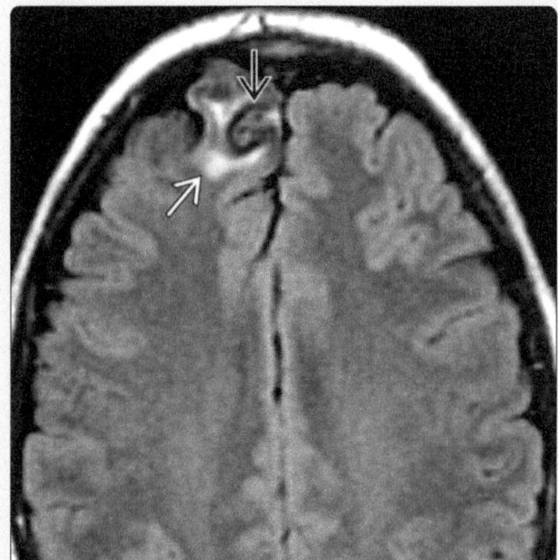
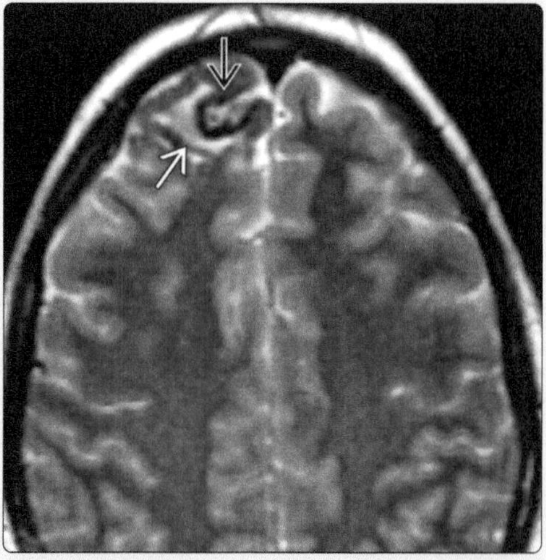

(Left) *Axial FLAIR MR in a pediatric patient with longstanding intractable seizures demonstrates subcortical gyriform hyperintensity* ➡ *with gyral distortion and linear hypointensity* ⇨ *representing* Ca^{++}. **(Right)** *Axial T2 MR in the same patient confirms a serpiginous peripheral right frontal lobe mixed signal intensity lesion* ➡ *with cortical hypointensity and subcortical hyperintensity. The hypointense region* ⇨ *corresponds to* Ca^{++} *detected on NECT (not shown).*

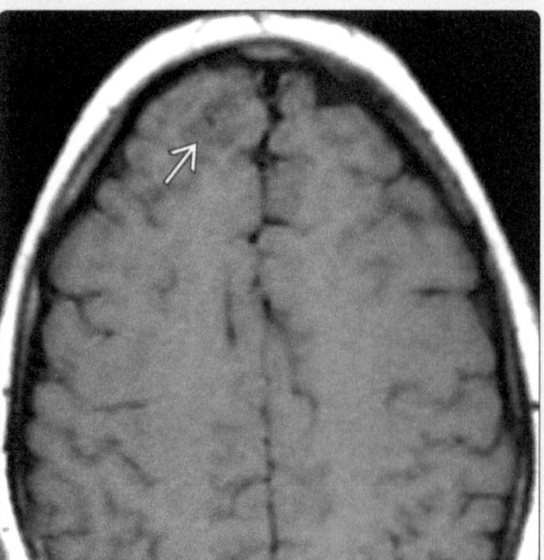
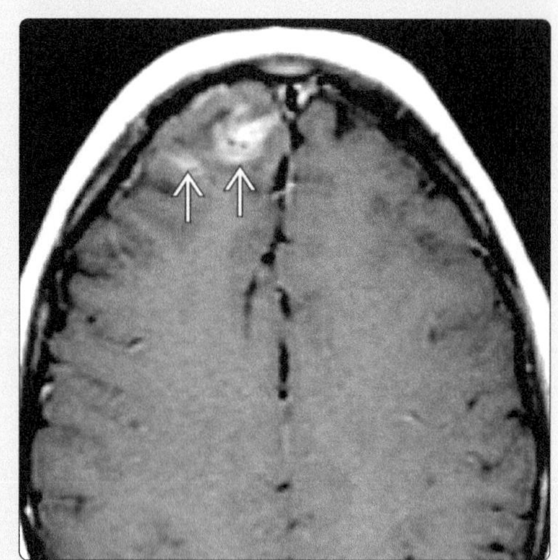

(Left) *Axial T1 MR in the same patient reveals hypointense subcortical signal with distorted cortical morphology* ➡. *The lesion is relatively subtle on T1 MR compared to FLAIR and T2 MR.* **(Right)** *Axial T1 C+ MR in the same patient confirms serpentine and nodular cortical and meningeal enhancement* ➡ *corresponding to the gyriform lesion demonstrated on nonenhanced imaging.*

TERMINOLOGY

Abbreviations

- Meningioangiomatosis (MA)

Definitions

- Benign hamartomatous cortical, subcortical white matter (WM) lesion with meningovascular proliferation
- Types
  - Sporadic MA
  - Neurofibromatosis (NF)-associated MA
  - Multifocal MA
  - Cystic MA
  - Meningioma-associated MA (MA-M)
  - MA with focal cortical dysplasia
  - MA associated with other neoplasms

IMAGING

General Features

- Best diagnostic clue
  - Cortical/subcortical WM mass with Ca^{++}, enhancing meningovascular proliferation
- Location
  - ~ 90% involve subcortical WM
  - 50% involve cortex (frontal, temporal lobes most common)

CT Findings

- NECT
  - Solitary, hyperdense, frequently calcified mass

MR Findings

- T1WI
  - Cortical component isointense to gray matter (GM); WM component hypointense
- T2WI
  - Cortex hypointense, WM hyperintense
  - ± hyperintense cysts, hypointense calcium
- FLAIR
  - Cortex hypointense, WM hyperintense
- T2* GRE
  - Hypointense susceptibility effects (blooms)
- T1WI C+
  - Cortex: Slight enhancement (gyriform)
  - WM: No enhancement
  - Leptomeninges variable fine linear to nodular enhancement

Imaging Recommendations

- Best imaging tool
  - Multiplanar MR best to demonstrate cortical abnormality, WM T2 hyperintensity, search for associated lesion
  - NECT best to demonstrate calcification

DIFFERENTIAL DIAGNOSIS

Lesions With Calcification and Cysts

- Meningioma
- Oligodendroglioma
- Granulomatous meningitis
  - Sarcoid, tuberculosis
- Parasitic diseases (cysticercosis)
- Ganglioglioma
- Sturge-Weber syndrome
- Dysembryoplastic neuroepithelial tumor (DNET)

PATHOLOGY

General Features

- Etiology
  - Theories include developmental, dysplastic, hamartoma, meningioma invading brain, or vascular malformation
    - Probably multiple etiologies depending on presence/absence of associated lesion
- Associated abnormalities
  - NF found in 1/2 of patients, particularly NF2
  - Meningioma (25%)
  - Other
    - Cortical dysplasia
    - Arteriovenous malformation
    - Encephalocele
    - Oligodendroglioma
    - Meningeal hemangiopericytoma

Gross Pathologic & Surgical Features

- Vascular-appearing cortical/subcortical mass
  - Serpentine pial vessels overlying lesion
- Psammomatous or serpentine Ca^{++}

Microscopic Features

- Proliferation of meningothelial cells, irregularly branched blood vessels in both cortex, subcortical WM
- Mass may invade underlying brain by infiltrating along perivascular spaces

CLINICAL ISSUES

Presentation

- Most common signs/symptoms
  - Asymptomatic, found incidentally (especially with NF)
  - Intractable seizures
  - Headaches
- Clinical profile
  - Classic presentation is child or young adult presenting with intractable seizure disorder

Treatment

- Antiepileptic drugs (AEDs)
- Gross total resection for treatment of seizure disorder
  - Excellent prognosis following complete surgical excision

DIAGNOSTIC CHECKLIST

Image Interpretation Pearls

- Calcified cortical/subcortical WM mass ± gyriform enhancement

SELECTED REFERENCES

1. Mansour MA et al: Meningioangiomatosis: a rare epileptogenic brain lesion. J Clin Neurosci. 110:4-6, 2023
2. Zhang GB et al: Pure and non-pure meningioangiomatosis of 36 Chinese patients: an analysis of clinical presentation, diagnosis, histopathology and prognosis. Neurosurg Rev. 45(5):3405-15, 2022

Basal Cell Nevus Syndrome

KEY FACTS

TERMINOLOGY

- Basal cell nevus syndrome (BCNS), nevoid basal cell carcinoma syndrome (NBCCS), Gorlin syndrome, Gorlin-Goltz syndrome
- BCNS: Hereditary tumor syndrome characterized by multiple basal cell epitheliomas (BCEs)/basal cell carcinomas (BCCs), odontogenic keratocysts (OKCs), palmoplantar pits, dural Ca^{++}, ± medulloblastoma

IMAGING

- Multiple jaw cysts, prominent dural Ca^{++}, macrocephaly
- Keratocystic odontogenic tumors (OKCs) in 80-90%
  - Most patients with BCNS have OKC; 5% of patients with OKC have BCNS
- Large, uni-/multilocular, sharply marginated cysts containing unerupted teeth
- Early Ca^{++} of falx cerebri, tentorium, periclinoid ligaments (dural bridging), dura, pia, choroid plexus, and basal ganglia

TOP DIFFERENTIAL DIAGNOSES

- Prominent dural Ca^{++} (physiologic, metabolic)
- Maxillary/mandibular cyst(s)
  - Ameloblastoma
  - Dentigerous or aneurysmal bone cyst
  - Cherubism
  - Giant reparative granuloma
  - Odontogenic myxoma
  - Maxillary sinus mucocele

PATHOLOGY

- Desmoplastic medulloblastoma seen in 4-20% (1-2% of patients with medulloblastomas have BCNS)
- Mutation of inactivated tumor suppressor gene *PTCH1*
  - < 2% risk of medulloblastoma
- *SUFU* mutations common in patients without *PTCH1* mutation
  - Risk of medulloblastoma 20x higher than *PTCH1*

(Left) *Coronal T2WI MR of basal cell nevus syndrome (BCNS) shows T2-hyperintense cysts ⇨ arising from the maxillary alveolar ridges. The left-sided cyst bulges into the maxillary sinus, displacing the sinus floor superiorly. A retention cyst is seen in the right maxillary sinus ⇨. Distinguishing a retention cyst from an alveolar ridge/dental cyst is best done with coronal images.* **(Right)** *Coronal NECT in an 11-year-old with BCNS & multiple OKCs ⇨ in the bilateral maxilla & left mandible involving unerupted teeth ⇨ is shown.*

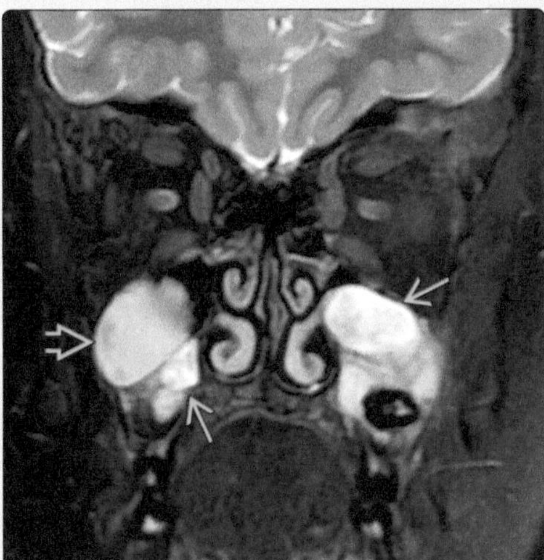

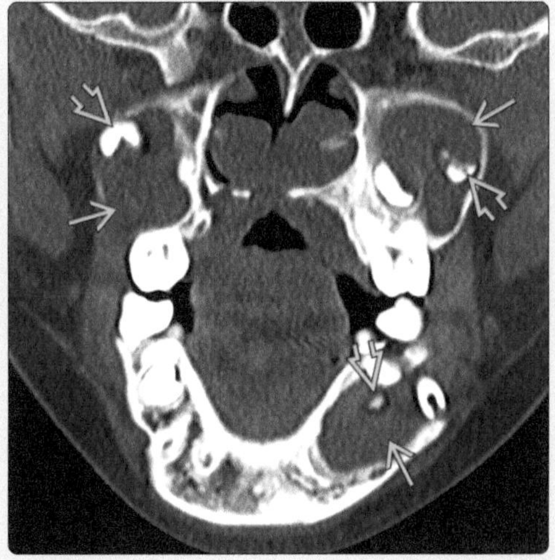

(Left) *Coronal NECT in a 16-year-old with BCNS & a left maxillary OKC ⇨ is shown. This lesion is centered about the roots of an erupted maxillary molar. OKCs usually involve roots of erupted teeth & the crowns of unerupted teeth. Note the protrusion into the maxillary sinus, a common feature of maxillary OKCs.* **(Right)** *Coronal NECT in a teen with BCNS & bilateral maxillary OKCs ⇨ is shown. Note prominent Ca^{++} within falx cerebri ⇨. The combination of dural Ca^{++} & OKCs should strongly suggest a diagnosis of BCNS.*

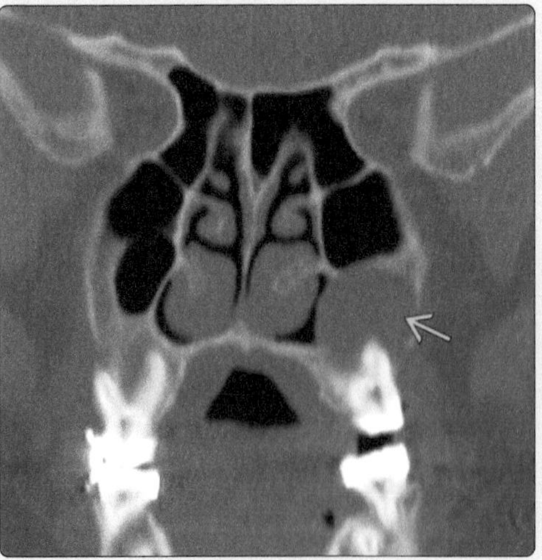

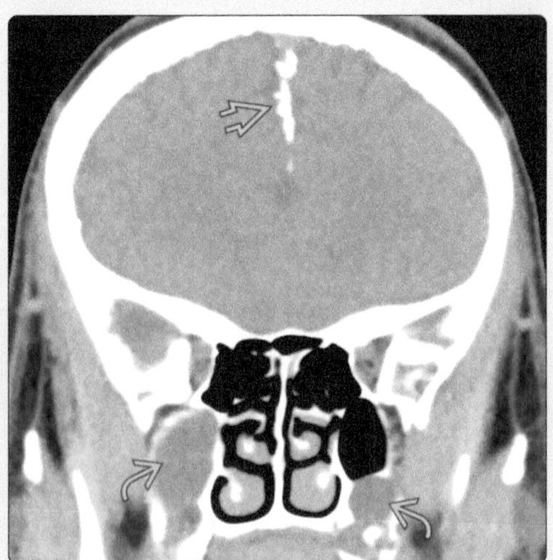

TERMINOLOGY

Abbreviations

- Basal cell nevus syndrome (BCNS)

Synonyms

- Nevoid basal cell carcinoma syndrome (NBCCS), Gorlin syndrome, Gorlin-Goltz syndrome

Definitions

- Hereditary tumor syndrome characterized by multiple basal cell epitheliomas (BCEs)/basal cell carcinomas (BCCs), odontogenic keratocysts (OKCs), palmoplantar pits, dural Ca^{++}, ± medulloblastoma
  - OKCs: Previously known as keratocystic odontogenic tumor (KCOT) prior to 2017

IMAGING

General Features

- Best diagnostic clue
  - Multiple jaw cysts, prominent dural Ca^{++}, macrocephaly
  - Other skeletal features: Hyperaerated paranasal sinuses, splayed/fused/bifid ribs, kyphoscoliosis, platybasia, Sprengel deformity of scapulae
- Location
  - Cysts: Mandible, maxilla
  - Ca^{++}: Intracranial dura
- Size
  - Variable enlargement of mandible, maxilla

Radiographic Findings

- Radiography
  - Diffuse, tiny, lytic (kerato-) cysts of bones (35%), especially jaws

CT Findings

- NECT
  - OKCs in 80-90%
    - Large, uni-/multilocular, sharply marginated cysts containing teeth
      - Surround roots in erupted teeth
      - Surround crowns of unerupted teeth
    - Mandible > maxilla
  - Early Ca^{++} of falx cerebri, tentorium, periclinoid ligaments (dural bridging), dura, pia, choroid plexus, and basal ganglia
  - ± ventriculomegaly
  - ± callosal dysgenesis
  - Cysts of all kinds common
- CECT
  - Look for
    - Medulloblastoma in cerebellar hemisphere [sonic hedgehog (SHH) subtype]
    - Meningioma
    - Colloid cyst

MR Findings

- T1WI
  - OKCs are hypointense to isointense, contain hypointensity representing unerupted tooth
  - Look for perineural spread as loss of perineural fat
- T2WI
  - OKCs are hyperintense, contain hypointensity representing associated tooth
- T2* GRE
  - GRE/SWI most sensitive for detection of dural Ca^{++}
- T1WI C+
  - Cysts may show thin, peripheral enhancing rim
  - Look for perineural spread of head and neck BCC using fat-saturated images

Nuclear Medicine Findings

- Bone scan
  - May show ↑ uptake

Imaging Recommendations

- Best imaging tool
  - MR to screen for medulloblastoma [especially if *SUFU* (+)], cystic jaw lesions
  - CT of face for oral surgery planning
- Protocol advice
  - Low mA 2- to 3-mm axial CT of face, including mandible, coronal reformats
  - Fat-saturated T2 and T1 C+ to diagnose jaw OKCs, perineural BCC spread

DIFFERENTIAL DIAGNOSIS

Prominent Dural Calcifications

- Physiologic (usually less striking than BCNS)
- Metabolic (hyperparathyroidism, long-term hemodialysis)

Keratocystic Odontogenic Tumors (Maxillary/Mandibular Cysts)

- Best clue to differentiate OKCs in BCNS from other maxillary/mandibular cysts is multiplicity
  - OKCs are multiple in most cases of BCNS
  - Other jaw cysts listed are typically solitary
- Ameloblastoma
  - Bubbly-appearing, solitary lesion may contain unerupted tooth
  - When large, associated enhancing soft tissue mass nearly always present
  - May have enhancing solid mural nodule
- Dentigerous cyst
  - Unilocular cyst surrounding tooth crown
  - No enhancing soft tissue
- Cherubism
  - Symmetrical cystic fibrous dysplasia of mandible
- Aneurysmal bone cyst
  - Multilocular, multiseptated mass in mandible
  - Enhancing soft tissues inside and outside of bony rim
- Giant reparative granuloma
  - Solitary mass, generally solid, does not contain unerupted tooth
- Odontogenic myxoma
  - Radiolucent areas with bony trabeculations
  - Well- or poorly defined margins, aggressive growth; benign histology
- Miscellaneous maxillary masses
  - Maxillary sinus mucocele: Contains no cysts or septa; smooth expansion of sinus walls

- Incisor canal cyst: Small; found in midline anterior maxilla, posterior to incisors; water density/intensity
- Globulomaxillary cyst: Small; located between lateral incisor and canine

PATHOLOGY

General Features

- Etiology
  - PATCHED (*PTCH1*) gene encodes SHH receptor and tumor suppressor protein defective in BCNS
- Genetics
  - Autosomal dominant: Complete penetrance, variable expression
  - De novo mutations (40%)
    - New mutations ↑ with advanced paternal age
  - Mutation of inactivated tumor suppressor gene *PTCH1*
    - < 2% risk of medulloblastoma
  - *SUFU* mutations common in patients without *PTCH1* mutation
    - Risk of medulloblastoma 20x higher than *PTCH1*
- Associated abnormalities
  - Neoplasms (mutation-inactivated tumor suppressor genes)
    - Rare ameloblastoma and squamous cell cancer
    - SHH medulloblastoma: Seen in 4-20% (1-2% of patients with medulloblastomas have BCNS)
    - Cardiac, abdominal, and pelvic mesenchymal tumors
- 3x more common in mandible than in maxilla
  - Mainly in premolar and retromolar triangle area
- Usually multiple, small or large, unilocular or multilocular
- May cross midline

Staging, Grading, & Classification

- Need either 2 major or 1 major/2 minor criteria for diagnosis
- Major criteria: > 2 (or 1 < 30 years) BCCs; > 10 basal cell nevi; OKC or polyostotic bone cyst; ≥ 3 palmar/plantar pits; lamellar or (< 20 years) falx Ca^{++}; family history
- Minor criteria: Rib or vertebral anomalies, macrocrania/frontal bossing; cardiac or ovarian fibromas; mesenteric cysts; facial clefting (5-13%), hand (long fingers, short 4th metacarpal, polydactyly) or ocular anomalies; bridging of sella turcica, medulloblastoma

Gross Pathologic & Surgical Features

- OKC: Expansile mandible &/or maxillary cysts with unerupted tooth
  - Satellite cyst formation is common; may involve coronoid process
  - Maxillary canine/premolar area > retromolar

Microscopic Features

- OKC: Parakeratinized lining and ↑ epithelial growth factor receptor

CLINICAL ISSUES

Presentation

- Most common signs/symptoms
  - Jaw and maxilla deformity with pain
- Desmoplastic medulloblastoma in boys 2 years of age and younger (before syndrome apparent)
  - Beware: Irradiation induced ↑ number of BCC
- BCE (75%) onset at puberty, resemble nevi or skin tags; BCC by 40 years of age
- Skin (other): Epidermal (kerato-) cysts (55%), milia, fibromas, lipomas
- Palmar and plantar pits (> 85%): Usually noticed after childhood
- Multiple OKCs that may fracture or become infected
- Dysmorphic facies, large head/brow, everted mandibular angle, hypertelorism, lip clefts common, macrosomia, tall stature
- Cognition normal if no malformations/tumors and no prior irradiation (intellectual disability in 5%)

Demographics

- Age
  - Usually diagnosed during 1st decade of life
    - OKC usually forms before 7 years of age
- Sex
  - No predilection
- Ethnicity
  - No predilection
- Epidemiology
  - 1 in 57,000 (1 in 200 with BCC have BCNS, 1 in 5 if < 19 years old)
  - Most patients with BCNS have OKC; 5% of patients with OKC have BCNS

Natural History & Prognosis

- Develop enormous numbers of BCCs
  - Especially lighter skin, sun exposure, irradiation
  - Darkly pigmented skin is protective, has smaller numbers of BCCs

Treatment

- Surgery for OKC; surgery/chemotherapy, avoid radiotherapy for medulloblastoma
- Vismodegib: New targeted medical therapy that inhibits hedgehog pathway
  - Reduction in basal cell tumor burden in BCNS patients

DIAGNOSTIC CHECKLIST

Consider

- When precocious dural Ca^{++} and OKC are detected

Image Interpretation Pearls

- Multiple mandibular cysts containing teeth or parts of teeth

SELECTED REFERENCES

1. Verkouteren BJA et al: A guideline for the clinical management of basal cell naevus syndrome (Gorlin-Goltz syndrome). Br J Dermatol. 186(2):215-26, 2022
2. Kloth K et al: Defining the spectrum, treatment and outcome of patients with genetically confirmed Gorlin syndrome from the HIT-MED cohort. Front Oncol. 11:756025, 2021
3. Verkouteren BJA et al: Prevalence of medulloblastoma in basal cell nevus syndrome patients with a PTCH1 mutation. Neuro Oncol. 23(6):1035-6, 2021
4. Sivapathasundharam B et al: The World Health Organization classification of odontogenic and maxillofacial bone tumors: an appraisal. J Oral Maxillofac Pathol. 23(2):178-86, 2019
5. Akbari M et al: Basal cell nevus syndrome (Gorlin syndrome): genetic insights, diagnostic challenges, and unmet milestones. Pathophysiology. 25(2):77-82, 2018

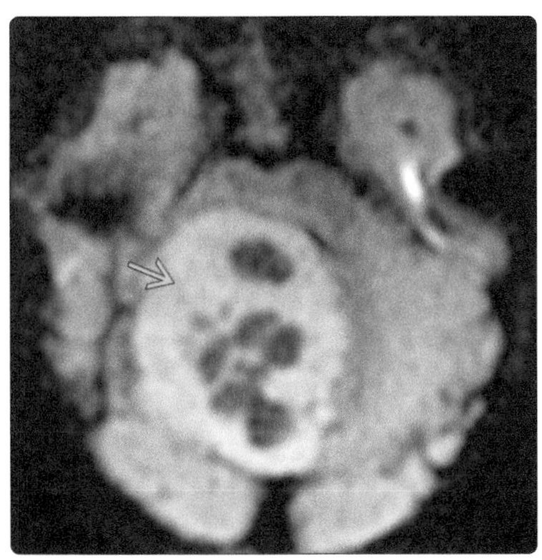

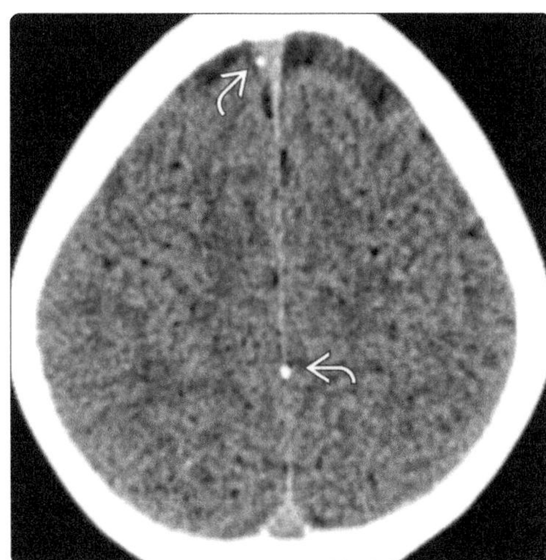

(Left) *Axial DWI MR in a 1-year-old with BCNS & medulloblastoma shows a highly cellular mixed solid & cystic tumor arising from the right cerebellar hemisphere. Medulloblastoma is highly associated with BCNS patients with SUFU gene mutation & is typically of the SHH molecular subtype.* **(Right)** *Axial NECT in a patient with medulloblastoma reveals 2 small dural-based Ca^{++}. Such Ca^{++} are not normal in a child of this age & should prompt a BCNS work-up.*

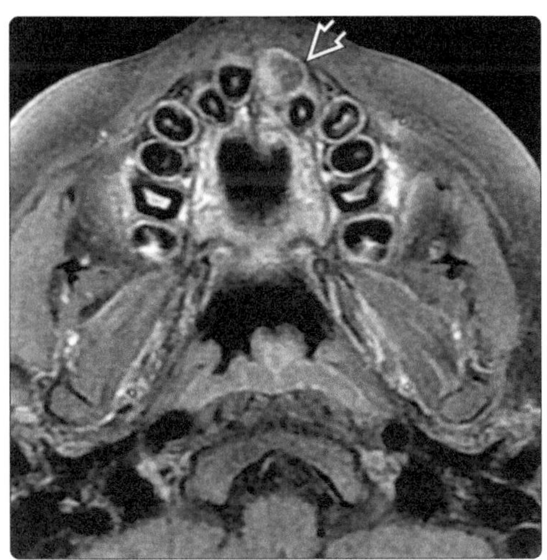

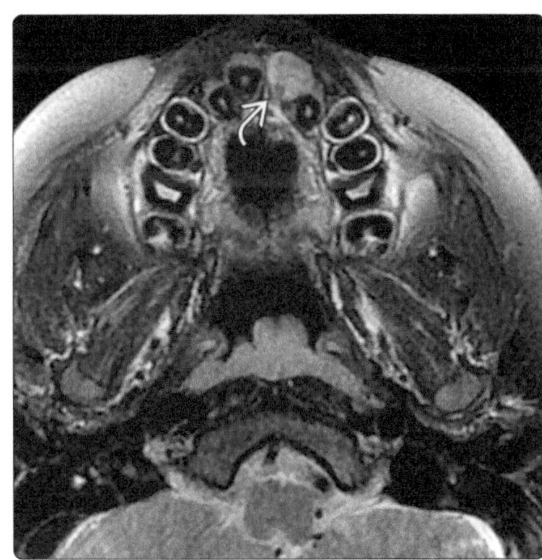

(Left) *Axial T1WI C+ FS MR in a 6-year-old child with known BCNS shows a small cystic mass in the anterior left maxillary ridge, consistent with an OKC. The cyst has a thin, faintly enhancing rim & an unerupted tooth medially. The MR was performed as a screening test for medulloblastoma.* **(Right)** *Axial T2WI FS MR in the same patient shows moderate hyperintensity of the lesion contents & a hypointense unerupted tooth medial to the lesion.*

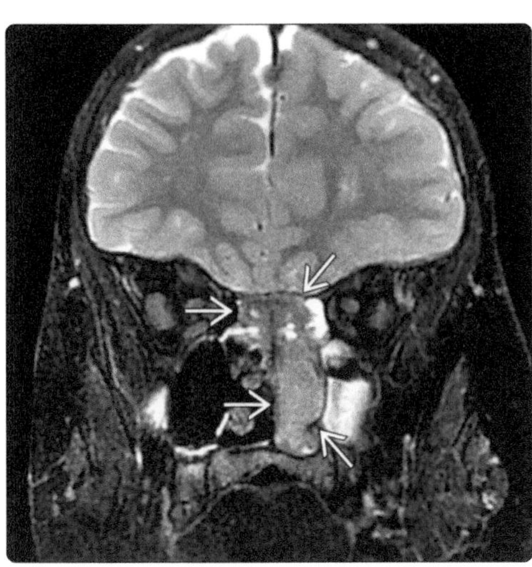

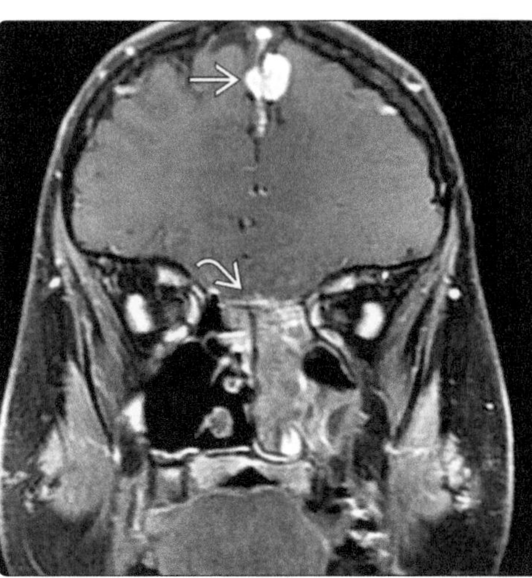

(Left) *Coronal T2WI FS MR reveals a T2-hypointense mass filling the left nasal cavity & extending into ethmoid air cells. This 19-year-old with BCNS was radiated for medulloblastoma & developed a radiation-induced rhabdomyosarcoma.* **(Right)** *Coronal T1WI C+ FS MR shows moderate enhancement of the nasal mass, which infiltrates the dura above the roof of the ethmoid air cells. A falx meningioma is also evident.*

Neurocutaneous Melanosis

KEY FACTS

TERMINOLOGY

- Neurocutaneous melanosis (NCM): Congenital phakomatosis characterized by giant or multiple cutaneous melanocytic nevi (CMN) + benign & malignant melanotic lesions of CNS
  - Parenchymal melanosis: Nonmalignant intraparenchymal foci
  - Leptomeningeal (LM) melanosis (LMs): Excess of benign melanotic cells in leptomeninges
  - LM melanoma (LMm): Malignant melanoma (MM) of leptomeninges
  - Primary CNS MM: Focal MM of CNS

IMAGING

- Parenchymal melanosis: CMN + foci of intraaxial T1 MR hyperintensity (hyperdense on CT, echogenic on US)
  - Medial temporal lobe, cerebellum, pons, thalami, base of frontal lobes
- LMs & LMm: CMN + diffuse LM enhancement
  - Typically develop communicating hydrocephalus
- MM: Focal intraparenchymal enhancing mass

PATHOLOGY

- Focal or diffuse proliferation of melanin-producing cells in both skin & leptomeninges
- Associated cerebellar hypoplasia in ~ 10%

CLINICAL ISSUES

- Only ~ 10-15% of CMN patients have NCM
  - ~ 80-90% have parenchymal melanosis
  - ~ 10% have LMs or LMm
  - ~ 1-5% have MM
- Screening recommended for CMN patients < 6 months
- Poor prognosis with LMs, LMm, or MM

DIAGNOSTIC CHECKLIST

- Normal MR does not exclude diagnosis of NCM
- LMs cannot be distinguished from LMm by imaging

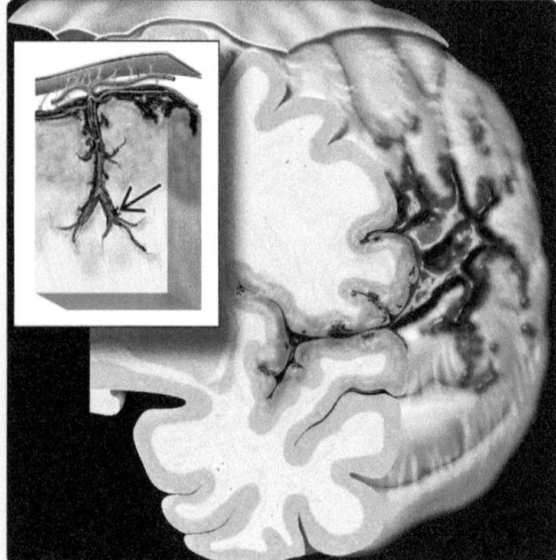

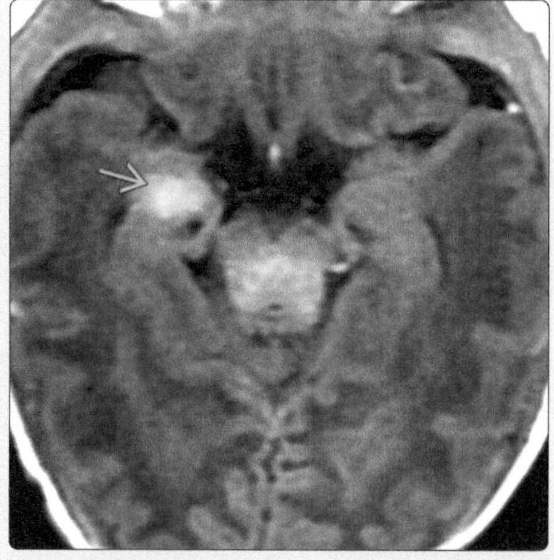

(Left) *Graphic shows localized dark (melanotic) pigmentation of the leptomeninges. Inset demonstrates extension of melanosis into the brain substance along the Virchow-Robin spaces ➞.* **(Right)** *Axial T1 MR in a 4-day-old with multiple large congenital cutaneous nevi shows a single focus of intraparenchymal hyperintense signal ➞ in the right medial temporal lobe. The medial temporal lobe is the most common location for parenchymal melanosis.*

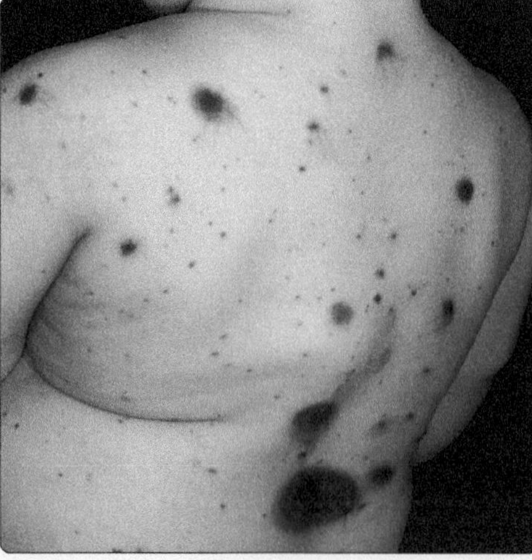

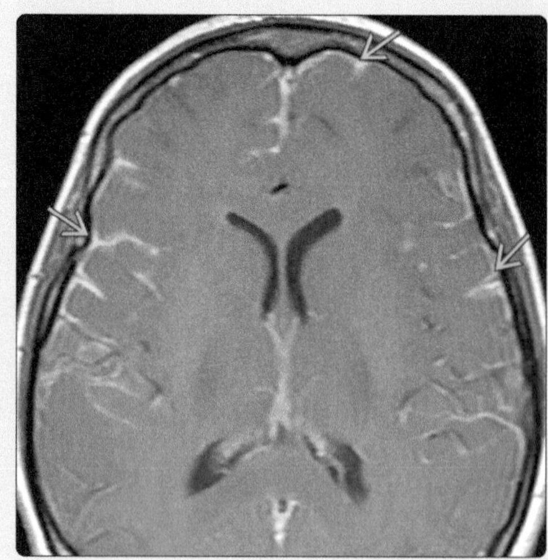

(Left) *Photograph of the back of a young child with neurocutaneous melanosis shows numerous cutaneous melanocytic nevi, many of which are several cm in size, qualifying for the distinction of "giant" nevi.* **(Right)** *Axial T1 C+ MR in a patient with headache & seizures shows extensive bilateral leptomeningeal (LM) enhancement ➞, consistent with LM melanocytosis. When LM enhancement is evident, this typically reflects a progressive disease process & poor prognosis.*

TERMINOLOGY

Abbreviations

- Neurocutaneous melanosis (NCM)

Definitions

- Congenital phakomatosis characterized by multiple congenital melanocytic nevi (CMN) + benign or malignant melanotic lesions of CNS
  - Parenchymal CNS disease
    - Melanosis: Focal collection of benign melanotic cells
    - Malignant melanoma (MM)
  - Leptomeningeal (LM) CNS disease
    - LM melanosis (LMs): Excess of benign melanotic cells in leptomeninges
    - LM melanoma (LMm): MM of leptomeninges

IMAGING

General Features

- Best diagnostic clue
  - CMN + intraparenchymal foci of T1 MR hyperintensity
  - CMN + diffuse LM enhancement
- Location
  - Parenchymal melanosis: Medial temporal lobe, cerebellum, pons, thalami, base of frontal lobes
  - LMs or LMm: Diffuse LM involvement; rarely focal
  - MM: Temporal lobe most common
- Size
  - Parenchymal melanosis: Foci usually < 1 cm
  - MM: Foci typically several cm
- Morphology
  - Parenchymal melanosis: Round or oval lesions, sometimes curvilinear in cortex
  - LMs/LMm: Linear or nodular (bulky)
  - MM: Large, round mass
- Patients with LMs & LMm typically develop communicating hydrocephalus
- Spinal involvement (LM enhancement, intra- or extramedullary cyst, syrinx, arachnoiditis) in ~ 20%
- Associated abnormalities: Hindbrain involvement is associated with cerebellar & brainstem hypoplasia

CT Findings

- NECT
  - Parenchymal melanosis: Normal or hyperdense foci
  - MM: Hyperdense mass with edema, mass effect; frequent necrosis/hemorrhage
- CECT
  - Parenchymal melanosis: No enhancement
  - LMs: Normal or diffuse LM enhancement
  - LMm: Diffuse LM enhancement
  - MM: Typically avid enhancement, often heterogeneous

MR Findings

- T1WI
  - Parenchymal melanosis: Hyperintense
  - LMs/LMm: Sulci/cisterns normal or iso- or hyperintense
  - MM: Mixed signal intensity; frequently hyperintense
- T2WI
  - Parenchymal melanosis: Mixed signal intensity, frequently hypointense; no edema or mass effect
  - LMs/LMm: Sulci/cisterns normal or iso- or hypointense
  - MM: Mixed signal intensity with edema, mass effect; frequent necrosis, hemorrhage
- FLAIR
  - LMm/LMs: Variable LM hyperintensity
- T2* GRE
  - Blooming of hemorrhage > melanin
- T1WI C+
  - Parenchymal melanosis: No enhancement
  - LMs: Normal or diffuse LM enhancement
  - LMm: Diffuse LM enhancement
  - MM: Typically avid enhancement, often heterogeneous
  - May see cutaneous enhancement of melanotic lesions
- Stable free radicals in melanin responsible for MR appearance

Ultrasonographic Findings

- Hyperechoic foci of parenchymal melanosis

Imaging Recommendations

- Best imaging tool
  - C+ MR brain & spine before 6 months of age
    - If normal: No routinely scheduled MR exams
    - Parenchymal melanosis only: Yearly clinical follow-up, MR if neurologic symptoms arise
    - LMs: Multidisciplinary clinical care
- Protocol advice
  - MR screening for asymptomatic infants with multiple large CMN
  - Parenchymal melanosis more conspicuous prior to myelination

DIFFERENTIAL DIAGNOSIS

T1-Hyperintense Mass

- Lipoma: Chemical shift artifact, extraaxial (subarachnoid) location, drops signal with fat suppression
- Dermoid: Chemical shift artifact, extraaxial location, sharply demarcated, exerts mass effect, drops signal with fat suppression
- Acute/subacute hemorrhage: Marked T2 hypointensity, mass effect/edema, neurologic deficit
- Hemorrhagic, nonmelanotic neoplasms: Areas of marked T2 hypointensity, mass effect/edema

Diffuse Leptomeningeal Enhancement

- Carcinomatous meningitis/CSF seeding: History of primary malignancy, linear/nodular LM enhancement
- Infectious meningitis (bacterial, TB, coccidioidomycosis): Basal cisterns, linear enhancement, signs/symptoms of meningitis; (+) CSF cultures
- Noninfectious inflammation (sarcoidosis, Wegener granulomatosis): Linear/nodular enhancement

PATHOLOGY

General Features

- Etiology
  - Focal or diffuse proliferation of melanin-producing cells in both skin & leptomeninges

- Pathologic presence of melanotic cells in Virchow-Robin (VR) spaces
- Results from error in morphogenesis of embryonic neuroectoderm
- LMm/MM: Degeneration (anaplasia) of melanotic cells
- Hydrocephalus found in 2/3 of symptomatic NCM: Obstruction of CSF flow at basal cisterns & arachnoid granulations
- Genetics
  - Majority sporadic: May survive autosomal lethal gene by somatic mosaicism
  - Deregulation of hepatocyte growth factor/scatter factor receptor may play role
  - Caused by postzygotic mutations in codon 61 of *NRAS* gene
- Associated abnormalities
  - Cerebellar hypoplasia (< 10%)
    - Abnormal meningeal cells causally related to hindbrain malformations
- Embryology
  - Neural crest-derived primordial cells migrate & differentiate into melanocytes in pia mater & basal layer of epidermis
- Anatomy
  - Melanocytes normally present in pia mater over convexities, base of brain, ventral brainstem, upper cervical cord, & lumbosacral spinal cord
  - Melanocytes normally surround blood vessels but do not extend into VR spaces

Staging, Grading, & Classification

- Criteria for diagnosis
  - Giant or multiple (≥ 3) cutaneous melanocytic nevi
    - Child: 6-cm body, 9-cm head maximal diameter
    - Adult: 20-cm maximal diameter

Gross Pathologic & Surgical Features

- Parenchymal melanosis: Focal, abnormal pigmentation within brain
- LMs/LMm: Darkly pigmented, thickened pia mater
- MM: Pigmented mass, ± necrosis, hemorrhage
- CMN: Giant or multiple pigmented, hairy nevi

Microscopic Features

- Parenchymal melanosis: Melanotic cells & melanin-laden macrophages in VR spaces & parenchyma
- Benign LMs difficult to differentiate from LMm histologically
  - Indicators of malignancy: Necrosis, hemorrhage, basal lamina invasion, cellular atypia, frequent mitoses, presence of annulate lamellae

CLINICAL ISSUES

Presentation

- Most common signs/symptoms
  - Parenchymal melanosis: Most asymptomatic; 25% with seizures; 30% with developmental delay
  - LMs, LMm: Seizures & symptoms of ↑ intracranial pressure (vomiting, headache, macrocranium, lethargy)
    - Almost uniformly symptomatic
- CSF (symptomatic NCM): ↑ protein, ↓ glucose, ± benign/malignant melanotic cells

Demographics

- Age
  - Symptomatic NCM typically manifests by 2-3 years of age
- Epidemiology
  - CMN: 1 in 20,000-500,000 live births
    - Parenchymal melanosis: ~ 10% of patients with CMN
    - LMs, LMm: ~ 1-2% of patients with CMN
    - CNS MM: < 1%

Natural History & Prognosis

- Natural history
  - CMN (isolated or with NCM): ~ 5% lifetime risk of malignant degeneration (melanoma)
  - Parenchymal melanosis: Typically stable over time
    - Few reports of regression or degeneration into MM
- Prognosis
  - Parenchymal melanosis: Good prognosis (death related to NCM rare)
  - LMs or LMm: Poor prognosis
  - CNS MM: Poor prognosis

Treatment

- Parenchymal melanosis: No treatment or follow-up imaging recommended unless patient becomes symptomatic
- LMs: Often requires ventricular shunting for hydrocephalus
- LMm: Shunting, XRT, ± systemic/intrathecal chemotherapy
- CNS MM: Surgery, XRT, ± systemic/intrathecal chemotherapy

DIAGNOSTIC CHECKLIST

Image Interpretation Pearls

- Normal MR does not exclude diagnosis of NCM
- LMs cannot be distinguished from LMm by imaging
  - Both carry poor prognosis

SELECTED REFERENCES

1. Neale H et al: Central nervous system magnetic resonance imaging abnormalities and neurologic outcomes in pediatric patients with congenital nevi: a 10-year multi-institutional retrospective study. J Am Acad Dermatol. 87(5):1060-8, 2022
2. Qazi SS et al: Primary leptomeningeal melanoma in association with neurocutaneous melanosis: a case report. Surg Neurol Int. 13:547, 2022
3. Rahman RK et al: Neurosurgical management of patients with neurocutaneous melanosis: a systematic review. Neurosurg Focus. 52(5):E8, 2022
4. Mormina E et al: Imaging and clinical features of neurocutaneous melanosis in the pediatric population. Curr Med Imaging. 17(12):1391-402, 2021
5. Chen L et al: Neurocutaneous melanosis in association with large congenital melanocytic nevi in children: a report of 2 cases with clinical, radiological, and pathogenetic evaluation. Front Neurol. 10:79, 2019
6. Jakchairoongruang K et al: New insights into neurocutaneous melanosis. Pediatr Radiol. 48(12):1786-96, 2018
7. Sharouf F et al: Neurocutaneous melanosis presenting with hydrocephalus and malignant transformation: case-based update. Childs Nerv Syst. 34(8):1471-7, 2018
8. Bekiesińska-Figatowska M et al: Age related changes in brain MR appearance in the course of neurocutaneous melanosis. Eur J Radiol. 85(8):1427-31, 2016
9. Barbarot S: Revisiting neurocutaneous melanosis spectrum: do we have to undertake systematic magnetic resonance imaging in children with congenital melanocytic naevi? Br J Dermatol. 173(3):639-40, 2015
10. Sibbald C et al: Neurocutaneous melanosis and congenital melanocytic naevi: a retrospective review of clinical and radiological characteristics. Br J Dermatol. 173(6):1522-4, 2015

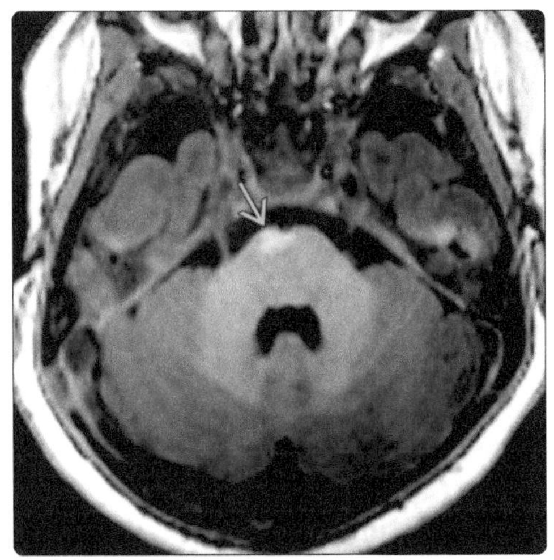

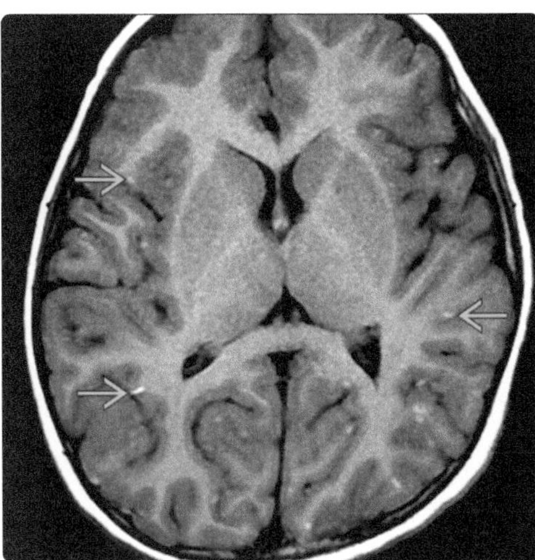

(Left) *Axial T1 MR in a 2-year-old girl shows a hyperintense focus ➡ in the anterior pons. After the amygdala, the pons is one of the more common locations for parenchymal neurocutaneous melanosis.* **(Right)** *Axial T1 MR in a 4-year-old boy with multiple large congenital cutaneous nevi shows innumerable tiny hyperintense foci ➡ within the superficial cerebrum, consistent with parenchymal melanosis.*

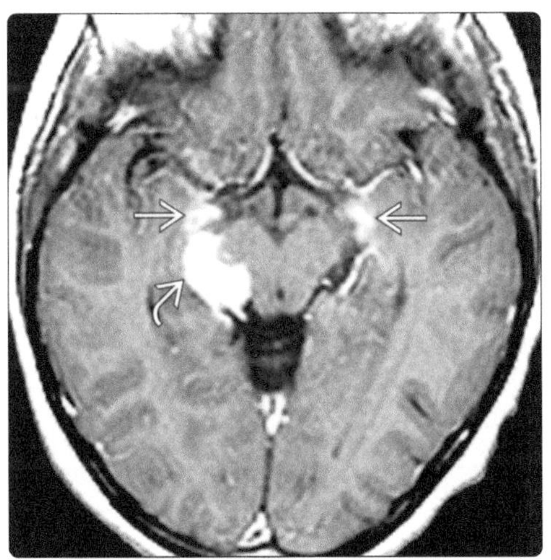

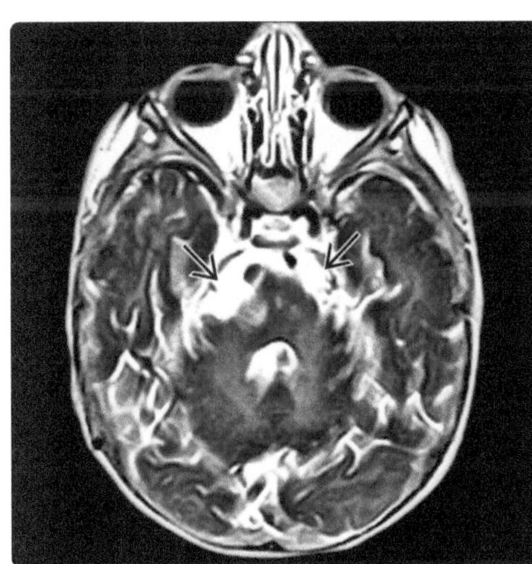

(Left) *Axial T1 C+ MR in a patient with neurocutaneous melanosis demonstrates enhancement of a LM lesion ➡. Parenchymal melanosis lesions ➡ do not enhance & are actually slightly less conspicuous, as is often the case following contrast injection.* **(Right)** *Axial T1 C+ MR in a symptomatic patient shows diffuse LM enhancement, consistent with LM melanosis or LM melanoma. Note the bulky LM enhancement in the prepontine cistern ➡.*

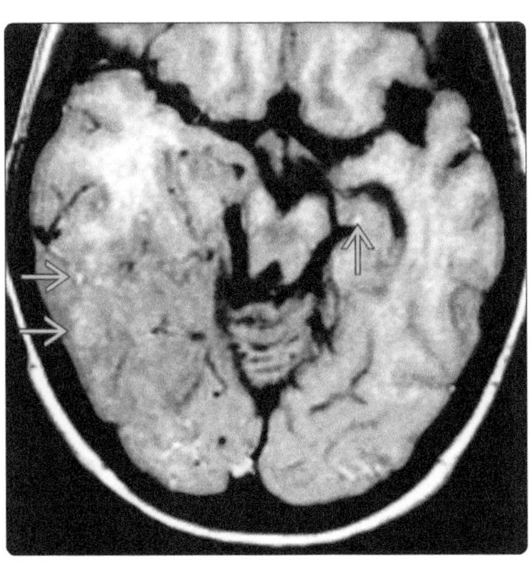

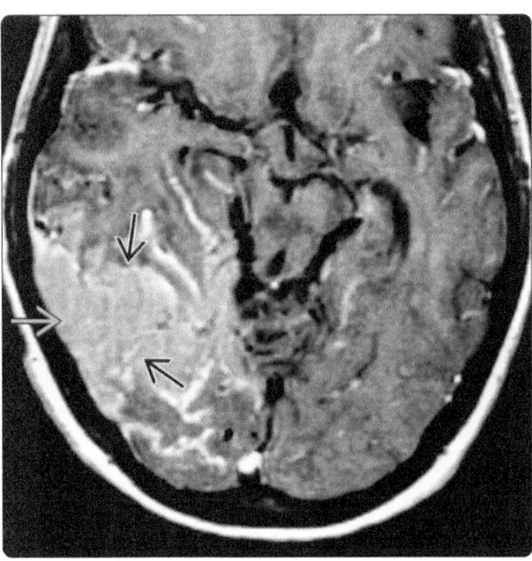

(Left) *Axial T1 MR shows significant mass effect in the right posterior temporal & occipital lobes with effacement of the surface sulci. Only minimal hyperintensity is evident, though other foci of T1 hyperintensity are seen ➡.* **(Right)** *Axial T1 C+ MR in the same patient shows a strongly enhancing superficial mass ➡ that fills the adjacent sulci & extends deeply into the underlying brain parenchyma ➡. Surgery disclosed extensive melanosis that had invaded the brain via the perivascular spaces.*

Hereditary Hemorrhagic Telangiectasia

KEY FACTS

TERMINOLOGY

- Hereditary hemorrhagic telangiectasia (HHT)
- Autosomal dominant disorder with widely distributed, multisystem angiodysplastic lesions

IMAGING

- Best diagnostic clue
  - Multiple pulmonary (pAVMs) or cerebral arteriovenous malformations (cAVMs) with recurrent epistaxis
- MR
  - Blooming of capillary telangiectasias (SWI > GRE)
    - "Fluffy" enhancement on T1 C+
  - cAVM: Nest (tangle) of flow voids, gliosis
- Useful: Multislice CT/CTA of lungs and liver

PATHOLOGY

- Genetically heterogeneous disorder caused by mutations in TGF-β/BMP signaling pathway
- 3 types of vascular malformations in HHT
  - Most common: Capillary vascular malformation (53-61%)
    - Tangle of abnormal vessels
    - No shunt, dilated feeding artery, or draining vein
  - Nidus-type AVM: (43-46%)
    - Dilated network of abnormal vessels
    - Ateriovenous (AV) shunting (early draining vein)
  - Direct high-flow AVF: (1-12%)
    - AV shunt with absence of intervening nidus

CLINICAL ISSUES

- Recurrent epistaxis from nasal mucosal telangiectasias
  - Intracranial bleed from AVM/arteriovenous fistula
  - TIA, stroke, abscess secondary to pAVMs

DIAGNOSTIC CHECKLIST

- Most common cerebral vascular malformation in HHT patients = AVM (not telangiectasia)
- Brain abscess, ischemia uncommon but serious complications in HHT patients with pAVMs

(Left) *Clinical photograph of an older adult patient with hereditary hemorrhagic telangiectasia (HHT) shows the purplish discoloration of the scalp and cheek with small mucosal telangiectasias of the nose and lip.* **(Right)** *Axial T1 C+ MR in a child with recurrent epistaxis shows an avidly enhancing lesion in the left frontal lobe.*

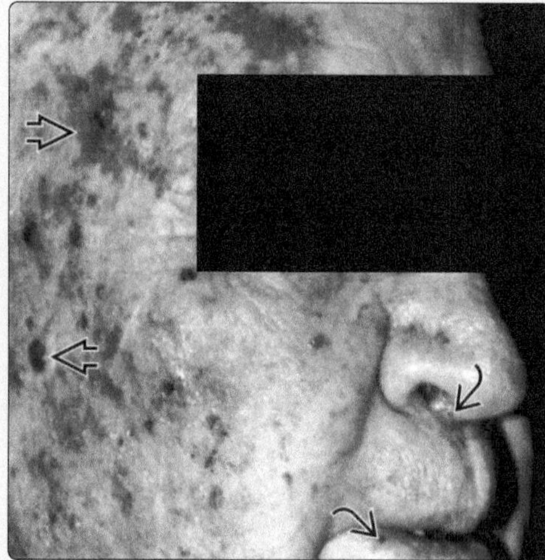

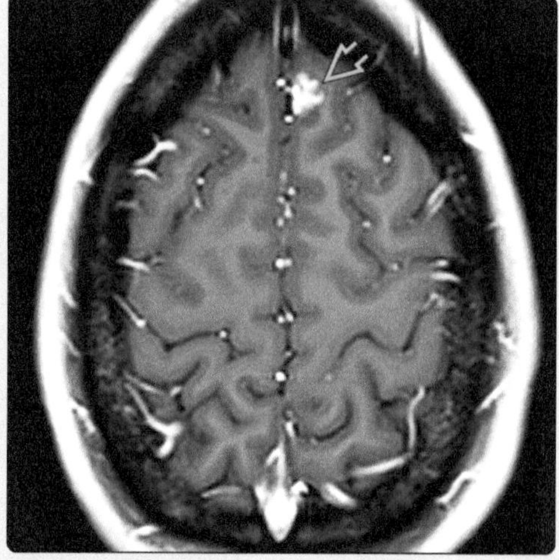

(Left) *Coronal T1 C+ MR in the same patient shows the lesion has a somewhat speckled appearance.* **(Right)** *Lateral DSA of the left internal carotid artery in the same patient shows a small arteriovenous malformation (AVM) nidus with an early draining vein, consistent with an arteriovenous (AV) shunt lesion. Genetic profiling showed ENG mutation in this patient with HHT.*

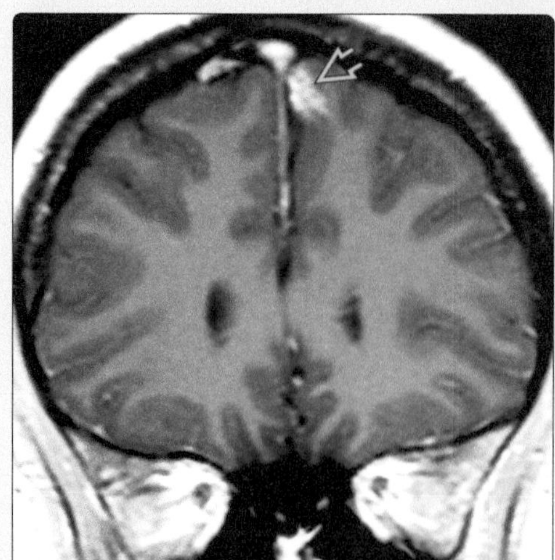

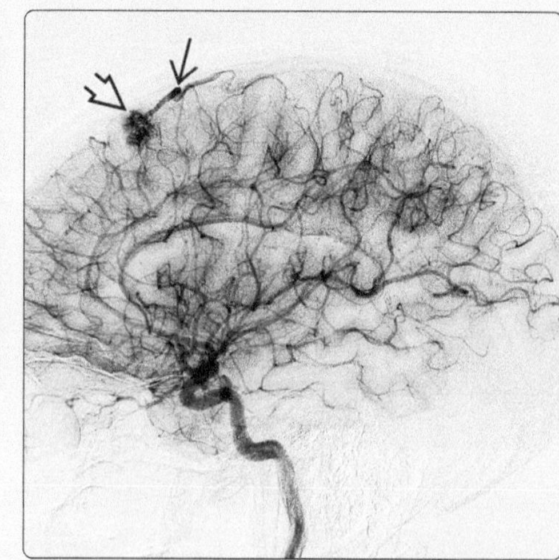

TERMINOLOGY

Abbreviations

- Hereditary hemorrhagic telangiectasia (HHT)

Synonyms

- Rendu-Osler, Rendu-Osler-Weber, Osler-Weber-Rendu syndrome

Definitions

- Autosomal dominant disorder with widely distributed, multisystem angiodysplastic lesions
  - Mucocutaneous telangiectasias and arteriovenous malformations (AVMs) in visceral organs (primarily lungs, brain, liver)

IMAGING

General Features

- Best diagnostic clue
  - Multiple pulmonary (pAVMs) or cerebral arteriovenous malformations (cAVMs) in patient with recurrent epistaxis
- Location
  - Capillary telangiectasias: Scalp, nasopharynx, orbit
  - Intracranial and spinal vascular malformations most often superficially located
- Size
  - Vascular malformations in HHT usually small (micro-AVMs or capillary vascular malformations)
    - Nidal AVMs are usually Spetzler-Martin grade 1 (~ 70-75%) or grades 2/3 (~ 20-25%)
- Morphology
  - Dilated tangle of vessels, blooming artifacts
- Number
  - Multiple vascular malformations: 44%

CT Findings

- NECT
  - Brain
    - AVM: Isodense serpentine vessels
    - Abscess: Low-density mass, iso-/hyperdense rim
- CECT
  - Brain
    - Strong, uniform vascular nidus enhancement
    - Ring enhancement of abscesses (late cerebritis, early capsule stage)
- CTA
  - Demonstrates feeders and draining veins of AVMs, arteriovenous fistulas (AVFs)
  - Visceral evaluation also needed

MR Findings

- T1WI
  - Nidus-type AVM: Flow voids common, ± hemorrhage
  - Capillary vascular malformations, developmental venous anomaly not visualized
  - Look for associated polymicrogyria, heterotopic gray matter
- T2WI
  - cAVM: Flow voids ± hemorrhage, gliosis
- FLAIR
  - cAVM: Nest (tangle) of flow voids, gliosis
- T2* GRE
  - Blooming of capillary malformations (SWI > GRE)
- PWI
  - ASL helps ↑ conspicuity of small AVMs and to distinguish capillary malformations from high-flow AVMs
- T1WI C+
  - Most sensitive sequence for vascular malformations
  - Capillary vascular malformation
    - Subcentimeter "fluffy" blush of enhancement without abnormal vascular dilation
    - Usually supratentorial, superficial
  - Delineates cAVM nidus, feeding arteries, draining veins
- MRA
  - Demonstrates intermediate to large cAVMs
  - Capillary vascular malformations usually not visualized

Angiographic Findings

- Vascular malformations shown in brain and nasal mucosa
  - Only 10-20% > 10 mm

Imaging Recommendations

- Best imaging tool
  - Brain: MR C+, T2* (SWI > GRE), ASL perfusion
    - Baseline screening in all patients with HHT or family history highly recommended (cAVMs may be devastating)
- Protocol advice
  - ASL perfusion ↑ conspicuity of small AVMs

DIFFERENTIAL DIAGNOSIS

Nasal Mucosal "Blush"

- Prominent but normal nasal mucosal "blush" can mimic capillary telangiectasia

Multiple Intracranial Arteriovenous Malformations Without Hereditary Hemorrhagic Telangiectasia

- 50% associated with other vascular neurocutaneous syndrome (Wyburn-Mason, etc.)

Multiple Intracranial Developmental Venous Anomaly

- Less common than in blue rubber bleb nevus syndrome (BRBN)

Multiple Capillary Telangiectasias

- Can be found incidentally without HHT
- Capillary telangiectasias in HHT more common outside brain (e.g., mucosa)

Multiple Cavernous Malformations

- Familial cavernous malformation syndrome
- No enhancement, marked blooming on SWI/GRE
- Unless very small, should have associated cystic change and hemosiderin ring

PATHOLOGY

General Features

- Etiology
  - Genetically heterogeneous disorder caused by mutations in TGF-β/BMP signaling pathway

- TGF-β regulates cell proliferation, differentiation, apoptosis, migration
- Abnormal TGF-β signal transduction affects
  - Vasculogenesis, angiogenesis, endothelial cell properties
- Genetics
  - Endoglin (*ENG*) mutations cause HHT1
  - Activin A receptor type II-like 1 (*ACVRL1/ALK1*) mutations cause HHT2
    - *ENG, ACVRL1* mutations detected in 85% of HHT cases (roughly = percentages)
  - *SMAD4* mutations cause combined juvenile polyposis/HHT syndrome
  - Mutations in growth differentiation factor-2 (GDF-2) cause HHT5
  - 15% of patients with HHT have no mutation in *ENG, ACVRL1*, or *SMAD4*
- Associated abnormalities
  - Malformations of cortical development (usually polymicrogyria) can be found in ~ 4-12% of cases
    - ↑ incidence of schizencephaly also recently reported

Staging, Grading, & Classification

- Most cAVMs in HHT are low grade (Spetzler-Martin 1 or 2)

Gross Pathologic & Surgical Features

- Multiple telangiectasias of mucosa, dermis, viscera
- 3 types of vascular malformations in HHT
  - Most common: Capillary vascular malformations (53-61%)
    - Tangle of abnormal vessels but no shunt, dilated feeding artery, or draining vein
  - Nidus-type AVM: 43-46%
    - Dilated network of abnormal vessels
    - Arteriovenous shunting (early draining vein)
  - Direct high-flow AVF: 1-12%
    - Shunt with absence of intervening nidus between feeding artery and draining vein
- Other associated vascular anomalies
  - Aneurysms: 2.4%
  - Cavernous malformation: 1%

Microscopic Features

- Smallest telangiectasias = focal dilatations of postcapillary venules that enlarge and extend through capillaries toward arterioles → AVF/AVM

CLINICAL ISSUES

Presentation

- Most common signs/symptoms
  - Recurrent epistaxis from nasal mucosal telangiectasias
    - 50% have nosebleeds by 10 years, 80-90% by 21 years; 95% lifetime
    - Wide variation in severity
- Other signs/symptoms
  - Telangiectasia locations
    - Lips, mouth, tongue, around nails
- Clinical profile
  - HHT diagnosis based on combination of findings (Shovlin criteria)
    - Mucocutaneous telangiectasias
    - Spontaneous/recurrent episodes of epistaxis
    - Visceral involvement
    - Family history
  - Significant phenotypic variability
    - 70% of patients with pAVMs have HHT
      - Pulmonary, brain AVMs more common in HHT1
      - 5-15% of HHT patients have pAVMs
    - > 50% of patients with multiple cAVMs have HHT
      - 5-13% of HHT patients have cAVMs (usually late in life)
    - 2-17% of HHT patients have hepatic AVMs
      - Hepatic AVMs more common in HHT2
- Neurologic symptoms common
  - Intracranial bleed from AVM/AVF
  - TIA, stroke, abscess secondary to pAVMs

Demographics

- Age
  - Epistaxis typically begins by age 10
  - Most HHT patients are symptomatic by age 21
  - Skin lesions appear later (most by age 40)
- Epidemiology
  - Rare: 1-2:10,000

Natural History & Prognosis

- Epistaxis
  - ↑ in frequency and severity
- HHT cAVMs have lower bleeding risk than sporadic AVMs
  - Rare cases may regress spontaneously
  - ↑ risk of brain abscess or stroke if pAVM present
- GI bleeding limits lifespan when < 50 years old
  - Many require multiple transfusions and endoscopies
  - Heart failure with hepatic AVM: Poor prognosis

Treatment

- pAVMs: Excellent results with embolization
  - Prophylactic antibiotics prior to all dental work
- cAVMs: Embolization vs. radiosurgery depending on size and location
- Mucosal telangiectasias (nose, GI tract): Laser coagulation
- IV iron useful if oral iron fails to maintain satisfactory level

DIAGNOSTIC CHECKLIST

Consider

- Screening brain MR in family members of HHT patients

Image Interpretation Pearls

- Most common cerebral vascular malformation in HHT patients = AVM (not telangiectasia)
- Brain abscess and ischemia uncommon but serious complication in HHT patients with pAVMs

SELECTED REFERENCES

1. Gaines JJ et al: Schizencephaly in hereditary hemorrhagic telangiectasia. AJNR Am J Neuroradiol. 43(11):1603-7, 2022
2. Hetts SW et al: Hereditary hemorrhagic telangiectasia: the convergence of genotype, phenotype, and imaging in modern diagnosis and management of a multisystem disease. Radiology. 300(1):17-30 2021
3. Kolarich AR et al: Imaging manifestations and interventional treatments for hereditary hemorrhagic telangiectasia. Radiographics. 41(7):2157-75, 2021
4. Vella M et al: Comparison of MRI, MRA, and DSA for detection of cerebral arteriovenous malformations in hereditary hemorrhagic telangiectasia. AJNR Am J Neuroradiol. 41(6):969-75, 2020

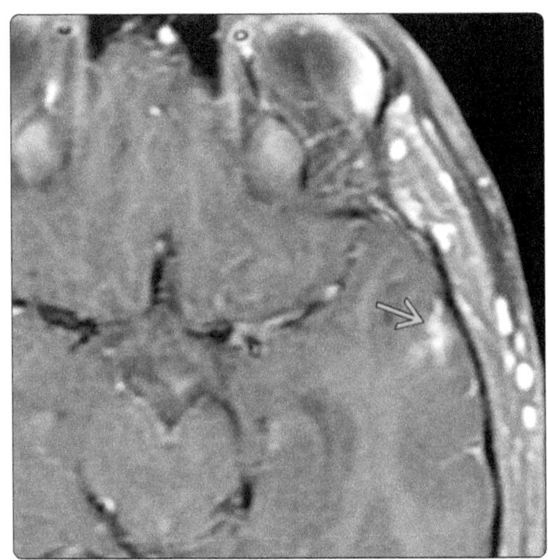

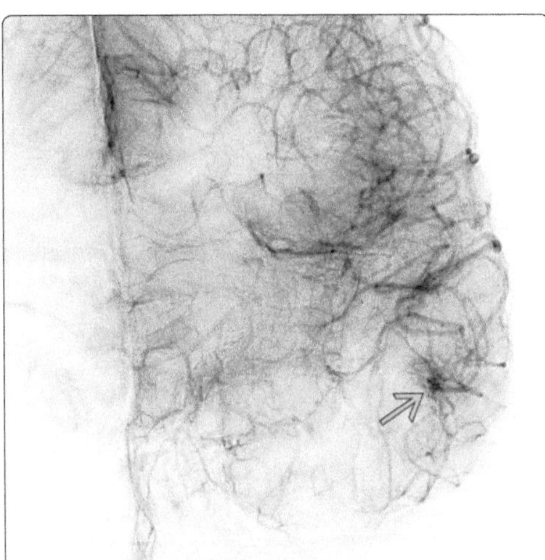

(Left) *Axial T1 C+ MR in a 14-year-old with HHT shows a hazy blush of contrast enhancement in the left superficial temporal lobe. This may represent a capillary telangiectasia or a small AVM.* **(Right)** *Frontal DSA in the same patient shows no AV shunting with the vascular lesion in the left temporal lobe opacifying at the same time as all other cerebral venous structures. These findings are consistent with a capillary malformation without AV shunting, the most common malformation seen in HHT.*

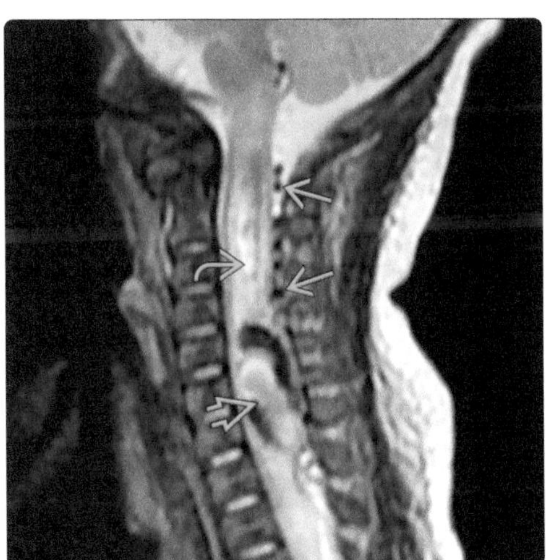

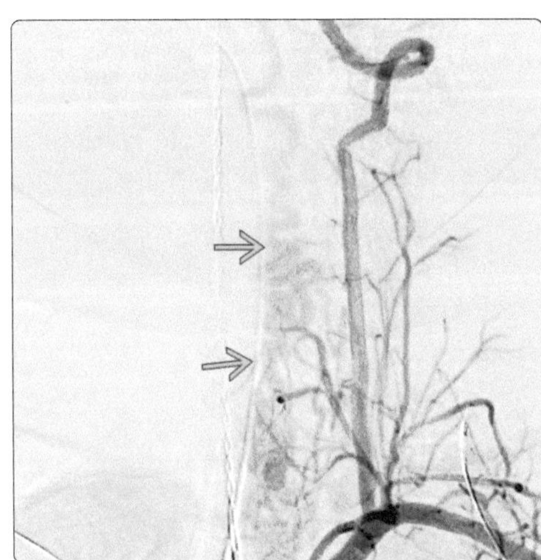

(Left) *Sagittal T2 MR in a 2-week-old with HHT shows multiple prominent flow voids along the dorsal spinal cord. Inferiorly, there is a large hemorrhagic lesion causing cord signal abnormality. Findings suggest a dural arteriovenous fistula (AVF), the least common of the vascular malformations in HHT.* **(Right)** *Frontal DSA with a left brachiocephalic injection in the same patient shows filling of the enlarged and tortuous paraspinal veins during arterial phase without an intervening nidus, confirming an AVF.*

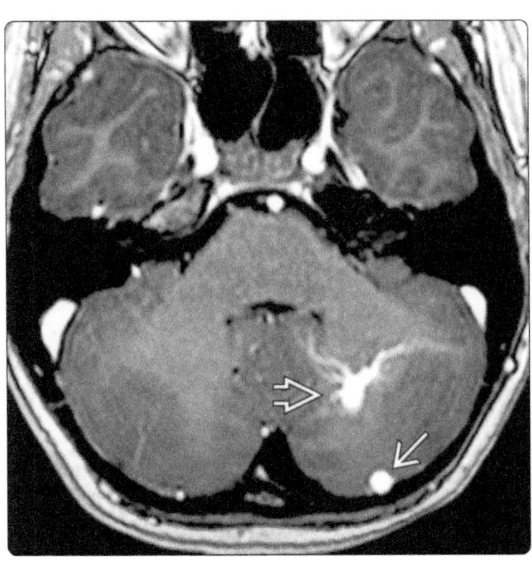

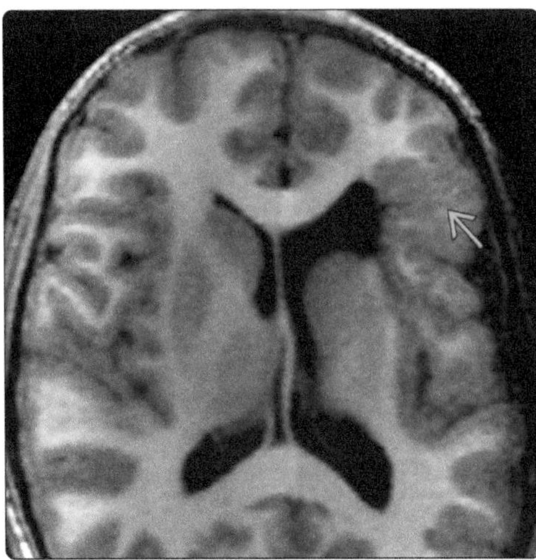

(Left) *Axial T1 C+ SPGR MR in a child with HHT shows a left cerebellar developmental venous anomaly (DVA) draining into a posterior pial vein. Although not specific, DVAs are more common in HHT than in the general population.* **(Right)** *Axial T1 MR in a 14-year-old with HHT shows left frontal closed-lip schizencephaly. Malformations of cortical development, such as schizencephaly and polymicrogyria, are reported in 4-12% of patients with HHT.*

Encephalocraniocutaneous Lipomatosis

KEY FACTS

TERMINOLOGY

- Rare congenital neurocutaneous syndrome characterized by ipsilateral scalp, eye, and brain abnormalities

IMAGING

- Cerebral hemispheric atrophy ipsilateral to scalp lipoma
- Intracranial (IC) lipomas in ~ 2/3 of patients
- Spinal lipomas/lipomatosis frequent
- Polymicrogyria of temporal, parietal, &/or occipital lobes
- ± diffuse, ipsilateral leptomeningeal enhancement
- Often associated with calvarial defects or medullary expansion

TOP DIFFERENTIAL DIAGNOSES

- Sturge-Weber syndrome
- Oculocerebrocutaneous syndrome
- Epidermal nevus syndrome
  - Ipsilateral epidermal nevus, hemimegalencephaly, facial lipoma, and hemihypertrophy
- Proteus syndrome
  - Progressive asymmetric, bilateral trunk/limb hypertrophy

PATHOLOGY

- Defect in development of mesenchymal tissues

CLINICAL ISSUES

- Newborn with nevus psiloliparus, scleral mass, and periocular papules
- Nevus psiloliparus: Sharply demarcated focus of scalp alopecia overlying scalp lipoma
  - Hallmark of encephalocraniocutaneous lipomatosis (ECCL)
- Rare; ~ 54 reported cases (likely underreported)

DIAGNOSTIC CHECKLIST

- Look carefully at scalp and calvarium when IC lipomas with associated hemicerebral atrophy/malformation are encountered

(Left) *Clinical photograph of a scalp shows the typical appearance of nevus psiloliparus, a well-circumscribed area of scalp alopecia. The nevus overlies a lipoma and is the clinical hallmark of encephalocraniocutaneous lipomatosis (ECCL).* **(Right)** *Axial NECT in a 2-year-old with ECCL shows focal lipomas in both cerebellopontine angle (CPA) cisterns ➔ and the cisterna magna ➔. Intracranial lipomas are seen in most patients with ECCL.*

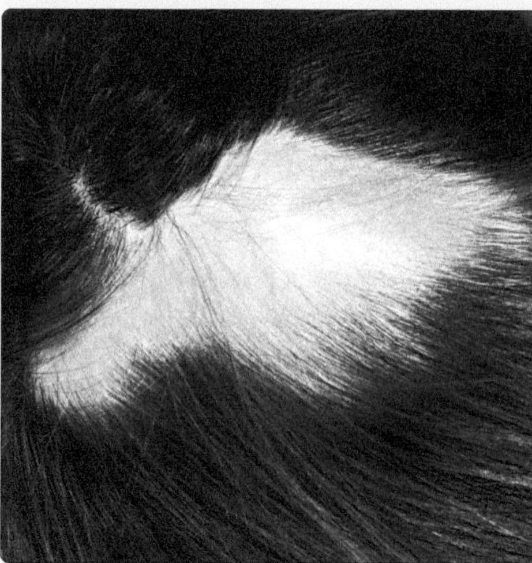

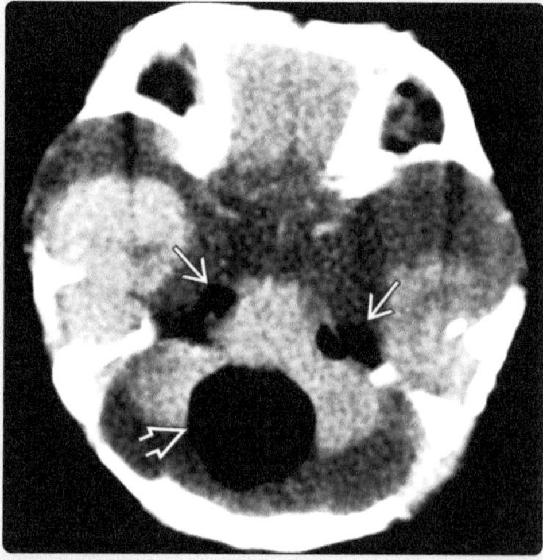

(Left) *Sagittal T1WI MR in the same patient obtained 3 years later shows a very large suboccipital lipoma ➔. The foramen magnum lipoma has massively increased in size and now occupies most of the posterior fossa ➔. The foramen magnum lipoma now extends inferiorly into the upper cervical spine ➔.* **(Right)** *Axial T1WI MR in the same patient shows how much the posterior fossa lipoma ➔ has increased in size compared to the baseline NECT. The CPA lipomas extend into Meckel caves ➔.*

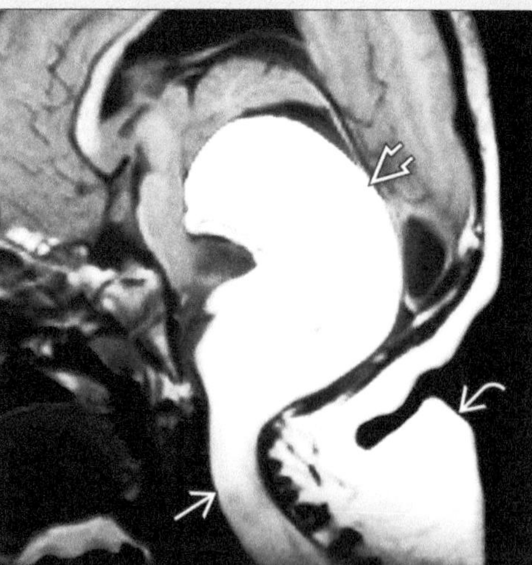

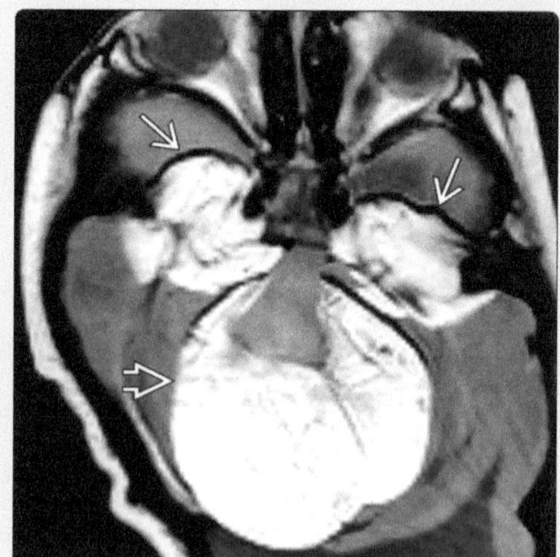

TERMINOLOGY

Abbreviations

- Encephalocraniocutaneous lipomatosis (ECCL)

Synonyms

- Haberland syndrome, Fishman syndrome

Definitions

- Rare congenital neurocutaneous syndrome characterized by ipsilateral scalp, eye, and brain abnormalities
- First described in 1970 by Catherine Haberland

IMAGING

General Features

- Best diagnostic clue
  - Unilateral cerebral hemispheric atrophy ipsilateral to scalp lipoma
  - Other frequent ipsilateral CNS abnormalities
    - Middle cranial fossa arachnoid cyst
    - Malformation of cortical development
    - Cortical Ca^{++}
  - Intracranial (IC) lipomas in ~ 2/3 of patients
  - Spinal lipomas/lipomatosis frequent; cervicothoracic > lumbar
  - Rarely, CNS abnormalities limited to IC lipoma
- Location
  - Affects skin, calvarium, and ipsilateral cerebral hemisphere
  - IC lipomas: Cerebellopontine angle (CPA), Meckel cave, foramen magnum
    - Usually ipsilateral to scalp lipoma; occasionally contra- or bilateral
  - All other CNS anomalies ipsilateral to scalp lipoma
- Morphology
  - Focal occipital lobe atrophy and occipital horn enlargement characteristic

CT Findings

- NECT
  - Hemispheric atrophy, ventriculomegaly
    - Ventriculomegaly primarily due to volume loss, although hydrocephalus occasionally present
  - Low-density scalp lipoma (may be difficult to identify, particularly if at vertex)
  - ± cortical Ca^{++}
    - Identified as early as 1st month of life, progressive
  - ± focal absence or enlargement of calvarium
    - Usually underlies scalp lipoma
- CECT
  - ± diffuse, ipsilateral leptomeningeal (LM) enhancement
- CTA
  - Arterial ectasias, pouches, and aneurysms described in older patients

MR Findings

- T1WI
  - Scalp/IC lipomas
  - Polymicrogyria of temporal, parietal, &/or occipital lobes
  - Scleral choristoma occasionally visible; heterogeneous with focal areas of hyperintensity
- T2WI
  - Cortical Ca^{++} hypointense
  - Lipomas hyperintense on T2 FSE
  - Arachnoid cysts isointense to CSF
- FLAIR
  - Nulling of signal from arachnoid cyst
- T2* GRE
  - Blooming of cortical Ca^{++}
- DWI
  - Arachnoid cyst isointense to CSF
- T1WI C+
  - ± diffuse, ipsilateral LM enhancement
- MRA
  - Arterial ectasias, pouches, and aneurysms described in older patients

Ultrasonographic Findings

- Ventriculomegaly reported on 3rd-trimester US

Angiographic Findings

- Conventional
  - Arterial ectasias, pouches, and aneurysms described in older patients

Imaging Recommendations

- Best imaging tool
  - Contrast-enhanced MR
- Protocol advice
  - Multiplanar MR with fat saturation to identify scalp lipoma (may be missed on CT)
  - MRA may disclose vascular abnormalities

DIFFERENTIAL DIAGNOSIS

Sturge-Weber Syndrome

- Unilateral hemispheric cerebral atrophy and cortical Ca^{++}, LM enhancement ipsilateral to forehead port-wine nevus
- Typically has dilated medullary veins draining to deep venous system
- Skin findings help discriminate
  - ECCL: Nevus psiloliparus; Sturge-Weber syndrome (SWS): Port-wine stain

Oculocerebrocutaneous Syndrome

- Characterized by unique cutaneous striated muscle hamartoma, cystic microphthalmia, and giant tectum absent vermis malformation
- Cortical dysplasia, agenesis of corpus callosum, and Dandy-Walker malformation frequently present
- Cutaneous, eye, and CNS anomalies usually ipsilateral but less consistently than ECCL

Epidermal Nevus Syndrome

- Ipsilateral epidermal nevus, hemimegalencephaly, facial lipoma, and hemihypertrophy
- Occasional scleral choristoma

Proteus Syndrome

- Progressive, asymmetric, bilateral trunk/limb hypertrophy
- Osteomas, lipomas, and pigmented nevi common
- CNS anomalies uncommon; hemimegalencephaly most common

PATHOLOGY

General Features

- Etiology
  - Defect in development of mesenchymal tissues
    - Affects mostly neural crest cells surrounding brain and forming vessels
- Genetics
  - Sporadic
  - May survive autosomal lethal gene by somatic mosaicism
  - Mosaic *FGFR1* and *KRAS* mutations have been reported
- ECCL considered distinct entity; however, some clinical/imaging overlap with SWS, oculocerebrocutaneous syndrome (OCCS), epidermal nevus syndrome (ENS), and proteus syndrome
- Embryology/anatomy
  - 3rd-week gestation: Embryonic disc consists of ectoderm, mesoderm, entoderm
  - Neural tube develops from ectoderm during 3rd-week gestation
  - 4th- and 5th-week gestation: Mesoderm forms mesenchymal sheath over brain and spinal cord → precursor blood vessels, bone, cartilage, and fat

Gross Pathologic & Surgical Features

- Brain: Cortical atrophy, white matter hypoplasia, ventriculomegaly, polymicrogyria, wallerian degeneration in brainstem
  - Arterial ectasias, pouches, aneurysms described in older patients
- Leptomeninges: Thick, gray, gelatinous with excess underlying arteries, veins, and varicose capillaries
- Skull: Macrocranium with focal hyperostosis
- Scalp: Focal lipomatous thickening with overlying circumscribed alopecia
- Face: Multiple tiny white/purple/yellow periocular > perinasal papules

Microscopic Features

- Brain: Abnormal 4-layered cytoarchitecture, mineral concretions outer cortical lamina, scattered glial nodules
- Leptomeninges: Lipoangiomatosis
- Skull: Diploic replacement with mature fat cells
- Scalp: Benign lipoma > fibrolipoma expanding into dermis; absent hair follicles with preserved erector pili muscles
- Skin: Subcutaneous angiofibroma, fibrolipoma, or lipoma
- Eye: Corneal limbus/scleral choristoma
  - Other ocular abnormalities: Persistent hyaloid vasculature, coloboma, cloudy cornea, lens dislocation, ectopic pupils

CLINICAL ISSUES

Presentation

- Most common signs/symptoms
  - Nevus psiloliparus: Sharply demarcated focus of scalp alopecia overlying scalp lipoma
    - Hallmark of ECCL
- Other signs/symptoms
  - Ipsilateral ocular choristomas and periocular > perinasal papules; epibulbar dermoid
  - Macrocranium (unrelated to hydrocephalus)
  - Seizures, psychomotor delay, spastic hemiparesis
  - Infrequent scoliosis, foot deformities, sensorimotor deficits (2° to spinal lipoma)
- Clinical profile
  - Newborn/infant with nevus psiloliparus, scleral mass, and periocular papules; seizures in infants

Demographics

- Age
  - Newborn > infant presentation
  - Rare presentation in teen/adult patients with cutaneous, ocular lesions
- Sex
  - M = F
- Ethnicity
  - No racial or geographic predilection
- Epidemiology
  - Rare; ~ 54 reported cases (likely underreported)

Natural History & Prognosis

- Reported growth of lipomas and ocular choristomas; remaining congenital abnormalities static
- Abnormal vasculature, aneurysms later in life
- Majority with variable degrees of psychomotor impairment and dependency
- Few reports of neurologically normal patients with nevus psiloliparus; nonsyndromic nevus psiloliparus vs. ECCL with minimal CNS involvement

Treatment

- Antiepileptics
- Shunt placement for hydrocephalus

DIAGNOSTIC CHECKLIST

Image Interpretation Pearls

- Considerable imaging overlap with SWS → search for scalp lipoma
- Low-density IC lipoma may be difficult to distinguish from CSF on CT

SELECTED REFERENCES

1. Machnikowska-Sokołowska M et al: Encephalocraniocutaneous lipomatosis, a radiological challenge: two atypical case reports and literature review. Brain Sci. 12(12), 2022
2. Moog U et al: Encephalocraniocutaneous Lipomatosis. Genereviews, 2022
3. de Moraes MPM et al: Clinical and neuroimaging features of encephalocraniocutaneous lipomatosis. Neurology. 97(16):785-6, 2021
4. McDonell LM et al: Mosaic KRAS mutation in a patient with encephalocraniocutaneous lipomatosis and renovascular hypertension. Am J Med Genet A. 176(11):2523-7, 2018
5. Siddiqui S et al: Encephalocraniocutaneous lipomatosis: a case report with review of literature. Neuroradiol J. 30(6):578-82, 2017
6. Bennett JT et al: Mosaic activating mutations in FGFR1 cause encephalocraniocutaneous lipomatosis. Am J Hum Genet. 98(3):579-87, 2016
7. Bieser S et al: Grade II pilocytic astrocytoma in a 3-month-old patient with encephalocraniocutaneous lipomatosis (ECCL): case report and literature review of low grade gliomas in ECCL. Am J Med Genet A. 167(4):878-81, 2015
8. Lin AW et al: Characteristic imaging findings in encephalocraniocutaneous lipomatosis. Neurology. 84(13):1384-5, 2015
9. Michael GA et al: Neuroimaging findings in encephalocraniocutaneous lipomatosis. Pediatr Neurol. 53(5):462-3, 2015
10. Chiang CC et al: Clinical manifestation and neurosurgical intervention of encephalocraniocutaneous lipomatosis–a case report and review of the literature. Childs Nerv Syst. 30(1):13-7, 2014

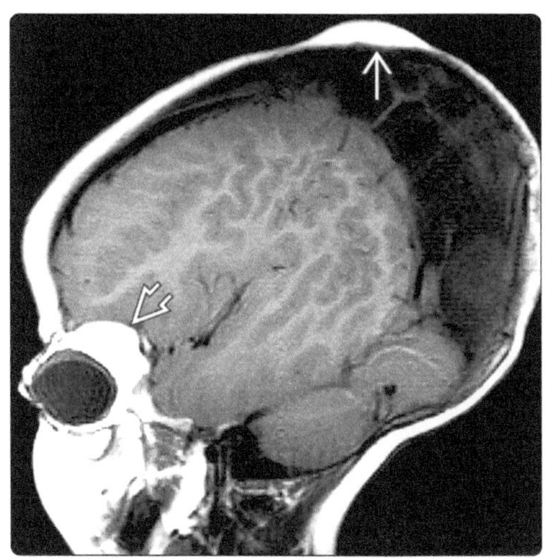
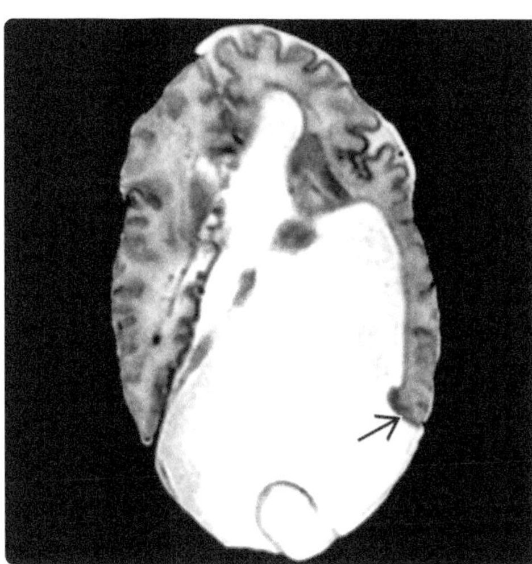

(Left) *Sagittal T1WI MR shows an ipsilateral scalp ➡ and orbital ➡ lipoma. The globe is buphthalmic with a scleral lipodermoid.* **(Right)** *Axial T2WI MR shows marked left ventriculomegaly with herniation of the ventricle through the choroidal fissure and hemispheric volume loss. The herniated ventricle is displacing the posterior aspect of the cerebral hemisphere ➡ anteriorly, thereby compressing and distorting the hemispheric parenchyma.*

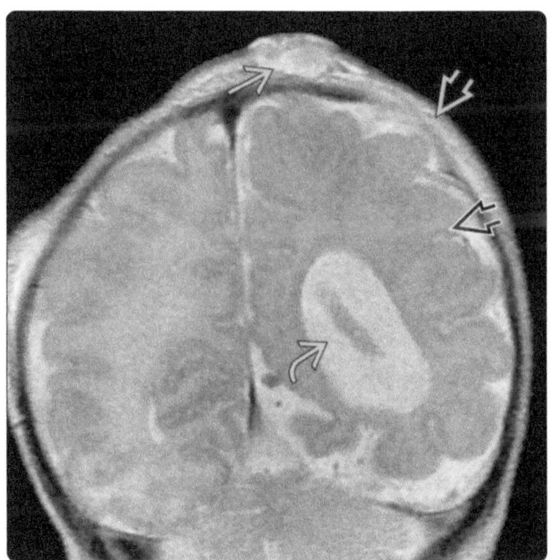
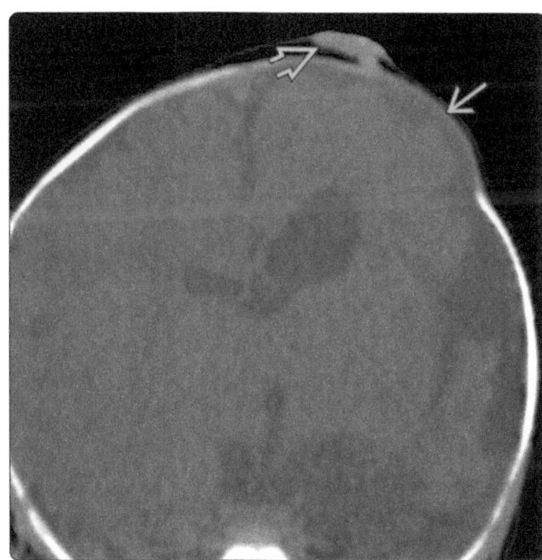

(Left) *Coronal T2WI MR in a neonate shows absence of a portion of the left parietal calvarium ➡ and a nodular scalp lesion ➡, characteristic findings in ECCL. Also note the left parietal cortical malformation ➡ and brain parenchymal volume loss, resulting in passive ventricular enlargement ➡.* **(Right)** *Coronal NECT in the same patient at 1 month of age shows the absent calvarium ➡ and the soft tissue nodule ➡ associated with the dermis. Again, note the underlying brain abnormalities.*

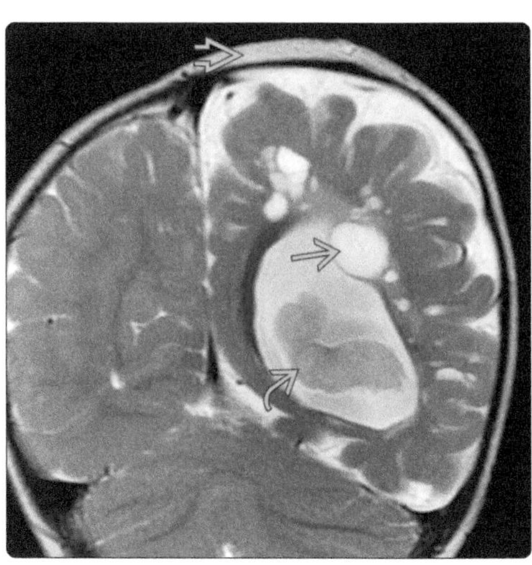
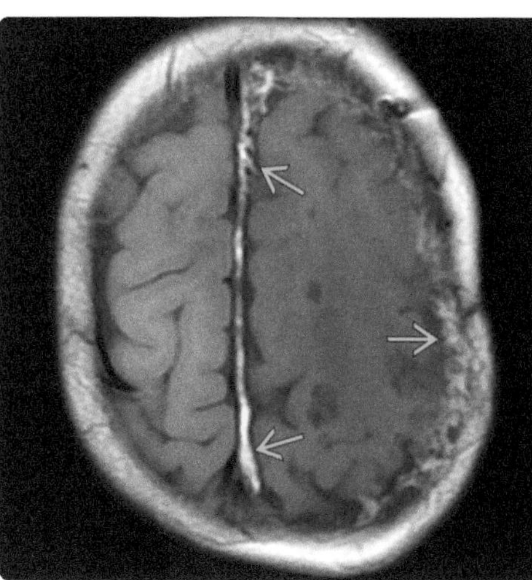

(Left) *Coronal T2WI MR (same patient) shows progressive left hemispheric volume loss with development of large perivascular spaces ➡ and hypertrophied choroid plexus ➡. Also note the increase in the fatty scalp mass ➡.* **(Right)** *Axial T1WI MR in the same patient at 4 years of age shows linear intracranial fat ➡ extending along nearly the entire left subdural space. This intracranial fat was not evident at birth or during the 1st year of life. Such lipomatous lesions often grow over the course of the patient's life.*

Neonatal Subpial Hemorrhage

KEY FACTS

TERMINOLOGY

- Neonatal hemorrhage into potential space between brain surface, pia mater

IMAGING

- Blood products constrained under pia that conform to gyral surface and spread sulci
- Size variable: May be large
- Adjacent scalp soft tissue swelling, contiguous parenchymal hemorrhage common
- Blood frequently located near suture
- CT/MR vascular imaging frequently negative but may reveal occluded ipsilateral vein of Labbé

TOP DIFFERENTIAL DIAGNOSES

- Subarachnoid hemorrhage
- Subdural hematoma
- Epidural hematoma

PATHOLOGY

- Parenchymal hemorrhage contiguous with subpial blood
- Fragility of neonatal pia-brain adhesion makes it particularly susceptible to injury → subpial hemorrhage
    - Pia more easily separated from immature than mature brain parenchyma
    - Blood in SpS compresses cortical veins (compartment syndrome) → parenchymal venous infraction

CLINICAL ISSUES

- Otherwise healthy term neonate presents with apnea or seizures 2-3 days after birth
- Typically vaginal delivery ± forceps or vacuum assistance

DIAGNOSTIC CHECKLIST

- Subpial hemorrhage in otherwise healthy term neonate presenting with seizures or apnea
- Subpial blood conforms to gyri, appears constrained, and spreads sulci

(Left) *Coronal NECT in a newborn with seizures after vaginal delivery demonstrates a left medial temporal lobe parenchymal hemorrhage ➡ with extension ➡ into the subpial space ➡. The subpial blood follows and expands the sulci.* **(Right)** *Coronal T2 MR in the same patient confirms parenchymal hemorrhage and delineates mass effect from subpial hemorrhage on the left temporal lobe. There is also retrograde interventricular blood extension ➡.*

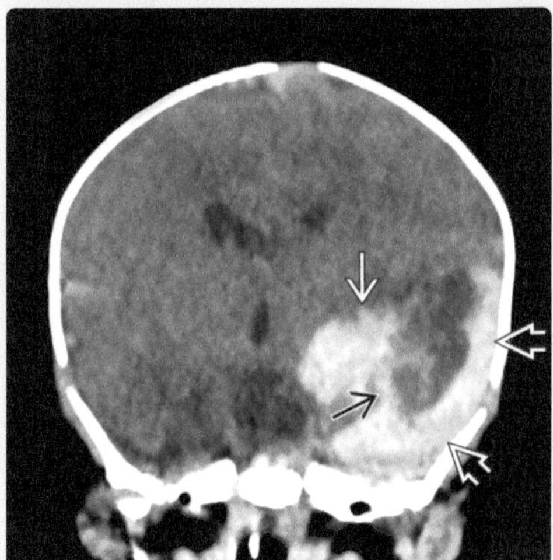

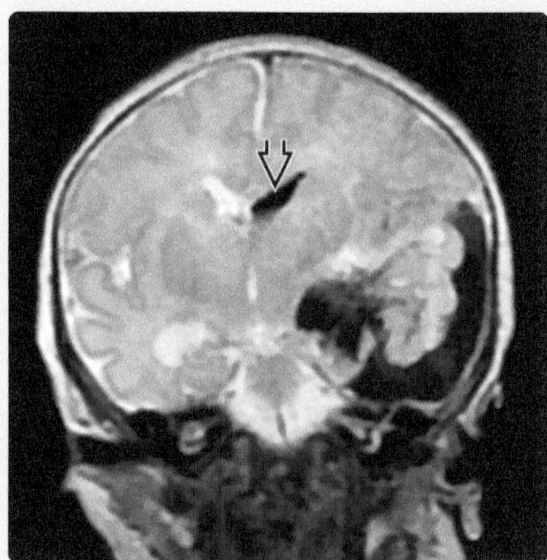

(Left) *Axial T1 MR in a newborn with Chiari 2 malformation reveals a small, T1-hyperintense (early subacute) parenchymal hemorrhage ➡ with subpial extension ➡. Note the blood-fluid level ➡ in the subpial hematoma. The cause of the hemorrhage was not determined.* **(Right)** *Axial T2 MR in the same patient confirms subacute parenchymal blood ➡ within a parenchymal cavitation with subpial ➡ extension.*

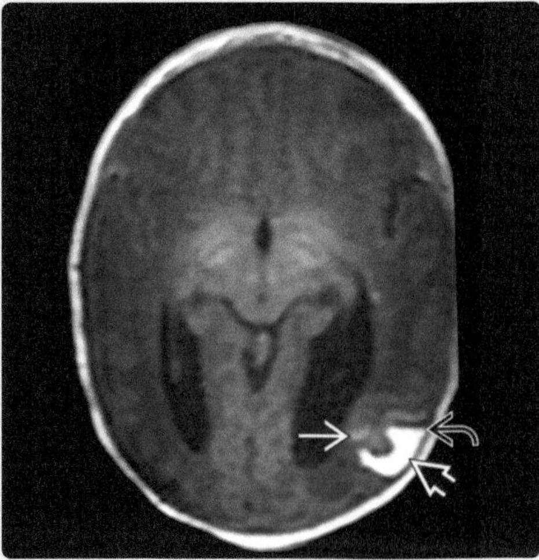

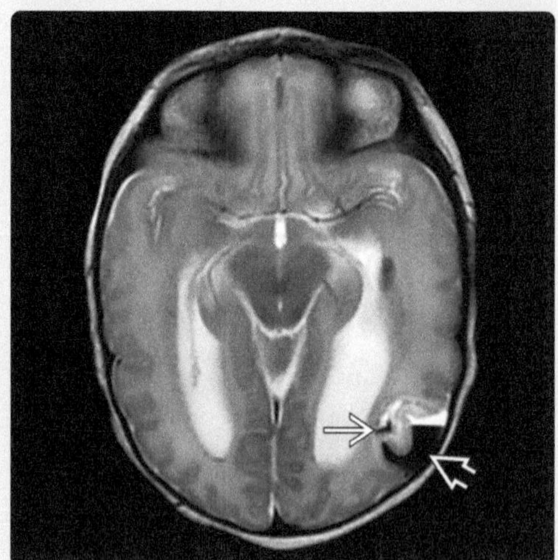

TERMINOLOGY

Definitions

- Neonatal patient presenting with hemorrhage into potential space between brain surface and pia mater [subpial space (SpS)]

IMAGING

General Features

- Best diagnostic clue
  - Blood products constrained under pia that conform to gyral surface and spread sulci
  - Contiguous underlying parenchymal hemorrhage very common
- Location
  - Subpial
  - Most commonly occurs in anterolateral temporal lobe, adjacent to pterion
  - Less commonly occurs in parietal lobe, frontal lobe, or lateral temporal lobe under squamosal suture
  - May be multiple and multifocal
- Size
  - Variable: May be very large
- Morphology
  - Extraaxial blood constrained over surface of brain with local sulcal spreading
  - Adjacent parenchymal hemorrhage common
  - Adjacent blood collections described as having Yin and Yang configuration

CT Findings

- NECT
  - Parenchymal + subpial hyperdensity
  - Blood frequently found near cranial suture
  - Often adjacent scalp swelling
- Bone CT
  - Adjacent fracture uncommon
- CTA
  - CTA/CTV often negative for source
  - Rarely detect local cortical venous thrombosis

MR Findings

- T1WI
  - Contiguous parenchymal and subpial blood
  - Signal variable depending on blood age
  - Adjacent scalp soft tissue swelling
- T2WI
  - Contiguous parenchymal and subpial blood
  - Signal variable depending on blood age
  - Yin and Yang shape of adjacent blood collections
- T2* GRE
  - Hypointense blood signal with blooming
- DWI
  - ± diffusion restriction within parenchyma adjacent to hemorrhage ubiquitous
  - Hypointensity on ADC map confirms true diffusion restriction
- T1WI C+
  - Subacute parenchymal infarct may enhance
  - Generally not useful addition to MR protocol
- MRA
  - Normal
- MRV
  - Usually normal
  - Rare patients with temporal lobe hemorrhage demonstrate ipsilateral vein of Labbé occlusion

Ultrasonographic Findings

- Parenchymal and subpial hyperechogenicity
  - Look for crescentic shape of subpial blood spreading sulci
  - Subpial blood may be hypoechoic if acute
- May be difficult to distinguish parenchymal from subpial hemorrhage

Imaging Recommendations

- Best imaging tool
  - Cranial sonography for initial screening
  - MR provides best delineation of brain injury and relationship to subpial hemorrhage
  - CT permits adequate characterization if MR not available or possible
- Protocol advice
  - Multiplanar brain MR with T1, T2, GRE/SWI, and DWI sequences
  - Consider MRA/MRV (usually negative)

DIFFERENTIAL DIAGNOSIS

Subarachnoid Hemorrhage

- Does not usually conform to gyri or spread sulci
- Disperses with time

Subdural Hematoma

- External to subarachnoid space
- Effaces rather than spreading sulci

Epidural Hematoma

- Bilenticular shape, external to subarachnoid space
- Effaces rather than spreads sulci

PATHOLOGY

General Features

- Etiology
  - Fragility of neonatal pia-brain adhesion (compared to mature brain) makes it particularly susceptible to injury → subpial hemorrhage
    - Pia more easily separated from immature than mature brain parenchyma
  - Current leading theory proposes that subpial hemorrhage results from primary insult to glia limitans membrane, astrocytic end-feet at interface of parenchymal cortex and pia
    - Insult leads to focal disruption of basement membrane and astrocytic endfeet
    - Rupture of perforating cortical vessels
    - Pooling of blood in adjacent SpS
    - Local mass effect → secondary compression of subpial vessels ("compartment syndrome")
    - Venous hypertension, subcortical parenchymal venous infarction

Gross Pathologic & Surgical Features

- Parenchymal hemorrhage contiguous with subpial blood

Microscopic Features

- Exact nature of subpial potential space debated
  - Electron micrographs show no true well-defined SpS in normal brain
  - Potential SpS consists of small intercellular clefts located between astrocytic processes and between glial footplates, brain basement membrane
- Histopathology reveals outer layer glial swelling and vacuolization in subpial hemorrhages
  - Correlates with edema, restricted diffusion in brain tissue adjacent to superficial parenchymal and leptomeningeal hemorrhage

CLINICAL ISSUES

Presentation

- Most common signs/symptoms
  - Seizure
  - Apnea
- Other signs/symptoms
  - Hypovolemia
- Clinical profile
  - Otherwise healthy term neonate presents with apnea or seizures 2-3 days after birth
  - Typically vaginal delivery ± forceps or vacuum assistance
  - Can rarely occur after caesarean section
    - Trial of unsuccessful labor often precedes caesarean section

Demographics

- Age
  - Neonates: Preterm or term infants
- Epidemiology
  - Not truly known because recording of neonatal leptomeningeal hemorrhage in databases not sufficiently granular
  - Proposed risk factors
    - Neonatal asphyxia
    - Birth trauma
    - Sutural overlap/distortion
    - Clotting disorders
    - Venous sinus compression
    - Variations in intracranial pressure

Natural History & Prognosis

- Term patients generally higher survival than preterm
- Neurologic outcome may be poor depending on multiplicity and severity
- Many patients with smaller bleeds recover with mild or no sequelae

Treatment

- Primarily supportive
- Early neurodevelopmental assessment and follow-up
- No role for surgical management in most patients

DIAGNOSTIC CHECKLIST

Consider

- Subpial hemorrhage in otherwise healthy neonate presenting with seizures or apnea
- Hemorrhage most often in temporal lobe and in proximity to sutures, accompanied by overlying soft tissue swelling

Image Interpretation Pearls

- Subpial blood conforms to gyri, appears constrained, and spreads sulci

SELECTED REFERENCES

1. Cyr PEP et al: Neonatal motor functional connectivity and motor outcomes at age two years in very preterm children with and without high-grade brain injury. Neuroimage Clin. 36:103260, 2022
2. Pinto C et al: Subpial hemorrhage: a distinctive neonatal stroke pattern. Clin Neuroradiol. 32(4):1057-65, 2022
3. Sandoval Karamian AG et al: Intracranial hemorrhage in term and late-preterm neonates: an institutional perspective. AJNR Am J Neuroradiol. 43(10):1494-9, 2022
4. Srivastava R et al: Perinatal stroke in fetuses, preterm and term infants. Semin Pediatr Neurol. 43:100988, 2022
5. Assis Z et al: Idiopathic neonatal subpial hemorrhage with underlying cerebral infarct: imaging features and clinical outcome. AJNR Am J Neuroradiol. 42(1):185-93, 2021
6. Dabrowski AK et al: Neonatal subpial hemorrhage: clinical factors, neuroimaging, and outcomes in a quaternary care children's center. Pediatr Neurol. 120:52-8, 2021
7. Hausman-Kedem M et al: Monogenic causes of apparently idiopathic perinatal intracranial hemorrhage. Ann Neurol. 89(4):813-22, 2021
8. Cain DW et al: Subpial hemorrhage of the neonate. Stroke. 51(1):315-8, 2020
9. Larsen KB et al: The pathology and aetiology of subcortical clefts in infants. Forensic Sci Int. 296:115-22, 2019
10. Huang AH et al: Spontaneous superficial parenchymal and leptomeningeal hemorrhage in term neonates. AJNR Am J Neuroradiol 2004, 25:469-75
11. Sandberg DI et al: Spontaneous intraparenchymal hemorrhage in full-term neonates. Neurosurgery. 48(5):1042-8; discussion 1048-9, 2001
12. Marín-Padilla M: Developmental neuropathology and impact of perinatal brain damage. I: hemorrhagic lesions of neocortex. J Neuropathol Exp Neurol. 55(7):758-73, 1996
13. Hanigan WC et al: Symptomatic intracranial hemorrhage in full-term infants. Childs Nerv Syst. 11(12):698-707, 1995
14. Hanigan WC et al: Lobar hemorrhages in full-term neonates. Childs Nerv Syst. 11(5):276-80, 1995

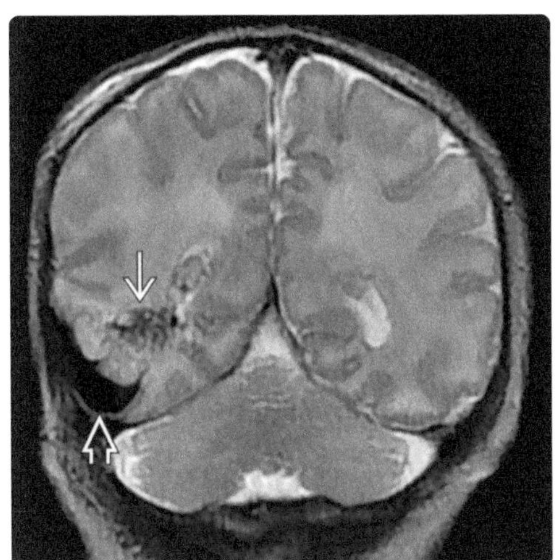
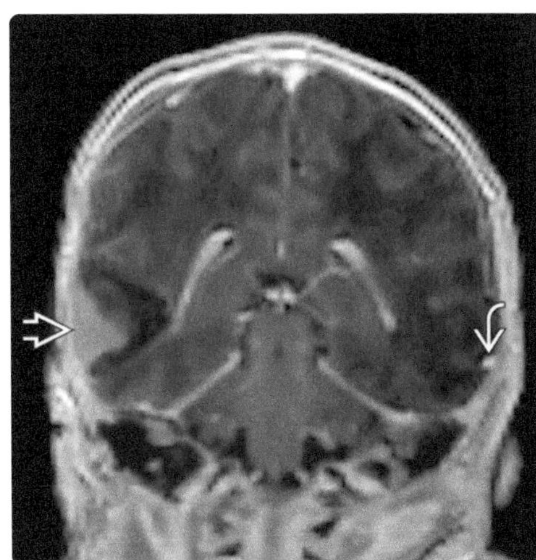

(Left) *Coronal T2 MR in a term infant with seizures demonstrates temporal lobe parenchymal hemorrhage → with subpial extension ⇨.* **(Right)** *Coronal C+ SPGR MR shows subacute subpial blood ⇨ splaying the inferior temporal sulcus. The left vein of Labbé ↷ is clearly seen but the right vein is occluded, resulting in a venous infarct with subpial extension.*

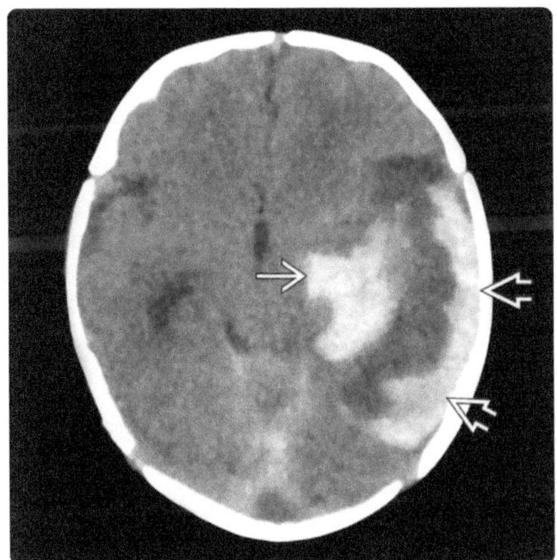
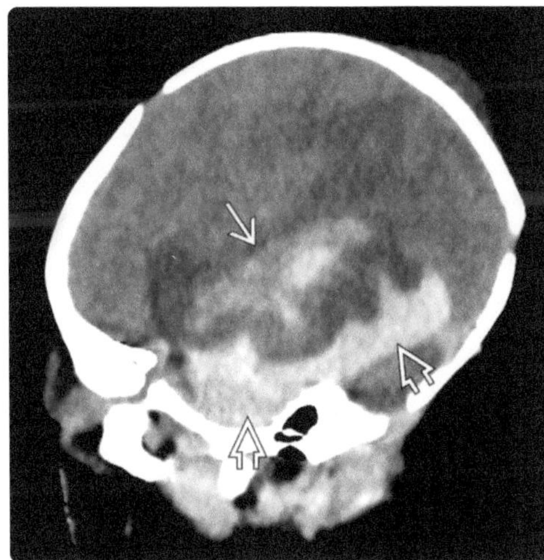

(Left) *Axial NECT in a seizing newborn after a vaginal delivery demonstrates parenchymal → and subpial ⇨ hemorrhage. In this location, one could consider venous infarct from vein of Labbé occlusion.* **(Right)** *Sagittal NECT in the same patient shows longitudinal extent of the parenchymal → and subpial ⇨ hemorrhage. Subpial hemorrhage can be extensive in a newborn and can result in hypovolemia and cardiovascular collapse.*

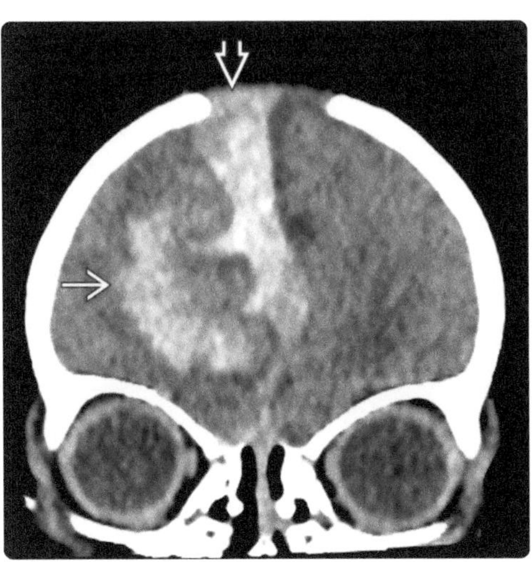
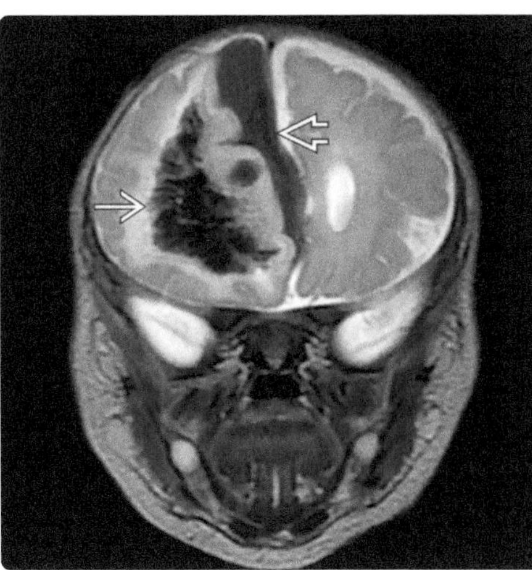

(Left) *Coronal NECT in a neonate with seizures following forceps-assisted vaginal delivery reveals parenchymal hemorrhage → and adjacent extraaxial blood ⇨ that widens the sulci and is constrained along the medial frontal lobe surface.* **(Right)** *Coronal T2 MR in the same patient depicts hypointense blood in both the frontal lobe parenchyma → as well as the subpial potential space ⇨. Other images (not shown) clearly demonstrated that the blood originated in the parenchyma and dissected into the subpial space.*

Epidural Hematoma, Classic

KEY FACTS

TERMINOLOGY

- Epidural hematoma (EDH)
  - Blood collection between skull and dura

IMAGING

- NECT
  - Hyperdense, biconvex, extraaxial collection
  - > 95% unilateral, supratentorial
  - Does not cross sutures unless venous or sutural diastasis/fracture is present
  - Compresses/displaces underlying brain, subarachnoid space
  - Low-density swirl sign: Active/rapid bleeding with unretracted clot
- Bone CT
  - Skull fracture in 90-95%

TOP DIFFERENTIAL DIAGNOSES

- Subdural hematoma
- Neoplasm
- Infection/inflammation
- Extramedullary hematopoiesis

PATHOLOGY

- Arterial (90-95%)
  - Arterial EDH is most often near middle meningeal artery groove fracture
- Venous EDH (5-10%)
  - Fracture is adjacent to dural sinus
  - Common sites: Vertex, anterior middle cranial fossa

CLINICAL ISSUES

- Classic "lucid interval" ~ 50% of cases
- Good outcome if promptly recognized and treated
- Some EDHs < 1 cm may be managed nonoperatively

DIAGNOSTIC CHECKLIST

- NECT is highly sensitive for detection

(Left) *Coronal graphic illustrates swirling acute hemorrhage from a laceration of the middle meningeal artery by an overlying skull fracture. The epidural hematoma displaces the dura inward as it expands.* **(Right)** *Axial NECT in 4-year-old girl who fell from a trampoline demonstrates a mixed-density, lentiform-shaped parietal epidural hematoma ➡. Dense blood represents acute hemorrhage, and lower density represents unclotted blood or ongoing hemorrhage.*

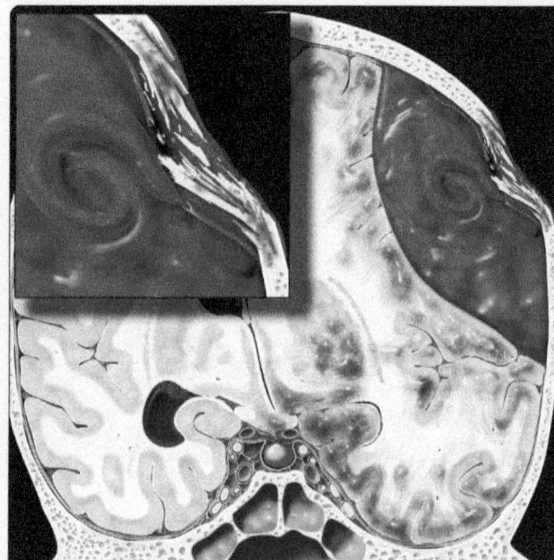

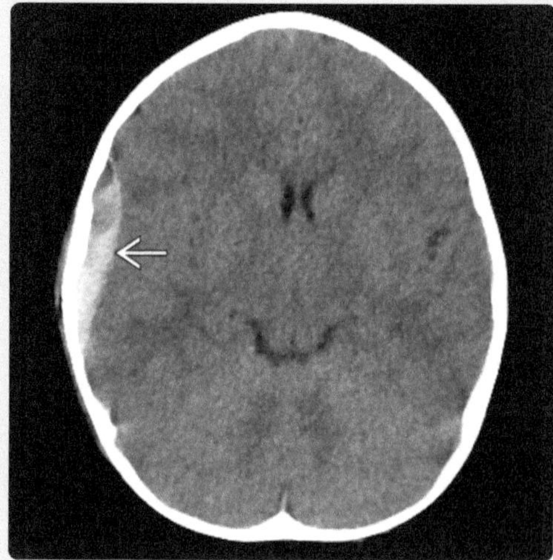

(Left) *Coronal NECT in the same patient confirms the lentiform shape and well demonstrates a mixture of clotted and unclotted blood ➡.* **(Right)** *Lateral 3D surface rendering in the same patient reveals a nondepressed, linear parietal bone fracture ➡, the source of epidural hemorrhage.*

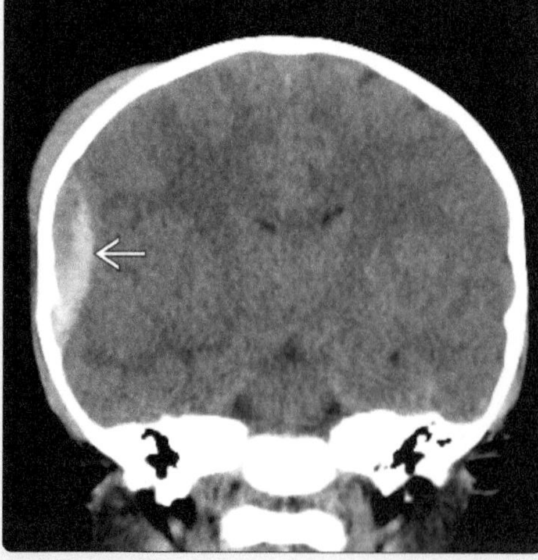

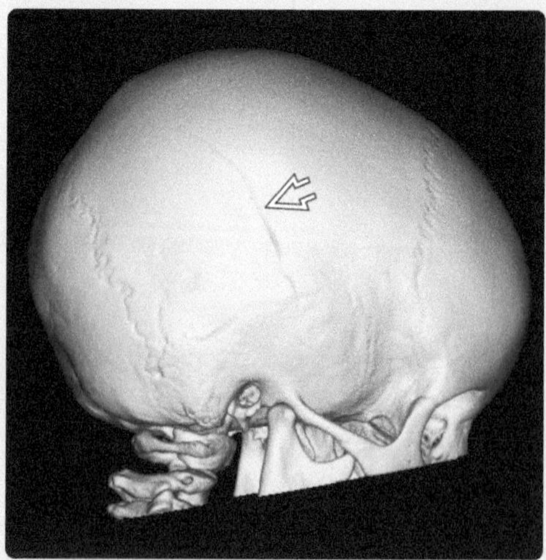

TERMINOLOGY

Abbreviations

- Epidural hematoma (EDH)

Definitions

- Blood collection between inner table of skull and outer (periosteal) layer of dura

IMAGING

General Features

- Best diagnostic clue
  - Hyperdense, biconvex, extraaxial collection on NECT
- Location
  - Epidural space (between skull and dura)
  - Nearly all EDHs occur at impact (coup) site
    - 90-95% arterial
    - 90-95% adjacent to skull fracture
    - 90-95% unilateral (bilateral rare)
  - Supratentorial (90-95%)
    - 65% temporoparietal, 35% frontal/parietooccipital
  - 5-10% in posterior fossa
  - Venous EDH (5%)
- Size
  - Variable; rapid expansion is typical
    - Attains maximum size within 36 hours
  - Slower accumulation of blood in venous EDH
- Morphology
  - Biconvex or lentiform extraaxial collection
  - Arterial EDHs usually do not cross sutures
    - Exception: If sutural diastasis/fracture is present
    - Compresses/displaces underlying brain, subarachnoid space
  - Venous EDH
    - Adjacent to venous sinus crossed by fracture
      - Skull base, vertex
      - Anterior middle fossa
    - May "straddle" sutures, dural attachments
      - Can cross falx, tentorium
    - Dural sinus displaced, usually not occluded
  - 1/3-1/2 have other significant lesions
    - Mass effect, secondary herniations common
    - Contrecoup subdural hematoma (SDH)
    - Cerebral contusions

CT Findings

- NECT
  - Acute: 2/3 hyperdense, 1/3 mixed density
    - Acute EDH with retracted clot = 60-90 HU
    - Low-density swirl sign: Active/rapid bleeding with unretracted clot
    - Medial hyperdense margin: Displaced dura
  - Air in EDH (20%) suggests sinus or mastoid fracture
  - Vertex EDH is easily overlooked
  - Chronic EDH → hypo-/mixed density
  - CT comma sign
    - EDH + SDH
    - Often temporoparietal or temporoparietooccipital
    - Important to identify → treated as 2 separate surgical entities
- CECT
  - Acute: May show contrast extravasation (rare)
  - Chronic: Peripheral dural enhancement from neovascularization, granulation
- Bone CT
  - Skull fracture in 95%

MR Findings

- T1WI
  - Acute: Isointense with brain
  - Subacute/early chronic: Hyperintense
  - Black line between EDH and brain: Displaced dura
- T2WI
  - Acute: Variable hyper- to hypointense
  - Early subacute: Hypointense
  - Late subacute/early chronic: Hyperintense
  - Black line between EDH and brain: Displaced dura
- T1WI C+
  - Venous EDH: Look for displaced dural sinus by hematoma
  - Spontaneous (nontraumatic) EDH: Enhancement of hemorrhagic epidural mass
- MRV
  - Assess venous sinus integrity
  - Hematoma may displace venous sinus, impede flow

Angiographic Findings

- Diagnostic
  - Avascular mass effect; displaced cortical arteries
  - If middle meningeal artery (MMA) laceration present
    - May form arteriovenous fistula → tram-track sign
      - Simultaneous opacification of MMA, both middle meningeal veins
  - Venous EDH: Look for displaced dural sinus

Imaging Recommendations

- Best imaging tool
  - NECT with bone CT for traumatic cases
  - MR + MRV if venous EDH suspected
- Protocol advice
  - Consider MR if EDH "straddles" dural compartments or sinuses on NECT

DIFFERENTIAL DIAGNOSIS

Acute Subdural Hematoma

- EDH and acute SDH may coexist
- Acute SDH is usually crescentic (occasionally biconvex)
- Crosses sutures but limited by dural attachments

Neoplasm

- Meningioma
- Soft tissue component (subperiosteal) of osseous mass
  - Metastasis, lymphoma, primary sarcoma
- Dural-based mass
  - Metastases, lymphoma, mesenchymal tumor

Infection/Inflammation

- Subperiosteal extension of osseous inflammatory lesion
- Epidural empyema secondary to osteomyelitis
- Soft tissue from granulomatous osseous lesion
  - Tuberculosis

Extramedullary Hematopoiesis

- History of blood dyscrasia

PATHOLOGY

General Features

- Etiology
  - Trauma most common
    - Fracture lacerates vessel
      - Arterial (90-95%), venous (5-10%)
    - Arterial EDH is most often near MMA groove fracture
    - Venous EDH is usually near fracture that crosses dural sinus
  - Nontraumatic
    - Coagulopathy, thrombolysis, vascular malformation, neoplasm, epidural anesthesia, Paget disease of skull
    - Spontaneous EDH is rare; may arise from skull metastases
- Associated abnormalities
  - Skull fracture in 95%; may cross MMA groove
  - Subdural/subarachnoid hemorrhage, contusion

Gross Pathologic & Surgical Features

- EDH is subperiosteal hematoma
  - Outer dural layer functions as periosteum of inner calvarium
- Hematoma collects between calvarium and outer dura
  - Rarely crosses sutures
    - Exception: Venous EDH, large hematoma with diastatic fracture
- Vertex EDH (rare)
  - Usually venous: Linear or diastatic fracture crosses superior sagittal sinus
- 20% have blood in both epidural and subdural spaces at surgery or autopsy

CLINICAL ISSUES

Presentation

- Most common signs/symptoms
  - Classic "lucid interval" ~ 50% of cases
    - Initial brief LOC; subsequent asymptomatic time between LOC and symptom/coma onset
  - Headache, nausea, vomiting, seizures, focal neurologic deficits (e.g., field cuts, aphasia, weakness)
  - Mass effect/herniation common
    - Pupil-involving CNIII palsy, somnolence, ↓ consciousness, coma
- Clinical profile
  - Alcohol and other intoxications are associated with ↑ incidence of EDH

Demographics

- Age
  - More common < 20 years; extremely rare in older adults
  - Uncommon in infants
- Sex
  - M:F = 4:1
- Epidemiology
  - 1-4% of imaged head trauma patients
  - 5-15% of patients with fatal head injuries

Natural History & Prognosis

- Factors affecting rate of growth
  - Arterial vs. venous, rate of extravasation
  - Occasionally decompresses through fracture into scalp
  - Tamponade
- Delayed development or enlargement common
  - 10-25% of cases within first 36 hours
- Good outcome if promptly recognized and treated
  - Overall mortality is ~ 5%
  - Bilateral EDHs have higher mortality and morbidity
    - 15-20% mortality rate
- ↑ mortality in posterior fossa EDH (26%)
  - Can have delayed symptom onset secondary to slower expansion from lower venous pressure

Treatment

- Prompt recognition and appropriate treatment are essential
  - Poor outcome often related to delayed referral, diagnosis, or operation
- Most EDHs are surgically evacuated
  - Options: Endovascular/endoscopic if poor surgical candidate
  - Mixed-density acute EDHs require earlier, more aggressive treatment
- Some EDHs < 1 cm with no cerebral edema are managed nonoperatively
  - Traditional approach suggests repeat CT in first 36 hours to monitor for change
    - 23% enlarge within 36 hours
    - Mean enlargement: 7 mm
  - Anterior middle fossa EDHs are venous and usually do not require surgery
- More recent reports suggest that subset of EDH with minimal mass effect and smaller size can be observed without repeat imaging
- Complications: Mass effect, edema, herniations

DIAGNOSTIC CHECKLIST

Image Interpretation Pearls

- NECT is highly sensitive
  - Coronal CT reconstructions to evaluate vertex EDH
- Use bone CT to look for fracture
- Consider CTV if fracture is near venous sinus

SELECTED REFERENCES

1. Goubran D et al: Initial CT imaging predicts mortality in severe traumatic brain injuries in pediatric population-a systematic review and meta-analysis. Tomography. 9(2):541-51, 2023
2. Jamous MA et al: Management of traumatic posterior fossa epidural hematomas in pediatrics: our experience and review of the literature. Childs Nerv Syst. 37(9):2839-46, 2021
3. Caruso G et al: Unusual case of posterior fossa extradural hematoma in a child: review of the literature. Pediatr Neurosurg. 55(6):399-403, 2020
4. Flaherty BF et al: Repeat head CT for expectant management of traumatic epidural hematoma. Pediatrics. 142(3):e20180385, 2018
5. Orlando A et al: Isolated subdural hematomas in mild traumatic brain injury. Part 1: the association between radiographic characteristics and neurosurgical intervention. J Neurosurg. 1-10, 2018
6. Flaherty BF et al: Pediatric patients with traumatic epidural hematoma at low risk for deterioration and need for surgical treatment. J Pediatr Surg. 52(2):334-9, 2017

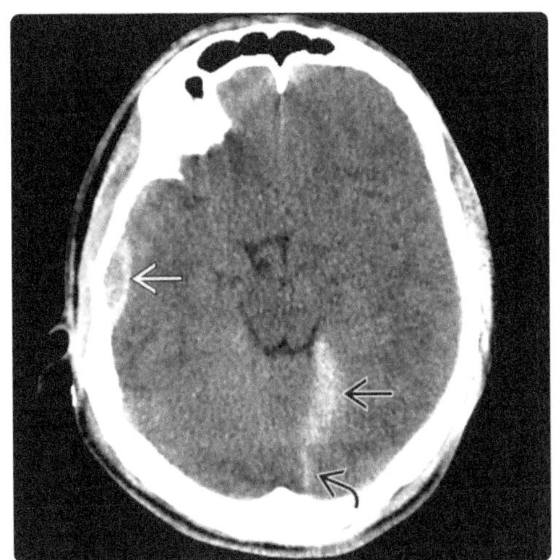

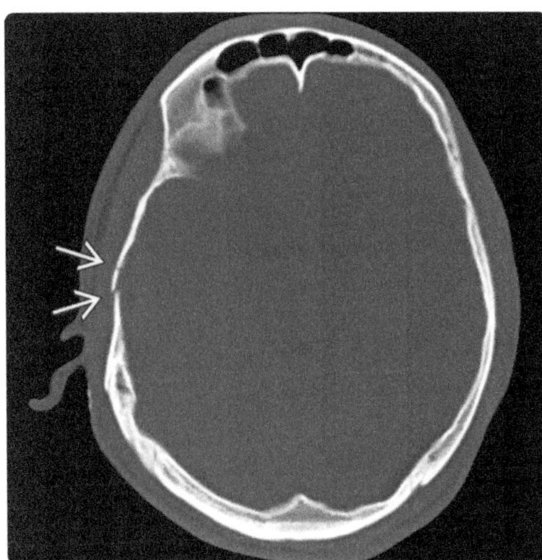

(Left) *Axial NECT reveals a small yet classic biconvex epidural hematoma* ➡ *underlying a linear skull fracture. There is also a posterior falcine traumatic subdural hematoma tracking along the tentorium* ➡ *and superior sagittal sinus* ↗. **(Right)** *Axial bone CT in the same patient demonstrates a portion of a comminuted fracture about the pterion* ➡ *that resulted in an arterial injury, resulting in an epidural hematoma.*

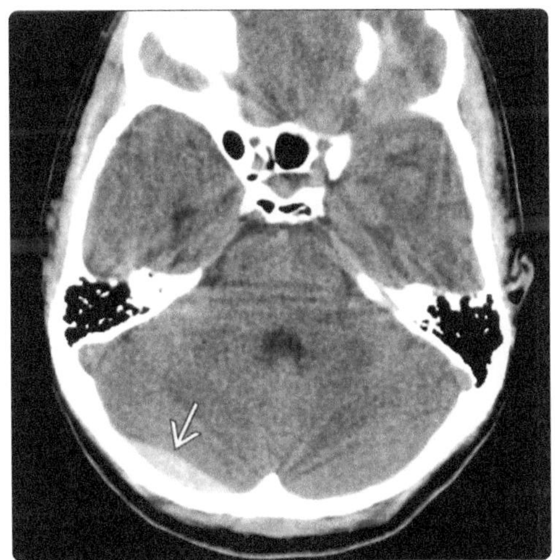

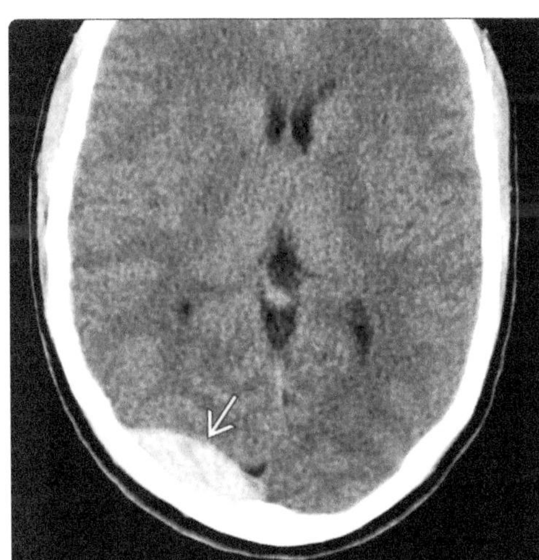

(Left) *Axial NECT demonstrates the infratentorial component of a biconvex venous epidural hematoma that extends both below the tentorium* ➡ *as well as above it. These small hematomas frequently do not require operative management.* **(Right)** *Axial NECT in the same patient demonstrates the supratentorial component of a biconvex venous epidural hematoma* ➡ *that extends both above and below the tentorium.*

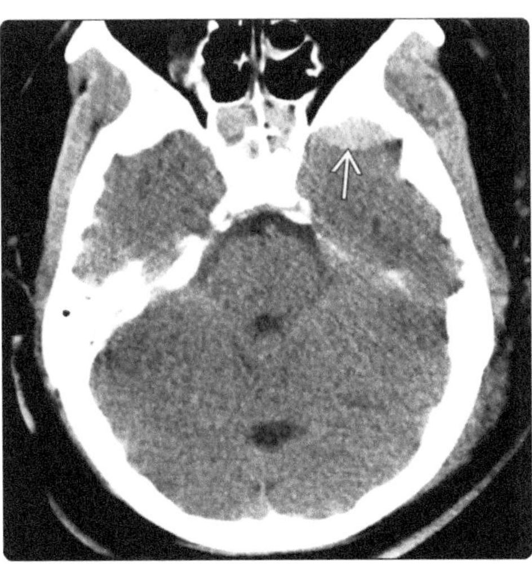

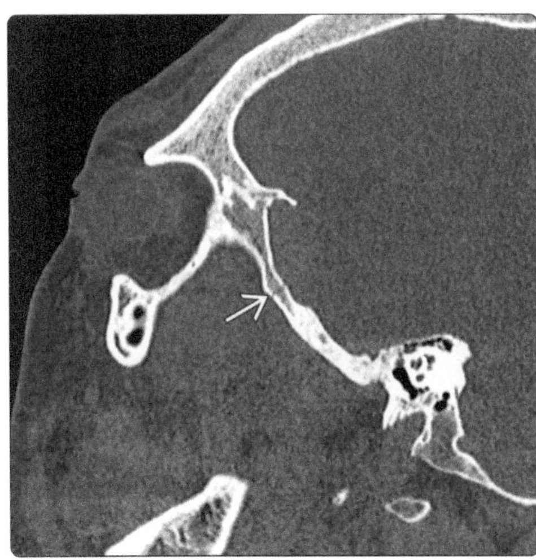

(Left) *Axial NECT demonstrates a small middle cranial fossa epidural hematoma* ➡ *adjacent to the temporal lobe tip. This is a common location for a venous epidural hematoma that can often be watched without surgical intervention.* **(Right)** *Sagittal bone CT reformat in the same patient shows a nondisplaced linear fracture* ➡ *that crosses the greater sphenoid wing. Such epidural hematomas that cross the sphenoparietal sinus are usually venous and typically do not require surgery.*

Acute Subdural Hematoma

KEY FACTS

TERMINOLOGY

- Acute blood in/between inner border cell layer of dura, arachnoid

IMAGING

- CT: Crescentic hyperdense extraaxial collection spread diffusely over convexity
- Between arachnoid and inner layer of dura
- Supratentorial convexity most common
- May cross sutures, not dural attachments
- NECT as initial screening study
- Inward displacement of cortical veins
- Presence of tears in pia-arachnoid membrane can lead to CSF leakage into subdural hematoma (SDH) collections; may also alter signal intensity by CSF dilution

TOP DIFFERENTIAL DIAGNOSES

- Hygroma
  - Clear CSF, no encapsulating membranes
- Effusion
  - Xanthochromic fluid secondary to extravasation of plasma from membrane; 1-3 days post trauma; near CSF density/intensity
- Empyema
  - Peripheral enhancement, hyperintensity on FLAIR and DWI; restricted diffusion
- Acute epidural hematoma
  - Biconvex extraaxial collection, may cross dural attachments, limited by sutures

PATHOLOGY

- Trauma most common cause

DIAGNOSTIC CHECKLIST

- Important to inform responsible clinician if unsuspected finding
- Wide window settings for CT ↑ conspicuity of subtle SDH

(Left) *Axial graphic shows an acute subdural hematoma (aSDH) compressing the left hemisphere and lateral ventricle, resulting in midline shift. Note also the hemorrhagic contusions and diffuse axonal injuries. Additional traumatic lesions are common in patients with subdural hematomas (SDHs).* **(Right)** *Axial NECT in a 3-year-old with altered mental status after a fall demonstrates a hyperdense right SDH. The heterogeneous attenuation is attributed to acute clotted and unclotted blood.*

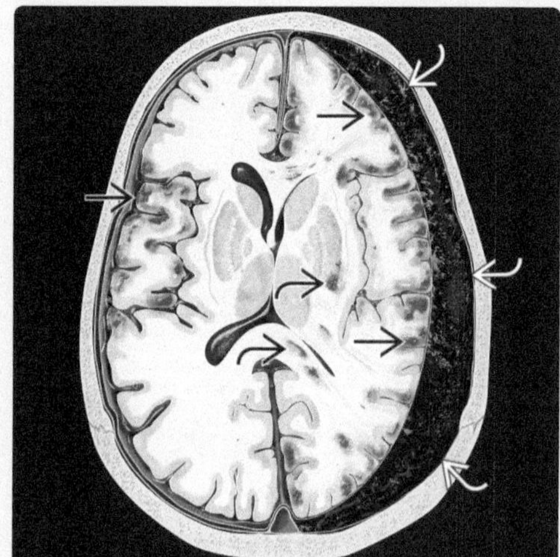

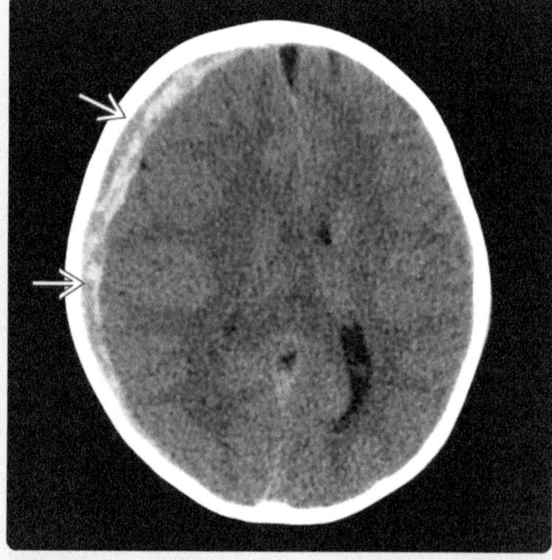

(Left) *Occasionally, aSDHs are isodense with underlying brain. This aSDH has mass effect, inward displacement of the underlying gray matter-white matter interface, and left-to-right subfalcine herniation of lateral ventricles.* **(Right)** *More cephalad NECT in the same patient shows the isodense aSDH effacing the underlying sulci (compare with the normal-appearing CSF-filled sulci over the right hemisphere).*

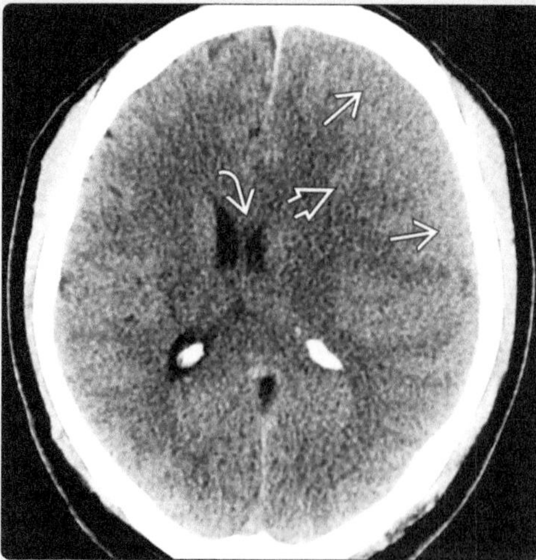

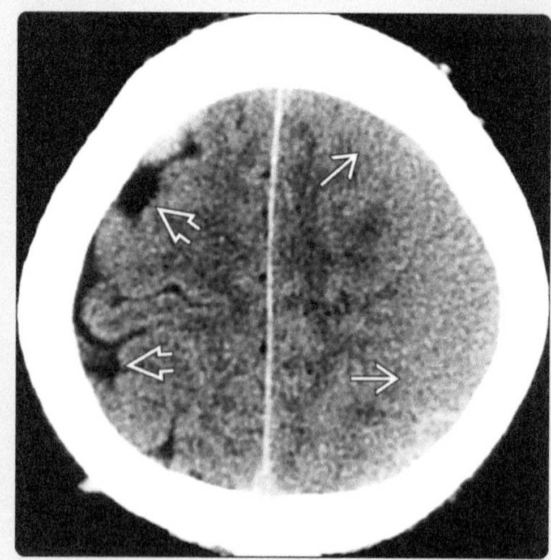

TERMINOLOGY

Abbreviations

- Acute subdural hematoma (aSDH)

Definitions

- Acute blood in or between inner border cell layer of dura and arachnoid

IMAGING

General Features

- Best diagnostic clue
  - CT: Crescentic, hyperdense, extraaxial collection spread diffusely over affected hemisphere
- Location
  - Between arachnoid and inner border cell layer of dura
  - Supratentorial convexity > interhemispheric, peritentorial
  - Uni- or bilateral
- Size
  - Variable
- Morphology
  - Crescent-shaped extraaxial fluid collection
  - May cross sutures, not dural attachments
  - May extend along falx, tentorium, and anterior and middle fossa floors

CT Findings

- NECT
  - Hyperacute subdural hematoma (SDH) (≤ 6 hours) may have heterogeneous density or hypodensity
  - aSDH (6 hours to 3 days)
    - aSDH: 60% homogeneously hyperdense
    - 40% mixed hyper-, hypodense with active bleeding (swirl sign), torn arachnoid with CSF accumulation, clot retraction
    - Rare: Isodense aSDH (coagulopathy, anemia with Hgb < 8-10 g/dL)
    - If no new hemorrhage, density ↓ ± 1.5 HU/day
- CECT
  - Inward displacement of cortical veins, gray matter-white matter interface
  - Dura and membranes enhance when subacute

MR Findings

- T1WI
  - Hyperacute (< 12 hours): Iso- to mildly hyperintense
  - Acute (12 hours to 2 days): Mildly hypointense
- T2WI
  - Hyperacute: Mildly hyperintense
  - Acute: Hypointense
- FLAIR
  - Typically hyperintense to CSF
  - Signal intensity varies depending on relative T1 and T2 effects
    - Acute hematomas can be isointense to CSF due to T2 shortening effects of intracellular methemoglobin
  - Often most conspicuous sequence
- T2* GRE
  - Hypointense unless hyperacute
- DWI
  - Heterogeneous signal (nonspecific)
  - May differentiate extraaxial empyema (marked central hyperintensity) from hemorrhage
- T1WI C+
  - Enhancement of displaced cortical veins
  - Enhancement within SDH predictive of subsequent growth
- MR signal of SDH quite variable
  - Often evolves in similar fashion to intraparenchymal hemorrhage
  - Recurrent hemorrhage common; results in acute and chronic blood products even at initial exam
  - SDH signal is variable due to recurrent hemorrhage; difficult to age accurately
  - Pia-arachnoid membrane tears can lead to CSF leakage into SDH collections and may alter signal intensity by CSF dilution
  - When chronic, SDHs may undergo fibrosis and enhance after contrast administration

Angiographic Findings

- Conventional
  - Mass effect from extraaxial collection; veins displaced from inner table of skull
  - Perform if underlying vascular lesion suspected

Imaging Recommendations

- Best imaging tool
  - NECT as initial screening study
  - MR more sensitive to detect and determine extent of SDH and additional findings of traumatic brain injury

DIFFERENTIAL DIAGNOSIS

Other Subdural Collections

- Subdural hygroma
  - Clear CSF, no encapsulating membranes
- Subdural effusion
  - Xanthochromic fluid secondary to extravasation of plasma from membrane or meningitis
  - Near CSF density
- Empyema: Peripheral enhancement, hyperintensity on FLAIR; restricted diffusion on DWI

Epidural Hematoma

- Biconvex extraaxial collection
- Often associated with fracture
- May cross dural attachments, limited by sutures

Pachymeningopathies (Thickened Dura)

- Chronic meningitis (may be indistinguishable)
- Neurosarcoid: Nodular, "lumpy-bumpy"
- Postsurgical (e.g., shunt)
- Intracranial hypotension
  - "Slumping" midbrain, tonsillar herniation

Tumor

- Meningioma, lymphoma, leukemia, metastases
- Dural-based enhancing masses
- ± skull and extracranial soft tissue involved

Peripheral Infarct

- Cortex involved, not displaced

- Hyperintense DWI

Chemical Shift Artifact

- Marrow or subcutaneous fat may "shift"; can appear intracranial, mimic T1-hyperintense SDH
  - Seen with ↑ field of view or ↓ bandwidth
  - Worse with higher field strength MR

PATHOLOGY

General Features

- Etiology
  - Trauma most common cause
    - Tearing of bridging cortical veins as they cross subdural space to drain into dural sinus
    - Nonimpact (falls) as well as direct injury
    - Trauma may be minor; often recurrent with initial episodes subclinical
  - Less common etiologies
    - Shunted hydrocephalus with ventricular decompression
    - Dissection of intraparenchymal hematoma into subarachnoid, then subdural space
    - Vascular malformations: Dural arteriovenous fistula, arteriovenous malformation (AVM), cavernoma
      - Typically, other hemorrhages present (parenchymal &/or subarachnoid)
    - Aneurysm rupture
    - Moyamoya (greater propensity for hemorrhage in adults, ischemia in children)
    - Spontaneous hemorrhage with severe coagulopathy
  - Predisposing factors
    - Atrophy
    - Shunting (→ ↑ traction on superior cortical veins)
    - Coagulopathy and anticoagulation
- Associated abnormalities
  - > 70% have other significant associated traumatic lesions
  - If mass effect, shift > aSDH thickness, suspect underlying edema/excitotoxic injury

Gross Pathologic & Surgical Features

- "Currant jelly," crescent-shaped hematoma
- Membranes/granulation tissue develop later
- Chronic SDHs may undergo fibrosis

Microscopic Features

- Outer membrane of proliferating fibroblasts and capillaries
- Fragile capillaries hypothesized as source of recurrent hemorrhage (chronic SDH)
- Inner membrane (made up of dural fibroblasts or border cells) forms fibrocollagenous sheet

CLINICAL ISSUES

Presentation

- Most common signs/symptoms
  - Most commonly following trauma
  - Varies from asymptomatic to loss of consciousness
    - "Lucid" interval in aSDH: Initially awake, alert patient loses consciousness few hours after trauma
    - Patients with early symptomatic presentation (< 4 hours) and advanced age have poor prognosis
  - Other symptoms (focal deficit, seizure) from mass effect, diffuse brain injury, secondary ischemia
  - Coagulopathy or anticoagulation ↑ risk and extent of hemorrhage

Demographics

- Any age, spontaneous SDH more common in older adults
- No sex predilection
- Epidemiology
  - Found in 30% of autopsy cases following craniocerebral trauma
  - In children, often seen after shunting for hydrocephalus

Natural History & Prognosis

- Can grow slowly with ↑ mass effect if untreated
- Compresses and displaces underlying brain
- Recurrent hemorrhage common; in children, raises suspicion of nonaccidental trauma

Treatment

- Poor prognosis (35-90% mortality)
  - Emergency preoperative high-dose mannitol may improve outcome
- Hematoma thickness, midline shift > 20 mm correlate with poor outcome
- Lethal if hematoma volume > 8-10% of intracranial volume

DIAGNOSTIC CHECKLIST

Consider

- NECT initial screen
- MR if degree of mass effect &/or symptoms > expected for size of SDH
  - Helps identify extent of traumatic brain injury
  - MR to evaluate nontraumatic causes
- In child with recurrent or mixed-age hemorrhage, suspect nonaccidental trauma

Image Interpretation Pearls

- Wide window settings for CT ↑ conspicuity of subtle SDH
- FLAIR, T2* usually most sensitive sequences for SDH
- CT density and MR intensity vary with age and degree of recurrent hemorrhage and contribution of CSF (arachnoid tears)

SELECTED REFERENCES

1. Aydın SO et al: Factors associated with non-traumatic spontaneous subdural hematomas in pediatric patients. Neuropediatrics. 54(4):239-43, 2023
2. Feldman KW et al: Short falls in childhood occasionally cause major brain injuries because of unusual circumstances. Pediatr Emerg Care. 39(5):335-41, 2023
3. Hahnemann ML et al: Characterization of subdural collections in initial neuroimaging of abusive head trauma: Implications for forensic age diagnostics and clinical decision-making. Eur J Radiol. 159:110652, 2023
4. Lee HC et al: Benign extracerebral fluid collection complicated by subdural hematoma and fluid collection: clinical characteristics and management. Childs Nerv Syst. 34(2):235-45, 2018
5. McLean LA et al: Does intracranial venous thrombosis cause subdural hemorrhage in the pediatric population? AJNR Am J Neuroradiol. 33(7):1281-4, 2012

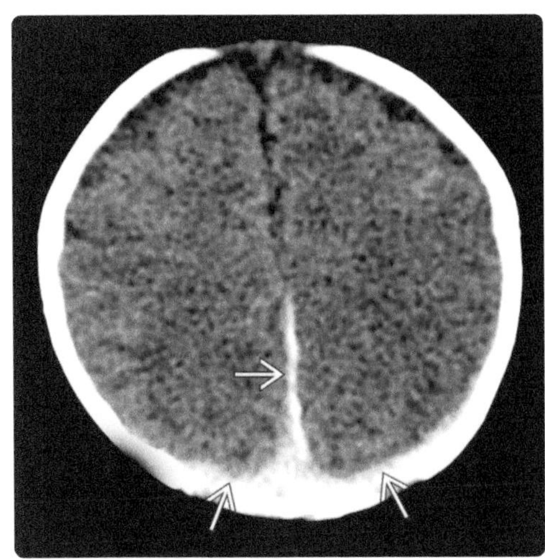

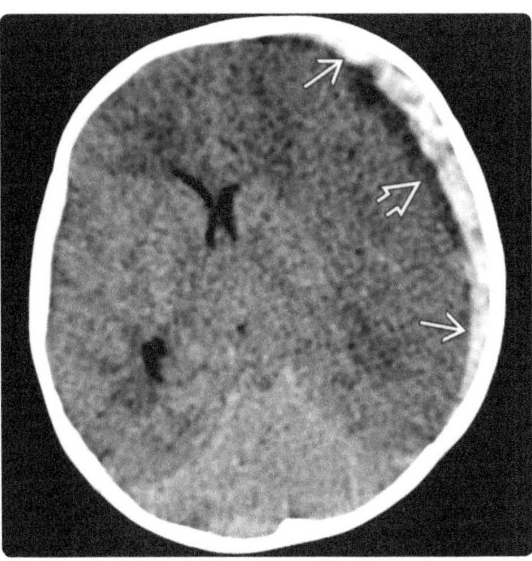

(Left) *Axial NECT in an infant with lethargy shows hyperdense subdural blood along the falx cerebri ➡ and dependently over the parietal lobes. An interhemispheric SDH is suspicious for abusive head trauma.* **(Right)** *Axial NECT shows an aSDH ➡ superimposed on a chronic SDH ➡ in an infant with nonaccidental trauma. Hypodensity in the left hemisphere and mass effect suggest underlying cerebral edema.*

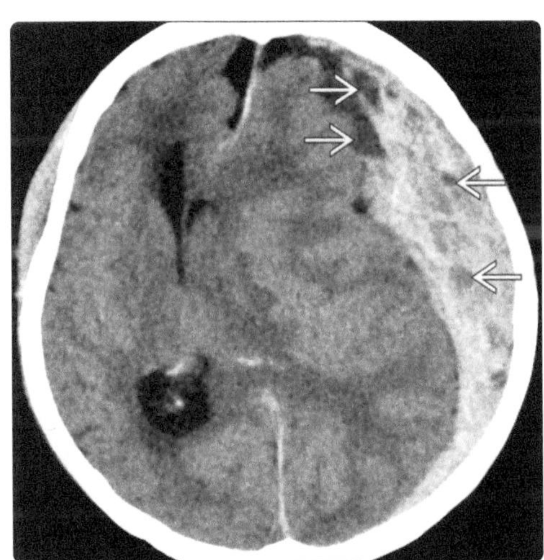

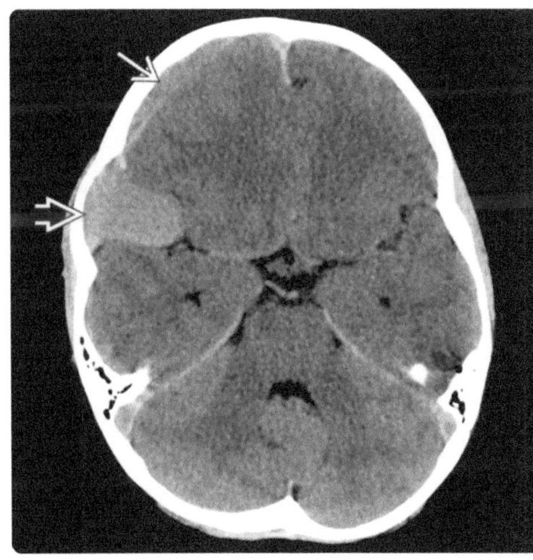

(Left) *Axial NECT shows a large, heterogeneous, acute left hemispheric SDH that is predominantly hyperdense but also contains irregular hypodense areas ➡, indicative of active bleeding (swirl sign).* **(Right)** *Axial NECT in a pediatric patient with headache after trivial trauma reveals an unusual mildly hyperdense SDH in the right middle cranial fossa ➡ continuing over the right frontal lobe ➡. This represents hemorrhage into a preexisting arachnoid cyst with CSF-blood mixing.*

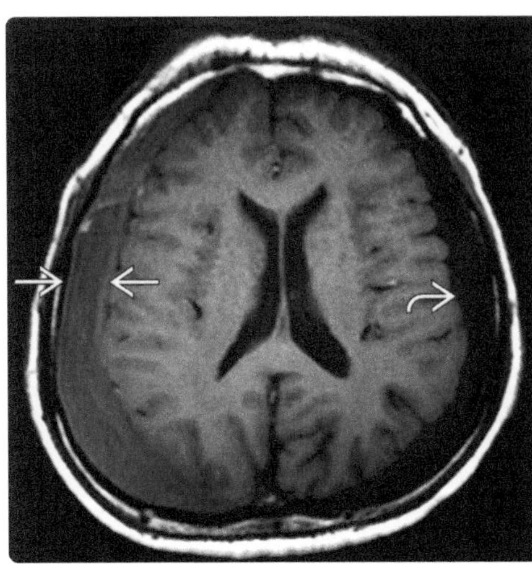

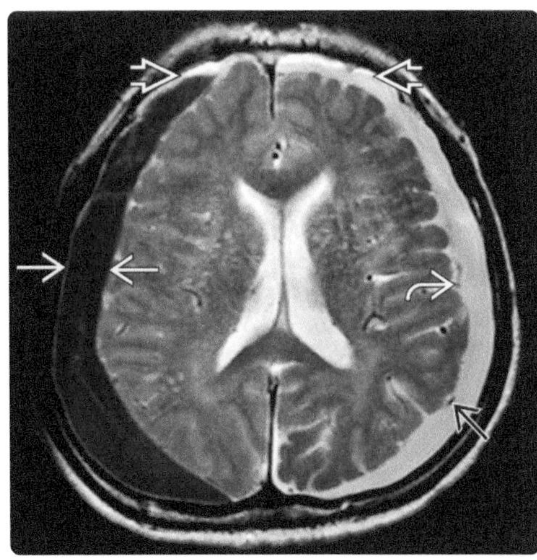

(Left) *Axial T1WI MR shows a right aSDH with early mild T1 hyperintensity ➡. The left-sided SDH ➡ is hyperacute and more closely follows CSF signal intensity.* **(Right)** *Axial T2WI MR of an aSDH in the same patient shows marked hypointensity ➡, typical for deoxyhemoglobin. The left-sided SDH ➡ is hyperacute, close to CSF signal. Pial vessels are displaced inward ➡ by the collection. Note layering fluid levels ➡ anteriorly in both.*

KEY FACTS

TERMINOLOGY

- Diverse presentations of subdural hematoma (SDH) according to timing, dilution, recurrence of bleed

IMAGING

- Crescent-shaped extraaxial collection that spreads diffusely over affected hemisphere with various densities/signals
- Within 1 or several cleavage planes within innermost cell layer of dura
- Crosses sutures, not dural attachments; may extend along falx, tentorium
- CT density & MR signal intensity vary with timing, dilution, organization, recurrence of bleed

PATHOLOGY

- Traumatic stretching & tearing of bridging cortical veins as they cross meninges
- Staging
    - Acute blood (< 7 days)
    - Subacute blood (7-22 days): Rapid, variable changes
    - Hygroma: CSF-like/CT, high T2/MR; may develop within days, either directly from trauma or from CSF ingress, into acute SDH
    - Chronic blood (> 22 days): Features relate to aging collection & to rebleeds from neomembranes

CLINICAL ISSUES

- Presentation ranges from asymptomatic to coma
- ↑ intracranial pressure, seizures, irritability, neurologic deficit, developmental delay
- Tends to resolve spontaneously after acute stage
- Prognosis depends on trauma severity & presence of associated lesions

DIAGNOSTIC CHECKLIST

- Guessing age of SDH from CT/MR appearance is highly deceptive
- Age of blood not necessarily same as age of hematoma or trauma

(Left) *Axial graphic shows a large convexity subdural hematoma (SDH) ➡ with traversing septations ➡ and compression of brain parenchyma. Magnified insert shows 2nd juxtaosseous SDH compartment ➡.* **(Right)** *Axial NECT shows a huge collection 3 months post surgery (no recorded intervening trauma) with 1 isodense ➡ and 1 hypodense ➡ component in 2 adjacent "subdural" (really dural) clefts.*

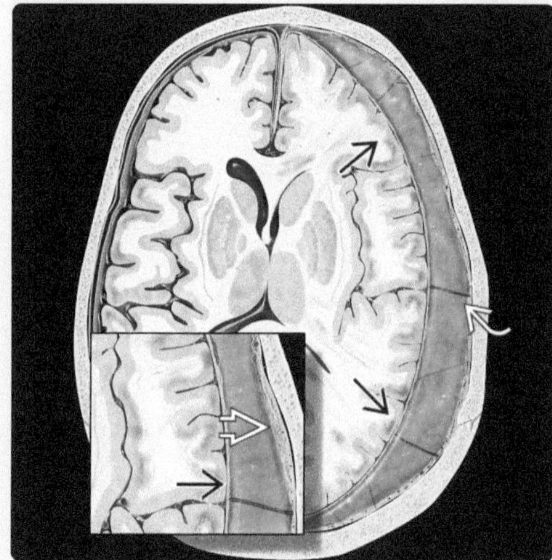

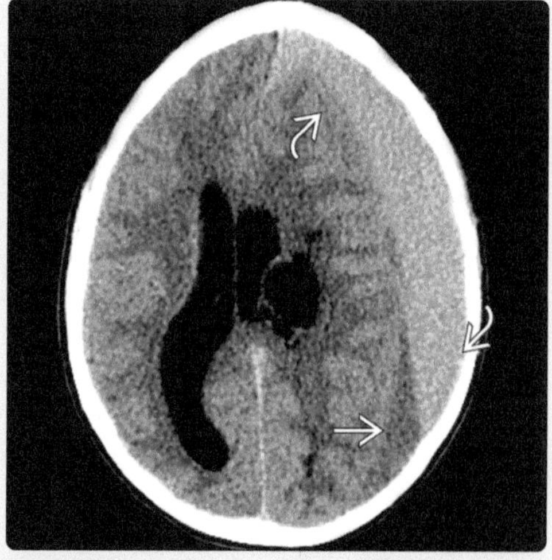

(Left) *Axial CECT shows large, bilateral, CSF-like subdural collections ➡ displacing the cortical vein ➡ inward. This collection developed over a period of 13 days after trauma and a minimal posterior SDH.* **(Right)** *Axial bone CT shows calcification of the inner membrane of an SDH ➡ in an infant who presented with an acute SDH right after birth.*

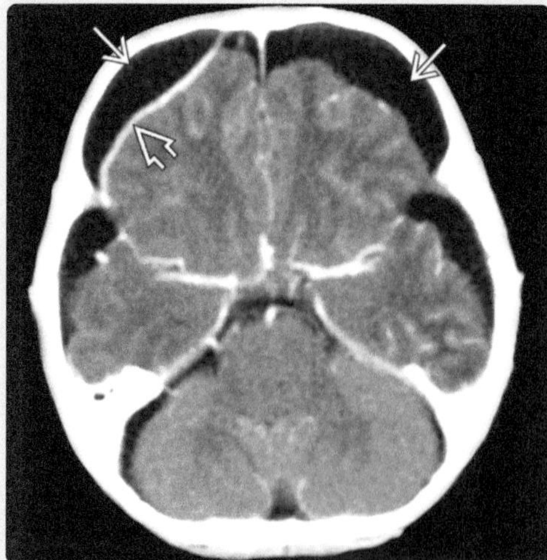

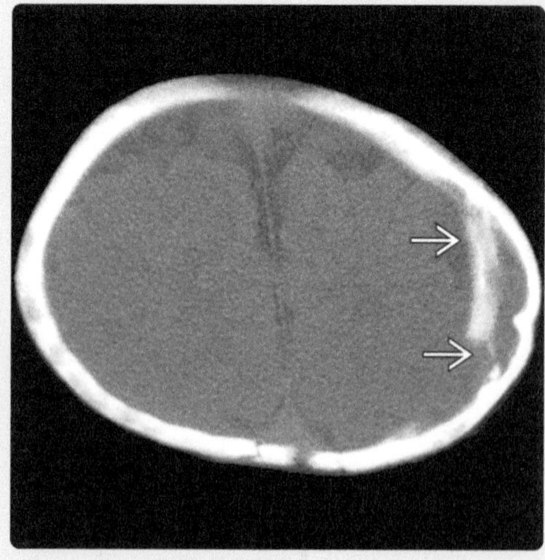

TERMINOLOGY

Abbreviations

- Evolving subdural hematoma (SDH)

Definitions

- Diverse presentations of SDH according to timing, dilution, recurrence of bleed

IMAGING

General Features

- Best diagnostic clue
  - Crescent-shaped extraaxial collection that spreads diffusely over affected hemisphere with various densities/signals
- Location
  - Within 1 or several cleavage planes within innermost cell layer of dura
- Morphology
  - Crescent-shaped extraaxial fluid collection
  - Crosses sutures, not dural attachments; may extend along falx, tentorium
  - Displaces underlying cortex
  - CT density & MR signal intensity vary with timing, dilution, organization, recurrence of bleed

CT Findings

- NECT
  - May be iso-, hyper-, or hypodense, or mixed in relation to cortex, at any stage of evolution
    - May be diverse in different locations
    - May be diverse in same location, in laminar way (typically acute stage)
    - May be diverse in same location, in patchy way (chronic, multiloculated SDH)
    - May be diverse in same location with dependent layering (chronic, bleed in hygroma)
  - May be CSF clear: Proteinaceous/xanthochromic hygroma (a.k.a. hydroma or sometimes effusion)
    - Directly from trauma or from aging acute SDH
    - May develop early; evolves to chronic SDH with subsequent bleed in 20-50%
  - Late calcification of inner membrane possible
  - Gray-white junction displaced medially; may see line of displaced/compressed sulci as "dots" of CSF
  - Low-dose CT detects large SDHs that need draining
- CECT
  - Dura, membranes enhance after acute stage
  - Inward displacement of enhanced cortical vessels

MR Findings

- T1WI
  - Diverse signals depending on age, hemoglobin (Hb) oxidation, CSF dilution
- T2WI
  - Usually hyperintense to CSF, layering possible
  - Very low intensity for recent blood or late hemosiderin
  - Vascular flow voids displaced inward
- FLAIR
  - Most conspicuous sequence; hyperintense compared to CSF
- T1WI C+
  - Dura, membranes enhance after acute stage

Imaging Recommendations

- Best imaging tool
  - Low-dose NECT initial screen; consider CECT for membranes/loculations
  - MR more sensitive for thin SDH & additional findings of traumatic brain injury

DIFFERENTIAL DIAGNOSIS

Other Pericerebral Hemorrhages

- Epidural hemorrhage (EDH): May be isodense, limited by sutures; may cross insertion of falx, tentorium
- Acute subdural hemorrhage: May be of mixed density on CT
- Subarachnoid hemorrhage (SAH): Cisternographic appearance; often associated with EDH, SDH, contusions

Other Subdural Collections

- Empyema: Pericerebral abscess, restricted diffusion

Clear, CSF-Like Pericerebral Collections

- Benign subarachnoid enlargement (benign idiopathic external hydrocephalus)
  - Crossed by bridging veins; macrocephaly; infants to toddlers (not so benign if due to ↑ venous pressure)
  - Controversial: Predisposing factor for SDH
- Subdural effusion: CSF-like, typically associated with meningitis; may be initial stage for empyema

Subdural Collections in Metabolic Diseases

- Menkes disease, glutaric aciduria type 1: Hygroma, hematoma

Pachymeningopathies: Thickened Enhancing Dura

- Postsurgical (shunt, etc.)
- Intracranial hypotension
- Diffuse dural thickening & enhancement from chronic venous thrombosis
- Subdural fibrosis after severe hydrocephalus

Tumors, Hemopathies

- Sarcoma, lymphoma, leukemia, extramedullary hematopoiesis
  - Dural-based, enhancing mass ± skull involvement

PATHOLOGY

General Features

- Etiology
  - Traumatic stretching & tearing of bridging cortical veins as they cross meninges
    - Anatomically, there is no subdural space, even virtual, between arachnoid & dura
    - Blood dissects innermost cell layer of dura into 1 or several cleavage planes
    - Meningeal tears allow CSF to develop similar collections as well or to mix with hemorrhages
  - Past acute stage, vascularized membranes/septa develop that may bleed spontaneously
- Associated abnormalities

- Be it nonaccidental or accidental, SDH commonly associated with other intracranial lesions

Gross Pathologic & Surgical Features

- CT, MR appearances: Depend on various factors
  - Clotted blood hyperdense to unclotted
  - Oxidation of Hb: Oxy-Hb (iso T1, high T2) vs. deoxy-Hb (iso T1, low T2)
  - Transition from ferrous Fe2+ to ferric Fe3+: Met-Hb (high T1, T2)
  - Late residual: Insoluble hemosiderin & soluble ferritin (low T2)
  - Fresh CSF mixing brings O2+ to Hb
  - CSF/blood dilution (secondary ingress of CSF in hemorrhage or secondary bleed in hygroma)
- Staging
  - Acute blood (< 7 days)
    - "Hyperacute" fresh unclotted blood: Isodense on CT; isointense T1, high T2 on MR
    - Acute clotted blood: Hyperdense on CT; isointense T1, low T2 on MR
    - Dilution apparent on CT mostly
    - Association common (laminar SDH)
  - Subacute blood (7-22 days): Rapid, variable changes
    - CT: Hypodensity more common (50%) than isodensity (40%); hyperdensity possible (10%)
    - MR: Classically high T1, low T2 early, turning high T1, high T2
    - Neomembranes, septations develop
  - Hygroma: CSF-like/CT, high T2/MR, may develop within days, either directly from trauma or from CSF ingress into acute SDH
  - Chronic blood (> 22 days): Features relate to aging collection & to rebleeds from neomembranes
    - Mostly secondary bleed in aging SDH/hygroma
    - Predominantly isodense (87%), uncommonly hypodense (13%)
    - Mixed loculated: Bleeds into septated collection
    - Mixed with dependent layering: Bleed into preexisting hygroma
    - CT/MR changes further dependent on age of rebleeds
- Acute SDH made of acute blood, but older SDH made of blood/fluid of various ages

Microscopic Features

- Membranes composed of hemorrhagic granulation tissue with resorbing blood products

CLINICAL ISSUES

Presentation

- Most common signs/symptoms
  - From asymptomatic to coma
  - ↑ intracranial pressure, seizures, irritability, neurologic deficit, developmental delay

Demographics

- Age
  - Teenagers: Sports, traffic accidents, violence
  - Infants: Abusive head injury, mostly
  - Neonate: Perinatal injury
- Sex
  - Among teenagers, boys > girls
- Epidemiology
  - SDH found in 10-20% of imaged & 30% of autopsy cases following craniocerebral trauma
    - Accidental trauma (high-velocity injury): Intensity & time of trauma well established
    - Nonaccidental injury (NAI): Unclear circumstances; evolving subdural more common; prognosis often poor
    - Untreated neonatal acute SDHs tend to evolve into chronic SDH
  - Uncommon complication of surgery: Craniectomy, shunting

Natural History & Prognosis

- Tends to resolve spontaneously after acute stage but not always
- Prognosis depends on trauma severity, presence of associated lesions
  - Death uncommon past acute period
  - Morbidity: 30-40%
- Developmental delay may result from neonatal SDH & associated injuries

Treatment

- Surgical evacuation/drainage if growing/symptomatic

DIAGNOSTIC CHECKLIST

Consider

- Guessing age of SDH from CT/MR appearance is highly deceptive
- Age of blood not necessarily same as age of hematoma or trauma

SELECTED REFERENCES

1. Dasgupta D et al: Utility of balanced steady-state field precession sequence in the evaluation of retinal and subdural hemorrhages in patients with abusive head trauma. Pediatr Radiol. 53(9):1842-53, 2023
2. Doswell A et al: Examining diagnostic variability among pediatric subspecialists using case examples of infant head injury. Child Abuse Negl. 144:106371, 2023
3. Raissaki M et al: Benign enlargement of the subarachnoid spaces and subdural collections-when to evaluate for abuse. Pediatr Radiol. 53(4):752-67, 2023
4. Asan Z: Growth potential of subdural hematomas under clinical observation: which subdural hematomas tend to grow and why they do. World Neurosurg. 113:e598-603, 2018
5. Gekat W et al: SDH and EDH in children up to 18 years of age-a clinical collective in the view of forensic considerations. Int J Legal Med. 132(6):1719-27, 2018
6. Pasarikovski CR et al: Delayed chronic subdural hematoma after total cranial vault reconstruction for sagittal synostosis. Pediatr Neurosurg. 53(3):200-4, 2018
7. Kpelao E et al: Clinical profile of subdural hematomas: dangerousness of subdural subacute hematoma. Neurosurg Rev. 39(2):237-40; discussion 240, 2016
8. Foster KA et al: Factors associated with hemispheric hypodensity after subdural hematoma following abusive head trauma in children. J Neurotrauma. 31(19):1625-31, 2014
9. Sieswerda-Hoogendoorn T et al: Age determination of subdural hematomas with CT and MRI: a systematic review. Eur J Radiol. 83(7):1257-68, 2014
10. Bradford R et al: Serial neuroimaging in infants with abusive head trauma: timing abusive injuries. J Neurosurg Pediatr. 12(2):110-9, 2013
11. Chotai S et al: Brain herniation induced by drainage of subdural hematoma in spontaneous intracranial hypotension. Asian J Neurosurg. 8(2):112-5, 2013
12. McKeag H et al: Subdural hemorrhage in pediatric patients with enlargement of the subarachnoid spaces. J Neurosurg Pediatr. 11(4):438-44, 2013

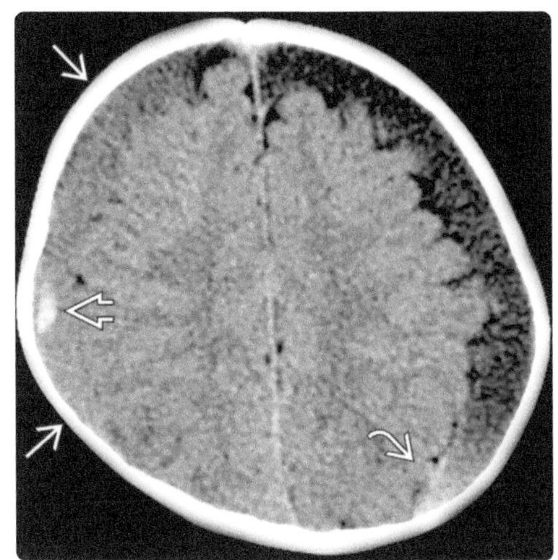

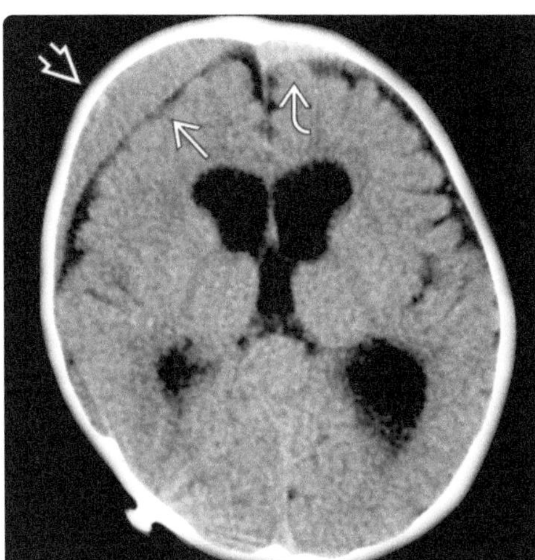

(Left) *Axial NECT in a 10-month-old infant with new neurologic symptoms shows large subdural collections, isodense ➡ with focal clot ➡ on the right and with layering on the left ➡.* **(Right)** *Axial NECT in the same child 2 months after evacuation of SDHs shows residual collections, larger on the right ➡ than on the left ➡, isodense to cortex with a tiny focal bleed on the right ➡.*

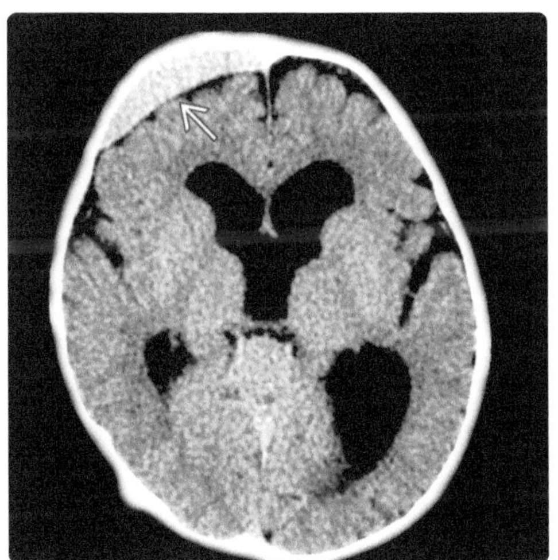

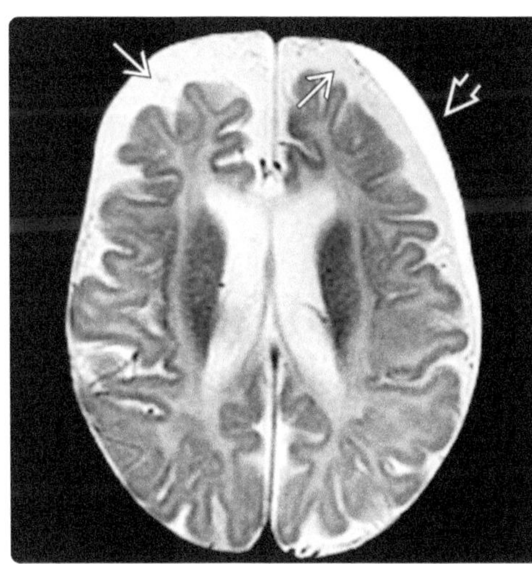

(Left) *Axial NECT in the same child after 1 month shows that the SDH has disappeared on the left while decreasing and becoming hyperdense on the right ➡; this disappeared altogether at 18 months.* **(Right)** *Axial T2 MR in an infant shows large, idiopathic, benign bilateral subarachnoid enlargement ➡ associated with a small left SDH ➡, possibly facilitated by venous stretching (controversial).*

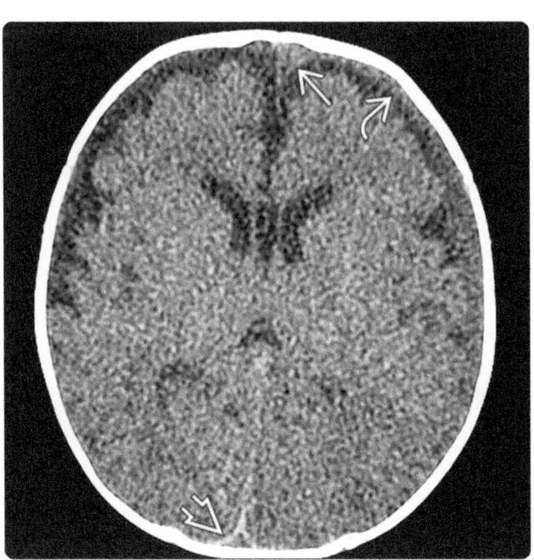

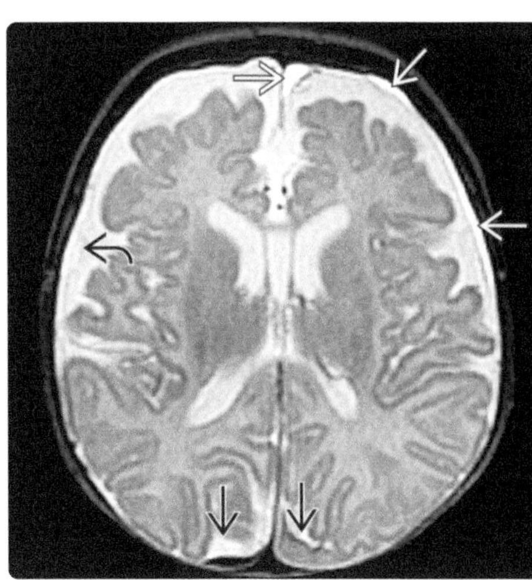

(Left) *Low-dose axial NECT shows subtle subacute SDH as hyperdensity to the left of the anterior falx cerebri ➡ and over the left frontal convexity ➡ as well as layering anterior to the superior sagittal sinus ➡.* **(Right)** *Axial T2 MR in the same patient 1 day later shows the anterior subdural collections ➡, larger posterior subdural collections ➡, and a small right-sided collection ➡. MR can be very useful in detecting SDH in the subacute phase.*

Cerebral Contusion

KEY FACTS

TERMINOLOGY

- Brain surface injuries involving gray matter and contiguous subcortical white matter

IMAGING

- Best diagnostic clue: Patchy hemorrhages within edematous background
- Characteristic locations: Adjacent to irregular bony protuberance or dural fold
- Anterior inferior frontal lobes and anterior inferior temporal lobes most common
- FLAIR: Best for hyperintense cortical edema and subarachnoid hemorrhage
- GRE: Hypointense hemorrhagic foci bloom
- Best imaging tool
  - CT to detect acute hemorrhagic contusions, other intracranial lesions, and herniations
  - MR to detect presence and delineate extent of lesions
    - MR is most sensitive for detection of associated DAI
- Coup: Direct injury to brain beneath impact site
- Contrecoup: Injury opposite impact site; usually more severe than coup

TOP DIFFERENTIAL DIAGNOSES

- Infarct
- Venous sinus thrombosis
- Cerebritis
- Low-grade neoplasm
- Transient postictal changes

CLINICAL ISSUES

- Initial symptom: Confusion → obtundation
- Central goal: Prevent and treat secondary injury
- Mass effect and herniation may require evacuation

DIAGNOSTIC CHECKLIST

- Perform multiplanar CT reconstructions for most sensitive detection
- Look for associated fractures or diastatic sutures

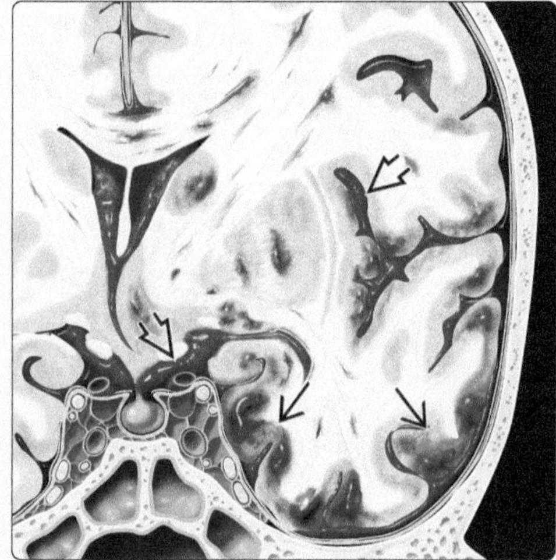

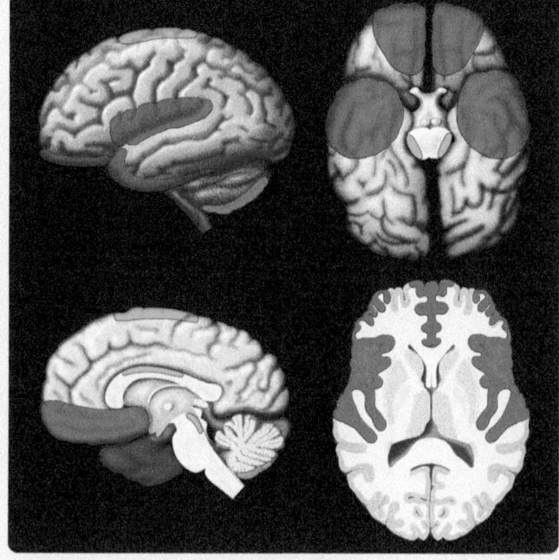

(Left) *Coronal graphic illustrates the pathology of a closed head injury. Note the hemorrhagic foci involving gray matter of several contused gyri ⇒, axonal and deep gray injuries, and traumatic subarachnoid hemorrhage ⇒ in the basal cisterns and sylvian fissure.* **(Right)** *Graphics depict the most common sites of cerebral contusions in red. Less common sites are shown in green. The most common locations of all are the anteroinferior frontal and temporal lobes.*

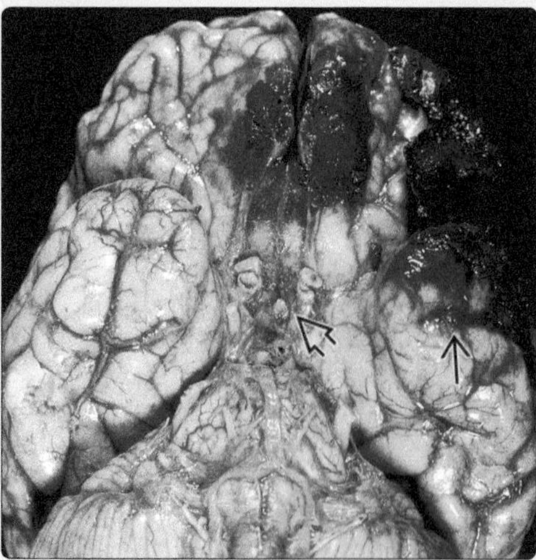

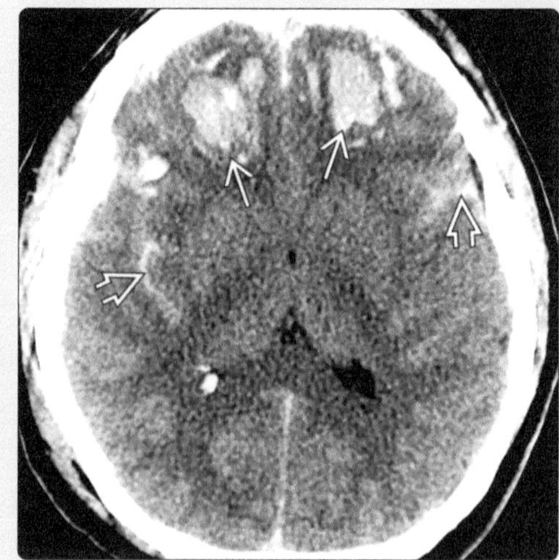

(Left) *Gross pathology of the brain from a patient who died from a severe closed head injury shows bifrontal and left temporal hemorrhagic contusions ⇒ as well as traumatic subarachnoid hemorrhage in the suprasellar cistern ⇒. (Courtesy R. Hewlett, MD.)* **(Right)** *Axial NECT shows extensive hemorrhagic contusions ➡ in the bilateral inferior frontal lobes. Also note the subarachnoid hemorrhage ➡ in the sylvian fissures in this patient with severe traumatic brain injury.*

TERMINOLOGY

Definitions

- Brain surface injuries involving gray matter and contiguous subcortical white matter

IMAGING

General Features

- Best diagnostic clue
  - Patchy hemorrhages within edematous background
- Location
  - Characteristic locations: Adjacent to irregular bony protuberance or dural fold
    - Anterior inferior frontal lobes and anterior inferior temporal lobes most common
    - 25% parasagittal ("gliding" contusions)
  - Less common locations
    - Parietal/occipital lobes, posterior fossa
  - Coup: Direct injury to brain beneath impact site
  - Contrecoup: Injury opposite impact site; usually more severe than coup
- Morphology
  - Early: Patchy, ill-defined, superficial foci of punctate or linear hemorrhage along gyral crests
  - 24-48 hours: Existing lesions enlarge and become more hemorrhagic; new lesions may appear
  - Chronic: Encephalomalacia with volume loss
  - Multiple bilateral lesions in 90% of cases

CT Findings

- NECT
  - Early: Patchy, ill-defined, low-density edema with small foci of hyperdense hemorrhage
  - 24-48 hours
    - Edema, hemorrhage, and mass effect often ↑
    - New foci of edema and hemorrhage may appear
    - Petechial hemorrhage may coalesce
  - Chronic
    - Become isodense, then hypodense
    - Encephalomalacia with volume loss
  - Secondary lesions
    - Herniations/mass effect with secondary infarction
    - Hydrocephalus due to hemorrhage
- Perfusion CT
  - More sensitive than NECT in detection of cerebral contusions (87.5% vs. 39.6%, respectively)

MR Findings

- T1WI
  - Acute: Inhomogeneous isointensity and mass effect
  - Chronic: Focal or diffuse atrophy
- FLAIR
  - Acute: Best for hyperintense cortical edema and subarachnoid hemorrhage (SAH)
  - Chronic
    - Hyperintense demyelination and microglial scarring
    - Hypointense hemosiderin staining
    - Hypointense cavitation (cystic encephalomalacia)
- T2* GRE
  - Acute: Hypointense hemorrhagic foci bloom
  - Chronic: Hypointense hemosiderin deposits
- DWI
  - Hyperintense in areas of cell death
  - ↓ apparent diffusion coefficient (ADC) correlates with poor outcome
  - Diffusion tensor imaging sometimes shows white matter damage when CT, routine MR appear normal
- MRS
  - ↓ NAA, ↑ choline

Nuclear Medicine Findings

- SPECT Tc-99m HMPAO imaging
  - Depicts focal changes in 53% with mild injury
  - Negative in 1st month predicts good outcome
    - Positive can predict poor clinical outcome

Imaging Recommendations

- Best imaging tool
  - CT to detect acute hemorrhagic contusions, other intracranial lesions, and herniations
  - MR to detect presence and delineate extent of lesions
- Protocol advice
  - CT: Perform multiplanar reconstructions for accurate detection
  - FLAIR for edema and SAH; GRE for hemorrhagic foci

DIFFERENTIAL DIAGNOSIS

Infarct

- No trauma history
- Characteristic acute-onset focal neurologic deficit
- Vascular distribution: Spares frontal and temporal poles

Venous Sinus Thrombosis

- Edema and hemorrhage adjacent to occluded sinus

Cerebritis

- No trauma history
- Herpes typically involves medial temporal lobe

Low-Grade Neoplasm

- No trauma history
- Solitary nonhemorrhagic lesion
- No predilection for anterior frontal or temporal lobes

Transient Postictal Changes

- No trauma history
- Preceding or ongoing seizure activity
- May be hyperintense on DWI; can enhance acutely

PATHOLOGY

General Features

- Etiology
  - Stationary head struck by object
    - Direct injury beneath impact site
    - Contusion is rare without fracture
  - Moving head: Motor vehicle crash, falls
    - Differential accel-/deceleration and rotational forces on portions of brain with different densities
    - Gliding injury: Cortex anchored to dura by arachnoid granulations; subcortical tissue glides more than cortex

- Traffic injuries are main cause in young adults (20-40 years of age)
- Falls are main cause in infants (0-4 years of age) and older adults (≥ 70 years of age)
- Associated abnormalities
  - Soft tissue injuries in 70% of patients
  - Subdural hematoma (SDH), traumatic SAH, intraventricular hemorrhage
  - Skull fracture at coup site

Gross Pathologic & Surgical Features

- Contusions
  - Edema along gyral crests
  - Petechial hemorrhages (most evident in 24-48 hours)
  - Small hemorrhages may coalesce into hematoma
  - Delayed hematomas may develop 24-48 hours later
- Lacerations
  - Intracerebral hematoma with "burst" lobe
  - SDH communicates with hematoma via lacerated brain, torn pia-arachnoid
- Liquefaction and encephalomalacia in chronic phase

Microscopic Features

- Capillary disruption → blood extravasation: RBCs cause visible hemorrhage, plasma leads to edema
- Perivascular hemorrhage, ↑ pinocytic activity of endothelial cells, and cytotoxic edema of astroglial cells
- Higher levels of serum protein S100B and IL-6 correlate with ultrastructural changes of endothelial cells

Cellular Features

- Chemokine, nitric oxide activation occurs early
  - Inflammatory response → neutrophil oxidative burst → proteolytic and neurotoxic enzyme release
  - Neuroinflammation mediated by cyto-/chemokines, complement
    - Contributes to secondary ischemic damage, contusion enlargement
  - CNS cells synthesize distinct chemokines
    - Chemokine CCL2 is highly expressed early in pericontusional area
    - Chemokine CXCL8 (a.k.a. IL-8) is highly expressed as late inflammatory mediator
  - Inflammatory processes contribute to pericontusional cytotoxic injury via astrocytic activation with capillary vessel compression and leukocyte accumulation → microvascular occlusion
- Blood-brain barrier failure aided by proinflammatory factor activation and matrix metalloproteinases
- Injured cortex upregulates peroxisome proliferator-activated receptor α (PPAR-α) binding activity and protein expression
  - Peaks 24-72 hours post injury; PPAR-α agonists protect against excessive oxidative stress and inflammation in traumatic brain injury (TBI) and stroke

CLINICAL ISSUES

Presentation

- Most common signs/symptoms
  - Varies with severity, from mild confusion to obtundation
    - ± cerebral dysfunction, seizures

Demographics

- Age
  - Children:adults = 2:1; highest risk between 15-24 years
- Sex
  - M:F = 3:1
- Epidemiology
  - Annual cerebral contusion incidence is 200 per 100,000 brain trauma-related hospitalizations
  - Contusion 2nd most common primary traumatic neuronal injury (44%); diffuse axonal injury (DAI) most common
  - 1.4 million suffer TBIs each year in USA; 50,000 die and 80,000 experience long-term disability
  - TBI causes 6.5% of deaths in USA (32 per 100,000)

Natural History & Prognosis

- Varies with extent of primary injury
- Outcome is critically dependent on extent of brain damage that evolves after initial insult
  - Secondary lesions: Hypoxia, hypotension, ischemia, brain edema, and ↑ intracranial pressure
- Highest mortality rate: Older adult population
  - Linear ↑ of 40-50% in odds of poor outcome for every 10 years of age
- 90% of patients survive injury
  - ~ 25% have significant residual complaints
- Temporal and especially brainstem contusions are independent risk factors for poor outcome
- In severe TBI, 63% have good clinical outcome, 32% have excellent clinical outcome

Treatment

- Central goal: Prevent or rapidly treat secondary injury
- Mitigate secondary effects of ↑ intracranial pressure, perfusion disturbances

DIAGNOSTIC CHECKLIST

Consider

- Repeat exam recommended if initial exam negative but symptoms persist for 24-48 hours

Image Interpretation Pearls

- Inferior anterior frontal lobes most often injured
- Mixed-density contusions can be mistaken for common artifacts caused by orbital roof

SELECTED REFERENCES

1. Branson HM et al: Conventional MR Imaging in trauma management in pediatrics. Neuroimaging Clin N Am. 33(2):251-60, 2023
2. Churchill NW et al: Perfusion imaging of traumatic brain injury. Neuroimaging Clin N Am. 33(2):315-24, 2023
3. Lin S et al: Establishment and validation of PTE prediction model in patients with cerebral contusion. Sci Rep. 12(1):20574, 2022
4. Zhang L et al: Combined radiomics model for prediction of hematoma progression and clinical outcome of cerebral contusions in traumatic brain injury. Neurocrit Care. 36(2):441-51, 2022
5. Ferrazzano PA et al: Use of magnetic resonance imaging in severe pediatric traumatic brain injury: assessment of current practice. J Neurosurg Pediatr. 8:1-9, 2019
6. Frey C et al: Essentials of head trauma imaging. Semin ultrasound CT MR. 39(5):469-40, 2018
7. Haghbayan H et al: The prognostic value of MRI in moderate and severe traumatic brain injury: a systematic review and meta-analysis. Crit Care Med. 45(12):e1280-8, 2017

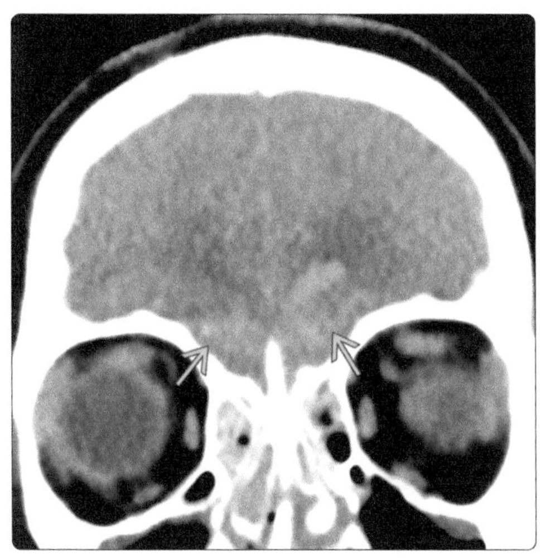

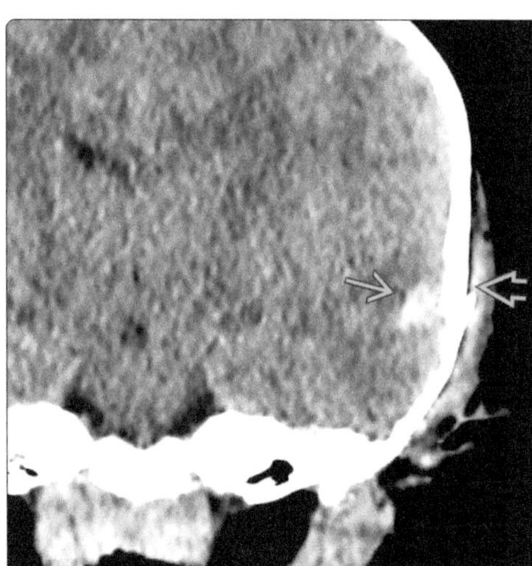

(Left) *Coronal NECT in a teenager involved in an MVA shows bilateral areas of high attenuation in the inferior frontal lobes, consistent with hemorrhagic contusions ➡. The inferior frontal lobes are a very common location for hemorrhagic contusion.* **(Right)** *Coronal NECT in a 3-year-old involved in an ATV accident shows a hemorrhagic contusion ➡ in the left temporal lobe deep to a diastatic squamosal suture ⇨. Younger children are at risk for sutural diastasis, which can result in underlying hemorrhagic contusion.*

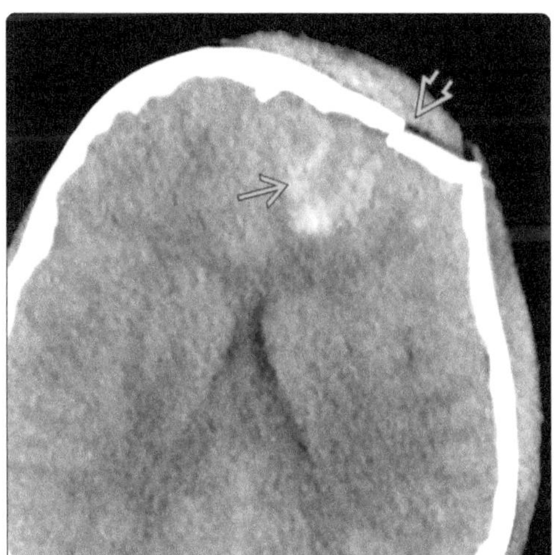

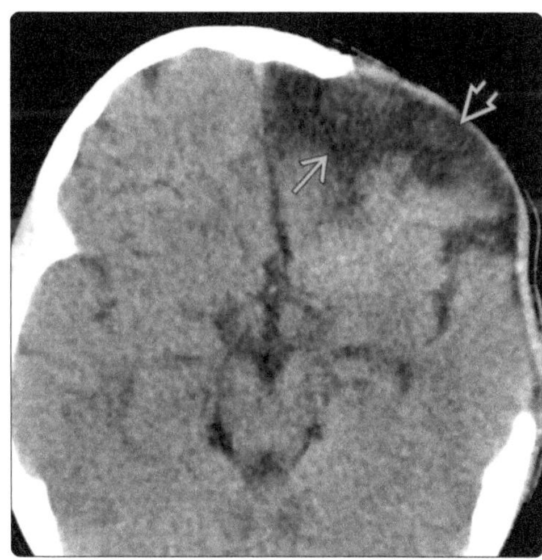

(Left) *Axial NECT in an 8-year-old shows a depressed frontal bone fracture ⇨ with large left frontal hemorrhagic contusion ➡. Large hemorrhagic contusions are often associated with overlying skull fractures.* **(Right)** *Axial NECT in the same patient following craniectomy ⇨ is shown. Months later, the high-attenuation blood products are no longer evident, and there are areas of low attenuation and volume loss ➡ consistent with encephalomalacia, a typical outcome for hemorrhagic contusions.*

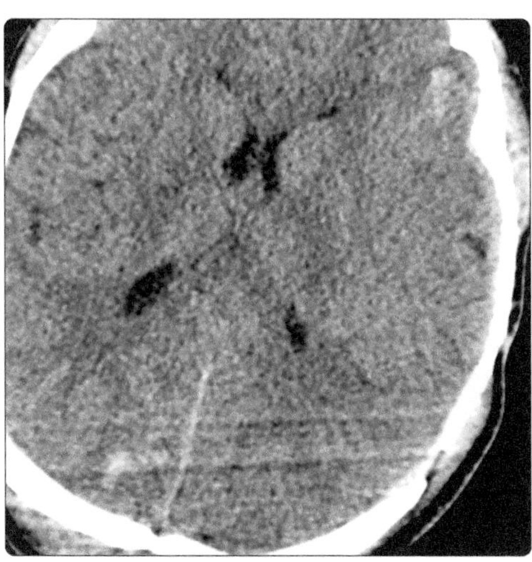

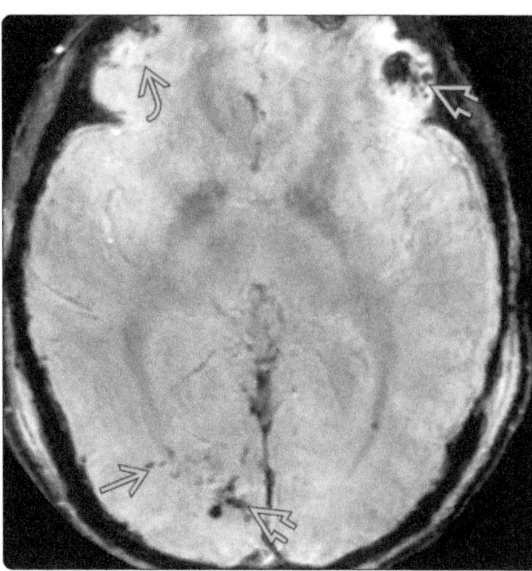

(Left) *Axial NECT in a teenager involved in an MVA shows hemorrhagic cortical contusions in the left frontal and right occipital lobes, consistent with contrecoup injury. Whenever a cortical contusion is identified, always look for a contrecoup injury.* **(Right)** *Axial SWI in the same patient shows the contrecoup injuries ⇨ but also shows small adjacent areas of injury in the occipital lobe ➡ and a 3rd area of injury in the right frontal lobe ↪, not seen on CT. SWI is the most sensitive sequence for detection of hemorrhagic brain injury.*

Diffuse Axonal Injury

KEY FACTS

TERMINOLOGY

- Diffuse axonal injury (DAI): Traumatic axonal stretch injury

IMAGING

- General features
  - Can be hemorrhagic or nonhemorrhagic
    - Hemorrhagic DAI: Microhemorrhages are important imaging biomarker for axonal injury
    - Nonhemorrhagic DAI: Stretch injury without associated microhemorrhage
  - Location
    - Subcortical/deep white matter (WM), corpus callosum
    - Deeper brain involvement = poor prognosis
- NECT often normal (50-80%)
- MR: Most sensitive imaging modality
  - FLAIR: Hyperintense foci
  - T2*GRE: Hypointense blooming foci (hemorrhage)
  - SWI: Depicts significantly more DAI foci than GRE
  - DWI: May show restricted diffusion

TOP DIFFERENTIAL DIAGNOSES

- Familial multiple cavernous malformations
- Prior cardiothoracic surgery
- Radiation-induced small vessel damage

PATHOLOGY

- Closed head injury (CHI)
  - Sudden deceleration, abrupt changes in angular momentum
- Cortex, WM have different densities, rotate at different speeds in CHI
  - Axons stretched (rarely disconnected or "sheared")
  - Occurs at interfaces between tissues of differing density
- 80% of lesions are microscopic, nonhemorrhagic

DIAGNOSTIC CHECKLIST

- Consider DAI if low GCS, normal NECT
- Deeper the abnormalities, more severe the brain injury
- Visible lesions are "tip of iceberg"

(Left) *Sagittal graphic shows multiple diffuse axonal injury (DAI) hemorrhagic foci within the corpus callosum and brainstem. Also note the hemorrhage levels in the ventricles. Intraventricular hemorrhage is often associated with more severe injury.* **(Right)** *Graphics depict the most common sites of DAI in red. Frequent but relatively less common locations are shown in green. Injury to the midbrain/upper pons (purple) is uncommon but often lethal. In general, the deeper the abnormalities, the more severe the injury.*

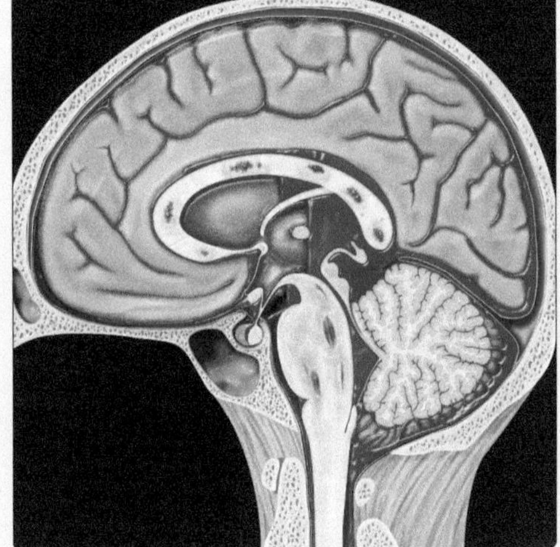

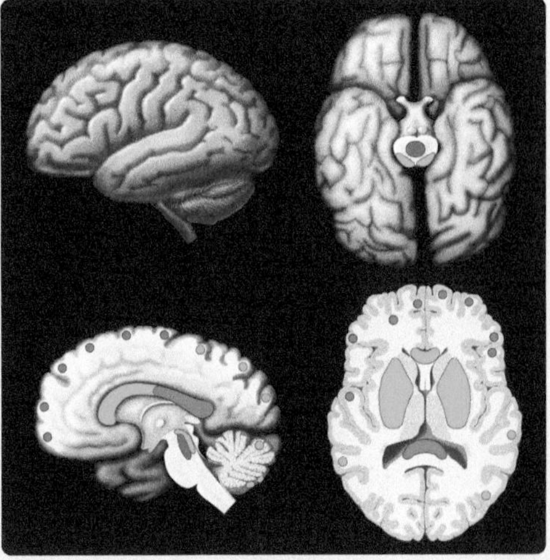

(Left) *Axial NECT in a 25-year-old man involved in a high-impact MVA shows multiple hemorrhagic foci in the subcortical WM, external and internal capsules, basal ganglia, and thalami. Blood is also present in the 3rd and lateral ventricles.* **(Right)** *Sagittal DWI MR in a 14-year-old involved in an MVA shows extensive diffusion restriction (↓ ADC not shown) throughout the body & anterior splenium of the corpus callosum. Diffusion restriction may be associated with hemorrhagic & nonhemorrhagic shear injury.*

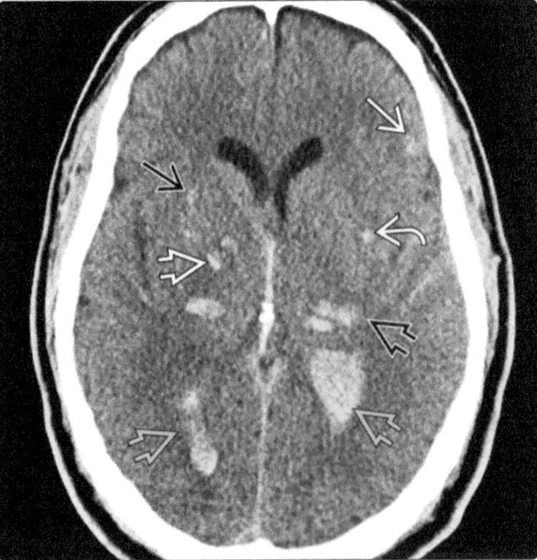

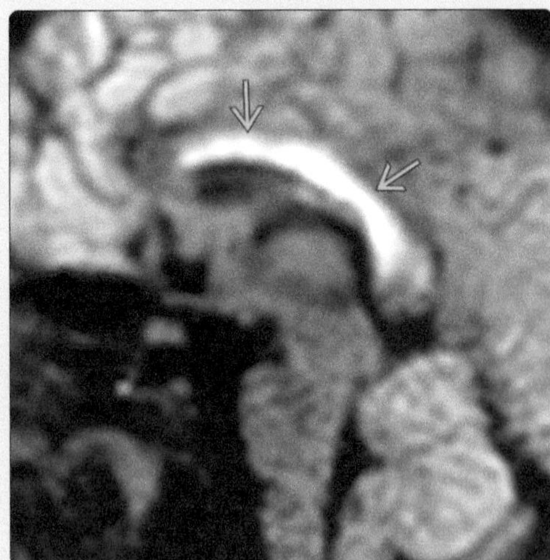

TERMINOLOGY

Abbreviations

- Diffuse axonal injury (DAI)

Definitions

- Traumatic axonal stretch injury

IMAGING

General Features

- Best diagnostic clue
  - Microbleeds (important imaging marker for DAI)
  - Punctate lesions at corticomedullary junction, corpus callosum, deep gray matter (GM), brainstem
  - Diffusion restriction is common associated finding
- Location
  - GM-white matter (WM) interface (67%), especially frontotemporal lobes
  - Corpus callosum (20%); 75% involve splenium, posterior body
  - Brainstem, especially dorsolateral midbrain and upper pons (poor prognosis)
  - Less common
    - Deep GM, internal/external capsule, tegmentum, fornix, corona radiata, cerebellar peduncles
- Size
  - Punctate to 15 mm
- Morphology
  - Punctate, round, ovoid foci; often hemorrhagic
  - Usually multifocal, often bilateral

CT Findings

- NECT
  - Often normal (50-80%)
    - > 30% with negative CT have positive MR
  - Nonhemorrhagic: Small, hypodense foci
  - Hemorrhagic: Small, hyperdense foci (20-50%)
    - 10-20% evolve to focal mass lesion
    - Lesions often more conspicuous on follow-up days later

MR Findings

- T1WI
  - Usually normal
  - If > 1 cm and hemorrhagic, hyperintense in acute phase
- T2WI
  - Nonhemorrhagic: Hyperintense foci
  - Hemorrhagic: Hypointense foci
- FLAIR
  - Nonhemorrhagic DAI: Hyperintense foci
  - Hemorrhagic DAI: Hypointense foci
- T2* GRE
  - Most sensitive "routine" sequence
    - Microbleeds may be visible only on GRE
    - Hypointense foci (susceptibility from blood products)
  - SWI
    - More sensitive detection of DAI compared to GRE
- DWI
  - May show foci of restricted diffusion, especially in WM and corpus callosum
  - Diffusion tensor imaging (DTI)
    - Fractional anisotropy (FA) maps document integrity and direction of WM tracts
    - Damage to WM may be visible on FA maps
    - DTI "tractograms" allow delineation of WM tract disruption pattern
      - Detect abnormalities when routine imaging, including GRE, is normal
- MRS
  - Normal-appearing brain
    - ↓ N-acetyl aspartate in WM 2° to neuronal injury
    - ↑ choline in GM suggestive of inflammation
  - Abnormal NAA/Cr and Cho/Cr accurately predicts outcomes in
    - Normal-appearing brain (85%)
    - Visibly injured brain (67%)

Nuclear Medicine Findings

- PET
  - Hypometabolism in cingulate gyrus, lingual gyrus, and cuneus
    - Dysfunction of above regions plays key role in neuropsychologic deficits
- SPECT
  - May show focal perfusion abnormalities

Imaging Recommendations

- Best imaging tool
  - MR with DTI
- Protocol advice
  - Nonhemorrhagic: FLAIR + DWI ± DTI tractography
  - Hemorrhagic: SWI best (use T2* GRE if not available)

DIFFERENTIAL DIAGNOSIS

Familial Multiple Cavernous Malformations

- Typically have numerous small foci of SWI/GRE signal loss randomly scattered throughout brain parenchyma
- Typically have some larger associated lesions evident on T1/T2 MR (mixed-age hemorrhages)

Prior Cardiothoracic Surgery

- Multifocal punctate foci of SWI/GRE signal loss are common following cardiothoracic bypass
- Likely etiology are small microemboli during bypass

Radiation-Induced Small Vessel Damage

- Whole-brain or focal radiation often results in multiple tiny foci of SWI/GRE signal loss
- Likely etiology is tiny microhemorrhages that may develop into cavernous malformations

PATHOLOGY

General Features

- Etiology
  - Overlying cortex moves at different speed in relation to underlying deep brain structures
    - Results in axonal stretching, particularly where brain tissues of different density intersect
  - Trauma-induced forces of inertia
    - Differential acceleration/deceleration and rotational/angular forces

- Head impact not required
- Axons stretched, rarely disconnected or "sheared" (only in most severe injury)
- Effect on nondisruptively injured axons
  - Traumatic depolarization, ion fluxes, spreading depression, and excitatory amino acid release
  - Metabolic alterations with accelerated glycolysis and lactate accumulation
  - Cellular swelling, cytotoxic edema, and apoptosis
- Corpus callosum injury
  - Believed due to rotational shear/strain forces
  - Posterior falx prevents tissue displacement, allowing greater tensile stresses locally

Staging, Grading, & Classification

- Adams and Gennarelli staging
  - Stage 1: Frontal and temporal lobe GM-WM interface lesions [mild traumatic brain injury (TBI)]
  - Stage 2: Lesions in lobar WM and corpus callosum (moderate TBI)
  - Stage 3: Lesions of dorsolateral midbrain and upper pons (severe TBI)
- Increasing severity of traumatic force correlates with deeper brain involvement

Microscopic Features

- 80% of lesions are microscopic, nonhemorrhagic
  - Visible lesions are "tip of iceberg"
- Impaired axoplasmic transport, axonal swelling
- Axonal swelling 2° to "axotomy" and "retraction" balls
- Microglial clusters
- Macro-, microbleeds (torn penetrating vessels = diffuse vascular injury)

CLINICAL ISSUES

Presentation

- Most common signs/symptoms
  - Transient LOC, retrograde amnesia in mild TBI
  - LOC at moment of impact: Moderate to severe TBI
  - Immediate coma typical
    - Persistent vegetative state in severe cases
    - Slow recovery in many cases
  - Greater impairment than with cerebral contusions, intracerebral hematoma, extraaxial hematomas
- Clinical profile
  - Suggestive in patient with clinical symptoms disproportionate to imaging findings
  - Most common primary traumatic neuronal injury (48%)
    - Usually in setting of high-velocity MVA
    - Admission Glasgow Coma Scale (GCS) may not correlate with outcome

Demographics

- Age
  - Any but most common in 15-24 year olds
  - May occur in utero if pregnant woman subjected to sufficient force
- Sex
  - Men 2x as likely to sustain TBI; peaks at 20-24 years
- Epidemiology
  - 2 million TBIs annually in USA
  - Leading cause of death/disability in children and young adults
  - ~ 50% of all primary intraaxial traumatic brain lesions in moderate and severe TBI
  - 80-100% autopsy prevalence in fatal injuries

Natural History & Prognosis

- Spectrum of severity: Mild to severe
  - Mild TBI most common: Clinical abnormalities may persist for months or longer
    - Headache, memory and mild cognitive impairment, personality change (postconcussion syndrome)
- Severe DAI rarely causes death
  - > 90% remain in persistent vegetative state (brainstem spared)
  - Prognosis worsens as number of lesions increases
- 10% of patients who return to normal function do so within 1 year
  - May experience prolonged symptoms
- Extent of DAI on MR correlates with functional outcome
  - Involvement of corpus callosum correlates with poor outcome
- Brainstem damage (pontomedullary rent) associated with immediate or early death
- Neurocognitive deficits thought to persist in 100% of severe, 67% of moderate, and 10% of mild TBI
  - Figures may significantly underestimate sequelae of mild and moderate TBI

Treatment

- No real treatment; supportive therapy
- Treatment of comorbidities: Herniation, hemorrhage(s), hydrocephalus, seizures

DIAGNOSTIC CHECKLIST

Consider

- Consider DAI if symptoms are disproportionate to imaging findings

Image Interpretation Pearls

- Best detected by FLAIR and DWI (nonhemorrhagic) or SWI (hemorrhagic)

SELECTED REFERENCES

1. Branson HM et al: Conventional MR Imaging in trauma management in pediatrics. Neuroimaging Clin N Am. 33(2):251-60, 2023
2. Sriyook A et al: Imaging of head trauma: pearls and pitfalls. Radiol Clin North Am. 61(3):535-49, 2023
3. Dahl J et al: Cerebral microbleeds and structural white matter integrity in patients with traumatic brain injury-a diffusion tensor imaging study. Front Neurol. 13:888815, 2022
4. Ferguson NM et al: Magnetic resonance imaging findings in infants with severe traumatic brain injury and associations with abusive head trauma. Children (Basel). 9(7), 2022
5. Janas AM et al: Diffuse axonal injury grade on early MRI is associated with worse outcome in children with moderate-severe traumatic brain injury. Neurocrit Care. 36(2):492-503, 2022
6. Ferrazzano PA et al: Use of magnetic resonance imaging in severe pediatric traumatic brain injury: assessment of current practice. J Neurosurg Pediatr. 1-9, 2019
7. van Eijck MM et al: Diffuse axonal injury after traumatic brain injury is a prognostic factor for functional outcome: a systematic review and meta-analysis. Brain Inj. 32(4):395-402, 2018

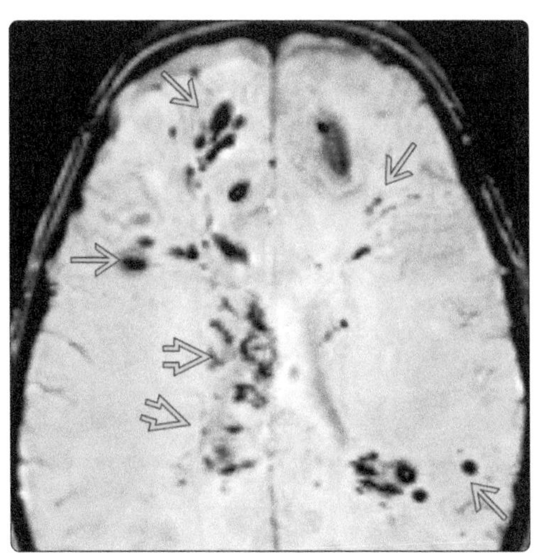

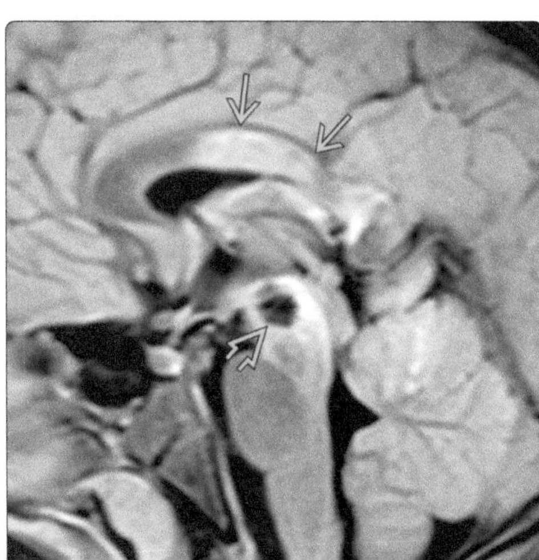

(Left) *Axial SWI MR in a teenager involved in an MVA shows extensive DAI in the periphery of the hemispheres near the gray-white junction ➔ as well as the right corpus callosum ⇨.* **(Right)** *Midline FLAIR MR in the same patient shows extensive signal abnormality throughout the corpus callosum ➔. Also note the hemorrhage/DAI within the midbrain ⇨. Involvement of DAI in critical structures, such as the corpus callosum and brainstem, portends a very poor prognosis in traumatic brain injury (TBI) patients.*

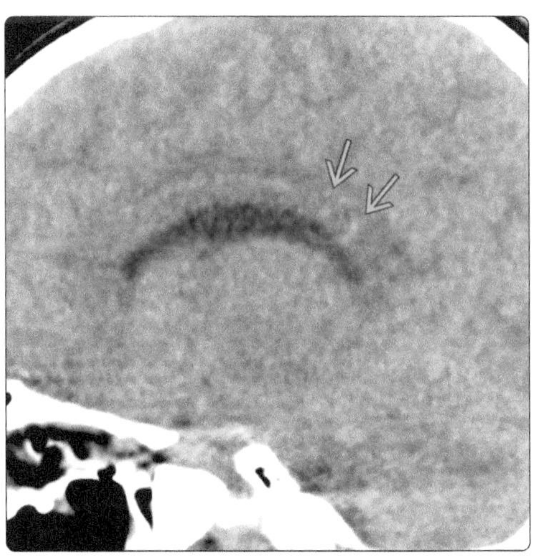

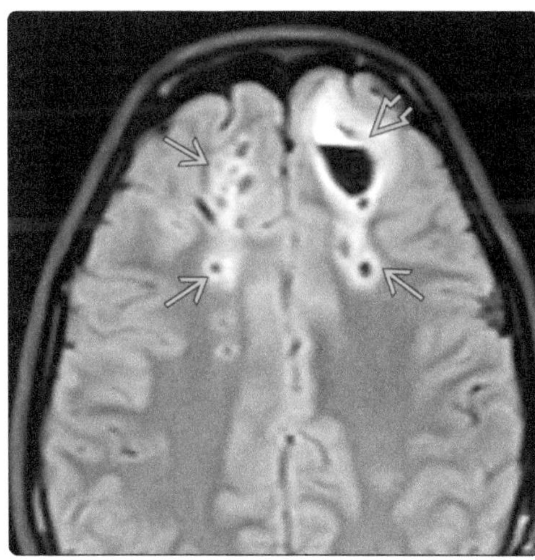

(Left) *Sagittal NECT in a 6-year-old involved in an MVA with DAI shows small, linear areas of increased attenuation ➔ in the posterior body & splenium, consistent with hemorrhagic axonal shear injury.* **(Right)** *Axial FLAIR MR in a teenager involved in an MVA shows bilateral parasagittal DAI ➔, a common location for DAI. Also note the associated parenchymal laceration in the left frontal lobe with the characteristic hematocrit level ⇨. Lacerations accompany a minority of TBI patients with DAI.*

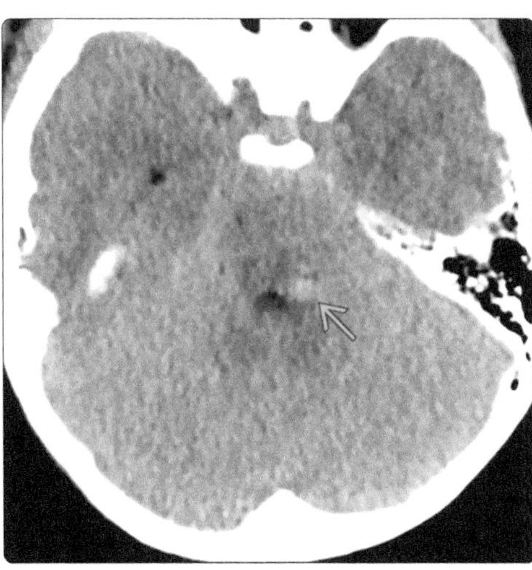

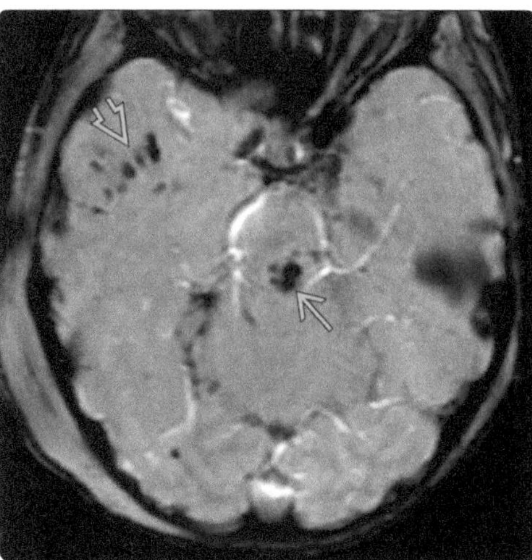

(Left) *Axial NECT in a 6-year-old involved in an MVA shows hyperattenuation within the dorsal midbrain ➔, the most likely brainstem location. Also note the loss of normal posterior fossa cisterns around the brainstem, consistent with cerebral swelling & herniation.* **(Right)** *Axial SWI MR in the same patient shows the hemorrhagic DAI ➔ in the posterior brainstem as well as additional foci of axonal shear injury ⇨ at the the GW-WM junction in the right temporal lobe.*

KEY FACTS

TERMINOLOGY

- Subcortical injury (SCI): Deep diffuse axonal injury lesions of brainstem, basal ganglia, thalamus, and regions around 3rd ventricle
- Intraventricular hemorrhage (IVH): Hemorrhage within ventricular system
- Choroid hemorrhage (CH): Hemorrhage localized to choroidal plexus

IMAGING

- SCI: SWI is most sensitive for detection; DWI helpful in detection of nonhemorrhagic axonal injury
- IVH: Hyperdense intraventricular blood; fluid-heme level common
- CH: Localized hyperdense choroidal hemorrhage

TOP DIFFERENTIAL DIAGNOSES

- SCI: Cavernous malformation, lacunar infarcts, small vessel ischemia
- IVH: None
- CH: Normal calcification may mask small hemorrhages

PATHOLOGY

- SCI: Most commonly induced by shear-strain forces that disrupt penetrating &/or choroidal vessels
- IVH: Disruption of subependymal veins
- CH: Traumatic shear forces damage to choroid tissue

CLINICAL ISSUES

- SCI: Profound neurologic deficits
- IVH: Obtundation, seizures
- CH: Can lead to IVH

DIAGNOSTIC CHECKLIST

- Delayed development of deep lesions common
  - Initial scan may show only diffuse brain swelling
  - Focal lesions often appear 24-48 hours later
- Remember: Deeper lesion indicates more severe injury

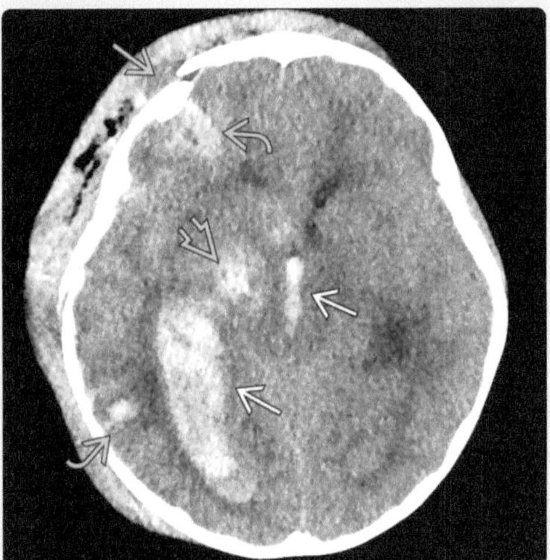

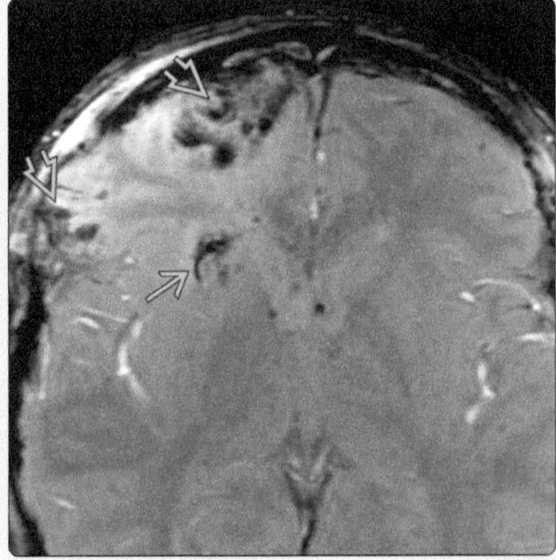

(Left) *Axial NECT in a 3-year-old with severe traumatic brain injury (TBI) after falling from a 2nd story shows a depressed skull fracture ➡, hemorrhagic contusions ➡, basal ganglia hemorrhage ➡, and intraventricular hemorrhage (IVH)* ➡. **(Right)** *Axial SWI MR in the same patient shows the right basal ganglia hemorrhage ➡ but also more extensive right frontal cortical contusion ➡, which was not well visualized on CT. SWI is the most sensitive exam for detection of subcortical hemorrhage and associated parenchymal injury.*

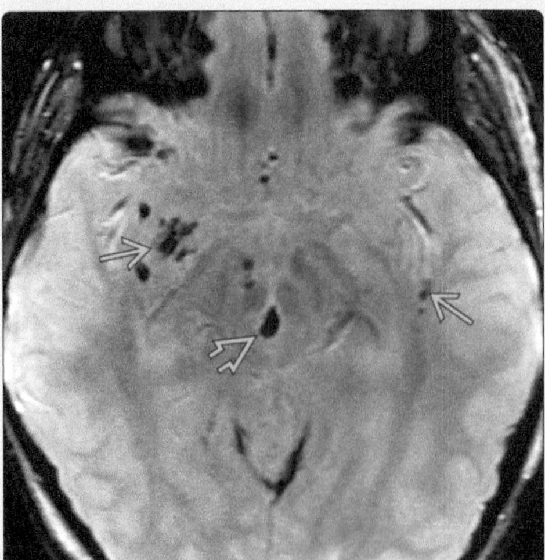

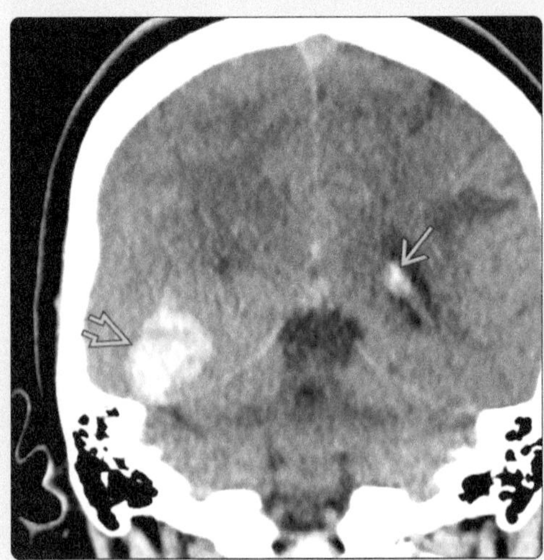

(Left) *Axial SWI MR in a 12-year-old in a severe bike accident shows multifocal areas of axonal shear injury in the cerebral hemispheres ➡ as well as the midline midbrain ➡. Deep hemorrhagic brain injury involving the brainstem carries a poor prognosis.* **(Right)** *Coronal NECT in a 12-year-old with chronic renal failure, HTN, and spontaneous right temporal hemorrhage ➡ shows increased attenuation in the left choroid glomus ➡, consistent with choroid plexus hemorrhage.*

TERMINOLOGY

Abbreviations

- Subcortical injury (SCI)

Definitions

- Traumatic lesions of brainstem (BS), basal ganglia (BG), thalamus, and ventricles, composed of
  - Deep diffuse axonal injury (DAI)-type SCI lesions
  - Intraventricular hemorrhage (IVH)
  - Choroid hemorrhage (CH)

IMAGING

General Features

- Best diagnostic clue
  - SCI: Punctate hemorrhages
  - IVH: Hyperdense intraventricular CSF on NECT, fluid-heme level common
  - CH: Hyperdense, enlarged choroid on NECT
- Location
  - SCI: BS, BG, thalamus, and regions around 3rd ventricle
    - Most within thalamus and putamen
  - IVH: Intraventricular spaces
  - CH: Localized within choroid tissue
- Size
  - SCI: Limited to size of structure involved
  - IVH: Can fill/expand ventricles
  - CH: Limited to size of choroid involved
- Morphology
  - SCI: Petechial, linear, globular
  - IVH: Can cast ventricle
  - CH: Shape of choroid involved

CT Findings

- NECT
  - SCI: Often normal; petechial hyperdense foci
    - Deep nuclei, dorsolateral BS, periaqueductal
    - Rarely overt hemorrhage
  - IVH
    - Hyperdense intraventricular blood
    - May fill, even expand, ventricle
    - Fluid-heme level common
  - CH: Localized hyperdense choroidal hemorrhage

MR Findings

- T1WI
  - SCI: Acutely isointense
  - IVH: Fluid-heme level common
- T2WI
  - SCI: Acutely hyperintense
  - IVH: Fluid-heme
- FLAIR
  - SCI: Most sensitive sequence → hyperintense foci
  - IVH: Detection comparable to CT in acute stage
- T2* GRE
  - SCI: Susceptibility of petechial hemorrhage
- DWI
  - SCI: Foci of restricted diffusion
    - ↓ apparent diffusion coefficient (ADC)
    - Damage to white matter reduces anisotropy: Visible on fractional anisotropy (FA) maps
    - DTI "tractograms" allow delineation of pattern of white matter tract disruption
    - Detects abnormalities when routine imaging, including GRE, are normal
- SWI
  - More sensitive than GRE for detection of DAI

Imaging Recommendations

- Best imaging tool
  - SCI: MR > > > CT
    - Protocol analogous to DAI
  - ICH/CH: NECT > MR
    - Protocol analogous to subarachnoid hemorrhage (SAH)
- Protocol advice
  - SCI: FLAIR and GRE
  - ICH/CH
    - CT = NECT
    - MR = FLAIR and GRE

DIFFERENTIAL DIAGNOSIS

Subcortical Injury

- Cavernous malformation: Symptoms without trauma
- Lacunar infarcts: Located in central tegmentum of pons/BS
- Small vessel ischemia

Intraventricular Hemorrhage

- ± choroid plexus hemorrhage

Choroid Hemorrhage

- Normal calcification may mask small hemorrhages

PATHOLOGY

General Features

- Etiology
  - SCI: Most commonly induced by shear-strain forces that disrupt penetrating &/or choroidal vessels
    - Usually very small, typically nonhemorrhagic
  - SCI: Less commonly
    - Dorsolateral BS impacts tentorial incisura with violent brain motion
    - Anterorostral BS damaged with sudden craniocaudal brain displacement
  - IVH
    - Disruption of subependymal veins (most common)
    - Bleeding from choroid plexus
    - Shearing injuries
    - BG/intracerebral hemorrhage with rupture into ventricles
    - Isolated IVH in absence of parenchymal hematoma is unusual
  - CH: Traumatic shear forces damage to choroid tissue
- Associated abnormalities
  - SCI: All stages of DAI present (without exception), cerebral contusion, intracranial hemorrhages
  - IVH: DAI, deep GM/BS/intracerebral hemorrhage, SAH, cerebral contusion, hydrocephalus
  - CH: DAI, SAH, cerebral contusion

Staging, Grading, & Classification

- SCI: BS injury (BSI)
  - Primary injury: Direct result of trauma
    - DAI; most common primary BSI
    - Direct laceration/contusion; rare
    - Multiple primary petechial hemorrhages; not associated with more superficial DAI
    - Pontomedullary rent or separation; may occur without widespread brain injury
  - Secondary injury: Indirect result of trauma, most common cause of BSI; usually herniation
- SCI: When BSI → BS hemorrhage
  - Group 1: Midline rostral anterior BS, posterior to interpeduncular cistern (69%)
    - Associated with anterior impact; 71% survival
  - Group 2: Misc foci of acute BS hemorrhage (18%)
    - Associated with transtentorial herniation and BS compression; 88% survival
  - Group 3: Any BS hemorrhage
    - Associated with transtentorial herniation and BS compression; 100% mortality

Gross Pathologic & Surgical Features

- SCI
  - Usually nonhemorrhagic, yet more often hemorrhagic than other primary intraaxial injuries
  - 2° to rich network of perforating vessels in BG and thalamus
- IVH
  - Gross blood collected within ventricular system
  - Blood-CSF level common
    - Layering, rather than clot formation, likely relates to intrinsic antithrombotic CSF properties due to high concentrations of fibrinolytic activators
  - May cast/expand involved ventricle
- CH: Hemorrhagic choroid tissue

CLINICAL ISSUES

Presentation

- Most common signs/symptoms
  - SCI: Profound neurologic deficits
    - Low initial Glasgow coma scale scores; coma
  - IVH: Obtundation, seizures

Demographics

- Age
  - Any, but most common in 15- to 24-year-old patients
- Sex
  - Men 2x as likely to sustain traumatic brain injury (TBI); peaks at 20-24 years
- Epidemiology
  - SCI: In 5-10% of TBI, 3rd most common primary traumatic neuronal injury
  - IVH: Present in 60% of patients with corpus callosal DAI, 12% in patients without

Natural History & Prognosis

- SCI: Severely injured patients
  - Poor prognosis, often die soon after trauma
  - Regain consciousness very slowly and retain permanent neurologic impairment/disability
- SCI: May proceed to BS hemorrhage
  - Associated with high mortality
- IVH
  - Gradually clears as resorbed, although patients > 20 cc of blood do poorly
  - Hydrocephalus rare manifestation
    - Early: CSF outlet obstruction
      - □ Obstructive, noncommunicating
      - □ Asymmetric ventricular dilatation
    - Late: Arachnoid dysfunction of CSF resorption
      - □ Obstructive, communicating hydrocephalus
      - □ Symmetric ventricular dilatation
  - Hemorrhagic dilation of 4th ventricle: Ominous predictor with 100% reported mortality
  - At baseline, predicts 2x ↑ in mortality
    - Does not predict functional outcome
- CH: Can lead to IVH

Treatment

- SCI
  - Supportive therapy
  - Treatment considerations of indirect/associated abnormalities: Herniation, hematoma, hydrocephalus, seizures, etc.
- IVH
  - Ventriculostomy
  - Excellent results following r-TPA thrombolytic therapy
    - Effective and safe, despite preexisting multiple hemorrhagic intracranial injuries
  - Repeat NECT to evaluate for hydrocephalus, treatment complications

DIAGNOSTIC CHECKLIST

Consider

- SCI results from severe trauma: Often highly complex cases with multitude of abnormal findings
  - Before finishing review of case, look at everything 1 more time

Image Interpretation Pearls

- Delayed development of visible lesions common

SELECTED REFERENCES

1. Janas AM et al: Diffuse axonal injury grade on early MRI is associated with worse outcome in children with moderate-severe traumatic brain injury. Neurocrit Care. 36(2):492-503, 2022
2. Bruggeman GF et al: Traumatic axonal injury (TAI): definitions, pathophysiology and imaging-a narrative review. Acta Neurochir (Wien). 163(1):31-44, 2021
3. Ferrazzano PA et al: Use of magnetic resonance imaging in severe pediatric traumatic brain injury: assessment of current practice. J Neurosurg Pediatr. 1-9, 2019
4. Moe HK et al: Association of cause of injury and traumatic axonal injury: a clinical MRI study of moderate and severe traumatic brain injury. J Neurosurg. 1-9, 2019
5. Schweitzer AD et al: Traumatic brain injury: imaging patterns and complications. Radiographics. 39(6):1571-95, 2019
6. O'Phelan KH et al: Common patterns of regional brain injury detectable by diffusion tensor imaging in otherwise normal-appearing white matter in patients with early moderate to severe traumatic brain injury. J Neurotrauma. 35(5):739-49, 2018
7. Haghbayan H et al: The prognostic value of MRI in moderate and severe traumatic brain injury: a systematic review and meta-analysis. Crit Care Med. 45(12):e1280-8, 2017

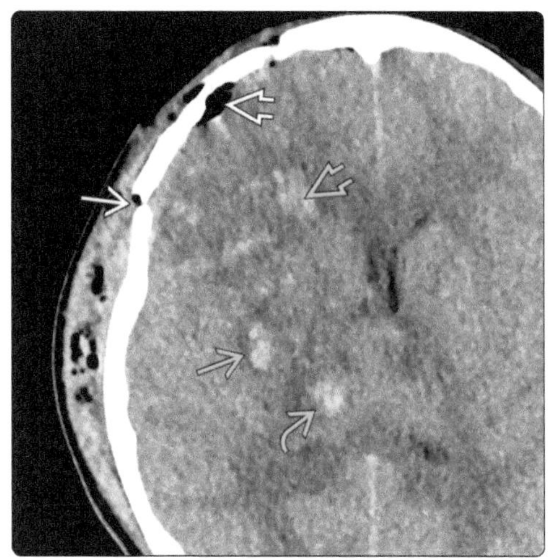

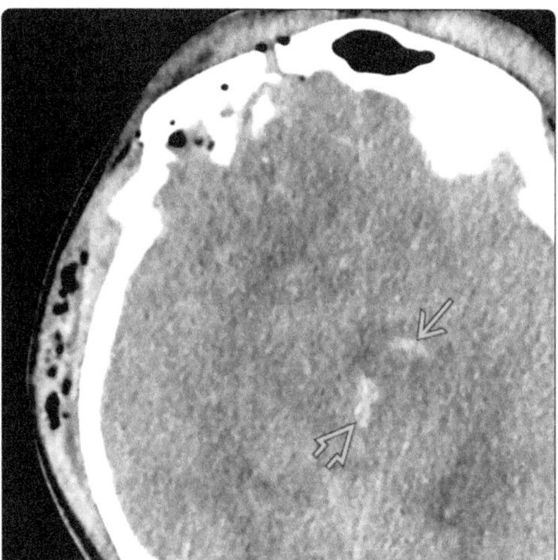

(Left) *Axial NECT in a 12-year-old with severe TBI shows extensive right frontal lobe hemorrhagic contusions as well as deep basal ganglia and thalami hemorrhages. Note the extensive right frontal bone fractures and intracranial gas.* **(Right)** *Axial NECT in the same patient with severe TBI shows a left basal ganglia hemorrhage and a hemorrhage within the midline midbrain, consistent with a Duret hemorrhage. Also note effacement of the basilar cisterns.*

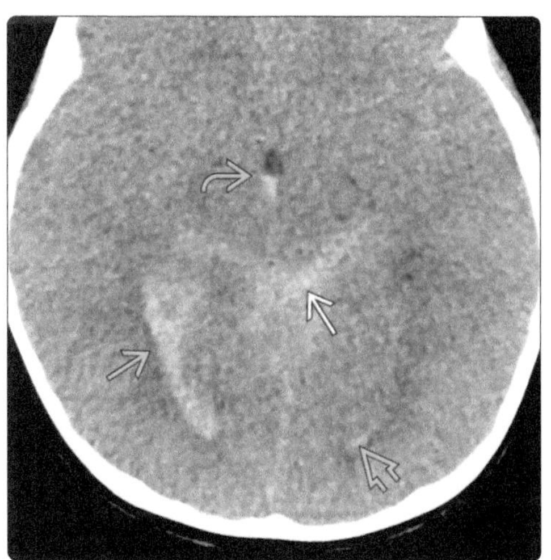

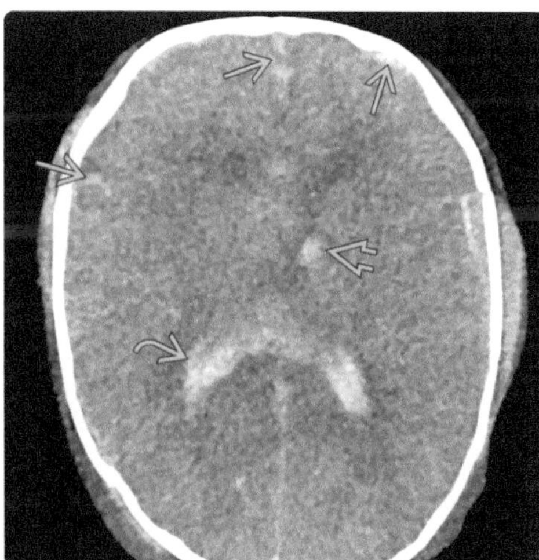

(Left) *Axial NECT in a 2-year-old with a gunshot wound shows IVH in the right atrium and occipital horn, left occipital horn, and 3rd ventricle. Also note the extensive basilar subarachnoid hemorrhage.* **(Right)** *Axial NECT in a 6-month-old with a history of fall and severe TBI shows extensive areas of superficial hemorrhage, left caudate nucleus hemorrhage, and IVH. Such a pattern of deep intracranial hemorrhage suggests severe brain injury and portends a poor prognosis.*

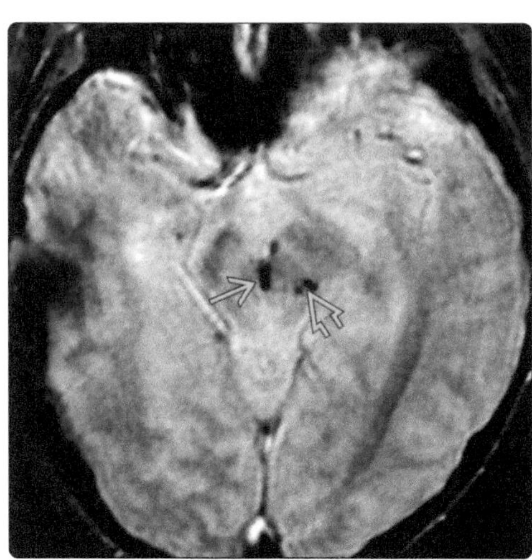

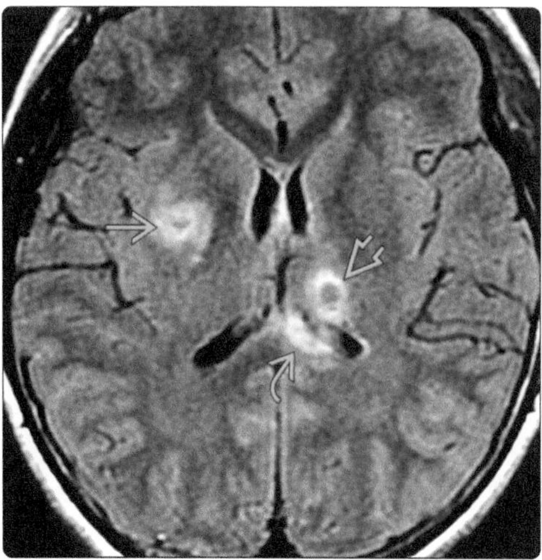

(Left) *Axial T2* GRE MR shows signal loss in the midline midbrain (Duret hemorrhage) and left cerebral peduncle (axonal injury). The patient had corresponding hemiplegia.* **(Right)** *Axial FLAIR MR in the same patient reveals more extensive subcortical injury (SCI) involving the right lentiform nuclei, left thalamus, and corpus callosum. These findings most likely reflect axonal injury.*

Abusive Head Trauma

KEY FACTS

TERMINOLOGY

- Abusive head trauma (AHT)
- Traumatic injury inflicted on infants & children by adults

IMAGING

- Direct impact injury: Direct blow to cranium
  - Calvarial (often complex) & skull base fractures
  - Focal brain injury deep to impact
- Shaking injury: Result of violent to-&-fro motion of head
  - Subdural hematomas (SDHs) in 90-98%
  - Generalized parenchymal injuries (cytotoxic edema, lacerations, axonal injury)
  - Bridging vein injury & thrombosis common
- CT primary imaging tool in initial evaluation of AHT
  - Multiplanar reconstructions improve detection of
    - Small intracranial hemorrhages (ICHs)
    - Fractures (with bone algorithm & 3D reformats)
- MR best for determining full extent of injury
  - DWI paramount for parenchymal injury
  - SWI/T2* GRE for hemorrhage
  - T2/T1/FLAIR for detection of subdural collections
  - T1 C+ for chronic SDH membranes
- Avoid speculation regarding timing & specific source of injury in report

TOP DIFFERENTIAL DIAGNOSES

- Accidental trauma
- Benign macrocrania of infancy
- Mitochondrial encephalopathies
- Bleeding disorders

CLINICAL ISSUES

- Discordance between stated history & degree of injury
  - "Killer couch": Injuries blamed on infant rolling off couch
- Retinal hemorrhages in ~ 75%
- #1 cause of brain injury death in children < 2 years of age
  - 17-25:100,000 annual incidence
  - Cause of death in 80% of fatalities is brain swelling

(Left) *Axial NECT in a 9-week-old with seizures shows bilateral mixed attenuation subdural fluid collections with predominantly low attenuation anteriorly & high attenuation posteriorly, consistent with a hematohygroma. This should not be described as "acute on chronic" subdural hemorrhage.* **(Right)** *Coronal NECT in the same patient shows the bilateral subdural collections as well as globular areas of hemorrhage in the parasagittal regions, consistent with bridging vein injuries/avulsions.*

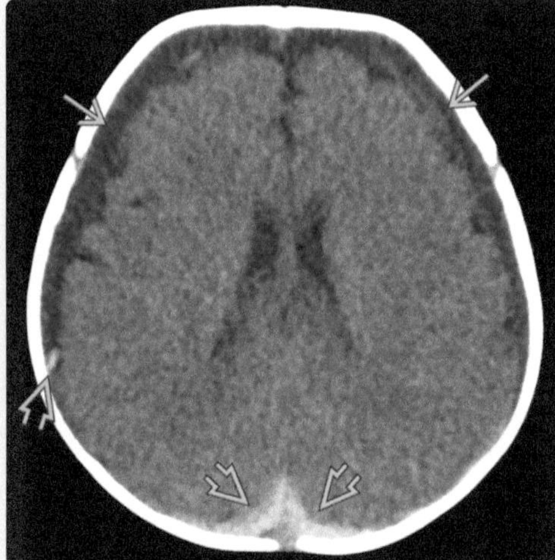

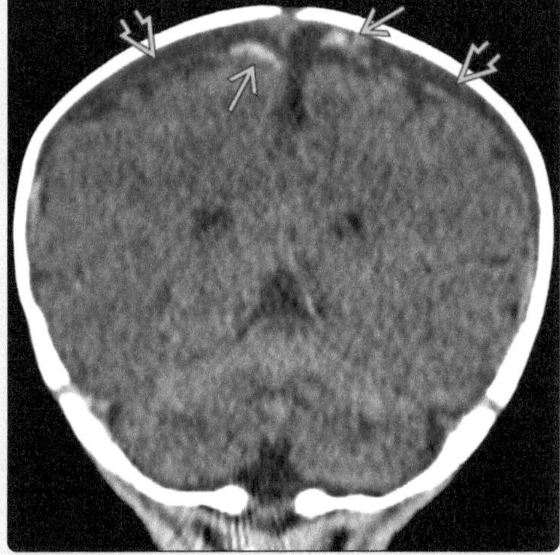

(Left) *Axial DWI MR in the same patient performed 3 days after presentation shows asymmetric (right > left) diffusion restriction, consistent with brain parenchymal injury. MR is the best exam for detection & characterization of brain injury in accidental head trauma.* **(Right)** *Coronal SSFSE in the same patient 6 weeks later shows a membrane separating loculated hyperintense & hypointense subdural components, a finding that suggests some component of chronicity.*

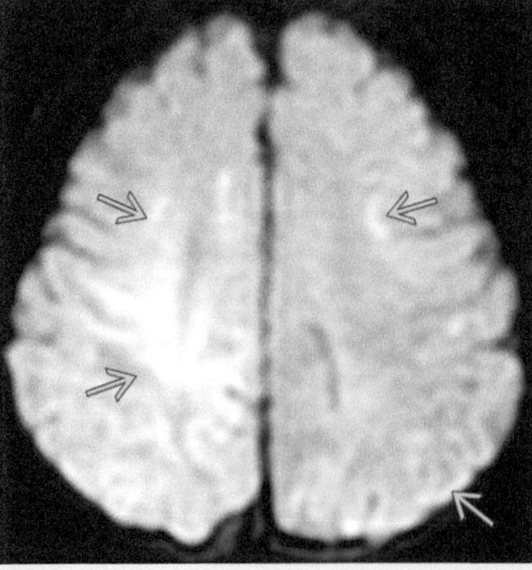

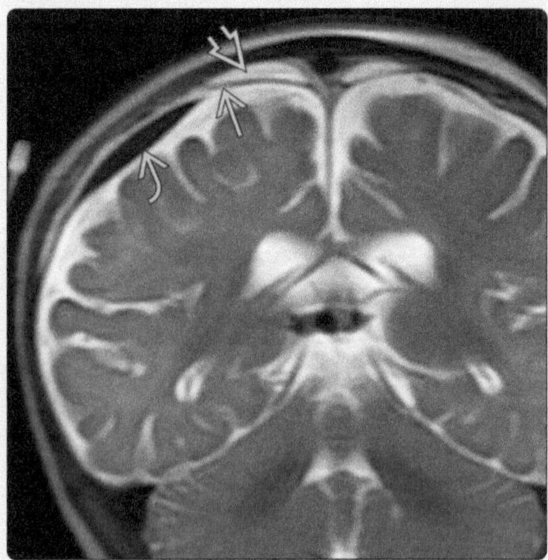

TERMINOLOGY

Abbreviations

- Abusive head trauma (AHT)

Synonyms

- Battered child syndrome, whiplash shaken infant syndrome, trauma-X, Caffey-Kempe syndrome, shaken-baby syndrome, nonaccidental head injury
- Multiple alternate titles have been suggested in attempt to minimize accusatory labeling in clinical setting
  - May do more harm than good by causing confusion & hampering communication

Definitions

- Traumatic injury inflicted on infants & children by adults
  - This discussion centers on head injury

IMAGING

General Features

- Multiple brain injuries disproportionately severe relative to offered history
- 2 major groupings of injuries (but can occur together)
  - Direct impact injury: Result of direct blow to cranium or impact of skull on object
  - Shaking injury: Result of violent to-&-fro head motion
- Direct impact injury typified by skull fractures & injury to immediately underlying brain
  - Scalp laceration, hematoma, swelling strongly associated
  - High association with injuries to other organs
- Shaking injury typified by subdural hemorrhage (SDH) & generalized brain parenchymal injury
  - Cytotoxic brain injury not conforming to arterial territories
    - Exact etiology of parenchymal injury uncertain but usually permanent
      - Hypoxic-ischemic vs. direct traumatic brain injury
  - May see bridging vein injury ± thrombosis
  - Imaging findings may suggest injuries of differing ages

Radiographic Findings

- Sensitive in detection of linear skull fractures
  - Fracture detection key component in forensic evaluation of suspected nonaccidental trauma (NAT)
  - CT (with appropriate techniques) better characterizes fractures; often being obtained to evaluate for intracranial hemorrhage (ICH)
- Some fractures considered more suspicious for NAT
  - Evidence does not support this
    - Multiple compound, diastatic fractures, & fractures crossing sutures imply significant trauma but are not specific for NAT
  - Discordance with provided history best indicator

CT Findings

- NECT primary imaging tool for initial evaluation of AHT
- ICH
  - SDH most common (90-98%)
    - Dominant feature of shaking injury
    - Overlying cerebral convexities, in interhemispheric fissure, overlying tentorium
    - Normal density of subarachnoid space (SAS) stands out next to ↑ density of SDH
  - Subarachnoid hemorrhage common (> 50%)
  - Epidural hemorrhage uncommon but may occur
    - More characteristic of accidental trauma
  - Use great caution if attempting to estimate "age" of ICH
    - Blood density based upon multiple factors: CSF dilution, hematocrit, coagulation status
    - SDHs of same age can have significantly different densities
    - Acute SDHs likely to have hyperdense component but usually have associated low-attenuation component from CSF admixture (i.e., hematohygroma)
    - Most specific findings for chronic SDHs are compartmentalization/loculation & membrane formation
- Bridging vein injury ± thrombosis common (40-50%)
  - Areas of ↑ density in paramedian high convexities
    - Tadpole & lollipop signs
    - May occur in accidental injury but more common in AHT
- Parenchymal ischemic injury often seen in shaking injuries
  - Areas of ↓ density (with loss of gray matter-white matter differentiation) & sulcal effacement not confined to arterial territories; may be diffuse
  - ↓ density of cerebrum vs. cerebellum: "Bright cerebellum"
  - May be evident within several hours after injury
- Parenchymal laceration in 10-15%
  - More commonly seen in AHT vs. accidental injury
- Shear injury (axonal injury) in ~ 15%
- Retinal hemorrhages uncommonly visualized on CT
- **CTA**: Detectable vascular injury relatively uncommon in child abuse

MR Findings

- **DWI**: Key for parenchymal injury
  - Patterns of parenchymal injury are variable, including diffuse symmetric, multifocal, & focal
- **T1WI**: Bright foci of hemorrhage or evolving cortical injury
- **T2WI**: Loss of cortical ribbon & deep nuclei in neonates
  - Coronal T2 often helpful to identify bridging vein injury
  - Lacerations are characterized by fluid clefts with hematocrit levels
- **FLAIR**: Very sensitive for detection of small subdural collections
- **SWI/T2* GRE**: Detects small ICH ± retinal hemorrhages
  - SWI is ~ 50% sensitive & 100% specific for retinal hemorrhage
  - Best sequence for detecting & characterizing bridging vein injury
- **T1WI C+**: Enhancing membranes best sign of chronic SDH
- **MRA**: Proximal vascular correlate (dissection, spasm) rarely shown in association with parenchymal injury

Imaging Recommendations

- Best imaging tool
  - NECT for acute evaluation
    - Sensitive in detection & characterization of fractures
    - Sensitive in detection & characterization of most ICH, but small low attenuation subdurals can be missed

- MR after 48-72 hours
  - Best exam for characterizing brain injury
  - Helpful to further characterize subdural collections (CT & MR are complementary)
- Protocol advice
  - NECT: Multiplanar & 3D reconstructions improve detection of
    - Small ICHs
    - Fractures (especially with bone algorithm & 3D)
    - Consider imaging down to C2 to detect atlantooccipital injuries
  - MR: DWI to assess parenchymal injury; FLAIR/SWI sequence to detect subtle SDH/subdural hygroma

DIFFERENTIAL DIAGNOSIS

Accidental Trauma

- Appropriate history for degree of injury

Benign Macrocrania of Infancy

- Self-limited communicating hydrocephalus
- Prominence of extraaxial spaces → isodense to CSF

Mitochondrial Encephalopathies

- May cause atrophy with subdural collections
  - Glutaric acidurias (types I & II), Menkes syndrome
  - Rare diseases with preexisting neurologic symptoms

Overshunting

- "Passive" subdurals can develop from ↓ volume associated with CSF shunting

Subdural Empyema

- Febrile, sinusitis, meningitis

Bleeding Disorders

- von Willebrand, thrombocytopenia
- Intracranial bleeding with minor trauma

PATHOLOGY

General Features

- ↑ vulnerability in infants due to
  - Large head:body ratio + weak neck muscles
  - Developing brain has less structural integrity prior to myelination, greater susceptibility to injury
- 85% of fatal child abuse victims have evidence of impact head injury at postmortem examination
- Retinal hemorrhage in ~ 75% (50-100% in literature)
  - Much less common in accidental head trauma (~ 6%)
- Retroclival collections can be seen in ~ 30% of AHT victims

CLINICAL ISSUES

Presentation

- Most common signs/symptoms
  - Discordance between stated history & degree of injury
    - Attempt by perpetrator to minimize suspicion
    - "Killer couch": Severe injuries blamed on infant rolling off couch onto floor by perpetrator
      - Frequently in infants too young to roll over at all
  - Unprovoked seizures & apnea raise suspicion for AHT
- Other signs/symptoms
  - Poor feeding, vomiting, irritability, seizures, lethargy, coma, apnea
  - Retinal hemorrhage
    - Can be missed on cursory exam
    - Can be seen in glutaric acidurias
  - Cause of death in 80% of fatalities is brain swelling
    - Severe hypoxic ischemic encephalopathy > diffuse axonal injury
- Clinical profile
  - Perpetrators are often direct caretakers: Parents, babysitters, mother's boyfriend
  - Developmentally delayed, "colicky," premature or low-birth-weight infants at higher risk
  - Psychosocial stressors & poor coping mechanisms in family environment

Demographics

- Most common from 1-6 months of age
- 17-25:100,000 annual incidence
  - Almost certainly underreported
  - #1 cause of brain injury death in children < 2 years of age
- M > F

Natural History & Prognosis

- Mortality rate: 20-25%
- High rates of impairment for survivors
  - Psychomotor delay, epilepsy, visual impairment, cognitive/behavioral disorders

Treatment

- Notification of local Child Protection Agency
  - Mandated in USA/Canada/Australia/some European countries
- Multidisciplinary child abuse & neglect team intervention

DIAGNOSTIC CHECKLIST

Image Interpretation Pearls

- Avoid temptation to precisely time ICH
- Accurate descriptions & detailed report are most helpful

Reporting Tips

- Avoid use of vague, oblique, obscuring language in reports
  - Can hamper care of child & legal investigation
  - May ↑ likelihood of interpretation being challenged in legal proceedings
- Avoid speculation regarding timing & specific source of injury in report
  - Appropriate to raise concern for abusive head injury
  - More can always be said about timing & mechanism in legal setting, but once statement is made in report, it is difficult to retract

SELECTED REFERENCES

1. Dias MS et al: Neuroradiologic timing of intracranial hemorrhage in abusive head trauma. Pediatr Radiol. 51(6):911-7, 2021
2. Oates AJ et al: Parenchymal brain injuries in abusive head trauma. Pediatr Radiol. 51(6):898-910, 2021
3. Sidpra J et al: Abusive head trauma: neuroimaging mimics and diagnostic complexities. Pediatr Radiol. 51(6):947-65, 2021

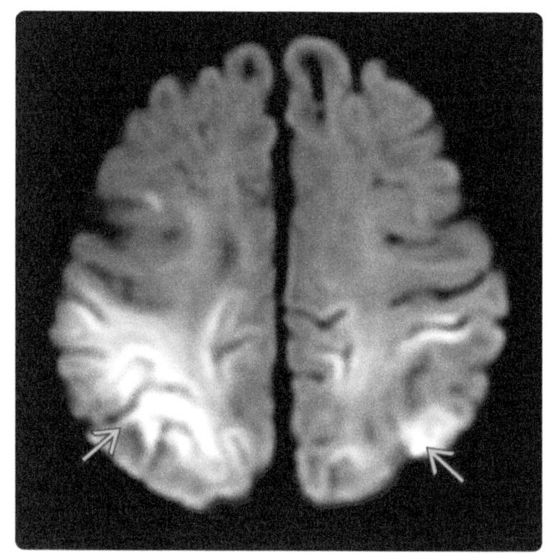

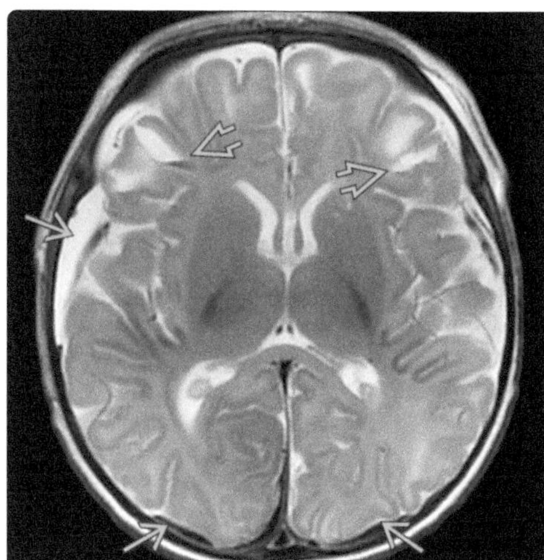

(Left) *Axial DWI MR in a 2-month-old with unexplained altered mental status & seizure shows nearly symmetric diffusion restriction → in the bilateral parietooccipital regions.* **(Right)** *Axial T2 MR in the same patient shows bilateral clefts with hematocrit levels, consistent with lacerations →. Also note the bilateral subdural hemorrhages →. This constellation of parenchymal injury, brain lacerations, & bilateral subdural hemorrhages is highly suspicious for abusive head trauma (AHT).*

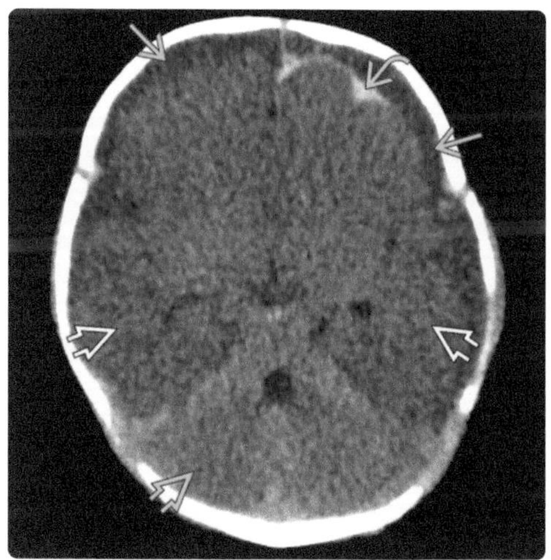

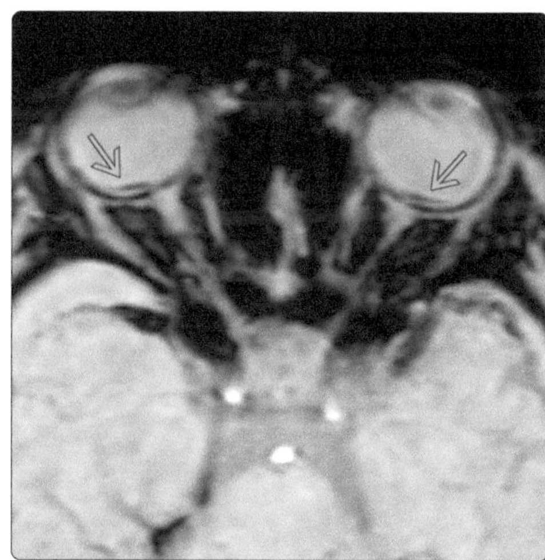

(Left) *Axial NECT in a 6-week-old with AHT shows hypodense subdural collections → & left frontal arachnoid hemorrhage →. ↓ attenuation throughout the cerebrum → with loss of gray matter-white matter differentiation is consistent with injury. Compare to the normal cerebellum →.* **(Right)** *Axial SWI in a 3-month-old with AHT shows thin areas of ↓ signal →, consistent with bilateral retinal hemorrhages. MR is insensitive for detection of retinal hemorrhages, but they should be reported when present.*

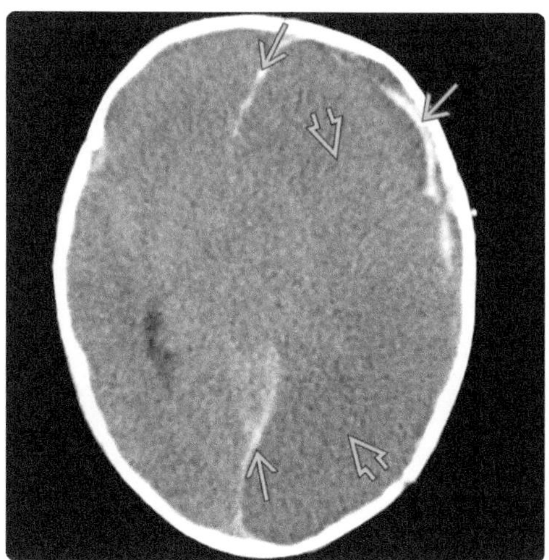

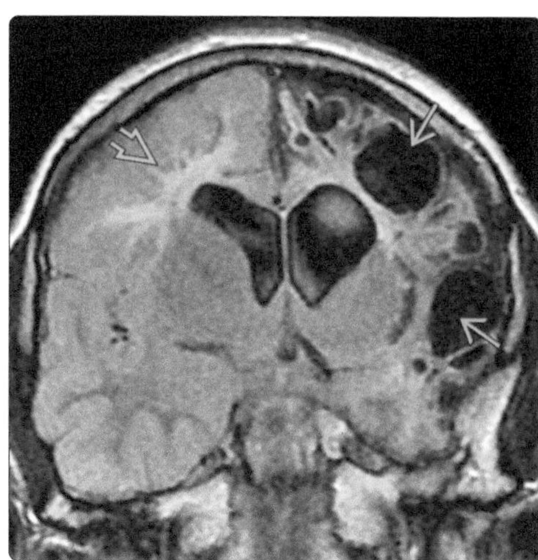

(Left) *Axial NECT in a 2-month-old with AHT shows subdural hemorrhage → over the left frontal lobe & along the falx. Note the extensive areas of ↓ attenuation → & loss of gray matter-white matter differentiation with significant left-to-right midline shift.* **(Right)** *Coronal FLAIR MR in the same patient 7 years later shows development of extensive areas of cystic → & noncystic → encephalomalacia affecting the left > right cerebral hemispheres.*

Germinal Matrix Hemorrhage

KEY FACTS

TERMINOLOGY

- Hemorrhage that occurs in richly vascular but fragile germinal matrix in premature infants

IMAGING

- Can occur anywhere along germinal matrix
  - Most common at caudothalamic groove
- Look for intraventricular extension, ventriculomegaly, & secondary intraparenchymal hemorrhage
- US: Globular echogenic focus in caudothalamic groove
  - Acute blood echogenic; later clot retracts & becomes iso- to hypoechoic
  - May appear as abnormally thick choroid plexus but of slightly different echogenicity & lacking vascularity
  - Fluid-debris levels may be visible in dependent ventricles
  - Coronal & sagittal cine clips sweeping though ventricles help differentiate hemorrhage from normal choroid
- MR: Sensitive for detection of germinal matrix hemorrhage (GMH) & intraventricular hemorrhage (IVH)
  - ↑ T1 signal; ↓ SWI/T2* GRE
  - Best imaging modality for detection of associated parenchymal abnormalities

PATHOLOGY

- Germinal matrix transiently present as region of fragile, thin-walled vessels & migrating neuronal components
  - Peaks at 23-25 weeks gestation, then begins involution
- In premature infants, perinatal stresses + poor cerebral autoregulation + germinal matrix → hemorrhage
- GMH-IVH grading system
  - Grade 1: GMH only
  - Grade 2: GMH + IVH, normal ventricle size
  - Grade 3: GMH + IVH + ventricular expansion
  - Grade 4: GMH-IVH + intraparenchymal hemorrhage
    - Venous compression leads to venous infarction

CLINICAL ISSUES

- Most common < 32-weeks gestation & < 1,500 g

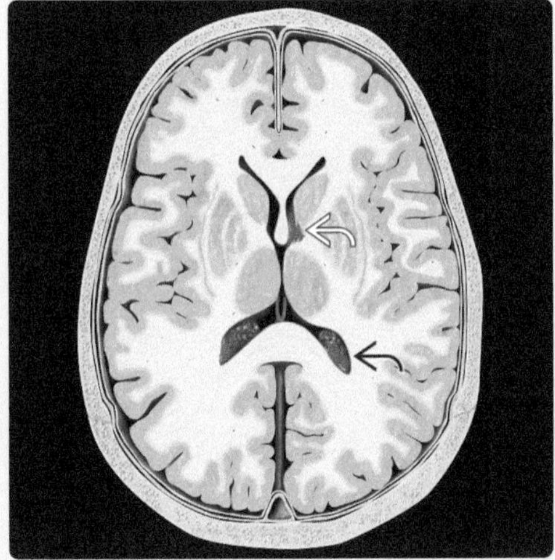

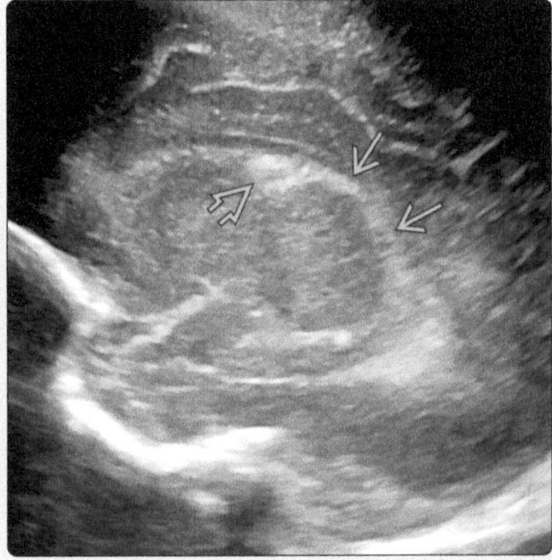

(Left) *Axial graphic shows a germinal matrix hemorrhage (GMH) (red) within the left caudothalamic groove* ➡. *There is associated intraventricular hemorrhage (IVH)* ➡ *without ventriculomegaly, consistent with a grade 2 IVH.* **(Right)** *Coronal US in a 1-day-old, 34-week gestational age newborn shows increased echogenicity in the left caudothalamic groove* ➡, *consistent with a grade 1 hemorrhage. Note the normal echogenic choroid plexus* ➡ *tapering up to the caudothalamic groove.*

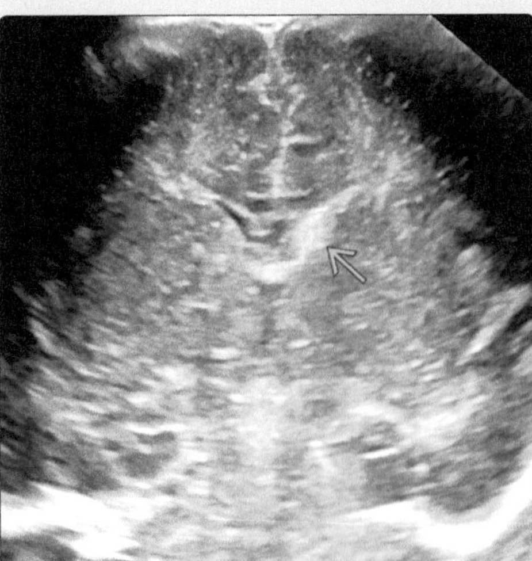

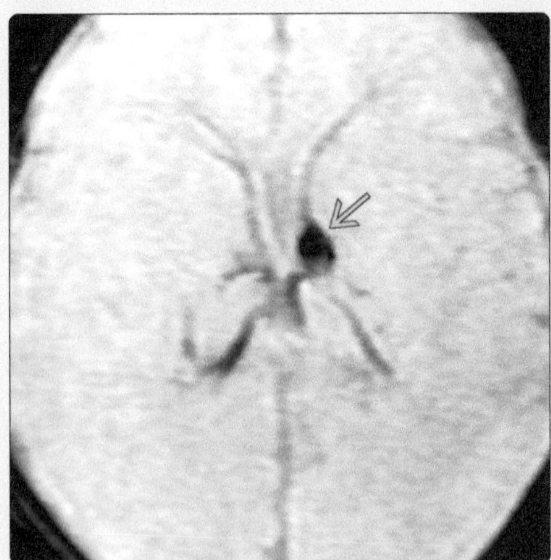

(Left) *Coronal US in the same premature neonate shows an asymmetric globular echogenic focus in the left caudothalamic groove* ➡, *consistent with a GMH. The lack of IVH makes this a grade 1 hemorrhage.* **(Right)** *Axial SWI MR in the same patient at 8 days of age shows a focus of signal loss in the left caudothalamic groove* ➡, *consistent with a remote GMH. There is no signal loss in the ventricles otherwise to suggest a component of IVH.*

TERMINOLOGY

Abbreviations

- Germinal matrix hemorrhage (GMH)

Synonyms

- Germinal matrix bleed, preterm caudothalamic hemorrhage, GMH-intraventricular hemorrhage (IVH)

Definitions

- Hemorrhage that occurs in very specific, richly vascular, stress-sensitive areas of brain

IMAGING

General Features

- Best diagnostic clue
  - Globular echogenic focus in caudothalamic groove, clearly asymmetric from contralateral normal choroid plexus
- Location
  - Most common in caudothalamic groove
    - But can occur anywhere along anatomic distribution of fetal germinal matrix
  - May extend posteriorly into ventricular system
    - Adherent to choroid plexus or layering in occipital horns
- Size
  - Variable
- Morphology
  - Globular & rounded when limited to caudothalamic groove (grade 1)
  - Lobulated or amorphous with posterior intraventricular extension (grade 2)

Ultrasonographic Findings

- Grayscale ultrasound
  - Hyperechoic acute hemorrhage; evolving clot retracts & becomes iso- to hypoechoic
  - IVH often adherent to choroid plexus
    - Fluid-debris levels may be visible in dependent ventricular occipital horns
    - Chemical ventriculitis in 2-3 days after IVH
      - Ependymal lining becomes thick & echogenic
  - Larger IVH will expand ventricle(s) (grade 3)
    - Further ventriculomegaly gradually develops due to
      - Posthemorrhagic hydrocephalus from obstruction of ventricular outlets & arachnoid granulations
      - White matter volume loss
  - Fan-shaped, echogenic parenchymal focus next to site of grade 3 IVH due to venous hemorrhagic infarction (grade 4)
  - Examine remainder of brain for
    - Associated white matter injury
    - Lack of congenital anomalies
- Color Doppler
  - Useful to differentiate avascular hemorrhage from vascular choroid plexus

MR Findings

- Very helpful in identifying
  - Associated brain parenchymal injury that often accompanies GMH-IVH
    - White matter injury of prematurity
    - Cerebellar microhemorrhage
  - Underlying congenital anomalies
- Variable signal intensity based on age of blood
  - **T1WI**: ↑ signal in subacute blood, ↓ signal in chronic hemosiderin
  - **T2WI**: ↓ hypointense signal in most phases of hemorrhage evolution
  - **SWI**: Most sensitive sequence for identifying small or remote GMH-IVH

CT Findings

- Not typically used in premature neonate due to availability of US & superior soft tissue resolution of MR

Imaging Recommendations

- Best imaging tool
  - US primary imaging modality
    - Portability allows US to go to patient in NICU
    - Available sonographic window of anterior fontanelle
    - Lack of ionizing radiation
    - High sensitivity & specificity for GMH-IVH
  - MR useful adjunctive imaging modality
    - More sensitive, specific, & reproducible than US but not always practical in critically ill premature infants
    - MR rarely performed acutely; usually performed to evaluate extent of parenchymal injury
- Protocol advice
  - US: Use small-footprint, high-frequency linear transducer with multiple focal zones
    - Coronal & sagittal cine clips through ventricles particularly helpful in separating hemorrhage from normal choroid plexus
  - MR: Include SWI or T2* GRE to identify hemorrhage

DIFFERENTIAL DIAGNOSIS

Hypoxic-Ischemic Encephalopathy

- Deep or peripheral patterns of parenchymal injury due to perinatal insult to preterm or term infant
- Abnormal echogenicity of affected deep gray structures &/or white matter
- Typically bilateral, often asymmetric

Hemorrhage Infarction From Venous Thrombosis

- Superficial or deep venous thrombosis may lead to echogenic parenchyma ± discrete hematoma in neonate
  - Can liquefy & mimic abscess
- May be isolated or secondary to infection or other systemic processes

Choroid Plexus Cysts or Hematoma

- Small cysts &/or hemorrhages may occur in choroid plexus, sparing germinal matrix
- Often without consequence

Ventriculitis

- May be seen from infectious, toxic, & metabolic disorders without bleeding
- May lead to communicating hydrocephalus

Periventricular Calcifications

- Not typically seen in caudothalamic groove
- Most commonly related to TORCH infections

Periventricular Gray Matter Heterotopia

- Nodular heterotopia less echogenic than blood, isoechoic to brain
- Follows gray matter on all sequences

Tuberous Sclerosis

- Echogenic nodular periventricular foci
- Echogenic cortical/subcortical tubers distorting overlying gyri

PATHOLOGY

General Features

- Etiology
  - Germinal matrix only transiently present as region of thin-walled vessels, migrating neuronal components, & vessel precursors
    - Involutes by ~ 34-weeks gestation, such that hemorrhage becomes less likely with ↑ gestational age
      - May occur later in gestation but typically requires significant physiologic stressor (e.g., infection, hypoxia-ischemia)
    - Most GMHs occur in 1st week of life
  - Germinal matrix prone to hemorrhage in premature infants due to
    - High density of fragile vascularized tissue
    - Poor cerebral autoregulation in premature infants
  - Hemorrhage occurs secondary to perinatal stresses: Labile blood pressure, hypoxia, hypercarbia, etc.

Staging, Grading, & Classification

- Germinal matrix grading system created by Burstein et al in 1979
  - Performed on initial head US within days of delivery
  - Grading not changed on follow-up exams (even with progression)
- Grade 1: GMH only
- Grade 2: GMH, IVH, normal ventricle size
- Grade 3: GMH, IVH, & ventricular expansion from IVH
  - Secondary hydrocephalus occurring several days after grade 2 IVH should not be mislabeled as grade 3 IVH
- Grade 4: IVH + intraparenchymal hemorrhage
  - Intraparenchymal hemorrhage represents hemorrhagic venous infarction, not extension of GMH or IVH into parenchyma
    - Deep draining vein compression → venous congestion → venous infarction → hemorrhagic infarction
    - Debated whether or not ventricular dilation necessary
      - Is periventricular hemorrhagic infarction of premature infant with grade 1 or 2 GMH actually due to GMH vs. discrete focus of hypoxic-ischemic injury or venous thrombosis?
  - Grade 4 may be called posthemorrhagic venous infarction

CLINICAL ISSUES

Presentation

- Most common signs/symptoms
  - Variable: Hypotonia, seizures, hyperreflexia, falling hematocrit, irritability, failure to thrive, paresis, acidosis, feeding difficulties
- Other signs/symptoms
  - GMH may occur in utero & follow same pathway of evolution & complications

Demographics

- Age
  - Premature infants in 1st week of life
  - 1/3-1/2 of all GMHs occur on 1st day of life
- Ethnicity
  - No predisposition
- Epidemiology
  - Most common in infants < 32-weeks gestation & < 1,500 g
  - Higher risk of GMH in premature infants with congenital heart disease, surgical procedures, severe respiratory distress
  - Incidence of GMH-IVH: 50% from 1975-1980 & then ↓ to ~ 15% after 2005
    - Improved modern outcomes attributed to prenatal steroids & surfactant, among other therapies

Natural History & Prognosis

- GMHs may progress or rebleed
- In general, clot retracts, lyses, & becomes hypoechoic, leaving behind cyst or area of porencephaly
- Prognosis
  - Grades 1 & 2 bleeds generally have good prognosis
  - Grades 3 & 4 bleeds have variable long-term deficits
    - Spastic diplegia, seizures, developmental delay

Treatment

- Prenatal
  - Prevent preterm delivery
  - Prenatal steroids
- Postnatal
  - Optimize neonatal resuscitation
  - Reduce fluctuations in cerebral blood flow
    - Minimize handling, gentle/synchronized ventilation, prompt treatment of patent ductus arteriosus, maintain normal oxygenation
- Posthemorrhagic hydrocephalus often requires CSF shunting

SELECTED REFERENCES

1. You SK: Neuroimaging of germinal matrix and intraventricular hemorrhage in premature infants. J Korean Neurosurg Soc. 66(3):239-46, 2023
2. Epstein KN et al: Prenatal evaluation of intracranial hemorrhage on fetal MRI: a retrospective review. AJNR Am J Neuroradiol. 42(12):2222-8, 2021
3. Parodi A et al: Cranial ultrasound findings in preterm germinal matrix haemorrhage, sequelae and outcome. Pediatr Res. 87(Suppl 1):13-24, 2020
4. Klebe D et al: Posthemorrhagic hydrocephalus development after germinal matrix hemorrhage: established mechanisms and proposed pathways. J Neurosci Res. 98(1):105-20, 2019
5. Coskun Y et al: A clinical scoring system to predict the development of intraventricular hemorrhage (IVH) in premature infants. Childs Nerv Syst. 34(1):129-36, 2018

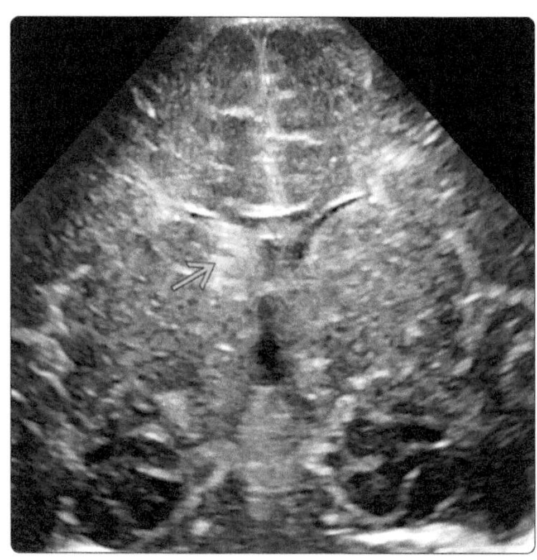

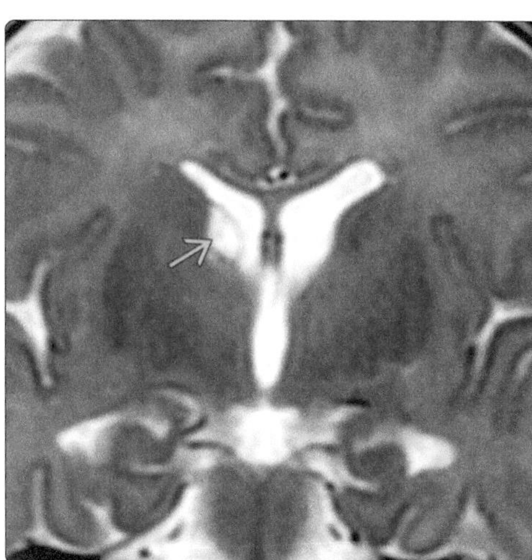

(Left) *Coronal US in a 1-day-old, 36-week gestational age newborn shows an asymmetric area of increased echogenicity* ➙ *in the right caudothalamic groove, consistent with a grade 1 GMH.* **(Right)** *Coronal T2 MR in the same patient 8 weeks later shows interval development of a germinolytic cyst* ➙ *in place of the prior GMH. This is the typical evolution of a GMH.*

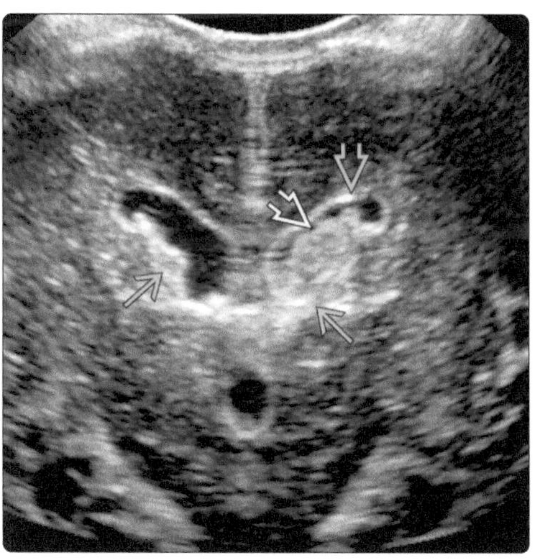

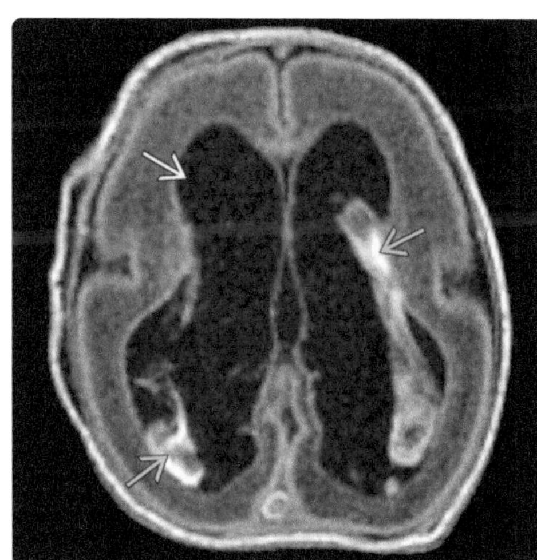

(Left) *Coronal head US in a former 24-week gestational age premature infant (now 6 days old) shows bilateral GMHs* ➙*. There is left intraventricular extension of the hemorrhage* ➡ *with expansion of the left frontal horn* ⇨*, consistent with a grade 3 IVH. A grade 2 IVH was seen on the right.* **(Right)** *Axial T1 MR 3 weeks later in the same patient shows foci of T1 shortening from the prior IVHs* ➙*. Further ventriculomegaly* ➡ *has developed, consistent with posthemorrhagic hydrocephalus.*

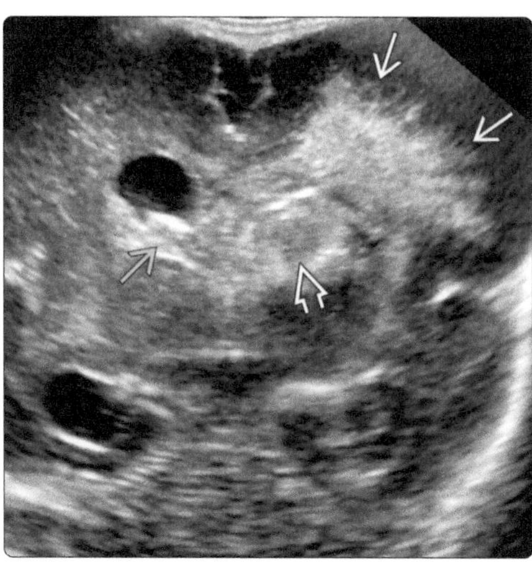

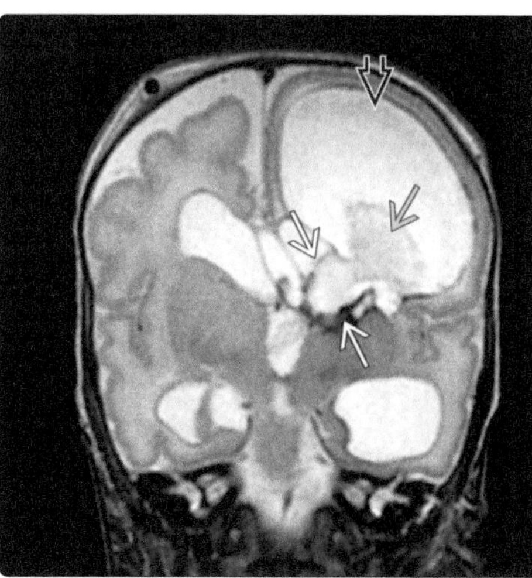

(Left) *Coronal head US in a former 28-week gestational age premature infant (now 3 days old) shows a right GMH* ➙ *and a left IVH, which fills and expands the lateral ventricle* ⮕*. There is a fan-shaped hemorrhagic infarction* ➡ *in the left centrum semiovale, consistent with a grade 4 IVH.* **(Right)** *Coronal T2 MR in the same infant 6 weeks later shows residua of the left-sided IVH* ➡ *and intraparenchymal hemorrhage* ➙ *with the development of cystic encephalomalacia* ⇨*, an expected evolution of grade 4 IVH.*

Hydranencephaly

KEY FACTS

TERMINOLOGY

- Absence of cerebral hemispheres with intact thalamus, brainstem, cerebellum, skull/meninges
  - Associated space filled with CSF ("water bag" brain)
  - Probably caused by in utero vascular occlusion, infection, or trauma after 1st trimester

IMAGING

- Absent cerebrum with fluid-filled cranial vault
- Thalamus, cerebellum, brainstem, falx intact
- Temporal, occipital lobe remnants common
- Macrocephaly

TOP DIFFERENTIAL DIAGNOSES

- Severe hydrocephalus
- Alobar holoprosencephaly (HLE)
- Severe bilateral open-lip schizencephaly
- Cystic encephalomalacia

PATHOLOGY

- In utero compromise of anterior cerebral circulation
- Implicated: Anoxia, infection, thrombophilia, maternal toxin exposure, radiation, genetic factors, twin-twin transfusion

CLINICAL ISSUES

- Newborn with macrocephaly, developmental failure, calvarial transillumination
  - Hyperirritability, hyperreflexia, seizures
- Neurologic function limited to brainstem
- Prognosis: Death in infancy; prolonged survival rare
- Ventricular shunt treats macrocephaly
- Choroid plexus cauterization: Alternative treatment to shunting

DIAGNOSTIC CHECKLIST

- Intact falx distinguishes hydranencephaly from alobar HLE
- Thin cortical mantle along inner table distinguishes severe hydrocephalus from hydranencephaly

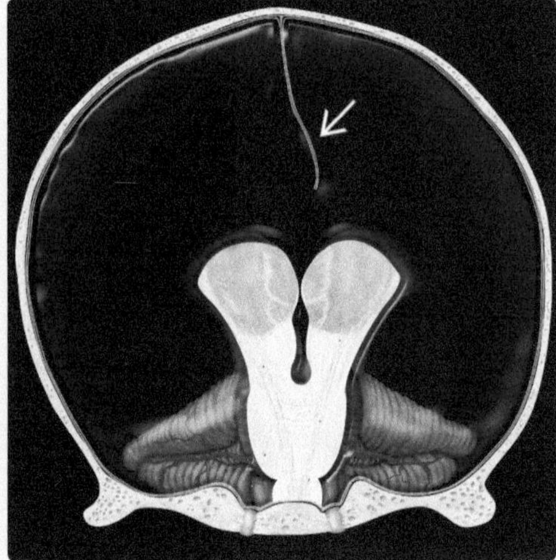

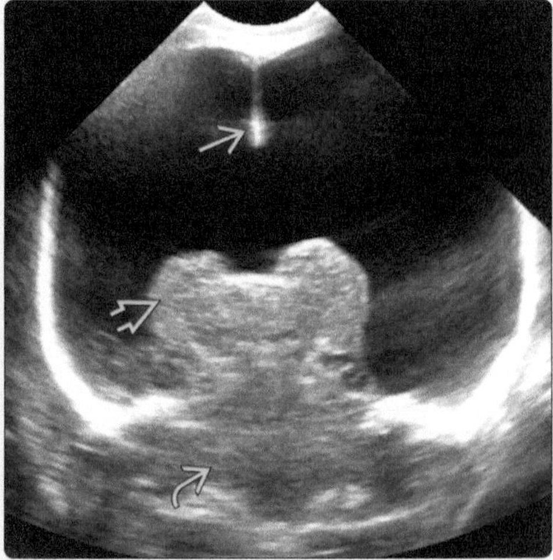

(Left) *Coronal graphic shows the classic features of hydranencephaly. The cerebral hemispheres are nearly absent, but the thalami, brainstem, and cerebellum are intact. The falx cerebri ➔ appears to float in a CSF-filled rostral cranial vault.* **(Right)** *Coronal ultrasound in a newborn with hydranencephaly shows near-complete absence of the cerebral hemispheres with residual brainstem, thalami ⇨, and cerebellum ↗ supplied by the vertebrobasilar system. Note the presence of the falx →.*

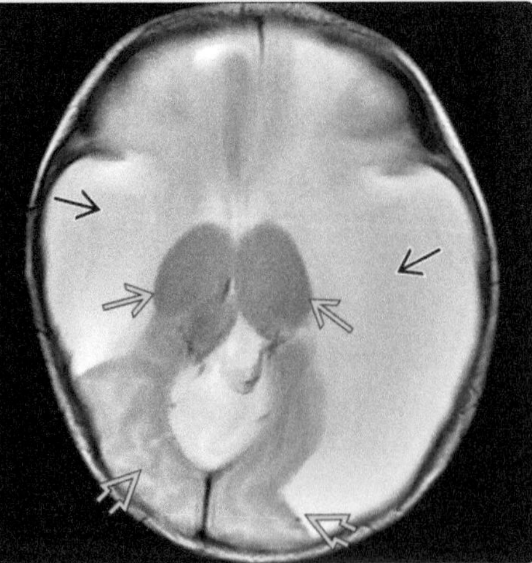

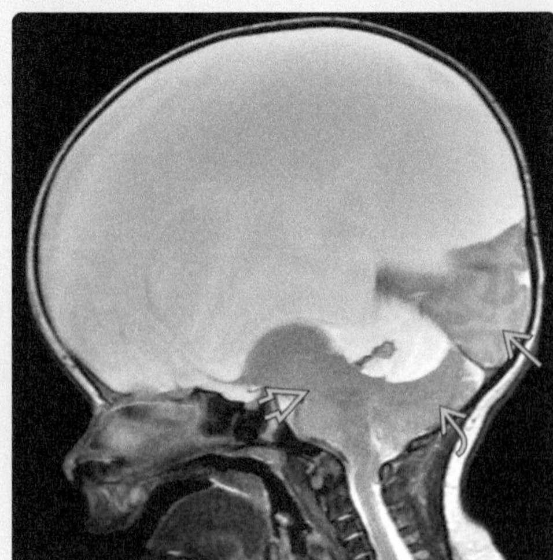

(Left) *Axial T2 MR in a 1-month-old shows complete absence of brain parenchyma ➔ supplied by the internal carotid artery (ICA) with preservation of brain supplied by the vertebrobasilar system (thalami ⇨ and posterior cerebral artery territories ⇨).* **(Right)** *Sagittal T2 MR in the same patient shows absence of the brain parenchyma in the ICA territories and preservation of occipital lobes ⇨, brainstem ⇨, and cerebellum ↗ in the posterior cerebral artery territory. Note the macrocephaly, a common feature in hydranencephaly.*

TERMINOLOGY

Definitions

- Absence of cerebral hemispheres with intact thalamus, brainstem, cerebellum, skull/meninges
  - Associated space filled with CSF
  - Probably caused by in utero vascular occlusion, infection, or trauma after 1st trimester
- Hemihydranencephaly: Rare unilateral form

IMAGING

General Features

- Best diagnostic clue
  - Absent cerebrum with fluid-filled cranial vault
  - Falx cerebri and posterior fossa structures intact
- Location
  - Cerebral hemispheres
- Morphology
  - "Water bag" brain
- Thalamus, cerebellum, brainstem, falx intact
- Medial temporal, occipital lobe remnants common

CT Findings

- Fluid-filled cranial vault; macrocephaly

MR Findings

- Absent cerebral mantle
- Falx cerebri partially/completely intact
- No gliosis in remaining brain structures

Ultrasonographic Findings

- Anechoic cranial vault

Other Modality Findings

- CTA, MRA: Atretic, stenotic, occluded, malformed or normal supraclinoid carotids and branch vessels
- Prenatal US/MR: Severe hemorrhage may precede hydranencephaly

Imaging Recommendations

- Best imaging tool
  - Prenatal US allows therapeutic intervention
  - Postnatal MR best delineates extent of destruction

DIFFERENTIAL DIAGNOSIS

Severe Hydrocephalus

- Thin cortical mantle compressed against inner table

Alobar Holoprosencephaly

- Fused midline structures; absent falx

Severe Bilateral Open-Lip Schizencephaly

- Perisylvian transmantle cleft lined by abnormal gray matter

Cystic Encephalomalacia

- Scattered cerebral cavities, gliosis

PATHOLOGY

General Features

- Etiology
  - In utero compromise of anterior cerebral circulation
  - Brain injury results in liquefactive necrosis by 20- to 27-weeks gestation
  - Implicated: Anoxia, infection, thrombophilic states, maternal toxin exposure, radiation, genetic factors, twin-twin transfusion
  - *COL4A1* mutations with large prenatal hemorrhages
- Genetics
  - Sporadic
  - Rare autosomal recessive syndromes
    - Fowler: Hydranencephaly, fetal akinesia, CNS vasculopathy
    - Microhydranencephaly: Hydranencephaly, microcephaly, small body (Chr 16p13.3-12.1)
- Associated abnormalities
  - Few reports: Vascular malformations, renal dysplasia

Gross Pathologic & Surgical Features

- Leptomeningeal-lined, fluid-filled "sacs" in lieu of cerebral hemispheres

Microscopic Features

- Hemosiderin-laden macrophages over remnant brain

CLINICAL ISSUES

Presentation

- Most common signs/symptoms
  - Microcephaly (initially) with development of macrocephaly over time (poor CSF regulation)
- Other signs/symptoms
  - Hyperirritability, hyperreflexia, seizures
- Clinical profile
  - Newborn with microcephaly/macrocephaly, developmental failure, calvarial transillumination

Demographics

- Age: Diagnosis usually made in 1st few weeks of life
- Epidemiology: < 1:10,000 births; 10x ↑ teenage mothers

Natural History & Prognosis

- Neurologic function limited to brainstem
- Progressive hydrocephalus requiring CSF diversion

Treatment

- Ventriculoperitoneal shunt treats macrocephaly → microcephaly after shunting
- Endoscopic coagulation of choroid plexus

DIAGNOSTIC CHECKLIST

Image Interpretation Pearls

- Intact falx distinguishes hydranencephaly from alobar holoprosencephaly
- Thin cortical mantle along inner table distinguishes severe hydrocephalus from hydranencephaly

SELECTED REFERENCES

1. Egger C et al: A forensic case of hydranencephaly in a preterm neonate fully documented by postmortem imaging techniques. Forensic Sci Res. 8(1):79-83, 2023
2. Huang J et al: Systematic Approach to pediatric macrocephaly. Radiographics. 43(5):e220159, 2023
3. Thiong'o GM et al: Hydranencephaly treatments: retrospective case series and review of the literature. J Neurosurg Pediatr. 26(3):228-31, 2020

White Matter Injury of Prematurity

KEY FACTS

TERMINOLOGY

- White matter (WM)
- Brain injury occurring before 37-weeks gestation, resulting in loss of periventricular WM

IMAGING

- **US**: Reliable for more severe or late disease, less reliable for mild/moderate or early disease
  - Acute findings
    - Patchy, globular foci of ↑ echogenicity in periventricular/deep WM
  - Subacute/chronic findings
    - Clusters of periventricular cysts
- **MR**: Reliable for entire spectrum of disease
  - Acute findings
    - T1-hyperintense, T2-hypointense foci
    - Hypointense SWI/GRE foci with hemorrhage
    - ↓ ADC (may miss if imaging < 24 hours or > 5 days)
    - MRS: Lactate peak or ↑ excitatory neurotransmitters
  - Subacute findings
    - Periventricular cysts
  - Chronic finding
    - Periventricular/deep WM volume loss
    - Typically minimal associated gliosis

TOP DIFFERENTIAL DIAGNOSES

- Normal periventricular halo (on US)
- Infection
- Shunted hydrocephalus

PATHOLOGY

- Wide variety of underlying causes, including pre-/peri-/postnatal insults
- Characteristic pattern of injury reflects distribution of immature oligodendrocytes during vulnerable period

CLINICAL ISSUES

- Motor & visual impairment most common neurologic sequelae of WM injury

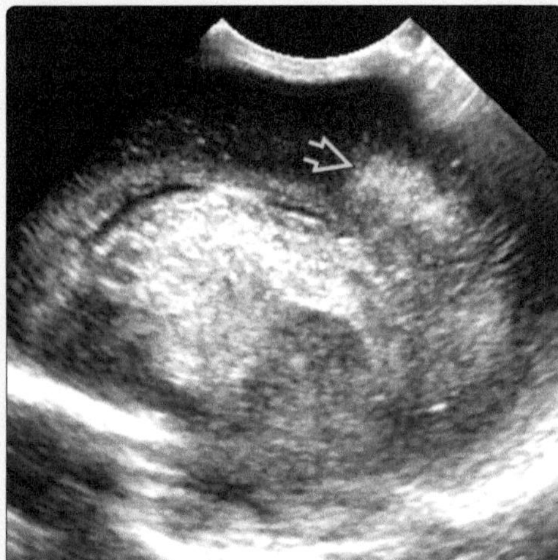

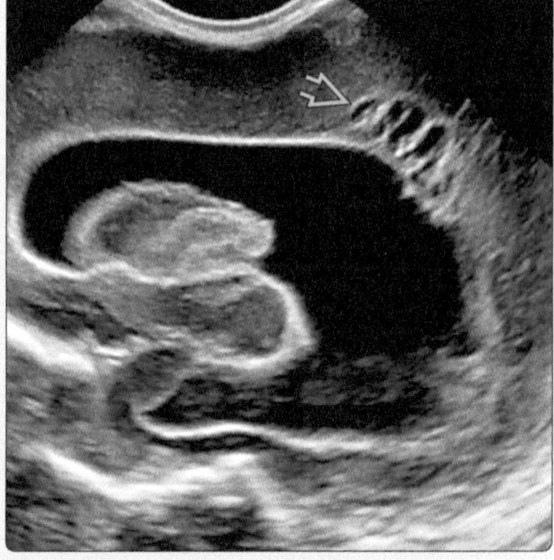

(Left) *Sagittal US of a 5-day-old, former 27-week gestational age newborn shows globular ↑ echogenicity ➔ in the periventricular white matter (WM), consistent with ischemic injury. Intraventricular hemorrhage and deep gray nuclei insult were also noted.* **(Right)** *Sagittal US in the same infant 1 month later reveals the previously seen focus of ↑ echogenicity has now evolved into cystic encephalomalacia ➔. The new ventriculomegaly is likely due to volume loss and obstruction by blood products.*

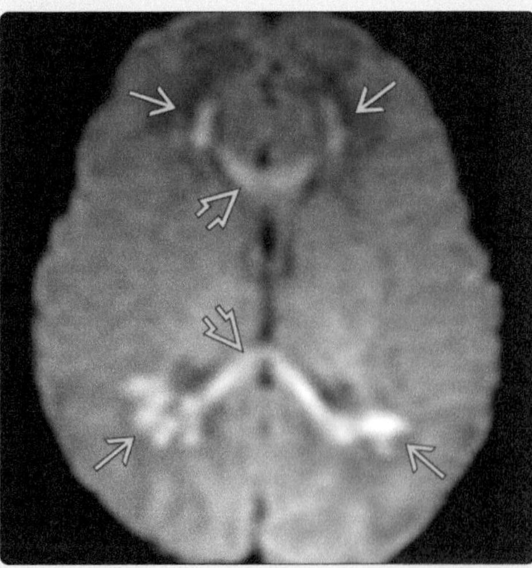

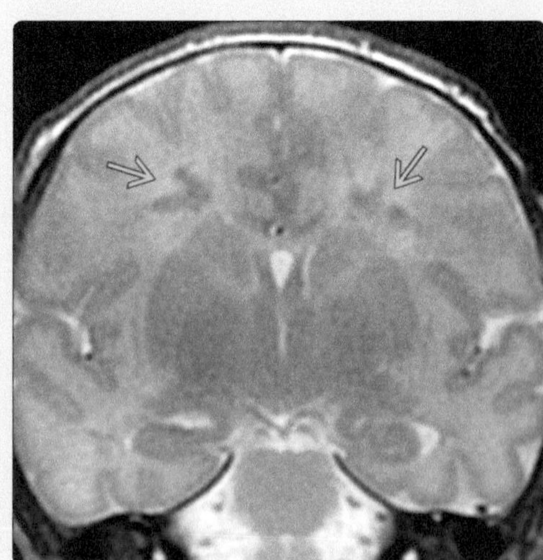

(Left) *Axial DWI MR in a 4-day-old, former 36-week gestational age infant with acute WM injury shows nearly symmetric diffusion restriction in deep and periventricular WM ➔ as well as corpus callosum ➔. Diffusion restriction is important in establishing acuity of injury.* **(Right)** *Coronal T2 MR in the same patient shows fan-shaped areas of T2 signal hypointensity ➔ corresponding to areas of diffusion restriction. Acute WM injury in neonate typically presents with ↓ T2 and ↑ T1 signal in affected areas.*

TERMINOLOGY

Abbreviations

- White matter (WM)

Synonyms

- Periventricular leukomalacia (PVL)
  - Cystic PVL; noncystic PVL
- Punctate WM lesions

Definitions

- Perinatal WM injury occurring before 34-weeks gestation
  - Affected WM not always periventricular/deep

IMAGING

General Features

- Best diagnostic clue
  - Acute: Patchy ↑ echogenicity in periventricular WM on US
  - Chronic: WM volume loss & angular ventricular margins on MR

Ultrasonographic Findings

- Grayscale ultrasound
  - 1st-line test due to portability & ease of US in NICU
  - Reliable for more severe or late disease, less reliable for mild/moderate or early injury
  - Acute findings
    - Patchy, globular foci of ↑ echogenicity in periventricular/deep WM
    - Loss of normal WM echotexture
  - Subacute findings
    - Periventricular cysts
  - Chronic findings: WM volume loss

CT Findings

- CT rarely used in neonatal setting but may be used later in life
- Reliable for more severe or late disease; less reliable for mild/moderate or early injury
  - Due to high water content of normal newborn brain
- Acute findings
  - ↓ attenuation in periventricular/deep WM
- Chronic findings
  - WM volume loss → angular ventricular margins
  - Cystic changes often difficult to distinguish from ventriculomegaly

MR Findings

- T1WI
  - Acute: Areas of T1 hyperintensity
  - Subacute: Cystic changes in periventricular WM
  - Chronic: WM volume loss, callosal thinning
- T2WI
  - Acute: Areas of T2 hypointensity
    - Represents astrogliosis & coagulative necrosis; blood has much shorter T2 relaxation time
  - Subacute: Cystic changes in periventricular WM
  - Chronic: WM volume loss, ventriculomegaly
    - Cortical ribbon extending down to ventricular margin
    - Angular ventricles with squared-off trigones
- FLAIR
  - Not usually performed in newborn period due to high water content in normal neonatal brain
  - Typically, minimal gliosis with injury that occurs in extreme prematurity
  - Chronic: Hyperintense signal in periventricular/deep WM
    - Represents gliosis or coagulation necrosis ± liquefaction
    - Also look for bright FLAIR signal in brainstem, thalamus, striatum, amygdala
- T2* GRE
  - Hypointense SWI/GRE foci in areas of hemorrhage
  - May see associated germinal matrix & intraventricular hemorrhage
- DWI
  - Reduced diffusion can precede US & T1/T2 abnormalities; ADC values may "normalize" after 7-10 days
  - May miss or underestimate WM injury if DWI is performed < 24 hours or > 7-10 days after injury
  - ↓ ADC signal/values in acute phase, ↑ ADC signal/values in chronic phase
  - DTI: Patients with WM injury have ↓ anisotropy
- MRS
  - Lactate peak, ↓ NAA, ↑ excitatory neurotransmitters; alterations may antedate MR abnormalities
  - ↑ Cho/Cr & ↓ NAA/Cho in posterior periventricular WM
    - MRS performed at term-equivalent age is predictive of motor outcome at 1 year in infants born at < 32-weeks gestation

Imaging Recommendations

- Best imaging tool
  - US in perinatal period
    - Convenient & well tolerated by neonates
    - Poor sensitivity/specificity for WM injury, especially for mild, early, or noncavitary lesions
    - Serial US exams are more sensitive for detection of cystic PVL
  - MR (including DWI & MRS)
    - Best performed ~ 5 days after suspected injury
- Protocol advice
  - US: Coronal & sagittal video clips helpful to ↑ confidence

DIFFERENTIAL DIAGNOSIS

Normal Periventricular Halo

- Specular reflections of normal WM tract condensations
- Visualized in posterior periventricular WM but less echogenic than choroid plexus
- Typically, uniform echogenicity rather than patchy or focal

Infection

- Human parechovirus meningoencephalitis: Symmetric WM & thalamic diffusion restriction, usually presents after 1st week of life
- CMV: Microcephaly, periventricular Ca^{++}, ± periventricular WM abnormalities, ± polymicrogyria
- Citrobacter: Squared-off abscesses
- Neonatal herpes simplex encephalitis: Early diffusion restriction, neuronal necrosis, ± hemorrhage

Shunted Hydrocephalus

- Ventricular distortion ± abnormal WM after shunting

Peroxisomal Disorders

- e.g., Zellweger syndrome
- Subependymal germinolytic cysts, microgyria, profound hypomyelination

PATHOLOGY

General Features

- Etiology
  - Predisposing factors of premature brain: Unique cellular vulnerability, impaired cerebrovascular autoregulation, periventricular arterial end zones
  - Common underlying etiologies
    - Hypoxia-ischemia → WM uniquely susceptible to ischemic injury in premature brain
    - Chorioamnionitis → vasculitis of chorionic plate → ↑ inflammatory cytokines
    - Other potentiating conditions: Severe premature lung disease, necrotizing enterocolitis, congenital heart disease
  - Characteristic pattern of injury reflects distribution of immature oligodendrocytes during vulnerable period
    - Selective injury to immature oligodendrocytes dramatically reduces WM volume in affected areas
- Associated abnormalities
  - Germinal matrix hemorrhage, intraventricular hemorrhage, cerebellar microhemorrhage

Staging, Grading, & Classification

- Sonographic grading of WM injury
  - Grade 1: ↑ periventricular echoes for ≥ 7 days
  - Grade 2: Periventricular echoes evolve into small frontoparietal cysts
  - Grade 3: Extensive periventricular cystic lesions

Gross Pathologic & Surgical Features

- Autopsy: Pontosubicular necrosis (59%), germinal matrix hemorrhage (50%), WM injury (24-50%)

Microscopic Features

- Focal WM injury: Reactive gliosis, coagulative necrosis, ± infarction, ± hemorrhage → tissue dissolution ± cavitation
- Diffuse WM injury: Hypoxic-ischemic injury affects differentiating oligodendroglia, causing more diffuse infarction of periventricular WM

CLINICAL ISSUES

Presentation

- Most common signs/symptoms
  - Acute: May be clinically silent initially ± EEG findings
  - Chronic: Spastic diplegia, visual & cognitive impairment
- Other signs/symptoms
  - ± hydrocephalus (essential to know head size before making diagnosis in order to differentiate ex vacuo ventriculomegaly)
- Clinical profile
  - Risk factors for WM injury of prematurity
    - Pregnancy: Low gestational age/weight, previous preterm birth, spontaneous preterm labor
    - Intrapartum: Preeclampsia, premature rupture of membranes, chorioamnionitis, group B streptococcus infection
    - Perinatal: Respiratory distress, PDA, ↓ PaCO2, sepsis, anemia, apnea, bradycardia, cardiac arrest
    - Postnatal: Severe premature lung disease, necrotizing enterocolitis

Demographics

- Age
  - < 37-weeks gestation with median age of 30-weeks gestation
  - Susceptibility of brain to WM injury ↓ with ↑ gestational age
- Sex
  - Not independent risk factor for WM injury
- Ethnicity
  - Poor antepartum care: ↑ fetal risk for WM injury
- Epidemiology
  - Recent studies suggest ↓ incidence of cerebral palsy & cystic PVL
    - Cerebral palsy: **6.5%** in 1990-1993 vs. **2.2%** in 2002-2005
    - Cystic PVL: **3.3%** in 1990-1993 vs. **1.3%** in 2002-2005
  - > 50% of patients with cystic WM injury develop cerebral palsy

Natural History & Prognosis

- Motor & visual impairment most common neurologic sequelae of WM injury
- Punctate WM lesions associated with psychomotor developmental delay, motor delay, & cerebral palsy

Treatment

- Improved outcomes have coincided with ↑ use of antenatal steroids, antenatal antibiotics, arterial line placement, & surfactant use

DIAGNOSTIC CHECKLIST

Consider

- Prior WM injury when US, CT, or MR shows unexplained ventricular dilation
- Look for gliosis & other findings of volume loss

Image Interpretation Pearls

- US may underestimate WM injury in very low-birth-weight preterm newborn
- MR is most sensitive & specific examination for evaluating WM injury in preterm newborn
  - However, may not be safe or feasible in NICU patient

SELECTED REFERENCES

1. Zhu J et al: White matter injury detection based on preterm infant cranial ultrasound images. Front Pediatr. 11:1144952, 2023
2. Buchmayer J et al: Routine use of cerebral magnetic resonance imaging in infants born extremely preterm. J Pediatr. 248:74-80.e1, 2022
3. Guillot M et al: Comparative performance of head ultrasound and MRI in detecting preterm brain injury and predicting outcomes: a systematic review. Acta Paediatr. 110(5):1425-32, 2021
4. Barnett ML et al: Exploring the multiple-hit hypothesis of preterm white matter damage using diffusion MRI. Neuroimage Clin. 17:596-606, 2018
5. Back SA: White matter injury in the preterm infant: pathology and mechanisms. Acta Neuropathol. 134(3):331-49, 2017

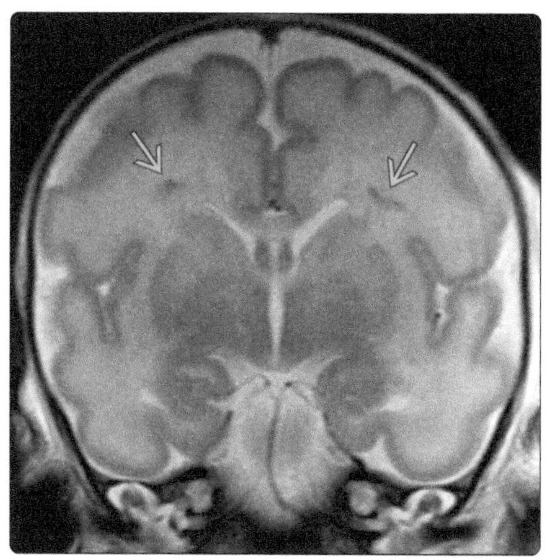

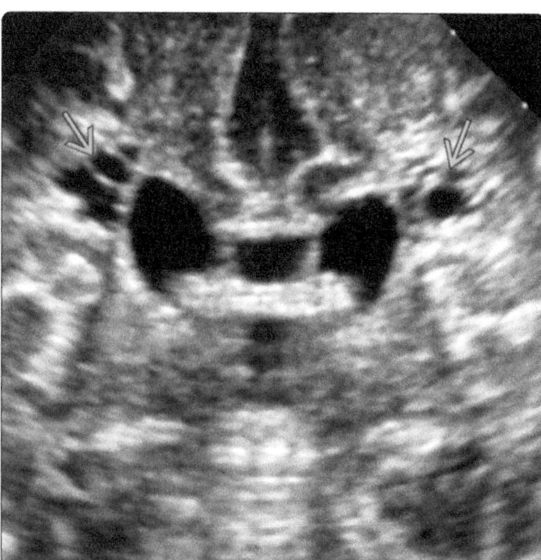

(Left) *Coronal T2 MR in an 18-day-old, former 33-week gestational age infant with tricuspid atresia demonstrates patchy, hypointense signal ⇒ in the bilateral periventricular/deep WM, consistent with ischemic injury.* **(Right)** *Coronal US in a premature infant shows bilateral periventricular WM cystic leukomalacia ⇒ adjacent to the frontal horns. Note mild frontal horn dilatation secondary to early WM volume loss.*

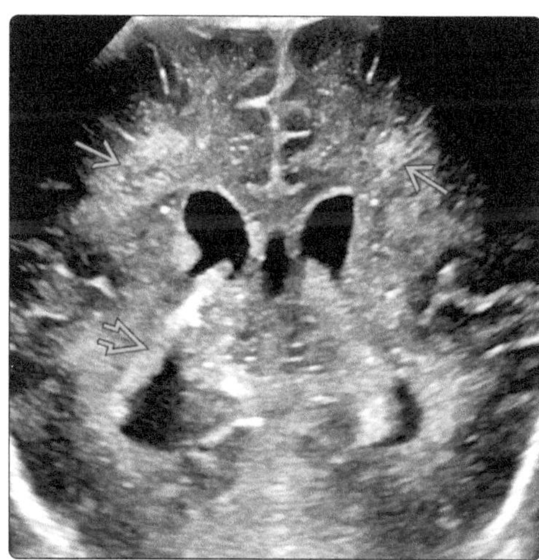

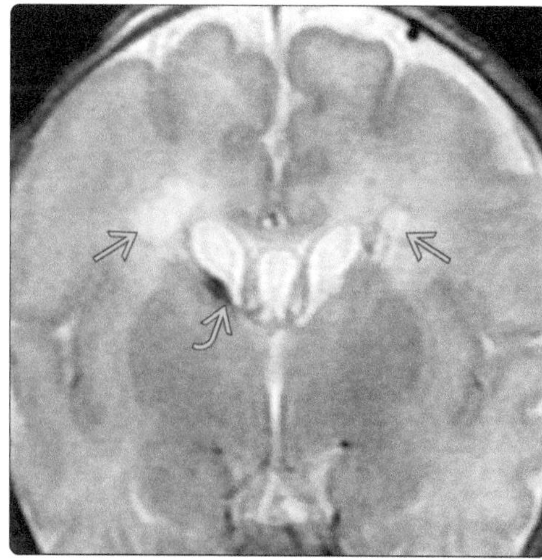

(Left) *Coronal US in a 13-day-old, former 24-week gestational age infant with WM injury shows patchy areas of ↑ echogenicity ⇒ within the periventricular and deep WM of the frontal lobes. Note how the injury is equal in brightness to the choroid plexus ⇒.* **(Right)** *Coronal T2 MR in the same patient at 5 weeks of age shows development of cystic leukomalacia within the areas of injury ⇒. Note the associated germinal matrix hemorrhage ⇒ in this extremely premature infant.*

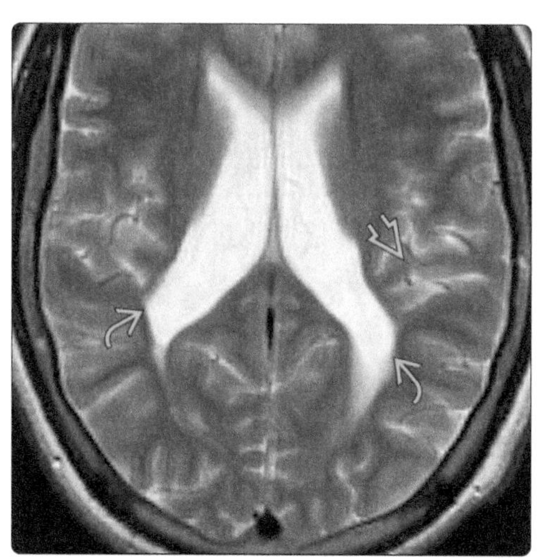

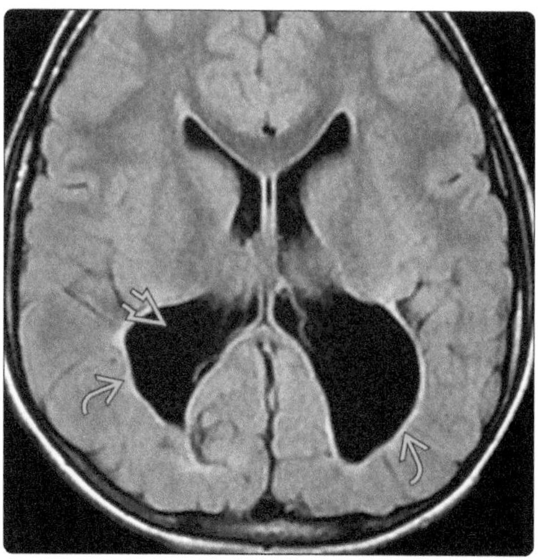

(Left) *Axial T2 MR in an infant with periventricular leukomalacia (PVL) shows the characteristic squared-off, angular morphology of the ventricular trigones ⇒. Note that the parietal lobe gyri ⇒ extend all the way down to the margin of the ventricles.* **(Right)** *Axial FLAIR MR in a 7-year-old with severe PVL shows thinning of posterior periventricular WM bilaterally ⇒ with ex vacuo expansion of the posterior lateral ventricles ⇒. Note the relative lack of signal abnormality (i.e., gliosis), characteristic of PVL.*

KEY FACTS

TERMINOLOGY

- Brain injury in neonate caused by hypoxic-ischemic insult

IMAGING

- US may be used for screening, particularly in acute setting or with concern for hemorrhage
- MR best imaging test for parenchymal injury
- Acute profound (a.k.a. "deep") pattern
  - Basal ganglia, thalami, ± perirolandic cortex, ± hippocampi
- Partial prolonged (peripheral) pattern of injury
  - Injury to cortex, especially watershed regions
- Mixed pattern common, especially in severe hypoxic-ischemic injury (HII)
- **T1WI & T2WI**: Usually normal in 1st day(s) following injury
  - T1WI: ↑ or ↓ signal in affected regions
  - T2WI: ↑ or ↓ signal in affected regions
- **DWI**: Best sequence to define extent of injury
  - ↑ DWI, ↓ ADC; pseudonormalization at ~ 8-10 days
- **MRS**: ↓ NAA & ↑ lactate in affected areas

PATHOLOGY

- Acute profound (deep) pattern: Short duration severe HII
  - Injury to regions of greatest metabolic demand
- Partial prolonged (peripheral) pattern: Less severe hypoxia, longer time period
  - Regions of greatest metabolic demand protected
- Preterm neonates likely to have associated white matter injury & gray matter hemorrhage

CLINICAL ISSUES

- Symptoms vary depending on severity of hypoxic-ischemic encephalopathy
- Sarnat grading based on signs, seizures, & duration
- Most common outcome: Cerebral palsy

DIAGNOSTIC CHECKLIST

- Findings may be inapparent/subtle in first 24 hours
- Image at 4-5 days for best MR evaluation of injury extent

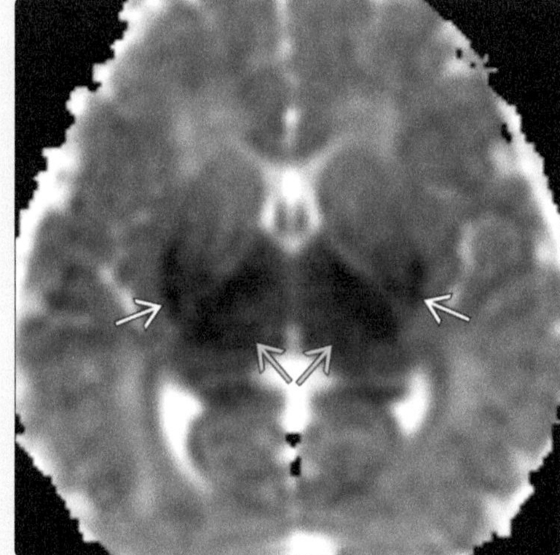

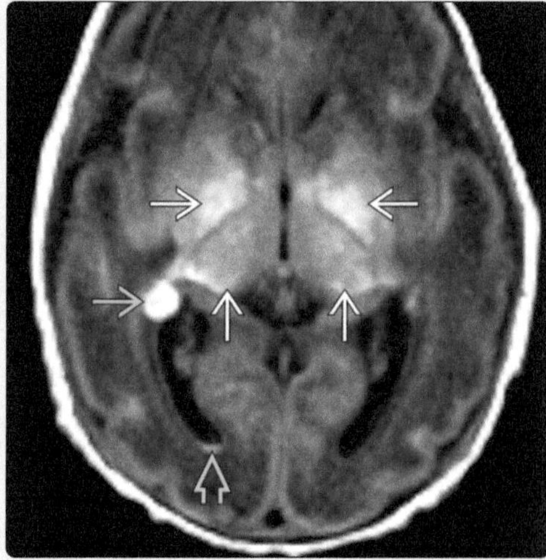

(Left) *Axial ADC MR in a 3-day-old term infant boy delivered via emergent C-section (with Apgar scores of 1, 1, & 1) shows diffusion restriction in the thalami ➙ & putamina ➙, consistent with the deep injury pattern of profound HIE.* **(Right)** *Axial T1 MR in a 31-weeks premature infant 11 days following placental abruption shows irregular hyperintense signal ➙ in the bilateral thalami & globus pallidus. Also note germinal matrix hemorrhage ➙ & small layering interventricular blood ➙, findings often seen in premature infants with HIE.*

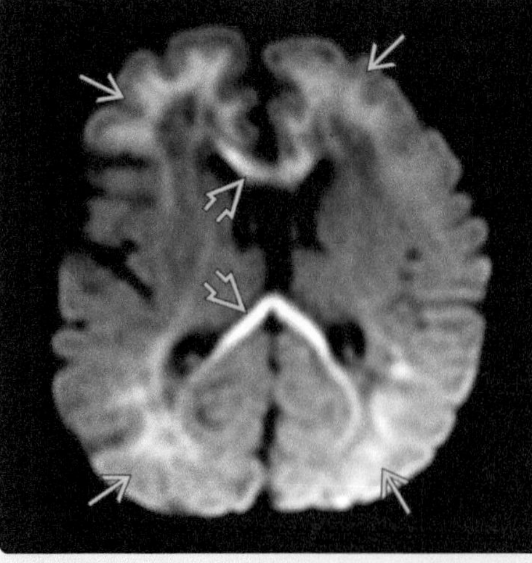

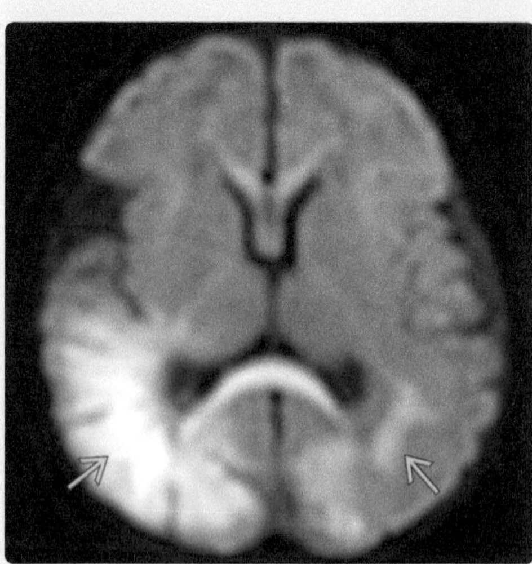

(Left) *Axial DWI in a 4-day-old with neonatal seizures shows symmetric diffusion restriction in the bilateral cerebral hemispheres, most severely affecting the watershed regions ➙. The diffusion restriction in the corpus callosum ➙ represents secondary neuronal injury.* **(Right)** *Axial DWI in a 4-day-old term neonate shows asymmetric (R > L) diffusion restriction ➙ in the bilateral temporal-occipital regions. Most HII are fairly symmetric, but asymmetry does occur & may reflect differences in cerebrovascular anatomy.*

TERMINOLOGY

Synonyms

- Hypoxic-ischemic injury (HII)
- Neonatal asphyxia or birth asphyxia

Definitions

- Hypoxic-ischemic encephalopathy (HIE): Constellation of clinical & imaging findings resulting from neonatal brain injury secondary to perinatal hypoxic-ischemic insult

IMAGING

General Features

- 2 main patterns of injury have been described
  - Acute profound pattern (a.k.a. deep or central pattern)
    - Injury to deep gray nuclei (basal ganglia & thalami), ± perirolandic cortex, ± hippocampi
    - Profound HII (e.g., asystole)
    - Associated with more severe encephalopathy
  - Partial prolonged pattern (a.k.a. peripheral pattern)
    - Injury to cortex & associated white matter (WM), usually most severely affecting watershed regions
    - Prolonged partial ischemia (e.g., fetal bradycardia)
    - Associated with seizures & less severe encephalopathy
  - Mixed pattern also frequently encountered
    - Involvement of both cortex & deep gray nuclei
    - Usually seen in most severe cases of HIE
- Chronic findings: Atrophy, gliosis/encephalomalacia

CT Findings

- Acute
  - Loss of gray-white differentiation
  - Indistinct, hypodense deep gray nuclei
  - Bright cerebellum sign due to supratentorial edema/ischemia
- Chronic
  - Parenchymal Ca^{++} & volume loss months after injury
  - ± ↑ ventricles & ↑ extraaxial CSF spaces

MR Findings

- T1WI
  - Usually normal during 1st day(s) following injury
  - ↑ or ↓ signal in areas of injury depending on anatomy involved
  - ↑ signal in deep gray nuclei & cortex (cortical laminar necrosis) may develop
  - Loss of normal bright T1 signal in posterior limb of internal capsule
- T2WI
  - Usually normal during 1st day(s) following injury
  - Indistinct deep gray nuclei & loss of cortical ribbon
  - ↑ signal in affected areas becomes more conspicuous over days
    - Some areas of injury may show ↓ signal beginning in latter 1/2 of 1st week
  - Late findings: ↑ signal & volume loss in affected areas
- PD/intermediate
  - ↑ signal in affected areas
  - May be more conspicuous than T1 & T2
- T2* GRE
  - Term neonates: Hemorrhage less common
  - Preterm neonates: Associated germinal matrix/intraventricular hemorrhage common
- DWI
  - Most important sequence
  - Restricted diffusion within 1-10 days, depending on anatomic area
    - Anatomic areas with diffusion restriction evolves over time
      - e.g., primary cortical injury & secondary WM injury
  - Pseudonormalization begins at ~ 8-10 days in most areas
    - Pseudonormalization (DWI & ADC similar to normal brain)
    - May be delayed in patients (> 10 days) treated with hypothermia
- PWI
  - ↑ ASL in affected deep gray nuclei during 1st week
  - ↑ ASL correlates with more severe injury
  - Cerebral oxygen metabolism more disturbed in severe vs. moderate HIE
- MRS
  - ↓ NAA & ↑ lactate in affected areas
  - ↑ lactate:NAA ratio correlates with more severe injury

Ultrasonographic Findings

- Findings often less conspicuous compared to MR
- Patchy ↑ echogenicity in WM
- Accentuated gray matter-WM differentiation
- ↑ echogenicity in deep gray nuclei
- Slit-like lateral ventricles & sulcal effacement: Not indicative of injury
  - Typical appearance for newborn who has undergone labor &/or born vaginally, so not helpful to suggest HIE

Imaging Recommendations

- Best imaging tool
  - MR with DWI & MRS
- Protocol advice
  - Findings may be inapparent/subtle in first 24 hours
  - Image at 4-5 days for best MR evaluation of injury extent
    - ADC changes peak at ~ 4-5 days

DIFFERENTIAL DIAGNOSIS

Metabolic Disorders

- Nonketotic hyperglycinemia
- Sulfite oxidase deficiency
- Molybdenum cofactor deficiency

Urea Cycle Disorders

- Ornithine transcarbamylase deficiency
- Elevated ammonia, present at 24-28 hours

Maple Syrup Urine Disease

- Edema in myelinated areas
- Brainstem, perirolandic, & cerebellar WM

Kernicterus

- Hyperbilirubinemia ± sepsis, hypoxia
- Mimics profound deep injury on T1WI
  - Globus pallidus (not putamen or thalamus)

Hypoglycemia

- Characteristic occipital cortex injury
- May potentiate HII

Perinatal Arterial Ischemic Stroke

- Focal arterial territory injury without hypoxic event

Venous Injury

- Edema, hemorrhage, or ischemia in venous distribution

TORCH Infections

- May mimic chronic findings of HIE
- Microcephaly, migration anomalies, Ca^{++}

Human Parechovirus Meningoencephalitis

- Symmetric WM & posterior thalami diffusion restriction
- Typically presents after 1st week of life

PATHOLOGY

General Features

- Etiology
  - Acute profound (deep) pattern associated with severe hypoxia of relatively brief (10-25 minutes) duration
    - Causative (sentinel) event usually identifiable
    - Injury to regions of greatest metabolic demand
  - Partial prolonged (peripheral) pattern associated with less severe hypoxia over longer period (15 minutes, up to hours)
    - Causative event may be cryptic
    - Regions of greatest metabolic demand protected
    - Watershed regions most susceptible
  - Preterm infants more susceptible to equivalent ischemic injury as compared to term infants
    - Preterm neonates more likely to have associated WM injury & germinal matrix hemorrhage
  - Asphyxia triggers cascade of cellular biochemical events → abnormal function, edema, or cell death
    - Extracellular glutamate accumulates, activates postsynaptic excitatory amino acid receptors
    - Postsynaptic receptor distribution changes with ↑ age; different injury patterns based on age
- Associated abnormalities
  - Maternal: Infection, preeclampsia, diabetes, drug use
  - Infant: Anemia, growth restriction, hypoglycemia, sepsis, seizures
  - Placental abnormalities: Chorioamnionitis, placental abruption
  - Ischemia, often multiorgan (e.g., cardiac, renal, liver)

Staging, Grading, & Classification

- Sarnat stage (based on clinical & EEG findings)
  - I (mild): Hyperalert/irritable, mydriasis, ↑ heart rate, EEG normal
  - II (moderate): Lethargy, hypotonia, miosis, ↓ heart rate, seizures common
  - III (severe): Stupor, flaccid, reflexes absent, seizures uncommon

Gross Pathologic & Surgical Features

- Acute profound pattern: Hippocampal, basal ganglia, thalamic, perirolandic atrophy
- Partial prolonged pattern: Ulegyria, gliosis, & atrophy with spared perirolandic region

CLINICAL ISSUES

Presentation

- Most common signs/symptoms
  - Symptoms depend on severity of HIE
    - Altered consciousness
    - Abnormal muscle tone
    - Respiratory & heart rate changes
    - Cranial nerve dysfunction
    - Seizures
- Other signs/symptoms
  - Low Apgar scores
  - Laboratory findings
    - Cord blood gases: Metabolic acidosis (↓ pH, ↓ HCO_3^-)
    - ± abnormal renal, liver, & heart labs
  - EEG findings
    - Mild: Normal/↓
    - Moderate: ↓ voltage (delta & theta waves), focal seizures
    - Severe: Isopotential or infrequent periodic discharges

Demographics

- Age
  - Ischemia may occur in immediate prenatal, intrapartum, & immediate postnatal periods
- Sex
  - M > F
- Epidemiology
  - 1-8/1,000 live births in resource-rich countries & ≤ 26/1,000 live births in resource-limited countries

Natural History & Prognosis

- Deep pattern associated with dyskinetic cerebral palsy
- Peripheral pattern associated with spastic cerebral palsy
- Burst suppression EEG is poor prognostic factor

Treatment

- Resuscitation, correction of fluid & electrolyte imbalance
- Therapeutic hypothermia
- Treat seizures
- Erythropoietin (EPO) therapy may improve outcome

DIAGNOSTIC CHECKLIST

Image Interpretation Pearls

- DWI is most critical sequence but evolves over time
  - Can be normal < 1 day, ↑ in severity over days, then pseudonormalization begins at ~ 8-10 days
- US: Slit-like lateral & 3rd ventricles are normal in 1st days of life following labor
  - Should not be mistaken for cerebral edema

SELECTED REFERENCES

1. Guarnera A et al: Predictive value of MRI in hypoxic-ischemic encephalopathy treated with therapeutic hypothermia. Children (Basel). 10(3):446, 2023
2. Parmentier CEJ et al: Magnetic resonance imaging in (near-)term infants with hypoxic-ischemic encephalopathy. Diagnostics (Basel). 12(3):645, 2022
3. Bach AM et al: Early magnetic resonance imaging predicts 30-month outcomes after therapeutic hypothermia for neonatal encephalopathy. J Pediatr. 238:94-101.e1, 2021

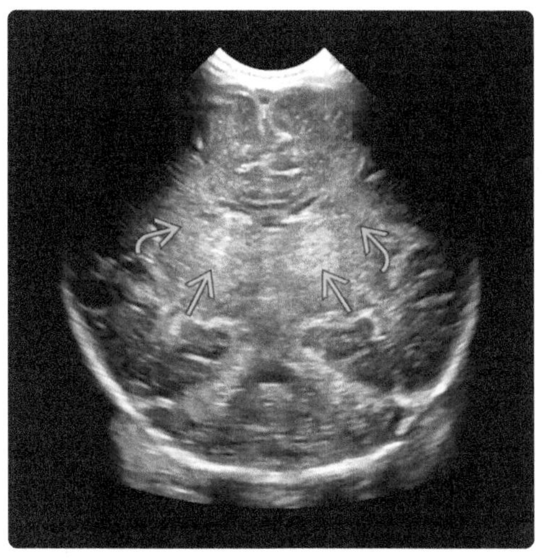

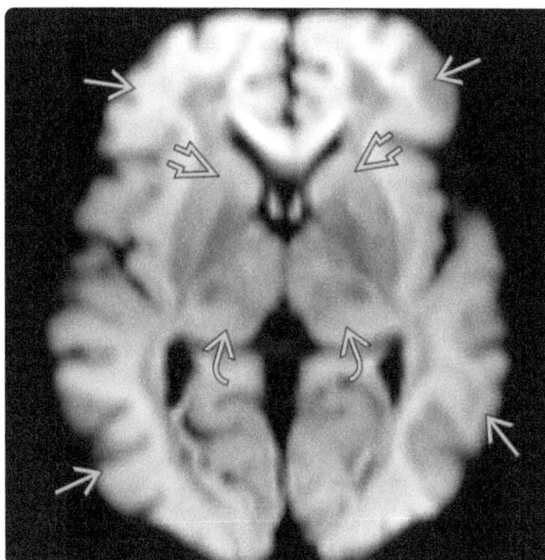

(Left) *Coronal US performed at ~ 1 hour of life in a newborn with polyhydramnios & mother with previous term stillborn shows mild ↑ echogenicity in the thalami ↪ & white matter →. The presence of these findings at 1 hour of life suggests a global HII occurred many hours or days prior to birth.* **(Right)** *Axial DWI MR in the same newborn at 4 days of life shows symmetric marked diffusion restriction in the cerebral hemispheres →, basal ganglia ⇒, & thalami ↪, consistent with a severe mixed pattern of HII.*

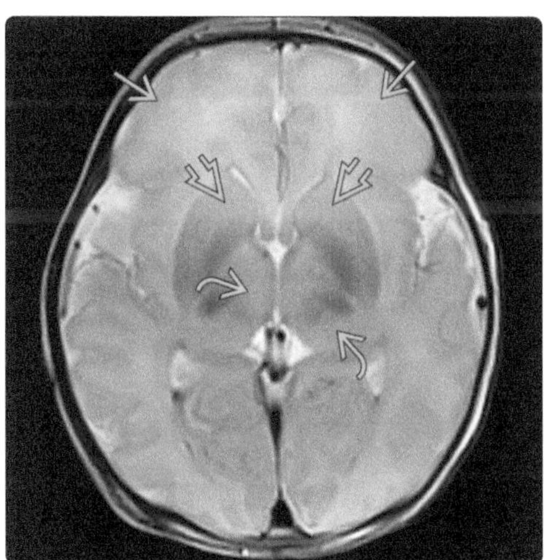

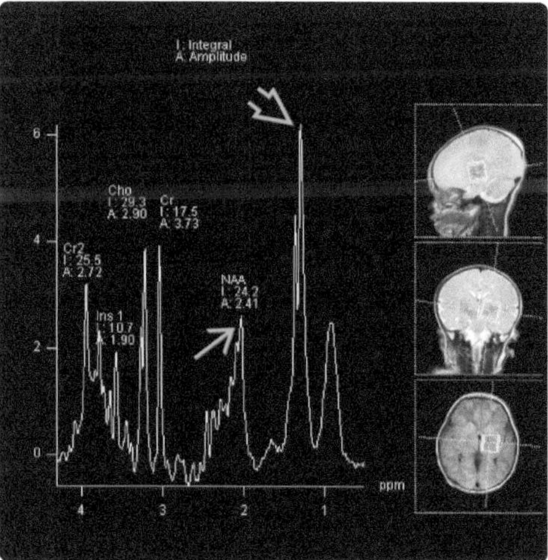

(Left) *Axial T2 MR in the same 4-day-old shows ↑ T2 signal within the affected cerebral hemispheres with loss or decrease of gray-white differentiation →. Note the ↑ signal in the basal ganglia ⇒ & thalami ↪ as well.* **(Right)** *Single-voxel short echo MR spectroscopy centered in the left basal ganglia & thalami shows a markedly ↑ doublet lactate peak ⇒ at 1.3 ppm & ↓ NAA peak → at 2.0 ppm. These findings support the diagnosis of HII.*

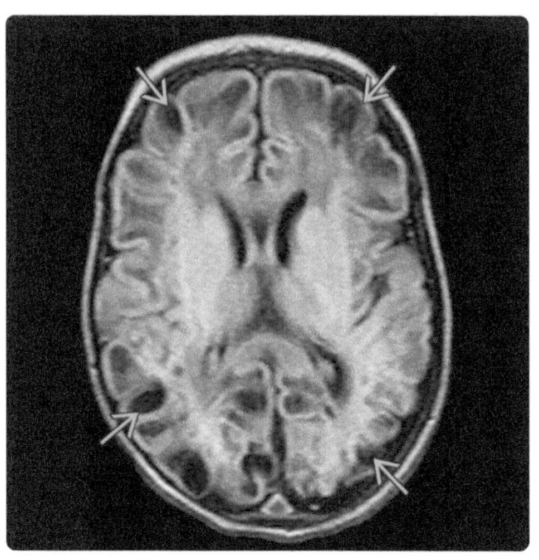

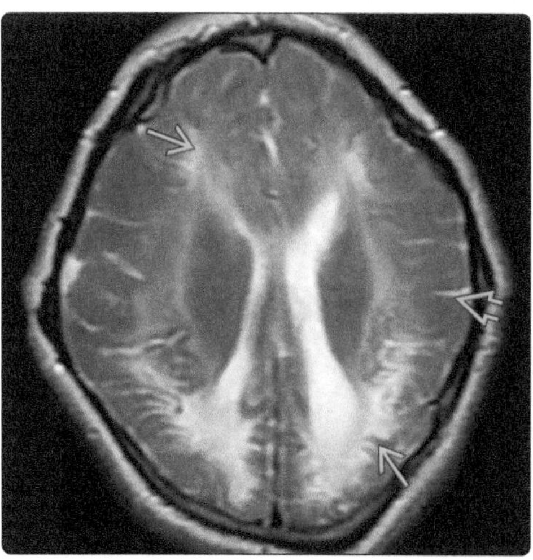

(Left) *Axial FLAIR in a 2-week-old with HIE → shows early evolution of cystic encephalomalacia in a symmetric watershed pattern.* **(Right)** *Axial T2WI MR in the same patient at 10 years of age shows the significant encephalomalacia & gliosis → in a symmetric watershed pattern with relative preservation of the perirolandic cortex ⇒. This anatomic distribution of injury suggests a partial prolonged pattern of HII.*

KEY FACTS

TERMINOLOGY

- Acute neurologic dysfunction due to loss of vascular integrity

IMAGING

- NECT: ↓ attenuation of affected gray matter
  - Insular ribbon sign → loss of distinct insular cortex
  - Hyperdense MCA sign → thrombosed MCA
- MR: ↓ diffusion within ~ 30 minutes of arterial occlusion
  - Cytotoxic edema evident in affected territory on FLAIR/T2 by 4-6 hours after arterial occlusion
  - Enhancement of infarct typically occurs after 5-7 days
- CTA/MRA: Critical for early evaluation & identification of possible etiology (e.g., dissection, arteriopathy)
  - CTA 1st line for rapid identification of large vessel occlusion amenable to catheter-directed thrombectomy
- MR perfusion imaging can provide valuable information regarding region at risk in setting of acute stroke

TOP DIFFERENTIAL DIAGNOSES

- Seizure-related injury
- Acute encephalitis
- Mitochondrial encephalopathies
- Posterior reversible encephalopathy syndrome (PRES)

PATHOLOGY

- Major causes: Cardiac disease (~ 25%), moyamoya, dissection, vasculitis, RCVS, hematologic

CLINICAL ISSUES

- Children typically present later than adults (> 24 hours)
- Focal deficit may be masked by lethargy, coma, irritability
- Catheter-based thrombectomy increasingly used in children
- Capacity for recovery in children much > adults

DIAGNOSTIC CHECKLIST

- When stroke is suspected clinically or by imaging, do not hesitate to perform vessel imaging

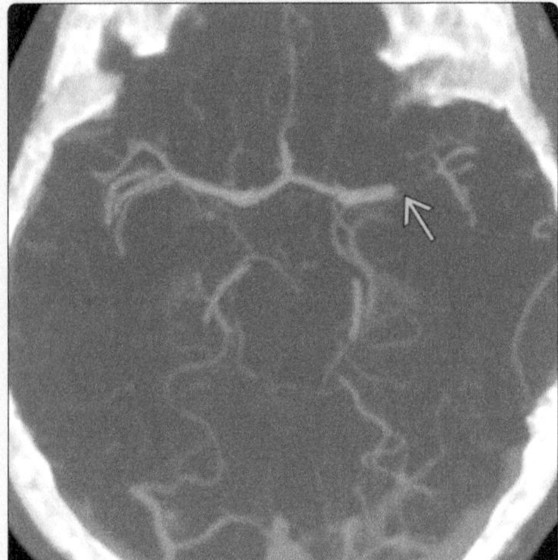

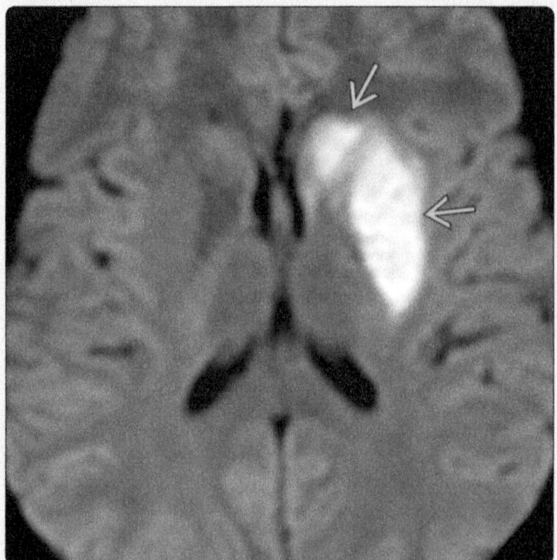

(Left) *Axial CTA MIP in a 14-year-old with right-sided weakness and history of congenital heart disease shows abrupt cutoff ⇒ of the M1 segment of the left middle cerebral artery (MCA). MIP imaging is particularly helpful to identify vessel occlusion in stroke. This patient was treated with catheter-directed thrombectomy.* **(Right)** *Axial DWI in the same patient after thrombectomy shows restricted diffusion ⇒ in the left basal ganglia, consistent with acute infarction. Note preservation of the remainder of the left MCA territory.*

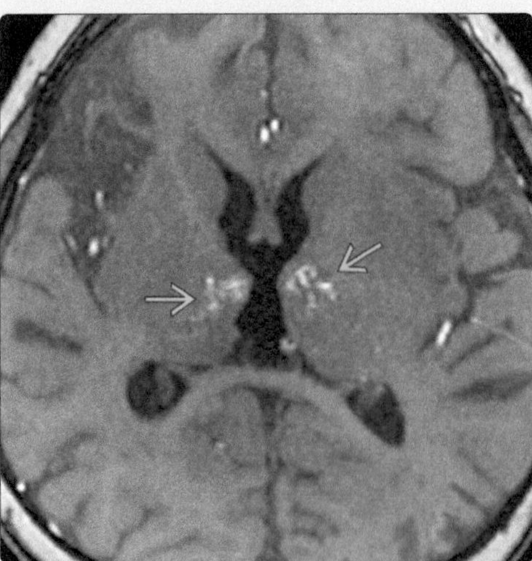

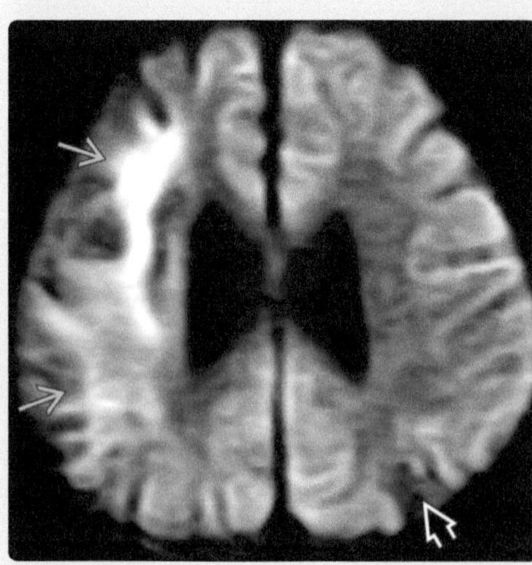

(Left) *Axial time-of-flight MRA in a 2-year-old with multiple infarcts of various ages shows multiple small areas of flow-related signal ⇒ in the bilateral thalami, consistent with lenticulostriate collaterals of moyamoya.* **(Right)** *Axial DWI MR in the same patient with moyamoya-type vasculopathy shows diffusion restriction in the right frontoparietal foci of signal abnormality ⇒, suggesting an acute/subacute infarct. However, there is no diffusion restriction in the left parietal region ➡, suggesting this infarct is of an older age.*

TERMINOLOGY

Synonyms

- Cerebrovascular accident, cerebral infarct, cerebral ischemia

Definitions

- Acute alteration of neurologic function due to loss of vascular integrity
  - This document specifically addresses arterial ischemia beyond perinatal period

IMAGING

General Features

- Best diagnostic clue
  - Cytotoxic edema & restricted diffusion (acutely) in affected vascular territory
- Location
  - Proximal & distal middle cerebral artery (MCA) territory most commonly affected
- Morphology
  - Stroke caused by arterial occlusion typically conforms to 1 arterial territory

CT Findings

- NECT
  - ↓ attenuation of affected gray matter with loss of normal gray matter-white matter differentiation
    - ↓ in white matter attenuation less pronounced
    - Often wedge-shaped & localized to 1 arterial territory
    - Diffuse ischemic injury can lead to reversal sign with gray matter diffusely ↓ in attenuation relative to white matter
  - Insular ribbon sign → loss of distinct of insular cortex
  - Hyperdense MCA sign → ↑ density of acutely thrombosed MCA
  - Hemorrhagic transformation (HT)
    - Symptomatic HT in 3%; asymptomatic HT in 30%
      - Asymptomatic HT usually parenchymal
    - White matter or deep nuclear hemorrhage often mass-like → hematoma within infarcted tissue
- CECT
  - Enhancement of infarcted territory typically occurs after 5-7 days
- CTA
  - Invaluable for demonstrating focal vascular abnormalities in acute setting
    - CTA 1st line for rapid identification of large vessel occlusion amenable to catheter-directed thrombectomy
    - Intimal flap in acutely dissected vessel

MR Findings

- **T1WI**: Acute: ↓ signal with gyral swelling
  - Chronic: ± ↑ signal in cortical laminar necrosis
- **T1WI FS**: Allows identification of mural hematoma (↑ signal) in dissected vessel
- **T2WI**: Loss of flow void in thrombosed vessel
- **FLAIR**: ↑ signal with gyral swelling (within ~4-6 hours)
  - Abnormal sulcal ↑ signal (climbing ivy sign) of chronic, slow-flow collaterals in setting of longstanding proximal vascular occlusion
- **DWI**: Most sensitive for early detection of ischemia
  - Acute: Restricted diffusion (↑ DWI, ↓ ADC signal) ≤ 30 minutes after ischemic insult
  - Subacute (7-14 days): Pseudonormalization of signal
    - ↑ DWI, ADC ~ brain parenchyma
  - Chronic: Facilitated diffusion in gliotic brain
    - ↑/~ DWI, ↑ ADC
- **SWI/T2* GRE**: May see ↑ size & number of cortical vessels
  - Suggests ↑ extraction fraction & possibly recoverable brain
- **T1WI C+**: Cortical & leptomeningeal enhancement seen after ~5-7 days following acute infarct
  - Enhancing climbing ivy sign
- **MRA**: Can detect arterial occlusion & stenosis in large- & medium-sized cerebral vessels
  - Important to identify underlying dissection or arteriopathy
- **PWI**: Provides valuable information about affected brain
  - Ischemic penumbra: ↓ perfusion, no DWI change (PWI-DWI mismatch)
    - May define brain salvageable with acute stroke therapy
  - Arterial spin labeling can provide useful perfusion information without contrast administration
- **MRS**: ↑ lactate hallmark of ischemia/infarct
  - Not specific
- **Vessel wall imaging**: Vessel wall enhancement patterns improve discrimination of underlying stroke etiology

Ultrasonographic Findings

- Grayscale ultrasound
  - Affected territory hyperechoic in acute/subacute stage
- Color Doppler
  - Direct Doppler evaluation ideal for surveillance of vascular occlusion in neonate with open sutures
  - Transcranial Doppler evaluation of circle of Willis through temporal squamosa
    - ↑ velocities can predict stenoses detectable by MRA
    - Used as screening tool in children with sickle cell anemia

Angiographic Findings

- Catheter angiography rarely necessary in acute evaluation of childhood stroke
  - Justified if contemplating endovascular therapy
- Best modality for detailed evaluation of primary arteriopathies

Imaging Recommendations

- Best imaging tool
  - CT initial imaging test for signs/symptoms of stroke; excellent for excluding hemorrhagic stroke (more common in children vs. adults)
  - MR with DWI, MRA, PWI
- Protocol advice
  - Contrast can help in assessing timing of injury & performing perfusion imaging
  - Dedicated vessel wall MR imaging to define underlying etiology [e.g. focal cerebral arteriopathy (FCA)]

DIFFERENTIAL DIAGNOSIS

Seizure-Related Injury

- Swelling & restricted diffusion secondary to persistent seizure activity
- Differentiation by clinical presentation & EEG

Acute Encephalitis

- Acute parenchymal inflammation secondary to infectious agents, typically viral
- Slower onset with encephalopathy

Mitochondrial Encephalopathies

- Symmetric basal ganglia involvement common
- Usually have manifestations beyond CNS

Posterior Reversible Encephalopathy Syndrome (PRES)

- Patchy cortical/subcortical edema most common in parietal & occipital lobes, typically in setting of hypertension
- Diffusion restriction uncommon

Neonatal Herpes Encephalitis

- Infant with seizures 2-5 weeks after birth
- DWI most sensitive for detection in early disease
- Often bilateral with temporal predominance but can occur anywhere

MELAS

- **M**itochondrial **e**ncephomyopathy, **l**actic acidosis, **s**troke-like episodes
- Areas of ischemia crossing arterial territories, often parietal
- MRS: ↑ lactate in normal-appearing brain

Group B Strep Meningitis

- Associated vasculitis causes ischemia in small perforating arteries
- Unilateral or bilateral deep gray nuclei ischemia

PATHOLOGY

General Features

- 6 major causes of arterial stroke in children
  - Cardiac disease (~ 25%)
    - Congenital heart disease, valvular heart disease, arrhythmias, & cardiomyopathies
  - Moyamoya-type arteriopathy
    - Sickle cell disease
    - Neurofibromatosis type 1
    - Radiation therapy
    - Trisomy 21
    - Alagille syndrome
  - Arterial dissection (e.g., trauma)
  - FCA of childhood
  - Reversible cerebral vasoconstriction syndrome (RCVS)
  - Hematologic/metabolic (e.g., coagulopathy)
  - Idiopathic (~ 25%)

CLINICAL ISSUES

Presentation

- Most common signs/symptoms
  - Depends on patient age, etiology, & involved artery
    - < 1 year: Seizures, encephalopathy > focal neurologic
    - > 1 year: Usually focal neurologic (e.g., hemiplegia, early hand preference)
    - Speech difficulties, gait abnormality, seizure
      - Seizure → deficit often attributed to postictal state (Jacksonian paralysis)
    - Embolic cause: Sudden onset of symptoms
    - Stenoocclusive cause: Gradual/intermittent (e.g., TIA)
  - Focal deficit may be masked by lethargy, coma, irritability
- Children typically present later than adults (> 24 hours)
  - Poor recognition/understanding of symptoms by child, caregiver, physician
  - Uncommon diagnosis in children, requires high degree of suspicion

Demographics

- Age
  - Incidence/mortality greatest < 1 year
  - Large percentage occur in perinatal period
    - Perinatal arterial ischemic stroke (PAIS)
- Epidemiology
  - Incidence: 2-3/100,000 per year in USA
    - Mortality: 0.6/100,000
  - Underrecognized as significant source of morbidity in pediatric population

Natural History & Prognosis

- Capacity for recovery better than in adults, due to
  - Better compensatory mechanisms, collateral recruitment, neuronal plasticity
  - Fewer concomitant risk factors

Treatment

- Mechanical thrombectomy frequently employed for acute large vessel occlusion
- Mainstay of chronic therapy for fixed vascular lesions & vasculopathies: Aspirin
- Transfusion therapy for at-risk children with sickle cell
- Dissection: Anticoagulation, vessel occlusion, or stenting

DIAGNOSTIC CHECKLIST

Image Interpretation Pearls

- Use same imaging signs as adults
- Have low threshold for use of CTA
- Dedicated vessel wall MR imaging often helpful to identify underlying etiology

SELECTED REFERENCES

1. Jiang B et al: Neuroimaging in pediatric stroke. Semin Pediatr Neurol. 43:100989, 2022
2. Chabrier S et al: Hyperacute recanalization strategies and childhood stroke in the evidence age. Stroke. 52(1):381-4, 2021
3. Oesch G et al: Focal cerebral arteriopathy of childhood: clinical and imaging correlates. Stroke. 52(7):2258-65, 2021
4. Visser MJ et al: Automated perfusion-diffusion magnetic resonance imaging in childhood arterial ischemic stroke. Stroke. 52(10):3296-304, 2021
5. Fearn ND et al: Focal cerebral arteriopathy and childhood stroke. Curr Opin Neurol. 33(1):37-46, 2020
6. Donahue MJ et al: Neuroimaging advances in pediatric stroke. Stroke. 50(2):240-8, 2019
7. Dlamini N et al: Arterial wall imaging in pediatric stroke. Stroke. 49(4):891-8, 2018
8. Khalaf A et al: Pediatric stroke imaging. Pediatr Neurol. 86:5-18, 2018

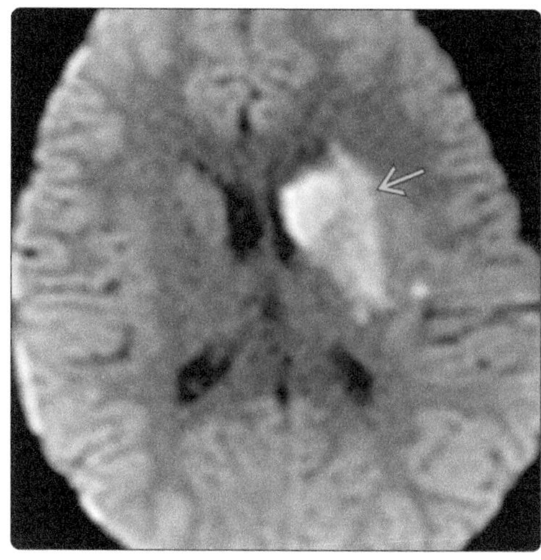

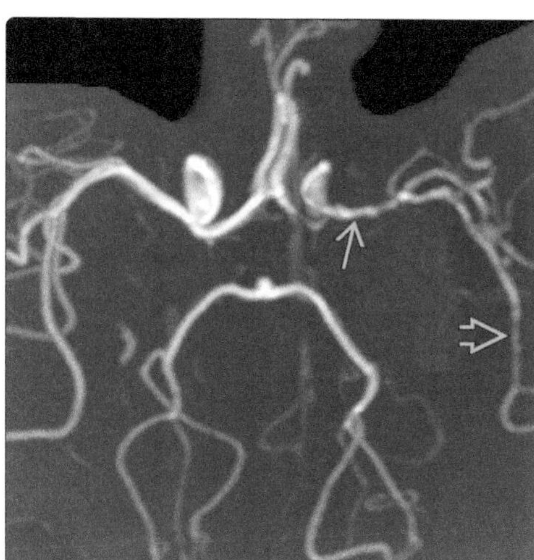

(Left) *Axial DWI MR in a 6-year-old with imbalance and acute infarct of the left basal ganglia ➡ shows diffusion restriction (↓ ADC not shown). Acute infarct in a child should prompt further evaluation with MRA or CTA to detect an underlying vessel abnormality.* **(Right)** *3D MRA of the circle of Willis in the same patient shows irregular narrowing of the left proximal ➡ and distal ➡ segments of the MCA, consistent with vasculitis.*

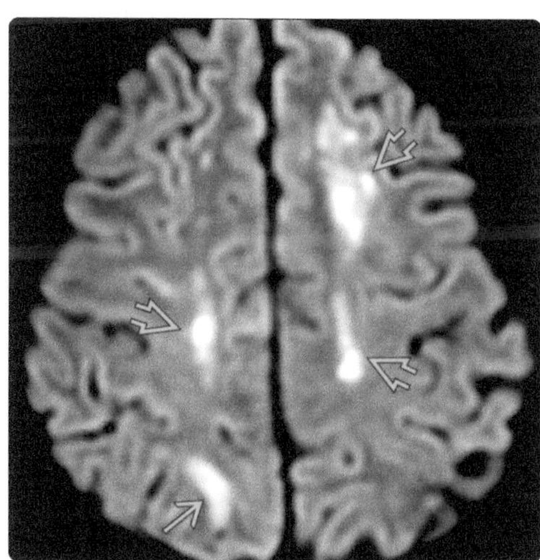

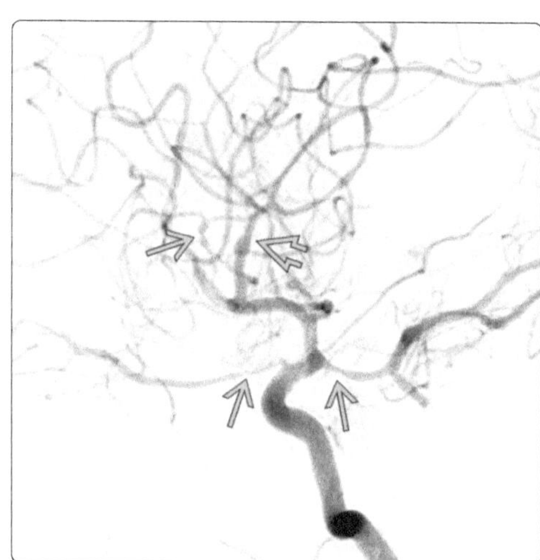

(Left) *Axial DWI MR in a 12-year-old with reversible cerebral vasoconstriction syndrome (RCVS) who recently started mycophenolate and presented with acute onset of left-sided weakness shows multifocal cortical ➡ and subcortical ➡ infarcts.* **(Right)** *Lateral projection DSA from an internal carotid artery (ICA) injection in the same patient shows multifocal areas of medium vessel narrowing ➡ and irregularity ➡, a common feature of RCVS. The spectrum of underlying etiologies for childhood stroke is diverse.*

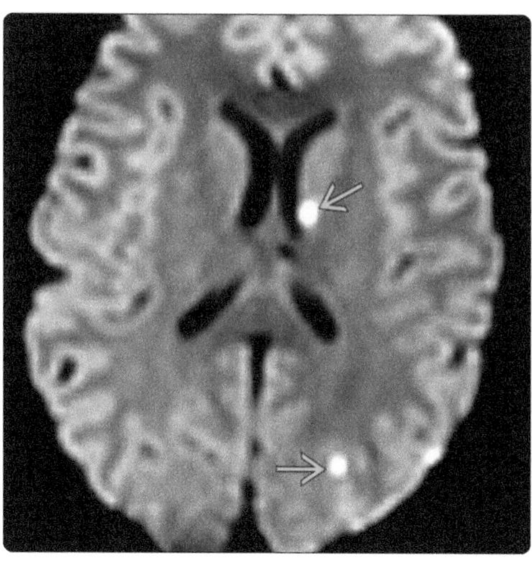

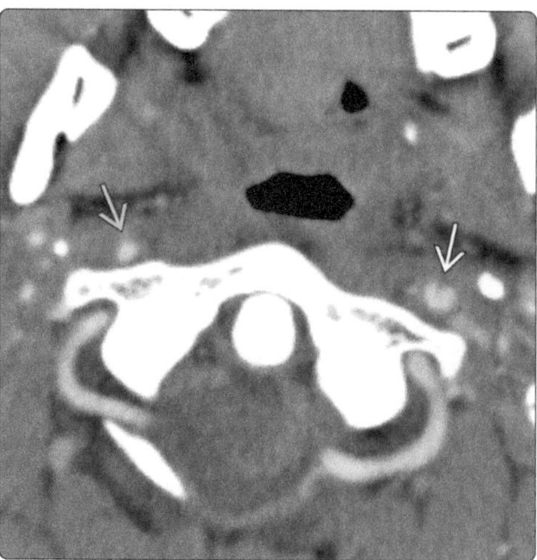

(Left) *Axial DWI MR in a 16-year-old boy involved in a motor vehicle accident shows multiple small foci of diffusion restriction ➡, consistent with small infarcts. Multiple infarcts should raise concern for dissection, especially when confined to a single arterial territory.* **(Right)** *Axial CTA in the same patient shows vessel wall irregularity and an intimal flap in the left ICA ➡. The right ICA ➡ is small and revealed areas of irregularity on other images (not shown). These findings are consistent with bilateral ICA dissections.*

KEY FACTS

TERMINOLOGY

- Abnormality in hemoglobin (Hgb) → change in shape (sickling) → ↑ "stickiness" of erythrocytes (RBCs) → capillary occlusions, ischemia, infarctions, premature RBC destruction (hemolytic anemia)

IMAGING

- Best diagnostic clue
  - Cerebral infarct(s) in Black child
  - Moyamoya (MM; secondary)

TOP DIFFERENTIAL DIAGNOSES

- Vasculitis
- Other causes of MM (inherited and secondary)

PATHOLOGY

- Point mutation of Hgb β gene, Chr 11p15.5: Glutamate → valine substitution
- Sickled RBCs adhere to endothelium → fragmentation of internal elastic lamina, degeneration of muscularis → large-vessel vasculopathy ± aneurysm formation

CLINICAL ISSUES

- Stroke
  - 17-26% of all patients with sickle cell disease (SCD)
  - 18x ↑ risk if transcranial Doppler velocity of internal carotid/middle cerebral arteries > 200 cm/s
  - Peak incidence: 1st decade of life
- 20% of children have white matter infarcts on MR without overt neurologic deficits = silent infarcts
  - 14x ↑ risk of stroke
- Regular blood transfusions keep Hgb S < 30%
  - ↓ stroke by up to 75%

DIAGNOSTIC CHECKLIST

- Always consider SCD in Black child with cerebral infarction

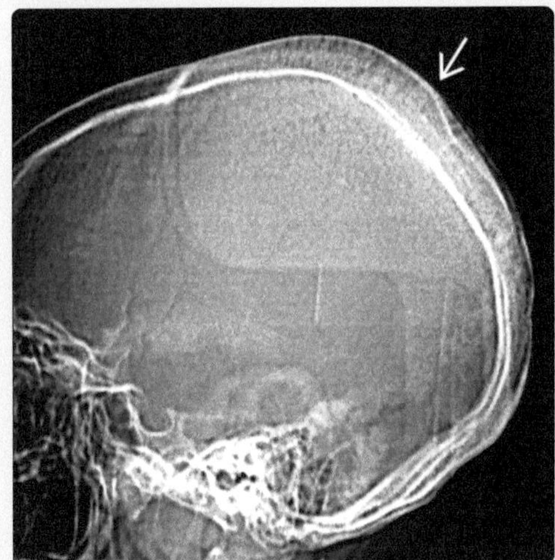

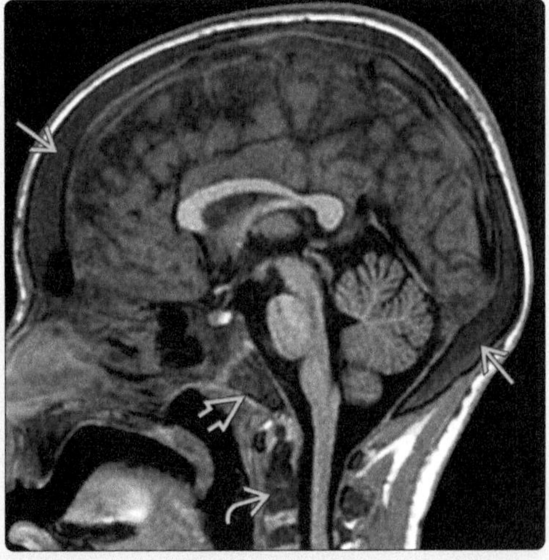

(Left) *Lateral scout image from a CT examination shows marked diploic thickening ➡ due to red marrow hyperplasia, causing a hair-on-end appearance.* **(Right)** *Midline sagittal T1 MR in an 8-year-old with sickle cell disease (SCD) shows calvarial thickening and marrow expansion ➡ with replacement of fatty marrow with hypointense red marrow due to marrow hyperplasia secondary to chronic anemia. Areas that would typically have bright fatty marrow, such as the clivus ➡ and spine ➡, are dark.*

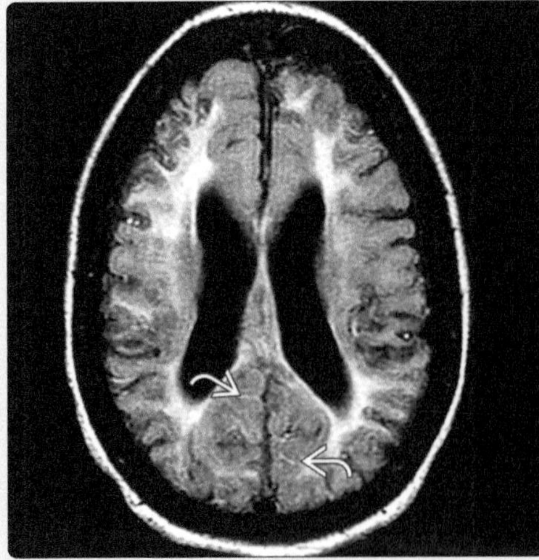

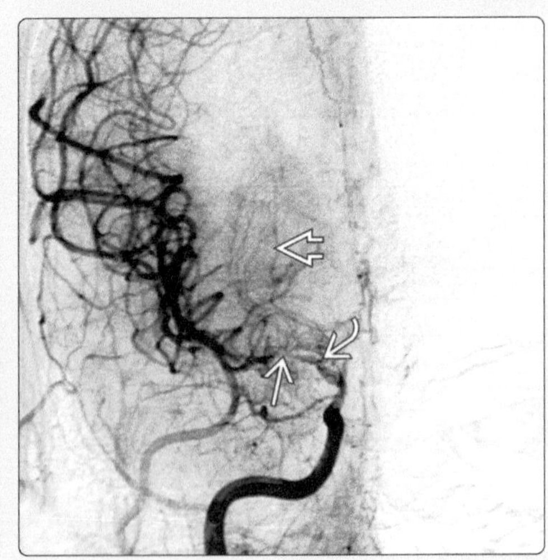

(Left) *Axial FLAIR MR shows considerable brain atrophy and signal hyperintensity due to chronic ischemic brain injury. Note presence of the ivy sign ➡, branching abnormal hyperintensity in the cerebral sulci. The ivy sign is thought to occur secondary to slow collateral flow in engorged pial vessels.* **(Right)** *DSA AP view from a right internal carotid artery (ICA) injection shows secondary moyamoya with enlarged lenticulostriate arteries ➡, resulting in a "puff of smoke" in this SCD patient with severe MCA ➡ and distal ICA ➡ stenosis.*

TERMINOLOGY

Abbreviations

- Sickle cell disease (SCD)

Definitions

- Abnormality in hemoglobin (Hgb) → change in shape (sickling) → ↑ "stickiness" of erythrocytes (RBCs) → capillary occlusions, ischemia, infarctions, premature RBC destruction (hemolytic anemia)

IMAGING

General Features

- Best diagnostic clue
  - Cerebral infarct(s) in Black child
  - Secondary moyamoya (MM)
    - Narrowing of distal internal carotid arteries (ICAs) or proximal anterior cerebral arteries (ACAs), middle cerebral arteries (MCAs)
    - Lenticulostriate collaterals in basal ganglia (BG)
- Location: ICAs, deep white matter (WM), cortex, bone marrow
- Cognitive impairment does not correlate with imaging findings
- ↓ gray matter (GM) volume in SCD children

Radiographic Findings

- Radiography
  - Thick skull with expanded diploic space
  - Opacified paranasal sinuses

CT Findings

- NECT
  - Hypodense GM or WM infarct(s) → diffuse atrophy
  - Rare: Subarachnoid (SAH) or intraventricular hemorrhage (IVH) from SCD-related aneurysm or MM
- CECT: Punctate enhancement BG from MM collaterals
- CTA: Stenosis of distal ICA, proximal circle of Willis (COW)

MR Findings

- T1WI
  - Hemorrhagic infarcts may be seen
  - Punctate flow voids in BG correspond to MM collaterals
  - ↓ signal, expanded marrow (↑ red marrow)
- T2WI
  - Cortical, deep WM infarcts
    - Often in ACA/MCA watershed distribution
    - Associated with reduced subcortical volumes
- FLAIR
  - Multifocal hyperintensities ± ivy sign of MM
- DWI
  - Diffusion restriction in acute infarcts
- PWI
  - ↑ cerebral blood flow (CBF) early: Adaptive response to anemia
  - ↓ CBF, ↑ mean transit time (MTT), ↑ time to peak (TTP) with arterial sludging, progressive COW narrowing
  - Arterial spin labeling (ASL) may be useful; assess CBF without use of contrast material
- T1WI C+
  - Vascular stasis and leptomeningeal collaterals in MCA territory with proximal MCA stenosis
- MRA
  - Enlarged, tortuous arteries early
    - Theory: Adaptive response to anemia and ↑ cerebral perfusion
  - Frequent eventual development of MM stenoocclusive arteriopathy
  - Aneurysms in atypical locations
- MRS
  - ↑ lactate, ↓ NAA, ↓ Cho, ↓ Cr in areas of infarction (lactate seen only in acute infarctions)

Ultrasonographic Findings

- Transcranial Doppler (TCD): Hyperdynamic flow distal ICA/MCA secondary to proximal stenosis
  - Time-averaged mean velocities > 200 cm/s → high risk of ischemic stroke
  - Velocities between 170-200 cm/s, conditional

Angiographic Findings

- MM: Stenosis of distal ICA, proximal COW with BG and external carotid artery (ECA) → ICA collaterals
  - Association between MM with persistent primitive carotid-basilar arterial communications
- Fusiform aneurysms
- Periprocedural risk of stroke higher than other populations: Hydrate, transfuse before catheter study

Nuclear Medicine Findings

- PET, SPECT: Focal areas of ↓ brain perfusion described

Imaging Recommendations

- Best imaging tool
  - MR/MRA ± DSA
- Protocol advice
  - DWI differentiates acute infarcts from chronic
  - Turbulent dephasing due to anemia, rapid flow can mimic stenosis on bright-blood MRA: Use lowest possible TE (< 5 ms) for bright-blood MRA or black-blood MRA if stenosis suspected

DIFFERENTIAL DIAGNOSIS

Vasculitis

- Idiopathic, infectious, autoimmune, substance abuse
- Classic imaging findings: Cortical and deep WM infarcts and parenchymal hemorrhage

Moyamoya

- Primary MM
  - Idiopathic, inherited
- Other causes of secondary MM
  - Neurofibromatosis 1 (NF1), Down syndrome, radiation therapy, connective tissue disease, prothrombotic states

Thick Skull With Expanded Diploë

- Other chronic anemias (thalassemia)

PATHOLOGY

General Features

- Etiology

- Abnormal Hgb (Hgb S) becomes "stiff" when deoxygenated → RBCs become sickle-shaped
- Sickled RBCs lose pliability to traverse capillaries → vascular occlusion (crisis), cell destruction (hemolysis)
- Sickled RBCs adhere to endothelium → fragments internal elastic lamina, degenerates muscularis → large-vessel vasculopathy ± aneurysm formation

- Genetics
  - Point mutation of Hgb β gene, Chr 11p15.5: Glutamate → valine substitution
  - SCD: Autosomal recessive, both β-globin affected
  - Sickle cell trait: 1 β-globin affected → mild disease
    - Carrier
    - ↑ resistance to malaria (hence prevalence)
- Associated abnormalities
  - Anemia, reticulocytosis, granulocytosis
  - Susceptibility to pneumococcal infection (due to malfunctioning spleen)
  - Occasionally causes pseudotumor cerebri

Gross Pathologic & Surgical Features

- Bone, brain, renal, and splenic infarcts; hepatomegaly

Microscopic Features

- Severe anemia with sickled cells on smear
- Vascular occlusions due to masses of sickled RBCs

CLINICAL ISSUES

Presentation

- Most common signs/symptoms
  - Focal neurologic deficit
- Other signs/symptoms
  - Children: Learning difficulties, headaches, psychiatric symptoms
- Clinical profile
  - Black child with stroke
- Stroke
  - 17-26% of all patients with SCD
  - 11% by age 20, 24% by age 45
  - 75% ischemic, 25% hemorrhagic
  - 20% of children have WM infarcts on MR but no overt neurologic deficit = silent infarcts
    - TCD usually normal
    - Associated with mild cognitive impairment
    - 14x ↑ risk of stroke consistent with patients with normal MR
  - 18x ↑ risk of stroke if TCD velocity of ICA or MCA > 200 cm/s
- Bone infarcts, avascular necrosis during crisis
- Osteomyelitis, especially *Salmonella*
- Gross hematuria from renal papillary necrosis and ulceration
- Splenic infarction from exposure to high altitude (e.g., flying)
- Infections common, especially *Pneumococcus* after splenic infarction

Demographics

- Age
  - Children = adults
  - Stroke risk highest from 2-5 years of age
- Sex: No predilection
- Ethnicity: Primarily Black people and their descendants
- Epidemiology
  - Birth prevalence in Black people: 1/375
  - Birth prevalence of sickle cell trait: 1/12
  - Primary cause of stroke in Black children
  - Incidence of cerebral lesions (MR) in patients with sickle cell trait: 10-19%

Natural History & Prognosis

- Unrelenting, severe hemolytic anemia beginning at few months of age after Hgb S replaces Hgb F (fetal)
- Cognitive dysfunction occurs even in absence of cerebral infarctions
- Repeated ischemic events → strokes with worsening motor and intellectual deficits
- Patients usually live to adulthood, albeit with complications
- Prognosis poor for SCD without transfusions

Treatment

- Screening TCD
  - Detection ↑ velocity (> 200 cm/s) prompts brain MR and treatment with regular blood transfusions
  - Regular blood transfusions keep Hgb S < 30%
    - ↓ incidence of stroke by up to 75%
    - ↓ intimal hyperplasia COW vessels
- Hydroxyurea: ↓ incidence of painful crises and acute chest syndrome; may improve TCD velocities
  - Induces Hgb F, which ↓ vasoocclusion and hemolysis
- Penicillin prophylaxis; pneumococcal vaccine
- Bone marrow transplantation only curative therapy
  - Available only to few who have human leukocyte antigen (HLA)-matched donor
- On horizon: Stem cell-based therapies

DIAGNOSTIC CHECKLIST

Image Interpretation Pearls

- Always consider SCD in Black child with cerebral infarction

SELECTED REFERENCES

1. Abdi SS et al: Neuroimaging and cognitive function in sickle cell disease: a systematic review. Children (Basel). 10(3):532, 2023
2. Abreu VS et al: Neuroimaging findings in paediatric patients with sickle cell disease. Clin Radiol. 78(7):509-17, 2023
3. Strumph K et al: Impact of magnetic resonance angiography parameters on stroke prevention therapy in pediatric patients with sickle cell anemia. Pediatr Blood Cancer. 70(2):e30109, 2023
4. Issar P et al: Conventional and advanced brain MR imaging in patients with sickle cell anemia. Indian J Radiol Imaging. 28(3):305-11, 2018
5. Miao X et al: Increased brain iron deposition in patients with sickle cell disease: an MRI quantitative susceptibility mapping study. Blood. 132(15):1618-21, 2018
6. Green NS et al: Enhanced long-term brain magnetic resonance imaging evaluation of children with sickle cell disease after hematopoietic cell transplantation. Biol Blood Marrow Transplant. 23(4):670-6, 2017
7. Kawadler JM et al: Brain atrophy in paediatric sickle cell anaemia: findings from the silent infarct transfusion (SIT) trial. Br J Haematol. 177(1):151-3, 2017
8. Chen R et al: A prospective longitudinal brain morphometry study of children with sickle cell disease. AJNR Am J Neuroradiol. 36(2):403-10, 2014
9. Helton KJ et al: Magnetic resonance imaging/angiography and transcranial Doppler velocities in sickle cell anemia: results from the SWiTCH trial. Blood. 124(6):891-8, 2014
10. Thust SC et al: Neuroimaging findings in sickle cell disease. Br J Radiol. 87(1040):20130699, 2014

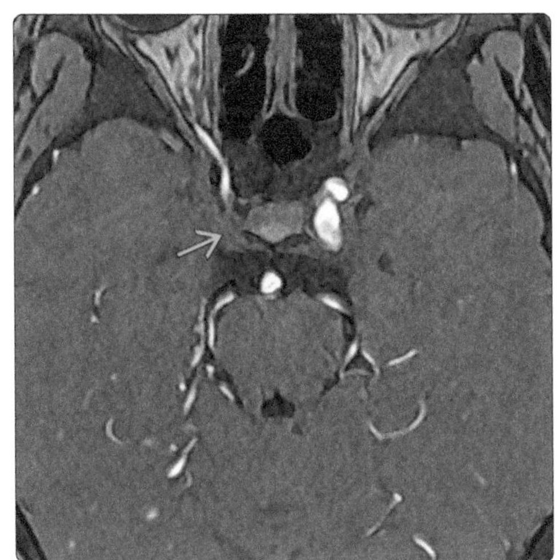

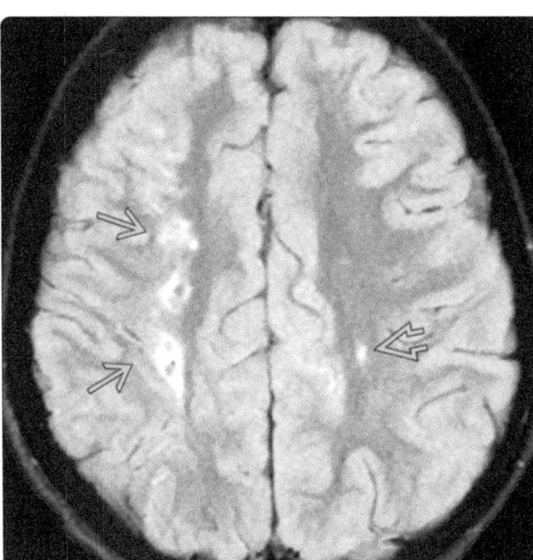

(Left) *Source images from a TOF MRA in an 8-year-old with SCD shows absence of the right carotid terminus →, a characteristic appearance for moyamoya stenoocclusive arteriopathy.* **(Right)** *Axial FLAIR MR in the same patient shows patchy leukomalacia → in the right centrum semiovale. Watershed cortex and white matter are common locations for ischemic injury in SCD patients without or with moyamoya arteriopathy. Note the small area of leukomalacia ⇨ on the left with no evidence of major vessel stenosis proximally.*

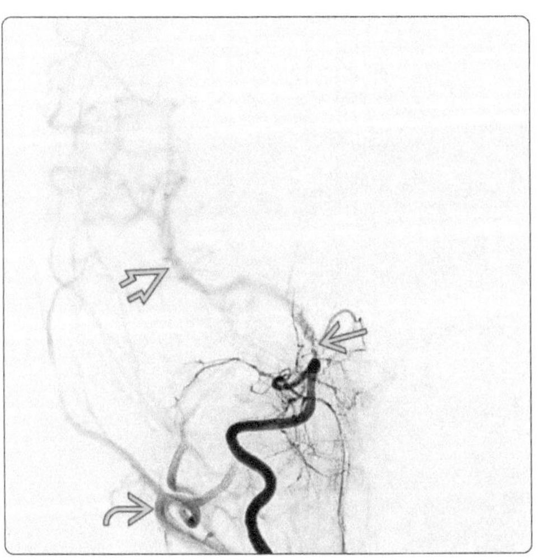

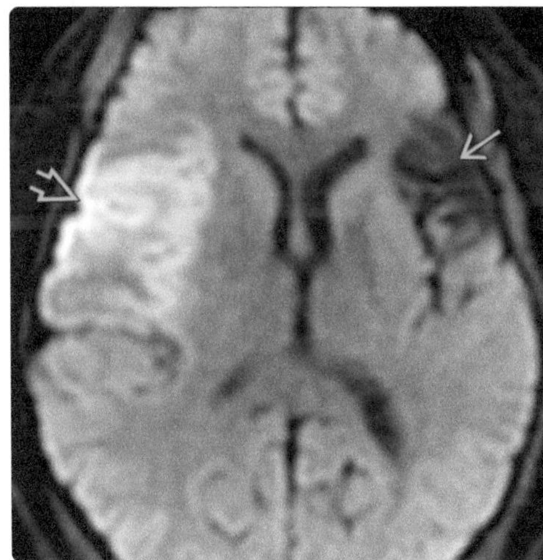

(Left) *Frontal DSA with a right ICA injection in the same 8-year-old with right MCA ischemia shows occlusion of the distal ICA → with slow collateral filling of the right MCA ⇨. Note the reflux of contrast into the ECA ↗ due to the severe ICA stenosis.* **(Right)** *Axial DWI MR in a 16-year-old with SCD and moyamoya arteriopathy shows acute infarct ⇨ of the right operculum. Note the prior chronic infarct → in the left operculum/insula. Infarcts of multiple ages are a typical finding in moyamoya arteriopathy.*

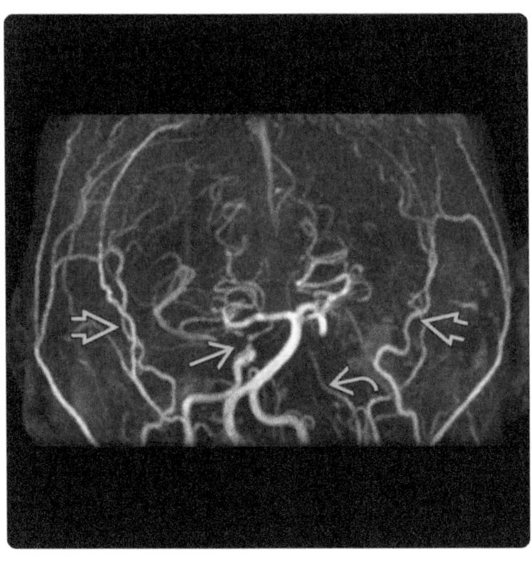

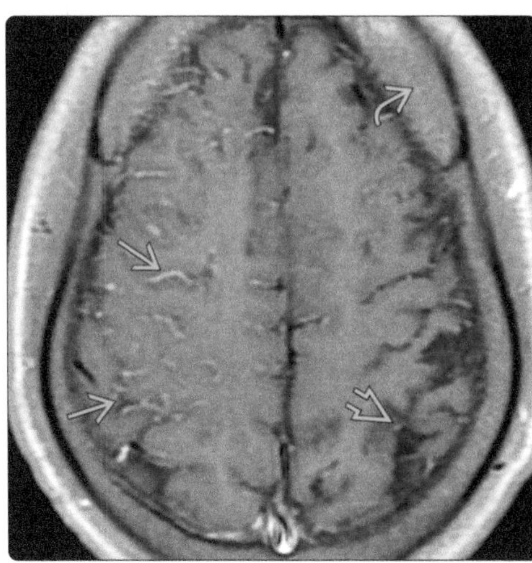

(Left) *Frontal projection of a 3D TOF MRA in the same patient shows complete occlusion of the right terminal ICA → and extremely small left ICA ↗. Note the enlarged middle meningeal arteries ⇨ providing collateral flow to the cerebral hemispheres.* **(Right)** *Axial T1 C+ MR in the same patient shows extensive right cerebral leptomeningeal enhancement →, consistent with pial collateral formation. Also note the prior left parietal infarct ⇨ and calvarial thickening ↗, consistent with the diagnosis of SCD.*

KEY FACTS

TERMINOLOGY

- Progressive narrowing of distal internal carotid artery (ICA) & proximal circle of Willis (COW) vessels → characteristic adjacent clusters of collateral flow appearing as "puff of smoke" on real-time angiography
- Moyamoya disease = primary (idiopathic) moyamoya
- Moyamoya arteriopathy (a.k.a. moyamoya syndrome or secondary moyamoya) due to other disorders

IMAGING

- Absent or narrowed distal ICA & abnormal COW
- Excessive tiny collaterals in basal ganglia & cisterns
  - "Puff of smoke" (moyamoya in Japanese) of lenticulostriate & thalamoperforator collaterals
- Prominent collaterals in sulci
  - Ivy sign on FLAIR & T1 C+ MR
- Acute & chronic infarcts
- CT/CTA: Acute use for ischemia or hemorrhage
- MR C+/MRA: Vascular protocol with DWI & perfusion
  - DWI: Helpful to identify "acute on chronic" injury

PATHOLOGY

- Moyamoya disease: Inherited idiopathic disorder
- Moyamoya arteriopathy: Secondary process
  - Sickle cell disease, trisomy 21, neurofibromatosis type 1, radiation therapy, Alagille syndrome, morning glory syndrome, TB meningitis, among others

CLINICAL ISSUES

- Bimodal age peaks: 6 & 35 years
- Presentation (children): Transient ischemic attacks (TIAs), alternating hemiplegia (exacerbated by crying), headache
- Presentation (adults): TIAs, hemorrhage (~ 30%), & cerebral infarct
- Prognosis depends on etiology, ability to form collaterals, age/stage at diagnosis

DIAGNOSTIC CHECKLIST

- Seek underlying causes of secondary moyamoya

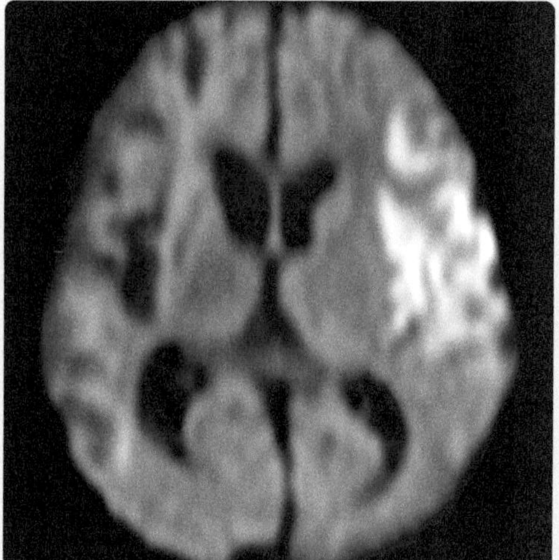

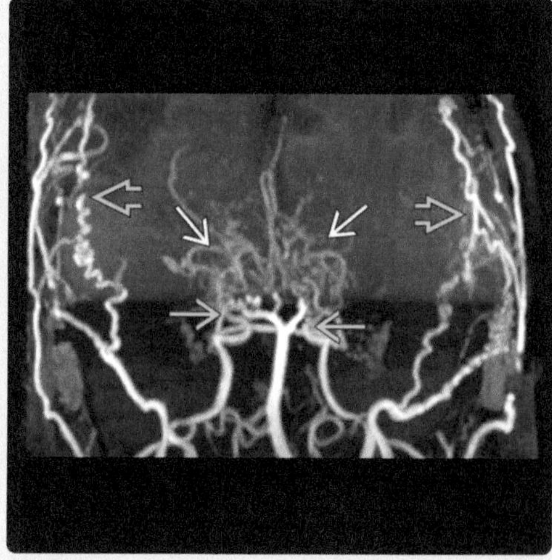

(Left) *Axial DWI MR in a 13-month-old with increasing seizures shows left MCA distribution ischemia as well as a remote infarct in the right MCA territory. This is a typical acute on chronic ischemic pattern of moyamoya.* **(Right)** *Anterior 3D TOF MRA in the same patient at 8 years of age shows occlusions of the terminal ICAs ➡, absence of the MCAs, & numerous lenticulostriate collaterals ➡ forming a "puff of smoke." The PCAs are also occluded. Note the enlarged ECA collaterals ➡ status post synangiosis & dural inversion.*

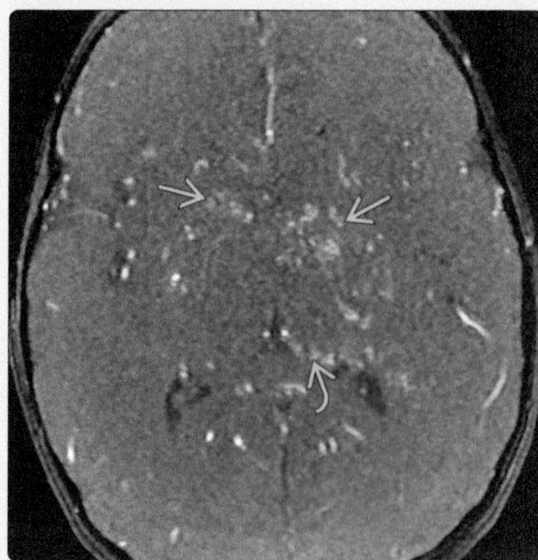

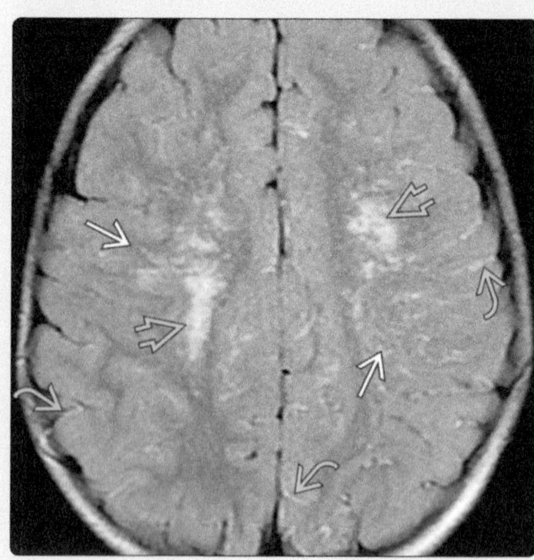

(Left) *Axial 3D TOF MRA in a 5-year-old with idiopathic moyamoya arteriopathy shows multiple small lenticulostriate ➡ and thalamostriate ➡ vessels within the deep nuclear structures.* **(Right)** *Axial FLAIR MR in the same patient shows areas of gliosis ➡ from vascular insufficiency, linear hyperintensities ➡ representing deep medullary collateral vessels, and hyperintensities ➡ conforming to the surface of the sulci representing pial collaterals (the leptomeningeal ivy sign).*

TERMINOLOGY

Synonyms

- Progressive stenoocclusive arteriopathy; spontaneous occlusion of circle of Willis (COW)

Definitions

- Progressive narrowing of distal internal carotid artery (ICA) & proximal COW vessels → characteristic adjacent clusters of collateral flow appearing as "puff of smoke" on real-time angiography
- Moyamoya disease: Primary (idiopathic) moyamoya
  - More common in Japan, Korea
- Moyamoya arteriopathy (a.k.a. moyamoya syndrome or secondary moyamoya) occurs in association with other disorders or after radiation treatment

IMAGING

General Features

- Best diagnostic clue: Multiple enhancing punctate dots (CECT) & flow voids (MR) in basal ganglia & cisterns
- Arterial occlusions: Distal ICA, COW, branches
  - Anterior > posterior circulation
    - Posterior circulation affected in ~ 25%
- Leads to prominent clusters of nearby collaterals
  - "Cloud-like" lenticulostriate & thalamoperforator collaterals on angiography: "Puff of smoke" (moyamoya in Japanese)
- Also leads to prominent sulcal collaterals distally

CT Findings

- NECT
  - Children: Acute ischemia ± old infarcts
  - Older children/adults: Usually ischemia but may present with intracranial hemorrhage
- CTA: Abnormal COW + basilar net-like collaterals
- Xe-133 CT: ↓ cerebral reserve with acetazolamide challenge

MR Findings

- T2WI
  - ↑ signal in gliotic areas from prior infarcts
  - Collateral vessels: Net-like cisternal flow voids
- FLAIR
  - Bright sulci = leptomeningeal ivy sign
    - Slow-flowing engorged pial collateral vessels, thickened arachnoid membranes
    - Correlates with ↓ cerebral vascular reserve
- T2* GRE
  - Hemosiderin if prior hemorrhage
- DWI
  - Very useful for "acute on chronic" infarcts
- PWI
  - ↓ cerebral blood flow (CBF) (ASL) in affected territories
  - ↑ MTT in affected territories
  - Variable rCBV depending on degree of collateral formation
  - May be used to measure response to revascularization
- T1WI C+
  - Lenticulostriate collaterals → enhancing "dots" in basal ganglia & net-like thin vessels in cisterns
  - Leptomeningeal enhancement (ivy sign)
  - Vessel wall imaging
    - Most consistent finding is negative remodeling (local shrinkage of vessel size) of affected vessels
    - Variable enhancement of affected vessel segments
      - ↑ wall thickening and ↑ stenosis correlates with ↑ wall enhancement
    - May help distinguish from other vasculopathies
- MRA
  - Narrowed/occluded distal ICA & COW vessels
- MRS
  - Lactate in acutely infarcted tissue
  - NAA:Cr & Cho:Cr ratios in frontal white matter improve ↑ after revascularization

Ultrasonographic Findings

- Grayscale: Reduction of ICA lumen size
- Pulsed Doppler
  - Spectral waveforms in ICA show no flow (occluded) or proximal high-resistance flow pattern
  - ↑ end-diastolic flow velocity, ↓ vascular resistance in external carotid artery (ECA) collaterals
- Color Doppler: Aliasing suggests stenoses
- Power Doppler: Improves visualization of slow-flow stenotic vessels & collaterals
- Can be used for vessel mapping prior to revascularization surgery

Angiographic Findings

- Predominantly (not exclusively) anterior circulation
  - Narrow proximal COW & ICA (early phase)
  - Lenticulostriate & thalamoperforator collaterals (intermediate phase)
  - Transdural/transosseous ECA-ICA collaterals (late phase)
- Dilation & branch extension of anterior choroidal artery predict adult hemorrhagic events

Nuclear Medicine Findings

- PET: ↓ hemodynamic reserve capacity
- SPECT I-123-iomazenil: Neuronal density preserved if asymptomatic, ↓ if symptomatic

Imaging Recommendations

- Best imaging tool: MR C+/MRA
- Catheter angiography defines anatomy prior to bypass
- Protocol advice
  - Acetazolamide challenge with ASL has been performed to measure cerebrovascular reserve, but Xe-133 CT is gold standard

DIFFERENTIAL DIAGNOSIS

Ivy Sign

- Leptomeningeal metastases, subarachnoid hemorrhage, meningitis, ↑ inspired oxygen, collateral veins of Sturge-Weber or other chronic venous occlusion

Large Vessel Inflammatory Vasculitis

- Postvaricella vasculitis, lupus, & other CNS vasculitides
- May be reversible with treatment

Cerebral Arterial Atherosclerosis

- Very rare in children & young adults

Severely Attenuated Circle of Willis

- Subarachnoid hemorrhage (spasm), meningitis, tumor encasement

PATHOLOGY

General Features

- Etiology
  - Moyamoya disease
    - Inherited polygenic or autosomal dominant
      - Low penetrance
    - Gene loci: 3p26-p24.2, 17q25, 8q23
    - ↑ in growth factors, cytokines, adhesion molecules in CSF implicates inflammation
  - Moyamoya arteriopathy (a.k.a. moyamoya syndrome or secondary moyamoya)
    - Sickle cell disease, neurofibromatosis type 1 (NF1), radiation therapy, trisomy 21, Alagille syndrome, morning glory syndrome, tuberculous meningitis, many others
      - NF1 + suprasellar tumor + radiation can be disastrous
- Epidemiology: Moyamoya disease
  - Incidence in Japan: 1:100,000
  - Incidence in North America, Europe: 0.1:100,000
  - 10-15% familial

Staging, Grading, & Classification

- Staging criteria (Suzuki)
  - Stage 1: Narrowing of ICA bifurcation
  - Stage 2: Anterior, middle, and posterior cerebral arteries (ACA, MCA, PCA) dilated
  - Stage 3: Maximal basal collaterals; small ACA/MCA
  - Stage 4: Fewer collaterals (vessels); small PCA
  - Stage 5: Further ↓ in collaterals; absent ACA/MCA/PCA
  - Stage 6: Extensive ECA-pial collaterals

Gross Pathologic & Surgical Features

- ↑ perforating (early) & ECA-ICA (late) collaterals in atrophic brain
- Hemorrhage (subarachnoid, intraventricular > parenchymal) in adults
- ↑ saccular aneurysms in adults (especially basilar)

Microscopic Features

- Intimal thickening & hyperplasia
- Excessive infolding & thickening of internal elastic lamina
- Periventricular pseudoaneurysms (cause of hemorrhage)

CLINICAL ISSUES

Presentation

- Most common signs/symptoms
  - Children: Transient ischemic attacks (TIAs), alternating hemiplegia (exacerbated by crying), headache
  - Adults: TIAs, hemorrhage (~ 30%), cerebral infarct
    - Hemorrhagic presentation more common in Asian adults
- Other signs/symptoms
  - Children: Developmental delay, poor feeding, chorea

Demographics

- Age
  - Bimodal age peaks
    - Japan, Korea: 6 years > 35 years
    - North America, Europe: 35 years > 6 years
- Sex
  - M:F = 1:1.8; in familial cases, M:F = 1:5
- Epidemiology
  - Most frequent cause of stroke in Asian children

Natural History & Prognosis

- Progressive narrowing, collateralization, & ischemia
- Prognosis depends on etiology, ability to form collaterals, age/stage at diagnosis
- Pediatric cases usually advance to stage 5 in < 10 years
  - Infantile moyamoya progresses faster
- Hemorrhagic moyamoya more common in older patients
  - May be due to large collateral vessels
  - Has poorer outcome

Treatment

- Aspirin therapy
- Direct bypass: Superficial temporal artery (STA)-MCA more common in adults
- Indirect bypass
  - Pial synangiosis & encephaloduroarteriosynangiosis with STA more common in children
    - 5-year risk of ipsilateral stroke post encephaloduroarteriosynangiosis = 15%
  - Dural inversion with middle meningeal artery
- Correct/control prothrombotic states & inflammatory etiologies
- Transfusion therapy for sickle cell-related moyamoya

DIAGNOSTIC CHECKLIST

Consider

- Seek underlying causes of secondary moyamoya

Image Interpretation Pearls

- Enhanced asymmetric atrophy found on childhood CT; look for abnormal vascular pattern
- Adult moyamoya can present with intracranial hemorrhage

Reporting Tips

- Successful revascularization = ↓ basal collaterals, ↑ flow in MCA branches, ↑ caliber of STA (direct bypass)

SELECTED REFERENCES

1. Larson AS et al: Vessel wall imaging features of moyamoya disease in a North American population: patterns of negative remodelling, contrast enhancement, wall thickening, and stenosis. BMC Med Imaging. 22(1):198, 2022
2. Larson AS et al: Implementation and rationale for a unified clinical and imaging protocol for evaluation and treatment of moyamoya angiopathy: a single institutional experience. Front Neurol. 12:662393, 2021
3. Wang LX et al: Ivy sign in moyamoya disease: a comparative study of the FLAIR vascular hyperintensity sign against contrast-enhanced MRI. AJNR Am J Neuroradiol. 42(4):694-700, 2021
4. Lehman VT et al: Contemporary and emerging magnetic resonance imaging methods for evaluation of moyamoya disease. Neurosurg Focus. 47(6):E6, 2019
5. Lee S et al: Monitoring cerebral perfusion changes after revascularization in patients with moyamoya disease by using arterial spin-labeling MR imaging. Radiology. 288(2):565-72, 2018

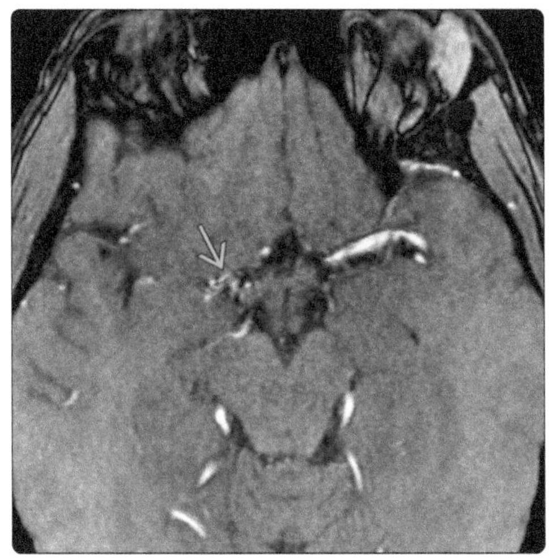

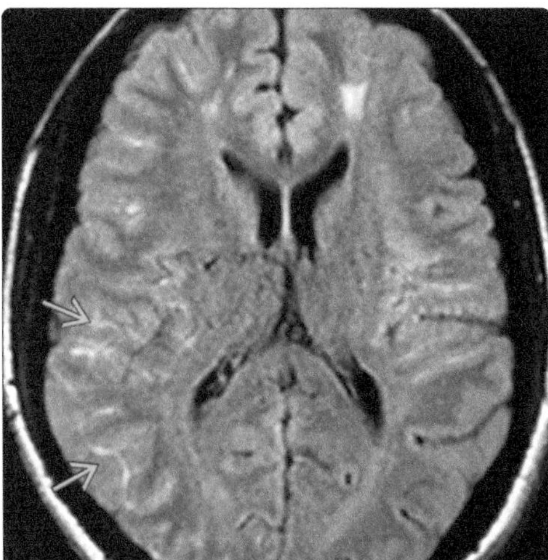

(Left) *Axial TOF MRA in a 14-year-old with neurofibromatosis type 1 shows absence of the right internal carotid terminus & MCA. In the expected location of the carotid terminus & MCA, there are multiple small leptomeningeal collaterals ➙.* **(Right)** *Axial FLAIR MR in a 21-year-old with sickle cell disease shows high signal ➙ within the right MCA distribution sulci, the so-called ivy sign. This abnormal signal corresponds to engorged pial collateral vessels & is often seen in moyamoya.*

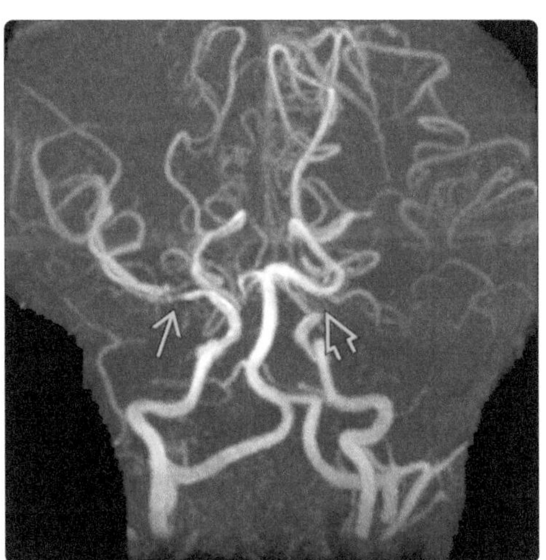

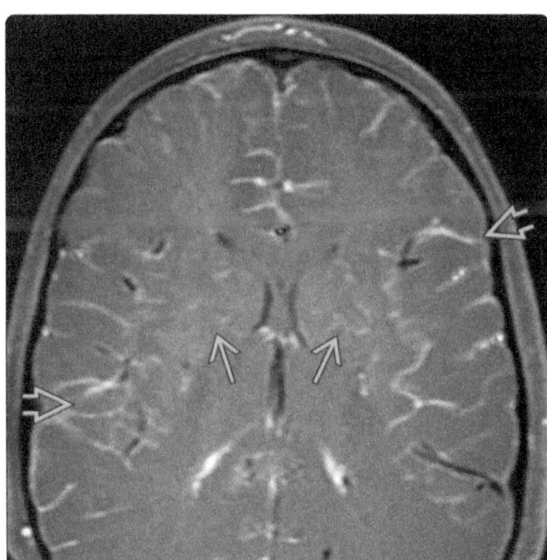

(Left) *Frontal 3D TOF MRA in a 10-year-old with history of nasal rhabdomyosarcoma at age 3 treated with XRT shows absence of flow in the left distal ICA ➙, severe narrowing of the right MCA ➙, & absent right ACA. Terminal ICA & proximal MCA are the most common locations for moyamoya arteriopathy.* **(Right)** *Axial T1 C+ MR in the same patient shows extensive leptomeningeal enhancement ➙ in the bilateral ICA territories with prominent vessel enhancement ➙ in the basal ganglia.*

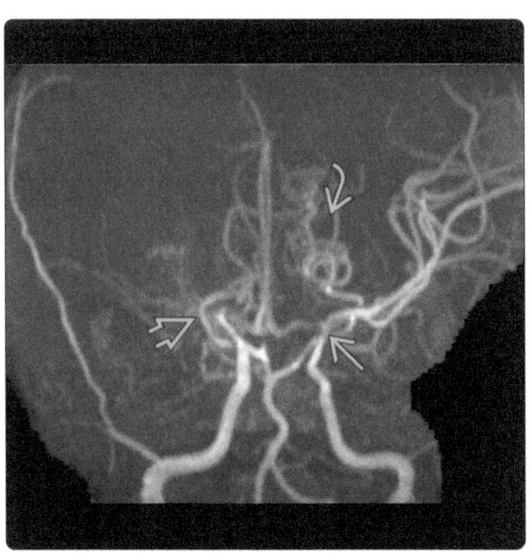

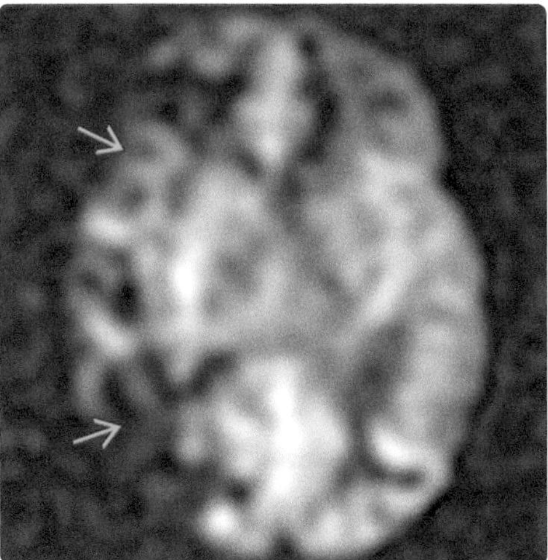

(Left) *3D TOF MRA in a 6-year-old with trisomy 21 and severe moyamoya arteriopathy shows marked narrowing of the left ICA terminus ➙ & complete occlusion of the right MCA origin ➙. Deep moyamoya collaterals ➙ have formed in the left basal ganglia.* **(Right)** *Axial ASL MR perfusion in the same patient shows near absence of signal ➙ in the right MCA territory, consistent with dramatically reduced blood flow, corroborating the findings on MRA.*

Arteriovenous Malformation

KEY FACTS

TERMINOLOGY

- Arteriovenous malformation (AVM): Vascular malformation with arteriovenous shunting through complex nidus of arterioles & venules (without intervening capillary bed)

IMAGING

- **NECT**: Parenchymal hematoma most common
  - Small unruptured AVMs often not visible; may see Ca^{++}
- **CTA**: Enhancing feeding arteries, nidus, & draining veins
  - May be negative if AVM compressed by hematoma
- **MR**
  - T1WI: Bright hemorrhage
  - T2WI: Prominent dark flow voids
  - T1 C+ (volumetric gradient): Enhancing abnormal vessels; important for micro-AVMs
  - ASL: High signal in nidus & draining veins
- **MRA**: Gross depiction of AVM components
  - Flow-related signal in draining veins reflects AV shunt
- **Digital subtraction catheter angiography**
  - Gold standard with high temporal & spatial resolution
  - Best identifies all 3 components of AVM
    - Multiple arterial feeding vessels (internal-external carotid & vertebrobasilar arteries)
    - Deep vs. superficial venous drainage
    - Associated arterial/nidus aneurysms, venous stenoses

PATHOLOGY

- Most AVMs sporadic; small percentage related to hemorrhagic telangiectasia
- Spetzler-Martin surgical risk grading system (1-5 points)
  - Size: < 3 cm (1 point), 3-6 cm (2 points), > 6 cm (3 points)
  - Location: Eloquent (1 point) vs. noneloquent (0 points)
  - Venous drainage: Deep (1 point) vs. superficial (0 points)

CLINICAL ISSUES

- Spontaneous parenchymal hemorrhage in child should be considered AVM until proven otherwise
- Annual bleeding risk = 2-4%

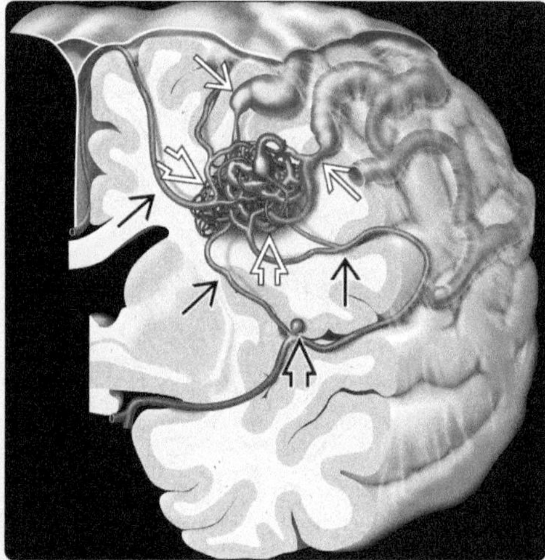

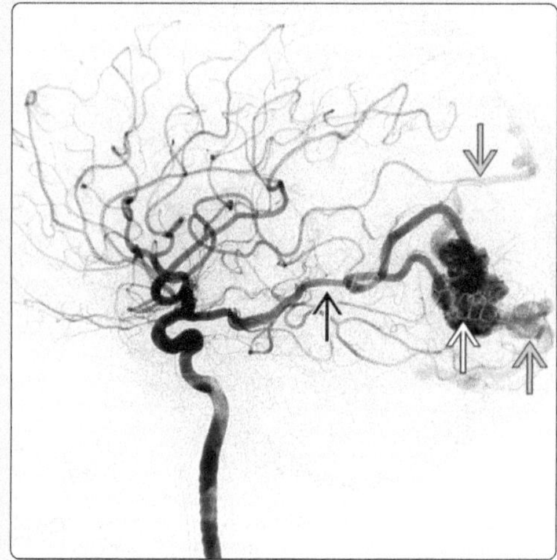

(Left) *Graphic shows cerebral arteriovenous malformation (AVM) with a centrum semiovale nidus ➡ fed from cortical & central arteries ➡ (with a proximal flow-related aneurysm ➡) & drained by enlarged cortical veins ➡.* **(Right)** *Lateral DSA (right ICA injection) in a 15-year-old girl shows an enlarged arterial feeder ➡ arising from the right ICA via the posterior communicating artery. The tightly packed nidus ➡ is well defined. Note 2 separate superficial draining veins that opacify early during arterial phase ➡, typical of an AVM.*

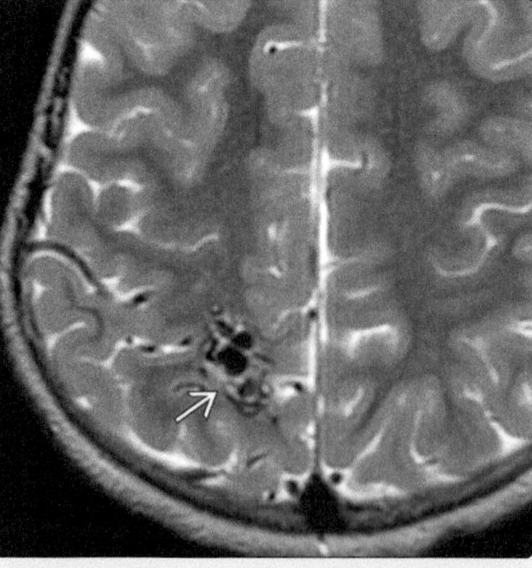

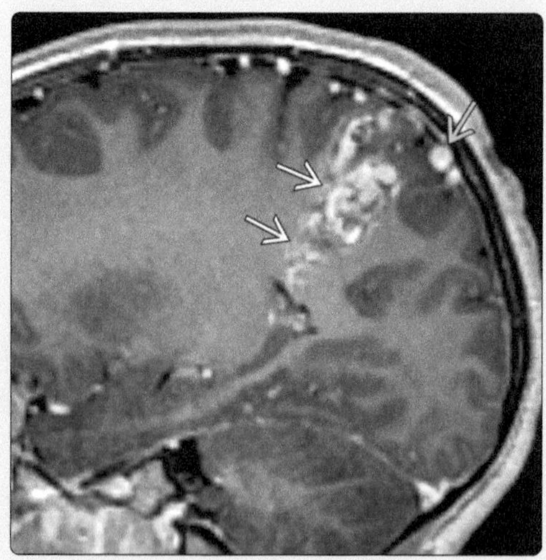

(Left) *Axial T2 MR in an 8-year-old girl with headaches shows multiple enlarged flow voids & tangles of vessels ➡ in the right parietal lobe. There is no adjacent parenchymal abnormality, consistent with an unruptured AVM. On routine noncontrast MR, flow voids on T2 may be the only clue to an AVM diagnosis.* **(Right)** *Volumetric sagittal T1 C+ MR in the same patient shows a wedge-shaped focus of tortuous, enhancing vessels in the AVM nidus ➡ as well as dilated superficial draining veins ➡.*

TERMINOLOGY

Definitions

- Arteriovenous malformation (AVM): High-flow vascular malformation with AV shunting through complex nidus of arterioles & venules (without intervening capillary bed)

IMAGING

General Features

- Best diagnostic clue
  - Parenchymal hemorrhage with extension into ventricle & cluster of adjacent abnormal vessels (nidus) with enlarged draining veins
- Location
  - Anywhere in brain tissue (including choroid plexus)
  - Typically solitary (sporadic) but also (rarely) multiple (syndromic)
- Size
  - From tiny/small (common in children) to giant
- Ruptured AVM
  - Parenchymal hematoma
    - Typically centered in white matter with extension into ventricle
  - Adjacent abnormal vessels
    - Multiple small & tortuous arteries
      - Can be seen on CTA, MRA, T2 MR
      - Difficult to appreciate on NECT
    - Enlarged draining veins
      - Typically obvious on CTA, T2 MR
      - Well demonstrated on SWI
    - May be compressed by hematoma
  - Bleeding typically from rupture of draining vein; rupture of flow-related aneurysm less common in children
- Unruptured AVM
  - Tightly packed mass of enlarged vascular channels with flow voids
    - Subtle on NECT, obvious on CTA
    - Well demonstrated on MRA, T2 MR
  - Mild enlargement of feeding arteries
  - Moderate enlargement of draining veins
    - Well demonstrated on T2, SWI MR
    - Identify if drainage deep or superficial
  - No mass effect (replaces rather than displaces parenchyma if unruptured)
  - Little or no abnormal signal in adjacent brain
  - Arteriovenous shunting
    - Time-resolved MRA can show AV shunting
    - SWI signal in draining veins may be bright

CT Findings

- **NECT**: Unruptured AVM often occult, unless large; ± Ca^{++}
  - Ruptured AVM: Spontaneous parenchymal hemorrhage
    - Subarachnoid & intraventricular hemorrhage may also be seen but less commonly
- **CTA**: Enlarged feeding arteries, nidus, draining veins
  - Nidus may be compressed by hematoma
- **CECT**: Strong vascular enhancement in dilated vascular bed

MR Findings

- **T1WI**: Hematoma in ruptured AVM typically of ↑ signal
  - Critical sequence for follow-up to distinguish (1) enhancing residual AVM, &/or (2) ↑ MRA flow signal vs. (3) intrinsic T1 signal from prior hemorrhage
- **T2WI**: Arterial feeder, nidal, & draining vein flow voids
  - Best sequence to identify AVM on routine brain MR
- **FLAIR**: May see adjacent gliosis, especially if prior bleed
  - Normal adjacent brain parenchyma in unruptured AVMs
- **SWI/T2* GRE**: Blooming with hemorrhagic blood products
  - Hyperintense (arterial) SWI signal in draining veins
    - Reflects rapid arteriovenous shunting
- **DWI**: Usually normal on initial imaging studies
  - ± ischemic complications following intervention
- **T1WI C+**: Avid enhancement of nidus & draining veins with GRE T1 (not spin echo)
  - Important for small peripheral AVMs
    - e.g., hereditary hemorrhagic telangiectasia (HHT)
- **MRA/MRV**: Gross depiction of AVM components
  - Flow-related signal in draining veins reflects AV shunt
- **ASL**: High signal in AVM nidus & draining veins
  - Sensitive sequence for detection of micro-AVMs or small residual AVMs after treatment
- **Vessel wall imaging**
  - Recent study suggests draining veins of hemorrhagic &/or high-flow AVMs are more likely to enhance

Angiographic Findings

- Evaluates shunt: Size of nidus & related vessels, flow speed
- Localizes AVM
  - Structure, lobe (lateral, medial, inferior aspects), gyrus/sulcus; neighboring eloquent areas
  - Superficial (pial fistula in neonates, infants), deep, central nuclei, choroid plexus, cerebellum
- Perform bilateral internal-external carotid & vertebrobasilar angiograms to detect multiple feeding arteries
- DSA depicts 3 components of AVMs with high spatial & temporal resolution
  - Arterial feeders
    - Enlarged; often from multiple arteries (internal-external carotid, vertebrobasilar)
    - Feeding artery aneurysms in 10-15%
  - AVM nidus
    - Central tangle of vessels where AV shunting occurs
    - Small aneurysms within nidus (~ 50%)
  - Venous drainage
    - Enlarged, tortuous veins
    - Must identify drainage as deep &/or superficial
      - Deep drainage has ↑ risk of rupture
    - ± venous varix, which indicates distal stenosis
      - Venous stenosis has ↑ risk of rupture

Imaging Recommendations

- Best imaging tool
  - CTA rapidly obtained with acute presentation; typically provides diagnosis & adequate detail to direct therapy
  - Lesions not requiring urgent intervention should have MR with SWI & MRA with time-resolved techniques
  - Catheter angiography allows for possible intervention
- Protocol advice
  - If initial study negative, repeat when hematoma resolves
    - Small AVM may be compressed by initial hematoma

- ASL & volumetric T1 C+ MR sensitive for detecting micro-AVMs, such as in HHT
- Recent literature has investigated use of 4D blood flow MR to characterize AVM hemodynamics

DIFFERENTIAL DIAGNOSIS

Cavernous Malformation

- "Angiographically occult" lesion
- Popcorn appearance on MR with blood-fluid levels, hemosiderin staining, ± Ca^{++}
- Associated with DVA in ~ 25%

Hemorrhagic Tumor

- Often enhances on MR; tumor blush on DSA
- No enlarged draining veins

Arteriovenous Fistula

- Direct AV shunting without nidus
- Congenital
  - High flow with dramatic venous enlargement
- Acquired
  - Low flow from small external carotid artery feeders
  - Often develop following sinus venous thrombosis

Arterial Aneurysm

- No nidus or enlarged draining veins
- Subarachnoid blood common
- Aneurysm typically seen on CTA/MRA

PATHOLOGY

General Features

- Etiology
  - Most AVMs sporadic; can develop in previously normal regions of brain
    - ↑ incidence with ↑ age
- Associated abnormalities
  - Syndromic AVMs (2% of cases)
    - HHT: 40-50% are micro-AVMs of brain
      - Additional lung & hepatic AVMs; cutaneous & mucosal telangiectasias

Staging, Grading, & Classification

- Spetzler-Martin scale predicts surgical morbidity: ↑ score = ↑ risk of open surgery
  - Size: < 3 cm (1 point), 3-6 cm (2 points), > 6 cm (3 points)
  - Location: Noneloquent (0 points) or eloquent (1 point)
  - Drainage: Superficial (0 points) or deep (1 point)

Microscopic Features

- Vascular changes
  - Nidus
    - Conglomeration of numerous AV shunts without interposed brain tissue & no capillary bed
  - Perinidal capillary network (may cause recurrence of surgically resected AVMs)
    - Dilated capillaries (10-25x larger than normal capillaries) form ring (1-7 mm thick) surrounding nidus
  - Adjacent gliosis, atrophy, blood residues

CLINICAL ISSUES

Presentation

- ~ 50% acute hemorrhage (headache, ↓ consciousness)
  - Spontaneous parenchymal hemorrhage in child should be considered AVM until proven otherwise
- ~ 25% seizure; ~ 15% focal neurologic findings; ~ 10% incidental
- Epilepsy & progressive neurologic deficits typically occur in setting of large lesions

Demographics

- Global prevalence of sporadic AVMs = 0.02-0.20%

Natural History & Prognosis

- Annual bleeding risk = 2-4%
- Factors that ↑ annual bleeding risk
  - Prior AVM rupture; exclusive deep venous drainage; deep brain location
- Possible factors that ↑ annual bleeding risk
  - Arterial or intranidal aneurysms
  - Venous outflow stenosis
- Recurrent complications
  - Vascular steal can only become worse
- Fatality rate for AVM rupture = 5-25%
- Disability rate for AVM rupture = 10-40%

Treatment

- Acute surgical decompression often required for mass effect from hematoma
  - May or may not resect malformation
- Optimal treatment for underlying AVM based on variety of factors; options include
  - Microsurgical resection
    - Ability to resect depends upon Spetzler-Martin grade
  - Endovascular embolization
    - Minimally invasive technique but often incomplete
  - Stereotactic radiosurgery
    - May take years to reach effect → risk of rebleed during this time
    - Can only be used for small AVMs
- ARUBA-2014 trial suggests medical management may be superior to interventional therapy
  - Follow-up trial data over 5 years showed persistent death and disability advantage of medical management
  - Best therapy approach likely dependent on number of AVM & patient factors

DIAGNOSTIC CHECKLIST

Image Interpretation Pearls

- Dilated vessels may be compressed by adjacent hematoma
- Tiny AVMs common in children; isolated early filling vein may be only clue to diagnosis

SELECTED REFERENCES

1. McGuire LS et al: Vessel wall imaging and quantitative flow assessment in arteriovenous malformations: a feasibility study. Interv Neuroradiol. 15910199221143189, 2022
2. Expert Panel on Neurological Imaging et al: ACR Appropriateness Criteria® cerebrovascular diseases-aneurysm, vascular malformation, and subarachnoid hemorrhage. J Am Coll Radiol. 18(11S):S283-304, 2021

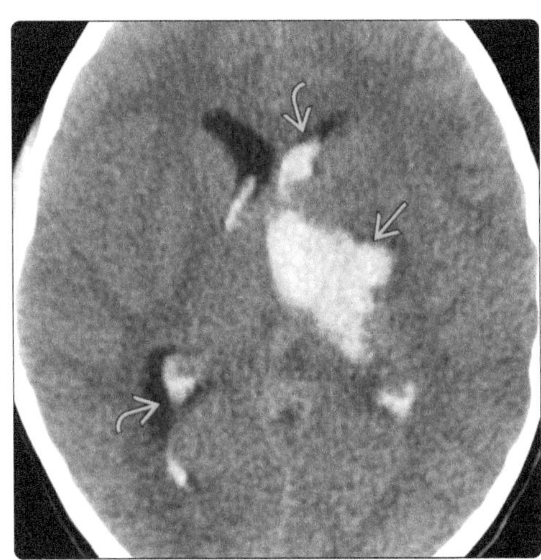

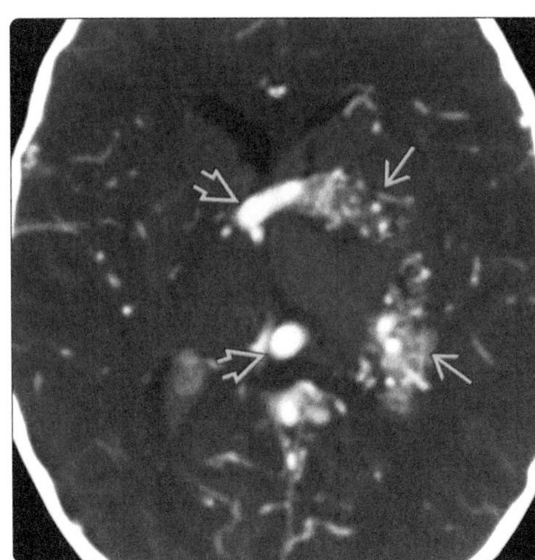

(Left) *Axial NECT in a 8-year-old with sudden onset of altered mental status shows a hyperdense hemorrhage ➔ in the left thalamus & basal ganglia with extension into the lateral ventricles ➔.* **(Right)** *Axial CTA in the same patient shows an extensive AVM nidus ➔ with deep venous drainage into a dilated internal cerebral vein ➔. Given the large size, deep venous drainage, and eloquent anatomy, this AVM has a high Spetzler-Martin grade and potential surgical morbidity. This AVM was treated with XRT.*

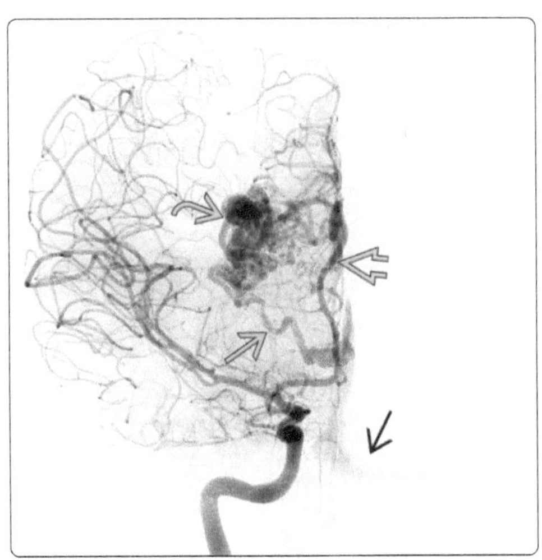

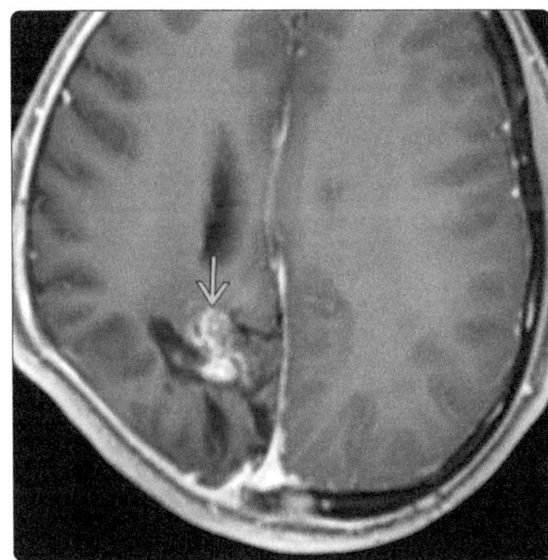

(Left) *Frontal DSA from a right ICA injection shows large right anterior cerebral artery feeding vessel ➔, the AVM nidus ➔, & draining vein ➔. Note the early filling of the torcula & left transverse sinus ➔ during arterial phase, consistent with a high-flow AVM.* **(Right)** *Axial T1 C+ MR in the same patient after hematoma evacuation & initial embolization shows a residual area of enhancement ➔ suspicious for residual AVM. Advanced imaging, such as ASL perfusion, can detect even small residual AVM components.*

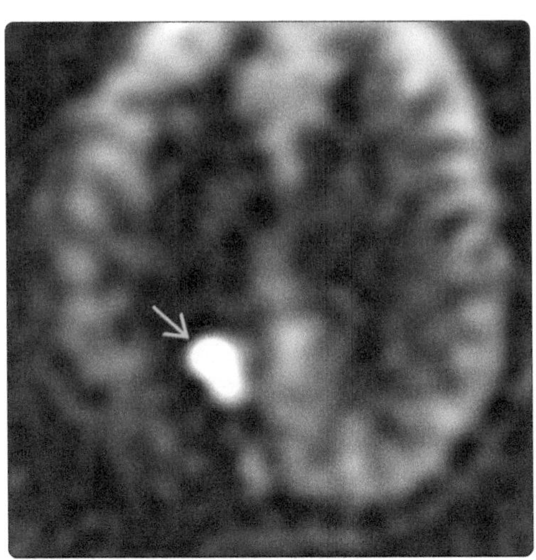

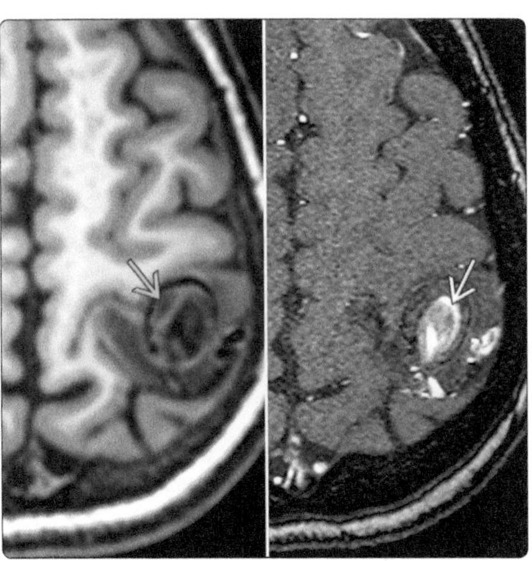

(Left) *Axial ASL MR perfusion in the same patient shows markedly increased cerebral blood flow ➔ in the area of enhancement, confirming residual high-flow AVM.* **(Right)** *Axial T1 MR (left) & 3D TOF MRA (right) in a 13-year-old girl show flow-related enhancement ➔ in the ovoid lesion, confirming an associated aneurysm. Note the absence of significant lesion ➔ hyperintensity on T1, confirming that the hyperintense signal on MRA is due to actual flow-related signal & not intrinsic T1 shortening.*

KEY FACTS

IMAGING

- Location: Dural sinus wall
  - Posterior fossa > > supratentorial; can involve any dural sinus (transverse sinus/sigmoid sinus most common)
- NECT
  - Usually normal
  - Intracranial hemorrhage (ICH) if outlet vein thrombosed or flow-related aneurysm, venous pouch ruptures
  - Dilated transosseous calvarial vascular channels
  - ± enlarged foramen spinosum
- MR
  - T2/T1 C+: Involved dural venous sinus usually enlarged
    - May have areas of stenosis distally due to shear injury
  - GRE/SWI: ↓ signal may represent Ca^{++} or hemorrhage
  - MRA/PWI: ↑ signal in dural venous sinuses at location of arteriovenous fistula (AVF)
- MRA/CTA: Network of tiny (crack-like) vessels in wall of dural venous sinus
- Angiography
  - Best study to characterize arterial feeders & reverse flow in dural venous sinuses (aggressive clinical course)

TOP DIFFERENTIAL DIAGNOSES

- Hypoplastic transverse-sigmoid sinus
- Sigmoid sinus-jugular foramen pseudolesion
- Thrombosed dural sinus
- Dural sinus stenosis

PATHOLOGY

- May be congenital, iatrogenic, or related to sinus venous thrombosis
- Pathologic activation of neoangiogenesis

CLINICAL ISSUES

- Adult > > child
- < 10% of high-flow, artery to vein shunt lesions in children
- Prognosis depends on location, venous drainage pattern
- Treatment options: Endovascular, surgery, stereotaxic XRT

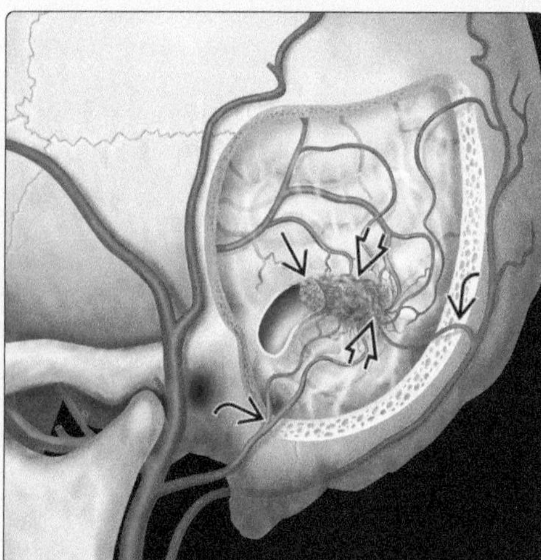

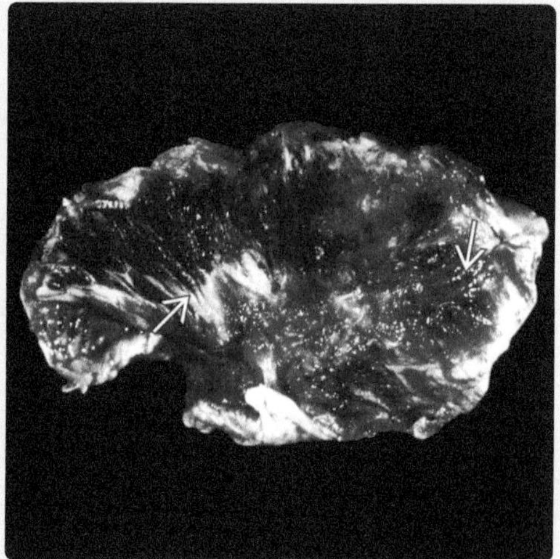

(Left) *Graphic depicts a dural arteriovenous fistula (dAVF) with a thrombosed transverse sinus ➔. Multiple transosseous branches ➔ from the external carotid artery supply innumerable tiny arteriovenous fistulae ➔ in the dural wall.* **(Right)** *Mass-like surgical specimen from a resected dAVF in the transverse sinus wall shows innumerable crack-like vessels ➔. (Courtesy R. Hewlett, MD.)*

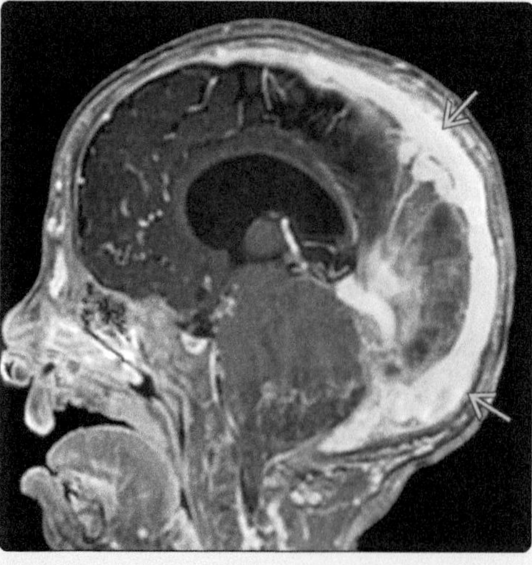

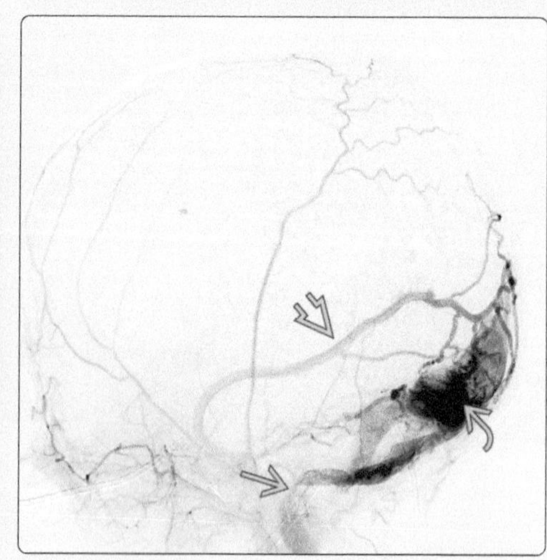

(Left) *Sagittal T1 C+ MR in a 10-month-old with an infantile dAVF shows marked enlargement of the dural venous sinuses ➔ due to increased venous pressure from the high arterial flow and outflow stenosis. When very large dural venous sinuses are encountered, additional signs of dAVF should be sought.* **(Right)** *Lateral DSA (same patient) shows a very large middle meningeal artery ➔ with direct filling of the torcular Herophili ➔. Note the narrowing of the jugular bulb ➔, causing increased venous pressures.*

TERMINOLOGY

Abbreviations

- Dural arteriovenous fistula (dAVF)

Synonyms

- Dural arteriovenous (AV) shunt

Definitions

- Heterogeneous group of lesions with common angioarchitecture (AV shunts in dural venous sinus wall)

IMAGING

General Features

- Best diagnostic clue
  - MR/CTA: Network of tiny (crack-like) vessels in wall of thrombosed or enlarged dural venous sinus
  - DSA: Predominant arterial supply from meningeal arteries
  - Bone CT: Dilated transosseous calvarial vascular channels, enlarged foramen spinosum
- Location
  - Posterior fossa > > supratentorial
  - Can involve any dural venous sinus
    - Most common (35-40%) = transverse sinus (TS) + sigmoid sinus (SS)
    - Other common sites = cavernous sinus (CS), superior sagittal sinus (SSS), superior petrosal sinus (SPS)

CT Findings

- NECT
  - May see dilated vascular channels in skull from transosseous feeding arteries
  - Ipsilateral enlargement of foramen spinosum; contains middle meningeal artery that commonly supplies dAVFs
  - Look for complications: Subarachnoid hemorrhage, cerebral edema (venous hypertension)
- CECT
  - Look for dilated dural venous sinuses and cortical veins
  - May see tortuous feeding arteries ± flow-related aneurysms (uncommon), draining veins
  - Involved dural sinus may be thrombosed/stenotic
- CTA
  - Standard 3D CTA may be useful in depicting gross angioarchitecture
  - 320-row detector dynamic 4D-CTA allows volumetric imaging, detailed spatial/temporal resolution

MR Findings

- T1WI
  - Isointense thrombosed dural sinus ± flow voids
- T2WI
  - Look for enlarged dural sinuses
  - Isointense thrombosed sinus ± flow voids
  - Areas of gliosis in chronic venous insufficiency
    - Look for retrograde leptomeningeal venous drainage
- FLAIR
  - Isointense thrombosed sinus ± adjacent edema (if venous ischemia/congestion)
- T2* GRE
  - Thrombosed dural sinus blooms
  - Areas of signal loss may represent Ca^{++} or hemorrhage
    - Ca^{++} from chronic venous insufficiency
    - Hemorrhage from venous hypertension
- DWI
  - Normal unless venous infarct or ischemia present
- PWI
  - Arterial spin labeling (ASL): Look for ↑ signal within venous structures to identify location of dAVF
- T1WI C+
  - Chronically thrombosed sinus usually enhances
- MRA
  - Look for flow-related signal in venous structures to suggest high-flow AV shunt
  - Useful for gross depiction of angioarchitecture, dynamics
  - TOF MRA may be negative with small or slow-flow shunts
- MRV
  - Depicts occluded parent sinus, collateral flow

Angiographic Findings

- Conventional angiography
  - Multiple arterial feeders are typical
    - Dural/transosseous branches from external carotid artery (ECA) most common
    - Tentorial/dural branches from internal carotid artery (ICA), vertebral artery (VA)
    - Parasitization of pial arteries with larger dAVFs
  - Involved dural sinus may be thrombosed/stenotic or enlarged
  - Flow reversal in dural sinus/cortical veins correlates with progressive symptoms, risk of hemorrhage
  - Tortuous engorged pial veins (pseudophlebitic pattern) with ↑ venous pressure (clinically aggressive)
  - High-flow venopathy → progressive stenosis, outlet occlusion, hemorrhage

Imaging Recommendations

- Best imaging tool
  - DSA ± superselective catheterization of dural, transosseous feeders
- Protocol advice
  - Screening MR, contrast-enhanced MRA
  - DSA to delineate vascular supply, venous drainage

DIFFERENTIAL DIAGNOSIS

Pial Arteriovenous Malformation

- Congenital vascular lesion with intraaxial nidus and no intervening normal brain parenchyma
- Predominant pial arterial supply, parasitization of dural supply possible (opposite to dAVF)

Sigmoid Sinus-Jugular Foramen Pseudolesion

- Slow or asymmetric flow creates variable signal on MR sequences
- Use MRV with multiple encoding gradients to clarify

Thrombosed Dural Sinus

- Collateral/congested venous drainage can mimic dAVF
- Can be spontaneous, traumatic, infectious (thrombophlebitis)

Dural Sinus Stenosis

- May have prominent collateral draining veins

PATHOLOGY

General Features

- Etiology
  - Adult dAVFs are usually acquired, not congenital
    - Often idiopathic; can occur in response to trauma, venous sinus thrombosis
  - Infant dAVFs are congenital and usually associated with enlargement of dural venous sinuses
  - Pathologic activation of neoangiogenesis
    - Proliferating capillaries within granulation tissue in dural sinus obliterated by organized thrombi
    - Budding/proliferation of microvascular network in inner dura connects to plexus of thin-walled venous channels, creating microfistulae
    - High basic fibroblast growth factor, vascular endothelial growth factor expression in dAVFs
- Associated abnormalities
  - Cortical venous drainage associated with edema, encephalopathy
  - Venous hypertension may lead to developmental delay in children
  - Arterialized flow in cortical veins/dural sinuses → high-flow venopathy, ↑ risk of intracranial hemorrhage (ICH), encephalopathy

Staging, Grading, & Classification

- Cognard classification of intracranial dAVFs correlates venous drainage pattern with risk of ICH
  - Grade 1: In sinus wall, normal antegrade venous drainage (low risk; benign clinical course)
  - Grade 2A: In wall, reflux into sinus (but not cortical veins)
  - Grade 2B: Retrograde drainage into cortical veins (10-20% hemorrhage)
  - Grade 3: Direct cortical venous drainage, no venous ectasia (40% hemorrhage)
  - Grade 4: Direct cortical venous drainage, venous ectasia (65% hemorrhage)
  - Grade 5: Spinal perimedullary venous drainage (progressive myelopathy)
- Indirect carotid-cavernous fistula (CCF) = 2nd most common dAVF site
  - Barrow classification based on arterial supply
    - Type A: Direct ICA-CS high-flow shunt (not dAVF)
    - Type B: Dural ICA branches-cavernous shunt
    - Type C: Dural ECA-cavernous shunt
    - Type D: ECA/ICA dural branches shunt to CS

Gross Pathologic & Surgical Features

- Multiple enlarged dural arteries converge on wall of thrombosed dural sinus
- Cortical draining veins enlarged (± stenoses, dilatation, tortuosity)

Microscopic Features

- Arterialized veins with irregular intimal thickening, variable loss of internal elastic lamina

CLINICAL ISSUES

Presentation

- Most common signs/symptoms
  - Clinical manifestations related to location, presence/absence of venous hypertension
    - TS-SS = pulsatile tinnitus
    - CS = pulsatile exophthalmos, cranial nerves (CNs) III, IV, VI neuropathy
    - Infant dAVF: Developmental delay, ↑ head circumference
  - Uncommon: Encephalopathic symptoms (venous hypertension, ischemia/thrombosis)
- Clinical profile
  - Infants and young children: Macrocephaly with cardiopulmonary symptoms
  - Older children: More likely to have focal neurologic deficits

Demographics

- Age
  - Adult > > child: Usually presents in middle-aged patients; pediatric dAVFs rare, high mortality
- Epidemiology
  - 10-15% of all cerebrovascular malformations with AV shunting

Natural History & Prognosis

- Depends on location, venous drainage pattern
  - 98% of dAVFs without retrograde venous drainage have benign course
  - dAVFs with retrograde venous drainage have aggressive clinical course
- dAVFs in children have lower rates of angiographic obliteration and poorer outcomes compared to other pediatric high-flow AV shunt lesions (e.g., AV malformation)

Treatment

- Conservative: Observation ± carotid compression technique
- Treatment options if (1) hemorrhage risk exists, or (2) for types 1 and 2A with debilitating pulsatile tinnitus
  - Embolization of arterial feeders with particulate or liquid agents, coil embolization of recipient venous pouch/sinus
  - Surgical skeletonization of involved dural venous sinus

DIAGNOSTIC CHECKLIST

Consider

- dAVF in patient with enlarged dural venous sinuses, particularly with history of venous thrombosis

Image Interpretation Pearls

- MR + MRA may be normal in small dAVF
- Use ASL perfusion to detect small dAVF

SELECTED REFERENCES

1. Chen X et al: Overview of multimodal MRI of intracranial dural arteriovenous fistulas. J Interv Med. 5(4):173-9, 2022
2. Hou K et al: Brain arteriovenous malformations and dural arteriovenous fistulas with extensive venous congestive encephalopathy. Acta Neurol Belg. 122(1):1-9, 2022
3. Martín-Noguerol T et al: Conventional and advanced MRI evaluation of brain vascular malformations. J Neuroimaging. 31(3):428-45, 2021

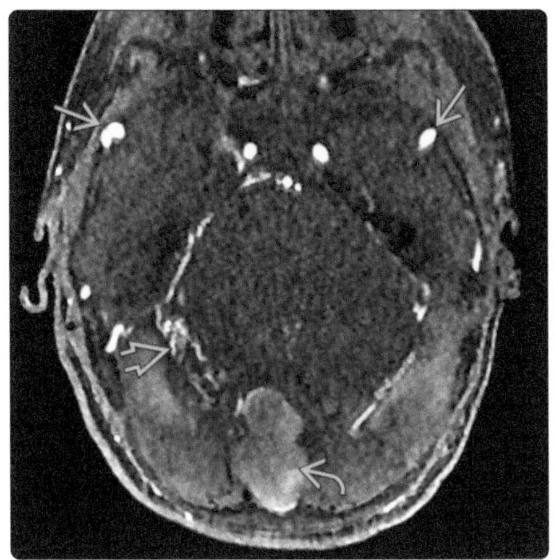

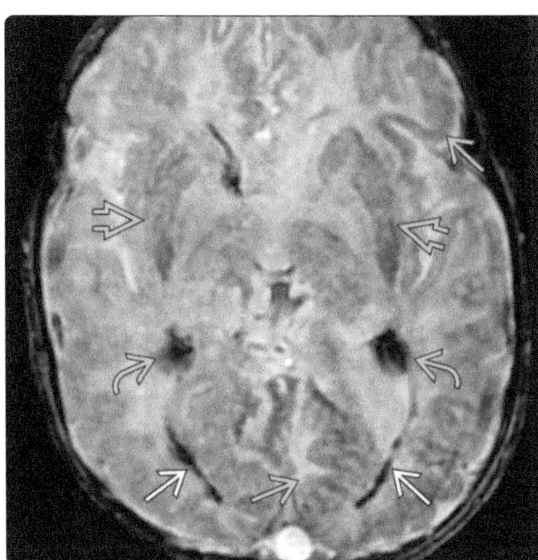

(Left) *Axial TOF MRA (same patient) shows enlargement of the bilateral middle meningeal arteries* ➙ *and multiple small arteries* ➙ *that communicate directly with the torcular Herophili* ➙*, which also contains some flow-related signal.* **(Right)** *Axial SWI MR (same patient) shows signal loss in the cortex* ➙ *and deep gray matter* ➙*, consistent with mineralization. Venous hypertension in dAVFs can lead to mineral deposition in the brain. Also note prior germinal matrix* ➙ *and intraventricular hemorrhage* ➙.

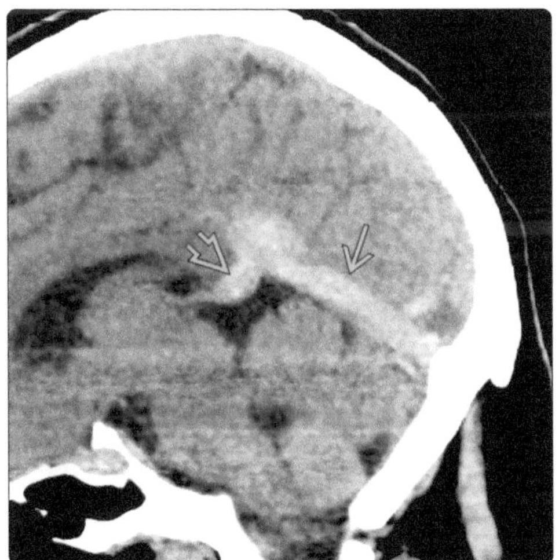

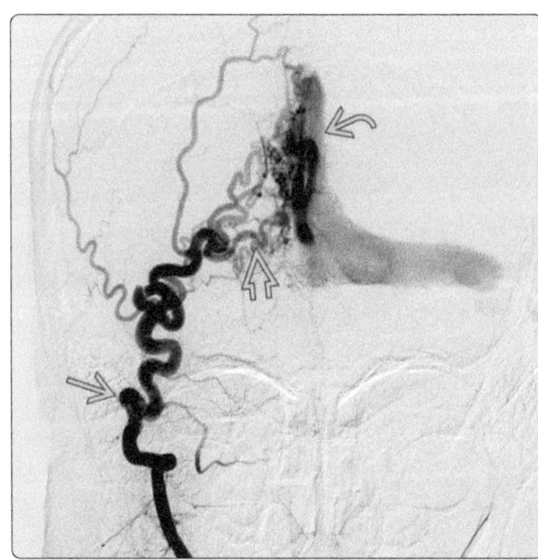

(Left) *Sagittal NECT in a teenager shows high attenuation within the vein of Galen* ➙ *and straight sinus* ➙*, consistent with acute thrombosis. Dural venous sinus thrombosis is the most common cause of dAVF.* **(Right)** *Frontal projection DSA (right external carotid artery injection) in the same patient 10 months later shows development of a dAVF. The middle meningeal artery* ➙ *is markedly enlarged and tortuous with multiple small feeding arterial vessels* ➙ *opacifying the straight sinus* ➙ *during the arterial phase.*

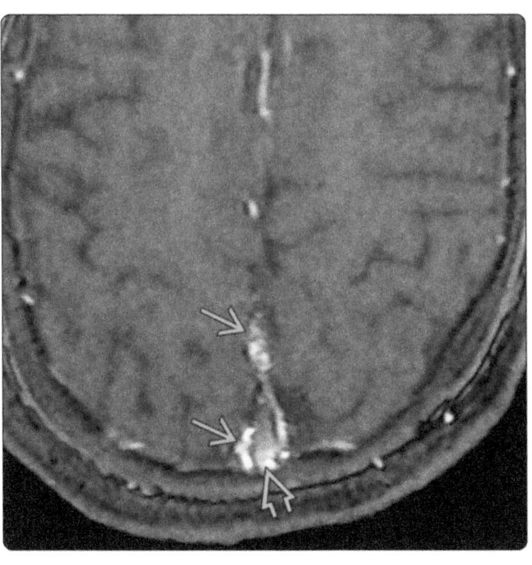

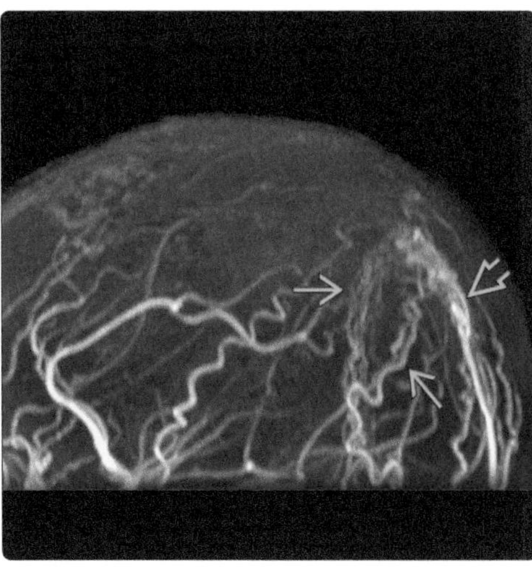

(Left) *Axial 3D TOF MRA in a 12-year-old with a history of corpus callosotomy shows multiple small arterial vessels* ➙ *along the margins of the superior sagittal sinus (SSS), as well as flow-related signal within the SSS* ➙*.* **(Right)** *Lateral view of a 3D TOF MRA in the same patient shows numerous small arterial vessels* ➙ *coursing toward the posterior aspect of the SSS* ➙ *with flow-related signal in the SSS, consistent with a high-flow dAVF.*

Vein of Galen Aneurysmal Malformation

KEY FACTS

TERMINOLOGY

- High-flow arteriovenous (AV) fistula between deep choroidal arteries & median prosencephalic vein (MPV)

IMAGING

- 2 major goals of imaging: Assess degree of brain injury, define vein of Galen aneurysmal malformation (VGAM) architecture to help plan embolization
- Some degree of ventriculomegaly typical
  - ↓ CSF resorption due to venous hypertension
  - Chronic volume loss
  - Obstruction from compression of tectum
- Venous outflow stenosis affects end-organ damage
  - Sigmoid/jugular stenoses protect heart, harm brain
- Classification system for VGAMs (Lasjunias)
  - Choroidal type: Multiple primitive choroidal arteries pass through nidus before entering MPV
  - Mural type: 1 or more (usually multiple) direct AV fistulas within wall of MPV

PATHOLOGY

- Flow through fistula prevents normal regression of MPV

CLINICAL ISSUES

- Most common extracardiac cause of high-output heart failure in newborn
- Preferred treatment: Transcatheter embolization at 4-6 months with occlusion of fistula, ideally from arterial side
- Bicêtre neonatal evaluation score guides therapy
  - Assesses end-organ damage
- Prognosis related to timing/success of treatment
  - High-volume shunts requiring treatment in newborn period have worse prognosis
  - Ability to delay treatment until 4-6 months associated with better outcome

DIAGNOSTIC CHECKLIST

- Always perform 3D imaging with MPR & 3D reconstruction
- Look for venous outflow stenosis: ↑ risk of brain damage

(Left) *Sagittal graphic shows medial & lateral posterior choroidal arteries with a fistulous connection to an enlarged midline vein [median prosencephalic vein (MPV)], which drains through a persistent falcine sinus to the superior sagittal sinus. This would be a mural-type vein of Galen aneurysmal malformation (VGAM).* **(Right)** *Lateral 3D MRA with contrast in a neonate with high-output cardiac failure shows enlarged choroidal ➡ & pericallosal ➡ arteries feeding a large MPV ➡ & straight sinus. No venous outflow stenosis is identified.*

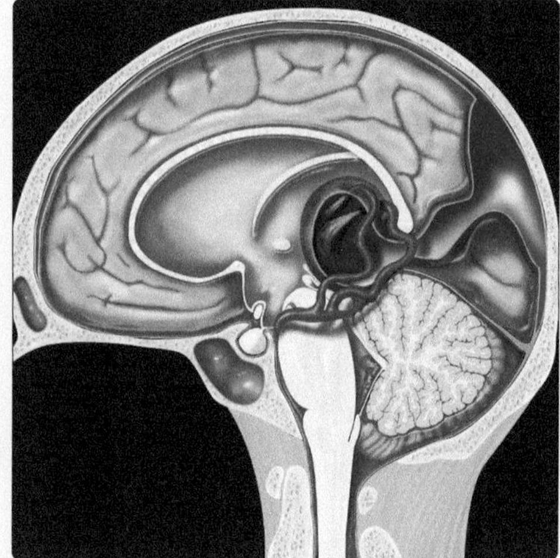

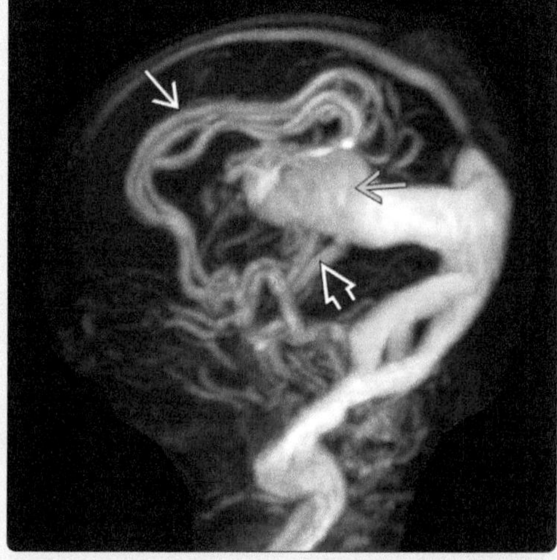

(Left) *Coronal T2 MR in the same neonate shows a large MPV ➡ & multiple enlarged, tortuous feeding arteries ➡. The brain parenchyma is thinned with loss of normal gray matter-white matter differentiation, a poor prognostic sign.* **(Right)** *Axial DWI MR in the same neonate shows extensive right ➡ & focal left ➡ cerebral diffusion restriction, representing severe brain injury ("melting brain") related to venous hypertension & arterial steal from the VGAM. No treatment was recommended for this patient.*

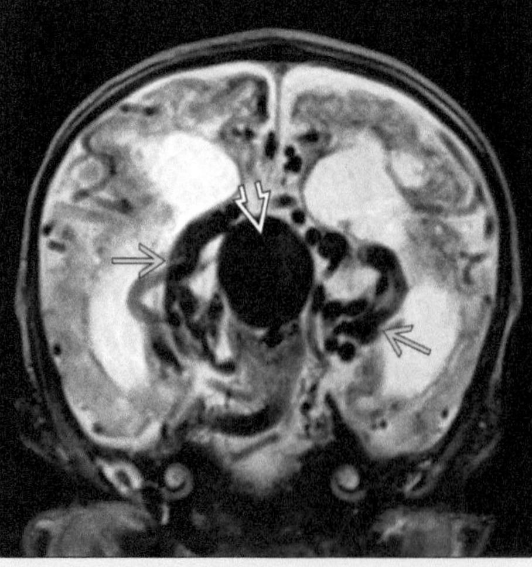

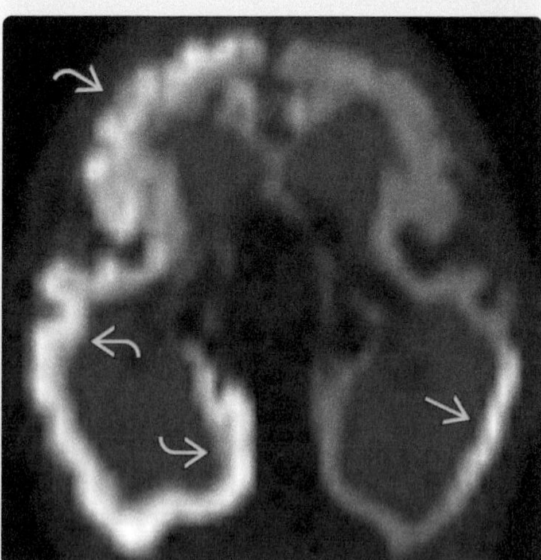

TERMINOLOGY

Abbreviations

- Vein of Galen aneurysmal malformation (VGAM)

Synonyms

- Vein of Galen malformation, vein of Galen aneurysm, galenic varix

Definitions

- High-flow arteriovenous (AV) fistula between deep choroidal arteries & median prosencephalic vein (MPV) of Markowski
  - Not actually aneurysm of true vein of Galen, which fails to form because of fistula

IMAGING

General Features

- Best diagnostic clue
  - Large midline varix in neonate/infant
- Location
  - Quadrigeminal plate cistern
- Size
  - Varix can be several centimeters in diameter
- Morphology
  - Spherical or tubular varix
- Diagnosis typically obvious on cross-sectional imaging
- 2 major goals of imaging
  - Assess brain injury to determine if treatment warranted
  - Delineate malformation architecture for embolization

Radiographic Findings

- Radiography
  - ± cardiomegaly & edema from CHF on chest radiograph

CT Findings

- NECT
  - Venous pouch follows density of blood elsewhere
  - Hydrocephalus
  - White matter Ca^{++} from chronic venous ischemia
  - Streak artifact from coils or glue make CT poor choice for posttreatment imaging
- CECT
  - Strong enhancement of feeding arteries & varix
- CTA
  - Excellent preangiography delineation of vessels
    - Streak artifact from embolics severely degrades posttreatment imaging

MR Findings

- T1WI
  - Phase-encoding pulsation artifact from varix
- T2WI
  - Large flow void of varix (unless slow/turbulent flow)
  - Prominent flow voids of feeding arteries around varix
  - Some degree of ventriculomegaly typical; ± ↑ T2 signal of white matter
    - ↓ CSF resorption due to venous hypertension
    - Obstruction from compression of tectum
    - Chronic volume loss
    - Overproduction from ↑ choroidal blood flow
- DWI
  - Restricted diffusion in areas of acute ischemia/infarction
    - Due to venous hypertension & arterial steal phenomenon
    - ± focal or extensive loss of cortical ribbon on T2WI
- PWI
  - Arterial spin labeling (ASL) can assess AV shunt reduction following embolization
- T1WI C+
  - Nicely shows overall morphology of VGAM
  - 3D acquisitions with reconstructions are ideal
- MRA
  - Key to define architecture of lesion
  - Major arterial feeders: Targets for embolization
  - Unaffected by embolics (ideal for posttreatment evaluation)
- MRV
  - Map out potential venous access to lesion for treatment
  - High flow through veins → venous stenoses
    - Affects end-organ damage
      - Venous stenosis protects heart at expense of brain
      - Jugular stenosis/atresia associated with poor outcome
- SWI: May show ↑ signal in veins related to AV shunt
- Fetal MR
  - Can identify malformation in 2nd & 3rd trimesters & provide information about end-organ injury
  - Width of straight or falcine sinus is best fetal MR outcome predictor (larger diameter = worse prognosis)
  - Contraindication to aggressive treatment: Significant antenatal end-organ injury

Ultrasonographic Findings

- Prenatal studies identify malformation in 2nd & 3rd trimesters
  - Cardiac dilation, hydrops fetalis = poor prognosis
- If not identified prenatally, postnatal head US often 1st test to make diagnosis
  - Venous aneurysm appears identical to cyst on grayscale imaging: Anechoic with posterior acoustic enhancement
  - Use color Doppler on any midline cystic lesion to detect flow

Angiographic Findings

- Choroidal or mural classification (Lasjunias) based on angioarchitecture of VGAM
  - Choroidal type: Primitive vessel morphology with multiple choroidal feeding arteries passing through nidus network before draining into MPV
  - Mural type: 1 or more (usually multiple) direct AV fistulas within wall of MPV
- Frequent venous abnormalities
  - Embryonic falcine sinus drains MPV in ~ 50%
  - Stenoses at sigmoid-jugular junction

Imaging Recommendations

- Best imaging tool
  - MR with MRA & MRV
  - Diagnostic arteriography performed in concert with embolization
- Protocol advice

- Maximize MRA evaluation
  - 3D reconstructions can provide valuable insight

DIFFERENTIAL DIAGNOSIS

Secondary Vein of Galen Aneurysmal Dilation

- AV malformation drains into true vein of Galen
- Looks like choroidal type of VGAM
  - Much less common than VGAM

Childhood Dural Arteriovenous Fistula

- High-flow fistula with venous varices
  - Typically in transverse sinuses
- Massive torcular enlargement may thrombose spontaneously before/after delivery

Giant Aneurysm

- Not associated with venous abnormalities
- "Onion skin" layers of blood products in wall

Complex Developmental Venous Anomaly

- "Umbrella" of medullary veins draining normal brain

Pial Arteriovenous Malformation

- Distinguished by true nidus at transition; large venous varices less common
- Rarely presents before 3 years of age

PATHOLOGY

General Features

- Etiology
  - Venous occlusion or stenosis
    - Primary atresia vs. occlusion 2° to ↑ pressure & flow
    - Provides some protection for right heart
  - Cerebral ischemia/atrophy
    - Arterial steal &/or chronic venous hypertension
  - Hydrocephalus
    - ↓ CSF resorption 2° to elevated venous pressure
    - ± cerebral aqueduct obstruction
- Genetics
  - Majority sporadic
- Embryology
  - Abnormal connection of choroidal arteries to MPV occurs at 6- to 11-weeks gestation
  - Flow through fistula prevents normal regression of MPV

CLINICAL ISSUES

Presentation

- Most common signs/symptoms
  - Neonate: High-output CHF, cranial bruit
  - Infant: Macrocrania (hydrocephalus), seizures, or neurocognitive delay
  - Older children/adults: Usually compensated, may present with hemorrhage
- Other signs/symptoms
  - Developmental delay, failure to thrive, hydrocephalus, seizure, headache, hepatic failure

Demographics

- Age: Neonatal period most common, but many now identified on routine fetal US
  - Rarely diagnosed after 3 years of age
- Sex: M:F = 2:1
- Epidemiology: Most common extracardiac cause of high-output heart failure in newborn

Natural History & Prognosis

- Prognosis related to volume of shunt & timing/success of treatment
  - High-volume shunts requiring treatment in newborn period have worse prognosis
  - Ability to delay treatment until 4-6 months associated with better outcome
- Severe cases → ischemia & cerebral atrophy: "Melting brain"
  - Due to venous insufficiency & arterial steal
  - Can occur even after unsuccessful treatment

Treatment

- Treatment in neonatal period based upon Bicêtre neonatal evaluation score
  - 21-point system based upon cardiac (5), cerebral (5), respiratory (5), hepatic (3), & renal (3) function
  - High score = good function; low score = poor function
    - < 8: No treatment
    - 8-12: Emergent embolization
    - > 12: Medical management initially followed by delayed embolization at 4-6 months
      - Medical therapy for CHF until 4-6 months of age
- Transcatheter embolization (TCE)
  - Failure of temporizing medical therapy warrants earlier neurointervention
  - Permanent occlusion of fistula, ideally from arterial side
    - Liquid agents or coils
  - Outcome following embolization
    - ~ 75% normal, ~ 10-15% moderate mental restrictions, ~ 5-10% severe mental restrictions, ~ 5% death
  - Incomplete closure of fistula can be associated with good outcome
- Potential future direction: Transuterine fetal US-guided VGAM embolization
- Treatment for hydrocephalus controversial
  - Shunt placement associated with exacerbation of venous ischemia
  - Hemorrhage risk from engorged subependymal veins
  - Reserved for refractory hydrocephalus after all TCEs performed

DIAGNOSTIC CHECKLIST

Image Interpretation Pearls

- Meticulous evaluation of MRA can identify essentially all feeders to VGAM
- MRA C+ can show arterial & venous anatomy together

SELECTED REFERENCES

1. Orbach DB et al: Transuterine ultrasound-guided fetal embolization of vein of Galen malformation, eliminating postnatal pathophysiology. Stroke. 54(6):e231-2, 2023
2. Arko L et al: Fetal and neonatal MRI predictors of aggressive early clinical course in vein of Galen malformation. AJNR Am J Neuroradiol. 41(6):1105-11, 2020
3. Berenstein A et al: Vein of Galen aneurysmal malformation: advances in management and endovascular treatment. Neurosurgery. 84(2):469-78, 2019

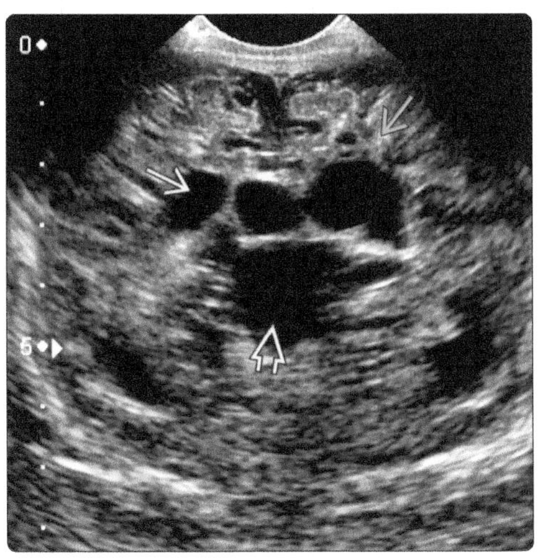

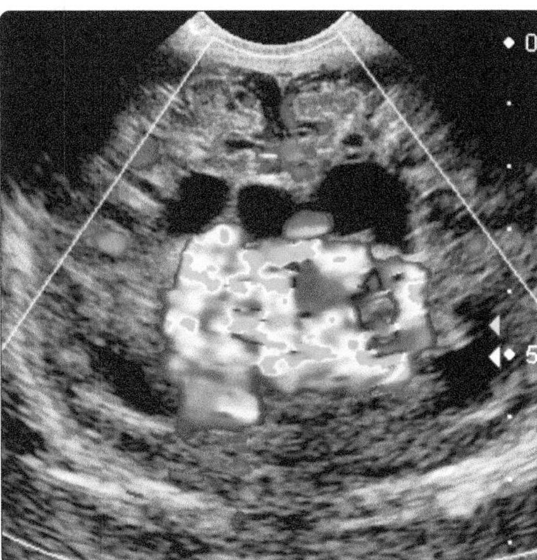

(Left) *Coronal US in a neonate with high-output cardiac failure shows a midline anechoic lesion. Also visible are the enlarged lateral ventricles & thin, heterogeneous parenchyma. These findings are suspicious for a VGAM with significant brain injury.* **(Right)** *Coronal color Doppler US in the same neonate shows turbulent vascular flow centrally, confirming that the anechoic lesion is a vessel & strongly suggesting the diagnosis of a VGAM.*

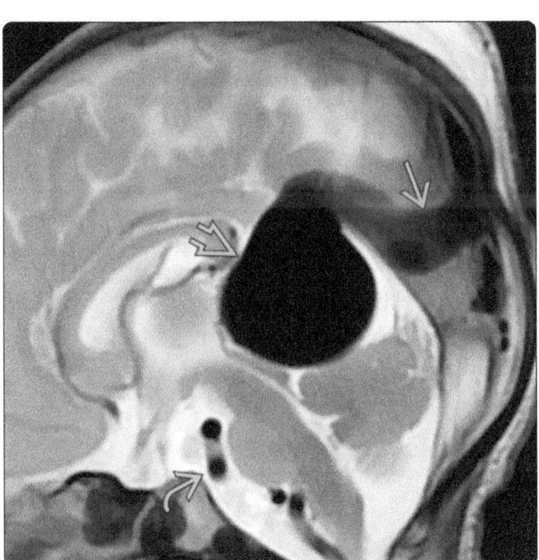

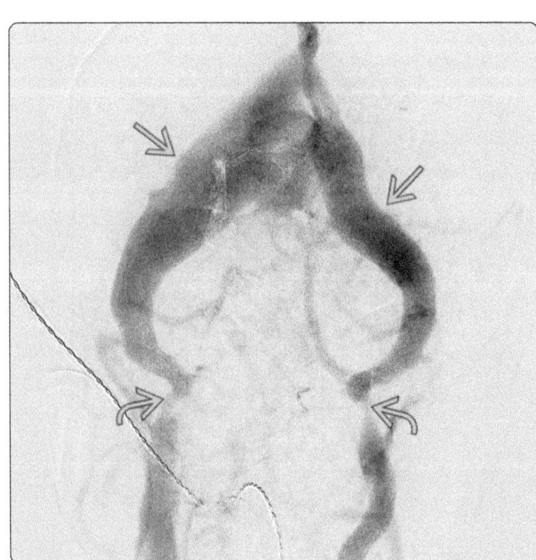

(Left) *Sagittal T2 MR in a newborn shows a markedly enlarged MPV draining into a prominent persistent falcine sinus. Note the markedly enlarged basilar artery.* **(Right)** *Frontal DSA projection in the same patient shows enlarged transverse & sigmoid sinuses with narrowing or stenosis at the level of the jugular bulbs. Outflow stenosis such as this typically reduces the risk of high-output cardiac failure but increases the risk of brain injury due to venous hypertension.*

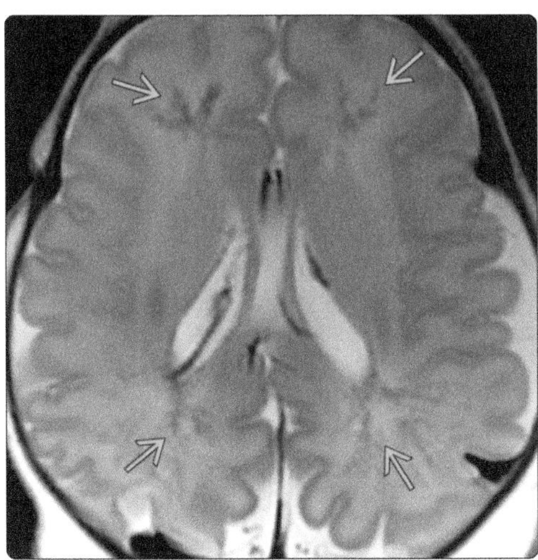

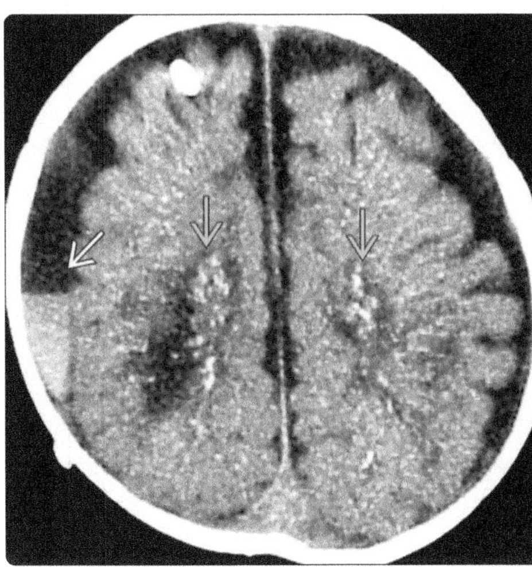

(Left) *Axial T2 MR in the same newborn shows areas of perimedullary hemorrhage due to venous hypertension from venous outflow stenosis.* **(Right)** *Axial NECT 18 months after the unsuccessful treatment of a VGAM shows the effects of chronic venous hypertension with extensive parenchymal Ca^{++}, volume loss, & development of a subdural hematoma. If complete closure cannot be achieved, shunting must be reduced enough to match venous capacity.*

Developmental Venous Anomaly

KEY FACTS

TERMINOLOGY

- Developmental venous anomaly (DVA): Congenital cerebral vascular malformation with mature venous elements
- Embryology: Compensatory adaptation to early fetal disruption of medullary venous development

IMAGING

- General features
  - Umbrella-like collection of enlarged medullary (white matter) veins ("Medusa head")
  - Numerous linear or dot-like enhancing foci
  - Converge on single enlarged collector vein
  - Collector vein drains into dural sinus/deep ependymal vein
  - Hemorrhage can occur with associated CM; rarely with thrombosis or "arterialized" DVA
- CT usually normal; enlarged collector vein can appear hyperdense
- MR
  - Variable signal depending on size, flow
  - Hypointense on SWI [blood oxygenation level-dependent (BOLD) effect in draining veins]
  - Strong enhancement

TOP DIFFERENTIAL DIAGNOSES

- Capillary telangiectasia, Sturge-Weber syndrome, intracranial hemorrhage

PATHOLOGY

- < 5% of DVAs have associated CM; ~ 25% of CMs have associated DVA
- ~ 5% of DVAs have associated FLAIR signal in adjacent brain
- Associated with orbitofacial vascular malformations & blue rubber bleb nevus syndrome
  - Often with large, holohemispheric DVAs

DIAGNOSTIC CHECKLIST

- DVAs provide only venous drainage pathway to brain within their drainage territory

(Left) *Coronal oblique graphic shows a classic development vein anomaly (DVA) with umbrella-like "Medusa head" of enlarged medullary [deep white matter (WM)] veins ➡ converging on a dilated transcortical collector vein ➡, which drains into the superior sagittal sinus ➡.* **(Right)** *Gross pathology shows an incidental finding of DVA, seen here as scattered enlarged venous channels ➡ near the frontal horn of the lateral ventricle. Normal WM is seen between the venous tributaries. Note the absence of hemorrhage. (Courtesy R. Hewlett, MD.)*

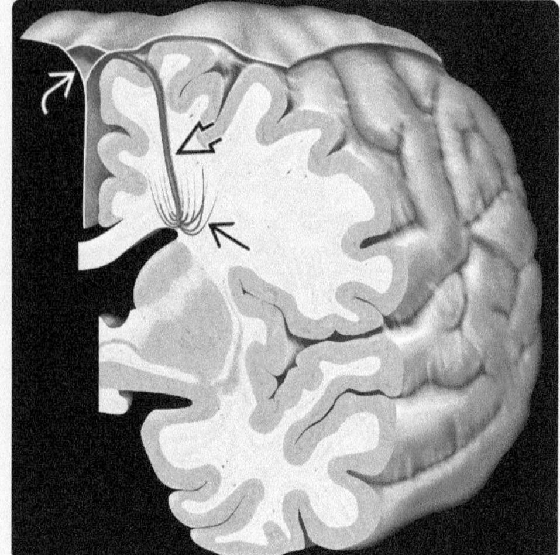

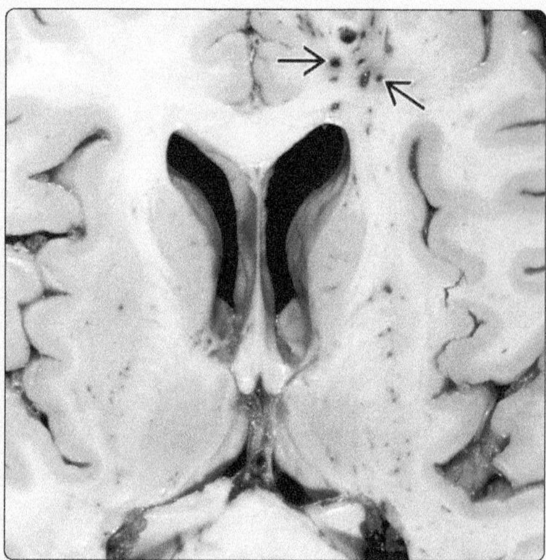

(Left) *Lateral venous-phase DSA shows the classic "Medusa head" of a DVA with numerous enlarged medullary venous radicles ➡ converging on an enlarged transcortical collector or drainage vein ➡.* **(Right)** *3D shaded surface rendering in the same patient elegantly depicts the classic "Medusa head" of a DVA ➡. (Courtesy P. Lasjaunias, MD.) The brain territory drained by DVAs has no collateral drainage pathways, thus DVAs are "do not touch" lesions due to the venous ischemia caused by obstructing or ligating the DVA.*

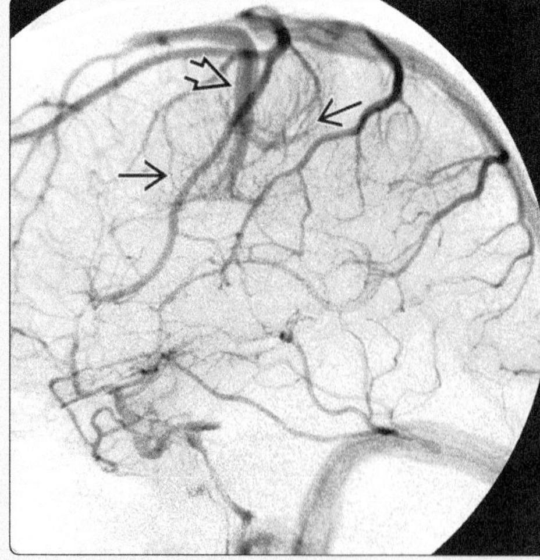

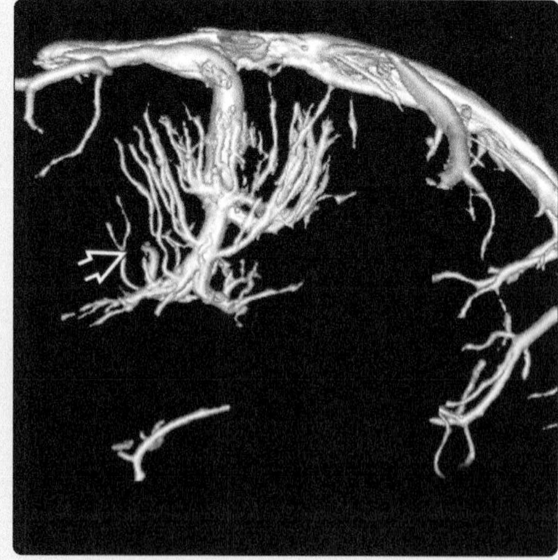

TERMINOLOGY

Abbreviations

- Developmental venous anomaly (DVA)

Synonyms

- Venous angioma

Definitions

- Congenital cerebral vascular malformation with mature venous elements
- Represents only drainage pathway for brain within drainage territory (i.e., no collaterals)
  - Surgical sacrifice of collecting vein will result in infarct

IMAGING

General Features

- Best diagnostic clue
  - "Medusa head" [dilated medullary white matter (WM) veins]
- Location
  - Frontal (36-56%), parietal (12-24%), temporal (2-19%), occipital (4%), cerebellum (14-29%), & brainstem (< 5%)
- Size
  - Varies (may be extensive), but usually < 3 cm
- Morphology
  - Umbrella-like collection of enlarged medullary venous radicles ("caput medusa")
  - Medullary veins drain into larger collecting vein
  - Drainage may be to superficial (~ 60%) or deep (~ 40%) venous system or both (< 5%)
  - Usually solitary; can be multiple & holohemispheric in syndromes (e.g., blue rubber bleb nevus syndrome)

CT Findings

- NECT
  - Usual: Enlarged collector vein may appear hyperdense; this is not pathological
  - Occasional: If associated Ca^{++} present, should raise concern for associated cavernous malformation (CM)
  - Rare: Acute parenchymal hemorrhage (if draining vein spontaneously thromboses)
- CECT
  - Numerous linear or dot-like enhancing foci
    - Well-circumscribed, round/ovoid enhancing areas on sequential sections
    - Converge on single enlarged tubular draining vein
    - Occasionally seen as linear structure in single slice

MR Findings

- T1WI
  - Usually normal when DVA is small; flow void when large
  - Variable signal depending on size, flow
- T2WI
  - ± flow void; more common when larger
- FLAIR
  - Usually normal; may show hyperintense signal within venous radicles
  - Subtle associated hyperintense signal in adjacent brain parenchyma (~ 5%)
    - Etiology uncertain: gliosis, demyelination, etc.
- T2* GRE
  - Most sensitive noncontrast sequence for DVA detection
  - Globular areas of hypointense signal (blooming) with associated T1 or T2 signal changes in drainage territory of DVA suggests associated CM
  - Punctate foci of signal loss have been seen in adjacent brain in up to 60% of adults in one study
    - Anecdotally, much less common in children
    - May represent microhemorrhage or CM precursor
  - Hypointense on SWI [blood oxygenation level-dependent (BOLD) effect in draining veins]
    - If high flow, deoxyhemoglobin reduced; may be isointense
- DWI
  - Almost always normal, except in cases of associated venous infarction (very rare)
- PWI
  - Nearly 80% of DVAs with perfusion abnormalities on bolus contrast PWI; < 10% on arterial spin labeling (ASL)
    - ↑ cerebral blood flow (CBF); ↑ cerebral blood volume (CBV); ↑ mean transit time (MTT)
- T1WI C+
  - Strong enhancement
    - Stellate tubular vessels converge on collector vein
    - Collector vein drains into dural sinus or ependymal vein
  - 3D FSPGR with contrast is most sensitive sequence for DVA detection
- MRA
  - TOF: Arterial phase usually normal
    - Rare: Flow-related signal in venous structures in "arterialized DVAs"
- MRV
  - Flow-related modalities (TOF or phase-contrast MRV) usually normal, except in larger DVAs
- MRS
  - Normal

Ultrasonographic Findings

- Brain parenchyma within DVA drainage territory is often hyperechoic
  - May mimic ischemia or intraparenchymal hemorrhage

Angiographic Findings

- DSA
  - Arterial phase normal in nearly all cases
  - Uncommon: Atypical "arterialized DVA" (transitional form of venous-arteriovenous malformation with enlarged feeders, arteriovenous shunting)
  - Venous phase: "Medusa head"

Nuclear Medicine Findings

- PET
  - ~ 70% of cases show hypometabolism in adjacent brain parenchyma
  - Rarely associated with ↑ metabolism

Imaging Recommendations

- Best imaging tool
  - T1 C+ MR plus SWI, MRV
- Protocol advice
  - Include T2* sequence (GRE, SWI) in noncontrast imaging

DIFFERENTIAL DIAGNOSIS

Capillary Telangiectasia

- Most often confused with DVA when small
- Typically more confluent blush of contrast without well-defined venous radicles or collecting vein

Sturge-Weber Syndrome

- May develop strikingly enlarged medullary, subependymal, choroid plexus veins
- Large or holohemispheric DVA may mimic Sturge-Weber syndrome (SWS) but should not have leptomeningeal enhancement
- Coexisting facial angioma

Intracranial Hemorrhage

- Large, dense collecting vein can mimic intracranial hemorrhage

Mixed Vascular Malformation (Usually Cavernoma)

- Hemorrhage often associated
- Typically should demonstrate signal loss on SWI/GRE & T1/T2 signal alterations

Vascular Neoplasm

- Must have well-defined associated lesion, usually with mass effect

Dural Sinus Thrombosis (Chronic)

- Chronic thrombosis → venous stasis
- Medullary veins enlarge as collateral drainage

Venous Varix (Isolated)

- Should not have numerous venous radicles (caput medusae)

PATHOLOGY

General Features

- Etiology
  - Embryology
    - Arrested medullary vein development at time when normal arterial development nearly complete
    - Developmental arrest results in persistence of large, primitive, embryonic deep WM veins
- Genetics
  - ~ 50% inherited as autosomal dominant
  - Mutations in chromosome 9p
    - Segregates pedigrees with skin, oral & GI mucosa, brain venous malformations
- Associated abnormalities
  - ≤ 5% of children with DVAs will have associated CM
  - 25% of all CMs associated with DVA
  - Blue rubber bleb nevus syndrome more often associated with large, holohemispheric DVAs
  - Sinus pericranii (cutaneous sign of underlying venous anomaly)
  - 60% of orbital slow-flow vascular malformations have associated DVAs
  - Cervicofacial venous or lymphatic malformation [cerebrofacial arterial/venous metameric syndrome 3 (CAMS-3)]

Gross Pathologic & Surgical Features

- Radially oriented dilated medullary veins
- Venous radicals are separated by normal brain
- Enlarged transcortical or subependymal draining vein

Microscopic Features

- Dilated, thin-walled vessels diffusely distributed in normal WM (no gliosis)
- Occasional: Thickened, hyalinized vessel walls

CLINICAL ISSUES

Presentation

- Most common signs/symptoms
  - Vast majority are asymptomatic & incidental
  - Uncommon: Hemorrhage with focal neurologic deficit (if associated with CM, thrombosis, or "arterialized" DVA)
- Clinical profile
  - Asymptomatic patient with incidental DVA found on MR

Demographics

- Age
  - All ages
- Sex
  - M = F
- Ethnicity
  - No known predilection
- Epidemiology
  - Most common cerebral vascular malformation at autopsy; 5-9% prevalence on contrast-enhanced MR scans; 60% of cerebral vascular malformations

Natural History & Prognosis

- Hemorrhage risk: 0.15% per lesion per year
  - Probably attributable mostly to associated CMs &, rarely, associated thrombosis or "arterialized" DVA

Treatment

- Solitary DVA: No treatment
- Associated CM: If symptomatic, CM may be resected
  - Important to identify associated DVA so surgeon can preserve sole venous drainage to adjacent brain

DIAGNOSTIC CHECKLIST

Consider

- DVAs provide only venous drainage pathway to brain within their drainage territory

Image Interpretation Pearls

- If DVA is not seen on daily basis in usual outpatient setting, it is probably being overlooked

SELECTED REFERENCES

1. Agosti E et al: Developmental venous anomaly associated with dural arteriovenous fistula: etiopathogenesis and hemorrhagic risk. Front Surg. 10:1141857, 2023
2. Hsu CC et al: Symptomatic developmental venous anomaly: state-of-the-art review on genetics, pathophysiology, and imaging approach to diagnosis. AJNR Am J Neuroradiol. 44(5):498-504, 2023
3. Chang SJ et al: COVID-19-associated cerebral developmental venous anomaly thrombosis with hemorrhagic transformation. Stroke. 53(7):e255-6, 2022

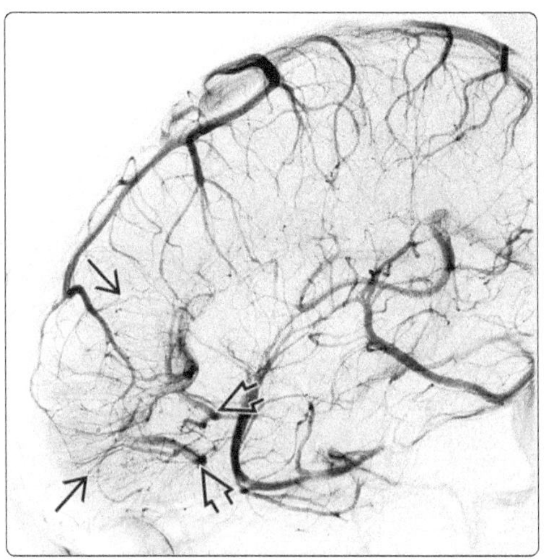

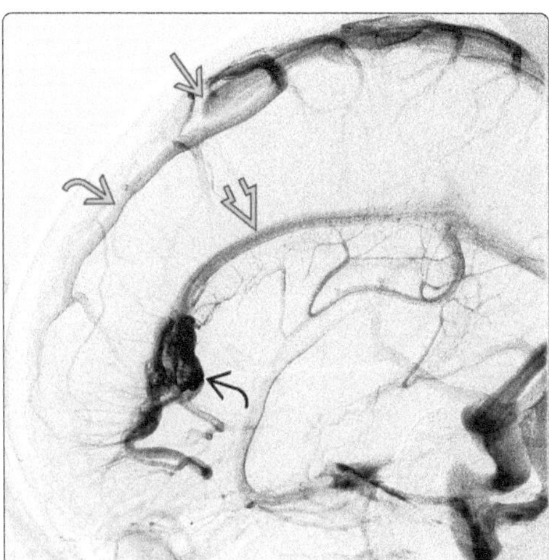

(Left) *Lateral early venous-phase DSA in the same patient shows the enlarged medullary veins → ("Medusa head") of the DVA. The large collector veins → are beginning to fill with contrast.* **(Right)** *Late venous-phase DSA shows the giant varix → draining the DVA and empties into a markedly enlarged inferior sagittal sinus →. The entire anterior 1/3 of the superior sagittal sinus is hypoplastic or absent, with the superior sagittal sinus originating → near the coronal suture at the confluence of a prominent cortical vein →.*

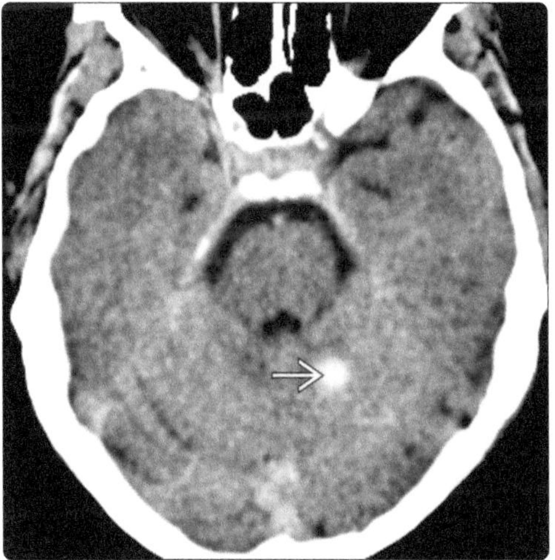

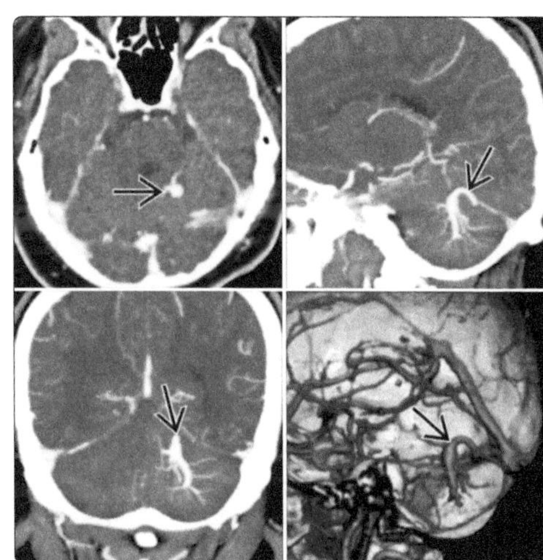

(Left) *Axial NECT shows a well-delineated hyperdensity in the left cerebellar hemisphere →. The large collecting vein can mimic intracranial hemorrhage on CT, particularly in the setting of elevated hematocrit.* **(Right)** *CTA with axial, sagittal, and coronal views as well as a 3D reconstruction in the same patient shows that the parenchymal hyperdensity corresponds to the large collector vein of the DVA → rather than hemorrhage.*

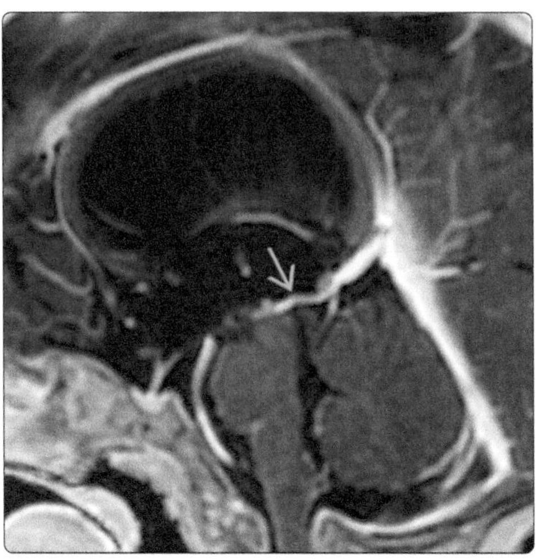

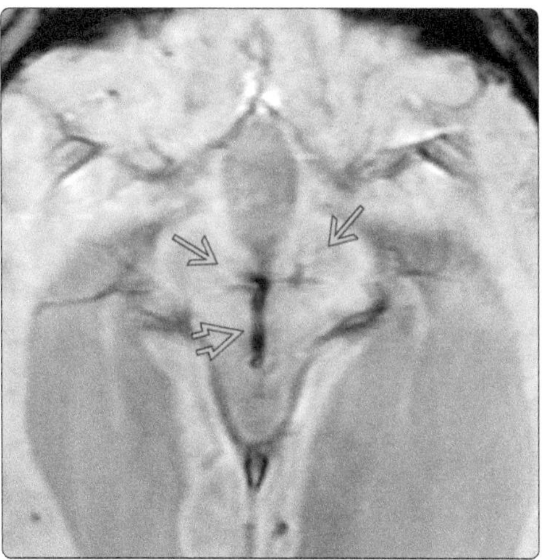

(Left) *Midline sagittal T1 C+ MR in a 7-month-old with obstructive hydrocephalus shows a central draining vein → of a DVA coursing across and obstructing the cerebral aqueduct.* **(Right)** *Axial SWI MR in the same patient shows the small venous radicles → in the midbrain draining into the midline draining vein →, obstructing the cerebral aqueduct and leading to hydrocephalus. This patient was treated with a 3rd ventriculostomy. Almost all DVAs are incidental but occasionally can cause pathology.*

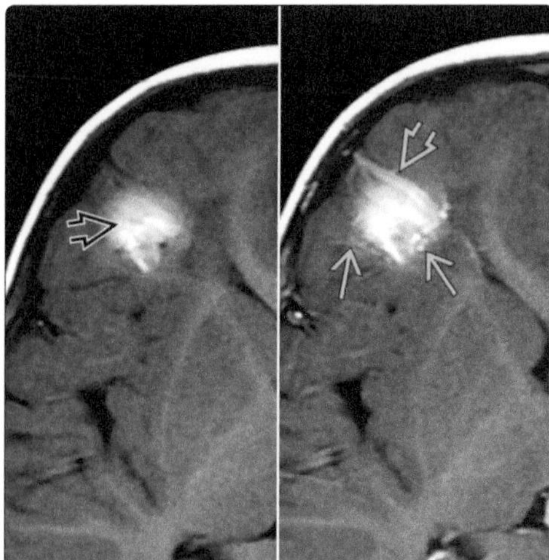

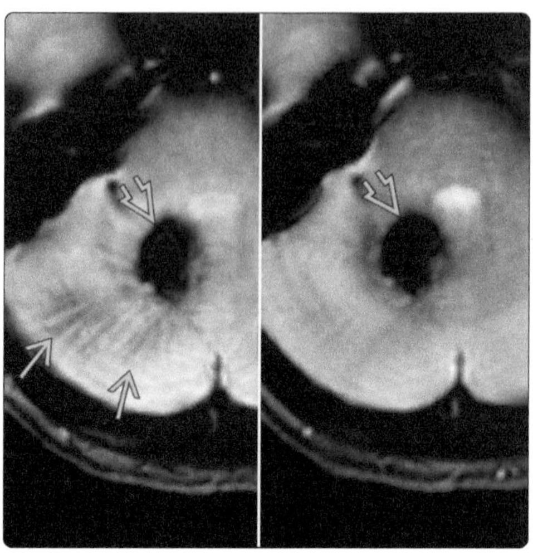

(Left) *Axial T1 MR (left) shows a T1-hyperintense cavernous malformation ⇒. T1 C+ MR (right) shows an associated DVA with small venous radicles → draining into a large collecting vein ⇒ that drains superficially. Contrast may be helpful in addition to SWI in identifying an associated DVA.* **(Right)** *Axial SWI (left) and GRE (right) MR images show a cavernous malformation ⇒ with an associated DVA →. The comparison demonstrates that SWI is more sensitive than GRE for the detection of DVAs.*

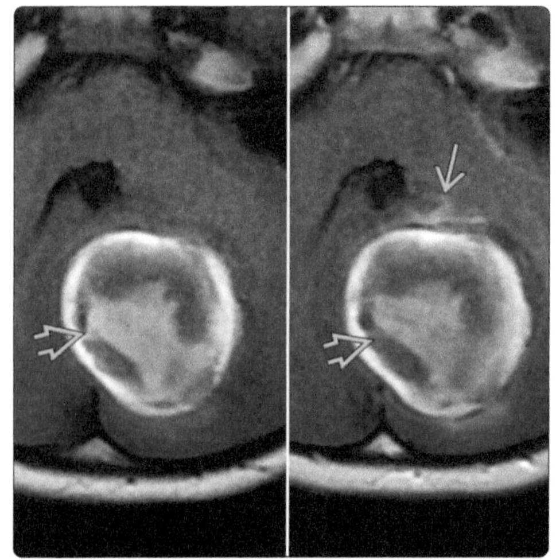

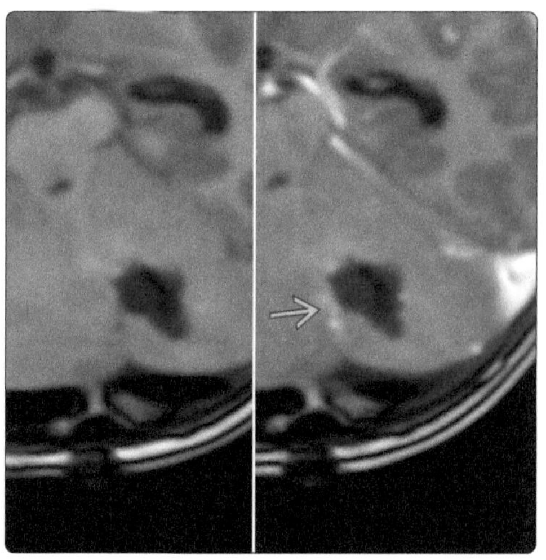

(Left) *Axial T1 (left) and T1 C+ (right) MR images show the importance of contrast administration in identifying the associated DVA →. Identifying a DVA strongly supports that the heterogeneously T1-hyperintense lesion ⇒ is a cavernous malformation.* **(Right)** *Axial T1 (left) and T1 C+ (right) MR images following resection of the cavernous malformation show intentional preservation of the DVA → by the neurosurgeon. Ligation of a DVA collecting vein will lead to venous infarction.*

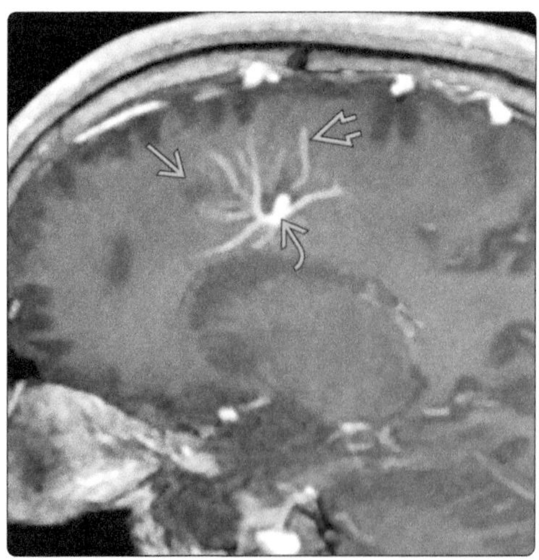

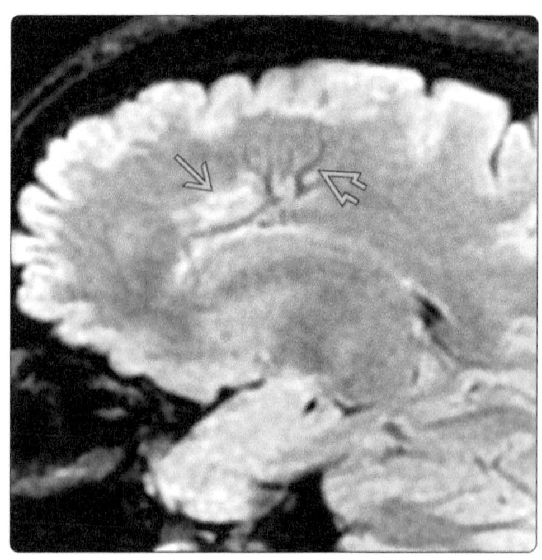

(Left) *Sagittal T1 C+ MR MIP in a 15-year-old boy with a frontal lobe DVA shows the venous radicles → draining into a central vein ↗. Note the area of decreased signal ⇒ along the anterior DVA territory.* **(Right)** *Sagittal FLAIR MR in the same patient more clearly shows the signal abnormality → in the drainage territory of the DVA ⇒. Signal abnormality is seen in ~ 5% of all DVAs but is usually less obvious than in this case. The etiology of this signal remains uncertain but may represent gliosis demyelination, edema, etc.*

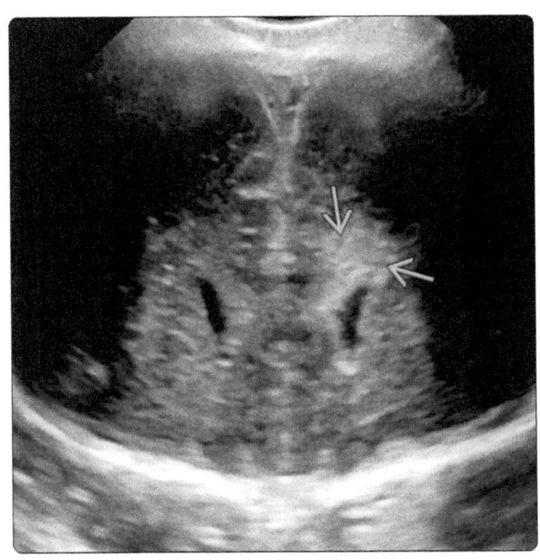

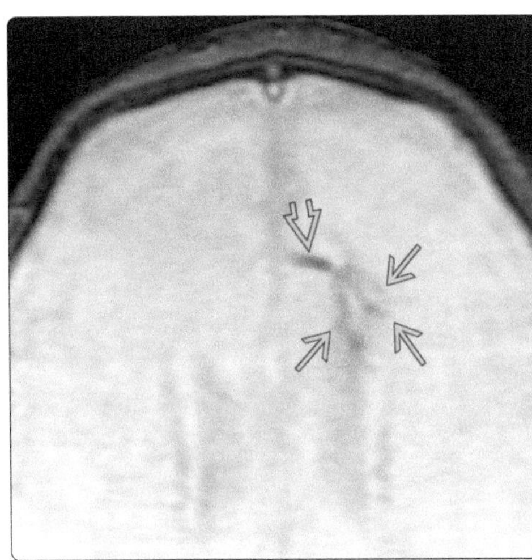

(Left) *Coronal US in a neonate shows an asymmetric area of increased echogenicity ➡ in the left frontal periventricular WM. Although hemorrhage &/or ischemia should be primary concerns, DVA is an important differential diagnosis. This is a common appearance for DVA on US.* **(Right)** *Axial SWI MR in the same neonate shows multiple venous radicles ➡ within the periventricular WM coalescing into a prominent draining vein ⇨, consistent with a DVA. The area of increased echogenicity on US corresponds to the drainage territory of the DVA.*

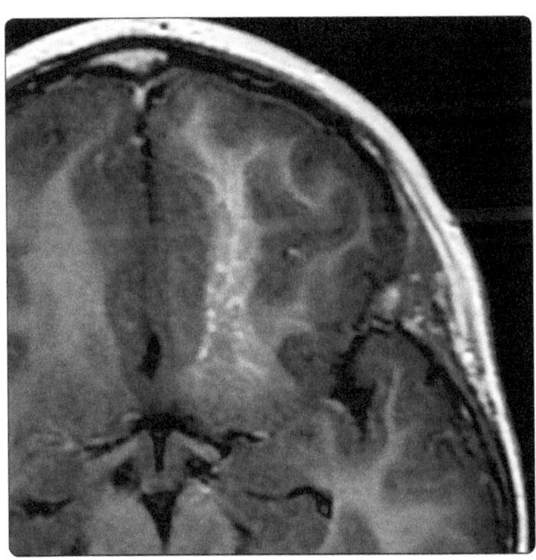

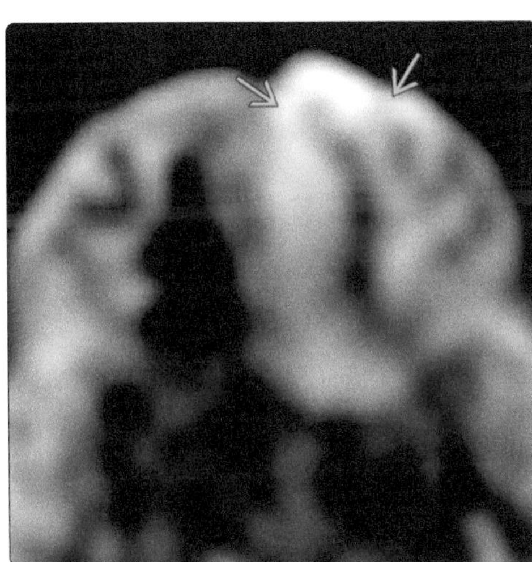

(Left) *Axial T1 C+ MR shows an extensive left frontal DVA. Companion ASL perfusion shows increased signal throughout the drainage territory of this DVA.* **(Right)** *Axial ASL in the same patient shows increased signal ➡ within the drainage territory of a large DVA. Perfusion abnormalities are common in the drainage territory of moderate to large DVAs. The most common ASL finding is increased cerebral blood flow. The most common contrast-enhanced perfusion finding is increased mean transit time and cerebral blood volume.*

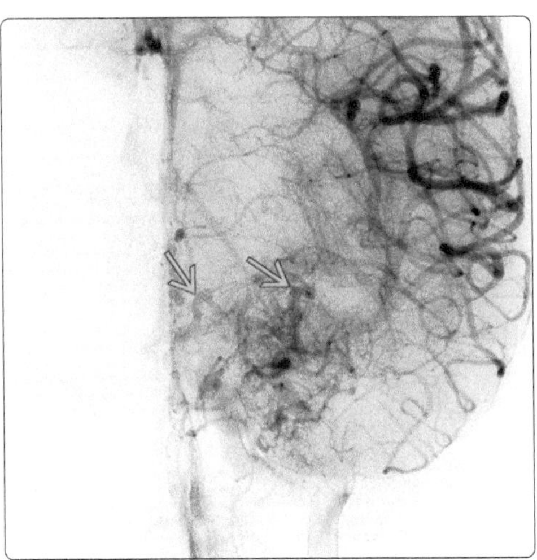

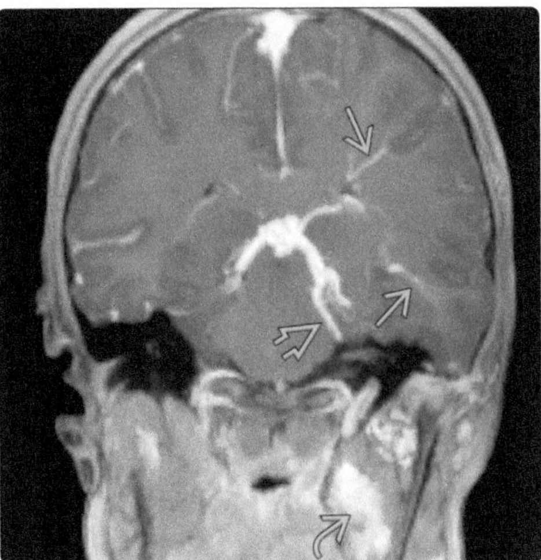

(Left) *AP view of a left internal carotid artery injection DSA shows opacification of the collecting vein ➡ of a DVA during the later arterial phase. Such findings are consistent with an arterialized DVA.* **(Right)** *Coronal T1 C+ MR in a teen with vascular malformation syndrome shows a holohemispheric DVA and left pterygoid venous malformation ↗. Note the venous radicles ➡ in the left cerebral hemisphere and a central vein ⇨ draining a left cerebellar DVA. Large DVAs are associated with venous malformation syndromes.*

Cavernous Malformation

KEY FACTS

TERMINOLOGY

- Benign vascular lesion with dilated sinusoids lined by thin, immature walls & containing blood products of various ages

IMAGING

- Cavernous malformations (CMs) occur throughout CNS
- Vary in size from microscopic to giant (> 6 cm)
- **CT**: Hyperdense lesion ± Ca^{++}; 50% not visible
- **MR**: Heterogeneous core with T2-hypointense rim
  - Popcorn ball appearance with internal fluid-fluid levels
  - Adjacent ↑ FLAIR signal suggests recent hemorrhage
  - SWI/T2* GRE most sensitive for small lesions

TOP DIFFERENTIAL DIAGNOSES

- Diffuse axonal injury
- Intracerebral hematoma
- Neoplasm
- Neurocysticercosis
- Capillary telangiectasia

PATHOLOGY

- Etiology: Initial parenchymal microhemorrhage followed by neoangiogenesis & recurrent hemorrhage
  - ↑ size from recurring intralesional hemorrhages
- Multiple (familial) CM syndrome: Autosomal dominant
  - *KRIT1*, *CCM2*, *PDCD10* genes; variable penetrance
- 25% of CMs associated with DVAs

CLINICAL ISSUES

- 0.6% incidence in children undergoing brain MR
- Symptoms: 1/2 incidental; 1/4 seizures; 1/4 neurologic deficits
- 70% solitary; 30% multiple (in familial & prior XRT)
- Treatment: Total surgical excision, sparing DVA

DIAGNOSTIC CHECKLIST

- Use SWI or T2* GRE for detection of small lesions
- Contrast administration will show associated DVA
- Imaging pearl: Giant CMs can mimic neoplasm

(Left) *Axial NECT in a 1-year-old with focal facial seizures shows heterogeneous high attenuation ➔ in right frontal lobe with low attenuation (edema) ⇨ deep to the lesion.* **(Right)** *Axial T1 (L) and T1 C+ (R) MRs in the same patient demonstrate intrinsically high signal ⇨ (Zabramski type I) in the lesion with multiple small vessels ➔ along the medial margin coalescing into a draining vein ➔, consistent with a developmental venous anomaly (DVA). 25% of cavernous malformations (CMs) are associated with DVAs.*

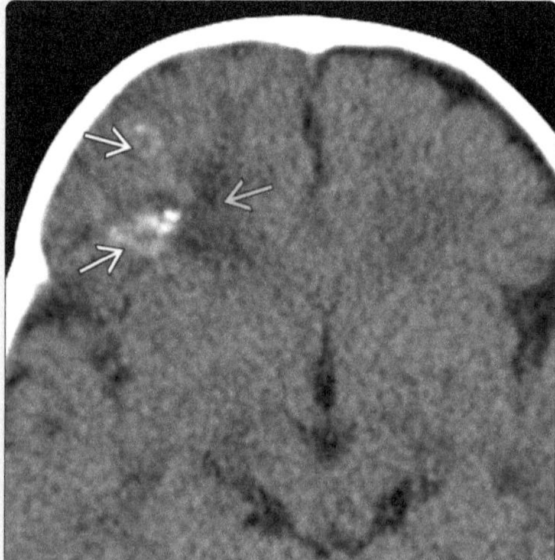

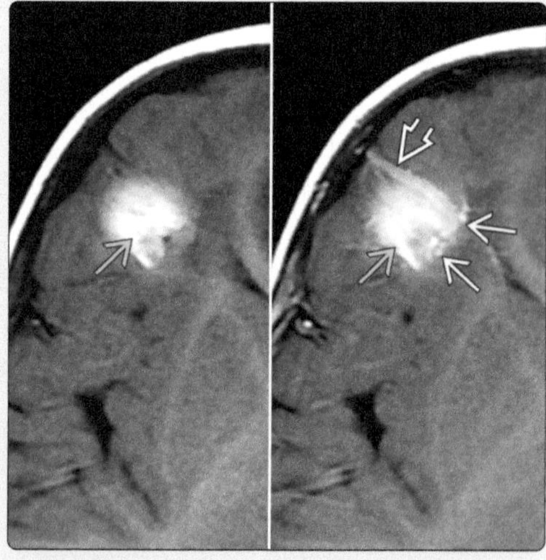

(Left) *Axial T2 MR in a 16-year-old with a severe headache shows the typical appearance of CM with heterogeneously hyperintense signal centrally with an incomplete rim of dark hemosiderin ⇨. The adjacent brain edema ⇨ suggests recent hemorrhage.* **(Right)** *Axial SWI MR in a 15-year-old with multiple familial CM syndrome shows 4 small areas of signal loss, consistent with CMs. Some of these lesions are only subtly visible on T2 (not shown). Note the DVA ⇨ associated with the right frontal CM ⇨.*

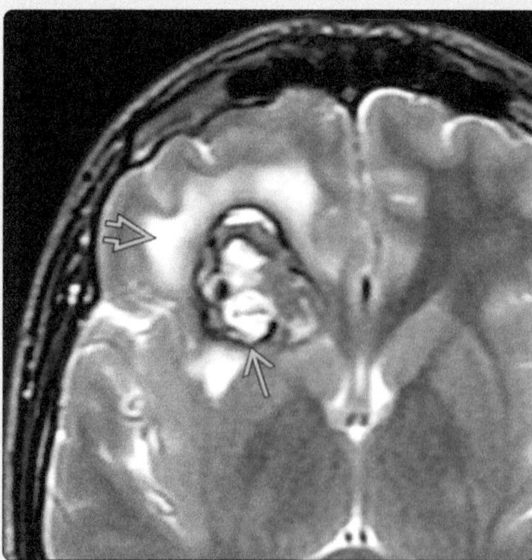

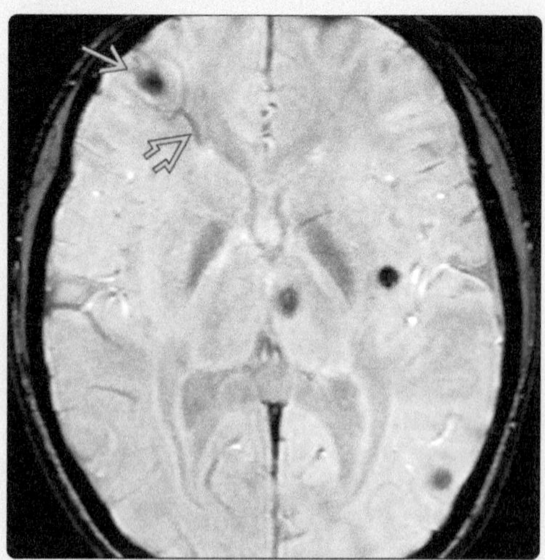

TERMINOLOGY

Abbreviations

- Cavernous malformation (CM)

Synonyms

- Cavernoma, cavernous hemangioma, cavernous angioma, angiographically occult vascular malformation

Definitions

- Benign vascular lesion arising in CNS
- Consists of dilated sinusoids containing blood products of various ages & lined by thin, immature walls

IMAGING

General Features

- Best diagnostic clue
  - Popcorn ball appearance with hypointense hemosiderin rim on T2 MR
- Morphology
  - Discrete, lobulated mass of interwoven vessels
  - Locules of variable size containing blood products at different stages of evolution
  - Complete hemosiderin rim surrounds lesion
  - Fluid-fluid levels often seen
- Location: Can be found throughout CNS
  - Supratentorial in ~ 80%
    - Frontal (26%), parietal (23%), temporal (15%), occipital (13%), basal ganglia/thalamus (5%)
  - Infratentorial in ~ 20%
    - Brainstem (10%), cerebellum (10%)
  - Rarely in spinal cord, except in multiple CMs
  - Extraaxial CMs rare
    - Can originate from within any venous sinus
    - Cavernous sinus most common site
    - May attain large size before becoming symptomatic
- Vary in size from microscopic to giant (> 6 cm)

CT Findings

- **NECT**: Round or irregular hyperdense lesion
  - ± hemorrhage & associated perilesional edema
  - Often shows small areas of Ca^{++}
  - CT negative in up to 50%, especially for small lesions
- **CECT**: No enhancement of actual lesion
  - ± associated developmental venous anomaly (DVA)
- **CTA:** CM itself should appear identical to NECT
  - CMs angiographically occult

MR Findings

- **T1WI**: Heterogeneous with blood of varied ages & Ca^{++}
  - Common: Popcorn ball appearance of mixed hyper- & hypointense blood-containing locules
  - Less common: Acute hemorrhage (nonspecific)
- **T2WI**: Mixed-signal core with complete hypointense rim corresponding to hemosiderin
  - Numerous septations or locules
  - ± fluid-fluid levels of layering blood products
  - Small lesions may appear as focal hypointensities
- **FLAIR**: Surrounding edema suggests recent hemorrhage
- **SWI/T2* GRE**: Exaggerated signal loss (blooming)
  - Most sensitive for detection of small CMs
    - Numerous punctate hypointense foci (black dots)
- **DWI**: Usually normal; may show susceptibility effect
- **T1WI C+**: Minimal or no enhancement
  - Associated enhancing DVA in ~ 25%
- **MRA**: Normal
  - CMs angiographically occult

Angiographic Findings

- DSA usually normal: Angiographically occult lesions

Imaging Recommendations

- Best imaging tool
  - MR is most sensitive for detection (SWI or GRE)
- Protocol advice
  - Use SWI or T2* GRE for detection of small lesions
  - Contrast administration will show associated DVA
    - SWI also often demonstrates associated DVA

DIFFERENTIAL DIAGNOSIS

Diffuse Axonal Injury

- Multiple small foci of hemosiderin deposition
- History of prior trauma with severe neurologic impairment

Venous Infarction

- More often hemorrhagic compared to arterial infarction
- Less complex-appearing; no hemosiderin ring if acute
- Old venous infarct may mimic Zabramski type III CM

Intracerebral Hematoma

- Usually more simple-appearing
- No hemosiderin at acute presentation
- Predisposing risk factors
  - Trauma; hypertension

Neoplasm

- Hemorrhage or Ca^{++} in primary brain tumor
- Often has enhancing soft tissue component
  - Pre- & postcontrast subtraction imaging can be helpful

Neurocysticercosis

- Chronic calcific phase mimics familial CM with many small CNS Ca^{++}

Capillary Telangiectasia

- Low signal on SWI/T2* GRE but no blooming
- Subtle enhancement following contrast administration

Hemorrhagic Metastases

- Rare in children & young adults
- Typically in patient with known primary tumor
- Usually show some degree of tumoral enhancement

PATHOLOGY

General Features

- Etiology
  - Initial microhemorrhage from variety of conditions followed by neoangiogenesis & recurrent hemorrhage
    - ↑ vascular permeability (familial CMs); ↑ venous flow/pressure (CMs associated with DVAs); small vessel injury (CMs associated with XRT)
  - May be congenital but usually acquired lesion with ↑ incidence in older patients

- Genetics
  - Sporadic CM
    - No *KRIT1* mutation
    - *PTEN* promoter methylation mutation common (also in familial CM syndrome)
  - Multiple (familial) CM syndrome: Autosomal dominant
    - Nonsense, frame-shift, or splice-site mutations consistent with 2-hit model for CM
    - Variable penetrance
      - Tend to present earlier than sporadic
    - 3 separate loci implicated: *KRIT1* (CCM1), *CCM2*, *PDCD10* (CCM3) genes
- Associated abnormalities
  - DVA: 25% of CMs have associated DVA; < 5% of DVAs have associated CM
    - Spontaneous CMs much more likely to be associated with DVAs
      - May be secondary to ↑ pressure or blood flow in DVA
    - No association between familial CMs & DVAs
  - Superficial siderosis

Staging, Grading, & Classification

- Zabramski classification of CMs
  - Type I: Subacute hemorrhage (↑ T1; ↑ or ↓ T2)
  - Type II: Reticulated mixed T1 & T2 with ↓ T2 rim
    - Classic popcorn ball appearance
  - Type III: Chronic hemorrhage (iso/↓ T1; ↓ T2)
    - Blooming on SWI/T2* GRE
  - Type IV: Tiny microhemorrhages only seen on SWI/T2*
    - Black dots appearance

Gross Pathologic & Surgical Features

- Discrete, lobulated, bluish purple (mulberry-like) nodule
  - Well-delineated collection of endothelial-lined, hemorrhage-filled vessels without intervening normal brain
  - Pseudocapsule of gliotic, hemosiderin-stained brain

Microscopic Features

- Angioarchitecture
  - Bland regions within thin-walled caverns
  - Honeycombed regions with notable capillary proliferation
- Dilated sinusoidal vessels lined by flattened endothelium
  - Absent smooth muscle layer & fibrous adventitia
  - Hemorrhage in different stages of evolution
  - Embedded in collagenous matrix; ± Ca^{++}
  - Does not contain normal brain tissue

CLINICAL ISSUES

Presentation

- Most common signs/symptoms
  - Identified incidentally (40-50%)
  - Seizures (20-25%)
    - Supratentorial more likely to present with seizures
  - Neurologic deficit from hemorrhage (20-25%)
    - Infratentorial more likely to have neurologic deficit

Demographics

- ~ 0.6% prevalence in all children undergoing brain MR
  - 0.2% in infants; ↑ with age
- ~ 70% solitary, 30% multiple
  - Multiple, typically familial CMs & XRT induced

Natural History & Prognosis

- Broad range of dynamic behavior (may progress, enlarge, regress)
- De novo lesions may develop, typically in setting of familial CMs, radiation therapy, & DVAs
  - Familial CMs at high risk of forming new lesions
    - Estimated 1% risk of hemorrhage per lesion per year
- Factors that ↑ risk of symptomatic hemorrhage in children
  - Prior hemorrhage: 11.3% annually
    - 18.2% within 3 years; 4.8% thereafter
  - Brainstem location: 16.7% annually
  - Associated DVA: 9.7% annually
- Annual risk of hemorrhage also predicted by MR
  - Zabramski I & II: 23.4% (5-60% in literature)
  - Zabramski III: 3.4% (0-6% in literature)
  - Zabramski IV: 1.3%

Treatment

- Total removal via microsurgical resection
  - Decision for surgery involves weighing risks of rehemorrhage against surgical risks
  - Gamma knife radiosurgery for nonresectable lesions controversial
- If DVA present, venous drainage should be preserved
  - DVA represents only venous drainage pathway for brain within DVA drainage territory
  - DVA removal → venous injury & venous infarct

DIAGNOSTIC CHECKLIST

Consider

- Perform SWI/T2* GRE MR to look for additional lesions in patients with spontaneous intracranial hemorrhage

Image Interpretation Pearls

- Giant CMs can mimic neoplasm

SELECTED REFERENCES

1. Kuroedov D et al: Cerebral cavernous malformations: typical and atypical imaging characteristics. J Neuroimaging. 33(2):202-17, 2023
2. Kurihara N et al: Hemorrhage owing to cerebral cavernous malformation: imaging, clinical, and histopathological considerations. Jpn J Radiol. 38(7):613-21, 2020
3. Zhang S et al: A rupture risk analysis of cerebral cavernous malformation associated with developmental venous anomaly using susceptibility-weighted imaging. Neuroradiology. 62(1):39-47, 2020
4. Flemming KD et al: Baseline and evolutionary radiologic features in sporadic, hemorrhagic brain cavernous malformations. AJNR Am J Neuroradiol. 40(6):967-72, 2019
5. Neu MA et al: Susceptibility-weighted magnetic resonance imaging of cerebrovascular sequelae after radiotherapy for pediatric brain tumors. Radiother Oncol. 127(2):280-6, 2018
6. Brinjikji W et al: Prevalence of cerebral cavernous malformations associated with developmental venous anomalies increases with age. Childs Nerv Syst. 33(9):1539-43, 2017
7. Young A et al: Sensitivity of susceptibility-weighted imaging in detecting developmental venous anomalies and associated cavernomas and microhemorrhages in children. Neuroradiology. 59(8):797-802, 2017
8. Gross BA et al: The natural history of cerebral cavernous malformations in children. J Neurosurg Pediatr. 1-6, 2015
9. Nikoubashman O et al: Prospective hemorrhage rates of cerebral cavernous malformations in children and adolescents based on MRI appearance. AJNR Am J Neuroradiol. 36(11):2177-83, 2015

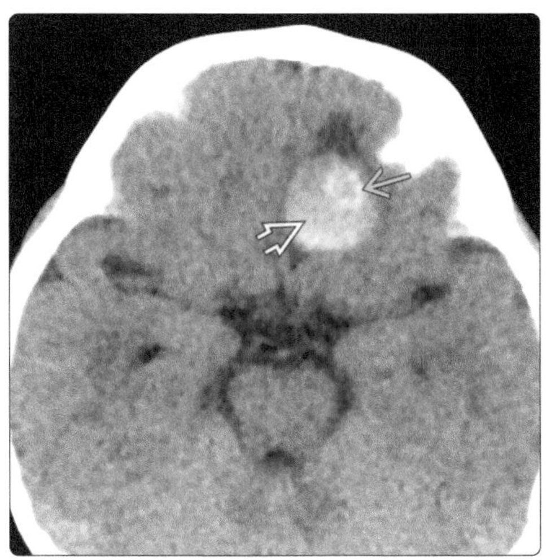

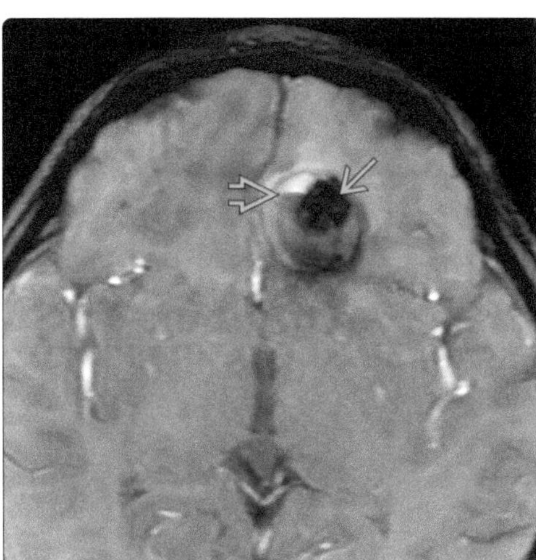

(Left) *Axial NECT in a 9-month-old with acute intraparenchymal hemorrhage ➡ shows a round calcific focus ➡ anteriorly within the hemorrhage, suggesting the source of the hemorrhage is a CM. Also note the vasogenic edema anteriorly, a common finding in hemorrhagic CMs.* **(Right)** *Axial SWI MR in the same patient shows an area of blooming ➡ in the region of the CM, a typical finding in CMs. Note the hematocrit level ➡ within the acute intraparenchymal hemorrhage.*

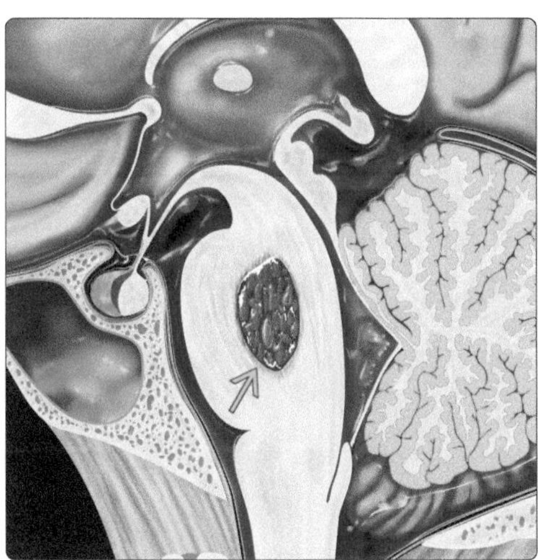

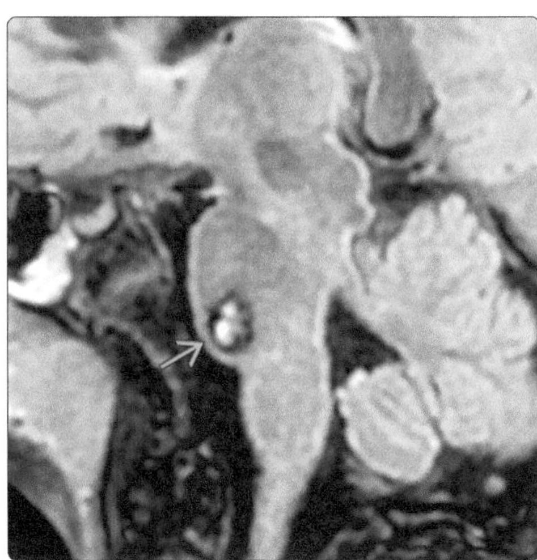

(Left) *Sagittal graphic shows a CM of the brainstem with multiple locules filled with blood in different stages of degradation. Note the orange hemosiderin ring ➡ along the margins of the CM.* **(Right)** *Sagittal FLAIR MR in a 13-year-old boy with familial multiple CMs shows a CM ➡ within the anterior pons. The appearance is typical with heterogeneously hyperintense central signal with a rim of dark hemosiderin. Most brainstem CMs present with cranial nerve dysfunction.*

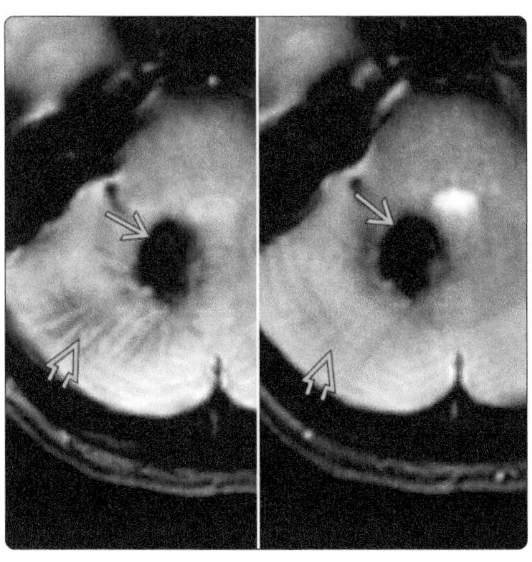

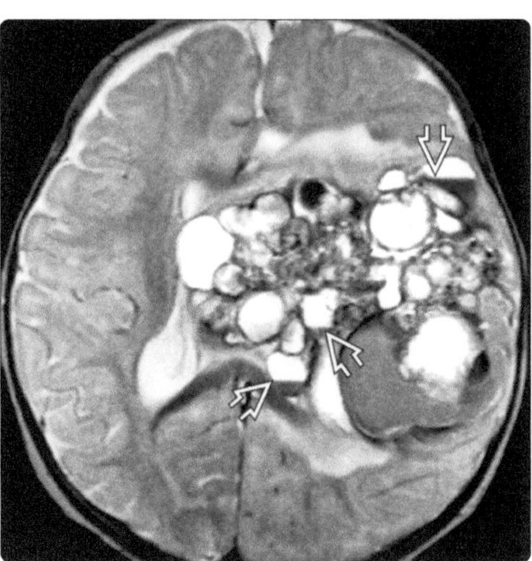

(Left) *Axial SWI (L) & T2* GRE (R) MR images in a 17-year-old boy with a right cerebellar CM ➡ show that the associated DVA ➡ is more conspicuous on SWI as compared to T2* GRE. SWI is the most sensitive sequence for detection of small Zabramski type IV CMs and associated DVAs.* **(Right)** *Axial T2 MR shows a giant CM in a young child. Note the fluid-fluid levels ➡ that confirm blood-filled caverns or locules. Giant CMs are often mistaken for CNS neoplasms.*

Capillary Telangiectasia

KEY FACTS

TERMINOLOGY

- Brain capillary telangiectasia (BCT)
- Cluster of enlarged, thin-walled capillaries surrounded and separated by normal brain [usually white matter (WM)]

IMAGING

- General features
  - Common sites: Pons, cerebellum, spinal cord
  - Usually < 1 cm
- CT
  - Usually normal
- MR
  - T1WI usually normal
  - T2WI
    - 50% normal on T2WI
    - 50% show faint stippled foci of hyperintensity
  - Large BCTs may show ill-defined FLAIR hyperintensity
  - Moderately hypointense on GRE; profoundly hypointense on SWI
  - T1 C+ shows faint stippled or speckled brush-like enhancement
  - Large BCTs typically contain prominent linear draining vein(s)

TOP DIFFERENTIAL DIAGNOSES

- Developmental venous anomaly
- Metastasis
- Cavernous malformation
- Capillary hemangioma

CLINICAL ISSUES

- BCTs represent 15-20% of all intracranial vascular malformations
- Usually found incidentally at autopsy or imaging
- Clinically benign, quiescent

DIAGNOSTIC CHECKLIST

- Faintly enhancing pontine lesion that becomes moderately hypointense on T2* is usually BCT

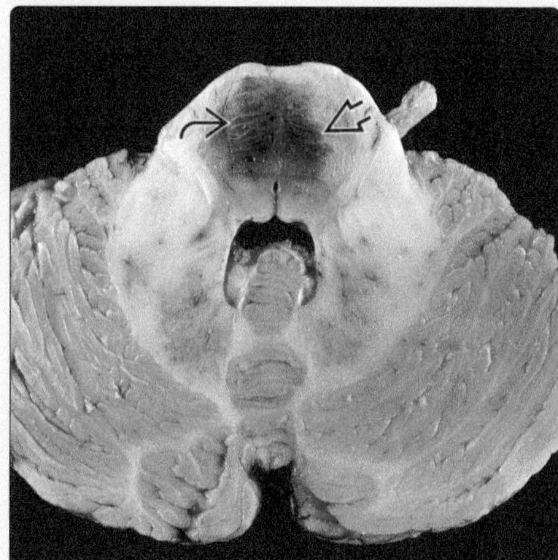

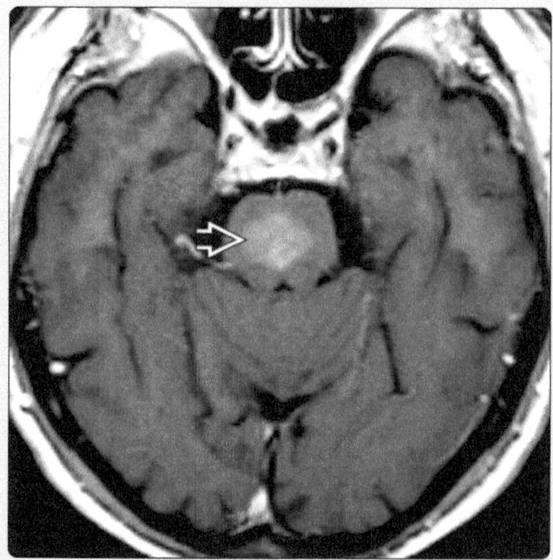

(Left) *Axial gross pathology shows a large capillary telangiectasia of the pons. The dusky color ➡ is caused by deoxygenated blood, not frank hemorrhage. Note undisturbed transverse pontine tracts ➡ crossing the telangiectasia.* **(Right)** *Axial T1 C+ MR in the same patient shows faint brush-like enhancement ➡ in the central pons, characteristic of a large capillary telangiectasia. (Courtesy P. Rodriguez, MD.)*

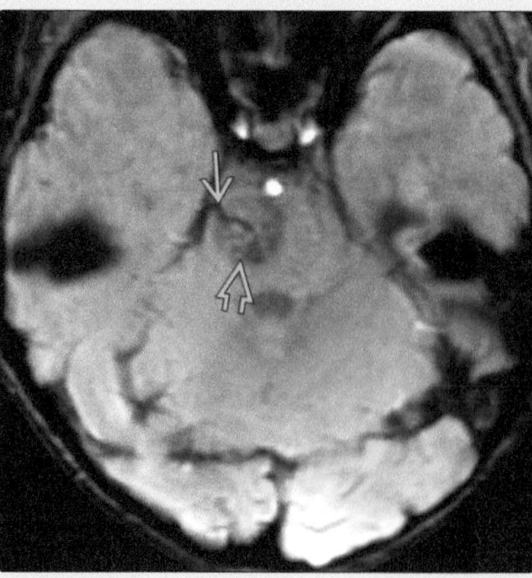

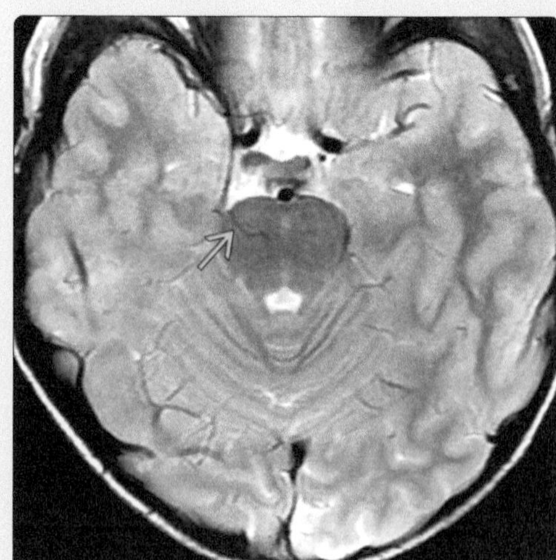

(Left) *Axial SWI in an 8-year-old shows a large pontine lesion with mild hypointensity throughout the round capillary telangiectasia ➡ with a prominent central draining vein ➡. SWI is a very sensitive sequence for detection of capillary telangiectasias.* **(Right)** *Axial T2 MR in the same patient shows no signal alteration within the right pons to correspond to the capillary telangiectasia other than the small flow void ➡ of the central draining vein. Lack of signal change on T2/FLAIR is typical for brain capillary telangiectasias (BCTs).*

TERMINOLOGY

Abbreviations

- Brain capillary telangiectasia (BCT)

Synonyms

- Capillary malformation
- **Not** capillary "hemangioma"
  - Hemangiomas are true benign vasoformative neoplasms
  - Usually in face, scalp, back, chest, orbit
  - Less common: Dura, venous sinuses
  - Exceptionally rare in brain parenchyma

Definitions

- Cluster of enlarged, thin-walled capillaries surrounded and separated by normal brain [usually white matter (WM)]

IMAGING

General Features

- Best diagnostic clue
  - Hypointense lesion on T2* with faint brush-like enhancement
- Location
  - Can be found anywhere
  - Most common sites
    - Pons
    - Cerebellum
    - Medulla
    - Spinal cord
  - Up to 1/3 in cerebral hemispheres
    - WM
    - Cortex
- Size
  - Usually < 1 cm
  - Occasionally "giant" (> 1 cm)
  - Solitary > > multiple
- Morphology
  - Small, poorly marginated
  - No mass effect
  - No edema

CT Findings

- NECT
  - Usually normal
  - Occasionally may show Ca^{++}
    - Usually only if mixed histology [most commonly cavernous malformation (CM)]
- CECT
  - Usually normal

MR Findings

- T1WI
  - Usually normal
  - May be hyperintense or hypo-/hyperintense (popcorn appearance) if mixed with CM
- T2WI
  - 50% normal
  - 50% show faint stippled foci of hyperintensity
- FLAIR
  - Usually normal
  - If large, may show ill-defined hyperintensity
  - No mass effect, edema
- T2* GRE
  - GRE
    - Lesion moderately hypointense
      - **Not** hemorrhage (unless mixed with CM)
      - Sluggish blood flow allows oxy- → deoxyhemoglobin
      - Do not typically bloom as would focal hemorrhage or CM
    - Occasionally multifocal BCTs seen as black or gray dots if mixed with CMs
  - SWI
    - SWI even more sensitive than standard T2*GRE
    - Lesion may be profoundly hypointense
- DWI
  - Usually normal
- PWI
  - Shows profound drop in signal intensity with relatively rapid recovery to baseline
- T1WI C+
  - Faint stippled or mild speckled brush-like enhancement
    - May have enlarged central draining vein with prominent linear enhancement
  - Large BCTs
    - Usually contain punctate, linear/branching vessel(s)
      - Represent radicles of draining veins
      - Larger "collector" vein often present
    - Mixed BCT with developmental venous anomaly (DVA) may occur
- DTI
  - BCTs are interspersed with normal WM tracts
  - No alteration of fractional anisotropy (FA)
  - No disturbance/displacement of WM tracts

Angiographic Findings

- Conventional
  - Usually normal
  - Faint vascular "stain" ± draining vein
  - Look for associated DVA

Imaging Recommendations

- Best imaging tool
  - MR with T2*, T1 C+ sequences
- Protocol advice
  - Include SWI

DIFFERENTIAL DIAGNOSIS

Developmental Venous Anomaly

- Often mixed with BCT
- Typically fan- or umbrella-shaped with distinct venous radicles draining to large central vein
- Typically does not have round or ovoid area of signal loss on SWI

Metastasis

- Strong > > faint enhancement
- Pons/cerebellum rare locations
- Associated with parenchymal signal changes on T2 and FLAIR

Cavernous Malformation

- Blood locules with fluid-fluid levels
- Complete hemosiderin rim
- Can be mixed with BCTs, cause hemorrhage
- CMs bloom with exaggerated loss of GRE/SWI signal
- CMs do not enhance

Capillary Hemangioma

- Vasoformative neoplasms, not congenital cerebrovascular malformations (CVMs)
- Dura, venous sinuses > > brain parenchyma

PATHOLOGY

General Features

- Etiology
  - Precise etiology of sporadic BCTs unknown
  - May develop as complication of radiation
    - 20% of children after whole-brain irradiation
- Genetics
  - May be related to mutated *SLPI*
    - ↑ perfusion → upregulated VEGF → ↑ capillary dysplasia
  - Capillary density increases with nonischemic venous hypertension
    - Hypoxia-inducible factor-1-α (HIF-1-α), downstream target VEGF upregulated
- Associated abnormalities
  - Often mixed with other vascular malformations (CMs, DVAs)
  - Hereditary hemorrhagic telangiectasia
    - a.k.a. Osler-Weber-Rendu disease
    - Autosomal dominant disorder
    - Often complicated by vascular malformations in brain, lung, GI tract, liver
      - Brain capillary vascular malformations most common phenotype in HHT
      - CTs also common in nasal mucosa (epistaxis, hemoptysis may be life threatening)
      - No correlation between HHT gene mutation, lesion type, or number
    - HHT-associated strokes usually secondary to pulmonary arteriovenous malformation (AVM)/AV, brain AVM with bleed, subarachnoid hemorrhage (SAH) with saccular aneurysm
  - Macrocephaly capillary malformation (MCM) syndromes
    - a.k.a. macrocephaly-cutis marmorata telangiectatica congenita (M-CMTC)
      - Facial nevus flammeus, cutis marmorata
    - Rapid brain growth during infancy
      - Megalencephaly, polymicrogyria
      - Tonsillar herniation
      - Ventriculomegaly, dilated dural venous sinuses
      - Prominent perivascular spaces (PVSs)
      - Skin > > brain capillary malformations

Gross Pathologic & Surgical Features

- Most BCTs found incidentally
  - Large BCTs may appear pinkish or slightly dusky
  - No hemorrhage unless other vascular malformation (e.g., CM) present

Microscopic Features

- Cluster of dilated but histologically normal capillaries
  - Thin-walled, endothelial-lined vascular channels
  - Largest channels may represent draining veins
- Normal brain interspersed between dilated capillaries
- Uncomplicated BCTs have no surrounding gliosis, hemorrhage, Ca^{++}

CLINICAL ISSUES

Presentation

- Most common signs/symptoms
  - Usually found incidentally at autopsy or imaging
  - Rare: Headache, vertigo, tinnitus
- Clinical profile
  - Asymptomatic, middle-aged patient with poorly delineated, enhancing brainstem lesion

Demographics

- Age
  - Any; 30-40 years most common
  - Rarely identified in children but does occur
- Epidemiology
  - 15-20% of all intracranial vascular malformations
  - Most common vascular malformation in HHT

Natural History & Prognosis

- Clinically benign, quiescent unless histologically mixed
- Rare reports of aggressive course

Treatment

- None

DIAGNOSTIC CHECKLIST

Image Interpretation Pearls

- Faintly enhancing pontine lesion that becomes moderately hypointense on T2* is usually BCT

SELECTED REFERENCES

1. Martín-Noguerol T et al: Conventional and advanced MRI evaluation of brain vascular malformations. J Neuroimaging. 31(3):428-45, 2021
2. Larson AS et al: Brain capillary telangiectasias: from normal variants to disease. Acta Neurochir (Wien). 162(5):1101-13, 2020
3. Brinjikji W et al: Natural history of brain capillary vascular malformations in hereditary hemorrhagic telangiectasia patients. J Neurointerv Surg. 9(1):26-8, 2016
4. Kalani MY et al: Developmental venous anomaly, capillary telangiectasia, cavernous malformation, and arteriovenous malformation: spectrum of a common pathological entity? Acta Neurochir (Wien). 158(3):547-50, 2016
5. Orgun LT et al: Symptomatic capillary telangiectasia of the pons: three pediatric cases diagnosed by suspectibility-weighted imaging. Childs Nerv Syst. 32(11):2261-4, 2016
6. Andrade CS et al: Giant symptomatic capillary telangiectasia of the brain. Arq Neuropsiquiatr. 73(1):66-7, 2015
7. Krings T et al: Neurovascular manifestations in hereditary hemorrhagic telangiectasia: imaging features and genotype-phenotype correlations. AJNR Am J Neuroradiol. 36(5):863-70, 2015
8. Chaudhry US et al: Susceptibility-weighted MR imaging: a better technique in the detection of capillary telangiectasia compared with T2* gradient-echo. AJNR Am J Neuroradiol. 35(12):2302-5, 2014
9. Gelal F et al: Capillary telangiectasia of the brain: imaging with various magnetic resonance techniques. JBR-BTR. 97(4):233-8, 2014
10. Gross BA et al: Cerebral capillary telangiectasias: a meta-analysis and review of the literature. Neurosurg Rev. 36(2):187-93; discussion 194, 2013
11. Ozcan HN et al: MRI findings in giant pontine capillary telangiectasis associated with a developmental venous anomaly. JBR-BTR. 94(5):293-4, 2011

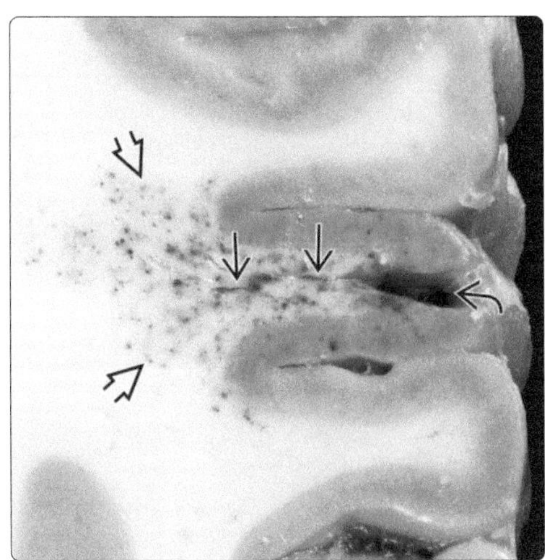

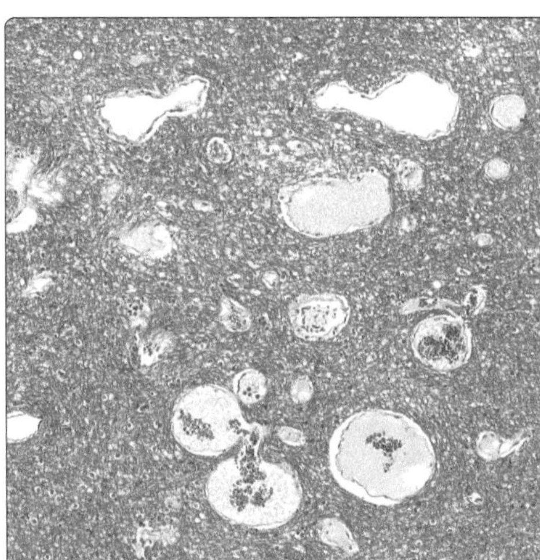

(Left) *Gross pathology shows a typical capillary hemangioma ⇨. Note normal-appearing white matter interspersed between the dilated capillaries. Many capillary telangiectasias have a prominent central vein → that drains into a cortical vein ↩.* **(Right)** *Luxol fast blue microscopic pathology in the same patient shows normal white matter (blue-stained tissue) between the dilated but histologically normal capillaries. (Courtesy P. Burger, MD.)*

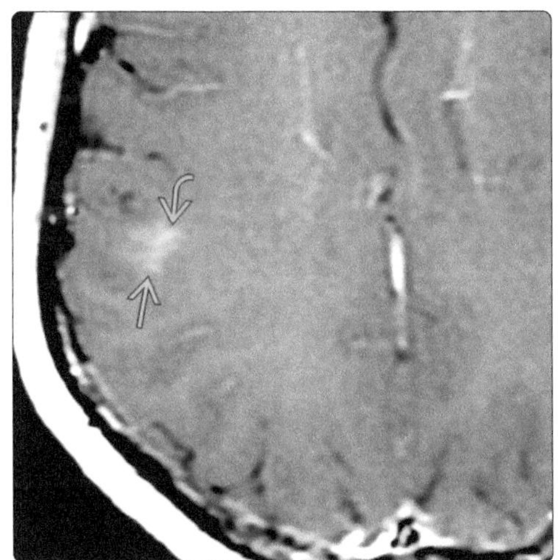

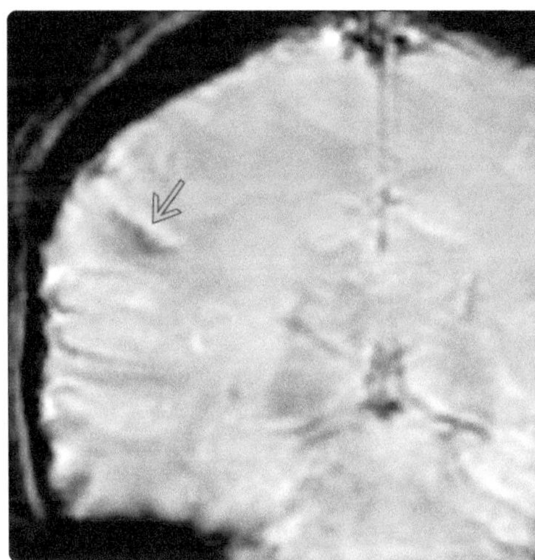

(Left) *Axial T1 C+ MR shows a blush of contrast → in the right parietal lobe with a central draining vein ↩, consistent with a capillary telangiectasia.* **(Right)** *Coronal SWI in the same patient shows signal loss without blooming →, characteristic for a capillary telangiectasia. While the pons is the most common location, capillary telangiectasia may occur anywhere in the brain, such as in this case.*

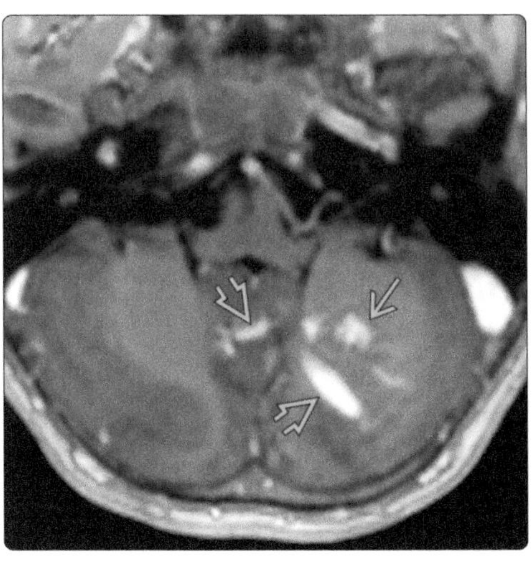

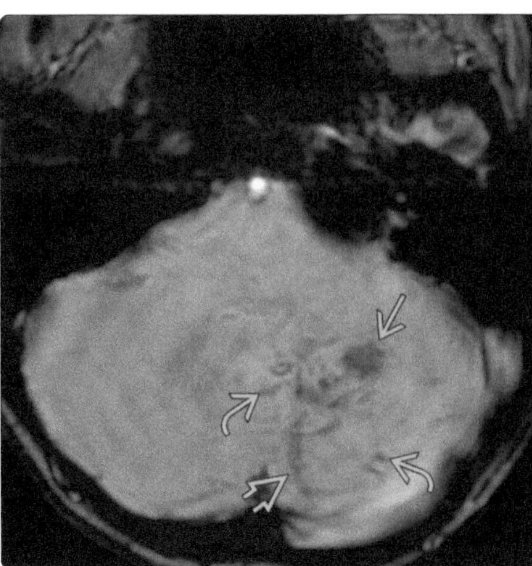

(Left) *Axial T1 C+ MR shows an enhancing area → within the drainage territory of a large cerebellar developmental venous anomaly (DVA). Note the large draining veins of the DVA ⇨. Although rare, capillary telangiectasias are found in association with DVAs.* **(Right)** *Axial SWI shows the capillary telangiectasia → to be hypointense without blooming, as is typical in capillary telangiectasia. Note the venous radicles ↩ and draining vein ⇨ of the DVA.*

KEY FACTS

TERMINOLOGY

- Anomalous communication between intracranial dural venous sinus (DVS), extracranial venous circulation

IMAGING

- CTV, MRV delineate all vascular components of sinus pericranii (SP)
  - Bone defect visualized on CT
  - 95% midline or parasagittal
    - Superior sagittal sinus most commonly involved

TOP DIFFERENTIAL DIAGNOSES

- Atretic cephalocele
  - Main DDx for SP is atretic cephalocele with herniated DVS
- Dermoid cyst
- Hemangioma

CLINICAL ISSUES

- Child with long history of painless, reducible scalp mass
- Excellent prognosis following surgical removal
- Surgery contraindicated if SP serves as major intracranial venous outflow or drains developmental venous anomaly (DVA)

DIAGNOSTIC CHECKLIST

- Describe contribution of SP to intracranial venous drainage
- Assess for associated DVA, other congenital venous variants
- Entire DVS network must be evaluated prior to SP removal (CTV/MRV)
- DSA may be required to delineate intracranial venous outflow, differentiate SP from atretic cephalocele with herniated DVS
  - 25% dominant (drain majority of intracranial venous outflow)
  - 75% accessory (drain only minority of outflow)

(Left) *Coronal graphic shows parasagittal sinus pericranii (SP). SP is composed of an intracranial varix ⮳, transosseous vein ➔, and developmental venous anomaly (DVA) ⇨ plus a scalp varix ➡. SPs are typically midline/paramedian scalp varices that communicate with superior sagittal sinus (SSS) via a transosseous vein &/or cortical vein.* **(Right)** *Axial CTV shows a small SP, seen here as a calvarial defect ➔ through which a scalp venous varix ⇨ drains into the SSS. No associated intracranial anomalies are present.*

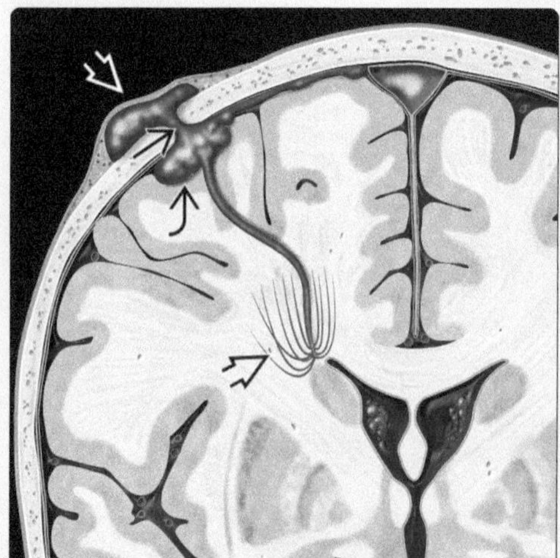

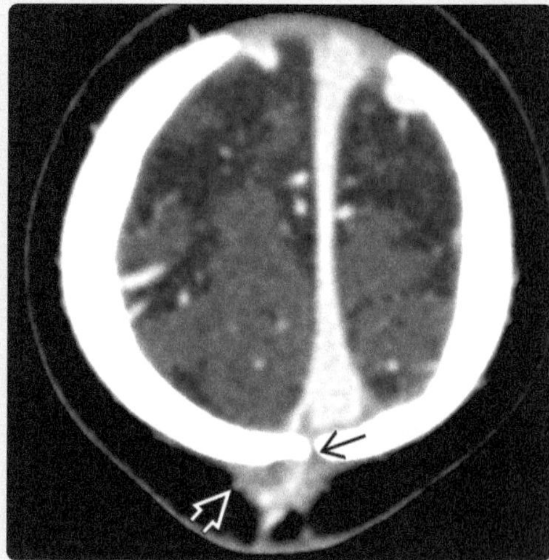

(Left) *Sagittal reformatted CTV in the same patient nicely shows the scalp varix ⇨ communicating through a calvarial defect ➔ with the underlying SSS.* **(Right)** *Late venous-phase DSA shows a small SP with a venous varix ⇨ communicating with the SSS via a tiny transosseous vein ➔. This is an accessory-type SP.*

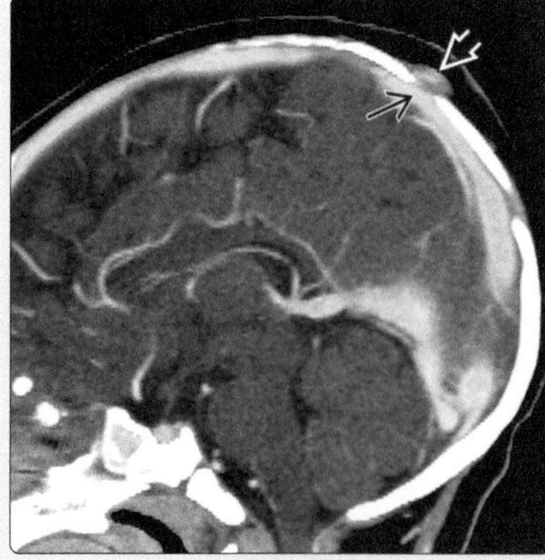

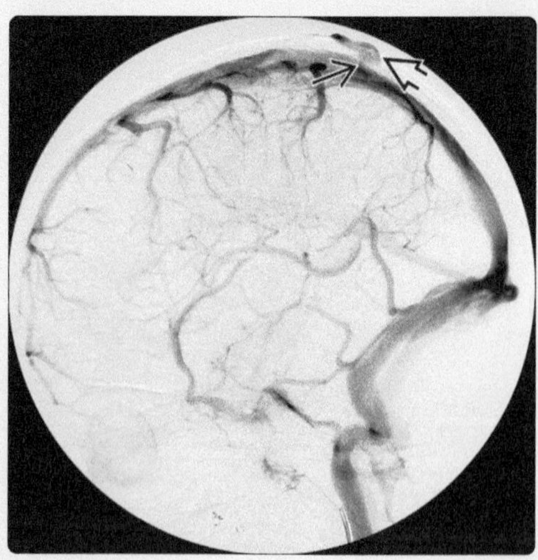

TERMINOLOGY

Abbreviations

- Sinus pericranii (SP)

Definitions

- Anomalous communication between intracranial dural venous sinus (DVS), extracranial venous circulation

IMAGING

General Features

- Best diagnostic clue
  - Vascular scalp lesion communicating with underlying DVS
- Location
  - 95% midline/parasagittal
    - Frontal (40%), parietal (34%), occipital (23%), temporal (4%)
  - Superior sagittal sinus (SSS) most commonly involved
    - Transverse sinus, torcular Herophili uncommon
- Size
  - Scalp lesion: 1-13 cm; most 2-6 cm
  - Bone defect: 1-4 mm (large defect rare)
- Morphology
  - Extracranial component
    - Most common = variably sized venous varix
    - Single or multiple enlarged vein(s)
    - True scalp venous malformation (VM) or arteriovenous malformation rare
  - Intracranial component
    - Midline SP: Direct transosseous communication with SSS
    - Parasagittal SP: Prominent cortical/scalp vein(s) connects with DVS
    - ± associated developmental venous anomaly (DVA)

CT Findings

- NECT
  - Homogeneous soft tissue density scalp mass
    - Septations, cysts, phleboliths rare (usually with VM)
  - Bone algorithm
    - Single/multiple, well-defined bone defect(s)
    - Pressure erosion from overlying varix/VM
- CECT
  - Intense, well-delineated enhancement
    - Heterogeneous if thrombus present or VM
- CTV: Best for delineating vascular components

MR Findings

- T1WI
  - Most iso-, hypo-, or mixed iso-/hypointense
    - Hyperintense if subacute thrombus present
    - Flow void if rapidly flowing varix/VM
- T2WI
  - Most hyperintense
    - Mixed signal in large varix/VM secondary to turbulent flow
    - Flow voids in rapidly flowing varix/VM
- T1WI C+
  - Intense, sharply demarcated enhancement
    - Heterogeneous if thrombus present
    - Peripheral/solid enhancement if VM
- MRV
  - Delineates all vascular components of SP

Ultrasonographic Findings

- Grayscale ultrasound
  - Hypoechoic scalp mass and transosseous feeder(s)
  - Shadowing from skull limits intracranial evaluation
- Color Doppler
  - Demonstrates direction of flow

Angiographic Findings

- Late venous phase delineates connection between DVS, extracranial veins

Other Modality Findings

- Percutaneous venography (PV)
  - Visualization of scalp veins
  - Visualization of transosseous vein, DVS inconstant

Imaging Recommendations

- Best imaging tool
  - CTV, T1 C+ MR/MRV
    - Both suitable for delineation of SP, associated intracranial anomalies
    - Bone defect best visualized on CT
- Protocol advice
  - DSA may be required to assess intracranial venous drainage preoperatively

DIFFERENTIAL DIAGNOSIS

Atretic Encephalocele

- Small herniation of intracranial contents through skull defect
- No enhancement unless vessels/DVS also herniate
- May be difficult to distinguish from SP on MR alone

Dermoid Cyst

- Well-defined fluid or fat density lesion
- Anterior fontanelle/bregma location classic

Hemangioma

- Intensely enhancing mass with flow voids
- Characteristic evolution

Rhabdomyosarcoma, Langerhans Cell Histiocytosis, Neuroblastoma Metastases

- Enhancing, destructive mass
- Invasion of DVS appears as filling defect

PATHOLOGY

General Features

- Etiology
  - Majority congenital
    - Probable anomalous venous development during late embryogenesis
    - Incomplete sutural fusion over prominent/abundant diploic or emissary veins
    - In utero DVS thrombosis
  - Traumatic

    - Disruption of emissary veins at outer table
    - Laceration or DVS thrombosis
  - Spontaneous
    - Secondary to remote, "forgotten" trauma
    - Subclinical, postnatal DVS thrombosis
- Associated abnormalities
  - DVA
  - Systemic VMs
  - Blue rubber bleb nevus syndrome
  - Multisutural craniosynostosis
    - SP forms secondary to DVS/internal jugular vein hypoplasia/atresia or intracranial hypertension
  - Isolated reports of cutis aplasia congenita

Staging, Grading, & Classification

- Based on intracranial venous outflow
  - 25% dominant (drain majority of intracranial venous outflow)
  - 75% accessory (drain only minority of outflow)

Gross Pathologic & Surgical Features

- Scalp varix/VM: Bluish, blood-filled sac or network of sacs beneath > above calvarial periosteum

Microscopic Features

- Scalp varix/VM: Nonmuscular venous channel(s)
  - Endothelial lining = congenital origin
  - Fibrous lining/capsule = traumatic origin
  - ± hemosiderin-laden macrophages, thrombus

CLINICAL ISSUES

Presentation

- Most common signs/symptoms
  - Painless nonpulsatile forehead/scalp mass (10% bluish discoloration)
    - Reduces in upright position
    - Distends when prone, with Valsalva, or crying
  - Rare: Pain, headache, nausea, dizziness
- Clinical profile
  - Child with long history of painless, reducible scalp mass

Demographics

- Age
  - Range: 0-70 years
    - Usually discovered in children, young adults
- Sex
  - Slight female predominance
- Epidemiology
  - Rare
    - 11% of patients presenting for treatment of craniofacial VMs

Natural History & Prognosis

- Not clearly understood
  - Usually stable, benign; rare spontaneous regression
  - Potential lifetime risk of hemorrhage, air embolus if SP injured is unknown
- Prognosis excellent following surgical removal

Treatment

- Observation may be appropriate in some cases
- Evaluate entire DVS network to ensure feasibility of SP removal
  - Surgery contraindicated if SP is dominant type
- Surgery
  - Ligation of transosseous emissary vein(s), removal of scalp lesion, closure of bone hole(s) with bone wax
- Endovascular therapy
  - Suitable for accessory SP
  - Transvenous or direct percutaneous embolization (coils, glue)

DIAGNOSTIC CHECKLIST

Consider

- Blue rubber bleb nevus syndrome if SP associated with multiple intracranial DVAs

Image Interpretation Pearls

- Assess for associated intracranial venous anomalies (DVA), congenital venous variants
- Entire DVS network must be evaluated prior to SP removal
- Diagnostic imaging appearance characteristic
  - Unless thrombosed, main DDx is cephalocele with herniated DVS

Reporting Tips

- Describe contribution of SP to intracranial venous drainage

SELECTED REFERENCES

1. Sharma A Sr et al: Sinus pericranii (parietal and occipital) with epicranial varicosities in a case of craniosynostosis. Cureus. 14(2):e21891, 2022
2. Khodarahmi I et al: Imaging spectrum of calvarial abnormalities. Radiographics. 41(4):1144-63, 2021
3. Ryu JY et al: Combined treatment of surgery and sclerotherapy for sinus pericranii. Arch Craniofac Surg. 21(2):109-13, 2020
4. Manjila S et al: A review of extraaxial developmental venous anomalies of the brain involving dural venous flow or sinuses: persistent embryonic sinuses, sinus pericranii, venous varices or aneurysmal malformations, and enlarged emissary veins. Neurosurg Focus. 45(1):E9, 2018
5. Ryorin M et al: Dynamic morphological changes of thrombosed lateral sinus pericranii revealed by serial magnetic resonance images. Childs Nerv Syst. 34(1):143-8, 2018
6. Bouali S et al: Spontaneous involution of a sinus pericranii. Childs Nerv Syst. 33(9):1435-7, 2017
7. Sanders FH et al: Extremely large sinus pericranii with involvement of the torcular and associated with Crouzon's syndrome. Childs Nerv Syst. 33(9):1445-9, 2017
8. Pavanello M et al: Sinus pericranii: diagnosis and management in 21 pediatric patients. J Neurosurg Pediatr. 15(1):60-70, 2015
9. Saba R et al: Sinus pericranii in a young adult with chronic headache. BMJ Case Rep, 2013
10. Akram H et al: Sinus pericranii: an overview and literature review of a rare cranial venous anomaly (a review of the existing literature with case examples). Neurosurg Rev. 35(1):15-26; discussion 26, 2012
11. Kanavaki A et al: Sinus pericranii: a scalp mass in a 6-month-old boy. Pediatr Neurosurg. 48(2):126-8, 2012
12. Kim YJ et al: Sonographic features of sinus pericranii in 4 pediatric patients. J Ultrasound Med. 2011 Mar;30(3):411-7. Erratum in: J Ultrasound Med. 30(5):684, 2011
13. Rozen WM et al: Spontaneous involution of two sinus pericranii - a unique case and review of the literature. J Clin Neurosci. 15(7):833-5, 2008
14. Gandolfo C et al: Sinus pericranii: diagnostic and therapeutic considerations in 15 patients. Neuroradiology. 49(6):505-14, 2007
15. Nomura S et al: Association of intra- and extradural developmental venous anomalies, so-called venous angioma and sinus pericranii. Childs Nerv Syst. 22(4):428-31, 2006

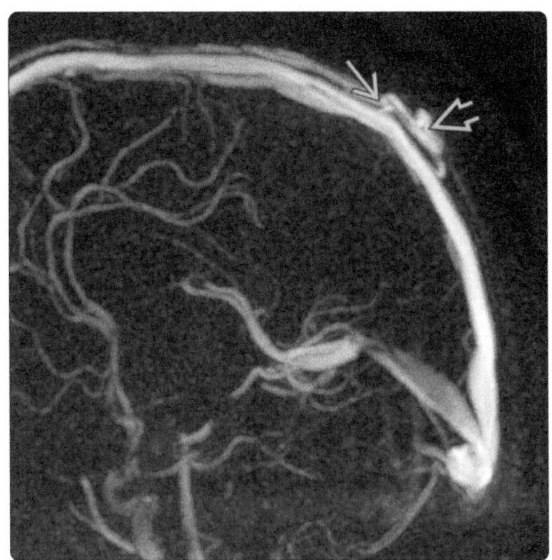

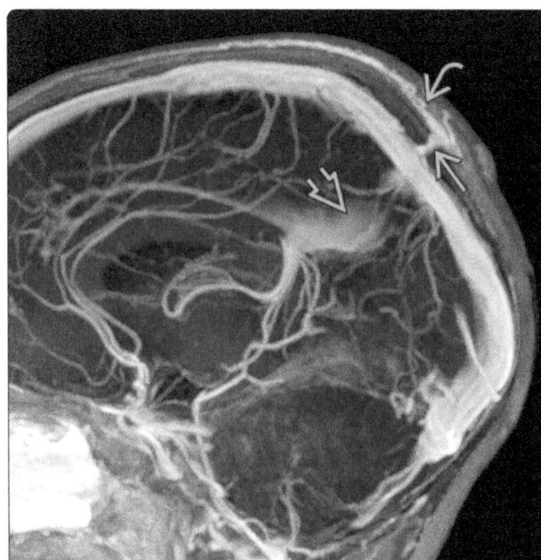

(Left) *Sagittal MRV in a 7-month-old with SP shows direct communication ➡ of a prominent collection of scalp veins ⇨ with the underlying SSS, consistent with SP.* **(Right)** *Sagittal T1 C+ MR MIP in a 5-year-old shows a persistent falcine sinus ⇨ with a direct communication ➡ from the SSS to a prominent collection of scalp veins ↷. Findings are consistent with an SP.*

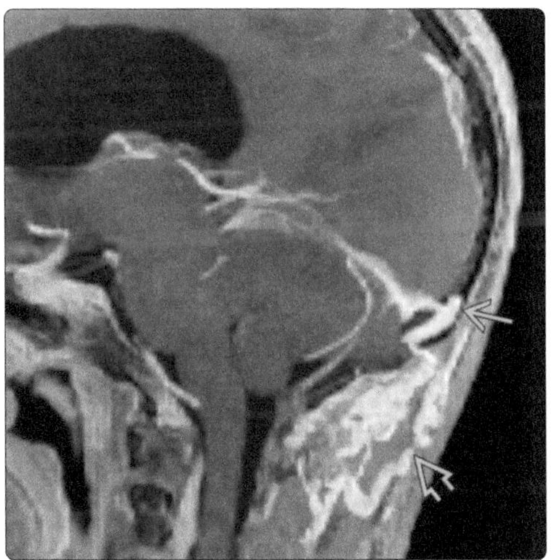

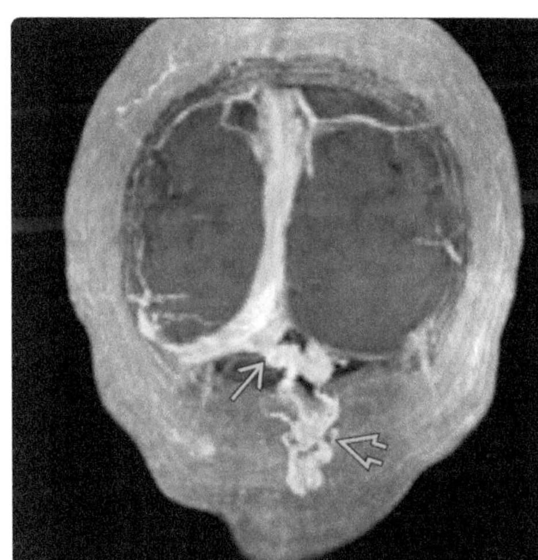

(Left) *Sagittal T1 C+ MR MIP in a 16-year-old boy with occipital SP shows a transcalvarial venous connection ➡ between the torcular Herophili and a tangle of tortuous veins ⇨ in the occipital scalp soft tissues.* **(Right)** *Coronal T1 C+ MR MIP in the same patient nicely shows the clear connection ➡ between the intracranial venous system and the prominent tortuous scalp veins ⇨.*

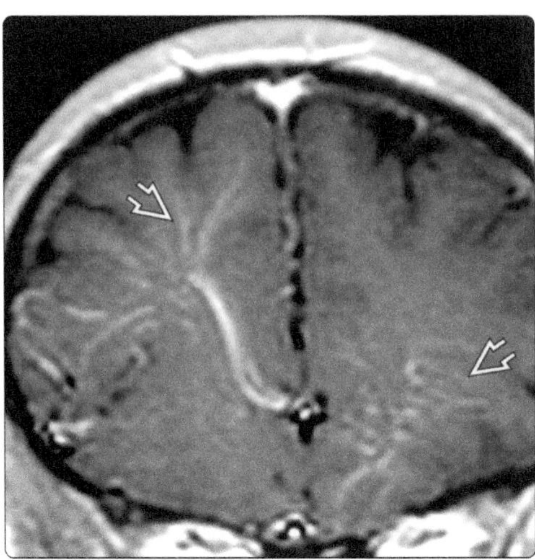

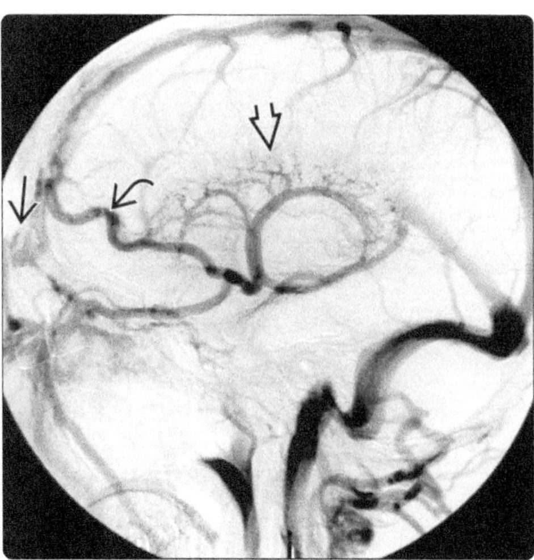

(Left) *Coronal T1 C+ MR in the same patient shows bilateral developmental venous anomalies ⇨.* **(Right)** *Lateral venous-phase DSA shows a huge DVA ⇨ and a large draining vein ↷ that communicates with the SP ➡. This is a dominant-type SP. (Courtesy J. Rees, MD.)*

Pilocytic Astrocytoma

KEY FACTS

TERMINOLOGY

- Pilocytic astrocytoma (PA)
  - WHO grade 1 astrocytic tumor
  - Most common primary brain tumor of children

IMAGING

- Location
  - Without neurofibromatosis type 1 (NF1): Cerebellum (midline or off-midline) > hypothalamus, brainstem, cerebral hemispheres > optic pathway (OP)
  - With NF1: OP most common
- Size: Cerebellar & cerebral lesions often > 5 cm
- > 95% enhance (patterns vary)
  - Nonenhancing cyst with enhancing mural nodule: 50%
  - Heterogeneous enhancement with smaller cysts: 40%
  - Solid, (typically) avid enhancement: 10%
- Ca^{++} in 20%; hemorrhage uncommon
- May show little surrounding vasogenic edema
- Often cause obstructive hydrocephalus
- ↑ diffusivity typical (unlike highly cellular tumors)
- Paradoxical aggressive-appearing MR spectroscopy
  - High choline, low NAA, ± lactate

TOP DIFFERENTIAL DIAGNOSES

- Posterior fossa: Medulloblastoma, ependymoma
- Hypothalamus/OP: Pilomyxoid astrocytoma, optic neuritis

PATHOLOGY

- Sporadic > syndromic
  - 15% of NF1 patients develop PAs: OP > brainstem
    - 50-60% of patients with OP PAs have NF1

CLINICAL ISSUES

- Location determines presentation, treatment, prognosis
  - Headaches, nausea/vomiting, cerebellar signs, visual loss
  - Cerebellar & cerebral lesions cured with total resection; OP lesions (especially NF1) may be observed for growth or visual loss prior to chemotherapy or radiation
- 10-year survival > 90%

(Left) *Axial T1 C+ MR in a 5-year-old shows a predominantly cystic lesion ➙ with a solid nodule ➙ centrally located in the right cerebellar hemisphere.* **(Right)** *Axial ADC (top) and ASL perfusion (bottom) MR images in the same patient show hyperintense signal in the solid component ➙, consistent with the paucicellularity of a pilocytic astrocytoma (PA). The ASL perfusion image shows low perfusion in the solid component ➙, typical for a PA. Perfusion imaging is helpful to differentiate a PA from hemangioblastoma.*

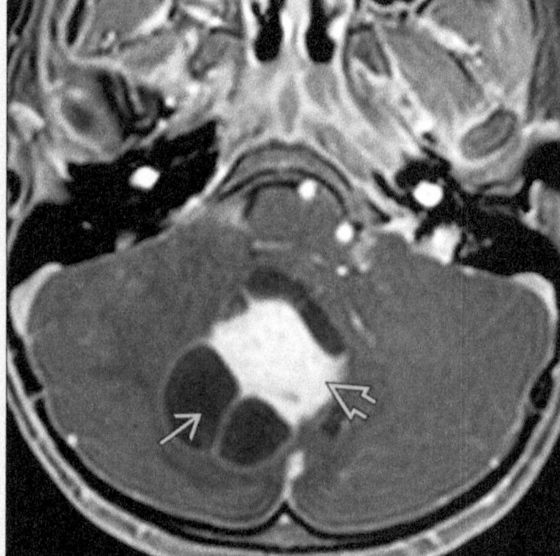

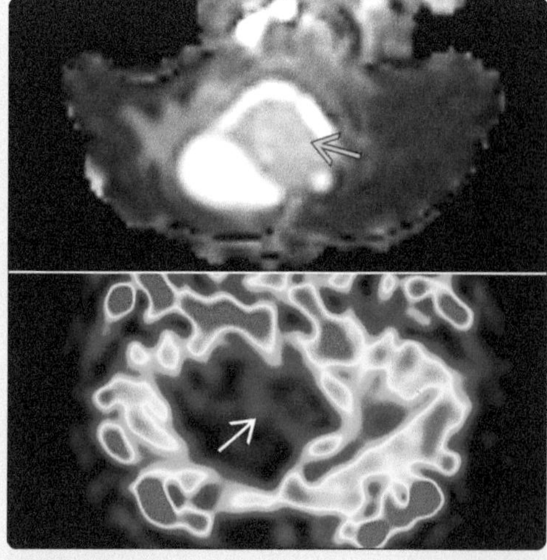

(Left) *Axial T2WI MR in a 9-year-old girl with headaches shows a solid-appearing midline mass ➙ with increased signal intensity that is slightly lower than CSF, typical for a PA.* **(Right)** *Axial ADC map in the same patient shows signal intensity in the mass ➙ that is much greater than the adjacent brain parenchyma. This increased diffusivity is typical of a PA. Diffusion characteristics can be helpful in distinguishing a PA from medulloblastoma, especially with midline tumors extending into the 4th ventricle.*

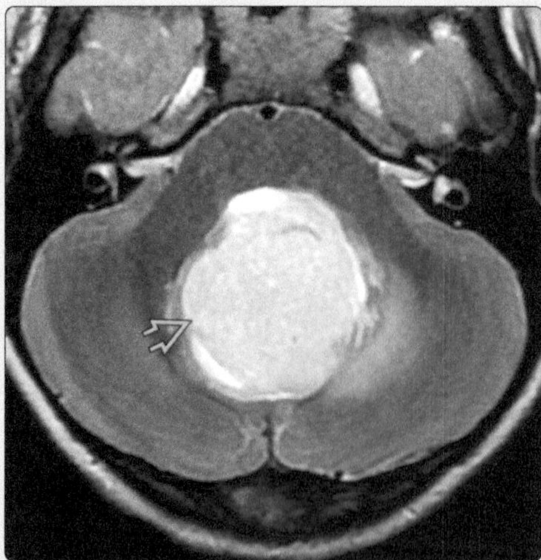

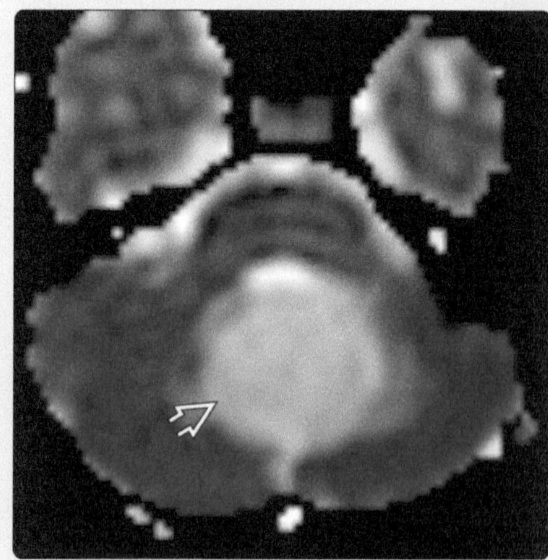

TERMINOLOGY

Abbreviations

- Pilocytic astrocytoma (PA)

Synonyms

- Juvenile pilocytic astrocytoma (JPA)

IMAGING

General Features

- Location
  - In patients without neurofibromatosis type 1 (NF1): Cerebellum > hypothalamus, brainstem, cerebral hemispheres > optic pathway (OP)
  - With NF1: OP most common
- Size
  - Cerebellar & cerebral lesions often > 5 cm
  - OP lesions typically smaller
- Morphology
  - Classic description: Cystic mass with enhancing mural nodule
  - OP lesions typically cause fusiform optic nerve enlargement & tortuosity

CT Findings

- Mixed cystic/solid mass
  - Solid component: Iso- or hypoattenuating to white matter
  - Cystic component: Similar attenuation to CSF
- Ca^{++} in 20%; hemorrhage rare
- Frequently cause obstructive hydrocephalus

MR Findings

- T1WI
  - Cyst contents iso- to slightly hyperintense to CSF
- T2WI
  - Solid portions hyperintense to gray matter (GM)
  - Cystic components usually equal to CSF
- FLAIR
  - Solid portions hyperintense to GM
  - Cyst contents iso- to hyperintense to nulled CSF
    - Can help determine relationship to 4th ventricle
  - May cause only mild surrounding vasogenic edema
- DWI
  - Variable, but classically bright on ADC (↑ diffusivity)
    - ↑ diffusivity typical in PA
- PWI
  - ASL: Cerebral blood flow (CBF) within tumor usually < GM
- T1WI C+
  - > 95% enhance (with exception of OP glioma)
    - 50% with large cyst & enhancing mural nodule
      - ± cyst wall enhancement
    - 40% with heterogeneous enhancement & small cysts
    - 10% with solid homogeneous enhancement
  - Many OP gliomas show no enhancement, especially when small
  - Leptomeningeal spread of tumor rare
- MRS
  - Paradoxical aggressive-appearing pattern
    - High Cho, low NAA ± lactate

Ultrasonographic Findings

- Grayscale ultrasound
  - Solid components hyperechoic relative to brain parenchyma
  - Cysts may contain debris

Imaging Recommendations

- Best imaging tool
  - Contrast-enhanced MR with DWI
- Protocol advice
  - Multiplanar or 3D volume postcontrast imaging key to showing point of origin & degree of extension
  - MRS pattern contradicts clinical behavior
  - Perfusion imaging helpful to distinguish pilomyxoid astrocytoma & hemangioblastoma

DIFFERENTIAL DIAGNOSIS

Medulloblastoma

- Midline posterior fossa mass with hyperattenuation (CT) & diffusion restriction (MR)
- Younger patient age (median: 6 years)
- Leptomeningeal metastases in ~ 1/3

Ependymoma

- "Plastic" tumor: Extends out 4th ventricle foramina
- Ca^{++}, cysts, hemorrhage common

Pilomyxoid Astrocytoma

- More aggressive, less common tumor; usually suprasellar
- Hemorrhage & ↑ arterial spin labeling perfusion suggestive
- More likely to disseminate in CSF

Atypical Teratoid-Rhabdoid Tumor

- Medulloblastoma mimic
  - Supra- or infratentorial mass with diffusion restriction but in younger patients (peak between 2-4 years of age)
  - Variable enhancement pattern

Ganglioglioma

- Solid/cystic, cortically based mass
- Ca^{++} common

Dysembryoplastic Neuroepithelial Tumor

- Cortical lesion, often cystic; enhancement uncommon
- May remodel overlying skull

Pleomorphic Xanthoastrocytoma

- Enhancing nodule abuts pia
- May remodel overlying skull

Hemangioblastoma

- Large cyst with small enhancing mural nodule
- Associated with von Hippel-Lindau disease
- May be distinguished from PA by ↑ relative cerebral blood volume (rCBV) & CBF in solid portion

Demyelination/Inflammation

- Optic neuritis can mimic optic nerve glioma
  - Will not cause ↑ optic nerve tortuosity

PATHOLOGY

General Features

- WHO grade 1, localized astrocytic neoplasm
  - Progression to higher grades uncommon
- Genetics
  - Sporadic (majority): *BRAF* gene (at chromosome 7q34) mutations most common, leading to activation of RAS/ERK/MAPK pathways
  - Syndromic: Loss of neurofibromin protein (*NF1* gene at 17q11.2) activates RAS pathway
    - 15-21% of NF1 patients develop PAs, usually of OP
      - 50-60% of OP PAs occur in NF1
      - 30% of all PAs occur in NF1

Gross Pathologic & Surgical Features

- Well-circumscribed, soft gray mass ± cyst

Microscopic Features

- Typically biphasic histologic pattern
  - Dense fibrillar piloid with Rosenthal fibers
    - Rosenthal fibers: Electron-dense GFAP staining cytoplasmic inclusions
  - Hypofibrillar spongy tissue
- Ki-67/MIB-1 indices usually 1-4%
- May infiltrate into parenchyma
- Rare development of malignant transformation
  - Some association with prior radiation therapy

CLINICAL ISSUES

Presentation

- Most common signs/symptoms
  - ↑ intracranial pressure: Headaches, nausea, vomiting
  - Cerebellar lesions: Ataxia, dysdiadochokinesia
  - OP lesions: Visual loss
- Clinical profile
  - Most common primary CNS tumor in children
    - Peak incidence in non-NF1: 5-15 years of age
  - Most common posterior fossa tumor in ages 5-19 years

Demographics

- Age
  - > 80% under 20 years old
- Sex
  - M = F

Natural History & Prognosis

- Typically slow growing
  - Mass effect tolerated due to accommodation
  - Some tumors may spontaneously regress
    - Especially lesions of OP, diencephalon, & tectum in NF1
- > 90% survival at 10 years
- Poorer prognosis: Solid lesions, brainstem extension, hypothalamic location, leptomeningeal spread, anaplasia
  - Pathology still demonstrates WHO grade 1 tumor

Treatment

- Cerebellar or cerebral locations: Surgical
  - Prognosis related to success of total resection
    - Complete resection curative
    - Tumor location primary determinant of resectability
  - Adjuvant chemotherapy or radiation only with residual progressive unresectable tumor
  - Molecular diagnosis is increasingly important for treatment
    - e.g., BRAF inhibitors in tumors with *BRAF* V600E mutations
  - Laser ablation increasingly used to treat nonresectable or recurrent PA
- OP: Often none
  - Stable or slowly progressive tumors observed, especially in NF1
  - Decision to treat driven by vision loss & tumor growth
  - Radiation or chemotherapy for progressive disease

DIAGNOSTIC CHECKLIST

Consider

- May rarely present with subarachnoid metastatic disease or as hemorrhagic mass

Image Interpretation Pearls

- Enhancing intraaxial tumor with cyst in 5-20 year old: Most likely PA
- Differentiating PA from other posterior fossa tumors
  - DWI key as PA shows ↑ (not restricted) diffusivity
  - PA more likely off-midline vs. ependymoma & medulloblastoma (centered in 4th ventricle)
  - Paradoxically aggressive MRS & PET imaging patterns

SELECTED REFERENCES

1. Cler SJ et al: Genetic and histopathological associations with outcome in pediatric pilocytic astrocytoma. J Neurosurg Pediatr. 29(5):504-12, 2022
2. Dury RJ et al: Meta-analysis of apparent diffusion coefficient in pediatric medulloblastoma, ependymoma, and pilocytic astrocytoma. J Magn Reson Imaging. 56(1):147-7, 2022
3. Kurokawa R et al: Differentiation of pilocytic astrocytoma, medulloblastoma, and hemangioblastoma on diffusion-weighted and dynamic susceptibility contrast perfusion MRI. Medicine (Baltimore). 101(44):e31708, 2022
4. Louis DN et al: The references 2021 WHO Classification of Tumors of the Central Nervous System: a summary. Neuro Oncol. 23(8):1231-51, 2021
5. Pehlivan KC et al: Clinical and neuroimaging features of magnetic resonance-guided stereotactic laser ablation for newly diagnosed and recurrent pediatric brain tumors: a single institutional series. World Neurosurg. 150:e378-87, 2021
6. Zhou X et al: Differentiation between supratentorial pilocytic astrocytoma and extraventricular ependymoma using multiparametric MRI. Acta Radiol. 63(12):1661-8, 2021
7. Ho CY et al: Differentiation of pilocytic and pilomyxoid astrocytomas using dynamic susceptibility contrast perfusion and diffusion weighted imaging. Neuroradiology. 62(1):81-8, 2020
8. McAuley E et al: The benefit of surveillance imaging for paediatric cerebellar pilocytic astrocytoma. Childs Nerv Syst. 35(5):801-5, 2019
9. Tabash MA: Characteristics, survival and incidence rates and trends of pilocytic astrocytoma in children in the United States; SEER-based analysis. J Neurol Sci. 400:148-52, 2019
10. Gaudino S et al: MR imaging of brain pilocytic astrocytoma: beyond the stereotype of benign astrocytoma. Childs Nerv Syst. 33(1):35-54, 2017
11. Alkonyi B et al: Differential imaging characteristics and dissemination potential of pilomyxoid astrocytomas versus pilocytic astrocytomas. Neuroradiology. 57(6):625-38, 2015
12. Collins VP et al: Pilocytic astrocytoma: pathology, molecular mechanisms and markers. Acta Neuropathol. 129(6):775-88, 2015
13. Nabavizadeh SA et al: High accuracy of arterial spin labeling perfusion imaging in differentiation of pilomyxoid from pilocytic astrocytoma. Neuroradiology. 57(5):527-33, 2015
14. Chourmouzi D et al: Manifestations of pilocytic astrocytoma: a pictorial review. Insights Imaging. 5(3):387-402, 2014
15. de Fatima Vasco Aragao M et al: Comparison of perfusion, diffusion, and MR spectroscopy between low-grade enhancing pilocytic astrocytomas and high-grade astrocytomas. AJNR Am J Neuroradiol. 35(8):1495-502, 2014

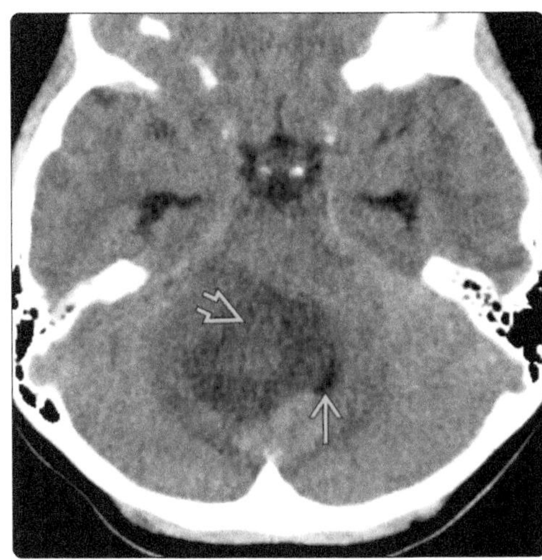

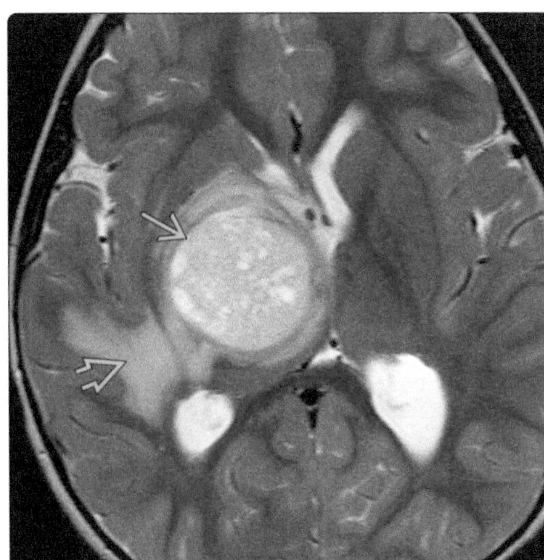

(Left) *Axial NECT of a cerebellar PA shows mass effect on the 4th ventricle ➔ from the hypodense tumor ➔. PAs will typically compress and displace the 4th ventricle, whereas medulloblastomas will fill and enlarge it.* **(Right)** *Axial T2WI MR in a patient with a PA shows a very hyperintense right basal ganglia mass ➔ with adjacent vasogenic edema ➔. PAs can arise anywhere in the supratentorial brain but are most often centered in the deep gray nuclei or white matter.*

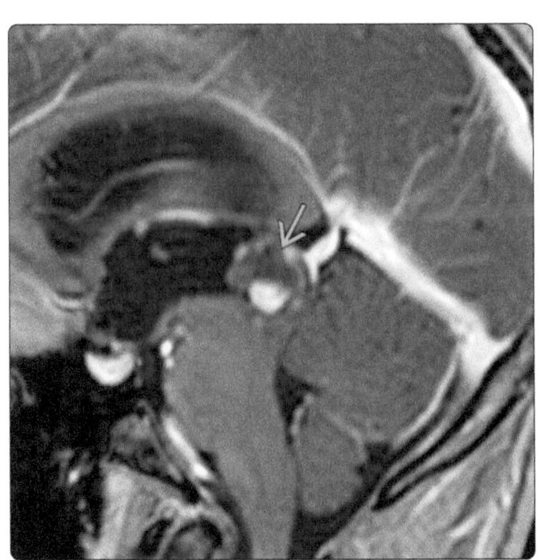

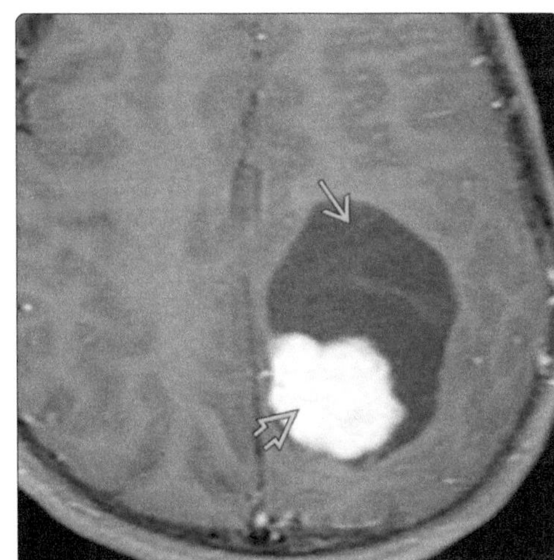

(Left) *Sagittal T1 C+ MR in a 12-year-old girl shows a partially enhancing mass centered in the tectal plate. Partially enhancing ➔ tectal plate masses are very likely to be PAs histologically.* **(Right)** *Axial T1 C+ MR in an 11-year-old shows a large cystic lesion ➔ with an avidly enhancing mural nodule ➔. This is the classic imaging appearance for a PA, but these imaging features are only seen in a minority of PAs. The spectrum of imaging appearance of a PA is quite broad.*

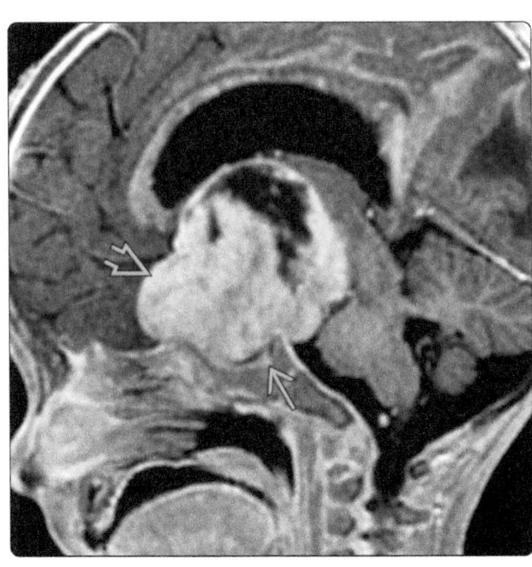

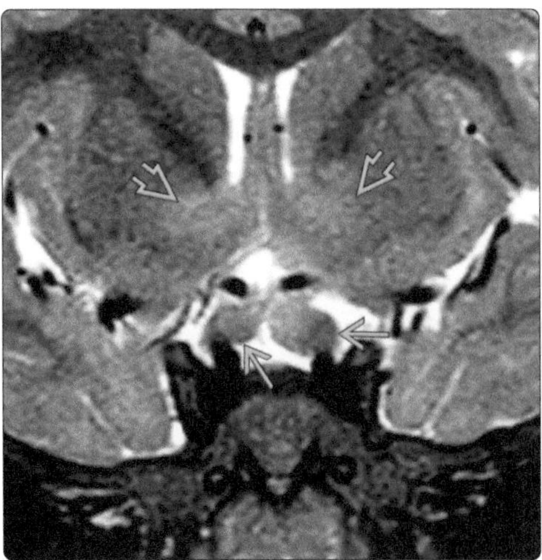

(Left) *Sagittal T1 C+ MR in a 22-month-old shows a homogeneously enhancing mass ➔ centered in the hypothalamus/optic chiasm, consistent with a hypothalamic glioma (histology showed a PA). Note the normal pituitary ➔ caudal to the lesion, flattened along the floor of the sella turcica.* **(Right)** *Coronal T2WI FS MR in a 2-year-old boy with NF1 and an optic pathway glioma is shown. The bilateral optic nerves ➔ are enlarged. Note the abnormal hyperintense signal in the pallidal nuclei ➔, characteristic of NF1.*

KEY FACTS

TERMINOLOGY

- Pilomyxoid astrocytoma (PMA): More aggressive, myxoid variant of pilocytic astrocytoma (PA)
  - High risk of local recurrence, CSF dissemination

IMAGING

- 60% suprasellar (large, bulky, H-shaped mass in hypothalamus/optic chiasm, medial temporal lobes)
- 40% outside diencephalon (hemisphere, ventricles)
- Grossly well circumscribed, little/no edema
- Enhances strongly
- 20% show intratumoral hemorrhage

TOP DIFFERENTIAL DIAGNOSES

- PA
- High-grade glioma
- Germinoma

PATHOLOGY

- WHO grade 2 (typical PA is WHO grade 1)

CLINICAL ISSUES

- Typical: Infants, young children (< 4 years)
- Less common: Older children, young adults
- 5-10% of cases initially diagnosed as PAs may actually be PMAs
  - Especially if tumor is hemorrhagic, presents in very young child, or shows CSF dissemination

DIAGNOSTIC CHECKLIST

- Consider PMA if
  - Infant or young child has large/bulky or hemorrhagic H-shaped suprasellar mass
  - Presumed PA in any patient who has atypical imaging (e.g., hemorrhage, metastases)

(Left) *Coronal graphic depicts a pilomyxoid astrocytoma (PMA). Note the large, bulky, H-shaped mass ⇒ centered in the hypothalamic/chiasmatic region and extending into both temporal lobes. The tumor is relatively well circumscribed and shows little/no edema. Glistening myxoid matrix is typical. Hemorrhage ⇒ occurs in ~ 20% of PMAs but is unusual in pilocytic astrocytoma (PA).* **(Right)** *Coronal T1 C+ MR in a 20-month-old with a PMA shows a large, heterogeneously enhancing hypothalamic mass ⇒.*

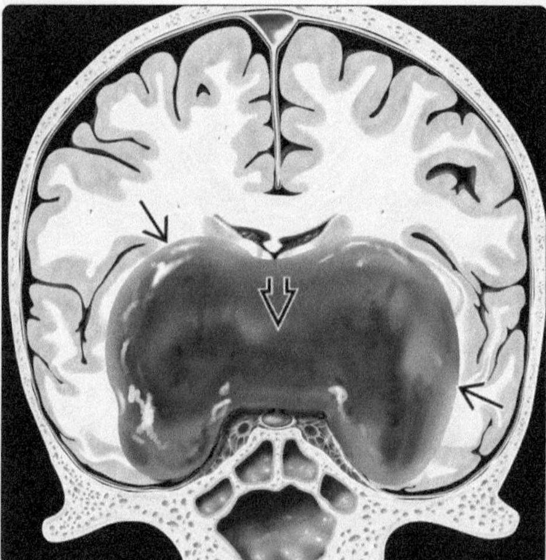

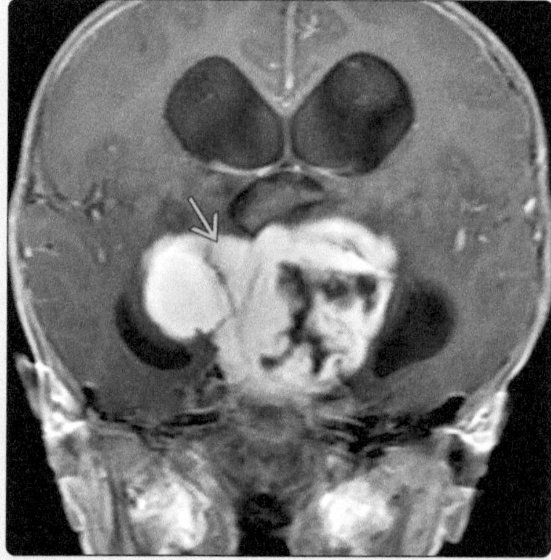

(Left) *Sagittal T2 MR in a 7-month-old with a PMA shows a large mass ⇒ centered in the hypothalamus and optic chiasm. Note the pituitary ⇒ pressed down along the floor of the sella. The large size of the tumor and the very young age of the patient are typical of a PMA.* **(Right)** *Axial ADC MR in the same patient shows almost universal increased signal in the tumor ⇒ compared to brain parenchyma, which is typical for low-grade astrocytic tumors, such as PMAs.*

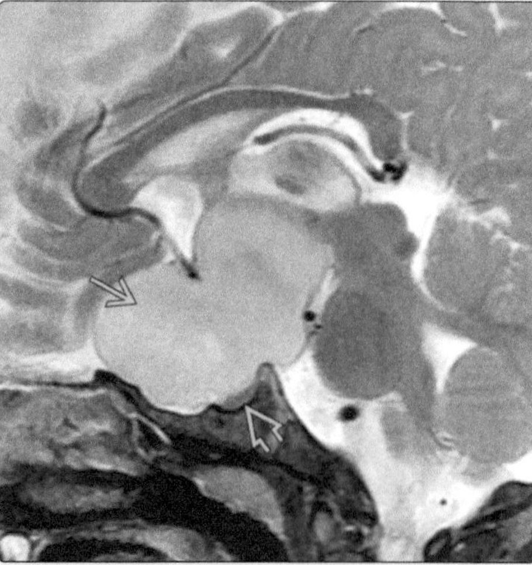

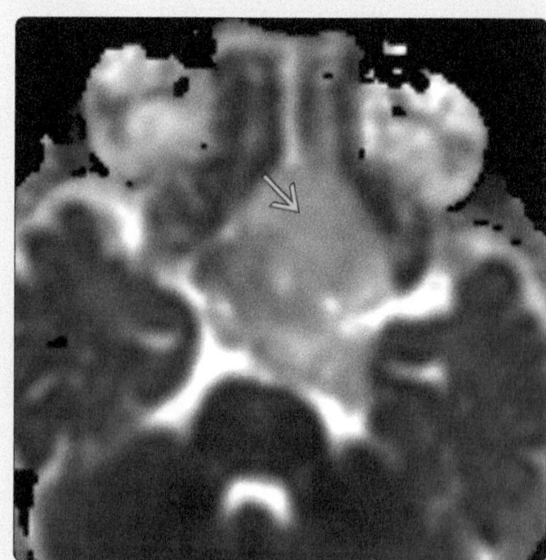

TERMINOLOGY

Abbreviations

- Pilomyxoid astrocytoma (PMA)

Synonyms

- Myxoid variant of pilocytic astrocytoma (PA)

Definitions

- Tumor with monomorphic piloid cells dispersed in mucopolysaccharide-rich matrix
  - More aggressive tumor than PA with high risk of local recurrence, dissemination

IMAGING

General Features

- Best diagnostic clue
  - Infant or young child with large, bulky, H-shaped mass in hypothalamus/optic chiasm, medial temporal lobes
- Location
  - 60% suprasellar
    - Optic chiasm, hypothalamus
    - Extension into adjacent structures is common with larger tumors
    - Deep gray nuclei, temporal lobes, adjacent white matter often involved
  - 40% centered **outside** diencephalon
    - Cerebral hemispheres
      - 2nd most common general location
      - Temporal lobe most common
      - May be purely cortical
    - Less common sites reported
      - Midbrain
      - Cerebellum
      - 4th ventricle
      - Spinal cord
- Size
  - Variable
    - Mean: 4 cm
    - Often large, bulky (up to 12 cm)
- Morphology
  - Grossly well circumscribed

CT Findings

- NECT
  - Uniform hypodensity most common
  - 20% show intratumoral hemorrhage
    - Hyperdense; mixed hypo-/hyperdense
  - Ca^{++} occurs but uncommon
- CECT
  - Strong, but inhomogeneous enhancement
  - Irregular central nonenhancing area in 1/3

MR Findings

- T1WI
  - Typical: Uniformly hypointense (almost 2/3 of cases)
  - Less common: Mixed hypo-/hyperintensity (10-15%)
  - Uncommon: Blood-fluid level
- T2WI
  - 70% uniformly hyperintense
  - 15% inhomogeneously hyperintense
  - 10% hypointense center, hyperintense rim
- FLAIR
  - 50% uniformly hyperintense
  - 33% heterogeneously hyperintense
  - Relatively well-demarcated margins
  - Little or no peritumoral edema
- T2* GRE
  - Intratumoral hemorrhage in 20%
  - May be strikingly hypointense
- DWI
  - Typically does not restrict
  - ADC signal in solid component usually significantly ↑ compared to brain parenchyma
- PWI
  - ASL and DSC PWI may help distinguish PMA from PA
    - ASL: Mean tumor:GM cerebral blood flow (CBF) ratio = 1.3 in PMA vs. 0.4 in PA
    - DSC: Relative cerebral blood volume (rCBV) is 2 in PMA vs. 1.5 in PA
- T1WI C+
  - Strong but heterogeneous enhancement
    - 50% heterogeneous (i.e., rim)
    - 40% solid, homogeneous
    - 10% no enhancement
  - Basilar/spinal meningeal enhancement is common and indicates CSF dissemination

Other Modality Findings

- MRS
  - ↑ Cho, ↓ Cr and NAA ± lactate
  - Some authors report low-metabolite pattern with ↓ Cho, Cr, NAA

Imaging Recommendations

- Best imaging tool
  - MR with T1 C+, DWI, T2* (GRE or SWI), MRS
- Protocol advice
  - Thin-section sagittal, coronal pre- and postcontrast T1WI
  - Whole-brain FLAIR
  - Thin-section T2WI through hypothalamus, chiasm
  - GRE or SWI (to look for hemorrhage)
  - Optional: Add DWI, MRS

DIFFERENTIAL DIAGNOSIS

Pilocytic Astrocytoma

- Older children (mean age at diagnosis: 6 years)
- In hypothalamus, typically enhances strongly/uniformly
- PMA usually more hyperintense on T2/FLAIR (mucoid matrix)
- Hemorrhage, CSF dissemination uncommon
- Paradoxically aggressive MRS pattern: ↑ Cho, ↓ Cr, ↓ NAA
  - Some PMAs show low metabolite concentrations

High-Grade Glioma (Anaplastic Astrocytoma, Glioblastoma)

- Hemorrhage, necrosis common
- Hypothalamus rare location
- Patients usually older
- May arise from lower grade astrocytoma

Germinoma

- Most often in suprasellar, pineal, or basal ganglia regions
- Numerous microcysts common
- Diffusion restriction of solid components reflects high cellularity

PATHOLOGY

General Features

- Etiology
  - Unknown
  - Some tumors demonstrate synaptophysin reactivity, suggesting PMAs may be of mixed glioneuronal origin
  - May also originate from tanycytic cells
- Genetics
  - PMA has significant differences in gene expression vs. PA
    - *H19*, *DACT2*, extracellular matrix collagens, *IGF2BP3* (*IMP3*) overexpressed in PMAs
    - Variable tendencies toward maturation to PA
- Associated abnormalities
  - Few cases associated with neurofibromatosis type 1 have been reported

Staging, Grading, & Classification

- WHO grade 2 (PA is WHO grade 1)
  - Grade 3 if anaplastic features
  - Malignant transformation to glioblastoma (grade 4) rare but does occur
- *MIB1* generally low (1-2%) but higher in anaplastic pleomorphic xanthoastrocytomas

Gross Pathologic & Surgical Features

- Large, grossly well-circumscribed mass
- Necrosis, hemorrhage may be present

Microscopic Features

- Lacks classic biphasic pattern seen in PAs
  - Alternating solid and loose areas interspersed with microcysts not seen
  - Rosenthal fibers, eosinophilic granular bodies absent
- Consists of monomorphic piloid tumor cells
  - Embedded in myxoid (mucopolysaccharide-rich) matrix
  - GFAP (+), vimentin (+)
- Conspicuous angiocentric growth pattern (perivascular rosettes)
  - Vascular proliferation may be marked
  - Infiltration of tumor cells into adjacent brain common
  - Necrosis rare

CLINICAL ISSUES

Presentation

- Most common signs/symptoms
  - Signs of ↑ intracranial pressure
    - Headache
    - Nausea, vomiting
  - Delayed development
  - Failure to thrive (so-called diencephalic syndrome)
  - Visual disturbances
  - Hypothalamic dysfunction
- Other signs/symptoms
  - Seizures
  - Focal neurologic deficit

Demographics

- Age
  - Typical: Infants, young children (< 4 years)
  - Less common: Older children, young adults
  - Rare: Middle-aged adult (up to 46 years)
- Sex
  - Slight male predominance (M:F = 4:3)
- Epidemiology
  - Rare; represent < 1% of astrocytomas
  - 5-10% of cases initially diagnosed as PAs may be PMAs, especially if hemorrhage is present or tumor presents in very young child

Natural History & Prognosis

- Higher recurrence rate than PA
- CSF dissemination common
- Bimodal pattern
  - Can mature to PA
  - May dedifferentiate into GBM

Treatment

- Partial resection with adjuvant therapy may prolong survival

DIAGNOSTIC CHECKLIST

Consider

- PMA if
  - Infant or young child has large/bulky or hemorrhagic suprasellar mass
  - Imaging atypical for PA (i.e., hemorrhage)
- If PA with repeated recurrences, CSF dissemination, review histopathology and consider PMA

Image Interpretation Pearls

- H-shaped suprasellar mass may be PMA

SELECTED REFERENCES

1. AlShail E et al: A molecular study of pediatric pilomyxoid and pilocytic astrocytomas: genome-wide copy number screening, retrospective analysis of clinicopathological features and long-term clinical outcome. Front Oncol. 13:1034292, 2023
2. Mbekeani JN et al: Pediatric pilomyxoid astrocytoma - ophthalmic and neuroradiologic manifestations. Eur J Ophthalmol. 32(5):2604-14, 2022
3. Benson JC et al: Hypothalamic pilomyxoid astrocytoma in a child with lipodystrophy. AJNR Am J Neuroradiol. 42(8):1370-4, 2021
4. Gader G et al: Pediatric cerebellar pilomyxoid astrocytoma: clinical and radiological findings in three cases. Asian J Neurosurg. 15(2):262-5, 2020
5. Ho CY et al: Differentiation of pilocytic and pilomyxoid astrocytomas using dynamic susceptibility contrast perfusion and diffusion weighted imaging. Neuroradiology. 62(1):81-8, 2020
6. He J et al: Posterior fossa pilomyxoid astrocytoma with spontaneous hemorrhage in pediatric patients. Childs Nerv Syst. 34(1):149-53, 2018
7. Louis DN et al: The 2016 World Health Organization classification of tumors of the central nervous system: a summary. Acta Neuropathol. 131(6):803-20, 2016
8. Wang Z et al: Spontaneous intratumoural and intraventricular haemorrhage associated with a pilomyxoid astrocytoma in the hypothalamic/chiasmatic region. J Clin Neurosci. 33:217-20, 2016
9. Alkonyi B et al: Differential imaging characteristics and dissemination potential of pilomyxoid astrocytomas versus pilocytic astrocytomas. Neuroradiology. 57(6):625-38, 2015
10. Nabavizadeh SA et al: High accuracy of arterial spin labeling perfusion imaging in differentiation of pilomyxoid from pilocytic astrocytoma. Neuroradiology. 57(5):527-33, 2015
11. Linscott LL et al: Pilomyxoid astrocytoma: expanding the imaging spectrum. AJNR Am J Neuroradiol. 29(10):1861-6, 2008

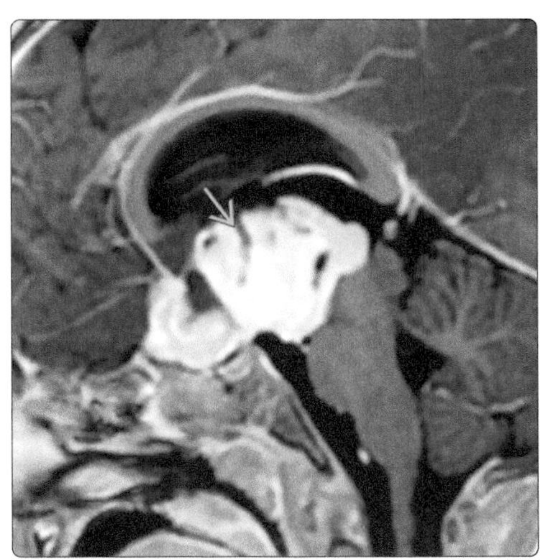

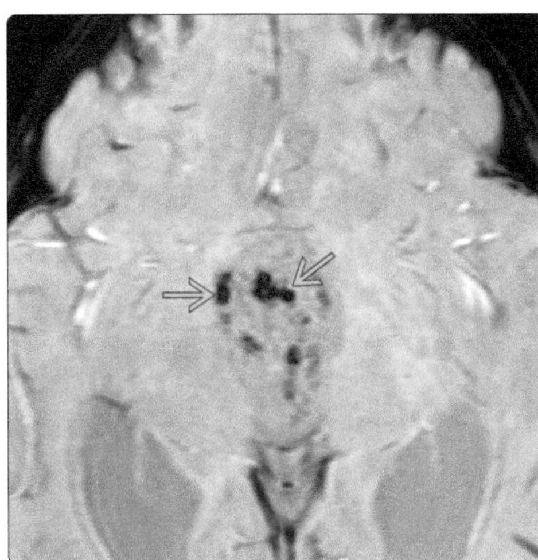

(Left) *Sagittal T1 C+ MR in a 2-year-old shows an avidly enhancing hypothalamic tumor ➡. This is a typical appearance for PMA.* **(Right)** *Axial SWI in the same patient shows multifocal areas of signal loss ➡, consistent with intratumoral microhemorrhage. Microhemorrhage is more common in PMAs compared to PAs. For this reason, it is helpful diagnostically to include SWI in evaluation of hypothalamic tumors.*

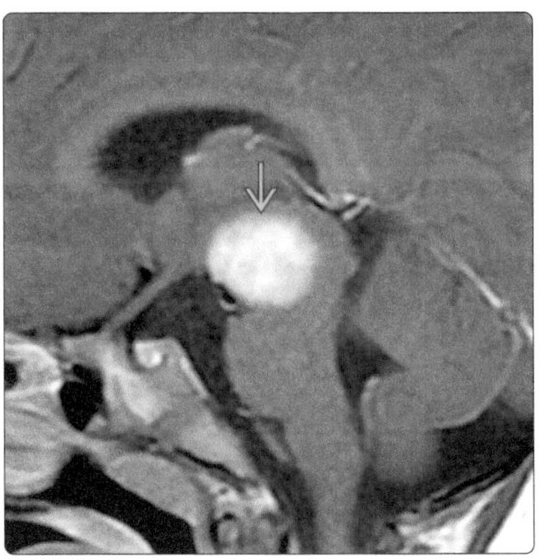

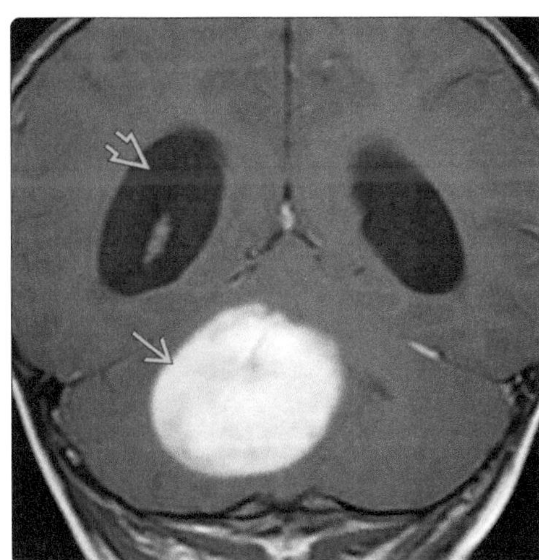

(Left) *Sagittal T1 C+ MR in a 23-month-old demonstrates a homogeneously enhancing midbrain lesion ➡. Pathology revealed a PMA. Regardless of location, PMAs should be considered for any likely low-grade glioma in a very young child.* **(Right)** *Coronal T1 C+ MR in a 2-year-old with a uniformly enhancing mass ➡ centered in the right cerebellar hemisphere is shown. Note the associated hydrocephalus ➡. While the cerebellum is the most common location for PAs, it is an uncommon location for PMAs.*

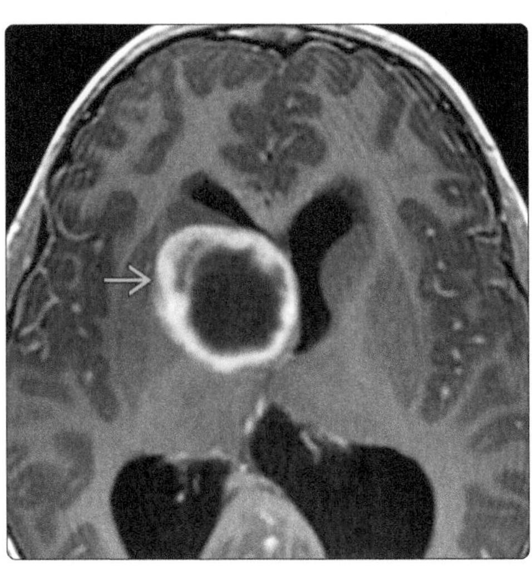

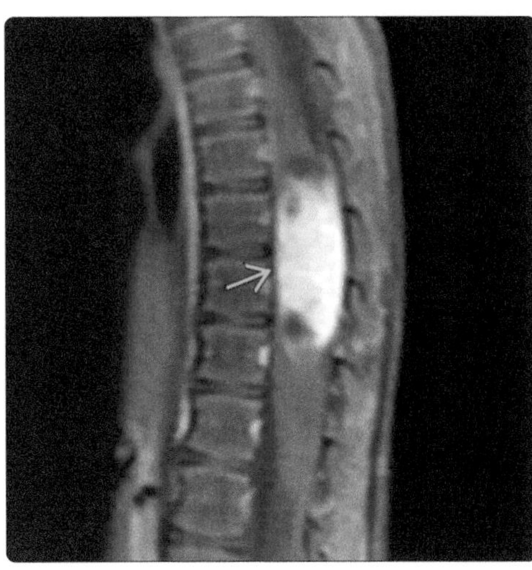

(Left) *Axial T1 C+ MR in 9-year-old shows a rim-enhancing mass ➡ with lack of adjacent edema. Enhancement patterns of PMAs vary greatly from solid homogeneous enhancement to peripheral enhancement, as seen here. Some degree of enhancement is almost universally present.* **(Right)** *Sagittal T1 C+ MR in a 3-year-old with an avidly enhancing intramedullary tumor ➡, found to be a PMA on pathology, is shown. While uncommon, PMAs have been reported to occur in the spine.*

Subependymal Giant Cell Astrocytoma

KEY FACTS

TERMINOLOGY

- Subependymal giant cell astrocytoma (SGCA, SEGA)
- Benign, slow-growing glioneuronal tumor in patient with tuberous sclerosis complex (TSC)

IMAGING

- Enlarging, enhancing mass near foramen of Monro in patient with TSC
- Other findings of tuberous sclerosis (TS) [cortical tubers, subependymal nodules (SENs)]

TOP DIFFERENTIAL DIAGNOSES

- Choroid plexus tumors
    - Choroid plexus papilloma > atypical choroid plexus papilloma, carcinoma
- Central neurocytoma
    - Body of lateral ventricle
- Astrocytoma
    - Pilocytic astrocytoma, chordoid glioma (rare)
- Subependymoma
    - Middle-aged, older adults
- Supratentorial primitive neuroectodermal tumors (rare)
    - Cellular tumor (↑ DWI/↓ ADC) in very young child

PATHOLOGY

- SEGA probably arises from SEN in region of germinal matrix
- Likely represents disordered neuronal migration
- WHO grade 1, curable with complete resection

CLINICAL ISSUES

- Most common CNS neoplasm in TSC
    - SEGA in up to 15% of patients with TSC
    - Rarely (if ever) arises in absence of TSC
- Treatment with mTOR inhibitors (everolimus)
    - Most TS patients have 50% ↓ in SEGA within 9 months

DIAGNOSTIC CHECKLIST

- Enlarging, enhancing intraventricular mass near foramen of Monro in TSC patient

(Left) *Coronal graphic demonstrates hydrocephalus secondary to a subependymal giant cell astrocytoma (SGCA, SEGA) arising near the left foramen of Monro. Note the subependymal tubers.* **(Right)** *Axial section through the ventricles in a patient with tuberous sclerosis complex (TSC) shows a large SGCA obstructing the foramen of Monro. Note the well-delineated tumor margins and cortical tuber. Despite emergent ventricular shunting, the ventricles were not decompressed successfully. (Courtesy R. Hewlett, MD.)*

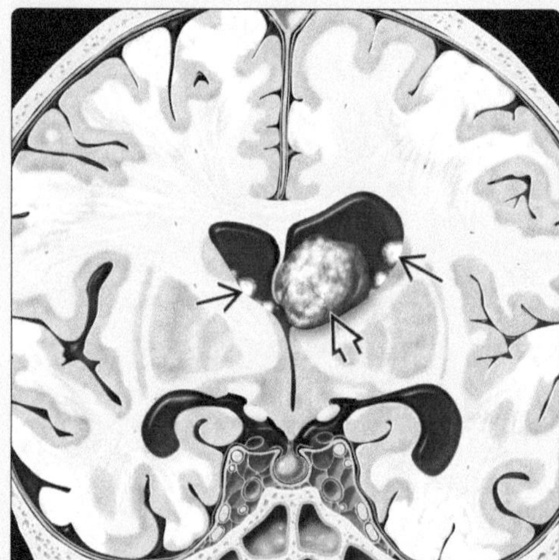

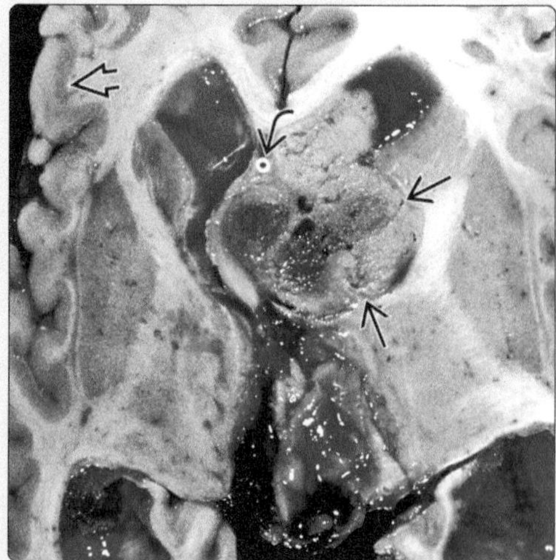

(Left) *Axial T1 C+ MR in a 2-year-old boy shows a prominent enhancing mass in the right caudothalamic groove. Also note the small lesion in the left caudothalamic groove (subependymal nodule) and the cortical/subcortical signal abnormalities in the left frontal lobe (cortical tubers) and white matter signal change. These findings are consistent with TSC.* **(Right)** *Axial FLAIR MR in the same patient at 5 years shows increased size of the SEGA and the full extent of cortical tubers in this TSC patient.*

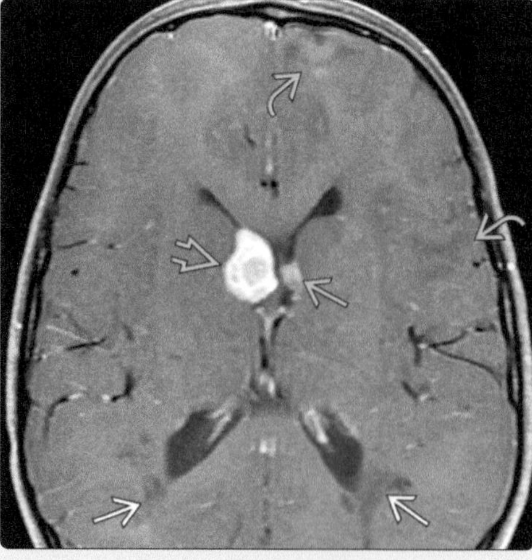

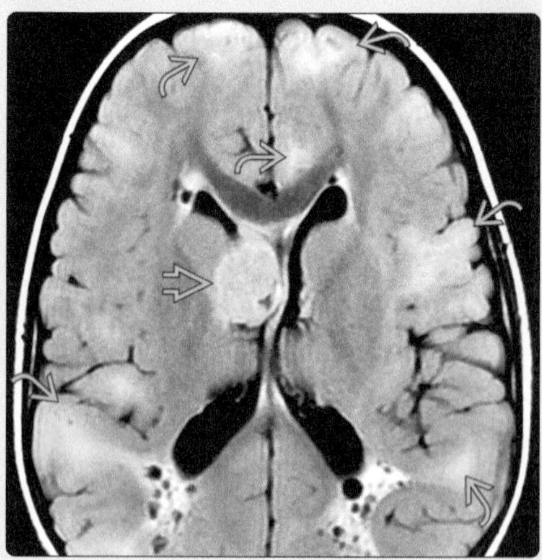

TERMINOLOGY

Abbreviations

- Subependymal giant cell astrocytoma (SGCA, SEGA)

Definitions

- Benign, slow-growing glioneuronal tumor usually arising adjacent to foramen of Monro in TSC

IMAGING

General Features

- Best diagnostic clue
  - Enlarging, enhancing foramen of Monro mass in patient with TSC
    - Other imaging findings of TSC [cortical tubers, subependymal nodules (SENs)]
    - SGCA in absence of clinical/genetic evidence of TSC reported but very rare
- Location
  - SENs in > 90% of tuberous sclerosis (TS) patients
    - Lateral ventricles adjacent to caudate nuclei
  - SEGAs may arise from SENs
    - Almost always near foramen of Monro
- Size
  - SEGAs variable, slowly growing
    - Often presents when 2-3 cm; causes obstructive hydrocephalus
  - SENs typically 5-10 mm
    - Larger SENs near foramen of Monro should be followed with serial imaging
      - SEGAs usually grow slowly while SENs remain stable
- Morphology
  - Well marginated
  - Often with lobulated contour

CT Findings

- NECT
  - Hypo- to isodense; heterogeneous
  - Ca^{++} variable
  - Hydrocephalus
- CECT
  - Heterogeneous, strong enhancement
  - Presence of interval growth suggests SGCA
  - Initially, tumor is typically > 1 cm
- CT perfusion
  - May be mildly hypervascular

MR Findings

- T1WI
  - Hypointense to isointense to gray matter (GM)
  - ± Ca^{++} (hyperintense to hypointense)
- T2WI
  - Heterogeneous
    - Isointense to hyperintense
  - Ca^{++} foci hypointense
  - Hydrocephalus
- PD/intermediate
  - Hyperintense
- FLAIR
  - Heterogeneously hyperintense
  - Periventricular interstitial edema from ventricular obstruction
- T2* GRE
  - Low signal from Ca^{++}
- DWI
  - Apparent diffusion coefficient (ADC) values are < parenchymal hamartomas of TS
- T1WI C+
  - Robust enhancement
    - Enhancement alone does not allow discrimination from hamartoma
  - Enlarging, enhancing foramen of Monro mass > 1.2 cm suggests SEGA
  - CSF dissemination not seen
- MRS
  - Less than expected ↓ in NAA due to some neuronal elements in this primarily glial neoplasm

Imaging Recommendations

- Best imaging tool
  - MR demonstrates extent of mass, delineates associated TSC features
- Protocol advice
  - FLAIR MR to detect subtle CNS features of TSC
  - Recommend brain MR every 1-2 years for SEGA follow-up
    - IV contrast may not be necessary for follow-up

DIFFERENTIAL DIAGNOSIS

Choroid Plexus Papilloma

- Atrium of lateral ventricle
- Foramen of Monro rare

Astrocytoma

- Origin: Septum pellucidum fornices or medial basal ganglia
  - Common pediatric intraaxial neoplasm
  - Variable enhancement, Ca^{++} rare

Germinoma

- Hugs midline; often arises near 3rd ventricle
- May originate from basal ganglia, resemble SEGA
- Early CSF spread

Subependymoma

- Tumor of middle-aged, older adults
- Inferior 4th/frontal horn of lateral ventricle

Central Neurocytoma

- Well-defined, variably vascularized, lobulated mass
- Body of lateral ventricle > foramen of Monro or septum pellucidum
- Necrosis, cyst formation are common
- Seen in young adults

Supratentorial Primitive Neuroectodermal Tumors

- May exophytically extend into ventricle
- Lack of peritumoral edema
- Highly cellular tumor → diffusion restriction

PATHOLOGY

General Features

- Etiology
  - SEGA probably arises from SEN in region of germinal matrix
  - Likely represents disordered neuronal migration complex
- Genetics
  - 50% of TSC patients have positive family history
    - High rate of de novo mutations
    - Inheritance: Autosomal dominant
    - High penetrance
    - Considerable phenotypic variability
  - Molecular genetics
    - Typically show biallelic inactivation of *TSC1* (15%) or *TSC2* (56%)
    - 2 distinct TSC loci (chromosome 9q on *TSC1* and 16p on *TSC2*)
    - Protein products of *TSC1* (hamartin) and *TSC2* (tuberin)
      - Suppress mammalian target of rapamycin (mTOR), major cell growth and proliferation controller
    - Mutation results in activation of mTOR
- Associated abnormalities
  - Other CNS, extraneural manifestations of TSC

Staging, Grading, & Classification

- WHO grade 1

Gross Pathologic & Surgical Features

- Well-marginated mass arising from lateral ventricular wall near foramen of Monro
  - ± cysts, Ca^{++}, and hemorrhage
- Does not seed CSF pathways

Microscopic Features

- Tumor cells of SEGAs show wide spectrum of astroglial phenotypes
  - Giant pyramidal ganglioid astrocytes
  - Perivascular pseudopalisading
- Histology may be indistinguishable from SENs
  - Diagnosis based on size and growth
- Immunohistochemistry
  - Variable immunoreactivity for GFAP, S100
  - Glial, neuronal antigen expression variable

CLINICAL ISSUES

Presentation

- Most common signs/symptoms
  - ↑ intracranial pressure secondary to tumor obstructing foramen of Monro
    - Headache, vomiting, loss of consciousness
  - Other signs/symptoms
    - Worsening epilepsy
    - Massive spontaneous hemorrhage
- Clinical profile
  - Patient with TSC develops signs and symptoms of ventricular obstruction
  - Worsening of epilepsy

Demographics

- Age
  - SEGA typically occurs during first 2 decades
    - Mean age: 11 years
    - Rarely arises after 20-25 years of age
- Epidemiology
  - 1.4% of all pediatric brain tumors
  - Most common CNS neoplasm in TSC
    - Incidence of SGCA: 10-20% of patients with TSC
    - Rarely occurs in absence of TSC
- Uncommon reports of congenital cases
- No race or sex predilection

Natural History & Prognosis

- Solitary, slow-growing, benign tumor
- Symptoms from ventricular obstruction
- Good outcome and low recurrence rate with complete resection
- Rarely, massive spontaneous hemorrhage

Treatment

- Randomized controlled trials have shown mTOR inhibitors (e.g., everolimus) to be highly effective at reducing size of SEGAs
  - Part of mTORC1 pathway
  - Restores pathway after inhibition by *TSC1* or *TSC2* mutation
  - Surgery is no longer necessary in many cases
  - Tangential benefits include ↓ seizure frequency and ↓ size of renal angiomyolipomas

DIAGNOSTIC CHECKLIST

Consider

- SEGA in TSC patient with worsening seizures &/or symptoms of ventricular obstruction

Image Interpretation Pearls

- Enlarging, enhancing intraventricular mass near foramen of Monro in TSC patient

SELECTED REFERENCES

1. Cobourn KD et al: Isolated subependymal giant cell astrocytoma (SEGA) in the absence of clinical tuberous sclerosis: two case reports and literature review. Childs Nerv Syst. ePub, 2023
2. Bobeff K et al: Maintenance therapy with everolimus for subependymal giant cell astrocytoma in patients with tuberous sclerosis - final results from the EMINENTS study. Front Neurol. 12:581102, 2021
3. Louis DN et al: TheReferences 2021 WHO classification of tumors of the central nervous system: a summary. Neuro Oncol. 23(8):1231-51, 2021
4. Northrup H et al: Updated international tuberous sclerosis complex diagnostic criteria and surveillance and management recommendations. Pediatr Neurol. 123:50-66, 2021
5. Wang MX et al: Tuberous sclerosis: current update. Radiographics. 41(7):1992-2010, 2021
6. WHO Classification of Tumours Editorial Board: WHO Classification of Tumours: CNS. 5th ed. IARC, 2021
7. Trelinska J et al: Maintenance therapy with everolimus for subependymal giant cell astrocytoma in patients with tuberous sclerosis (the EMINENTS study). Pediatr Blood Cancer. 64(6), 2017
8. French JA et al: Adjunctive everolimus therapy for treatment-resistant focal-onset seizures associated with tuberous sclerosis (EXIST-3): a phase 3, randomised, double-blind, placebo-controlled study. Lancet. 388(10056):2153-63, 2016
9. Kwiatkowski DJ et al: Response to everolimus is seen in TSC-associated SEGAs and angiomyolipomas independent of mutation type and site in TSC1 and TSC2. Eur J Hum Genet. 23(12):1665-72, 2015

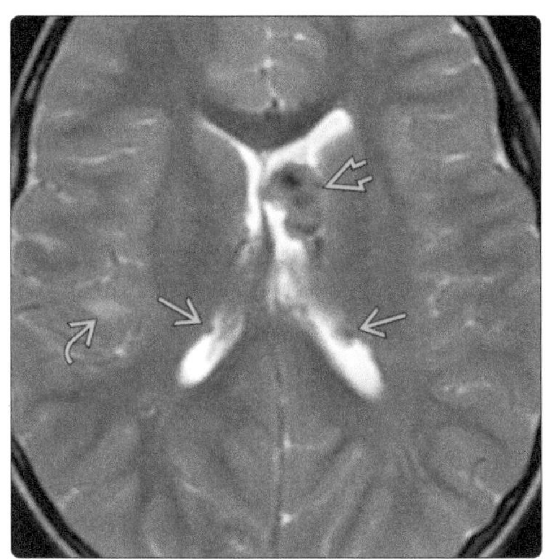

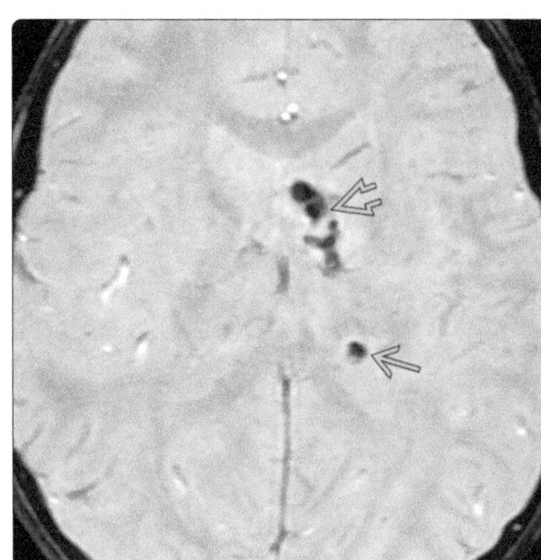

(Left) *Axial T2 MR in the same 7-year-old with TSC shows the left frontal SEGA ⇨ as well as multiple small subependymal nodules ➡. Note how dysplastic tubers ↷ are evident but much less conspicuous than on FLAIR.* **(Right)** *Axial SWI MR shows signal loss in the left frontal SEGA ⇨, consistent with Ca^{++}. Also note the Ca^{++} within the more posterior subependymal nodule ➡. Both SEGAs and subependymal nodules are frequently calcified, but SEGAs typically have a large amount of noncalcified soft tissue.*

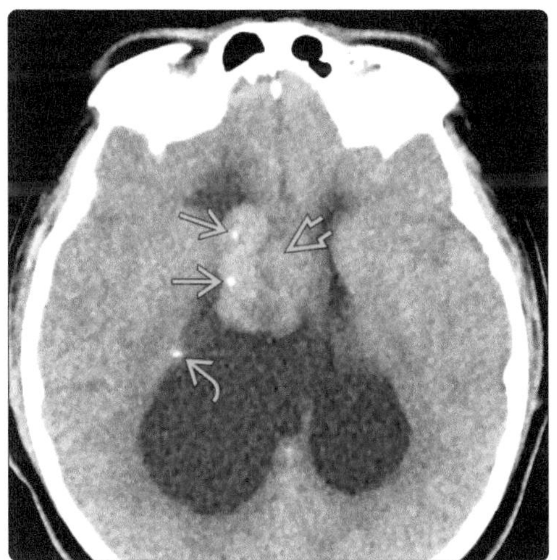

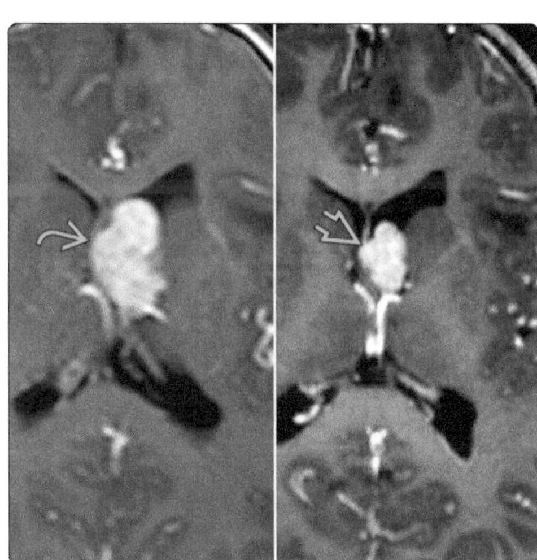

(Left) *Axial NECT in a 15-year-old with TSC shows a large mass ⇨ with punctate Ca^{++} ➡, consistent with a SEGA. Also note the small Ca^{++} ↷ associated with a subependymal nodule.* **(Right)** *Axial T1 C+ MR in a 4-year-old girl shows a large SEGA ↷ in the left caudothalamic groove (left). Three months after initiation of an mTOR inhibitor (right), the SEGA ⇨ has substantially decreased in size. mTOR inhibitors are often used as 1st-line therapy for symptomatic SEGAs and have secondary benefits of decreased seizure frequency.*

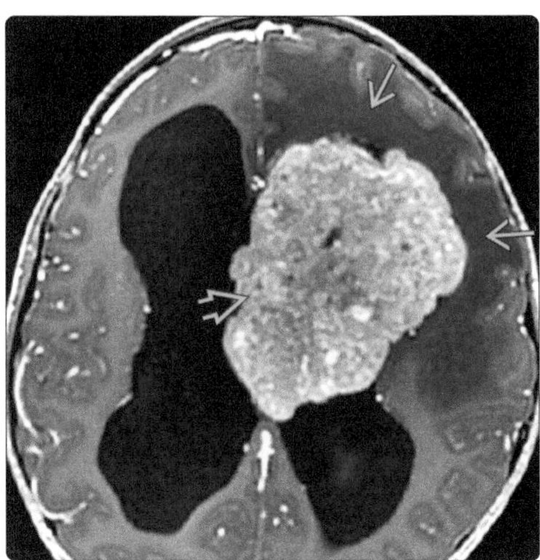

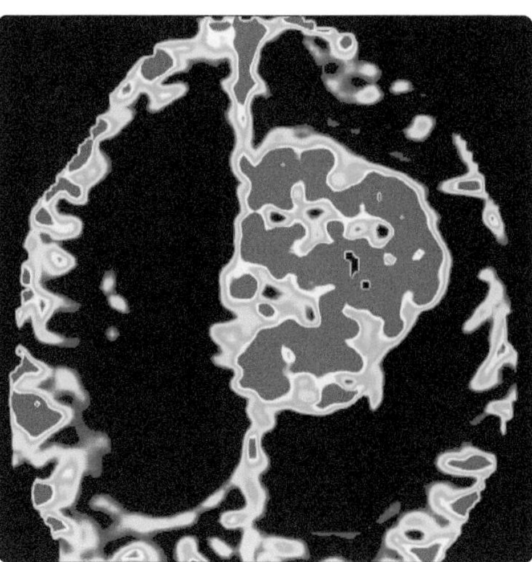

(Left) *Axial T1 C+ MR in a 7-year-old shows a large enhancing mass ⇨ centered in the left frontal horn with peritumoral edema ➡ and severe obstructive hydrocephalus. Pathology revealed a SEGA.* **(Right)** *Axial contrast perfusion MR in the same patient shows markedly increased rCBV in this tumor. There were no additional imaging signs of TSC, and genetic testing was negative. It is unusual for SEGA to arise in the absence of TSC, but it does occur and has been reported broadly in the literature.*

KEY FACTS

TERMINOLOGY

- Pleomorphic xanthoastrocytoma (PXA): Astrocytic neoplasm with generally favorable prognosis in children and young adults

IMAGING

- Peripherally located hemispheric mass, often involves cortex and meninges
  - Temporal lobe most common
- Supratentorial cortical mass with enhancing dural tail
  - Cyst and enhancing mural nodule typical
  - Enhancing nodule often abuts pial surface

TOP DIFFERENTIAL DIAGNOSES

- Ganglioglioma
- Pilocytic astrocytoma
- Dysembryoplastic neuroepithelial tumor
- Oligodendroglioma
- Meningioma

PATHOLOGY

- WHO grade 2
- "PXA with anaplastic features" also described

CLINICAL ISSUES

- Majority of patients have longstanding epilepsy, often partial complex seizures (temporal lobe)
  - Rare but important cause of temporal lobe epilepsy
- Tumor of children and young adults; majority < 18 years
- Represents < 1% of all astrocytomas
- Surgical resection is treatment of choice
- Survival 70% at 10 years
- Extent of resection and mitotic index are most significant predictors of outcome

DIAGNOSTIC CHECKLIST

- If cortical mass and meningeal thickening in young adult with long seizure history, think PXA
- Ganglioglioma may mimic PXA clinically and by imaging

(Left) *Coronal graphic shows a cystic and solid cortical mass ➡ with thickening of the adjacent meninges ➢, characteristic of pleomorphic xanthoastrocytoma (PXA). The mural nodule often abuts the pial surface and may result in a dural tail. Thinning of the adjacent bone is rare.* **(Right)** *Coronal T1 C+ MR depicts a classic PXA as an enhancing cystic and solid temporal lobe mass ➡ in a young seizure patient. Note that the mass touches the dura, and there is a subtle dural tail ➢. Surgical resection is the treatment of choice.*

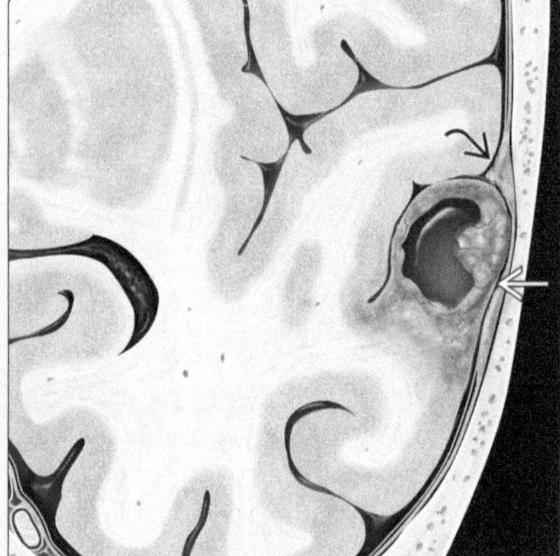

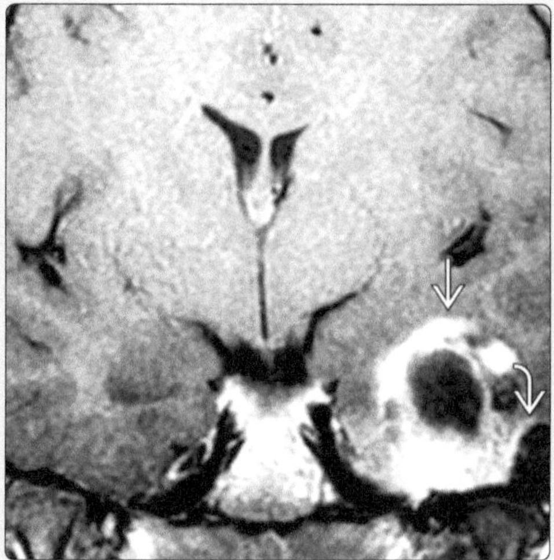

(Left) *Axial T2 MR reveals a large cystic and solid intraaxial temporal lobe mass ➡ in a 6-year-old girl presenting with epilepsy.* **(Right)** *Axial T1 C+ MR in the same patient confirms marked enhancement of the solid portions of the mass. Note the relative lack of surrounding edema and mass effect, characteristic of PXA. The imaging differential diagnosis includes ganglioglioma and pilocytic astrocytoma. Enhancement along the meninges, when present, helps make an accurate preoperative diagnosis.*

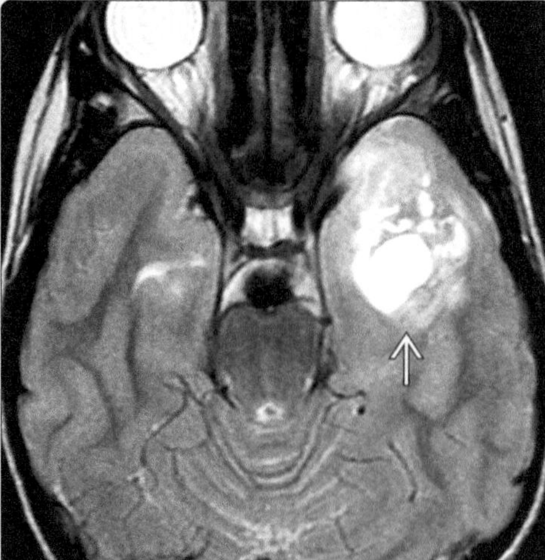

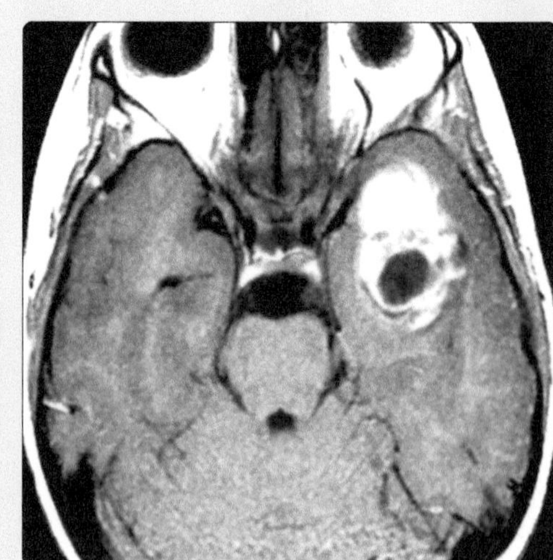

TERMINOLOGY

Abbreviations

- Pleomorphic xanthoastrocytoma (PXA)

Definitions

- Astrocytic neoplasm with generally favorable prognosis in children and young adults
  - Superficial location in cerebral hemispheres with involvement of meninges

IMAGING

General Features

- Best diagnostic clue
  - Supratentorial cortical mass with adjacent enhancing dural tail
  - Cyst and enhancing mural nodule typical
- Location
  - Peripherally located hemispheric mass, often involves cortex and meninges
    - 98% supratentorial
  - Temporal lobe most common (40-50%) in grade 2 PXA
    - Frontal and parietal > occipital lobes
  - Grade 3 PXA may have deeper location, no preference for temporal lobe, and more likely show peritumoral edema
  - Rarely found in cerebellum, sella, spinal cord, retina
- Size
  - Variable
- Morphology
  - 50-60% cyst with mural nodule that abuts meninges (may be solid)
  - Discrete, round to oval mass typical (may be ill defined)
  - Despite circumscribed appearance, tumor often infiltrates into brain and perivascular spaces

CT Findings

- NECT
  - Cystic/solid mass: Hypodense with mixed-density nodule
  - Solid mass: Variable; hypodense, hyperdense, or mixed
  - Minimal or no edema is typical
  - Ca^{++}, hemorrhage, frank skull erosion (rare)
- CECT
  - Strong, sometimes heterogeneous enhancement of tumor nodule

MR Findings

- T1WI
  - Mass is hypo- or isointense to gray matter
  - Mixed signal intensity may be seen
  - Cystic portion isointense to CSF
  - Associated cortical dysplasia may be seen (rare)
- T2WI
  - Hyperintense or mixed signal intensity mass
  - Cystic portion isointense to CSF
  - Surrounding edema (rare)
- FLAIR
  - Hyperintense or mixed signal intensity mass
  - Cystic portion isointense to CSF
- DWI
  - May show apparent diffusion coefficient (ADC) hypointensity in solid portions
  - Relatively low ADC values and ADC ratios (compared with pilocytic astrocytoma and ganglioglioma)
  - Mean ADC ratio of tumor to normal brain: 1.14 ± 0.26
- T1WI C+
  - Enhancement usually moderate/strong, well delineated
  - Enhancement of adjacent meninges, dural tail common (~ 70%)
    - Enhancing nodule often abuts pial surface
  - Rare: Deep tumor extension, distant metastases

Angiographic Findings

- Typically avascular
- Vascular blush may indicate necrotic or aggressive PXA

Nuclear Medicine Findings

- PET
  - FDG PET may show hypermetabolic foci even in low-grade PXA

Imaging Recommendations

- Best imaging tool
  - Multiplanar MR is most sensitive
  - CT may be helpful for calvarial changes
- Protocol advice
  - Contrast-enhanced MR, including coronal images to better evaluate temporal lobes

DIFFERENTIAL DIAGNOSIS

Ganglioglioma

- Cortically based, solid/cystic or solid hemispheric mass
- Mural nodule typical, often not adjacent to meninges
- Variable enhancement, no enhancing dural tail
- Ca^{++} common; may remodel calvarium

Pilocytic Astrocytoma

- Supratentorial location other than hypothalamus/chiasm is rare
- Typically solid and cystic or solid mass
- Enhancement but no dural tail

Dysembryoplastic Neuroepithelial Tumor

- Superficial cortical tumor, well demarcated
- Multicystic bubbly appearance
- T2-hyperintense mass with rare, mild enhancement
- May remodel

Oligodendroglioma

- Heterogeneous, Ca^{++} mass
- Typically larger and more diffuse than PXA
- May remodel/erode

Meningioma

- Diffusely enhancing, dural-based mass with dural tail
- Usually older patients

Low-Grade Astrocytoma (Grade 2)

- Demarcated but infiltrative white matter mass
- No enhancement

PATHOLOGY

General Features

- Etiology
  - May originate from cortical (subpial) astrocytes
  - May arise from multipotential neuroectodermal precursor cells common to both neurons and astrocytes or from preexisting hamartomatous lesions
- Genetics
  - No definite association with hereditary tumor syndromes
  - Rare reports of PXA in neurofibromatosis type 1 and Sturge-Weber patients
  - PXA with *TP53* mutations reported (low incidence)
  - Tumors with *BRAF* mutation associated with overall longer survival
  - Frequent loss of chromosome 9
- Associated abnormalities
  - PXA may occur with ganglioglioma and oligodendroglioma (rare)
  - PXA reported with dysembryoplastic neuroepithelial tumor and atypical teratoid-rhabdoid tumor
  - Synchronous, multicentric PXA lesions are rare
  - May be associated with cortical dysplasia

Staging, Grading, & Classification

- WHO grade 2
- PXA with anaplastic features (10-15%)
  - Significant mitoses (≥ 5 per 10 HPF) &/or necrosis
  - Has been associated with poorer prognosis
    - Increased recurrence and decreased survival
  - Some classify these PXAs as WHO grade 3

Gross Pathologic & Surgical Features

- Cystic mass with mural nodule abutting meninges
- May be completely solid
- Leptomeningeal adhesion/attachment is common
- Dural invasion is rare
- Deep margin may show infiltration of parenchyma

Microscopic Features

- Superficial, circumscribed astrocytic tumor noted for cellular pleomorphism and xanthomatous change
- Pleomorphic appearance
  - Fibrillary and giant multinucleated neoplastic astrocytes
  - Large xanthomatous (lipid-containing) cells are GFAP positive
  - Dense reticulin network
  - Lymphocytic infiltrates
- Tumor sharply delineated from cortex, but infiltration may be seen
- Some positive for synaptophysin, neurofilament proteins, S100 protein
- CD34 antigen may help differentiate PXA from other tumors
- Necrosis, mitotic figures rare/absent
  - *MIB1* index generally < 1%

CLINICAL ISSUES

Presentation

- Most common signs/symptoms
  - Majority with longstanding epilepsy, often partial complex seizures (temporal lobe)
  - Other signs/symptoms: Headache, focal neurologic deficits

Demographics

- Age
  - Tumor of children and young adults
    - Typically first 3 decades
    - 2/3 < 18 years
    - Range: 2-82 years; mean: 26 years
- Sex
  - No definite predominance
- Epidemiology
  - < 1% of all astrocytomas
  - Rare but important cause of temporal lobe epilepsy

Natural History & Prognosis

- Usually circumscribed, slow growing
- Recurrence of tumor is uncommon
- Hemorrhage is rare complication
- Survival 70% at 10 years
- 5-year survival 75-80%
- Malignant transformation in 10-25% of cases
- Extent of resection and mitotic index are most significant predictors of outcome
- Younger age at diagnosis portends better overall survival
- Aggressive PXA with malignant progression, dissemination may occur

Treatment

- Surgical resection is treatment of choice
- Repeat resection for recurrent tumors
- Radiation therapy and chemotherapy show mild improvement in outcome in some cases
- *BRAF*-mutation patients may respond to targeted inhibitor
  - 2/3 of PXA tumors harbor *BRAF* gene mutation

DIAGNOSTIC CHECKLIST

Consider

- If cortical mass and meningeal thickening in young adult with long seizure history, think PXA
- Ganglioglioma may mimic PXA clinically and by imaging

Image Interpretation Pearls

- Meningioma-like lesion in young patient should raise suspicion of PXA

SELECTED REFERENCES

1. Park YW et al: The 2021 WHO classification for gliomas and implications on imaging diagnosis: part 3-summary of imaging findings on glioneuronal and neuronal tumors. J Magn Reson Imaging. 58(6):1680-702, 2023
2. Zhang H et al: Clinical, morphological, and molecular study on grade 2 and 3 pleomorphic xanthoastrocytoma. Curr Oncol. 30(2):2405-16, 2023
3. Kata K et al: BRAF/MEK dual inhibitors therapy in progressive and anaplastic pleomorphic xanthoastrocytoma: case series and literature review. J Natl Compr Canc Netw. 20(11):1193-202.e6, 2022
4. Lundar T et al: Neurosurgical treatment of pediatric pleomorphic xanthoastrocytomas: long-term follow-up of a single-institution, consecutive series of 12 patients. J Neurosurg Pediatr. 1-5, 2019
5. Thomas AA et al: Anaplastic pleomorphic xanthoastrocytoma with leptomeningeal dissemination responsive to BRAF inhibition and bevacizumab. Pediatr Blood Cancer. 66(1):e27465, 2019
6. Mallick S et al: Grade II pleomorphic xanthoastrocytoma; a meta-analysis of data from previously reported 167 cases. J Clin Neurosci. 54:57-62, 2018

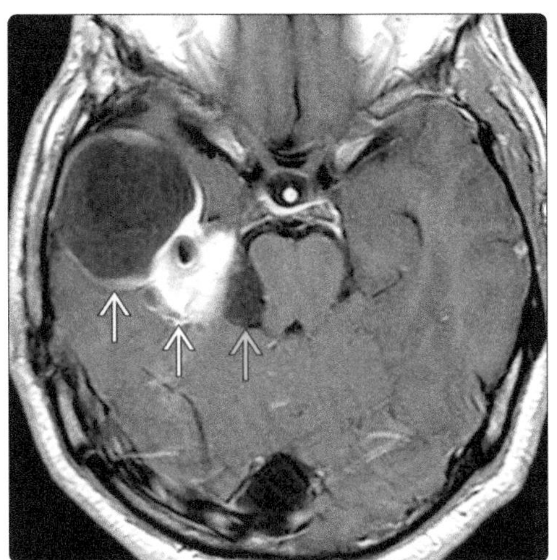

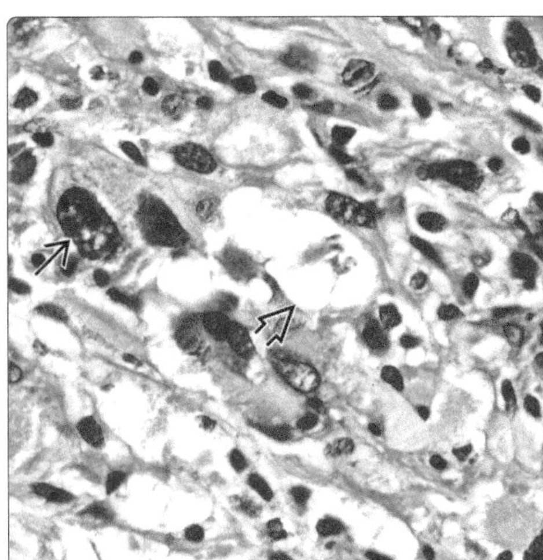

(Left) *Axial T1 C+ MR shows a solid and cystic temporal lobe mass ➡ related to a recurrent PXA. Note the cystic extraaxial portion ⇨ with mass effect on the adjacent midbrain.* **(Right)** *H&E micropathology from the same patient reveals conspicuous pleomorphism of the tumor with multinucleated giant cells ⇨ and vacuolation ➪, characteristic of PXA, WHO grade 2. Malignant transformation occurs in 10-25% of cases. (Courtesy R. Hewlett, MD.)*

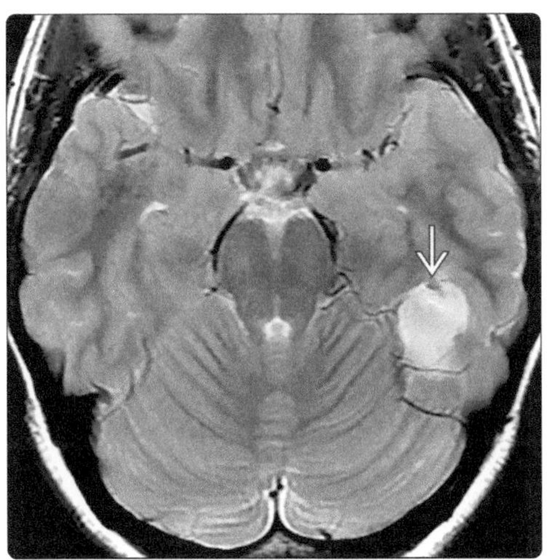

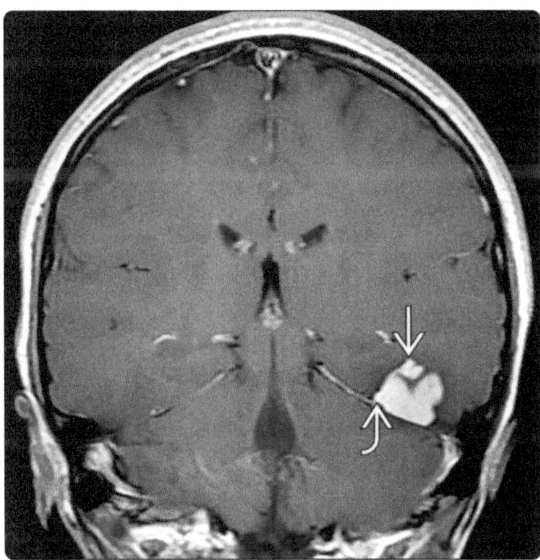

(Left) *Axial T2 MR in a 15-year-old patient presenting with seizures demonstrates a predominantly solid left inferior temporal lobe mass ➡.* **(Right)** *Coronal T1 C+ MR in the same patient confirms avid enhancement of the intraaxial mass ➡ abutting the dura. A small tail ➡ extends medially along the dura. In variation to the most common appearance, there was no significant cystic component in this pathology-proven WHO grade 2 PXA.*

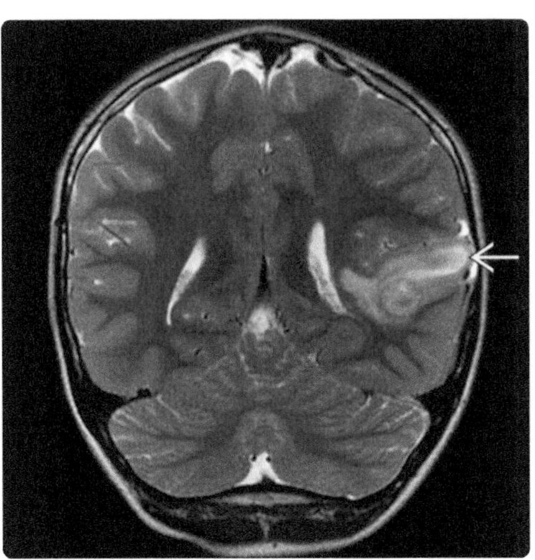

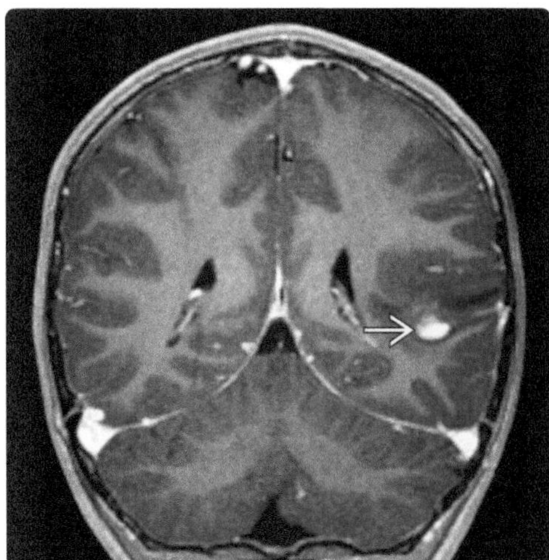

(Left) *Coronal T2 MR in a 9-year-old patient with seizures shows an ill-defined mass ➡ in the left temporal lobe. Pathology revealed a grade 3 anaplastic PXA. There is more T2 signal in the adjacent brain than usual for PXA, perhaps reflecting its anaplastic histology.* **(Right)** *Coronal T1 C+ MR in the same patient confirms an enhancing nodule ➡ that contacts a pial surface (sylvian fissure).*

Ganglioglioma

KEY FACTS

TERMINOLOGY

- Well-differentiated, slowly growing neuroepithelial tumor composed of neoplastic ganglion & glial cells

IMAGING

- Best imaging clue: Partially cystic, partially enhancing, cortically based mass in child/young adult with temporal lobe epilepsy
- Most commonly involves cerebral cortex, especially temporal lobe (~ 50%)
- Ca^{++} common (up to 50%), enhancement in ~ 50%
- Superficial lesions may remodel overlying calvarium
- Ill-defined, adjacent cortical signal abnormality suggests associated focal cortical dysplasia (FCD)

TOP DIFFERENTIAL DIAGNOSES

- Dysembryoplastic neuroepithelial tumor
- FCD
- Pleomorphic xanthoastrocytoma
- Pilocytic astrocytoma
- Diffuse astrocytoma (grade II)
- Oligodendroglioma

PATHOLOGY

- WHO grade 1 (80%) or 2
- Uncommon: Anaplastic ganglioglioma (GG) (WHO grade 3)
- Rare: Malignant with glioblastoma multiforme-like glial component (WHO grade 4)

CLINICAL ISSUES

- Most common glioneuronal tumor; 1-4% of all pediatric CNS neoplasms
- Most common neoplastic cause of temporal lobe epilepsy
- Excellent prognosis with complete resection

DIAGNOSTIC CHECKLIST

- GG in young patient with history of complex partial epilepsy
- Look for abnormal adjacent cortex that may suggest associated FCD

(Left) *Coronal T2 MR in a 5-year-old boy with episodes of eyelid fluttering & left arm dystonia shows a well-defined, hyperintense solid mass in the right mesial temporal lobe causing enlargement of the hippocampus ➔. This is a common location & appearance for ganglioglioma (GG).* **(Right)** *Axial T1 C+ MR in the same patient shows a lack of enhancement within the lesion. There is mass effect upon the adjacent vessels ➔ & brainstem ➔. Up to 50% of GG will demonstrate no enhancement.*

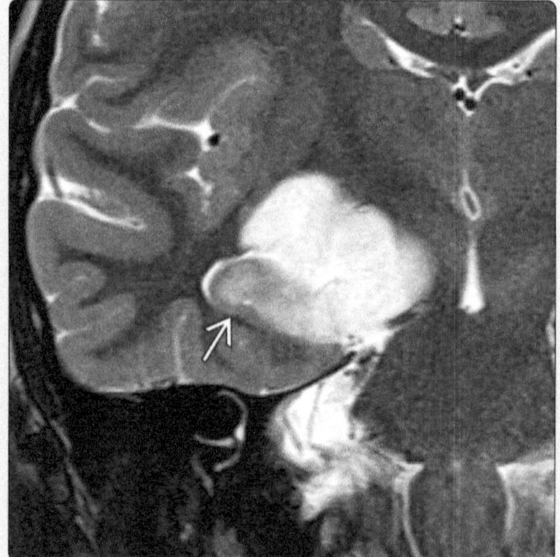

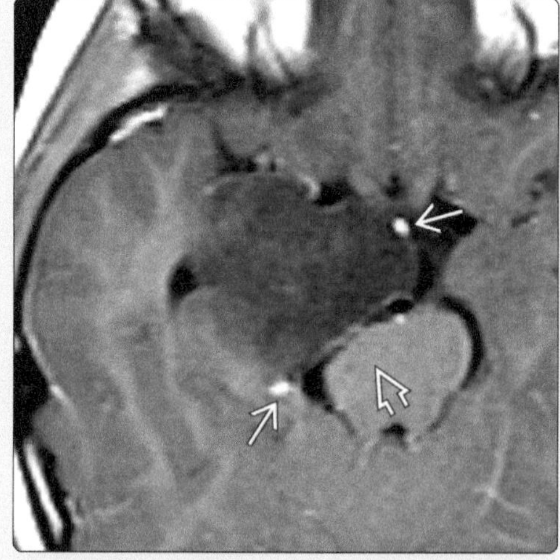

(Left) *Coronal T1 C+ MR in a 12-year-old girl with new onset of nocturnal partial seizures shows a well-defined, round area of enhancement ➔ in the right posterior temporal lobe.* **(Right)** *Coronal reconstruction of 3D FLAIR MR in the same patient shows abnormal signal within the adjacent cortex ➔, a finding that suggests associated focal cortical dysplasia (FCD). Pathology confirmed dysplastic neurons of FCD in this adjacent cortex.*

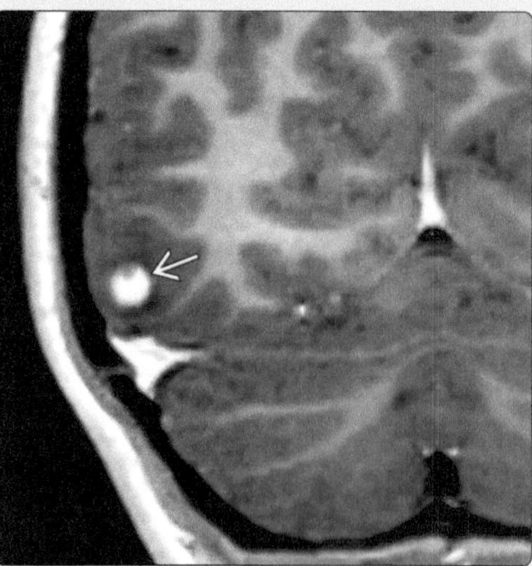

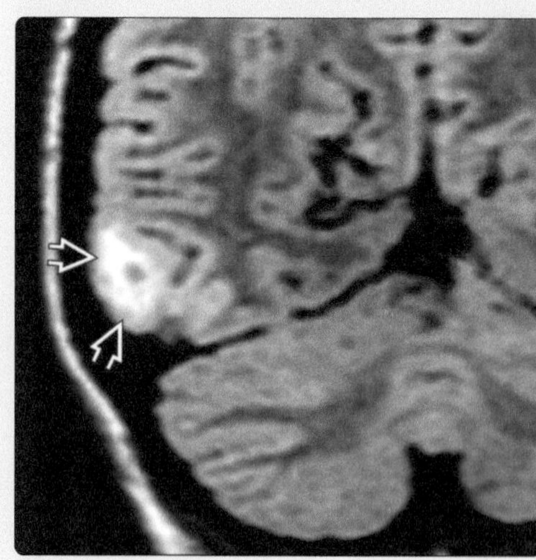

TERMINOLOGY

Abbreviations

- Ganglioglioma (GG)

Definitions

- Slow-growing neuroepithelial tumor composed of neoplastic ganglion & glial cells

IMAGING

General Features

- Best diagnostic clue
  - Partially cystic, calcified, cortically based mass in child/young adult with temporal lobe epilepsy
- Location
  - Temporal lobe most common (~ 50%)
  - Frontal & parietal lobes next most common
  - Less common: Cerebellum, brainstem, intraventricular, spinal cord, optic nerve/chiasm, hypothalamus, & cranial nerves
- Size
  - Variable, typically 1-7 cm
    - May present when small due to epileptogenic nature
- Morphology
  - 3 patterns
    - Solid tumor: 43-50%
    - Mixed solid & cystic: 38-52%
    - Predominantly cystic: 5-17%
  - Surrounding vasogenic edema uncommon
  - Adjacent cortical/subcortical signal abnormality suggests associated focal cortical dysplasia (FCD)
    - Type IIIb FCD

CT Findings

- NECT
  - Variable density
    - Ca^{++} common (up to 50%)
    - Hemorrhage rare
  - Superficial lesions may remodel overlying bone
- CECT
  - Up to 50% enhance
    - May be solid, nodular, or thin & rim-like
    - May show cystic lesion with enhancing mural nodule

MR Findings

- T1WI
  - Solid components typically hypointense to isointense to gray matter
  - Cystic components typically equal to CSF
- T2WI
  - Solid tumor component variable but usually hyperintense to gray matter
  - Cystic components typically near CSF signal
  - Foci of very hypointense signal due to Ca^{++}
- FLAIR
  - Cystic areas more variable in signal intensity as compared to T2
  - Surrounding vasogenic edema uncommon
  - Adjacent indistinct, hyperintense signal suggests possible associated FCD
- T2* GRE
  - Foci of exaggerated, hypointense signal (blooming) suggest Ca^{++}
- DWI
  - Solid components typically show ↑ ADC relative to adjacent brain
    - Due to ↓ cellularity & ↑ extracellular spaces
- T1WI C+
  - Variable enhancement (up to 50%)
    - May be homogeneous, nodular, heterogeneous, or rim-like
- MRS
  - Nonspecific: ↑ Cho & ↓ NAA
- Perfusion imaging
  - Higher cerebral blood volume (CBV) compared to low-grade astrocytomas & oligodendrogliomas

Nuclear Medicine Findings

- PET
  - Typically ↓ activity on FDG PET due to tumor hypometabolism
  - May have some hypermetabolic foci
- 201Tl-SPECT
  - Most GGs have ↓ uptake or activity similar to cerebrum
  - ↑ activity in high-grade GGs (grades III, IV)

Imaging Recommendations

- Best imaging tool
  - Brain MR with contrast
- Protocol advice
  - Seizure protocol to include 3D isotropic T1 & coronal oblique FLAIR MR sequences
    - Helpful to detect associated FCD & hippocampal sclerosis

DIFFERENTIAL DIAGNOSIS

Dysembryoplastic Neuroepithelial Tumor

- Wedge-shaped, multicystic, cortically based tumor in child/young adult
- Less likely to enhance or have Ca^{++} compared to GG
- More likely to have cystic components, especially multiple small cysts

Focal Cortical Dysplasia

- Ill-defined cortical thickening with blurring of gray matter-white matter junction; "tail" of abnormal signal extending toward ventricle
- Should not have mass effect, enhancement, or growth over time

Pleomorphic Xanthoastrocytoma

- Supratentorial cortical mass with enhancing nodule abutting pial surface
- Temporal lobe most common location

Pilocytic Astrocytoma

- Cortical location (other than hypothalamus/chiasm) less common
- Solid components typically enhance avidly
- Consider for cystic lesion with enhancing mural nodule

Diffuse Astrocytoma (Low Grade)

- Consider for cortically based mass with infiltrative margins
- Enhancement less common
- Usually involves deeper hemispheric structures (white matter & deep gray nuclei)

Oligodendroglioma

- Uncommon in children
- Calcified, heterogeneous mass
- Typically less well defined than GG
- May remodel/erode calvarium

PATHOLOGY

General Features

- Etiology
  - Cellular origin from pluripotent progenitor cells capable of divergent differentiation to glial & neuronal cells
  - Associated FCD suggests that GGs may be developmental lesions
- Associated abnormalities
  - FCD commonly associated
    - International League Against Epilepsy (ILAE) type IIIb FCD
  - GGs have been found in association with oligodendroglioma, dysembryoplastic neuroepithelial tumor (DNET), tanycytic ependymoma
  - Malignant transformation into glioblastoma & neuroblastoma has been reported

Staging, Grading, & Classification

- WHO grade 1 (80%) or 2
  - No established criteria differentiating grade 1 vs. 2
- Uncommon: Anaplastic GG (WHO grade 3)
  - Frequent mitoses & foci of necrosis
- Rare: Malignant with glioblastoma-like glial component (WHO grade 4)

Gross Pathologic & Surgical Features

- Solid or cystic mass, sometimes with mural nodule
- Firm, well-circumscribed mass, often expanding cortex

Microscopic Features

- Mix of mature but neoplastic ganglion cells & neoplastic glial cells (usually astrocytes)
- Dysmorphic, occasionally binucleate neurons
  - Immunohistochemistry of neuronal cells
    - Synaptophysin & neurofilament protein positive
    - Majority exhibit CD34 immunoreactivity (70-80% of GGs)
  - Immunohistochemistry of glial component & intermediate cells
    - GFAP & S100 positive
- Mitoses rare; low Ki-67
- Electron microscopy shows dense core granules, variable synapses
- *BRAF* V600E point mutation in up to 50%

CLINICAL ISSUES

Presentation

- Most common signs/symptoms
  - Supratentorial cortical tumors
    - Majority present with seizures (complex partial seizures most common)
    - Uncommon signs/symptoms: Headache & focal neurologic deficits
  - Infratentorial tumors
    - Majority present with manifestations of ↑ intracranial pressure secondary to obstructive hydrocephalus

Demographics

- Age
  - Mean: 10-20 years
  - 80% of patients < 30 years
- Sex
  - M:F = 3:2
- Epidemiology
  - Represents 1-4% of pediatric CNS neoplasms
  - Most common glioneuronal tumor
  - Most common tumor to cause temporal lobe epilepsy
    - GG > DNET > pilocytic astrocytoma > low-grade astrocytoma > oligodendroglioma > pleomorphic xanthoastrocytoma

Natural History & Prognosis

- Well-differentiated tumor with slow growth pattern
- Excellent prognosis if surgical resection complete
- 94% have 7.5-year recurrence-free survival
- Majority of patients (80%) seizure-free after surgery

Treatment

- Treatment of choice: Surgical resection
- 3 factors shown to favorably impact long-term seizure freedom
  - Gross total resection
  - Early operative intervention (< 1 year of epilepsy)
  - Extended resection for temporal lobe tumors to include amygdalohippocampectomy
- Radiation therapy &/or chemotherapy only for aggressive or unresectable tumors

DIAGNOSTIC CHECKLIST

Consider

- GG in young patient with history of complex partial epilepsy
- GGs larger & more cystic in children < 10 years of age

Image Interpretation Pearls

- Look for abnormal adjacent cortex that may suggest associated FCD

SELECTED REFERENCES

1. Agarwal A et al: Value of quantitative apparent diffusion coefficients in differentiating low-grade gliomas from mixed neuronal-glial tumors. World Neurosurg X. 18:100159, 2023
2. Jiang B et al: MRI characteristics predict BRAF V600E status in gangliogliomas and pleomorphic xanthoastrocytomas and provide survival prognostication. Acta Radiol. 2841851231183868, 2023
3. Vaz A et al: Uncommon glioneuronal tumors: a radiologic and pathologic synopsis. AJNR Am J Neuroradiol. 43(8):1080-9, 2022
4. WHO Classification of Tumours Editorial Board: WHO Classification of Central Nervous System Tumours. 5th ed. IARC, 2021
5. Ramaglia A et al: Role of diffusion weighted imaging for differentiating cerebral pilocytic astrocytoma and ganglioglioma BRAF V600E-mutant from wild type. Neuroradiology. 62(1):71-80, 2020

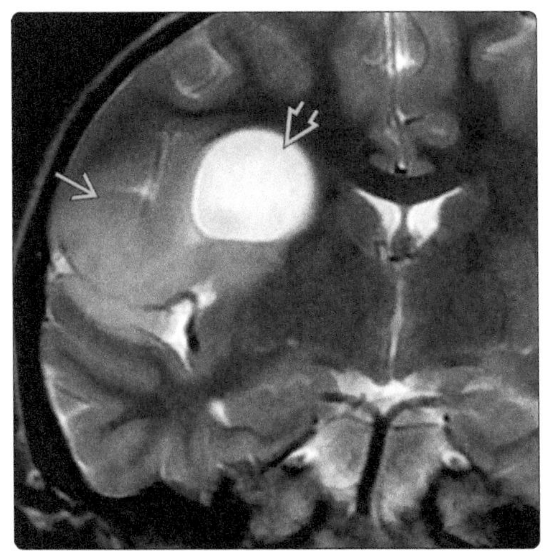

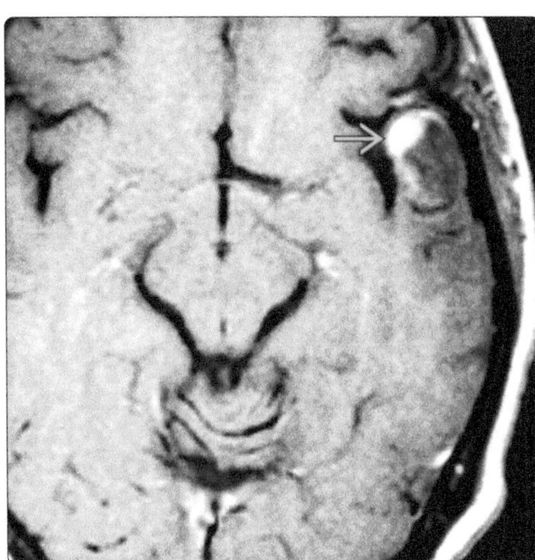

(Left) *Coronal T2 MR in a 6-year-old with GG shows a mixed solid ⇒ & cystic ⇒ lesion diffusely involving the cortex with extension to the underlying white matter. Somewhere between 25-50% of GG will have a cystic component.* **(Right)** *Axial T1 C+ MR in the same patient shows a cystic & solid temporal lobe mass with enhancement of the solid portion ⇒, a common pattern for GG. The patient was seizure free after resection of this mass.*

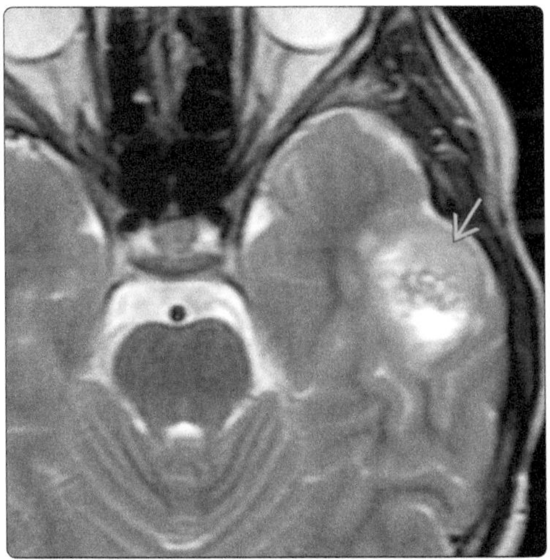

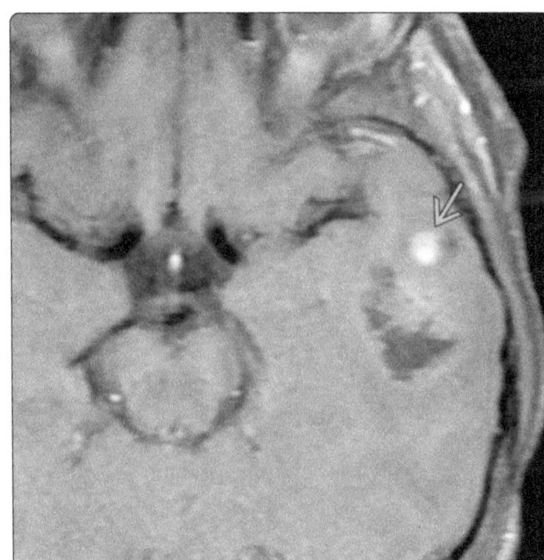

(Left) *Axial T2 MR in a 13-year-old with seizures shows a heterogeneous lesion ⇒ involving the cortex & subcortical white matter of the left lateral temporal lobe. The temporal lobe is the most common location for GG.* **(Right)** *Axial T1 C+ MR shows the mass lesion to be mostly nonenhancing with a small enhancing nodule ⇒ along the anterior margin of the tumor. Contrast enhancement is seen in ~ 50% of GGs.*

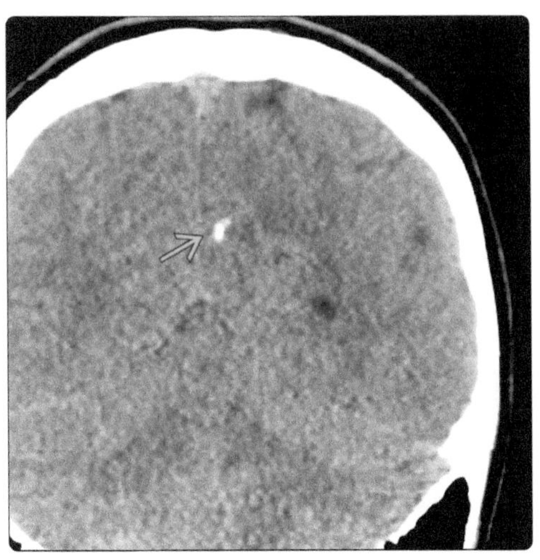

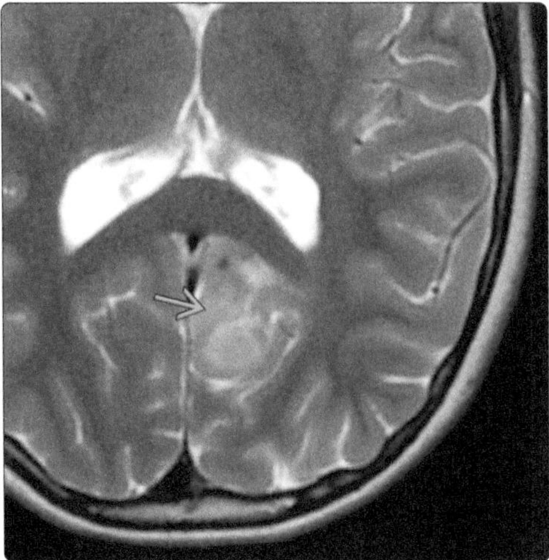

(Left) *Coronal NECT in an 11-year-old with seizures shows coarse Ca^{++} ⇒ in the left medial parietooccipital cortex. Sometimes, Ca^{++} may be the only clue to an underlying lesion, such as a GG. Ca^{++} are seen in ~ 50% of GGs.* **(Right)** *Axial T2 MR in the same patient shows ill-defined signal hyperintensity ⇒ in the left medial parietooccipital cortex with minimal associated mass effect. GG tumor margins vary tremendously from sharply marginated to hazy and ill defined.*

KEY FACTS

TERMINOLOGY

- Dysembryoplastic neuroepithelial tumor (DNET)
  - Benign, mixed glial-neuronal neoplasm
  - Adjacent cortical dysplasia frequently present

IMAGING

- May occur in any region of supratentorial cortex
  - Medial temporal lobe most common
- Typically sharply demarcated, wedge-shaped
  - Often cystic ("bubbly")
  - Minimal or no mass effect
  - No peritumoral edema
- Some DNETs have less distinct margins
  - Associated cortical dysplasia more likely in these cases
- Faint focal punctate or ring enhancement in 20-30%
- Ca^{++} in 6-36%
- Slow or no growth over years
- Remodel overlying bone in 20-44%

TOP DIFFERENTIAL DIAGNOSES

- Ganglioglioma
- Focal cortical dysplasia
- Neuroepithelial cyst
- Pleomorphic xanthoastrocytoma
- Angiocentric glioma

PATHOLOGY

- WHO grade 1
- Pathologic hallmark: Specific glioneuronal element
- Histologic subtypes: Simple, complex, and nonspecific
  - Complex: Associated cortical dysplasia present

CLINICAL ISSUES

- Typical history: Child or young adult with seizures
- Gross total resection (including adjacent dysplasia) usually curative and most important factor for seizure freedom
- Histology usually remains benign even with enhancing tumor recurrence

(Left) *Coronal oblique graphic shows an intracortical DNET. The gyrus is expanded by the characteristic multicystic-appearing tumor. Note how the tumor replaces normal cortex rather than displacing it (resulting in little to no mass effect).* **(Right)** *Axial NECT in a 13-year-old with seizures and DNET shows a geographic area of low attenuation ⮕ involving both cortex and underlying white matter in the right occipital lobe. Such an appearance is often incorrectly presumed to represent an infarct on CT.*

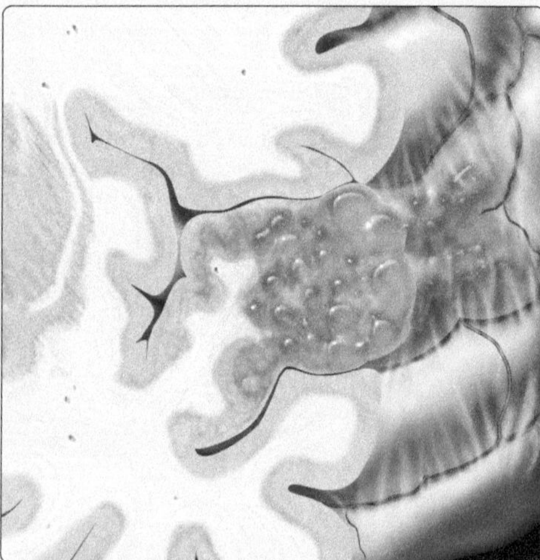

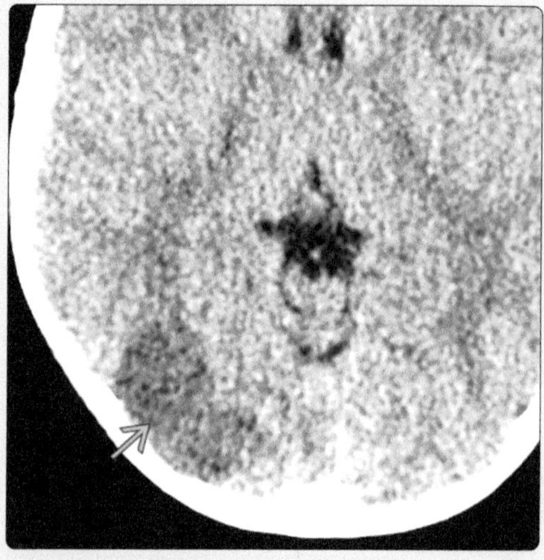

(Left) *Axial T2 MR in the same patient shows infiltrative "bubbly" hyperintense signal ⮕ replacing both cortex and subcortical white matter. Note the relative lack of mass effect, given the size of the lesion, which is common with DNET. DNETs often appear to replace rather than displace brain parenchyma.* **(Right)** *Axial T1 C+ MR in the same patient shows lack of contrast enhancement within the mass lesion ⮕. This is a typical appearance for a DNET, especially when they demonstrate a multicystic bubbly appearance on T2.*

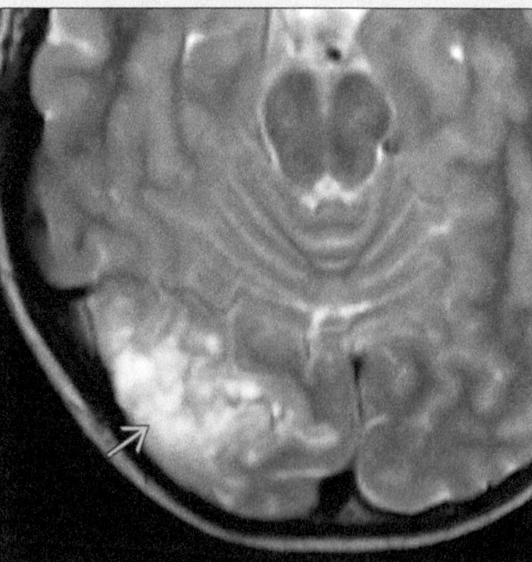

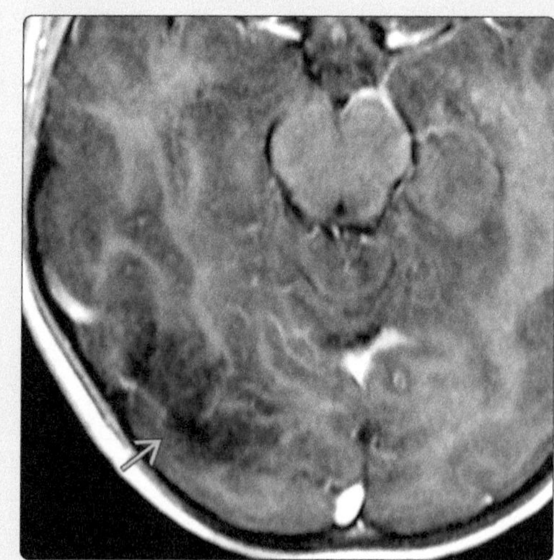

TERMINOLOGY

Abbreviations

- Dysembryoplastic neuroepithelial tumor (DNET)

Definitions

- Benign, mixed glial-neuronal neoplasm
- Epileptogenic tumor often associated with cortical dysplasia

IMAGING

General Features

- Best diagnostic clue
  - Multicystic cortical mass in young patients with seizures
- Location
  - Almost exclusively cortical
    - Temporal: 50-80%
      - Often located medially (involving amygdala and hippocampus)
    - Frontal: 15-25%
    - Parietal: 5-15%
    - Occipital: 5-15%
  - Rare: Basal ganglia, septum pellucidum, and ventricles
    - Previously described septal DNET is now classified as myxoid glioneuronal tumor in 2021 WHO CNS classification
- Size
  - Variable; may involve large portions of lobe
    - 1-7 cm (mean: 3 cm)
  - Often small at presentation due to epileptogenic nature
- Morphology
  - Often circumscribed, wedge-shaped, cystic
    - Cysts occur in majority of DNETs
  - Noncystic DNETs often less well circumscribed
    - More likely to have associated peritumoral cortical dysplasia
    - More likely to have mixed or nonspecific histology
    - More likely to be located in temporal lobe
  - Minimal mass effect, even with larger lesions
    - Replaces, rather than displaces, brain parenchyma
  - No peritumoral edema
  - Slow growth or no growth over many years
    - Often remodel overlying bone (20-44%)

CT Findings

- NECT
  - Wedge-shaped focus of cortical/subcortical hypoattenuation
    - May mimic acute processes, such as ischemia or infection (such as herpes encephalitis)
  - Scalloping of inner table of calvariae
  - Ca^{++} in 6-36%
  - Hemorrhage rarely reported
- CECT
  - Faint nodular or patchy enhancement in 20%

MR Findings

- T1WI
  - Multilobular, hypointense, "bubbly" mass
  - Noncystic component typically isointense to cortex
- T2WI
  - Large, septated cyst(s) or many small cysts
    - Not true cysts but "pseudocysts" (due to lack of epithelial lining)
  - Noncystic component typically appears mildly hyperintense to cortex (but variable)
- FLAIR
  - Appearance of cystic component variable
    - Fluid often suppresses like CSF
    - Fluid may be isointense or hyperintense to adjacent solid component
  - Noncystic component also variable but usually hyperintense to cortex
  - Best sequence to detect possible adjacent cortical dysplasia
- T2* GRE
  - Hemorrhage rarely reported
  - Hypointense areas often correspond to Ca^{++}
- DWI
  - Typically high ADC signal/values relative to normal brain parenchyma
    - High diffusivity, low cellularity
- T1WI C+
  - Enhancement in 20-30%
    - Nodular, ring-like, or heterogeneous
    - Nodular enhancement common in recurrent tumor
- MRS
  - Nonspecific, but relatively normal MRS may help distinguish from higher grade tumor (such as oligodendroglioma)
- Perfusion
  - Typically decreased cerebral blood flow (CBV) compared to contralateral normal brain parenchyma

Nuclear Medicine Findings

- PET
  - Hypometabolism with FDG-18 PET
  - Relatively low 11C-methionine uptake in DNETs compared to ganglioglioma or gliomas

Imaging Recommendations

- Best imaging tool
  - MR with T1WI C+, FLAIR
    - Most sensitive sequences for small tumor identification: 3D and coronal oblique FLAIR

DIFFERENTIAL DIAGNOSIS

Ganglioglioma

- Ca^{++} and enhancement more common
- More often noncystic

Focal Cortical Dysplasia

- Nonenhancing, noncystic lesion
- Resembles cortical tuber of tuberous sclerosis without gyral enlargement

Neuroglial Cyst

- Nonenhancing single or complex cystic lesion
- Suppresses on FLAIR MR with no abnormal adjacent signal

Pleomorphic Xanthoastrocytoma

- Enhancing nodule abuts pia with variable pial enhancement
- Look for dural tail

Angiocentric Glioma (Angiocentric Neuroepithelial Tumor)

- Rare, cortically based, low-grade neoplasm, typically nonenhancing
- Similar age group to DNET

PATHOLOGY

General Features

- Etiology
  - Embryology: Likely dysplastic cells in germinal matrix
  - Extend along migratory path of neurons toward cortex
    - Accounts for wedge-shaped morphology of tumor
  - Contain gelatinous cysts
  - Associated with cortical dysplasia
- Genetics
  - Sporadic

Staging, Grading, & Classification

- WHO grade 1

Gross Pathologic & Surgical Features

- Neocortical lesion
- Thick gyrus
- Viscous consistency of glioneuronal component of tumor
- Firm nodules represent more stromal components

Microscopic Features

- Hallmark: Specific glioneuronal element (SGNE)
  - Characterized by columns of bundled axons oriented perpendicular to cortex
  - Columns lined by oligodendroglia-like cells
  - Other cells show astrocytic and neuronal differentiation
- Several histologic types
  - Simple DNET: Classic form with SGNE
  - Complex DNET: Simple form plus
    - Associated glial nodules (oligodendroglial, astrocytic, or both)
    - Associated cortical dysplasia
  - Nonspecific DNET: Controversial (not true histopathologic entity)
    - SGNE absent, but glial and dysplastic components of complex form present
    - Overlaps with other glial and glioneuronal tumors
    - By imaging, cysts uncommon, and tumor margins may be indistinct
- Microcystic degeneration
  - Neurons "float" in pale, eosinophilic, mucoid matrix
- Low proliferative potential with variable MIB-1 index

Molecular Features

- *BRAF* V600E mutations frequently identified (~ 50%)
- *FGFR1* alterations in ~ 40-80%
  - Septal DNET with *PDGFRA* alterations is now classified as myxoid glioneuronal tumor

CLINICAL ISSUES

Presentation

- Most common signs/symptoms
  - Partial complex seizures

Demographics

- Age
  - Children and young adults
    - Mean age of seizure onset: ~ 10 years
    - Majority present by 20 years
- Sex
  - Slight male predominance
- Ethnicity
  - None established
- Epidemiology
  - ~ 1% of primary neuroepithelial brain tumors in patients < 20 years of age

Natural History & Prognosis

- Benign lesions
  - Rare, malignant transformation or spinal drop metastases
- Slow growth or stability over time
- Rarely recur status post resection, but imaging follow-up recommended in most cases
  - Recurrent tumor commonly presents as nodular enhancement
  - Histology of recurrent tumor usually remains benign but may have features of other low-grade tumors (such as astrocytoma)
  - Malignant transformation described but very rare

Treatment

- Seizures may become intractable
  - Glutamate receptors shown within tumor and margins may explain typical, difficult to control seizures
- Most important factors for long-term seizure freedom: Gross total resection of tumor and adjacent cortical dysplasia

DIAGNOSTIC CHECKLIST

Consider

- DNET with T2-hyperintense, "bubbly" cortical mass in child/young adult with partial complex epilepsy

Image Interpretation Pearls

- Beware of enhancing lesions, which may be more ominous than DNET

SELECTED REFERENCES

1. Agarwal A et al: Value of quantitative apparent diffusion coefficients in differentiating low-grade gliomas from mixed neuronal-glial tumors. World Neurosurg X. 18:100159, 2023
2. Vaz A et al: Uncommon glioneuronal tumors: a radiologic and pathologic synopsis. AJNR Am J Neuroradiol. 43(8) 1080-9, 2022
3. WHO Classification of Tumours Editorial Board: WHO Classification of Tumours: Central Nervous System Tumours. 5th ed. IARC, 2021
4. Onishi S et al: T2-FLAIR mismatch sign in dysembryoplasticneuroepithelial tumor. Eur J Radiol. 126:108924, 2020
5. Chiang JCH et al: Septal dysembryoplastic neuroepithelial tumor: a comprehensive clinical, imaging, histopathologic, and molecular analysis. Neuro Oncol. 21(6):800-8, 2019

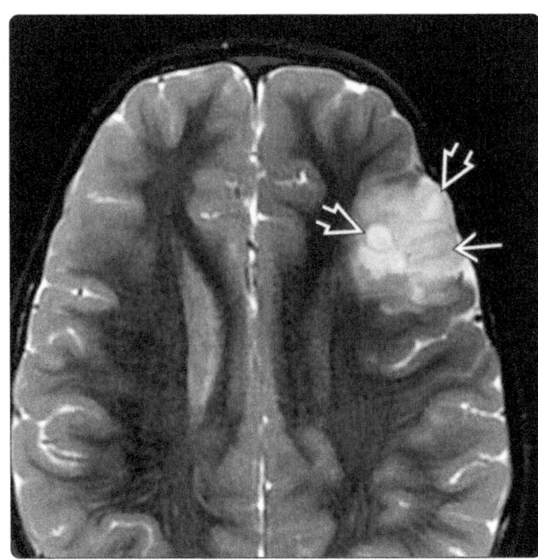

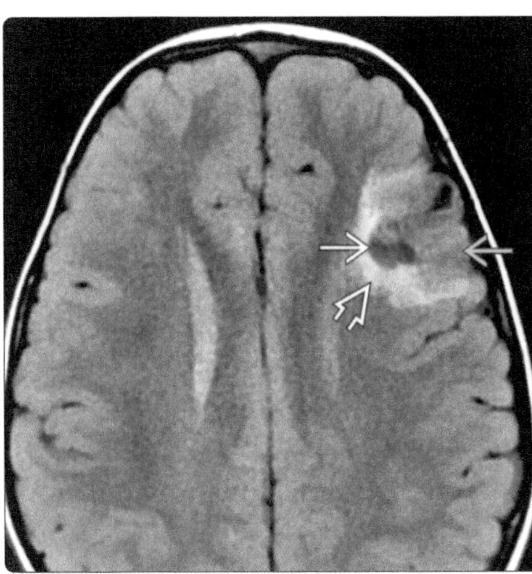

(Left) *Axial T2 MR in a 6-year-old boy with rapid eye movements and lip smacking shows a tumor with mixed solid ➡ and cystic ➡ components. Note the replacement of normal cortex with hyperintense tumor as well as the lack of mass effect.* **(Right)** *Axial FLAIR MR in the same patient shows that the high T2 signal within the cystic components has now suppressed ➡. The noncystic component ➡ of a DNET is typically hyperintense to gray matter but can be isointense or even hypointense ➡.*

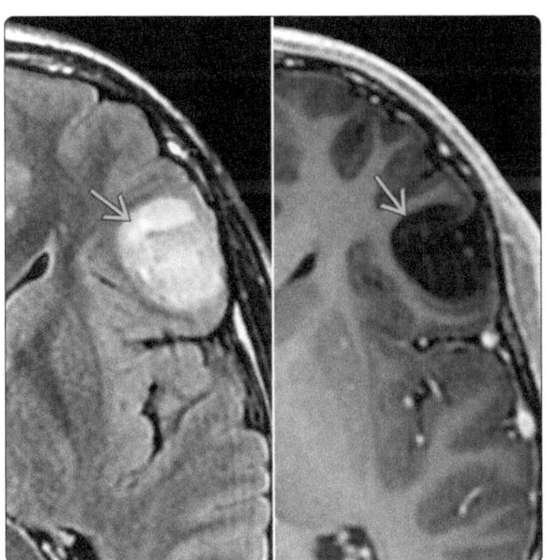

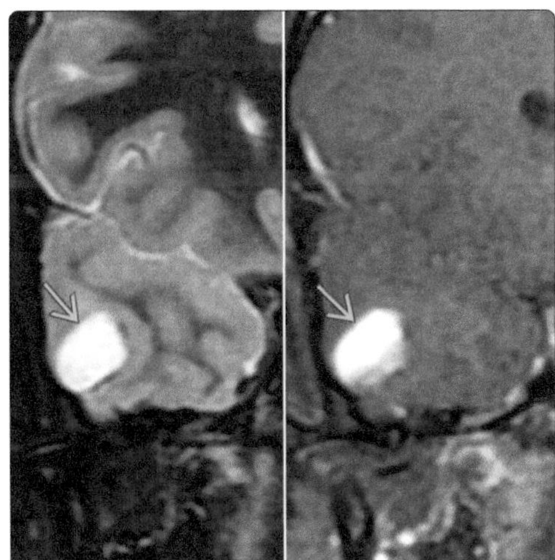

(Left) *Axial FLAIR (left) and T1 C+ (right) MR in a 14-year-old with a DNET show a well-defined lesion ➡ involving both cortex and underlying white matter. The margins of DNETs are highly variable from sharp, well-delineated margins, such as this case, to hazy, ill-defined margins. Lack of contrast enhancement is most common.* **(Right)** *Coronal STIR (left) and T1 C+ (right) MR in an 11-year-old with new-onset seizures show avid enhancement throughout the majority of the tumor ➡. Enhancement is seen in ~ 20-30% of DNETs.*

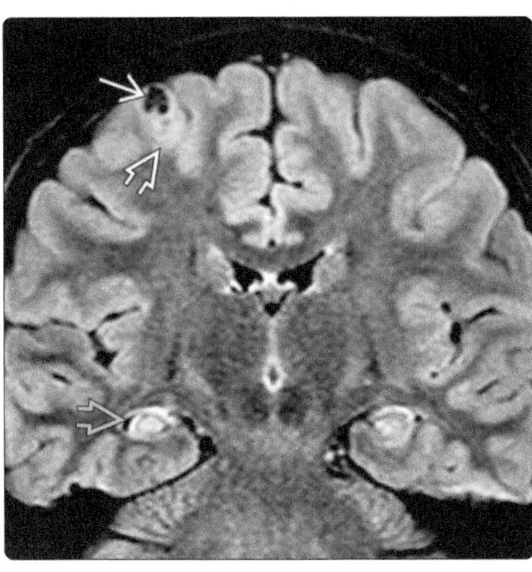

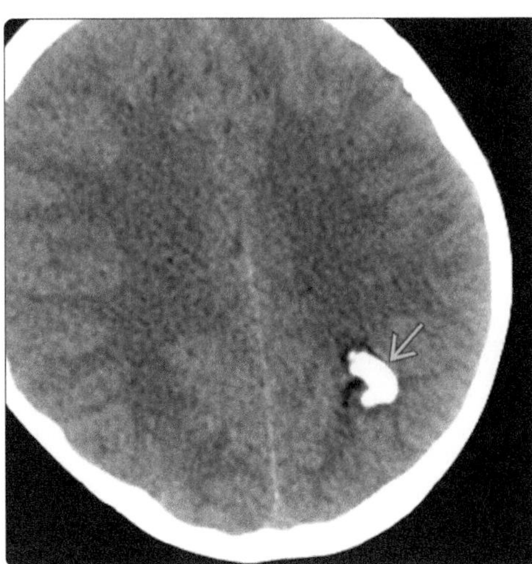

(Left) *Coronal oblique FLAIR MR in a 12-year-old girl with intractable epilepsy for 2 years shows a small DNET with complete signal suppression of the cystic component ➡. The noncystic component ➡ shows subtle hyperintensity. Note the associated right hippocampal sclerosis ➡.* **(Right)** *Axial NECT in a 10-year-old boy with a DNET shows thick, chunky Ca^{++} ➡ within the subcortical white matter. Ca^{++} can occur in DNET but is less common in DNET compared to another common cortical tumor, ganglioglioma.*

Desmoplastic Infantile Tumors

KEY FACTS

TERMINOLOGY

- Large, cystic tumors of infants involving superficial cerebral cortex & leptomeninges
- Desmoplastic infantile ganglioglioma (DIG)
  - Prominent desmoplastic stroma + neoplastic astrocytes & variable neuronal component
- Desmoplastic infantile astrocytoma (DIA)
  - Desmoplastic stroma + neoplastic astrocytes

IMAGING

- Peripheral supratentorial tumor with large cyst(s) & cortically based solid nodule/plaque in child < 2 years of age
- Variable T2 signal of solid component, often markedly ↓
  - Peritumoral edema may be vasogenic or interstitial from obstructive hydrocephalus
- May have diffusion restriction despite low histologic grade
- Peripheral solid component often avidly enhances
- Broad dural base + enhancement of adjacent meninges
- Hemorrhage & Ca^{++} uncommon

TOP DIFFERENTIAL DIAGNOSES

- Embryonal tumor with multilayered rosettes
- Infantile glioblastoma
- Atypical teratoid/rhabdoid tumor (AT/RT)
- Supratentorial ependymoma
- Pleomorphic xanthoastrocytoma
- Pilocytic astrocytoma

PATHOLOGY

- WHO grade 1
- Areas of cellular proliferation, mitoses, & necrosis may cause misdiagnosis as higher grade tumor

CLINICAL ISSUES

- Most found at 1-24 months of age (peak: 3-6 months)
- 16% of intracranial tumors in 1st year of life
- Median survival rate > 75% at 15 years
- Complete surgical resection typically curative
  - 40% require additional therapy beyond surgery

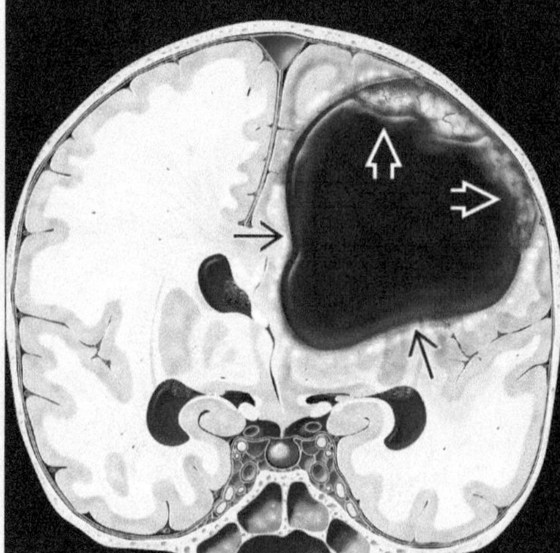

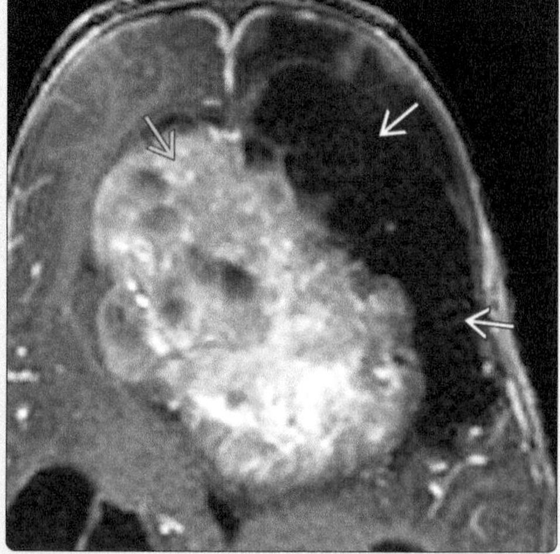

(Left) *Graphic shows desmoplastic infantile ganglioglioma/astrocytoma (DIG/DIA). Note the dominant cystic component ⇨ with a dural-based plaque of desmoplastic stroma ➡. Mild surrounding edema and hydrocephalus is present.* **(Right)** *Axial T1 C+ MR in a 15-month-old with loss of developmental milestones shows a large, central supratentorial mass with enhancing solid ⇨ & complex cystic ➡ areas. DIG arising from paracentral cortex may appear central rather than peripheral in location.*

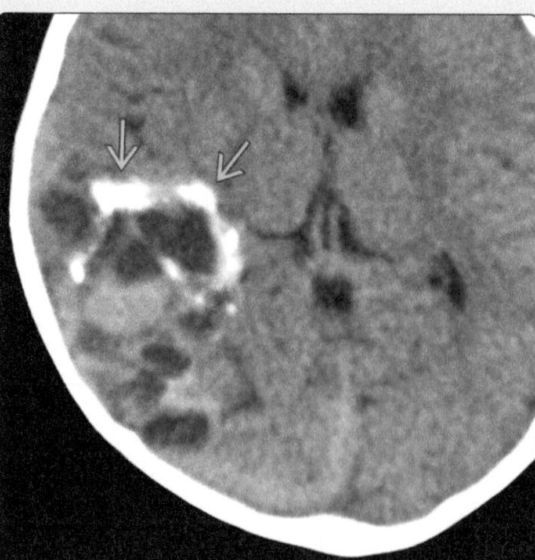

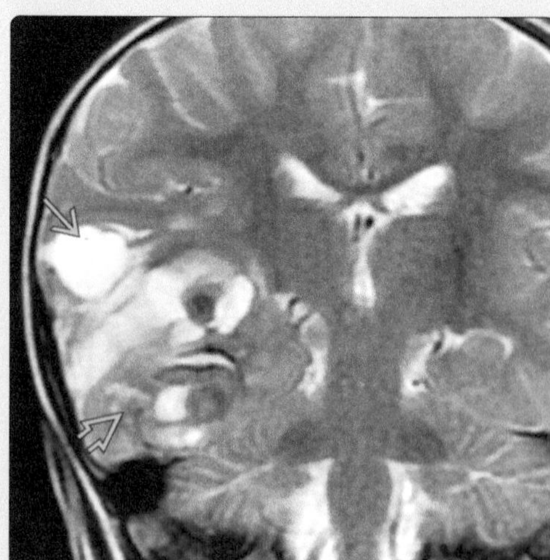

(Left) *Axial NECT in a 20-month-old with DIG shows chunky peripheral Ca^{++} ⇨ anteriorly with heterogeneous attenuation elsewhere amongst the cysts and solid tumor components. Ca^{++} and hemorrhage is commonly seen on CT in DIG/DIA.* **(Right)** *Coronal T2 MR in the same patient shows mixed solid ⇨ and cystic ⇨ components of the tumor, common in DIG/DIA. Common appearances include multiple prominent cysts as well as a single large cyst with a solid, peripheral component.*

TERMINOLOGY

Abbreviations

- Desmoplastic infantile ganglioglioma (DIG)
- Desmoplastic infantile astrocytoma (DIA)

Synonyms

- Desmoplastic supratentorial neuroepithelial tumors of infancy
- Superficial cerebral astrocytoma ± neuronal elements attached to dura

Definitions

- Large WHO grade 1 cystic tumors of infants involving superficial cerebral cortex & leptomeninges, often attached to dura
- DIG: Prominent desmoplastic stroma + neoplastic astrocytes, variable neuronal component
- DIA: Desmoplastic stroma + neoplastic astrocytes

IMAGING

General Features

- Best diagnostic clue
  - Large, cystic mass with cortically based, enhancing solid nodule/plaque in child < 2 years of age
  - Enhancement of adjacent pia + reactive dural thickening
  - Solid portion may have hypointense T2 signal
- Location
  - Supratentorial: Frontal/parietal > temporal > occipital
- Size
  - Cysts may be very large & cause macrocephaly with bulging fontanelle in infants
- Morphology
  - Solid & cystic mass, usually with dural attachment
    - Solid components typically concentrated at superficial location
  - Minority of tumors (~ 20%) may be completely solid

CT Findings

- NECT
  - Large, heterogeneous, solid & cystic mass
  - Well-demarcated hypodense cysts (isodense to CSF)
  - Solid tumor nodule(s) isodense/slightly hyperdense to gray matter (GM)
  - Ca^{++} & hemorrhage uncommon
- CECT
  - Large cysts ± rim enhancement
  - Solid component typically shows marked enhancement
- CTA
  - Vessels often significantly displaced by large tumors

MR Findings

- T1WI
  - Cysts: Hypointense, often multilobulated
    - May contain septations
  - Solid portion: Heterogeneous nodule or plaque-like areas in periphery
- T2WI
  - Cysts hyperintense
  - Solid components variable but sometimes markedly hypointense [< myelinated white matter (WM)]
  - Peritumoral edema often present, particularly with larger masses
- FLAIR
  - Cysts isointense to CSF
  - Solid portions usually isointense to GM
  - Hyperintense WM signal (transependymal or vasogenic edema) often seen with larger masses
- T2* GRE
  - Hemorrhage & Ca^{++} uncommon
- DWI
  - DWI & ADC signal typically equal to GM in solid component despite low grade
- T1WI C+
  - Solid tumor nodule/plaque markedly enhances
  - Enhancement of leptomeninges & dura adjacent to solid tumor typical
  - Cysts typically more central than enhancing solid nodule
    - ± wall enhancement of cysts
  - Leptomeningeal spread of disease may occur (but uncommon)
- MRS
  - ↓ NAA, ↑ choline
  - No significant alterations in myoinositol/Cr

Ultrasonographic Findings

- Grayscale ultrasound
  - Large, multicystic mass
  - Hypo- to isoechoic solid tumor nodule/plaque
    - May be difficult to see on US due to typical superficial location

Imaging Recommendations

- Best imaging tool
  - Multiplanar contrast-enhanced MR

DIFFERENTIAL DIAGNOSIS

Embryonal Tumor With Multilayered Rosettes

- Formerly known as primitive neuroectodermal tumor (PNET)
- Solid tumor, hyperdense on CT, very low ADC values, Ca^{++} in 50-70%
- Large, heterogeneously enhancing hemispheric mass
- Large cyst less common than in DIG/DIA

Infantile Glioblastoma

- Less commonly contain cystic components (~ 30%)
- Typically lower ADC values with more heterogeneous enhancement of solid component

Atypical Teratoid/Rhabdoid Tumor

- Large, solid/cystic/necrotic tumors
- Similar imaging characteristics: Solid portion with hypointense T2 & reduced diffusion
- Infra- or supratentorial
- Found in infants & young children

Supratentorial Ependymoma

- Nonspecific imaging findings but commonly contains Ca^{++}
- Solid portion usually less peripherally located than DIG
- Cysts often less complex than DIG

Pleomorphic Xanthoastrocytoma

- May appear identical to DIG
- Temporal lobe most common location
- Occurs in older children & young adults

Pilocytic Astrocytoma

- Uncommon in cerebral hemispheres
- Cyst usually smaller than DIG/DIA with enhancing nodule
- Rare in infancy

PATHOLOGY

General Features

- Etiology
  - Possibly related to progenitor cells in subcortical zone along with mature subpial astrocytes
- Genetics
  - No consistent chromosomal alterations
  - *BRAF* V600D & V600E mutations occur in ~ 40% of tumors
  - DIA & DIG share similar molecular profiles, suggesting they represent histologic spectrum of same tumor rather than 2 separate entities

Staging, Grading, & Classification

- WHO grade 1
- Small subset of tumors show anaplasia & have more aggressive course

Gross Pathologic & Surgical Features

- 2 distinct components
  - Cortically based solid tumor nodule with adjacent dural thickening
    - Firm attachment to dura & brain parenchyma
  - Large associated cysts compress adjacent ventricular system
    - Large cyst contains xanthochromic fluid

Microscopic Features

- DIA: Astrocytes only tumor cell
- DIG: Astrocytes + neoplastic neurons
  - Intense desmoplasia with mixture of astroglial & immature neuronal cells
- Spindle cells in collagenous stroma forming whorled patterns
- Areas of cellular proliferation, mitoses, & necrosis may cause misdiagnosis as higher grade tumors
  - Mitoses rare
- Ki-67 (MIB-1) proliferation indices < 2-5%

Immunohistochemistry

- GFAP & vimentin positive
- Synaptophysin positive if neuronal elements present (DIG)

CLINICAL ISSUES

Presentation

- Most common signs/symptoms
  - ↑ head size, bulging fontanelles, paresis, seizures
  - Older children: Seizures & focal neurologic signs/symptoms
- Clinical profile
  - Infant with rapidly progressive macrocephaly

Demographics

- Age
  - Most found at 1-24 months (peak: 3-6 months)
  - ~ 20% occur in older children & adults
- Sex
  - M:F = 2:1
- Epidemiology
  - 1.25% of intracranial tumors in childhood
  - 16% of intracranial tumors in 1st year of life

Natural History & Prognosis

- Median survival rate > 75% 15 years after diagnosis
  - 40% require additional therapy beyond surgery

Treatment

- Surgical resection curative (no recurrence with complete resection)
- Chemotherapy if brain invasion or recurrence
- Targeted BRAF inhibitors may work in *BRAF* V600 mutants

DIAGNOSTIC CHECKLIST

Consider

- DIG/DIA: Large, cystic mass in infant with plaque-like or nodular component along meninges
  - Important to mention DIG/DIA in report as pathologists may initially misinterpret as highly malignant tumor

Image Interpretation Pearls

- Solid peripheral portion involves cortex, often invades adjacent meninges
- Solid portion may be markedly hypointense (< myelinated WM)

SELECTED REFERENCES

1. Dias DJL et al: MRI Findings of desmoplastic infantile ganglioglioma: a case report and analysis. Cureus. 15(8):e43770, 2023
2. Louis DN et al: The 2021 WHO classification of tumors of the central nervous system: a summary. Neuro Oncol. 23(8):1231-51, 2021
3. WHO Classification of Tumours Editorial Board: WHO Classification of CNS Tumours. 5th ed. IARC, 2021
4. Benson JC et al: Mixed solid and cystic mass in an infant. AJNR Am J Neuroradiol. 40(11):1792-5, 2019
5. Cohen AR: The great neurosurgical masquerader: 3 cases of desmoplastic infantile ganglioglioma. J Neurosurg Pediatr. 1-9, 2019
6. van Tilburg CM et al: Response in a child with a BRAF V600E mutated desmoplastic infantile astrocytoma upon retreatment with vemurafenib. Pediatr Blood Cancer. 65(3), 2018
7. Wang AC et al: Desmoplastic infantile ganglioglioma/astrocytoma (DIG/DIA) are distinct entities with frequent BRAFV600 mutations. Mol Cancer Res. 16(10):1491-8, 2018
8. Bianchi F et al: Supratentorial tumors typical of the infantile age: desmoplastic infantile ganglioglioma (DIG) and astrocytoma (DIA). A review. Childs Nerv Syst. 32(10):1833-8, 2016
9. Bader A et al: Radiological features of infantile glioblastoma and desmoplastic infantile tumors: British Columbia's Children's Hospital experience. J Neurosurg Pediatr. 1-7, 2015
10. Jurkiewicz E et al: MR imaging, apparent diffusion coefficient and histopathological features of desmoplastic infantile tumors-own experience and review of the literature. Childs Nerv Syst. 31(2):251-9, 2015
11. Kralik SF et al: Diffusion imaging for tumor grading of supratentorial brain tumors in the first year of life. AJNR Am J Neuroradiol. 35(4):815-23, 2014
12. Romero-Rojas AE et al: Desmoplastic infantile ganglioglioma with late presentation. A clinical, radiological and histopathological analysis. Neuroradiol J. 26(6):649-54, 2013
13. Balaji R et al: Imaging of desmoplastic infantile ganglioglioma: a spectroscopic viewpoint. Childs Nerv Syst. 25(4):497-501, 2009

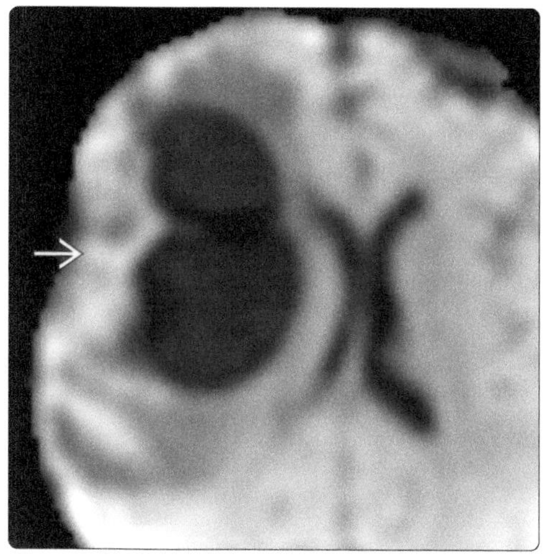

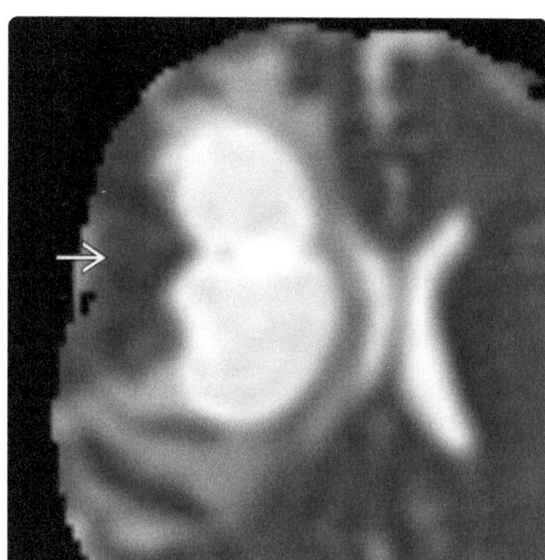

(Left) *Axial DWI MR in a 5-month-old girl with DIG shows the peripheral solid component* ➡ *to be iso- to hyperintense to brain parenchyma. Diffusion within the solid component is highly variable but is most often equal to gray matter. For this reason, more cellular tumors are often included in the DDx.* **(Right)** *Axial ADC map in the same patient shows the peripheral solid component* ➡ *to be isointense to brain parenchyma. ADC signal in the solid component is variable but most often is isointense to gray matter.*

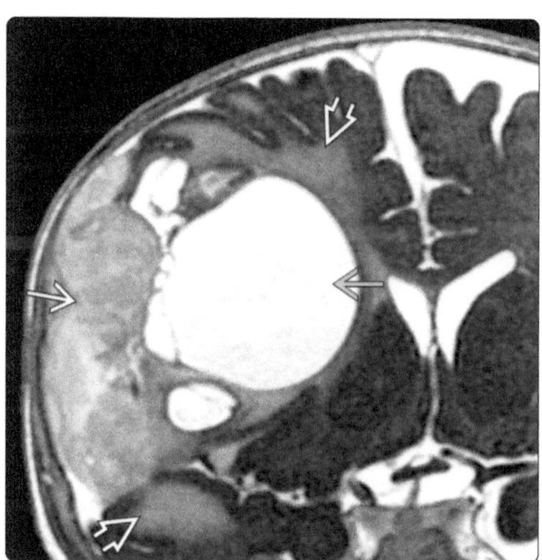

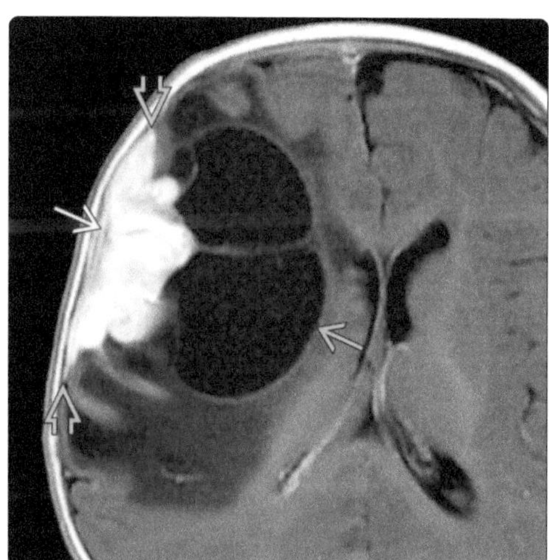

(Left) *Coronal 3D FIESTA MR in a 5-month-old girl with increasing head circumference shows a large, right cerebral mass with a peripheral hyperintense solid component* ➡ *& a more central cystic component* ➡*. Note also the peritumoral vasogenic edema* ➡*.* **(Right)** *Axial T1 C+ MR in the same patient shows homogeneous enhancement of the peripheral solid component* ➡ *& no significant enhancement along the margins of the central cystic component* ➡*. Note the broad-based dural attachment* ➡ *of this DIG.*

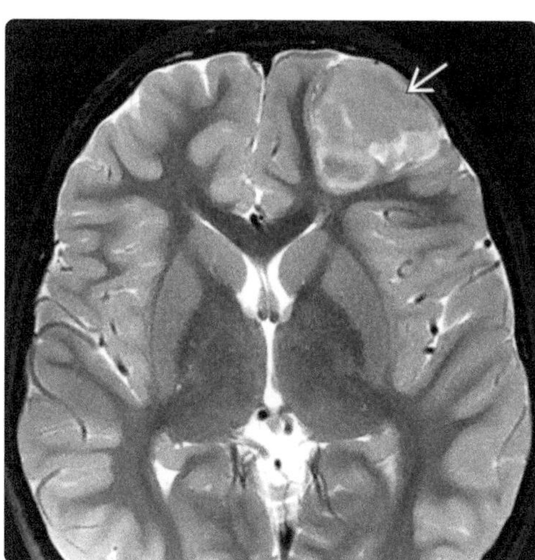

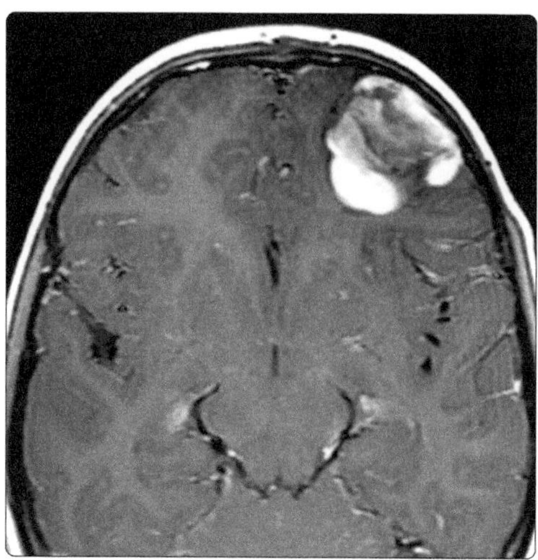

(Left) *Axial T2 MR in a 10-year-old boy with headache shows a left frontal lobe, cortically based, solid mass with signal intensity predominantly equal to gray matter* ➡*. Pathology revealed a DIG. DIG is uncommon in older children & adults but can occur in these age groups.* **(Right)** *Axial T1 C+ MR in the same patient shows a cortically based, solid mass with avid but heterogeneous enhancement. Pathology revealed a DIG. A minority of DIG tumors are completely solid (as in this case).*

Dysplastic Cerebellar Gangliocytoma

KEY FACTS

TERMINOLOGY

- Benign cerebellar lesion; controversial whether neoplastic or hamartomatous; WHO grade 1
- Multiple hamartoma syndrome (MHAM) → autosomal dominant, mutation in *PTEN* gene, associated with ↑ incidence of malignancy
- Lhermitte-Duclos disease (LDD) now considered neurologic manifestation of MHAM and part of new neurocutaneous syndrome
- MHAM = Cowden syndrome; Cowden-Lhermitte-Duclos (COLD) = MHAM + LDD

IMAGING

- Unilateral mass-like widening of multiple cerebellar folia
- T2/FLAIR hyperintensity in white matter with normal cortex
  - Striated/corduroy/tigroid/gyriform pattern
- LDD always in cerebellum and may be large → mass effect, tonsillar herniation, hydrocephalus

TOP DIFFERENTIAL DIAGNOSES

- Subacute cerebellar infarction
- Cerebellitis
- Unclassified cerebellar dysplasias
- Pilocytic astrocytoma
- Ganglioglioma
- Medulloblastoma
- Meningeal metastases
- Meningeal granulomatous disease

CLINICAL ISSUES

- Most common presentation: Headache, nausea and vomiting, ataxia, blurred vision
  - Can present in coma
- Surgical resection is treatment of choice
- If LDD, screen for MHAM; if MHAM, screen for LDD
- Long-term cancer screening needed, especially thyroid and breast (↑ malignancy in MHAM)

(Left) *Axial graphic shows thickened and irregular cerebellar folia in the right cerebellar hemisphere. This results in the enlargement of the hemisphere and mass effect upon the brainstem, which is typical of Lhermitte-Duclos disease (LDD).* **(Right)** *Coronal T2 MR shows striated thickening of isointense cortex with hyperintense intervening white matter composing the right cerebellar mass ➡ that extends into the vermis and herniates ⮫ across the cerebellar midline.*

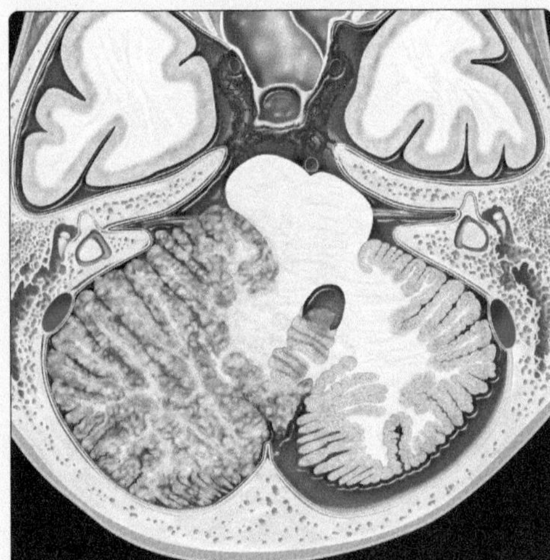

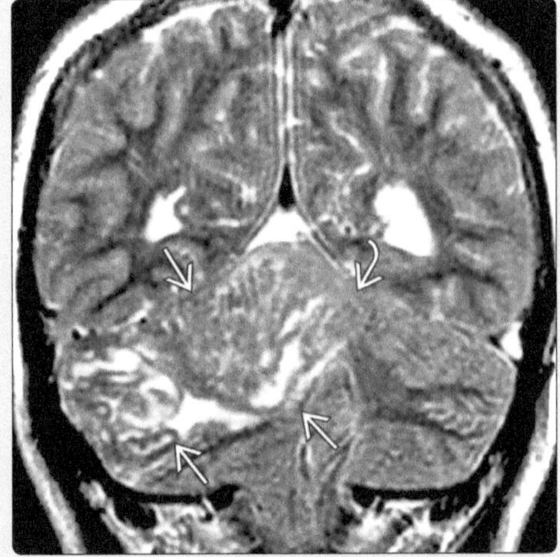

(Left) *Axial T2 MR in an adult with dysplastic gangliocytoma shows a hyperintense mass lesion ➡ in the left posterior cerebellar hemisphere. Note the partial maintenance of cerebellar sulci and folia with expansion of the folia. This is a characteristic appearance for dysplastic gangliocytoma and is sometimes described as the corduroy or tigroid pattern.* **(Right)** *Axial T1 C+ MR in the same patient shows no intrinsic enhancement within the lesion. Multiple linear and punctate areas of enhancement ➡ correspond to vessels.*

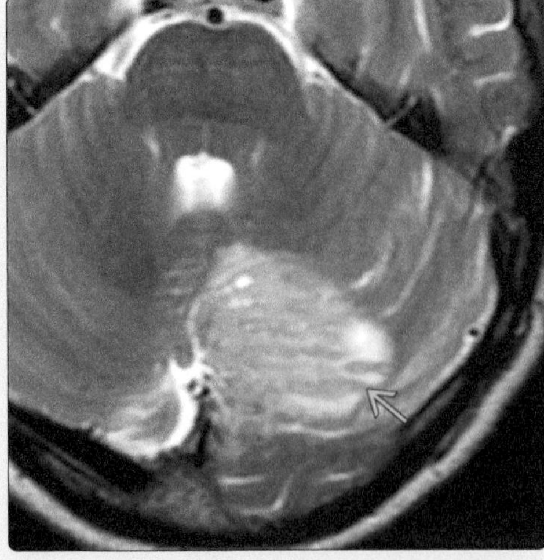

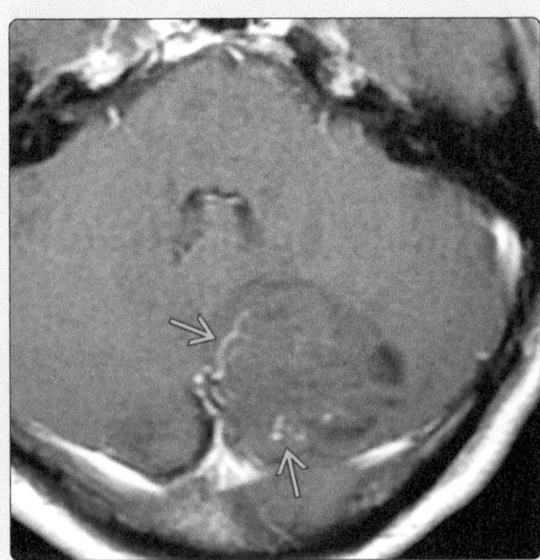

TERMINOLOGY

Synonyms

- Lhermitte-Duclos disease (LDD)
  - Dysplastic cerebellar gangliocytoma, gangliocytoma dysplasticum, hamartoma of cerebellum
  - Hamartoblastoma, cerebelloparenchymal disorder 6, granule cell hypertrophy, granular cell hypertrophy, granulomolecular hypertrophy
  - Diffuse ganglioneuroma of cerebellar cortex, diffuse cerebellar hypertrophy, neurocytic blastoma, myelinated neurocytoma, purkinjeoma
- Multiple hamartoma syndrome (MHAM)
  - Multiple hamartoma-neoplasia syndrome, Cowden disease, Cowden syndrome (CS), Cowden-Lhermitte-Duclos (COLD) syndrome

Definitions

- LDD → neurologic manifestation of MHAM
  - Benign cerebellar lesion with some controversy about whether it represents neoplastic or hamartomatous lesion
    - Considered WHO grade 1 tumor of ganglion cell origin in 2021 WHO Classification of CNS Tumours
    - Recurrent growth and development of this lesion in patients with previously normal MR findings suggest some component of neoplasia
  - Association between LDD and MHAM probably represents new neurocutaneous syndrome
- MHAM: Autosomal dominant, variable expression, typically mutation in *PTEN* gene
  - *PTEN* is part of mTORC1 pathway, involved in cell proliferation and neoplasia
  - Hamartomatous neoplasms of skin (90-100%), mucosa, GI tract, bones, CNS, eyes, and GU tract
  - Associated with ↑ incidence of malignancy
  - Other types of tumors and vascular malformations may be present on MR

IMAGING

General Features

- Best diagnostic clue
  - Widened cerebellar folia, gyriform pattern
  - Widened folia are typically hyperintense on T2/FLAIR
- Location
  - Always in cerebellum, usually unilateral
  - Often involves vermis, rarely brainstem
- Size
  - Variable, may be large → mass effect, tonsillar herniation, hydrocephalus
- Morphology
  - Margins are typically well demarcated but may sometimes be indistinct

Radiographic Findings

- ± thinning of skull

CT Findings

- NECT
  - Normal to high attenuation with striations
  - Occasionally, cystic areas &/or calcifications
- CECT
  - ± enhancement

MR Findings

- T1WI
  - Iso- to hypointense with striations
  - Calcifications may rarely cause ↑ signal
- T2WI
  - ↑ signal in expanded white matter (WM) with darker cortex
    - Results in striated corduroy or tigroid pattern
  - May have bizarre gyriform appearance
  - Newborns may not have obvious striations since cerebellar WM not fully myelinated
- FLAIR
  - ↑ signal within WM of expanded folia
  - May have hypointense cysts
- T2* GRE
  - Veins between folia
- DWI
  - ↑ signal on DWI usually due to T2 hyperintensity
  - Low to ↑ ADC; ↑ ADC in WM, cysts
  - May have ↑ fractional anisotropy (FA) in WM
- PWI
  - May show areas of ↑ relative cerebral blood volume (rCBV) and regional cerebral blood flow (rCBF)
- T1WI C+
  - No or mild enhancement is typical but can vary
    - ↑ vascularity peripherally in molecular layer and leptomeninges
- MRS
  - ↓ NAA, ↓ choline, ↓ myoinositol
  - Variable lactate, may be ↑

Nuclear Medicine Findings

- PET
  - ↑ uptake FDG PET and 11C-methionine PET
  - Report of ↑ CBF, ↓ OEF, and similar $CMRO_2$ compared to normal cerebral hemisphere

Imaging Recommendations

- Best imaging tool
  - MR with DWI, MRS, and contrast
- Protocol advice
  - Coronal T2WI may be helpful
  - If LDD, initiate work-up for MHAM and screen for malignancies
  - If lesion enhances, consider differential diagnosis carefully

DIFFERENTIAL DIAGNOSIS

Subacute Cerebellar Infarction

- Diffusion restriction, typically in wedge-shaped or vascular distribution
- Acute onset of cerebellar symptoms typical

Cerebellitis/Vasculitis

- Acute onset of symptoms
- Can be very difficult to distinguish, but follow-up imaging should help delineate
  - Cerebellitis will mostly resolve on follow-up

Unclassified Cerebellar Dysplasias

- Do not progress; hydrocephalus rare
- Affected cerebellum usually smaller rather than large

Pilocytic Astrocytoma

- May be difficult to distinguish on imaging features alone
- Typically more well defined with robust enhancement
- More likely to have cystic components

Ganglioglioma

- May have bizarre appearance simulating LDD
- More likely to have areas of nodular enhancement and cyst formation

Tuberous Sclerosis Complex

- Typically demonstrate wedge-shaped volume loss with enhancement and ↓ SWI/GRE signal

Medulloblastoma

- Lateral sonic hedgehog (SHH) molecular subtype may have somewhat striated appearance
- Typically demonstrates diffusion restriction

Meningeal Metastases

- Nodular leptomeningeal enhancement
- Look for involvement elsewhere (basilar cisterns)

Meningeal Granulomatous Disease

- Nodular leptomeningeal enhancement
- Typically shows involvement in suprasellar and basilar cisterns

PATHOLOGY

General Features

- Etiology
  - Unclear, but evidence of nonproliferation/absence of malignant transformation favors hamartomatous nature
  - Can develop in patients with previously normal MR exams
- Genetics
  - Many have mutations of *PTEN* (MMAC1) gene at 10q23.31 (tumor suppressor gene)
  - Activation of PTEN/AKT/mTOR molecular pathway suggests role for mTOR in pathogenesis
- Associated abnormalities
  - Most patients with LDD likely have MHAM

Staging, Grading, & Classification

- WHO grade 1

Gross Pathologic & Surgical Features

- Markedly enlarged cerebellar hemisphere/vermis with thick folia
- Mass appears pale

Microscopic Features

- Widening of molecular cell layer → occupied by abnormal ganglion cells
- Absence of Purkinje cell layer
- Hypertrophy of granule cell layer
- ↓ volume of WM
- Histologically may be confused with ganglion cell tumor

CLINICAL ISSUES

Presentation

- Most common signs/symptoms
  - Headache, nausea and vomiting, papilledema, unsteady gait, upper limb ataxia and dysmetria, blurred vision, lower cranial nerve palsies
- Other signs/symptoms
  - Sensory motor deficits, vertigo, neuropsychologic deficits
- Clinical profile
  - If LDD, screen for MHAM; if MHAM, screen for LDD

Demographics

- Age
  - Any; presentation most common from 20-40 years
- Sex
  - M ~ F
- Ethnicity
  - No known predilection
- Epidemiology
  - ↑ degree of penetrance in family members

Natural History & Prognosis

- Many do not grow or grow only slowly
- If mass effect is not relieved, prognosis is poor
- Postsurgery recurrences are rare but do occur

Treatment

- Options, risks, complications
  - Borders of lesion blend into normal surrounding cerebellum → total resection difficult
  - Surgical resection in symptomatic patients

DIAGNOSTIC CHECKLIST

Consider

- Search for other features of MHAM when LDD is diagnosed and vice versa
- Long-term cancer screening needed (especially breast in women, thyroid in men and women)

Image Interpretation Pearls

- Relatively well-defined cerebellar mass with striated tigroid or gyriform pattern

SELECTED REFERENCES

1. Zhang HW et al: MR imaging features of Lhermitte-Duclos disease: case reports and literature review. Medicine (Baltimore). 101(4):e28667, 2022
2. Puiseux C et al: Dysplastic gangliocytoma of the cerebellum (Lhermitte-Duclos disease) presenting as a prenatally heterotopic hamartoma. Childs Nerv Syst. 37(3):1017-20, 2020
3. Dhamija R et al: Updated imaging features of dysplastic cerebellar gangliocytoma. J Comput Assist Tomogr. 43(2):277-81, 2019
4. WHO Classification of Tumours Editorial Board: WHO Classification of CNS Tumours. 5th ed. IARC, 2021
5. Ma J et al: Clinical perspective on dysplastic gangliocytoma of the cerebellum (Lhermitte-Duclos disease). World Neurosurg. 122:16-23, 2019
6. Jiang T et al: Lhermitte-Duclos disease (dysplastic gangliocytoma of the cerebellum) and Cowden syndrome: clinical experience from a single institution with long-term follow-up. World Neurosurg. 104:398-406, 2017
7. Bosemani T et al: Pseudotumoral hemicerebellitis as a mimicker of Lhermitte-Duclos disease in children: does neuroimaging help to differentiate them? Childs Nerv Syst. 32(5):865-71, 2016
8. Cianfoni A et al: Morphological and functional MR imaging of Lhermitte-Duclos disease with pathology correlate. J Neuroradiol. 35(5):297-300, 2008

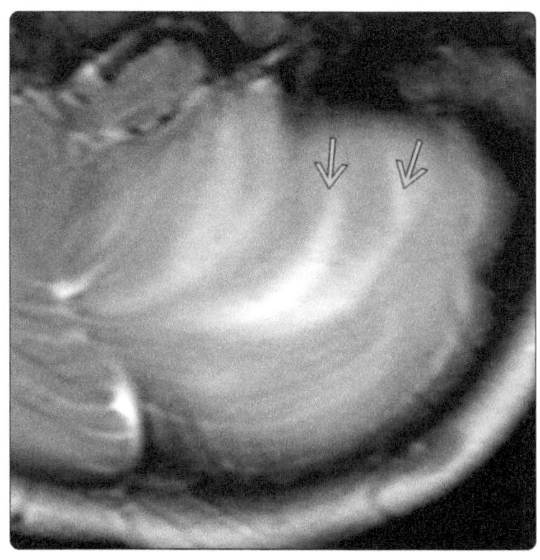

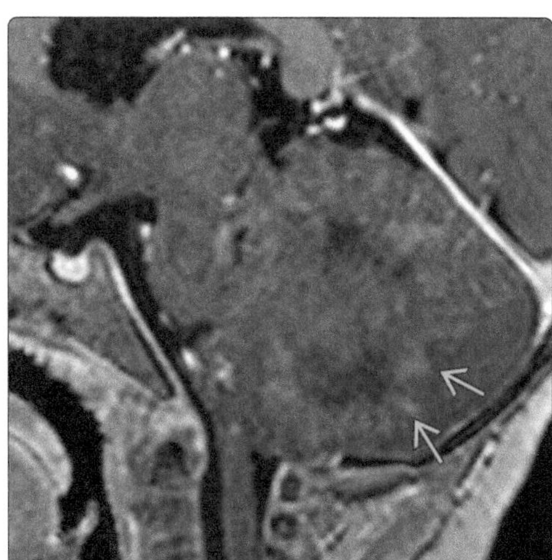

(Left) *Axial T2 MR in an 18-month-old with dysplastic gangliocytoma localized to the left cerebellar hemisphere shows the distinct enlargement and increased signal of the multiple cerebellar folia ➡, resulting in a striated or tiger stripes pattern.* **(Right)** *Sagittal T1 C+ MR in the same patient shows mild enhancement ➡ along the margins of the mass. Minimal or no enhancement is the most typical pattern for dysplastic gangliocytoma. If there is significant enhancement, consider pilocytic astrocytoma.*

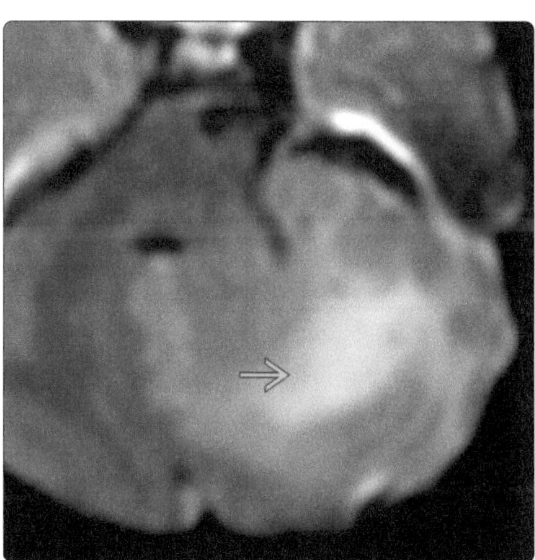

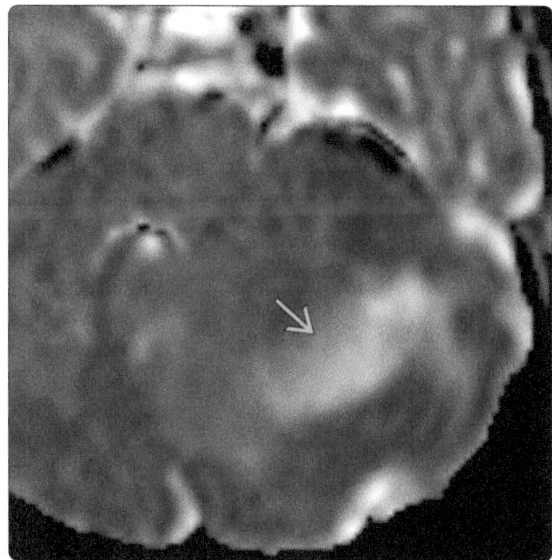

(Left) *Axial DWI MR in the same patient shows increased signal within the mass ➡ and enlarged, hyperintense cerebellar folia; however, this represents T2 shine-through rather than diffusion restriction, as evidenced by the following image.* **(Right)** *Axial ADC map in the same patient shows hyperintense signal in the areas of DWI signal intensity ➡, consistent with T2 shine-through. Diffusion restriction is atypical for dysplastic gangliocytoma. If present, one should consider an alternate diagnosis, such as a higher grade astrocytoma.*

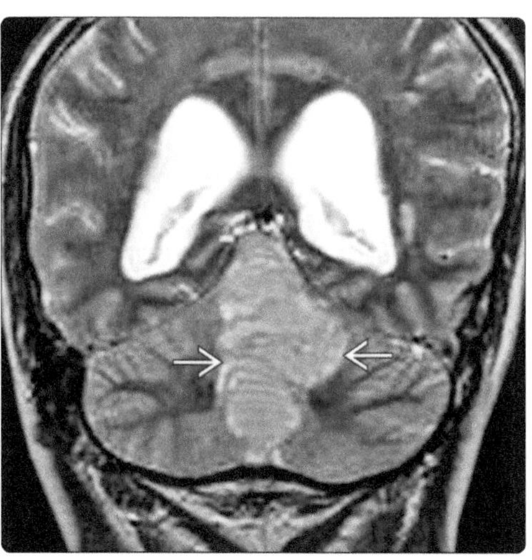

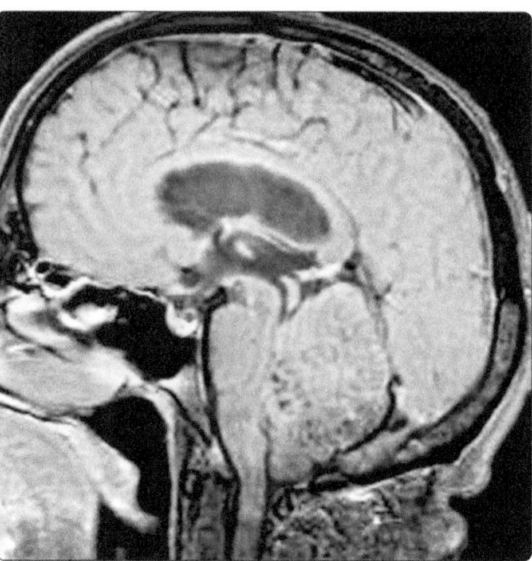

(Left) *Coronal T2 MR shows involvement largely limited to the cerebellar vermis ➡. As is typical in LDD, the involved region of the cerebellum is sharply marginated, striated in appearance, and demonstrates moderate mass effect.* **(Right)** *Sagittal T1 MR in the same patient shows effacement of the 4th ventricle and mass effect on the brainstem with effacement of the prepontine cistern. The cerebellar tonsils are herniated through the foramen magnum.*

Choroid Plexus Papilloma

KEY FACTS

TERMINOLOGY

- Intraventricular, papillary neoplasm derived from choroid plexus epithelium (WHO grades 1 & 2)

IMAGING

- Child with avidly enhancing, lobulated, ventricular mass
- Choroid plexus papillomas (CPPs) occur in proportion to amount of normally present choroid plexus
    - ~ 70-75% in lateral ventricle
    - ~ 10-15% in 3rd ventricle (roof)
    - ~ 10-15% in 4th ventricle & foramina of Luschka
- Choroidal artery enlargement for lateral ventricular (trigonal) CPPs
- Hydrocephalus common
- Consider advanced imaging modalities (DWI, ASL, MRS) to distinguish CPP & higher grade choroid plexus tumors

TOP DIFFERENTIAL DIAGNOSES

- Choroid plexus carcinoma (CPC)
- Medulloblastoma
- Infratentorial ependymoma
- Intraventricular metastasis
- Meningioma
- Physiologic choroid plexus enlargement

CLINICAL ISSUES

- Most common brain tumor in children < 1 year
    - 13.1% of all brain tumors in 1st year of life
    - 7.9% of fetal brain tumors diagnosed by ultrasound
- Rarely seed CSF pathways
- Excellent prognosis for grade 1 CPP

DIAGNOSTIC CHECKLIST

- Consider CPP in intraventricular mass with frond-like margins in child
- Imaging alone cannot reliably distinguish CPP from CPC
    - Although some features (e.g., brain invasion) & advanced imaging (e.g., ASL, MRS) may help distinguish

(Left) *Axial graphic shows a choroid plexus papilloma (CPP) arising from the glomus of the left lateral ventricular trigone. Note the characteristic frond-like surface projections. CPPs are most common in the lateral ventricles of a child.* **(Right)** *Axial T1 C+ MR in the same patient shows avid enhancement of the tumor, characteristic of CPP. In addition to enhancement, choroid plexus tumors (CPTs) tend to be quite vascular.*

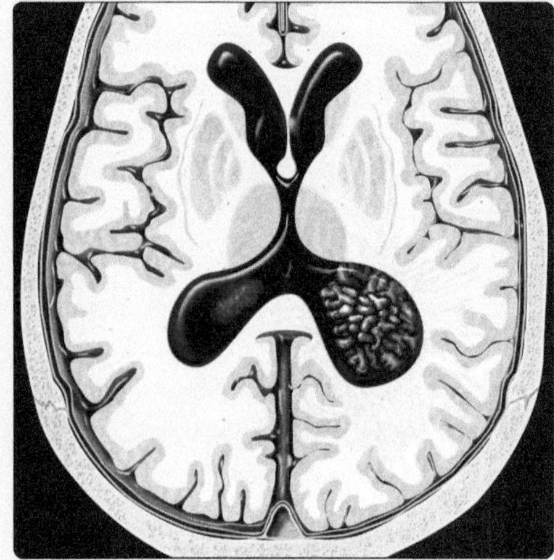

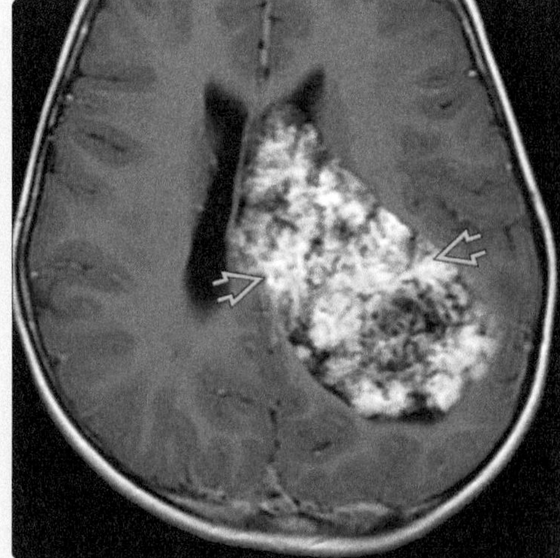

(Left) *Axial NECT in a 21-month-old child with macrocephaly and grade 1 CPP shows an isodense mass centered in the atrium of the left lateral ventricle with lobulated margins. Note the small punctate Ca^{++}, which are seen in ~ 25% of CPPs.* **(Right)** *Coronal T2 MR in the same patient shows a heterogeneous mass lesion in the atrium of left lateral ventricle. Note the central flow void. The ventricles are enlarged due to overproduction of CSF by the tumor.*

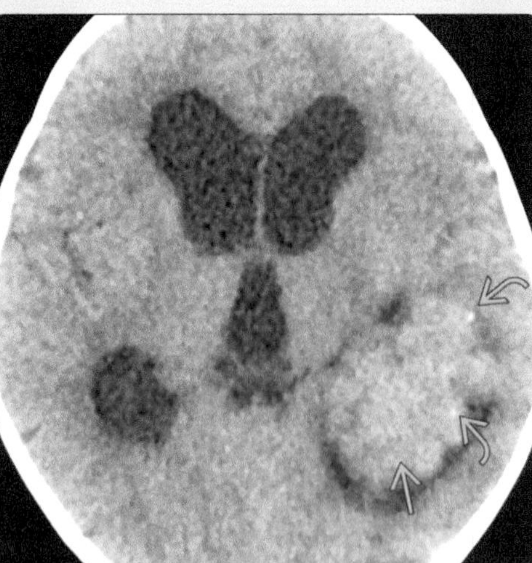

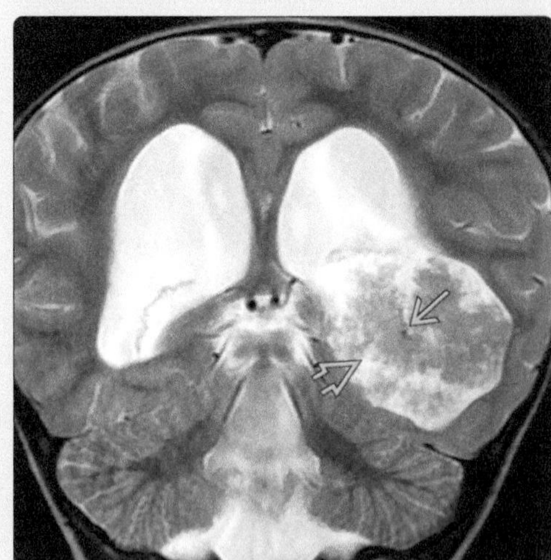

TERMINOLOGY

Abbreviations

- Choroid plexus papilloma (CPP)
  - Atypical CPP (aCPP)
- Choroid plexus tumor (CPT)
- Choroid plexus carcinoma (CPC)

Definitions

- Intraventricular, papillary neoplasm derived from choroid plexus epithelium (WHO grade 1 or 2)

IMAGING

General Features

- Best diagnostic clue
  - Child with avidly enhancing, lobulated, ventricular mass
- Location
  - CPPs in children occur much more commonly in lateral/3rd ventricles compared to adults
    - 70-75% in atrium of lateral ventricle, left > right
    - ~ 10-15% in 3rd ventricle
    - ~ 10-15% in 4th ventricle (posterior medullary velum) & foramina of Luschka
    - ~ 5% in extraventricular sites [e.g., cerebellopontine angle (CPA)]
    - Rare: CPA, suprasellar, intraparenchymal
- Size
  - Often of remarkable size at diagnosis
- Morphology
  - Well-defined, lobulated (frond-like) margins
  - Cauliflower-like mass

CT Findings

- NECT
  - Intraventricular lobular mass
  - 75% iso- or hyperattenuating
  - Ca^{++} in 25%
  - Hydrocephalus
    - Often related to overproduction of CSF by tumor
- CECT
  - Intense, homogeneous enhancement
    - Heterogeneous enhancement suggests CPC
  - Occasionally, minimal parenchymal invasion
  - Rarely, vascular pedicle twists, leading to CPP infarction & dense Ca^{++} ("brain stone")
- CTA: Choroidal artery enlargement for lateral ventricular (trigonal) CPPs

MR Findings

- T1WI
  - Well-delineated iso- to hypointense lobular mass
- T2WI
  - Iso- to hyperintense mass
  - ± internal linear & branching vascular flow voids
  - Large CPP may bury itself within brain parenchyma
    - Extensive invasion suggests CPC
  - Hydrocephalus common
- FLAIR
  - Bright periventricular signal
    - Transependymal interstitial edema due to ventricular obstruction
    - Asymmetric ipsilateral T2 hyperintensity may suggest invasion & CPC
- T2* GRE
  - ± foci of diminished signal if Ca^{++} &/or blood products are present
- PWI
  - ASL may be helpful in distinguishing CPC & CPP
    - ↑ cerebral blood flow (CBF) much higher in CPC
- T1WI C+
  - Robust homogeneous enhancement
  - Occasional cysts & small foci of necrosis
  - ± CSF seeding lesions
- MRA
  - Flow-related signal within mass
  - Enlarged choroidal artery (trigonal mass)
- MRS
  - NAA absent, mild ↑ choline,
    - ↑ choline greater in CPC vs. CPP
    - ↑ myoinositol more characteristic of CPP

Ultrasonographic Findings

- Grayscale ultrasound
  - Hyperechoic mass with frond-like projections
  - Mass echogenicity similar to normal choroid plexus (CP)
  - Hydrocephalus
- Pulsed Doppler
  - Vascular pedicle & internal sampling of mass
    - Bidirectional flow through diastole
    - Arterial tracing shows low impedance
- Color Doppler
  - Hypervascular mass with bidirectional flow

Angiographic Findings

- Conventional
  - Enlarged anterior or posterior choroidal artery
  - Prolonged vascular stain
  - Arteriovenous shunting

Nuclear Medicine Findings

- PET
  - 11C-methionine → high tumor:normal brain ratios in CPP compared to gliomas
  - FDG → unable to distinguish between CPP & glioma

Imaging Recommendations

- Best imaging tool
  - MR with contrast
- Protocol advice
  - Perform contrast-enhanced MR of entire neuraxis before surgery

DIFFERENTIAL DIAGNOSIS

Choroid Plexus Carcinoma

- Difficult to distinguish from CPP by imaging
- More likely to invade brain
- May see heterogeneous enhancement
- ↑ cerebral blood flow, diffusion restriction more common in CPC

Medulloblastoma
- Hyperdense 4th ventricular mass in child
- More spherical than CPP

Infratentorial Ependymoma
- More common in 4th ventricle in children
- Heterogeneous enhancing mass

Intraventricular Metastasis
- Known history of primary tumor
- Rare in children

Meningioma
- Enhancing, circumscribed intraventricular mass
- Consider neurofibromatosis type 2
- Older adults

Physiologic Choroid Plexus Enlargement
- Collateral venous drainage (Sturge-Weber)
- Enlargement of choroid following hemispherectomy

Subependymoma
- Nonenhancing intraventricular mass

Villous Hypertrophy
- Many presumed villous hypertrophy (VH) cases may be bilateral CPPs
- Proliferation index (MIB-1) is useful to distinguish

Intraventricular Ependymoma
- Most common in trigones
- CSF spread may occur
- Differentiation is histologic

PATHOLOGY

General Features
- Genetics
  - DNA sequences from simian virus 40 (SV40) have been found in CPTs
  - High expression of *TWIST1* (transcription factor that inhibits p53)
  - Association with Aicardi & Li-Fraumeni syndromes
  - Duplication of short arm of chromosome 9 reported
- Associated abnormalities
  - Diffuse hydrocephalus from
    - CSF overproduction
    - Mechanical obstruction
    - Impaired CSF resorption (due to hemorrhage)

Staging, Grading, & Classification
- WHO grade 1 (CPP) & grade 2 (aCPP)

Gross Pathologic & Surgical Features
- Well-circumscribed, lobulated intraventricular mass
- ± cysts, necrosis, & hemorrhage

Microscopic Features
- Fibrovascular connective tissue fronds
  - Covered by cuboidal or columnar epithelium
- Mitotic activity, necrosis, & brain invasion typically absent
- Resembles nonneoplastic CP
- Immunohistochemistry
  - Transthyretin may help distinguish from normal CP
  - GFAP reactivity can distinguish from normal CP
  - Kir7.1 & stanniocalcin-1 reactivity differentiates normal CP & CPT from other cell origins
- aCPP: Greater cytologic atypia, pseudostratification, nonpapillary areas, & ≥ 2 mitoses per 10 HPF

CLINICAL ISSUES

Presentation
- Most common signs/symptoms
  - Macrocrania, bulging fontanelle, vomiting, headache, ataxia, seizure
- Clinical profile
  - Child < 2 years with signs & symptoms of elevated intracranial pressure

Demographics
- Age
  - Tumor grade
    - CPP: 49% < 5 years; 26% < 1 year
    - CPC: 75% < 5 years; 33% < 1 year
  - Location
    - Lateral ventricular CPPs: Much more common in children
    - 4th ventricular CPPs: More common in adults
- Sex
  - M > F: ~ 1.5:1.0
- Epidemiology
  - 0.5% of all adult brain tumors
  - 2-3% of all pediatric brain tumors
  - Most common brain tumor in children < 1 year
    - 50% manifest in 1st decade
    - 86% present by 5 years
    - 13.1% of all brain tumors in 1st year of life
    - 7.9% of fetal brain tumors diagnosed by ultrasound

Natural History & Prognosis
- Benign, slowly growing; rarely seed CSF pathways
- 5-year survival: ~ 100%

Treatment
- Total surgical resection: Recurrence rare

DIAGNOSTIC CHECKLIST

Consider
- CPP if lobulated intraventricular mass in young child

Image Interpretation Pearls
- Imaging alone cannot reliably distinguish CPP from CPC
  - Although some features (e.g., brain invasion) & advanced imaging (e.g., ASL, MRS) may help distinguish
  - Final diagnosis is histologic

SELECTED REFERENCES

1. WHO Classification of Tumours Editorial Board: WHO Classification of Tumours: CNS Tumours. 5th ed. IARC, 2021
2. Thomas C et al: Epigenetics impacts upon prognosis and clinical management of choroid plexus tumors. J Neurooncol. 148(1):39-45, 2020
3. Trybula SJ et al: Infratentorial choroid plexus tumors in children. Childs Nerv Syst. 36(8):1761-6, 2020
4. Dangouloff-Ros V et al: Choroid plexus neoplasms: toward a distinction between carcinoma and papilloma using arterial spin-labeling. AJNR Am J Neuroradiol. 36(9):1786-90, 2015

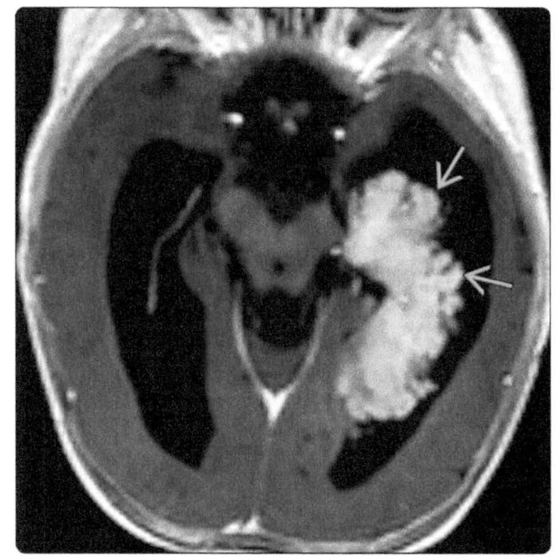

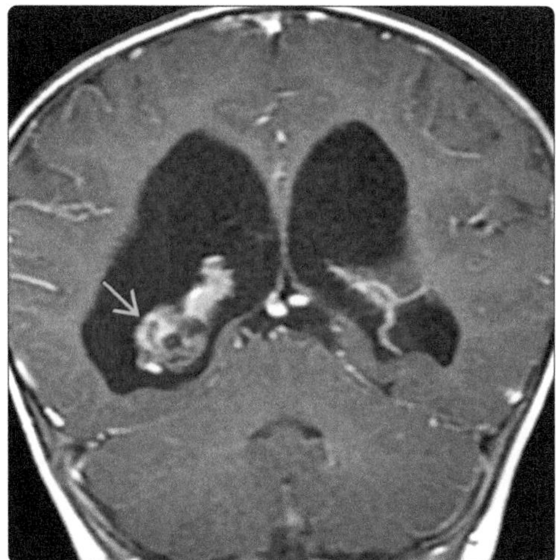

(Left) *Axial T1 C+ MR in a 7-month-old with macrocephaly shows a lobulated mass in the dilated temporal horn and atrium of the left lateral ventricle. Note the frond-like lobulated borders →, typical for CPTs, especially CPP.* **(Right)** *Coronal T1 C+ MR in a 1-year-old with macrocephaly shows a small mass → in the right choroid plexus and moderate enlargement of the lateral ventricles. This case and the case in the prior image demonstrate how CPTs, even when small, may overproduce CSF, causing hydrocephalus.*

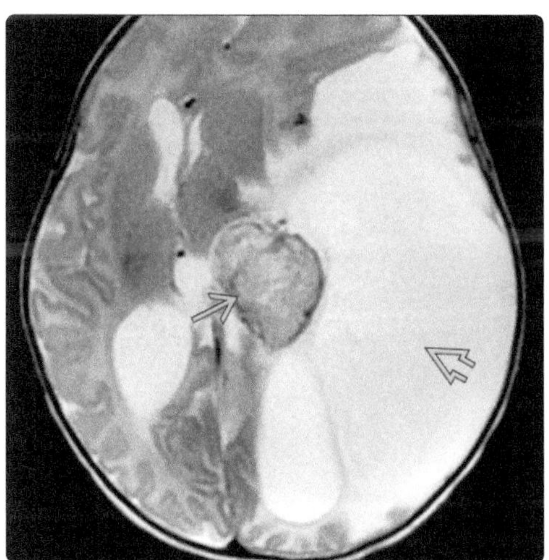

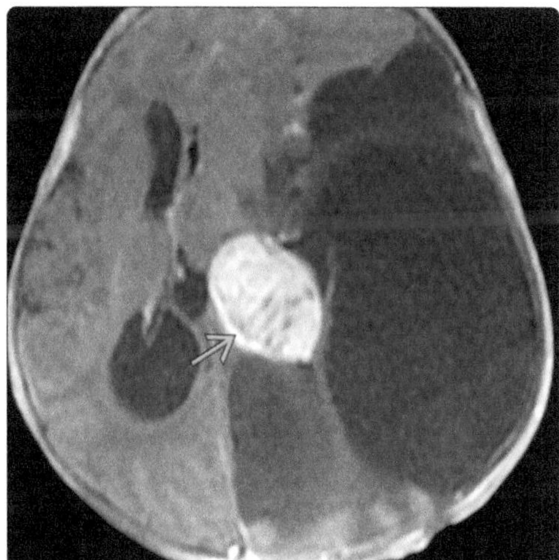

(Left) *Axial T2 MR in a 7-week-old infant with grade 1 CPP shows a mixed solid and cystic mass in the left cerebral hemisphere. ASL perfusion imaging (not shown) showed increased vascularity within the solid component →. Note the large cystic component ⇨ laterally.* **(Right)** *Axial T1 C+ MR in the same patient shows that the solid component → is avidly enhancing. CPPs are usually solid masses, but cystic components (often large) do occur, and CPP is an important DDx for large supratentorial mixed solid and cystic masses.*

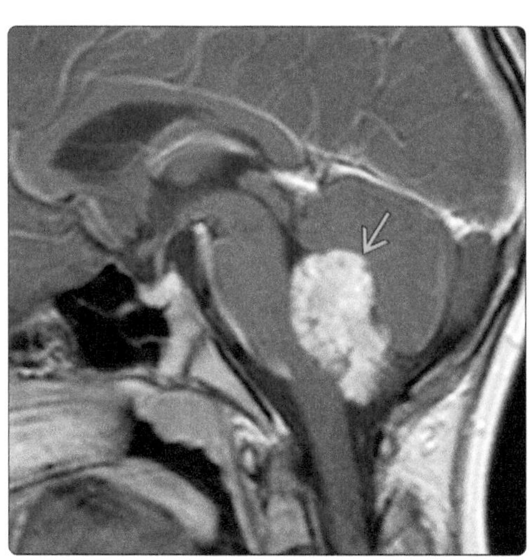

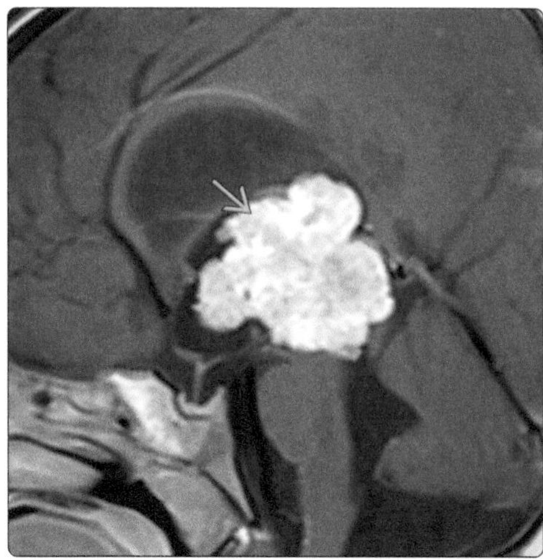

(Left) *Sagittal T1 C+ MR shows a brightly enhancing 4th ventricle CPP →. This location for a CPT is more common in adults than in children where medulloblastoma and ependymoma are more common. However, a CPT should be considered in any avidly enhancing 4th ventricular mass.* **(Right)** *Coronal T1 C+ MR in a 2-year-old with grade 1 CPP shows a lobulated mass → centered in the 3rd ventricle. The 3rd ventricle is a less common location for CPP given the small amount of choroid plexus in this location.*

Choroid Plexus Carcinoma

KEY FACTS

TERMINOLOGY

- Malignant tumor originating from epithelium of choroid plexus (WHO grade 3)

IMAGING

- Best imaging clue: Child < 5 years with enhancing intraventricular mass & ependymal invasion, ± prominent flow voids
    - Asymmetric periventricular white matter edema suggests invasion
- MR may not distinguish papilloma from carcinoma
    - Heterogeneity, brain invasion, CSF spread favors CPC
    - ↑ size & ↓ ADC values correlate with higher grade
- Important to image spine prior to surgery

TOP DIFFERENTIAL DIAGNOSES

- Choroid plexus papilloma
- Ependymoma
- Subependymal giant cell astrocytoma

PATHOLOGY

- WHO grade 3
- Microscopic features: Hypercellularity, pleomorphism, ↑ mitotic activity
    - Cysts, necrosis, hemorrhage, microcalcifications
    - Brain invasion common
- ↑ incidence in Li-Fraumeni & Aicardi syndromes

CLINICAL ISSUES

- Occurs in infants & young children
    - 70% occur before 2 years of age
- Nausea, vomiting, headache, obtundation most common presenting features
- CPC represents 20-40% of all choroid plexus tumors
- Poor outcome with brain invasion or CSF seeding

DIAGNOSTIC CHECKLIST

- CPC in child with invasive intraventricular mass & focal neurologic signs

(Left) *Axial graphic demonstrates a lobular mass centered in the atria of the left lateral ventricle ➡. Note the invasion and expansion of the surrounding parenchyma ➡, more characteristic of a choroid plexus carcinoma (CPC). There is associated midline shift ➡ and entrapment of the right lateral ventricle ➡.* **(Right)** *Axial NECT in a 2-year-old girl with a large head and papilledema shows a predominately hyperdense mass ➡ in the left cerebral hemisphere.*

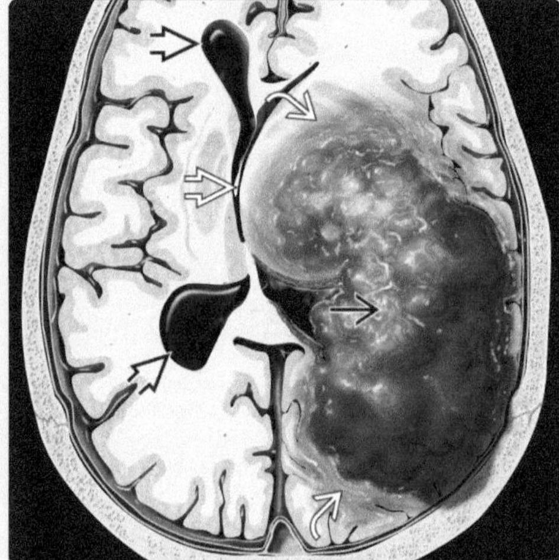

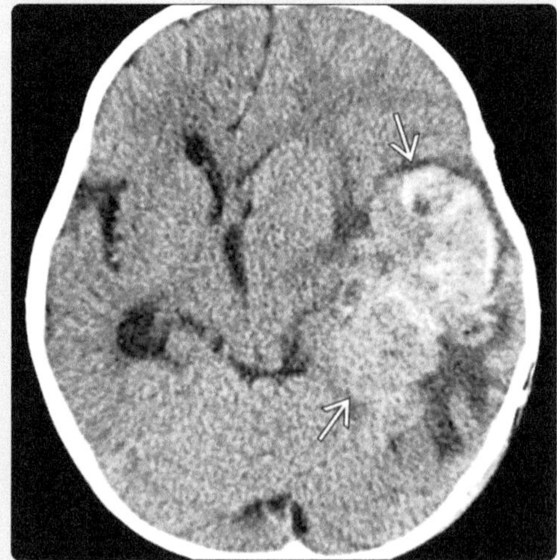

(Left) *Axial NECT in a 9-month-old with macrocephaly and vomiting shows a large, hyperdense mass ➡ centered in the atrium of the lateral ventricle with associated hydrocephalus. Density of CPC can vary, but hyperdensity raises concern for a higher grade tumor, such as a CPC rather than a choroid plexus papilloma (CPP).* **(Right)** *Axial T2 MR (same patient) shows areas of brain parenchymal invasion with vasogenic edema along anterior ➡ and posterior ➡ margins of the mass. Brain invasion is more likely in CPC compared to CPP.*

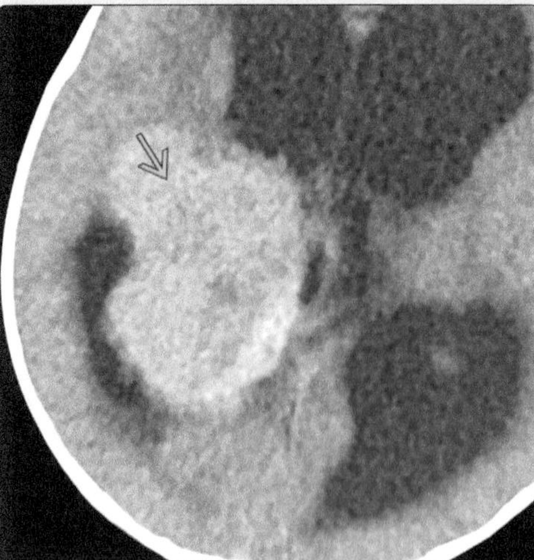

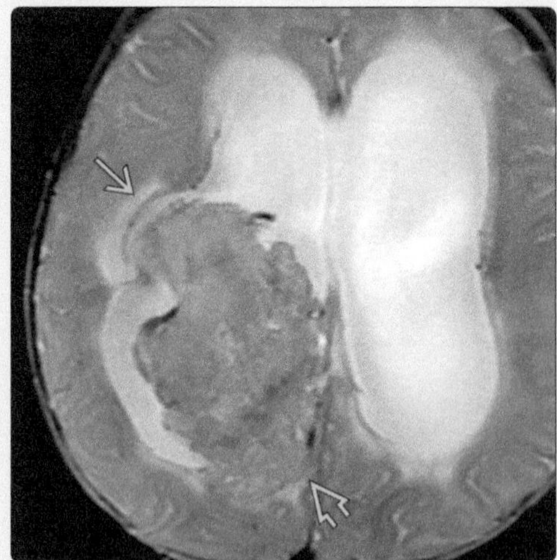

TERMINOLOGY

Abbreviations

- Choroid plexus carcinoma (CPC)

Definitions

- Malignant tumor originating from epithelium of choroid plexus

IMAGING

General Features

- Best diagnostic clue
  - Child (< 5 years) with enhancing intraventricular mass & ependymal invasion
  - Differentiation of CPC from choroid plexus papilloma (CPP) is often not possible, but some imaging features are more suggestive of CPC
- Location
  - Vast majority arise in lateral ventricles
- Size
  - Variable
  - Larger size correlates with higher grade in choroid plexus tumors (CPTs)
- Morphology
  - Well-defined, lobulated margins
  - Necrosis, cysts, & hemorrhage common

CT Findings

- NECT
  - Iso- to hyperattenuating mass with irregular contours
  - Necrosis, cysts, & hemorrhage common
  - Hydrocephalus common
  - Ca^{++} in 20-25%
- CECT
  - Heterogeneous, often strong enhancement
  - Peritumoral edema
  - ± CSF tumor seeding

MR Findings

- T1WI
  - Iso- to hypointense intraventricular mass
  - Well-defined, lobulated margins
  - Heterogeneous (necrosis, cysts, hemorrhage)
- T2WI
  - Mixed-signal mass, hypo-/iso-/hyperintense
  - Heterogeneous (necrosis, cysts, hemorrhage, Ca^{++})
  - ± prominent flow voids
  - Many invade brain & cause edema
- PD/intermediate
  - Heterogeneous mass with vascular flow voids
- FLAIR
  - Heterogeneous intraventricular mass
  - Periventricular white matter edema suggests invasion
  - Transependymal CSF flow from hydrocephalus
- T2* GRE
  - Low signal from hemorrhage or Ca^{++}
- DWI
  - Low ADC values in solid portions of tumor
  - Lower ADC values correlate with higher grade & poorer outcome in CPTs
- PWI
  - ASL may be helpful for distinguishing CPC & CPP
    - ↑ cerebral blood flow (CBF) much higher in CPC vs. CPP
- T1WI C+
  - Heterogeneous enhancement, ± CSF seeding
- MRS
  - NAA absent; ↑ choline ± ↑ lactate
    - ↑ choline greater in CPC vs. CPP
    - ↑ myoinositol more characteristic of CPP

Angiographic Findings

- Conventional
  - Enlarged choroidal artery & vascular stain

Nuclear Medicine Findings

- PET
  - 11C-methionine → ↑ tumor: Normal brain ratios
- Tc-99m sestamibi → ↑ in CPTs

Imaging Recommendations

- Best imaging tool
  - Contrast-enhanced MR of brain & spine
- Protocol advice
  - Enhanced MR of entire neuraxis prior to surgery

DIFFERENTIAL DIAGNOSIS

Choroid Plexus Papilloma

- MR may not distinguish CPC from typical or atypical CPP
- Aggressive CPP may seed through CSF pathways
- CPP rarely shows minimal brain invasion
- Advanced imaging: ASL, DWI, & MRS may help to distinguish CPC from CPP

Ependymoma

- Heterogeneous 4th ventricular mass
- Classically squeezes out 4th ventricular foramina
- Supratentorial ependymoma often extraventricular

Subependymal Giant Cell Astrocytoma

- Associated CNS findings of tuberous sclerosis
- Characteristic location near foramen of Monro
- Rarely cause edema

Astrocytic Tumors

- May arise from periventricular tissues (e.g., thalamus)
- Smooth or lobular masses, no papillary margins
- High-grade tumor may cause periventricular edema

Medulloblastoma

- Hyperdense, round 4th ventricular mass
- Arises from roof of 4th ventricle (superior medullary velum)

Central Neurocytoma

- "Bubbly" intraventricular mass in adult
- Often attached to septum pellucidum

Meningioma

- Delineated, oval enhancing mass
- Uncommon in children, associated with neurofibromatosis type 2

Primitive Neuroectodermal Tumor

- Heterogeneous tumor can be lobulated within lateral ventricle
- May arise deep in hemisphere
- Peritumoral edema often minimal

Atypical Teratoid/Rhabdoid Tumor

- Heterogeneous tumor with cysts or hemorrhage
- Common in posterior fossa; may occur in lateral ventricle, often intraaxial
- Typically present in patients < 2 years of age
- INI1 protein negative on immunohistochemistry
  - Most CPC positive

Vascular Lesions

- Arteriovenous malformation
- Cavernous malformation

Metastases

- History of previous tumor often known
- Multiple lesions common
- Rare in children

PATHOLOGY

General Features

- Etiology
  - Simian virus 40 (SV40) DNA sequences in 50% of CPTs
- Genetics
  - ↑ incidence in Li-Fraumeni & Aicardi syndromes
    - Li-Fraumeni TP53 mutation/deletion accounts for ~ 40% of CPCs
    - Autosomal dominant tumor predisposition syndrome
  - Overlap with rhabdoid tumors & *SMARCB1* (SNF5, INI1) mutation
  - ↑ copy number of *TP53* mutation associated with ↓ survival
- Associated abnormalities
  - Diffuse hydrocephalus → mechanical obstruction, ↑ CSF production, ↓ resorption

Staging, Grading, & Classification

- WHO grade 3

Gross Pathologic & Surgical Features

- Well-circumscribed, lobulated intraventricular mass
- Ependymal invasion

Microscopic Features

- Hypercellular, pleomorphic, ↑ mitotic activity
- Cysts, necrosis, hemorrhage, microcalcifications
- Brain invasion common
- May have CSF seeding
- ↑ Ki-67/MIB-1 proliferation index (~ 20%; range 7.8-42.5%)

Immunochemistry

- Kir7.1 & stanniocalcin-1 may distinguish choroid plexus origin from other tumors
- CPC express cytokeratins
- Transthyretin, S100 positive (< CPP)

Genetic Alterations

- Recurrent copy number losses & gains of multiple chromosomes, varying with age

CLINICAL ISSUES

Presentation

- Most common signs/symptoms
  - Nausea, vomiting, headache, obtundation
  - Focal neurologic signs & symptoms
- Clinical profile
  - Infant or child with elevated ICP & focal neurologic deficits

Demographics

- Age
  - Infants & young children (typically < 5 years)
  - Median: 26-32 months
- Sex
  - M = F
- Epidemiology
  - 80% arise in children
  - 70% before 2 years of age
  - 20-40% of all CPTs
  - ~ 5% of supratentorial tumors in children
  - < 1% of all pediatric intracranial tumors

Natural History & Prognosis

- Small percentage may be malignant progression from WHO grades 1 & 2 papillomas
- Grows rapidly
- ~ 60% 5-year survival in modern era
- Poor outcome with brain invasion, CSF seeding

Treatment

- "Head Start" (HS) irradiation-avoiding strategy has improved survival, minimized neurocognitive sequelae
  - Maximal surgical resection first
    - High-dose consolidation myeloablative chemotherapy next
      - With autologous hematopoietic stem cell rescue
  - ± postchemotherapy irradiation (based on patient age, evidence of residual disease)

DIAGNOSTIC CHECKLIST

Consider

- CPC in child with invasive intraventricular mass & focal neurologic signs

Image Interpretation Pearls

- MR may not distinguish papilloma from carcinoma
- Heterogeneity, brain invasion, CSF spread favors CPC
- Image spine prior to surgery

SELECTED REFERENCES

1. Takaoka K et al: Incidence and survival of choroid plexus tumors in the United States. Neurooncol Pract. 10(1):41-9, 2023
2. Louis DN et al: The references 2021 WHO Classification of Tumors of the Central Nervous System: a summary. Neuro Oncol. 23(8):1231-51, 2021
3. Thomas C et al: Epigenetics impacts upon prognosis and clinical management of choroid plexus tumors. J Neurooncol. 148(1):39-45, 2020
4. Lin H et al: Choroid plexus tumours on MRI: similarities and distinctions in different grades. Cancer Imaging. 19(1):17, 2019

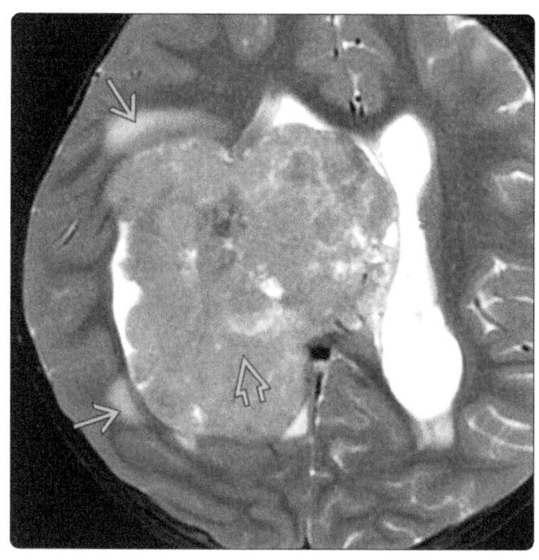

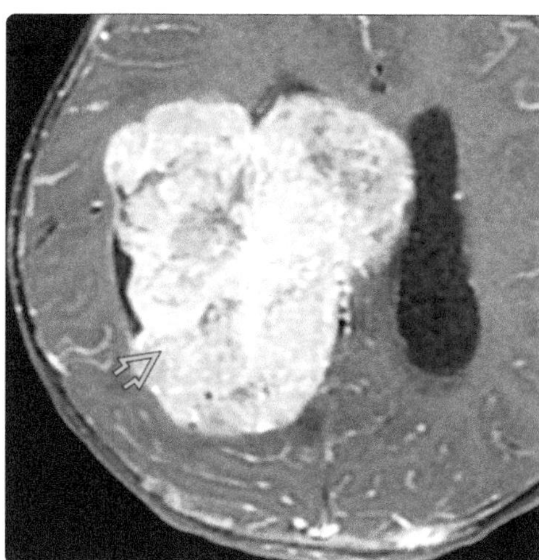

(Left) *Axial T2 MR in a 2-year-old shows a large, heterogeneous mass ⇨ centered in the atrium of the right lateral ventricle with extension into the adjacent brain parenchyma and associated vasogenic edema →. Brain invasion and edema are found more commonly in CPC compared to CPP.* **(Right)** *Axial T1 C+ MR in the same patient shows avid enhancement of the mass lesion ⇨. CPCs typically show avid contrast enhancement, although the patterns may vary with central necrosis sometimes evident.*

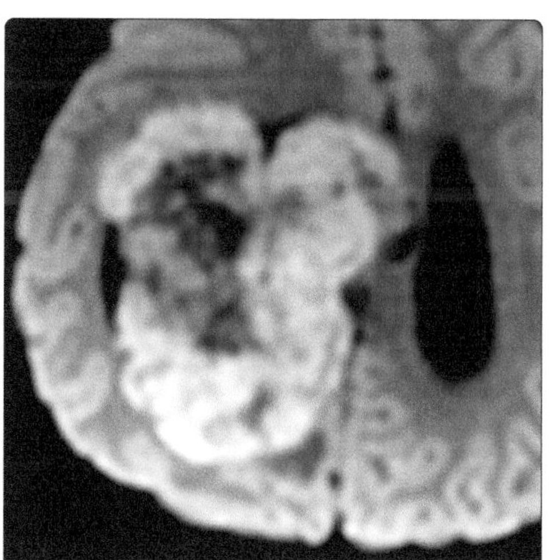

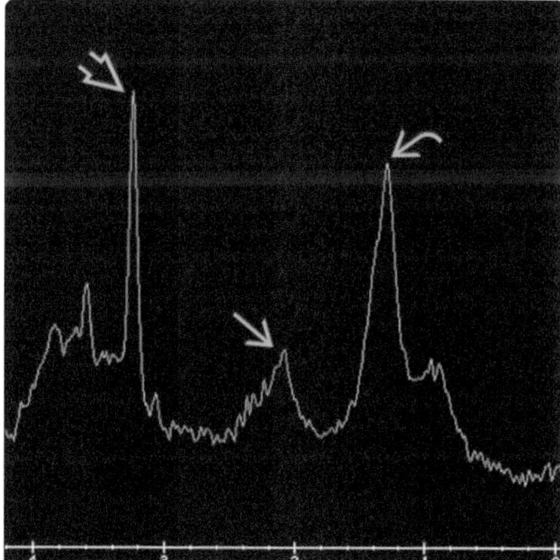

(Left) *Axial DWI MR in the same patient shows DWI ↑ signal and ↓ ADC signal, consistent with ↑ cellularity. While DWI is variable in CPTs, diffusion restriction within the solid components should raise additional concern for a high-grade tumor, such as CPC.* **(Right)** *Single voxel short-echo MR spectroscopy in a 3-year-old patient with CPC shows marked ↓ NAA →, marked ↑ Cho ⇨, and marked ↑ lactate peak ↷. This spectrum is typical for CPC.*

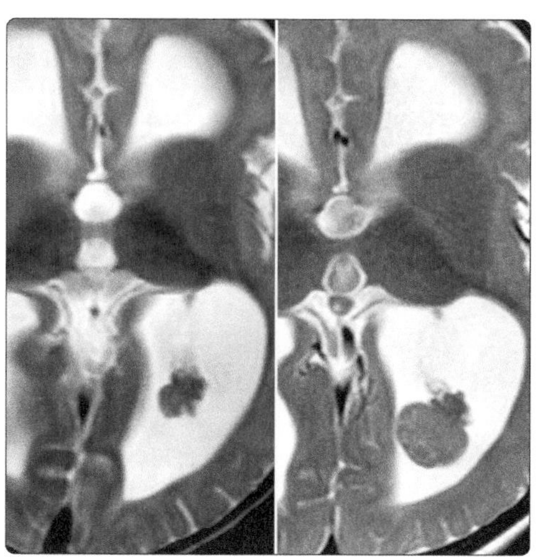

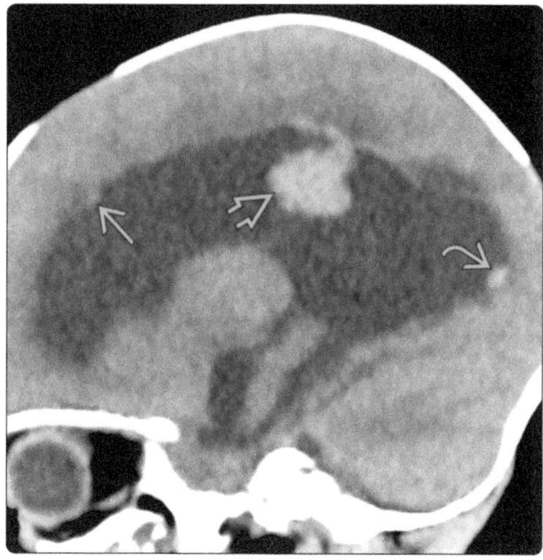

(Left) *Axial T2 MR in an 11-month-old boy with a suspected TP53 mutation presents with an incidental left choroid plexus mass that substantially enlarged between the initial imaging study (left) and follow-up study (right) performed 4 months later. Pathology revealed a CPC.* **(Right)** *Sagittal NECT in a 4-month-old with CPC shows a primary mass lesion ⇨ in the choroid plexus. Note the associated lesions in the right frontal → and occipital ↷ horns, consistent with CSF metastases.*

Infratentorial Ependymoma

KEY FACTS

TERMINOLOGY

- Posterior fossa ependymoma (PF-EPN)

IMAGING

- PF (2/3 of CNS EPNs)
  - Lobulated mass in body/inferior 4th ventricle
    - Soft or "plastic" tumor
      - Accommodates to shape of ventricle
      - ± extension through foramina of Luschka into cerebellopontine angle cisterns
  - 3-17% CSF dissemination at diagnosis
- NECT
  - Fine, stippled Ca^{++} common (50%)
  - ± cysts, hemorrhage
  - Obstructive hydrocephalus common
- MR
  - Variable enhancement
  - Iso- to hyperintense on ADC compared to brain

TOP DIFFERENTIAL DIAGNOSES

- Medulloblastoma (MB)
- Cerebellar pilocytic astrocytoma

PATHOLOGY

- PF-EPN subtype A
  - Most common (~ 80% of PF-EPNs)
  - Foramen of Luschka invasion common
  - Predominately infants & young children
  - Poor prognosis
- PF-EPN subtype B
  - 10% of PF-EPNs
  - Usually midline 4th ventricle without lateral extension
  - Older children, adults
  - Better prognosis

DIAGNOSTIC CHECKLIST

- Best clue: "Plastic" tumor that expands 4th ventricle, extends through outlet foramina

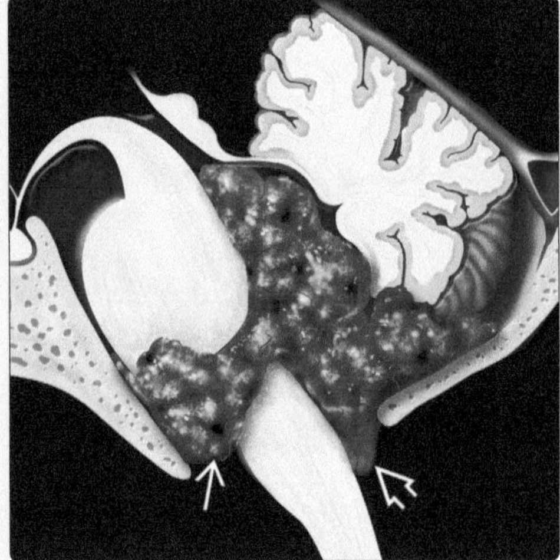

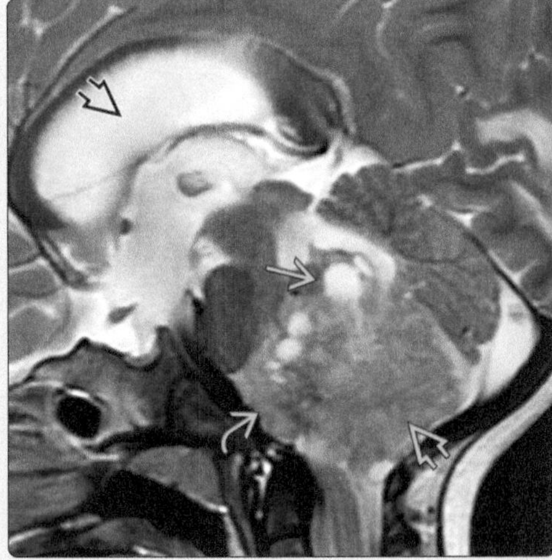

(Left) *Sagittal graphic shows a posterior fossa ependymoma (PF-EPN) extending through the 4th ventricle outlet foramina into the cisterna magna ➡ and cerebellopontine angle (CPA) cistern ➡. This plastic pattern of growth is typical of an ependymoma.* **(Right)** *Parasagittal T2 MR in a 2-year-old with grade 2 PF-EPN subtype A (PF-EPN-A) (1Q gain) shows a large, predominantly solid lesion ➡ with peripheral cysts ➡ in the lower 4th ventricle extending into the CPA cistern ➡. Note associated hydrocephalus ➡.*

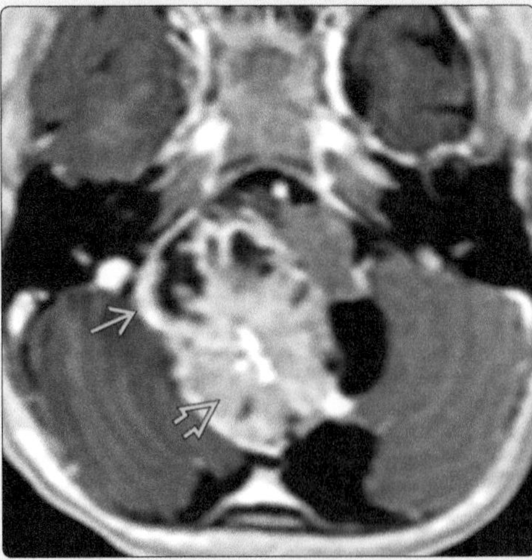

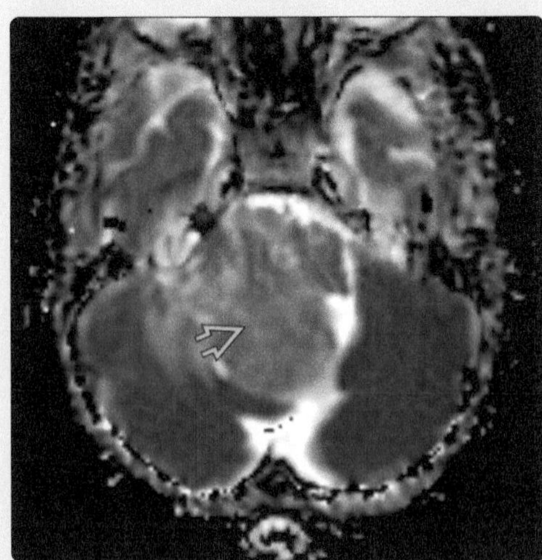

(Left) *Axial T1 C+ MR in the same 2-year-old shows heterogeneous enhancement of the tumor ➡. Note the extension into the right foramen of Luschka ➡. The young age, large size, heterogeneous enhancement, and foramen of Luschka extension are all characteristic imaging features of PF-EPN-A.* **(Right)** *Axial ADC MR in the same patient ➡ shows signal slightly brighter than adjacent brain. PF-EPNs typically have ADC values between the primary DDx lesions, pilocytic astrocytoma and medulloblastoma.*

TERMINOLOGY

Definitions

- Posterior fossa ependymoma (PF-EPN)
  - Slow-growing tumor of ependymal cells

IMAGING

General Features

- Best diagnostic clue
  - Soft "plastic" tumor squeezes out through 4th ventricle foramina into cisterns
  - Heterogeneous density, signal intensity
  - ± indistinct interface with floor of 4th ventricle
- Location
  - PF-EPN subtype A (PF-EPN-A) often invade foramina, especially Luschka
  - PF-EPN subtype B (PF-EPN-B) usually confined to midline 4th ventricle
- Size
  - 1-4 cm
  - PF-EPN-A larger on average compared to PF-EPN-B
- Morphology
  - Accommodates to shape of ventricle
  - Typical = lobulated inferior 4th ventricle mass
    - Anterolateral extension through recess(es) into cerebellopontine angle (CPA) cistern
      - Usually PF-EPN-A
    - Posteroinferior extension through foramen of Magendie into cisterna magna

CT Findings

- NECT
  - 4th ventricle mass
  - Fine, stippled Ca^{++} common
    - More common in PF-EPN-A (~ 90%)
  - ± cysts, hemorrhage
  - Hydrocephalus common
- CECT
  - Variable enhancement

MR Findings

- T1WI
  - Heterogeneous, usually iso- to hypointense
  - Cystic foci slightly hyperintense to CSF
  - Hyperintense foci (Ca^{++}, blood products)
- T2WI
  - Heterogeneous, usually iso- to hyperintense
  - Hyperintense cystic foci
    - PF-EPN-B more commonly cystic, sometimes with soap bubble appearance
  - Hypointense foci (Ca^{++}, blood products)
- FLAIR
  - Can show sharp interface between tumor, CSF
  - Tumor cysts very hyperintense to CSF
- T2* GRE
  - Hypointense blooming of Ca^{++} & blood products
- DWI
  - Iso- to hypointense ADC compared to gray matter
  - Diffusion restriction depends on tumor grade
    - Diffusion restriction typically less than medulloblastoma (MB) but greater than pilocytic astrocytoma (PA)
    - Therefore, higher ADC signal than MB but less intense than PA (which often has ↑ diffusivity)
- T1WI C+
  - Enhancement
    - Highly variable
    - PF-EPN-A more often heterogeneous enhancement
    - PF-EPN-B more often homogeneous enhancement
- MRS
  - ↓ NAA; ↑ Cho, lipid/lactate peaks
  - MRS not reliable for distinguishing PF tumors

Angiographic Findings

- Findings vary from avascular to hypervascular with arteriovenous shunting

Nuclear Medicine Findings

- ↓ FDG uptake on PET
- May help differentiate recurrent tumor from radiation necrosis

Imaging Recommendations

- Best imaging tool
  - MR of brain & spine with contrast
    - Spine imaging necessary for complete staging
- Protocol advice
  - Sagittal imaging may distinguish point of origin as floor vs. roof of 4th ventricle
  - High-resolution SSFP MR can visualize cranial nerve involvement by tumor extending into cisterns
  - MR angiography can delineate involvement of PF vessels by tumor extending into cisterns

DIFFERENTIAL DIAGNOSIS

Medulloblastoma

- Hyperdense on NECT
- Diffusion restriction (↑ DWI, ↓ ADC)
- Arises from roof of 4th ventricle, 90% midline
- More distinct interface with floor

Cerebellar Pilocytic Astrocytoma

- Arises from cerebellar parenchyma
- 90% off-midline
- Most have cystic component
- Enhancing portion enhances vigorously in > 90%

Choroid Plexus Papilloma

- Vigorously enhancing intraventricular tumor
- 4th ventricle location more common in adults
- Look for lobulated, frond-like border

Atypical Teratoid/Rhabdoid Tumor

- Cellular mass with diffusion restriction (↑ DWI, ↓ ADC)
- More likely to be off-midline compared to MB
- More likely to have cysts & hemorrhage, compared to MB
- Most common in very young children

Brainstem Glioma

- Infiltrating mass expanding brainstem
- Homogeneous signal on MR

- May project dorsally into 4th ventricle

PATHOLOGY

General Features

- Etiology
  - Recent studies suggest radial glial cells as cells of origin
    - Radial glial cells located primarily in subventricular zone
- Genetics
  - Supratentorial, infratentorial, & spinal EPNs genetically distinct
  - 3 PF-EPN subgroups
    - Sub-EPN (PF-SE)
    - PF-EPN-A
      - ~ 80% of PF tumors
      - Location: Foramen of Luschka & CPA common
      - More common in younger children
      - M:F = 2:1
      - 1q gain or 6q loss are high risk prognostic factors
      - Highly malignant with poor response to surgery, radiation therapy
    - PF-EPN-B
      - ~ 10-20% of all cases
      - Location: Midline 4th ventricle
      - Older children, adults
      - M:F = 1:1
      - CpG island methylator phenotype (CIMP) (-)
      - Better prognosis
  - DNA methylation profiling identifies 9 molecular EPN subgroups
  - Risk stratification by molecular subgrouping superior to histologic grading

Staging, Grading, & Classification

- WHO grade 2 (low grade, well differentiated)
  - Cellular: Most common type in PF
  - Papillary: Extensive epithelial surface
  - Clear cell: Microscopic features of oligodendroglioma
  - Tanycytic: Elongated cells resembling PA
- WHO grade 3 (high grade, anaplastic)
  - Anaplastic EPN

Gross Pathologic & Surgical Features

- Well demarcated
- Soft, lobulated, grayish red mass
- ± cysts, necrosis, hemorrhage
- Extrudes through 4th ventricle outlet foramina into "plastic development"
- Typically displaces, rather than invades, adjacent brain parenchyma

Microscopic Features

- Despite being histologically similar, EPNs from different anatomic regions are biologically & clinically distinct

CLINICAL ISSUES

Presentation

- Most common signs/symptoms
  - ↑ intracranial pressure: Headache, nausea, vomiting
- Clinical profile
  - Age 1-5 years; headache, vomiting
- Other
  - Ataxia, hemiparesis, visual disturbances, neck pain, torticollis, dizziness
  - Infants: Irritability, lethargy, developmental delay, vomiting, macrocephaly

Demographics

- Age
  - PF-EPN-A
    - 1-5 years (mean: 3 years)
  - PF-EPN-B
    - Mean at diagnosis: 30 years
- Sex
  - Slight male predominance, especially in PF-EPN-A
- Epidemiology
  - 3-5% of all intracranial tumors
  - 15% of PF tumors in children
    - 3rd most common PF tumor in children
      - Most common are PA & MB

Natural History & Prognosis

- Prognosis highly variable
  - PF-EPN-A: 50-60% 5-year survival
  - PF-EPN-B: 90-95% 5-year survival
- 3-17% CSF dissemination
- 15% 5-year survival after recurrence

Treatment

- Maximal safe surgical resection, then XRT
  - Surgical resection often difficult due to adherence & infiltrating nature of tumor
  - Gross total resection + XRT correlates with improved survival
- Chemotherapy does not improve survival

DIAGNOSTIC CHECKLIST

Consider

- Much less common than MB or PA
- Gross total resection has greater impact on survival than in MB or PA
- Surveillance imaging to detect asymptomatic recurrence can ↓ survival

Image Interpretation Pearls

- When tumor is small, location can help delineate EPN from MB
  - With **floor** of 4th ventricle = EPN
  - With **roof** of 4th ventricle = MB

SELECTED REFERENCES

1. Jin Y et al: "Soap bubble" sign as an imaging marker for posterior fossa ependymoma Group B. Neuroradiology. 65(12):1707-14, 2023
2. Leclerc T et al: Imaging features to distinguish posterior fossa ependymoma subgroups. Eur Radiol. ePub, 2023
3. Cui Z et al: MRI-based texture analysis for differentiate between pediatric posterior fossa ependymoma type A and B. Eur J Radiol. 152:110288, 2022
4. Osborn AG et al: The 2021 World Health Organization classification of tumors of the central nervous system: what neuroradiologists need to know. AJNR Am J Neuroradiol. 43(7):928-37, 2022
5. Zhang M et al: Radiomic signatures of posterior fossa ependymoma: molecular subgroups and risk profiles. Neuro Oncol. 24(6):986-94, 2022

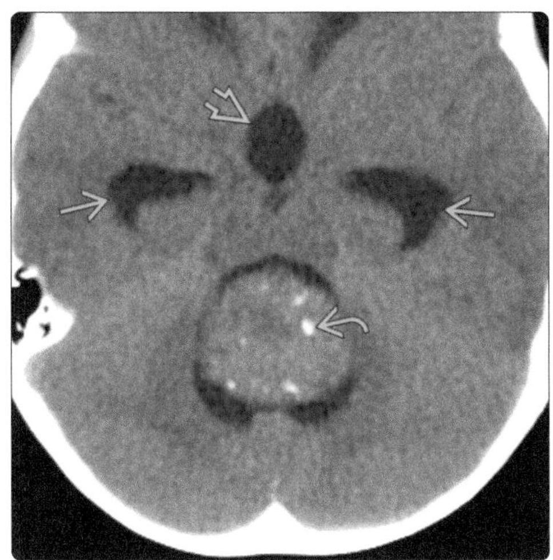

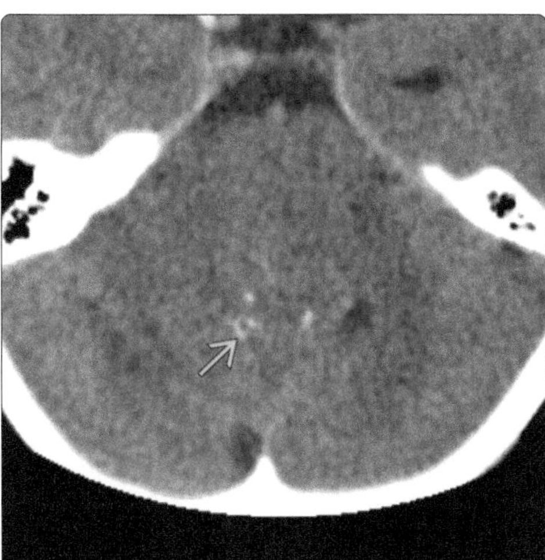

(Left) *Axial NECT in a 2-year-old girl shows a mass centered in the 4th ventricle containing scattered fine, stippled Ca⁺⁺ ➩. Note the enlargement of the temporal horns ➔ and 3rd ventricle ➪, consistent with obstructive hydrocephalus.* **(Right)** *Axial NECT in a young child with ependymoma shows obliteration of the 4th ventricle with a mass. Note the associated fine, stippled Ca⁺⁺ typical of ependymoma ➔. Such Ca⁺⁺ can be seen in up to ~ 50% of ependymomas.*

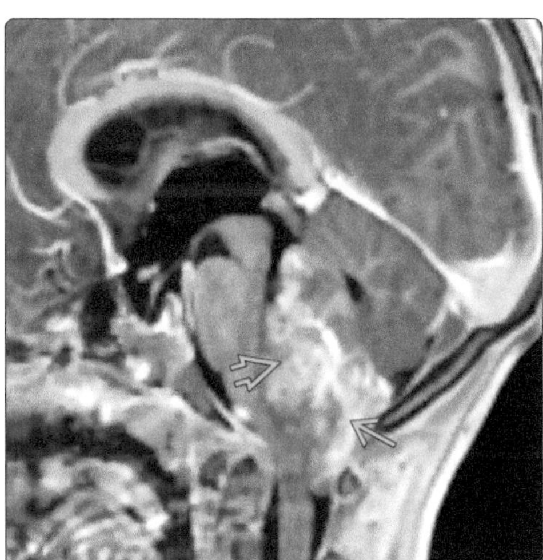

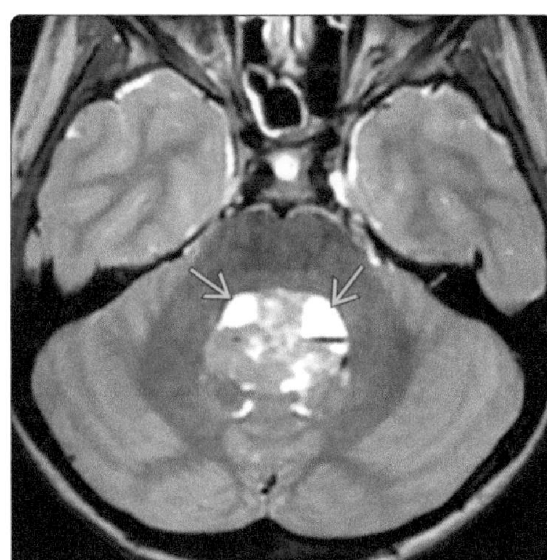

(Left) *Midline sagittal T1 C+ MR in a 9-year-old with grade 2 PF-EPN type B (PF-EPN-B) shows a heterogeneously enhancing lesion ➪ centered in the lower 1/2 of the 4th ventricle with extension into the foramen of Magendie ➔.* **(Right)** *Axial T2 MR in the same patient shows the tumor centered in the midline 4th ventricle with multiple cysts ➔. This midline location is typical for PF-EPN-B. On average, PF-EPN-B is more likely to have cystic components.*

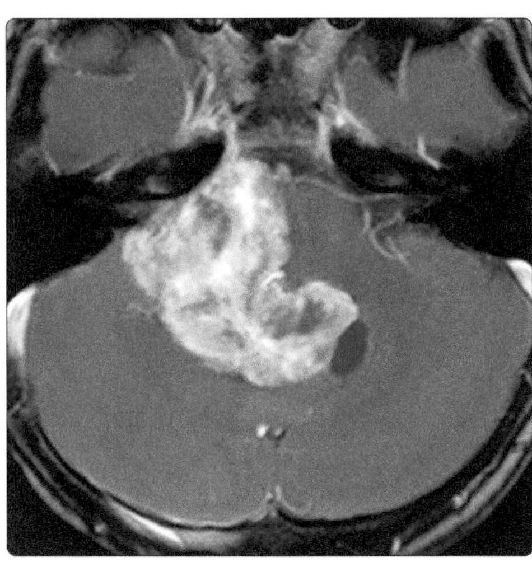

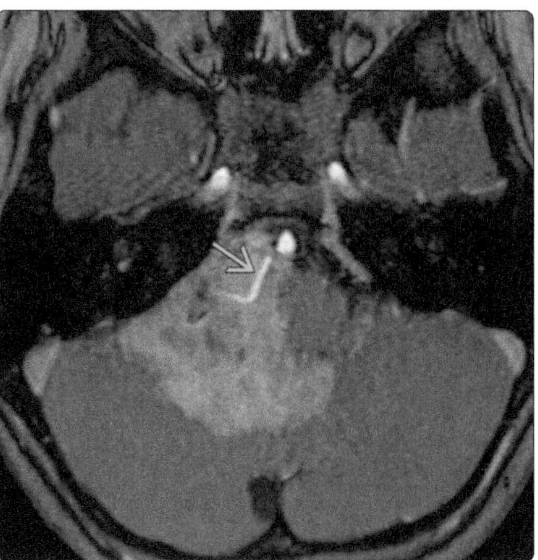

(Left) *Axial T1 C+ MR in a 2-year-old girl shows a mass centered in the right foramen of Luschka with extension to the 4th ventricle and CPA. Involvement of the CPA and the many cranial nerves and vessels that course through it often makes complete resection difficult.* **(Right)** *3D time-of-flight MRA in the same patient shows that the right posterior inferior cerebellar artery ➔ is encased by the mass. MRA is very helpful for delineating vascular involvement of masses extending into the basilar cisterns.*

Supratentorial Ependymoma

KEY FACTS

IMAGING

- Most supratentorial ependymomas (STEs) are **extraventricular**
- Common locations of STEs: Cerebral hemisphere > 3rd ventricle > lateral ventricle
- Imaging features
  - Large, complex-appearing mixed solid/cystic hemispheric mass
  - CT
    - Heterogeneous, cystic, & solid mass ± Ca^{++}
  - MR
    - Complex mixed solid & cystic mass
    - SWI/GRE: Foci of ↓ signal → hemorrhage or Ca^{++}
    - DWI: Often shows ↑ DWI ↓ ADC
    - Moderate but inhomogeneous enhancement

TOP DIFFERENTIAL DIAGNOSES

- High-grade glioma
- Embryonal tumor with multilayered rosettes
- Atypical teratoid/rhabdoid tumor
- Ganglioglioma
- Astrocytoma (other)
- Oligodendroglioma, anaplastic oligodendroglioma
- Pleomorphic xanthoastrocytoma

PATHOLOGY

- Most STEs WHO grade 3 tumors (anaplastic ependymoma)
- ZFTA fusion (+) (> 90% include RELA fusion)
  - Most common with worse prognosis
- YAP1 fusion (+)
  - Uncommon (≤ 10% of STEs) with better prognosis

CLINICAL ISSUES

- Treatment: maximal safe resection + radiation therapy

DIAGNOSTIC CHECKLIST

- If large, mixed solid-cystic, calcified hemispheric/cortical mass in child, think STE

(Left) *Graphic depicts supratentorial ependymoma (STE) as a large, hemorrhagic hemispheric mass with multiple cysts, fluid-fluid levels ➡, Ca^{++} ➡, significant mass effect, and peritumoral edema ➡.* **(Right)** *Axial T2 MR in a 2-year-old patient demonstrates a large, mixed cystic ➡ and solid ➡ mass with peritumoral edema ➡. The large size, heterogeneous solid component, and cysts are typical of STE.*

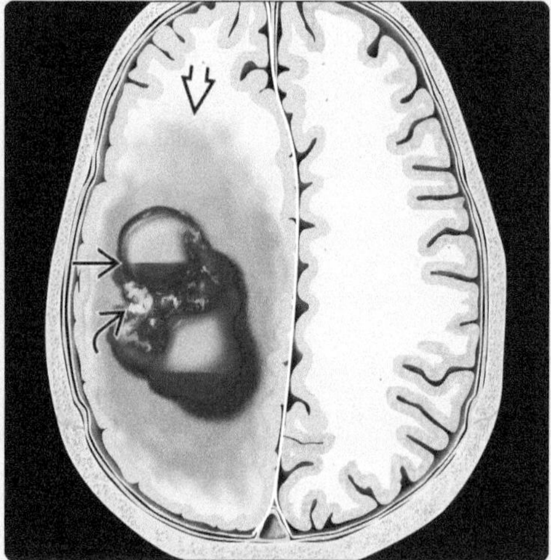

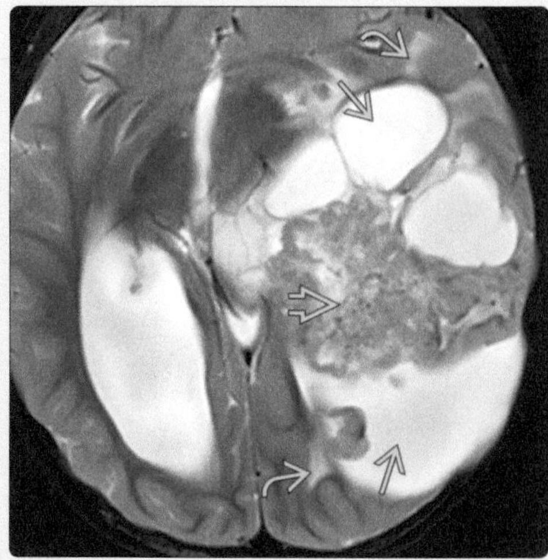

(Left) *Coronal T2 MR in a 4-year-old with ZFTA fusion STE shows a large, heterogeneous tumor ➡ in the left cerebral hemisphere with cystic and solid components and peritumoral edema ➡.* **(Right)** *Axial T1 C+ MR in the same patient shows heterogeneous enhancement of the solid components of the tumor ➡ with a large cystic component along the posterior aspect of the tumor ➡. Note the obstructed right lateral ventricle ➡.*

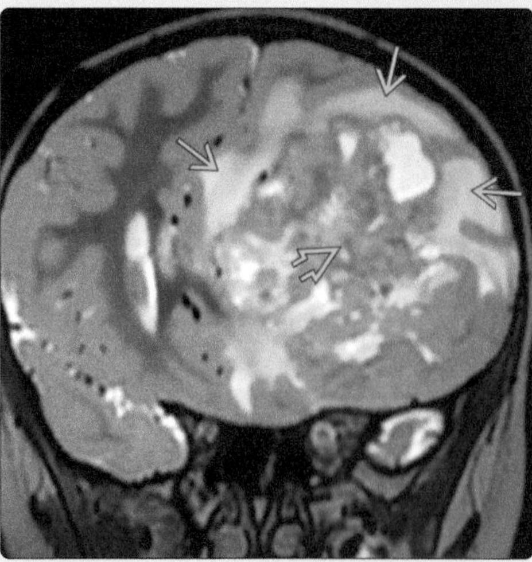

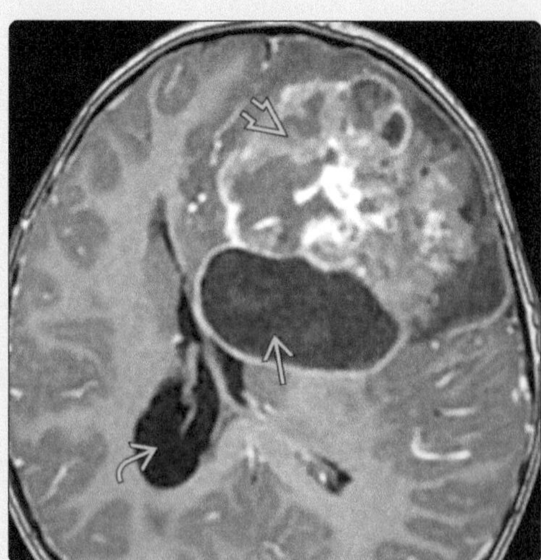

TERMINOLOGY

Abbreviations

- Supratentorial ependymoma (STE)

Synonyms

- Hemispheric STE (a.k.a. brain surface ependymoma)
- Supratentorial ectopic cortical ependymoma
- Cortical ependymoma

Definitions

- Ependymoma in supratentorial location

IMAGING

General Features

- Best diagnostic clue
  - Large, complex-appearing, mixed solid/cystic hemispheric mass
- Location
  - Majority of STEs are **extraventricular**
    - Hemispheric white matter or cortex
      - Frontal lobe most common location of cortical STEs
      - In cortex or infiltrating cortex from white matter
    - Rare: Suprasellar region
  - Less common location = intraventricular
    - 3rd ventricle > lateral ventricle
- Size
  - STEs often very large in size
    - 95% > 4 cm

CT Findings

- NECT
  - Mixed iso-/hypodense
    - Hyperdense = solid portion
    - Hypodense = cystic component
    - Ca^{++} (44%)
      - Can be small scattered foci or very extensive
  - May show bone destruction (tumor invades meninges, dura, & bone)

MR Findings

- T1WI
  - Iso-/hypointense
  - Cysts follow CSF
- T2WI
  - Variable morphologic features
    - Cystic with mural nodule
    - Solid mass
    - Huge, partially necrotic mass
  - Variable signal
    - Hyper to hypointense (high cellularity, Ca^{++})
    - Cysts hyperintense (CSF)
- T2* GRE
  - Low signal indicates hemorrhage or Ca^{++}
- DWI
  - Variable but often with ↑ DWI & ↓ ADC in hypercellular solid portions
- PWI
  - Increased perfusion correlates with higher grade & worse prognosis
- T1WI C+
  - Moderately intense enhancing tumor (solid parts) with necrotic foci
  - Rarely nonenhancing
  - Pattern
    - Cystic + mural nodule appearance (often in hemispheric location)
      - Mural nodule moderate or intensely enhancing
      - Nonenhancing or rim-enhancing cysts
  - Continuity with ventricle may be present
  - Continuity with surface present in cortical STE
- MRS
  - Generally show ↓ NAA, ↑ Cho, & occasional ↑ lactate

Imaging Recommendations

- Best imaging tool
  - MR with contrast of brain & spine
    - Image entire neuraxis for metastatic disease
  - SWI/GRE: (hemorrhage, Ca^{++})

DIFFERENTIAL DIAGNOSIS

High-Grade Glioma

- Less common in children vs. adults
- Cellular, heterogeneous supratentorial mass
- Look for central necrosis to suggest diagnosis
- Less common: Low-grade anaplastic astrocytoma

Embryonal Tumor With Multilayered Rosettes

- Usually in children < 5 years of age
- Significant imaging overlap with STE

Atypical Teratoid/Rhabdoid Tumor

- Very young children
- Cellular tumor: Look for ↑ DWI & ↓ ADC

Ganglioglioma

- Most common in temporal lobe
- May be complex-appearing
- Consider desmoplastic infantile ganglioglioma (DIG) in infant/young child

Astrocytoma (Other)

- Anaplastic astrocytoma, anaplastic pleomorphic xanthoastrocytoma can be very complex, heterogeneous-appearing

Oligodendroglioma, Anaplastic Oligodendroglioma

- Much less common in children
- Cerebral hemispheres
- Cortical & subcortical locations
- Scalloping of inner table of skull

Pleomorphic Xanthoastrocytoma

- Cortically based enhancing mass with dural tail
- Temporal lobe most common
- May be cystic with solid enhancing components

Astroblastoma

- Older children & young adults
- Solid cystic mass
- Supratentorial location
- Ca^{++}

PATHOLOGY

General Features

- Etiology
  - General: Ependymoma is glial-based neoplasm arising from ependymal lining of ventricular system
  - Extraventricular STEs arise either from
    - Fetal rests of ependymal cells located at angle of ventricles
    - Random distribution of fetal ependymal rests located periventricularly
- Genetics
  - 2021 WHO CNS tumor classification using molecular/genetic diagnosis for tumor classification
    - Previous 2016 WHO nomenclature of RELA fusion no longer used
  - ZFTA fusion (+) STEs
    - Most (but not all) contain RELA fusion, which was former 2016 WHO molecular designation
    - Represent majority of STEs
    - Occur in both children & adults
    - Poor prognosis
  - YAP1 fusion (+) STEs
    - Represent minority (≤ 10%) of STEs
    - Occur in young children
    - Better prognosis compared to ZFTA fusion (+) STE

Staging, Grading, & Classification

- Molecular diagnosis (ZFTA & YAP1 fusion) is primary classification
- Grading should also be included as part of integrated diagnosis
- WHO grade 2 ependymoma
  - 4 variants: Cellular, papillary, clear cell, & tanycytic
- WHO grade 3 anaplastic ependymoma
  - Majority of adult STEs are WHO grade 3 tumors
  - Defined by presence of any 2 of 4 + factors
    - 4 mitoses per 10 HPF (brisk mitotic activity)
    - Hypercellularity
    - Endothelial proliferation
    - Necrosis (pseudopalisading necrosis)

Gross Pathologic & Surgical Features

- Well-delineated tumors
- Lobulated mass, grayish-red surface, hemorrhagic & calcified parts

Microscopic Features

- Histologic hallmarks
  - Perivascular rosettes
  - Ependymal rosettes
  - GFAP (+)
- Nonrosetting angiocentric growth pattern
- Variable amount of solid tumor growth
- Low proliferative index
- Infiltrating brain parenchyma
  - Infiltration along axonal tracts, perineuronal satellitosis, subpial mounding

CLINICAL ISSUES

Presentation

- Most common signs/symptoms
  - Seizures most common symptom
  - Focal motor or sensory deficit, headache
  - When large, may cause increased intracranial pressure & obstructive hydrocephalus

Demographics

- Age
  - Bimodal
    - Most in children 1-5 years old; smaller peak: 20-30 years old
    - ZFTA fusion (+) STE occur in children & adults
    - YAP1 fusion (+) STE occurs in young children
- Sex
  - M > F
- Epidemiology
  - Uncommon tumor in children

Natural History & Prognosis

- ZFTA fusion (+) STE: Poor prognosis
- YAP1 fusion (+) STE: Better prognosis
- Higher recurrence rate for 3rd ventricular tumors (compared to hemispheric tumors)

Treatment

- Gross total resection with adjuvant radiotherapy

DIAGNOSTIC CHECKLIST

Consider

- STE: Large, heterogeneous, solid-cystic, calcified hemispheric mass in child

SELECTED REFERENCES

1. Osborn AG et al: The 2021 World Health Organization classification of tumors of the central nervous system: what neuroradiologists need to know. AJNR Am J Neuroradiol. 43(7):928-37, 2022
2. Safai A et al: Developing a radiomics signature for supratentorial extra-ventricular ependymoma using multimodal MR imaging. Front Neurol. 12:648092, 2021
3. Tauziède-Espariat A et al: Supratentorial non-RELA, ZFTA-fused ependymomas: a comprehensive phenotype genotype correlation highlighting the number of zinc fingers in ZFTA-NCOA1/2 fusions. Acta Neuropathol Commun. 9(1):135, 2021
4. Kuai XP et al: MRI features of intracranial anaplastic ependymomas: a comparison of supratentorial and infratentorial lesions. Front Oncol. 10:1063, 2020
5. Lillard JC et al: Pediatric supratentorial ependymoma: surgical, clinical, and molecular analysis. Neurosurgery. 85(1):41-9. 2018
6. Nowak J et al: MRI phenotype of RELA-fused pediatric supratentorial ependymoma. Clin Neuroradiol. 29(4):595-604, 2018
7. Onishi S et al: RELA fusion-positive anaplastic ependymoma: molecular characterization and advanced MR imaging. Brain Tumor Pathol. 35(1):41-5, 2018
8. Sun S et al: Clinical, radiological, and histological features and treatment outcomes of supratentorial extraventricular ependymoma: 14 cases from a single center. J Neurosurg. 128(5):1396-402, 2018
9. Witt DA et al: Specific expression of PD-L1 in RELA-fusion supratentorial ependymoma: implications for PD-1-targeted therapy. Pediatr Blood Cancer. 65(5):e26960, 2018
10. Gessi M et al: Role of immunohistochemistry in the Identification of supratentorial C11ORF95-RELA fused ependymoma in routine neuropathology. Am J Surg Pathol. 43(1):56-63, 2017

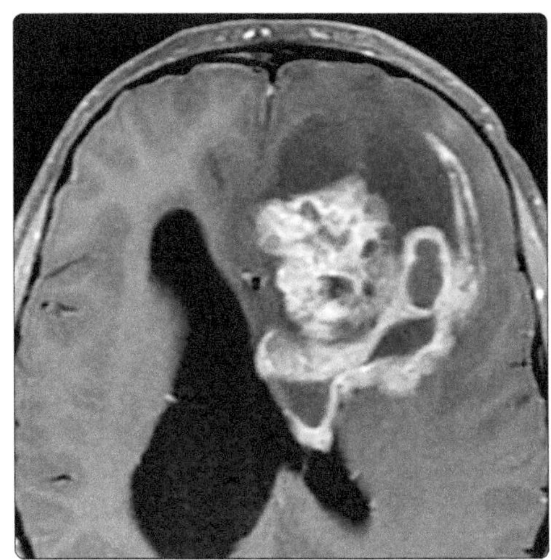

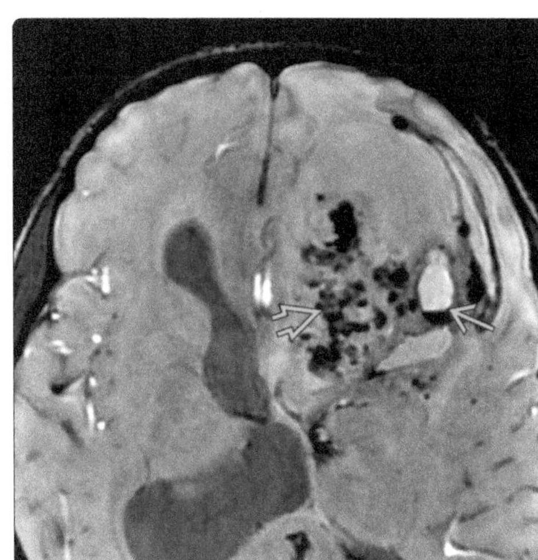

(Left) *Axial T1 C+ MR in an 11-year-old with grade 2 STE shows a heterogeneously enhancing, mixed solid and cystic mass centered in left frontal white matter with extension to the left lateral ventricle. The lesion causes obstructive hydrocephalus.* **(Right)** *Axial SWI in the same patient shows multiple foci of signal loss ⇒, which may represent Ca^{++} or hemorrhage. Note the hemorrhage level → within an intratumoral cyst. Ca^{++} &/or hemorrhage are common findings in STE.*

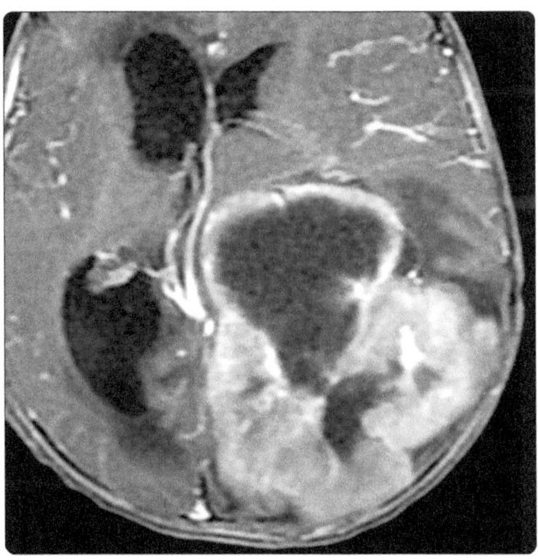

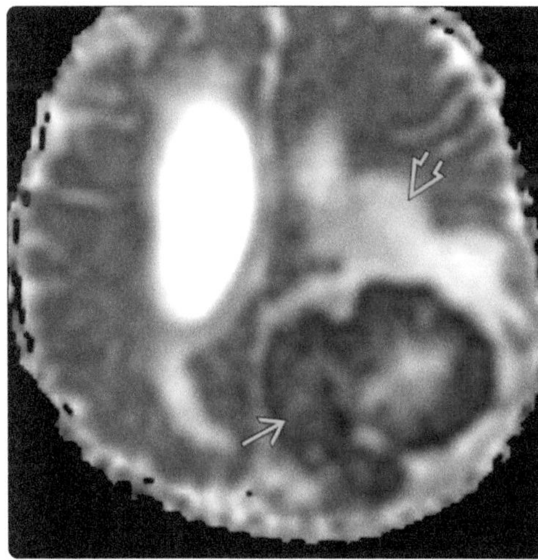

(Left) *Axial T1 C+ MR in a 4-month-old with WHO grade 2 STE shows a large, mixed solid and cystic mass in the left parietal region, causing obstructive hydrocephalus.* **(Right)** *Axial ADC map in the same patient shows decreased signal within the solid components of the mass →, suggesting increased cellularity. Also note the increased signal in adjacent brain, representing vasogenic edema ⇒. Diffusion restriction is often seen within the solid components of STE.*

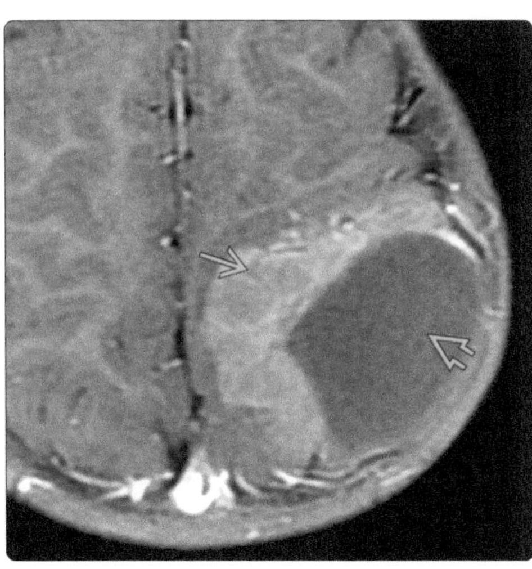

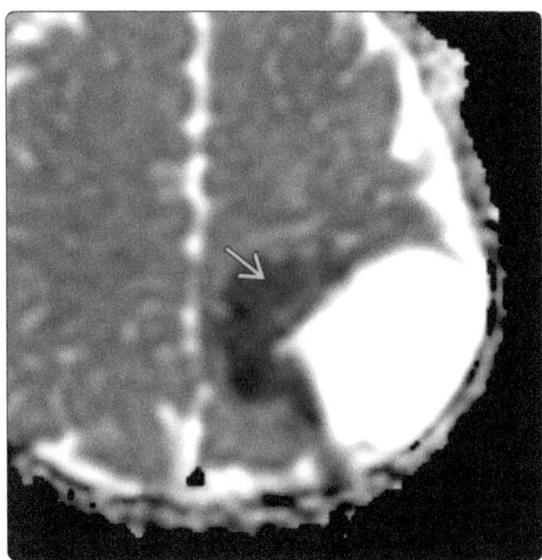

(Left) *Axial T1 C+ MR in a 10-month-old with left parietal STE shows a predominantly enhancing → lesion with a single large peripheral cyst ⇒. This is a nonspecific pattern that can be seen in STE.* **(Right)** *Axial ADC map in the same patient shows decreased signal in the solid component → of the tumor, suggesting increased cellularity. Signal on diffusion-weighted imaging is highly variable in STE.*

KEY FACTS

TERMINOLOGY

- Malignant (WHO grade 4), invasive, highly cellular embryonal tumor

IMAGING

- Round cellular mass in midline 4th ventricle
  - ~ 10% cerebellar hemisphere → sonic hedgehog (SHH) subtype
  - < 5% cerebellopontine angle → WNT subtype
- Obstructive hydrocephalus in 95%
- **CT**: 90% hyperattenuating (due to ↑ cellularity)
  - Ca^{++} in up to 20%; hemorrhage rare
- **MR**: Restricted diffusion reflects ↑ cellularity
  - C+ of entire neuraxis to detect CSF spread
- 33% have subarachnoid metastatic disease at diagnosis

TOP DIFFERENTIAL DIAGNOSES

- Atypical teratoid/rhabdoid tumor (AT/RT)
- Ependymoma
- Pilocytic astrocytoma

PATHOLOGY

- 4 major molecular subgroups
  - Non-WNT, non-SHH (most common): Group 3, group 4
  - SHH activated, TP53-wildtype
  - SHH activated, TP53-mutant
  - WNT (least common)

CLINICAL ISSUES

- Most common posterior fossa tumor in ages 0-4 years
- Prognosis dependent on (1) metastatic disease, (2) molecular subgroup, and (3) other molecular markers

DIAGNOSTIC CHECKLIST

- Location and enhancement are imaging biomarkers for medulloblastoma subtype
  - Cerebellar hemisphere (SHH), cerebellopontine angle (WNT)
- Remember AT/RT in DDx in patients < 3 years old

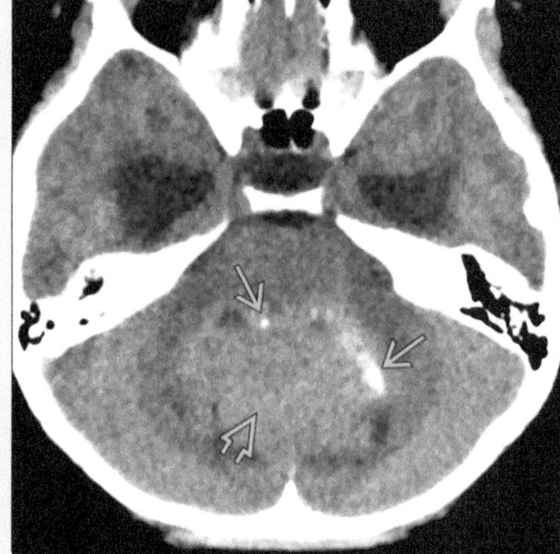

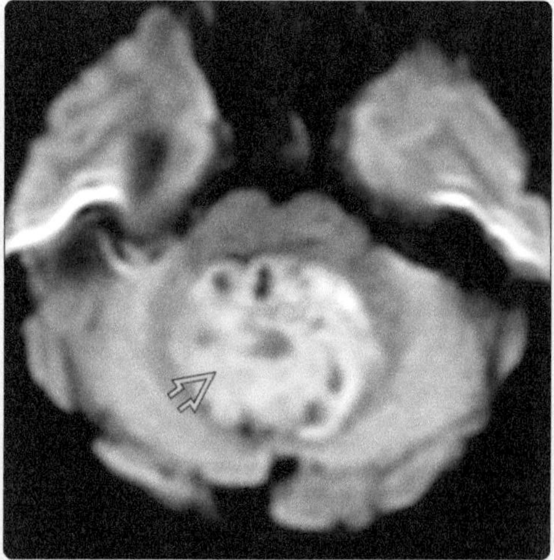

(Left) *Axial NECT in a 7-year-old with group 4 medulloblastoma (MB) shows a hyperdense mass ⇨ centered in the 4th ventricle with some chunky and punctate peripheral Ca^{++} ⇨. The hyperdensity of MB corresponds to its high cellularity.* **(Right)** *Axial DWI MR in the same patient shows diffusion restriction in the tumor ⇨, also a reflection of the high cellularity of these grade 4 tumors. This is the key distinguishing feature of MB.*

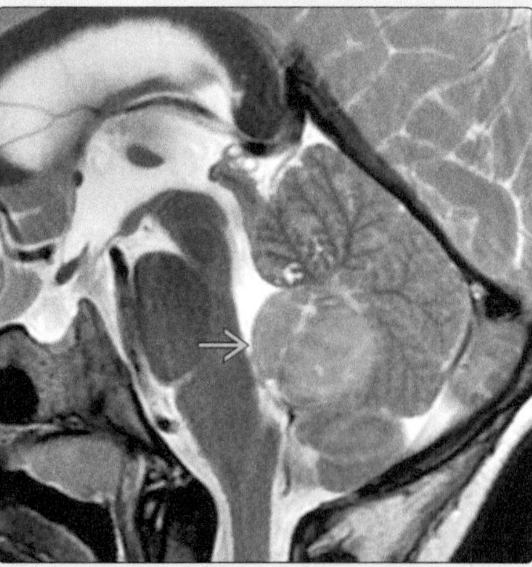

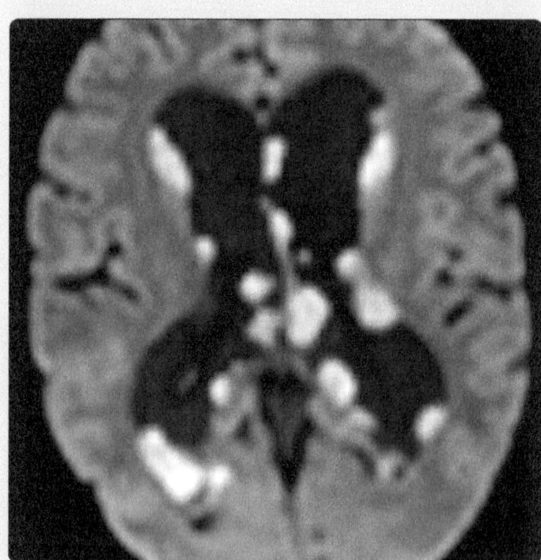

(Left) *Sagittal T2WI MR in a 4-year-old shows a midline mass ⇨ arising from the roof of the 4th ventricle with signal equal to gray matter. When small, most MBs clearly arise from the roof of the 4th ventricle. When larger, the origin of 4th ventricle tumors can be difficult to determine.* **(Right)** *Axial DWI MR in a 13-year-old with MB status post gross total resection 3 years ago shows CSF dissemination of recurrent tumor along the ependymal lining of the lateral ventricles.*

TERMINOLOGY

Abbreviations

- Medulloblastoma (MB)

Synonyms

- Previously referred to as posterior fossa primitive neuroectodermal tumor (PNET), PNET-MB
  - PNET no longer used in CNS terminology, replaced by molecularly defined tumors under umbrella of embryonal tumors

Definitions

- Malignant (WHO grade 4), invasive, highly cellular embryonal tumor

IMAGING

General Features

- Best diagnostic clue
  - Midline 4th ventricular mass in 1st decade of life
  - Hyperattenuating (CT), diffusion restricting (MR)
- Location
  - 75-90% occur in midline; 4th ventricular mass arising from roof (dorsal 4th ventricle)
    - Superior medullary velum
    - Group 3 and group 4 subtypes are exclusively located in midline/4th ventricle
  - Cerebellar hemisphere more frequent location in older children and adults
    - Hemispheric location strongly suggests sonic hedgehog (SHH) subtype
  - Small percentage occurs in cerebellopontine angle (CPA) cistern; CPA cistern locations suggest WNT molecular subtype
  - ~ 33% have subarachnoid metastatic disease at diagnosis
  - Bony metastases may occur in ~ 5%; usually sclerotic
    - Spread to lymph nodes, liver, lung less frequent
- Size
  - Variable but often large since usually clinically silent until causing obstructive hydrocephalus
- Morphology
  - Usually round
    - Unlike ependymoma, which often protrudes through 4th ventricle foramina
  - Predominantly solid but may have associated cysts

CT Findings

- NECT
  - Hyperattenuation (90%) reflects high cellularity
  - Ca^{++} in up to 20%
  - Hemorrhage is uncommon
  - Obstructive hydrocephalus in up to 95%
  - May see scattered hypodense cysts, especially in larger tumors
- CECT
  - Enhancement is variable

MR Findings

- T1WI
  - Hypointense to gray matter (GM)
- T2WI
  - Iso- to hyperintense to GM
- FLAIR
  - Hyperintense to brain
- T2* GRE
  - Hypointense foci reflect Ca^{++} or, less likely, hemorrhage
- DWI
  - Hyperintense on DWI; hypointense on ADC
    - Reflects high cellularity
  - Very helpful for detecting small leptomeningeal metastases and early recurrence
- PWI
  - Arterial spin labeling (ASL) can discriminate high- and low-grade tumors but is not very helpful for discriminating specific histologies
    - MB typically has ↑ cerebral blood flow (CBF) compared to low-grade tumors (e.g., pilocytic astrocytoma)
- T1WI C+
  - Variable enhancement of primary tumor
    - Contrast improves detection of CSF dissemination
  - No/minimal or central stellate enhancement is most common in group 4 subtype
- MRS
  - ↑ Cho, ↓ NAA, ↓ Cr, ± ↑ lipid/lactate typical but not specific for MB
  - Taurine peak may be detected on MRS at 3.4 ppm

Nuclear Medicine Findings

- PET
  - Uniform ↑ FDG uptake is typical

Imaging Recommendations

- Best imaging tool
  - MR with DWI and postcontrast sequences
- Protocol advice
  - Sagittal images pre- and postcontrast often show site of origin (roof vs. floor of 4th ventricle) in smaller tumors
  - Appropriate staging requires total spine imaging
  - bSSFP (e.g., FIESTA, CISS) very helpful for detection of small spinal leptomeningeal metastases

DIFFERENTIAL DIAGNOSIS

Atypical Teratoid/Rhabdoid Tumor

- No consistently differentiating imaging features; often more heterogeneous than MB
- Younger children (usually < 3 years of age)

Ependymoma

- Punctate Ca^{++} and hemorrhage more common than MB
- Extension through 4th ventricle foramina: "Plastic tumor"
- Less likely to have diffusion restriction (except anaplastic ependymoma)

Pilocytic Astrocytoma

- Cerebellar hemispheric lesion; often cystic
- Solid portion: ↑ ADC signal (↑ diffusivity, not ↓)

Choroid Plexus Papilloma

- 4th ventricle and CPA location less common
- Vigorous enhancement typical
- No diffusion restriction unless higher grade (carcinoma)

PATHOLOGY

General Features

- Most common posterior fossa tumor in ages 0-4 years
- Associated with many familial cancer syndromes
  - Li-Fraumeni syndrome
  - Gorlin (nevoid basal cell carcinoma) syndrome
  - Turcot syndrome
  - Gardner syndrome
  - Cowden syndrome
- Also associated with Rubenstein-Taybi syndrome

Staging, Grading, & Classification

- WHO grade 4
- Molecular subgroups defined in WHO 2021 CNS Tumor Classification
  - WNT (least common)
    - *CTNNB1* mutation
    - Often located in CPA
  - SHH activated, TP53-wildtype
    - 4 subtypes
    - *PTCH1* and *SUFU* mutations common
    - Often nodular/desmoplastic histology
    - Better prognosis compared to TP53 mutant
  - SHH activated, TP53 mutant
    - U1, snRNA, and *GLI2* mutations common
    - Worse prognosis compared to TP53-wildtype
  - Non-WNT, non-SHH (most common)
    - Group 3
      - *MYC* amplification common
      - Located in midline/4th ventricle
    - Group 4
      - i17q mutation common
      - Located in midline/4th ventricle
      - Often with minimal enhancement

Microscopic Features

- Densely packed hyperchromatic cells with scant cytoplasm
- Frequent mitoses
- Anaplasia in 24%
- Desmoplastic subtype has abundant connective tissue between tumor cells
- Immunohistochemistry: ± synaptophysin, vimentin
  - Some have glial differentiation (positive GFAP staining)
- Histologic subtypes (still applicable and important in treatment decisions)
  - Classic (~ 70%)
  - Nodular/desmoplastic (~ 20%)
  - Anaplastic/large cell (~ 10%)
    - Puts patient in high-risk category
    - More likely to have ring enhancement reflecting tumor necrosis

CLINICAL ISSUES

Presentation

- Ataxia, signs of ↑ intracranial pressure
  - Relatively short duration (weeks) of symptoms

Demographics

- M > F = 2-4:1
- 75% of patients < 10 years of age
  - Molecular subgroups/types cluster by age
    - 0-3: SHH-1, SHH-2, group 3
    - 4-10: Group 3, group 4, SHH-3, WNT
    - 11-16: Group 4, SHH-3, WNT
    - 17+: SHH-4, WNT

Natural History & Prognosis

- Rapid growth seen with early subarachnoid spread
- Initial positive response to treatment reflects high mitotic activity
- Prognosis depends on number of risk factors
  - Metastatic disease
  - Molecular subgroup
  - Other molecular markers (e.g., *MYC* amplification status)
- Long-term survival in resourced countries
  - Average risk: > 80%
  - High risk: > 60%

Treatment

- Surgical excision, adjuvant chemotherapy
- Craniospinal irradiation if > 3 years of age

DIAGNOSTIC CHECKLIST

Consider

- Key imaging factors to determine therapy and prognosis: Identifying metastatic disease and defining residual tumor status post resection
  - High quality imaging is key to identifying metastatic disease and appropriate risk stratification
- Machine learning radiogenomics approach may improve imaging discernment of MB molecular subgroups

Image Interpretation Pearls

- Classic teaching regarding posterior fossa tumors based on location in 4th ventricle
  - Arising from roof: MB
  - Arising from floor: Ependymoma
  - Distinction difficult in larger tumors
- Remember atypical teratoid/rhabdoid tumor in DDx when patient < 3 years old

SELECTED REFERENCES

1. Funakoshi Y et al: Recent advances in the molecular understanding of medulloblastoma. Cancer Sci. 114(3):741-9, 2023
2. Jackson K et al: Recent advances in pediatric medulloblastoma. Curr Neurol Neurosci Rep. 23(12):841-8, 2023
3. Dasgupta A et al: Magnetic resonance imaging in the contemporary management of medulloblastoma: current and emerging applications. Methods Mol Biol. 2423:187-214, 2022
4. Luo Y et al: The diagnostic efficiency of quantitative diffusion weighted imaging in differentiating medulloblastoma from posterior fossa tumors: a systematic review and meta-analysis. Diagnostics (Basel). 12(11):2796, 2022
5. Osborn AG et al: The 2021 World Health Organization classification of tumors of the central nervous system: what neuroradiologists need to know. AJNR Am J Neuroradiol. 43(7):928-37, 2022
6. Zhang M et al: MRI radiogenomics of pediatric medulloblastoma: a multicenter study. Radiology. 304(2):406-16, 2022
7. Dangouloff-Ros V et al: Imaging features of medulloblastoma: conventional imaging, diffusion-weighted imaging, perfusion-weighted imaging, and spectroscopy: from general features to subtypes and characteristics. Neurochirurgie. 67(1):6-13, 2021
8. Reddy N et al: Pediatric posterior fossa medulloblastoma: the role of diffusion imaging in identifying molecular groups. J Neuroimaging. 30(4):503-11, 2020

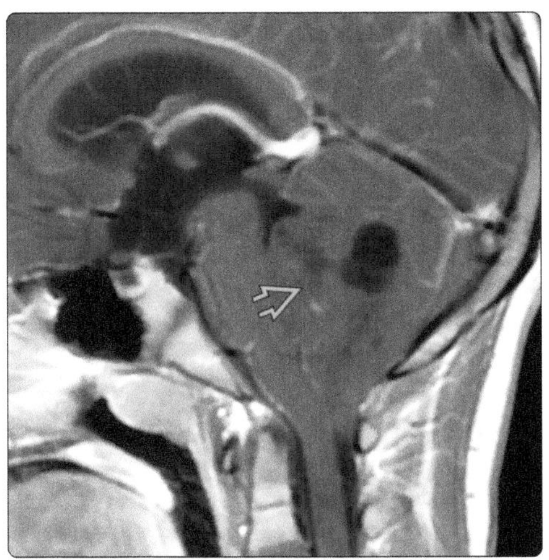

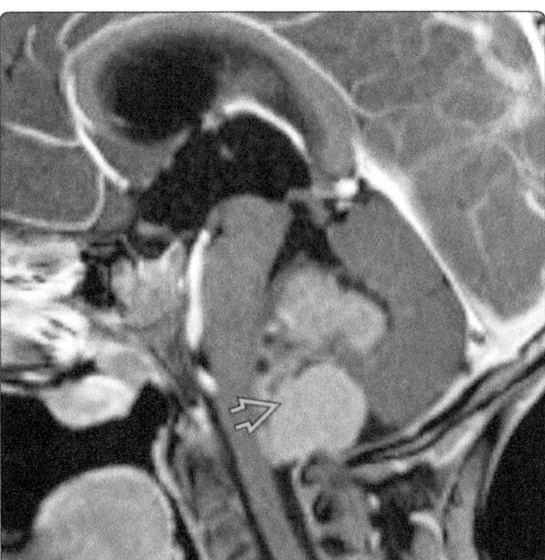

(Left) *Sagittal T1WI C+ MR in a 10-year-old group 4 MB shows lack of contrast enhancement of the tumor ➡ arising from the roof of the 4th ventricle. Lack of, or decreased, enhancement is a characteristic finding of group 4 MB.* **(Right)** *Sagittal T1WI C+ MR in a 4-year-old with group 3 MB shows avid enhancement of the tumor ➡, which is characteristic of group 3 MB. Both group 3 and 4 MBs occur almost exclusively in the midline 4th ventricle, so enhancement is the best discriminating imaging finding.*

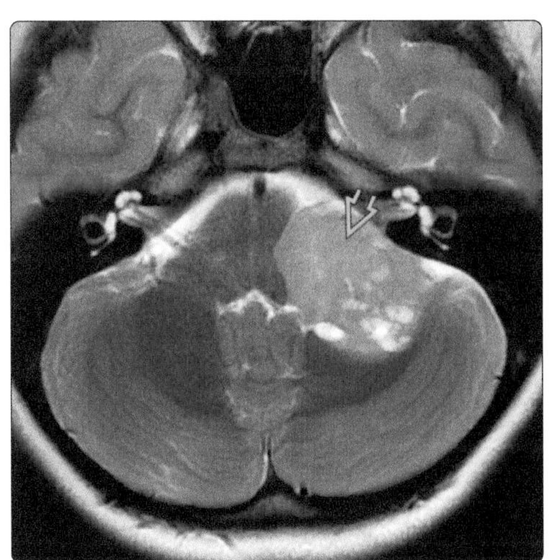

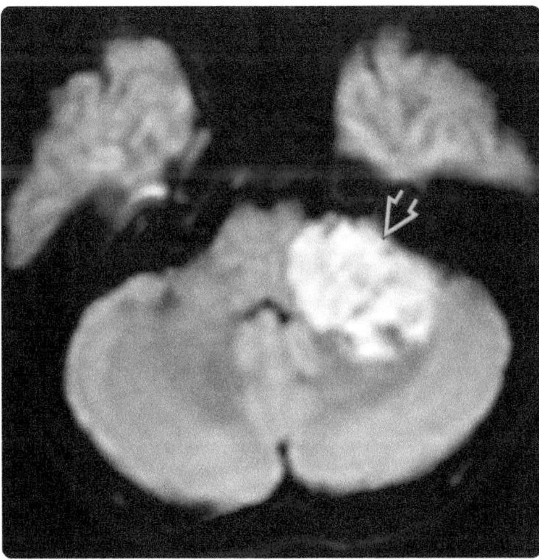

(Left) *Axial T2WI MR in a 10-year-old with WNT molecular subtype MB shows a predominantly solid mass ➡ centered in the left cerebellopontine angle (CPA) cistern with a few peripheral cysts. WNT MB can occur anywhere in the posterior fossa, but this CPA location is quite characteristic for WNT MB.* **(Right)** *Axial DWI MR in the same patient with WNT subtype MB shows diffusion restriction within the CPA mass ➡, characteristic for MB.*

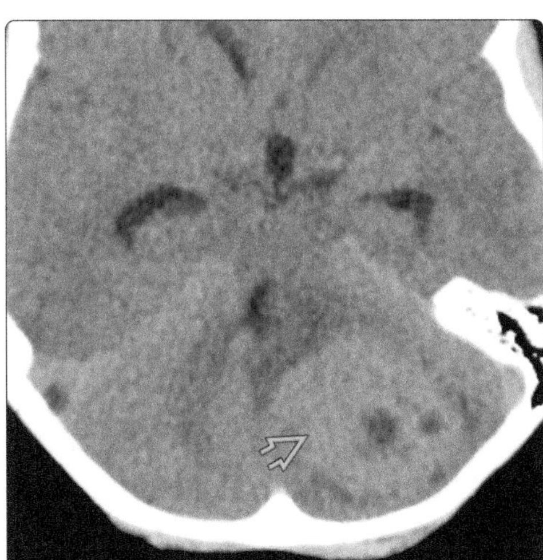

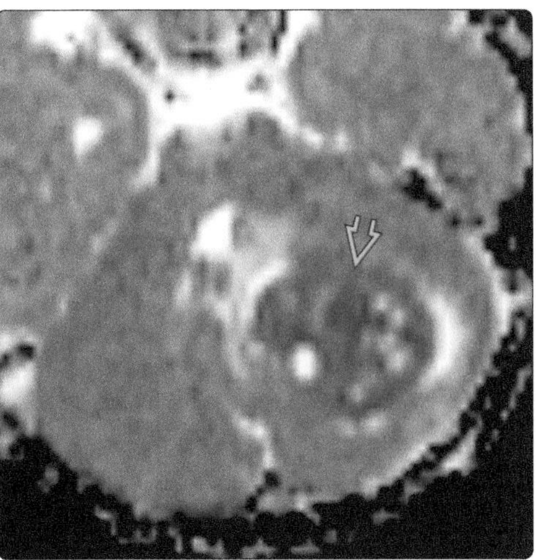

(Left) *Axial NECT in a 9-year-old with sonic hedgehog (SHH) subtype MB shows a hyperdense mass ➡ centered in the left cerebellar hemisphere with a few small hypoattenuated cysts.* **(Right)** *Axial ADC map MR in the same patient shows dark signal in the mass ➡, consistent with the high cellularity of MB. Approximately 50% of SHH MB occur in the cerebellar hemispheres but is the only subtype to occur regularly in this location. Key point: A highly cellular tumor in the cerebellar hemisphere should specifically suggest SHH MB.*

Atypical Teratoid/Rhabdoid Tumor

KEY FACTS

TERMINOLOGY

- Highly malignant (WHO grade 4) embryonal neoplasm

IMAGING

- Heterogeneous intracranial mass in infant/young child
  - Commonly contains cysts or hemorrhage
  - Solid components show ↑ attenuation on CT & restricted diffusion on MR due to high cellularity
- 47% infratentorial, 41% supratentorial, 12% both
- Often causes obstructive hydrocephalus
- Leptomeningeal spread common (15-20%)

TOP DIFFERENTIAL DIAGNOSES

- Medulloblastoma (MB)
- Supratentorial primitive neuroectodermal tumor (PNET)
- Ependymoma
- Desmoplastic infantile tumor
- Teratoma
- Choroid plexus tumor

PATHOLOGY

- Morphologic & immunophenotypic heterogeneity
- Divergent differentiation accounts for teratoid label
  - Sheets of primitive cells separated by fibrovascular septa
  - Large rhabdoid cells with eosinophilic cytoplasm
- Most rhabdoid tumors show lack of INI1 immunostain due to *SMARCB1* (hSNF5/INI1) mutation (22q11.2)
- Histology similar to renal & soft tissue rhabdoid tumors
  - May be concurrent with CNS AT/RT

CLINICAL ISSUES

- Child < 3 years old with increasing head size, vomiting
- Median survival: 12-18 months; overall survival rate: 23-37%

DIAGNOSTIC CHECKLIST

- Always consider AT/RT in young child (< 3 years old) if
  - Large, heterogeneous CNS tumor
  - MB or PNET being considered
  - Infant with new cranial nerve palsy + cisternal mass

(Left) *Axial NECT in a 4-month-old shows a mixed solid ⇨ & cystic ⇨ mass with central Ca^{++} ⇨ centered in the left cerebellopontine angle with marked mass effect on the brainstem & 4th ventricle. AT/RT is much more likely to be centered off-midline in the cerebellopontine angle than its more common posterior fossa embryonal tumor mimic, medulloblastoma.* **(Right)** *Axial DWI MR in the same patient shows increased signal within the solid component ⇨ of the tumor, a characteristic finding in this highly cellular tumor.*

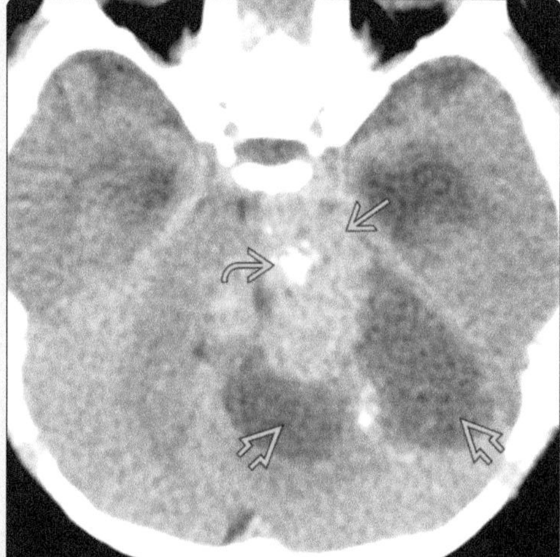

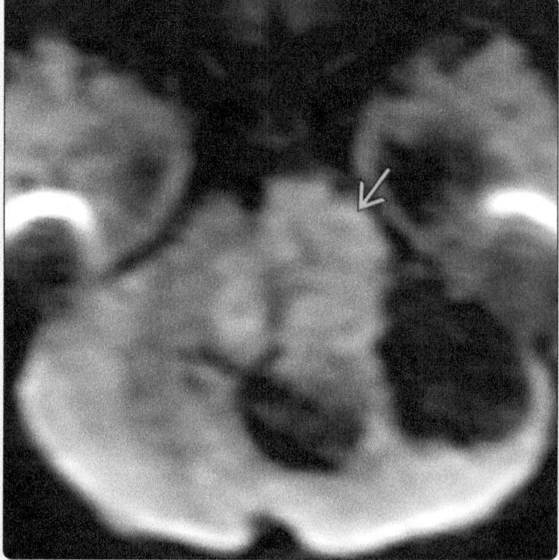

(Left) *Axial T2 MR in a 2-year-old boy demonstrates a large intraventricular AT/RT with nodular masses along the ependyma of both lateral ventricles ⇨, consistent with CSF spread of disease.* **(Right)** *Axial T2 MR in an 11-month-old boy demonstrates a large, heterogeneous mass centered in the left frontotemporal region. The fluid levels ⇨ suggest prior intratumoral hemorrhage. AT/RT should be considered for any large hemorrhagic CNS mass in an infant or young child.*

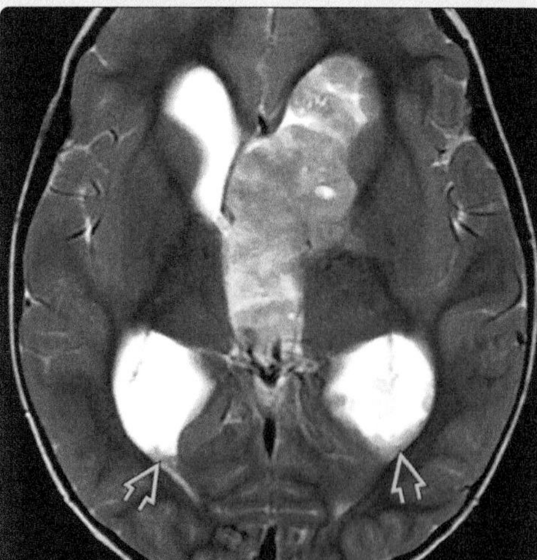

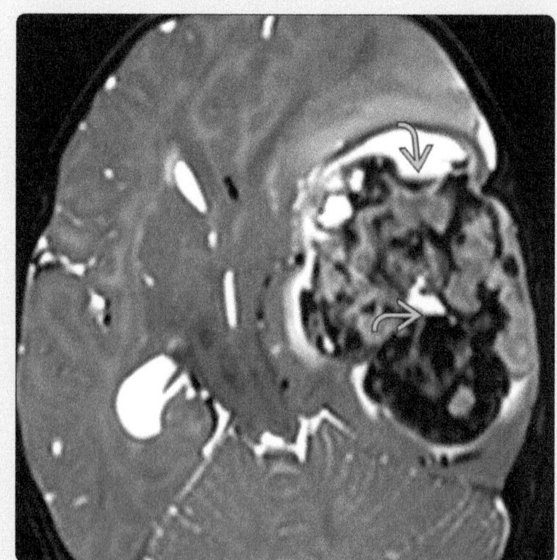

Atypical Teratoid/Rhabdoid Tumor

TERMINOLOGY

Synonyms

- Malignant rhabdoid tumor of brain
- Intracranial rhabdoid tumor

Definitions

- Atypical teratoid/rhabdoid tumor (AT/RT): Malignant embryonal tumor of CNS in early childhood
  - Closely related to renal & soft tissue rhabdoid tumors

IMAGING

General Features

- Best diagnostic clue
  - Large solid & cystic tumor (± hemorrhage) with diffusion restriction in infant/young child
- Location
  - Infratentorial (47%)
    - Often off-midline
      - Cerebellopontine angle
      - Cerebellum &/or brainstem
      - Individual cranial nerves
  - Supratentorial (41%)
    - Hemispheric or intraventricular
  - Both infra- & supratentorial (12%)
  - May occur in spine but uncommon
  - 15-20% have disseminated tumor at initial diagnosis
- Size
  - Usually 1-4 cm at presentation (can be very large)
- Morphology
  - Roughly spherical, but margins may be irregular/lobulated

CT Findings

- NECT
  - Hyperattenuating mass
  - Commonly contains cysts &/or hemorrhage
  - May contain Ca^{++}
  - Obstructive hydrocephalus common
- CECT
  - Strong but heterogeneous enhancement typical

MR Findings

- T1WI
  - Heterogeneous ± hyperintense hemorrhage
- T2WI
  - Heterogeneous signal ± hyperintense cystic foci
- FLAIR
  - Hyperintense cysts ± peritumoral edema
- T2* GRE
  - Hemorrhagic foci causing exaggerated signal loss (blooming)
    - Hemorrhage is seen in most tumors on SWI
- DWI
  - Positive diffusion restriction (↓ ADC signal) due to high cellularity
    - Similar to other embryonal tumors [medulloblastoma (MB), embryonal tumor with multilayered rosettes (ETMR), pineoblastoma]
- T1WI C+
  - Heterogeneous but avid enhancement most common
    - Important in detecting local recurrence & CSF dissemination
  - Less commonly, no enhancement
- MRA
  - Helpful to identify vessel involvement for surgical planning
- MRS
  - Aggressive metabolite pattern

Imaging Recommendations

- Best imaging tool
  - MR of brain & spine with contrast
- Protocol advice
  - Image entire neuraxis
    - Leptomeningeal spread common (15-20%)

DIFFERENTIAL DIAGNOSIS

Medulloblastoma

- ~ 90% are midline; AT/RT more likely to be off-midline
- AT/RT on average more heterogeneous & more likely to have cysts than MB
- MB in younger & older children; AT/RT rare in older children

CNS Embryonal Tumor (Formerly Primitive Neuroectodermal Tumor)

- Cellular supratentorial tumor with diffusion restriction
- Typically in slightly older children compared to AT/RT

Ependymoma

- Infratentorial tumor often extending out 4th ventricular foramina
- Supratentorial tumor often large & cystic
- Ca^{++}, cysts, hemorrhage common
- Diffusion restriction less common compared to AT/RT

Desmoplastic Infantile Ganglioglioma/Astrocytoma

- Very young children (peak age: 3-6 months)
- Very large cystic components

Teratoma

- More often pineal or parasellar in location
- Heterogeneous due to Ca^{++}, ± fat

Choroid Plexus Tumors

- Centered in ventricle
- Vigorous, homogeneous enhancement
- Lobulated, frond-like margins
- Diffusion restriction much less common compared to AT/RT

Glioblastoma

- Variety of appearances; frequently with necrosis

PATHOLOGY

General Features

- Genetics
  - Loss of tumor suppressor gene *SMARCB1* (hSNF5/INI1) in most rhabdoid tumors, including CNS, renal, extrarenal
    - Gene located at chromosome 22q11.2
    - Mutation at 19p13.2 less common (*SMARCA4*)

- Germline mutation tumors present earlier than somatic
  - Rhabdoid tumor predisposition syndrome
    - Synchronous renal & CNS or bilateral renal tumors

Staging, Grading, & Classification

- WHO grade 4
- 2021 WHO molecular subgroups
  - Studies suggest imaging biomarkers for subgroups
  - AT/RT-SHH
    - Most common (44%)
    - Toddlers 1-5 years (median: 20 months)
    - Supratentorial (65%), intratentorial (35%); often crosses incisura
    - Imaging features: Often minimal/no enhancement; hemorrhage common
  - AT/RT-TYR
    - 2nd most common (34%)
    - Infants/toddlers 0-2 years (median: 12 months)
    - Infratentorial (75%), supratentorial (25%)
    - Imaging features: Peritumoral edema common; strong enhancement common
  - AT/RT-MYC
    - Least common (22%)
    - Toddlers/children (median age: 27 months)
    - Supratentorial (50%), infratentorial (38%), spinal (12%)
    - Imaging features: Peripheral cysts very common; strong enhancement common

Microscopic Features

- Hypercellular with morphologic & immunophenotypic heterogeneity
  - Divergent differentiation accounts for teratoid label: Neuroectodermal, mesenchymal, epithelial, & rhabdoid
    - Rhabdoid cells large with eosinophilic cytoplasm
      - Very similar cells in malignant rhabdoid tumor of kidney & soft tissue (extrarenal) rhabdoid tumor
      - Rhabdoid cells may be sparse despite high tumor cellularity
- Lack of immunostaining for INI1 protein correlates with *SMARCB1* (hSNF5/INI1) mutation
  - Most discriminating finding for diagnosing AT/RT
- ↑ expression of *CLDN6* gene (encodes claudin-6 tight junction protein) compared to other CNS tumors
- Highly proliferative tumor

CLINICAL ISSUES

Presentation

- Most common signs/symptoms
  - Signs of ↑ intracranial pressure
    - Lethargy, vomiting, ↑ head circumference
  - Other signs/symptoms: Torticollis, seizure, developmental regression, new cranial nerve palsy
    - Most commonly involves cranial nerves VII, VI, or III
- Clinical profile
  - Child < 3 years (70-80%); median age: 1 year

Demographics

- Sex
  - M > F; 1.2:1
- Epidemiology
  - < 2% of all pediatric CNS tumors
  - Up to 20% of primitive CNS tumors in children < 3 years of age

Natural History & Prognosis

- Aggressive tumor with poor prognosis in absence of intensive therapy
- Prognosis depends upon age at diagnosis, presence of metastatic disease, & molecular subtype
  - Age < 3 years carries worse prognosis (~ 30% 5-year survival)
  - Metastases: < 20% 5-year survival
  - ASCL-1-negative tumors: < 20% 5-year survival

Treatment

- Gross total resection alone: Early recurrence
- Intensive trimodal therapy has ↑ survival
  - Maximal resection with high-dose systemic & intrathecal chemotherapy + radiation
  - Localized disease + trimodal therapy: ~ 50% 5-year survival

DIAGNOSTIC CHECKLIST

Consider

- AT/RT in young children (usually < 3 years of age) with tumor otherwise suggestive of primitive neuroectodermal tumor (PNET) or MB by imaging

Image Interpretation Pearls

- Hemorrhage, diffusion restriction (reflecting cellularity) suggest diagnosis in young child

SELECTED REFERENCES

1. Calandrelli R et al: Atypical teratoid rhabdoid tumor: proposal of a diagnostic pathway based on clinical features and neuroimaging findings. Diagnostics (Basel). 13(3):475, 2023
2. Wu HW et al: MRI features of pediatric atypical teratoid rhabdoid tumors and medulloblastomas of the posterior fossa. Cancer Med. 12(9):10449-61, 2023
3. WHO Classification of Tumours Editorial Board: WHO Classification of Tumours: Central Nervous System Tumours. 5th ed. IARC, 2021
4. Zhang M et al: Radiomic phenotypes distinguish atypical teratoid/rhabdoid tumors from medulloblastoma. AJNR Am J Neuroradiol. 42(9):1702-8, 2021
5. Zhang M et al: Machine assist for pediatric posterior fossa tumor diagnosis: a multinational study. Neurosurgery. 89(5):892-900, 2021
6. Tamrazi B et al: Pediatric atypical teratoid/rhabdoid tumors of the brain: Identification of metabolic subgroups using in vivo 1H-MR spectroscopy. AJNR Am J Neuroradiol. 40(5):872-7, 2019
7. Nowak J et al: Magnetic resonance imaging surrogates of molecular subgroups in atypical teratoid/rhabdoid tumor. Neuro Oncol. 20(12):1672-9, 2018
8. Fischer-Valuck BW et al: Assessment of the treatment approach and survival outcomes in a modern cohort of patients with atypical teratoid rhabdoid tumors using the National Cancer Database. Cancer. 123(4):682-7, 2017
9. Katz JS et al: Cerebellopontine angle tumors in young children, displaying cranial nerve deficits, and restricted diffusion on diffusion-weighted imaging: a new clinical triad for atypical teratoid/rhabdoid tumors. Childs Nerv Syst. 33(5):833-8, 2017
10. Frühwald MC et al: Atypical teratoid/rhabdoid tumors-current concepts, advances in biology, and potential future therapies. Neuro Oncol. 18(6):764-78, 2016
11. Johann PD et al: Atypical teratoid/rhabdoid tumors are comprised of three epigenetic subgroups with distinct enhancer landscapes. Cancer Cell. 29(3):379-93, 2016
12. Ho DM et al: Integrated genomics has identified a new AT/RT-like yet INI1-positive brain tumor subtype among primary pediatric embryonal tumors. BMC Med Genomics. 8:32, 2015
13. Torchia J et al: Molecular subgroups of atypical teratoid rhabdoid tumours in children: an integrated genomic and clinicopathological analysis. Lancet Oncol. 16(5):569-82, 2015

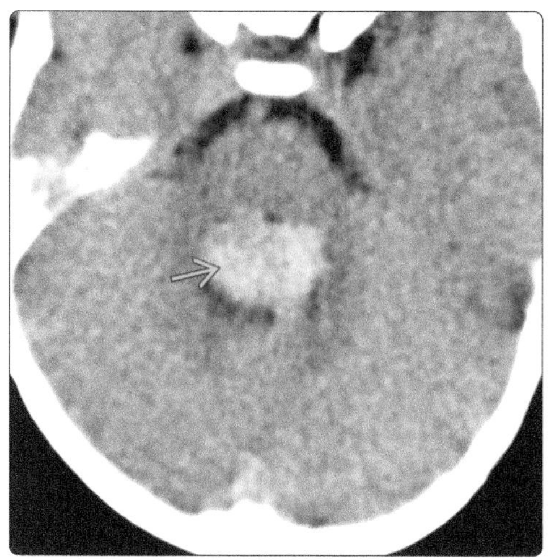

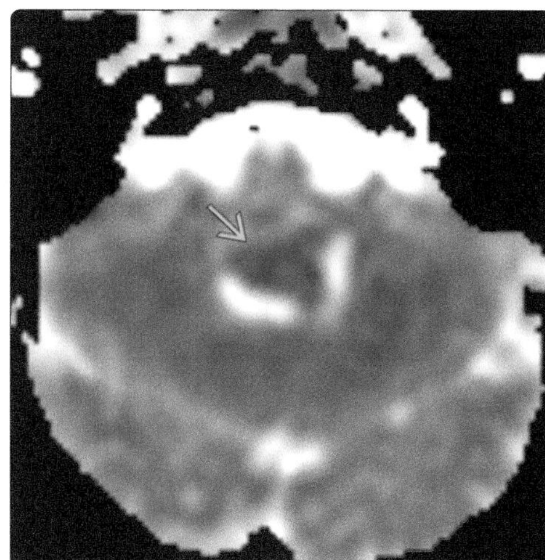

(Left) *Axial NECT in a 15-month-old with AT/RT shows a hyperdense mass ➡ lesion centered in the 4th ventricle. The increased attenuation is reflective of the high cellularity of this WHO grade 4 tumor. DDx would also include medulloblastoma.* **(Right)** *Axial ADC in the same patient shows the 4th ventricular mass ➡ to be markedly decreased in signal. DWI/ADC is the most reliable MR imaging marker of increased cellularity & is a critical sequence in narrowing the DDx.*

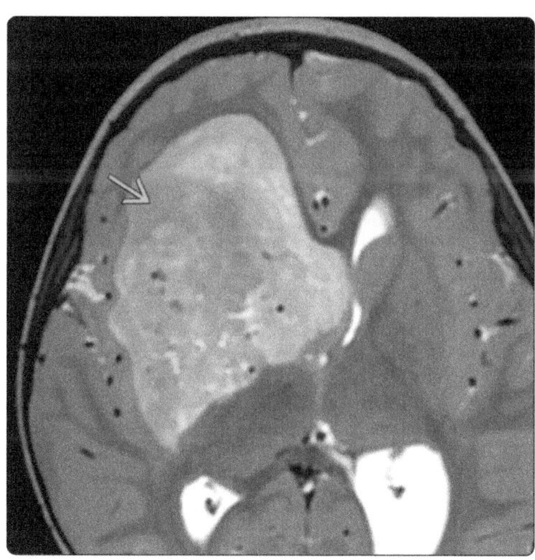

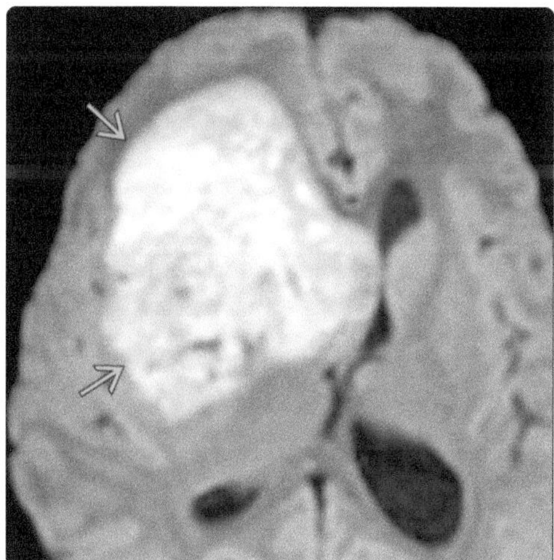

(Left) *Axial T2 MR in a 4-year-old with AT/RT (SHH molecular subgroup) shows a well-defined mass lesion ➡ centered in the right frontal lobe causing obstructive hydrocephalus. The SHH molecular subgroup of AT/RT is most likely to be located in supratentorial compartment.* **(Right)** *Axial DWI MR (same patient) shows homogeneous hyperintensity consistent with increased cellularity in this high-grade tumor ➡. AT/RT can occur anywhere along neuraxis & should be included in DDx of any cellular tumor in a young child.*

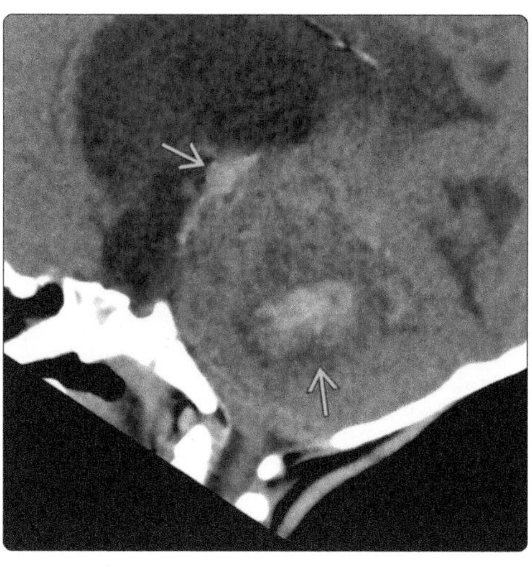

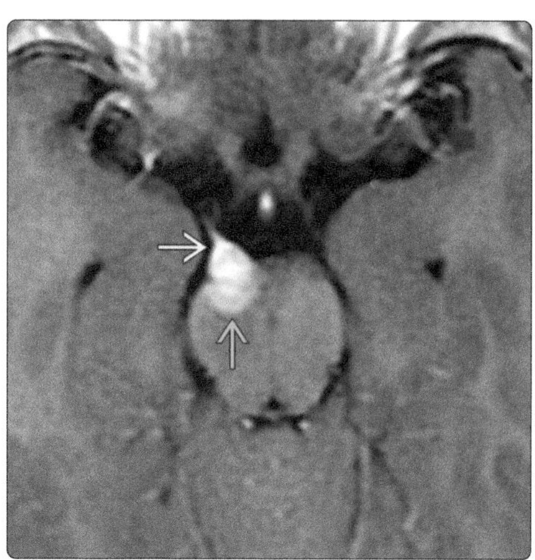

(Left) *Sagittal NECT in a 7-month-old with a posterior fossa AT/RT shows multiple areas of high attenuation ➡, consistent with hemorrhage. The majority of AT/RT will show evidence of intratumoral hemorrhage.* **(Right)** *Axial T1 C+ MR in a nearly 2-year-old patient with right ptosis & left hemiparesis shows a lobular, enhancing mass of the right cerebral peduncle ➡ with bulbous involvement of the proximal right 3rd cranial nerve ➡. Restricted diffusion was seen in the lesion (not shown). AT/RT was confirmed at subtotal resection.*

KEY FACTS

TERMINOLOGY

- Embryonal tumor with multilayered rosettes (ETMR)
- Includes former histologic diagnoses: Ependymal tumor with abundant neuropil & true rosettes (ETANTR) & ependymoblastoma
- Now molecularly & genetically distinct entities considered under embryonal tumors (all WHO grade 4) include
  - Medulloblastoma
  - Atypical teratoid/rhabdoid tumor (AT/RT)
  - ETMR
  - CNS neuroblastoma, *FOXR2* activated
  - CNS tumor with *BCOR* internal tandem duplication

IMAGING

- Large (mean: 5 cm), complex-appearing hemispheric mass in infant/young child
- ~ 50% well defined with minimal peritumoral edema
- Ca^{++} in 50-70%; hemorrhage common
- Heterogeneous enhancement
- Restricted diffusion of solid highly cellular components
- Subarachnoid spread common at presentation
  - Perform MR of entire neuraxis before surgery

TOP DIFFERENTIAL DIAGNOSES

- AT/RT
- Supratentorial ependymoma
- Pediatric-type diffuse high-grade gliomas
- Dysembryoplastic infantile ganglioglioma/astrocytoma
- Choroid plexus carcinoma

PATHOLOGY

- Most common (90-95%) genetic alteration at 19q13.42 (C19MC amplification)
  - 5-10% harbor *DICER1* mutation, usually germline

CLINICAL ISSUES

- Most common in younger children
- Treatment: Aggressive surgical resection, chemotherapy, craniospinal radiation (if of tolerable age)

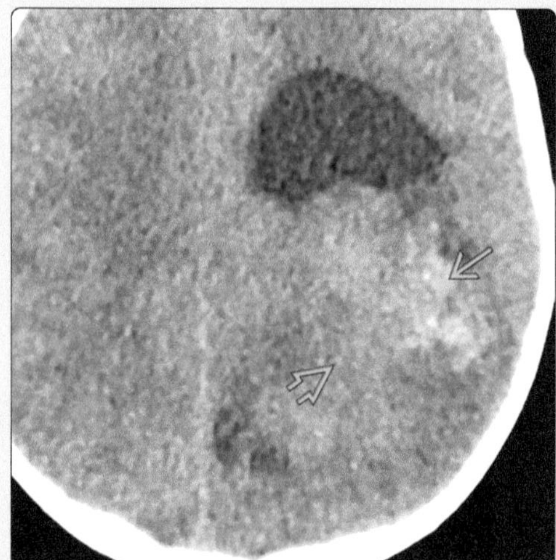

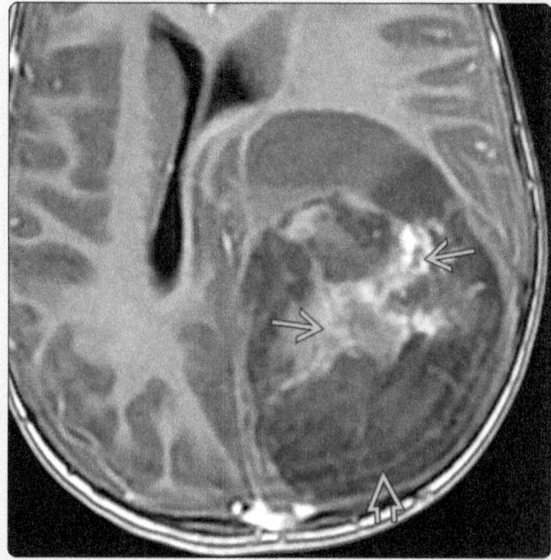

(Left) *Axial NECT in a 2-year-old with ETMR shows a predominantly isodense mixed solid and cystic mass lesion ⇨ with some areas of high-attenuation hemorrhage or Ca^{++} ⇨ in the lateral aspect of the mass.* **(Right)** *Axial T1 C+ MR in the same patient shows no significant enhancement in the solid portions of the mass ⇨. The areas of high signal ⇨ were similar on the precontrast T1 MR (not shown), likely representing hemorrhage or Ca^{++}. Lack of contrast enhancement is common in ETMR.*

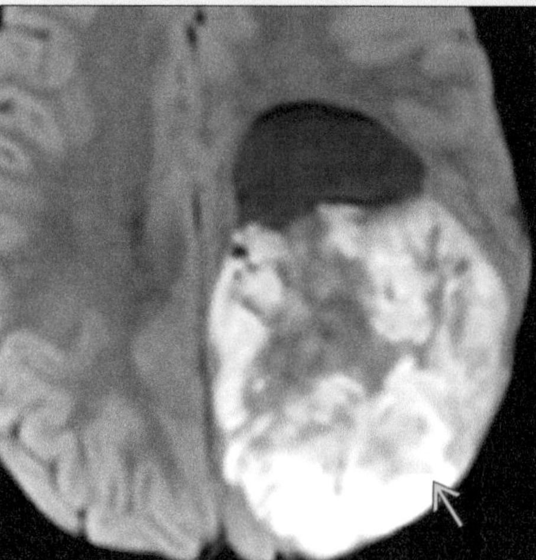

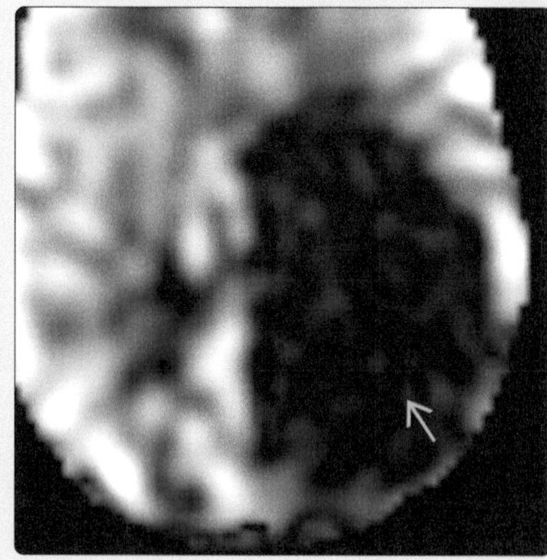

(Left) *Axial DWI MR in the same patient shows diffusion restriction within the solid portion of the mass ⇨, reflecting the high cellularity of this grade 4 embryonal tumor. ETMR should be at the top of the DDx in any well-defined supratentorial cellular tumor.* **(Right)** *Axial ASL perfusion-weighted MR in the same patient shows decreased cerebral blood flow (CBF) within the tumor ⇨. Small case series suggest that ETMR typically shows decreased CBF on ASL and increased cerebral blood volume (CBV) on DSC.*

TERMINOLOGY

Abbreviations

- Embryonal tumor with multilayered rosettes (ETMR)

Synonyms

- Includes former histologic diagnoses: Ependymal tumor with abundant neuropil & true rosettes (ETANTR) & ependymoblastoma

Definitions

- CNS primitive neuroectodermal tumor (CNS-PNET): Antiquated term for primitive cerebral embryonal tumor; no longer in WHO 2016
  - Umbrella term formerly containing CNS neuroblastoma, ependymoblastoma, medulloepithelioma, & ETANTR
- Now molecularly & genetically distinct entities considered under embryonal tumors (all WHO grade 4) include
  - Medulloblastoma
  - Atypical teratoid/rhabdoid tumor (AT/RT)
  - ETMR
  - CNS Neuroblastoma, *FOXR2* activated
  - CNS tumor with *BCOR* internal tandem duplication
  - CNS embryonal tumor, not otherwise specified (NOS)

IMAGING

General Features

- Best diagnostic clue
  - Large, complex-appearing hemispheric mass with diffusion restriction in infant/young child
- Location
  - Most often hemispheric in location
    - Other less common locations include thalamus, brainstem, & suprasellar
- Size
  - Variable, based on location
    - Cerebral hemispheric embryonal lesions larger at diagnosis (mean diameter: ~ 5 cm)
      - Hemispheric lesions in infants often huge
    - Brainstem embryonal lesions tend to be smaller at presentation
- Morphology
  - Vast majority are sharply delineated from adjacent brain

Radiographic Findings

- Macrocephaly & widened sutures (in neonate & infant)

CT Findings

- NECT
  - Iso- to hyperattenuating mass
  - Ca^{++} (50-70%)
  - Hemorrhage & necrosis common
  - Large cystic components may be present
  - Usually has little, if any, adjacent edema
- CECT
  - Heterogeneous enhancement
  - Prone to subarachnoid tumor seeding

MR Findings

- T1WI
  - Hypo- to isointense to gray matter
  - Homogeneous to heterogeneous
- T2WI
  - Solid elements isointense to slightly hyperintense to gray matter
  - ~ 50% with no peritumoral edema
  - Ca^{++} → hypointense foci
  - Blood products → mixed signal intensity
- FLAIR
  - Solid components typically hyperintense
  - ≥ 50% with no peritumoral edema
  - Postcontrast FLAIR particularly sensitive for leptomeningeal metastases
- T2* GRE
  - Dephasing from blood products
  - Blood products & Ca^{++} common
- DWI
  - Restricted diffusion common
- PWI
  - Small case series suggest ↓ cerebral blood flow (CBF) (ASL) & ↑ cerebral blood volume (CBV) (DSC)
- T1WI C+
  - Heterogeneous enhancement
  - Subarachnoid seeding common
- MRS
  - ↓ ↓ NAA, ↓ creatine, ↑ ↑ choline, + lipid & lactate

Ultrasonographic Findings

- Congenital embryonal tumor (antenatal sonography)
  - Large hyperechoic hemispheric mass
  - Hydrocephalus

Imaging Recommendations

- Best imaging tool
  - MR with T1WI C+, FLAIR, DWI
- Protocol advice
  - Image entire neuraxis for complete staging prior to surgery
  - Postcontrast FLAIR may improve sensitivity for leptomeningeal metastases

DIFFERENTIAL DIAGNOSIS

Atypical Teratoid/Rhabdoid Tumor

- Posterior fossa > 50%, supratentorial 39%
- Necrosis, cysts, & vasogenic edema common
- Subarachnoid seeding common

Supratentorial Ependymoma

- Usually intraaxial when supratentorial (30%)
- Necrosis & hemorrhage common
- Often with multiple cystic spaces

Pediatric-Type Diffuse High-Grade Gliomas

- e.g., diffuse midline glioma (DMG) H3K27M altered, diffuse hemispheric glioma H3G34 mutant, diffuse pediatric-type high-grade glioma, infant-type hemispheric glioma
- Typically ↑ peritumoral edema & indistinct margins
- Often shows facilitated diffusion (e.g., DMG H3K27M altered)
- Ca^{++} less common compared with embryonal tumors

Dysembryoplastic Infantile Ganglioglioma/Astrocytoma

- Also occurs in infants & very young children
- Typically with large cystic components
- Solid components typically do not restrict diffusion but varies

Choroid Plexus Carcinoma

- Lobulated intraventricular mass with avid enhancement
- Parenchymal invasion can be dramatic
- Extensive vasogenic edema

Other Rare Embryonal Tumors

- CNS neuroblastoma, *FOXR2* activated
- CNS tumor with *BCOR* internal tandem duplication

Oligodendroglioma

- Frontotemporal peripheral tumor with coarse Ca^{++}
- More common in teenagers & adults

Giant Cavernous Malformation

- Can be huge in newborn, infant
- Hemosiderin rim with locules of fluid-fluid levels
- $\pm Ca^{++}$

PATHOLOGY

General Features

- Etiology
  - Tumor suppressor gene aberrations may play role
- Genetics
  - Regardless of histology, if 19q13.42 (C19MC amplification) is present, diagnosis is ETMR
  - 90-95% harbor mutations in C19MC
  - 5-10% harbor *DICER1* mutations
    - Almost all *DICER1* ETMR patients harbor *DICER1* germline mutation & should have genetic testing/counseling

Staging, Grading, & Classification

- WHO grade 4

Gross Pathologic & Surgical Features

- Variable consistency
  - Solid & homogeneous → cystic, necrotic, hemorrhagic, & partially calcified
  - Solid portions & soft, pink-red coloration, unless prominent desmoplasia
  - Demarcation between tumor & brain may range from indistinct to sharp

Microscopic Features

- Biphasic histologic pattern featuring
  - Cellular areas of small round blue cells with numerous mitoses & apoptosis (blast cells) that are often arrayed in multilayered rosettes
  - Paucicellular neuropil-rich areas with fewer blast cells often containing larger more differentiated neuronal cells
- Immunohistochemical marker LIN28A has been found to be highly sensitive marker for ETMR
  - However, recent studies suggest small percentage of AT/RT also shows LIN28A positivity

CLINICAL ISSUES

Presentation

- Most common signs/symptoms
  - Vary with site of origin & size of tumor
    - Hemispheric → seizures, altered mental status, motor deficit, elevated intracranial pressure
- Other signs/symptoms
  - Cranial neuropathies due to herniation or diffuse CSF metastases
- Clinical profile
  - Infant presenting with macrocephaly, seizures, & large hemispheric mass

Demographics

- Age
  - Most common in younger children
    - Median age at diagnosis: 2.9 years
- Sex
  - M:F = 1:1
- Ethnicity
  - No predilection

Natural History & Prognosis

- Compared with histologically similar medulloblastoma, ETMR carries poor prognosis
  - ETMR → median survival: 10 months
  - Medulloblastoma → 5-year survival: 80-85%
- Critical survival factors include
  - Complete surgical resection
  - Absence of metastases

Treatment

- Aggressive surgical resection, chemotherapy, craniospinal radiation (if of acceptable age)

DIAGNOSTIC CHECKLIST

Image Interpretation Pearls

- Large cellular hemispheric mass with sparse peritumoral edema

SELECTED REFERENCES

1. Chadda KR et al: Embryonal tumor with multilayered rosettes: overview of diagnosis and therapy. Neurooncol Adv. 5(1):vdad052, 2023
2. Sugawa M et al: Prognostic impact of the multimodal treatment approach in patients with C19MC-altered embryonal tumor with multilayered rosettes. J Neurosurg Pediatr. 1-7, 2022
3. Gupta K et al: Clinicopathological characteristics and outcomes in embryonal tumor with multilayered rosettes: a decade long experience from a tertiary care centre in North India. Ann Diagn Pathol. 53:151745, 2021
4. WHO Classification of Tumours Editorial Board: WHO Classification of Tumours: Central Nervous System Tumours. 5th ed. IARC, 2021
5. Dangouloff-Ros V et al: CT and multimodal MR imaging features of embryonal tumors with multilayered rosettes in children. AJNR Am J Neuroradiol. 40(4):732-6, 2019
6. Hwang EI et al: Extensive molecular and clinical heterogeneity in patients with histologically diagnosed CNS-PNET treated as a single entity: a report from the Children's Oncology Group randomized ACNS0332 trial. J Clin Oncol. JCO2017764720, 2018
7. Wang B et al: Embryonal tumor with multilayered rosettes, C19MC-altered: clinical, pathological, and neuroimaging findings. J Neuroimaging. 28(5):483-9, 2018

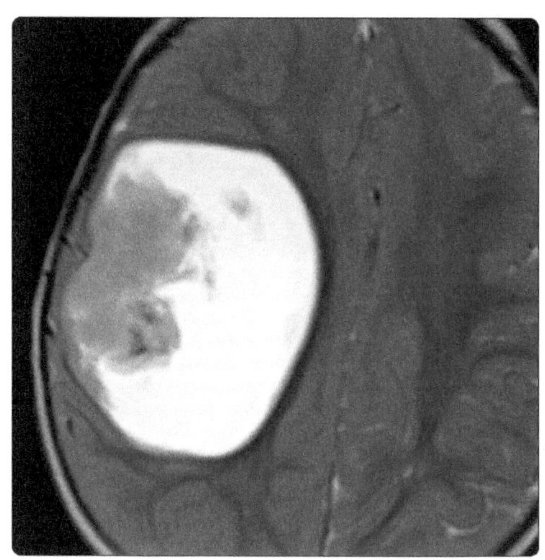

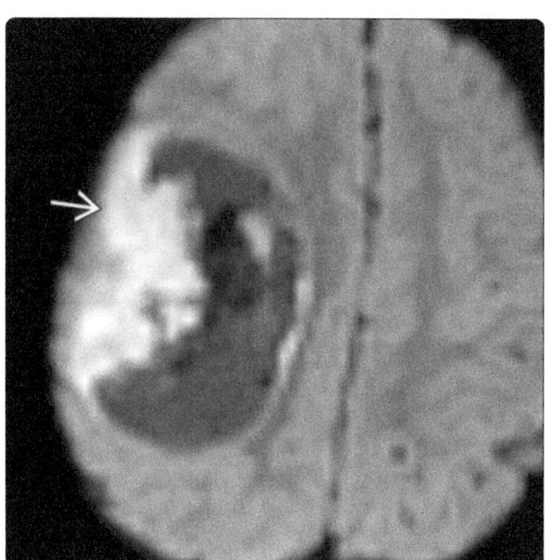

(Left) *Axial T2 MR in a 3-year-old male patient with left-sided weakness and difficulty walking shows a well-demarcated, mixed solid and cystic mass in the right cerebral hemisphere. Note the lack of surrounding vasogenic edema.* **(Right)** *Axial DWI MR in the same patient shows mildly high signal ➔ within the solid portions of the mass, consistent with diffusion restriction from the high cellularity of embryonal tumors. Restricted diffusion is a key diagnostic clue to making this diagnosis.*

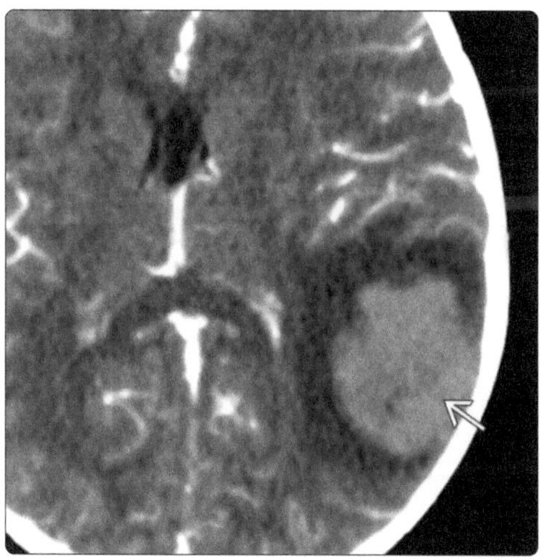

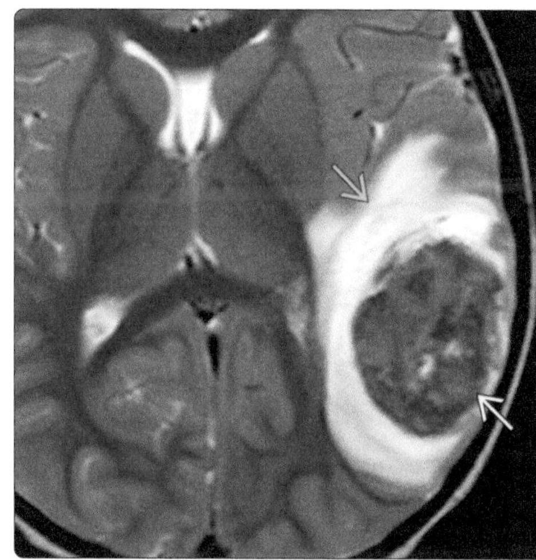

(Left) *Axial CECT in a 4-year-old girl with new-onset seizures shows a superficial hyperdense mass ➔. This high attenuation may represent hemorrhage or contrast enhancement. Follow-up MR confirmed this high-attenuation focus to be very hemorrhagic.* **(Right)** *Axial FLAIR MR in the same 4-year-old girl shows heterogeneously hypointense signal within the mass ➔ and moderate peritumoral vasogenic edema ➔. The presence of peritumoral edema should not exclude the diagnosis of embryonal tumor.*

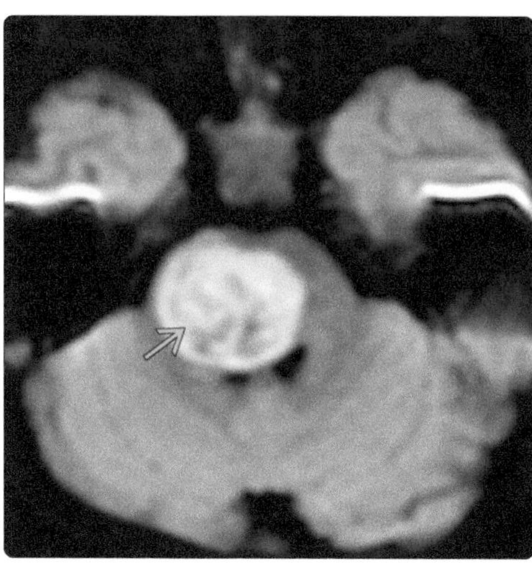

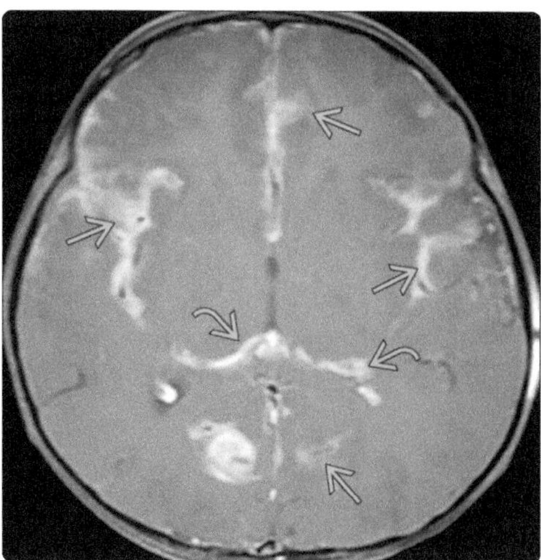

(Left) *Axial DWI in a 2-year-old male patient with ETMR shows a well-defined mass ➔ centered in the pons with marked diffusion restriction. This tumor should not be mistaken for a DIPG, which usually shows facilitated diffusion.* **(Right)** *Axial T1 C+ MR in the same patient 8 months after diagnosis shows extensive leptomeningeal enhancement and mass effect within the sulci ➔ and ventricles ➔, consistent with leptomeningeal disease. Like many high-grade embryonal tumors, leptomeningeal spread of disease is common.*

Pineoblastoma

KEY FACTS

TERMINOLOGY

- Pineoblastoma (PB)
  - Highly malignant embryonal tumor of pineal gland

IMAGING

- General features
  - Large, heterogeneous pineal mass
  - Lobulated with poorly delineated margins
- Solid portion
  - NECT
    - Hyperdense with peripheral or scattered Ca^{++}
  - MR
    - Iso- to hypointense on T2WI
    - Diffusion restriction common
    - Variable heterogeneous enhancement

TOP DIFFERENTIAL DIAGNOSES

- Germ cell tumors
- Other pineal parenchymal tumors

PATHOLOGY

- WHO grade 4: Embryonic precursors of pineal parenchymal cells (pinealocytes)
- Common phylogenetic origin of retina and pineal gland
- Germline mutations in *DICER1* → distinctive autosomal dominant tumor predisposition syndrome (DICER1 syndrome)
- Germline mutations in retinoblastoma gene *RB1* → trilateral retinoblastomas
- *MYC-I/FOXR2*-activated tumors (usually in very young)

CLINICAL ISSUES

- ↑ intracranial pressure (hydrocephalus)
- Parinaud syndrome, ataxia
- Mean age at diagnosis in children: 3 years

DIAGNOSTIC CHECKLIST

- Image **entire neuraxis** preoperatively
  - Up to 45% CSF dissemination on MR or in CSF

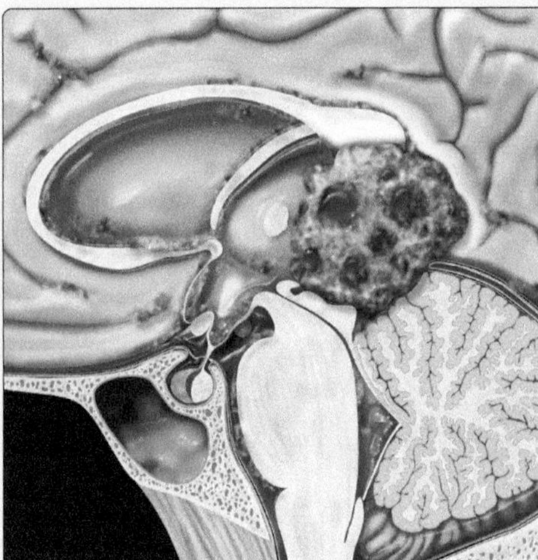

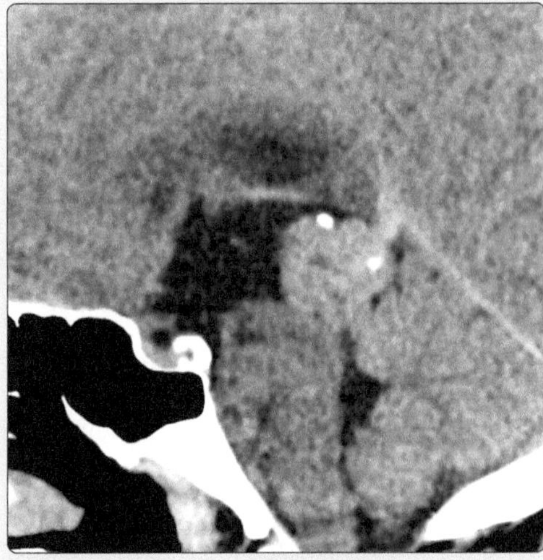

(Left) *Sagittal graphic shows a large, heterogeneous pineal mass with areas of hemorrhage and necrosis. Note the compression of adjacent structures, hydrocephalus, and diffuse CSF seeding, which is typical of pineoblastoma (PB).* **(Right)** *Sagittal NECT in a 26-year-old man with PB shows a hyperdense mass centered in the pineal gland with peripheral Ca^{++}. Germinomas may have a similar appearance, but Ca^{++}, when identified, is more often central (engulfed).*

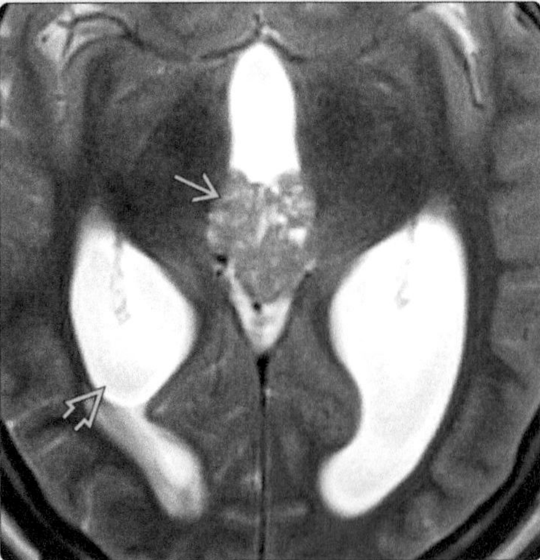

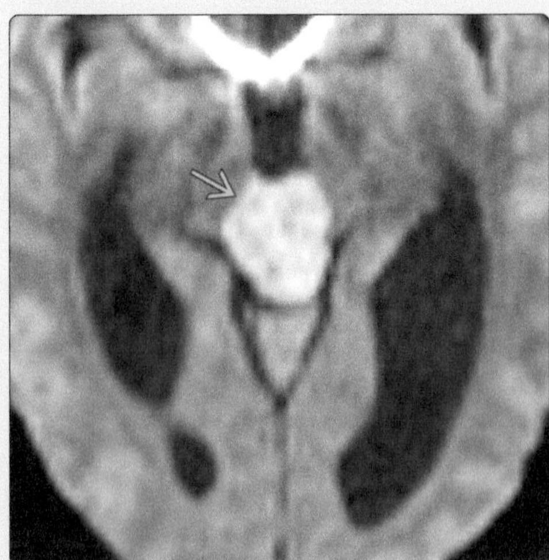

(Left) *Axial T2 MR in the same patient shows a heterogeneously hypointense pineal region mass ⇨ with multiple small, microcystic spaces scattered about the tumor. Note the associated obstructive hydrocephalus ⇨.* **(Right)** *Axial DWI MR in the same patient shows a pineal mass ⇨ with diffusion restriction, reflecting the highly cellular nature of PB. Unfortunately, DWI does not help to distinguish the most likely DDx of germinoma, which is also very cellular and typically shows diffusion restriction.*

TERMINOLOGY

Abbreviations

- Pineoblastoma (PB)

Synonyms

- Primitive neuroectodermal tumor (PNET) of pineal gland

Definitions

- Highly malignant embryonal tumor of pineal gland
- Pineal parenchymal tumor (PPT) [not germ cell tumor (GCT)]

IMAGING

General Features

- Best diagnostic clue
  - Child with large, heterogeneous, hyperdense pineal mass with peripheral Ca^{++}
- Location
  - Pineal gland
    - Pineal masses lie below corpus callosum splenium
    - Elevate internal cerebral veins (ICVs)
    - Flatten/compress tectal plate
  - Frequent invasion of adjacent brain common
    - Corpus callosum, thalami, midbrain, vermis
- Size
  - Medium sized (often ≥ 3 cm)
- Morphology
  - Irregular, lobulated mass with poorly delineated margins

CT Findings

- NECT
  - Mixed density; solid portion frequently hyperdense
  - Peripheral and scattered Ca^{++} common
  - Nearly 100% have obstructive hydrocephalus
- CECT
  - Weak to avid but heterogeneous enhancement

MR Findings

- T1WI
  - Heterogeneous; solid portion iso-/hypointense
- T2WI
  - Heterogeneous
    - Solid portion iso-/hypointense more common than minimally hyperintense to cortex
    - Frequent necrosis/hemorrhage, cysts
  - Mild peritumoral edema characteristic
- T2* GRE
  - Ca^{++} and hemorrhage may bloom
- DWI
  - Solid portion frequently restricts
  - ADC values, on average, are lower than other pineal tumors (except germinoma, which is also highly cellular)
- T1WI C+
  - Heterogeneous enhancement
- MRS
  - ↑ Cho, ↓ NAA
  - Prominent glutamate and taurine peak (~ 3.4 ppm) described at TE 20 ms

Nuclear Medicine Findings

- PET
  - ↑ F-18 FDG

Other Modality Findings

- No elevation of serum tumor markers

Imaging Recommendations

- Best imaging tool
  - T1WI C+, DWI MR
- Protocol advice
  - Image entire neuraxis preoperatively
    - 15-45% present with **CSF dissemination**
  - Sagittal images ideal for pineal region anatomy

DIFFERENTIAL DIAGNOSIS

Germ Cell Tumors

- M > > F; 2nd decade most common
- Germinoma: Very difficult to distinguish from PB
  - Peritumoral edema and bithalamic extension much more common
  - Localized Ca^{++} more common
- Mature teratoma: 2nd most common GCT and pineal region tumor; heterogeneous, multicystic mass with foci of Ca^{++} and fat
- Choriocarcinoma, endodermal sinus tumor, embryonal cell carcinoma
  - Uncommon, highly malignant
  - Characteristic elevation of serum tumor markers
    - Choriocarcinoma: β-hCG
    - Endodermal sinus tumor: α-fetoprotein (AFP)
    - Embryonal cell carcinoma: β-hCG and AFP
- 10% of GCTs are of mixed histology (mixed GCT)

Other Pineal Parenchymal Tumors

- Pineocytoma (PC) (WHO grade 1), PPT of intermediate differentiation (PPTID; WHO grades 2-3)
- Arise from pineal gland parenchymal cells
- Well-defined mass "explodes" pineal Ca^{++}
- Older age group compared to PBs
- Cone-rod homeobox gene (*CRX*) expressed in PPTs and retinoblastomas as well as some medulloblastomas and PNETs

Papillary Tumor of Pineal Region

- Rare; usually older patients

Trilateral Retinoblastoma

- PB and retinoblastoma are histologically and molecularly identical
- Most consider them to be same tumor
- Look for ocular lesions

Astrocytoma

- Rarely arise from pineal gland
- More commonly from thalamus or midbrain tectum
- Pilocytic astrocytoma (WHO grade 1) most common
- Tectal astrocytoma
  - Nonenhancing, well-defined, expansile tectal mass
- Thalamic astrocytoma: T2-hyperintense, paramedian mass or cyst with enhancing mural nodule

Meningioma

- Female patients (5th-7th decades)
- Well-defined, round, dural-based mass isointense to cortex on all sequences with intense, homogeneous enhancement
- Pineal region meningiomas arise from tentorium cerebelli, falx
- Dural tail (35-80%)

Metastases

- Pineal gland metastases uncommon
- Adenocarcinoma reported

PATHOLOGY

General Features

- Etiology
  - Derived from embryonic precursors of pineal parenchymal cells (pinealocytes)
  - Pinealocytes have photosensory and neuroendocrine function
  - Common phylogenetic origin of retina and pineal gland as light-sensing organs
- Genetics
  - Germline mutations in *DICER1* → distinctive autosomal dominant tumor/dysplasia predisposition syndrome (DICER1 syndrome)
    - *DICER1* is important susceptibility gene for PB, ciliary body medulloepithelioma
  - *MYC-I/FOXR2*-activated tumors occur in younger patients
  - Germline mutations in retinoblastoma gene *RB1* → trilateral retinoblastomas
    - Bilateral retinoblastomas + PB
    - Incidence of PB 10x in bilateral vs. unilateral retinoblastomas

Staging, Grading, & Classification

- WHO grade 4
- New prognostic grading system for PPTs
  - Grade 1 = PC
  - Grades 2 and 3 = PPTs with intermediate differentiation
    - Grade 2 if < 6 mitoses and immunolabeling positive for neurofilaments
    - Grade 3 if ≥ 6 mitoses or if < 6 mitoses but immunolabeling negative for neurofilaments
  - Grade 4 = PB

Gross Pathologic & Surgical Features

- Soft, friable, poorly marginated, infiltrative
- Compresses/invades cerebral aqueduct, leading to hydrocephalus
- CSF dissemination at autopsy frequent

Microscopic Features

- Highly cellular tumor
  - Sheets of packed, small, undifferentiated cells
  - Mitoses common; MIB-1 elevated

CLINICAL ISSUES

Presentation

- Most common signs/symptoms
  - ↑ intracranial pressure (hydrocephalus)
    - Headache, nausea, vomiting, lethargy
    - Papilledema, abducens nerve palsy
- Other signs/symptoms: Parinaud syndrome, ataxia
- Clinical profile: Toddler with Parinaud syndrome, signs/symptoms of ↑ intracranial pressure

Demographics

- Age
  - Children > young adults (rare tumors up to 5th decade)
  - Mean age at diagnosis in children = 3 years
- Sex
  - M:F = 1:2
- Epidemiology
  - PPTs comprise 0.5-1.0% of primary brain tumors and 15% of pineal region neoplasms
  - PBs comprise 30-45% of PPTs

Natural History & Prognosis

- CSF seeding common: Up to 45% of patients present with spinal dissemination on MR &/or CSF analysis
- Rare reports of hematogenous metastases to bone
- 5-year survival ~ 60%; younger age and larger tumor size have poorer prognosis
- Prognosis better in *DICER1* syndrome (68-100%) vs. *RB1* altered (29%) and *MYC-I/FOXR2* activated (23%)

Treatment

- Surgical resection plus cranial/spinal radiation and chemotherapy

DIAGNOSTIC CHECKLIST

Consider

- Could pineal region mass be GCT (more common than PPTs)?
  - Does patient have elevated serum tumor markers?
  - Is patient male?
  - Is there coexistent suprasellar mass (germinoma)?
- Are there associated retinal lesions → trilateral retinoblastoma?

Image Interpretation Pearls

- Both PBs and germinomas frequently hyperdense on CT, hypointense on T2WI, and prone to CSF dissemination
- Significant peritumoral edema and bithalamic extension much more common in germinoma

SELECTED REFERENCES

1. Nandoliya KR et al: Post-surgical prognosis of patients with pineoblastoma: a systematic review and individual patient data analysis with trends over time. Cancers (Basel). 15(13):3374, 2023
2. Osborn AG et al: The 2021 World Health Organization Classification of Tumors of the Central Nervous System: what neuroradiologists need to know. AJNR Am J Neuroradiol. 43(7):928-37, 2022
3. WHO Classification of Tumours Editorial Board: WHO classification of tumors of the central nervous system. 5th ed. IARC, 2021
4. Jaju A et al: MRI features of histologically diagnosed supratentorial primitive neuroectodermal tumors and pineoblastomas in correlation with molecular diagnoses and outcomes: a report from the Children's Oncology Group ACNS0332 Trial. AJNR Am J Neuroradiol. 40(11):1796-803, 2019
5. Choudhri AF et al: Diffusion characteristics of pediatric pineal tumors. Neuroradiol J. 28(2):209-16, 2015

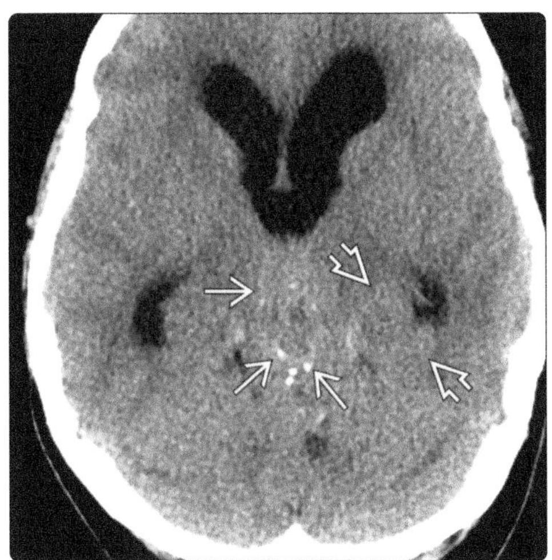

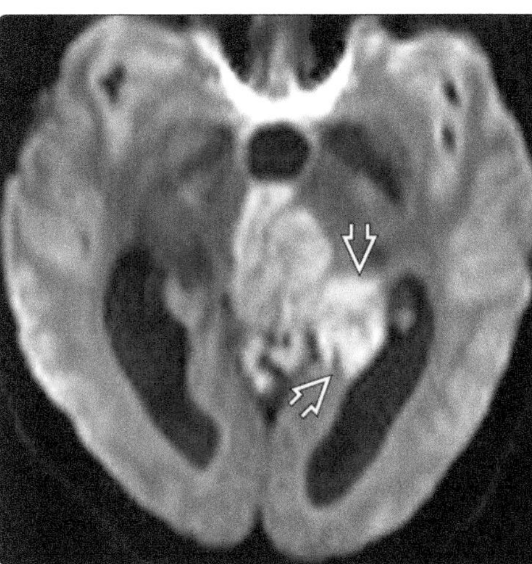

(Left) *Axial NECT shows a poorly demarcated, infiltrative, mildly hyperdense mass centered in the pineal region. Note the peripheral* Ca^{++} ➡. *On close evaluation, there is invasion of the adjacent brain parenchyma* ➡. *There is compression of the aqueduct of Sylvius and resultant hydrocephalus.* **(Right)** *Axial DWI MR shows restricted diffusion in the solid mass and better delineates the neoplasm and the invasion of the adjacent brain parenchyma* ➡.

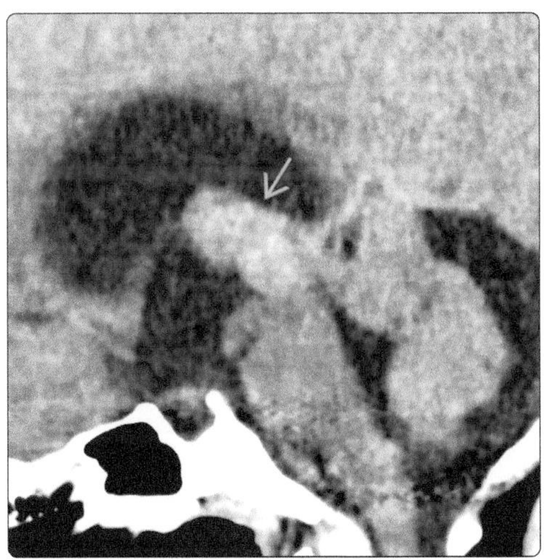

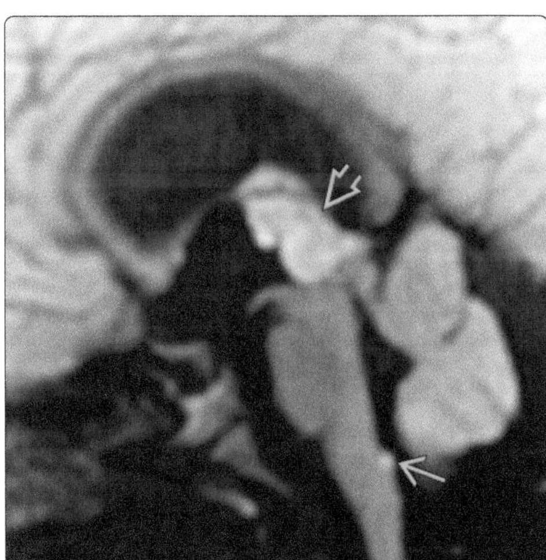

(Left) *Midline sagittal NECT in a 4-year-old boy with DICER1-mutant PB shows a hyperdense mass* ➡ *arising from the pineal region and extending anteriorly along the roof of the 3rd ventricle.* **(Right)** *Midline sagittal DWI MR in the same patient shows diffusion restriction in the mass* ➡, *consistent with a highly cellular tumor. Also note the small leptomeningeal metastatic deposit along the dorsal medulla* ➡. *Metastatic disease is seen in ~ 1/3 of PB tumors at diagnosis.*

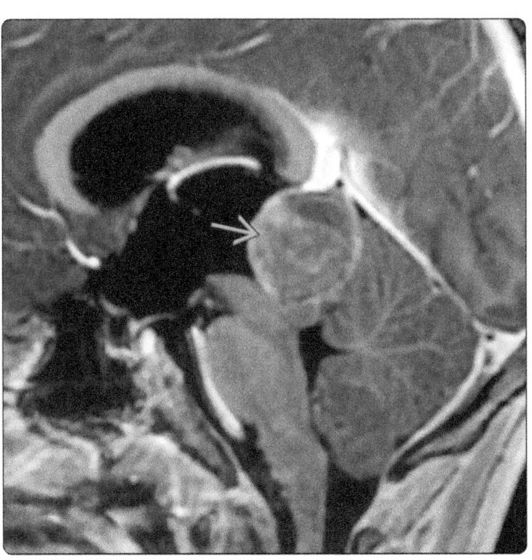

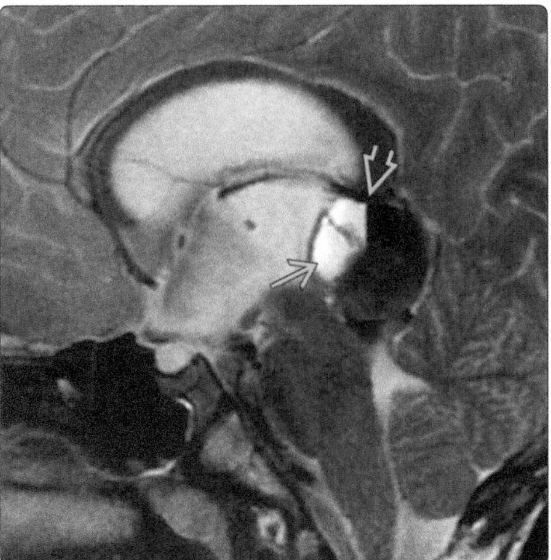

(Left) *Sagittal T1 C+ MR in an 11-year-old boy with DICER1-mutant PB shows a heterogeneously hypoenhancing mass* ➡ *in the pineal region. The enhancement pattern of PB is highly variable.* **(Right)** *Sagittal T2 MR in the same patient shows a sizable cystic component* ➡ *with a hematocrit level* ➡. *Cystic components and hemorrhage can be seen in PB. Significant intratumoral hemorrhage can make evaluation of tumor cellularity on DWI difficult.*

Pediatric-Type Diffuse High-Grade Gliomas

KEY FACTS

TERMINOLOGY

- Term glioblastoma no longer used in 2021 WHO pediatric CNS tumor classification scheme
  - Replaced by pediatric-type diffuse high-grade glioma (HHG)
  - Diffuse midline glioma, H3K27-altered (DMG)
  - Diffuse hemispheric glioma, H3G34-mutant (DHG)
  - Diffuse pediatric-type HGGs, H3, wildtype and IDH wildtype (pHGG)
  - Infant-type hemispheric glioma (IHG)

IMAGING

- DMG: Ill-defined, nonenhancing or minimally enhancing hypocellular thalamic or pontine mass
- DHGs: Glioblastoma-like cellular tumor with enhancement and necrosis in cerebral hemisphere
- pHGG: Ill-defined, nonenhancing mass or glioblastoma-like mass
- IHG: Large, heterogeneous mass ± hemorrhage in infant

TOP DIFFERENTIAL DIAGNOSES

- Embryonal tumor with multilayered rosettes
- Atypical teratoid/rhabdoid tumor
- Supratentorial ependymoma
- Ganglioglioma
- Desmoplastic infantile ganglioglioma/astrocytoma
- Pilocytic astrocytoma

PATHOLOGY

- DMG: Alteration of H3K27M or EGFR
- DHG: Mutation of H3G34
- pHGG: Diffuse glioma wildtype for H3, *IDH1*, and *IDH2*
- IHG: High-grade astrocytoma with frequent RTK fusions
- All except IHG are WHO grade 4 tumors

CLINICAL ISSUES

- DMG: Poor prognosis (2-year overall survival < 10%); Tx-XRT
- DHG + pHGG: Poor prognosis; Tx-Sx + chemo + XRT
- IHG: Better prognosis compared to most pediatric HGG

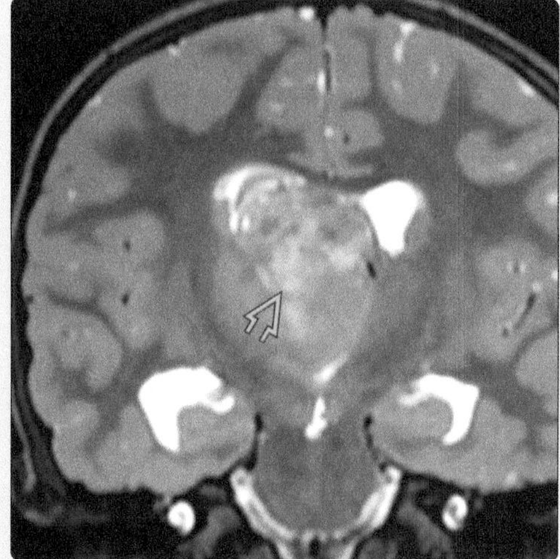

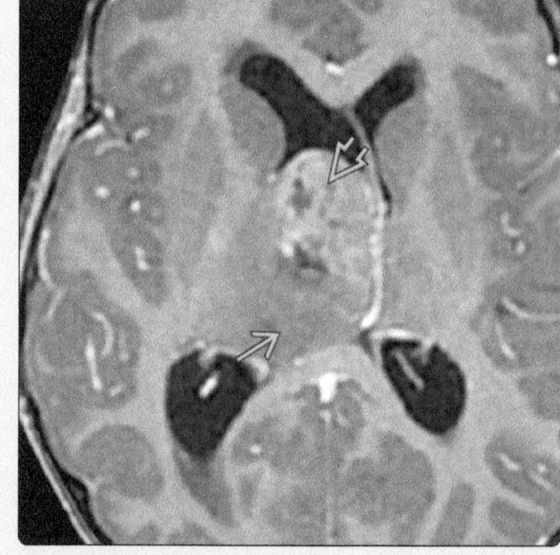

(Left) *Coronal T2 MR in a 6-year-old with a diffuse midline H3K27M-altered diffuse midline glioma (DMG) shows a heterogeneously hyperintense mass centered in the right thalamus causing obstructive hydrocephalus.* **(Right)** *Axial T1 C+ MR in the same patient shows both enhancing and nonenhancing components of the right thalamic tumor. Enhancement is variable in DMG, but these tumors often demonstrate no enhancement at time of diagnosis*

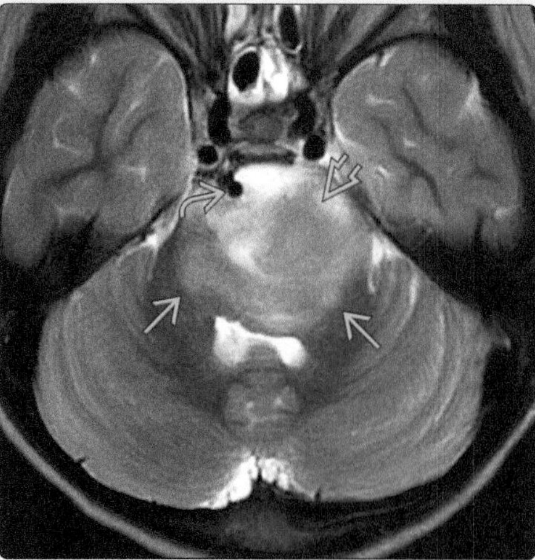

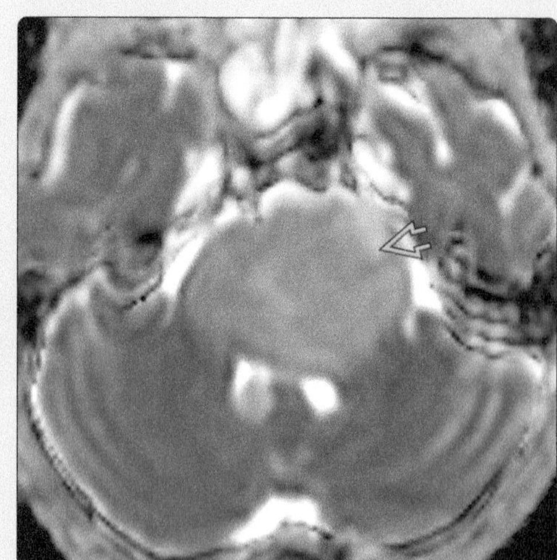

(Left) *Axial T2 MR in 5-year-old with DMG shows expansile T2 signal centered in the pons with irregular margins and encasement of the basilar artery. When located in the pons, DIPG terminology is often appropriately used to describe this tumor.* **(Right)** *Axial ADC image in the same patient shows intratumoral hyperintense signal (facilitated diffusion), which is typical for diffuse intrinsic pontine glioma (DIPG). Despite being a high-grade glioma, DIPGs often have a hypocellular imaging appearance.*

TERMINOLOGY

Definitions

- In 2021 WHO CNS tumor classification scheme, term glioblastoma is no longer used in children and has been supplanted with umbrella diagnostic category pediatric-type diffuse high-grade gliomas (HGGs)
  - Diffuse midline glioma (DMG), H3K27-altered
  - Diffuse hemispheric glioma (DHG), H3G34-mutant
  - Diffuse pediatric-type HGG, H3 wildtype, and IDH wildtype (pHGG)
  - Infant-type hemispheric glioma (IHG)

IMAGING

General Features

- Best diagnostic clue
  - DMG: Ill-defined, nonenhancing or minimally enhancing hypocellular thalamic or pontine mass
  - DHGs: Glioblastoma-like cellular tumor with enhancement and necrosis in cerebral hemisphere
  - pHGG: Ill-defined, nonenhancing mass or glioblastoma-like mass
  - IHG: Large, heterogeneous cellular mass ± hemorrhage in infant
- Location
  - DMGs occur mostly in pons (diffuse intrinsic pontine glioma) or thalami (sometimes bithalamic)
  - DHGs and IHGs arise in cerebral hemispheres
  - pHGGs mostly arise in supratentorial brain (80-90%) with minority being infratentorial
- Size
  - Varies depending on location
  - Hemispheric tumors in young patients are often very large
- Morphology
  - DMGs typically have infiltrative appearance, facilitated diffusion, and usually do not enhance
  - DHGs, IHGs, and pHGGs often have glioblastoma-like appearance with cellular-enhancing solid components and often cysts, necrosis, and hemorrhage when large
    - pHGGs and DHGs may sometimes have morphology of DMG but in more peripheral cerebral hemispheres

CT Findings

- DMG
  - Expansile low attenuation in pons or thalami
  - Ca^{++} and hemorrhage uncommon
- DHG, pHGG, and IHG
  - Vary from ill-defined, low-attenuation to more well-defined, hypercellular mass
  - Iso- to hyperattenuation of solid cellular components
  - Areas of intratumoral low attenuation may correspond to cysts/necrosis
  - Ca^{++} and hemorrhage common
  - ± peritumoral edema

MR Findings

- T1WI
  - DMG: Ill-defined, mass-like low signal
  - DGH, pHGG: Vary from ill-defined ↓ signal to heterogeneous mass
  - IHG: Heterogeneous; ↑ signal may reflect Ca^{++}/hemorrhage
- T2WI
  - DMG: Ill-defined, expansile high signal
  - DHG, pHGG: Varies from ill-defined ↑ signal to heterogeneous mass
  - IHG: Heterogeneous; ↓ signal may reflect Ca^{++}/hemorrhage
- T2* GRE
  - DMG: Ca^{++}/hemorrhage uncommon
  - DHG, pHGG, IHG: Ca^{++}/hemorrhage common
- DWI
  - DMG: Majority show facilitated diffusion (↑ ADC signal)
    - Diffusion restriction, when present, correlates with worse prognosis
  - DHG, pHGG: Varies from ill-defined facilitated diffusion (↑ ADC signal) to solid hypercellular (↓ ADC signal)
- PWI
  - DMG: Typically iso- or hypoperfusion compared to adjacent brain
    - Hyperperfusion is associated with worse prognosis
  - DHG, IHG, pHGG: Variable, but generally ↑ perfusion (cerebral blood flow and relative cerebral blood volume) compared to low-grade tumors
- T1WI C+
  - DMG: Most tumors are nonenhancing
    - Enhancement suggests more aggressive tumor
  - DHG, pHGG: Variable from no enhancement to avid/heterogeneous
  - IHG: Majority of tumors show heterogeneous enhancement

Imaging Recommendations

- Best imaging tool
  - MR ± contrast
- Protocol advice
  - Image entire neuraxis to evaluate for leptomeningeal metastatic disease
  - Use DWI and PWI to help distinguish from lower grade tumors

DIFFERENTIAL DIAGNOSIS

Embryonal Tumor With Multilayered Rosettes

- Solid or mixed solid/cystic tumor with highly cellular (↓ ADC) solid components
- Frequently show minimal enhancement and peritumoral edema
- Usually in young patients (early 1st decade)

Atypical Teratoid/Rhabdoid Tumor

- Heterogenous tumor with highly cellular (↓ ADC) solid components
- Hemorrhage common
- Usually in patients ≤ 3 years

Supratentorial Ependymoma

- Solid or mixed solid/cystic tumor with highly cellular (↓ ADC) solid components
- Ca^{++}/hemorrhage common

Ganglioglioma

- Solid or mixed solid/cystic tumor, usually cortically based
- Solid components typically are hypocellular (↑ ADC) solid components
- Majority enhance, Ca^{++} common

Desmoplastic Infantile Ganglioglioma/Astrocytoma

- Large mixed solid/cystic hemispheric tumor in infants

Pilocytic Astrocytoma

- Solid or mixed solid/cystic enhancing tumor, usually in deep gray nuclei, cerebellum, or white matter
- Solid components typically are hypocellular (↑ ADC) solid components

Uncommon and Rare High-Grade Pediatric Tumors

- CNS Neuroblastoma, *FOXR2* activated
- CNS Tumor with *BCOR* internal tandem duplication

PATHOLOGY

General Features

- DMG: Diffuse infiltration of small monomorphic cells; necrosis and microvascular proliferation are rare
- DHG: Glioblastoma-like pattern with highly cellular infiltrative astrocytic tumor with high mitotic activity
- pHGG: Glioblastoma-like pattern (vascular proliferation, high mitotic activity, and necrosis or undifferentiated morphology)
- IHG: Usually cellular and well-demarcated from brain parenchyma

Staging, Grading, & Classification

- DMG: Alteration of H3K27M or EGFR
  - Grade 4 regardless of histology
- DHG: Mutation of H3G34
  - Grade 4 regardless of histology
- pHGG: Diffuse glioma wildtype for H3, *IDH1*, and *IDH2*
  - Grade 4 regardless of histology
  - Subtypes: RTK1, RTK2, and MYCN
- IHG: High-grade cellular astrocytoma with frequent RTK fusions
  - Not assigned WHO grade
  - Subtypes: NTRK altered, *ROS1* altered, *ALK* altered, and *MET* altered

Gross Pathologic & Surgical Features

- Diffuse infiltration of brain parenchyma with enlargement and distortion of brain structures
- Softening and discoloration of brain with hemorrhagic &/or necrotic zones

CLINICAL ISSUES

Presentation

- Most common signs/symptoms
  - DMG: DIPG presents with cranial nerve deficits (82%) and ataxia (62%), among others
    - Thalamic DMG presents with intracranial hypertension and motor/sensory deficits
  - DHG, pHGG: Seizures, motor/sensory deficits
  - IHG: Macrocephaly, altered mental status

Demographics

- DMG: Median age: ~ 5 years
  - DIPGs account for 10-15% of pediatric CNS tumors
- DHG: Median age: 15-19 years
- IHG: Median age: 3 months

Natural History & Prognosis

- DMG: Poor prognosis (2-year overall survival: < 10%)
  - Limited surgical options due to midline locations
- DHG: Median overall survival: 18-22 months
- pHGG: 2-year overall survival: ~ 25%
- IHG: Better prognosis than most HGGs
  - Small studies suggest 5-year overall survival ~ 25-50%

Treatment

- DMG: XRT remains primary therapy
- DHG: Surgical resection + chemotherapy; ± XRT
- pHGG: Surgical resection + chemotherapy + XRT
- IHG: Surgical resection + chemotherapy

DIAGNOSTIC CHECKLIST

Consider

- DMG: Ill-defined, nonenhancing or minimally enhancing hypocellular thalamic or pontine mass
- DHGs: Glioblastoma-like cellular tumor with enhancement and necrosis in cerebral hemisphere
- pHGG: Ill-defined, nonenhancing mass or glioblastoma-like mass
- IHG: Large, heterogeneous cellular mass ± hemorrhage in infant

Image Interpretation Pearls

- Most nonenhancing, ill-defined DMGs and some pHGGs show facilitated diffusion (↑ ADC signal)
  - Despite this paucicellular appearance on DWI, these are HGGs with poor prognosis
- ↑ CT attenuation and diffusion restriction of solid components should prompt consideration of pediatric-type diffuse HGG in addition to other DDx

Reporting Tips

- Use term pediatric HGG rather than glioblastoma

SELECTED REFERENCES

1. Park YW et al: The 2021 WHO classification for gliomas and implications on imaging diagnosis: part 2-summary of imaging findings on pediatric-type diffuse high-grade gliomas, pediatric-type diffuse low-grade gliomas, and circumscribed astrocytic gliomas. J Magn Reson Imaging. 58(3):690-708, 2023
2. Thomas DL: 2021 updates to the World Health Organization classification of adult-type and pediatric-type diffuse gliomas: a clinical practice review. Chin Clin Oncol. 12(1):7, 2023
3. Osborn AG et al: The 2021 World Health Organization classification of tumors of the central nervous system: what neuroradiologists need to know. AJNR Am J Neuroradiol. 43(7):928-37, 2022
4. Gonçalves FG et al: Advanced magnetic resonance imaging in pediatric glioblastomas. Front Neurol. 12:733323, 2021
5. WHO Classification of Tumours Editorial Board: WHO Classification of Tumours: CNS Tumours. 5th ed. IARC, 2021

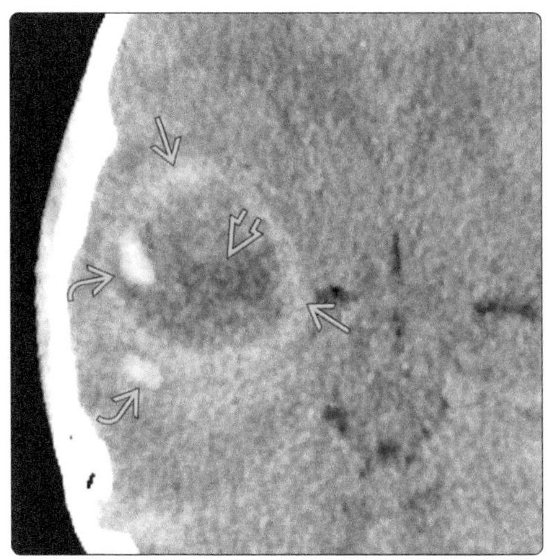

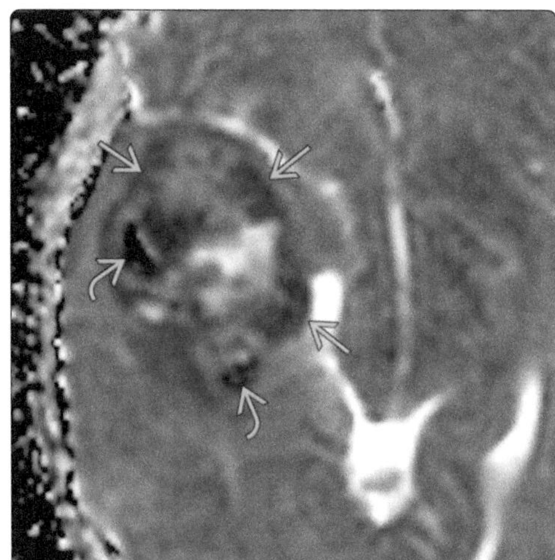

(Left) *Axial NECT in an 8-year-old with H3G34-mutant diffuse hemispheric glioma (DHG) shows hyperattenuation in the solid tumor ➡ with central necrosis ➡ and few peripheral areas of intratumoral hemorrhage ➡.* **(Right)** *Axial ADC MR in the same patient shows decreased signal (diffusion restriction) within the solid peripheral tumor components, consistent with hypercellular tumor ➡. Areas of ADC signal loss correspond to hemorrhage ➡.*

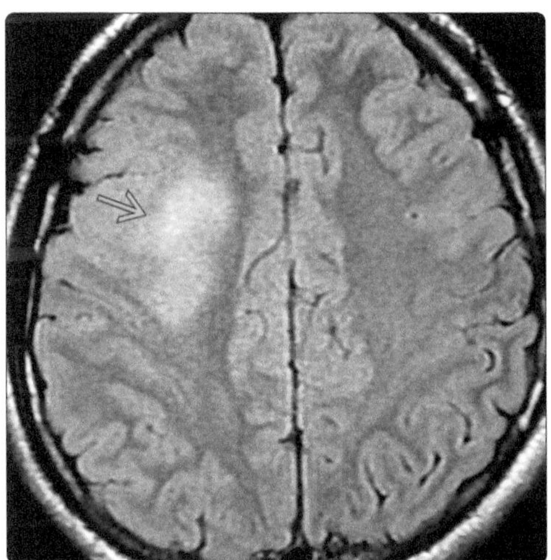

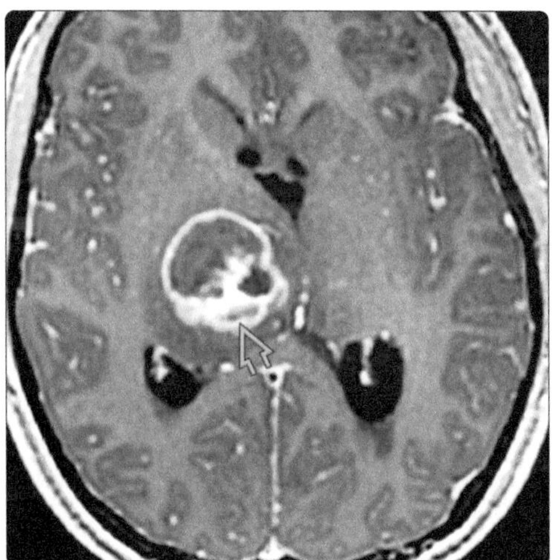

(Left) *Axial FLAIR MR in a patient with pHGG H3 and IDH wildtype shows indistinct mass-like signal hyperintensity ➡ in the right frontal lobe. Postcontrast images (not shown) showed no associated enhancement.* **(Right)** *Axial T1 C+ MR in a patient with pHGG H3 and IDH wildtype tumor with EGFR alteration shows a rim-enhancing tumor ➡ in the right thalamus with adjacent peritumoral edema. PWI (not shown) showed increased cerebral blood flow within the solid enhancing component.*

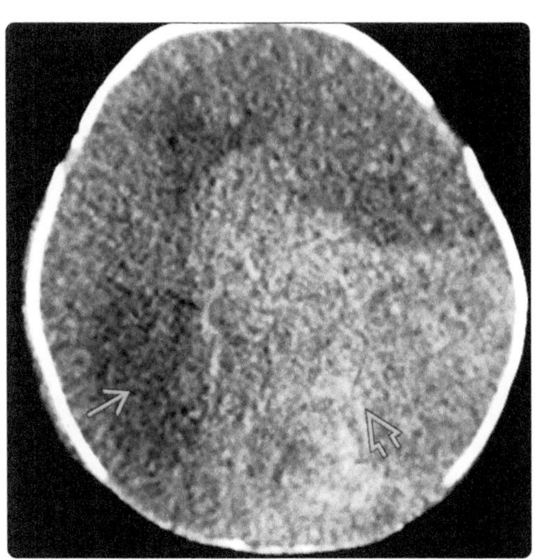

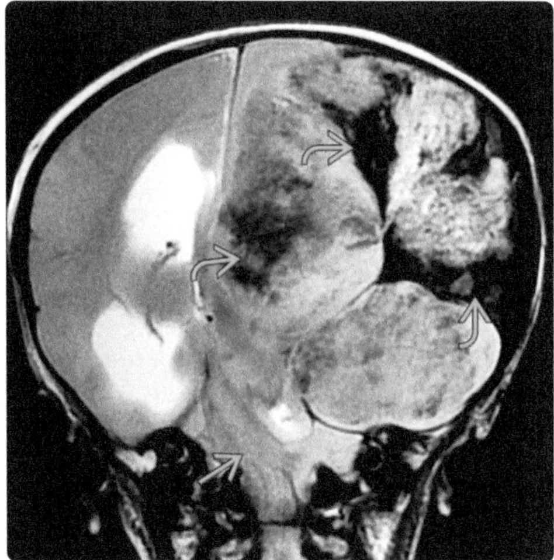

(Left) *Axial NECT in a newborn with an infantile hemispheric glioma (IHG) shows a very large, hyperintense mass ➡ occupying much of the left cerebral hemisphere, causing significant midline shift and right lateral ventricular hydrocephalus ➡.* **(Right)** *Coronal T2 MR in the same patient shows heterogeneous signal intensity in the mass, including areas of low signal corresponding to hemorrhage ➡. Note the severe mass effect on the brainstem ➡.*

Diffuse Intrinsic Pontine Glioma

KEY FACTS

TERMINOLOGY

- Diffuse intrinsic pontine glioma (DIPG)

IMAGING

- Expansile tumor centered in pons, effacing CSF cisterns & 4th ventricle; often encases basilar artery
  - Vast majority do not enhance at diagnosis
  - Most tumors have ↑ ADC signal
- Best imaging study: MR with contrast
  - Advanced techniques ± helpful in DIPG prognosis
    - ↓ ADC, ↑ rCBV, ↑ Cho:NAA suggest ↓ survival

TOP DIFFERENTIAL DIAGNOSES

- Pilocytic astrocytoma
- Autoimmune white matter disease (acute disseminated encephalomyelitis & multiple sclerosis)
- Neurofibromatosis type 1
- Osmotic demyelination syndrome
- Brainstem abscess

PATHOLOGY

- Astrocytomas of varying grades (WHO 2-6)
- Vast majority (80-90%) harbor mutation in H3K27M
  - Defined as diffuse midline glioma (grade 6) in 2021 WHO CNS Tumor Classification

CLINICAL ISSUES

- Presentations include cranial nerve palsies, hemiparesis, gait disturbance, ataxia, headache, nausea, vomiting
- Poor prognosis: Median survival ~ 1 year
- Tumor biopsy now universal for molecular diagnosis/treatment
- XRT remains backbone of current treatment

DIAGNOSTIC CHECKLIST

- Perform MR imaging of entire neuraxis to detect mets
- Negative prognostic imaging features: Extrapontine extension, larger size, enhancement, necrosis, diffusion restriction, & distant disease

(Left) *Axial NECT in a 7-year-old with H3K27M mutant diffuse midline glioma (DMG) shows a diffusely hypoattenuating expansile mass ⇨ centered in the pons, resulting in obliteration of the prepontine cisterns ⇨ and near-complete effacement of the 4th ventricle ⇨.* **(Right)** *Sagittal T2 MR in the same patient shows the mass ⇨ to be centered within and expanding the pons. This particular tumor has sharply delineated margins ⇨, but diffuse midline gliomas (DIPGs) often have very indistinct margins.*

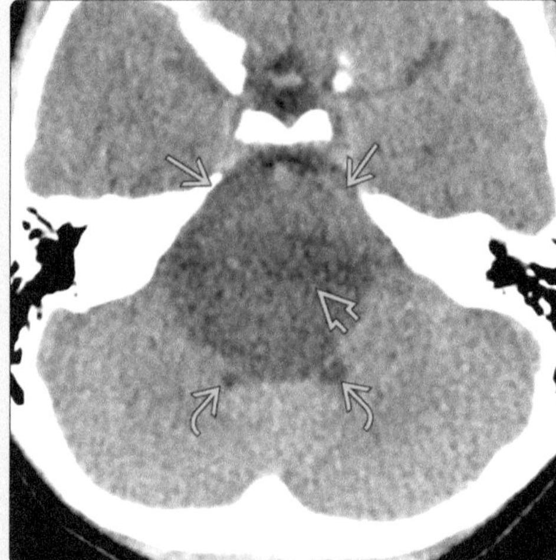

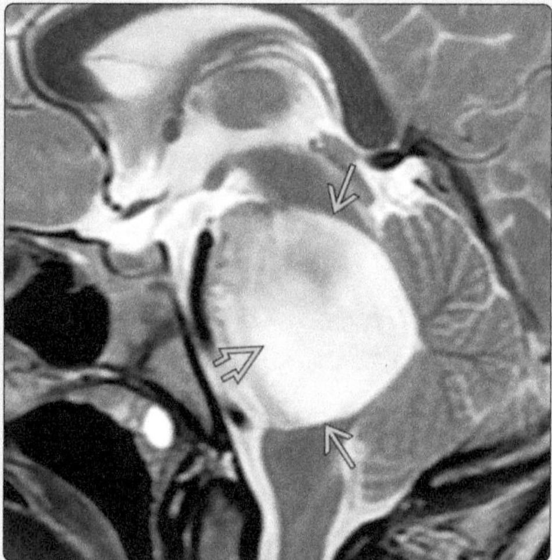

(Left) *Axial T1 C+ MR in the same patient shows no significant enhancement of the pontine mass ⇨, which is typical for most DIPGs at time of diagnosis. Following XRT, heterogeneous enhancement becomes common.* **(Right)** *Axial ADC map in the same patient shows this tumor ⇨ to be very hyperintense compared to brain parenchyma. Despite the grade 6 designation and aggressive clinical course of H3K27M-mutant DMG, these tumors typically have a paucicellular appearance.*

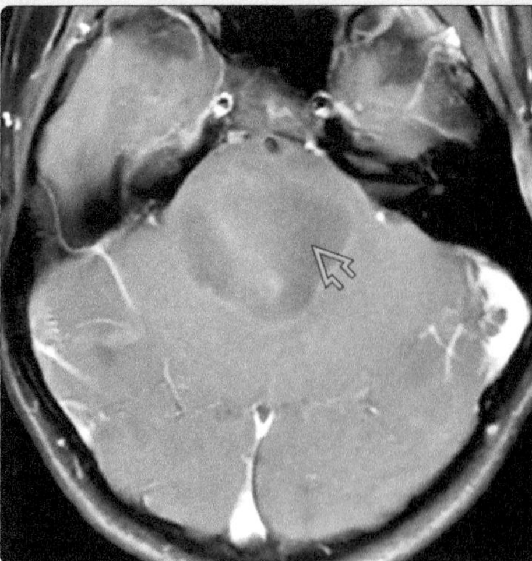

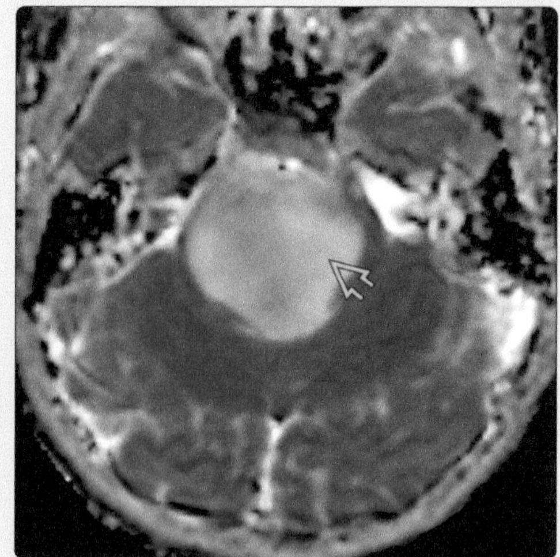

TERMINOLOGY

Abbreviations

- Diffuse intrinsic pontine glioma (DIPG)

Synonyms

- Diffuse midline glioma (DMG)
- Pontine glioma

Definitions

- Glial tumor centered in pons (WHO grades 2-6)
  - Expansile, often poorly marginated, typically lacks enhancement
  - Glioblastoma shows focal enhancement & central necrosis

IMAGING

General Features

- Best diagnostic clue
  - Expansile mass centered in pons with indistinct margins & no enhancement
- Location
  - Lesion must be centered in pons to be considered DIPG
  - Tumor often extends into brainstem/medulla or middle cerebellar peduncle
- Size
  - Varies, but typically occupies majority of pons at time of diagnosis
- Morphology
  - Expansile with poorly defined margins
  - Often will have exophytic projections anteriorly, which may surround basilar artery
  - Usually effaces posterior fossa cisterns & distorts 4th ventricle

CT Findings

- NECT
  - Brainstem enlargement with ↓ attenuation
  - Often difficult to identify on CT due to frequent low attenuation in pons from skull base beam hardening artifact
  - Best clue on CT is effacement or asymmetry of posterior fossa cisterns &/or distortion of 4th ventricle
  - In advanced cases, hydrocephalus may be present
  - Hemorrhage & Ca^{++} rare
- CECT
  - Typically no enhancement
    - Focal areas of enhancement, often with central necrosis → poor prognostic sign

MR Findings

- T1WI
  - Mild to moderate hypointensity
  - Central areas of normal signal may represent relatively preserved white matter (WM) tracts
- T2WI
  - Hyperintense mass (homogeneous to heterogeneous) & margins (edema vs. infiltrating tumor)
    - Treatment often results in ↑ heterogeneity
  - Basilar artery flow void may be partially engulfed by tumor
- FLAIR
  - Hyperintense mass, ± better defined than on T2
- T2* GRE
  - Areas of signal loss typically represent intratumoral hemorrhage
    - More common in posttreatment setting
- DWI
  - Diffusion restriction uncommon; ADC signal usually much brighter than adjacent brain
    - ↓ ADC values associated with shorter survival time & higher grade tumor
  - Diffusion tractography (DTI) can show displacement of WM tracts by tumor
    - WM tracts typically infiltrated or displaced by DIPG (but not interrupted)
- PWI
  - ↑ relative cerebral blood volume (rCBV) associated with ↓ survival time
- T1WI C+
  - Vast majority do not enhance at time of diagnosis
  - Enhancement change during treatment of unclear etiology
    - Altered enhancement during therapy may reflect steroid effect on blood-brain barrier, not necessarily change in tumor
  - Metastatic disease more common than initially reported
    - Especially late in disease or post bevacizumab therapy
- MRA
  - Basilar artery often engulfed by tumor but not typically narrowed
- MRS
  - ↑ Cho:NAA ratio associated with shorter survival
  - Presence of lactate implies necrosis & poor prognosis in some studies

Nuclear Medicine Findings

- PET/CT: FDG uptake in ≥ 50% of tumor area → shorter survival
  - Hypermetabolic tumors more likely to be glioblastoma multiforme

Imaging Recommendations

- Best imaging tool
  - MR with contrast
- Protocol advice
  - PWI & MRS helpful to distinguish progression from pseudoprogression following XRT
  - Perform imaging of entire neuraxis to detect metastatic disease

DIFFERENTIAL DIAGNOSIS

Low-Grade Astrocytoma (e.g., Pilocytic Astrocytoma)

- Usually arise from medulla & are mostly exophytic
- Typically demonstrate avid enhancement

Autoimmune White Matter Disease (Acute Disseminated Encephalomyelitis & Multiple Sclerosis)

- Supratentorial & spinal sites often affected as well
- Delayed onset after viral prodrome or vaccination
- Typically does not have same degree of mass effect as DIPG

Neurofibromatosis Type 1

- Asymptomatic, poorly defined T2-hyperintense foci in brainstem, cerebellum, globus pallidus
  - Develop in early childhood, diminish with age
  - Thought to represent areas of myelin vacuolization
- Look for additional findings of neurofibromatosis type 1 (e.g., optic pathway glioma, neurofibromas)

Osmotic Demyelination Syndrome

- Central pontine T2 hyperintensity with sparing of periphery
- Classic clinical setting: Rapid correction of hyponatremia

Brainstem Abscess

- More acute clinical course; often febrile
- *Listeria monocytogenes* often implicated
- Look for central areas of nonenhancement with diffusion restriction

Viral Encephalitis

- More acute clinical course; often febrile
- Viral agents → West Nile virus, adenovirus, EBV, herpes simplex virus

Cavernous Malformation

- Low-flow vascular malformation with locules containing fluid-fluid levels
- SWI/T2* GRE hypointensity classic
- Often associated with other sites of disease

PATHOLOGY

General Features

- Genetics
  - Vast majority (80-90%) harbor mutation in H3K27M
    - Defined as DMG (grade 6) in 2021 WHO CNS Tumor Classification
  - Mutations of *TP53* tumor suppressor gene (42-71%)
  - Progression to higher grade gliomas associated with
    - Inactivation of tumor suppressor gene (*TP53*)
    - Loss of heterozygosity of chromosomes 10, 17p

Staging, Grading, & Classification

- Astrocytomas of varying grades (WHO 2-6)
  - In past decade, diagnosis was often made solely on imaging without biopsy
  - Molecular diagnosis more important than histology in 2021 WHO CNS tumor classification
  - Biopsy is now universal in order to determine molecular subtype
    - Molecular subtyping helps with prognosis & identifying targeted therapy

Gross Pathologic & Surgical Features

- Diffuse tumor infiltration; craniocaudal extension along fiber tracts

Microscopic Features

- Variable cellularity & mitoses with pleomorphism & nuclear atypia, necrosis, & endothelial proliferation

CLINICAL ISSUES

Presentation

- Most common signs/symptoms
  - Cranial nerve palsies with long tract signs
  - Hemiparesis, ataxia, gait disturbance
  - Headache, nausea, vomiting
- Other signs/symptoms
  - Dysarthria, nystagmus, sleep apnea

Demographics

- Age
  - Peak incidence: ~ 3-10 years old
- Sex
  - M = F
- Epidemiology
  - ~ 10-15% of childhood CNS cancers
  - ~ 25-30% of pediatric posterior fossa tumors

Natural History & Prognosis

- Poor prognosis
  - Median survival: ~ 1 year
  - 20% survival at 2 years
  - CSF dissemination in 50% prior to death

Treatment

- Radiation therapy if > 3 years old
- Chemotherapy, though not particularly effective

DIAGNOSTIC CHECKLIST

Consider

- Fever & rapid symptom onset: Encephalitis or abscess
- Blood products: Cavernous malformation (look for associated developmental venous anomaly)
- Lesions in other locations: Infection or demyelination
- Atypical appearance → consider biopsy

Image Interpretation Pearls

- Sagittal T2/FLAIR helpful to show extent of lesion
- Hydrocephalus usually late finding

Reporting Tips

- Pontine tumor signal extending to cerebellum, midbrain, or medulla suggests higher grade

SELECTED REFERENCES

1. Osborn AG et al: The 2021 World Health Organization Classification of Tumors of the Central Nervous System: what neuroradiologists need to know. AJNR Am J Neuroradiol. 43(7):928-37, 2022
2. Chang PD et al: Predictive values of location and volumetric MRI injury patterns for neurodevelopmental outcomes in hypoxic-ischemic encephalopathy neonates. Brain Sci. 10(12), 2020
3. Giagnacovo M et al: Retrospective analysis on the consistency of MRI features with histological and molecular markers in diffuse intrinsic pontine glioma (DIPG). Childs Nerv Syst. 36(4):697-704, 2020
4. Pfaff E et al: Brainstem biopsy in pediatric diffuse intrinsic pontine glioma in the era of precision medicine: the INFORM study experience. Eur J Cancer. 114:27-35, 2019
5. Harward S et al: T2-weighted images are superior to other MR image types for the determination of diffuse intrinsic pontine glioma intratumoral heterogeneity. Childs Nerv Syst. 34(3):449-55, 2018
6. Hoffman LM et al: Clinical, radiologic, pathologic, and molecular characteristics of long-term survivors of diffuse intrinsic pontine glioma (DIPG): a collaborative report from the International and European Society for Pediatric Oncology DIPG Registries. J Clin Oncol. 36(19):1963-72, 2018
7. Mackay A et al: Integrated molecular meta-analysis of 1,000 pediatric high-grade and diffuse intrinsic pontine glioma. Cancer Cell. 32(4):520-37.e5, 2017
8. Tisnado J et al: Conventional and advanced imaging of diffuse intrinsic pontine glioma. J Child Neurol. 31(12):1386-93, 2016

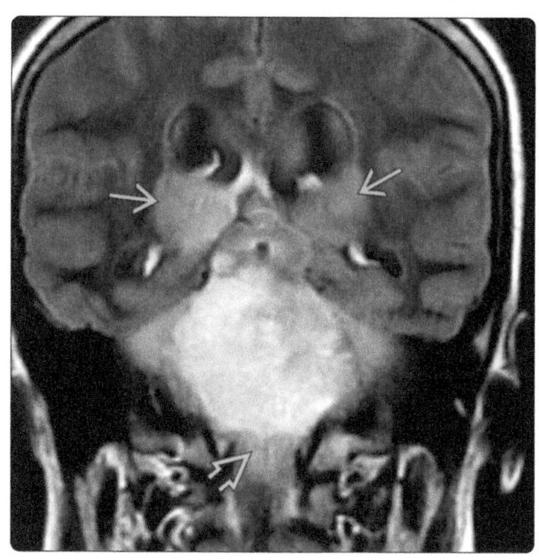

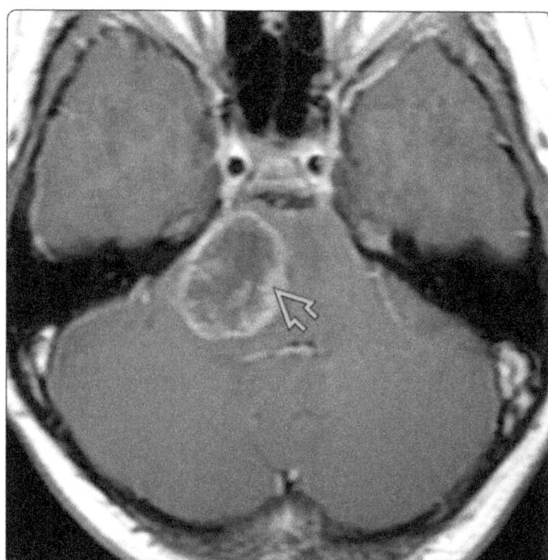

(Left) *Coronal FLAIR MR in a 9-year-old girl with a DIPG shows extension of abnormal signal into the bilateral thalami ➡ and medulla ⇨. Such distant extension of signal abnormality typically suggests an infiltrative, higher grade tumor.* **(Right)** *Axial T1 C+ MR at the time of diagnosis in a 12-year-old boy with H3K27M mutant DMG shows rim enhancement with central necrosis ⇨. Enhancement and necrosis at the time of initial diagnosis are poor prognostic imaging markers.*

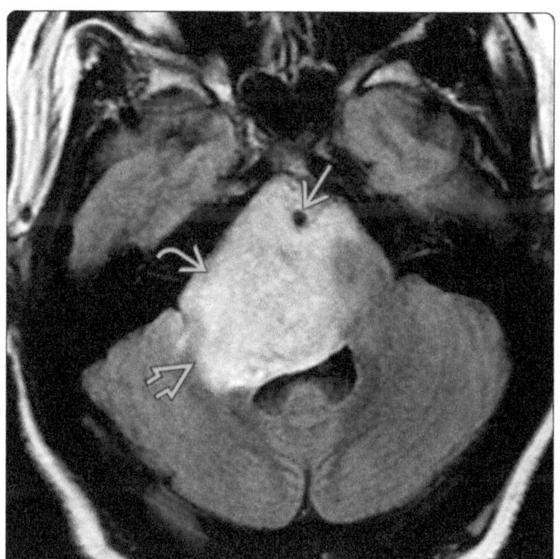

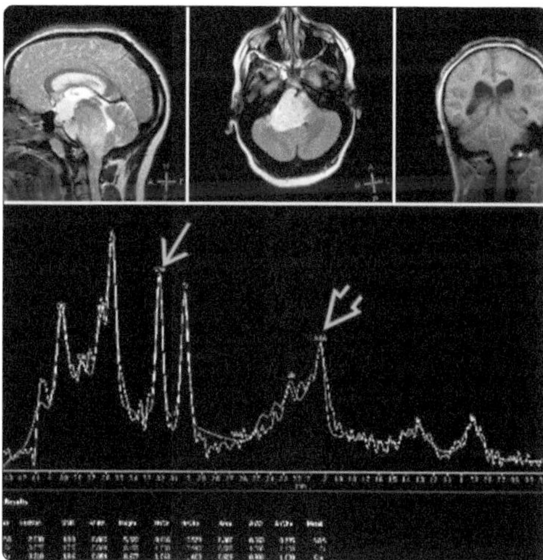

(Left) *Axial FLAIR MR in a 13-year-old girl with downbeat nystagmus shows a hyperintense expansile mass centered in the pons, consistent with a DIPG. Note how the mass has poorly defined margins ⇨, extends into the right middle cerebellar peduncle ↷, and encases the basilar artery ➡, all typical findings of DIPGs.* **(Right)** *Short-echo single voxel MRS in the same patient shows decreased NAA ⇨ and increased Cho ➡. Increasing Cho:NAA ratios are associated with shorter survival time in a DIPG.*

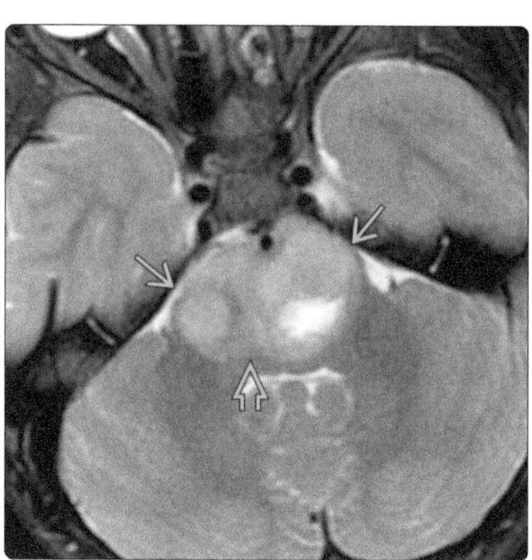

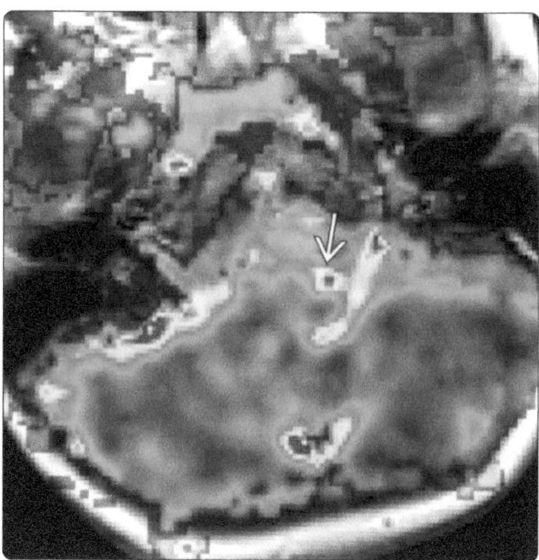

(Left) *Axial T2WI MR in a 4-year-old girl with a DIPG shows a heterogeneously hyperintense expansile mass ⇨ centered in the pons, the typical location and appearance for a DIPG. Note the effacement of the cerebellopontine angle cisterns ➡.* **(Right)** *Axial rCBV MR fused with a T1WI C+ MR in a 4-year-old girl shows areas of increased perfusion ➡ corresponding to areas of enhancement. This feature has been shown to be associated with higher grade tumors and shorter survival time.*

Brainstem Tumors

KEY FACTS

TERMINOLOGY

- Brainstem tumors (BSTs) distinguished by location, imaging appearance, & histology

IMAGING

- Diffuse intrinsic pontine glioma (DIPG): Expansile tumor centered in pons, effacing CSF cisterns & 4th ventricle; often encases basilar artery
  - Vast majority (80-90%) harbor mutation in H3K27M
  - Most tumors show ↑ ADC signal and no enhancement
- Pilocytic astrocytoma: Exophytic enhancing tumor anywhere in brainstem
- Tectal plate glioma: Nonenhancing mass in tectum
- Midbrain tumors: Heterogeneous group of tumors
- Best imaging study: MR with contrast
  - Advanced techniques ± helpful in DIPG prognosis
    - ↓ ADC, ↑ rCBV, ↑ Cho:NAA suggest ↓ survival

TOP DIFFERENTIAL DIAGNOSES

- Brainstem abscess, acute disseminated encephalomyelitis, NF1, osmotic demyelination syndrome, cavernous malformation

PATHOLOGY

- BSTs ~ 15% of pediatric brain tumors, 20-30% of pediatric posterior fossa tumors
  - Astrocytomas (WHO grades 1-6), embryonal tumors (embryonal tumor with multilayered rosettes & atypical teratoid/rhabdoid tumor), rare gangliogliomas

CLINICAL ISSUES

- Presentations: Cranial nerve palsies, hemiparesis, gait disturbance, ataxia, headache, nausea, vomiting
- Prognosis depends on location & histology: Pons: Poor prognosis (unresectable); DIPG: Median survival ~ 1 year; emdulla or midbrain: Variable prognosis; tectum: Good prognosis (only requires CSF diversion)

(Left) *Axial T2 MR in a 5-year-old girl with a H3K27M mutant diffuse midline glioma (DMG) [also called a diffuse intrinsic pontine glioma (DIPG)] shows the tumor is T2 hyperintense with somewhat indistinct margins ⇨, expands the pons, and encases the basilar artery ⇨.* **(Right)** *Axial ADC map in the same patient shows this tumor ⇨ to be very hyperintense compared to brain parenchyma. Despite the grade 4 designation and aggressive clinical course of H3K27M mutant DMG, these tumors typically have a paucicellular appearance.*

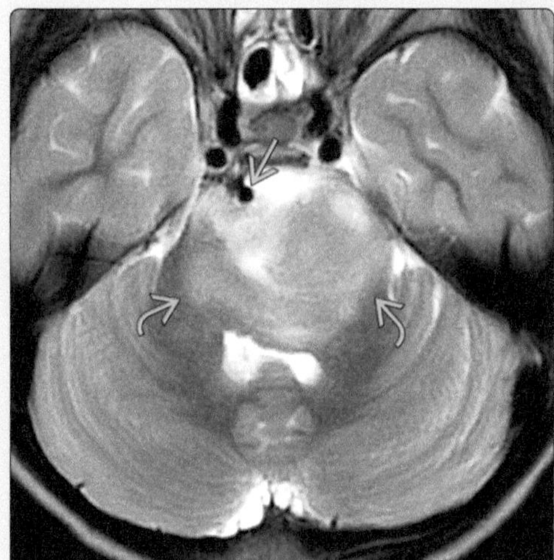

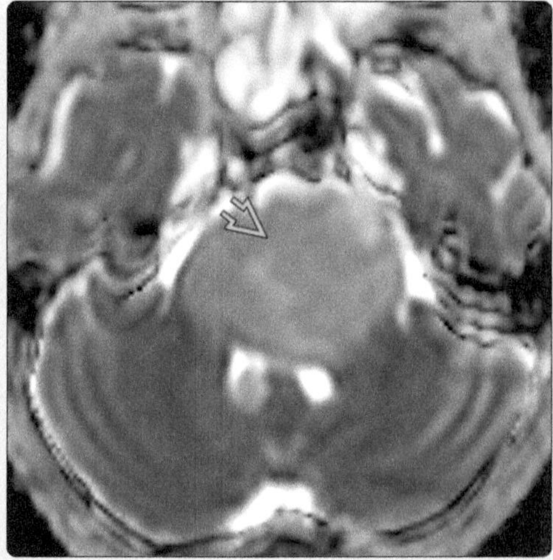

(Left) *Axial T1 C+ MR in a 9-year-old with H3K27M-mutant DMG shows no significant enhancement of the pontine mass ⇨, which is typical for most DIPGs at time of diagnosis. Following XRT, heterogeneous enhancement becomes common.* **(Right)** *Coronal FLAIR MR in a 9-year-old girl with a DIPG shows extension of abnormal signal into the bilateral thalami ➡ and medulla ⇨. Such distant extension of signal abnormality typically suggests an infiltrative, higher grade tumor.*

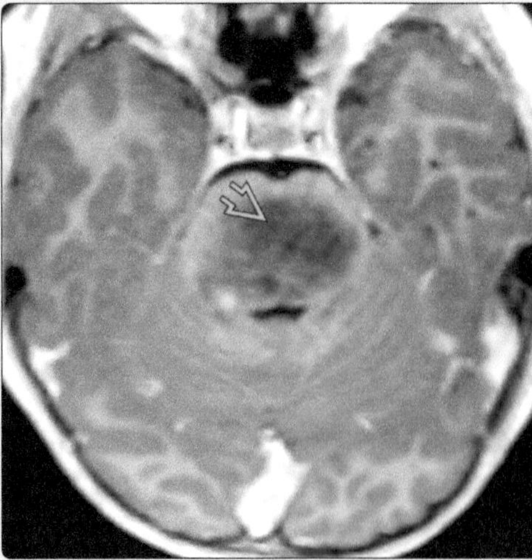

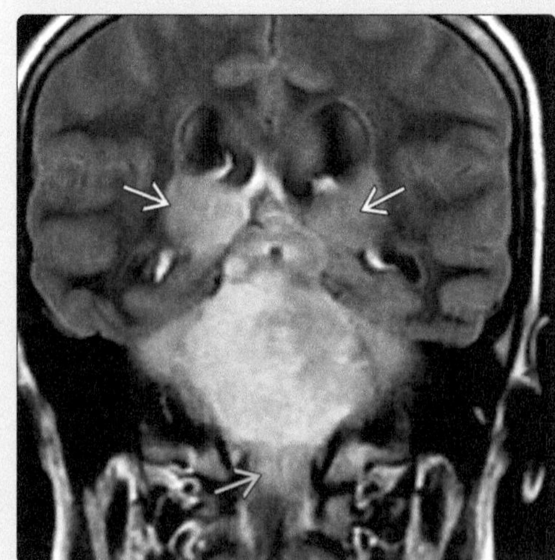

TERMINOLOGY

Abbreviations

- Brainstem tumors (BSTs)

Synonyms

- Pontine glioma, midbrain glioma, medullary glioma, dorsally exophytic medullary glioma

Definitions

- BSTs distinguished by location & imaging/histologic characteristics of tumor
  - Diffuse intrinsic pontine glioma (DIPG): Glial tumor centered in pons
    - Expansile, often poorly marginated, often lack enhancement
    - Vast majority (80-90%) harbor mutation in H3K27M
      - Defined as diffuse midline glioma (DMG) (grade 6) in 2021 WHO CNS Tumor Classification
  - Tectal gliomas
    - Present with hydrocephalus in 6-10 year olds
    - Rarely progressive
    - CSF diversion often only treatment required
  - Midbrain or mesencephalic tumors
    - All histologies occur (including PNET, atypical teratoid/rhabdoid tumor)
  - Medullary tumors
    - Pilocytic astrocytoma (PA) most likely histology
    - Usually dorsally exophytic & solidly enhancing
  - BSTs associated with neurofibromatosis type 1 (NF1) → another distinct group
    - Rarely enlarge, often asymptomatic

IMAGING

General Features

- Best diagnostic clue
  - DIPG: Expansile lesion in pons
  - PA: Exophytic enhancing lesion anywhere in brainstem
  - Tectal plate glioma: Nonenhancing lesion in tectum
- Location
  - Cervicomedullary junction to cerebral peduncles
    - Medullary, pontine, midbrain, tectal
  - DIPG: By definition, must be centered in pons
- Size
  - Varies greatly, partly related to location
    - DIPG often very large at presentation
    - Tectal plate gliomas often small
- Morphology
  - Depends on histology; focal vs. large/infiltrative
    - Sometimes exophytic
    - DIPG: Signal extension into cerebellar peduncles, midbrain, or medulla → higher grade

CT Findings

- NECT
  - Brainstem enlargement with ↓ attenuation & effacement of adjacent CSF cisterns
    - Streak artifact from skull base can mimic tumor
  - Pontine tumors → flattening of anterior 4th ventricle
- CECT
  - Variable enhancement
    - PA in any region of brainstem usually enhancing

MR Findings

- T1WI
  - Mild to moderate hypointensity
  - Central areas of preserved signal may represent relatively preserved white matter (WM) tracts
- T2WI
  - Hyperintense mass (homogeneous to heterogeneous) & margins (edema vs. infiltrating tumor)
    - Treatment often results in ↑ heterogeneity
  - Basilar artery flow void engulfed by DIPG
- FLAIR
  - Hyperintense mass, ± better defined than on T2
- T2* GRE
  - Areas of signal loss usually represent intratumoral hemorrhage
    - Mineralization uncommon in BST
- DWI
  - DIPG typically does not show diffusion restriction; ADC signal usually greater than brain
    - ↓ ADC values associated with shorter survival time & higher grade tumor
  - DTI can show displacement of WM tracts by tumor
    - WM tracts typically infiltrated or displaced by DIPG (but not interrupted)
- PWI
  - ↑ relative cerebral blood volume (rCBV) associated with ↓ DIPG survival time
- T1WI C+
  - DIPG: Usually no enhancement at diagnosis
    - Focal areas of enhancement → worse prognosis (higher grade)
  - PA: Solid portion enhances
    - ± solid, cystic with nodule, or rim enhancing; most often located dorsally with exophytic component
  - T1 C+ changes in DIPG treatment of unclear etiology
    - May reflect steroid effect on blood-brain barrier, not necessarily change in tumor
  - Metastatic disease more common than initially reported
    - Especially late in disease or post bevacizumab therapy
- MRA
  - Basilar artery engulfed by DIPG, but not typically narrowed
- MRS
  - ↑ Cho:NAA ratio associated with shorter survival
  - Lactate implies necrosis & poor prognosis in some studies

Nuclear Medicine Findings

- PET/CT: FDG uptake in ≥ 50% of tumor → shorter survival
  - Hypermetabolic tumors more likely to be GBM

Imaging Recommendations

- Best imaging tool
  - MR with contrast
- Protocol advice
  - DTI, PWI, & MRS have prognostic significance in DIPG & may help prognosticate

DIFFERENTIAL DIAGNOSIS

Brainstem Abscess

- *Listeria monocytogenes* often implicated
  - Viral agents: West Nile virus, adenovirus, EBV, HSV
- More acute clinical course; often febrile

Acute Disseminated Encephalomyelitis/Other Autoimmune Inflammation

- Supratentorial & spinal sites often affected as well
- Delayed onset after viral prodrome or vaccination
- Behçet disease causes marked midbrain edema/swelling

Neurofibromatosis Type 1

- Asymptomatic, poorly defined T2-hyperintense foci in brainstem, cerebellum, globus pallidus
  - Develop in early childhood, diminish with age
- Cerebellar WM involvement more common than pons
  - Look for additional findings of NF1

Osmotic Demyelination Syndrome

- Central pontine T2 hyperintensity with sparing of periphery
- Classic clinical setting: Rapid correction of hyponatremia

Cavernous Malformation

- Low-flow vascular malformation with locules containing fluid-fluid levels
- SWI/T2* GRE hypointensity classic
- Often associated with developmental venous anomaly (DVA)

Histiocytosis

- Langerhans cell histiocytosis, hemophagocytic lymphohistiocytosis
- May cause signal abnormalities in pons & cerebellum
- Often associated with other sites of disease

PATHOLOGY

General Features

- Genetics
  - Mutations of *TP53* tumor suppressor gene (42-71%)
  - Histone-H3 mutations carry worse prognosis, regardless of histologic grade
- Associated abnormalities
  - Better prognosis of BST when associated with NF1
    - Medulla most common site in NF1

Staging, Grading, & Classification

- DIPG: Astrocytomas of varying grades (WHO 1-6)
  - Biopsy of presumed DIPG now standard of care
    - Vast majority harbor H3K27M mutation
    - Molecular subtyping allows improved prognostication & potential targeted therapy
- PAs, embryonal tumors, rare gangliogliomas
  - If suspected based on imaging, recommend biopsy

Gross Pathologic & Surgical Features

- Pontine swelling in DIPG
  - Diffuse tumor infiltration; craniocaudal extension along fiber tracts

Microscopic Features

- Variable cellularity & mitoses with pleomorphism & nuclear atypia, necrosis, & endothelial proliferation

CLINICAL ISSUES

Presentation

- Most common signs/symptoms
  - Cranial nerve palsies with long tract signs
  - Hemiparesis, ataxia, gait disturbance
  - Headache, nausea, vomiting

Demographics

- Age
  - Peak incidence ~ 3-10 years old
- Sex
  - M = F
- Epidemiology
  - ~ 15% of pediatric brain tumors
  - 20-30% of pediatric posterior fossa tumors

Natural History & Prognosis

- DIPG: Very poor prognosis
  - CSF dissemination in 50% prior to death
  - Median survival ~ 1 year
  - 20% survival at 2 years
- PA (dorsally exophytic): Fair to good prognosis, especially in setting of NF1
- Tectal plate gliomas: Good prognosis

Treatment

- DIPG: Radiation therapy if > 3 years old
  - Chemotherapy, though not particularly effective
- PA: Consider surgical resection based upon location
- Tectal plate glioma: Often only requires 3rd ventriculostomy followed by observation

DIAGNOSTIC CHECKLIST

Consider

- Rapid onset of symptoms: Abscess
- Blood products: Cavernous malformation (look for associated DVA)
- Lesions in other locations: Infection or demyelination
- Atypical appearance → consider biopsy

Image Interpretation Pearls

- Sagittal T2/FLAIR helpful to show extent of lesion
- Hydrocephalus usually late finding

Reporting Tips

- Pontine tumor signal extending to cerebellum, midbrain, or medulla suggests higher grade
- Solid exophytic enhancement most common in PA; may suggest better prognosis

SELECTED REFERENCES

1. Osborn AG et al: The 2021 World Health Organization Classification of Tumors of the Central Nervous System: what neuroradiologists need to know. AJNR Am J Neuroradiol. 43(7):928-37, 2022
2. Chiang J et al: Clinical, imaging, and molecular analysis of pediatric pontine tumors lacking characteristic imaging features of DIPG. Acta Neuropathol Commun. 8(1):57, 2020

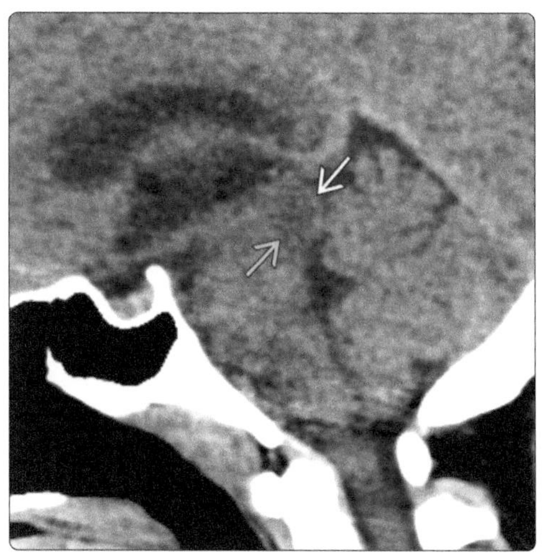

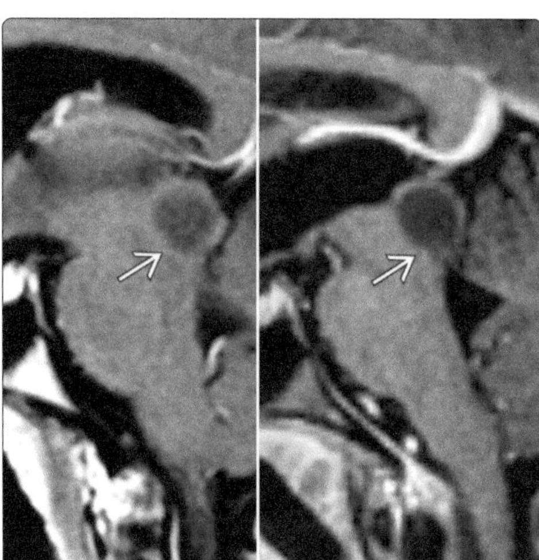

(Left) *Midline sagittal NECT in a 16-year-old girl involved in a motor vehicle collision shows a low-attenuation expansile mass centered in the tectum ➡ with obliteration of the cerebral aqueduct ⇨.* **(Right)** *Midline sagittal T1 C+ MR in the same patient at diagnosis (left) and 16 months later (right) shows a nonenhancing, expansile mass centered in the tectum ➡. The lack of enhancement and lack of interval growth (or very slow growth over time) is typical for a tectal plate glioma.*

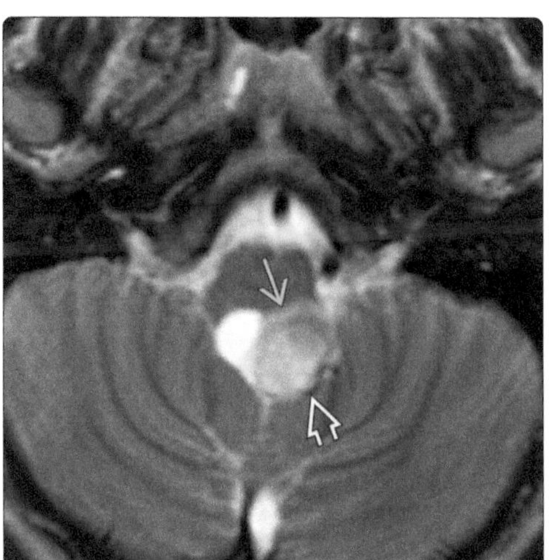

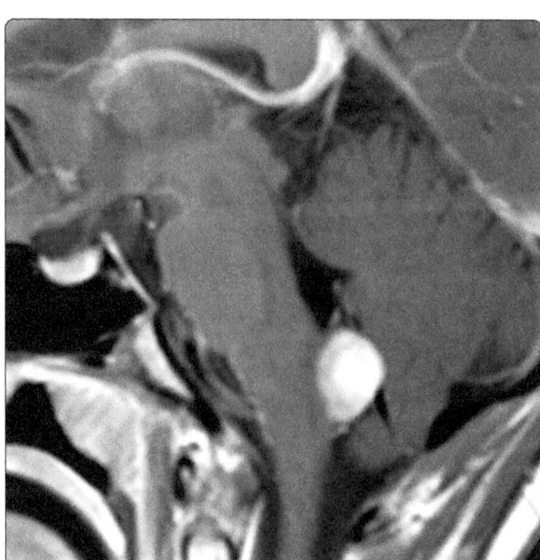

(Left) *Axial T2 MR in an 11-year-old with a heterogeneously hyperintense mass at the inferior 4th ventricle shows an indistinct border ⇨ of the mass with the medulla, but a distinct border ➡ with the cerebellum, suggesting an exophytic origin from the dorsal medulla.* **(Right)** *Sagittal T1 C+ MR in the same patient shows homogeneous enhancement of the mass arising from the dorsal medulla, a typical pattern of enhancement for a pilocytic astrocytoma (confirmed histologically).*

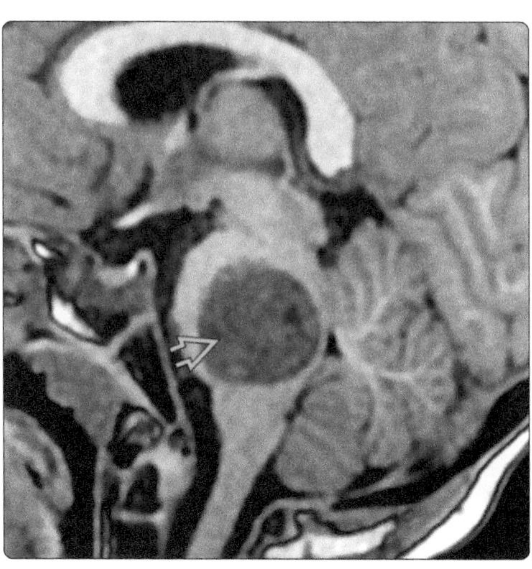

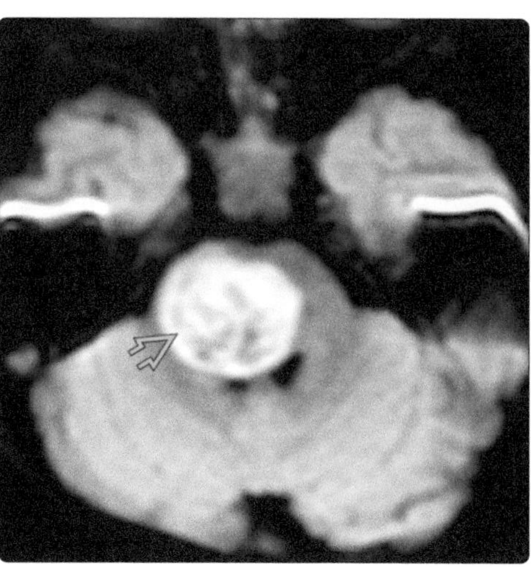

(Left) *Sagittal T1 MR in a 2-year-old with embryonal tumor with multilayered rosettes (ETMR) shows a well-delineated tumor ⇨ centered in the pons.* **(Right)** *Axial DWI MR in the same patient shows marked diffusion restriction throughout the well-defined tumor ⇨, which would suggest a highly cellular tumor, such as an ETMR. ETMRs usually occur in the supratentorial compartment, but may occur anywhere in the CNS. This would be a very unusual appearance on DWI for a DIPG.*

KEY FACTS

TERMINOLOGY

- Tumor of primordial germ cells, histologically identical to gonadal & nongonadal seminoma or dysgerminoma

IMAGING

- CT: Hyperattenuating solid components
  - Pineal region: Localized "engulfed" Ca^{++}
  - Other sites: Ca^{++} rare but hemorrhage may occur
- MR: Mass in suprasellar, pineal, or basal ganglia regions
  - T2: Multiple small cysts not unusual (~ 25%)
  - DWI: Diffusion restriction in solid components
  - T1 C+: Avid enhancement, often speckled pattern
  - Pineal: Bithalamic extension, peritumoral edema
  - Suprasellar: Absent T1 posterior pituitary "bright spot"
  - Metastatic CSF dissemination common (25-40%)

TOP DIFFERENTIAL DIAGNOSES

- Pineal region
  - Pineoblastoma
  - Nongerminomatous germ cell tumors (teratoma, etc.)
  - Tectal plate glioma
- Suprasellar
  - Craniopharyngioma
  - Hypothalamic/chiasmatic astrocytoma
  - Langerhans cell histiocytosis

CLINICAL ISSUES

- M > F, especially in pineal region
- Mean age: 10-15 years
- Pineal: Headache, paralysis of upward gaze
- Suprasellar: Diabetes insipidus (DI), vision changes
- ± ↑ serum & CSF human chorionic gonadotropin
- Favorable prognosis (5-year survival > 90%)

DIAGNOSTIC CHECKLIST

- Image entire neuraxis to detect CSF dissemination
- Occult germinoma possible in child with DI & normal MR
  - Repeat MR in 3-6 months to assess for growing mass

(Left) *Midline sagittal graphic shows a pineal region germinoma ➡ with subarachnoid spread of tumor to the hypothalamus, infundibulum, anterior 3rd ventricle, frontal horn, & 4th ventricle.* **(Right)** *Sagittal T1 C+ MR in a teenager with diabetes insipidus (DI) shows a multifocal germinoma with masses in the pineal region ➡, infundibulum ➡, & genu/body of the corpus callosum ➡. This sort of multisite involvement is considered metastatic in the United States but synchronous in Canada & Europe.*

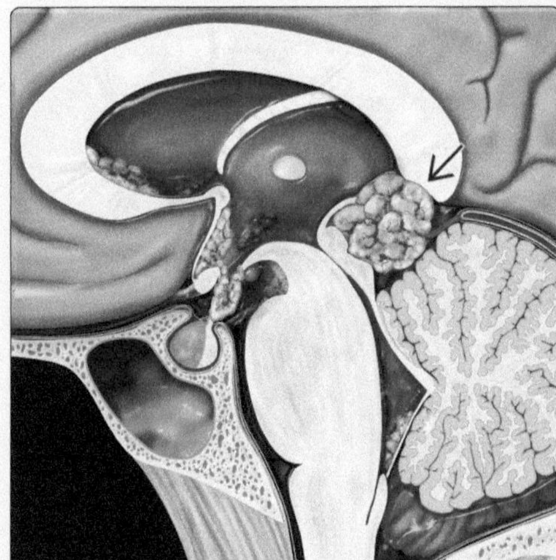

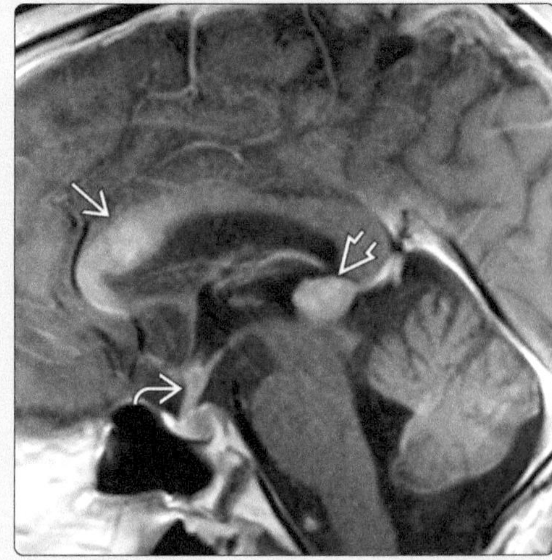

(Left) *Midline sagittal NECT in an 18-year-old man with DI shows a hyperdense mass ➡ centered on the pituitary infundibulum. The hyperdensity is a reflection of the ↑ cellularity of germinoma. Associated involvement of the pineal gland ➡ was seen on MR (not shown).* **(Right)** *Axial DWI MR in a 12-year-old boy with daily headaches & ↓ vision demonstrates hyperintense signal ➡ (↓ ADC not shown) within the solid portions of the mass, consistent with high tumor cellularity.*

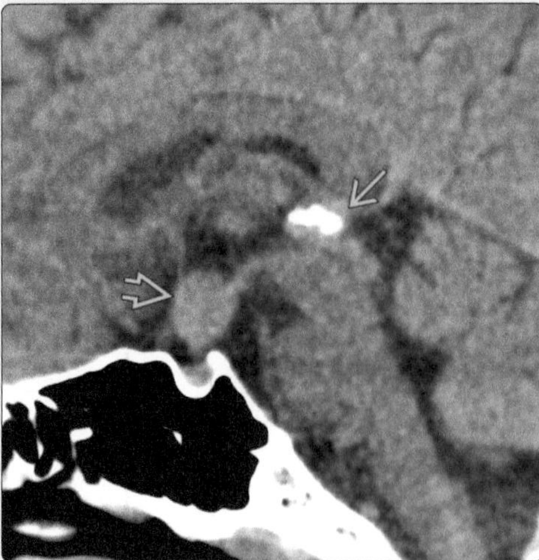

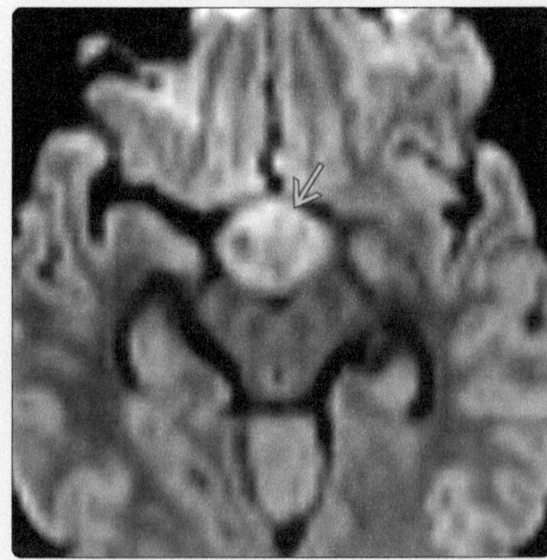

TERMINOLOGY

Definitions

- Tumor of primordial germ cells, essentially identical to gonadal or extragonadal seminoma & dysgerminoma

IMAGING

General Features

- Best diagnostic clue
  - Pineal mass with localized Ca^{++} & bithalamic extension
  - Suprasellar mass with diabetes insipidus (DI)
- Location
  - CNS germinomas typically occur in midline near 3rd ventricle
    - Pineal region (40-50%)
      - Majority (~ 80%) extend into bilateral thalami ± 3rd ventricle
      - Minority extend posteriorly into quadrigeminal plate cistern
    - Suprasellar (30-40%)
      - May have intrasellar, infundibular, &/or hypothalamic involvement
    - Basal ganglia (BG) tumors less common (5-15%)
    - Thalamic tumors rare
  - CSF spread of metastases common (25-40%)
- Size
  - Typically small (1-3 cm)
  - Tiny or inapparent suprasellar germinoma may cause DI
  - Relatively small pineal region germinoma may present with ventricular obstruction
  - BG tumors may be large at presentation
- Morphology
  - Often well delineated, lobular
  - Peritumoral edema common (~ 40%)
  - Invasive tumor more likely to recur after treatment

Radiographic Findings

- Radiography
  - Pineal Ca^{++} on skull radiographs before age 10: Not useful in CT era
    - Physiologic pineal Ca^{++} reported in children younger than 6 years of age

CT Findings

- Sharply circumscribed, heterogeneously hyperdense mass
  - Solid components usually hyperattenuating to gray matter (GM)
- Localized ("engulfed") Ca^{++} common in pineal tumors
  - Represent residual pineal gland Ca^{++}
  - Pineal parenchymal tumors more often have scattered ("exploded") Ca^{++}
- Ca^{++} rare in suprasellar tumors
- Hemorrhage uncommon, mostly seen in larger suprasellar & BG lesions
- Primary tumors & metastases usually enhance avidly

MR Findings

- **T1WI**: Isointense to hypointense
- **T2WI**: Hyperintense cystic components
- **FLAIR**: Sensitive for peritumoral edema
- **DWI**: Solid components typically show diffusion restriction
- **GRE/SWI**: Hypointense signal may represent Ca^{++} (pineal) or hemorrhage (suprasellar & BG)
- **T1 C+**: Most tumors show marked enhancement
  - Speckled pattern in tumors with small cysts
  - Most sensitive sequence for CSF metastases
- **PWI**: Lower cerebral blood flow (CBF) values compared to NGGCTs
- **MRS**: ↑ choline, ↓ NAA, ± lactate

Imaging Recommendations

- Best imaging tool
  - Contrast-enhanced MR of brain & spine
- Protocol advice
  - MR evaluation of entire neuraxis before surgery
  - Negative brain MR exam in child with DI does not exclude germinoma
    - Repeat study in 3-6 months to assess for growing suprasellar tumor
  - Optional brain sequences
    - Sagittal DWI, bSSFP (e.g., FIESTA)
    - ASL or other perfusion imaging

DIFFERENTIAL DIAGNOSIS

Pineal Region Masses

- Pineoblastoma
  - Highly cellular pineal mass in young child
  - Scattered ("exploded") Ca^{++} rather than localized ("engulfed") Ca^{++} in germinoma
  - Less common than germinoma & typically younger age
- Pineocytoma
  - Very uncommon in children
- Pineal cyst
  - Atypical features: > 1 cm, enhancement, ± tectal compression
  - Repeat imaging in 9-12 months to show stability if no other findings
- Tectal plate glioma
  - Little or no enhancement
  - Cysts rare
  - High ADC signal (no diffusion restriction)

Sellar/Suprasellar Masses

- Craniopharyngioma
  - Dominant cystic components ± T1 shortening, Ca^{++}
  - DI not usually present until after surgery
- Hypothalamic/chiasmatic astrocytoma
  - No diffusion restriction
  - Rarely associated with DI
- Langerhans cell histiocytosis (LCH)
  - Thickened infundibulum; look for osseous lesions
- Pituitary macroadenoma
  - Unlikely to cause DI
  - No normal pituitary tissue
- Hypothalamic hamartoma
  - Nonenhancing mass isointense to GM
  - Classic history: Gelastic seizures
- Teratoma
  - Intratumoral fat essentially pathognomonic

PATHOLOGY

General Features

- Etiology
  - Germ cell tumors (GCTs) found in gonads, mediastinum, & intracranial (parasellar & pineal) locations
    - Regions where primordial germ cells migrate during embryogenesis
  - Primordial germ cells persist & maldifferentiate into germinoma
- Genetics
  - ↑ risk of CNS germ cell neoplasms
    - Klinefelter syndrome (47 XXY)
      - Other sex chromosome aneuploidies
    - Cytogenetics
      - Alterations of chromosome 1 (1q21-qter region)
      - Overrepresentation of chromosome 12 (12p duplication)
    - Molecular genetics
      - *TP53* tumor suppressor gene mutations (exons 5-8)
      - *MDM2* gene amplification
- Associated abnormalities
  - ± ↑ serum & CSF human chorionic gonadotropin
    - Controversial whether HCG positivity affects prognosis
  - Other laboratory derangements
    - Elevated placental alkaline phosphatase

Staging, Grading, & Classification

- Involvement of multiple sites (pineal, suprasellar, BG, thalamus) considered metastatic in United States but synchronous in Canada & Europe

Gross Pathologic & Surgical Features

- Unencapsulated solid mass, soft & friable, tan-white coloration, ± cystic foci

Microscopic Features

- Sheets of large, polygonal primitive germ cells
  - Large vesicular nuclei & prominent nucleoli
  - Clear, glycogen-rich cytoplasm (PAS positive)
- Lymphocytic inflammatory component common

CLINICAL ISSUES

Presentation

- Most common signs/symptoms
  - Pineal region germinoma
    - Headache secondary to aqueduct obstruction & hydrocephalus
    - Parinaud syndrome (paralysis of upward gaze)
    - Ataxia
    - Precocious puberty
  - Suprasellar germinoma
    - DI
      - Can be present for extended period of time prior to MR abnormalities
    - Hypothalamic-pituitary dysfunction (↓ growth, precocious puberty)
    - Visual symptoms
  - BG
    - Pyramidal (e.g., Babinski) & extrapyramidal (e.g., dystonia, dyskinesia) symptoms
    - Headache

Demographics

- Age
  - Mean in most studies: 10-15 years
- Sex
  - M > F, especially in pineal region
- Ethnicity
  - CNS GCTs much more prevalent in Asia
    - 9-15% of all CNS tumors in Japan
    - BG & thalamic germinomas more common in Japan & Korea
- Epidemiology
  - 3-8% of pediatric CNS tumors
    - 9-15% of CNS tumors in Japanese children
  - 40% of pineal region neoplasms in children & young adults
  - 65-70% of all CNS GCTs

Natural History & Prognosis

- Pure germinoma has favorable prognosis
  - Very radiosensitive
- Treatment with radiotherapy ± adjuvant chemotherapy
  - 5-year survival > 90%

Treatment

- Biopsy to confirm histology; pure germinomas have best outcome

DIAGNOSTIC CHECKLIST

Image Interpretation Pearls

- Child or adolescent with DI
  - Expect absence of posterior pituitary "bright spot"
  - Lobular, enhancing suprasellar mass = germinoma
  - Thick, enhancing infundibulum = LCH or germinoma
  - No enhancing lesion = could be occult germinoma
- Adolescent with pineal mass = germinoma or nongerminomatous germ cell tumor (NGGCT)
- Child with pineal mass
  - Complex, cystic = also consider NGGCT
  - Homogeneous with restricted diffusion = germinoma vs. pineoblastoma

Reporting Tips

- Repeat MR imaging with contrast in 3-6 months in children with DI & no identified lesion

SELECTED REFERENCES

1. Kremenevski N et al: Intracranial germinomas: diagnosis, pathogenesis, clinical presentation, and management. Curr Oncol Rep. 25(7):765-75, 2023
2. Yang M et al: Update on MRI in pediatric intracranial germ cell tumors-The clinical and radiological features. Front Pediatr. 11:1141397, 2023
3. Takano M et al: Detecting non-germinomatous germ cell tumor component by arterial spin labeling perfusion-weighted MR imaging in central nervous system germ cell tumor. Eur J Radiol. 136:109523, 2021
4. Choudhri AF et al: Diffusion characteristics of pediatric pineal tumors. Neuroradiol J. 28(2):209-16, 2015
5. Awa R et al: Neuroimaging diagnosis of pineal region tumors-quest for pathognomonic finding of germinoma. Neuroradiology. 56(7):525-34, 2014

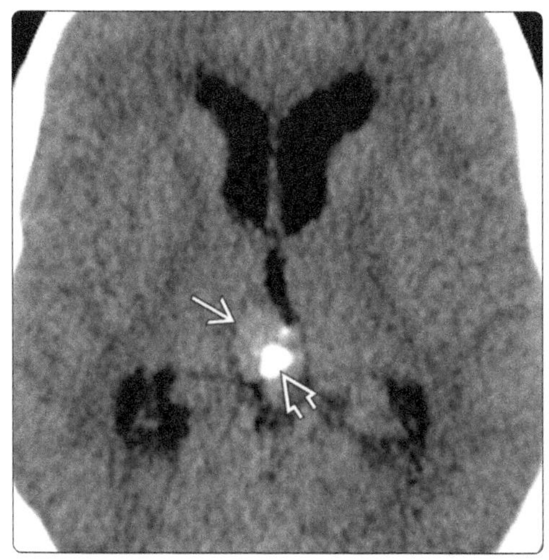

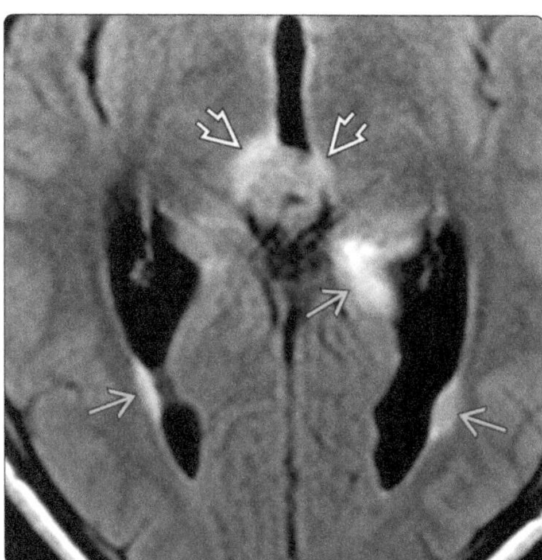

(Left) *Axial NECT in a 14-year-old boy with worsening headaches shows a hyperattenuating mass ➡ with localized calcifications ➡. Calcifications are common in a pineal germinoma & are thought to represent pineal calcifications "engulfed" by tumor.* **(Right)** *Axial FLAIR MR in the same patient shows parenchymal edema ➡ within the bilateral thalami (right > left). Peritumoral edema is a common finding (~ 40%) in a germinoma. Also note multiple ependymal metastases ➙, a common finding in a germinoma.*

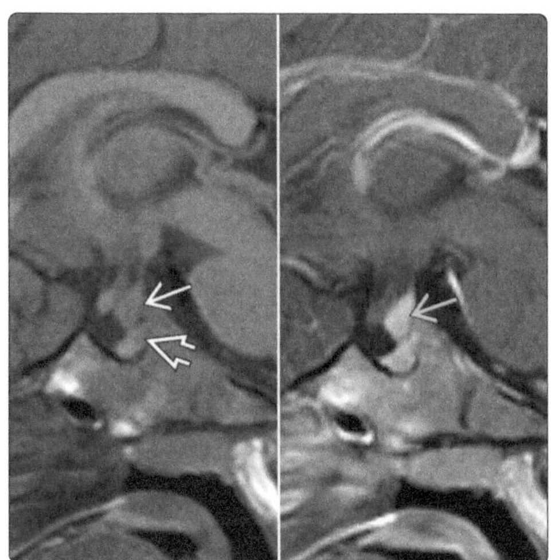

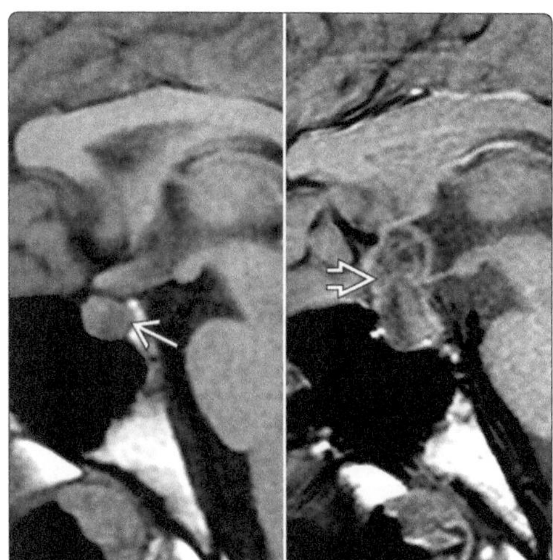

(Left) *Sagittal T1 C+ MR in a 4-year-old boy with central DI shows an infundibular mass ➡ & absence of the posterior pituitary "bright spot" ➡. After contrast, the mass enhances homogeneously ➙.* **(Right)** *Sagittal T1 MR in a 17-year-old boy with DI shows initial absence of the posterior pituitary "bright spot" ➡ with interval development of a large sellar & suprasellar mass ➡ 2 months later. Patients with DI & an absent posterior pituitary "bright spot" require follow-up imaging to detect an occult germinoma.*

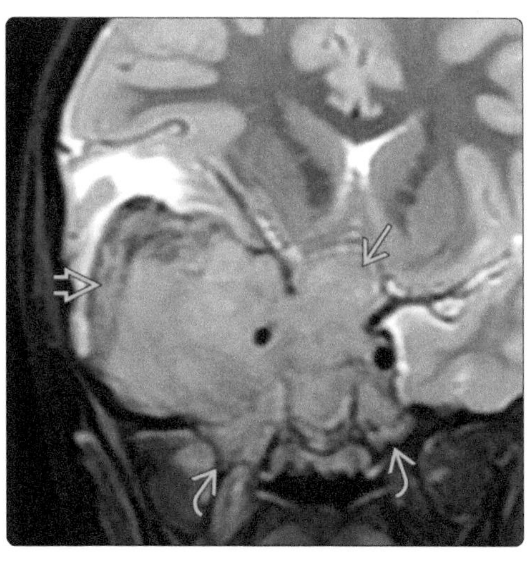

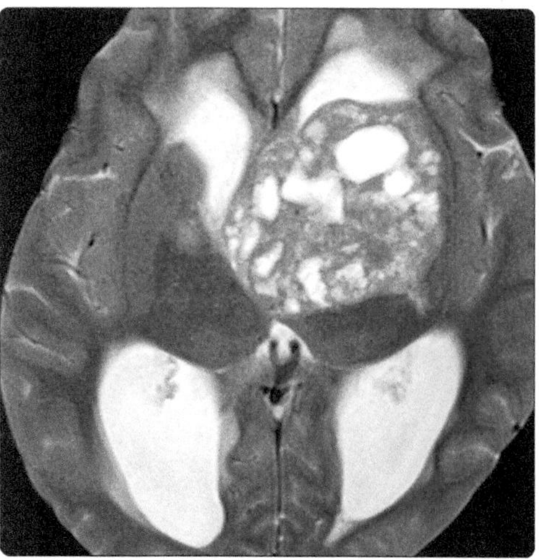

(Left) *Coronal T2 FS MR in a 9-year-old girl shows a large suprasellar mass ➙ with extension into the right middle cranial fossa ➙ with invasion of the skull base ➙. This is an atypical presentation, but germinoma should be considered in any skull base mass that involves the sella.* **(Right)** *Axial T2 MR in a 10-year-old girl with fatigue, headaches, & vomiting shows a large, solid, & cystic mass centered in the left basal ganglia. The basal ganglia is a less common (5-15%) location for a germinoma, & they are often large at presentation.*

KEY FACTS

TERMINOLOGY

- Teratoma: Nongerminomatous germ cell tumor
  - Arises from multipotential germ cells
  - Tridermic (contains tissues derived from all 3 germ cell layers)
- Types
  - Mature teratoma (most common; well differentiated)
  - Immature teratoma (some incompletely differentiated tissue)
  - Teratoma with malignant transformation

IMAGING

- NECT
  - Midline mass containing Ca^{++}, soft tissue, cysts, and fat
- T1WI
  - Fat → increased signal, Ca^{++} → variable signal
  - Soft tissue components iso- to hyperintense, enhancing
- T2WI: Decreased signal from Ca^{++}
- DWI: Restriction in solid (high cellular) parts
- Anatomic location indeterminate in 50%
  - Huge holocranial mass in newborns or fetus
  - Anatomic landmarks effaced
- Fetal US: Macrocephaly
  - Rapidly increasing mass, mixed hyper-, hypoechoic features

TOP DIFFERENTIAL DIAGNOSES

- Germinoma
- Other nongerminomatous germ cell tumor
- Primitive neuroectodermal tumors; atypical teratoid/rhabdoid tumor
- Dermoid; craniopharyngioma

CLINICAL ISSUES

- Often detected in utero or as neonate
- M:F = 4:1

DIAGNOSTIC CHECKLIST

- If newborn with holocranial tumor, think teratoma

(Left) *Sagittal graphic shows a heterogeneous pineal teratoma with the characteristic 3 tissue types: Solid/cystic tissue ⇨, Ca^{++} ⇨, and fat ⇨. When all 3 tissue types are present in a mass, this is consistent with a teratoma, especially when located in the pineal or suprasellar regions.* **(Right)** *Sagittal gross pathology section shows a pineal teratoma with solid ⇨ and fatty ⇨ elements. Ca^{++} glioma are more difficult to see on this gross specimen but were present. (Courtesy B. Alvord, MD.)*

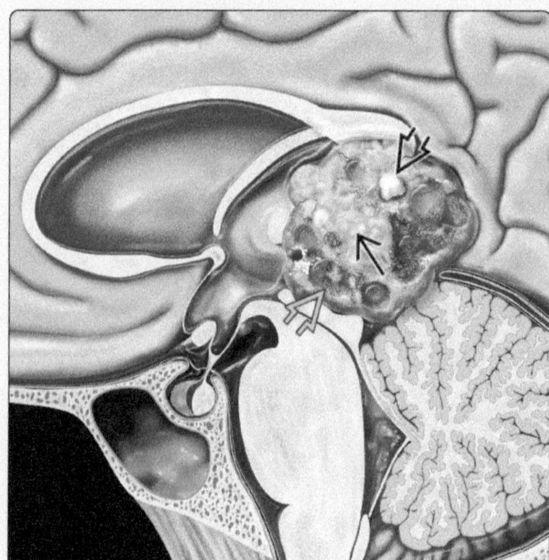

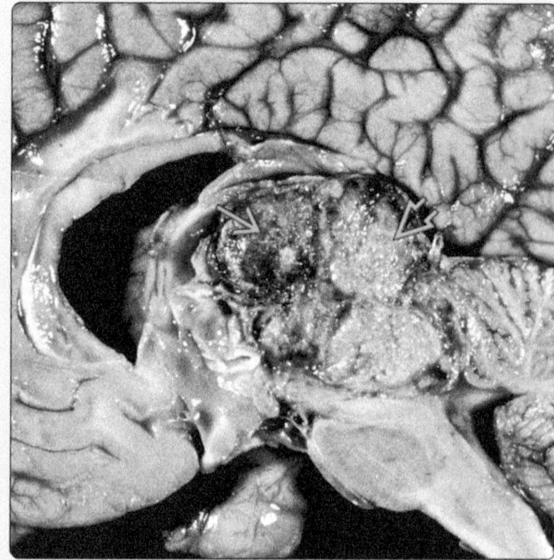

(Left) *Sagittal NECT in a 7-year-old boy shows all 3 characteristic tissue components of a mature teratoma: Fat ⇨, Ca^{++} ⇨, and soft tissue ⇨. These 3 components are often best demonstrated on CT.* **(Right)** *Axial T1 MR pre- (left) and post (right) contrast images in the same patient show the hyperintense fat ⇨ as well as enhancing soft tissue ⇨. A solid enhancing soft tissue component is common in teratomas and is helpful to distinguish from a lipoma and dermoid cyst.*

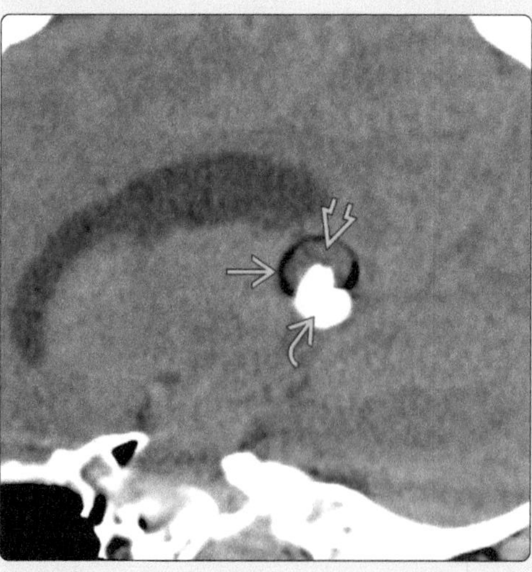

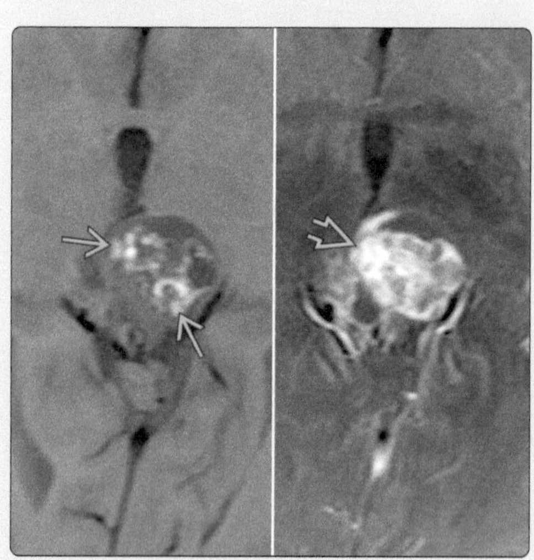

TERMINOLOGY

Definitions

- Teratoma: Nongerminomatous germ cell tumor (NGGCT)
  - Arises from multipotential germ cells
  - Tridermic (contains tissues derived from all 3 germ cell layers)
- Types
  - Mature teratoma (most common; well differentiated)
  - Immature teratoma (some incompletely differentiated tissue)
  - Teratoma with malignant transformation

IMAGING

General Features

- Best diagnostic clue
  - Midline mass containing Ca^{++}, soft tissue, cysts, fat
  - Huge holocranial mass in newborn or fetus
- Location
  - Midline
    - Pineal gland
      - Tectum, mesencephalon commonly involved
    - Sellar/suprasellar
      - Hypothalamus, optic chiasm
      - Less common: Parasellar (cavernous sinuses or mesial middle cranial fossa)
    - Basal ganglia, thalami
    - Spine (thoracolumbar junction)
  - Rare locations
    - Brain hemispheres
    - Ventricles
    - ~ 50% so large that anatomic origin indeterminate
- Size
  - Variable; infantile teratomas often huge (holocranial)

CT Findings

- NECT
  - Fat, soft tissue, Ca^{++}
  - Cystic components common
  - Often large (may fill entire cranium)
- CECT
  - Soft tissue components enhance
- Bone CT
  - Look for tooth-like configuration of Ca^{++}

MR Findings

- T1WI
  - Increased signal from fat
  - Variable signal from Ca^{++}
- T2WI
  - Soft tissue components iso- to hyperintense
  - Perifocal edema
    - Usually minimal or absent (mature teratoma)
    - Common in immature (malignant) teratoma
- FLAIR
  - ↓ signal from cysts, ↑ signal from solid tissue
- T2* GRE
  - ↓ signal from Ca^{++}
- DWI
  - Restricted diffusion in solid (high cellular) parts
  - Useful in differentiating high- vs. low-grade neoplasms for large, bulky supratentorial tumors in 1st year of life
    - ADC values negatively correlated with tumor grade
- PWI
  - NGGCTs (including teratomas) have higher cerebral blood flow values on ASL compared to pure germinomas
- T1WI C+
  - Soft tissue enhancement
- Fetal MR
  - Extremely heterogeneous mass containing fat, fluid, bone, and soft tissue
  - Usually midline, may fill and expand cranium
  - When small, often midline
    - Suprasellar vs. pineal region vs. 4th ventricle

Ultrasonographic Findings

- Neonates: Heterogeneous mass with internal shadowing (Ca^{++})
- Fetal ultrasound
  - Intracranial mass (often huge)
  - Hydrocephalus, polyhydramnios

Imaging Recommendations

- Best imaging tool
  - CT to demonstrate soft tissue, fat, Ca^{++}
  - MR best characterizes relationship of teratoma to midline structures
- Protocol advice
  - MR ± fat suppression
  - Optional brain sequences
    - Sagittal DWI, bSSFP (e.g., FIESTA)
    - Perfusion imaging (e.g., ASL)

DIFFERENTIAL DIAGNOSIS

Germinoma

- More homogeneous appearance compared to teratoma
- More cellular appearing on DWI (lower ADC values)

Other Nongerminomatous Germ Cell Tumor

- Includes embryonal carcinoma, yolk sac tumor, choriocarcinoma, mixed germ cell tumor
- Heterogeneous suprasellar or pineal mass

Craniopharyngioma

- Cystic and solid, Ca^{++}

Dermoid

- Minimal/no enhancement
- Ca^{++} common
- Look for rupture with fat "droplets"

Pineoblastoma

- Large pineal mass with "exploded" Ca^{++}
- Hydrocephalus present in 100%

Supratentorial Primitive Neuroectodermal Tumor

- Ca^{++}, hemorrhage, necrosis common
- Does not contain fat

Atypical Teratoid/Rhabdoid Tumor

- Large, bulky atypical teratoid/rhabdoid tumor in newborn difficult to distinguish

Astrocytoma

- Newborn glioblastoma can be large, bulky, very heterogeneous

Lipoma

- Contains fat, Ca^{++} but no soft tissue component
- Uncommon in suprasellar location

PATHOLOGY

General Features

- Etiology
  - Originates during 3rd or 4th week of fetal development
  - Anomalous development of primitive streak or its derivatives
- Genetics
  - Gains of hypomethylated, active X chromosomes occur in all intracranial germ cell tumors (ICGCTs)
- Associated abnormalities
  - Increased serum CEA
  - Increased α-fetoprotein if tumor contains enteric glandular elements (yolk sac cells)

Staging, Grading, & Classification

- WHO classification
  - Mature teratoma (WHO grade 1)
  - Immature teratoma
  - Teratoma with malignant transformation (TMT)
    - Usually arises from immature teratoma
    - Contains somatic-type cancers (e.g., rhabdomyosarcoma)

Gross Pathologic & Surgical Features

- Mature teratomas → fully differentiated tissue
  - Cystic component frequent in mature teratoma
- Immature or malignant teratoma → resembles fetal tissues
- Teratomas may be part of mixed tumors with germinomas or nongerminomatous ICGCTs

Microscopic Features

- Contain elements representing 3 germinal layers
  - Ectoderm
  - Mesoderm
  - Endoderm

CLINICAL ISSUES

Presentation

- Most common signs/symptoms
  - Macrocephaly → congenital teratoma
  - Parinaud syndrome → pineal lesions
- Other signs/symptoms
  - Increased serum CEA
- Clinical profile
  - In utero demonstration of hydrocephalus, macrocephaly, and heterogeneous mass
  - Congenital teratomas
    - Diffuse intracranial form: Large tumors replacing intracranial content
    - Small tumors causing hydrocephalus
    - Massive form: Extension in orbits, pharynx, neck

Demographics

- Age
  - Average age at diagnosis: 5 years
  - Range: Newborn to 6th decade
  - Often detected in utero or as neonate
- Sex
  - M > F
- Ethnicity
  - More common among Asian patients
- Epidemiology
  - 2-4% of intracranial tumors in children
  - Leading perinatal brain tumor (42%)

Natural History & Prognosis

- 5-year survival for malignant teratomas: 18%
- Congenital teratoma
  - May be seen on fetal ultrasound or MR
  - Majority stillborn or die within 1st week of life
- Lowest survival rate of all fetal brain tumors
- Pineal mature teratomas have good prognosis
- CSF metastases common in malignant (immature) teratoma

Treatment

- Surgical removal
  - Operative mortality in 1st year: 20%

DIAGNOSTIC CHECKLIST

Consider

- Think teratoma in newborn with holocranial tumor
- Heterogeneous midline mass, young age, male predominance, pineal preferential location

Image Interpretation Pearls

- Midline tumor predominantly in sellar and pineal region containing fat, soft tissue, and Ca^{++}

SELECTED REFERENCES

1. Yang M et al: Update on MRI in pediatric intracranial germ cell tumors- the clinical and radiological features. Front Pediatr. 11:1141397, 2023
2. Frappaz D et al: EANO, SNO and Euracan consensus review on the current management and future development of intracranial germ cell tumors in adolescents and young adults. Neuro Oncol. 24(4):516-27, 2022
3. Morana G et al: Imaging response assessment for CNS germ cell tumours: consensus recommendations from the European Society for Paediatric Oncology Brain Tumour Group and North American Children's Oncology Group. Lancet Oncol. 23(5):e218-28, 2022
4. Takano M et al: Detecting non-germinomatous germ cell tumor component by arterial spin labeling perfusion-weighted MR imaging in central nervous system germ cell tumor. Eur J Radiol. 136:109523, 2021
5. Venkatasai J et al: A pragmatic diagnostic approach to primary intracranial germ cell tumors and their treatment outcomes. CNS Oncol. 10(4):CNS79, 2021
6. Abdelmuhdi AS et al: Intracranial teratoma: imaging, intraoperative, and pathologic features: AIRP best cases in radiologic-pathologic correlation. Radiographics. 37(5):1506-11, 2017
7. Lagman C et al: Teratomas of the cranial vault: a systematic analysis of clinical outcomes stratified by histopathological subtypes. Acta Neurochir (Wien). 159(3):423-33, 2017
8. Robles Fradejas M et al: Fetal intracranial immature teratoma: presentation of a case and a systematic review of the literature. J Matern Fetal Neonatal Med. 1-8, 2016
9. Zygourakis CC et al: Management of central nervous system teratoma. J Clin Neurosci. 22(1):98-104, 2015
10. Kralik SF et al: Diffusion imaging for tumor grading of supratentorial brain tumors in the first year of life. AJNR Am J Neuroradiol. 35(4):815-23, 2014
11. Bohara M et al: Mature posterior fossa teratoma mimicking dermoid cyst. Brain Tumor Pathol. 30(4):262-5, 2013

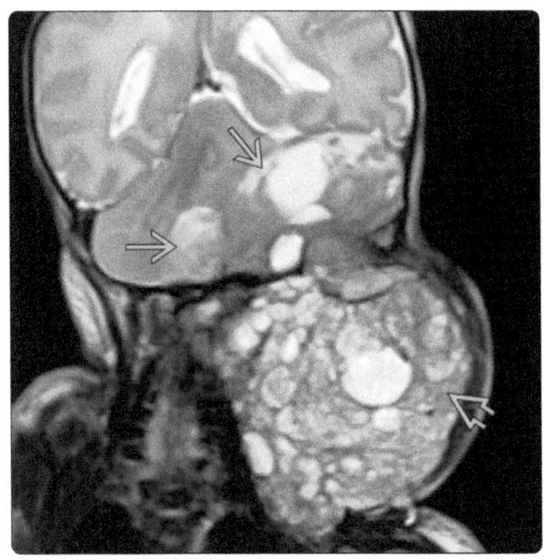

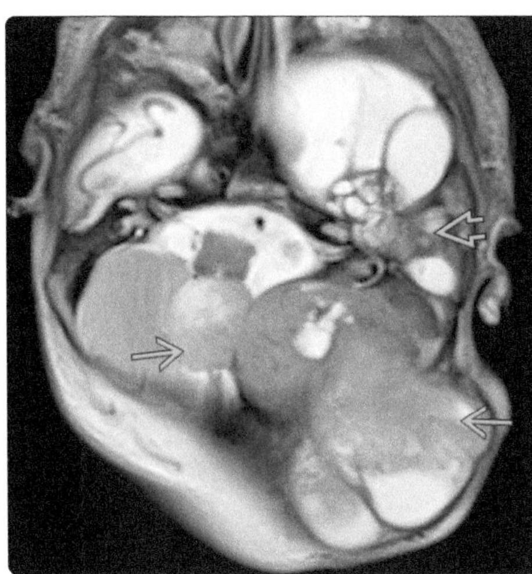

(Left) *Coronal T2WI MR in a neonate with a teratoma shows a mixed solid and cystic mass with a very large extracranial component ⇨ in the left neck and a large intracranial component ⇨, which exerts significant mass effect on the brain.* **(Right)** *Axial T2WI MR in the same patient shows the large size of the intracranial ⇨ and left temporal bone ⇨ components of the mass. It is not uncommon for teratomas to have both extracranial and intracranial components, as in this case. (Courtesy A. Carl Merrow, MD.)*

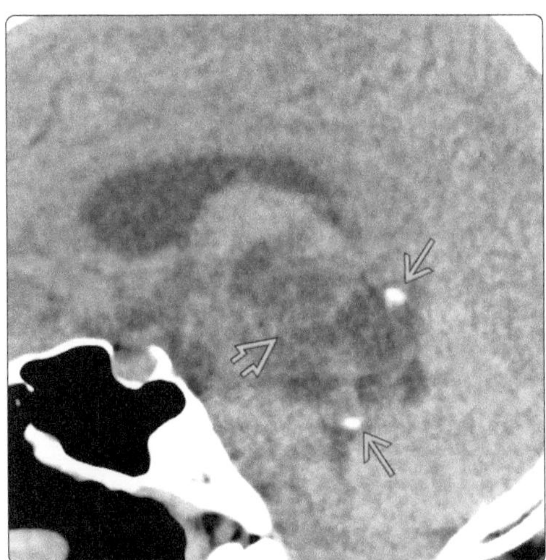

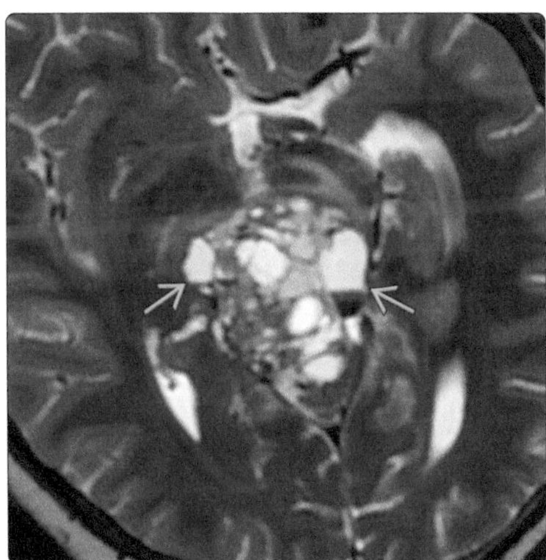

(Left) *Sagittal NECT in a 13-year-old with an immature teratoma shows a heterogeneously mixed solid and cystic mass ⇨ with scattered Ca^{++} ⇨ peripherally.* **(Right)** *Axial T2WI MR in the same patient shows the complexity of this mass lesion with multiple cystic components with fluid-fluid levels ⇨. Complex pineal region masses such as this should suggest nongerminomatous germ cell tumors, which includes teratomas.*

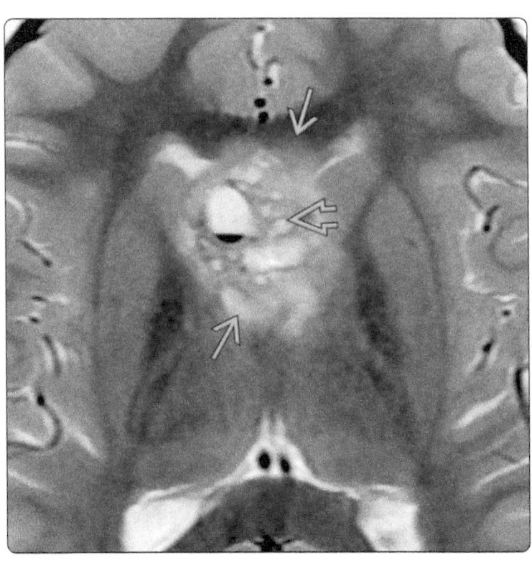

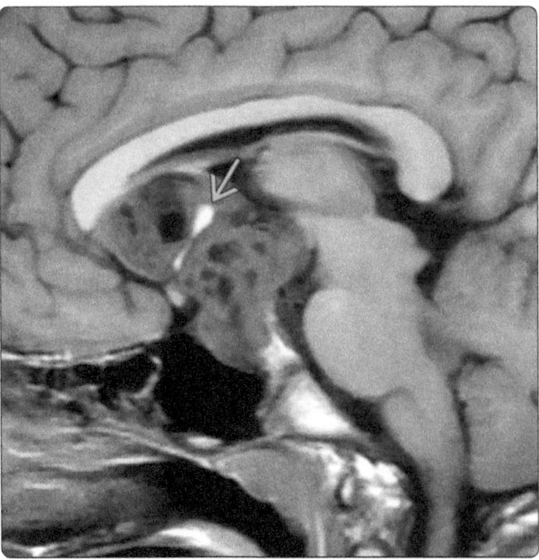

(Left) *Axial T2WI MR in a 6-year-old girl with a mature cystic teratoma shows a mixed solid and cystic suprasellar lesion ⇨ with adjacent edema ⇨ in the basal ganglia and corpus callosum.* **(Right)** *Sagittal T1WI MR in the same patient shows that the mass involves the sella and suprasellar regions. There is a T1-hyperintense area within the lesion, consistent with fat ⇨. The presence of fat would favor a mature teratoma, although immature elements may be present and may only be identified histologically.*

KEY FACTS

TERMINOLOGY

- Malignant tumor of sympathetic nervous system arising from embryonal neural crest cell derivatives

IMAGING

- Classic imaging appearance
  - "Hair on end" spiculated periostitis of orbits and skull ± bone destruction
- Cranial metastases
  - Nearly always extradural, calvarial-based mass
- Brain metastases rare
  - ↑ prevalence with improved treatment protocols, stage IV metastatic disease
  - Most parenchymal neuroblastoma mets supratentorial, hemorrhagic

TOP DIFFERENTIAL DIAGNOSES

- Leukemia
- Langerhans cell histiocytosis (LCH)
- Extraaxial hematoma
- Ewing sarcoma

PATHOLOGY

- Calvarial metastases indicate stage IV disease
  - 60-75% < 1-year survival
  - 15% > 1-year survival despite aggressive treatment

CLINICAL ISSUES

- Most common solid extracranial tumor in children < 5 years
- Most common tumor in neonates/infants < 1 month (congenital)
  - Ophthalmic manifestation in 20-55%
    - Proptosis and "raccoon eyes"
- Metastasis to bone most common (2/3 of patients at diagnosis)

DIAGNOSTIC CHECKLIST

- CT without contrast can help identify bone spicules, eliminating LCH from differential

(Left) *Coronal NECT in a child with an abdominal mass reveals orbital, facial bone, and calvarial spiculated periostitis giving rise to a hair on end appearance ➡ with associated large soft tissue masses. Note bilateral disease ⮚. Metastatic stage IV neuroblastoma typically involves the skull and bony orbits.* **(Right)** *Axial NECT in the same patient shows the hair on end appearance. Involvement of the orbits often gives rise to proptosis and ecchymosis "raccoon eyes," which may be mistaken for abuse.*

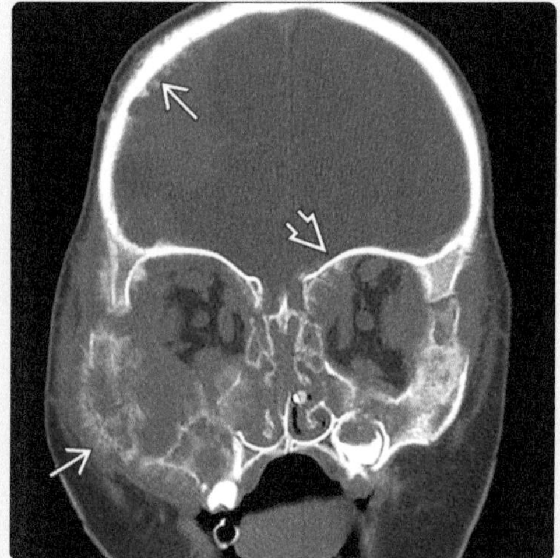

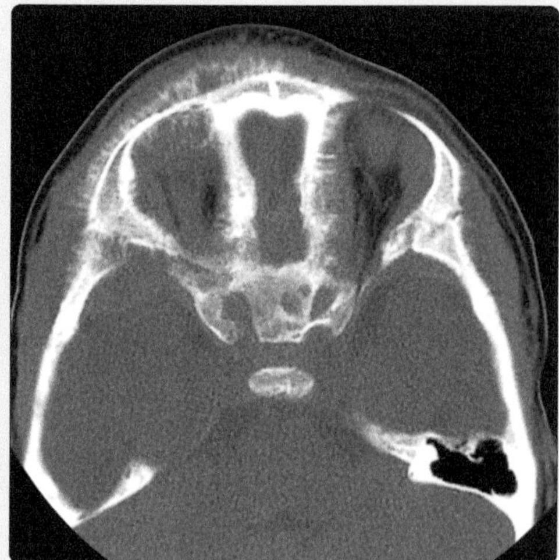

(Left) *Axial CECT in a 2-year-old boy with neuroblastoma shows strong, heterogeneously enhancing epidural masses ➡ with mass effect and edema in the frontal lobe.* **(Right)** *Cephalad CECT in the same patient shows strongly enhancing epidural masses ➡. Irregularity of overlying skull ⮚ indicates calvarial involvement. Intracranial involvement in neuroblastoma is typically from adjacent calvarial metastases with dural invasion. Brain parenchymal metastases are rare.*

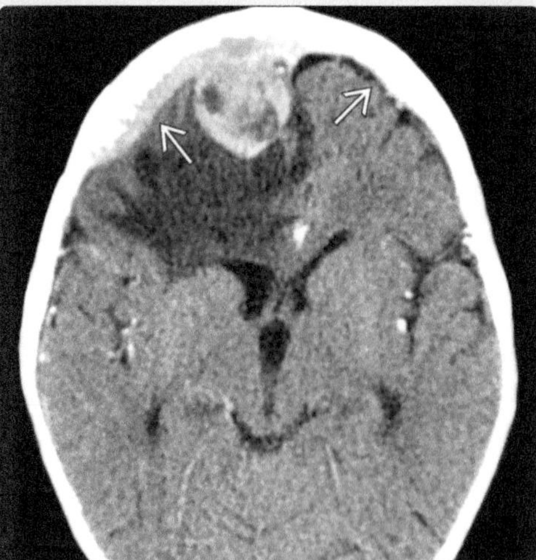

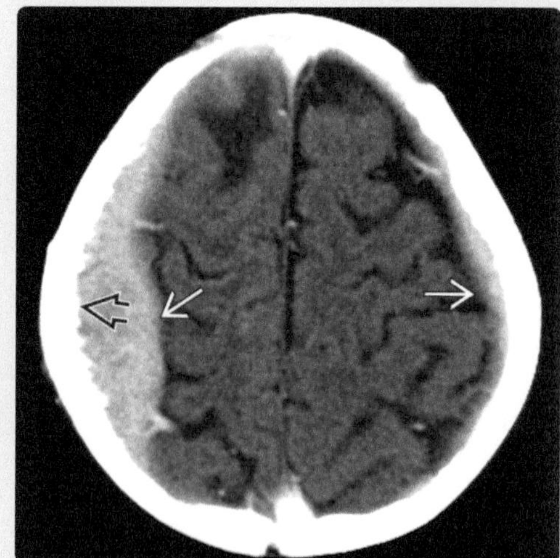

TERMINOLOGY

Abbreviations

- Neuroblastoma (NB)

Definitions

- Malignant tumor of sympathetic nervous system arising from embryonal neural crest cell derivatives

IMAGING

General Features

- Best diagnostic clue
  - Spiculated periorbital bone mass causing proptosis in child with "raccoon eyes"
- Location
  - Cranial metastases nearly always extradural calvarial-based masses
    - Calvarium, orbit, skull base
  - Brain metastases rare but ↑ with improved treatment protocols, stage IV metastatic disease
    - CNS NB is sole site of disease recurrence in 64% of high-risk patients
    - CNS may represent "sanctuary site" for NB
    - Most parenchymal NB metastases supratentorial, hemorrhagic
    - Leptomeningeal, intraventricular lesions also occur
- Classic imaging appearance: "Hair on end" spiculated periostitis of orbits and skull ± bony destruction

CT Findings

- NECT
  - Best for showing fine spicules of periosteal bone projecting off skull or sphenoid wings
  - Soft tissue mass typically iso- to hyperdense to brain
    - May mimic epidural or subdural hematoma
  - Mass projects into orbit (extraconal) with extension to surrounding spaces not preseptal space
  - May project through inner and outer tables of skull
- CECT
  - Enhancing dural metastasis if intracranial
  - Rare ring-enhancing brain parenchymal metastasis

MR Findings

- T1WI
  - Slightly heterogeneous
  - Hypointense to muscle
- T2WI
  - Heterogeneous
  - Hypointense to brain
  - Slightly hyperintense to muscle
- FLAIR: Heterogeneous; hyperintense to muscle
- T1WI C+: Vigorously enhances, may be heterogeneous

Nuclear Medicine Findings

- Bone scan
  - MIBG
    - Catecholamine analog
    - Labeled with iodine-131 or iodine-123
    - Avid uptake by neural crest tumors
      - NB, ganglioneuroblastoma, ganglioneuroma, carcinoid, medullary thyroid carcinoma
    - 99% specific for neuroblastic tumors (NBTs)
    - Caveat: Up to 30% of NB not MIBG positive
      - Misses 50% of recurrent tumors
    - Cannot distinguish marrow disease from bone disease
  - Tc-99m-MDP (methylene diphosphonate)
    - ↑ uptake from calcium metabolism of tumor not specific to neural crest tissue
    - 74% sensitivity for bony metastases
    - May distinguish marrow from bone disease
    - Bone scan essential for differentiating stage IV disease from stage IV-S in children < 1 year
  - In111 pentetreotide
    - Somatostatin analog
    - Not specific to NBT; not superior to MIBG
- PET
  - FDG PET has shown high sensitivity and specificity for recurrent tumor in small numbers of cases
  - FDG PET may identify recurrence when MIBG negative due to dedifferentiation

Imaging Recommendations

- Best imaging tool
  - CT/MR to evaluate primary tumor
  - Nuclear medicine MIBG & Tc-99m MDP bone scan
  - Brain/orbit CT if scintigraphy indicates metastases

DIFFERENTIAL DIAGNOSIS

Leukemia

- Dural- or calvarial-based masses
- More frequent parenchymal masses
- Less heterogeneous on MR

Langerhans Cell Histiocytosis

- Lytic bone lesions without periosteal new bone
- Often associated with diabetes insipidus

Extraaxial Hematoma

- Subdural or epidural hematoma
- Bleeding disorder or child abuse to be considered

Ewing Sarcoma

- < 1% of cases involve skull
- Aggressive bone destruction
- Spiculated periosteal reaction

Osteosarcoma

- Rarely primary in calvarium

Rhabdomyosarcoma

- Most common soft tissue malignancy of pediatric orbit
- Less likely bilateral; may invade preseptal space

Beta Thalassemia Major

- Classic "hair on end" calvarial expansion
- Not focal or destructive like NB

PATHOLOGY

General Features

- Etiology
  - Arises from pathologically maturing neural crest progenitor cells

- Primary tumors arise at sites of sympathetic ganglia
- No known causative factor
- Genetics
  - Multiple gene loci associated with NB: 1p, 4p, 2p, 12p, 16p, 17q
    - *Myc-N* oncogene (chromosome 2) important marker
    - 35% have chromosome 1 short arm deletion
  - 1-2% of cases inherited
- Associated abnormalities
  - Rarely associated with Beckwith-Wiedemann syndrome, neurofibromatosis type 1
  - Some association with neurocristopathy syndromes
    - Hirschsprung disease, congenital central hypoventilation, DiGeorge syndrome

Staging, Grading, & Classification

- Calvarial metastases indicate M stage disease (formerly stage IV)
- International Neuroblastoma Risk Group Staging System (INRGSS)
  - Developed to establish consensus approach for pretreatment risk stratification
    - L1: Localized tumor not involving vital structures as defined by list of image-defined risk factors and confined to 1 body compartment
    - L2: Locoregional tumor with presence of ≥ 1 image-defined risk factors
    - M: Distant metastatic disease (except stage MS)
    - MS: Metastatic disease in children < 18 months old with metastases confined to skin, liver, &/or bone marrow

Gross Pathologic & Surgical Features

- Grayish-tan soft nodules
- Infiltrating or circumscribed without capsule
- Necrosis, hemorrhage, and calcifications variable

Microscopic Features

- Undifferentiated round blue cells with scant cytoplasm, hyperchromatic nuclei
- May form Homer Wright rosettes
- Ganglioneuroblastoma has interspersed mature ganglion cells
  - Different regions of same tumor may have ganglioneuroblastoma or NB

CLINICAL ISSUES

Presentation

- Most common signs/symptoms
  - "Raccoon eyes" (periorbital ecchymosis)
  - Palpable calvarial masses
- Other signs/symptoms
  - Palpable abdominal or paraspinal mass
  - Cranial metastatic disease rarely occurs in isolation
- Clinical profile
  - Ophthalmic manifestation in 20-55% at presentation
    - Proptosis and "raccoon eyes," 50% bilateral
    - Horner syndrome
    - Opsoclonus, myoclonus, and ataxia
      - Myoclonic encephalopathy of infancy
      - Paraneoplastic syndrome (not metastatic)
      - Up to 2-4% of NB patients; more favorable prognosis
  - Elevated vasoactive intestinal peptides (VIP)
    - Up to 7% of NBT patients
    - Diarrhea, hypokalemia, achlorhydria
  - Elevated homovanillic acid and vanillylmandelic acid in urine (> 90%)

Demographics

- Age
  - Median at diagnosis: 22 months
  - 40% diagnosed by 1 year
  - 35% between 1-2 years
  - 25% > 2 years
  - 89% by 5 years
- Epidemiology
  - Most common solid extracranial tumor in patients < 5 years
  - 8-10% of all childhood cancers
  - Most common tumor in patients < 1 month (congenital)
  - Metastasis to bone most common (2/3 of patients at diagnosis)
  - 1-2% spontaneously regress in 6-12 months, mostly stage IV-S
  - NB is most common and aggressive of NBTs

Natural History & Prognosis

- Stages I, II, and IV-S have 3-year event-free survival (EFS) of 75-90%
- Stage III: < 1 year old (80-90%) 1-year EFS; > 1 year old (50%) 3-year EFS
- Stage IV: < 1 year old (60-75%) 1-year EFS; > 1 year old (15%) 3-year EFS
- Poor prognostic indicators: Deletion of 1p, translocation of 17q, *Myc-N* amplification
- Good prognostic indicators: Localized disease, stage IV-S, decreased *Myc-N* amplification

Treatment

- Surgical resection + chemotherapy, radiation, proton beam therapy
- Bone marrow transplant
- Stage IV-S may spontaneously regress

DIAGNOSTIC CHECKLIST

Consider

- Abdominal imaging to identify primary tumor site

Image Interpretation Pearls

- CT without contrast can help identify bone spicules, eliminating Langerhans cell histiocytosis from differential

SELECTED REFERENCES

1. Liu S et al: Metastasis pattern and prognosis in children with neuroblastoma. World J Surg Oncol. 21(1):130, 2023
2. Khoei S et al: An atypical imaging characteristic of calvarial metastasis of neuroblastoma as multiple multi-loculated cystic masses with internal blood-fluid levels: a case report. BMC Neurol. 22(1):471, 2022
3. Del Campo Braojos F et al: Practical application of the International Neuroblastoma Risk Group Staging System: a pictorial review. Curr Probl Diagn Radiol. 48(5):509-18, 2019
4. Monclair T et al: The International Neuroblastoma Risk Group (INRG) staging system: an INRG Task Force report. J Clin Oncol. 27(2):298-303, 2009

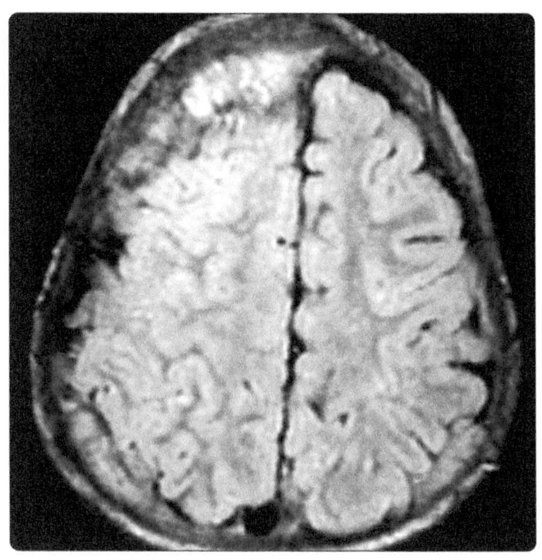

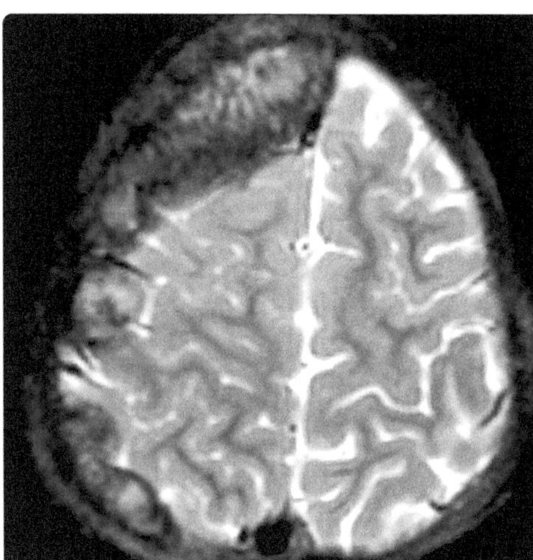

(Left) *Axial FLAIR MR shows heterogeneous signal in a patient with extradural metastatic neuroblastoma. Little reactive change is seen in the underlying brain parenchyma despite significant mass effect.* **(Right)** *Axial T2WI MR in the same patient shows a heterogeneous and hypointense signal in this metastatic neuroblastoma. T2 hypointensity is characteristic of densely cellular masses with high nuclear:cytoplasmic ratio.*

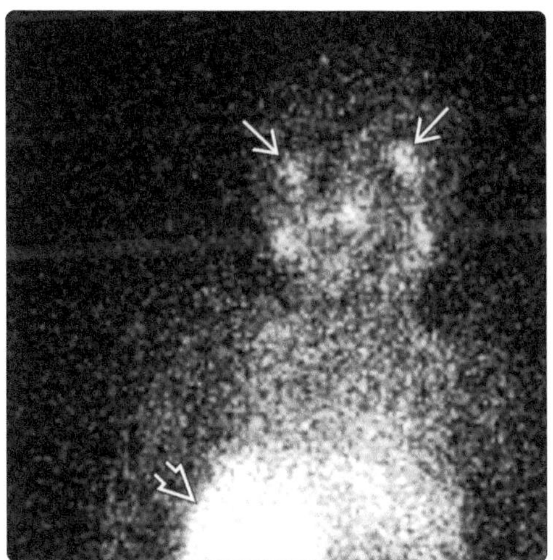

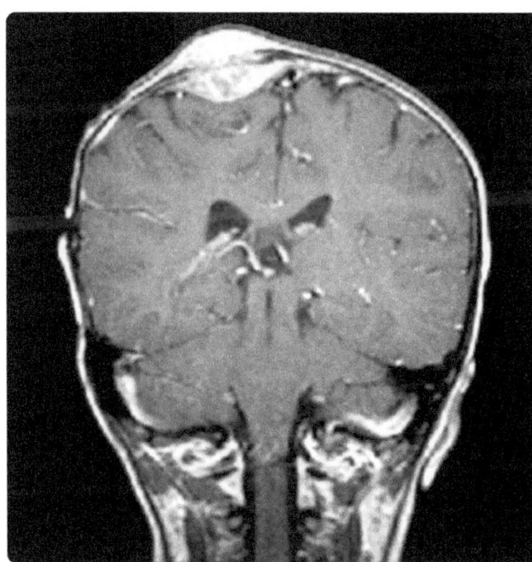

(Left) *Coronal I-123-labeled MIBG scan shows areas of increased uptake in the orbits ➔ related to neuroblastoma metastases. Note the large area of uptake in the right abdomen from the primary tumor ➔. Although MIBG scanning is highly specific for neuroblastic tumors, up to 30% of primary and 50% of recurrent neuroblastomas do not take up MIBG.* **(Right)** *Coronal T1WI C+ MR shows an enhancing convexity mass centered at the diploic space with subperiosteal and epidural components in a child with neuroblastoma.*

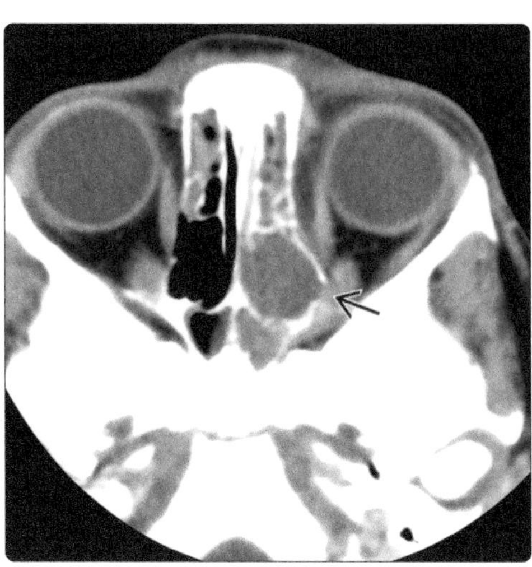

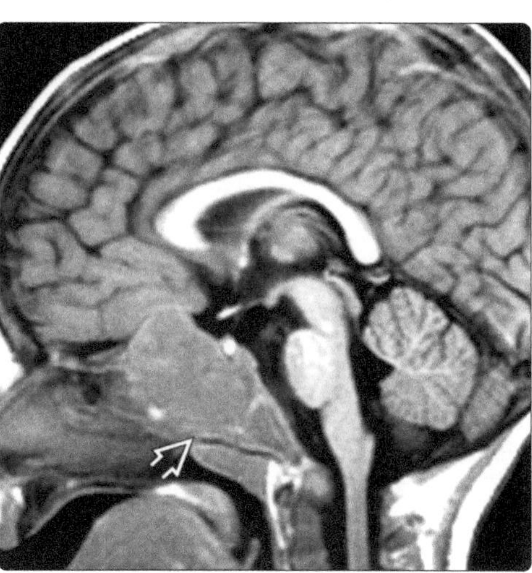

(Left) *Axial NECT in a child with neuroblastoma shows an ethmoid mass. There is a small focus of bony erosion ➔ suggesting the correct diagnosis of neuroblastoma metastasis.* **(Right)** *Sagittal T1WI MR shows a mildly heterogeneous, large, central skull base mass ➔ with marked expansion of the clivus in this 2-year-old with stage IV neuroblastoma. Imaging mimics other malignancies. Neuroblastoma metastases most commonly involve the calvariae or orbital region.*

Leukemia, Brain

KEY FACTS

TERMINOLOGY

- Extramedullary leukemic tumors; synonyms: Myeloid sarcoma, granulocytic sarcoma, chloroma
- Multiple other intracranial manifestations, complications of leukemia/treatment
  - Posterior reversible encephalopathy syndrome, invasive fungal infection
  - Late development of cavernous angiomas after radiation therapy
  - Posttransplantation lymphoproliferative disease after bone marrow transplantation
  - Venous thrombosis associated with chemotherapy

IMAGING

- Homogeneous enhancing tumor(s) in patients with known or suspected myeloproliferative disorder
- Cellular tumors: ↑ DWI/↓ ADC
- May present with/mimic hematoma
- Meningeal (dural-based or pial) > intraparenchymal lesions
- May present as primarily osseous lesions (e.g., diffuse calvarial involvement)

TOP DIFFERENTIAL DIAGNOSES

- Metastatic neuroblastoma; meningioma
- Extraaxial hematoma; extramedullary hematopoiesis
- Langerhans cell histiocytosis
- Rhabdomyosarcoma

PATHOLOGY

- CNS leukemia presents in 3 forms
  - Meningeal disease (usually with acute lymphoblastic leukemia)
  - Intravascular aggregates (leukostasis): Can rupture, hemorrhage with markedly ↑ leukocyte counts
  - Tumor masses (myeloid sarcoma)

DIAGNOSTIC CHECKLIST

- Hemorrhagic lesions in children with AML may represent myeloid sarcoma **or** complication of therapy

(Left) *Coronal graphic shows multiple leukemic infiltrates in the skull base/paranasal sinuses, hypothalamus/infundibulum, basal ganglia, and dura. The green color observed at pathology results in the name chloroma. The most common term now is myeloid sarcoma.* **(Right)** *Coronal T1WI C+ MR shows an enhancing myeloid sarcoma with a dural tail. Imaging signs of a high cellularity (e.g., diffusion restriction) should be looked for to differentiate from other dural-based lesions.*

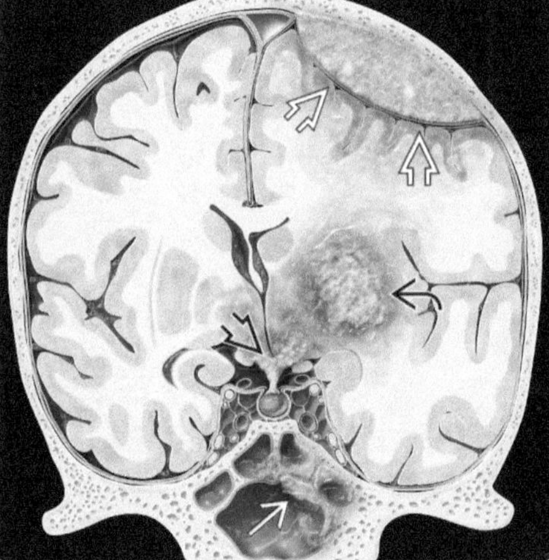

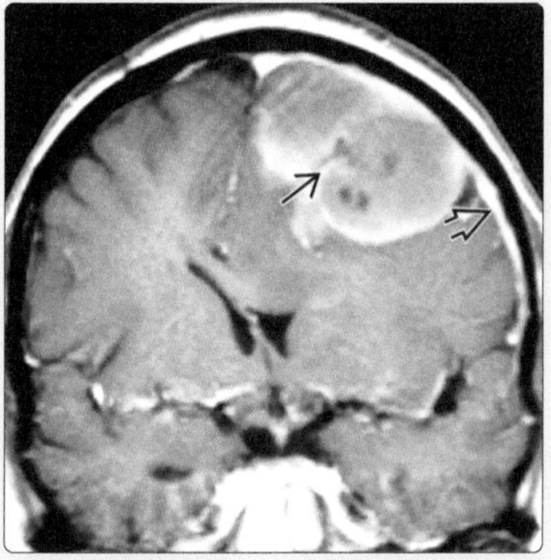

(Left) *Axial T2WI (left) and T1WI C+ (right) MR in 13-year-old with right parietooccipital chloroma show enhancing very hypointense lesion with surrounding vasogenic edema. The markedly decreased T2 signal corresponded to signal loss on SWI (not shown), suggesting a hemorrhagic component.* **(Right)** *Axial T1WI C+ FS MR in a 7-year-old with leukemia shows symmetric enlargement and enhancement of extraocular muscles and bilateral trigeminal nerves, representing leukemic infiltration.*

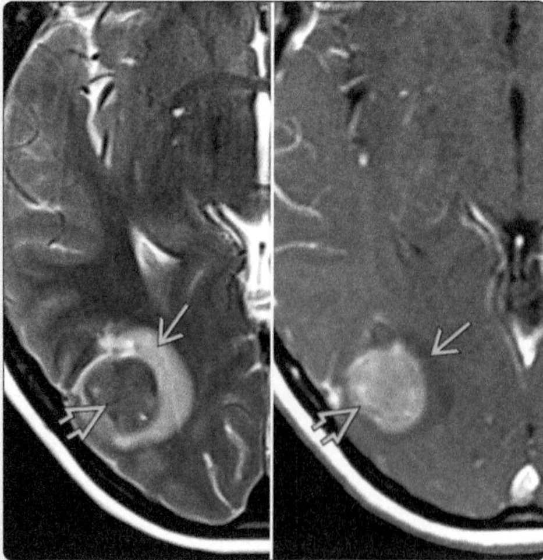

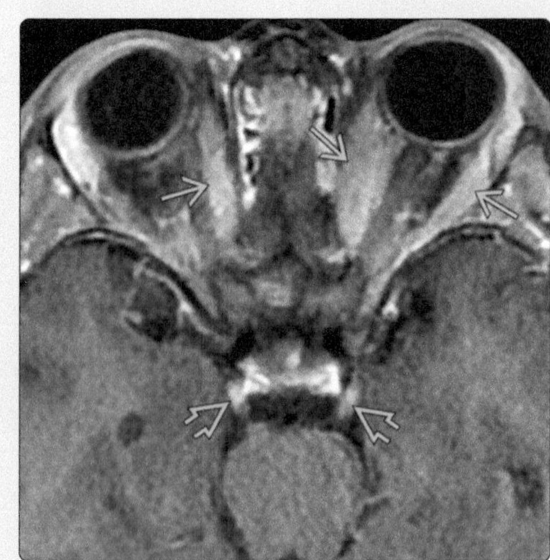

TERMINOLOGY

Synonyms

- Extramedullary leukemic tumors (EML)
- Extramedullary myeloblastoma, extramedullary myeloid cell tumors (EMMCT)
- Myeloid sarcoma, granulocytic sarcoma, chloroma
  - Leukemic masses first described in 1811
  - Chloroma coined in 1853
  - Renamed granulocytic sarcoma in 1966
  - Now most commonly termed myeloid sarcoma

Definitions

- Solid tumor of myeloblasts/myelocytes/promyelocytes
  - In patients with myeloproliferative disorder
- Multiple other intracranial manifestations of leukemia/treatment complications
  - Acute methotrexate toxicity
  - Posterior reversible encephalopathy syndrome (PRES)
  - Invasive fungal infection
  - Cavernous malformations after radiation therapy
  - Posttransplantation lymphoproliferative disease (PTLD) after bone marrow transplantation
  - Venous thrombosis associated with L-asparaginase
  - Spontaneous multifocal intraparenchymal hemorrhage in severe hyperleukocytosis
  - Vasculitis
    - Primary manifestation of leukemia
    - Secondary to treatment (transretinoic acid)
    - Secondary to infection (e.g., *Aspergillus*)

IMAGING

General Features

- Best diagnostic clue
  - Homogeneous enhancing tumor(s) in patients with known or suspected myeloproliferative disorder
  - Most often complication of acute myelogenous leukemia (AML)
- Location
  - Meningeal (dural-based) > intraparenchymal lesions

CT Findings

- NECT
  - Iso-/hyperdense to brain
    - May rapidly become hypodense (necrosis, liquefaction) with therapy
  - May present with (or mimic) hematoma
  - Look for skull base/paranasal sinus involvement
- CECT
  - Homogeneous enhancement
    - Hyperdensity or presence of hemorrhage may mask enhancement
  - May have rim enhancement, mimic abscess

MR Findings

- T1WI
  - Hypo-/isointense to brain
  - Can distinguish between acute hematoma, nonhemorrhagic mass
- T2WI
  - Heterogeneously hyper- to isointense
  - Pial disease may extend into perivascular spaces, appear as patchy white matter (WM) hyperintensities
- FLAIR
  - More sensitive than T2WI for leptomeningeal disease
- T2* GRE
  - Minority (15-20%) show areas of signal loss on SWI
- DWI
  - ~ 5% masses restrict (↑ DWI, ↓ ADC) due to ↑ cellularity
  - Helps distinguish ischemic complications from PRES
  - Best sequence for detecting acute methotrexate toxicity
- PWI
  - ASL: Most masses ≤ cerebral blood flow of brain
- T1WI C+
  - Homogeneous enhancement
    - May become heterogeneous with necrosis/liquefaction
  - Leptomeningeal or perivascular space enhancement
  - Fat-saturation technique essential for assessment of skull base disease
- MRA
  - May show vasospasm in cases of PRES
  - May identify medium-vessel vasculitis
- MRV
  - Essential in evaluation of hemorrhagic lesions
  - Identify presence or extent of venous thrombosis

Nuclear Medicine Findings

- Bone scan
  - Tc-99m MDP may be used for leukemic bone disease
- PET
  - Avid uptake on FDG PET exams

Imaging Recommendations

- Best imaging tool
  - MR with contrast
  - NECT provides additional information in hemorrhagic lesions
- Protocol advice
  - Use T1WI C+ FS
    - FS is important for detecting skull base disease

DIFFERENTIAL DIAGNOSIS

Metastatic Neuroblastoma

- Rarely occurs without extracranial disease
- Characteristic "raccoon eyes" clinical presentation
- Spiculated periostitis

Meningioma

- May be very difficult to distinguish
- Dural tail may be more common in meningioma

Extraaxial Hematoma

- Extracranial soft tissue swelling or skull fracture
- If no appropriate history, consider possibility of child abuse
- Does not enhance

Extramedullary Hematopoiesis

- Markedly hypointense on T2WI MR
- Patients with bone marrow dysfunction

Langerhans Cell Histiocytosis

- Destruction of adjacent bone without periosteal reaction
- Diabetes insipidus
- CT shows punched-out lytic lesions

Rhabdomyosarcoma

- Cellular tumor often found in head & neck
- Usually more heterogeneous than myeloid sarcoma

Ewing Sarcoma

- Aggressive pattern of growth
- Destruction of adjacent bone

Neurosarcoidosis

- Mimic of leptomeningeal disease
- Less commonly presents as dural-based masses

PATHOLOGY

General Features

- Etiology
  - CNS leukemia presents in 3 forms
    - Focal tumor masses (myeloid sarcoma)
    - Meningeal disease
      - Usually with acute lymphoblastic leukemia (ALL)
    - Intravascular aggregates (leukostasis)
      - May rupture, hemorrhage (especially with hyperleukocytosis)
- Genetics
  - Children with CNS leukemic infiltrates in AML have ↑ chromosome 11 abnormalities compared to those without CNS disease
- Associated abnormalities
  - Complications/diseases associated with leukemia and its treatment
  - Acute methotrexate toxicity
    - Restricted diffusion in unilateral or bilateral centrum semiovale
    - Nearly normal signal on FLAIR
  - Acute nelarabine toxicity
    - Nonspecific findings, including
      - ↑ FLAIR in WM, CN enhancement, and myelopathy
  - PRES
    - Signal abnormality in watershed cortex (often bilateral, symmetric)
    - May have associated hemorrhage; diffusion restriction less common
  - Invasive fungal infection
    - Usually paranasal sinuses
    - Look for invasion of paranasal fat
  - Venous thrombosis associated with L-asparaginase
    - Patients at much ↑ risk for venous thrombosis

Gross Pathologic & Surgical Features

- Called chloroma due to green color in 70% of cases
  - Caused by high levels of myeloperoxidase

Microscopic Features

- Moderate to large cells
- Pleomorphic nuclei
- Multiple mitoses give starry-sky appearance

CLINICAL ISSUES

Presentation

- Most common signs/symptoms
  - May precede marrow diagnosis of leukemia
  - 50% of cases diagnosed only at autopsy
  - CNS lesions more likely symptomatic
  - Focal signs from local mass effect
  - Headache from hemorrhage
- Clinical profile
  - Child with AML develops new neurologic symptoms

Demographics

- Age
  - 60% of patients < 15 years
- Sex
  - M:F = 1.4:1
- Epidemiology
  - 11% of patients with AML

Natural History & Prognosis

- Overall survival rates for AML (40-50%)
- Chloroma in setting of other myeloproliferative syndrome
  - Implies blastic transformation
  - Poor prognostic sign

Treatment

- Chemotherapy for induction
  - Cytarabine (Ara-C)
  - Anthracycline
- Bone marrow transplant for consolidation
- Intrathecal methotrexate treatment can cause stroke-like symptoms
  - Diffusion restriction in centrum semiovale with minimal FLAIR signal change

DIAGNOSTIC CHECKLIST

Consider

- Extramedullary hematopoiesis can present in same patient population with similar appearance
- Hemorrhagic lesions in children with AML may represent myeloid sarcoma **or** complication of therapy

Image Interpretation Pearls

- Best clue: Uniformly enhancing mass with ↑ DWI ↓ ADC
- Multiple lesions at multiple sites suggestive of diagnosis

SELECTED REFERENCES

1. Sastow D et al: Multi-institutional analysis of outcomes in acute myeloid leukemia patients with central nervous system involvement. Leuk Lymphoma. 1-6, 2023
2. Serrallach BL et al: Imaging findings in children presenting with CNS nelarabine toxicity. AJNR Am J Neuroradiol. 43(12):1802-9, 2022
3. Meyer HJ et al: Radiological and clinical patterns of myeloid sarcoma. Radiol Oncol. 53(2):213-8, 2019
4. Hou X et al: Use of magnetic resonance imaging for diagnosis and after treatment of patients with myeloid sarcoma of the brain. Oncotarget. 8(60):102581-9, 2017
5. Chaudhry AA et al: Qualitative assessment of diffusion weighted imaging and susceptibility weighted imaging of myeloid sarcoma involving the brain. J Comput Assist Tomogr. 40(1):61-6, 2016
6. Bhojwani D et al: Methotrexate-induced neurotoxicity and leukoencephalopathy in childhood acute lymphoblastic leukemia. J Clin Oncol. 32(9):949-59, 2014

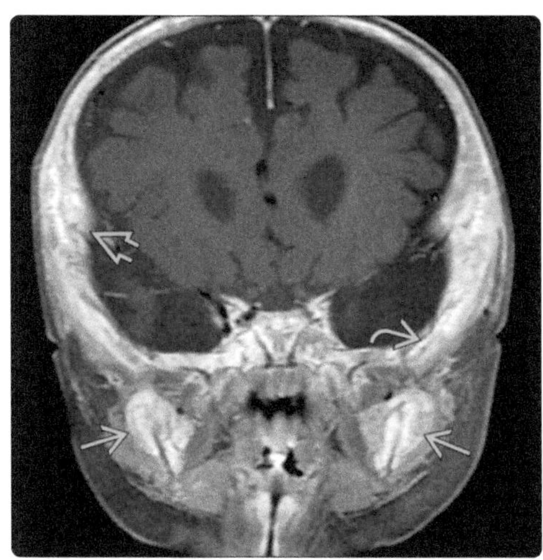

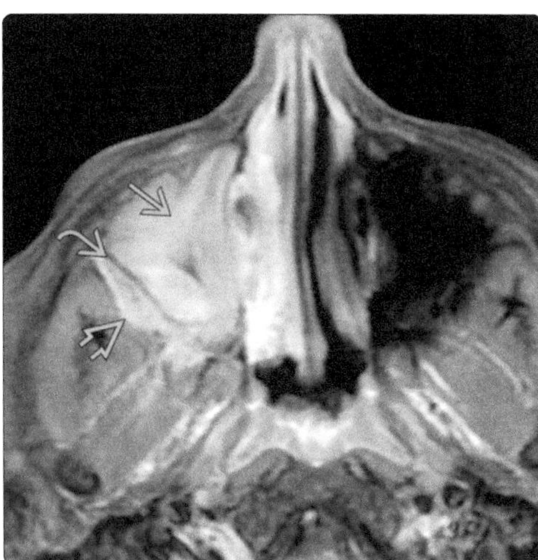

(Left) *Coronal T1WI C+ FS MR in a 6-month-old shows expansion of the calvarium ➡ and skull base ↪ with soft tissue extending beyond the bony margins, consistent with leukemic infiltration. Also note the symmetric leukemic lesions involving the mandibular condyles ➡.* **(Right)** *Axial T1WI C+ FS MR in a 12-year-old with myeloid sarcoma shows an enhancing lesion ➡ in the right maxillary sinus with enhancing soft tissue ➡ extending beyond the posterior maxillary sinus wall ↪.*

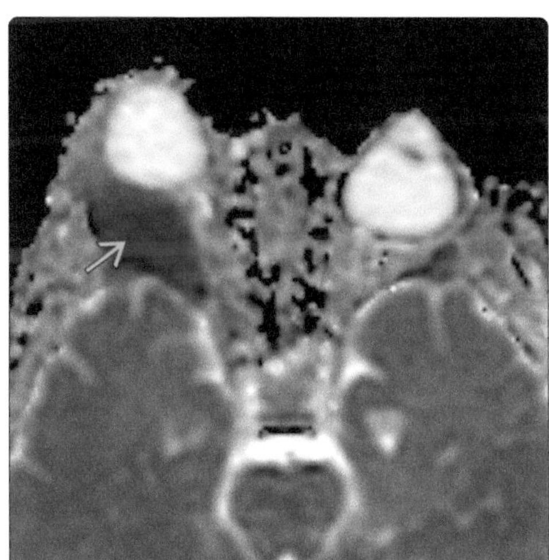

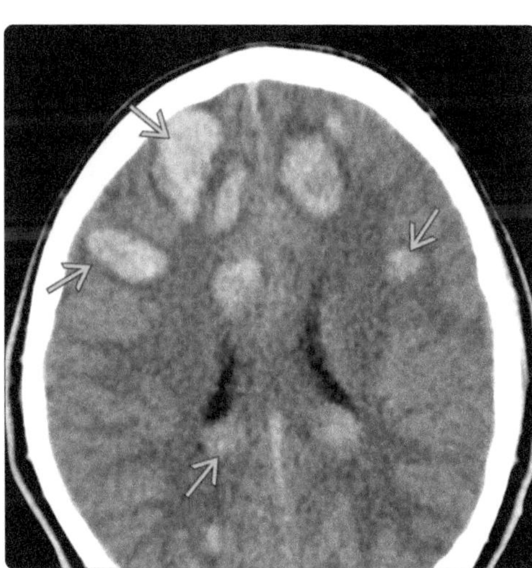

(Left) *Axial ADC map in an 8-year-old shows a large lesion ➡ in the right orbit causing proptosis. Note the dark ADC signal, consistent with a highly cellular lesion. T2WI and T1WI C+ MR (not shown) demonstrated very homogeneous signal and enhancement. Pathology confirmed myeloid sarcoma.* **(Right)** *Axial NECT in a teenager with leukemia and hyperleukocytosis (WBC-940k) shows multifocal brain hemorrhages ➡. Spontaneous intraparenchymal hemorrhage can occur with severe hyperleukocytosis.*

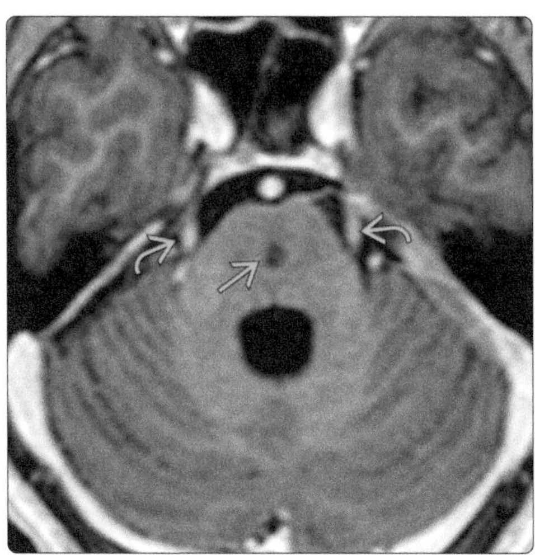

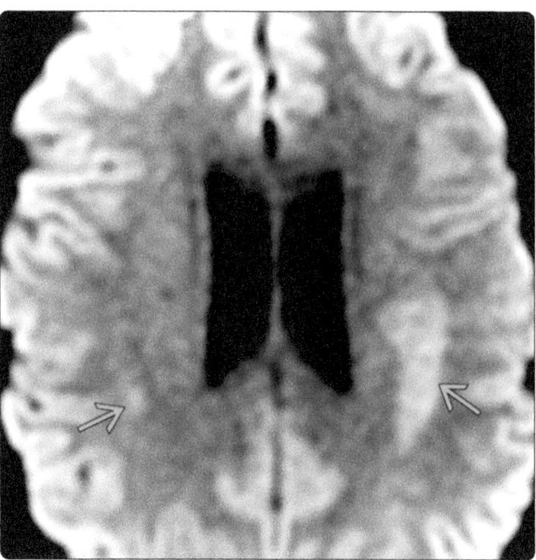

(Left) *Axial T1WI C+ MR in a 16-year-old with acute lymphoblastic leukemia (ALL) treated with nelarabine shows a focal area of ↓ signal in the central pons ➡ and cranial nerve enhancement ↪. Nelarabine toxicity findings are nonspecific but often involve myelopathy and cranial neuropathy.* **(Right)** *Axial DWI MR in teenager with ALL treated with intrathecal MTX presenting with stroke-like symptoms shows bilateral (L > R) diffusion restriction ➡ in the centrum semiovale white matter, consistent with acute MTX toxicity.*

Langerhans Cell Histiocytosis, Skull and Brain

KEY FACTS

TERMINOLOGY

- Langerhans cell histiocytosis (LCH)
- Now best understood as neoplastic disease
  - Activating somatic *BRAF* mutations, LCH cell clonality

IMAGING

- NECT
  - Sharply marginated lytic skull defect
    - Beveled edges
  - Mastoid: Geographic destruction, soft tissue mass
- MR
  - Absent posterior pituitary "bright spot" on T1WI
  - Thick, enhancing infundibulum
  - Enhancing masses in choroid plexus, leptomeninges, basal ganglia
  - Sometimes cerebellar white matter (WM) disease

TOP DIFFERENTIAL DIAGNOSES

- Lytic calvarial lesions
  - Surgical (burr hole, shunt, surgical defect)
  - Epidermoid
  - Dermoid
- Pituitary infundibular/hypothalamic thickening, enhancement
  - Germinoma
  - Metastasis
- Mastoid involvement
  - Severe otomastoiditis
  - Rhabdomyosarcoma

DIAGNOSTIC CHECKLIST

- Calvarium is most frequent bony site involved by LCH
- Thick, enhancing pituitary stalk is most common CNS manifestation of LCH
  - If initially "normal" MR in patient with diabetes insipidus, repeat in 2-3 months
- Consider LCH for ataxic patient with choroid plexus masses, cerebellar WM demyelination

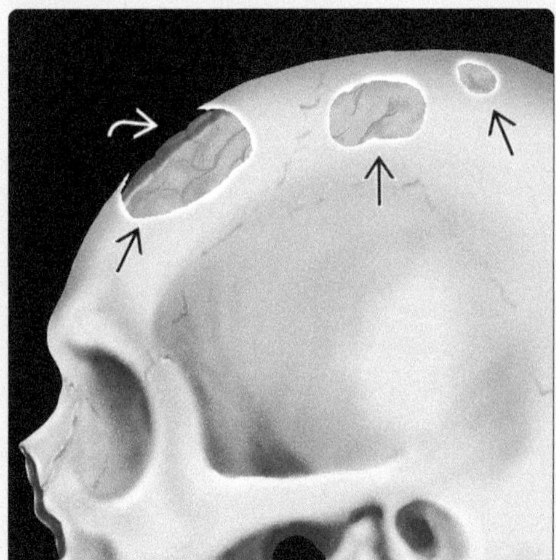

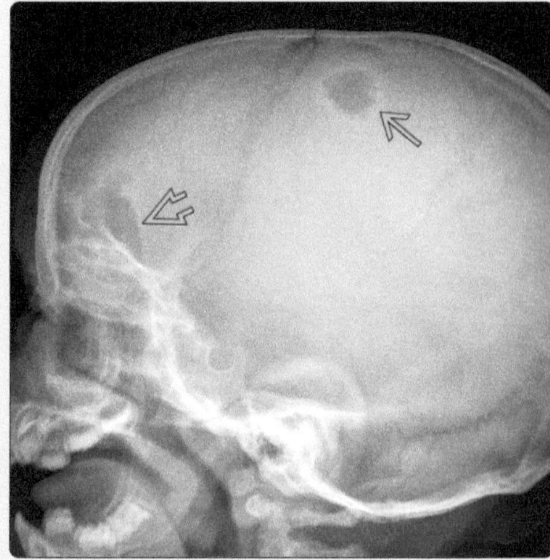

(Left) *Lateral graphic demonstrates 3 sharply defined lytic lesions ➡ of the membranous calvarium with geographic destruction. Note the beveled margins of the bony lysis ➦.* **(Right)** *Lateral radiograph in a 1-year-old shows multiple lytic lesions within the parietal ➡ and frontal calvarium ⇨. Multiple well-defined lytic bone lesions in a young child are most likely to represent Langerhans cell histiocytosis (LCH).*

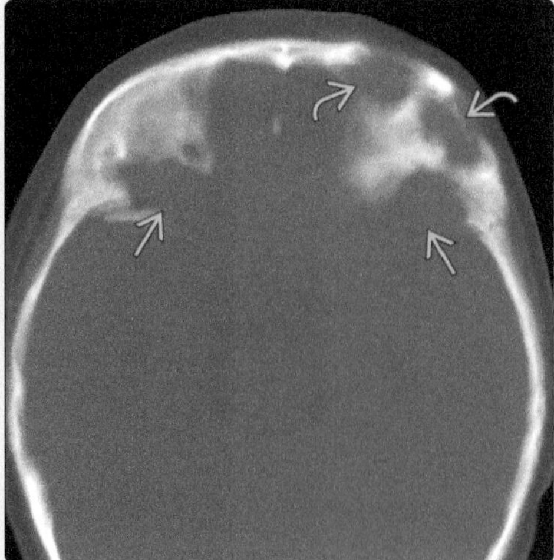

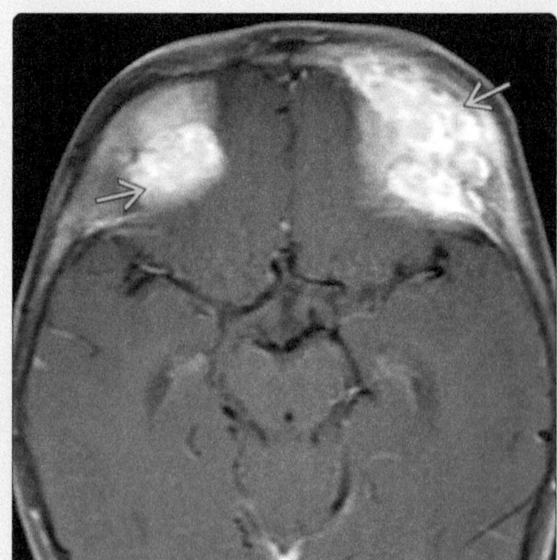

(Left) *Axial NECT in a 1-year-old shows bilateral, well-defined, punched-out lytic lesions involving the left supraorbital ➦ and bilateral orbital plates ➡ of the frontal bones.* **(Right)** *Axial T1 C+ FS MR in the same patient shows avidly enhancing soft tissue lesions ➡ in the location of the lytic defects on CT. The calvarium and skull base are frequently affected in LCH.*

TERMINOLOGY

Synonyms

- Langerhans cell histiocytosis (LCH)
  - Several entities (eosinophilic granuloma, Hand-Schüller-Christian disease, Letterer-Siwe disease, and histiocytosis X) now under single designation of LCH

Definitions

- LCH now best understood as neoplastic disease
  - Activating somatic *BRAF* mutations, LCH cell clonality
  - Inflammatory myeloid neoplasia
- Divided into 3 groups (based on number of lesions, systems involved)
  - Unifocal localized form (a.k.a. eosinophilic granuloma)
    - 70% of cases
    - Limited to single or few bones, may involve lung
  - Multifocal unisystem
    - 20% of cases
    - Chronic, recurring
    - Multiple bones, reticuloendothelial system, pituitary/hypothalamus
  - Multifocal, multisystem
    - 10% of cases
    - Fulminant (often fatal)

IMAGING

General Features

- Best diagnostic clue
  - Calvaria: Sharply marginated lytic skull defect with beveled margins
  - Skull base (mastoid most common): Geographic destruction ± soft tissue mass
  - Brain: Thick, enhancing infundibulum, absent posterior pituitary "bright spot" on T1WI
- Location
  - Calvarium
    - Most common bony site
      - Frontal, parietal bones > temporal, occipital
    - Also mastoid portion of temporal bone, mandible, orbit, facial bones
  - Brain: Pituitary gland/infundibulum, hypothalamus
    - Rare: Choroid plexus, leptomeninges, basal ganglia, cerebellar white matter (WM), and brain parenchyma
- Size
  - Skull and facial bones: May grow, coalesce
  - Pituitary infundibulum: Small lesions due to early endocrine dysfunction [central diabetes insipidus (DI)]
- Morphology
  - Variable patterns of bony lysis ("geographic" skull)
  - Soft tissue masses vary from discrete ↔ infiltrative

Radiographic Findings

- Radiography
  - Calvarium: Well-defined lytic lesion, beveled edge, lack of marginal sclerosis
    - ± button sequestra or sclerotic margins when healing
  - Mastoid: Geographic destruction, often bilateral, little regional adenopathy
  - Facial/orbital: More variable patterns of bony lysis, discrete ↔ permeative

CT Findings

- NECT
  - Calvarium
    - Lytic defect, "beveled" edge (inner table > outer table)
    - Small soft tissue mass, no periosteal reaction
  - Mastoid
    - Bone destruction, often bilateral, soft tissue mass
- CECT
  - Calvarium/mastoid: Enhancing soft tissue in lytic defect
  - Brain: Thick, enhancing pituitary stalk, ± hypothalamic mass or enhancement

MR Findings

- T1WI
  - Soft tissue mass at site of bony lysis (± T1 shortening due to lipid-laden histiocytes)
  - Brain
    - Pituitary/infundibulum: Absent posterior pituitary "bright spot," thick stalk, ± soft tissue mass
- T2WI
  - Skull, mastoid, orbital/facial lesions: Soft tissue masses show slight T2 hyperintensity
  - Brain
    - Infundibulum/hypothalamus: Slightly hyperintense
    - ± cerebellar WM hyperintensity (autoimmune-mediated demyelination)
- FLAIR
  - Rare: Hyperintense cerebellar WM demyelination
- T1WI C+
  - Skull, mastoid, orbital/facial: Enhancing soft tissue masses (defined or infiltrating)
  - Brain
    - Infundibulum: Thick, strongly enhancing stalk
    - Parenchyma: Enhancing masses in choroid plexus, leptomeninges, and basal ganglia

Nuclear Medicine Findings

- Bone scan
  - Tc-99m bone scan: Variable (cold ↔ warm)
- PET
  - F-18 FDG: ↑ uptake in proliferating lesions, ↓ uptake for "burned-out" lesions

Imaging Recommendations

- Best imaging tool
  - Skull: NECT (with CECT for mastoid disease)
  - Brain: MR with contrast
- Protocol advice
  - Skull: CT using bone algorithm; include coronal and sagittal reconstructions
  - Brain MR
    - Pituitary MR: Small field of view, thin section, no gap, sagittal and coronal T1WI with contrast
      - If initially normal in patient with DI, repeat in 2-3 months

DIFFERENTIAL DIAGNOSIS

Lytic Calvarial Lesions

- Surgical (burr hole, shunt, surgical defect)
- Epidermoid
- Dermoid
- Leptomeningeal cyst
- Metastases
- Enlarged parietal foramina
- Aneurysmal bone cyst

Temporal Bone Destructive Processes

- Severe otomastoiditis: Usually less lytic than LCH
- Rhabdomyosarcoma: Often with large cervical nodes
  - More often isolated to anterior temporal bone

Pituitary Infundibular/Hypothalamic Thickening or Masses

- Germinoma
- Metastasis
- Neurosarcoid
- Lymphocytic hypophysitis

Rare Histiocytic Diseases

- Rosai-Dorfman disease: Dural involvement common; cervical lymphadenopathy
- Erdheim-Chester disease: Rare in children

PATHOLOGY

General Features

- Genetics
  - Pathologic LCH cells are clonal
  - Activating *BRAF* mutations
  - Activation of ERK signaling pathway in myeloid differentiation as essential/universal driver of LCH pathology
- Associated abnormalities
  - ↑ risk of LCH: Family history of thyroid disease, underimmunization, penicillin use, solvent exposure

Staging, Grading, & Classification

- Formerly classified into 1 of 3 overlapping forms
  - Eosinophilic granuloma
    - Localized, calvarium most common (70%)
  - Hand-Schüller-Christian
    - Chronic disseminated form, multifocal (20%)
  - Letterer-Siwe
    - Acute disseminated form, onset at < 2 years of age, ± skeletal involvement (10%)
- Now classified according to risk factors: Young age, multifocal involvement, multiorgan dysfunction, relapse

Microscopic Features

- Monoclonality of Langerhans cells
  - Presence of CD1a and Birbeck granules needed to establish diagnosis
- Accumulation of CD1A(+)/CD207(+) mononuclear phagocytes in granulomatous lesions

CLINICAL ISSUES

Presentation

- Most common signs/symptoms
  - Calvarium: Pain, subscalp mass, bony defect
  - Mastoid destruction: Pain, chronic otitis externa, retroauricular subscalp mass
  - Retroorbital mass: Exophthalmos, ± painful ophthalmoplegia
  - Pituitary infundibular involvement: Central DI, ± visual disturbance, ± hypothalamic dysfunction
- Clinical profile
  - Child < 2 years with DI, ± lytic calvarial lesion

Demographics

- Age
  - LCH typically presents at < 2 years
- Sex
  - M:F = 2:1
- Ethnicity
  - More common among White patients
- Epidemiology
  - Affects 4 in 1 million
  - Peak age at onset: 1 year (isolated), 2-5 years (multifocal)
  - 50% of cases are monostotic
  - Familial LCH < 2%
  - Lytic bone lesions are most common manifestations of LCH (seen in 80-95% of children with LCH)

Natural History & Prognosis

- Variable depending on extent of involvement
  - Multifocal and systemic LCH: Mortality may approach 18%

Treatment

- Therapeutic options depend on symptoms, location, and extent of disease
  - Observation, excision/curettage, sclerotherapy/injection, radiation/chemotherapy
- Solitary eosinophilic granuloma has best prognosis with spontaneous remission common
- LCH patients with DI: Oral or nasal vasopressin, ± chemotherapy and radiation
- Targeted therapy for refractory cases with *BRAF* V600E mutations

DIAGNOSTIC CHECKLIST

Consider

- CNS LCH for ataxic patient with choroid plexus masses and cerebellar WM demyelination

Image Interpretation Pearls

- Skull is most frequent bony site involved by LCH
- Thick, enhancing pituitary stalk is most common CNS manifestation of LCH

SELECTED REFERENCES

1. Cohen Aubart F et al: Histiocytosis and the nervous system: from diagnosis to targeted therapies. Neuro Oncol. 23(9):1433-46, 2021
2. Dhar S et al: Langerhans cell histiocytosis in children: a retrospective case series of 126 cases. Pediatr Dermatol. 37(6):1085-9, 2020

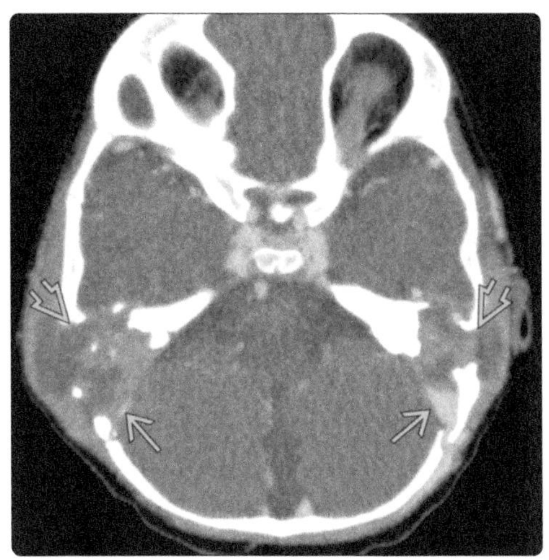

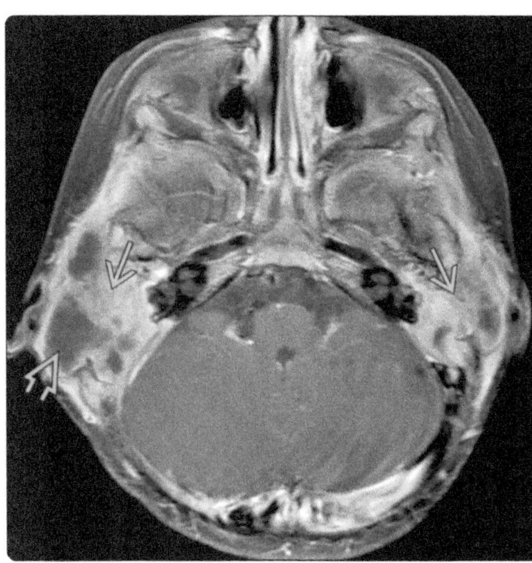

(Left) *Axial CECT in a 1-year-old with bilateral mastoid LCH shows heterogeneous lytic soft tissue masses in both mastoids ➡ with posterior displacement of the bilateral sigmoid sinuses ➡.* **(Right)** *Axial T1 C+ FS MR in the same patient shows bilateral enhancing mastoid masses ➡ with some central nonenhancement ➡. LCH can mimic acute otomastoiditis but should have more extensive soft tissue component and more lytic mastoid changes.*

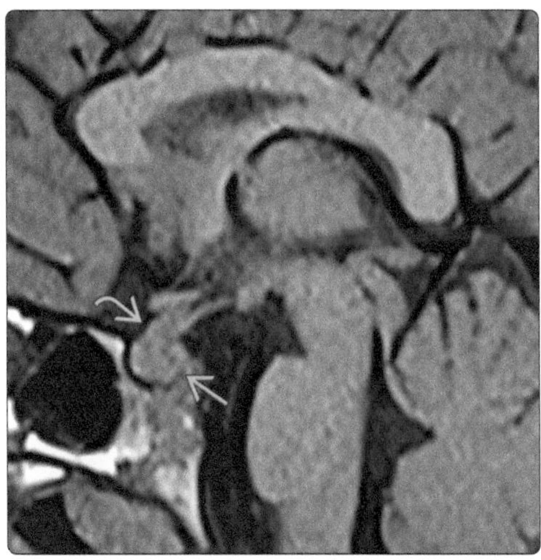

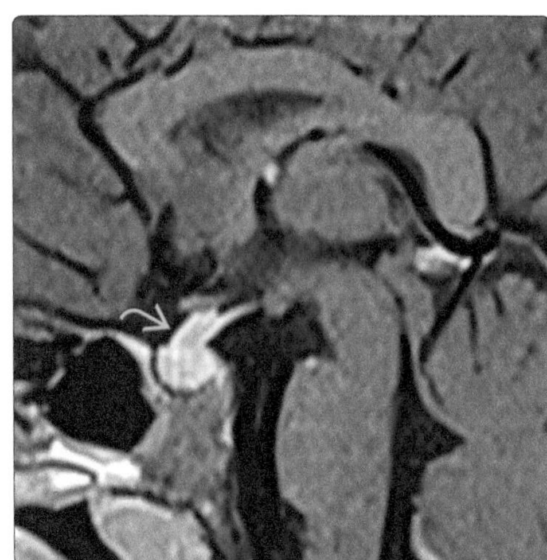

(Left) *Midline sagittal T1 MR in 4-year-old with central diabetes insipidus shows thickened infundibulum ➡ and absence of posterior pituitary "bright spot" ➡. Absence of pituitary "bright spot" is typically permanent even after LCH treatment.* **(Right)** *Midline sagittal T1 C+ MR in the same patient shows avid enhancement of the thickened infundibulum ➡. This appearance should invoke a primary DDx of LCH and germinoma. The presence of lytic bone lesions should be sought to clinch the diagnosis of LCH.*

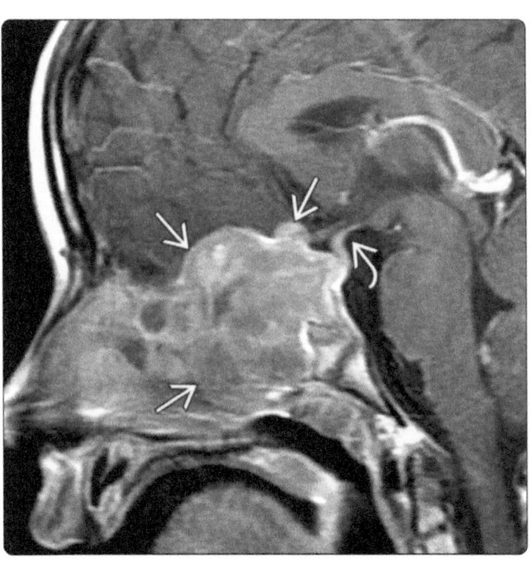

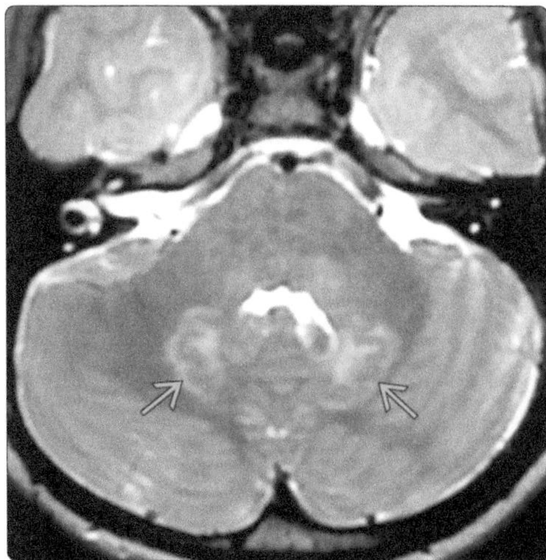

(Left) *Sagittal T1 C+ FS MR in a 5-year-old boy with chronic headaches and diabetes insipidus demonstrates a heterogeneously enhancing lesion ➡ of the central skull base. Note the thickening and displacement of the pituitary infundibulum ➡.* **(Right)** *Axial T2 MR in a 10-year-old with history of LCH for 7 years shows hyperintense signal ➡ adjacent to the dentate nuclei. Cerebellar involvement should be carefully sought out in every case of LCH. Cerebellar involvement often presents in a delayed fashion years after initial diagnosis.*

Arachnoid Cyst

KEY FACTS

TERMINOLOGY

- Focal extraaxial CSF collection lined by arachnoid

IMAGING

- Location
  - Middle cranial fossa: 50-70%
  - Retrocerebellar: 15-20%
  - Less common: Basilar cisterns, interhemispheric fissure, cerebral convexities
  - Rare: Intraventricular
- Displaces adjacent vessels & nerves
- Typically shows less mass effect than expected
  - Adjacent brain accommodates cyst
- Calvarial remodeling: Thinning/scalloping ± bulging
- **US**: Anechoic; no internal vascularity
- **NECT**: Isodense to CSF, unless hemorrhage occurs (rare)
- **MR**: Follows CSF signal intensity on all sequences
  - Fluid signal suppression on FLAIR
  - DWI/ADC signal equal to CSF

TOP DIFFERENTIAL DIAGNOSES

- Epidermoid cyst
- Chronic subdural hematoma
- Subdural hygroma
- Mega cisterna magna

PATHOLOGY

- Wall consists of flattened but normal arachnoid cells

CLINICAL ISSUES

- Asymptomatic in vast majority (typically found incidentally)
- More likely to grow in younger patients (< 4 years of age)
- In young children: 80% stable, 10% enlarge, 10% ↓
- Surgery only indicated if symptoms directly attributable to arachnoid cyst

DIAGNOSTIC CHECKLIST

- FLAIR, DWI best MR sequences for distinguishing cystic-appearing intracranial masses

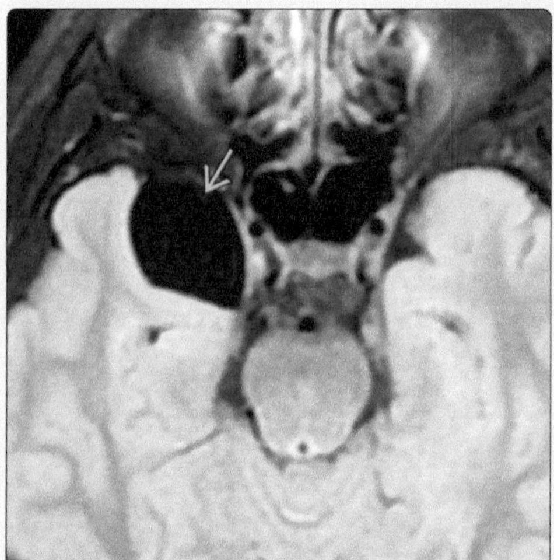

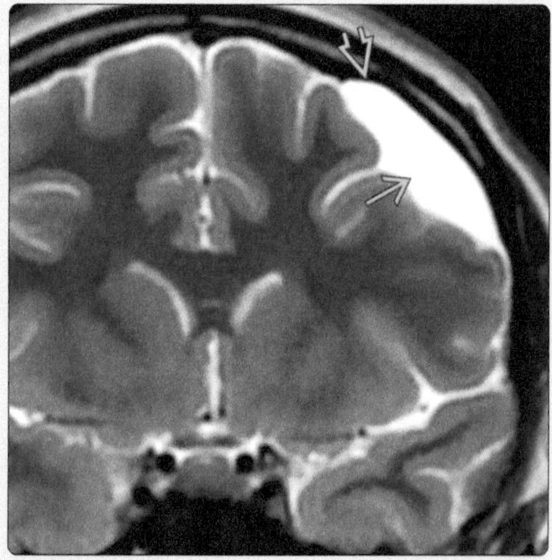

(Left) *Axial FLAIR MR in a 7-year-old shows an incidental arachnoid cyst (AC) ➡ in the right middle cranial fossa, the most common location to find ACs. Note the complete suppression of signal in this cyst on FLAIR.* **(Right)** *Coronal T2 MR in a teen shows a fluid-signal cyst ➡ overlying the left frontal lobe with mild mass effect on the underlying brain and scalloping/remodeling ➡ of the overlying calvarium, a characteristic appearance for an AC.*

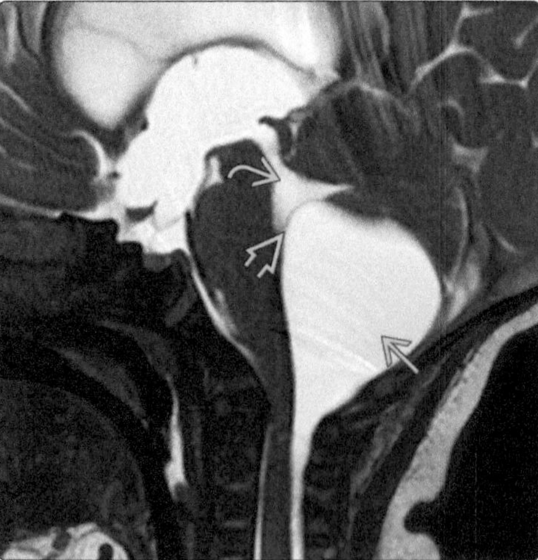

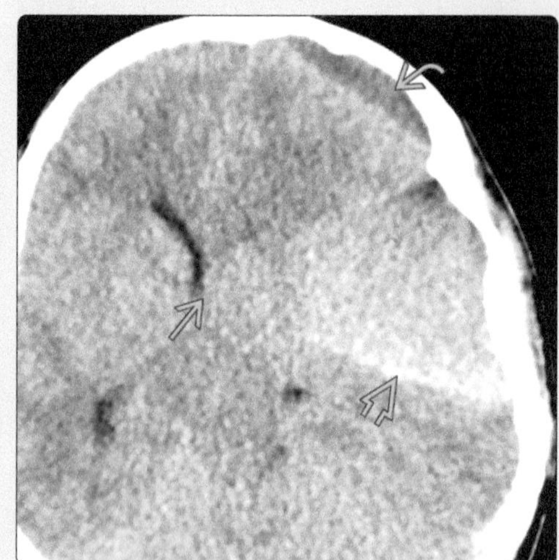

(Left) *Sagittal FIESTA MR in a 1-month-old shows a large posterior fossa AC ➡, which causes obstructive hydrocephalus. Note the barely perceptible septation ➡ between the cyst and the 4th ventricle ➡.* **(Right)** *Axial NECT in a teen with a ruptured left middle cranial fossa AC shows layering of hyperdense acute blood products ➡ within the large AC and extension of low attenuation fluid ➡ into the adjacent subdural space. Note the rightward midline shift ➡.*

TERMINOLOGY

Abbreviations

- Arachnoid cyst (AC)

Synonyms

- Subarachnoid cyst

Definitions

- Focal extraaxial CSF collection lined by arachnoid; generally lacks free communication with ventricles or subarachnoid space

IMAGING

General Features

- Best diagnostic clue
  - Focal extraaxial CSF collection with mass effect
- Location
  - Middle cranial fossa (MCF): 50-70%
  - Retrocerebellar: 15-20%
  - Less common locations: Cerebral convexities or interhemispheric fissure (5-10%), cerebellopontine angle (5-10%), quadrigeminal plate (1-5%), suprasellar (1-5%)
  - Rare locations: Intraventricular
- Size
  - Mean diameter: 3 cm; ~ 20% > 5 cm
  - Variable as likelihood of symptoms (&, therefore, detection) ↑ with cyst size
- Morphology
  - Sharply marginated extraaxial fluid collection
    - Lentiform, crescentic, ovoid, or lobular
    - Thin, nearly imperceptible wall
  - Less than expected mass effect
    - Adjacent brain accommodates cyst; parenchyma may be mildly hypoplastic
  - Thinning/scalloping ± bulging of overlying calvarium

CT Findings

- NECT
  - Isodense to CSF
    - Hemorrhage within cyst may (rarely) ↑ attenuation
- CECT
  - Nonenhancing cystic mass displaces vessels
- **CT cisternogram**: AC shows absent or delayed opacification relative to subarachnoid spaces

MR Findings

- T1WI
  - Isointense to CSF
- T2WI
  - Isointense to CSF
  - Displaced vascular flow voids; mild deformation of adjacent cortex
- PD/intermediate
  - Isointense to CSF
- FLAIR
  - Suppresses completely, similar to CSF
    - No edema in adjacent brain parenchyma
- DWI
  - Follows CSF signal
- T1WI C+
  - No cyst enhancement
- MRA
  - Cystic mass displaces adjacent vessels
- SSFP cine
  - Reduced/absent CSF flow compared to subarachnoid spaces (e.g., mega cisterna magna)
- **MR cisternography**: May distinguish communicating from noncommunicating ACs

Ultrasonographic Findings

- Grayscale ultrasound
  - Anechoic with ↑ posterior acoustic shadowing
- Color Doppler
  - No internal vascularity
- Only useful in young infants with open fontanelles
  - Complete visualization may still be difficult depending on AC location
  - Distinguishes midline ACs from venous varix (e.g., vein of Galen malformation)

Nuclear Medicine Findings

- SPECT: May show hypoperfusion in brain adjacent to cyst

Imaging Recommendations

- Best imaging tool
  - Noncontrast MR
- Protocol advice
  - Always use FLAIR & DWI on MR; use balanced SS-GRE sequence (e.g., FIESTA, CISS, b-FFE) to evaluate cyst walls & adjacent structures (e.g., cranial nerves)

DIFFERENTIAL DIAGNOSIS

Epidermoid Cyst

- Does not follow CSF on all modalities/sequences
  - Brighter on CT & T1 MR
  - Does not suppress on FLAIR MR
  - Markedly restricted diffusion (light-bulb bright) on MR
- Engulfs (rather than displaces) vessels & nerves

Chronic Subdural Hematoma

- Crescentic collection differing from CSF appearance
  - Hyperdense on CT/hyperintense on FLAIR, PD, & T1 MR relative to CSF (though difference may only be mild)
- May show enhancing membrane(s)

Subdural Hygroma

- CSF leak from subarachnoid space into subdural space
  - 2-7 days after trauma
- Crescentic, often bilateral
- Lack of overlying calvarial changes

Porencephalic Cyst

- Result of remote trauma or ischemic injury
- Surrounded by injured, chronically abnormal brain (vs. otherwise normal compressed/distorted brain)

Neuroepithelial Cyst

- Periventricular, intraventricular, or choroidal fissure cyst
  - Benign, lined by "epithelium"

Epidural Abscess

- Collection with enhancing wall & restricted diffusion

- Elevated lactate on MRS
- Typically with relevant causative findings (e.g., sinusitis, penetrating injury)

Pilocytic Astrocytoma

- Intraaxial cystic mass with enhancing mural nodule

Mega Cisterna Magna

- More posterior & central than retrocerebellar AC
- Communicates freely with subarachnoid space

PATHOLOGY

General Features

- Etiology
  - Old concept: "Split" or diverticulum of developing arachnoid
  - New concept (for MCF ACs)
    - Frontal & temporal embryonic meninges (endomeninx) fail to merge as sylvian fissure forms
      - Remain separate, forming "duplicated" arachnoid
  - May rarely form from shunt complication
- Associated abnormalities
  - In MCF ACs, adjacent temporal lobe often hypoplastic
  - ↑ prevalence of subdural hematomas (especially MCF ACs)
  - Found with some syndromes: Acrocallosal (ACs ~ 30%), Aicardi, Pallister-Hall
- Possible mechanisms for enlargement
  - Active fluid secretion by cyst wall
  - Slow distention by CSF pulsations
  - 1-way CSF intake/flow (ball-valve mechanism)

Staging, Grading, & Classification

- Noncommunicating vs. communicating
  - ACs may demonstrate varying degrees of communication with adjacent subarachnoid spaces
    - May be determined using CT or MR cisternography
  - Clinical significance uncertain; some authors suggest this feature may help determine need for surgical therapy
- Galassi classification for MCF AC (based on size/mass effect & communication with basal cisterns)
  - Type I: Small, spindle-shaped, limited to anterior MCF
    - Free communication with subarachnoid space on CT cisternogram
  - Type II: Superior extent along sylvian fissure; temporal lobe displaced
  - Type III: Huge, filling entire MCF; frontal/temporal/parietal lobe displacement
    - Minimal, if any, communication with subarachnoid space on CT cisternogram

Gross Pathologic & Surgical Features

- Bluish gray arachnoid bulges around CSF-filled cyst

Microscopic Features

- Wall consists of flattened but normal arachnoid cells
- No inflammation or neoplastic changes

CLINICAL ISSUES

Presentation

- Most common signs/symptoms
  - Vast majority asymptomatic & found incidentally
  - Associated symptoms vary with size & location of cyst
    - Headache, dizziness, sensorineural hearing loss, hemifacial spasm/tic
      - Smaller ACs in basilar cisterns most likely to be symptomatic due to mass effect on critical structures
      - Symptomatic ACs in MCF & over cerebral convexities typically very large
      - Suprasellar ACs may cause obstructive hydrocephalus, "bobble-head doll syndrome," precocious puberty

Demographics

- Age
  - Most symptomatic ACs diagnosed in children
  - Cysts in older children & adults usually incidental
- Sex
  - M:F = 2:1

Natural History & Prognosis

- More likely to enlarge in younger patients (< 4 years old)
  - In young children: 80% stable, 10% ↑, 10% ↓
- Stable, asymptomatic ACs more likely in adults (97%)

Treatment

- Typically none
  - Morbidity from treatment may be greater than symptoms attributed to cyst
- Treatment only indicated if symptoms directly attributable to AC & potential benefits of surgery outweigh risks
- Surgical options
  - Cyst location, patient age, surgical expertise, & patient preference all influence approach
    - Endoscopic cyst fenestration
    - Open microsurgical cyst resection/fenestration
    - Cystoperitoneal shunt
- Recent literature suggests no need to restrict participation in sports

DIAGNOSTIC CHECKLIST

Consider

- Epidermoid cyst when encountering midline & cerebellopontine angle cistern cystic lesions

Image Interpretation Pearls

- FLAIR, DWI best MR sequences for distinguishing cystic-appearing intracranial masses

SELECTED REFERENCES

1. Sahap SK et al: The unique features of middle cranial fossa and sylvian fissure arachnoid cysts in children: MRI evaluation. Childs Nerv Syst. 39(1):79-85, 2023
2. Carbone J et al: Intracranial arachnoid cysts: review of natural history and proposed treatment algorithm. Surg Neurol Int. 12:621, 2021
3. Amelot A et al: Microsurgical, endoscopic, and shunt management of pediatric temporosylvian arachnoid cysts: a comparative study. J Neurosurg Pediatr. 1-9, 2019
4. Yahal O et al: Prenatal diagnosis of arachnoid cysts: MRI features and neurodevelopmental outcome. Eur J Radiol. 113:232-7, 2019
5. Ali ZS et al: Pediatric intracranial arachnoid cysts: comparative effectiveness of surgical treatment options. Childs Nerv Syst. 30(3):461-9, 2014
6. Al-Holou WN et al: Prevalence and natural history of arachnoid cysts in children. J Neurosurg Pediatr. 5(6):578-85, 2010

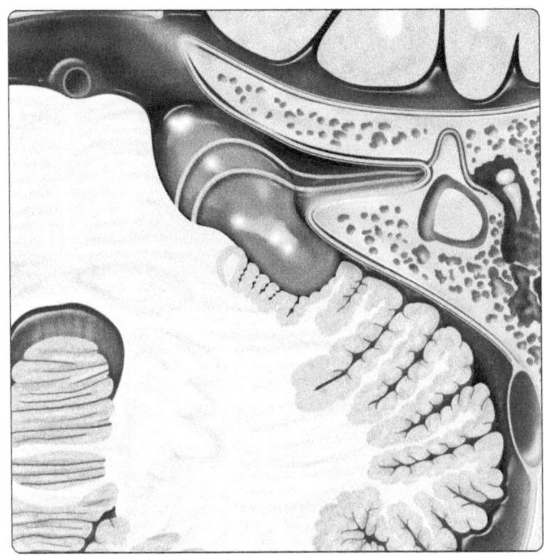

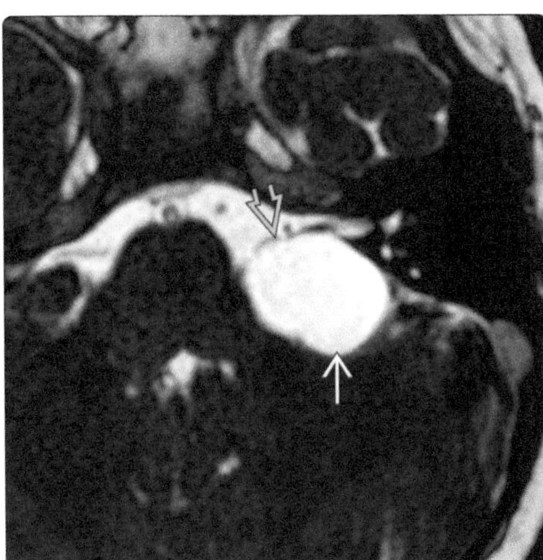

(Left) *Axial graphic shows an AC of the cerebellopontine angle (CPA) displacing cranial nerves VII and VIII superiorly with minimal mass effect on the adjacent cerebellum.* **(Right)** *Axial 3D FIESTA MR in a 3-year-old shows a left CPA AC ➔ with mass effect on cranial nerves VII and VIII complex ⇨. ACs may enlarge, especially in younger patients. Balanced SS-GRE (e.g., FIESTA, CISS) sequence is very helpful for defining the thin AC walls and adjacent structures (e.g., cranial nerves).*

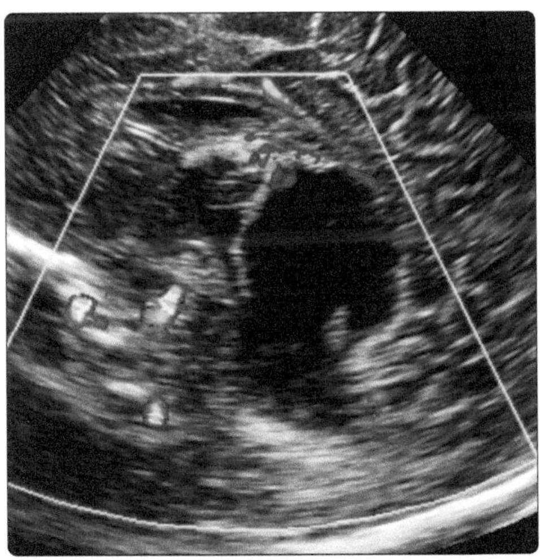

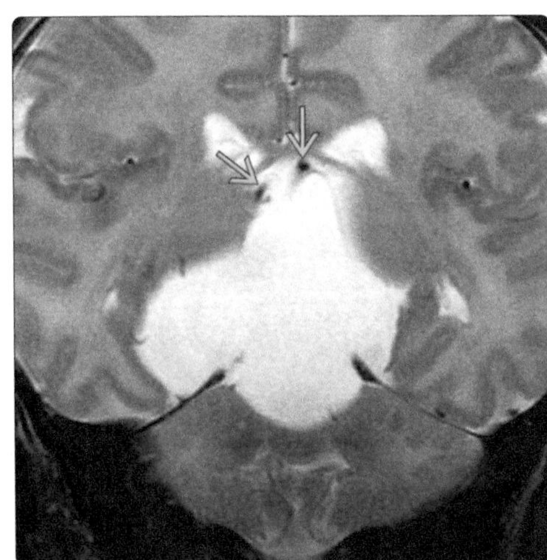

(Left) *Sagittal color Doppler ultrasound in a newborn demonstrates a lobulated anechoic mass in the quadrigeminal cistern. There is no flow within the lesion, excluding a vein of Galen aneurysm and making an AC the most likely diagnosis.* **(Right)** *Coronal T2 MR in the same newborn shows the full extent of the large, lobulated cyst in the quadrigeminal cistern. The cyst extends into the supratentorial compartment through the tentorial incisura, displacing the internal cerebral veins ➔ superiorly.*

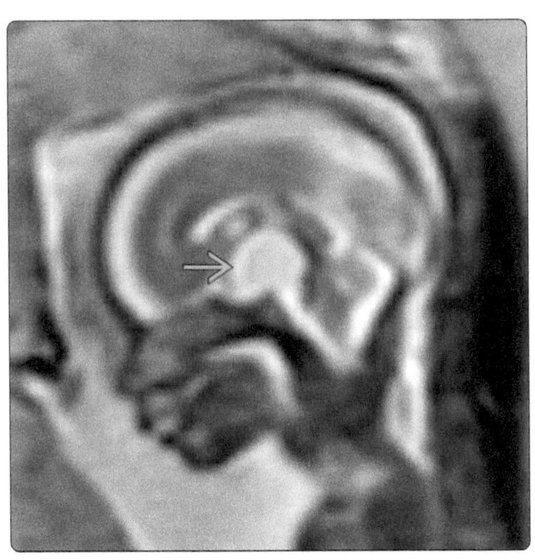

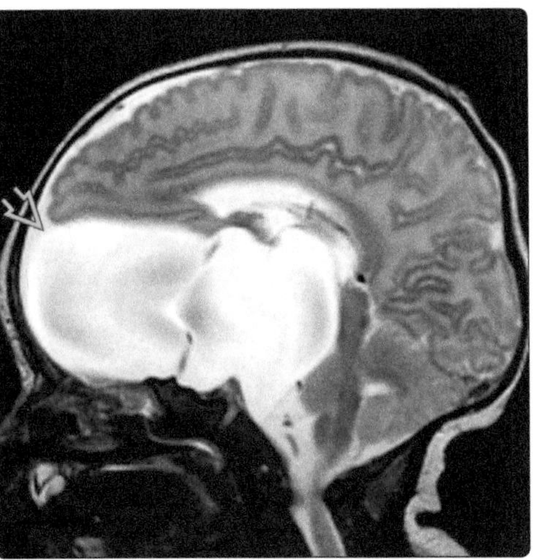

(Left) *Sagittal T2 SSFSE from a fetal MR in a 21-weeks-gestational age fetus shows a suprasellar cystic mass ➔ that followed CSF signal intensity on all sequences, consistent with an AC.* **(Right)** *Sagittal T2 MR in the same patient 3 days following birth shows a dramatic interval increase in the size of the lesion with extension from the suprasellar cistern into the inferior left anterior cranial fossa ⇨. ACs identified in fetuses and young children have a higher risk of growing.*

KEY FACTS

TERMINOLOGY

- Benign, ectopic, squamous epithelial cyst containing dermal elements, including hair follicles and sebaceous and sweat glands

IMAGING

- Midline unilocular cystic lesion with fat
    - Subarachnoid fatty droplets if ruptured
- Suprasellar or posterior fossa most common intracranial sites
- Extracranial sites = spine, orbit
    - May have fistulous connections to skin (dermal sinus tract)
- CT hypodensity and negative Hounsfield units (fat)
    - 20% capsular Ca^{++}
- MR: T1 hyperintense
    - Fat-suppression sequence confirms lipid elements
    - Fat-fluid level in cyst and in ventricles (if ruptured)
- With rupture: Extensive leptomeningeal enhancement possible from chemical meningitis

TOP DIFFERENTIAL DIAGNOSES

- Epidermoid cyst
- Craniopharyngioma
- Teratoma
- Lipoma

CLINICAL ISSUES

- Rare: < 0.5% of primary intracranial tumors
- Intradural dermoid cysts 4-9x less common than epidermoid cysts
- Rupture can cause significant morbidity/mortality
- Dermoid + dermal sinus may cause meningitis, hydrocephalus
- Treatment: Complete surgical excision ± shunt for hydrocephalus

(Left) *Sagittal graphic of an inferior frontal dermoid cyst* ➡ *shows a discrete, heterogeneous, fat-containing mass with squamous epithelium and dermal appendages. There is a ventricular fat-fluid level* ➡ *and fat within the subarachnoid spaces* ➡ *related to the rupture.* **(Right)** *Axial NECT shows a hypodense midline fatty mass with focal Ca^{++}* ➡*, characteristic for a ruptured dermoid cyst. Note fatty hypodense droplets in the sylvian fissures and subarachnoid spaces* ➡*.*

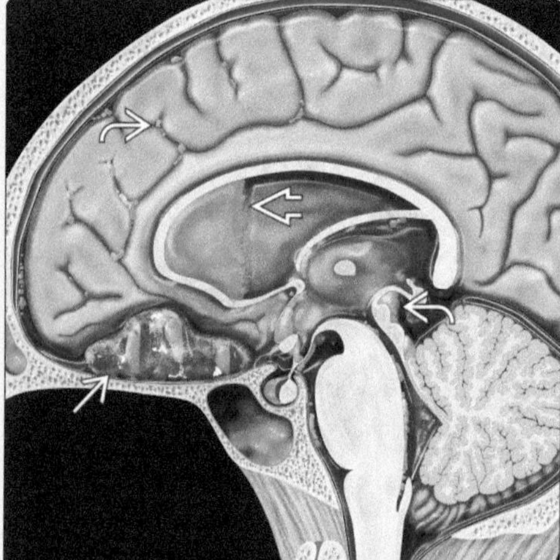

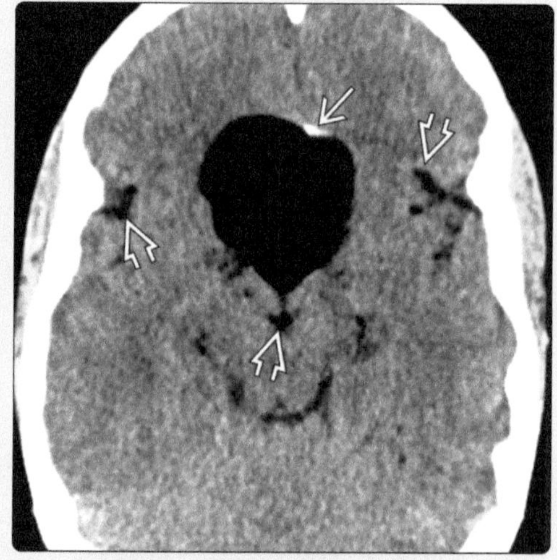

(Left) *Axial T1 MR shows a classic dermoid cyst with hyperintense T1 signal* ➡*. Note fatty droplets in the adjacent sylvian fissure* ➡*, consistent with prior rupture of the dermoid cyst.* **(Right)** *Sagittal T2 FS MR in a 9-month-old shows a nasal dermal cyst* ➡*, also along the deep sinus tract in the prenasal space* ➡*, with an intracranial dermoid component at the foramen cecum* ➡*. This case demonstrates the spectrum of regions that may be affected with a nasal dermal sinus and nasal dermoid.*

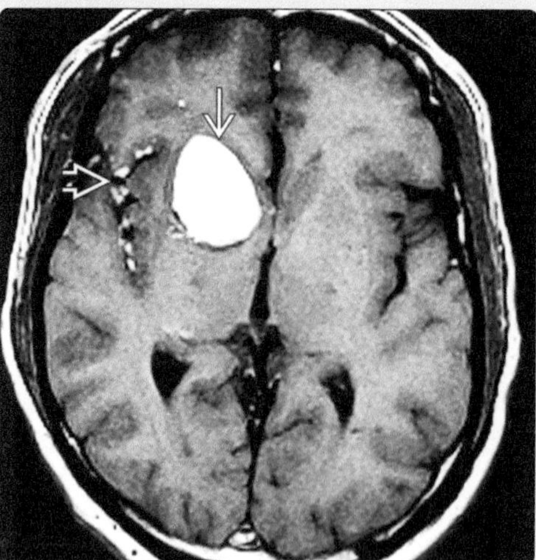

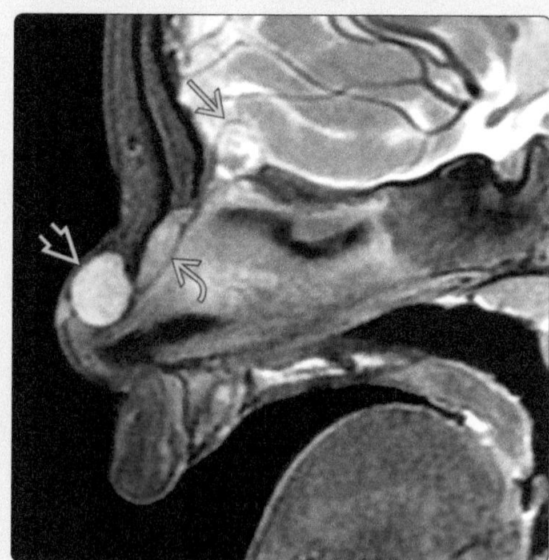

TERMINOLOGY

Synonyms

- Dermoid inclusion cyst, ectodermal inclusion cyst

Definitions

- Benign, ectopic, squamous epithelial cyst containing dermal elements, including hair follicles and sebaceous and sweat glands

IMAGING

General Features

- Best diagnostic clue
  - Midline, nonenhancing, unilocular cystic lesion with fat
    - Subarachnoid and intraventricular fatty droplets may occur with rupture
- Location
  - Suprasellar, parasellar
  - Less common in posterior fossa: Cisterna magna, 4th ventricle, basal cisterns, cavernous sinus
  - Extracranial sites = nose, spine, orbit
    - May have fistulous connections to skin (dermal sinus tract)
    - Orbit: Dermolipoma at zygomaticofrontal suture
  - Ruptured: Subarachnoid/intraventricular spread of contents
- Size
  - Variable
- Morphology
  - Well-circumscribed, lipid-containing mass
  - Fat is sometimes only small component

CT Findings

- NECT
  - Round/lobulated, well-delineated, unilocular cystic mass
  - Hypodensity and negative Hounsfield units from fat
  - Capsular Ca^{++} (20%)
  - With rupture, droplets of fat disseminate in cisterns, may cause fat-fluid level within ventricles
  - Skull/scalp dermoid expands diploë
  - Frontonasal dermoid sinus tract: Bifid crista galli; large foramen cecum + sinus tract
  - Rare, dense dermoid: Hyperattenuating
- CECT
  - Generally no enhancement in absence of infection

MR Findings

- T1WI
  - Unruptured: Hyperintense
  - Ruptured: Droplets very hyperintense
    - Fat-suppression sequence confirms lipid elements
    - Fat-fluid level in cyst; if ruptured, in ventricles as well
  - Rare, dense dermoid: Very hyperintense
- T2WI
  - Unruptured: Heterogeneous, hypo- to hyperintense
    - Chemical shift artifact in frequency encoding direction with long repetition time
  - Ruptured: Typically hyperintense droplets
  - Rare, dense dermoid: Very hypointense
  - With hair: Fine curvilinear hypointense elements
- DWI
  - Variable, diffusion restriction may occur in solid components
- T1WI C+
  - ± mild enhancement of capsule without central enhancement
  - With rupture: Extensive leptomeningeal enhancement possible from chemical meningitis
  - With infection: May see rim enhancement
- MRS
  - Elevated lipid peak from 0.9-1.3 ppm

Angiographic Findings

- Vasospasm with chemical meningitis from rupture
  - May relieve vasospasm with angioplasty
- Dermoid-encased vessels may have ↑ rupture risk

Imaging Recommendations

- Best imaging tool
  - MR with fat saturation
- Protocol advice
  - Use fat-suppression sequence to confirm diagnosis
  - Chemical shift-selective sequence useful to detect tiny droplets

DIFFERENTIAL DIAGNOSIS

Epidermoid Cyst

- Most epidermoid cysts resemble CSF, not fat
- Restricted diffusion on DWI is classic
- Cyst lined with squamous epithelium without dermal elements
- 4-9x more common than dermoid
- Off-midline > midline: In cerebellopontine angle (40-50%), parasellar/middle fossa (10-15%), diploic (10%)

Craniopharyngioma

- Also suprasellar/midline, often with intrasellar component
- Does not contain fat
- CT: Multilocular with solid enhancing tissue (> 90%), nodular Ca^{++} in majority
- MR: Commonly T1 hypointense, T2 hyperintense, enhances strongly
- More common than dermoid (3-5% of primary intracranial tumors)

Teratoma

- Location similar but usually pineal region
- 90% have all 3 embryologic layers: Ectoderm, mesoderm, endoderm
- Often multicystic/multiloculated
- Heterogeneous appearance containing Ca^{++}, CSF, lipid, and soft tissue components
- Does not have fat-fluid level

Lipoma

- Homogeneous midline fat
- Dermoids more likely heterogeneous
- Ca^{++} less frequent than in dermoid

PATHOLOGY

General Features

- Etiology
  - Embryology (2 theories)
    - Sequestration of surface ectoderm at lines of epithelial fusion/along course of normal embryonic invaginations
    - Inclusion of cutaneous ectoderm at time of neural tube closure; 3rd to 5th week of embryogenesis
  - Can also arise at any age from traumatic implantation (i.e., lumbar puncture)
  - Similar etiology with epidermoid, which is thought to be later in development and off-midline
- Genetics
  - Usually sporadic
  - Association with Goldenhar syndrome
  - Possible association with Klippel-Feil syndrome
- Associated abnormalities
  - Occipital/nasofrontal dermal sinus may be present; 89% of dermal sinuses associated with inclusion cysts
  - Goldenhar syndrome (a.k.a. oculoauriculovertebral dysplasia); congenital condition includes
    - Cranial lipomas and dermoids
    - Ocular dermoids
    - Anomalies of 1st and 2nd branchial arch derivatives
    - Cardiovascular, facial, oral, auricular, visceral, and spinal defects

Gross Pathologic & Surgical Features

- Unilocular cyst with thick wall
- Contents = lipid and cholesterol elements from sebaceous secretions floating on proteinaceous material

Microscopic Features

- Outer wall of squamous epithelium
- Inner lining contains dermal elements of hair follicles, sebaceous and apocrine glands
- Rare squamous cell carcinoma (SCCa) degeneration
  - Squamous cell predominance with some glandular differentiation
  - Suggestive of poorly differentiated SCCa with adenomatous component

CLINICAL ISSUES

Presentation

- Most common signs/symptoms
  - Uncomplicated dermoid: Headache (32%), seizure (30%) are most common symptoms
    - Large cyst can cause obstructive hydrocephalus
    - Less commonly hypopituitarism, diabetes insipidus, or cranial nerve (CN) defects
    - Suprasellar may present with visual symptoms
  - Cyst rupture causes chemical meningitis (6.9%)
- Other signs/symptoms
  - Recurrent meningitis when associated with sinus tract

Demographics

- Age
  - 2nd-3rd decades
- Sex
  - Slight male predilection
- Epidemiology
  - Rare: < 0.5% of primary intracranial tumors
  - Intradural dermoid cysts 4-9x less common than epidermoid cysts

Natural History & Prognosis

- Benign, slow growing
- Larger lesions associated with higher rupture rate
- Rupture can cause significant morbidity/mortality
  - Relatively rare and typically spontaneous
  - Seizure, coma, vasospasm, infarction, death
- Dermoid + dermal sinus may cause meningitis, hydrocephalus
- Rare malignant transformation into SCCa
  - Postulated prolonged or reparative process from foreign material leads to cellular atypia and neoplasia
  - May occur years after surgical resection

Treatment

- Complete surgical excision
  - Residual capsule may lead to recurrence
  - Rare SCCa degeneration within surgical remnants
- Subarachnoid dissemination of contents may occur during operative/postoperative course
  - Cause aseptic meningitis or other complications (hydrocephalus, seizures, CN deficits)
    - May require shunt placement for hydrocephalus
  - Alternatively, disseminated fat particles can remain silent without radiologic/neurologic change
    - Justifies "wait and see" approach
    - Regular MR and clinical exams are necessary to avoid complications

DIAGNOSTIC CHECKLIST

Consider

- When possible, dermoid is seen near glabella or crista galli; look for sinus tract

Image Interpretation Pearls

- Follows fat characteristics on NECT and T1WI fat-suppressed MR

SELECTED REFERENCES

1. Delgado-Muñoz P et al: A rare case of an intracranial dermoid cyst with atypical appearance on computed tomography and magnetic resonance imaging. Am J Case Rep. 23:e935115, 2022
2. Taha A et al: Traumatic rupture of a skull base dermoid cyst mimicking chronic meningitis. Cureus. 14(5):e25066, 2022
3. Balasundaram P et al: Evolution of epidermoid cyst into dermoid cyst: embryological explanation and radiological-pathological correlation. Neuroradiol J. 32(2):92-7, 2019
4. Akbari SHA et al: Focal traumatic rupture of a dermoid cyst in a pediatric patient: case report and literature review. Childs Nerv Syst. 34(12):2485-90, 2018
5. Giordano F et al: Interdural cavernous sinus dermoid cyst in a child: case report. J Neurosurg Pediatr. 19(3):354-60, 2017
6. Zhang YK et al: Association of craniovertebral junction anomalies, Klippel-Feil syndrome, ruptured dermoid cyst and mirror movement in one patient: a unique case and literature review. Turk Neurosurg. 26(1):153-65, 2016
7. Wang YM et al: Spontaneous rupture of intracranial dermoid cyst with chemical meningitis. J Emerg Med. 44(2):e275-6, 2013
8. Schneider UC et al: Intracranial, supratentorial dermoid cysts in paediatric patients–two cases and a review of the literature. Childs Nerv Syst. 28(2):185-90, 2012

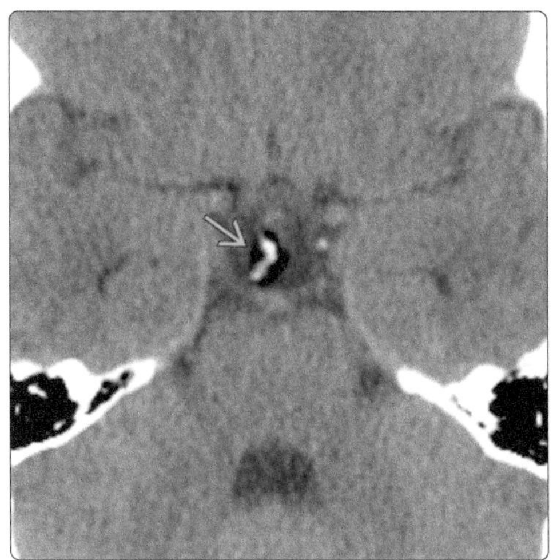

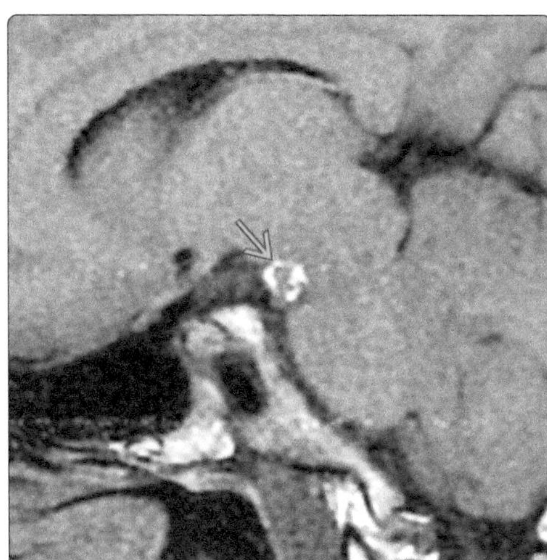

(Left) *Axial NECT in a teenage patient shows a small lesion ⇒ in the suprasellar cistern containing fat and* Ca^{++}. *Intracranial fat can mimic gas on brain windows so it is important to apply a narrow window (e.g., lung).* **(Right)** *Sagittal T1 MR in the same patient shows areas of hyperintense signal within the lesion ⇒, which suppressed on fat-saturation images, consistent with macroscopic fat. Postcontrast images showed no associated enhancement. The location and imaging appearance is typical for a dermoid cyst.*

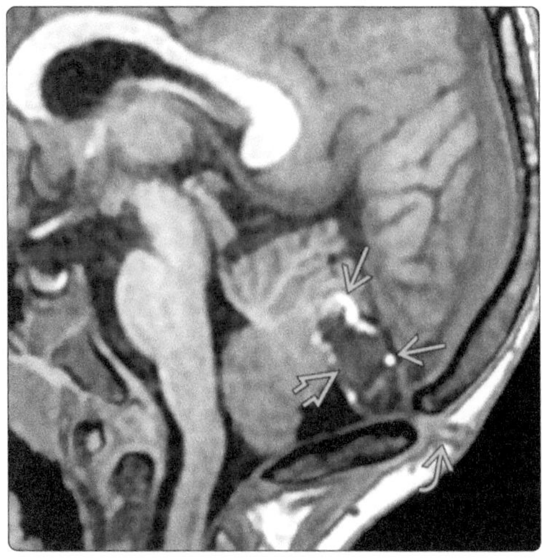

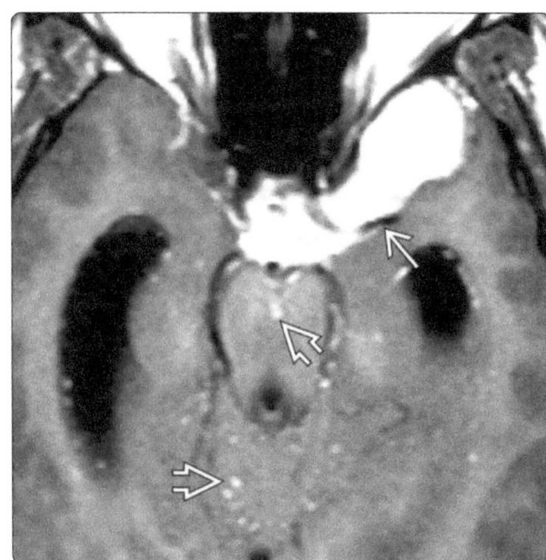

(Left) *Sagittal T1 MR in a 7-year-old with a dermoid cyst in the midline posterior fossa associated with cerebellar vermis shows hyperintense fat ⇒ along cyst margin, dermal sinus tract ⇒, and occipital bone defect ⇒.* **(Right)** *Axial T1 MR in the same patient shows a hyperintense mass ⇒ with scattered foci of hyperintensity throughout the subarachnoid space ⇒. Chemical meningitis from a ruptured dermoid, while uncommon, can cause significant morbidity from seizures, vasospasm, infarction, and even death.*

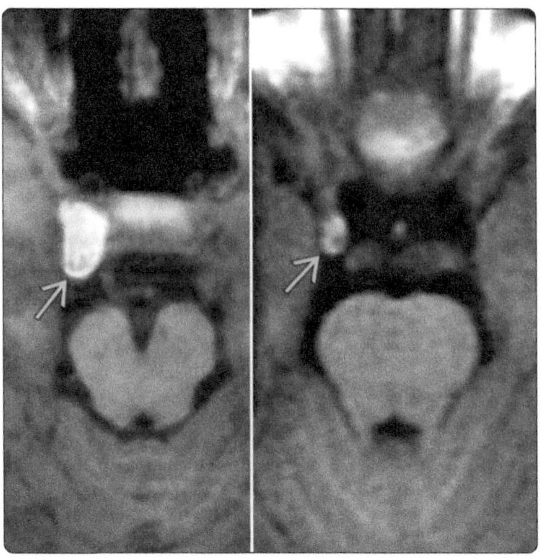

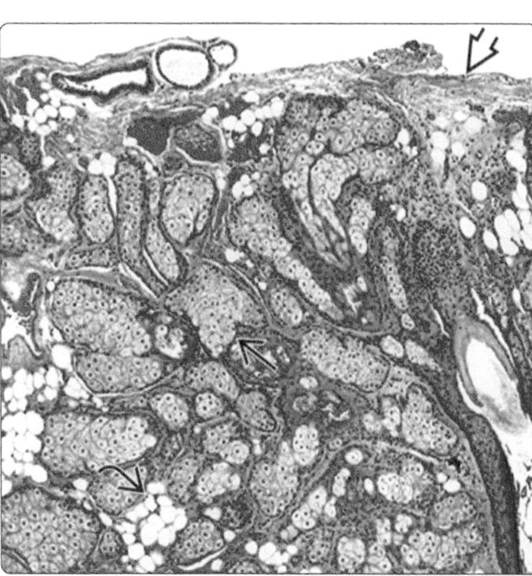

(Left) *Axial T1 MR images in a patient at 15 years (left) and 1 year (right) of age shows the slow growth of a hyperintense lesion ⇒ in the right cavernous sinus. The lesion demonstrated no associated enhancement. Overall, these findings are most suggestive of a dermoid cyst. Cysts in this location will typically present with cranial nerve deficits.* **(Right)** *High-power micropathology shows the typical dermoid cyst features with keratin lining ⇒, multiple sebaceous glands ⇒, and fat ⇒.*

KEY FACTS

TERMINOLOGY

- Intracranial epidermoids: Congenital ectodermal inclusion cysts

IMAGING

- CSF-like mass that insinuates cisterns and encases neurovascular structures
- Morphology: Lobulated, irregular, cauliflower-like mass with "fronds"
- CT: Hypodense (~ CSF), nonenhancing mass
- MR
    - T1/T2: Often nearly isointense to CSF
    - FLAIR: Usually does not completely null
    - T1 C+: No enhancement
    - DWI: Marked "light bulb bright" hyperintensity

TOP DIFFERENTIAL DIAGNOSES

- Arachnoid cyst
- Inflammatory cyst (e.g., neurocysticercosis)
- Cystic neoplasm
- Dermoid cyst

PATHOLOGY

- Arise from ectodermal inclusions during neural tube closure, weeks 3-5 of embryogenesis

CLINICAL ISSUES

- Symptoms depend on location and effect on adjacent neurovascular structures
    - Most common symptom: Headache
    - Cranial nerve V, VII, VIII neuropathy common
- 0.2-1.8% of all primary intracranial tumors
- Rare malignant degeneration into squamous cell carcinoma
- Treatment: Microsurgical resection
    - Recurrence common if incompletely removed

DIAGNOSTIC CHECKLIST

- Insinuates and surrounds rather than displaces
- Incomplete nulling on FLAIR; DWI hyperintense

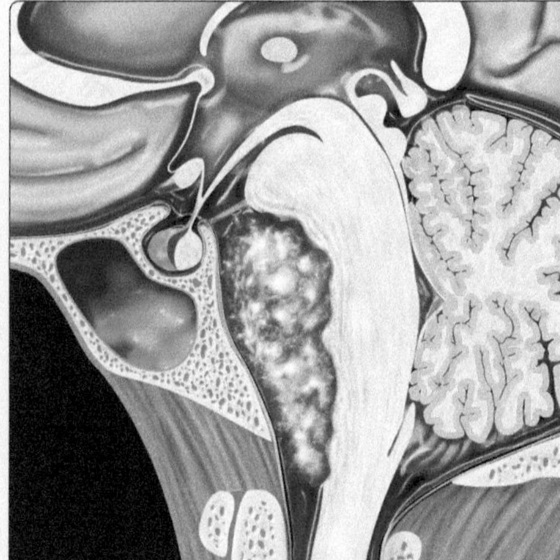

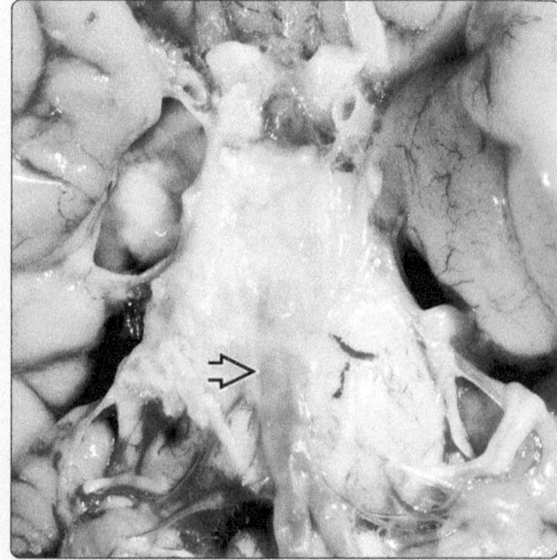

(Left) *Sagittal graphic illustrates a multilobulated epidermoid cyst primarily within the prepontine cistern. Significant mass effect displaces the pons, cervicomedullary junction, and upper cervical spine.* **(Right)** *Gross pathology shows an epidermoid cyst extending anterosuperiorly from the cerebellopontine angle (CPA) cistern, insinuating within the prepontine cistern, and encasing the basilar artery ➾. Note its typical pearly appearance. (Courtesy E. Hedley-Whyte, MD.)*

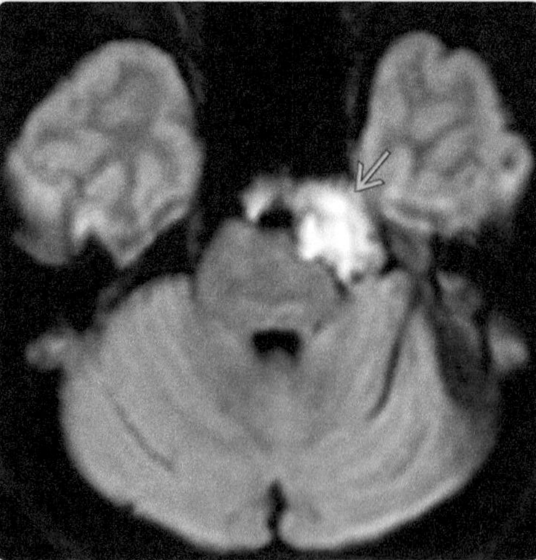

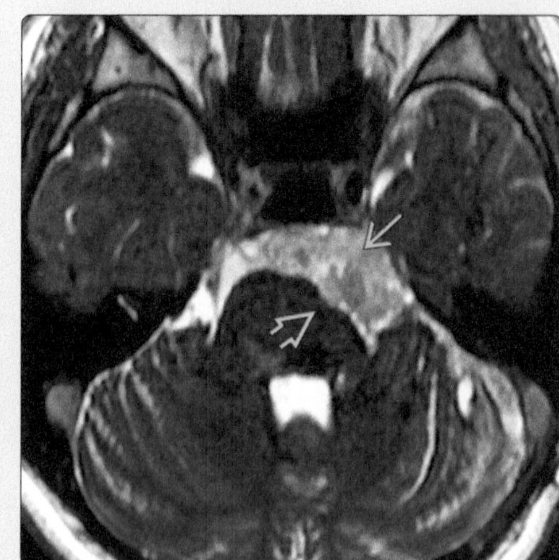

(Left) *Axial DWI MR in a teenager shows a lesion ➡ in the left CPA cistern with extension across midline. The marked ↑ DWI signal and location are characteristic of an epidermoid cyst. Epidermoid cysts in this location often cause cranial neuropathy over time as they grow.* **(Right)** *Axial FIESTA MR in the same patient shows the epidermoid ➡ causing mass effect on the brainstem ➾. FIESTA imaging is often helpful to evaluate for involvement of small structures, such as cranial nerves.*

TERMINOLOGY

Synonyms

- Ectodermal inclusion cyst

Definitions

- Intracranial epidermoids: Congenital ectodermal inclusion cysts

IMAGING

General Features

- Best diagnostic clue
  - CSF-like mass that insinuates cisterns and encases neurovascular structures
- Location
  - Extracranial and calvarial epidermoids are very common
  - Intracranial epidermoids are uncommon with lesions located primarily in basal cisterns
    - Cerebellopontine angle (CPA) (40-50%)
    - 4th ventricle (17%)
    - Parasellar/middle cranial fossa (10-15%)
    - Cerebral hemispheres (rare) (1.5%)
    - Brainstem location exceedingly rare
    - Intraventricular within tela choroidea of temporal horn, 3rd or 4th ventricles
- Morphology
  - Lobulated, irregular, cauliflower-like mass with "fronds"
  - Insinuates without mass effect unless large

Radiographic Findings

- Radiography
  - Diploic space epidermoids
    - May alter scalp, outer/inner skull tables, and epidural space appearance
    - Typically round or lobulated
    - Well delineated with sclerotic rim

CT Findings

- NECT
  - Round/lobulated mass
  - > 95% hypodense, resembling CSF
  - 10-25% contain Ca^{++}
  - Rare variant = "dense" epidermoid
    - 3% of intracranial epidermoids
    - Secondary to hemorrhage, high protein, saponification of cyst debris to calcium soaps or iron-containing pigment
- CECT
  - Usually none, though margin of cyst may show minimal enhancement
- Bone CT
  - May have bony erosion; sharply corticated margins when intradiploic

MR Findings

- T1WI
  - Often (~ 75%) slightly hyperintense to CSF
  - Lobulated periphery may be slightly more hyperintense than center
  - Uncommonly hyperintense to brain ("white epidermoid") due to high triglycerides and unsaturated fatty acids
  - Uncommonly hypointense to CSF ("black epidermoid")
    - Presence of solid crystal cholesterol and keratin
    - Lack of triglycerides and unsaturated fatty acids
- T2WI
  - Often isointense (65%) to slightly hyperintense (35%) to CSF
  - Very rarely hypointense due to Ca^{++}, ↓ hydration, viscous secretions, and iron pigments
- FLAIR
  - Usually does not completely null
- DWI
  - Characteristic hyperintensity
    - High fractional anisotropy due to diffusion along 2D geometric plane
      - □ Attributed to microstructure of parallel-layered keratin filaments and flakes
    - In comparison to white matter, which also shows high fractional anisotropy, due to diffusion along single direction
  - ADC = ~ brain parenchyma
- T1WI C+
  - Usually none, though margin of cyst may show minimal enhancement (25%)
  - Enhancing tumor is sign of malignant degeneration (very rare)
- MRS
  - Resonances from lactate; no NAA, choline, or lipid

Angiographic Findings

- Conventional
  - Depending on location and size, may show avascular mass effect

Nonvascular Interventions

- Myelography
  - Cisternography contrast delineates irregular lobulated tumor borders, extends into interstices

Imaging Recommendations

- Best imaging tool
  - MR with contrast
- Protocol advice
  - FLAIR and DWI are key to identification and discrimination, especially in small lesions
  - Diffusion hyperintensity definitively distinguishes from arachnoid cyst
  - Contrast may be helpful to distinguish from cellular tumor

DIFFERENTIAL DIAGNOSIS

Arachnoid Cyst

- Usually isointense to CSF on all standard sequences
  - Completely nulls on FLAIR
  - Hypointense diffusion: Contains highly mobile CSF, ADC = stationary water
- Rather than insinuate and engulf local structures, arachnoid cysts displace them
- Smooth surface, unlike lobulations of epidermoids

Inflammatory Cyst

- i.e., neurocysticercosis

- Often enhances
- Density/signal intensity usually not precisely like CSF
- Adjacent edema, gliosis common

Cystic Neoplasm

- Attenuation/signal intensity not that of CSF
- Often enhances

Dermoid Cyst

- Usually at or near midline
- Resembles fat, not CSF, and contains dermal appendages; often ruptured

PATHOLOGY

General Features

- Etiology
  - Congenital: Embryology
    - Arise from ectodermal inclusions during neural tube closure at weeks 3-5 of embryogenesis
    - Congenital intradural CPA epidermoids derived from cells of 1st branchial groove
  - Acquired: Develop as result of trauma
    - Uncommon etiology for intracranial tumors
    - More common as spine etiology following lumbar puncture
- Genetics
  - Sporadic
- Associated abnormalities
  - May have occipital/nasofrontal dermal sinus tract
  - Elevated CA19-9

Gross Pathologic & Surgical Features

- Outer surface often has shiny, glistening mother of pearl appearance ("beautiful tumor")
- Soft and pliable
  - Conforms to shape of adjacent local structures/spaces
- Lobulated excrescences
  - May invaginate into brain
- Insinuating growth pattern, extends through cisterns, surrounds and encases vessels/nerves
- Cyst filled with soft, waxy, creamy, or flaky material

Microscopic Features

- Cyst wall = internal layer of simple stratified cuboidal squamous epithelium covered by fibrous capsule
- Cyst contents = solid crystalline cholesterol, keratinaceous debris; no dermal appendages
- Grows by progressive desquamation with conversion to keratin/cholesterol crystals, forming concentric lamellae

CLINICAL ISSUES

Presentation

- Most common signs/symptoms
  - Symptoms depend on location and effect on adjacent neurovascular structures
    - Most common symptom: Headache
    - Cranial nerve V, VII, VIII neuropathy common
    - 4th ventricular cerebellar signs common, yet ↑ intracranial pressure rare
    - Less commonly hypopituitarism, diabetes insipidus
    - Seizures if in sylvian fissure/temporal lobe
  - May remain clinically silent for many years

Demographics

- Age
  - Presents between 20-60 years with peak at 40 years
  - Presentation is uncommon in childhood
- Sex
  - M = F
    - CT-hyperdense variant lesions have female predominance (M:F = 1.0:2.5)
- Epidemiology
  - Epidermoids make up 0.2-1.8% of all primary intracranial tumors
  - Much more common than dermoid cyst (4-9x higher incidence)
  - 3rd most common CPA/internal carotid artery (ICA) mass, after vestibular schwannoma and meningioma

Natural History & Prognosis

- Grows slowly: Epithelial component growth rate commensurate to that of normal epithelium
- Chemical meningitis possible from content leakage
- Rare malignant degeneration into squamous cell carcinoma (SCCa) reported
  - Postulated prolonged or reparative process from foreign material leads to cellular atypia and neoplasia
  - Often predated by frequent recurrences
  - May occur years after surgical resection
  - Mean age at presentation: 52 years with male preponderance

Treatment

- Microsurgical resection
  - Complicated by investment of local structures
  - Recurrence common if incompletely removed
  - Subarachnoid dissemination of contents may occur during operative/postoperative course
    - May cause chemical meningitis
    - CSF seeding and implantation reported
- Rare malignant degeneration of resection bed into SCCa reported

DIAGNOSTIC CHECKLIST

Consider

- Epidermoid if insinuates and surrounds rather than displaces

Image Interpretation Pearls

- Resembles CSF on imaging studies, except usually incomplete nulling on FLAIR
- DWI hyperintensity is diagnostic

SELECTED REFERENCES

1. Pop MM et al: Intracranial epidermoid cysts: benign entities with malignant behavior: experience with 36 cases. Sci Rep. 13(1):6474, 2023
2. Hasegawa H et al: Long-term surgical outcomes of intracranial epidermoid tumors: impact of extent of resection on recurrence and functional outcomes in 63 patients. J Neurosurg. 136(6):1592-600, 2022
3. Nitheesha Reddy V et al: Spectrum of intracranial and spinal epidermoids including unusual locations and imaging findings: a pictorial review. J Med Imaging Radiat Oncol. 67(1):65-76, 2022

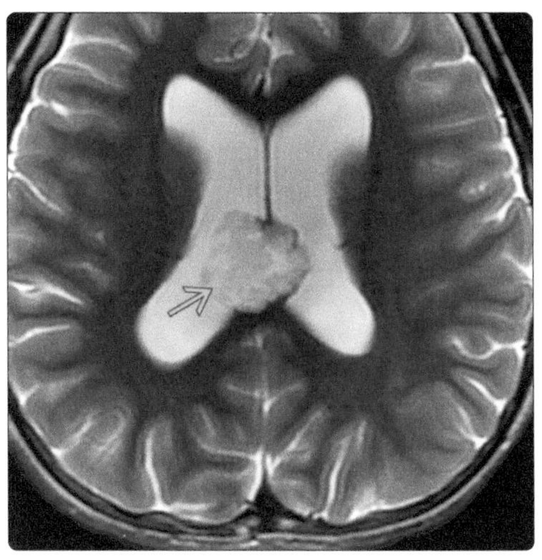

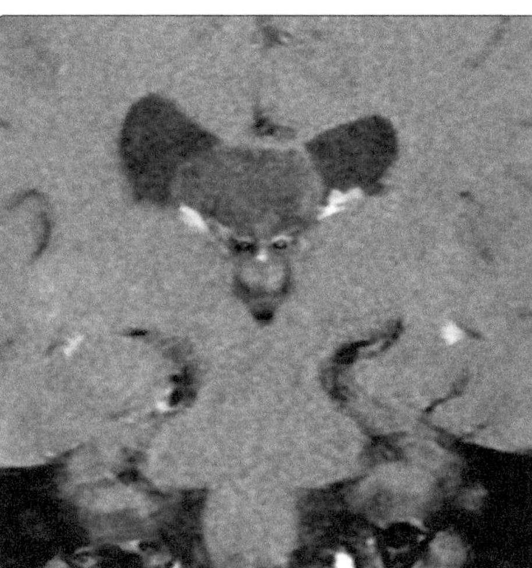

(Left) *Axial T2 MR in a 14-year-old boy with a slightly lobulated lesion ⇒ centered in the posterior septum pellucidum is shown. The lesion is very T2 hyperintense, nearly equal to CSF, common for epidermoid cysts.* **(Right)** *Coronal T1 C+ MR in the same patient shows a hypointense lesion with no associated enhancement. Depending on the imaging parameters, epidermoids may be invisible on T1, as they are isointense to CSF. DWI (not shown) showed markedly hyperintense signal, confirming an epidermoid.*

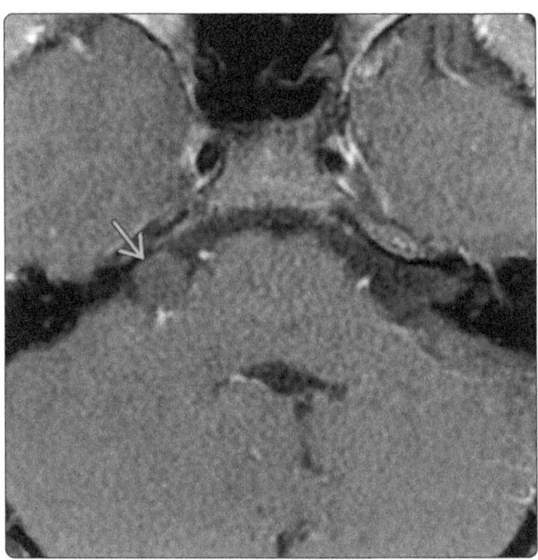

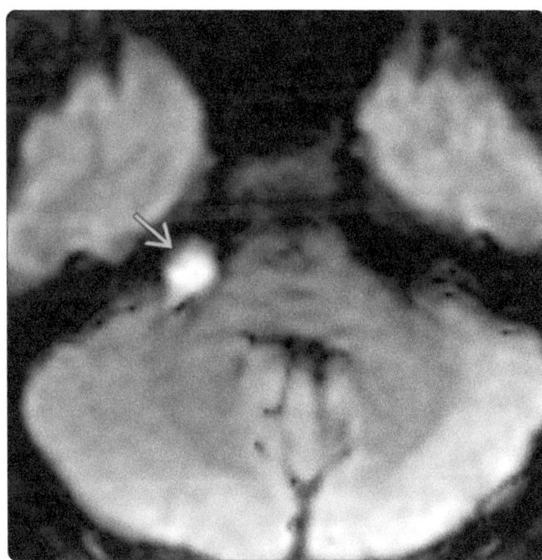

(Left) *Axial T1 C+ MR in a 9-year-old with a small lesion ⇒ in the right CPA shows the lesion to be very hypointense with no associated contrast enhancement. Nonenhancement is one of the hallmark findings of epidermoid cysts.* **(Right)** *Axial DWI MR in the same patient shows marked "light-bulb bright" hyperintense signal ⇒, characteristic of an epidermoid cyst. Small epidermoids may be inconspicuous on conventional imaging but very obvious on DWI.*

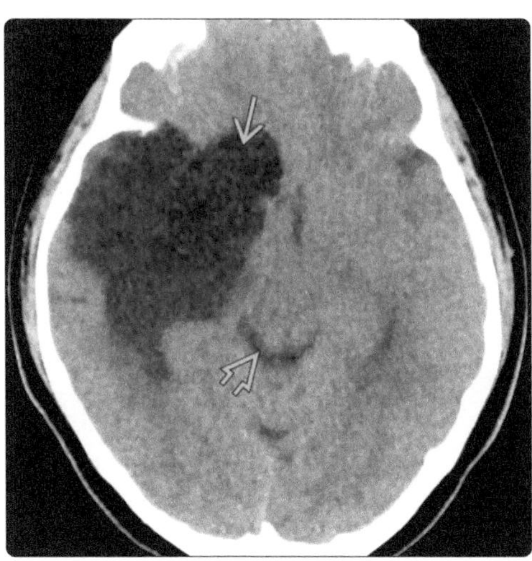

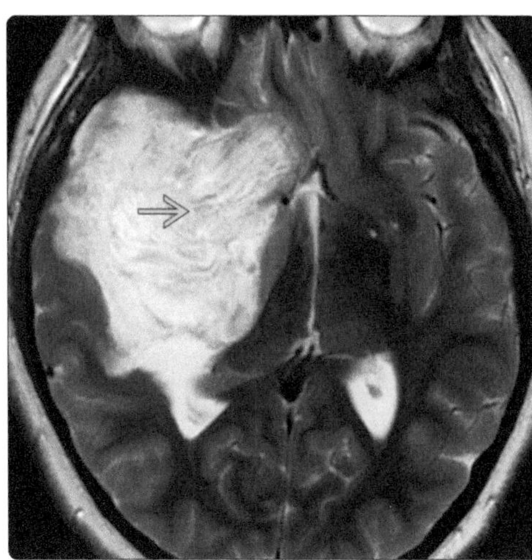

(Left) *Axial NECT in a 14-year-old with a very large hypointense lesion ⇒ centered in the right sylvian fissure is shown. The lesion causes scalloping of adjacent brain, and the density of the lesion is nearly that of CSF ⇒, which is characteristic of epidermoid cysts.* **(Right)** *Axial T2 MR in the same patient shows the lesion to be very hyperintense (nearly CSF signal) with internal sheets of isointense signal ⇒. Such large epidermoids are very uncommon and are often mistaken for primary CNS neoplasms.*

Neuroglial Cyst

KEY FACTS

TERMINOLOGY

- Neuroglial cyst (NGC), a.k.a. glioependymal cyst
- Benign, glial-lined, fluid-containing cavity buried within cerebral white matter
  - May occur anywhere throughout neuraxis
  - Frontal lobe most common site
  - Size varies from few mm up to several cm

IMAGING

- CT
  - Well-delineated, low-density, unilocular parenchymal cyst
  - No Ca^{++} or enhancement
- MR
  - T1 hypo-/T2 hyperintense (resembles CSF)
  - Suppresses on FLAIR
  - Does not restrict on DWI
  - No enhancement
  - Minimal/no surrounding signal abnormality

TOP DIFFERENTIAL DIAGNOSES

- Porencephalic cyst
- Enlarged perivascular spaces
- Arachnoid cyst
- Ependymal cyst
- Epidermoid cyst
- Infectious cyst (e.g., neurocysticercosis, echinococcosis)
- Low-grade neoplasm

DIAGNOSTIC CHECKLIST

- Parenchymal cysts that do not communicate with ventricular system and have minimal/no surrounding gliosis may be NGC
- Use FLAIR, DWI to help distinguish between different types of intracranial cysts
- If lesion does not suppress on FLAIR, must consider solid lesion (i.e., low-grade neoplasm)

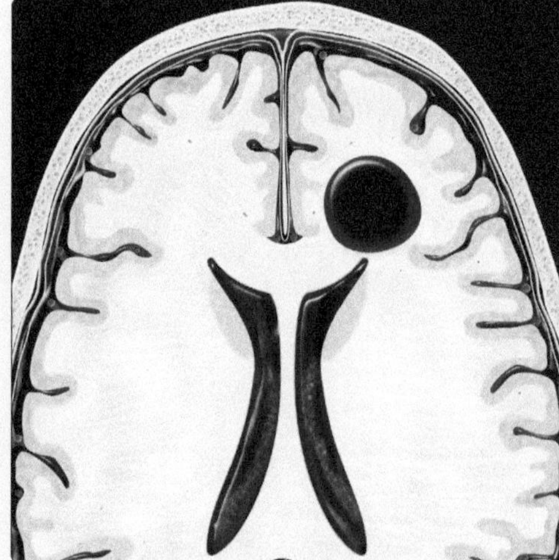

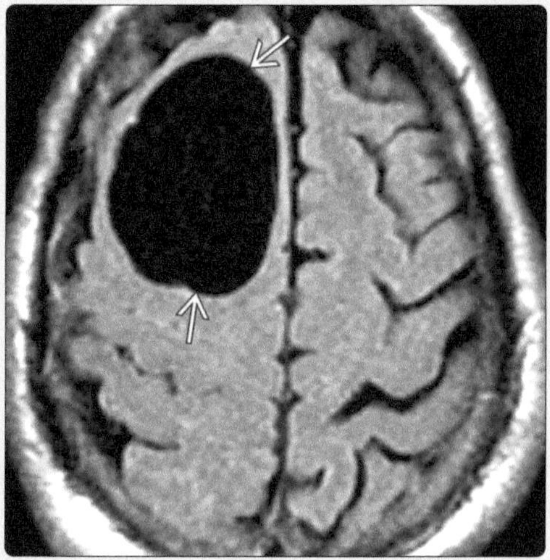

(Left) *Axial graphic shows a classic neuroglial cyst. This well-delineated, unilocular lesion does not communicate with the ventricles and contains clear fluid. The surrounding brain is normal. Neuroglial cysts are lined with glial cells, astrocytes, and, rarely, ependymal cells.* **(Right)** *Axial FLAIR MR in a young adult with headaches shows a large right frontal CSF-like cyst ➡.*

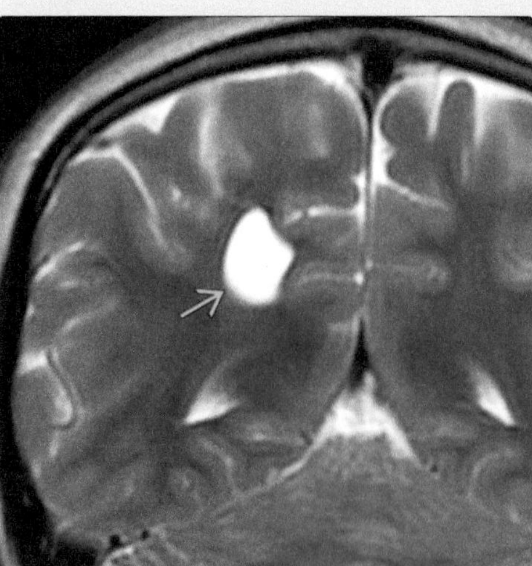

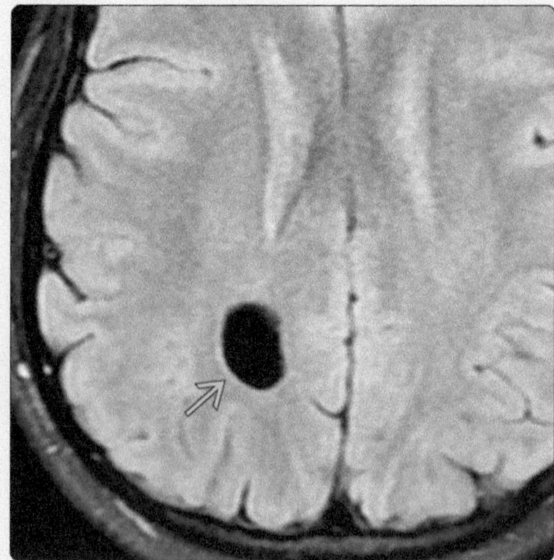

(Left) *Coronal T2 MR in a teenager with a headache shows a unilocular cyst ⇨ in the right parietal deep white matter.* **(Right)** *Axial FLAIR MR in the same patient shows the cyst ⇨ contents completely suppress similar to CSF, a characteristic finding in a neuroglial cyst. Also note the lack of any nodular soft tissue or parenchymal signal abnormality that would suggest an alternative diagnosis, such as a neoplasm.*

TERMINOLOGY

Abbreviations

- Neuroglial cyst (NGC)

Synonyms

- Glioependymal cyst

Definitions

- Benign, glial-lined, fluid-containing cavity buried within cerebral white matter

IMAGING

General Features

- Best diagnostic clue
  - Nonenhancing, CSF-like parenchymal cyst with minimal/no surrounding signal abnormality
- Location
  - May occur anywhere throughout neuraxis
    - Frontal lobe most common site
    - Intraparenchymal > extraparenchymal
- Size
  - Varies from few mm up to several cm
- Morphology
  - Smooth, rounded, unilocular, benign-appearing cyst

CT Findings

- NECT
  - Well-delineated, low-density cyst
    - Unilocular; no Ca^{++}
- CECT
  - Wall does not enhance

MR Findings

- T1WI
  - Usually hypointense, resembles CSF
- T2WI
  - Hyperintense
- PD/intermediate
  - May be slightly hyperintense to CSF
- FLAIR
  - Suppresses
- DWI
  - No diffusion restriction
- T1WI C+
  - No enhancement

Imaging Recommendations

- Best imaging tool
  - MR with T1 C+, FLAIR, DWI

DIFFERENTIAL DIAGNOSIS

Porencephalic Cyst

- Communicates with ventricles
- Adjacent brain usually shows gliosis, spongiosis

Enlarged Perivascular Spaces

- Clusters of variable-sized cysts > single, unilocular cyst

Arachnoid Cyst

- Extraaxial

Ependymal Cyst

- Intraventricular

Epidermoid Cyst

- Does not suppress on FLAIR, restricts on DWI

Infectious Cyst

- e.g., neurocysticercosis, echinococcosis

Low-Grade Neoplasm

- Must consider anytime "cystic" lesion does not suppress on FLAIR

PATHOLOGY

Gross Pathologic & Surgical Features

- Rounded, smooth, unilocular cyst usually containing clear fluid resembling CSF

Microscopic Features

- Varies from columnar (ependymal type) epithelium to low cuboidal cells resembling choroid plexus
  - Variable expression of GFAP
  - Cytokeratin, EMA expression absent

CLINICAL ISSUES

Presentation

- Most common signs/symptoms
  - Headache
- Other signs/symptoms
  - Seizures
  - Neurologic deficit (depends on cyst size, location)

Demographics

- Age
  - Any age; adults > children
- Sex
  - M = F
- Epidemiology
  - Uncommon (< 1% of intracranial cysts)

Natural History & Prognosis

- Varies with cyst size, location
- May be stable over many years

Treatment

- Observation vs. fenestration/drainage of cyst

DIAGNOSTIC CHECKLIST

Image Interpretation Pearls

- Use FLAIR, DWI to help distinguish between different types of intracranial cysts
- If lesion does not suppress on FLAIR, must consider solid lesion (i.e., low-grade neoplasm)

SELECTED REFERENCES

1. Pereira RG et al: Non-neoplastic intracranial cystic lesions: not everything is an arachnoid cyst. Radiol Bras. 54(1):49-55, 2021
2. Robles LA et al: Intracranial glioependymal (neuroglial) cysts: a systematic review. Acta Neurochir (Wien). 160(7):1439-49, 2018
3. Osborn AG et al: Intracranial cysts: radiologic-pathologic correlation and imaging approach. Radiology. 239(3):650-64, 2006

Enlarged Perivascular Spaces

KEY FACTS

TERMINOLOGY

- Perivascular space (PVS) fluid-filled channels in subpial space that accompany penetrating arteries into brain

IMAGING

- Found in virtually all locations; conspicuity ↑ at 3T MR
  - Most commonly within inferior basal ganglia
  - Cerebral hemisphere white matter
- ↑ size & number with ↑ age
- Round/oval in basal ganglia; tubular in white matter
- Giant or tumefactive clusters of PVSs most often located in midbrain; may have associated mass effect
- **CT**: Well-defined, low-attenuation lesion (~ CSF)
- **MR**: PVS contents follow CSF signal on all sequences
  - May see penetrating vessels within PVSs
  - No significant adjacent parenchymal signal abnormality

TOP DIFFERENTIAL DIAGNOSES

- Cystic neoplasms (e.g., DNET)
- Mucopolysaccharidoses
- Neurocysticercosis & other cyst-forming parasites
- Lacunar infarcts (typically in older patients)
- Cystic encephalomalacia

PATHOLOGY

- Actually contain interstitial fluid, not CSF
- Single or double layer of invaginated pia

CLINICAL ISSUES

- Most common history: Incidentally identified area of low attenuation or cystic neoplasm on CT
- PVSs provide entry site to CNS in infectious, inflammatory, & neoplastic disease

DIAGNOSTIC CHECKLIST

- Numerous prominent PVSs in child → consider mucopolysaccharidosis
- "Leave alone" lesion should be distinguished from more serious considerations; MR ± contrast often diagnostic

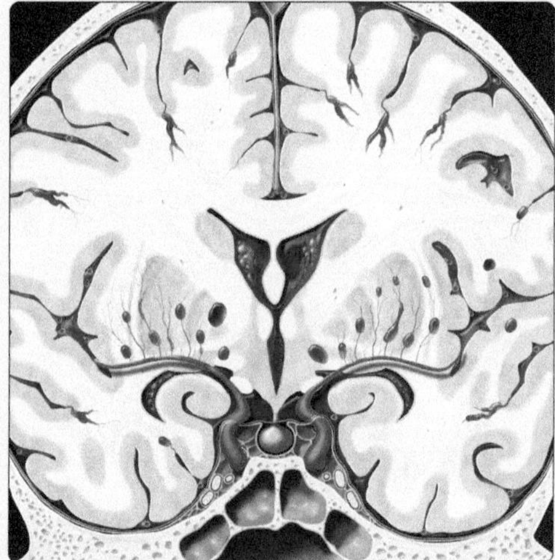

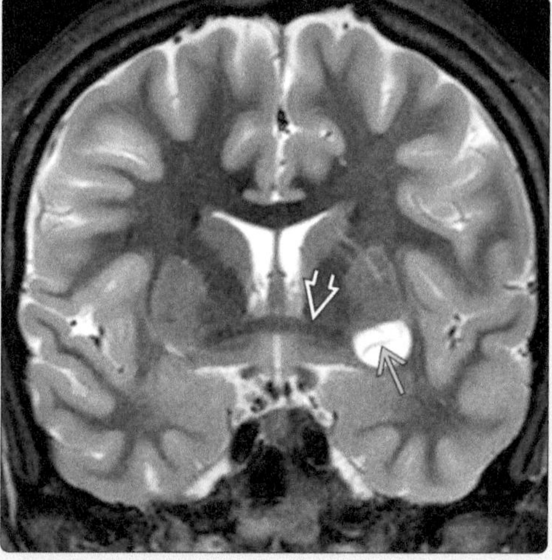

(Left) *Coronal graphic shows possible distributions & morphologies of normal perivascular spaces (PVSs) as they accompany penetrating arteries into the basal ganglia & subcortical white matter. Normal PVSs cluster around the anterior commissure but occur in all areas.* **(Right)** *Coronal T2 FS in the same child shows the small perforating lenticulostriate vessel ⇒ within this cyst-like PVS. This location, at the lateral margin of the anterior commissure ➡, is the most common location for PVSs.*

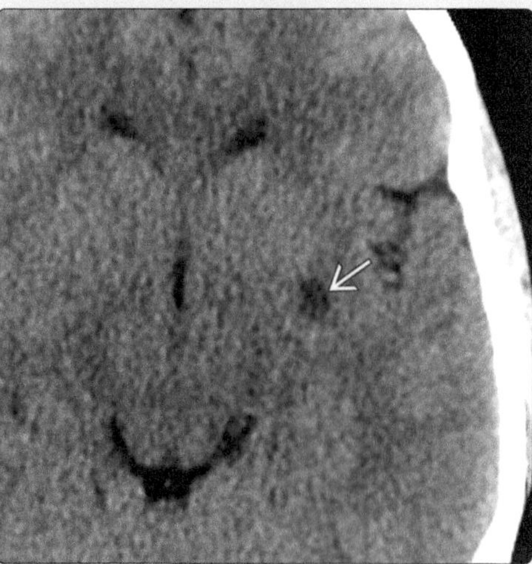

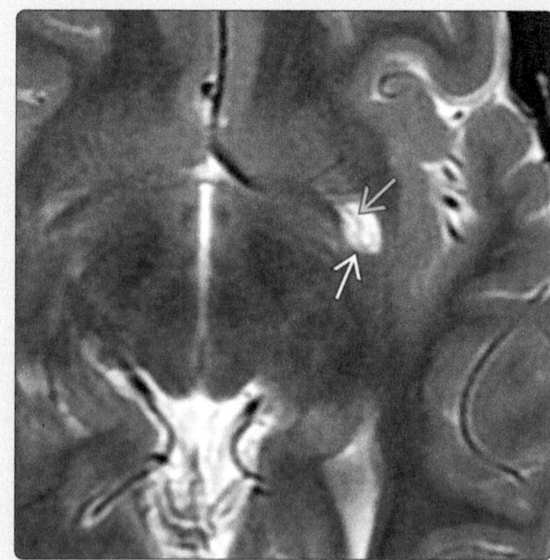

(Left) *Axial NECT in a 15-year-old girl with a headache shows a focus of low attenuation ➡ in the left basal ganglia. While statistically this most likely represents an enlarged PVS, the finding is nonspecific on CT & warrants MR.* **(Right)** *Axial T2 MR in the same patient further characterizes the lesion seen on CT as an ovoid focus ➡ isointense to CSF & centered around a vessel ⇒, consistent with a PVS. The inferior basal ganglia are the most common locations for PVSs.*

TERMINOLOGY

Synonyms

- Perivascular space (PVS)
- Virchow-Robin space (VRS)

Definitions

- Channels in subpial space that accompany penetrating arteries into brain

IMAGING

General Features

- Best diagnostic clue
  - Parenchymal cluster of fluid-filled spaces resembling CSF
    - Surround/accompany penetrating arteries
    - Found in virtually any location & in patients of all ages
- Location
  - Most common site for normal PVSs: Basal ganglia (clustered around anterior commissure)
  - Other common locations
    - Midbrain
    - Deep white matter
    - Subinsular & high cerebral subcortical white matter
  - Less common sites
    - Corpus callosum, cingulate gyrus
    - Thalami
    - Dentate nuclei
  - Giant or tumefactive PVSs
    - Most common location is midbrain but can occur anywhere
    - Almost never involve cortex (PVSs expand within subcortical white matter)
- Size
  - PVSs usually ≤ 5 mm
    - Rarely may expand, attain large size (up to several cm)
    - May cause focal mass effect, hydrocephalus
      - Expand overlying gyri
      - Midbrain enlarged PVSs may compress aqueduct/3rd ventricle, cause hydrocephalus
    - Widespread dilation of PVSs may look very bizarre
      - Often seen in association with mucopolysaccharidoses
- Morphology
  - Solitary or multiple clustered, well-demarcated, variable-sized parenchymal cysts
  - Circular, oval, or lobular in deep gray nuclei
  - Typically long & tubular in cerebral white matter

CT Findings

- NECT
  - Clusters of round/ovoid/linear/punctate cyst-like lesions
    - Low density (attenuation = CSF); no Ca^{++}
- CECT
  - Do not enhance but may see central enhancing vessel

MR Findings

- Follow CSF signal intensity on all sequences
- ± visualization of fluid-encircled penetrating arteries with contrast
- No significant edema in adjacent brain
  - 25% have minimal ↑ signal surrounding enlarged PVSs
- MRS in adjacent brain typically normal

Nuclear Medicine Findings

- Tc-99m HMPAO SPECT normal, shows no ischemic changes

Imaging Recommendations

- Best imaging tool
  - Routine MR with FLAIR, DWI
- Protocol advice
  - Contrast optional

DIFFERENTIAL DIAGNOSIS

Mucopolysaccharidoses

- Mucopolysaccharide collects in PVSs, enlarges them
- Supratentorial, hemispheric
- Other characteristic features present: Skull base, spine, musculoskeletal

Cystic Neoplasm

- Giant peripheral PVS may mimic dysembryoplastic neuroepithelial tumor (DNET)
- Most other cystic neoplasms have some solid component
- Signal within tumoral cysts typically differs slightly from CSF on some sequences
- Parenchymal signal abnormalities common

Multiple Sclerosis

- Chronic demyelinating lesions may mimic PVSs
- Typically do not follow CSF signal on all sequences, usually FLAIR hyperintense

Lacunar Infarcts

- Older patients, very rare in children
- Common in superior basal ganglia, white matter
- Adjacent parenchymal hyperintensity (MR)

Infectious/Inflammatory Cysts

- Neurocysticercosis
  - Cysts often have scolex
  - Cyst walls often enhance
  - ± Ca^{++}
  - Most < 1 cm
  - Can be multiple but do not typically occur in clusters
  - Surrounding edema often present
- Other parasites
  - Hydatid cysts often unilocular
  - Multilocular parasitic cysts typically enhance, mimic neoplasm more than PVSs

Cryptococcal Meningitis

- Organisms with gelatinous capsule fill & expand PVSs in immunocompromised patients

Cystic Encephalomalacia

- Often has some surrounding signal abnormality
- Typically has associated volume loss

Neuroglial Cyst

- Round or ovoid cyst lined with thin epithelium & with CSF-like content
- Differentiation between neuroepithelial cysts & enlarged VRSs can be made with certainty only by pathologic study

PATHOLOGY

General Features

- Etiology
  - Theory: Interstitial fluid (ISF) accumulates between penetrating vessel & pia
  - Recent investigations have shown PVSs to be critical part of glymphatic system
    - Glymphatic system acts as conduit allowing exchange between CSF & ISF for brain waste removal
    - ↑ size & number of PVSs may suggest dysfunction of glymphatic system
  - Egress of ISF blocked, causing cystic enlargement of PVS
    - Actually contain ISF, not CSF
  - Some studies in adults suggest they are related to small vessel disease
- Genetics
  - Usually normal unless PVSs expanded by undegraded mucopolysaccharides (Hurler, Hunter disease)
  - PVSs expand in some congenital muscular dystrophies
- Associated abnormalities
  - Hydrocephalus (midbrain expanding PVSs can obstruct aqueduct)
  - "Cysts" caused by enlarged/obstructed PVSs reported with pituitary adenomas, large aneurysms
  - PVSs provide entry site into CNS in inflammatory, neoplastic disorders
    - Transmigration across capillaries, venules into PVSs
    - Progress across glia limitans into parenchyma
  - ↑ size & number of PVSs are associated with many neurodegenerative diseases in older adults
    - Alzheimer disease, cerebral amyloid angiopathy, & cerebrovascular disease
    - Generally associated with declining cognition in older adults
    - Not well studied in children & young adults

Staging, Grading, & Classification

- Type I: PVS located along lenticulostriate arteries entering basal ganglia through anterior perforated substance
- Type II: PVS located along path of perforating medullary arteries within cerebral white matter
- Type III: PVS located in midbrain

Gross Pathologic & Surgical Features

- Smoothly demarcated, fluid-filled cyst(s)

Microscopic Features

- Single or double layer of invaginated pia
- Pia becomes fenestrated, disappears at capillary level
- PVSs usually very small in cortex, often enlarge in subcortical white matter
- Surrounding brain usually lacks gliosis

CLINICAL ISSUES

Presentation

- Most common signs/symptoms
  - Usually normal & discovered incidentally at imaging/autopsy
  - Nonspecific symptoms (e.g., headache)
  - Numerous large PVSs in children occurs almost exclusively in mucopolysaccharidoses

Demographics

- Age
  - Occur in all locations at all ages
    - 3T imaging ↑ conspicuity
  - ↑ size & number with ↑ age
  - Giant or tumefactive PVSs
    - Mean age: Mid-40s
    - Rarely occur in children
- Sex
  - Giant PVSs: M:F = 1.8:1.0
- Epidemiology
  - Common nonneoplastic brain "cyst"
  - Common cause of multifocal hyperintensities on T2 MR
  - Recent studies in adults suggests PVSs may be imaging markers of cerebral small vessel disease

Natural History & Prognosis

- Usually remain stable in size
- Occasionally continue to expand
- Studies in adults disagree on association of ↑ PVSs & ↓ cognition

Treatment

- "Leave alone" lesion that should not be mistaken for serious disease
- Shunt ventricles if midbrain lesions cause obstructive hydrocephalus

DIAGNOSTIC CHECKLIST

Consider

- Numerous prominent PVSs in child → consider mucopolysaccharidosis

Image Interpretation Pearls

- When imaging at 3T, normal PVSs can be identified in many patients

SELECTED REFERENCES

1. Moses J et al: Automated methods for detecting and quantitation of enlarged perivascular spaces on MRI. J Magn Reson Imaging. 57(1):11-24, 2023
2. Yang Y et al: Enlarged perivascular spaces and age-related clinical diseases. Clin Interv Aging. 18:855-67, 2023
3. Gouveia-Freitas K et al: Perivascular spaces and brain waste clearance systems: relevance for neurodegenerative and cerebrovascular pathology. Neuroradiology. 63(10):1581-97, 2021
4. Francis F et al: Perivascular spaces and their associations with risk factors, clinical disorders and neuroimaging features: a systematic review and meta-analysis. Int J Stroke. 4(4):359-71, 2019
5. Hilal S et al: Enlarged perivascular spaces and cognition: a meta-analysis of 5 population-based studies. Neurology. 91(9):e832-42, 2018
6. Laveskog A et al: Perivascular spaces in old age: assessment, distribution, and correlation with white matter gyperintensities. AJNR Am J Neuroradiol. 39(1):70-6, 2018
7. Niazi M et al: Quantitative MRI of perivascular spaces at 3T for early diagnosis of mild cognitive impairment. AJNR Am J Neuroradiol. 39(9):1622-8, 2018
8. Riba-Llena I et al: Arterial stiffness is associated with basal ganglia enlarged perivascular spaces and cerebral small vessel disease load. Stroke. 49(5):1279-81, 2018
9. Rudie JD et al: Neuroimaging of dilated perivascular spaces: from benign and pathologic causes to mimics. J Neuroimaging. 28(2):139-49, 2018
10. Zhang X et al: Brain atrophy correlates with severe enlarged perivascular spaces in basal ganglia among lacunar stroke patients. PLoS One. 11(2):e0149593, 2016

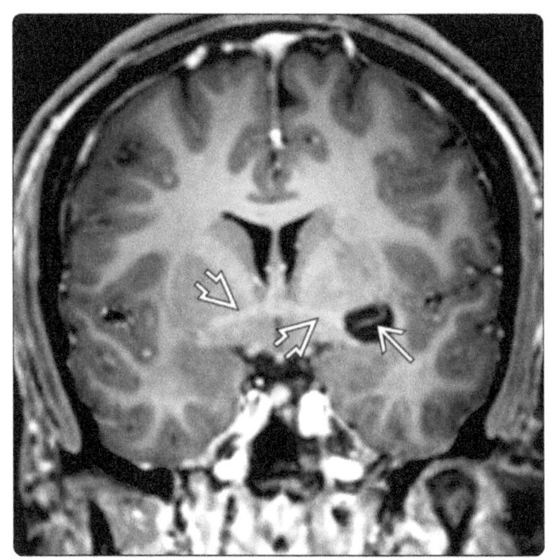

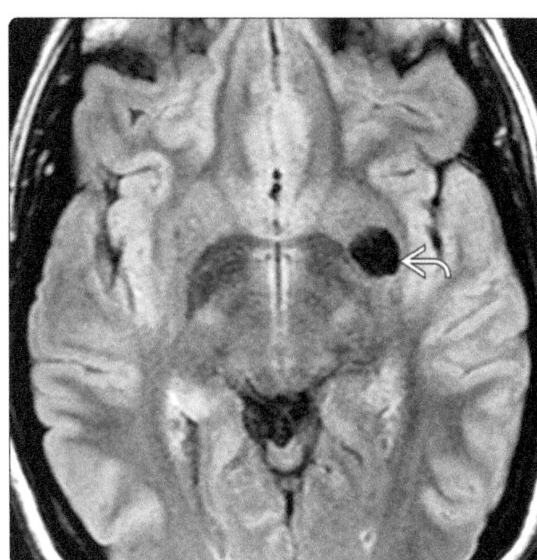

(Left) *Coronal T1 C+ MR in the same child shows the small perforating lenticulostriate vessel ➡ within this cyst-like PVS. This location, at the lateral margin of the anterior commissure ➡, is the most common site for PVSs.* **(Right)** *Axial FLAIR MR in a 9-year-old with headaches shows a round, cystic focus ➡ in the left basal ganglia. The content of the lesion is similar to CSF. Note the absence of gliosis or discernible mass effect in the surrounding parenchyma.*

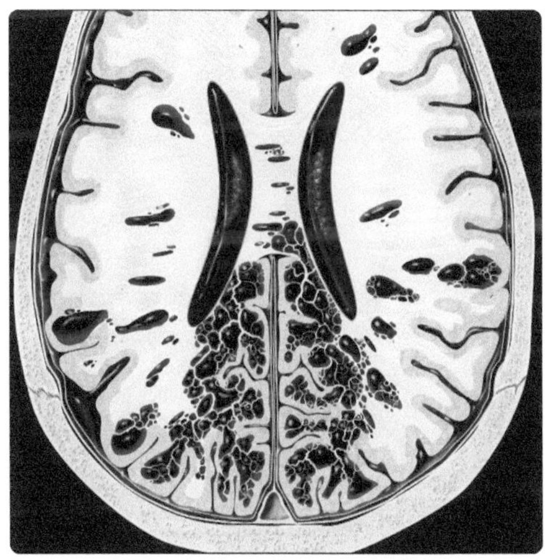

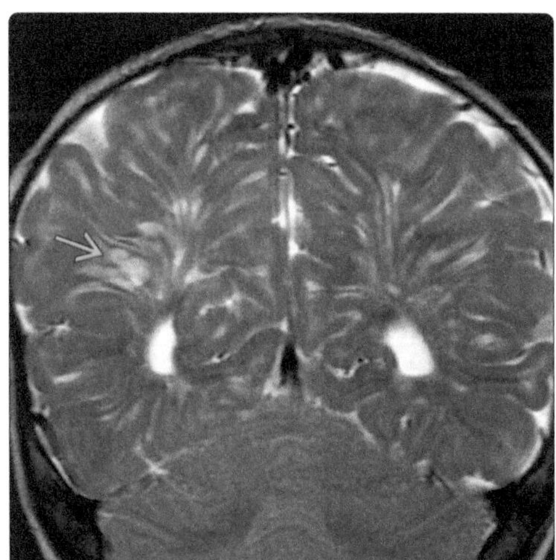

(Left) *Axial graphic shows enlarged PVSs in the white matter of the occipital lobe, centrum semiovale, corpus callosum, & cingulate gyrus. Note the focal expansion of the overlying cortex. The number of enlarged PVSs seen here would not be typical for a normal child.* **(Right)** *Coronal T2 MR in a 1-year-old boy with Hurler syndrome shows multiple enlarged PVSs within the cerebral white matter. Most of the PVSs are tubular (as is typical in this location), but some have become more bulbous & cystic ➡.*

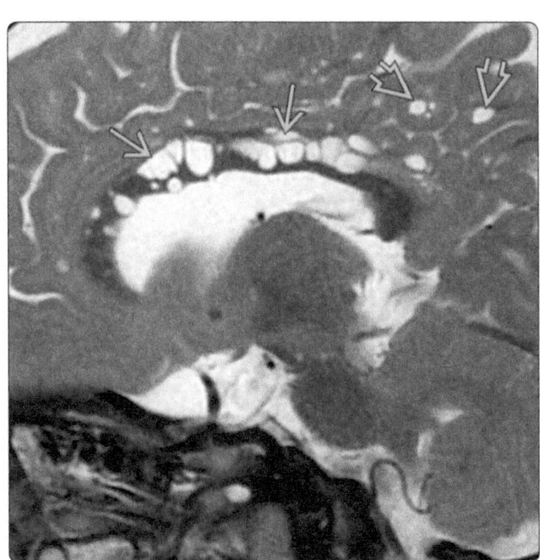

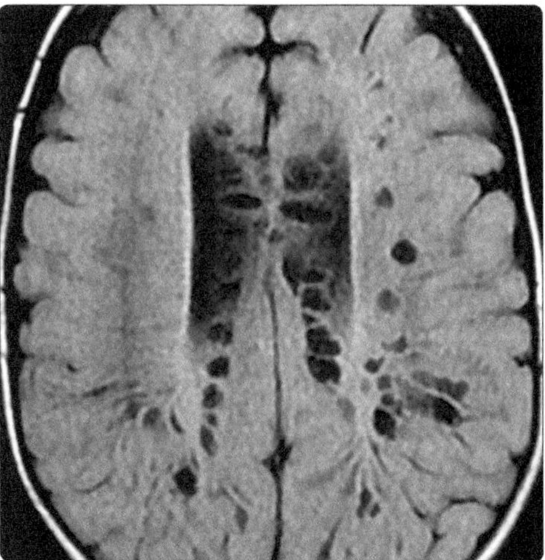

(Left) *Sagittal T2 MR in a 17-month-old with Hurler syndrome shows extensive cystic spaces within the corpus callosum ➡ & more peripheral subcortical white matter ➡.* **(Right)** *Axial FLAIR MR in the same patient shows that these cystic lesions suppress completely & follow CSF on all sequences. This extent of PVSs in a child is nearly pathognomonic for mucopolysaccharidosis (MPS). Solitary, small PVSs are common in children, but extensive PVSs are extremely rare outside of MPS.*

Pineal Cyst

KEY FACTS

TERMINOLOGY

- Nonneoplastic intrapineal glial-lined cyst

IMAGING

- Most common appearance: Single round/ovoid cyst < 1 cm
- Lobulated shape & internal septations common
- CT
  - Low-attenuation focus in pineal region
    - May be difficult to identify thin walls on CT
  - 25% with Ca^{++} in cyst wall; more common with ↑ age
- MR
  - Cyst contents typically similar to CSF on T1, T2
  - Cyst contents do not suppress on FLAIR
  - Cyst contents do not restrict diffusion
  - ~ 90% show wall enhancement
    - Most common pattern: Thin rim (≤ 2 mm)

TOP DIFFERENTIAL DIAGNOSES

- Arachnoid cyst
- Epidermoid cyst
- Velum interpositum cyst
- Pineocytoma

CLINICAL ISSUES

- Very common: > 50% prevalence with high-resolution MR
- Occur at all ages but prevalence ↓ in older adults
- Most commonly incidental
- Large cysts (> 1 cm) may become symptomatic
  - Headache (aqueduct compression → hydrocephalus)
  - Parinaud syndrome (due to tectal plate compression)
  - In absence of hydrocephalus & visual changes, symptoms unlikely to be related to cyst

DIAGNOSTIC CHECKLIST

- Development of pineal gland cyst considered normal
- Imaging follow-up typically not necessary in children
  - Unless size or degree of enhancement unusual
- Pineocytoma appearance overlaps but rare in children

(Left) *Sagittal graphic shows a small, cystic lesion within the pineal gland ➔. The presence of a pineal cyst should not be considered abnormal & generally does not require comment in the imaging report.* **(Right)** *Midline sagittal 3D SSFP MR in a 14-year-old with vision changes shows a simple pineal cyst ➔. The lesion is well defined, slightly hypointense to CSF, & contains no septations. There is mild mass effect on the tectum & cerebral aqueduct ➔. The visual symptoms could reflect Parinaud syndrome, which can occur with larger pineal cysts.*

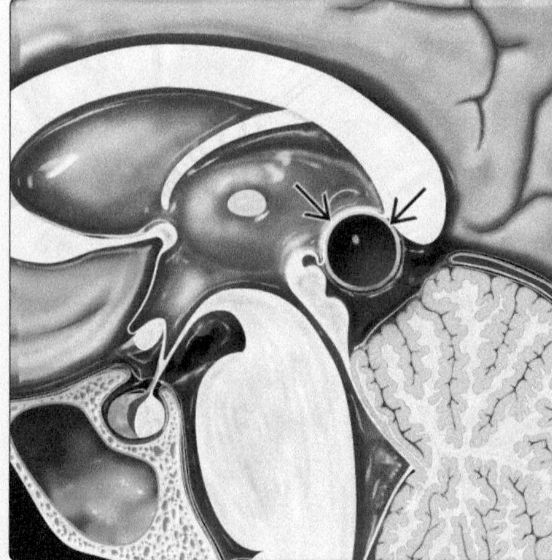

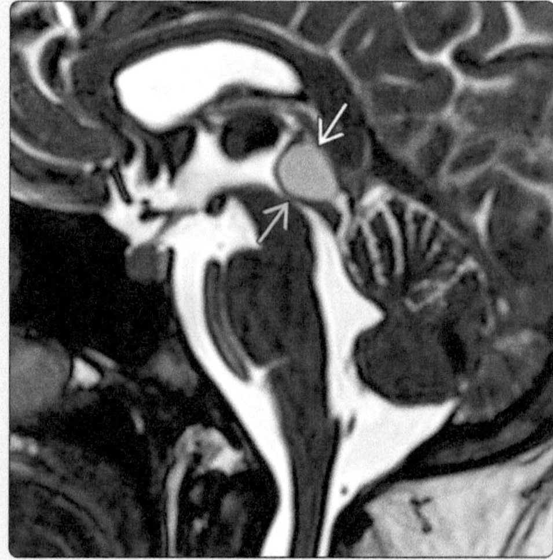

(Left) *Sagittal NECT in a 19-year-old with a large pineal cyst ➔ shows pineal Ca^{++} ➔ along the anterior margin of the cyst. There is no solid nodular components to suggest a pineal tumor.* **(Right)** *Sagittal T1 C+ MR in the same patient shows thin, smooth enhancement along the margins ➔ of the cyst. Such an appearance suggests a benign simple cyst. Peripheral enhancement is not always present, but when present, typically represents pineal parenchyma &/or vascular enhancement.*

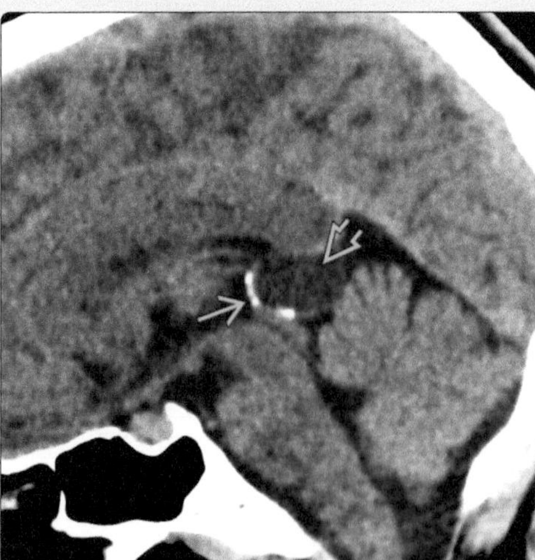

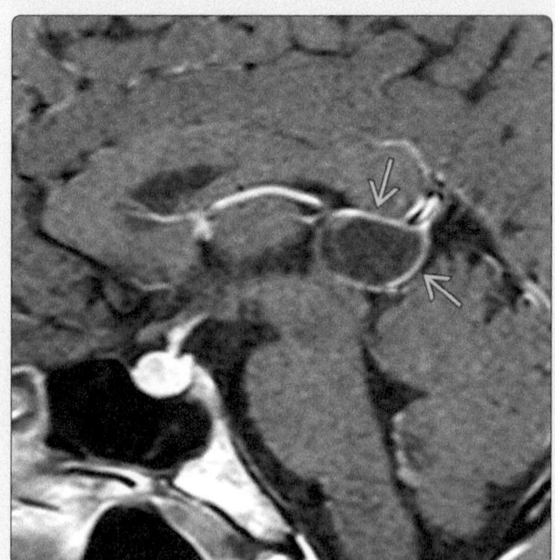

TERMINOLOGY

Abbreviations

- Pineal cyst (PC)

Synonyms

- Benign glial cyst of pineal gland

Definitions

- Nonneoplastic intrapineal glial-lined cyst

IMAGING

General Features

- Best diagnostic clue
  - Fluid-filled pineal region mass
- Location
  - Superior to & clearly distinct from tectum
  - Inferior to velum interpositum & internal cerebral veins
- Size
  - Typically small (< 1 cm); mean: 4 mm
  - ~ 2% of all children undergoing MR will have PC ≥ 1 cm
  - Occasionally up to 2 cm or more
- Morphology
  - 3T & 3D SSFP MR imaging has shown
    - Shape
      - Round or ovoid (60-85%)
      - Lobulated (15-40%)
    - Septations
      - 24-48%
    - Typically thin walled
      - However, residual normal pineal gland may cause thick-walled or nodular appearance

CT Findings

- NECT
  - Low attenuation in region of pineal gland
    - Fluid iso- or slightly hyperdense to CSF
    - Ca^{++} in cyst wall (25%), presumably representing intrinsic pineal Ca^{++}
    - Hyperdense cyst rare
      - Acute hemorrhage ("pineal apoplexy")
  - Can be difficult to clearly delineate cyst borders due to adjacent low-attenuation, CSF-filled cisterns
- CECT
  - Rim or nodular enhancement, presumably representing normal pineal tissue
  - Amount of enhancing tissue should not exceed expected pineal gland volume

MR Findings

- T1WI
  - Majority hypointense, nearly CSF signal
  - Hemorrhage with heterogeneous signal intensity (uncommon)
- T2WI
  - Iso- to slightly hyperintense to CSF
  - May show fluid-fluid levels after hemorrhage (uncommon)
- PD/intermediate
  - Hyperintense to CSF (85-90%)
- FLAIR
  - Cyst contents do not suppress like CSF
- T2* GRE
  - Usually normal
  - Blooming from old or recent hemorrhage (uncommon)
- DWI
  - No restricted diffusion within cyst
- T1WI C+
  - ~ 90% enhance, presumably representing normal pineal tissue
    - Most common pattern: Thin rim (≤ 2 mm)
      - Can be partial, eccentric, incomplete
    - Cystic areas may fill in on delayed scans, resembling solid tumor
    - Amount of enhancing tissue should not exceed expected pineal gland volume
      - If > expected soft tissue component, consider pineal region tumor
- MRV
  - Internal cerebral veins may be splayed or elevated by large lesions

Angiographic Findings

- Arterial phase almost always normal
- Venous phase may show elevation & displacement of internal cerebral veins if large PC present

Imaging Recommendations

- Best imaging tool
  - MR ± contrast
- Protocol advice
  - High-resolution imaging (3D SSFP) most sensitive for detection & characterization

DIFFERENTIAL DIAGNOSIS

Pineocytoma

- Rare in children (1-2% of pineal region tumors)
- Usually solid or partially solid/cystic
- Purely cystic form much less common
  - May be indistinguishable from PC on imaging studies
  - Requires histology for definitive diagnosis

Epidermoid Cyst

- Quadrigeminal cistern relatively rare location
- Cauliflower configuration
- Diffusion restriction on DWI (dark on ADC map)

Arachnoid Cyst

- No Ca^{++} or enhancement
- Follows CSF attenuation on CT & signal intensity on all MR sequences

Velum Interpositum Cyst

- Superior & anterior to pineal
- Inferiorly displaces internal cerebral veins

PATHOLOGY

General Features

- Etiology
  - Extremely common: PCs detected in > 50% of children using advanced MR imaging (3T & 3D SSFP)
    - 33-40% prevalence in autopsy series

- Etiology/pathogenesis: 3 major theories
  - Enlargement of embryonic pineal cavity
  - Ischemic glial degeneration ± hemorrhagic expansion
  - Small preexisting cysts enlarge with hormonal influences
- Genetics
  - None known
- Associated abnormalities
  - Hydrocephalus (rare)
- Embryology
  - Primitive pineal diverticulum divides into pineal recess, cavum pineal
  - Cavum pineal usually obliterated by glial fibers
  - Incomplete obliteration may leave residual cavity

Gross Pathologic & Surgical Features

- Smooth, soft, tan to yellow cyst wall
  - Cavity can be uni- or multilocular
  - Fluid contents vary
    - Clear yellow (most common) to hemorrhagic

Microscopic Features

- Delicate (usually incomplete) outer leptomeningeal layer
- Middle layer of attenuated pineal parenchyma
  - $\pm Ca^{++}$
- Inner layer of dense fibrillar glial tissue with
  - Variable granular bodies
  - ± hemosiderin-laden macrophages
- Compare with pineocytoma
  - Pseudolobular arrangement of small, round cells with pleomorphic nuclei
  - "Pinocytic" rosettes
  - Neuronal differentiation
    - NSE, synaptophysin (+) cells

CLINICAL ISSUES

Presentation

- Most common signs/symptoms
  - Vast majority clinically silent
    - Discovered incidentally at imaging/autopsy
    - If no associated hydrocephalus or visual symptoms, PC unlikely to be cause of symptoms
  - Large cysts (> 1 cm) may become symptomatic
    - Headache (aqueduct compression → hydrocephalus)
    - Parinaud syndrome (vertical gaze palsy due to tectal plate compression)
  - Rare: "Pineal apoplexy"
    - Severe headache (can be "thunderclap," mimicking aneurysmal subarachnoid hemorrhage)
    - Intracystic hemorrhage, acute hydrocephalus, sudden death (very rare)
  - Recent studies suggest that larger cysts (> 1 cm) are associated with sleep disturbances
- Clinical profile
  - Incidentally identified PC in setting of unrelated symptoms
  - Pineal gland is responsible for melatonin production

Demographics

- Age
  - Can occur at **any** age
  - Large studies suggest ↓ prevalence with ↑ age after first 2 decades
- Sex
  - M:F = 1:1
- Ethnicity
  - None known
- Epidemiology
  - Extremely common: PCs detected in > 50% of children using advanced MR imaging (3T & 3D SSFP)
    - 33-40% prevalence in autopsy series

Natural History & Prognosis

- Majority stable over time; gradual interval ↑ or ↓ in size may occur
- Rare: Sudden expansion, hemorrhage ("pineal apoplexy")

Treatment

- Usually none
- Atypical/symptomatic lesions may require biopsy/resection
- Surgical resection in absence of hydrocephalus or Parinaud syndrome remains controversial

DIAGNOSTIC CHECKLIST

Consider

- PCs almost always incidental on MR
  - Frequently discovered when thin-section imaging performed
- Heterogeneous, nodular, or ring-like enhancing pineal mass still most likely represents complex benign cyst rather than neoplasm
  - In absence of hemorrhage, restricted diffusion should suggest alternate pathology

Image Interpretation Pearls

- Cannot distinguish benign PC from neoplasm (pineocytoma) by imaging
  - However, pineocytomas rare in children (1-2% of pineal region tumors)

SELECTED REFERENCES

1. Hasegawa H et al: Pineal cyst: results of long-term MRI surveillance and analysis of growth and shrinkage rates. J Neurosurg. 138(1):113-9, 2023
2. McDowell MM et al: Clinical and radiographic features of pineal cysts in pediatric and young adult patients. World Neurosurg. 176:e719-27, 2023
3. Szathmari A et al: Pineal cysts in children: a paediatric series treated over the last twenty years in Lyon. Childs Nerv Syst. 39(12):3467-74, 2023
4. Tanaka T et al: Pineal cysts: does anyone need long-term follow up? J Clin Neurosci. 83:146-51, 2021
5. Gokce E et al: Evaluation of pineal cysts with magnetic resonance imaging. World J Radiol. 10(7):65-77, 2018
6. Jussila MP et al: Follow-up of pineal cysts in children: is it necessary? Neuroradiology. 59(12):1265-73, 2017
7. Nevins EJ et al: Incidental pineal cysts: is surveillance necessary? World Neurosurg. 90:96-102, 2016
8. Kahilogullari G et al: Pineal cysts in children: case-based update. Childs Nerv Syst. 29(5):753-60, 2013
9. Whitehead MT et al: Incidental pineal cysts in children who undergo 3-T MRI. Pediatr Radiol. 43(12):1577-83, 2013
10. Bumb JM et al: TrueFISP of the pediatric pineal gland: volumetric and microstructural analysis. Clin Neuroradiol. 22(1):69-77, 2012
11. Al-Holou WN et al: The natural history of pineal cysts in children and young adults. J Neurosurg Pediatr. 5(2):162-6, 2010
12. Al-Holou WN et al: Prevalence of pineal cysts in children and young adults. Clinical article. J Neurosurg Pediatr. 4(3):230-6, 2009

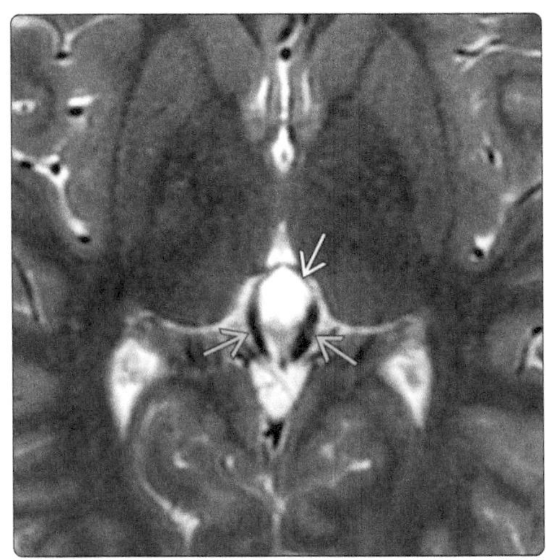

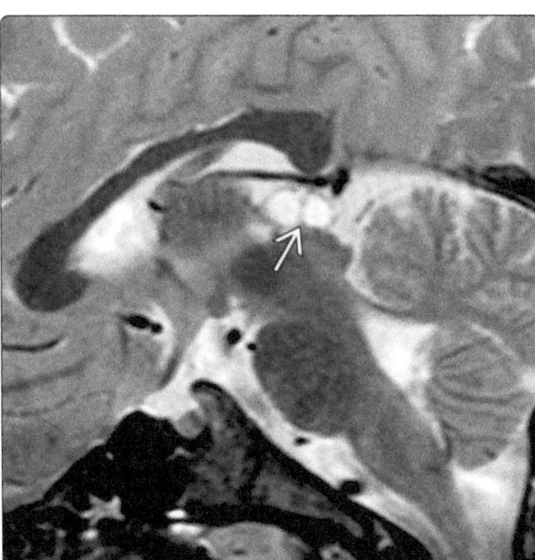

(Left) *Axial T2 MR in an 11-year-old boy with headache shows a pineal cyst ➡ splaying the flow voids of the internal cerebral veins ➡.* **(Right)** *Sagittal T2 MR in a 6-year-old with seizures shows a pineal cyst, either with a septation ➡ or representing 2 adjacent cysts. Septations are common, seen in 25% or more of pineal cysts, & are especially evident when using high-spatial-resolution MR. Septations or multiple cysts in the absence of increased soft tissue component should not raise alarm.*

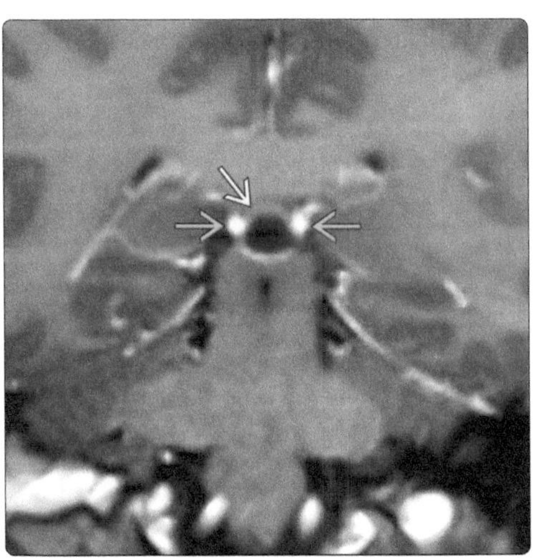

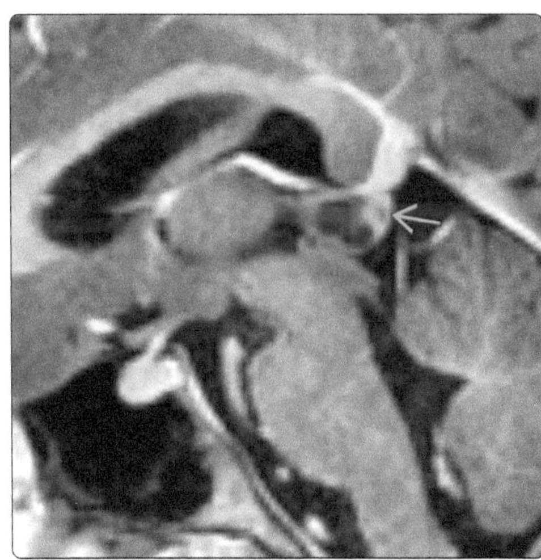

(Left) *Coronal T1 C+ MR shows a pineal cyst splaying the internal cerebral veins ➡. There is a typical thin rim of enhancement ➡ to the cyst.* **(Right)** *Sagittal T1 C+ MR in a 13-year-old shows a small focus of nodular enhancement ➡ along the posterior aspect of the pineal cyst. This is a common finding in pineal cysts & likely represents residual normal pineal tissue. If the volume of enhancing tissue is not greater than the expected volume of a normal pineal gland, this finding should not alarm the radiologist.*

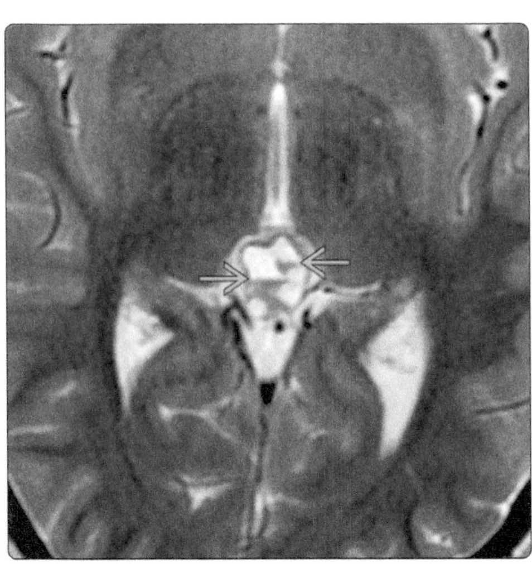

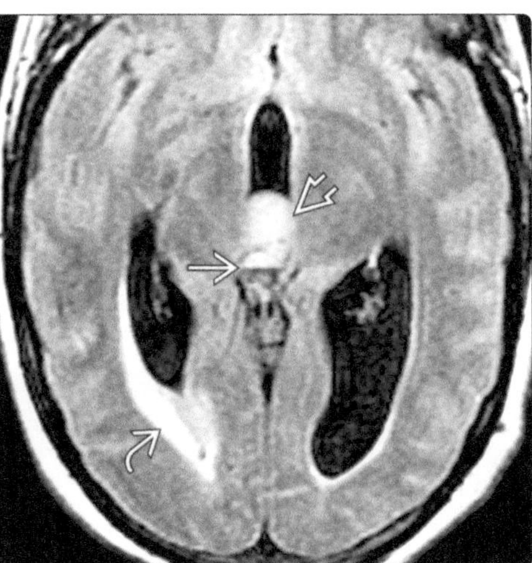

(Left) *Axial T2 MR shows a multicystic pineal gland with fluid-fluid levels ➡ within a few of the cystic compartments, suggesting hemorrhage.* **(Right)** *Axial FLAIR MR in a patient shows a hemorrhage level ➡ in the pineal cyst ➡. Note the ventricular enlargement & transependymal CSF flow ➡ due to obstructive hydrocephalus. A benign, nonneoplastic hemorrhagic cyst was found at surgery. Rarely, large pineal cysts can cause obstructive hydrocephalus, often following acute hemorrhage.*

KEY FACTS

TERMINOLOGY

- Nonneoplastic, noninflammatory cysts
  - Contained within choroid plexus
  - Lined by choroid plexus connective tissue

IMAGING

- General
  - Typically in atria of lateral ventricle
  - Usually small (2-8 mm)
  - Rare: Large cysts (> 2 cm)
  - Usually multiple, often bilateral
- CT
  - Isodense or slightly hyperdense to CSF
  - Irregular, peripheral Ca^{++} common in adults
- MR
  - Isointense or slightly hyperintense compared to CSF on T1WI
  - Usually hyperintense to CSF on FLAIR
  - Diffusion restriction → choroid plexus xanthogranuloma
  - Enhancement (ring, nodular, solid) varies from none to strong

TOP DIFFERENTIAL DIAGNOSES

- Ependymal cyst
- Neurocysticercosis
- Epidermoid cyst
- Choroid plexus papilloma (CPP)
  - Purely cystic CPP very rare

CLINICAL ISSUES

- Found at both ends of age spectrum
  - Common in fetus, infants, older adults
  - Less common in children, young adults
- Clinically silent; discovered incidentally
- Associations: Aicardi syndrome, trisomy 18

DIAGNOSTIC CHECKLIST

- Most common choroid plexus mass in adults = choroid plexus cyst

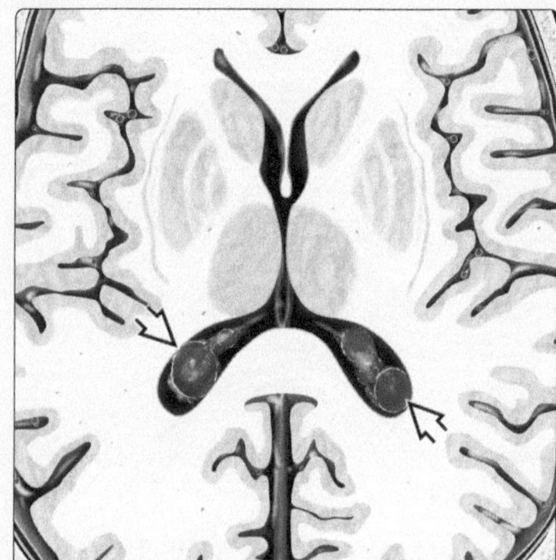

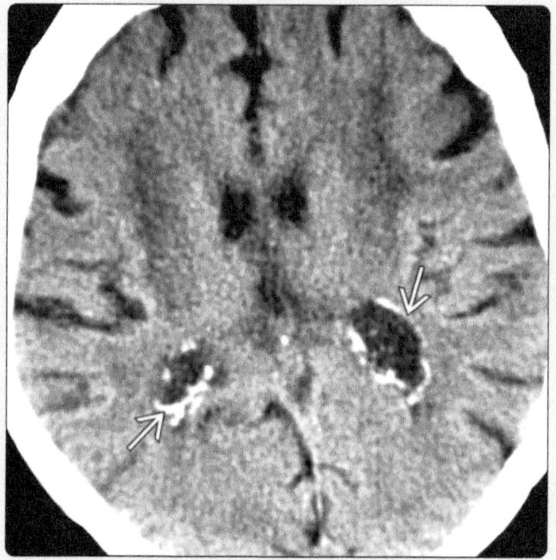

(Left) *Axial graphic shows multiple cystic masses in the choroid plexus glomi ➡, often seen incidentally on scans of middle-aged and older adults. Most are degenerative xanthogranulomas.* **(Right)** *Axial NECT obtained in an older adult with minor head trauma and a normal neurologic examination shows dense peripheral* Ca^{++} ➡ *around cystic masses in the atria of both lateral ventricles. This was an incidental finding with no clinical significance.*

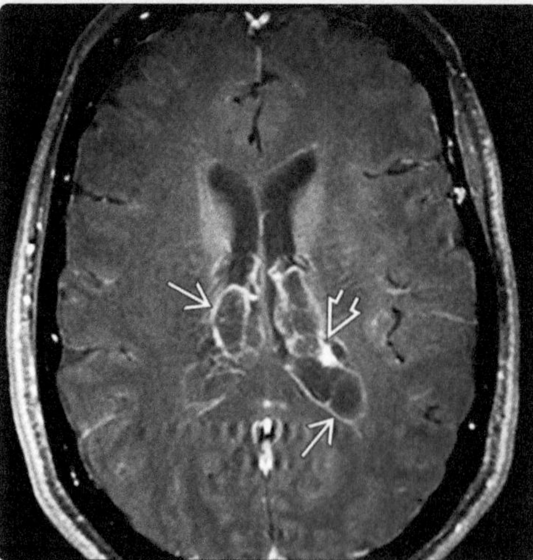

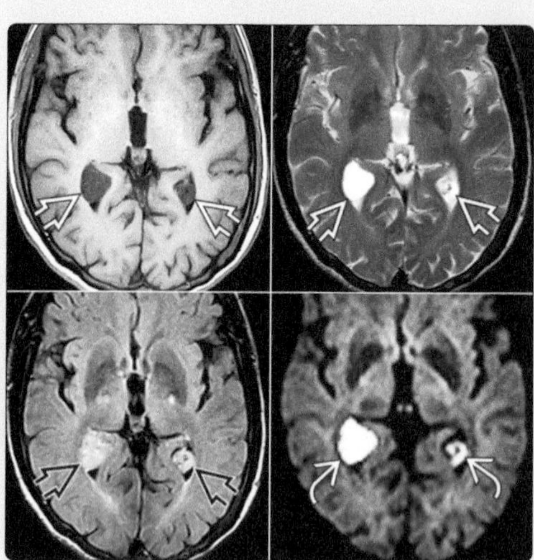

(Left) *Axial T1 C+ FS MR in the same patient shows that the choroid plexus cysts (CPCs) exhibit mixed rim ➡ and solid ➡ enhancement. These represent incidental CPCs (xanthogranulomas).* **(Right)** *Series of axial MR scans show an incidental finding of bilateral CPCs in an older patient. Cysts are slightly hyperintense to CSF on T1 and T2 ➡, typically do not suppress on FLAIR ➡, and frequently appear very bright on DWI ➡.*

TERMINOLOGY

Abbreviations

- Choroid plexus cyst (CPC)

Definitions

- Nonneoplastic, noninflammatory cysts of choroid plexus
  - Includes both simple cysts (CPC) and choroid plexus xanthogranuloma (CPX)
  - Lined by compressed connective tissue
  - Adult: CPC is common incidental finding on imaging studies in older patients (~ 40% prevalence)
  - Fetus: CPCs seen in 1-2% of routine 2nd-trimester US

IMAGING

General Features

- Best diagnostic clue
  - Older patient with "bright" cysts in choroid plexuses on T2WI
  - Fetus or newborn with large (> 2 mm) CPC(s) on US
- Location
  - Most common: Atria of lateral ventricles
    - Attached to or within choroid plexus
    - Often bilateral
  - Less common: 3rd and 4th ventricles
- Size
  - Variable
    - Usually small (2-8 mm)
    - Often multiple
    - Rare: Large cysts (> 2 cm)
- Morphology
  - Cystic or nodular/partially cystic mass(es) in choroid plexus glomi

CT Findings

- NECT
  - Iso-/slightly hyperdense (due to presence of increased protein) to CSF
  - Irregular, peripheral Ca^{++} in majority of adult cases
- CECT
  - Varies from none to rim of solid enhancement

MR Findings

- T1WI
  - Isointense or slightly hyperintense (due to presence of increased protein) compared to CSF
- T2WI
  - Hyperintense compared to CSF
- PD/intermediate
  - Hyperintense
- FLAIR
  - Variable, but usually hyperintense to CSF
- T2* GRE
  - Foci of blooming common
    - Ca^{++} (intracystic hemorrhage rare)
- DWI
  - Simple cysts (CPCs) show ↑ ADC
  - Diffusion restriction suggests XPC
- T1WI C+
  - Enhancement varies from none to strong
  - Variable pattern (solid, ring, nodular)
  - Delayed scans may show filling in of contrast within cysts

Ultrasonographic Findings

- Grayscale ultrasound
  - Prenatal US
    - Cyst > 2 mm surrounded by echogenic choroid
    - In absence of other abnormalities, low risk for chromosomal abnormalities

Imaging Recommendations

- Best imaging tool
  - Adults: MR ± contrast
  - Fetus, newborn
    - Antenatal: Maternal US or MR
    - Postnatal: US of infant with anterior, posterior, mastoid fontanelles as acoustic windows
- Protocol advice
  - MR with contrast, FLAIR, DWI
  - US transverse view of lateral ventricle at atrial level

DIFFERENTIAL DIAGNOSIS

Ependymal Cyst

- Does not enhance
- Usually unilateral
- Attenuation, signal more like CSF
- Immunohistochemistry differentiates

Neurocysticercosis

- Multiple cysts common (subarachnoid space, parenchyma ventricles)
- Not associated with choroid plexus
- Look for scolex, other signs of neurocysticercosis (NCC) (e.g., parenchymal Ca^{++})
- May be migratory

Epidermoid Cyst

- Intraventricular location rare (4th > > lateral ventricle)
- Cauliflower, insinuating pattern

Choroid Plexus Papilloma

- Children < 5 years of age
- Strong, relatively uniform enhancement
- Purely cystic choroid plexus papilloma (CPP) very rare

Villous Hyperplasia of Choroid Plexus

- Rare
- Often overproduces CSF
- Causes hydrocephalus

Ultrasound Pseudolesion

- Tiny, anechoic areas in fetal choroid are normal, not CPCs
- Normal, fluid-filled atria can be confused with CPC on transverse view
- "Split" or "truncated" choroid can mimic CPC

Neoplasm

- Meningioma (usually solid)
- Metastasis (rarely cystic)
- Cystic astrocytoma (rare in older patients)

Sturge-Weber Syndrome

- Enlarged, angiomatous, choroid plexus ipsilateral to malformation

Choroid Plexus Infarct

- Usually seen in choroid artery infarct
- May cause increased intraventricular signal on DWI

Choroid Plexus Cavernoma

- Rare mass most common in adults
- Mention when MR shows marked susceptibility

PATHOLOGY

General Features

- Etiology
  - CPCs
    - Lipid from desquamating, degenerating choroid epithelium accumulates in choroid plexus
    - Lipid provokes xanthomatous response
- Genetics
  - Large fetal CPCs associated with trisomy 21 or 18 in only 6% of cases
  - Presence of additional malformations increases risk factors for aneuploidy
- Associated abnormalities
  - Fetal CPC
    - Trisomy 18 (mildly increased risk < 2x baseline risk)
    - Trisomy 21 (only if other markers present)
  - Child/adult CPC: May cause obstructive hydrocephalus (rare)
  - Aicardi syndrome
    - Patients diagnosed by presence of retinal lacunae, severe corpus callosum hypo-/agenesis, polymicrogyria, heterotopia
    - Usually associated with CPPs, but CPCs may occur

Gross Pathologic & Surgical Features

- CPCs commonly found at autopsy in middle-aged, older adults
  - Nodular, partly cystic, yellowish-gray masses in choroid plexus glomus
  - Contents often gelatinous, highly proteinaceous
  - Rare: Hemorrhage

Microscopic Features

- Neuroepithelial microcysts
- Trapped choroid plexus epithelium often associated
- Cysts contain nests of foamy, lipid-laden histiocytes
- Foreign body giant cells
- Chronic inflammatory infiltrates (lymphocytes, plasma cells)
- Cholesterol clefts, hemosiderin
- Peripheral psammomatous Ca^{++} common
- Immunohistochemistry positive for prealbumin, cytokeratins, GFAP, EMA, S100

CLINICAL ISSUES

Presentation

- Most common signs/symptoms
  - Adult CPC
    - Typical: Clinically silent; discovered incidentally at autopsy/imaging
    - Rare: Headache

Demographics

- Age
  - Found at both ends of age spectrum
    - Adult CPC: Prevalence increases with age
    - Fetal CPC: Prevalence decreases with age
- Sex
  - No known prevalence
- Ethnicity
  - No known prevalence
- Epidemiology
  - Most common type of neuroepithelial cyst
    - 1-2% of all pregnancies on 2nd-trimester US
    - Small, asymptomatic CPCs found incidentally in > 1/3 of all autopsied adults

Natural History & Prognosis

- Fetal CPCs
  - Transient finding; typically resolve in 3rd trimester regardless of whether isolated or with associated anomalies
  - Clinical significance of fetal CPCs remains controversial, but weak association with aneuploidy is suggested in literature
- Adult CPCs
  - Usually remain asymptomatic, nonprogressive

Treatment

- Adult CPC: Usually none
  - Rare: Shunt for obstructive hydrocephalus
- Fetal CPC
  - In absence of other markers, none
  - With other markers, amniocentesis warranted

DIAGNOSTIC CHECKLIST

Consider

- Amniocentesis with karyotyping if CPCs + other anomalies (e.g., cardiac anomaly, clenched hands with overlapping fingers, clubfeet) present on fetal US

Image Interpretation Pearls

- Benign degenerative cyst (xanthogranuloma): Most common cause of choroid plexus mass in adults

SELECTED REFERENCES

1. Poyuran R et al: Nonneoplastic and noninfective cysts of the central nervous system: a histopathological study. Neuropathology. 43(3):221-32, 2022
2. Kürten C et al: A Bayesian risk analysis for trisomy 21 in isolated choroid plexus cyst: combining a prenatal database with a meta-analysis. J Matern Fetal Neonatal Med. 34(6):889-97, 2021
3. Maekawa T et al: Choroid plexus cysts analyzed using diffusion-weighted imaging with short diffusion-time. Magn Reson Imaging. 57:323-7, 2019
4. Winter TC et al: How to integrate cell-free DNA screening with sonographic markers for aneuploidy: an update. AJR Am J Roentgenol. 210(4):906-12, 2018
5. Zhang S et al: A retrospective study of cytogenetic results from amniotic fluid in 5328 fetuses with abnormal obstetric sonographic findings. J Ultrasound Med. 36(9):1809-17, 2017
6. Naeini RM et al: Spectrum of choroid plexus lesions in children. AJR Am J Roentgenol. 192(1):32-40, 2009

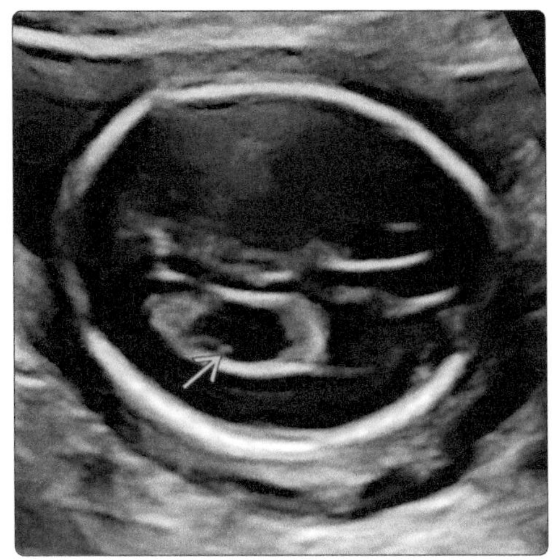

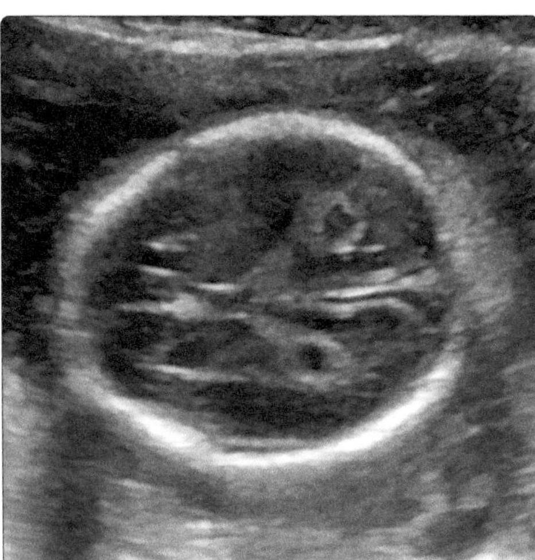

(Left) *Axial US in a 17-week gestational age fetus shows a prominent cyst ➡ within the choroid plexus.* **(Right)** *Axial fetal US in a 20-week gestational age fetus shows bilateral CPCs. CPCs are commonly encountered in fetal US with an incidence of ~ 1-2%. Such cysts usually resolve over time and are of no consequence. There may be a slight increased risk of trisomy 18 (< 1% chance), so such a finding should prompt a thorough anatomic evaluation.*

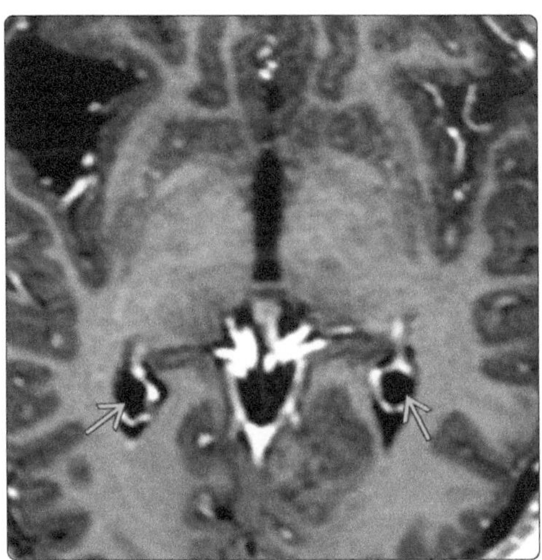

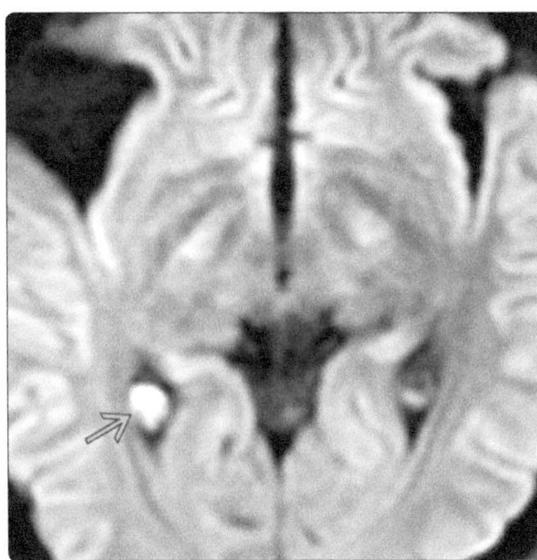

(Left) *Axial T1 C+ MR in a teenager shows bilateral CPCs ➡ within the bilateral choroid plexus glomus.* **(Right)** *Axial DWI MR in the same patient shows that the right CPC ➡ demonstrates diffusion restriction, consistent with a xanthogranuloma. This imaging appearance is thought to be related to degenerated desquamated epithelium within the CPC. The left CPC did not demonstrate associated diffusion restriction.*

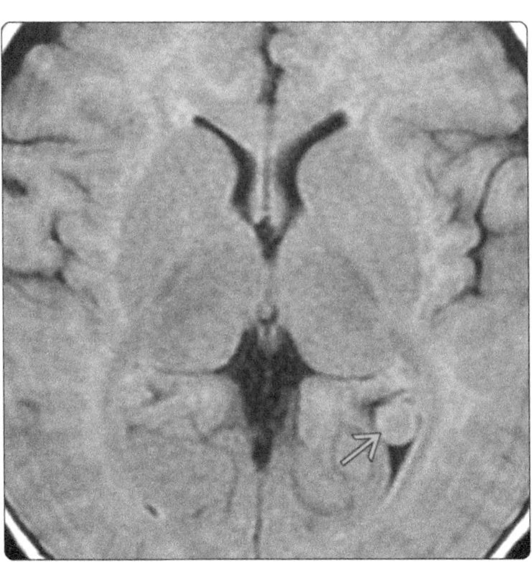

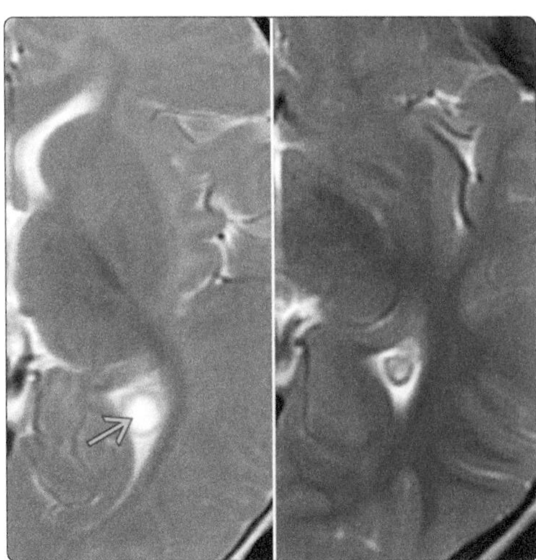

(Left) *Axial FLAIR MR in a 7-month-old shows a subcentimeter CPC ➡ in the left choroid plexus glomus. Most, but not all, CPCs do not suppress on FLAIR imaging.* **(Right)** *Axial T2 MR in the same patient at 7 months (left) and 4 years (right) of age shows a CPC ➡ in the left choroid plexus glomus, which resolves spontaneously over time. Fetal and infantile CPCs often resolved with increasing age.*

Ependymal Cyst

KEY FACTS

TERMINOLOGY

- Congenital, benign, ependymal-lined cyst of brain

IMAGING

- Nonenhancing, thin-walled cyst
  - CSF density/intensity
- Most common location = intraventricular (lateral; 3rd rare)
  - Less common: Parenchyma, subarachnoid space

TOP DIFFERENTIAL DIAGNOSES

- Asymmetric lateral ventricles (normal variant)
- Choroid plexus cyst
- Arachnoid cyst
- Epidermoid cyst
- Neurenteric cyst
- Porencephalic cyst
- Neurocysticercosis

PATHOLOGY

- Thin-walled cyst filled with clear serous liquid
- Fluid-filled space lined by columnar or cuboidal cells

CLINICAL ISSUES

- Typically asymptomatic
- Headache, seizure, gait disturbance, dementia
- Symptoms related to CSF obstruction/↑ ICP
- Young adults (typically < 40 years old)
- Interval follow-up typically shows no clinical or imaging changes in asymptomatic lesions
- Symptomatic intraventricular cysts treated via neuronavigation-assisted fenestration

DIAGNOSTIC CHECKLIST

- Ependymal cysts may be indistinguishable from other benign intracranial cysts
- Ependymal cysts follow CSF on all MR sequences, including DWI; no enhancement

(Left) *Axial graphic depicts a typical ependymal cyst of the lateral ventricle ➡, seen here as a CSF-containing simple cyst that displaces the choroid plexus around it. Ependymal cysts typically follow CSF signal on all sequences.* **(Right)** *Axial MR images demonstrate the typical appearance of an ependymal cyst in the atrium of the left lateral ventricle. Cyst ➡ behaves exactly like CSF on all sequences, suppressing completely on FLAIR ➡. Note choroid plexus ➡ displaced around the cyst. This was an incidental finding in this asymptomatic patient.*

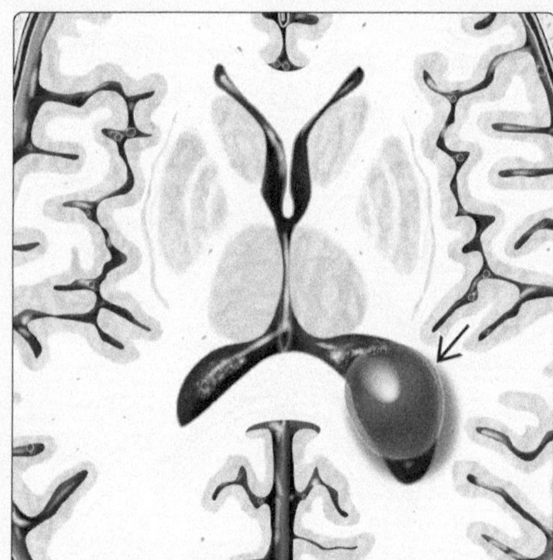

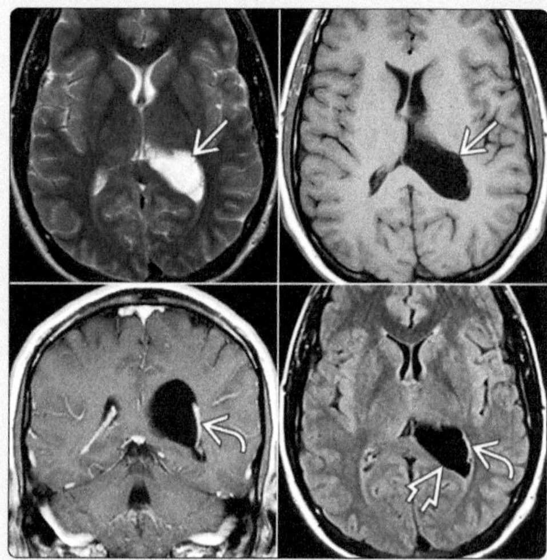

(Left) *Sagittal FIESTA MR in a 14-year-old shows an intraventricular cyst ➡ in the body of the lateral ventricle. High-resolution balanced FFE sequences, such as FIESTA, are excellent for depicting ependymal cysts due to high spatial resolution and elimination of CSF flow artifacts.* **(Right)** *Axial T1 C+ MR in a 3-month-old shows a pathology proven ependymal cyst ➡ associated with the left choroid plexus. The large size of the cyst causes entrapment of the left temporal horn ➡.*

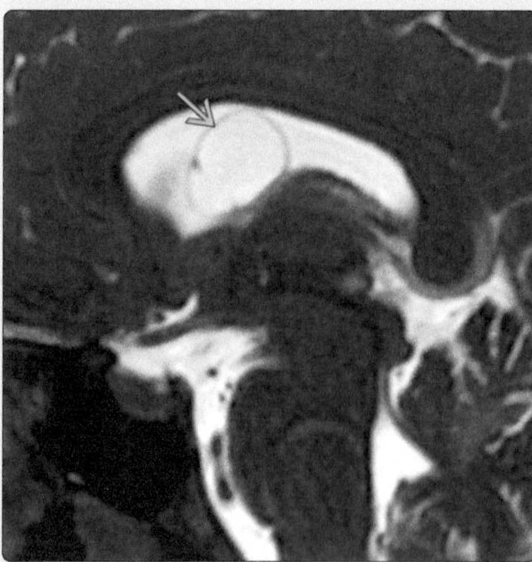

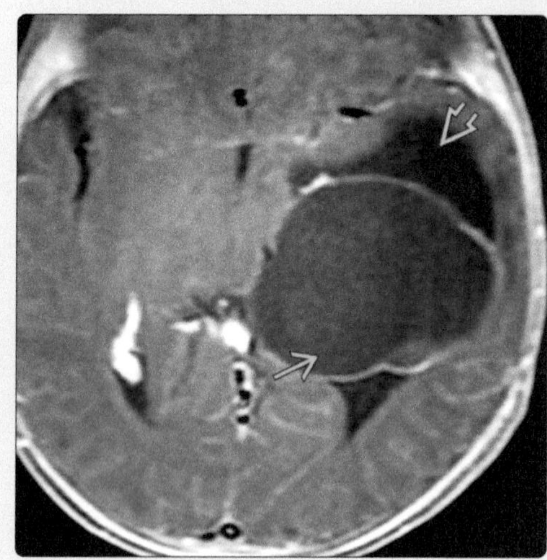

TERMINOLOGY

Abbreviations

- Ependymal cyst (EC)

Synonyms

- Neuroepithelial cyst, glioependymal cyst

Definitions

- Congenital, benign, ependymal-lined cyst of brain

IMAGING

General Features

- Best diagnostic clue
  - Nonenhancing, thin-walled, CSF density/intensity
- Location
  - Most common: Intraventricular (lateral > 3rd, 4th)
  - Less common: Cerebral parenchyma
- Size
  - Typically small (2-3 mm) but up to 8-9 cm reported
- Morphology
  - Smooth, thin-walled cyst

CT Findings

- NECT
  - Cyst is isodense to CSF; Ca^{++} extremely rare
- CECT
  - No enhancement

MR Findings

- T1WI
  - Isointense to CSF, cyst wall may be seen
- T2WI
  - Isointense to hyperintense to CSF (protein content)
- FLAIR
  - Isointense to CSF (suppresses)
- DWI
  - Isointense to CSF
- T1WI C+
  - No enhancement unless infected

Imaging Recommendations

- Best imaging tool
  - Multiplanar MR with T1 C+, DWI

DIFFERENTIAL DIAGNOSIS

Asymmetric Ventricles

- Lateral ventricle asymmetry, normal variant

Choroid Plexus Cyst

- Typically bilateral, arises in choroid plexus glomus

Neurocysticercosis

- Scolex present; does not suppress on FLAIR

Arachnoid Cyst

- May be indistinguishable; CSF intensity

Epidermoid Cyst

- Subarachnoid space > ventricles (4th most common)
- Heterogeneous on FLAIR, DWI hyperintensity

Neurenteric Cyst

- Extraaxial (typically posterior fossa) > parenchyma

PATHOLOGY

Gross Pathologic & Surgical Features

- Thin-walled cyst
- Filled with clear, serous liquid

Microscopic Features

- Fluid-filled space
  - May be lined by columnar or cuboidal cells

CLINICAL ISSUES

Presentation

- Most common signs/symptoms
  - Typically asymptomatic
- Other signs/symptoms
  - Rarely, headache, seizure, gait disturbance, dementia
  - Symptoms related to CSF obstruction/↑ intracranial pressure (ICP)

Demographics

- Age
  - Young adults (typically < 40 years old)
- Sex
  - M > F
- Epidemiology
  - Uncommon (< 25 symptomatic cases reported)

Natural History & Prognosis

- Uncommon so natural history unknown
- Follow-up typically shows no clinical or imaging changes in asymptomatic lesions
  - Imaging follow-up best with MR

Treatment

- If asymptomatic, conservative management
- Symptomatic intraventricular cysts treated via neuronavigation-assisted fenestration

DIAGNOSTIC CHECKLIST

Consider

- ECs may be indistinguishable from other benign intracranial cysts

Image Interpretation Pearls

- ECs follow CSF on all MR sequences, including DWI; no enhancement

SELECTED REFERENCES

1. Paulla Galdino Chaves J et al: Intracranial ependymal cyst - a modern systematic review with a pathway to diagnosis. J Clin Neurosci. 99:10-6, 2022
2. El-Ghandour NMF: Endoscopic treatment of intraventricular ependymal cysts in children: personal experience and review of literature. Childs Nerv Syst. 34(12):2441-8, 2018
3. Kutlay M et al: Endoscope-assisted microsurgical removal of an intraventricular ependymal cyst that manifested with tremor. World Neurosurg. 90:704.e11-8, 2016
4. Prieto R et al: Ependymal cyst of the midbrain. Clin Neuropathol. 32(3):183-8, 2013
5. Osborn AG, Preece MT. Intracranial cysts: radiologic-pathologic correlation and imaging approach. Radiology. 239(3):650-64, 2006

Porencephalic Cyst

KEY FACTS

TERMINOLOGY

- CSF-filled parenchymal cavity
  - Deep unilateral/bilateral cavity/excavation
  - Usually communicates with ventricle &/or subarachnoid space
  - Lined by reactive gliosis/astrocytic proliferation
- Congenital (perinatal brain destruction) or acquired (trauma, infection, etc.)

IMAGING

- Best diagnostic clue: CSF-filled cavities with enlarged adjacent ventricle
- MR: Smooth-walled cavity; CSF isointense; lined by gliotic white matter

TOP DIFFERENTIAL DIAGNOSES

- Consider arachnoid, ependymal, neoplastic, or inflammatory cyst
- Agenesis of corpus callosum
- Encephalomalacia
- Schizencephaly
- Dandy-Walker malformation
- Hydranencephaly

PATHOLOGY

- Brain injury in early intrauterine or postnatal premature timeframe
  - Common: Cerebral vascular event (e.g., hemorrhagic venous infarct: Grade 4 germinal matrix hemorrhage/intraventricular hemorrhage)
  - Rare: Infectious injury (e.g., CMV)

CLINICAL ISSUES

- Spastic hemiplegia most common symptom
- Indications for therapy: Mass effect, localized/generalized refractory symptoms

DIAGNOSTIC CHECKLIST

- Arachnoid cyst simulating porencephalic cyst

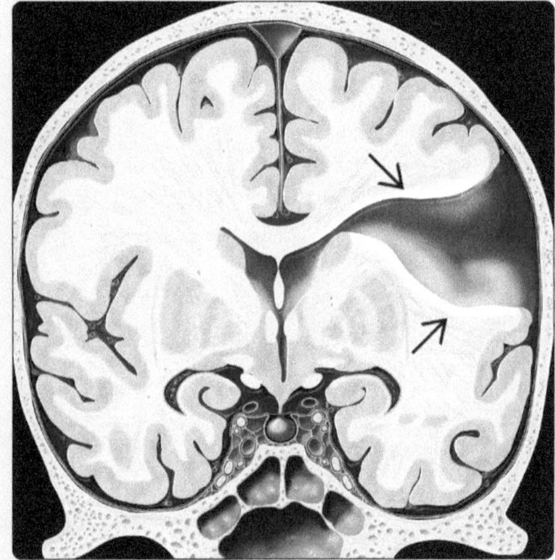

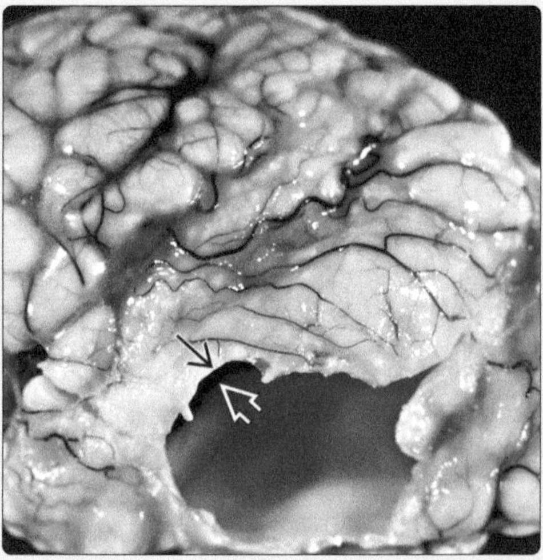

(Left) *Coronal graphic illustrates an intraparenchymal CSF-filled cavity that communicates with the left lateral ventricle and subarachnoid space. Note the classic porencephalic cyst is lined with gliotic white matter (WM) ➙.* **(Right)** *Lateral view of an autopsied brain with a porencephalic cyst in the temporal lobe shows a CSF-filled cavity that extends from the brain surface ➙ to the ventricular ependyma of the temporal horn ➙. The cyst is lined with gliotic WM. (Courtesy J. Townsend, MD.)*

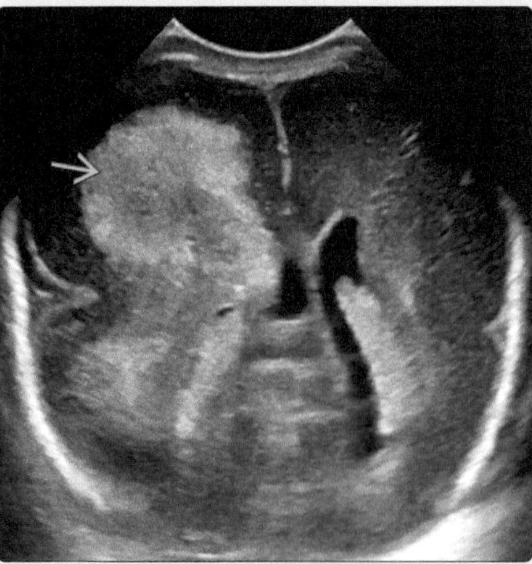

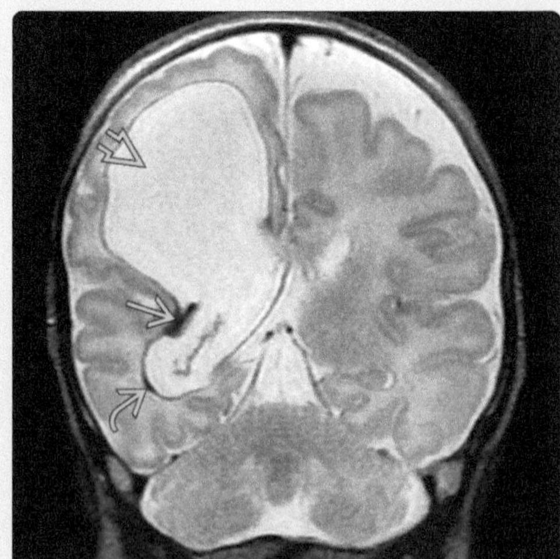

(Left) *Coronal US in an 8-day-old, former 24-week gestational age twin shows a large, fan-shaped area of ↑ echogenicity ➙ in the right frontal and temporal periventricular and deep WM, consistent with a hemorrhagic venous infarct [i.e., grade 4 germinal matrix hemorrhage (GMH)/intraventricular hemorrhage].* **(Right)** *Coronal T2 MR in the same patient at 3 months old shows interval development of porencephaly ➙ in location of hemorrhagic venous infarct. Note right GMH ➙ and hemosiderin ➙ lining right lateral ventricle.*

TERMINOLOGY

Synonyms

- Porencephaly

Definitions

- Various definitions of porencephaly
  - Congenital/acquired CSF-filled cavity that usually communicates with ventricular system
    - Deep unilateral/bilateral cavities or excavations
    - Lined by reactive gliosis/astrocytic proliferation
  - Presence of cysts/cavities in brain parenchyma
    - Communicating by "pore" with arachnoid space
  - Cavities arising in fetal life or early infancy
    - Brain destruction [e.g., hemorrhagic venous infarct: Grade 4 germinal matrix hemorrhage/intraventricular hemorrhage (IVH)] in early intrauterine development or postnatal injury of prematurity
    - Frequently communicate with subarachnoid space &/or lateral ventricles

IMAGING

General Features

- Best diagnostic clue
  - CSF-filled cavities; enlarged adjacent ventricle
- Location
  - Often corresponds to territories supplied by cerebral arteries (ischemic injury in midgestation)
  - Cortical/subcortical cavity, unilateral/bilateral
  - Usually connected with lateral ventricle
- Size
  - Varies from small to enormous

CT Findings

- NECT
  - Intraparenchymal smooth-walled cavity
    - Isodense with CSF
  - Directly communicates with ventricle
  - May see thin membrane separating cavity from ventricle
- CECT
  - No contrast enhancement of fluid-filled cavity
- Bone CT
  - Skull remodeling from chronic CSF pulsation
- CTA
  - Absence of vessels at site of porencephaly

MR Findings

- T1WI
  - Smooth-walled cavity; CSF isointense; lined by white matter (WM)
- T2WI
  - Brain atrophy, gliosis common; CSF isointense; lined by WM
- FLAIR
  - Accurately depicts CSF content of cyst and gliosis
- T1WI C+
  - Nonenhancing cyst

Ultrasonographic Findings

- Prenatal ultrasound for congenital porencephaly
  - Solitary or multiple echo-spared lesions(s)
  - Some cortical tissue may be preserved

Nonvascular Interventions

- Myelography
  - Contrast material injected into lumbar region may fill cystic space

Nuclear Medicine Findings

- PET
  - Area of absent glucose metabolism

Imaging Recommendations

- Best imaging tool
  - MR
- Protocol advice
  - FLAIR

DIFFERENTIAL DIAGNOSIS

Arachnoid Cyst

- CSF-isointense extraaxial cyst that exerts variable degrees of mass effect
- Unlike porencephalic cyst, extraaxial and displaces brain tissue away from adjacent skull

Ependymal Cyst

- Intraventricular; brain usually normal

Neoplastic Cyst

- Any cystic appearance of neoplastic processes

Inflammatory Cyst

- Mass effect, contrast enhancement if neoplastic

Agenesis of Corpus Callosum

- CSF-filled space extending cephalad from 3rd ventricle
- Parallel appearance of lateral ventricles
- Colpocephaly: Dilatation of occipital horns and posterior portions of temporal horns

Encephalomalacia

- Late gestational, perinatal, or postnatal injuries (thrombotic/embolic infarction, asphyxia, infection)
- May be slightly hyperdense/hyperintense to CSF (T1, T2, FLAIR)
- Cavity typically does not communicate with ventricle
  - Often contains septations and is lined by astrocytic proliferation

Schizencephaly

- Intraparenchymal cavity lined by gray matter, extending from ventricular surface to brain surface

Dandy-Walker Malformation

- Large median posterior fossa cyst widely communicating with 4th ventricle
- Rotated, raised, and small cerebellar vermis in contact with tentorium
- Upward displacement of tentorium and lateral sinuses

Hydranencephaly

- Early destructive process of developing brain caused by toxoplasmosis, CMV, or arterial occlusion
- Cortex and WM destroyed and replaced by thin-walled, CSF-filled sacs of leptomeninges

PATHOLOGY

General Features

- Etiology
  - Congenital: In utero destructive process caused by cerebral vascular events or infectious injury (CMV)
    - May be induced by antenatal trauma, even when mild or not directed at uterine wall
  - Perinatal: Most commonly occurs secondary to grade 4 IVH
  - Acquired: Injury later in life, following head trauma, surgery, vascular occlusion, or infection
- Genetics
  - Most cases are sporadic
  - Inherited cases often result from bleeding
    - Rare, autosomal dominant familial porencephaly
      - Chromosome 13qter → mutation of gene encoding procollagen type IV α1
      - Encodes basement membrane protein expressed in all tissues
      - ↑ intracerebral hemorrhage risk for life
    - COL4A mutation: Collagen disorder at ↑ risk of intracranial hemorrhage
    - Inherited thrombophilia, most often heterozygosity for factor V Leiden mutation (gene *F5*)
- Associated abnormalities
  - Amygdala-hippocampal atrophy often coexists with congenital porencephaly (95% in some reports)
    - May be bilateral despite unilateral cysts
  - Syndromes: Septo-optic dysplasia, orofaciodigital syndrome type I, encephalocraniocutaneous lipomatosis, Proteus syndrome, Delleman syndrome, DK-phocomelia
  - Alloimmune thrombocytopenia
  - Coagulopathies (e.g., von Willebrand disease), factor V or X deficiency, maternal warfarin use
  - Multiple gestation associated with vascular disruption defects: Large intestinal atresia, transverse limb deficiency, porencephaly, and renal agenesis

Gross Pathologic & Surgical Features

- CSF-filled cavity with smooth walls
  - Lined by gliotic or spongiotic WM
- Overlying skull
  - May be remodeled due to long-term transmission of CSF pulsations
  - May be thickened when intervening brain tissue precludes transmission of CSF pulsations

Microscopic Features

- Congenital porencephalic cyst
  - Gray matter and WM necrosis
  - Fluid-filled, focal cavity with smooth walls and minimal surrounding glial reaction
- Acquired porencephalic cyst
  - Mature brain reacts to injury by significant astrocytic proliferation
  - Resulting cavity often has septations and irregular wall composed primarily of reactive astrocytes

CLINICAL ISSUES

Presentation

- Most common signs/symptoms
  - Spastic hemiplegia most common feature
  - May be associated with severe neurologic deficits
    - Intellectual disabilities, medically intractable epilepsy
- Clinical profile
  - Cerebellar symptoms; ophthalmologic signs
  - Various forms of cerebral paralysis
  - Seizures, psychomotor restrictions

Demographics

- Age
  - Most commonly occurs in premature infants
    - Sequelae of grade 4 IVH (hemorrhagic venous infarct)
  - May occur to lesser degree in older children, but gliosis (without cyst formation) more common after term gestational age
- Sex
  - M > F infants, especially with mothers < 20 years
- Epidemiology
  - 2.5% incidence of porencephalic cysts among 1,000 congenital and acquired brain lesions
  - 0.035% prevalence per 10,000 live births

Natural History & Prognosis

- Narrow communication with ventricular system may ↑ pressure in cyst → mass effect
- Children with neonatal intraparenchymal echodensities and porencephaly have much worse long-term neurodevelopmental outcome

Treatment

- Usually no treatment required
- Indications for therapy: Mass effect, localized/generalized refractory symptoms
  - Cystoperitoneal shunt (preferred)
  - If no communication with ventricular system: Fenestration or partial resection of cyst wall
  - Children with intractable seizures benefit from uncapping and cyst fenestration to lateral ventricle
- Congenital porencephaly should prompt collagen *4A1* genetic screening

DIAGNOSTIC CHECKLIST

Consider

- Arachnoid cyst simulating porencephalic cyst

Image Interpretation Pearls

- Look for hemosiderin rim in younger patients to confirm prior cerebrovascular hemorrhage

SELECTED REFERENCES

1. AlGoraini Y et al: Post-traumatic cysts detected by ultrasound in infant presented with first-time seizures: Case report. Radiol Case Rep. 17(11):4128-31, 2022
2. Moradi B et al: Ultrasound and magnetic resonance imaging features of fetal intracranial cystic lesions: a pictorial essay. J Clin Ultrasound. 50(9):129731-1, 2022
3. Wynne D et al: Endoscopic fenestration of a symptomatic porencephalic cyst in an adult. World Neurosurg. 141:245-6, 2020

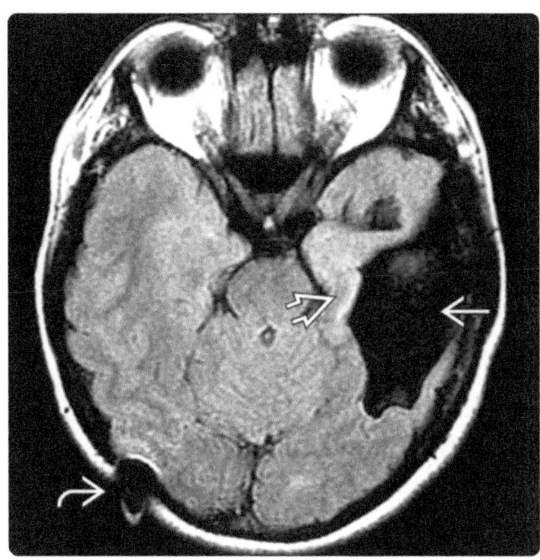

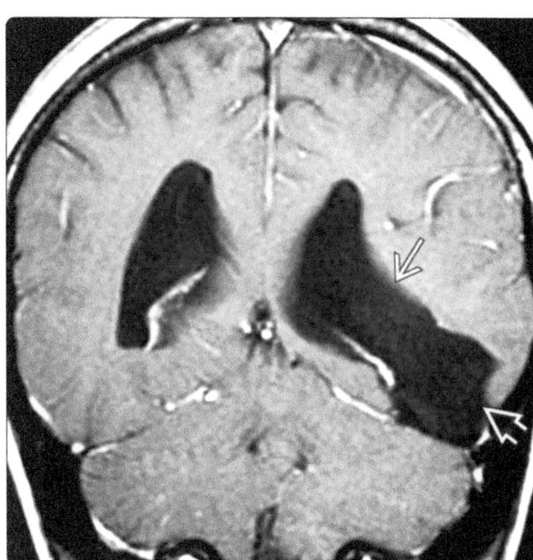

(Left) *Axial FLAIR MR of a porencephalic cyst reveals a CSF-intensity parenchymal defect, which was isointense to CSF on all sequences, including FLAIR nulling ➡. Also note the small amount of associated WM gliosis ➡. Susceptibility artifact is secondary to a ventriculostomy shunt ➡.* **(Right)** *Coronal T1 C+ MR in the same patient shows a CSF-density parenchymal defect ➡, which communicates with the atrium of the left lateral ventricle with dilatation of the occipital horn ➡. A classic porencephalic cyst is also seen.*

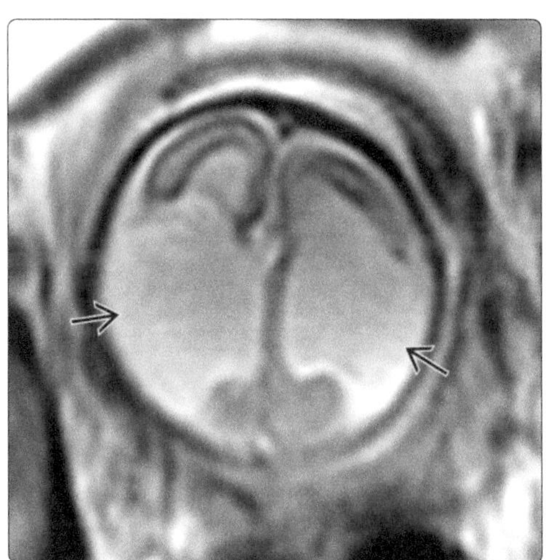

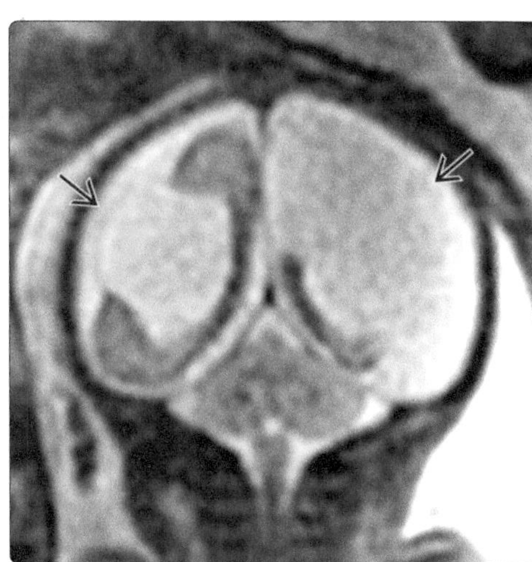

(Left) *Axial T2 fetal MR demonstrates bilateral supratentorial porencephalic cysts ➡ as CSF-isointense lesions communicating with dilated lateral ventricles.* **(Right)** *Coronal T2 fetal MR in the same patient nicely shows bilateral supratentorial porencephalic cysts ➡ with normal posterior fossa contents. Congenital porencephalic cysts are the result of an in utero destructive process, usually cerebral vascular events or infectious injury.*

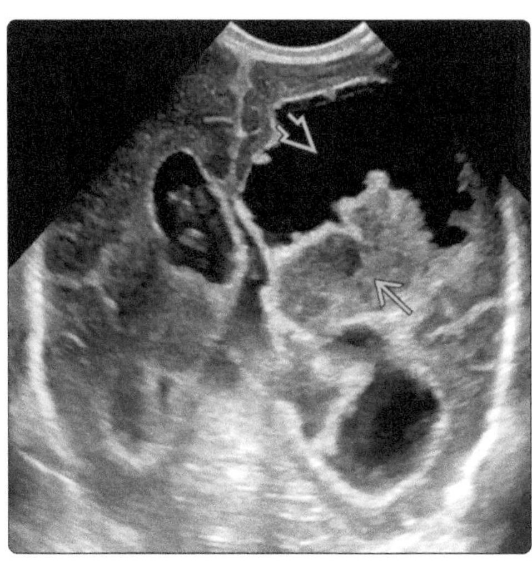

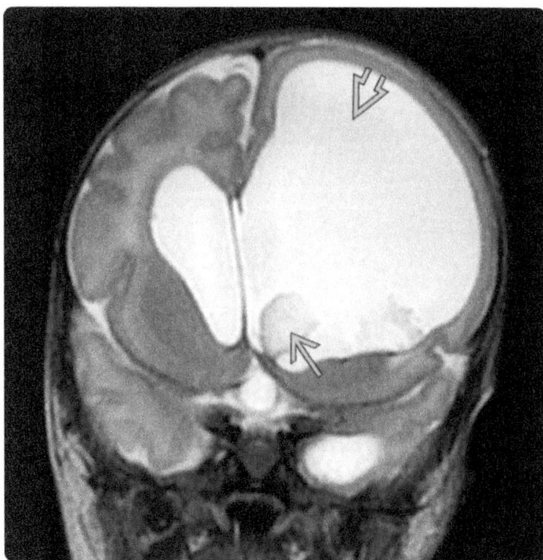

(Left) *Coronal US in a 2-month-old, former 26-week gestational age infant shows an evolving hemorrhagic venous infarct with retracting central clot ➡ and surrounding liquefaction ➡ of brain, which will eventually become a porencephalic cyst.* **(Right)** *Coronal T2 MR in the same patient at 3 months of age shows smooth margins of the porencephalic cyst ➡ now in continuity with the lateral ventricle. Note the much smaller central clot ➡ from prior hemorrhagic venous infarct.*

KEY FACTS

TERMINOLOGY

- Congenital endodermal cyst
  - Like Rathke cleft, colloid cysts

IMAGING

- General
  - Oblong, nonenhancing, slightly hyperintense (to CSF) mass in front of medulla
- Location
  - More common in spine than brain (3:1)
  - 70-75% of intracranial neurenteric cysts (NECs) infratentorial, extraaxial
  - Anterior/lateral to pontomedullary junction
  - 25-30% supratentorial (suprasellar, cerebral hemispheres)
- CT
  - Hypo-/iso-/hyperdense, no Ca^{++}
  - Bony anomalies usually absent
- MR
  - Almost always iso-/hyperintense to CSF on T1WI
  - 90% hyperintense to CSF, 10% hypointense on T2WI
  - Usually does not restrict on DWI
  - Usually no enhancement (mild rim in some)

TOP DIFFERENTIAL DIAGNOSES

- Most common
  - Epidermoid; arachnoid cyst
- Less common
  - Schwannoma (cystic)
- Rare
  - Ecchordosis physaliphora

PATHOLOGY

- Contents vary from clear, colorless fluid (like CSF) to thicker, more viscous/mucoid

DIAGNOSTIC CHECKLIST

- Mass in front of brainstem, hyperdense/hyperintense to CSF may be NEC

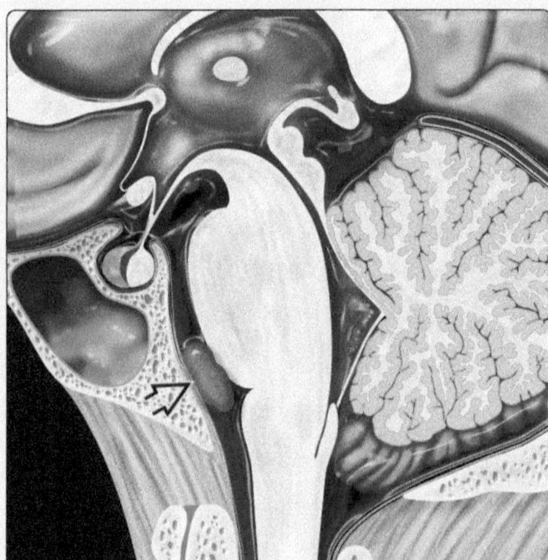

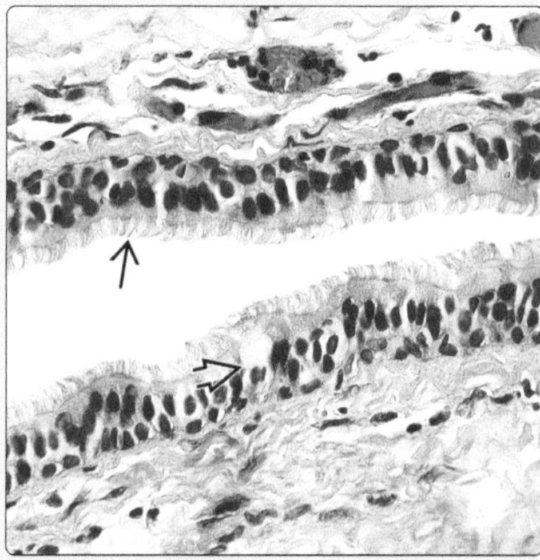

(Left) *Sagittal graphic shows a classic neurenteric cyst (NEC) ➾. Intracranial NECs are most often found near the midline, anterior to the brainstem.* **(Right)** *NECs (endodermal) are mostly lined with pseudostratified columnar epithelium with heavily ciliated cells ➾. Variable numbers of mucin-secreting goblet cells ➾ are present. (Courtesy P. Burger, MD.)*

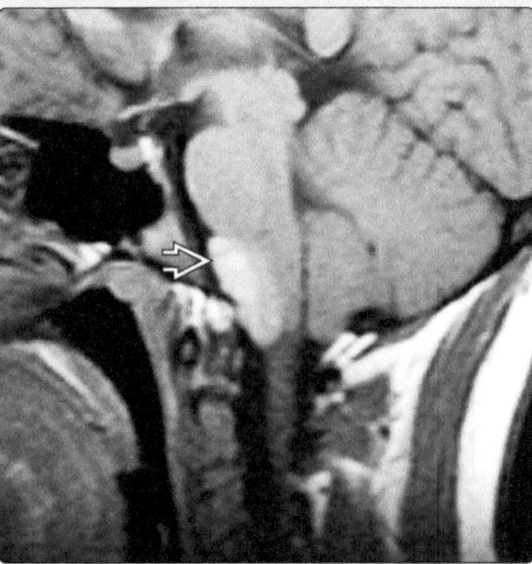

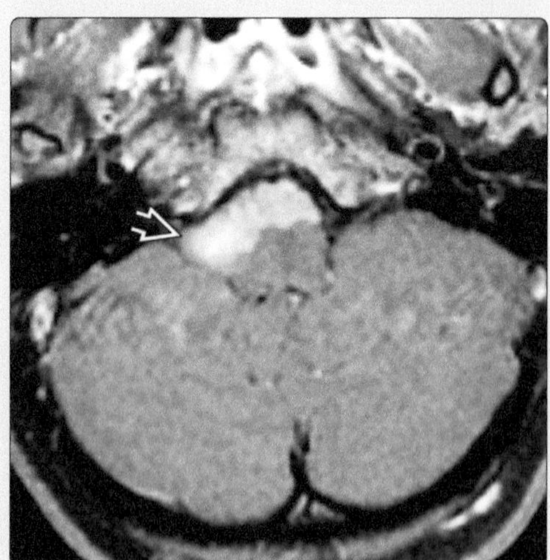

(Left) *Sagittal T1WI MR shows a typical NEC as a well-delineated, hyperintense, ovoid paramedian mass ➾ anterior to the pontomedullary junction.* **(Right)** *Axial T1 C+ FS MR in the same patient shows that the mass ➾ extends inferolaterally in front of the lower medulla. The center of the mass is slightly off-midline, a typical location for a posterior fossa NEC.*

TERMINOLOGY

Abbreviations

- Neurenteric cyst (NEC)

Synonyms

- Neuroepithelial cyst, enterogenous cyst, endodermal cyst, enteric cyst

Definitions

- Rare, benign, malformative endodermal CNS cyst

IMAGING

General Features

- Best diagnostic clue
  - Oblong, nonenhancing, slightly T1-/T2-hyperintense mass in front of medulla
- Location
  - More common in spine than brain (3:1)
  - 70-75% of intracranial NECs found in posterior fossa
    - > 95% extraaxial
    - Most anterior/lateral to pontomedullary junction
    - 70% extend to midline
      - Rarely posterior, mimicking arachnoid cyst
  - 25-30% supratentorial
    - Suprasellar, quadrigeminal cisterns
    - Cerebral hemispheres (frontal most common)
- Size
  - Posterior fossa usually < 2 cm; supratentorial often large
- Morphology
  - Smooth, lobulated, well demarcated

CT Findings

- NECT
  - Hypo-/iso-/hyperdense mass, no Ca^{++} or hemorrhage
  - Bony anomalies usually absent
- CECT
  - No enhancement

MR Findings

- T1WI
  - Almost always iso-/hyperintense to CSF
- T2WI
  - 90% hyperintense, 10% hypointense to CSF
- FLAIR
  - Hyperintense to CSF
- DWI
  - Usually none but may show mild restriction
- T1WI C+
  - Usually none; occasionally, mild rim

Imaging Recommendations

- Best imaging tool
  - MR with T1 C+, FLAIR, DWI

DIFFERENTIAL DIAGNOSIS

Epidermoid Cyst

- "White" epidermoid (rare) is hyperintense on T1WI
- Usually restricts on DWI

Dermoid Cyst

- Like fat; often Ca^{++}

Arachnoid Cyst

- Like CSF on all sequences

Schwannoma

- Enhances strongly; usually not midline

Other Endodermal Cysts

- Rathke cleft, colloid cysts
- Excluded by location

Ecchordosis Physaliphora

- Notochordal remnant
- Often involves clivus

PATHOLOGY

General Features

- Etiology
  - Congenital endodermal cyst
  - Probably arises from persistent neurenteric canal

Gross Pathologic & Surgical Features

- Transparent, thin-walled, smooth, round/lobulated cyst
- Contents vary from clear, colorless fluid (like CSF) to thicker, more viscous/mucoid

CLINICAL ISSUES

Presentation

- Most common signs/symptoms
  - Brain = asymptomatic or headache

Demographics

- Age
  - Any age; peak 34 years
- Sex
  - M:F = 1:3
- Epidemiology
  - Rare (only 75 intracranial cases reported)

Natural History & Prognosis

- May be stable for years or grow very slowly

Treatment

- Observation vs. total surgical excision

DIAGNOSTIC CHECKLIST

Consider

- Mass in front of brainstem, hyperdense/hyperintense to CSF may be NEC

SELECTED REFERENCES

1. Oppenhuizen B et al: Pediatric intracranial neurenteric cyst of the oculomotor nerve: a case-based review. Childs Nerv Syst. 37(12):3681-93, 2021
2. Kawamura Y et al: A dorsally located endodermal cyst in the foramen magnum mimicking an arachnoid cyst: a case report. Pediatr Neurosurg. 55(4):197-202, 2020
3. Menéndez RH et al: Neurenteric cyst of the ventral craniocervical junction: case report and a literature review. World Neurosurg. 125:257-60, 2019
4. Nunes Dias L et al: Supratentorial neuroenteric cyst in children: a case report and brief literature review. Childs Nerv Syst. 35(11):2227-31, 2019

Lipoma, Brain

KEY FACTS

TERMINOLOGY

- Intracranial lipoma (ICL)

IMAGING

- Well-delineated, lobulated, extraaxial mass with fat attenuation/intensity
- 80% supratentorial
  - 40-50% interhemispheric fissure (over corpus callosum; may extend into lateral ventricles, choroid plexus)
  - 15-20% suprasellar (attached to infundibulum, hypothalamus)
  - 10-15% tectal region (usually inferior colliculus/superior vermis)
- 20% infratentorial
- Cerebellopontine angle (may extend into internal auditory canal, vestibule)
- Lobulated, pial-based fatty mass that may encase vessels and cranial nerves
- CT: -50 to -100 Hounsfield units (fat density)
- Ca^{++} varies from none to extensive
- Standard spin-echo MR: Hyperintense on T1/T2WI
- Becomes hypointense with fat suppression

TOP DIFFERENTIAL DIAGNOSES

- Teratoma
- Dermoid cyst

PATHOLOGY

- Mass of mature, nonneoplastic adipose tissue
- CNS lipomas congenital malformations, not true neoplasms

CLINICAL ISSUES

- Usually incidental; may grow with child

DIAGNOSTIC CHECKLIST

- When in doubt, use fat-saturation sequence
- Consider whether high signal on T1WI is due to other substances with short T1 (e.g., subacute hemorrhage)
- NECT: Use bone windows to distinguish fat from air

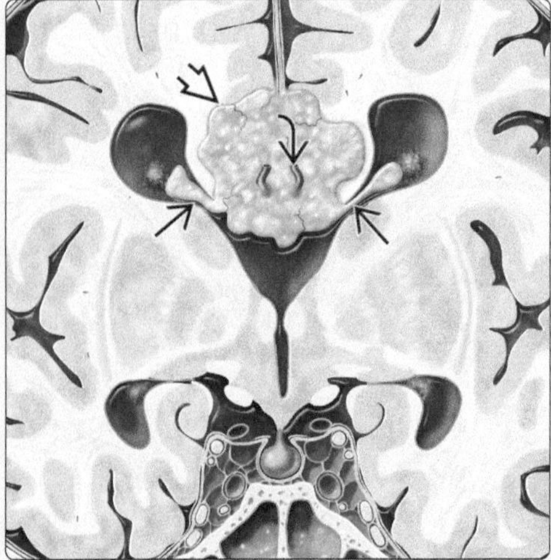

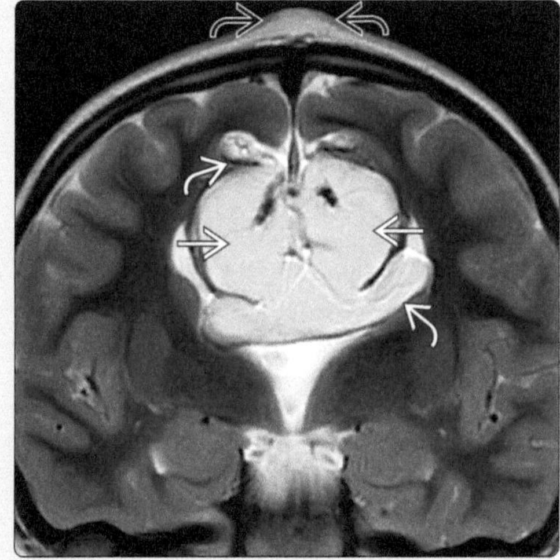

(Left) *Coronal graphic shows callosal agenesis with a bulky, interhemispheric lipoma ⇒ that encases arteries ➚ and extends into lateral ventricles ⇒.* **(Right)** *Coronal T2WI MR shows a large, hyperintense tubulonodular callosal lipoma ➡. Chemical shift artifacts are seen at the periphery ➡. Multiple hypointensities within the lipoma could be blood vessels or Ca^{++}, which will be SWI hypointense also. SWI signal of lipoma was predominantly isointense to brain with peripheral dark rim (not shown). Note small scalp lipoma ➚.*

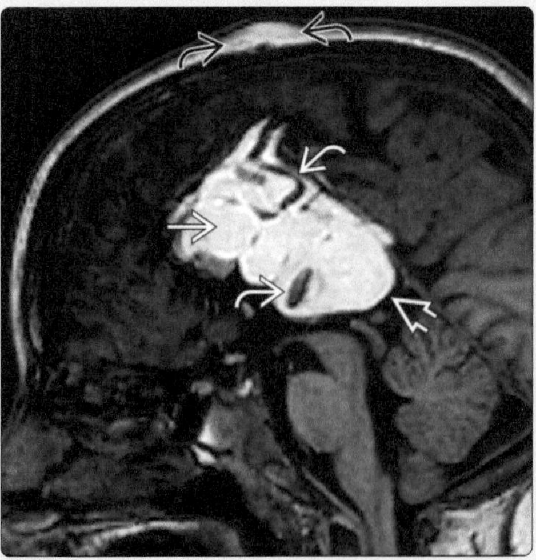

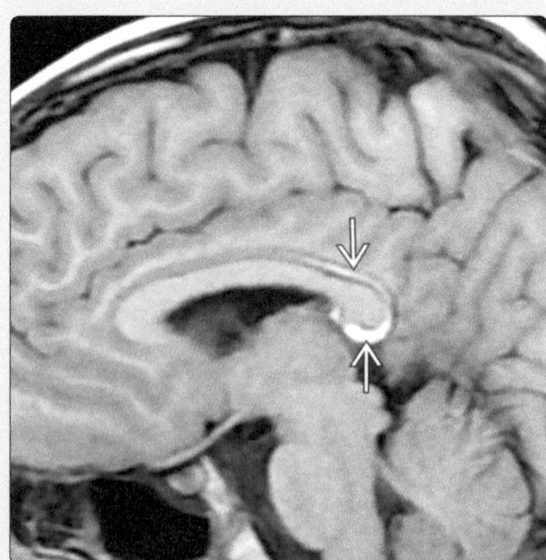

(Left) *Sagittal T1WI MR in the same patient shows that this large tubulonodular callosal lipoma ➡ is hyperintense on T1WI also. Tortuous blood vessels are seen within the lipoma ➡. Corpus callosum is dysgenetic with absence of splenium ➡. Note small scalp lipoma ➚.* **(Right)** *Sagittal T1WI MR in a 10-year-old with a thin, curvilinear pericallosal lipoma ➡ that curves around the splenium is shown. Many small linear lipomas have little or no associated callosal dysgenesis/agenesis, as in this case.*

TERMINOLOGY

Abbreviations

- Intracranial lipoma (ICL)

Synonyms

- Lipomatous hamartoma

Definitions

- Mass of mature nonneoplastic adipose tissue
  - CNS lipomas congenital malformations, not true neoplasms
  - Lipoma variants in CNS include angiolipoma, hibernoma, osteolipoma

IMAGING

General Features

- Best diagnostic clue
  - Well-delineated, lobulated, extraaxial mass with fat attenuation/intensity
- Location
  - Midline location common
  - 80% supratentorial
    - 40-50% interhemispheric fissure [over corpus callosum (CC)]; may extend into lateral ventricles, choroid plexus)
    - 15-20% suprasellar (attached to infundibulum, hypothalamus)
    - 10-15% tectal region (usually inferior colliculus/superior vermis)
    - Uncommon: Meckel cave, lateral cerebral fissures, middle cranial fossa, interpeduncular cistern
  - 20% infratentorial
    - Cerebellopontine angle (may extend into internal auditory canal, vestibule)
    - Uncommon: Jugular foramen, foramen magnum
- Size
  - Varies from tiny to very large
  - May grow as child grows
- Morphology
  - Lobulated, pial-based fatty mass that may encase vessels and cranial nerves
  - 2 kinds of interhemispheric lipoma
    - Curvilinear type (thin ICL curves around callosal body, splenium)
    - Tubulonodular type (bulky mass; frequent Ca^{++}, usually associated with callosal agenesis or severe dysgenesis)

Radiographic Findings

- Radiography
  - Usually normal
  - Very large interhemispheric lipomas may show low density
  - Tubulonodular lipomas may show rim Ca^{++}

CT Findings

- NECT
  - -50 to -100 Hounsfield units (HU); fat density
  - Ca^{++} varies from none to extensive
    - Present in 65% of bulky, tubulonodular CC lipomas
    - Rare in posterior fossa, parasellar lesions
- CECT
  - Does not enhance
- CTA
  - May demonstrate aberrant pericallosal artery (anterior cerebral artery division) course in interhemispheric lipoma associated with callosal dysgenesis

MR Findings

- T1WI
  - Hyperintense mass (occasionally, in fetal MR, will not be due to immature fat cells)
  - Becomes hypointense with fat suppression
  - Chemical shift artifact in frequency-encoding direction
- T2WI
  - Hypointense on conventional spin-echo with striking chemical shift artifact
    - Round/linear filling defects present where vessels and cranial nerves pass through lipoma
    - May show low signal intensity foci (Ca^{++})
  - FSE: Iso- to hyperintense (J-coupling)
- PD/intermediate
  - Iso- to hyperintense (depending on repetition and echo times)
    - Striking chemical shift artifact
- STIR
  - Hypointense
- FLAIR
  - Hyperintense
- T2* GRE
  - SWI: Predominantly isointense to brain with peripheral dark rim (chemical-shift artifact resultant from fat-water interface)
    - Ca^{++} and blood vessels coursing through lipoma SWI hypointense
- DWI
  - No diffusion restriction
  - Diffusion tensor imaging visualizes altered fiber connections if associated callosal dysgenesis present
- T1WI C+
  - Does not enhance

Ultrasonographic Findings

- Grayscale ultrasound
  - Fetal/neonatal mass, generally hyperechoic
  - May show other fetal anomalies (CC agenesis, etc.)

Imaging Recommendations

- Best imaging tool
  - MR
- Protocol advice
  - Add fat-suppression sequence for confirmation

DIFFERENTIAL DIAGNOSIS

Dural Dysplasia

- Fat often in falx, cavernous sinuses
- Metaplastic ossified dura may contain fat

Dermoid

- Density usually 20-40 HU
- Signal intensity usually more heterogeneous

- Rupture with cisternal fat droplets common
- Usually no associated malformations (common with lipoma)
- Dermoids often calcify, lipomas in locations other than interhemispheric typically do not

Teratoma

- Locations similar to lipoma
- Tissue from all 3 embryonic germ layers
- Imaging appearance usually more heterogeneous
  - May show foci of contrast enhancement

Lipomatous Differentiation of Neoplasm

- May occur occasionally in primitive tumors, ependymoma, gliomas
- Cerebellar liponeurocytoma
  - Primarily hypointense on T1WI, mixed with hyperintense foci
  - Patchy, irregular enhancement
- Meningiomas, schwannomas, metastases rarely have lipomatous transformation

Subacute Hemorrhage

- T1 shortening can be confused with lipoma
- Use T2* (hemorrhage blooms), fat saturation (hemorrhage does not suppress)

Encephalocraniocutaneous Lipomatosis

- Also known as Haberland syndrome/Fishman syndrome
- Eye anomalies, skin lesions, ILCs, cortical malformation mainly polymicrogyria
- ± diffuse, ipsilateral leptomeningeal enhancement (mimics Sturge-Weber syndrome)
- **Nevus psiloliparus**: Sharply demarcated focus of scalp **alopecia** overlying **scalp lipoma**

PATHOLOGY

General Features

- Etiology
  - Persistent maldevelopment of embryonic meninx primitiva
    - Normally differentiates into leptomeninges, cisterns
    - Maldifferentiates into fat instead
  - Developing pia-arachnoid invaginates through embryonic choroid fissure
    - Explains frequent intraventricular extension of interhemispheric lipomas
- Genetics
  - No known defects in sporadic ICL
- Associated abnormalities
  - Most common: Interhemispheric lipoma with CC anomalies
  - Other congenital malformations: Cephaloceles, closed spinal dysraphism
  - Encephalocraniocutaneous lipomatosis (Haberland/Fishman syndrome)
  - Pai syndrome → facial clefts, skin lipomas; occasional ICLs, usually interhemispheric

Gross Pathologic & Surgical Features

- Yellow, lobulated, fatty mass attached to leptomeninges, sometimes adherent to brain
- Cranial nerves, arteries/veins pass through lipoma

Microscopic Features

- Identical to adipose tissue elsewhere
- Cells vary in shape/size, measure up to 200 μm
- Occasional nuclear hyperchromasia; mitoses rare/absent
- Liposarcoma: Extremely rare malignant intracranial adipose tumor

CLINICAL ISSUES

Presentation

- Most common signs/symptoms
  - Usually found incidentally at imaging, autopsy
  - Rare: Cranial neuropathy (vestibulocochlear dysfunction, facial pain), seizures (associated with other congenital anomalies)
  - Seizures associated with lipomas over (dysmorphic) cortex

Demographics

- Age
  - Any age
- Sex
  - M = F
- Ethnicity
  - None known
- Epidemiology
  - < 0.5% of all intracranial masses (not true neoplasm)

Natural History & Prognosis

- Benign, usually stable
- May expand with corticosteroids
  - High-dose, long-term administration may result in neural compressive symptoms

Treatment

- Generally not surgical lesion
  - Surgery has high morbidity/mortality
  - May have arteries, veins, and nerves passing through lipoma
- Reduce/eliminate steroids

DIAGNOSTIC CHECKLIST

Consider

- Consider whether high signal on T1WI is due to other substances with short T1 (e.g., subacute hemorrhage)

Image Interpretation Pearls

- When in doubt, use fat-saturation sequence
- Beware: Lipoma can mimic intracranial air on NECT (use bone windows to distinguish)

SELECTED REFERENCES

1. Kashyap R et al: Susceptibility or chemical shift artifacts in intracranial lipomas mimicking hemorrhage - case series with review of the literature. J Neurosci Rural Pract. 13(4):759-63, 2022
2. Uysal E et al: Internal auditory canal lipoma: an unusual intracranial lesion. World Neurosurg. 135:156-9, 2020
3. Erbay MF et al: A pericallosal lipoma case with abnormal vasculature mimicking arteriovenous malformation. Neurol India. 67(5):1331-3, 2019
4. Atallah A et al: Limitations and pitfalls in prenatal diagnosis of pericallosal curvilinear lipoma based on a specific imaging pattern. Ultrasound Obstet Gynecol. 51(2):269-73, 2018
5. Chougar L et al: Variability of T1-weighted signal intensity of pericallosal lipomas in the fetus. Pediatr Radiol. 48(3):383-91, 2018

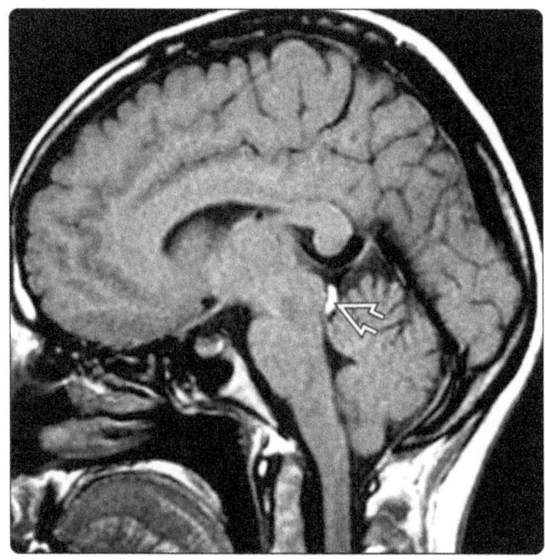

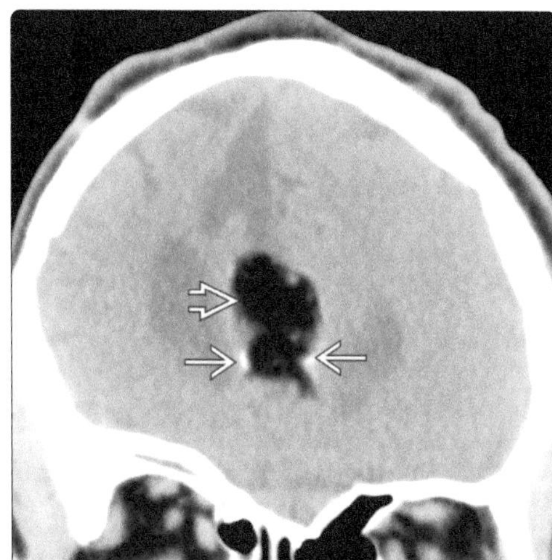

(Left) *Sagittal T1WI MR shows a tectal plate lipoma ➡ situated immediately posterior to the inferior tectum and between the inferior colliculus and the superior surface of the cerebellar vermis, a very common location for lipomas.* **(Right)** *Coronal NECT shows a midline hypodense pericallosal lipoma ➡ with density equal to orbital and scalp fat. Note the small Ca^{++} ➡, a finding often associated with pericallosal lipomas.*

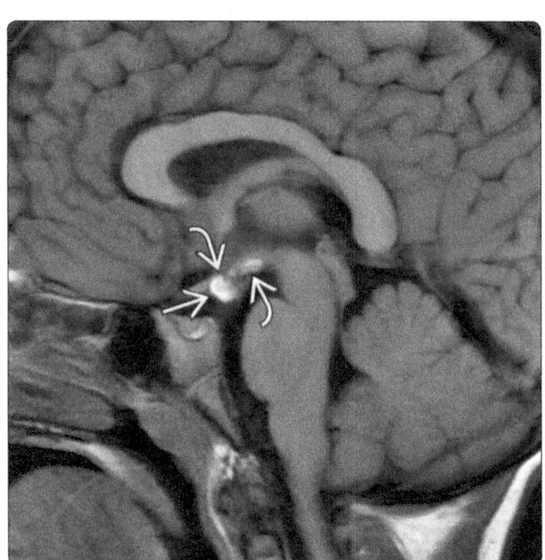

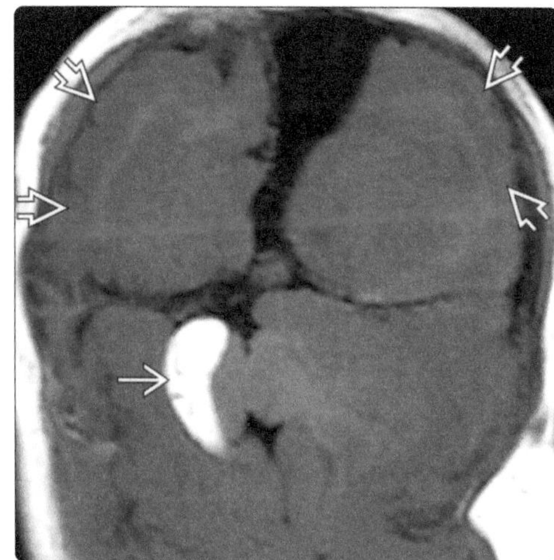

(Left) *Midline sagittal T1WI MR shows a T1-hyperintense lipoma arising from the hypothalamus ➡ and protruding into suprasellar cistern ➡. T1WI C+ MR showed no solid enhancement to suggest a dermoid (not shown).* **(Right)** *Axial T1WI MR in a 10-month-old shows right perimesencephalic lipoma ➡. Note bilateral frontoparietal polymicrogyria ➡. Lipomas are associated with many brain malformationsand syndromes, including Haberland/Fishman syndrome (encephalocraniocutaneous lipomatosis).*

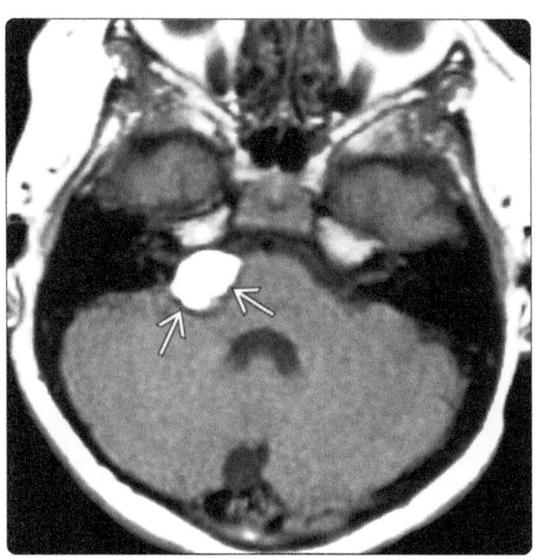

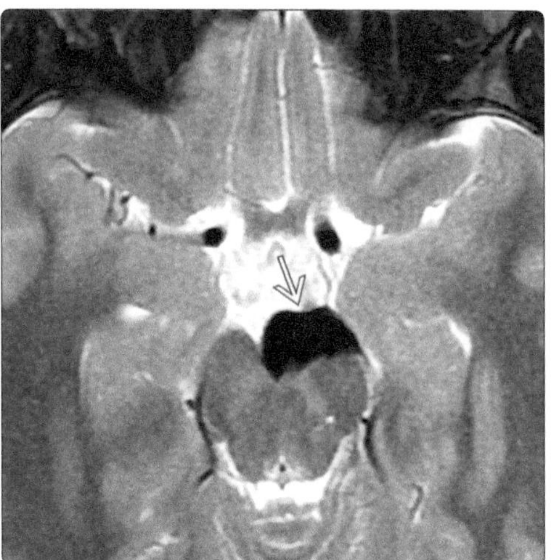

(Left) *Axial T1WI MR shows a round lipoma ➡ in the right cerebellopontine angle cistern, adjacent to internal auditory canal. Lipomas do not cause hearing loss, may have nerves and vessels passing through them, and should not be resected.* **(Right)** *Axial T2WI FS MR in a 10-year-old boy shows complete nulling of signal within an interpeduncular lipoma the lesion ➡. Non-fat-suppressed T1 and T2WI demonstrated bright signal of the lipoma (not shown). Note the mass effect on left anterior midbrain.*

Congenital CMV

KEY FACTS

TERMINOLOGY

- Congenital cytomegalovirus (CMV)

IMAGING

- Microcephaly: Spectrum and severity of brain injury depends on timing of fetal infection
- Cranial sonography
  - Periventricular hyperechoic foci
  - Branching basal ganglia hyperechogenicities (lenticulostriate vasculopathy)
  - Ring-like periventricular lucency may precede Ca^{++}
- NECT when clinically CMV &/or to complement brain MR
  - Intracranial Ca^{++} (40-70%): Periventricular (subependymal, germinolytic zones)
- MR brain to completely characterize abnormalities
  - Agyria ↔ pachygyria ↔ diffuse polymicrogyria ↔ focal cortical dysplasia ↔ schizencephalic clefting
  - White matter (WM) abnormalities: Periventricular germinolytic cysts, demyelination, gliosis

TOP DIFFERENTIAL DIAGNOSES

- Congenital lymphocytic choriomeningitis
- Toxoplasmosis
- Pseudo-TORCH syndromes

PATHOLOGY

- Ubiquitous DNA virus of herpesvirus family
- Hematogenously seeds choroid plexus, replicates in ependyma, germinal matrix, and capillary endothelia

CLINICAL ISSUES

- 55% with systemic disease have CNS involvement
- Sensorineural hearing loss common

DIAGNOSTIC CHECKLIST

- Microcephaly, migration anomalies, periventricular cysts/Ca^{++}, WM changes, cerebellar hypoplasia
- Look for periventricular cysts, particularly anterior to temporal horns

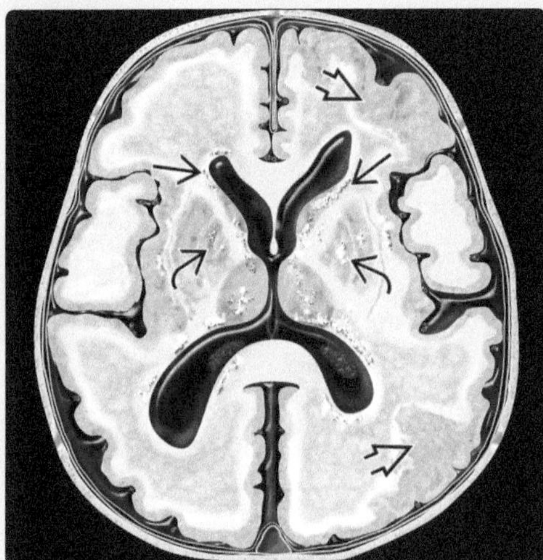

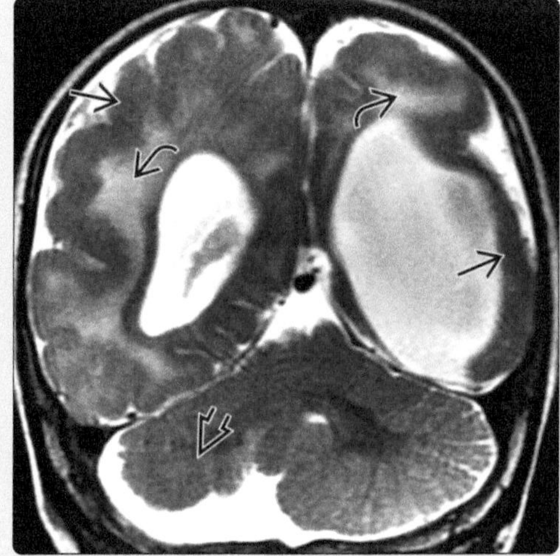

(Left) *Axial graphic shows numerous periventricular ➡ and basal ganglia ➡ Ca^{++}. Note regions of cortical malformation (polymicrogyria) ➡. Ventricular dilation reflects adjacent white matter (WM) volume loss. The yellowish WM abnormalities reflect regions of demyelination &/or gliosis.* **(Right)** *Coronal T2WI MR shows ex-vacuo ventriculomegaly due to central WM volume loss, WM hyperintensities due to gliosis/demyelination ➡, and polymicrogyria ➡. Note right cerebellar hypoplasia ➡.*

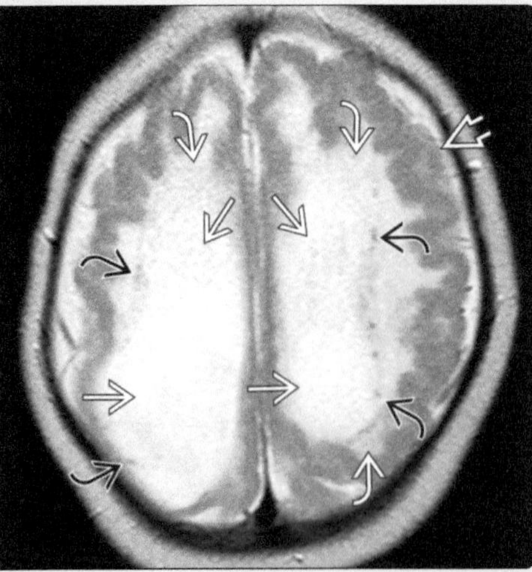

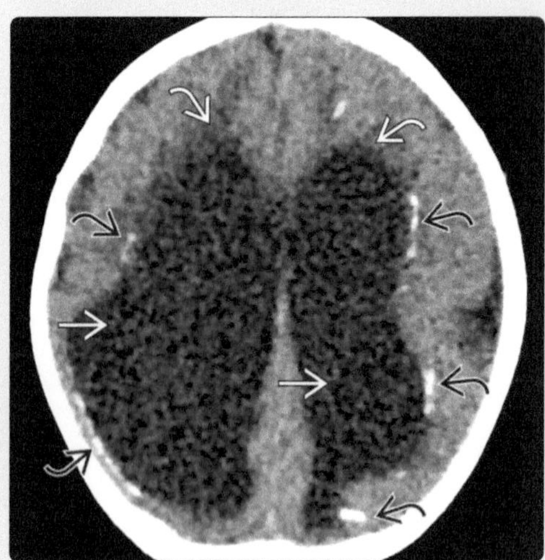

(Left) *Axial T2WI MR in congenital CMV shows ex-vacuo ventricular dilation ➡ due to WM volume loss. There are surrounding regions of abnormal WM signal ➡ due to gliosis &/or demyelination. Note pebbled cortical irregularities due to polymicrogyria ➡. Periventricular T2 hypointensities ➡ suggesting possible Ca^{++} are seen.* **(Right)** *Axial NECT in the same patient reconfirms periventricular Ca^{++} ➡. Ventricular dilation ➡ and periventricular WM hypodensities ➡ are also noted.*

TERMINOLOGY

Abbreviations

- Congenital cytomegalovirus (CMV)

Definitions

- Congenital infection caused by transplacental transmission of CMV; member of herpesvirus family
  - Most common cause of intrauterine infection in USA

IMAGING

General Features

- Best diagnostic clue
  - Microcephaly, spectrum of brain injury depending on timing of fetal infection
  - Intracranial Ca^{++} (40-70%); periventricular (subependymal germinal matrix zones)
  - Migration abnormalities: Lissencephaly ↔ pachygyria ↔ polymicrogyria ↔ schizencephalic clefting
  - White matter (WM) abnormality: Delayed myelination, dysmyelination
  - Cerebral, cerebellar atrophy
  - Periventricular cysts (particularly temporal), ventriculomegaly, ventricular adhesions, lenticulostriate vasculopathy
- Gestational age at time of infection determines pattern of CNS injury
  - Prior to 18 weeks → reduction in neurons and glia, lissencephaly, small cerebellum, ventriculomegaly
  - 18-24 weeks → migration anomalies, cerebellar hypoplasia, schizencephaly
  - 3rd trimester → delayed myelination, dysmyelination, periventricular cysts
  - Perinatal infection → delay in myelin maturation, focal WM injury (astrogliosis)

CT Findings

- NECT
  - Intracranial Ca^{++} (40-70%): Periventricular (subependymal, germinolytic zones)
  - WM volume loss, WM low attenuation, ± periventricular cysts, ventriculomegaly
  - Cortical gyral abnormalities
  - Cerebellar hypoplasia

MR Findings

- T1WI
  - Periventricular subependymal foci of T1 shortening secondary to Ca^{++}
  - Ventricular dilatation and periventricular WM volume loss ± periventricular cysts
  - Cerebellar hypoplasia
- T2WI
  - Migration abnormalities: Lissencephaly, pachygyria, diffuse or focal polymicrogyria, schizencephaly
  - Myelination delay or destruction ± periventricular cysts (often at temporal tip)
  - Focal WM ↑ T2 lesions (gliosis/demyelination) predominantly in parietal deep WM
  - Hippocampal dysplasia (vertical orientation)
- FLAIR
  - Focal, patchy, or confluent regions of ↑ signal due to gliosis ± periventricular hypointense cysts
- T2* GRE
  - Periventricular ↓ signal due to Ca^{++}, SWI shows better
- MRS
  - ↓ NAA:Cr ratio due to loss of neuronal elements, ↑ myoinositol (gliosis)

Ultrasonographic Findings

- Grayscale ultrasound
  - Ring-like regions of periventricular lucency may precede subependymal Ca^{++}
  - Branching basal ganglia and thalamic echoes (**lenticulostriate vasculopathy**)
  - Periventricular cysts and ventricular adhesions
  - Cerebellar hypoplasia

Imaging Recommendations

- Best imaging tool
  - Sonography for prenatal or neonatal screening
  - NECT rarely necessary
  - Brain MR to completely characterize abnormalities
  - Fetal MR can provide similar information as neonatal imaging
- Protocol advice
  - High-resolution neonatal neurosonography
  - NECT or T2* GRE/SWI to detect subtle Ca^{++} or hemorrhage

DIFFERENTIAL DIAGNOSIS

Congenital Lymphocytic Choriomeningitis

- Rodent-borne arenavirus: Carried by feral house mouse and hamster
- Necrotizing ependymitis leading to aqueductal obstruction (macrocephaly in 43%, microcephaly in 13%)
- Appearance on NECT may perfectly mimic CMV

Toxoplasmosis

- Protozoan parasite
  - Maternal risk factors include
    - Exposure to cat excreta during pregnancy
    - Eating raw or undercooked meat
- 1/10 as common as CMV, macrocrania > microcrania, cortical dysplasia less common, random cerebral Ca^{++}

Pseudo-TORCH Syndromes

- Baraitser-Reardon, Aicardi-Goutières (CSF pleocytosis, ↑ CSF α-interferon)
  - Autosomal recessive, progressive cerebral and cerebellar demyelination and degeneration
  - Basal ganglia and brainstem Ca^{++}, periventricular Ca^{++} less common
- Mutations of *OCLN* gene encoding occludin
  - Autosomal recessive microcephaly
  - Polymicrogyria with band of subcortical Ca^{++}

PATHOLOGY

General Features

- Etiology
  - CMV, ubiquitous DNA virus of herpesvirus family

- Neurotropic virus that replicates in ependyma, germinal matrix, capillary endothelium
- Chronic ischemia from placentitis leading to secondary perfusion insufficiency
- Most common cause of intrauterine infection
- Mechanisms of infection
  - Fetal infection
    - Mother with primary infection during pregnancy vs. mother with reactivation of latent infection
  - Neonatal infection
    - Mother infected at delivery, transmission of virus in breast milk, or by blood transfusion

Staging, Grading, & Classification

- Timing of gestational infection determines insult
  - Neuronal formation between 8-20 weeks
  - Neuron migration until 24-26 weeks
  - Astrocyte generation begins near end of neuronal production
  - Maximal size of germinal zones at 26 weeks
  - Oligodendrocytes produced during first 1/2 of 3rd trimester

Gross Pathologic & Surgical Features

- Microcephaly
- Early gestational infection
  - Germinal zone necrosis, diminished number of glia and neurons, WM volume loss

Microscopic Features

- Hallmark of CMV infection: Cytomegaly with viral nuclear and cytoplasmic inclusions
- Patchy and focal cellular necrosis (particularly germinal matrix cells)
- Vascular inflammation and thrombosis, vascular and subependymal dystrophic Ca^{++}

CLINICAL ISSUES

Presentation

- Most common signs/symptoms
  - Most infected newborns appear normal
  - 10% have systemic signs of disease
    - Hepatosplenomegaly, petechiae, chorioretinitis, jaundice, intrauterine growth restriction
  - 55% with systemic disease have CNS involvement
    - Microcephaly, seizures, hypotonia or hypertonia, chorioretinitis, sensorineural hearing loss [(SNHL) in 1/3 to 1/2 symptomatic infants]
- Clinical profile
  - Seronegative women are at greatest risk for vertical transmission
    - But prior maternal infection does not preclude infection in neonate
  - 1-4% of seronegative mothers acquire primary CMV infection during pregnancy
    - Risk of congenital CMV in infant 30-50% in these cases
  - ↑ susceptibility for congenital CMV in HIV-exposed neonates, ± antiretroviral therapy
  - CMV coinfection accentuates residual burden of in utero HIV transmission, even with antiretroviral therapy
- Methods of diagnosis
  - Shell vial assay for CMV (urine)
  - Late diagnosis with PCR for CMV-DNA from neonatal Guthrie card
  - Elevated CSF β-2 microglobulin levels, microcephaly, neuroimaging findings predictive of outcome

Demographics

- Epidemiology
  - Affects ~ 1% of all newborns (10% of whom have CNS or systemic signs and symptoms)

Natural History & Prognosis

- 3 prognostic groups
  - Newborns with CNS manifestations (microcephaly, periventricular Ca^{++})
    - Up to 95% have major neurodevelopmental sequelae
  - Newborns with only systemic manifestations (hepatosplenomegaly, petechiae, jaundice)
    - Have better prognosis but still significantly affected
  - Infected newborns with neither CNS nor systemic manifestations
    - Best prognosis yet still at risk for developmental delays, motor deficits, and SNHL
  - Overall mortality ~ 5%

Treatment

- Ganciclovir or valacyclovir therapy may benefit infected infants
- Antenatal therapy controversial
- Antenatal antivirals/CMV hyperimmune globulin given in research protocols

DIAGNOSTIC CHECKLIST

Consider

- Congenital CMV in developmentally delayed, microcephalic infant with SNHL

Image Interpretation Pearls

- Congenital CMV encephalitis should be considered when MR shows
  - Microcephaly, migration anomalies, periventricular cysts/Ca^{++}, WM lesions, cerebellar hypoplasia
- When NECT classic for CMV encephalitis but work-up for (S)TORCH infections negative, consider
  - Lymphocytic choriomeningitis and pseudo-TORCH syndromes

SELECTED REFERENCES

1. Kyriakopoulou A et al: Fetal brain imaging provides valuable information in cCMV infected infants. J Matern Fetal Neonatal Med. 36(1):2220564, 2023
2. Chebib E et al: Predictors of cochleovestibular dysfunction in children with congenital cytomegalovirus infection. Eur J Pediatr. 181(8):2909-18, 2022
3. Pesch MH et al: Cytomegalovirus infection in pregnancy: prevention, presentation, management and neonatal outcomes. J Midwifery Womens Health. 66(3):397-402, 2021
4. Pathirana J et al: Prevalence of congenital cytomegalovirus infection and associated risk of in-utero HIV acquisition in a high HIV prevalence setting, South Africa. Clin Infect Dis. 69(10):1789-96, 2019
5. Society for Maternal-Fetal Medicine (SMFM). et al: Diagnosis and antenatal management of congenital cytomegalovirus infection. Am J Obstet Gynecol. 214(6):B5-11, 2016
6. Capretti MG et al: Role of cerebral ultrasound and magnetic resonance imaging in newborns with congenital cytomegalovirus infection. Brain Dev. 36(3):203-11, 2014

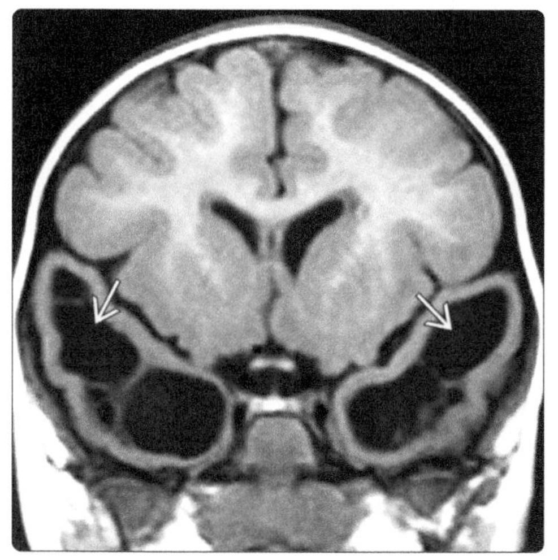

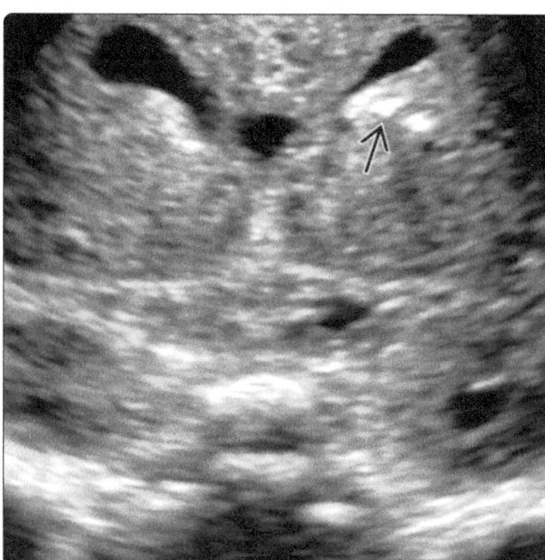

(Left) *Coronal T1WI MR in a microcephalic infant shows numerous periventricular cavitary germinolytic cysts ➡. Detecting these cysts (including anterior temporal lobe) on US, CT, or MR imaging should prompt the consideration of possible congenital CMV infection.* **(Right)** *Coronal cranial ultrasound in congenital CMV shows periventricular foci of echogenicity ➡, consistent with Ca^{++}.*

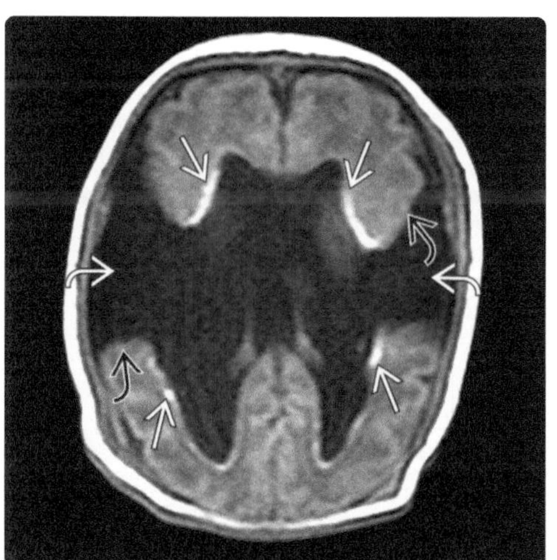

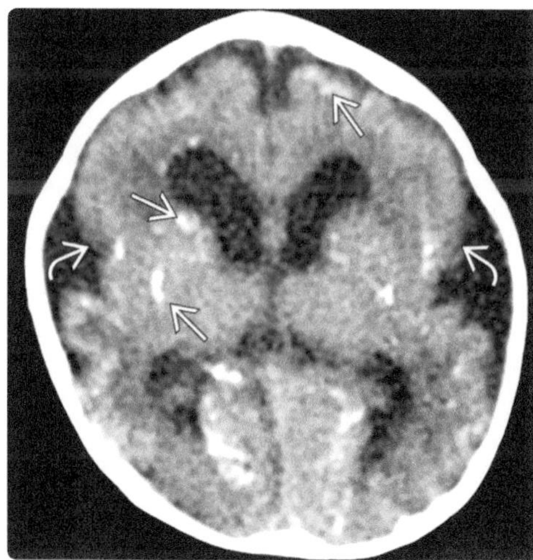

(Left) *Axial T1WI MR in an infant with congenital CMV demonstrates bilateral open lip schizencephaly ➡ lined by gray matter ➡. Note the periventricular T1-hyperintense signal ➡ due to Ca^{++}.* **(Right)** *Axial NECT shows extensive periventricular and parenchymal Ca^{++} ➡. Note the open sylvian fissures and simplified gyral pattern of perisylvian cortex ➡. MR confirmed polymicrogyria.*

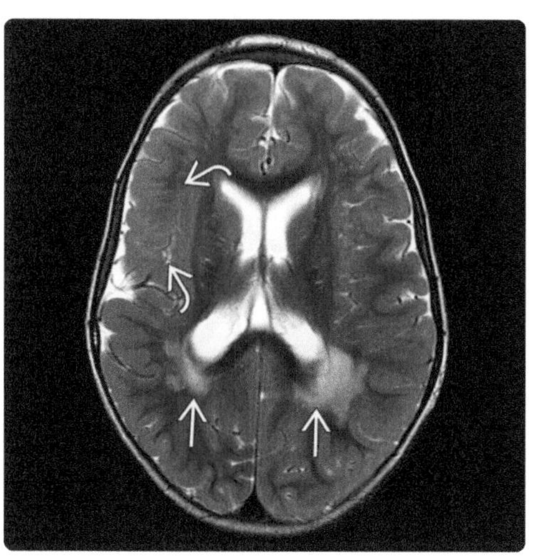

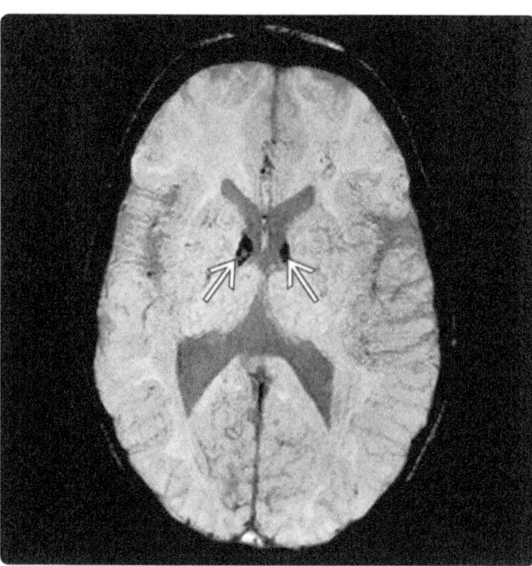

(Left) *Axial T2WI MR in a child with congenital CMV shows an abnormal, thick right perisylvian cortex ➡ (polymicrogyria) and regions of abnormal WM signal ➡ predominantly in the parietal lobes due to gliosis &/or demyelination. Ventricular dilation is secondary to WM volume loss.* **(Right)** *Axial SWI in the same patient shows foci of low signal ➡ in the frontal periventricular region due to subependymal Ca^{++}.*

Congenital HIV

KEY FACTS

TERMINOLOGY

- Congenital AIDS, maternally transmitted AIDS

IMAGING

- Basal ganglia (BG) Ca^{++} (develops months after birth)
- Cerebral atrophy, particularly frontal lobes
- Mineralizing microangiopathy: BG Ca^{++} (30-85%) > frontal white matter (WM) > cerebellum
- Atrophy, ± T1 shortening within BG due to Ca^{++}
- ± high signal in frontal subcortical WM, infarcts
- Fusiform vasculopathy (late)
- Include MRA with baseline NECT/MR

TOP DIFFERENTIAL DIAGNOSES

- CMV: Periventricular Ca^{++}, microcephaly, cortical dysplasia
- Toxoplasmosis: Scattered Ca^{++}, ± hydrocephalus
- Pseudo-TORCH: BG, brainstem, & parenchymal Ca^{++}, neurodegeneration

PATHOLOGY

- HIV in microglial cells & macrophages
- Fibrosing & calcific vasculopathy, aneurysms, strokes, demyelination, ± hemorrhage

CLINICAL ISSUES

- Developmental delay, progressive encephalopathy, ↓ motor milestones, stroke
- Pediatric HIV: HIV cases in USA (2%), worldwide (5-25%); 90% vertically transmitted
- Most acquired at birth, 3rd trimester, or via breastfeeding
- Opportunistic infections less common than in adult HIV

DIAGNOSTIC CHECKLIST

- Consider congenital HIV with bilateral symmetrical BG Ca^{++} in children > 2 months; (not feature of adult HIV)
- Consider congenital HIV when fusiform arteriopathy detected

(Left) *Axial NECT in a patient with congenital HIV shows bilateral symmetrical basal ganglia Ca^{++} ➔, predominantly in the globi pallidi.* **(Right)** *Axial T1WI MR in a patient with congenital HIV shows T1 shortening in the basal ganglia ➔ due to Ca^{++}. Cystic encephalomalacia ➔ due to old infarcts are also noted.*

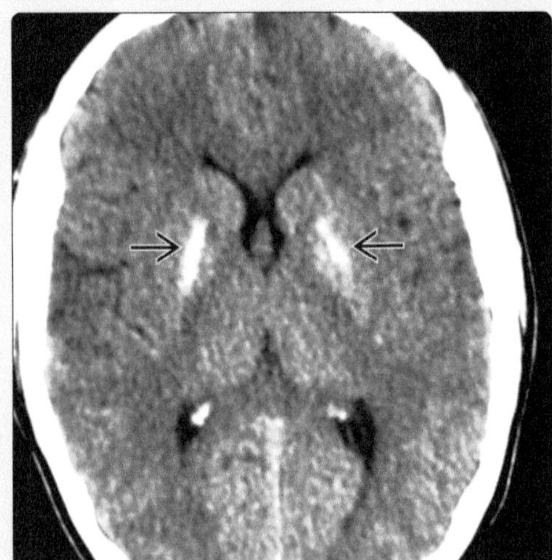

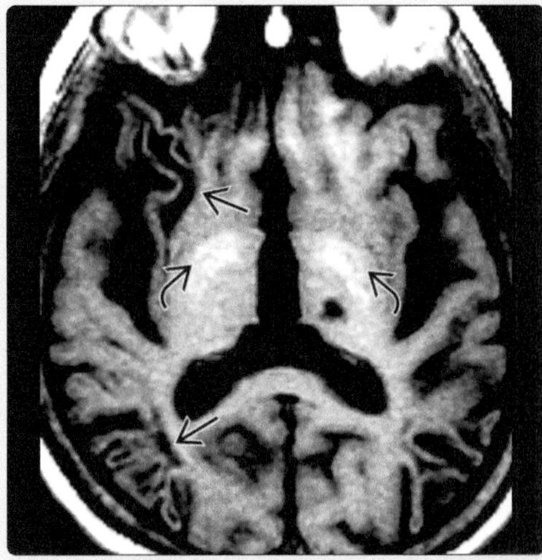

(Left) *Axial 3D TOF MRA without contrast in a 12-year-old boy with a history of previous strokes and congenital HIV infection demonstrates flow-related enhancement within the fusiform, aneurysmally dilated M1 segments of the middle cerebral arteries ➔.* **(Right)** *Axial T2WI MR in a 10-year-old with congenital HIV shows encephalomalacia due to old infarcts in the right frontal ➔ and both parietal lobes ➔. Note diffuse volume loss as well as ill-defined T2 signal change in the deep white matter ➔.*

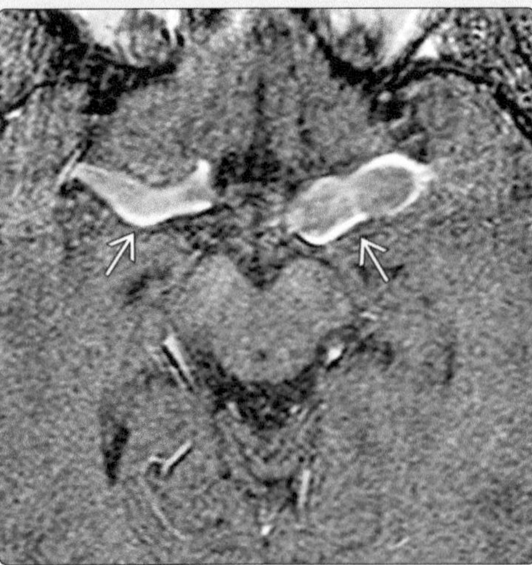

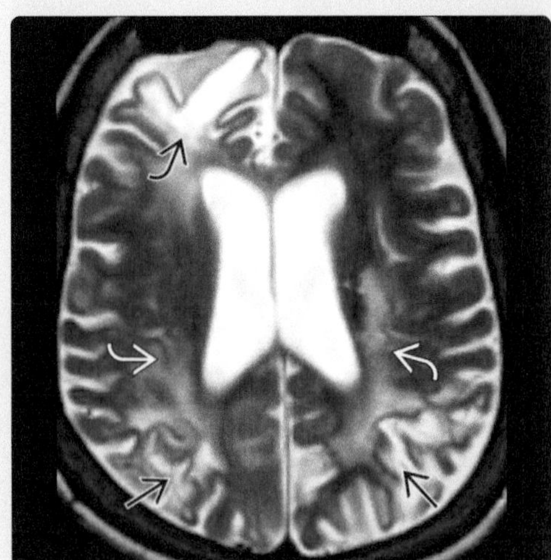

TERMINOLOGY

Definitions

- HIV-1 infection early in utero/late pregnancy, at delivery, or by breastfeeding

IMAGING

General Features

- Best diagnostic clue
  - Basal ganglia (BG) Ca^{++} in congenital HIV (not in adult)
  - Cerebral atrophy; fusiform vasculopathy, stroke, subarachnoid hemorrhage

CT Findings

- NECT
  - Atrophy, particularly frontal lobes
  - Mineralizing microangiopathy (not at birth): BG Ca^{++} (30-85%) > frontal white matter (WM) > cerebellum
- CECT
  - ± faint enhancement of BG prior to appearance of Ca^{++}; hemorrhage
- CTA
  - Ectasia/fusiform dilation of intracranial arteries (3-5%)

MR Findings

- T1WI
  - Atrophy, ± T1 shortening within BG due to Ca^{++}
- T2WI
  - ± high signal in frontal subcortical WM, infarcts
- T2* GRE
  - May accentuate Ca^{++}; detect hemorrhage
- DWI
  - ± restricted diffusion for patients presenting with stroke
- T1WI C+
  - ± faint BG enhancement initially
- MRA
  - Fusiform vasculopathy (late)
- MRS
  - ↓ NAA, ↑ Cho:Cr, presence of excitatory neurotransmitters

Imaging Recommendations

- Best imaging tool
  - NECT
- Protocol advice
  - Include MRA with baseline NECT/MR

DIFFERENTIAL DIAGNOSIS

CMV

- Periventricular Ca^{++}, microcephaly, cortical dysplasia

Toxoplasmosis

- Scattered Ca^{++}, ± hydrocephalus

PATHOLOGY

Gross Pathologic & Surgical Features

- Generalized brain volume loss
- Fibrosing & calcific vasculopathy, aneurysms, strokes, demyelination, ± hemorrhage
- Cerebrovascular disease 25% at autopsy (3-5% on imaging)

Microscopic Features

- HIV in microglial cells & macrophages
- HIV infects vascular endothelial cells → endothelial dysfunction
- Microglial nodules, multinucleated giant cells, Ca^{++} vasculopathy, myelin loss

CLINICAL ISSUES

Presentation

- Most common signs/symptoms
  - Unlike adults, pediatric CNS more vulnerable to HIV, & antiretroviral drugs poorly penetrate CNS
  - HIV encephalopathy due to direct action of virus in CNS → neuronal dysfunction & brain growth impairment
    - Encephalopathy, ↓ motor milestones, microcephaly
  - Later, vasculopathy, stroke, hemorrhage
- Clinical profile
  - Hepatomegaly, lymphadenopathy, pneumonitis, infections, encephalopathy
  - ↑ susceptibility for congenital CMV in HIV-exposed neonates, ± antiretroviral therapy
  - CMV coinfection accentuates residual burden of in utero HIV transmission, even with antiretroviral therapy

Demographics

- Age
  - Symptoms begin after 3rd month of life; some asymptomatic until 10 years
  - Cerebral aneurysmal arteriopathy usually seen at 8-13 years when meeting AIDS criteria
- Epidemiology
  - Pediatric HIV cases in USA (2%), worldwide (5-25%); 90% vertically transmitted

Natural History & Prognosis

- If symptomatic in 1st year of life → 20% die in infancy
- Opportunistic infections less common than in adult HIV
- Rare primary CNS leiomyosarcomas (dural-based intracranial or intraspinal tumors) in immunocompromised adult with history of congenital HIV reported
  - Associated with latent EBV infection

Treatment

- Confirm diagnosis with polymerase chain reaction, HIV blood culture, p24 antigen assay
- HAART ↑ survival
- Early diagnosis of vasculopathy in AIDS very important
  - Treatment could halt disease progression or induce regression, preventing complications
    - HAART, steroids, & neurovascular interventions

DIAGNOSTIC CHECKLIST

Image Interpretation Pearls

- Consider congenital HIV with bilateral symmetrical BG Ca^{++} in children > 2 months
- Consider HIV when fusiform arteriopathy detected

SELECTED REFERENCES

1. Scoco A et al: A curious cervical spine case: multiple, primary CNS leiomyosarcomas presenting with rapid growth in the immunocompromised patient. Spinal Cord Ser Cases. 9(1):35, 2023

Neonatal Herpes Encephalitis

KEY FACTS

TERMINOLOGY

- Neonatal HSV, HSV-2

IMAGING

- Early: Edema, DWI abnormality
- Late: Atrophy, cysts, ventriculomegaly, Ca^{++}
- Variable brain involvement, early DWI abnormality
- Variable: White matter, gray matter (cortical, basal ganglia), temporal lobe, brainstem, cerebellum, ± watershed
  - Unlike HSV encephalitis in adults & older children, infants with HSV have diffuse rather than temporal lobe predilection
- Early: CT normal (27%); variable distribution, low attenuation
- Early: Swelling, T1 hypointensity in affected regions
- Early: T2 hyperintensity (edema, neuronal necrosis), basal ganglia involved in ~ 57%
- Hemorrhage less common than with HSV-1

TOP DIFFERENTIAL DIAGNOSES

- Peripartum &/or postnatal infection
- Stroke/ischemia, arterial or venous
- Vertically transmitted infection, TORCH
  - CMV → microcephaly, Ca^{++}, cortical clefting or malformation
  - Toxoplasmosis → scattered Ca^{++}, hydrocephalus

PATHOLOGY

- Transmission: Peripartum (85%), postnatal (10%), in utero (5%)

CLINICAL ISSUES

- C-section if active maternal infection, intravenous acyclovir

DIAGNOSTIC CHECKLIST

- Suspect HSV-2 in neonates with unexplained DWI abnormality

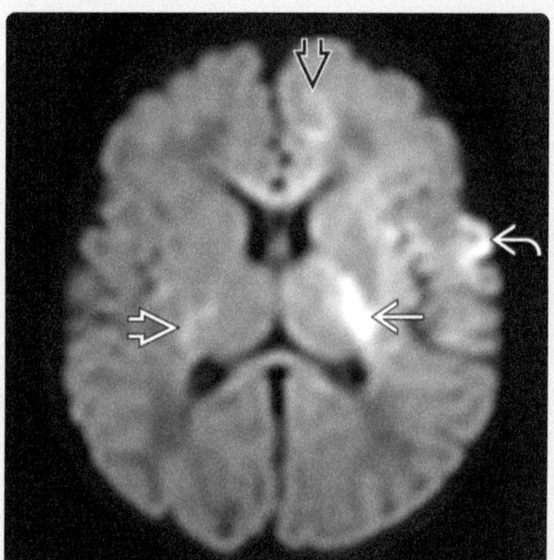

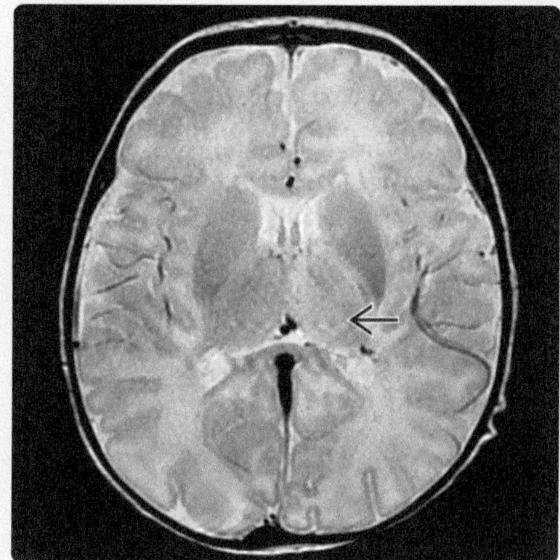

(Left) *Axial DWI MR in a 5-week-old infant with HSV2 infection who presented with seizures demonstrates relatively modest diffusion restriction (confirmed on ADC map, not shown) in the left posterior limb of internal capsule (PLIC), right PLIC, left temporal lobe, and left frontal lobe.* **(Right)** *Axial T2 MR in the same patient shows minimal T2 correlate to the areas of diffusion restriction. However, there is asymmetric T2 hyperintensity within the left thalamus that did not show restriction.*

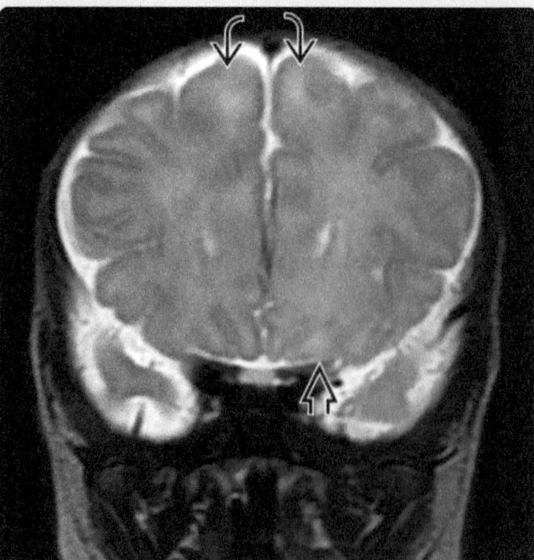

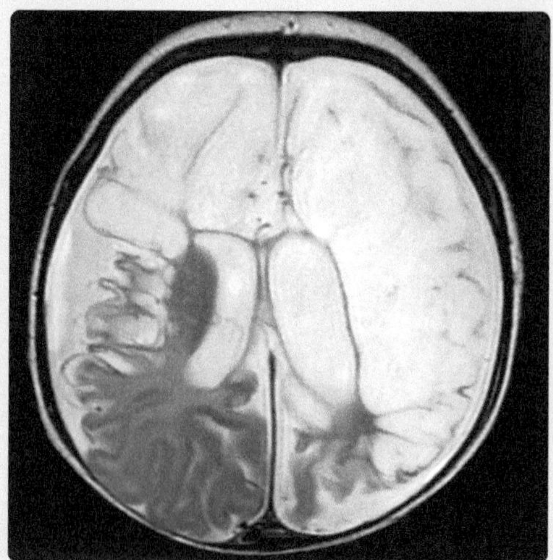

(Left) *Coronal T2 MR in the same patient shows abnormal white matter (WM) T2 hyperintensity in the left inferior frontal lobe with loss of normal gray matter-WM differentiation as well as abnormal T2 hyperintensity in the medial frontal subcortical WM bilaterally. All of these findings are subtle on T2 imaging.* **(Right)** *Axial T2 MR in the same patient at 4 months of age shows devastating extensive cystic encephalomalacia, indicating that brain injury far exceeds what was visible on early MR imaging.*

TERMINOLOGY

Abbreviations

- Neonatal HSV, HSV-2

IMAGING

General Features

- Best diagnostic clue
  - Variable brain involvement, early DWI abnormality
- Location
  - Variable: White matter (WM), gray matter (GM) [cortical, basal ganglia (BG)], temporal lobe, brainstem, cerebellum, ± watershed

CT Findings

- NECT
  - Early: Normal (27%), variable distribution, low attenuation
  - Late: Hydrocephalus, cysts, Ca^{++} (BG, thalami, cortex, or WM)

MR Findings

- T1WI
  - Early: Swelling, T1 hypointensity in affected regions
  - Late: Atrophy, cysts, ventriculomegaly, ± T1 shortening (Ca^{++})
- T2WI
  - Early: T2 hyperintensity (edema, neuronal necrosis), BG involved in ~ 57%
  - Late: Cystic encephalomalacia, atrophy, WM hyperintensity
- T2* GRE
  - Hemorrhage less common than with HSV-1
- DWI
  - Restricted diffusion in affected regions
- T1WI C+
  - Patchy enhancement in affected regions, ± meningeal enhancement
- MRS
  - Acute: ↑ Cho, Glx, glutamine, ± lipid lactate, ↓ NAA
  - Chronic: All metabolites ↓

Ultrasonographic Findings

- Early: Linear echoes in BG
- Late: Multicystic encephalomalacia, ± Ca^{++}

Imaging Recommendations

- Protocol advice
  - NECT, MR

DIFFERENTIAL DIAGNOSIS

Peripartum &/or Postnatal Infection

- Other bacterial and viral infections can mimic neonatal HSV

Stroke/Ischemia

- Arterial or venous infarction

Vertically Transmitted Infection, TORCH

- CMV → microcephaly, Ca^{++}, cortical clefting or malformation
- Toxoplasmosis → scattered Ca^{++}, hydrocephalus

PATHOLOGY

General Features

- Etiology
  - Transmission: Peripartum (85%), postnatal (10%), in utero (5%)

Staging, Grading, & Classification

- HSV infection acquired in intrauterine, peripartum, or postnatal period is classified into following types
  - Intrauterine infection
  - Disseminated disease
  - CNS disease

Gross Pathologic & Surgical Features

- Early: Meningoencephalitis, necrosis, ± hemorrhage, microglial proliferation
- Late: Atrophy, cysts, Ca^{++}, ± hydranencephaly

CLINICAL ISSUES

Presentation

- Most common signs/symptoms
  - Postnatal: Lethargy, apnea, poor feeding, ± seizures, bulging fontanelle
  - In utero: Low birth weight, microcephaly, microphthalmia, ± mucous membrane ulceration
- Clinical profile
  - CSF: Pleocytosis (mononuclear cells), ↑ protein
  - EEG: Nonspecific

Demographics

- Age
  - Onset for peripartum infection → 2-4 weeks
- Epidemiology
  - Uncommon, estimated 1 in 3,200 deliveries

Natural History & Prognosis

- Death in ~ 3 % of neonates with CNS disease and 29% with disseminated disease
- Survivors → cerebral palsy, seizures, intellectual disabilities

Treatment

- C-section if active maternal infection, intravenous acyclovir

DIAGNOSTIC CHECKLIST

Consider

- HSV-2 in neonates with unexplained MR diffusion abnormalities

Image Interpretation Pearls

- Postnatal: Varied distribution, + DWI, ± hemorrhage
- In utero: Atrophy, scattered brain Ca^{++}, cystic encephalomalacia, ventriculomegaly

SELECTED REFERENCES

1. D'Aiuto L et al: The impaired neurodevelopment of human neural rosettes in HSV-1-infected early brain organoids. Cells. 11(22), 2022
2. Qiao H et al: Herpes simplex virus type 1 infection leads to neurodevelopmental disorder-associated neuropathological changes. PLoS Pathog. 16(10):e1008899, 2020
3. Bajaj M et al: Clinical and neuroimaging findings in neonatal herpes simplex virus infection. J Pediatr. 165(2):404-7.e1, 2014

Parechovirus Encephalitis

KEY FACTS

TERMINOLOGY

- Neonatal meningoencephalitis caused by HPeV-3

IMAGING

- MR is best imaging modality
  - Acute phase
    - DWI: Restricted diffusion in white matter (WM) ± thalami
    - T1: Often normal; ± perimedullary ↑ signal
    - T2: Often normal; ± perimedullary ↓ signal
    - T1 C+: Typically no contrast enhancement
    - MRS: ± ↑ lactate, ↓ NAA, ↑ choline in affected areas
  - Chronic phase
    - T2/FLAIR: ↑ signal with volume loss
- US often abnormal
  - ↑ echogenicity within WM in acute phase

TOP DIFFERENTIAL DIAGNOSES

- Enterovirus, rotavirus, & chikungunya viral encephalitides
- Perinatal hypoxic-ischemic injury
- Metabolic brain disease
- WM injury of prematurity (acute)
- Periventricular leukomalacia (chronic)

PATHOLOGY

- Pathophysiology not well understood
- Diagnosis made by PCR of CSF & blood

CLINICAL ISSUES

- Median age: 23 days (range: 7-72 days)
- Supportive treatment
- Severity of imaging abnormalities correlates with neurodevelopmental outcomes

DIAGNOSTIC CHECKLIST

- DWI most sensitive sequence
  - Other sequences may be normal or only subtly abnormal
- Age at onset is one important discriminator of DDx
  - Symptom onset usually ≥ 7 days after birth

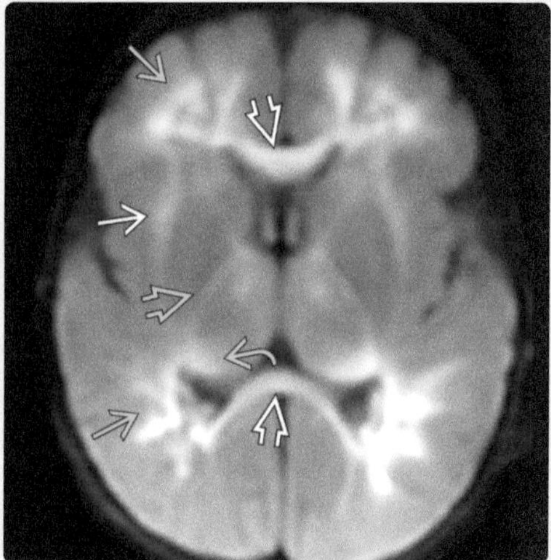

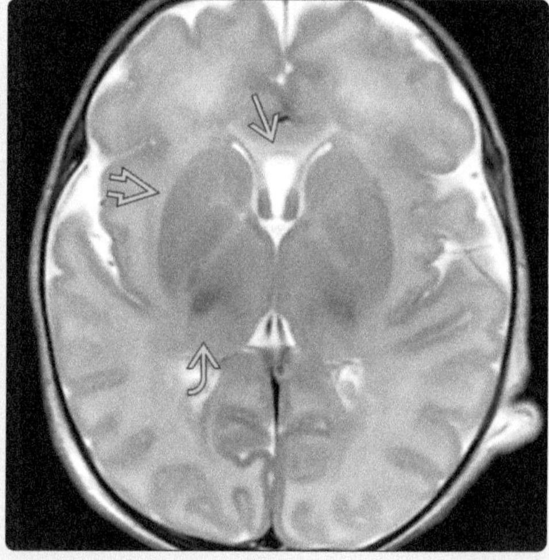

(Left) *Axial DWI MR in a 14-day-old with seizures shows symmetric diffusion restriction in the bilateral periventricular and deep white matter, internal capsules, external capsules, corpus callosum (CC), and thalami. Note the preservation of the basal ganglia.* **(Right)** *Axial T2 MR in the same patient is nearly normal. Careful review and comparison to the DWI shows subtle increased signal in the anterior genu of CC, external capsule, and posterior thalami. This case emphasizes the critical importance of DWI.*

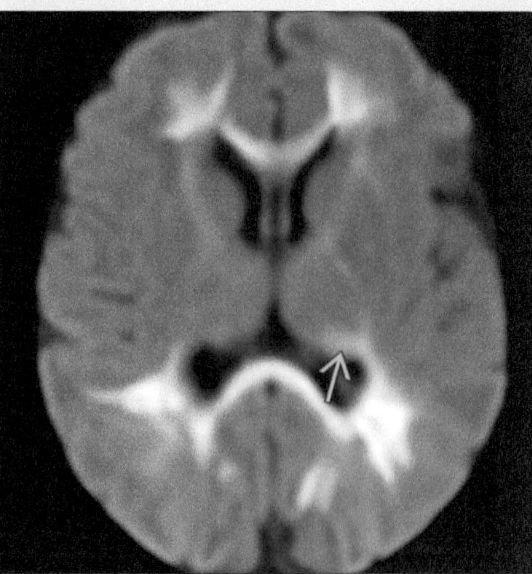

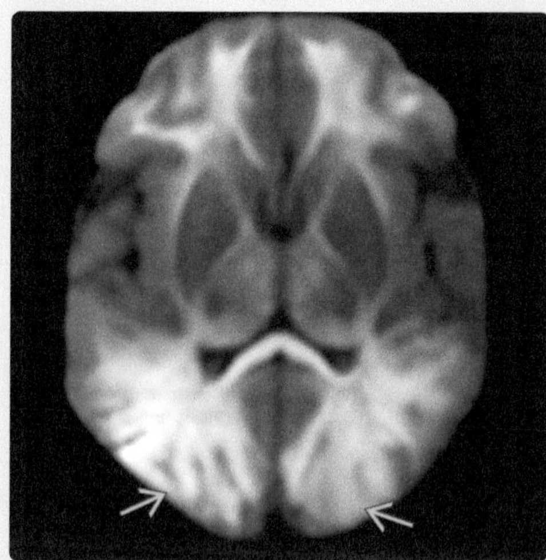

(Left) *Axial DWI MR in a 28-day-old with apnea and concern for meningitis shows a typical distribution of diffusion restriction involving white matter and, to a lesser degree, the left thalamus.* **(Right)** *Axial DWI MR in a 16-day-old with seizures shows a more severe distribution of diffusion restriction involving nearly all the white matter and thalami. In the most severely affected areas (e.g., occipital lobes), there is extension to the cortex. Again, note preservation of the basal ganglia.*

TERMINOLOGY

Definitions

- Human parechovirus (HPeV) is family of viruses closely related to enteroviruses
- Human parechovirus type 3 (HPeV-3) is emerging pathogen increasingly recognized as cause of neonatal meningoencephalitis

IMAGING

General Features

- Best diagnostic clue
  - Symmetric diffusion restriction within bilateral supratentorial white matter (WM) ± thalami
- Location
  - Supratentorial WM
    - Common: Centrum semiovale & corpus callosum
    - Less common: Internal/external capsule
  - ± thalamus
- Morphology
  - Often linear, flare-shaped signal abnormality & diffusion restriction along perimedullary vein distribution

CT Findings

- Difficult to detect on CT in neonates given already low attenuation of unmyelinated WM

MR Findings

- T1WI
  - Often normal or only subtly abnormal
  - ± scattered ↑ WM signal in perimedullary distribution in acute phase
  - ↓ signal in areas of leukomalacia in chronic phase
- T2WI
  - Often normal or only subtly abnormal
  - ± scattered ↓ WM signal in perimedullary distribution in acute phase
  - ↑ signal in areas of leukomalacia in chronic phase
- FLAIR
  - ↑ signal in areas of leukomalacia in chronic phase
- T2* GRE
  - Associated hemorrhage not reported
- DWI
  - Most important sequence
  - Diffusion restriction (usually symmetric) in supratentorial WM
    - Diffusion restriction in thalami also common
- T1WI C+
  - Usually normal
- MRS
  - ± ↑ lactate, ↓ NAA, ↑ choline in affected areas

Ultrasonographic Findings

- Variable ↑ echogenicity within WM

Imaging Recommendations

- Best imaging tool
  - MR with DWI

DIFFERENTIAL DIAGNOSIS

Other Viral Encephalitides

- Enterovirus, rotavirus, & chikungunya infection

Perinatal Hypoxic-Ischemic Injury

- Cortical involvement much more common
- Basal ganglia involvement in acute profound pattern
- Usually presents with symptoms at birth

White Matter Injury of Prematurity

- Occurs in premature infant
- Often involves clinically salient event

Metabolic Brain Disease

- Isolated sulfite oxide & molybdenum cofactor deficiencies
  - Basal ganglia & cortical involvement common

Periventricular Leukomalacia

- Difficult to distinguish chronic periventricular leukomalacia from HPeV

PATHOLOGY

General Features

- Pathophysiology poorly understood; 2 proposed theories
  - Intraneuronal viral growth & injury
  - Perivenular invasion &/or venous ischemia
- Diagnosis typically made by PCR testing of CSF & blood

CLINICAL ISSUES

Presentation

- Most common signs/symptoms
  - Fever, seizures, irritability, rash, apnea
- Other signs/symptoms
  - Poor feeding, diarrhea, lethargy, mottling

Demographics

- Median age: 23 days (range: 7-72 days)

Natural History & Prognosis

- Severity of imaging abnormalities correlates with neurodevelopmental outcomes, e.g., cerebral palsy

Treatment

- Supportive treatment
- No current antiviral therapy

DIAGNOSTIC CHECKLIST

Consider

- HPeV in weeks-old patient with WM injury

Image Interpretation Pearls

- DWI is most sensitive sequence

SELECTED REFERENCES

1. Alali M et al: Human parechovirus encephalitis in infants: a retrospective single-center study (2017-2022). Eur J Pediatr. 182(10):4457-65, 2023
2. Tierradentro-García LO et al: Neuroimaging findings in parechovirus encephalitis: a case series of pediatric patients. Pediatr Neurol. 130:41-5, 2022
3. Sarma A et al: Human parechovirus meningoencephalitis: neuroimaging in the era of polymerase chain reaction-based testing. AJNR Am J Neuroradiol. 40(8):1418-21, 2019

Group B Streptococcal Meningitis

KEY FACTS

TERMINOLOGY

- Group B β-hemolytic streptococcal (GBS) meningitis
- Leading newborn meningitis cause in developed countries

IMAGING

- Acute: Meningitis, cerebritis, vasculitis, ventriculitis, subdural effusion, empyema, arterial and venous infarction
- Arterial distributions often affected; variable dural, leptomeningeal, and parenchymal enhancement
- Ventriculitis: Ependymal enhancement, ventricular debris
- Missing neonatal T2 cortical ribbon (encephalitis or infarcts)
- Blurring/loss of gray matter-white matter junction → ± basal ganglia, thalamic, white matter hyperintensities
- ↑ FLAIR in cortex, subarachnoid space, and subdural, cisternal, and ventricular spaces
- Diffusion restriction within infarcts and empyema
- Rim enhancement with subdural effusion (thinner) and empyema (thicker)
- Arterial stenosis/occlusions; venous thrombosis

TOP DIFFERENTIAL DIAGNOSES

- Enteric, gram-negative meningitis
- *Escherichia coli*: Along with GBS meningitis, major cause of newborn meningitis in developed countries
- *Listeria monocytogenes*: Gram-positive rod
- *Enterobacter*: Most common cause of meningitis in 1st few months of life

PATHOLOGY

- Debris, exudates within subarachnoid spaces and ventricles
- Brain infarct/encephalomalacia; vasculitis &/or vasospasm

CLINICAL ISSUES

- Newborn with sepsis; typical signs/symptoms of meningitis subtle in neonate

DIAGNOSTIC CHECKLIST

- No imaging features distinguish GBS meningitis from other neonatal meningitides
- Do MR with IV contrast, DWI, MRA, and postcontrast MRV

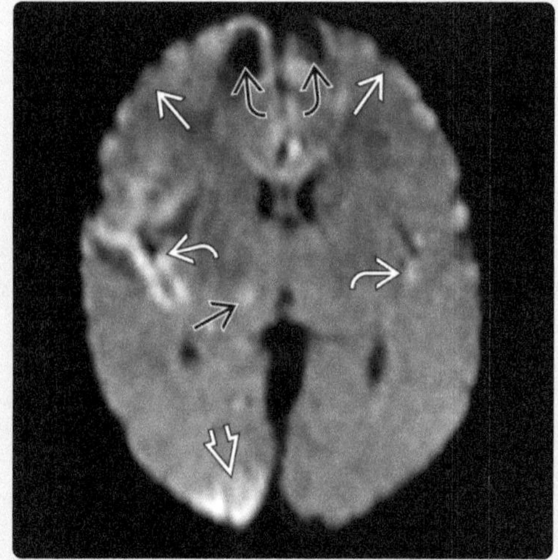

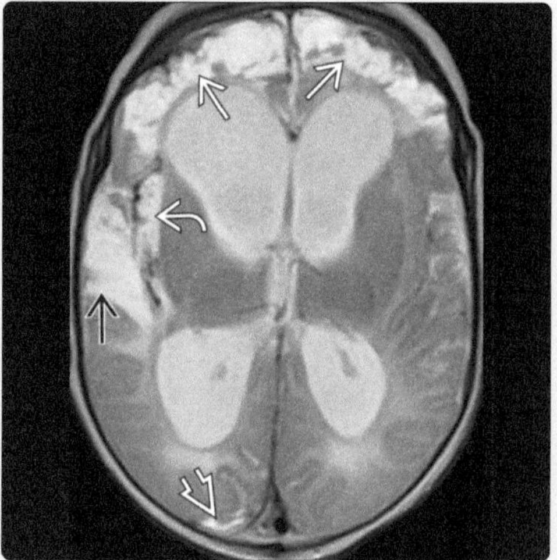

(Left) *Axial DWI MR in a 35-day-old infant with group B Streptococcal (GBS) meningoencephalitis shows bifrontal ➡, insular ➡, occipital ➡ cortical and right thalamic ➡ diffusion restricting encephalitis. Bifrontal hypointensities ➡ were blood products on SWI (not shown).* **(Right)** *Axial T2WI MR in the same patient at 55 days of age shows bifrontal ➡, right temporal ➡, insular ➡, and tiny focal right occipital ➡ cortical cystic encephalomalacia with volume loss and dilated ventricles.*

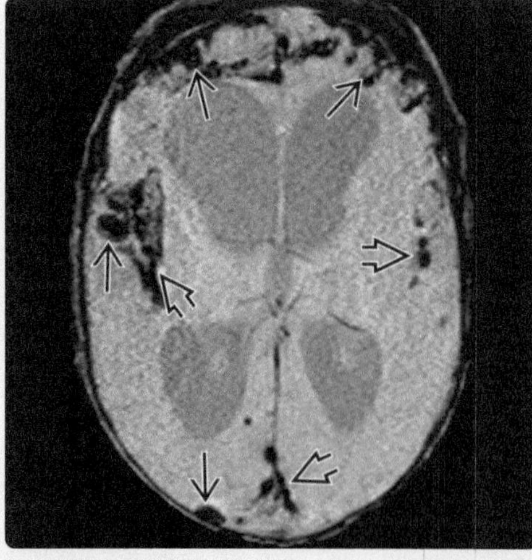

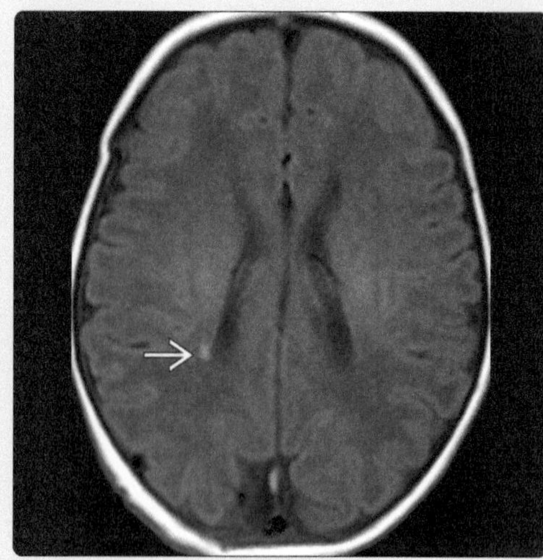

(Left) *Axial SWI MR at 55 days of age shows scattered, blooming, hypointense blood in cortical encephalomalacia ➡ and extraaxial spaces ➡.* **(Right)** *Axial T1WI MR in a 9-day-old infant with GBS meningoencephalitis shows a solitary tiny speck ➡ of right periventricular white matter (WM) T1 hyperintensity (prominently seen within unmyelinated T1-hypointense WM). This speck was hypointense on T2WI and diffusion restricting on DWI/ADC, suggesting periventricular WM injury due to ischemia.*

Group B Streptococcal Meningitis

TERMINOLOGY

Abbreviations

- Group B streptococcal (GBS) meningitis

Synonyms

- Group B β-hemolytic streptococcal meningitis

Definitions

- Leading cause of newborn meningitis in developed countries
  - Early-onset disease (EOD): GBS sepsis presenting in 1st week of life; 80% of GBS infections EOD
    - Meningitis complicates in 10%
  - Late-onset disease (LOD): GBS sepsis presenting between 1-4 weeks of life; 20% GBS infections LOD
    - Meningitis complicates in 40-60%

IMAGING

General Features

- Best diagnostic clue
  - Meningoencephalitis in newborn
- Location
  - Leptomeninges, cerebral hemispheres, and deep gray matter (GM)
- Morphology
  - Multifocal involvement
  - Arterial distributions often affected, particularly basal ganglia (BG) and thalami
- Acute: Meningitis, cerebritis, vasculitis, ventriculitis, subdural effusion, empyema, arterial and venous infarction
  - Occasional spinal cord involvement
- Chronic sequelae: Loculated hydrocephalus, cystic encephalomalacia

CT Findings

- NECT
  - Hydrocephalus ± dependent debris in ventricles
  - Hypodensities in arterial distributions, BG, thalami, white matter (WM)
  - Occasional hyperdense foci = hemorrhagic venous infarcts, laminar necrosis
  - Hypodense subdural collections (effusion vs. empyema)
- CECT
  - Variable: Dural, leptomeningeal, and parenchymal enhancement
    - Rim enhancement around subdural effusions and empyemas
  - Ependymal enhancement/ventricular debris

MR Findings

- T1WI
  - Hypo- and hyperintense foci common
    - Multifocal hypointensities = edema, ischemia, infarction
    - Hyperintense foci cortex, BG, and WM = laminar necrosis, hemorrhagic venous infarction
- T2WI
  - Blurring/loss of GM-WM junction, ± BG, thalamic, and WM hyperintensity
  - Focal cortical ↑ T2 in encephalitis (or infarcts) continuous with neonatal normally ↑ T2 subcortical WM looks like focally "missing cortical ribbon"
- FLAIR
  - Hyperintensity in cortex and subarachnoid, subdural, cisternal, and ventricular spaces
- T2* GRE
  - Blooming of hemorrhagic foci in brain or extraaxial spaces
  - SWI better demonstrates blood products
- DWI
  - Diffusion restriction in infarcts, pus collections
    - Extremely rare for abscess and empyema to have no restricted diffusion
  - Patterns of ischemic injury
    - Multiple punctuate infarcts in BG
    - Focal or diffuse cerebral infarcts
    - Focal periventricular or subcortical WM infarcts
- T1WI C+
  - Variable: Dural, leptomeningeal, parenchymal, and ependymal enhancement
  - Rim enhancement with subdural effusion (thinner) and empyema (thicker)
  - Postcontrast FLAIR better demonstrates abnormal meningeal enhancement
- MRA
  - Arterial narrowing (vasculitis &/or vasospasm) ± occlusions
- MRV
  - Dural venous sinus/cortical vein thrombosis (in up to 30%)
- MRS
  - ↑ choline, ↓ NAA; ↑ lactate in areas of ischemia/infarction

Ultrasonographic Findings

- Grayscale ultrasound
  - ↑ echogenicity of sulci and parenchyma → hydrocephalus → ventricular debris

Imaging Recommendations

- Best imaging tool
  - MR with IV contrast, DWI, MRA, and MRV
- Protocol advice
  - CECT for rapid initial assessment of hemodynamically unstable neonate

DIFFERENTIAL DIAGNOSIS

Other Neonatal Meningitides

- Enteric, gram-negative meningitis
  - Account for majority of early-onset meningitis in developing countries
  - Higher mortality than GBS meningitis
  - Specific pathogens
    - *Escherichia coli*: Major cause of newborn meningitis in developed countries (along with GBS meningitis)
    - *Enterobacter*: Most common cause of meningitis in 1st few months of life
    - *Citrobacter*: Rare; high morbidity/mortality secondary to frequent abscess (square morphology) formation
- Other meningitides

- *Listeria monocytogenes*: Gram-positive rod

Congenital Infections (TORCH)

- CMV, toxoplasmosis, rubella: Infection occurs in utero with chronic sequelae present in neonate/infant
  - CMV: Periventricular Ca^{++}, microcephaly, migrational abnormalities, encephalomalacia, cerebellar hypoplasia
  - Toxoplasmosis: Parenchymal Ca^{++}, encephalomalacia, microphthalmia
- HSV-2: Infection acquired during vaginal birth; presents in first 2-4 weeks of life
  - Meningoencephalitis with extensive edema, necrosis, late cystic encephalomalacia

Hypoxic-Ischemic Encephalopathy

- Preterm: Injury to periventricular WM (mild) or thalami, BG, brainstem (severe)
- Term: Injury to mature vascular watershed (mild) or areas of early myelination/metabolic activity (severe)

PATHOLOGY

General Features

- Etiology
  - EOD: Aspiration of infected amniotic fluid or birth canal secretions
  - LOD: Postnatal maternal contact, breast milk, nosocomial
  - Bacteremia facilitated by immature neonatal immune system
  - Development of meningitis related to magnitude/duration of bacteremia
  - Production of β-hemolysin facilitates access of GBS across blood-brain barrier
- GBS agalactiae serotype 3 responsible for majority of GBS meningitis
- GBS potent activator of neonatal immune/inflammatory response

Gross Pathologic & Surgical Features

- Debris, exudates within subarachnoid spaces and ventricles
- Parenchymal infarction/encephalomalacia; luminal narrowing of vessels

Microscopic Features

- Inflammation of adventitia and vaso vasorum = vasculitis

CLINICAL ISSUES

Presentation

- Most common signs/symptoms
  - Lethargy, poor feeding, irritability
  - Seizures (40%) and bulging fontanelle typically late findings
- Clinical profile
  - Newborn with sepsis
  - Typical signs/symptoms of meningitis subtle or absent in neonate
- CSF analysis: ↑ WBCs, ↑ protein, ↓ glucose
- CSF/blood Gram stain: Gram-positive diplococci
- Maternal risk factors for EOD
  - GBS colonization, GBS chorioamnionitis/bacteruria
  - Membrane rupture > 18 hours; intrapartum fever ≥ 38°C
  - Previous newborn with EOD; delivery at < 37 weeks

Demographics

- Age
  - 90% of newborns with GBS EOD present within first 24 hours of life
  - GBS LOD presents between 1-4 weeks after birth; occasionally up to 6 months
- Sex
  - Male, preterm infants (< 37 weeks) most at risk for EOD
- Ethnicity
  - Maternal GBS colonization rates highest in Black women
- Epidemiology
  - 10-30% of pregnant women have asymptomatic GBS colonization of genital/gastrointestinal tract
    - EOD in < 1% of newborns born to colonized women
  - EOD incidence: 0.5/1,000 live births
    - Incidence ↓ by > 50% as result of maternal screening and intrapartum chemoprophylaxis
    - ↓ incidence of GBS EOD accompanied by ↑ incidence of neonatal gram-negative sepsis
    - Term infants account for 50% of GBS EOD secondary to preterm intrapartum chemoprophylaxis

Natural History & Prognosis

- Prognosis
  - Mortality of EOD: Full-term newborns (2%), 34-36-weeks gestation (10%), < 33-weeks gestation (30%)
  - Morbidity of meningitis: Neurologic sequelae (12-30%) (cortical blindness, spasticity, global intellectual disability)
  - Preterm neonatal LOD significantly ↑ risk of cerebellar hemorrhage and lower motor scores by 3 years of age

Treatment

- Maternal
  - GBS screen: Rectovaginal swab at 35-37 weeks gestation
  - Positive maternal GBS screen or presence of other risk factors: Intrapartum IV penicillin
  - Future strategies
    - GBS PCR assay and rapid *Streptococcus* screen at onset of labor
    - GBS vaccine: Ideal prevention strategy; would prevent development of antibiotic-resistant pathogens
- Neonatal meningitis
  - High-dose IV penicillin → ± antiepileptics → CSF diversion may be required for complicated hydrocephalus

DIAGNOSTIC CHECKLIST

Image Interpretation Pearls

- No imaging features distinguish GBS meningitis from other neonatal meningitides

SELECTED REFERENCES

1. Mynarek M et al: Mortality and neurodevelopmental outcome after invasive group B streptococcal infection in infants. Dev Med Child Neurol. 66(1):125-33, 2023
2. Procter SR et al: Maternal immunisation against group B streptococcus: a global analysis of health impact and cost-effectiveness. PLoS Med. 20(3):e1004068, 2023
3. Kartam M et al: Late-onset sepsis in preterm neonates is associated with higher risks of cerebellar hemorrhage and lower motor scores at three years of age. Oman Med J. 37(2):e368, 2022

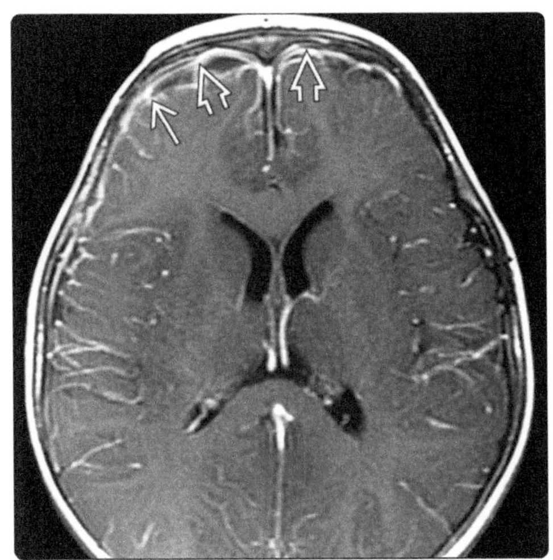

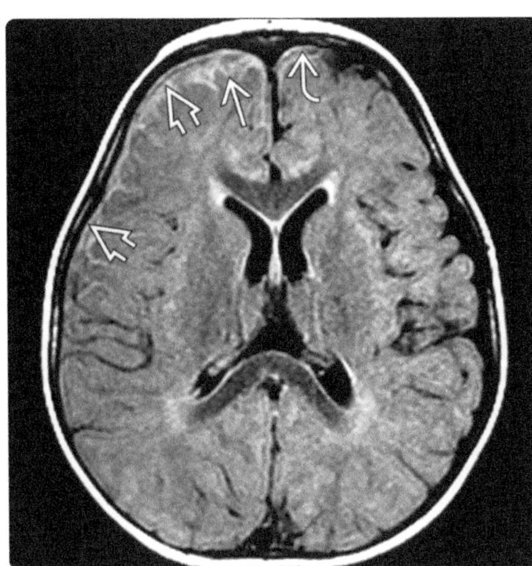

(Left) *Axial T1WI C+ MR in an infant with GBS meningitis shows cortical ➔ and leptomeningeal ➔ enhancement. CSF Gram stain showed gram-positive diplococci.* **(Right)** *Axial FLAIR MR shows hyperintensity in the right frontal cortex ➔ and within the right convexity subarachnoid spaces ➔. Note the early involvement of the left frontal subarachnoid space ➔. FLAIR MR is a sensitive tool to detect early complicated extraaxial fluid collections and FLAIR C+ for meningeal enhancement.*

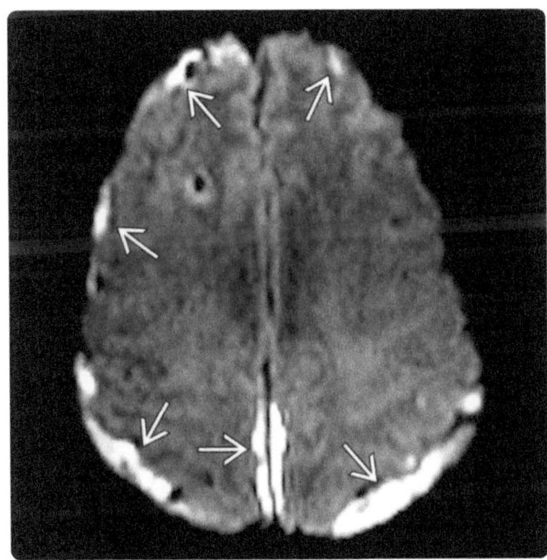

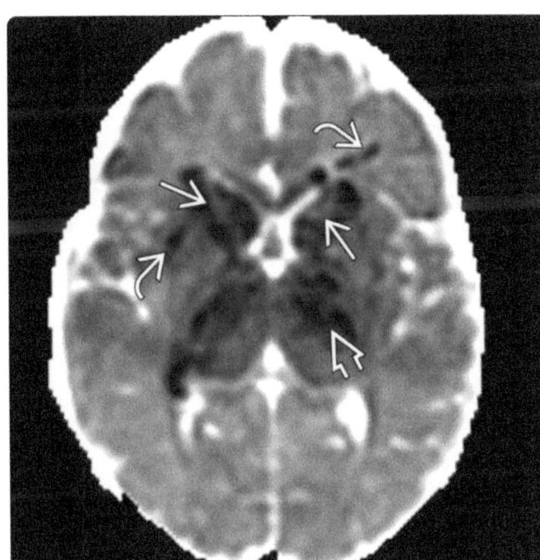

(Left) *Axial DWI MR in a patient with GBS meningitis shows restricted diffusion ➔ in the subdural collections, consistent with empyemas. DWI helps to differentiate reactive subdural effusions (facilitated diffusion) from empyemas (restricted diffusion).* **(Right)** *Axial ADC with GBS meningoencephalitis shows multiple basal ganglia ➔ and thalamic ➔ infarctions. Note the scattered WM infarctions ➔.*

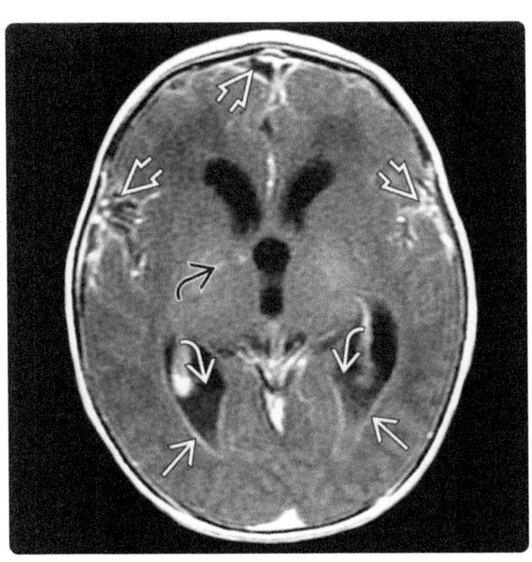

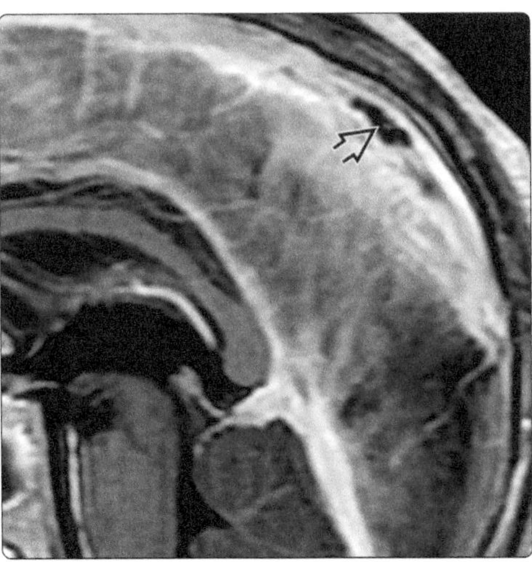

(Left) *Axial T1WI C+ MR shows extensive leptomeningeal enhancement ➔. Note the ventricular ependymal enhancement ➔, dependent ventricular debris ➔ (ventriculitis), and basal ganglia enhancement ➔ due to perivascular space inflammation/arteritis. Ventricular dilation reflects early hydrocephalus.* **(Right)** *Sagittal MRV with contrast shows a hypointense clot ➔ within the sagittal sinus, creating a partial occlusion. Small clots were also detected in the transverse sinuses.*

KEY FACTS

TERMINOLOGY

- *Citrobacter* species meningitis & encephalitis

IMAGING

- Multiple large & small cystic white matter (WM) lesions
- Predilection for lobar WM
- ± diffuse **pneumocephalus** (due to gas production)
- **Square (or polygonal) morphology** of abscesses
- "Rounding" of edges suggests increased pressure/active infection
- **Rim or dot**-like **septal** enhancement
- **Diffusion restriction** of **dependent** infected **debris**
- Subdural empyema &/or ventriculitis occasionally

TOP DIFFERENTIAL DIAGNOSES

- *Cronobacter sakazakii* has similar imaging
- Other bacterial brain infections
- Periventricular WM injury
- Cystic encephalomalacia
- WM lacerations in nonaccidental head injury

PATHOLOGY

- Infection acquired: Horizontally (nosocomial) or vertically (maternal)
- Colonization (skin, umbilicus stump) → bacteremia → meningitis

CLINICAL ISSUES

- Immunocompromised patients at higher risk
  - Sick preterms & some neonates
- Preterm newborns most susceptible
- 5% of neonatal (gram-negative) meningitis → **80% of neonatal brain abscesses**
- Abscesses may only appear near completion of therapy
- 80% of *Citrobacter* meningitis neonates develop abscesses

DIAGNOSTIC CHECKLIST

- Square or polygonal WM abscesses with rim or dot-like septal enhancement, often multiple

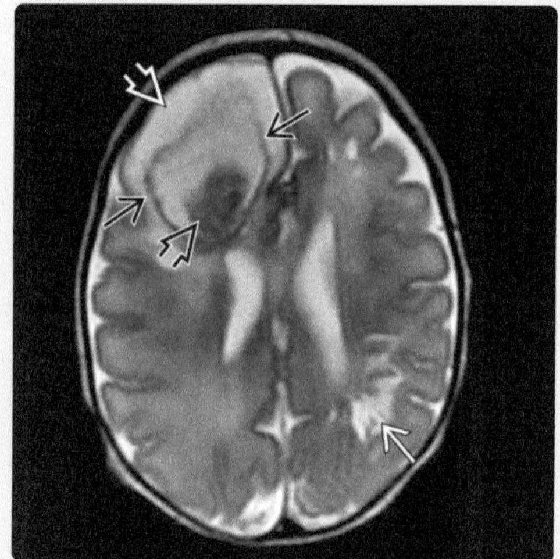

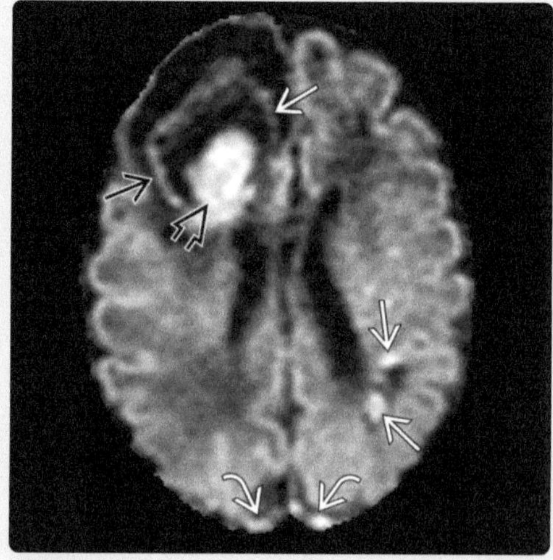

(Left) *Axial T2WI MR shows a large polygonal, almost square-shaped Citrobacter abscess in the right frontal white matter (WM). Note the T2 iso- to hypointensity of abscess wall ➡ & dependent debris ➡. Mild surrounding WM edema is seen ➡. Also note the smaller left parietal WM abscess ➡.* **(Right)** *Axial DWI MR in the same patient shows diffusion restriction of large right frontal abscess wall ➡ & dependent debris ➡ & in the small left parietal WM abscess ➡. Note bilateral diffusion restricting posterior subdural empyema ➡.*

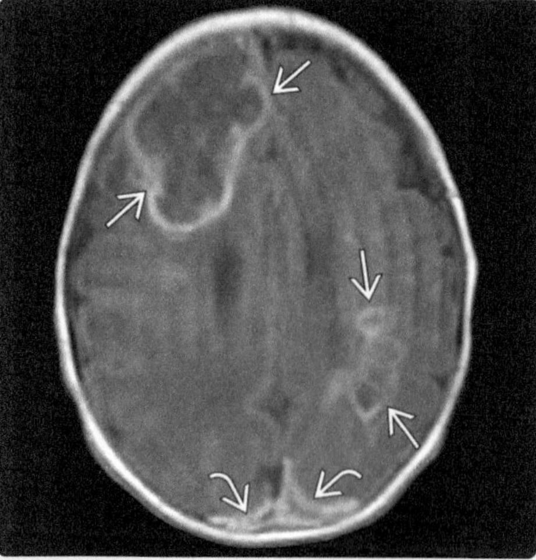

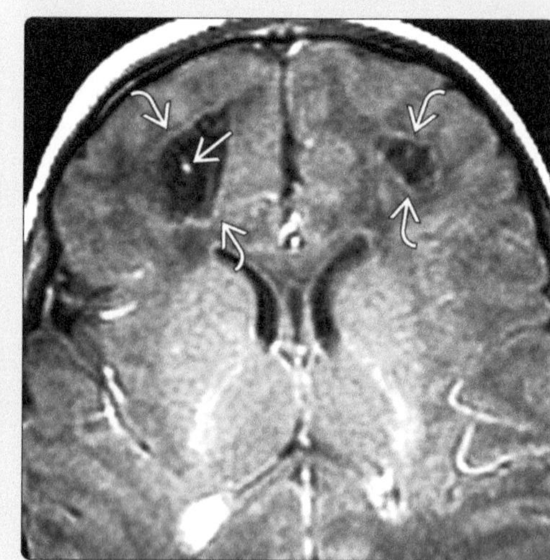

(Left) *Axial T1WI C+ MR shows ring enhancement of the bilateral abscess cavity walls ➡. Also note the peripheral enhancement surrounding the bilateral posterior parietooccipital subdural empyema ➡. (Courtesy T. J. E. Muttikkal, MD.)* **(Right)** *Axial T1WI C+ MR shows bilateral frontal lobe WM liquefying cavitary abscesses in a patient diagnosed with Citrobacter meningitis with faint ring enhancement ➡ and focal dot-like septal enhancement ➡ on the right side.*

TERMINOLOGY

Synonyms

- *Citrobacter* cerebritis

Definitions

- Gram-negative enteric bacterium infection

IMAGING

General Features

- Best diagnostic clue
  - **Multiple** large & small cystic white matter (WM) lesions
  - **Square (or polygonal)-shaped abscesses** from complete replacement of WM; border parallels cortex
    - Increasing mass effect/edema more likely to have infected contents
    - **"Rounding" of edges** suggests increased pressure/active infection
- Location
  - Predilection for lobar WM
  - Occasionally subdural empyema &/or ventriculitis
- Size
  - Multiple large WM cysts
- Morphology
  - Square or polygonal-shaped abscesses

CT Findings

- NECT
  - Early (cerebritis)
    - Patchy, multilobar WM lesions
    - Low attenuation compared to unmyelinated brain
    - ± diffuse **pneumocephalus** (due to gas production)
  - Late (abscess)
    - Lobar WM cavities with septations
    - Square or polygonal morphology of abscesses
    - Dot-like focus of septal Ca^{++}
- CECT
  - Early (cerebritis)
    - Variable, often subtle parenchymal enhancement
  - Late (abscess)
    - Rim or **dot-like septal enhancement**
    - Multiple large cavities (± septations) replace WM

MR Findings

- T1WI
  - Early (cerebritis)
    - Patchy, multilobar areas of T1 hypointensity
  - Late (abscess)
    - Multiple large cysts
    - Square morphology
    - Septations
    - T1 WM signal abnormality diminishes
- T2WI
  - Early (cerebritis)
    - Patchy, multilobar T2 hyperintensity
  - Late (abscess)
    - Multiple, often septated cavities
    - Usually bilateral, variably sized
    - T2 hyperintensity within WM
    - Variable edema, mass effect
    - Eventually, cavities may contract, causing profound WM loss
    - **T2 iso- to hypointensity** of abscess **wall** & **dependent debris**
- FLAIR
  - Increased signal within lobar WM
- T2* GRE
  - Dot-like Ca^{++} within septal walls shows diminished signal
- DWI
  - **Diffusion restriction** usually within **dependent** infected **debris**
  - Faint diffusion restriction of abscess wall may be seen
- T1WI C+
  - Early (cerebritis)
    - Subtle, patchy WM enhancement
  - Late (abscess)
    - Patchy WM enhancement
    - Rim or septal wall enhancement
    - Dot-like focus of septal enhancement
- MRS
  - Products of fermentation
    - Lactate (1.3 ppm), acetate (1.9 ppm), and succinate (2.4 ppm)
  - Proteolysis end products released from neutrophils
    - Valine and leucine (0.9 ppm)

Ultrasonographic Findings

- Grayscale ultrasound
  - Early (meningitis/cerebritis)
    - Sulcal thickening and increased sulcal echogenicity
    - Regions of WM hyperechogenicity
    - Loss of normal WM echo architecture
  - Late (abscess)
    - Multiple septated WM, anechoic or hypoechoic cavities
- Color Doppler
  - Subtle flow within abscess septal walls

Imaging Recommendations

- Best imaging tool
  - MR with contrast best depicts location and severity of involvement
- Protocol advice
  - MR with contrast
    - Shows early parenchymal enhancement of cerebritis
    - Reveals dot-like foci of septal enhancement of "squared" or polygonal abscesses
    - Detects complications of brain infection (vascular, extraaxial purulent collections)

DIFFERENTIAL DIAGNOSIS

Cronobacter sakazakii

- Opportunistic pathogen in powdered infant formula
- Can have similar imaging pattern of *Citrobacter*

Other Bacterial Brain Infections

- Usually with greater surrounding edema and mass effect
- Search for possible sinus, mastoid, or embolic/hematogenous sources of infection

Periventricular Leukomalacia

- Perifrontal and peritrigonal locations of WM cysts
- Slower progression of cystic change
- No rim or septal dot-like enhancement

Cystic Encephalomalacia

- Cortical and deep gray matter involved
- Cysts replace WM
- Passive ex-vacuo ventricular dilation

White Matter Lacerations in Nonaccidental Head Injury

- Frontal lobe WM
- Fluid level may be seen dependently within laceration
- Associated intracranial manifestations of nonaccidental head injury
  - Parafalcine/convexity subdural hematoma, subarachnoid hemorrhage

PATHOLOGY

General Features

- Etiology
  - Neurovirulence factors of *Citrobacter* species
    - Unique 32-kD outer membrane protein
    - Resistance to phagocytosis
  - *Citrobacter* invades (by transcytosis) microvascular endothelial cells
    - Leads to hemorrhagic necrosis and abscess
  - Intracellular replication of *Citrobacter* in microvascular endothelial cells
    - Contributes to persistence of brain infection and cavitation
- Associated abnormalities
  - Infection acquired: Horizontally (nosocomial) or vertically (maternal)
  - Colonization (skin, umbilicus stump) → bacteremia → meningitis
  - *Citrobacter* facultative anaerobe
    - Hydrolyzes urea and ferments glucose → produces gas

Gross Pathologic & Surgical Features

- Opaque leptomeninges, purulent exudate
- Diffuse ependymitis

Microscopic Features

- No well-formed fibrotic capsule
- Organisms in walls of congested vessels
- Neutrophils plus necrotic cell debris

CLINICAL ISSUES

Presentation

- Most common signs/symptoms
  - Septic newborn or preterm infant: Bulging fontanelle, apnea, seizures
- Clinical profile
  - In very premature neonates
    - Sepsis, irritability, poor feeding, bulging fontanelle
  - Immunocompromised patients at higher risk
    - Sick preterms and some neonates may be immunocompromised

Demographics

- Age
  - Predilection for very young, very old patients
    - Newborns → sepsis, meningitis, and cerebral abscesses
    - Older adults → urinary, upper respiratory tract infections
  - Mean age of sepsis onset: 5 days
  - Preterm newborns most susceptible
  - Citrobacter CNS infection beyond 1 month of age rare
- Epidemiology
  - *Citrobacter* infection
    - 5% of neonatal (gram-negative) meningitis → 80% of neonatal brain abscesses
    - Abscesses may only appear near completion of therapy
  - *Citrobacter* CNS infection
    - Most cases considered sporadic ↔ neonatal ICU outbreaks do occur

Natural History & Prognosis

- 30% of neonates & infants with *Citrobacter* CNS infection die
- 80% of neonates with *Citrobacter* meningitis develop brain abscesses
- 50% of *Citrobacter* meningitis/abscess survivors have significant CNS damage

Treatment

- Antibiotics mainstay of therapy
- Late abscesses occur; prolonged IV therapy as rule
- Adjunctive surgical drainage of abscesses
  - For enlarging cysts on optimized IV therapy
  - Poorly responsive to initial antibiotic therapy

DIAGNOSTIC CHECKLIST

Image Interpretation Pearls

- Minimal edema surrounding abscesses
- Square or polygonal abscesses with focal septal enhancement
- All rim-enhancing cavities not abscesses
  - Some represent WM necrosis and liquefaction
- *Citrobacter* species and *Cronobacter sakazakii* have similar imaging features

SELECTED REFERENCES

1. Yang M et al: Cronobacter brain abscess and refractory epilepsy in a newborn: role of epilepsy surgery. Illustrative case. J Neurosurg Case Lessons. 5(25), 2023
2. Chen D et al: New insights into Citrobacter freundii sepsis in neonates. Pediatr Int. 61(4):375-80, 2019
3. Lechowicz M et al: Multiple brain abscesses caused by Citrobacter koseri in a preterm neonate - case Report. Pol J Radiol. 82:837-41, 2017
4. Nuñez Cuadros E et al: Medical and neurosurgical management of Citrobacter koseri, a rare cause of neonatal meningitis. J Med Microbiol. 63(Pt 1):144-7, 2014
5. Plakkal N et al: Citrobacter freundii brain abscess in a preterm infant: a case report and literature review. Pediatr Neonatol. 54(2):137-40, 2013
6. Vaz Marecos C et al: Sepsis, meningitis and cerebral abscesses caused by Citrobacter koseri. BMJ Case Rep. 2012, 2012

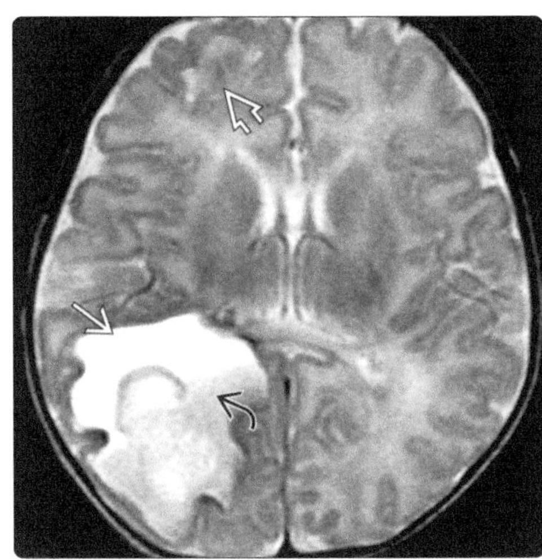

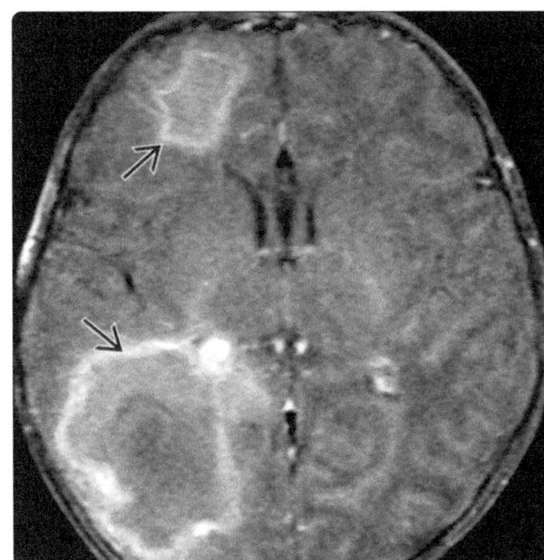

(Left) *Axial T2WI MR in a 1-month-old with neonatal Citrobacter sepsis demonstrates a large, cavitary right parietooccipital abscess ➔ with dependent debris ➔. Note the developing small right frontal lobe abscess ➔, which is just starting to cavitate. (Courtesy L. Lowe, MD.)* **(Right)** *Rim enhancement ➔ of a more mature parietooccipital and less mature frontal abscess is seen. Progression from meningitis to cerebritis to abscess is common (~ 80%). (Courtesy L. Lowe, MD.)*

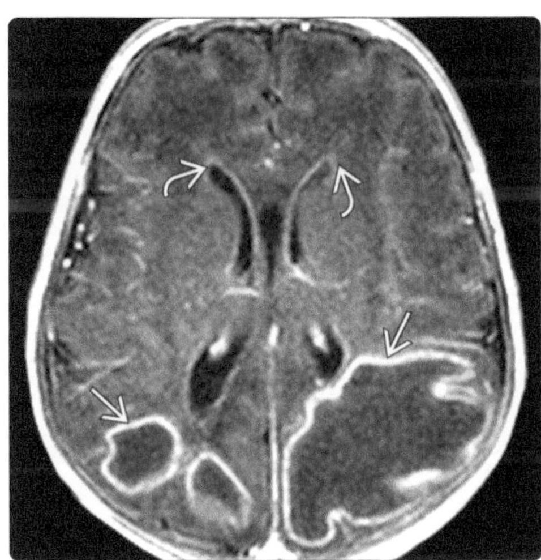

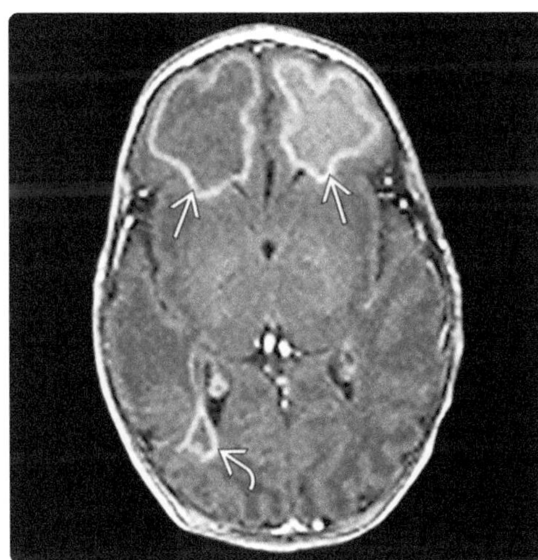

(Left) *Axial T1WI C+ MR in an infant with "treated" Citrobacter meningitis demonstrates large, bilateral, parietooccipital rim-enhancing abscesses ➔. Note the associated ependymal thickening and enhancement reflecting ventriculitis ➔. (Courtesy T. Booth, MD.)* **(Right)** *In this newborn with "treated" Citrobacter meningitis, bilateral frontal ➔ and right peritrigonal ➔ rim-enhancing abscesses are seen. Long-term IV therapy is the rule in such cases. (Courtesy T. Feygin, MD.)*

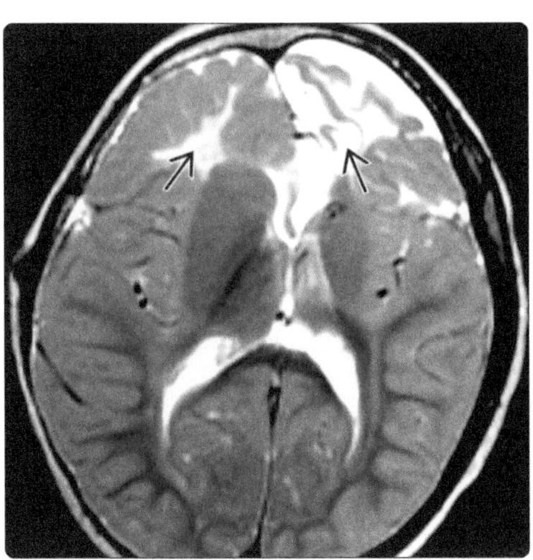

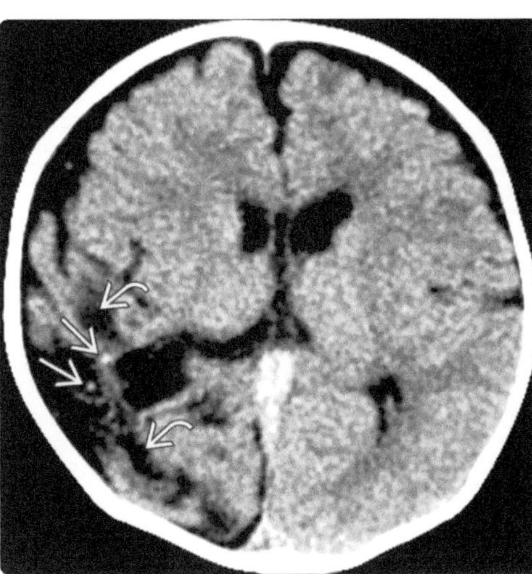

(Left) *Axial T2WI MR in a 1-year-old with refractory seizures remote from long-term IV therapy for Citrobacter brain abscesses shows bilateral frontal retraction cavities, gliosis, and atrophy ➔. (Courtesy C. Glasier, MD.)* **(Right)** *Axial NECT in another patient previously treated for Citrobacter brain abscesses demonstrates retraction of cavities ➔ with tiny residual "dot" of calcifications ➔ and significant local brain volume loss.*

Abscess, Brain

KEY FACTS

TERMINOLOGY

- Focal pyogenic infection of brain parenchyma, typically bacterial; fungal or parasitic less common
- 4 pathologic stages: Early cerebritis, late cerebritis, early capsule, and late capsule

IMAGING

- Ring-enhancing lesion with T2-hypointense rim and central diffusion restriction characteristic
- Imaging varies with stage of abscess development
- Findings with contrast enhancement
  - Early cerebritis: Patchy enhancement
  - Late cerebritis: Intense, irregular rim enhancement
  - Early capsule: Well-defined, thin-walled, enhancing rim
  - Late capsule: Cavity collapses, capsule thickens
- MRS: Central necrotic area may show presence of amino acids (0.9 ppm), lactate (1.3 ppm), acetate (1.9 ppm), succinate (2.4 ppm)

TOP DIFFERENTIAL DIAGNOSES

- Glioblastoma
- Parenchymal metastases
- Demyelinating disease
- Resolving intracerebral hematoma
- Subacute cerebral infarction

CLINICAL ISSUES

- Headache (up to 90%); may have seizures, altered mental status, focal deficits, nausea, vomiting
- Potentially fatal but treatable lesion

DIAGNOSTIC CHECKLIST

- DWI, MRS helpful to distinguish abscess from mimics
- T2-hypointense rim with surrounding edema suggests correct diagnosis
- Search for local cause (sinusitis, otitis media, mastoiditis)

(Left) *Axial graphic shows early cerebritis, the initial phase of abscess formation, in the right frontal lobe. There is a focal, unencapsulated mass of petechial hemorrhage, inflammatory cells, and edema.* **(Right)** *Axial T1 C+ MR in a patient with headache, fever, and altered sensorium shows an ill-defined, hypointense lesion ➙ with patchy peripheral enhancement, imaging findings compatible with early cerebritis.*

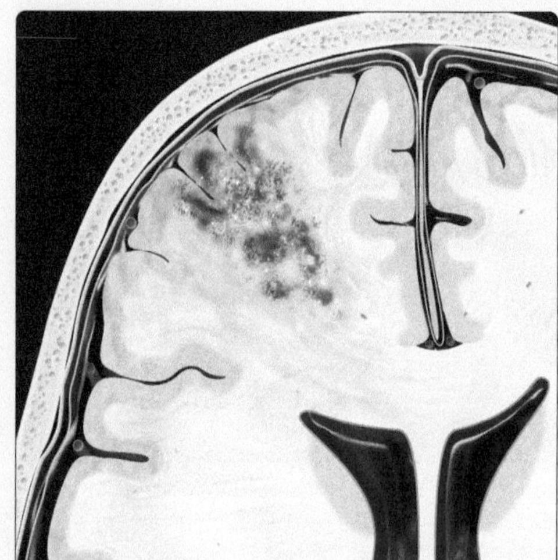

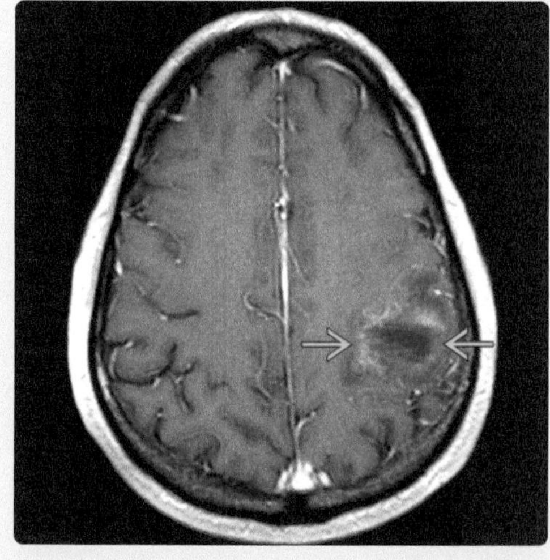

(Left) *Axial graphic shows the early capsule formation of an abscess with central liquified necrosis and inflammatory debris. Collagen and reticulin form the well-defined abscess wall. Note the surrounding edema in the frontal lobe.* **(Right)** *Axial T1 C+ MR demonstrates a large frontal lobe ring-enhancing abscess ➙ with a central necrotic core ➡ and surrounding edema ➚.*

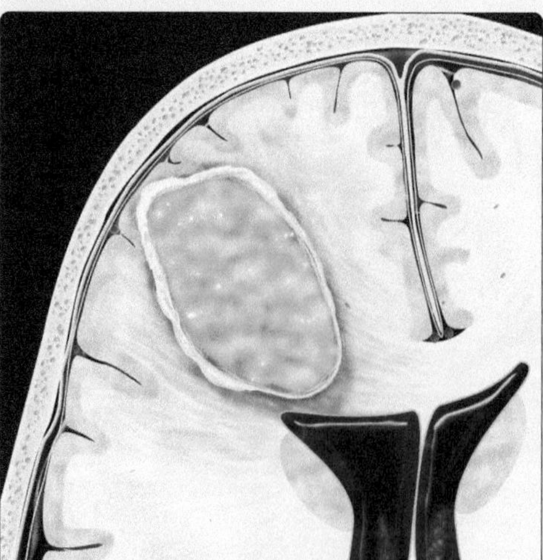

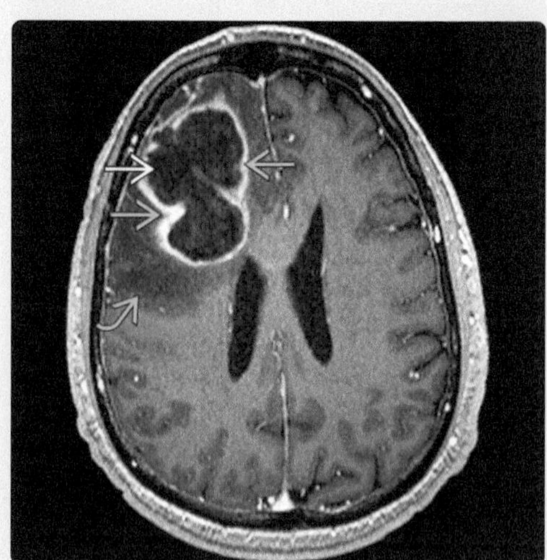

TERMINOLOGY

Definitions

- Localized infection of brain parenchyma, typically bacterial; fungal or parasitic less common
- 4 pathologic stages: Early cerebritis, late cerebritis, early capsule, and late capsule

IMAGING

General Features

- Best diagnostic clue
  - Imaging varies with stage of abscess development
  - Early capsule: Well-defined, thin-walled, enhancing rim
    - Ring-enhancing lesion: DWI high signal, low ADC
    - T2-hypointense rim with surrounding edema
- Location
  - Typically supratentorial; up to 14% infratentorial
  - Frontal lobe (sinusitis, odontogenic infection), temporal lobe (otomastoiditis)
  - Usually at gray matter-white matter junction (hematogenous)
  - Multiple lesions may represent septic emboli
- Size
  - 5 mm up to several cm
- Morphology
  - Thin-walled, well-delineated, ring-enhancing, cystic-appearing mass

CT Findings

- NECT
  - Early cerebritis: Ill-defined, hypodense subcortical lesion with mass effect; CT may be normal early
  - Late cerebritis: Central low-density area; peripheral edema, increased mass effect
  - Early capsule: Hypodense mass with moderate vasogenic edema and mass effect
  - Late capsule: Edema, mass effect diminish
  - Gas-containing abscess rare
- CECT
  - Early cerebritis: ± mild, patchy enhancement
  - Late cerebritis: Irregular rim enhancement
  - Early capsule: Low-density center with thin, distinct, enhancing rim
    - Medial or ventricular wall of capsule thinnest; thickest near cortex
  - Late capsule: Cavity shrinks, capsule thickens
    - May have "daughter" abscesses

MR Findings

- T1WI
  - Early cerebritis: Poorly marginated, mixed hypo-/isointense mass
  - Late cerebritis: Hypointense center, iso-/mildly hyperintense rim
  - Early capsule: Rim iso-/hyperintense to white matter; center hyperintense to CSF
  - Late capsule: Cavity shrinks, capsule thickens
- T2WI
  - Early cerebritis: Ill-defined, hyperintense mass
  - Late cerebritis: Hyperintense center, hypointense rim; hyperintense edema
  - Early capsule: Hypointense rim (due to collagen, hemorrhage, or paramagnetic free radicals)
  - Late capsule: Edema and mass effect diminish
- T2* GRE
  - Dual rim sign on SWI (hypointense outside, hyperintense inside) helpful in distinguishing from other ring-enhancing lesions
- DWI
  - Increased signal intensity in cerebritis and abscess
  - ADC map: Markedly decreased signal (low ADC) centrally within abscess
  - Elevated fractional anisotropy (FA) within abscess cavity
- T1WI C+
  - Early cerebritis: Patchy enhancement
  - Late cerebritis: Intense, irregular rim enhancement
  - Early capsule: Well-defined, thin-walled enhancing rim
  - Late capsule: Cavity collapses, capsule thickens
    - Capsule thinnest on ventricular side
- MRS
  - Central necrotic area may show presence of amino acids (0.9 ppm), lactate (1.3 ppm), acetate (1.9 ppm), succinate (2.4 ppm)
- PWI: Abscess capsule shows lower rCBV values than rims of enhancing tumors
- Resolving abscess: T2-hypointense rim resolves, central ADC increases, enhancement resolves last
  - Small ring/punctate enhancing focus may persist for months

Nuclear Medicine Findings

- PET: FDG and carbon-11-methionine show increased uptake in brain abscess

Imaging Recommendations

- Best imaging tool
  - Contrast-enhanced MR
- Protocol advice
  - Multiplanar MR ± contrast, DWI, ± MRS, PWI

DIFFERENTIAL DIAGNOSIS

Glioblastoma

- Thick, nodular > thin wall
- Low signal on DWI (rarely high, mimics abscess)
- Hemorrhage common
- Other cystic primary neoplasms can also mimic abscess

Parenchymal Metastases

- Thick-walled, centrally necrotic mass; often multiple; marked edema
- May be solitary ring-enhancing lesion
- DWI may be positive and mimic abscess

Demyelinating Disease

- Multiple sclerosis, acute disseminated encephalomyelitis (ADEM)
- Ring enhancement often incomplete ("horseshoe")
- Characteristic lesions elsewhere in brain
- Mass effect small for size of lesion

Resolving Intracerebral Hematoma

- History of trauma or vascular lesion
- Blood products present on MR

Subacute Cerebral Infarction

- History of stroke, vascular distribution
- Gyriform > > ring enhancement (rare)

PATHOLOGY

General Features

- Etiology
  - Hematogenous from extracranial location (pulmonary infection, endocarditis, urinary tract infections)
  - Direct extension from calvarial or meningeal infection
    - Paranasal sinus, middle ear, teeth infections (via valveless emissary veins)
  - Postoperative
  - Penetrating trauma (bone fragments > metal)
  - Right-to-left shunts (congenital cardiac malformations, pulmonary arteriovenous fistulas)
  - Neonatal: 2/3 associated with meningitis
    - "Square abscess" associated with *Citrobacter* meningitis
  - 20-30% have no identifiable source (cryptogenic)
    - Often polymicrobial (streptococci, staphylococci, anaerobes)

Gross Pathologic & Surgical Features

- Early cerebritis (3-5 days)
  - Infection focal but not localized
  - Unencapsulated mass of PMNs, edema, scattered foci of necrosis, petechial hemorrhage
- Late cerebritis (4-5 days to 2 weeks)
  - Necrotic foci coalesce
  - Rim of inflammatory cells, macrophages, granulation tissue, and fibroblasts surrounds central necrotic core
  - Vascular proliferation, surrounding vasogenic edema
- Early capsule (begins at ~ 2 weeks)
  - Well-delineated, collagenous capsule
  - Liquified necrotic core, peripheral gliosis
- Late capsule (weeks to months)
  - Central cavity shrinks; thick wall (collagen, granulation tissue, macrophages, gliosis)

Microscopic Features

- Early cerebritis: Hyperemic tissue with PMNs, necrotic blood vessels, microorganisms
- Late cerebritis: Progressive necrosis, inflammatory cells, fibroblasts deposit early reticulin matrix around periphery
- Early capsule: Granulation tissue proliferation around necrotic core
- Late capsule: Multiple layers of collagen and fibroblasts

CLINICAL ISSUES

Presentation

- Most common signs/symptoms
  - Headache (up to 90%); may have seizures, altered mental status, focal deficits, nausea, vomiting
  - Fever in only 50%
- Other signs/symptoms
  - Increased ESR (75%), elevated WBC count (50%), absence of leukocytosis does not exclude diagnosis

Demographics

- Age
  - Most common in 3rd, 4th decades; 25% in patients < 15
- Sex
  - M:F = 2:1
- Epidemiology
  - Uncommon; ~ 2,500 cases per year in USA
  - Bacterial: *Staphylococcus, Streptococcus, Pneumococcus*
  - Diabetic: *Klebsiella pneumoniae*
  - Posttransplant: *Nocardia, Aspergillus, Candida*
  - AIDS: *Toxoplasmosis, Mycobacterium tuberculosis*
  - Neonates: *Citrobacter, Proteus, Pseudomonas, Serratia, Staphylococcus aureus* (meningitis related)

Natural History & Prognosis

- Potentially fatal but treatable lesion
  - Stereotactic surgery + medical therapy have greatly reduced mortality
- Complications of inadequately or untreated abscesses
  - Meningitis, "daughter" lesions, mass effect, herniation
  - Intraventricular rupture, ventriculitis
    - Ventricular debris with irregular fluid level
    - Hydrocephalus and ependymal enhancement
- Factors affecting prognosis: Size, location, virulence of infecting organism(s), and immune status
- Variable mortality: 0-30%
- Epilepsy: Common complication in pediatric patients

Treatment

- Primary therapy: Surgical drainage favored over excision
- If < 2.5 cm or early-phase cerebritis, antibiotics only
- Steroids to treat edema and mass effect
- Lumbar puncture hazardous if findings of increased intracranial pressure; pathogen often cannot be determined from CSF unless related to meningitis

DIAGNOSTIC CHECKLIST

Consider

- DWI, MRS helpful to distinguish abscess from mimics
- Dual rim sign on SWI (hypo- outside, hyperintense inside) helpful in distinguishing from other ring-enhancing lesions

Image Interpretation Pearls

- Search for local cause (sinusitis, otitis media, mastoiditis)
- T2-hypointense abscess rim resolves before enhancement in successfully treated patients

SELECTED REFERENCES

1. Patel J et al: Is contrast-enhanced computed tomography redundant for suspected intracranial infection in the emergency setting? J Comput Assist Tomogr. 47(1):102-7, 2023
2. Lannon M et al: Surgical aspiration versus excision for intraparenchymal abscess: a systematic review and Meta-analysis. Br J Neurosurg. 36(6):743-9, 2022
3. Rollán-Martínez Herrera M et al: Central nervous system infection by Bacillus cereus: a case report and literature review. Rev Neurol. 75(8):239-45, 2022
4. Brouwer MC et al: Epidemiology, diagnosis, and treatment of brain abscesses. Curr Opin Infect Dis. 30(1):129-34, 2017
5. Rath TJ et al: Imaging of cerebritis, encephalitis, and brain abscess. Neuroimaging Clin N Am. 22(4):585-607, 2012

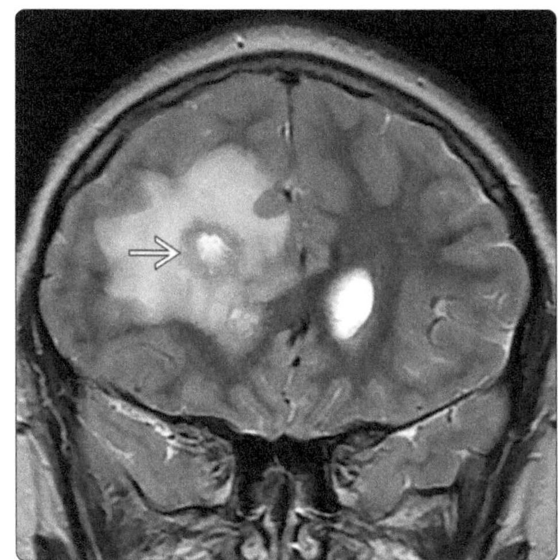

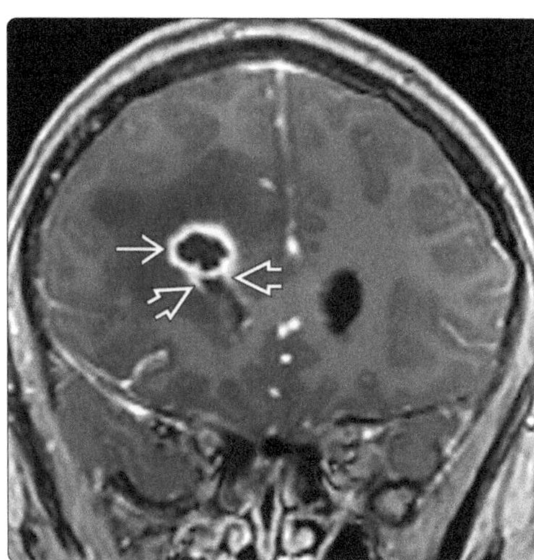

(Left) *Coronal T2 MR in a patient with headache and fever demonstrates a fluid-filled lesion with a hypointense peripheral rim and marked surrounding vasogenic edema relative to its size.* **(Right)** *Coronal T1 C+ MR in the same patient confirms robust peripheral rim enhancement of the abscess (Staphylococcus aureus). Note also the right lateral ventricle ependymal enhancement, reflecting ventriculitis from interventricular extension.*

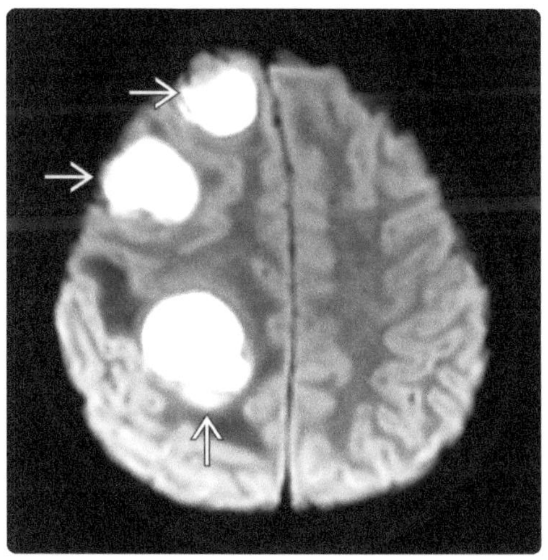

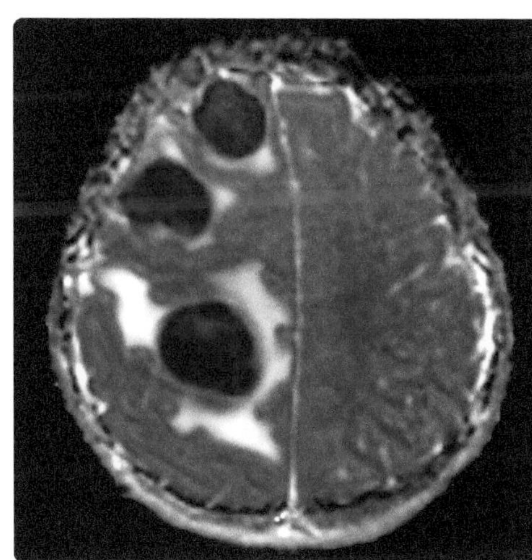

(Left) *Axial DWI MR in a pediatric patient reveals 3 separate large, diffusion-restricting abscesses. The patient had relatively minimal clinical symptoms. Gram stain revealed gram-positive cocci in chains after needle drainage.* **(Right)** *Axial ADC map in the same patient confirms marked hypointensity. All 3 lesions demonstrated a T2-hypointense rim, SWI double rim sign, and ring enhancement on other sequences (not shown), compatible with mature abscess.*

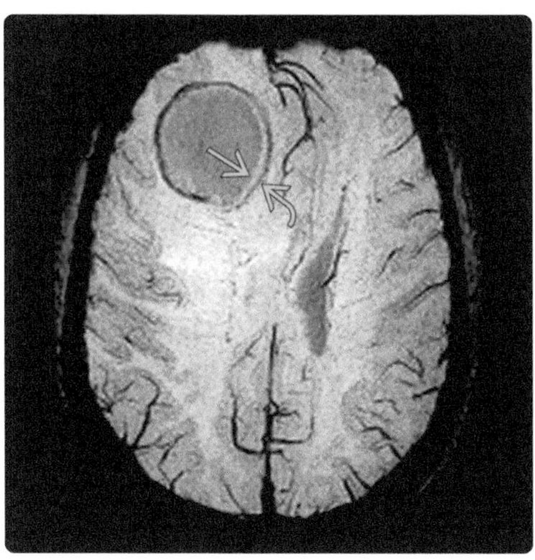

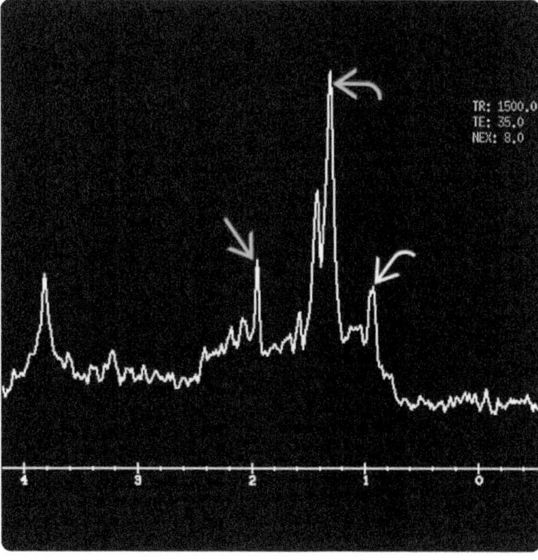

(Left) *Axial SWI MR in a patient with a large right frontal lobe abscess reveals the characteristic dual rim sign. The abscess is bordered by 2 concentric rims, the outer one hypointense and the inner one hyperintense relative to cavity content, forming the dual rim sign.* **(Right)** *MRS (TR 1500, TE 35) shows the typical spectrum for a bacterial brain abscess. There is a large lactate peak at 1.3 ppm and smaller peaks for acetate (1.9 ppm) and branch chain amino acids (valine, leucine, isoleucine) at 0.9 ppm.*

Ventriculitis

KEY FACTS

TERMINOLOGY

- Ventricular ependyma infection related to meningitis, ruptured brain abscess, or ventricular catheter

IMAGING

- Best imaging clue: Ventriculomegaly with debris level, abnormal ependyma, periventricular T2/FLAIR hyperintensity
- DWI MR: Diffusion restriction of layering debris
- T1WI C+ MR: Marked ependymal enhancement with ventriculomegaly
- Ultrasound: Ventriculomegaly with echogenic ependyma & debris in infant
    - Can play important role in detection of postinfectious hydrocephalus

TOP DIFFERENTIAL DIAGNOSES

- Intraventricular hemorrhage
- Ependymal tumor spread (e.g., medulloblastoma, ependymoma, pineal & choroid plexus tumors)
- Primary CNS lymphoma
- Prominent ependymal veins (e.g., arteriovenous malformation, developmental venous anomaly, Sturge-Weber)

CLINICAL ISSUES

- Bacterial ventriculitis may occur in healthy individuals after trauma or neurosurgical procedure
- Fungal or viral ventriculitis occurs most commonly in immunosuppressed patients
- Ventriculitis occurs in 30% of meningitis patients; up to 80-90% in neonates/infants
- High mortality rate: 40-80%
- Treatment: Surgical irrigation, drainage, &/or IV antibiotics

DIAGNOSTIC CHECKLIST

- Look carefully on DWI for small amount of pus in occipital horns

(Left) *Axial graphic shows a right frontal abscess that has ruptured into the ventricular system, resulting in ventriculitis. Note the characteristic debris level ⇒ within the ventricles & periventricular inflammation ⇒.* **(Right)** *Axial DWI MR in an infant with E. coli meningitis shows layering purulent material in the occipital horns ⇒ & diffusion restriction (pus) in the subarachnoid spaces ⇒. Diffusion restriction in the corticospinal tracts ⇒ is secondary injury from hemispheric cerebritis/ischemia.*

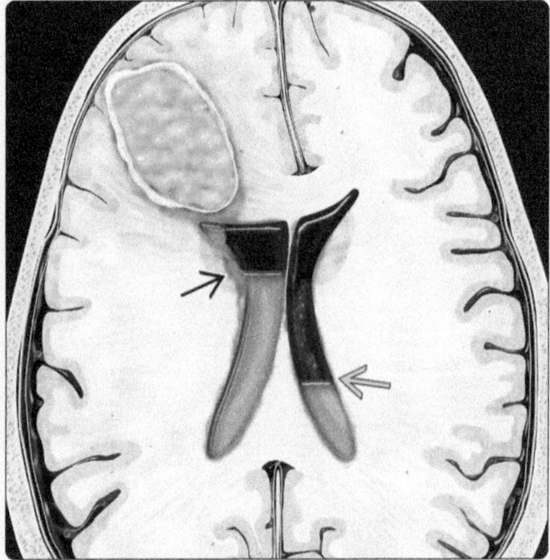

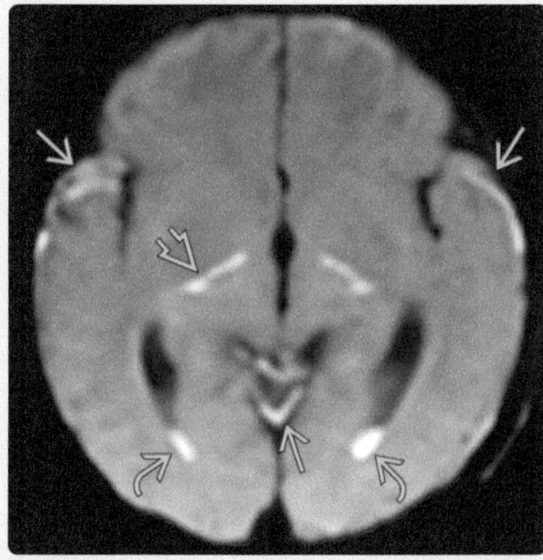

(Left) *Axial T1 C+ MR in a 12-day-old with Citrobacter infection shows intense ependymal enhancement ⇒ characteristic of ventriculitis. Bifrontal ⇒ & left posterior ⇒ brain abscesses have ruptured into & infected the ventricular system.* **(Right)** *Coronal ultrasound in a 3-week-old with staphylococcal sepsis & meningitis shows echogenic debris ⇒ within the ventricular atria with multiple intraventricular septations ⇒, findings that suggest associated ventriculitis.*

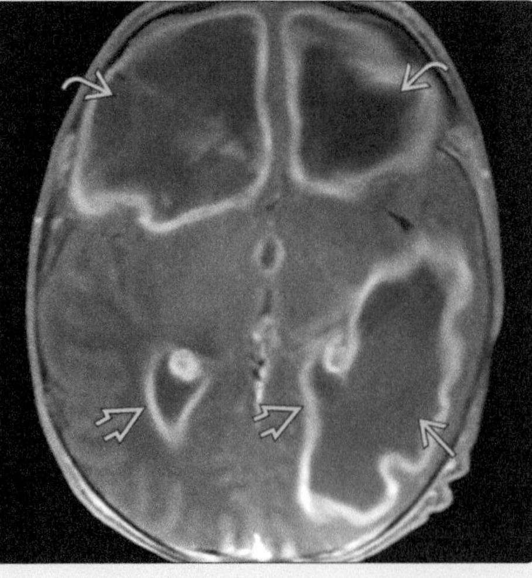

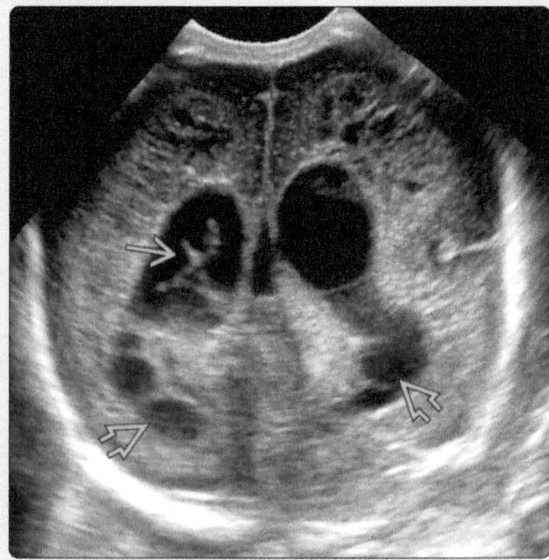

TERMINOLOGY

Synonyms

- Ependymitis, ventricular abscess, pyocephalus

Definitions

- Ventricular ependyma infection related to meningitis, ruptured brain abscess, or ventricular catheter

IMAGING

General Features

- Best diagnostic clue
  - Ventriculomegaly with debris level, abnormal ependymal enhancement, periventricular T2/FLAIR hyperintensity

CT Findings

- NECT
  - Ventriculomegaly with dependent debris level
  - Subtle low density along ventricular margins
- CECT
  - Enhancement of ventricular walls

MR Findings

- T1WI
  - Ventriculomegaly with hyperintense debris
  - Subtle periventricular hypointensity
- T2WI
  - May see hypointense debris layering dependently
- FLAIR
  - Hyperintensity along ventricular margins
  - Hyperintense debris layering dependently
- DWI
  - Diffusion restriction of layering debris
  - Most sensitive sequence for small amounts of intraventricular pus
- T1WI C+
  - Marked ependymal enhancement
  - May have associated choroid plexitis with enlarged, edematous choroid
  - Inflammatory septations & loculations (chronic)

Ultrasonographic Findings

- Ventriculomegaly with echogenic debris
- Echogenic ependyma ± ↑ periventricular echogenicity

Imaging Recommendations

- Best imaging tool
  - Ultrasound may be initial test in infants
  - MR with contrast is best test
- Protocol advice
  - Multiplanar MR with contrast, DWI, FLAIR

DIFFERENTIAL DIAGNOSIS

Intraventricular Hemorrhage

- History of prematurity or trauma
- Look for high attenuation (CT), SWI/GRE signal loss (MR)

Ependymal Tumor Spread

- Primary brain tumors: Medulloblastoma, pineal tumors, ependymoma, choroid plexus tumors

Primary CNS Lymphoma

- Rare in children
- Ependymal enhancement, typically nodular
- Parenchymal disease usually present

Prominent Ependymal Veins

- Vascular malformations: Arteriovenous malformation, developmental venous anomaly, cavernoma
- Abnormal venous drainage (i.e., Sturge-Weber)

PATHOLOGY

General Features

- Etiology
  - Complication of meningitis or cerebral abscess that ruptures into ventricular system
  - Complication of neurosurgical procedure, most commonly intraventricular catheter
  - Pathogens include bacteria, fungus, virus, parasites
    - Common bacterial organisms: *Staphylococcus, Streptococcus, Enterobacter*
    - Most common in neonates: *E. coli, Klebsiella, Enterobacter*, & group B Strep

Gross Pathologic & Surgical Features

- Intraventricular sedimentation levels with inflammation & proteinaceous debris

Microscopic Features

- Ependymal & subependymal inflammation with macrophages, lymphocytes

CLINICAL ISSUES

Presentation

- Most common signs/symptoms
  - Dependent on etiology; often indolent
- Clinical profile
  - CSF cytology, cultures may be normal

Demographics

- Epidemiology
  - Bacterial ventriculitis may occur in healthy individuals after trauma or neurosurgical procedure
  - Fungal or viral ventriculitis occurs most commonly in immunosuppressed patients
  - Ventriculitis occurs in 30% of meningitis patients; up to 80-90% in neonates/infants
  - Intrathecal chemotherapy, rarely associated

Natural History & Prognosis

- Mortality rate: 40-80%

Treatment

- Surgical irrigation, drainage, &/or IV antibiotics

SELECTED REFERENCES

1. Karvouniaris M et al: Current perspectives on the diagnosis and management of healthcare-associated ventriculitis and meningitis. Infect Drug Resist. 15:697-721, 2022
2. Luque-Paz D et al: Ventriculitis: a severe complication of central nervous system infections. Open Forum Infect Dis. 8(6):ofab216, 2021
3. Peros T et al: Neonatal bacterial meningitis versus ventriculitis: a cohort-based overview of clinical characteristics, microbiology and imaging. Eur J Pediatr. 179(12):1969-77, 2020

KEY FACTS

TERMINOLOGY

- Subdural empyema (SDE), epidural empyema (EDE)
- Collection of pus in subdural or epidural space or both (15%); subdural much more common

IMAGING

- Best diagnostic clue: Extraaxial collection with enhancing rim, DWI positive
- Supratentorial typical
  - EDE: Often adjacent to frontal sinus
  - SDE: Convexity in > 50%, parafalcine in 20%
- Infratentorial (up to 10%); related to mastoiditis
- **MR with DWI** best to demonstrate presence, nature, extent, and complications

TOP DIFFERENTIAL DIAGNOSES

- Chronic subdural hematoma
- Subdural effusion, subdural hygroma

PATHOLOGY

- Infants, young children: Complication of bacterial meningitis
- Older children, adults: Related to paranasal sinus disease

CLINICAL ISSUES

- EDE, SDE rare yet highly lethal
- Sinus or ear infection in > 75% of cases
- Complications common: Cerebritis, abscess, venous thrombosis, ischemia, hydrocephalus
- Surgical drainage by craniotomy is primary treatment
- Sinus drainage + antibiotics may be tried for small sinus-related EDE

DIAGNOSTIC CHECKLIST

- MR with contrast and **DWI** is most sensitive; CT may miss small collections
- Look for empyema in patient with sinusitis and neurologic symptoms

(Left) *Axial FLAIR MR in a 7-year-old with fever and headaches shows a right frontal epidural fluid collection ➡ associated with left frontal sinus opacification ⇨ and scalp fluid accumulation ↩. There is also right frontal cortical edema. Sinus CT (not shown) revealed complete sinus opacification.* **(Right)** *Axial DWI MR in the same patient confirms diffusion restriction in an epidural empyema (EDE) ➡ and a Pott puffy tumor ↩.*

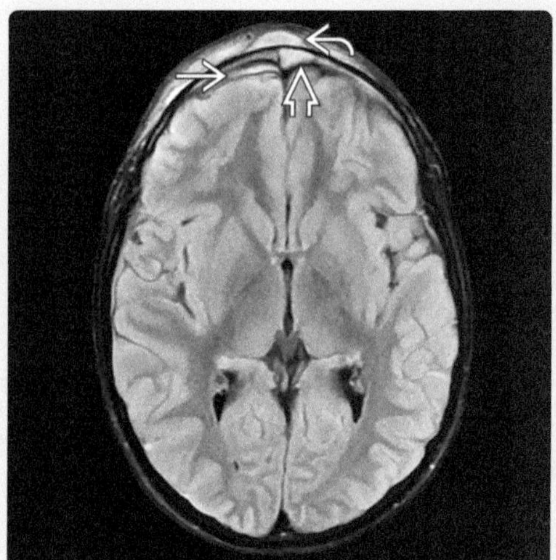

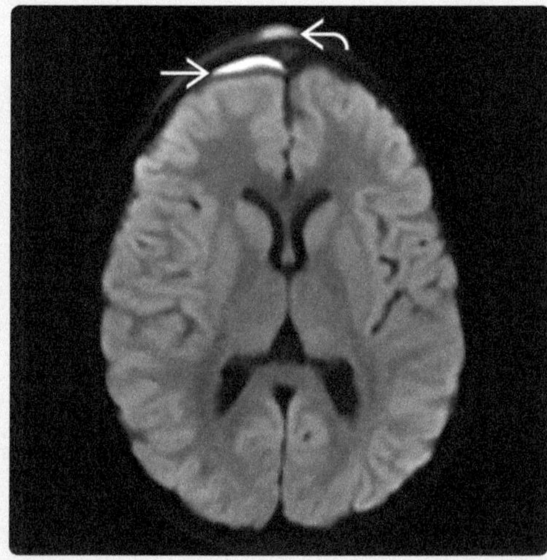

(Left) *Axial T2 MR in the same patient reveals, in addition, a "dirty," complex appearance in the right frontal subdural fluid collection ➡ with regional mass effect on the right frontal lobe.* **(Right)** *Axial T1 C+ FS MR in the same patient reveals thick dural and leptomeningeal enhancement around this subdural empyema (SDE). DWI MR (not shown) confirmed that this collection also restricted. It is not unusual to see both EDE and SDE in the same patient.*

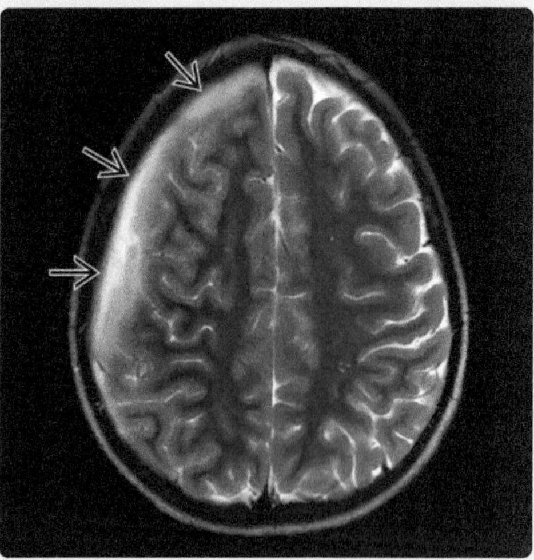

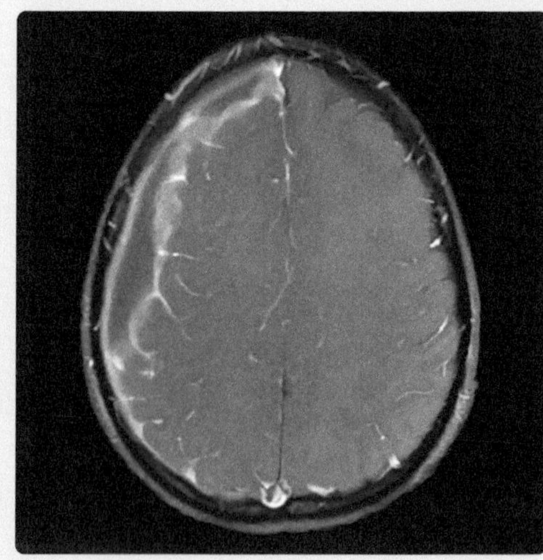

TERMINOLOGY

Synonyms

- Epidural empyema (EDE) = epidural abscess

Definitions

- Collection of pus in subdural or epidural space or both; subdural much more common

IMAGING

General Features

- Best diagnostic clue
  - Extraaxial collection with enhancing rim
- Location
  - Supratentorial typical
    - Subdural empyema (SDE): Convexity in > 50%, parafalcine in 20%
    - EDE: Often adjacent to frontal sinus
  - Infratentorial (up to 10%)
    - Often associated with mastoiditis
    - > 90% associated with hydrocephalus
- Morphology
  - SDE: Crescentic typical; may be lens-shaped (lentiform) on coronal images
    - Can spread diffusely over hemispheres, along tentorium/falx
  - EDE: Biconvex, lentiform

CT Findings

- NECT
  - Extraaxial collection, iso- to hyperdense to CSF
  - SDE: Crescentic iso- to hyperdense collection, limited by dural reflections
    - Frequently bilateral
    - Warning: Can be small, easily overlooked
  - EDE: Biconvex, low-density collection between dura, calvarium; contained by cranial sutures
    - Often continuous across midline
  - Posterior fossa EDE
    - Typically at sinodural angle
    - Tegmen tympani ± sigmoid plate eroded
    - Pus may extend into cerebellopontine angle
- CECT
  - Strong peripheral rim enhancement
  - Posterior fossa EDE: Look for venous thrombosis
- Bone CT
  - **Sinusitis** common in **supratentorial** SDE-EDE
  - **Otomastoiditis** common in **infratentorial** SDE-EDE

MR Findings

- T1WI
  - Extraaxial collection, hyperintense to CSF
  - SDE: Crescentic extraaxial collection
  - EDE: Lentiform bifrontal or convexity collection
    - May cross midline in frontal region
- T2WI
  - Iso- to hyperintense to CSF
  - SDE: Crescentic collection, underlying brain may be hyperintense
  - EDE: Lentiform bifrontal or convexity collection
    - Inwardly displaced dura seen as **hypointense line** between fluid and brain
- FLAIR
  - Hyperintense to CSF
  - SDE: Crescentic collection, underlying brain may be hyperintense
  - EDE: Lentiform bifrontal or convexity collection
  - Hyperintensity in underlying brain parenchyma may be caused by cerebritis or ischemia (venous or arterial)
- DWI
  - SDE: **Restricted diffusion** (↑ signal intensity) typical
  - EDE: Variable signal with some restricting components
- T1WI C+
  - Prominent enhancement at margin related to granulomatous tissue and inflammation
  - SDE: Encapsulating membranes enhance strongly, may be loculated with internal fibrous strands
  - EDE: Strong enhancement of collection margins
  - May see enhancement of adjacent brain parenchyma (cerebritis/abscess)
  - May see leptomeningeal enhancement due to associated meningitis
  - Frontal subgaleal phlegmon or abscess (Pott puffy tumor)
- MRV: Venous thrombosis, especially with SDE

Ultrasonographic Findings

- Useful in infants
- Heterogeneous echogenic convexity collection with mass effect
  - Hyperechoic fibrous strands
  - Thick, hyperechoic inner membrane
  - ↑ echogenicity of pia-arachnoid and exudates in subarachnoid space

Imaging Recommendations

- Best imaging tool
  - **MR with DWI** best to demonstrate presence, nature, extent, and complications
- Protocol advice
  - Contrast-enhanced multiplanar MR with DWI
  - **DWI** helpful to evaluate extent and complications

DIFFERENTIAL DIAGNOSIS

Chronic Subdural Hematoma

- MR shows blood products; may be loculated
- Often enhances along edge; enhancement usually thinner than SDE
- May be indistinguishable; history may help

Subdural Effusion

- Sterile, CSF-like collection associated with meningitis
- Follows CSF on all MR sequences
- Usually nonenhancing; may enhance mildly
- Frontal and temporal regions common, often bilateral

Subdural Hygroma

- Nonenhancing CSF collection, often trauma/surgical history

Dural Metastasis

- Primary tumor often known, typically breast, prostate

- Often diffuse, nodular enhancement
- May have associated bone metastases

PATHOLOGY

General Features

- Etiology
  - Infants, young children: Complication of **bacterial meningitis**
  - Older children, adults: Related to **paranasal sinus disease** (> 2/3)
    - Direct spread via posterior wall of frontal sinus
    - Retrograde spread through **valveless bridging emissary veins** of extra- and intracranial spaces
  - **Mastoiditis** (± cholesteatoma) in 20%
  - Complication of head trauma or neurosurgical procedure (rare)
  - Complication of meningitis in adults (very rare)
  - Causative organism: *Staphylococcus aureus*, *Staphylococcus epidermidis*, enteric gram-negative bacilli most common
  - Aerobic and microaerophilic streptococci (infection from paranasal sinuses)
- SDE much more common than EDE
- SDE more commonly complicated by abscess and venous thrombosis (> 10%)
- 15% of cases have both EDE and SDE

Gross Pathologic & Surgical Features

- Encapsulated, yellowish, purulent collection
- Spreads widely but may be loculated
- Often accompanying osteitis

Microscopic Features

- Inflammatory infiltrate and granulomatous tissue

CLINICAL ISSUES

Presentation

- Most common signs/symptoms
  - Majority have fever, headaches
  - Meningismus common, may mimic meningitis
  - Sinusitis often present
  - Cerebritis/brain abscess causes neurologic signs
- Clinical profile
  - Sinus or ear infection in > 75% of cases
  - Frontal subgaleal abscess (Pott puffy tumor) in up to 1/3; typically adolescent males
  - Periorbital swelling may be seen
  - Confused with meningitis; delayed diagnosis
  - EDE, SDE rare, yet highly lethal

Demographics

- Age
  - Can occur at any age
- Epidemiology
  - SDE: 15-22%, EDE: 2-5% of focal intracranial infections
  - SDE: Sinusitis (67%), mastoiditis (10%)

Natural History & Prognosis

- Progresses rapidly, **neurosurgical emergency**
- Rapidly evolving, fulminant course
- EDE may occasionally have indolent course as dura mater functions as barrier between infection and brain
  - Much better prognosis than SDE
- Can be fatal unless recognized and treated
  - **Lumbar puncture** can be **fatal**
  - CSF can be normal
- Complications common
  - Cerebritis and brain abscess: ~ 5%
  - Cortical vein, dural sinus thrombosis (venous ischemia)
  - Cerebral edema
  - Hydrocephalus (> 90% of infratentorial SDE)
- **Mortality: 10-15%**

Treatment

- Surgical drainage via wide craniotomy is gold standard
- Intravenous antibiotics
- Sinus drainage + antibiotics possible in small sinus-related EDE

DIAGNOSTIC CHECKLIST

Consider

- Chronic subdural hematoma may be difficult to differentiate from SDE; history may help
- Look for empyema in patient with sinusitis and neurologic symptoms
- If SDE or EDE discovered, look also for sinusitis, otomastoiditis, dural sinus thrombosis, brain abscess

Image Interpretation Pearls

- MR with contrast and **DWI** is most sensitive; CT may miss small collections
- DWI differentiates SDE from subdural effusions
- MR with DWI may be used to monitor treatment response

SELECTED REFERENCES

1. Yazar U et al: Subdural empyema in immunocompetent pediatric patients with recent SARS-CoV-2 positivity: case report. Childs Nerv Syst. 39(5):1335-9, 2023
2. Accorsi EK et al: Pediatric brain abscesses, epidural empyemas, and subdural empyemas associated with Streptococcus species - United States, January 2016-August 2022. MMWR Morb Mortal Wkly Rep. 71(37):1169-73, 2022
3. Agouzoul S et al: Intracranial empyema complicating sinusitis in childhood: epidemiology, imaging findings and outcome. Int J Pediatr Otorhinolaryngol. 162:111299, 2022
4. Gillard DM et al: Efficacy of endoscopic sinus surgery alone versus in combination with neurosurgical intervention for the treatment of pediatric subdural empyema. Int J Pediatr Otorhinolaryngol. 148:110836, 2021
5. Ziegler A et al: Neurological complications of acute and chronic sinusitis. Curr Neurol Neurosci Rep. 18(2):5, 2018
6. Rapalino O et al: Intracranial infectious and inflammatory diseases presenting as neurosurgical pathologies. Neurosurgery. 81(1):10-28, 2017
7. Patel NA et al: Systematic review and case report: intracranial complications of pediatric sinusitis. Int J Pediatr Otorhinolaryngol. 86:200-12, 2016
8. French H et al: Intracranial subdural empyema: a 10-year case series. Ochsner J. 14(2):188-94, 2014
9. Ouiminga HA et al: [Intracranial empyemas: epidemiological, clinical, radiological and therapeutic aspects. Retrospective study of 100 observations.] Neurochirurgie. 60(6):299-303, 2014
10. Salomão JF et al: Neurosurgical implications of Pott's puffy tumor in children and adolescents. Childs Nerv Syst. 30(9):1527-34, 2014
11. Sharma PK et al: Orbitocranial complications of acute sinusitis in children. J Emerg Med. 47(3):282-5, 2014
12. Nickerson JP et al: Neuroimaging of pediatric intracranial infection–part 1: techniques and bacterial infections. J Neuroimaging. 22(2):e42-51, 2012

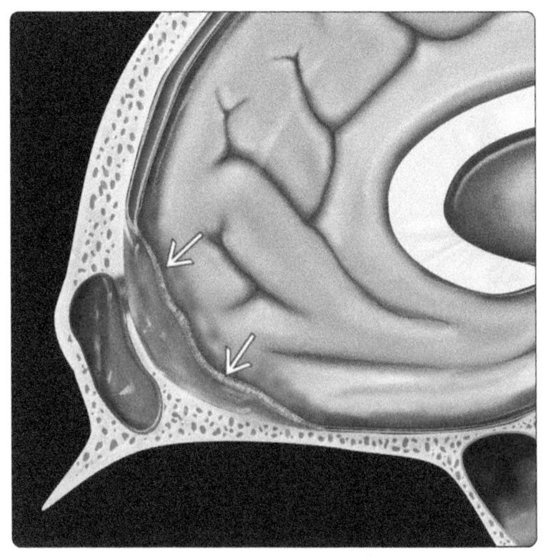

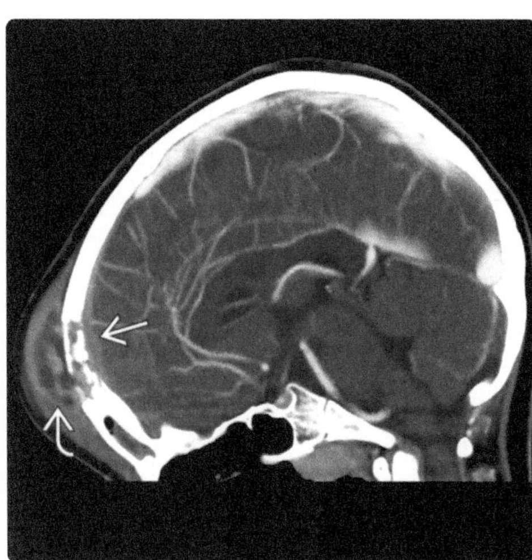

(Left) *Sagittal graphic shows frontal sinus purulence with direct extension into the epidural space, resulting in an EDE* ➡*. Note the displaced dura and inflammation in the adjacent frontal lobe. EDE is often located adjacent to the frontal sinus.* **(Right)** *Sagittal CECT demonstrates a large frontal soft tissue abscess (Pott puffy tumor)* ➡ *related to complicated frontal sinusitis. Note small frontal EDE* ➡*.*

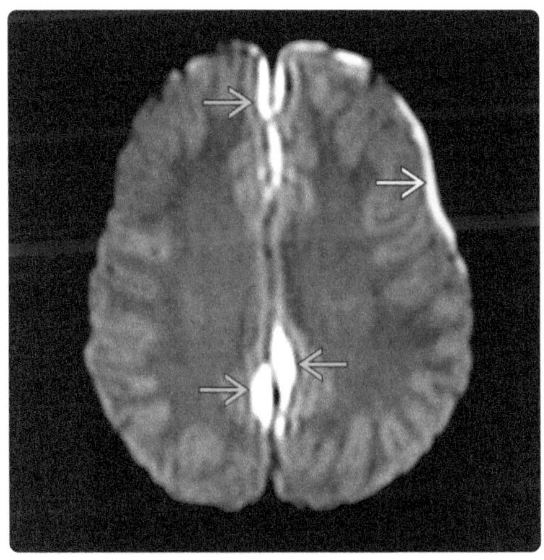

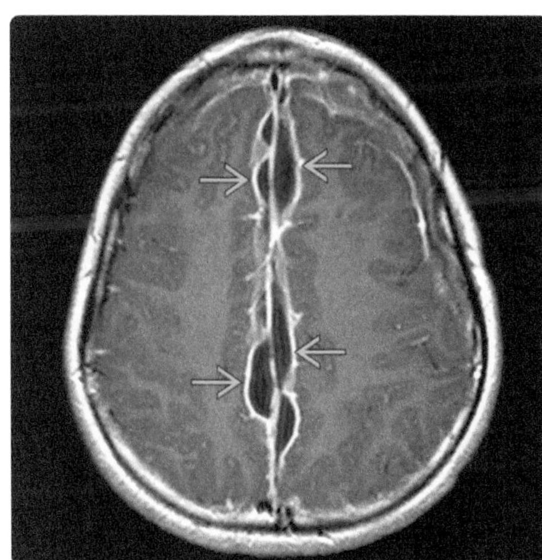

(Left) *Axial DWI MR in a patient presenting with headache and fever reveals bright diffusion restriction within parafalcine* ➡ *and left frontal* ➡ *SDEs. DWI is an important sequence to demonstrate the presence, extent, and complications of an SDE or EDE.* **(Right)** *Axial T1 C+ FS MR in the same patient confirms rim-enhancing parafalcine complex fluid collections* ➡ *reflecting SDEs.*

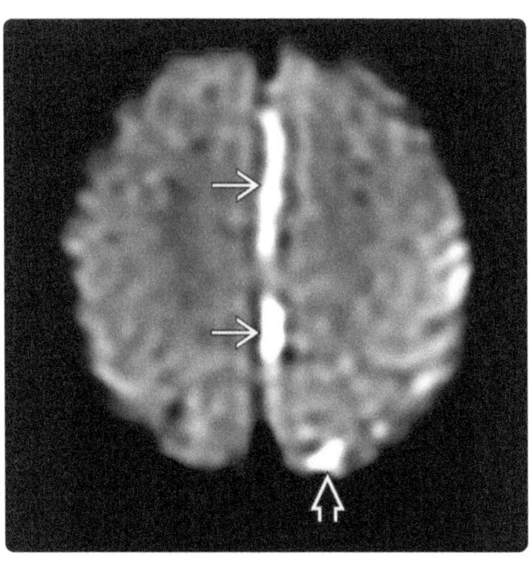

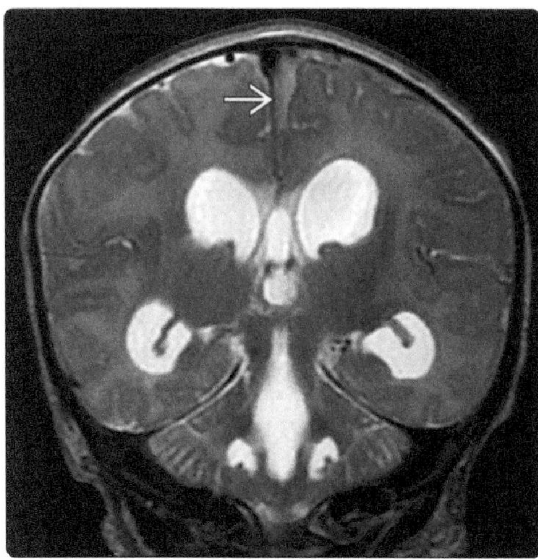

(Left) *Axial DWI MR in the same patient reveals markedly hyperintense diffusion restriction (ADC confirmed) along the falx* ➡ *as well as over the left parietal lobe* ➡ *and left hemispheric convexity.* **(Right)** *Coronal T2 MR in the same patient with Salmonella meningitis confirms complex "dirty" signal in the left parafalcine empyema* ➡ *with extension over the left parietal convexity. Note also hydrocephalus and partial obscuration of convexity sulci related to meningitis.*

Herpes Encephalitis Type 1

KEY FACTS

TERMINOLOGY

- **HSV1** brain infection
- Typically reactivation in immunocompetent patients
- **Different from neonatal (HSV2)** herpes encephalitis

IMAGING

- T2/FLAIR hyperintensity in **mesial temporal, subfrontal, insular, and cingular cortex** with DWI restriction
  - Typically **bilateral** disease **but asymmetric**
  - **Hemorrhage** typically subacute/**late**
- T2/FLAIR: Cortical, subcortical hyperintensity with relative white matter sparing
- GRE: If hemorrhagic, hypointensity blooms
- DWI: Restricted diffusion in limbic system
- T1WI C+: May see mild, patchy enhancement early
  - **Gyriform enhancement** usually **late**, after 1 week

TOP DIFFERENTIAL DIAGNOSES

- Acute cerebral ischemia-infarction
- Status epilepticus
- Limbic encephalitis
- Infiltrating neoplasm

PATHOLOGY

- Hemorrhagic, necrotizing HSV1 encephalitis

CLINICAL ISSUES

- Common presentation: Fever, headache, seizures, ± viral prodrome
- Children often present with nonspecific symptoms
- PCR of CSF most accurate diagnosis
- HSV1 causes 95% of all herpetic encephalitis
- Start IV acyclovir immediately if herpes simplex encephalitis suspected

DIAGNOSTIC CHECKLIST

- CT often normal early; MR with FLAIR/DWI most sensitive for early diagnosis

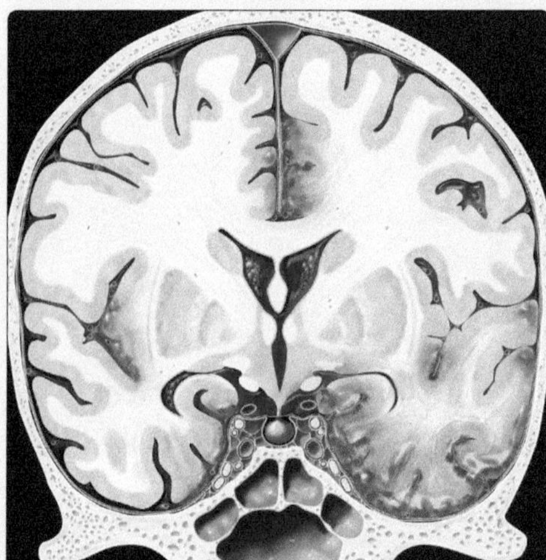

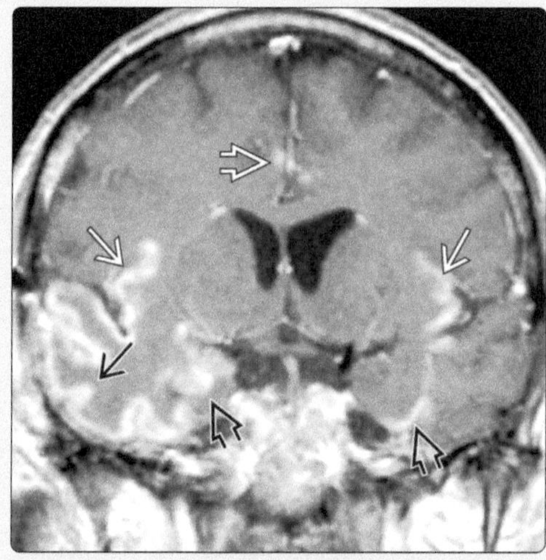

(Left) *Coronal graphic shows the classic features of herpes encephalitis with bilateral but asymmetric involvement of the limbic system. There is inflammation involving the temporal lobes, cingulate gyri, and insular cortices.* **(Right)** *Coronal T1 C+ MR in a subacute case of HSV1 herpes encephalitis shows striking bilateral but asymmetric enhancement in the mesial ➡ more than lateral temporal lobes ➡ and insular cortex ➡. Subtle lesions are seen in the cingulate gyri ➡.*

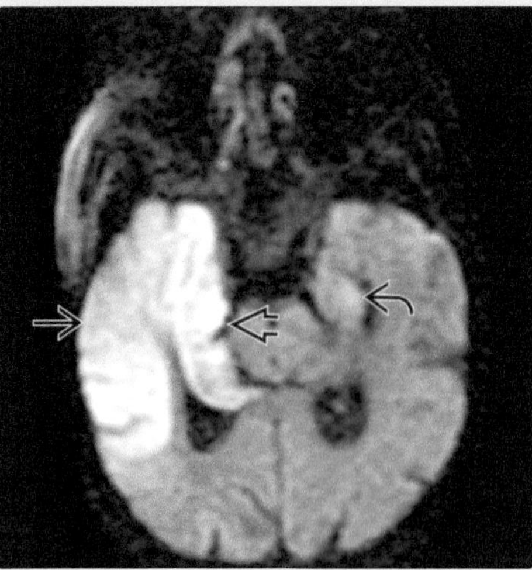

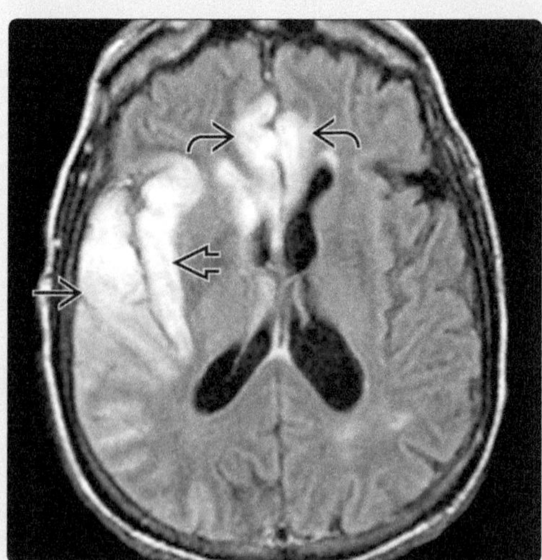

(Left) *Axial DWI MR in a patient with acute herpes encephalitis shows diffusion restriction in the right mesial ➡ and lateral temporal ➡ lobes. Subtle diffusion restriction of the left hippocampus ➡ is also seen.* **(Right)** *Axial FLAIR MR at a higher level in the same patient shows diffuse cortical swelling and hyperintensity in the right superior temporal lobe ➡, right insular cortex ➡, and bilateral cingulate gyri ➡. Note relative sparing of the underlying white matter.*

TERMINOLOGY

Abbreviations

- Herpes simplex encephalitis (HSE)

Definitions

- Older children and adults: Brain parenchyma infection caused by **HSV1**
- Typically reactivation in immunocompetent patients
- Different from neonatal herpes encephalitis
  - **Neonates and infants: HSV2**

IMAGING

General Features

- Best diagnostic clue
  - Abnormal signal in **mesial temporal, subfrontal, insular, and cingular cortex** with DWI restriction
  - **Bilateral but asymmetric** with **late hemorrhage**
- Location
  - HSV1: Limbic system: Temporal lobes, insula, subfrontal area, cingulate gyri typical
  - Cerebral convexity, posterior occipital cortex may become involved
  - Typically bilateral disease but asymmetric
  - Basal ganglia usually spared
  - Rarely in midbrain and pons (mesenrhombencephalitis)
  - Atypical patterns seen in infants and children (may be caused by HSV1 or HSV2)
    - May primarily affect cerebral hemispheres

CT Findings

- NECT
  - CT often normal early
    - Low attenuation, mild mass effect in medial temporal lobes, insula; hemorrhage typically late feature
  - Predilection for limbic system; basal ganglia spared
  - Earliest CT findings at 3 days after symptom onset
- CECT
  - Patchy or gyriform **enhancement** of temporal lobes (**late** acute/subacute feature)

MR Findings

- T1WI
  - Cortical swelling with loss of gray matter-white matter (WM) differentiation
  - May see subacute hemorrhage as ↑ signal within edematous brain
  - Atrophy, encephalomalacia in late subacute/chronic cases
- T2WI
  - Cortical and subcortical hyperintensity with relative WM sparing
  - May see subacute hemorrhage as ↑ signal within edematous brain
- FLAIR
  - Changes seen earlier than on T2WI
- T2* GRE
  - If hemorrhagic, hypointensity blooms within edematous brain
- DWI
  - **Restricted diffusion** in limbic system
  - Look for bilateral disease
  - DWI findings may precede T2/FLAIR changes
- T1WI C+
  - May see mild, patchy enhancement early
  - Gyriform enhancement usually seen 1 week after initial symptoms
  - Meningeal enhancement occasionally seen
  - Enhancement seen in temporal lobes, insular cortex, subfrontal area, cingulate gyrus
- MRS
  - ↓ NAA, prominent lipid-lactate peak

Imaging Recommendations

- Best imaging tool
  - MR (positive 24-48 hours earlier than CT)
- Protocol advice
  - Multiplanar MR with coronal T2 &/or FLAIR, DWI, T2* GRE, contrast

DIFFERENTIAL DIAGNOSIS

HSV2: Neonatal HSV encephalitis

- Neonates/infants with HSV2 have diffuse/scattered disease unlike HSV1 temporal lobe predilection
- Deep/periventricular WM &/or cortical early DWI restriction
- Early meningeal enhancement may be seen
- Congenital HSV2 may be transplacental or from exposure to maternal HSV2 genital lesions during vaginal birth
- Transplacental infection during 1st trimester: Cerebral and cerebellar necrosis, atrophy, microcephaly
  - Intracranial Ca^{++}, hydranencephaly, chorioretinitis, and cutaneous and systemic involvement
- Birth canal infection: Presents within first 3 weeks of life

Neurosyphilis

- Can affect medial temporal lobes; mimic HSE
- Involve meninges, blood vessels (obliterative endarteritis)

Other Encephalitides

- **Human herpesvirus 6 (HHV-6)** in transplant patients, can mimic HSE
- West Nile can mimic HSE clinically, but typically involves basal ganglia &/or thalami

Acute Cerebral Ischemia-Infarction

- Typical vascular distribution [middle cerebral artery, anterior cerebral artery (ACA), posterior cerebral artery]
- Hyperacute symptoms vs. 2-3 day history of flu-like illness
- Reduced diffusivity in acute infarct
- ACA distribution ischemia may mimic HSE

Status Epilepticus

- Active seizures may disrupt blood-brain barrier, cause signal abnormalities and enhancement
- Temporal lobe epilepsy hyperperfusion may mimic HSE
- No hemorrhage in status epilepticus

Limbic Encephalitis

- Rare autoimmune/paraneoplastic syndrome associated with primary tumor, often lung
- Predilection for limbic system, often bilateral
- Nonhemorrhagic; imaging may be indistinguishable
- Symptom onset weeks to months (vs. acute in HSE)

Infiltrating Neoplasm

- Low-grade gliomas may involve medial temporal lobe and cause epilepsy; onset usually indolent
- Gliomatosis cerebri may involve frontal and temporal lobes; may be bilateral

PATHOLOGY

General Features

- Etiology
  - Initial HSV1 infection usually occurs in oronasopharynx via contact with infected secretions
    - Invades along cranial nerves (via lingual nerve, division of trigeminal nerve) to ganglia
    - Remains dormant in trigeminal ganglion
    - Reactivation may occur spontaneously or be precipitated by various factors
      - Local trauma, immunosuppression, hormonal fluctuations, emotional stress

Staging, Grading, & Classification

- Herpesviruses include HSV1, HSV2, EBV, CMV, varicella-zoster virus (VZV), B virus, HHV-6, HHV-7, HHV-8
- HSV1 in adults, children
- HSV2 is more common in neonates
- HSV1 and HSV2 DNA viruses
- Viruses obligate intracellular pathogens

Gross Pathologic & Surgical Features

- Hemorrhagic, necrotizing encephalitis
  - Severe edema, massive tissue necrosis with hemorrhage
  - Involvement of temporal lobes, insular cortex, orbital surface of frontal lobes
  - Less frequent involvement of cingulate gyrus and occipital cortex

Microscopic Features

- Intense perivascular cuffing, interstitial lymphocytic inflammation
- Intranuclear inclusion bodies in infected cells (neurons, glia, endothelial cells)
  - Typically eosinophilic Cowdry A nuclear inclusions
- Immunohistochemistry shows viral antigens, HSV1 antibodies
- Chronic cases: Microglial nodules

CLINICAL ISSUES

Presentation

- Most common signs/symptoms
  - Fever, headache, seizures, ± viral prodrome
  - Children often present with nonspecific symptoms
    - Behavioral changes, fever, headaches, seizures
  - Patients typically immunocompetent
    - HSV1 uncommon in AIDS patients
- Other signs/symptoms
  - Altered mental status
  - Focal or diffuse neurologic deficit (< 30%)
- Clinical profile
  - CSF studies show lymphocytic pleocytosis, ↑ protein
  - PCR of CSF most accurate
    - Sensitivity/specificity nearly 95-100%
    - False-negative PCR possible if CSF obtained < 72 hours after clinical onset
  - EEG: Temporal high voltage discharges in background of generalized slowing
  - Brain biopsy may be required for diagnosis

Demographics

- Age
  - Highest incidence in adolescents and young adults
  - ~ 1/3 of all patients < 20 years old
- Sex
  - M = F
- Epidemiology
  - HSV1 causes 95% of all HSE
  - Most common cause of fatal sporadic encephalitis
  - Most common nonepidemic cause of viral meningoencephalitis

Natural History & Prognosis

- May progress to coma and death
  - 50-70% mortality rate
  - Rapid diagnosis, early treatment with antiviral agents can ↓ mortality, may improve outcome
- Nearly 2/3 of survivors have significant neurologic deficits despite acyclovir therapy
- Survival complicated by memory difficulties, hearing loss, intractable epilepsy, personality changes
- HSV encephalitis can initiate autoimmune reaction with antibodies to neuronal surface antigens
  - → **secondary autoimmune encephalitis**
  - Suspect if recurrence of neurologic symptoms after treated HSV encephalitis episode
  - After ~ 24 days in children and 40 days in adults
  - Mostly anti-N-methyl-d-aspartate receptor (**anti-NMDAR**)encephalitis
  - More frequency of **movement disorders** than seizures, especially in children
  - Psychiatric symptoms more in adults

Treatment

- Antiviral therapy with intravenous acyclovir
- Foscarnet may help in acyclovir unresponsive cases

DIAGNOSTIC CHECKLIST

Consider

- Start IV acyclovir immediately if HSE suspected
- Unilateral disease may mimic stroke or tumor
- Autoimmune limbic encephalitis if all clinical HSE tests negative and subacute onset of symptoms
- Acute onset of HSE helps differentiate from other etiologies

Image Interpretation Pearls

- CT often normal early; MR with FLAIR/DWI most sensitive for early diagnosis
- Imaging often key in diagnosis

SELECTED REFERENCES

1. Ayvacioğlu Çağan C et al: Life after tetra hit: anti-NMDAR encephalitis after HSV encephalitis in a NMOSD coexistent with Sjögren's syndrome. Noro Psikiyatr Ars. 59(2):161-3, 2022

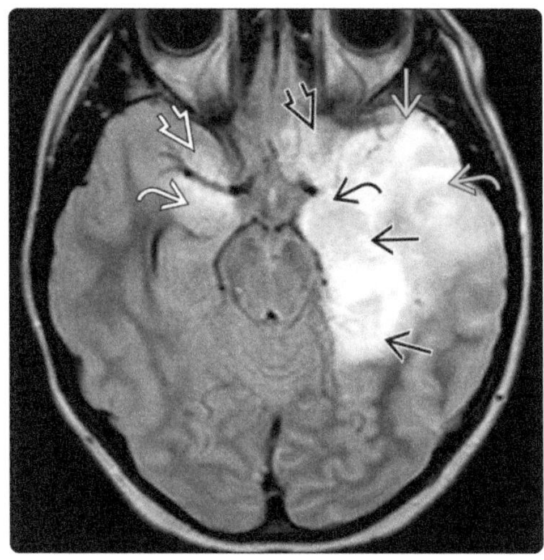

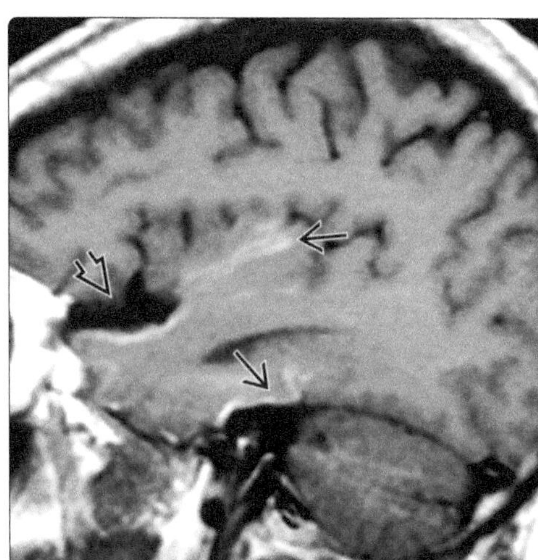

(Left) *Axial FLAIR MR in child with HSV-1 herpes encephalitis shows typical left temporal lobe hyperintensity, swelling of amygdala ▭, hippocampus ▭, uncus ▭, and (unusually) anterior temporal pole ▭ and lateral temporal lobe ▭. Note mild right amygdalar ▭, uncal ▭ involvement.* **(Right)** *Sagittal T1 MR in patient 2 weeks after initial presentation of herpes encephalitis shows volume loss in temporal lobe ▭, linear gyriform T1 hyperintensity ▭, characteristic of subacute cortical hemorrhage.*

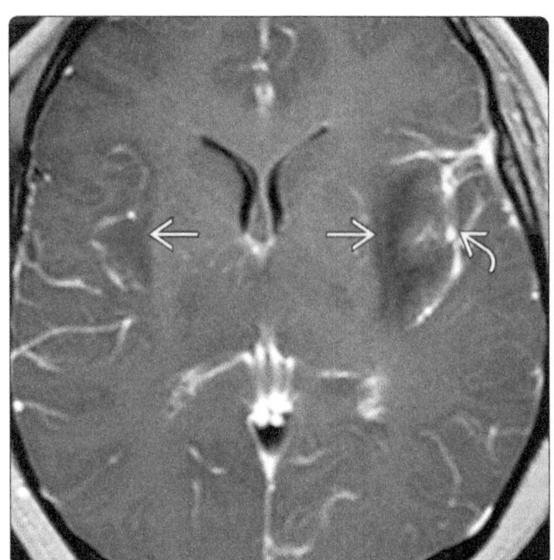

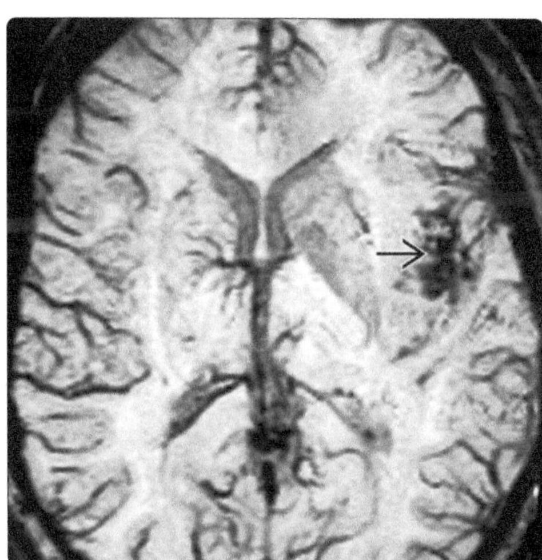

(Left) *Axial T1 C+ MR in the subacute stage of herpes encephalitis shows bilateral but asymmetric hypointensities ▭ in the insular regions. There is associated pial enhancement in the left insular region ▭. Pial, leptomeningeal, diffuse, ring-like enhancement patterns have been reported in herpes encephalitis.* **(Right)** *Axial SWI MR in the same patient shows patchy hypointense hemorrhage ▭ in the left insular region. MR is superior to CT in detecting subacute or chronic hemorrhage.*

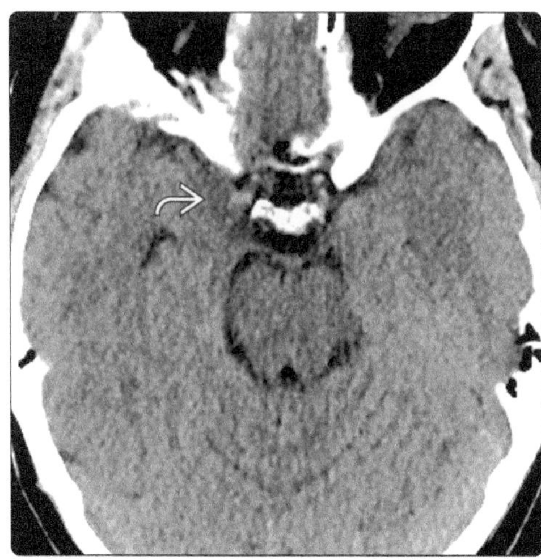

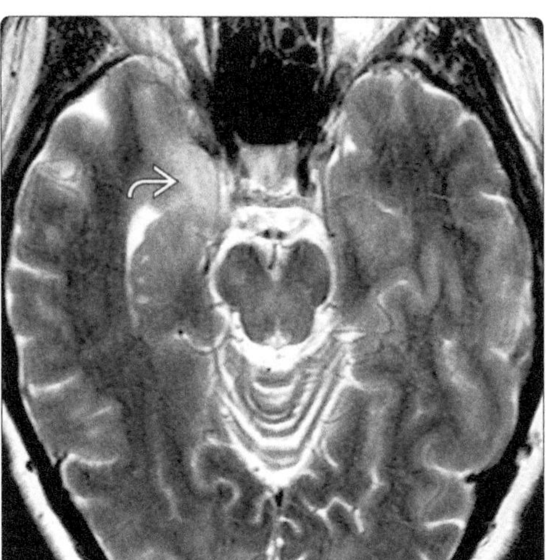

(Left) *Axial NECT in a 45-year-old with fever and altered mental status shows questionable, subtle low-density changes ▭ in the right medial temporal lobe.* **(Right)** *Axial T2 MR in the same patient shows signal abnormality ▭ in the right medial temporal lobe. CSF PCR was positive for HSV-1. CT study may be normal in early stages of herpes encephalitis.*

Miscellaneous Encephalitis

KEY FACTS

TERMINOLOGY

- Diffuse brain parenchymal inflammation caused by variety of pathogens, most commonly viruses
- Location dependent on etiology

IMAGING

- Abnormal T2 hyperintensity of gray matter ± white matter or deep gray nuclei
- Large, poorly delineated areas of involvement common, ± patchy hemorrhage
- Imaging often nonspecific, mimics other etiologies

TOP DIFFERENTIAL DIAGNOSES

- Acute ischemia
- Autoimmune encephalitis
- Herpes encephalitis
- Status epilepticus
- Toxic/metabolic lesions

PATHOLOGY

- Most (but not all) caused by viruses
- Spread of virus to CNS hematogenous or neural

CLINICAL ISSUES

- Herpes: Most common cause of sporadic (nonepidemic) viral encephalitis
- Japanese encephalitis: Most common endemic encephalitis in Asia
- Enterovirus D68: Pediatric acute flaccid paralysis
- Many encephalitides have high morbidity, mortality
- Rapid diagnosis and early treatment with antiviral or antibacterial agents
  - Decrease mortality, may improve outcome

DIAGNOSTIC CHECKLIST

- Clinical history often helpful for accurate diagnosis
- DWI may detect lesions earlier than conventional MR

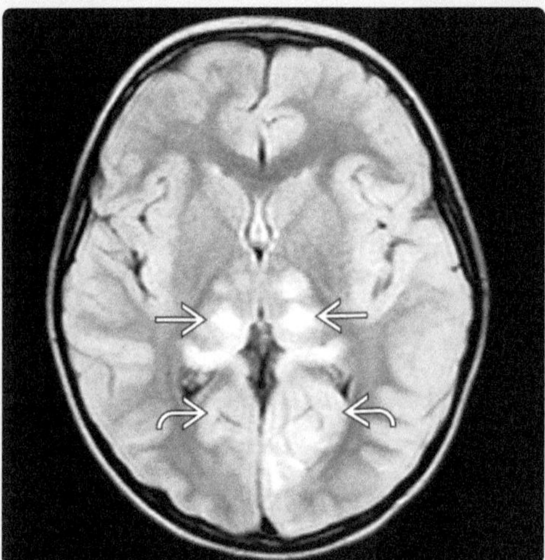
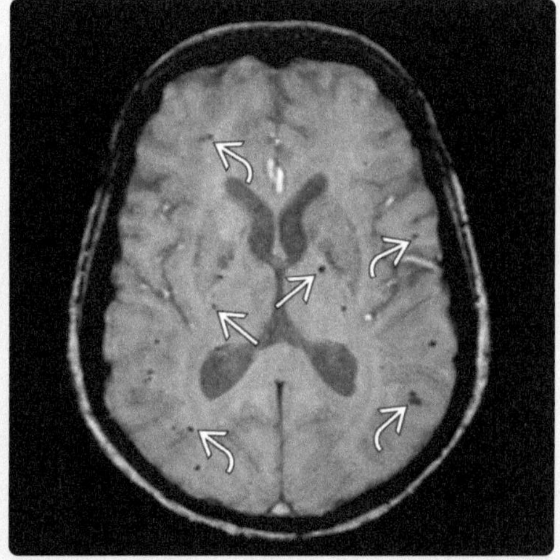

(Left) *Axial FLAIR MR in influenza encephalitis shows hyperintense, swollen bilateral thalami →, occipital lobes →. DWI MR (not shown) revealed diffusion restriction.* **(Right)** *Axial SWI MR in ventilated COVID-19 case shows critical illness-associated cerebral microbleeds (hypoxemia-induced hydrostatic/chemical effects on blood-brain barrier). This involves juxtacortical white matter (WM) →, corpus callosum, internal capsules →, brainstem, & middle cerebellar peduncles. Microbleeds spare deep/periventricular WM, basal ganglia, thalami, cortex.*

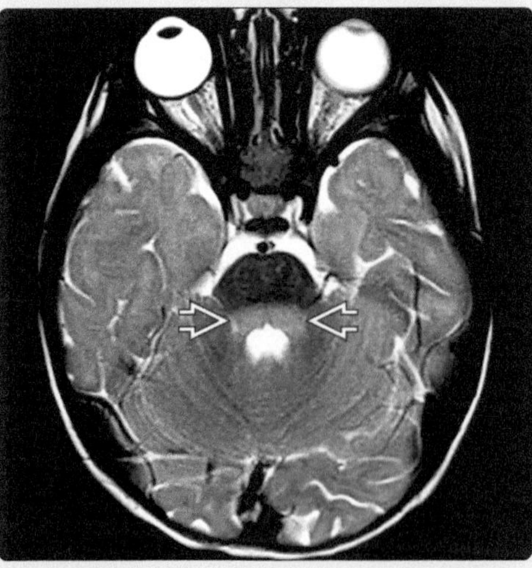
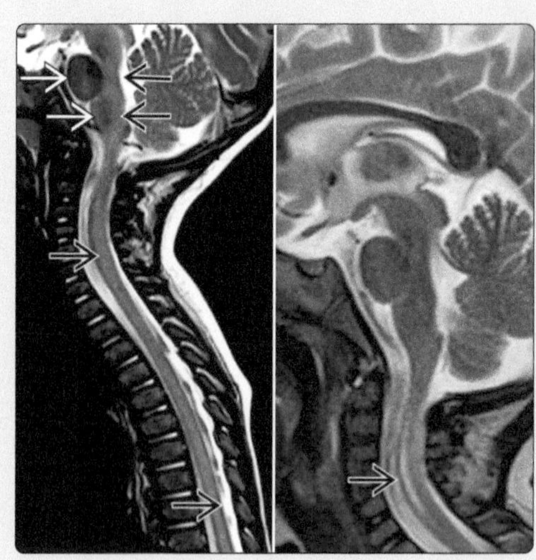

(Left) *Axial T2 MR in 13-month-old girl with enterovirus D68-associated acute flaccid paralysis shows hyperintense signal in dorsal pons →.* **(Right)** *Sagittal T2 MR during same scan (left) shows longitudinally extensive hyperintensity in cervicothoracic central cord gray matter (GM), extending into dorsal brainstem →, sparing ventral brainstem →. Sagittal T2 MR (right) after 10 days shows resolution of brainstem and posterior cord GM hyperintensity with lesions confined to cord of anterior horn.*

TERMINOLOGY

Definitions

- Diffuse brain parenchymal inflammation caused by variety of pathogens, most commonly viruses
- Location dependent on etiology

IMAGING

General Features

- Best diagnostic clue
  - Abnormal T2 hyperintensity of gray matter (GM) ± white matter (WM) or deep gray nuclei/basal ganglia (BG)
  - Large, poorly delineated areas of involvement common ± patchy hemorrhage
  - Imaging often nonspecific
- Location
  - Herpes simplex virus type 1 (**HSV1**): Limbic system
  - **CMV**: Deep periventricular WM
  - **EBV**: Multifocal, diffuse involvement of brain and spinal cord; splenium of corpus callosum
  - Varicella-zoster virus (**VZV**)
    - Varicella: Multifocal areas of cortex, cerebellum
    - Zoster: Brainstem/cortical GM, cranial nerves (CNs)
  - **Cerebellitis**: Bilateral cerebellar hemispheres
  - Eastern equine encephalitis (**EEE**): BG, thalami
  - **Enteroviral** encephalomyelitis
    - **Enterovirus (EV) 71**: Posterior medulla, pons, midbrain, dentate nuclei, spinal cord
    - **Polio, Coxsackie**: Midbrain, anterior spinal cord
    - **EV-D68**: Spinal cord GM ± dorsal brainstem
  - **Hantavirus**: Pituitary gland hemorrhage
  - **HIV-1**: Cerebral WM, brainstem, thalamus, BG
  - **Japanese encephalitis**: Bilateral thalami, brainstem, cerebellum, spinal cord, cerebral cortex
  - Murray Valley encephalitis (**MVE**): Bilateral thalami; may affect midbrain, cervical spinal cord
  - **Nipah viral encephalitis**: Multifocal WM
  - **Rabies encephalitis**: Brainstem, hippocampi, hypothalamus, WM, GM
  - **Rhombencephalitis**: Brainstem and cerebellum
  - **St. Louis encephalitis**: Substantia nigra
  - West Nile virus (**WNV**): BG &/or thalami; brainstem, cerebral WM, substantia nigra, cerebellum, cord
  - **Influenza encephalitis**: Reversible splenial lesion; thalamus, brainstem, cerebellum, or multifocal in brain
    - Rarely acute necrotizing encephalopathy (ANE)

CT Findings

- NECT: Initial CT negative in vast majority of patients
  - Japanese encephalitis: May see thalamic hemorrhage

MR Findings

- T1WI
  - **Japanese encephalitis**: Low-signal foci in WM, brainstem, BG, thalami bilaterally
  - **Rabies encephalitis**: Hyperintense bilateral BG (rare)
- T2WI
  - **CMV**: Deep periventricular WM patchy increased signal
  - **EBV**: Hyperintensity in BG, thalamus, cortex
  - **Varicella**: Multifocal increased cortical signal
  - **Zoster**: Increased signal in brainstem, cortex
  - **Cerebellitis**: Hyperintense cerebellar signal
  - **EEE**: Increased signal in BG and thalami; may involve brainstem, cortex, periventricular WM
  - Enteroviral encephalomyelitis (**EV71**): Hyperintense lesions in dorsal medulla, pons, midbrain, dentate nuclei
    - Less common: Cervical cord, thalamus, putamen
  - **EV-D68**: Longitudinally extensive cord hyperintensity
    - Acute: Entire cord GM hyperintensity; subacute: Confined to anterior horn
    - Brainstem lesions, most commonly pontine tegmentum
    - Bilateral facial nerve enhancement reported
  - **Japanese encephalitis**: High-signal foci in WM, brainstem, BG, thalami bilaterally
  - **MVE**: Hyperintensity in bilateral thalami; may involve midbrain, cerebral peduncles
  - **Nipah viral encephalitis**: Multifocal WM hyperintensities; may affect GM
  - **Rabies encephalitis**: Ill-defined mild hyperintensity in brainstem, hippocampi, thalami, WM, BG
    - Paralytic rabies: Medulla and spinal cord
  - **Rhombencephalitis**: Patchy hyperintensity in pons, medulla, midbrain
  - **St. Louis encephalitis**: May see hyperintensity of substantia nigra, often normal
  - **WNV**: Hyperintensity in deep gray nuclei ± cerebral WM
- FLAIR
  - **Nipah encephalitis**: Discrete high-signal lesions in subcortical, deep WM ± GM
    - Confluent cortical involvement in relapsed and late-onset encephalitis
- T2* GRE
  - Japanese encephalitis: Thalamic hemorrhage
- DWI: Diffusion restriction common/earliest finding
- T1 C+: Variable enhancement, none to intense
  - Meningeal enhancement can be seen
  - Herpes zoster oticus (Ramsay Hunt syndrome): Enhancing CNVII, CNVIII, membranous labyrinth
  - EV-D68: Ventral cauda equina and ventral cervical nerve root enhancement subacutely > 2 days
- MRS: May help distinguish encephalitis from infarct
- **MR Findings in COVID-19**
  - Infarcts: Thrombotic and vasculitis patterns
  - Hypoxic ischemic encephalopathy (HIE)
  - Delayed posthypoxic leukoencephalopathy (DPHL)
  - Cerebral venous sinus thrombosis
  - Brain hemorrhage
  - Hemorrhagic posterior reversible encephalopathy syndrome (PRES)
  - Critical illness-associated cerebral microbleeds
  - Acute hemorrhagic necrotizing encephalopathy (AHNE)
  - ANE
  - Acute hemorrhagic leukoencephalopathy (AHLE/Weston Hurst syndrome)
  - Meningoencephalitis
  - Leukoencephalopathy
  - Olfactory bulb signal abnormality
  - Miller Fisher syndrome
  - Acute disseminated encephalomyelitis (ADEM)

- Leukoencephalopathy with bilateral reticular formation involvement
- Collicular hyperactivation
- Virus-associated necrotizing disseminated acute leukoencephalopathy (VANDAL)
- Flare-up/exacerbation of infections (due to immunosuppression)

Imaging Recommendations

- Protocol advice
  - Multiplanar MR with FLAIR, DWI, and contrast

DIFFERENTIAL DIAGNOSIS

Acute Ischemia

- Typical vascular distribution, DWI positive

Autoimmune Encephalitis

- Subcortical WM, limbic encephalitis, or scattered

Herpes Encephalitis

- Limbic system and temporal lobe involvement

Status Epilepticus

- Active seizures with cerebral hyperperfusion, blood-brain barrier disruption cause abnormal signal and enhancement

Toxic/Metabolic Lesions

- Symmetric BG or thalamic involvement common

PATHOLOGY

General Features

- Etiology
  - Most (but not all) caused by viruses
    - Viruses obligate intracellular parasites
    - Replicate in skin or mucous membranes of respiratory, gastrointestinal tracts
    - Spread of virus to CNS hematogenous or neural
    - Some invade along CNS (i.e., HSV1 via lingual nerve to trigeminal ganglia)
    - Latent infections may reactivate, spread along meningeal branches
  - **Herpesviruses** include HSV1, HSV2, CMV, EBV, VZV, B virus, HHV6, HHV7, HHV8
    - HSV1: Encephalitis (adult/child); HSV2: Neonatal
  - **Varicella**: Meningoencephalitis, cerebellar ataxia, and aseptic meningitis (< 1% of patients)
  - **Zoster infection**: Encephalitis, neuritis, myelitis, or herpes ophthalmicus
    - Latent virus in ganglia of CN (often CNV and CNVII) can reactivate, spread to brainstem
    - Immunocompetent patients: Cranial and peripheral nerve palsies
    - Immunosuppressed patients: Diffuse encephalitis
    - Herpes zoster ophthalmicus can cause internal carotid artery necrotizing angiitis
  - **EBV**: Agent in infectious mononucleosis
    - Diffuse encephalitis seen in < 1% of patients
    - Associated with meningoencephalitis, Guillain-Barré syndrome, transverse myelitis
  - **EVs** include coxsackieviruses A and B, poliovirus, echoviruses, EVs 68-71
  - **Arboviruses** (arthropod-borne viruses) include Eastern, Western, and Venezuelan equine encephalitis, St. Louis encephalitis, Japanese B encephalitis, California encephalitis, tick-borne encephalitis
  - **Nipah encephalitis**: Paramyxovirus related to close contact with infected pigs
    - Consuming fruits or sap contaminated by *Pteropus* genus large fruit bats (natural reservoir of virus)
    - Close physical contact with Nipah virus patients
    - Nipah encephalitis: Inflammation of small blood vessels with thrombosis and microinfarction
  - **Rhombencephalitis**: Viruses (most common), *Listeria monocytogenes*, *Legionella*, *Mycoplasma*, Lyme disease
  - **Cerebellitis**: Viruses: EVs, EBV, varicella, Coxsackie, influenza A and B, mumps, measles
    - Other causes: Lead, cyanide, methadone, vasculitis, ADEM

Gross Pathologic & Surgical Features

- Vascular congestion, generalized or local edema ± hemorrhage, necrosis

CLINICAL ISSUES

Presentation

- Most common signs/symptoms
  - Varicella and herpes zoster: Different clinical manifestations of infection by same virus (VZV)
    - **Varicella encephalitis**: Fever, headache, vomiting, seizures, altered mental status
      - Days to weeks after onset of chicken pox rash
    - **Zoster**: Immunocompetent, CN and peripheral nerve palsies in dermatomes involved by skin lesions
      - CNV, ophthalmic branch most affected (herpes zoster ophthalmicus)
  - **Zoster**: Immunosuppressed patient with fever, meningismus, altered mental status
  - **Cerebellitis**: Sudden onset of limb &/or gait ataxia after infectious prodrome
  - EV encephalitis (**EV 71**)
    - Hand, foot, and mouth disease (HFMD): Fever, vesicles on hands, feet, elbows, knees, lips
    - Cranial neuropathies, ocular disturbance, dyspnea, tachycardia if brainstem involved
  - **EV-D68**-associated anterior myelitis: **Pediatric acute flaccid paralysis**
  - **Nipah virus**: Fever, headache, dizziness, vomiting, myoclonus, areflexia, hypotonia, hypertension
  - **MVE**: Fever, headache, confusion, tremors; may progress to paralysis, coma, respiratory failure
  - **Rabies** (encephalitic): Fever, malaise, altered mental status, limbic dysfunction, autonomic stimulation
    - Paralytic: Weakness of all extremities
  - **Rhombencephalitis**: Areflexia, ataxia, ophthalmoplegia
  - **St. Louis encephalitis**: Tremors, fever

SELECTED REFERENCES

1. Tan Y et al: Clinical and MRI differential analysis of autoimmune encephalitis and viral encephalitis. J Taibah Univ Med Sci. 18(2):271-8, 2023
2. El Beltagi AH et al: Spectrum of neuroimaging findings in COVID-19. Br J Radiol. 94(1117):20200812, 2021
3. Vattoth S et al: Critical illness-associated cerebral microbleeds in COVID-19. Neuroradiol J. 33(5):374-6, 2020

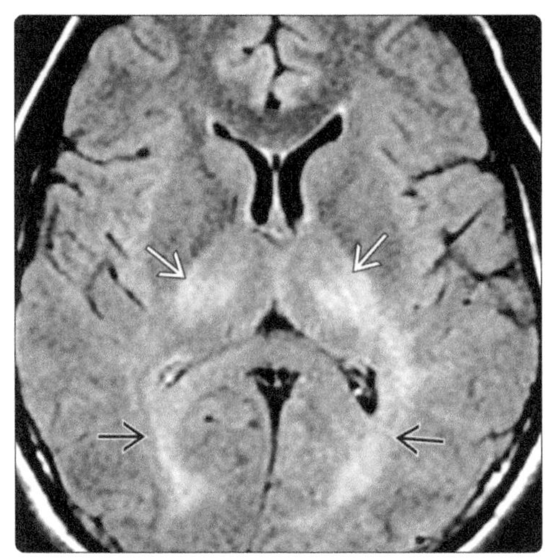

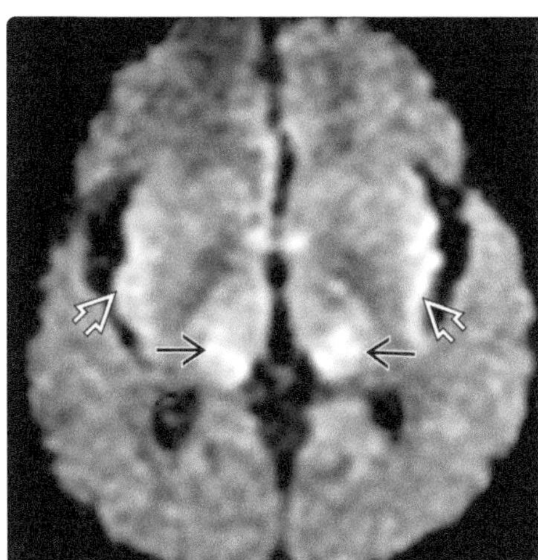

(Left) *Axial FLAIR MR shows symmetric hyperintense signal in the thalami ➡ and periventricular/deep WM ➡ in this patient with a history of infectious mononucleosis. EBV commonly involves the basal ganglia, thalami, cortex, &/or brainstem.* **(Right)** *Axial DWI MR shows symmetric diffusion restriction in the thalami ➡ and insula ➡ in a patient with West Nile virus encephalitis. Basal ganglia and thalamic involvement is classic for West Nile virus encephalitis. DWI detects lesions earlier than conventional MR.*

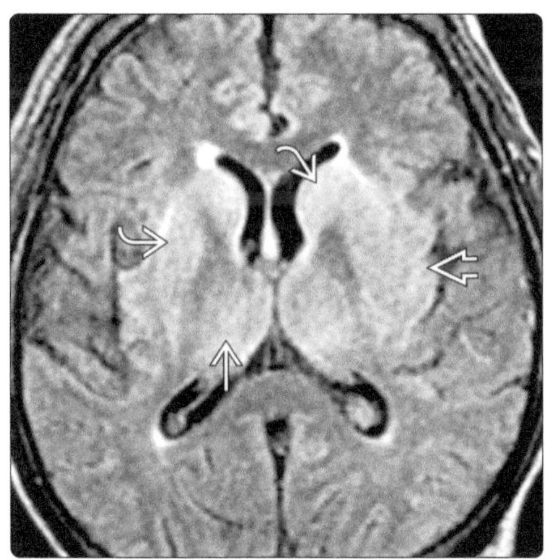

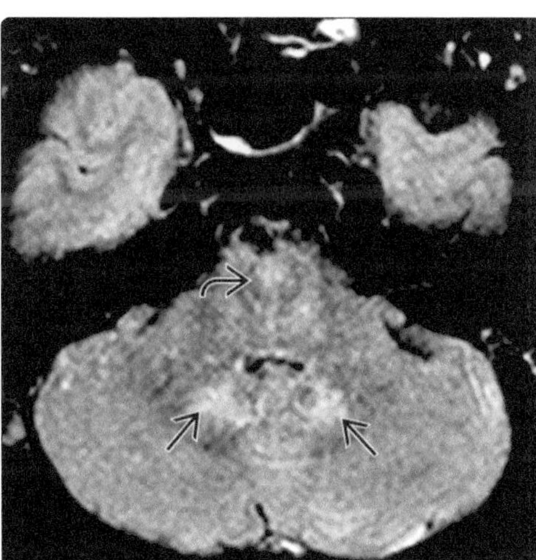

(Left) *Axial FLAIR MR in a patient with West Nile virus encephalitis shows symmetric abnormal hyperintensity in the basal ganglia ➡, thalami ➡, and insula ➡. The symmetric appearance of deep gray nuclei involvement mimics toxic and metabolic etiologies.* **(Right)** *Axial FLAIR MR of enterovirus encephalitis shows hyperintense signal in the medulla ➡ and dentate nuclei ➡. MR spine showed diffuse cervical cord involvement (not shown). Enteroviruses include coxsackieviruses, poliovirus, echovirus, and enteroviruses 68-71.*

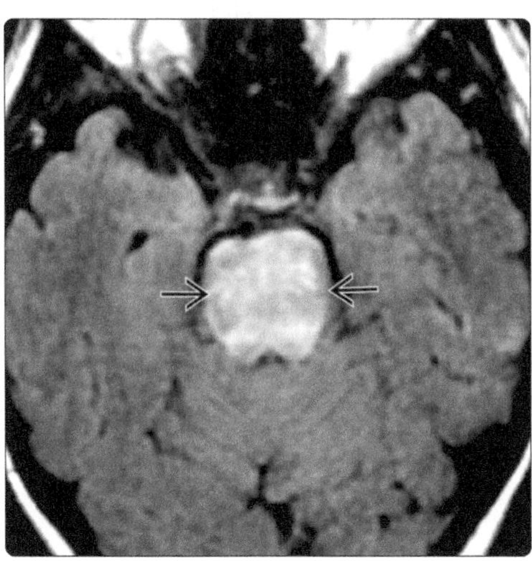

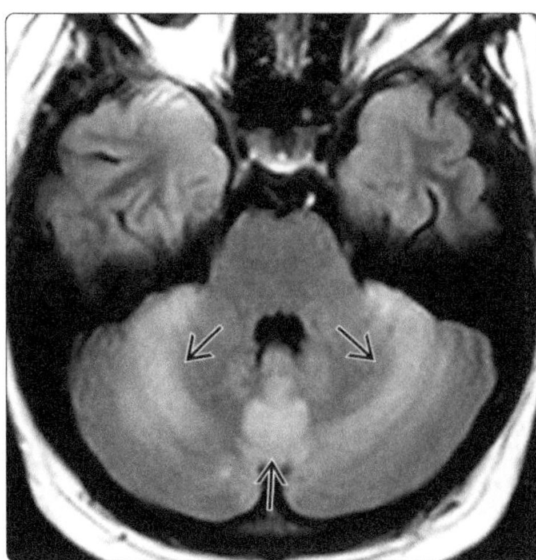

(Left) *Axial FLAIR MR in a patient with ataxia shows diffuse hyperintensity and enlargement of brainstem ➡. Rhombencephalitis is often caused by viruses; other pathogens include Listeria monocytogenes, Legionnaire, Mycoplasma, Lyme disease.* **(Right)** *Axial FLAIR MR shows hyperintensity in cerebellar hemispheres and vermis ➡, suggestive of cerebellitis. Usual etiology includes viruses (enteroviruses, EBV, varicella, Coxsackie, influenza, mumps, measles), intoxication (lead, cyanide, methadone), vasculitis, and ADEM.*

KEY FACTS

TERMINOLOGY

- Chronic focal (localized) encephalitis
- Chronic, progressive, unilateral brain inflammation of uncertain etiology
- Characterized by drug-resistant focal epilepsy, progressive hemiplegia, cognitive decline
- Classically considered to be childhood encephalopathy
  - Unusually, adolescent-/adult-onset variant forms seen

IMAGING

- Unilateral progressive cortical atrophy
- CT/MR: Normal → cortical swelling → atrophy
- Usually unilateral, predominantly frontoinsular/parietal
- Crossed cerebellar diaschisis
- Best imaging tools: MR with contrast, ± PET (FDG)

TOP DIFFERENTIAL DIAGNOSES

- Sturge-Weber syndrome
- Other autoimmune encephalitides (often bilateral)
- Dyke-Davidoff-Masson syndrome

PATHOLOGY

- Hemispheric cortical atrophy
- Cortical inflammation, neuronal loss, gliosis

CLINICAL ISSUES

- Intractable partial epilepsy, clonic movements
  - Other: Hemiparesis, visual and sensory deficits, dysarthria, dysphasia, personality changes
- Partial complex seizures that ↑ in frequency → 20% present in status epilepticus
- Surgery only definitive treatment of seizures in RE

DIAGNOSTIC CHECKLIST

- Consider RE when/if
  - ↑ frequency of partial complex seizures, postictal deficit in patients (1-15 years) with initial "normal" imaging
  - Intractable epilepsy with progressive atrophy of one hemisphere showing high T2 signal

(Left) *Coronal FLAIR MR in a patient with Rasmussen encephalitis shows right, predominantly perisylvian opercular/frontotemporal atrophy with dilated sylvian fissure ⇒ & temporal horn of right lateral ventricle ⇒. There is also atrophy of right basal ganglia with slightly increased FLAIR signal ⇒ & ex vacuo dilation of right frontal horn ⇒.* **(Right)** *Coronal FLAIR MR more posteriorly shows right temporoparietal atrophy ⇒ & left cerebellar atrophy & hyperintense signal (crossed cerebellar diaschisis) ⇒.*

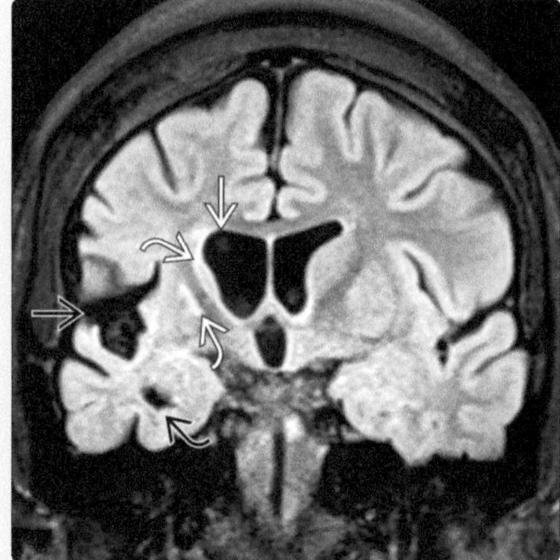

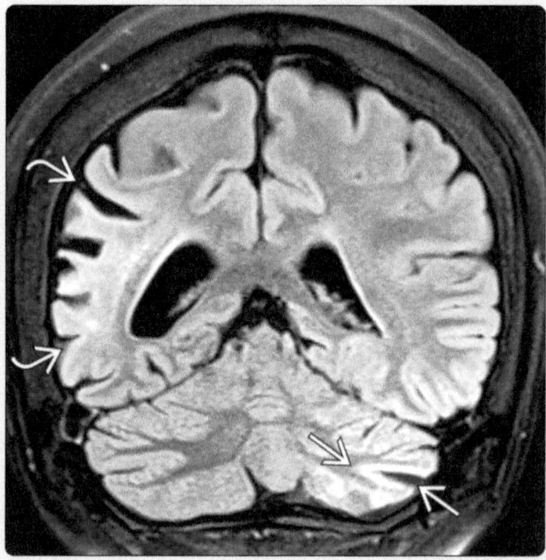

(Left) *Right lateral parasagittal FLAIR MR in the same patient shows the perisylvian atrophic changes with an enlarged right sylvian fissure ⇒. Note the normal right lateral cerebellar hemisphere ⇒.* **(Right)** *Left lateral parasagittal FLAIR MR in the same patient shows normal left cerebral hemisphere with a normal-sized left sylvian fissure ⇒. Note the left-sided crossed cerebellar diaschisis with an atrophic & slightly hyperintense left lateral cerebellar hemisphere ⇒.*

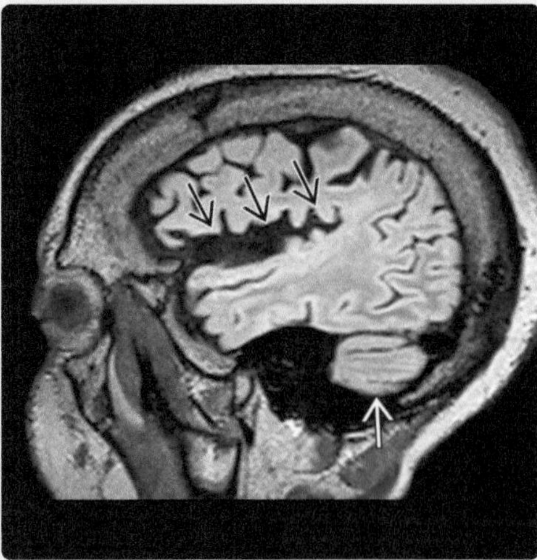

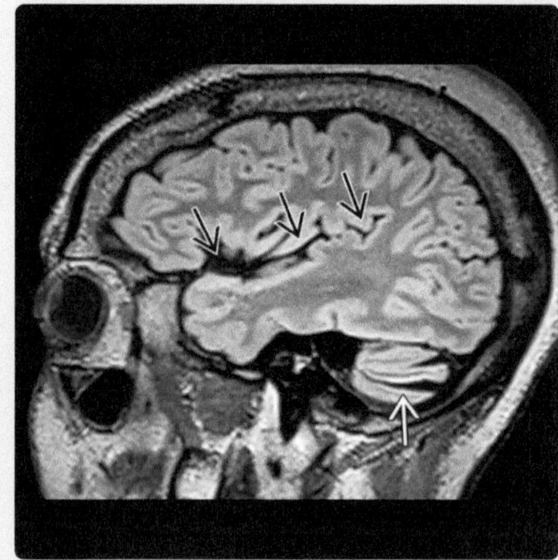

TERMINOLOGY

Abbreviations

- Rasmussen encephalitis (RE)

Synonyms

- Chronic focal (localized) encephalitis

Definitions

- Chronic, progressive, unilateral brain inflammation of uncertain etiology
- Characterized by hemispheric volume loss and difficulty controlling focal seizure activity

IMAGING

General Features

- Best diagnostic clue
  - Unilateral progressive cerebral atrophy
  - CT/MR often normal initially
    - Early cortical swelling, then cortical/subcortical T2/FLAIR hyperintensity with atrophy ensues
    - Most cerebral damage occurs in first 8-12 months after clinical onset of disease
- Location
  - Cerebral hemisphere
  - Usually unilateral, predominantly frontal/insular and parietal
    - Precentral, inferior frontal atrophy
      - Contralateral cerebellar volume loss (crossed cerebellar diaschisis)
- Size
  - Variable, usually lobar, occasionally entire hemisphere affected
- Morphology
  - Focal abnormality, "spreads across hemisphere"
  - Becomes progressively more diffuse

CT Findings

- NECT
  - Initially normal, → atrophy
- CECT
  - Usually no enhancement
  - **Rare** transient pial &/or cortical enhancement

MR Findings

- T1WI
  - Sulcal effacement due to early swelling
- T2WI
  - Early focal swelling of gyri
    - Gray matter-white matter (GM-WM) "blurring" and T2 prolongation
    - ± basal ganglia, hippocampi involvement
  - Late: Atrophy of involved cerebral hemisphere or lobe
- FLAIR
  - Cortical and subcortical areas of hyperintensity that progressively ↑ over time
  - Late: Atrophy, encephalomalacia/gliosis
- T2* GRE
  - Typically normal
  - Nonhemorrhagic
- DWI
  - Subtle high signal on trace images; ↑ diffusivity
- T1WI C+
  - Usually does not enhance
    - Occasionally, subtle pial &/or cortical enhancement
- MRS
  - ↓ NAA and choline; ↑ myoinositol, ↑ glutamine/glutamate

Nuclear Medicine Findings

- Tc-99m HMPAO scintigraphy: ↓ perfusion even if normal MR
- PET/SPECT
  - ↓ diffuse hemispheric metabolism/perfusion
  - Crossed cerebellar diaschisis
  - Transient hypermetabolism may be related to recent seizures (rare)
    - C-11 methionine shows ↑ multifocal uptake

Imaging Recommendations

- Best imaging tool
  - MR + clinical signs/symptoms + appropriate EEG findings
- Protocol advice
  - MR with contrast, ± PET (FDG)

DIFFERENTIAL DIAGNOSIS

Sturge-Weber Syndrome

- Port-wine facial nevus and enhancement of pial angioma
- Progressive hemispheric atrophy
- Cortical Ca^{++}

Mitochondrial Encephalopathy, Lactic Acidosis, and Stroke-Like Episodes

- Acute: May cause cortical hyperintensity (parietooccipital most common) + DWI
- Chronic: Cortical atrophy, lacunes (basal ganglia, thalami)

Dyke-Davidoff-Masson (Prenatal/Neonatal Hemispheric Insult)

- Unilateral brain atrophy following fetal/perinatal/early childhood infarct or other insult
- Compensatory calvarial thickening
- Elevated petrous ridge and hyperaerated paranasal sinuses

Focal Cortical Dysplasia

- May cause hemispheric status epilepticus, resulting in unilateral volume loss

Other Autoimmune Inflammatory Disorders

- Unilateral cerebral vasculitis, paraneoplastic syndromes, onconeural antibodies
- Rasmussen-like encephalitis in anti-NMDA receptor antibody-positive patients reported

PATHOLOGY

General Features

- Etiology
  - Etiology and pathogenesis of RE remains unknown
  - Evidence for immunopathologic basis growing
    - Antibody-mediated, T-cell cytotoxicity and microglial-induced degeneration
- Genetics

- Possibly viral trigger of genetic predisposition to immunodysfunction
- Associated abnormalities
  - 3 potentially overlapping factors may initiate or perpetuate events leading to injury
    - Viral infection
    - Autoimmune antibodies
    - Autoimmune cytotoxic T lymphocytes

Staging, Grading, & Classification

- 3 disease stages of RE
  - Prodromal stage: Nonspecific, low seizure frequency, and mild hemiplegia
  - Acute stage: Frequent seizures, often epilepsia partialis continua, progressive hemiparesis, cognitive decline
  - Residual stage: Permanent and stable neurologic deficits and continuing seizures
- Classification and staging: MR (T2WI)
  - Stage 1: Swelling/hyperintense signal
  - Stage 2: Normal volume/hyperintense signal
  - Stage 3: Atrophy/hyperintense signal
  - Stage 4: Progressive atrophy and normal signal

Gross Pathologic & Surgical Features

- Hemispheric cortical atrophy
- Area of damage often surrounded by normal cortex or mild inflammation
  - Biopsy can be misleading

Microscopic Features

- Robitaille classification describes cortical inflammation, neuronal loss, and gliosis confined to 1 hemisphere
  - Group 1 (pathologically active): Ongoing inflammatory process
    - Microglial nodules, ± neuronophagia, perivascular round cells
  - Group 2 (active and remote disease): Acute on chronic
    - Above + ≥ 1 gyral segment of complete necrosis and cavitation, including full-thickness cortex
  - Group 3 (less active "remote" disease)
    - Neuronal loss/gliosis and fewer microglial nodules
  - Group 4 (burnt out)
    - Nonspecific scarring with little active inflammation

CLINICAL ISSUES

Presentation

- Most common signs/symptoms
  - Intractable epilepsy, clonic movements
  - Progresses to epilepsia partialis continua
  - Other: Hemiparesis, visual and sensory deficits, dysarthria, dysphasia, personality changes
- Clinical profile
  - Young child with progressive partial epilepsy unresponsive to medical therapy
  - Unusual late-onset adolescent and adult forms described
- Clinical course
  - Partial complex seizures that ↑ in frequency
  - 20% present in status epilepticus
  - Followed by worsening seizures, progressive hemiparesis, cognitive deterioration, death
  - **Late-onset forms** show more frequent focal complex partial seizures and less frequent epilepsia partialis continua
  - T2/FLAIR hyperintensity in paramedian frontal or insular cortex may antedate or simultaneously occur with epilepsia partialis continua
- EEG: Initial normal to persistent unilateral slowing ± epileptiform activity
- CSF: ± oligoclonal bands

Demographics

- Age
  - Usually begins in childhood (6-8 years)
  - 10% present as late-onset adolescent or adult forms
- Sex
  - M = F; M:F = 4:1 in late-onset forms
- Ethnicity
  - No predilection
- Epidemiology
  - Preceded by inflammatory episode (50%)
    - Tonsillitis, upper respiratory infection, otitis media

Natural History & Prognosis

- Hemiplegia and cognitive deterioration in most cases
- Prognosis poor
- Hemiplegia inevitable ± treatment
- Late-onset forms have longer prodromal stage and delayed occurrence of cortical deficit
  - Less cognitive deterioration, better outcome

Treatment

- Refractory to antiepileptic medications
- ± transient improvement with plasma exchange, IVIG therapy, steroids, B-cell and T-cell directed agents
- Immunomodulatory treatment even in late stages improves 2/3 of late-onset cases
- Surgery only definitive treatment of seizures in RE
  - Functional hemispherectomy/central disconnection
  - Hemispherotomy
- Functional MR may demonstrate motor functions relocated to contralateral hemisphere after hemispherectomy

DIAGNOSTIC CHECKLIST

Image Interpretation Pearls

- Consider RE
  - ↑ frequency of partial complex seizures + postictal deficit in patients with **initial "normal" imaging**
  - Intractable epilepsy with progressive atrophy of one hemisphere showing high T2 signal

SELECTED REFERENCES

1. Jaafar F et al: Role of early intravenous immunoglobulins in halting clinical and radiographic disease progression in Rasmussen encephalitis. Pediatr Neurol. 145:30-5, 2023
2. Jagtap SA et al: Epilepsia partialis continua and unilateral cortical-subcortical FLAIR-hyperintense lesion in Rasmussen's encephalitis: is it diagnostic? Epileptic Disord. 25(3):321-30, 2023
3. Foster MT et al: Motor cortex relocation after complete anatomical hemispherectomy for intractable epilepsy secondary to Rasmussen's encephalitis. Br J Neurosurg. 1-3, 2019
4. Dupont S et al: Late-onset Rasmussen encephalitis: a literature appraisal. Autoimmun Rev. 16(8):803-10, 2017
5. Gurcharran K et al: Anti-N-methyl-D-aspartate receptor encephalitis and Rasmussen-like syndrome: an association? Pediatr Neurol. 66:104-7, 2017

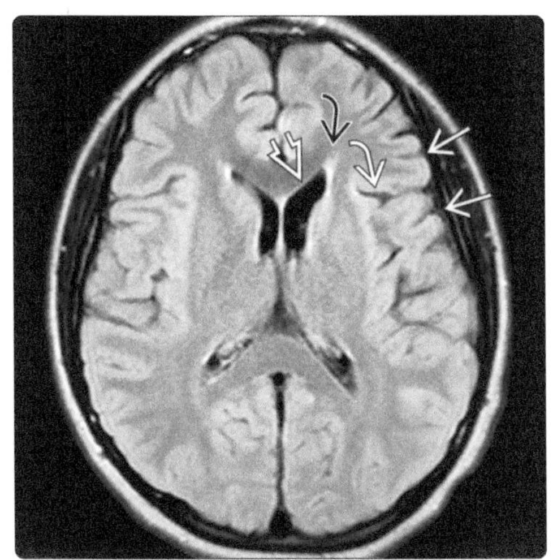

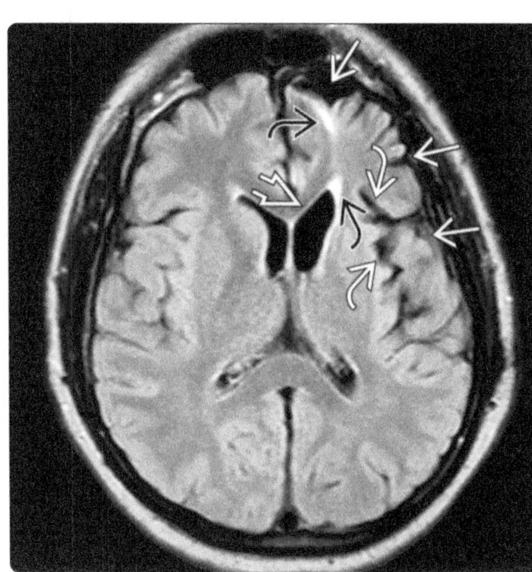

(Left) *Axial FLAIR MR in a child with Rasmussen encephalitis shows subtle prominence of left frontal sulci, adjacent left sylvian fissure, & the left lateral ventricle frontal horn. Subtle focal left periventricular hyperintensity is noted.* **(Right)** *Axial FLAIR MR in the same patient on follow-up shows further increased ex vacuo dilation of the left frontal sulci, adjacent left sylvian fissure, & left frontal horn. Also note the left frontal increasing hyperintense signal.*

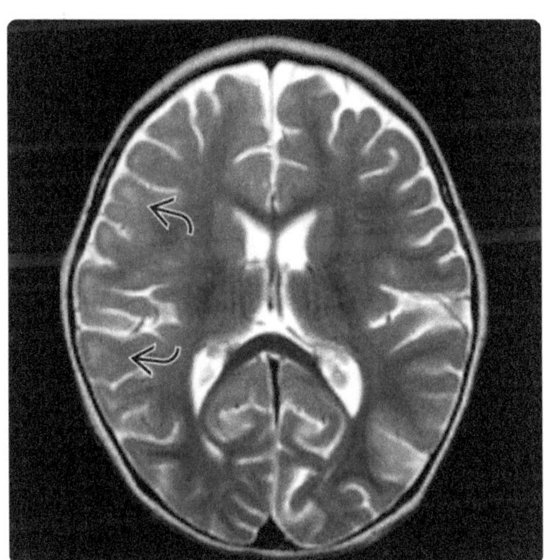

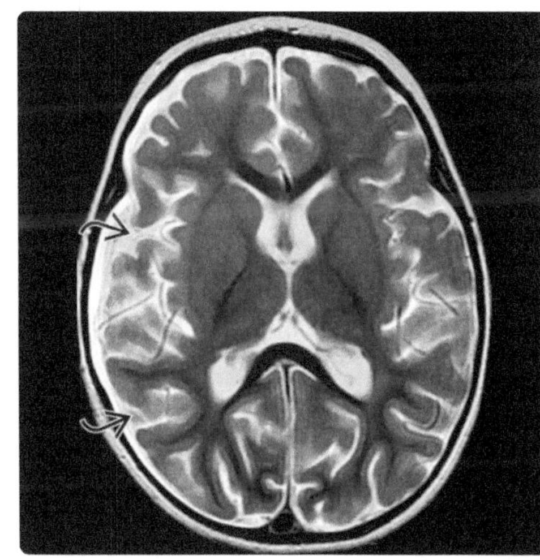

(Left) *Axial T2WI MR in a 1-year-old with drug-resistant focal seizures & progressive left hemiparesis demonstrates subtle T2 hyperintensity in the right frontoparietal subcortical white matter.* **(Right)** *Axial T2WI MR in the same patient after 1 month shows marked right hemisphere volume loss with prominence of the sulci. Serial MR in Rasmussen encephalitis shows progression of atrophy & cortical/subcortical signal change.*

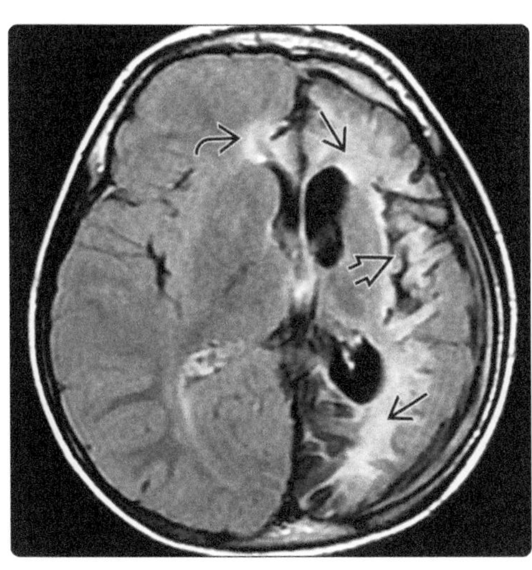

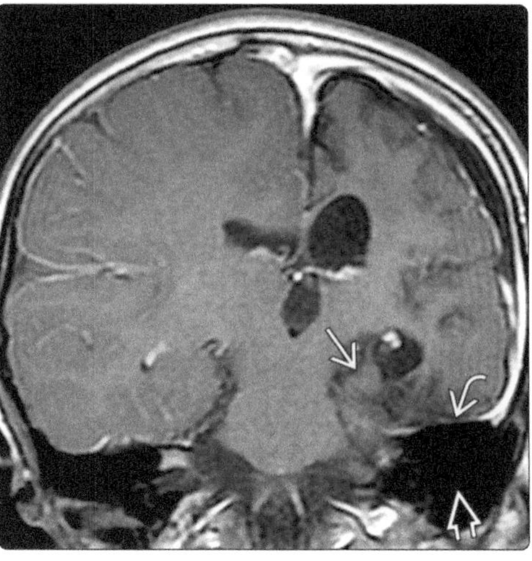

(Left) *Axial FLAIR MR shows atrophy of the left hemisphere & gliosis with FLAIR hyperintensity. Note the insular cortical & subcortical atrophy & involvement of the parasagittal right frontal cortex.* **(Right)** *Coronal T1 C+ MR shows extensive atrophy of the left hemisphere with profound left hippocampal volume loss. Note the compensatory hyperaeration of left mastoid air cells with elevation of the left middle cranial fossa floor in this chronic case of Rasmussen encephalitis.*

Subacute Sclerosing Panencephalitis

KEY FACTS

TERMINOLOGY

- Definition: Rare, progressive, measles virus-mediated encephalitis

IMAGING

- CT: Imaging often initially normal; cortical swelling, cortical/subcortical hypoattenuation
- MR: Ill-defined T2 hyperintensities in periventricular or subcortical white matter
    - Frontal > parietal > occipital; no mass effect
- MRS: ↑ choline and myoinositol; ↓ NAA (may precede MR abnormalities)

TOP DIFFERENTIAL DIAGNOSES

- Acute disseminated encephalomyelitis
- Tumefactive multiple sclerosis
- Human immunodeficiency virus
- Progressive multifocal leukoencephalopathy

PATHOLOGY

- Postinfectious progressive encephalitis years after measles infection

CLINICAL ISSUES

- Behavioral changes, mental deterioration, ataxia, myoclonus, and visual disturbances
- Begins insidiously; subacute course; death (1-3 years after symptom onset)
- Positive CSF, plasma complement fixation test for measles; CSF plus oligoclonal bands

DIAGNOSTIC CHECKLIST

- Consider subacute sclerosing panencephalitis (SSPE) in unvaccinated child with behavioral changes and multifocal white matter disease
- SSPE incidence may be underrecognized in context of ↓ vaccination rates

(Left) *Axial T2 MR in a 7-year-old boy with behavioral changes and mental deterioration reveals asymmetric right peritrigonal demyelination ➡.* **(Right)** *Axial T2 MR in the same patient 6 months later now demonstrates progressive demyelination involving the bilateral frontal and parietooccipital regions ➡.*

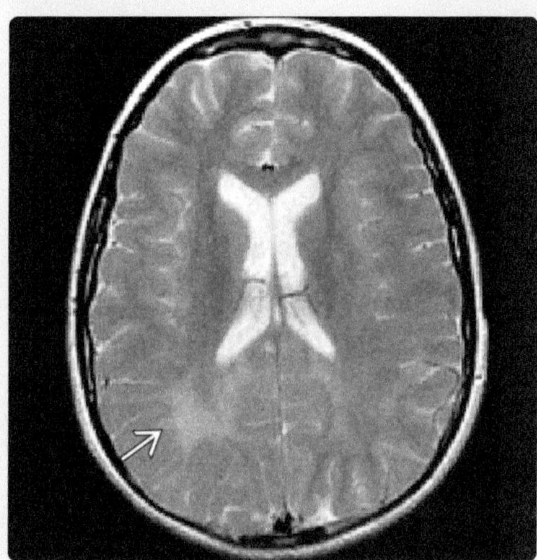

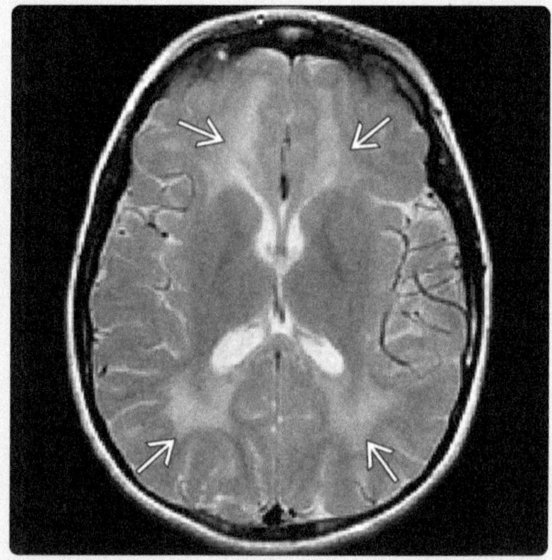

(Left) *Coronal FLAIR MR in the same patient 6 months after initial presentation demonstrates progressive frontal lobe white matter FLAIR hyperintensity ➡. CSF complement fixation test for measles confirmed the diagnosis.* **(Right)** *Axial FLAIR MR in the same patient 10 months after initial clinical presentation with progressive cognitive deterioration and worsening myoclonus shows bilateral frontal lobe white matter volume loss and FLAIR hyperintensity ➡ representing demyelination and gliosis.*

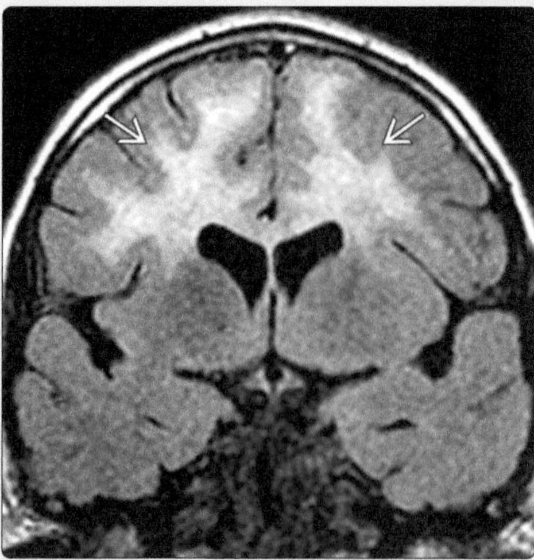

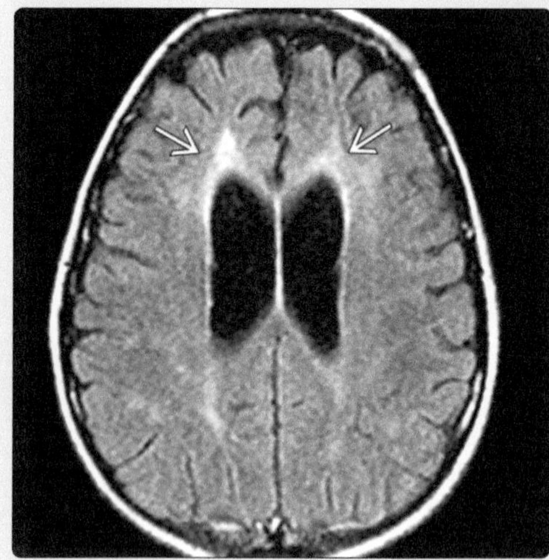

TERMINOLOGY

Abbreviations

- Subacute sclerosing panencephalitis (SSPE)

Definitions

- Progressive measles virus-mediated encephalitis

IMAGING

General Features

- Best diagnostic clue
  - T2 hyperintensities in periventricular, deep, or subcortical white matter (WM)
- Location
  - Frontal > parietal > occipital lobes

CT Findings

- NECT
  - Imaging often initially normal; later cortical swelling, cortical/subcortical hypoattenuation

MR Findings

- T1WI
  - Areas of ↓ signal in WM, corpus callosum
- T2WI
  - ↑ signal in WM, frontal > parietal > occipital, generally symmetric and eventually leading to diffuse atrophy
- DWI
  - Diffusion tensor imaging reveals ↓ anisotropy in associative tracts
- T1WI C+
  - No enhancement

Imaging Recommendations

- Best imaging tool
  - Brain MR + intravenous contrast

DIFFERENTIAL DIAGNOSIS

Acute Disseminated Encephalomyelitis

- Prior viral illness, peripheral areas of ↑ T2 signal
- Often deep nuclei gray matter involvement

Tumefactive Multiple Sclerosis

- Mass-like lesions in periventricular WM, perimeter enhancement

Human Immunodeficiency Virus

- Atrophy, ill-defined areas of ↑ T2 signal in WM
- ↑ attenuation of basal ganglia (NECT)

Progressive Multifocal Leukoencephalopathy

- WM areas of ↑ T2 signal (includes subcortical WM) in immunocompromised (AIDS, cancer) patients

PATHOLOGY

General Features

- Etiology
  - Postinfectious progressive encephalitis; commences years after measles infection

Gross Pathologic & Surgical Features

- Early diffuse cerebral swelling; subcortical and periventricular WM, basal ganglia
- Rapidly progressive diffuse cortical atrophy

Microscopic Features

- Leptomeningeal, parenchymal, and perivascular inflammation
- Reactive gliosis with WM demyelination, intranuclear inclusions in neurons, and oligodendroglia

CLINICAL ISSUES

Presentation

- Most common signs/symptoms
  - Behavioral changes, mental deterioration, ataxia, myoclonus, and visual disturbances
- Clinical profile
  - Positive CSF, plasma complement fixation test for measles; CSF plus oligoclonal bands
  - EEG: Periodic complexes with generalized polyspike, high-voltage slow waves

Demographics

- Age
  - Childhood, early adolescence; rare in adults
- Epidemiology
  - History of measles before age 2 in most patients → 18x risk of developing SSPE
  - Incidence may be underrecognized in context of decreasing vaccination rates

Natural History & Prognosis

- Minor behavioral changes initially → motor dysfunction (myoclonic jerks) → death (1-3 years after symptom onset)
- May be misdiagnosed as psychiatric disorder initially

Treatment

- No curative treatment, but there are some benefits from intraventricular α-interferon and isoprinosine

DIAGNOSTIC CHECKLIST

Consider

- SSPE in unvaccinated child with behavioral changes and multifocal WM disease
- Incidence seems to be increasing in conjunction with reduced vaccination rates, measles resurgence

Image Interpretation Pearls

- MR findings correlate poorly with clinical stage

SELECTED REFERENCES

1. Campbell H et al: A re-emergence of subacute sclerosing panencephalitis in the United Kingdom. Pediatr Infect Dis J. 42(1):82-4, 2023
2. Tomasino B et al: Dissociations in white matter tracts and neuropsychological findings in a 17 years old patient with subacute sclerosing panencephalitis. Brain Cogn. 165:105941, 2023
3. Rocke Z et al: Subacute Sclerosing Panencephalitis. StatPearls, 2022
4. Wendorf KA et al: Subacute sclerosing panencephalitis: the devastating measles complication that might be more common than previously estimated. Clin Infect Dis. 65(2):226-32, 2017

KEY FACTS

TERMINOLOGY

- Typically causes tuberculous meningitis (TBM) &/or localized CNS infection, tuberculoma

IMAGING

- Basilar meningitis + extracerebral TB (pulmonary)
- Meningitis + parenchymal lesions highly suggestive
- Tuberculomas
  - Supratentorial parenchyma most common
  - Usually T2 hypointense
  - Enhances strongly (solid or ring enhancing)
- Tuberculous abscess: Multiloculated ring enhancement
- MR with FLAIR, DWI, FLAIR C+, T1 C+, ± MRA, MRS
- TB abscess has prominent lipid & lactate but no amino acid

TOP DIFFERENTIAL DIAGNOSES

- Meningitis
- Neurosarcoidosis
- Abscess
- Neoplasm

PATHOLOGY

- CNS TB almost always secondary (often pulmonary source)
- Meningitis = most frequent manifestation of CNS TB
  - More common in children

CLINICAL ISSUES

- Varies from mild meningitis with no neurologic deficit to coma
- Long-term morbidity in up to 80%: Intellectual disabilities, paralysis, seizures, rigidity, speech or visual deficits
- Mortality in 25-30% of patients; higher in AIDS patients
- Reemerging disease (immigration from endemic areas, AIDS, drug-resistant strains)
- TB-associated IRIS: Increased size of lesions, edema, & symptoms

DIAGNOSTIC CHECKLIST

- TB often mimics other diseases, such as neoplasm

(Left) *Coronal graphic shows basilar tuberculous meningitis (TBM) and tuberculomas ➙, which often coexist. Note the vessel irregularity and early basal ganglia ischemia related to arteritis.* **(Right)** *Axial T1 C+ FS MR in a patient with disseminated Mycobacterium bovis infection shows abnormal cisternal, cerebellar fissural and cerebral sulcal enhancement ➡. Multiple tiny enhancing brain parenchymal granulomatous nodules ➡ are seen. Also note the nodular enhancement of pituitary stalk ➡.*

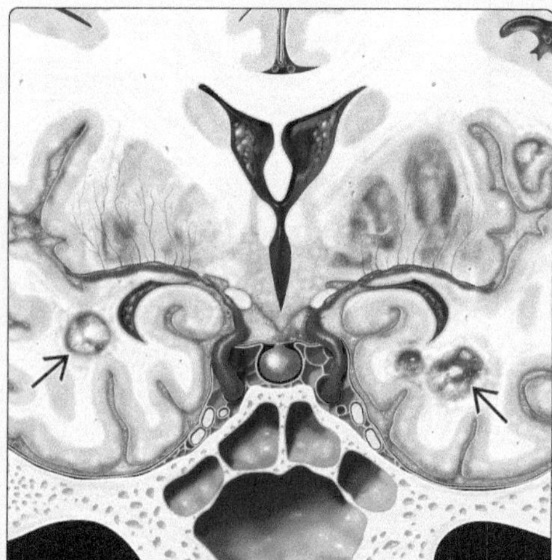

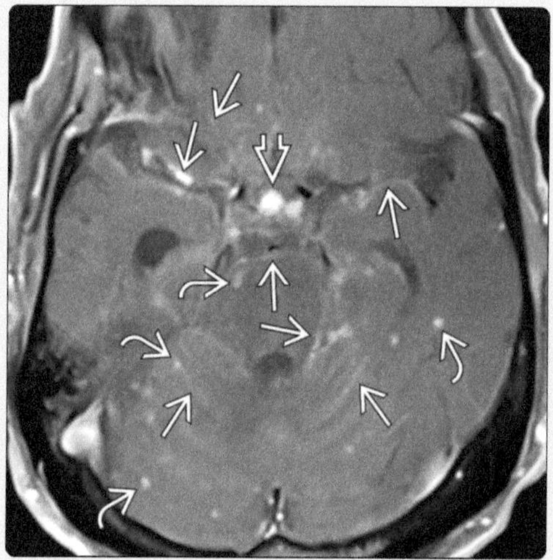

(Left) *Axial postcontrast FLAIR MR in a patient with TBM shows enhancement in the right sylvian cistern ➡ and adjacent sulci ➡. Note tiny hyperintense foci in the right insula ➙, external capsule ➙, and globus pallidus externa ➙, which could be tuberculomas or infarcts.* **(Right)** *Axial DWI MR in the same patient shows diffusion restriction in the areas of FLAIR hyperintensities, consistent with acute lacunar infarcts involving the right insula ➙, external capsule ➙, and globus pallidus externa ➙.*

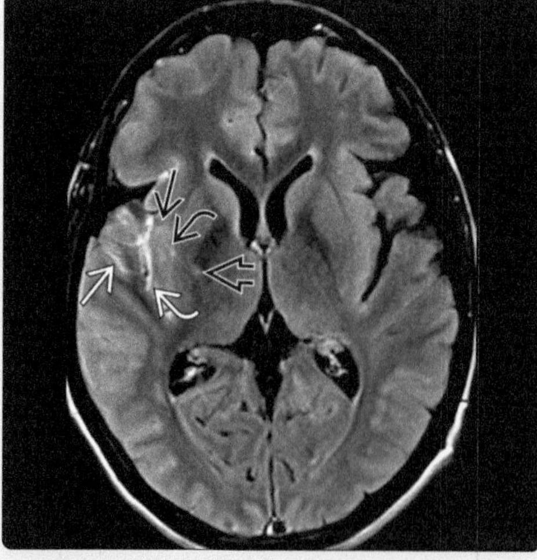

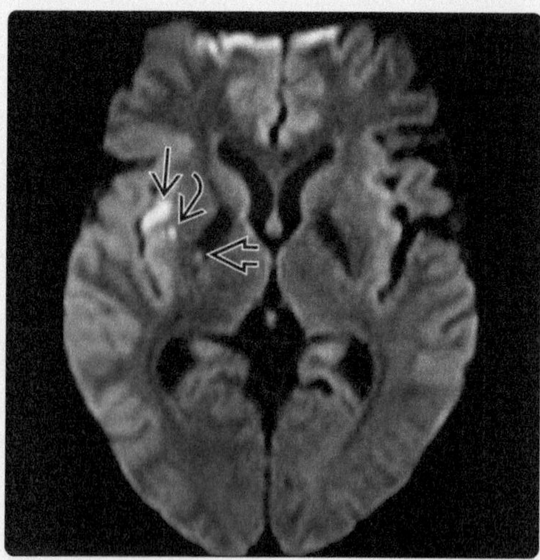

TERMINOLOGY

Abbreviations

- Tuberculosis (TB)

Definitions

- Infection by acid-fast bacillus *Mycobacterium tuberculosis*
- Other members of *M. tuberculosis* complex, such as *Mycobacterium bovis*, rarely cause CNS disease
- CNS TB almost always secondary to hematogenous spread (often pulmonary, rarely GI or GU tract)
  - Tuberculous meningitis (TBM) & parenchymal infection: Tuberculoma (common), TB abscess (rare)

IMAGING

General Features

- Best diagnostic clue
  - Basilar meningitis + extracerebral TB (pulmonary)
  - Meningitis + parenchymal lesions highly suggestive
- Location
  - Meningitis (basal cisterns > superficial sulci)
  - Tuberculomas
    - Typically parenchymal: Supratentorial most common
    - Cerebral hemispheres & basal ganglia
    - Cerebellum, brainstem, & hypothalamus can be involved
    - Dural tuberculomas may occur
    - Rarely, miliary pattern with innumerable tiny brain parenchymal lesions
    - Rarely, pituitary tuberculoma mimicking pituitary adenoma
- Size
  - Tuberculomas range from 1 mm to 6 cm
  - Rarely, giant tuberculoma mimicking tumor
  - Tuberculous abscess: Usually > 3 cm
  - **TB**-associated immune reconstitution inflammatory syndrome (**IRIS**)
    - Increased size of tuberculomas & edema
- Morphology
  - TBM: Thick basilar exudate
  - Tuberculoma: Round or oval mass
    - Solitary or multiple (more common)
  - Tuberculous abscess: Large, solitary, frequently multiloculated
- Associated findings
  - Spine most frequent osseous site: TB spondylitis (Pott disease)
  - Less common sites: Calvarium (± dura), otomastoid
  - TB cervical adenitis: Conglomerate nodal neck mass

CT Findings

- NECT
  - TBM: May be normal early (10-15%)
    - Isodense to hyperdense exudate effaces CSF spaces, fills basal cisterns, sulci
  - Tuberculoma
    - Hypodense to hyperdense round or lobulated nodule/mass with moderate to marked edema
    - Ca^{++} uncommon (~ 20%)
- CECT
  - TBM: Intense basilar meningeal enhancement
  - Tuberculoma: Solid or ring enhancing
    - Target sign: Central focus of enhancement + ring of peripheral enhancement
  - Tuberculous abscess: Solitary, often multiloculated ring enhancing

MR Findings

- T1WI
  - TBM: Exudate isointense or hyperintense to CSF
  - Tuberculoma
    - **Noncaseating** granuloma: Hypointense to brain
    - **Caseating** granuloma
      - **Solid center**: Hypointense or isointense
      - **Necrotic center**: Central hypointensity; may have hyperintense rim (paramagnetic material)
- T2WI
  - TBM: Exudate isointense or hyperintense to CSF; may see low-signal nodules (rare)
  - Tuberculoma
    - **Noncaseating** granuloma: Hyperintense to brain
    - **Caseating** granuloma: Hypointense rim
      - **Solid center**: Usually hypointense
      - **Necrotic center**: Hyperintense; may have hypointense rim
    - Surrounding edema common
  - Tuberculous **abscess**: Hyperintense lesion with hypointense rim & marked vasogenic edema
- FLAIR
  - TBM: Increased intensity in basal cisterns, sulci
  - Tuberculoma & tuberculous abscess: Similar to T2
  - **Postcontrast FLAIR** accentuates meningeal enhancement in meningitis due to any etiology
- DWI
  - May show hyperintense center of tuberculoma
  - **Restricted diffusion** in tuberculous **abscess**
  - Helpful for detecting complications (infarcts, cerebritis)
  - **Infarcts** most common in **basal ganglia**, cerebral cortex, pons, cerebellum
- PWI
  - Ring-enhancing **tuberculoma wall** shows mildly elevated mean relative cerebral blood volume (**rCBV**) values (2-3.3)
    - Also entire nodular enhancing tuberculoma
  - Helps differentiate from lower mean rCBV of neurocysticercosis (NCC) wall (1.3)
  - Cutoff value of **wall rCBV 1.965 for tuberculoma**: 90% sensitivity & 100% specificity
  - **Core** of tuberculoma & NCC rCBV < normal white matter (WM)
  - Metastasis wall show more elevated mean rCBV (5.43)
    - Cut-off value of ≥ **3.745 for** differentiating ring-enhancing **metastases** from tuberculomas
- T1WI C+
  - TBM: Marked meningeal enhancement, basilar prominence; may be nodular
    - Punctate/linear basal ganglia enhancement = vasculitis
    - Rare: Ventriculitis, choroid plexitis
    - Rare: Pachymeningitis with dural thickening, enhancement (may mimic meningioma)

- Tuberculomas
  - **Noncaseating** granuloma: Nodular, homogeneous enhancement
  - **Caseating** granuloma: Peripheral rim enhancement
    - Necrotic center shows low signal
- Tuberculous **abscess**: Multiloculated ring enhancement
- MRA
  - May see vessel narrowing, irregularity, occlusion
  - Due to **arteritis** or **vasospasm**
  - Lenticulostriate arteries, middle cerebral arteries, thalamoperforators
- MRS
  - TB abscess has prominent lipid & lactate but no amino acid resonances
    - Lipids at 0.9 ppm, 1.3 ppm, 2.0 ppm, 2.8 ppm
- **Complications**: Hydrocephalus, ischemia
- **Chronic changes**: Atrophy, Ca^{++}, chronic ischemia

Imaging Recommendations

- Best imaging tool
  - MR with FLAIR, DWI, T1 C+, ± MRA, MRS

DIFFERENTIAL DIAGNOSIS

Meningitis

- Infectious meningitis (bacterial, fungal, viral, parasitic)
  - Coccidioidomycosis, cryptococcosis often basilar
- Carcinomatous meningitis (CNS or systemic primary) or lymphoma

Neurosarcoidosis

- Typically leptomeningeal &/or dural enhancement
- Rarely causes parenchymal nodules

Abscess

- Pyogenic abscess more edema, MRS amino acid peaks

Neoplasm

- Primary or metastatic tumors
- Thick, nodular enhancing wall, variable diffusivity

PATHOLOGY

General Features

- Etiology
  - *M. tuberculosis* most common
  - In early 20th century, *M. bovis* caused ~ 25% of TBM cases, especially in young children
    - Transmission mainly from cattle by consumption of unpasteurized milk
    - Incidence dramatically decreased following milk pasteurization & bovine TB surveillance
  - TBM pathophysiology
    - Penetration of meningeal vessel walls by hematogenous spread
    - Ruptured subependymal/subpial granulomas into CSF
  - Tuberculoma pathophysiology
    - Hematogenous spread (gray matter-WM junction lesions)
    - Extension of meningitis into parenchyma via cortical veins or small penetrating arteries
  - Arteries directly involved by basilar exudate or indirectly by reactive arteritis/vasospasm

Gross Pathologic & Surgical Features

- TBM: Thick, gelatinous cisternal exudate
- Tuberculoma: Noncaseating, caseating with solid center, or caseating with necrotic center
  - Rarely progresses to TB abscess
- Tuberculous abscess: Rare encapsulated collection of pus with abundant viable tubercle bacilli

Microscopic Features

- TBM: Inflammatory cells, fragile neocapillaries
  - Caseous necrosis, chronic granulomas, endarteritis, perivascular inflammatory changes
- Tuberculoma
  - Early capsule: Peripheral fibroblasts, epithelioid cells, Langerhans giant cells, lymphocytes
  - Late capsule: Thick collagen layer, central liquefied caseating material in mature tuberculoma

CLINICAL ISSUES

Presentation

- Clinical profile
  - LP: Increased protein, pleocytosis (lymphocytes), low glucose, negative for organisms
    - CSF positive on initial LP in < 40%
    - Mycobacteria grow slowly; culture 6-8 weeks
    - PCR for TB may help confirm diagnosis earlier

Natural History & Prognosis

- Long-term morbidity in up to 80%: Intellectual disabilities, paralysis, seizures, rigidity, speech or visual deficits
- Mortality in 25-30% of patients; higher in AIDS patients
- Complications: Hydrocephalus (70%), stroke (up to 40%), cranial neuropathies (CNIII, CNIV, CNVI common), syrinx
- Tuberculomas may take months to years to resolve
- TB-associated IRIS shows worsening inflammatory response
  - While on antituberculous treatment after initiation of HIV antiretroviral therapy
- IRIS can occur with other HIV coinfections, e.g., progressive multifocal leukoencephalopathy (PML) & cryptococcosis
- Also reported in non-HIV immunocompromised states

Treatment

- Untreated TBM can be fatal in 4-8 weeks
- Multidrug therapy required: Isoniazid, rifampin, pyrazinamide, ± ethambutol or streptomycin
- Hydrocephalus typically requires CSF diversion
- Corticosteroids for IRIS

DIAGNOSTIC CHECKLIST

Image Interpretation Pearls

- Meningitis + parenchymal lesions: Consider TB

SELECTED REFERENCES

1. Aziz Khan A et al: Pituitary tuberculoma with panhypopituitarism masquerading as a pituitary adenoma. Neuropathology. 43(6):496-9, 2023
2. Mahomed N et al: Tuberculosis revisted: classic imaging findings in childhood. Pediatr Radiol. 53(9):1799-828, 2023
3. Clifford KM et al: Disseminated Mycobacterium bovis infection complicated by meningitis and stroke: a case report. Open Forum Infect Dis. 7(10):ofaa475, 2020
4. Ghosh RN et al: Perfusion magnetic resonance imaging in differentiation of neurocysticercosis and tuberculoma. Neuroradiology. 61(3):257-63, 2019

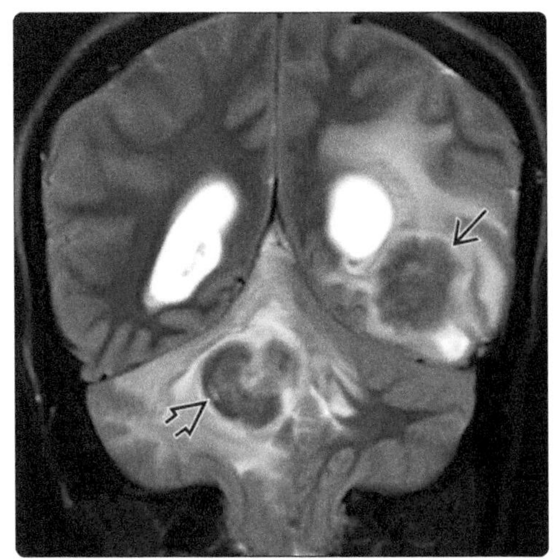

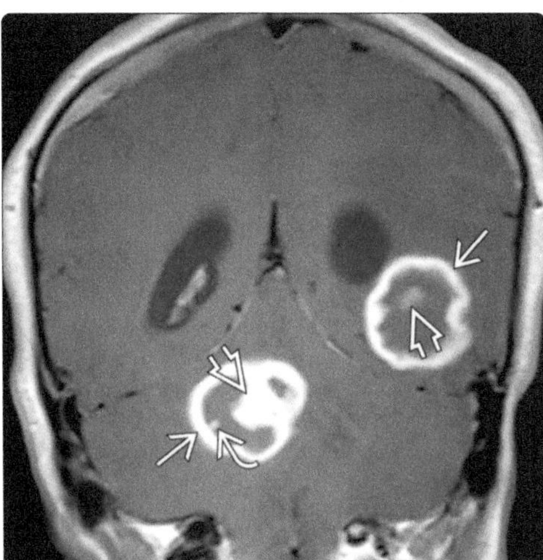

(Left) *Coronal T2 MR in a patient with left temporooccipital* ⇨ *and right cerebellar* ⇨ *tuberculomas shows large iso- to hypointense lesions with significant edema and hydrocephalus. There is mild right parietal WM edema due to another tuberculoma more anteriorly (not shown).* **(Right)** *Coronal T1 C+ MR in the same patient shows irregular, thick ring enhancement* → *with some internal punctate* ↷ *and nodular* ⇨ *enhancing foci. Giant tuberculomas can mimic primary or metastatic brain tumors on routine MR.*

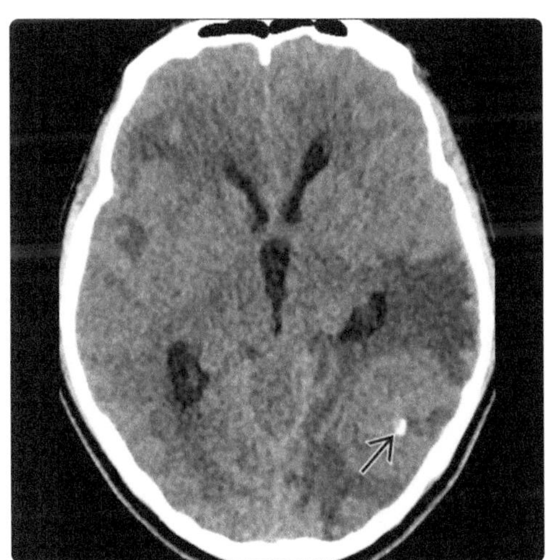

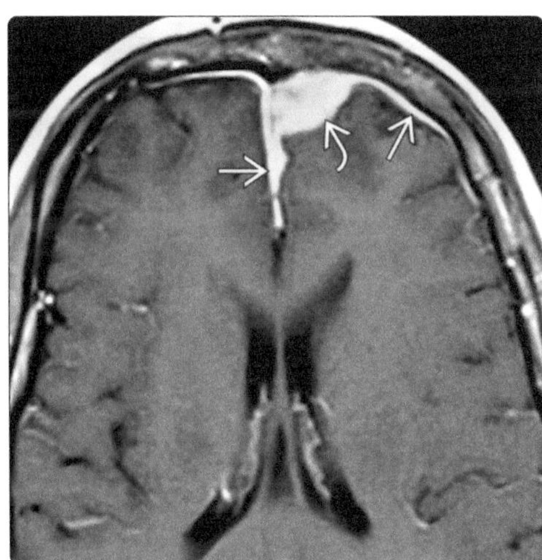

(Left) *Axial NECT in the same patient shows Ca^{++} in the left temporooccipital tuberculoma* →*.* **(Right)** *Axial T1 C+ MR demonstrates an enhancing dural-based mass* ↷ *with adjacent dural tails* →*. After surgical resection, the final diagnosis was a dural tuberculoma. CNS tuberculosis (TB) may involve the dura, causing a pachymeningitis, which may be focal or diffuse. MR imaging is nonspecific in TB pachymeningitis and may mimic a large number of inflammatory and noninflammatory conditions.*

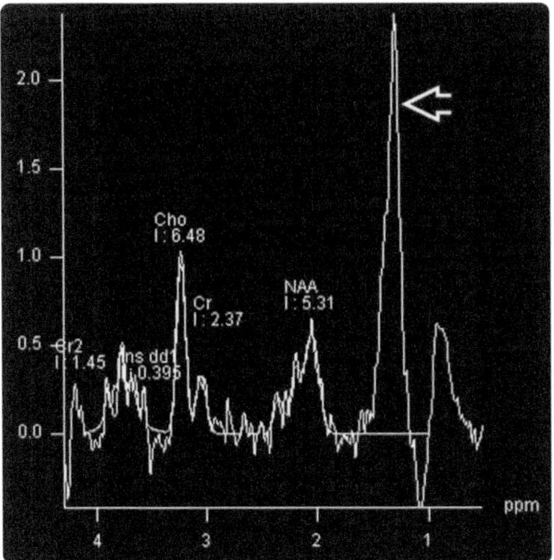

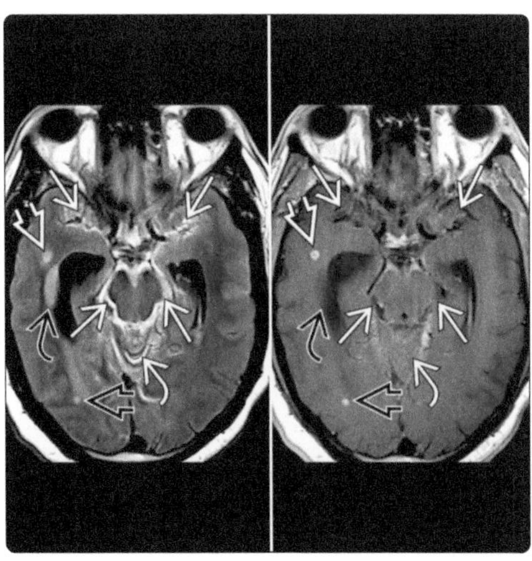

(Left) *MRS (PRESS, intermediate echo) from a brain parenchymal tuberculoma wall shows diminished NAA and a large lipid peak* ⇨ *(1.3 ppm), a common finding in TB.* **(Right)** *Axial FLAIR C+ MR (left) and axial T1 C+ MR (right) in a patient with TBM/ependymitis show that the basal cisternal* →*, sulcal* ↷*, and ventricular ependymal* ⇨ *abnormal enhancement is much better seen in FLAIR C+ images. Note right temporal ring-enhancing* ⇨ *and temporooccipital solid tuberculomas* ⇨*.*

Neurocysticercosis

KEY FACTS

TERMINOLOGY

- Neurocysticercosis (NCC): Intracranial parasitic infection caused by pork tapeworm *Taenia solium*

IMAGING

- Best diagnostic clue: Cyst with "dot" inside
- Convexity **subarachnoid spaces** most common location
  - Inflammatory response around cyst may **seal sulcus**, making lesions **appear intraaxial**
- May involve cisterns > parenchyma > ventricles
- Intraventricular cysts often isolated, 4th > 3rd ventricle
- **Racemose** (grape-like) NCC: In basal cisterns; no scolex
- Lesions may be at different stages in same patient
- GRE/SWI helpful in young adults presenting with seizures
- In children, may see "**encephalitic cysticercosis**": Multiple small, enhancing lesions (starry-sky) & diffuse edema

TOP DIFFERENTIAL DIAGNOSES

- Abscess, tuberculosis, neoplasm
- Epidermoid/arachnoid cyst (racemose NCC differential)
- Toxoplasmosis, enlarged perivascular spaces

PATHOLOGY

- 4 pathologic stages (2 vesicular & 2 nodular)
  - Vesicular, colloidal vesicular, granular nodular, & nodular calcified

CLINICAL ISSUES

- Seizures, headaches, hydrocephalus common
  - NCC asymptomatic until larvae degenerate
- Cysticercosis most common parasitic infection worldwide
- Most common cause of epilepsy in endemic areas
- Increased travel, immigration have spread disease
- Diagnosis confirmed by ELISA of serum or CSF
- Oral albendazole (reduces parasitic burden, seizures)
- Steroids often required to decrease edema

DIAGNOSTIC CHECKLIST

- Cyst with scolex & calcific foci in patients in endemic areas

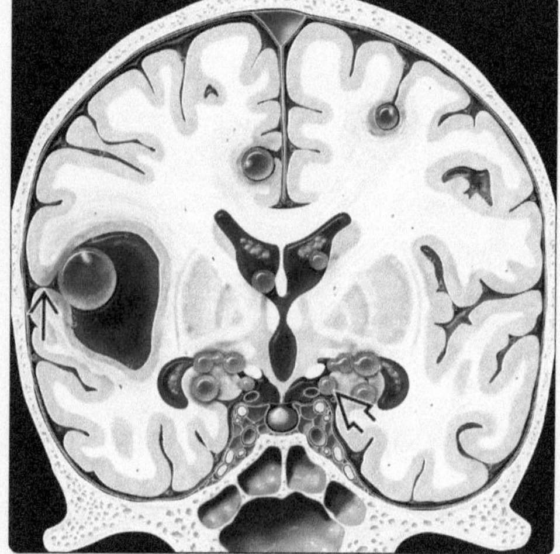

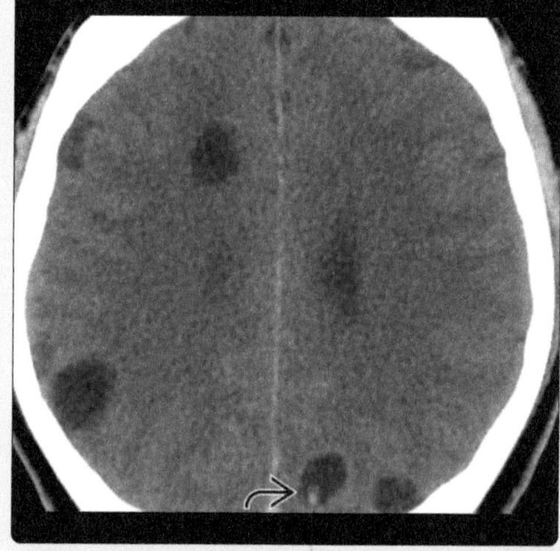

(Left) *Coronal graphic shows subarachnoid & ventricular neurocysticercosis (NCC). Convexity cysts have a scolex and surrounding inflammation. Note that inflammation around the largest cyst "seals" the sulcus ➡, making it appear parenchymal. Racemose cysts ➡ are multilocular, nonviable in the basal cisterns & typically lack scolex.* **(Right)** *Axial CECT shows bilateral frontoparietal nonenhancing cysts without edema. One left parietal lobe cyst shows hyperdense scolex ➡, suggesting NCC vesicular stage.*

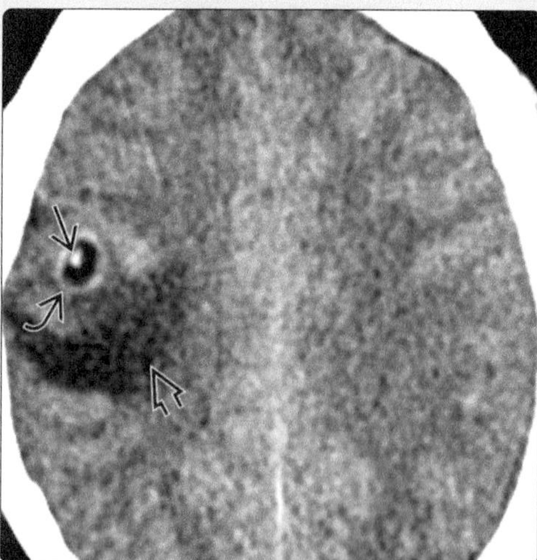

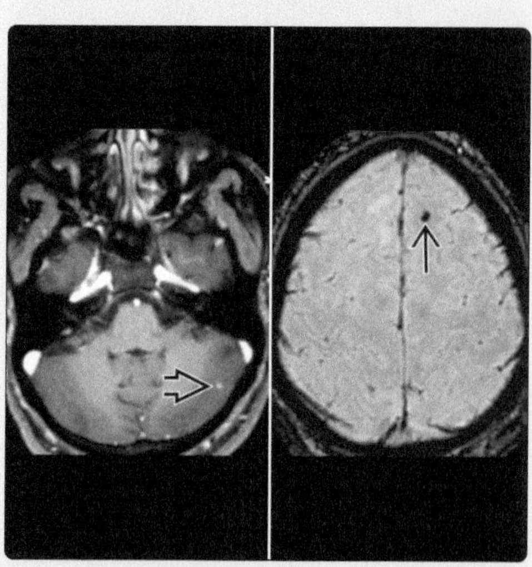

(Left) *Axial CECT in a young male patient with 1st episode of seizure demonstrates a ring-enhancing lesion ➡ with an eccentric hyperdense "dot" ➡ that denotes scolex. Note the edema ➡ surrounding this colloidal vesicular stage of NCC.* **(Right)** *Axial postcontrast MR (left) shows a tiny, solidly enhancing nodule in the left cerebellar hemisphere ➡ due to granular nodular stage of NCC. Axial SWI MR (right) in the same patient shows a blooming hypointense focus in the left frontal lobe ➡ due to nodular calcified stage of NCC.*

TERMINOLOGY

Abbreviations

- Neurocysticercosis (NCC)

Definitions

- Intracranial parasitic infection caused by pork tapeworm *Taenia solium*; 4 pathologic stages: 2 vesicular & 2 nodular

IMAGING

General Features

- Best diagnostic clue
  - Cyst with "dot" (scolex) inside
- Location
  - Convexity **subarachnoid spaces** most common
  - May involve cisterns > parenchyma > ventricles
  - Parenchymal cysts often at gray-white junction
  - Intraventricular cysts are often isolated
    - 4th ventricle most common, then 3rd ventricle
    - May migrate; causes ependymitis & hydrocephalus
  - Basal cistern cysts may be racemose (grape-like)
  - Rare head & neck/CNS locations: Sella, orbit (especially **extraocular muscles**), spinal **cord**
    - Ocular cysticercosis may present at diagnosis or later after commencing cysticidal treatment
  - Other sites: Skeletal/heart muscles, subcutaneous tissue
- Size
  - ~ 1-cm cysts; range: 5-20 mm; scolex (1-4 mm)
- Morphology
  - Round or ovoid cyst, solitary in 20-50%
  - Disseminated form (a.k.a. **miliary NCC**): Rare
- Imaging varies with development stage & host response
- Lesions may be at different stages in same patient
- Inflammatory response around cyst may **seal sulcus**, making lesions **appear intraaxial**
- In children &, occasionally, adults (usually young females, rarely males), may see "**encephalitic cysticercosis**"
  - Multiple small, enhancing lesions (**starry-sky** appearance) & diffuse edema

CT Findings

- NECT
  - **Vesicular** stage (viable larva): Smooth, thin-walled cyst, isodense to CSF, no edema
    - Hyperdense "dot" within cyst = protoscolex
  - **Colloidal vesicular** stage (degenerating larva): Hyperdense cyst fluid with surrounding edema
  - **Granular nodular** stage (healing): Mild edema
  - **Nodular calcified** stage (healed): Small, calcified nodule
- CECT
  - **Vesicular** stage: No (or mild) wall enhancement
  - **Colloidal vesicular** stage: Thick, ring-enhancing capsule
  - **Granular nodular** stage: Involuting, enhancing nodule
  - **Nodular calcified** stage: Shrunken, Ca^{++} nodule
- Intraventricular cysts not well seen on CT
- Subarachnoid NCC: Multiple isodense cysts without scolex; may cause meningitis, vasculitis, or hydrocephalus

MR Findings

- T1WI
  - **Vesicular** stage: Cystic lesion isointense to CSF
    - May see discrete, eccentric scolex (hyperintense)
  - **Colloidal vesicular** stage: Cyst mildly hyperintense
  - **Granular nodular** stage: Thickened, retracted cyst wall; edema ↓
  - **Nodular calcified** stage: Shrunken, Ca^{++} lesion
  - Useful to detect intraventricular cysts
- T2WI
  - **Vesicular** stage: Cystic lesion isointense to CSF
    - May see discrete, eccentric scolex
    - No surrounding edema
  - **Colloidal vesicular** stage: Cyst hyperintense
    - Surrounding edema, mild to marked
  - **Granular nodular** stage: Thickened, retracted cyst wall; edema ↓
  - **Nodular calcified** stage: Shrunken, Ca^{++} lesion
- FLAIR
  - **Vesicular** stage: Cystic lesion isointense to CSF
    - May see discrete, eccentric scolex (hyperintense to CSF); no edema
  - **Colloidal vesicular** stage: Cyst hyperintense
    - Surrounding edema, mild to marked
  - Useful to detect intraventricular cysts (hyperintense)
  - 100% inspired **oxygen** ↑ conspicuity
  - **Postcontrast FLAIR** best to detect abnormal meningeal enhancement
- T2* GRE
  - Useful to demonstrate calcified scolex; SWI better
  - May show multiple black dots appearance
- DWI
  - Cystic lesion typically isointense to CSF
  - Scolex detectable as hyperintense nodule
- PWI
  - Ring-enhancing NCC wall shows lower mean rCBV (1.3) compared with tuberculoma wall
    - Tuberculoma: Mild ↑ mean rCBV (2-3.3)
  - Cutoff value of wall rCBV 1.965 for tuberculoma: 90% sensitivity & 100% specificity
  - Core of both tuberculoma & NCC lower rCBV than normal white matter
- T1WI C+
  - **Vesicular** stage: No enhancement typical, may see mild enhancement/eccentric scolex enhancement
  - **Colloidal vesicular** stage: Thick cyst wall enhances
    - Enhancing marginal nodule (scolex)
  - **Granular nodular** stage: Thickened, retracted cyst wall; may have nodular or ring-like enhancement
  - **Nodular calcified** stage: Small calcified lesion, rare minimal enhancement
- MRS
  - ↑ lactate, alanine, succinate, choline; ↓ NAA & Cr
- Steady-state sequences (CISS) for intraventricular cysts
- **Cisternal** NCC may appear **racemose** (multilobulated, grape-like), typically **lacks scolex**
  - Complications: Meningitis, hydrocephalus, vasculitis

Imaging Recommendations

- Best imaging tool
  - MR most sensitive; SWI MR & CT for calcifications

DIFFERENTIAL DIAGNOSIS

Abscess

- Typically T2-hypointense rim & **DWI-restricting core**
- Multiple lesions may occur related to septic emboli

Tuberculosis

- Tuberculomas often occur with meningitis
- Nodular stages of NCC mimic tuberculoma

Neoplasm

- Primary or metastatic (primary often known)
- May have cyst & mural nodule (e.g., pilocytic astrocytoma, hemangioblastoma)
- Metastasis wall show more elevated mean rCBV (5.43)
  - Cut-off value of ≥ 3.745 for differentiating ring-enhancing metastases from tuberculomas

Arachnoid Cyst & Epidermoid Cyst

- **Arachnoid cyst**: CSF intensity on T2, FLAIR, & DWI
- **Epidermoid**: CSF intensity on T2, "dirty" on FLAIR, & shows diffusion restriction on DWI
- **Racemose NCC**: CSF intensity with septa on T2, "dirty" on FLAIR, but no diffusion restriction on DWI

Enlarged Perivascular Spaces

- Follow CSF on all MR sequences, no enhancement

Other Parasitic Infection

- **Toxoplasmosis** ring-enhancing cyst with enhancing **eccentric target sign** of nodule mimicking NCC scolex
- Other parasitic cysts, but no scolex seen

PATHOLOGY

General Features

- Etiology
  - Caused by larval form of pork tapeworm *T. solium*
  - Humans **intermediate hosts** in life cycle of tapeworm
    - **Fecal-oral** most common route of infection
    - **Ingestion** of **eggs** from contaminated water, food
    - From GI tract, primary larvae (**oncospheres**) disseminate into CNS & skeletal muscle
    - Once intracranial, primary develop into secondary larvae, **cysticerci**
  - Humans may also be **definitive hosts** (infected with tapeworm): Typically from **undercooked pork**
    - **Viable larvae ingested**, attach in GI tract

Staging, Grading, & Classification

- 4 pathologic stages (**2 vesicular** & **2 nodular**)
- **Vesicular** stage: Larva small with marginal nodule projecting into small cyst with clear fluid
  - Viable parasite with little or no inflammation
  - May remain in this stage for years or degenerate
- **Colloidal vesicular** stage: Larva begins to degenerate
  - Scolex shows hyaline degeneration, slowly shrinks
  - Cyst fluid becomes turbid, & capsule thickens
  - Surrounding edema & inflammation
- **Granular nodular** stage: Cyst wall thickens & scolex mineralized granule; surrounding edema regresses
- **Nodular calcified** stage: Lesion completely mineralized & small; no edema

CLINICAL ISSUES

Presentation

- Most common signs/symptoms
  - Seizure, headaches, hydrocephalus
- Clinical profile
  - Diagnosis confirmed by ELISA of serum or CSF

Demographics

- Epidemiology
  - Cysticercosis most common parasitic infection
  - CNS infection in 60-90% of cysticercosis cases
  - Endemic in many countries (Latin America, parts of Asia, India, Africa, Eastern Europe)
  - ↑ travel, immigration have spread disease
- Age: Any; commonly young, middle-aged adults
- Ethnicity: In USA, Latin American patients common

Natural History & Prognosis

- Most common cause of **epilepsy** in endemic areas
- Variable time from initial infection until symptoms: 6 months to 30 years; typically 2-5 years
- Variable time to progress through pathologic stages: 1-9 years; mean: 5 years
- Subarachnoid disease may be complicated by meningitis, vasculitis, & hydrocephalus
- Intraventricular NCC has ↑ morbidity & mortality (↑ morbidity related to **acute hydrocephalus**)
- High association of NCC **coinfection** with **Japanese encephalitis (JE)**
- JE lesions asymmetrically more at ipsilateral side of brain with more NCC lesions or NCC cyst with edema
- JE lesions in coinfections more florid, more common in children, & patients show altered immune status

Treatment

- Oral albendazole (reduces parasitic burden, seizures)
- Albendazole along with praziquantel if > 2 viable cysts
  - Steroids often required to ↓ edema
- Consider excision or drainage of parenchymal lesions
- Consider endoscopic resection of ventricular lesions
- CSF diversion often required to treat hydrocephalus
- **Encephalitic cysticercosis** in those without prior exposure, newly infected with heavy load *T. solium* eggs
  - Host immune system react actively: Acute encephalitis with multiple degenerating cysticerci & swollen brain
  - Antiparasitic drugs not needed, as most parasites die spontaneously from host response
  - Drugs can exacerbate inflammatory reaction turning harmful to patients
  - If antihelminthic drugs used, give under steroid cover

DIAGNOSTIC CHECKLIST

Image Interpretation Pearls

- Cyst with scolex & calcific foci in patients in endemic areas

SELECTED REFERENCES

1. Sakhuja A et al: Severe Neurocysticercosis in an immunocompetent male without travel to an endemic region: a case report. Cureus. 15(2):e34870, 2023
2. Ghosal A et al: Nightmares with a starry sky - treating neurocysticercal encephalitis, how far to go. Trop Parasitol. 10(2):158-62, 2020

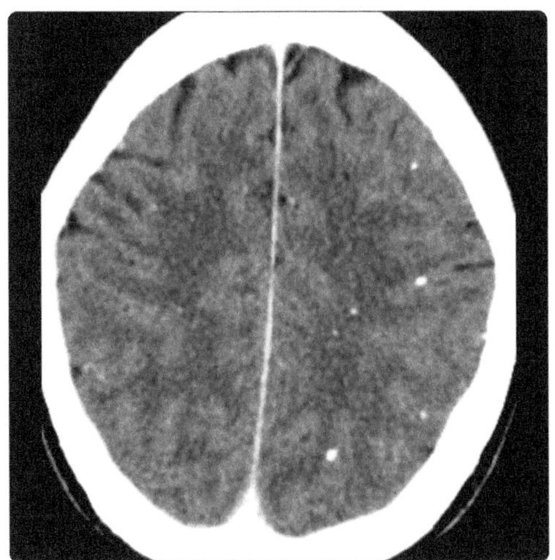

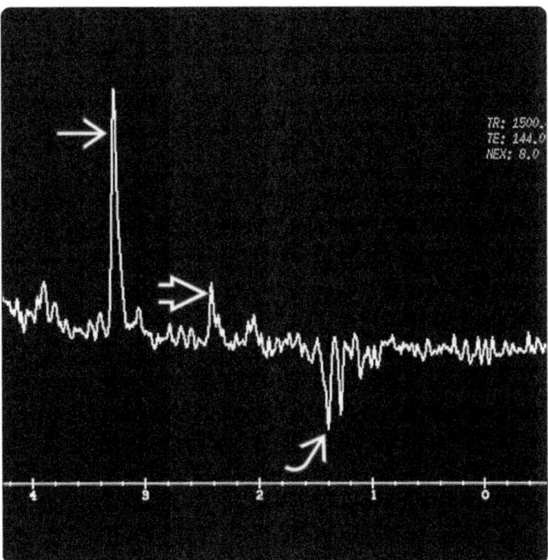

(Left) *Axial NECT in a patient with seizures shows multiple scattered, hyperdense, left more than right frontoparietal lobe calcifications. Perilesional gliosis contributes to the epileptogenicity of nodular calcified NCC.* **(Right)** *MRS at TR 1500, TE 144 within the cyst cavity of a colloidal vesicular NCC lesion in a patient (not shown) shows peaks of Cho (3.2 ppm), succinate (2.4 ppm), and lactate (1.3 ppm).*

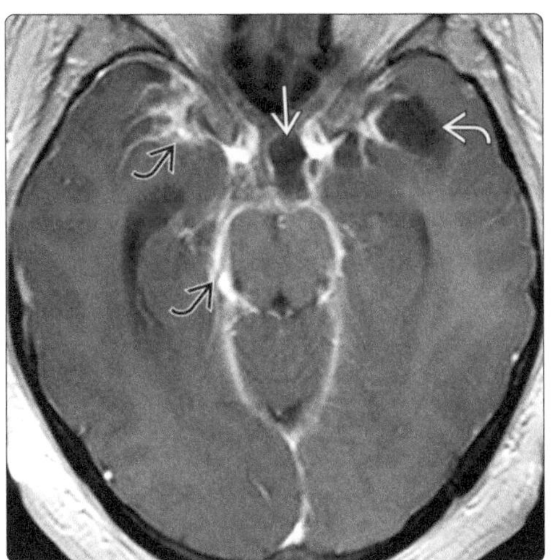

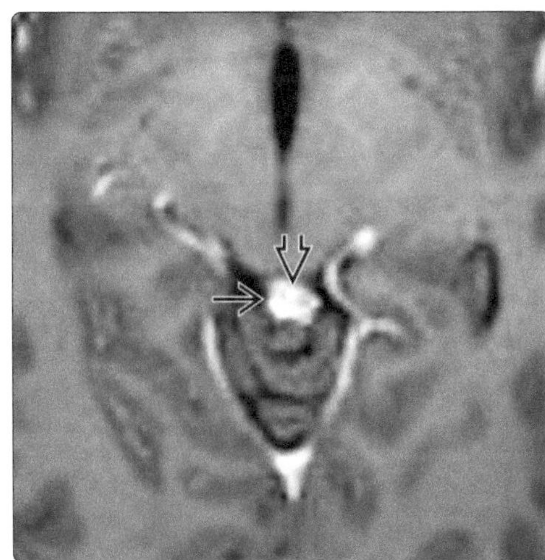

(Left) *Axial T1 C+ MR demonstrates multiple cysts in the suprasellar cistern and left sylvian fissure. There is extensive leptomeningeal enhancement in the basal cisterns and sylvian fissures. Cisternal NCC, also termed racemose (grape-like) if multiple cysts without scolex, may cause meningeal inflammation, communicating hydrocephalus, vasculitis, and infarcts.* **(Right)** *Axial T1 C+ MR in an NCC patient shows a ring-enhancing cyst with tiny scolex enhancement in the quadrigeminal cistern posterior to the midbrain.*

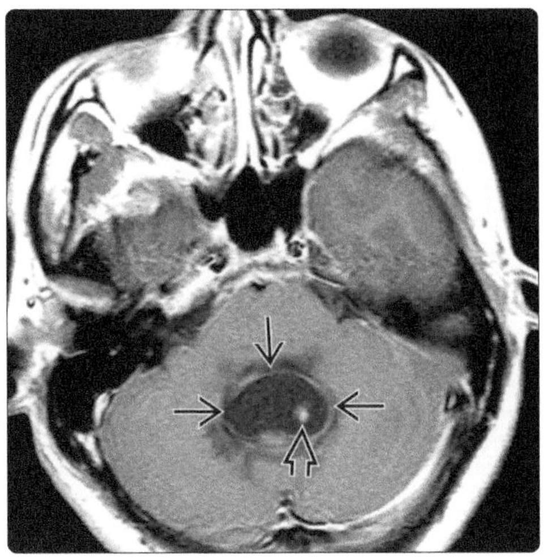

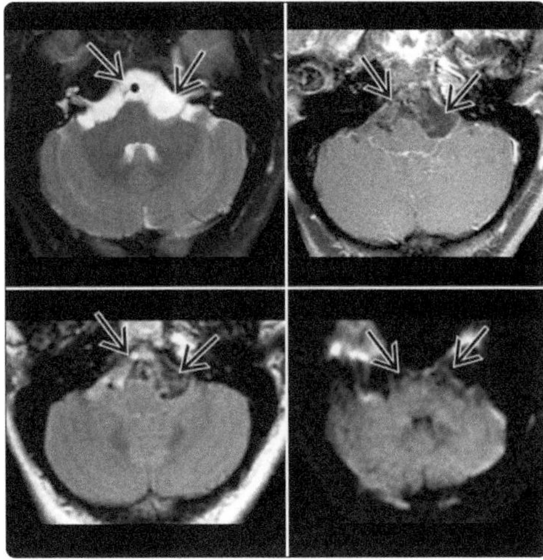

(Left) *Axial T1 C+ MR in a patient with hydrocephalus shows rim-enhancing isolated 4th ventricular NCC with enhancing scolex.* **(Right)** *Axial T2WI MR (top left) shows a CSF intensity cyst with septa in prepontine cistern/CP angles. Axial postcontrast T1WI MR (top right) shows no enhancement. Axial FLAIR (bottom left) shows a dirty appearance due to incomplete fluid suppression (excluding arachnoid cyst). Axial DWI (bottom right) shows no diffusion restriction (excluding epidermoid). Findings are consistent with racemose NCC.*

Miscellaneous Parasites

KEY FACTS

IMAGING

- **Amebic encephalitis**: Ring-enhancing lesions (*Entamoeba*)
- Primary amebic meningoencephalitis (*Naegleria*); granulomatous amebic encephalitis (*Acanthamoeba*)
- *Balamuthia mandrillaris* mimics tuberculosis
- **Echinococcosis**: Large, uni- or multilocular cyst ± detached germinal membrane, daughter cysts, no edema
- **Malaria**: Punctate & ring hemorrhages, infarcts, edema
- **Paragonimiasis**: Acutely may cause hemorrhage or infarct followed by granuloma formation; conglomerated, multiple ring-enhancing lesions
- **Schistosomiasis**: Granulomatous encephalitis, hyperintense mass, enhancing dots along linear area; central linear enhancement surrounded by multiple punctate nodules, **arborized** appearance
- **Sparganosis**: Conglomerate, multicystic ring enhancement
    - May cause **tunnel sign** (worm migration)
- **Trichinosis**: **Eosinophilic** meningoencephalitis, vascular thrombi, infarcts
- **Trypanosomiasis**: Meningoencephalitis, organisms in **perivascular spaces** → edema, congestion, petechial hemorrhages

TOP DIFFERENTIAL DIAGNOSES

- Neoplasms (glioblastoma multiforme, metastases), neurosarcoid

PATHOLOGY

- Cysts, edema, hemorrhage, infarct, meningeal exudates, & granulomatous encephalitis

CLINICAL ISSUES

- Variable, depending on etiology: Headache, fever, seizures, ↑ intracranial pressure, encephalopathy

DIAGNOSTIC CHECKLIST

- Complex, conglomerated lesions in patients from endemic areas/with history of travel to endemic areas

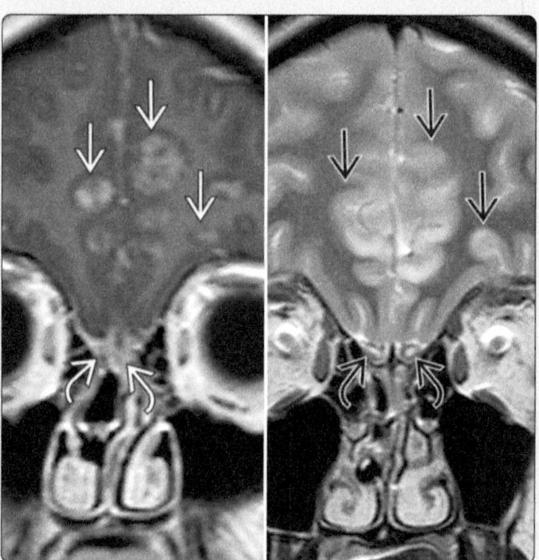

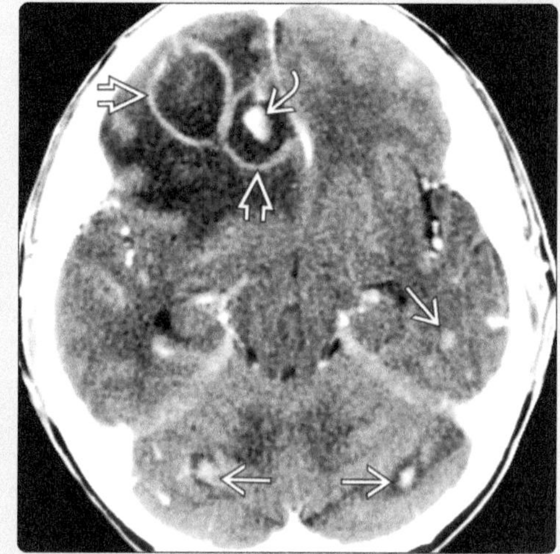

(Left) *Coronal T1WI C+ & T2WI MR show meningeal enhancement around the bilateral olfactory fossae with T2 hyperintensity of the olfactory bulbs in a child with Naegleria fowleri primary amebic meningoencephalitis. Also note bilateral frontal lobe thick leptomeningeal & cortical enhancement & T2 hyperintensity. (Courtesy R. H. Ramakrishnaiah, MD.)* **(Right)** *Axial CECT shows multiple nodular & ring-enhancing lesions with nodules, edema, & mass effect in amebic encephalitis.*

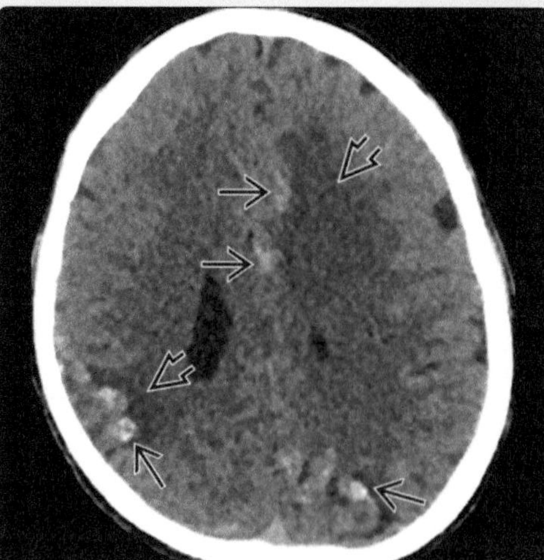

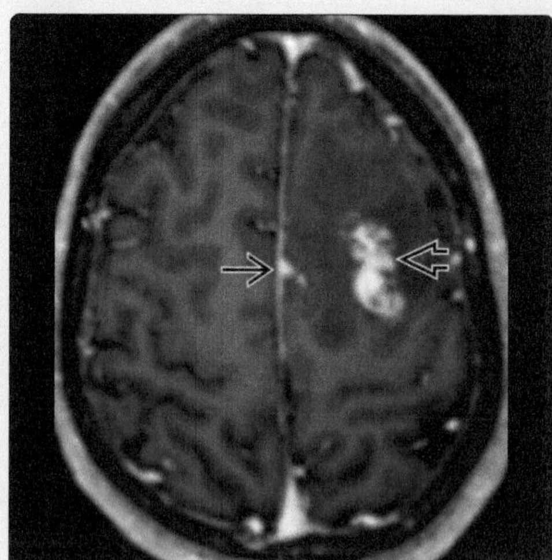

(Left) *Axial NECT shows bilateral parietal & left parasagittal frontal cortical/juxtacortical Ca^{++} in a patient with neuroschistosomiasis. Note white matter edema underlying the Ca^{++}, which is unduly prominent in the left frontal lobe.* **(Right)** *Axial T1 C+ MR in the same patient shows central linear enhancement surrounded by multiple punctate nodules (arborized pattern) within the left frontal lobe CT edema. Also note the tiny nodular cortical enhancing foci overlying left frontal Ca^{++}.*

TERMINOLOGY

Definitions

- Rare parasitic infections affecting CNS

IMAGING

General Features

- Location
  - Majority of parasitic infections supratentorial
  - **Amebic encephalitis**: *Entamoeba histolytica* (EH): Ring-enhancing meninges, cortex/subcortical, deep gray matter (GM)
    - *Naegleria fowleri* (NF): **Primary amebic meningoencephalitis (PAM)** in olfactory bulb region, frontal/temporal lobes
    - *Acanthamoeba* (AC): **Granulomatous amebic encephalitis (GAE)** in meninges, brain parenchyma
    - *Balamuthia mandrillaris* (BM): Mimics tuberculosis
  - **Echinococcosis**: Predilection for middle cerebral artery (MCA) territory, most commonly parietal (embolic)
    - Rarely intraventricular hydatid cyst
  - **Malaria**: Predilection for basal ganglia, cortex
  - **Paragonimiasis**: Hemispheric, commonly posterior
  - **Schistosomiasis**: Hemispheric & cerebellar
  - **Sparganosis**: Hemispheric
  - **Trichinosis**: Cerebral cortex & white matter (WM)
- Morphology
  - **Amebic encephalitis**: Meningoencephalitis; single or multiple focal, nodular, or ring-enhancing mass(es)
  - **Echinococcosis**: *Echinococcus granulosus*: Large, uni- or multilocular cyst; no edema
    - ± detached germinal membrane, daughter cysts
    - **Water lily sign (Camalote sign)**: Endocyst wall detached from pericyst & floats freely in cyst fluid
      - Very rare in brain hydatid cyst, more in lung/liver
    - *Echinococcus alveolaris/multilocularis*: Multivesicular cysts with edema; may enhance (nodular or ring)
  - **Malaria**: Punctate & ring hemorrhages, infarcts, edema
  - **Paragonimiasis**: Acutely may cause hemorrhage or infarct followed by granuloma formation
    - In chronic stage, round & ovoid Ca^{++} in mass
  - **Schistosomiasis**: Granulomatous encephalitis, hyperintense mass, enhancing dots along linear area
  - **Sparganosis**: Conglomerate, multicystic mass with surrounding edema
    - May cause tunnel sign related to worm migration
  - **Trichinosis**: Eosinophilic meningoencephalitis, vascular thrombi, infarcts
  - **Trypanosomiasis**: Meningoencephalitis, perivascular space organisms, congestion, petechial hemorrhages

CT Findings

- NECT
  - **Amebic encephalitis**: Diffuse edema
  - **Echinococcosis**: Unilocular or multilocular cyst, isodense to CSF, no edema; Ca^{++} rare, < 1%
  - **Malaria**: 4 patterns, correlate with disease severity
    - Normal, diffuse edema, focal infarct (cortex, basal ganglia, thalamus, pons, cerebellum; ± hemorrhage) & bilateral thalamic & cerebellar hypodensity
  - **Paragonimiasis**: Multiple conglomerated granulomas, ± hemorrhage
    - Multiple round or oval Ca^{++}, surrounding low density, cortical atrophy, ventriculomegaly
  - **Schistosomiasis**: Single or multiple hyperdense lesion(s) with edema, mass effect
    - Rarely cortical/gray-white junction Ca^{++}
  - **Sparganosis**: Conglomerate, multicystic mass with surrounding edema; ± Ca^{++}
    - Typically unilateral, hemispheric
    - Atrophy, ventricular dilatation in chronic cases
  - **Trichinosis**: Hypodense WM lesions, cortical infarcts
  - **Trypanosomiasis**: Edema with scattered petechial hemorrhage

MR Findings

- T1WI
  - Amebic encephalitis: Centrally hypointense mass
  - Echinococcosis: Cyst isointense to CSF
- T2WI
  - **Amebic encephalitis**: Hyperintense lesions, ± hemorrhage
    - May have hypointense rim
  - **Echinococcosis**: Cyst isointense to CSF with hypointense rim; no perilesional edema
  - **Paragonimiasis**: Heterogeneous mass with surrounding edema, ± hemorrhage
    - May have isointense or hypointense rim
  - **Malaria**: Cortical & WM ischemia, hyperintense
    - Deep gray nuclei & cerebellar hyperintensity
  - **Schistosomiasis**: Hyperintense mass with edema
  - **Sparganosis**: Conglomerate, multicystic mass with surrounding edema, ± hemorrhage
    - May see mixed signal lesion, central low signal, & peripheral high signal
    - Unilateral WM degeneration, cortical atrophy in chronic cases
- T1WI C+
  - **Amebic encephalitis**: Heterogeneous or ring enhancement
  - **Echinococcosis**: No enhancement typical; may see fine peripheral enhancement
  - **Paragonimiasis**: Conglomerated, multiple ring-enhancing lesions
    - Chronic: Atrophy & Ca^{++}
  - **Schistosomiasis**: Multiple punctate nodules, **arborized** around central linear enhancement
  - **Sparganosis**: Variable; pattern may change on follow-up related to worm migration
    - **Tunnel sign**: Peripherally enhancing hollow tube (also reported in **melioidosis & listeriosis**)
    - May see conglomerate ring enhancement with multiple rings (bead appearance)
- SWI
  - Ca^{++}; rare cortical Ca^{++} in schistosomiasis
  - Malaria: SWI may rarely show innumerous blooming hypointense specks scattered throughout brain
    - Parasitemia-induced capillary sludging & hemorrhage

Imaging Recommendations

- Best imaging tool

- Contrast MR is most sensitive for detection
- SWI MR & CT may be helpful to identify associated Ca^{++}

DIFFERENTIAL DIAGNOSIS

Glioblastoma Multiforme

- Thick, irregular margin enhancement with central necrosis
- Typically in older adult

Parenchymal Metastases

- Enhancing mass at corticomedullary junctions

Abscess

- T2-hypointense rim & DWI (+) typical
- Ring enhancement, thinner on ventricular margin

Neurocysticercosis

- Cyst with marginal scolex

Neurosarcoid

- Enhancing lesions involving dura, leptomeninges, & subarachnoid space
- Rarely affects brain parenchyma
  - Hypothalamus > brainstem > cerebral hemispheres > cerebellar hemispheres

PATHOLOGY

General Features

- Etiology
  - **Amebic encephalitis**: EH, NF, AC
    - Most transmitted by fecal-oral route; enter CNS hematogenously
    - NF found in stagnant fresh water; enter through nose to olfactory tract/CNS
  - **Echinococcosis (hydatid disease)**: *E. granulosus* & *E. alveolaris/multilocularis*
    - Dogs or other carnivores definitive hosts
    - Sheep or cattle intermediate hosts
    - Humans secondarily infected by ingestion of food or water contaminated with parasite eggs
    - Parasite from GI tract to portal system, lymphatics
    - Infection usually occurs in liver & lungs
  - **Malaria**: Infection of RBCs by *Plasmodium falciparum*
    - Humans infected by female anopheles mosquito bite
    - Vascular occlusion of capillaries by infected RBCs
  - **Paragonimiasis**: Ingestion of undercooked fresh water crabs/crayfish with *Paragonimus westermani* (lung fluke)
    - Worms penetrate skull base foramina & meninges & directly invade brain parenchyma
  - **Schistosomiasis**: Trematoda (fluke) *Schistosoma* species
    - Host is freshwater snail
    - Humans infected through skin
    - Migrate to lungs & liver, reach venous system
  - **Sparganosis**: Ingestion of water or food (snake, frogs) contaminated with larvae of *Spirometra mansoni*
  - **Trichinosis**: Ingestion of uncooked meat containing infective encysted *Trichinella spiralis* larvae
  - **Trypanosomiasis**: **African** (*Trypanosoma brucei*: **Sleeping** sickness); **American** (*Trypanosoma cruzi*: **Chagas** disease)
    - African: Transmitted to humans by tsetse fly; invade meninges, subarachnoid, perivascular spaces
    - American: Transmitted by reduviid bugs

CLINICAL ISSUES

Presentation

- Most common signs/symptoms
  - **Amebic encephalitis**: Headache, fever, seizures, ↑ intracranial pressure, coma
  - **Echinococcosis**: Mass effect related to lesion location
  - **Malaria**: Altered consciousness, seizures
  - **Paragonimiasis**: Headache, seizure, visual changes
  - **Schistosomiasis**: Encephalopathy, seizures, paresis, headache, visual changes
  - **Sparganosis**: Headache, seizure, neurologic signs
  - **Trichinosis**: Fever, headache, delirium, seizures, focal neurologic deficits
  - **African trypanosomiasis**: Behavior change, indifference, daytime somnolence
  - **American trypanosomiasis**: Acute (fever, swollen face, conjunctivitis), chronic (neurologic)
- Clinical profile
  - Varies with organism, development stage, host immune response
  - ELISA studies can be helpful in some diseases

Demographics

- Age
  - Most parasitic infections occur at all ages but commonly affect children & young adults

Natural History & Prognosis

- Some parasitic infections (e.g., echinococcosis) develop slowly over many years
- **Amebiasis**: 2nd most common cause of death from parasites
- **Echinococcosis**: Complicated by rupture, hemorrhage, secondary infection
- **Malaria**: Most common cause of death from parasites
  - 15-25% mortality despite appropriate therapy
- **Trichinosis**: Mortality in 5-10% of affected individuals
- **American trypanosomiasis**: Mortality in 2-10% of meningoencephalitis patients

Treatment

- Variable, ranges from oral therapy to lesion resection

DIAGNOSTIC CHECKLIST

Consider

- Complex conglomerated parasitic cysts of any etiology may mimic brain tumor
- Patient travel history is often key to diagnosis

SELECTED REFERENCES

1. Liu J et al: A clinical case report of Balamuthia granulomatous amoebic encephalitis in a non-immunocompromised patient and literature review. BMC Infect Dis. 23(1):245, 2023
2. Ono Y et al: Balamuthia mandrillaris amoebic encephalitis mimicking tuberculous meningitis. Neuropathology. ePub, 2023
3. Kaushik K et al: Camalote sign in intraventricular hydatid cyst: a rare presentation of uncommon disease. Surg Neurol Int. 12:541, 2021
4. Souza CA et al: Prevalence of urodynamic changes with risk for upper urinary tract damage in neuroschistosomiasis patients. Rev Soc Bras Med Trop. 52:e20180101, 2019

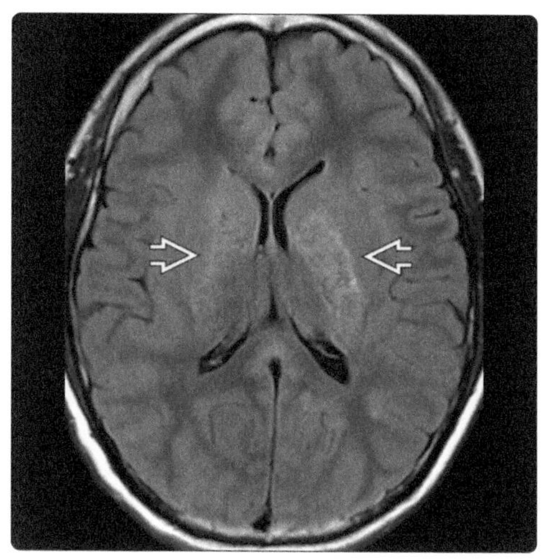

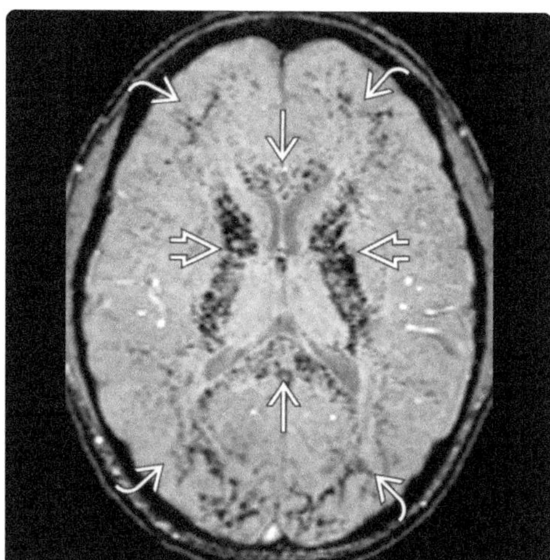

(Left) *Axial FLAIR MR in a patient with cerebral malaria shows ill-defined, feathery bilateral basal ganglia hyperintensities* ➡. **(Right)** *Axial SWI MR in the same patient shows much more dramatic, scattered, blooming hypointense foci in the basal ganglia* ➡ *cerebral white matter* ↪, *including the corpus callosum* ➡ *& the cerebellum (not shown). These findings are consistent with malarial parasitemia-induced capillary sludging & hemorrhage.*

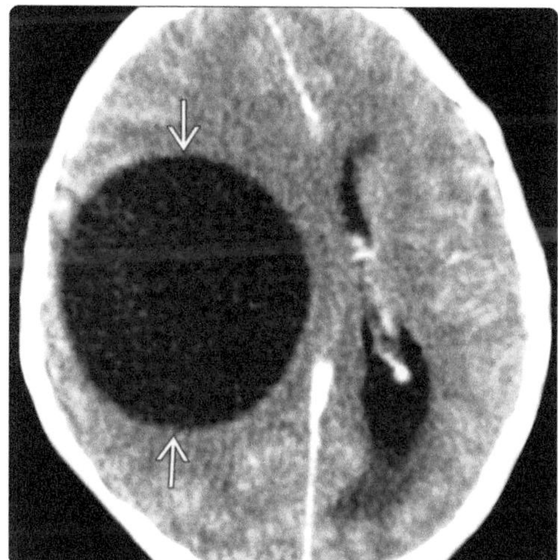

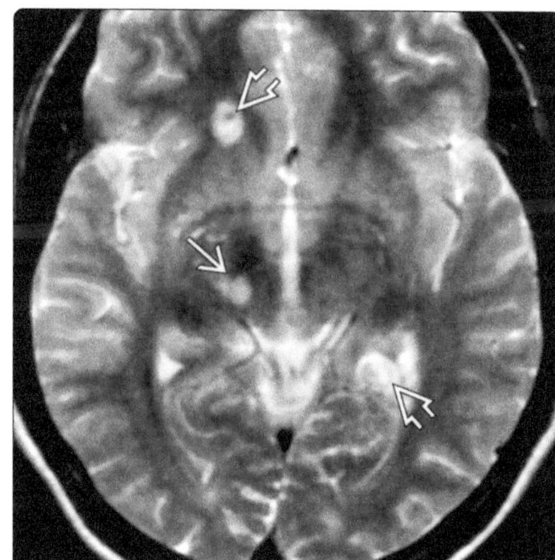

(Left) *Axial CECT in a patient from Turkey shows a right, frontoparietal unilocular cyst* ➡ *with no surrounding edema or enhancement, typical of Echinococcus granulosus (hydatid disease). Note the significant mass effect, midline shift, & left lateral ventricle dilation due to obstructive hydrocephalus.* **(Right)** *Axial T2WI MR in sparganosis shows round, hyperintense midbrain* ➡ *& other lesions with hypointense foci/rim* ➡. *Postcontrast MR showed ring enhancement (not shown). (Courtesy M. Castillo, MD.)*

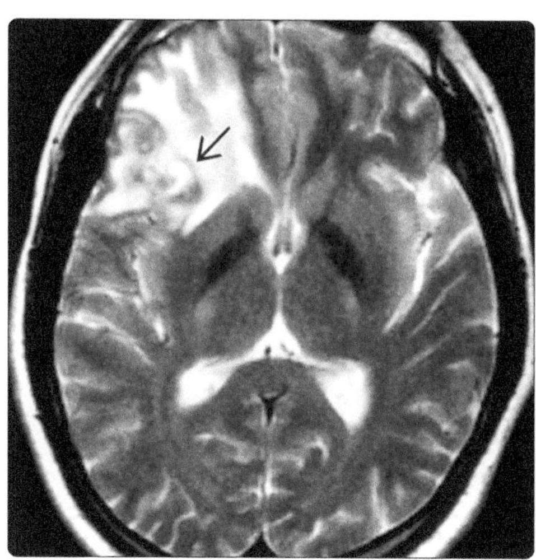

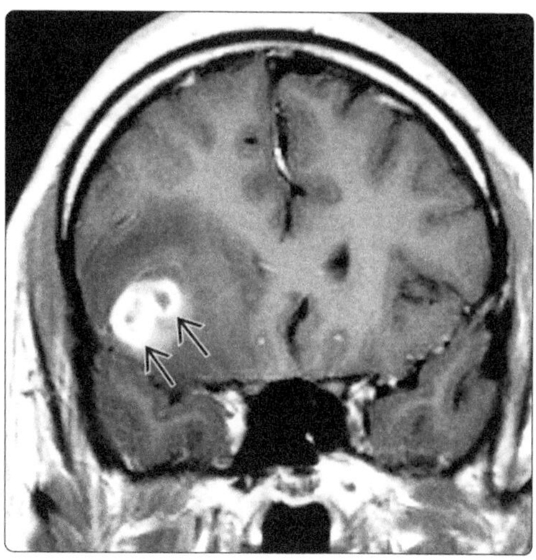

(Left) *Axial T2WI MR shows a heterogeneous lesion in the right frontal lobe with mass effect & surrounding edema in this patient from East Asia with paragonimiasis. Note the hypointense rim* ➡. **(Right)** *Coronal T1WI C+ MR in the same patient shows conglomerated, ring-enhancing lesions* ➡ *with marked surrounding edema. Paragonimiasis may acutely cause hemorrhage or infarct followed by granuloma formation. Imaging mimics a neoplasm. Chronically,* Ca^{++} *& atrophy will develop.*

Introduction

Differential diagnostic considerations for pediatric acute CNS demyelination include clinically isolated syndrome (CIS), optic neuritis (ON), transverse myelitis (TM), acute disseminated encephalomyelitis (ADEM), multiple sclerosis (MS), neuromyelitis optica spectrum disorders (NMOSD), and myelin oligodendrocyte glycoprotein antibody-associated disease (MOGAD). Various infectious and metabolic and rheumatologic conditions can mimic demyelinating processes. The wide spectrum of demyelinating diseases, which may have similar clinical presentations, has motivated interest in developing more specific diagnostic imaging criteria for demyelinating disorders.

Clinical Implications

Clinically Isolated Syndrome

A CIS is the 1st acute episode of clinical CNS symptoms in a child with a presumed inflammatory demyelinating process and no previous history of a CNS demyelinating event. Presenting symptoms may be either monofocal or multifocal. The most common CIS presentations are ON and TM. Imaging will frequently confirm an abnormality in the area of clinical symptoms but will not detect other areas of abnormality that would permit a more specific diagnosis. A CIS episode by definition is prognostically ambiguous. Many children will not recur after a single CNS demyelinating event, but recurrence risk has not yet been defined precisely enough to forgo clinical and imaging surveillance.

Optic Neuritis

ON refers to optic nerve inflammation. It is believed that ON demyelination is immune mediated, but the specific mechanism and target antigen(s) are as yet not defined. Pediatric ON often presents as a CIS with findings isolated to the optic nerves. ON can also present in conjunction with other demyelinating disorders, including ADEM, MS, NMOSD, and MOGAD. ON is usually monocular in older children and adults but bilateral in up to 50% of children younger than 12-15 years of age. Patients may report headache or painful eye movements prior to demonstrable vision loss.

Brain and orbit MR with contrast provides confirmation of the ON diagnosis and evaluates for concurrent brain demyelinating lesions that permit a more specific diagnosis of ADEM, MS, NMOSD, or MOGAD. ON in MOGAD tends to favor long-segment anterior optic nerve involvement with orbital perineuritis, sparing the chiasm and tracts. Involvement of the optic chiasm and retrochiasmatic tracts favors NMOSD over MOGAD. Unilateral ON is more likely to be MS than MOGAD or NMOSD. ON patients typically have normal or near-normal recovery of vision after convalescence. More severe vision impairment at onset results in a worse prognosis for vision recovery.

Transverse Myelitis

TM is defined as spinal cord dysfunction that develops over hours or days in patients without an extrinsic compressive lesion. Frequently, there is a clinical history of antecedent febrile viral illness. TM can present either as a CIS or as a manifestation of ADEM, MS, NMOSD, or MOGAD. Clinical presentation of TM is characterized by motor and sensory deficits, including motor weakness, sensory paresthesias, and anal/bladder sphincter dysfunction. TM typically progresses over several days with paresthesias preceding motor weakness and urinary retention.

MR imaging of the spine with contrast should be performed to rule out a spinal cord compressive mass, especially when presentation is rapidly progressive. Typical MR findings of TM include 1 or more geographically defined T2-hyperintense intramedullary spinal cord lesions that may enhance after contrast. Such lesions may be longitudinally short or long [longitudinally extensive TM (LETM)].

Acute Disseminated Encephalomyelitis

ADEM typically presents as an acute monophasic disorder with multifocal neurologic symptoms and encephalopathy. There is frequently an antecedent viral illness prior to development of ADEM, often a nonspecific upper respiratory infection. Neurologic symptoms typically appear 4-13 days after the preceding infection. Although early reports suggested that a minority of ADEM cases follow immunization (postvaccinal ADEM), subsequent studies have found little or no association between ADEM and immunizations. Pediatric ADEM is an uncommon illness; the estimated annual incidence is 0.2-0.5 per 100,000 children with an average age of onset between 3-7 years. ADEM pathogenesis is incompletely understood but is thought to be triggered by an environmental stimulus in genetically susceptible individuals.

Primary diagnostic criteria for pediatric ADEM diagnosis (International Pediatric Multiple Sclerosis Study Group, 2007 and 2012) include acute or subacute onset of multifocal neurologic deficits, including encephalopathy, headache, fever, vomiting, &/or meningismus. Encephalopathy is required for definitive pediatric ADEM diagnosis and usually develops rapidly in association with multifocal neurologic deficits. In addition to encephalopathy, the other most common neurologic features of ADEM include long-tract (pyramidal) signs, acute hemiparesis, cerebellar ataxia, cranial neuropathies (including ON), and myelopathy (TM).

MR imaging of the brain and spine with contrast frequently demonstrates widespread white and gray matter brain abnormalities. Lesions associated with ADEM are typically bilateral, asymmetric, and often poorly marginated. Almost all patients have multiple lesions in the deep and subcortical white matter with periventricular white matter sparing. Gray matter lesions most frequently affect the thalami and basal ganglia in children. Spinal cord lesions may be short and focal or extensive (LETM). Contrast enhancement varies from absent to prominent incomplete rim enhancement reflecting the advancing wave of demyelination.

Pediatric Multiple Sclerosis

Previously known as early-onset MS (EOMS) or juvenile MS, pediatric MS is a chronic demyelinating disease characterized by recurrent episodes of CNS demyelination separated in space and time in a genetically susceptible patient after an environmental stimulus. Pediatric MS is defined as onset of MS before 18 years of age, ~ 5% of MS patients. Less than 1% of patients have MS onset before 10 years of age. Acute demyelination in a critical area of brain, optic nerves, or spinal cord produces a corresponding clinically detectable neurologic deficit. Myriad proposed but unproven environmental triggers for MS include exposure to infectious agents (Epstein-Barr virus in particular) and low serum vitamin D levels (reflecting higher MS prevalence in northern latitudes). Young children with MS are more likely to present with isolated ON, brainstem syndrome, or encephalitic symptoms, such as headache, vomiting, seizure, or altered consciousness compared to adult patients.

Children being evaluated for MS should undergo brain MR with contrast. Spinal cord MR should be performed if there are spinal cord signs or symptoms or if brain MR findings are suggestive but inconclusive for MS. Typical brain MS imaging findings are multiple well-demarcated, T2-hyperintense lesions in the periventricular, cortical, juxtacortical, infratentorial, &/or spinal cord white matter. Rarely, children present with large, tumor-like demyelinating lesions but demonstrate only modest clinical neurologic deficits despite large lesion size. T1-weighted sequences may demonstrate "black holes," hypointense lesions representing complete tissue loss following a previous inflammatory injury. Contrast will frequently show enhancement of active areas of inflammation.

The McDonald criteria (2001, revised in 2005 and 2017) is widely used for adult MS diagnosis and is useful for pediatric MS diagnosis. The criteria can be satisfied by fulfilling any 1 of the following diagnostic criteria: (1) 2 or more nonencephalopathic clinical CNS events with presumed inflammatory cause, (2) separated by > 30 days (time), and (3) involving > 1 CNS area (space). Please see references for expanded discussion of the McDonald criteria.

More than 95% of children with MS initially have relapsing-remitting MS (RRMS), characterized by intermittent attacks of increased disability followed by either partial or complete recovery. Primary progressive MS (PPMS), characterized by continuous disability over time in the absence of specific attacks, is much less common than RRMS in pediatric patients. Some patients with RRMS eventually convert to secondary progressive MS (SPMS).

Neuromyelitis Optica Spectrum Disorders

NMOSD [previously Devic disease or neuromyelitis optica (NMO)] are CNS inflammatory disorders characterized by severe, immune-mediated demyelination and axonal damage predominantly targeting the optic nerves and spinal cord mediated by the NMOSD disease-specific aquaporin-4 (AQP4) autoantibody. AQP4 receptor, the target antigen of NMO-IgG, is a water channel protein abundant in blood-brain barrier astrocytic foot processes. It is highly concentrated in spinal cord gray matter, periaqueductal gray matter, and the periventricular regions, explaining lesion localization in those areas.

Clinical hallmark features of NMOSD include acute bilateral or rapidly sequential ON and TM causing limb weakness and urinary bladder dysfunction. Other manifestations of NMOSD include encephalopathy, intractable vomiting and hiccups (area postrema syndrome), narcolepsy with autonomic dysfunction (hypothalamic lesions), or seizures. In rare cases, severe diffuse cerebral edema from demyelination results in brain herniation or neurogenic respiratory failure leading to death.

Comprehensive imaging evaluation includes brain, orbit, and spinal cord MR imaging with contrast. At presentation, brain MR is normal in 55-84% of NMOSD patients with demonstrable optic nerve inflammation. Subsequently T2-hyperintense brain lesions develop in up to 85% of NMOSD patients, primarily in the central medulla, hypothalamus, and diencephalon as well as less frequently within subcortical white matter and corticospinal tracts. Optic nerve lesions tend to be extensive and in comparison to MS and MOGAD, extend more posteriorly to involve the optic chiasm and retrochiasmatic tracts. The inflamed nerves are enlarged with abnormal T2 hyperintensity and avid contrast enhancement. Longitudinally extensive T2-hyperintense spinal cord lesions ≥ 3 vertebral segments with primarily central cord gray matter involvement are highly suggestive of NMOSD. Acute lesions involve most of the cord cross-sectional area with cord swelling and contrast enhancement. Cervical cord is affected in ~ 60% of cases, and lesions may extend into medulla.

Laboratory evaluation for NMOSD includes determination of AQP4 antibody status and CSF examination. Patients who are seronegative for AQP4 antibodies should be tested for antibodies directed against myelin oligodendrocyte glycoprotein (MOG), as MOGAD may appear clinically similar to NMOSD at outset and generally has a more benign course.

Adult NMOSD diagnostic criteria are used for pediatric patients with the caveat that a longitudinally extensive spinal cord lesion on MR may be less specific for NMOSD in children compared with adults. Diagnostic criteria require presence of at least 1 core clinical characteristic (e.g., ON, TM, area postrema syndrome), a positive test for AQP4-immunoglobulin G (IgG), and exclusion of alternative diagnoses. Clinical prognosis is generally more severe than MS and MOGAD. Severe residual deficits generally follow initial and subsequent attacks leading to disability from blindness and paraplegia. Any child with a severe progressive disease course or severe attacks of TM or ON should raise suspicion for NMOSD.

Myelin Oligodendrocyte Glycoprotein Antibody-associated Disease

Like other pediatric demyelinating disorders, MOGAD is characterized by attacks of immune-mediated demyelination. MOG is a myelin protein expressed on the surface of oligodendrocytes (as opposed to astrocytes in NMOSD) and the in myelin sheath. MOG function has not been fully elucidated, but it is thought to act as a cell adhesion molecule, regulate microtubule stability, and modulate myelin immune interactions. MOGAD is considered to represent a distinct demyelinating disorder that is distinguishable clinically and in the laboratory from MS and NMOSD, although there is overlap of clinical findings with both at onset. MOGAD has a predilection for children (~ 50% of MOGAD cases) but can affect any age group. Presentation may be proceeded by a viral or febrile illness.

Most children with MOGAD present with a clinical phenotype of encephalopathy (similar to ADEM), ON, or combination of both. TM is next most commonly observed. Involvement of the brainstem, cerebellum, or both is common in MOGAD but usually occurs as a component of a multifocal CNS process rather than in isolation. ON may be unilateral or bilateral and is the most common clinical MOGAD manifestation at symptom onset and during relapses. ADEM-like encephalopathy is noted in 68% of all MOG-positive pediatric cases. A unique brain manifestation of MOGAD among pediatric demyelinating processes is cerebral cortical encephalitis, presenting with seizures, aphasia, stroke-like episodes, headache, &/or fever. Spinal signs and symptoms include weakness, sensory loss, and bowel, bladder, or sexual dysfunction.

Imaging protocols include MR of brain, spine, and orbits with intravenous contrast. Orbital MR typically shows a T2-hyperintense, enlarged, tortuous optic nerve. Unlike NMOSD, inflammation predominantly involves the anterior optic nerve segments, sparing the optic chiasm and retrochiasmatic pathways. Up to 84% of patients show bilateral optic nerve involvement on orbital MR during the 1st ON presentation. Perioptic nerve sheath enhancement adjacent orbital fat is present in 50-80% of patients. Brain lesions are typically seen in deep white matter, juxtacortical white matter, periventricular white matter, deep nuclei, including thalamus and basal ganglia, brainstem, and cerebellar peduncles. A minority of lesions show contrast enhancement. Typically, these demyelinating lesions are bilateral, T2 hyperintense, and "fluffy" or poorly demarcated. Compared to adults, children more frequently have bilateral, large, brainstem, cerebellar peduncle, and deep gray nuclei lesions. Cortical encephalitis demonstrates cortical swelling and T2 hyperintensity with adjacent leptomeningeal enhancement. Not all cases of cortical encephalitis show a radiologic correlate, but its presence strongly suggests a MOGAD diagnosis. Spinal cord findings are typically those of TM. Lesions are commonly longitudinally extensive (≥ 3 vertebral segments). Cord lesions tend to be central, involve gray matter, and may be multiple. Unlike other pediatric demyelinating diseases, MOGAD has a predilection for conus medullaris involvement. Cervical and thoracic cord involvement is more common than cervical or thoracic cord alone. Cervical lesions may extend rostral into the posterior medulla and area postrema region. Contrast enhancement is relatively uncommon and is typically patchy and faint when present. Laboratory assessment includes serum testing for MOG-IgG antibody and CSF analysis with testing for MOG and oligoclonal bands. Aquaporin-4 expression is preserved in MOGAD.

New diagnostic criteria for MOGAD proposed by an expert international consensus panel (March 2023) requires the following: (1) 1 of 6 core clinical demyelinating events (ON, TM, ADEM, cerebral monofocal or polyfocal deficits, brainstem or cerebellar deficits, or cerebral cortical encephalitis), (2) a positive MOG-immunoglobulin G (IgG) antibody test, (3) the exclusion of a better diagnosis. The new MOGAD criteria are intended to improve identification of patients with MOGAD and distinguish it from disorders with overlapping clinical features, such as MS and NMOSD.

Prognostically, MOGAD may have a monophasic or relapsing course. MOGAD generally responds well to steroid administration with rapid improvement of symptoms in many cases, and MOGAD long-term disability rates are lower than with NMOSD or MS. A subset of patients with ADEM-like attacks develop relapsing disease with multiple separate episodes. These previously were known as "multiphasic ADEM," but many of these patients may have actually had MOGAD prior to routine testing for MOG antibody.

Differential Diagnosis

Collagen Vascular Disorders

Collagen vascular disorders that may present in children with primarily CNS involvement include systemic lupus erythematosus (SLE), Sjögren syndrome, and neuro-Behçet disease. Elevated markers of systemic inflammation, such as abnormal antinuclear antibody profile, positive double-stranded DNA antibodies, elevated angiotensin converting enzyme, and positive antiphospholipid antibodies, can help to distinguish these entities from pediatric demyelinating disorders.

Neoplasms

Neoplasms that can mimic features of pediatric demyelinating processes include optic pathway neoplasms, primary brain tumors, and intramedullary spinal cord tumors. Specific imaging features and clinical history can help distinguish from pediatric demyelinating disorders, and the diagnosis confirmed in suspicious cases with tissue biopsy.

Hemophagocytic Lymphohistiocytosis

Hemophagocytic lymphohistiocytosis (HLH) with primary CNS involvement can rarely precede systemic HLH manifestations. Pediatric CNS-isolated HLH can mimic the clinical presentations of ADEM and chronic lymphocytic inflammation with pontine perivascular enhancement responsive to steroids (CLIPPERS).

Mitochondrial Diseases

Mitochondrial diseases may present acutely in the setting of an intercurrent acute infection. Typical brain MR features include symmetrical, T2-hyperintense signal in the basal ganglia or nonvascular distribution hemispheric T2-hyperintense lesions. Diffusion-weighted imaging may show acute restriction reflecting "metabolic stroke" that can be helpful to distinguish from nonrestricting demyelinating processes. Symmetry of imaging abnormalities should prompt strong consideration for an underlying metabolic disease. Other features of mitochondrial disorders include elevation of serum and CSF lactate levels.

Leukodystrophies

Genetic white matter diseases are typically symmetrical, sometimes with characteristic location or appearance. Examples include metachromatic leukodystrophy (MLD), X-linked adrenoleukodystrophy (ALD), Alexander disease (AD), or globoid cell leukodystrophy (Krabbe disease).

Imaging Pearls

There is substantial clinical overlap between the pediatric demyelinating processes, particularly on initial presentation.

Specific MR imaging features may help distinguish the different pediatric demyelinating processes.

Laboratory assessment for AQP4 antibodies, MOG antibodies, and oligoclonal bands in conjunction with imaging may allow a specific diagnosis.

Selected References

1. Banwell B et al: Diagnosis of myelin oligodendrocyte glycoprotein antibody-associated disease: International MOGAD Panel proposed criteria. Lancet Neurol. 22(3):268-82, 2023
2. Shahriari M et al: MOGAD: How it differs from and resembles other neuroinflammatory disorders. AJR Am J Roentgenol. 216(4):1031-9, 2021
3. Jeong A et al: Epidemiology of pediatric-onset multiple sclerosis: a systematic review of the literature. J Child Neurol. 34(12):705-12, 2019

Optic Neuritis

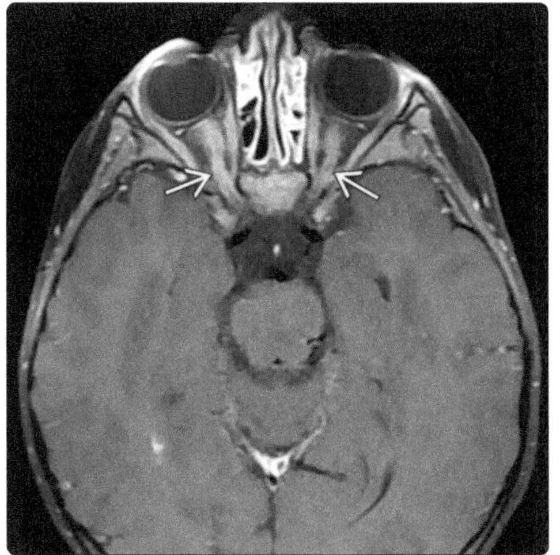

Optic Neuritis

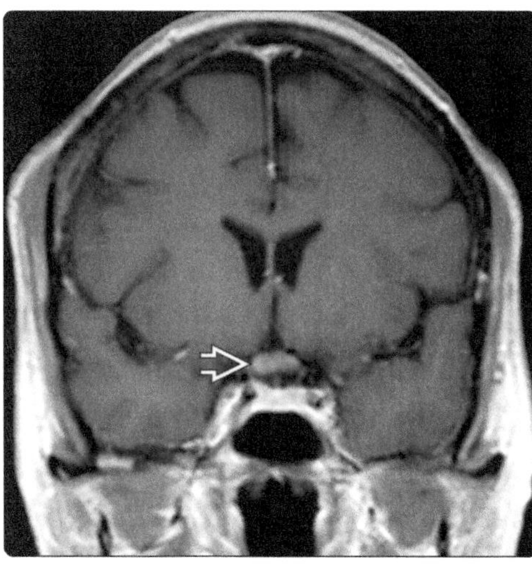

(Left) *Axial T1 C+ FS MR demonstrates abnormal bilateral optic nerve enhancement ➡ involving the anterior (orbital) segments in a 2.5-year-old patient with bilateral optic neuritis presenting as a clinically isolated syndrome (CIS).* **(Right)** *Coronal T1 C+ MR in a patient with neuromyelitis optica spectrum disorder (NMOSD) demonstrates abnormal enlargement and enhancement of the chiasmatic optic nerves ➡, more typical of NMOSD than multiple sclerosis.*

MOGAD

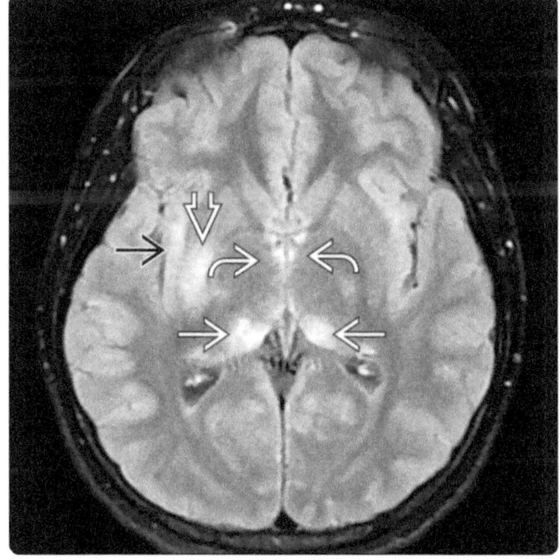

MOGAD

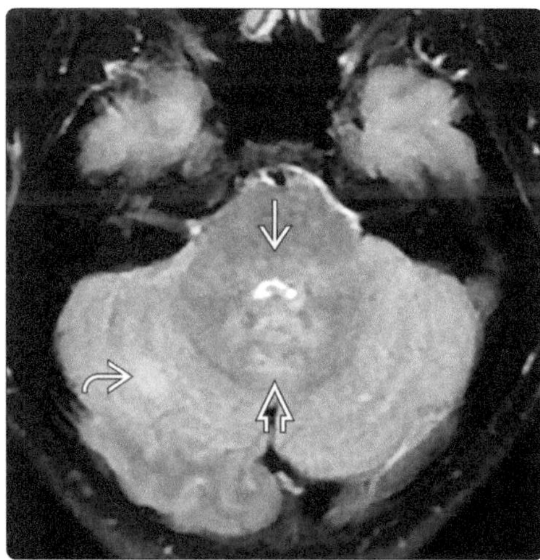

(Left) *Axial FLAIR MR in a 10-year-old with acute MOGAD demonstrates characteristic thalamic ➡, basal ganglia ➡, hypothalamic ➡, and insular cortex ➡ hyperintense lesions. The hypothalamic lesions are subtle on FLAIR but showed enhancement on T1 C+ MR (not shown).* **(Right)** *Axial FLAIR MR in the same patient additionally reveals brainstem/cerebellar peduncle ➡, deep cerebellar white matter ➡, and cerebellar hemisphere ➡ lesions as well.*

Transverse Myelitis (Short Segment)

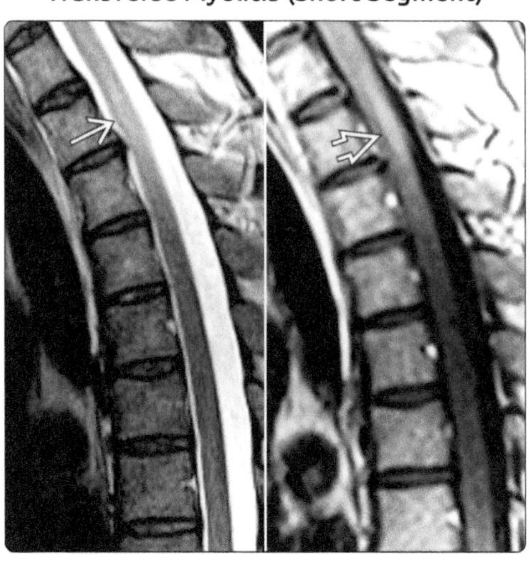

Transverse Myelitis (LETM)

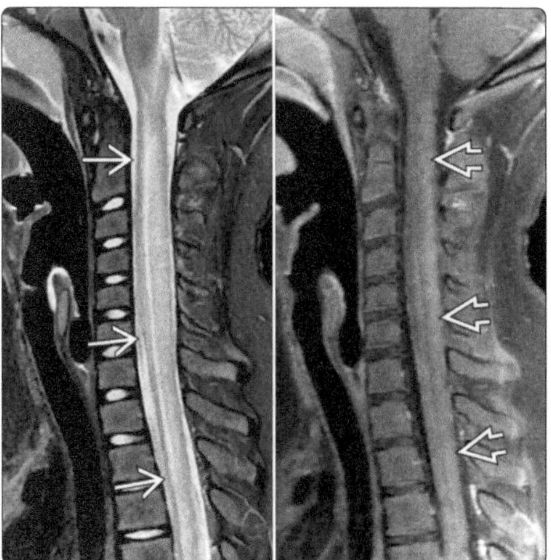

(Left) *Sagittal T2 (left) and T1 C+ MR (right) in a patient with acute ADEM demonstrate short-segment thoracic cord demyelination (~ 1 vertebra in length) with abnormal T2 hyperintensity ➡ and moderate contrast enhancement ➡.* **(Right)** *Sagittal STIR (left) and T1 C+ FS (right) MR in a pediatric MOGAD patient reveal a long-segment cord demyelinating lesion from medulla into thoracic spinal cord. Note abnormal T2 hyperintensity ➡, marked cord enlargement, and mild abnormal contrast enhancement ➡.*

KEY FACTS

TERMINOLOGY

- Probable autoimmune-mediated demyelination in which environmental factors act upon genetically susceptible individuals

IMAGING

- Multiple perpendicular callososeptal T2 hyperintensities characteristic of multiple sclerosis (MS)
  - Perivenular extension: Dawson fingers
- Bilateral, asymmetric, linear/ovoid FLAIR hyperintensities
  - > 85% periventricular/perivenular
  - 50-90% callososeptal interface
  - May also commonly involve subcortical U fibers, brachium pontis, brainstem, spinal cord
- Transient enhancement during active demyelination
- Rare: Large, tumefactive enhancing rings

TOP DIFFERENTIAL DIAGNOSES

- Acute disseminated encephalomyelitis
- Neuromyelitis optica
- Autoimmune-mediated vasculitis
- Leukodystrophies and mitochondrial diseases
- Lyme disease
- Susac syndrome

PATHOLOGY

- Pathogenesis requires combination of genetically susceptible individual and specific environmental trigger

CLINICAL ISSUES

- Pediatric MS defined as onset < 18 years
  - ≈ 5% of MS patients
- Most common disabling CNS disease of young adults; 1:1,000 in Western world

DIAGNOSTIC CHECKLIST

- Requires dissemination in time and space within CNS for diagnosis

(Left) *Sagittal graphic illustrates multiple sclerosis (MS) plaques involving the corpus callosum, pons, and spinal cord. Note the characteristic perpendicular orientation of the lesions ➔ at the callososeptal interface along penetrating venules.* **(Right)** *Sagittal T1 MR in a 14-year-old presenting with gait instability and facial numbness demonstrates T1-hypointense corpus callosum lesions ➔ that represent "black holes" of chronic demyelination. This was the initial clinical MS presentation for this patient.*

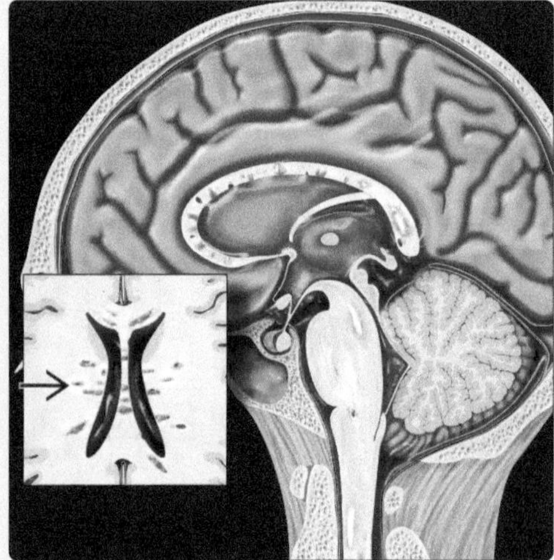

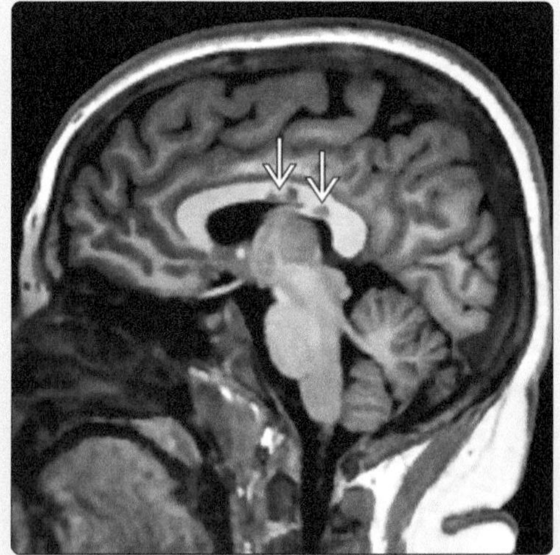

(Left) *Axial FLAIR MR in the same patient reveals larger lesions ➔ in the right frontal lobe and left periventricular white matter. Note surrounding edema in these more acute lesions.* **(Right)** *Axial T1 C+ FS MR in the same patient reveals the characteristic heterogeneous enhancement pattern for a demyelinating process in these more recent lesions ➔, meeting McDonald criteria for dissemination in space and time.*

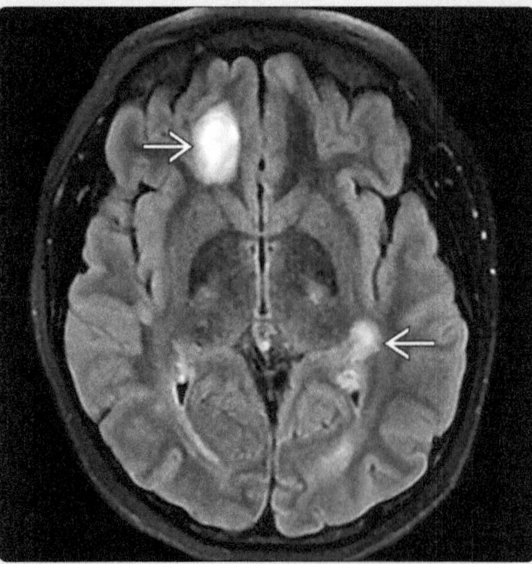

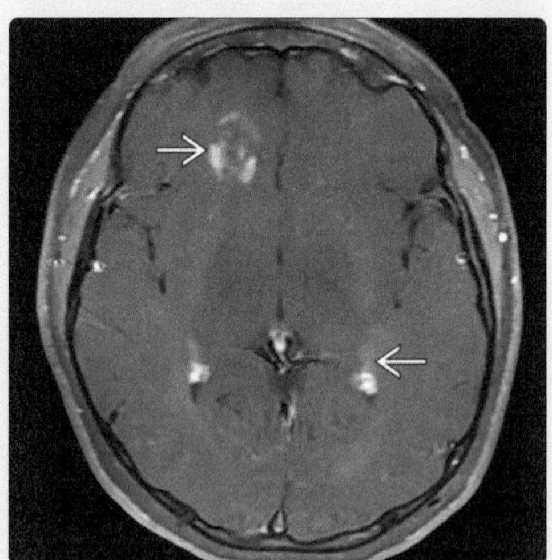

TERMINOLOGY

Abbreviations

- Multiple sclerosis (MS)

Synonyms

- Previously known as early-onset MS (EOMS) or juvenile MS

Definitions

- Chronic demyelinating disease characterized by recurrent episodes of CNS demyelination separated in space and time
- Pediatric MS defined as onset < 18 years
  - ≈ 5% of MS patients
  - < 1% of MS patients have onset < 10 years

IMAGING

General Features

- Best diagnostic clue
  - Multiple perpendicular callososeptal T2 hyperintensities
- Location
  - > 85% periventricular/perivenular
  - 50-90% callososeptal interface
  - Subcortical U fibers, brachium pontis, brainstem, spinal cord
  - Infratentorial (< 10% in adults, more common in children)
- Size
  - Small (5-10 mm); tumefactive lesions several cm
- Morphology
  - Linear, round, or ovoid; beveled, target, lesion-in-lesion appearance

CT Findings

- CECT
  - Iso-/hypodense ± mild/moderate enhancement
  - Both solid and ring enhancement patterns

MR Findings

- T1WI
  - Typically hypo- or isointense
  - Hypointensity correlates with axonal destruction (black holes)
    - Complete tissue loss following inflammatory injury
  - T1-hypointense lesions suggest worse prognosis
    - Correlated with disability, atrophy, progressive disease
- T2WI
  - Hyperintense, linear foci radiating from ventricles
  - Also prevalent in subcortical U fibers, brachium pontis, brainstem, and spinal cord
  - Lesions tend to be well demarcated
  - High cortical disease burden can be predictor of PPMS
- FLAIR
  - Most sensitive sequence for brain lesions but relatively unhelpful in spinal cord
  - Earliest finding: Alternating linear hyperintensity along ependyma on sagittal FLAIR
    - Ependymal dot-dash sign
  - Bilateral, asymmetric, linear/ovoid hyperintensities
  - Perivenular extension; Dawson fingers
    - Along path of deep medullary veins
  - Hyperintensities become confluent with ↑ severity
- DWI
  - Majority of acute plaques: Normal or ↑ diffusivity
  - Few acute MS plaques may show restricted diffusion
    - Often at margins of acute plaque
  - Subacute/chronic plaques: ↑ diffusivity
  - DTI: Reduced longitudinal diffusivity in areas of axonal injury
- T1WI C+
  - Transient enhancement during active demyelination (> 90% disappear within 6 months)
    - Nodular (68%) or ring (23%)
    - Semilunar, incomplete, horseshoe-shaped (9%)
    - Rare: Large, tumefactive enhancing rings
- Perfusion MR (contrast-enhanced T2*): Low rCBV
  - Can separate tumefactive MS from neoplasm
- Magnetization transfer (MT)
  - ↓ MT ratio (MTR) in lesions/normal-appearing white matter
- Functional connectivity MR (fcMR)
  - ↓ functional connectivity between right/left hemisphere primary visual and motor cortices
- 3.0 T vs. 1.5 T: 21% ↑ number of contrast-enhancing lesions, 30% ↑ enhancing lesion volume, 10% ↑ total lesion volume

Imaging Recommendations

- Protocol advice
  - Contrast-enhanced brain MR with FLAIR
  - Sagittal thin T2 FLAIR sequence in midline
  - Fat saturation to assess for optic neuritis (ON)

DIFFERENTIAL DIAGNOSIS

Acute Disseminated Encephalomyelitis

- Viral prodrome, monophasic illness; more common in children
- Can mimic MS; gray matter often involved

Neuromyelitis Optica

- ON and spinal cord lesions
- Brain lesions look atypical for MS, tend to border midline CSF spaces

Autoimmune-Mediated Vasculitis

- Enhancing lesions spare callososeptal interface
- Beaded angiogram appearance

Leukodystrophies and Mitochondrial Diseases

- Consider in younger patients and atypical presentations
- Genetic &/or laboratory confirmation

Lyme Disease

- Can be identical to MS (skin rash common)

Susac Syndrome

- Classic triad: Encephalopathy, branch retinal artery occlusions, hearing loss

PATHOLOGY

General Features

- Etiology
  - Unknown; probably virus &/or autoimmune mediated in genetically susceptible individuals

- Proposed environmental triggers for MS include exposure to infectious agents (Epstein-Barr virus in particular), low serum vitamin D levels
- To date, causation has not been proved for any of proposed pathogenic etiologies

- Genetics
  - Multifactorial; ↑ incidence in 1st-order relatives

Staging, Grading, & Classification

- Major clinical subtypes
  - **Relapsing-remitting** (RR) 85% initial presentation
  - **Secondary-progressive** (SP), a.k.a. relapsing progressive
    - By 10 years 50%; by 25 years 90% of RR patients enter SP phase
  - **Primary-progressive** (PP), a.k.a. chronic progressive
    - 5-10% of MS population progressive from start
  - **Progressive-relapsing** (PR)
    - Rare; defined as progressive disease with clear acute relapses ± full recovery
    - Periods between relapses characterized by continuing disease progression
  - **Radiologically isolated syndrome** (RIS)
    - MR findings satisfy criteria for dissemination in space, but with no attributable MS signs and symptoms
      - Increasingly recognized in pediatric population
      - Presumed that some will transition to formal MS diagnosis over time
- MS variants/subtypes
  - **Malignant/Marburg disease**: Younger patients, febrile prodrome, clinically fulminant, death in months
  - **Schilder** type (diffuse sclerosis): Extensive, confluent, asymmetric demyelination in bilateral supra-/infratentorial parenchyma
  - **Baló** type (concentric sclerosis): Large lesions with alternating zones of demyelinated/myelinated white matter
- **2017 revised McDonald criteria for MS diagnosis**
  - **Dissemination in space**
    - ≥ 1 T2-hyperintense lesion(s) characteristic of MS
    - In at least 2 of following 4 areas
      - Periventricular, juxtacortical, infratentorial, spinal cord
  - **Dissemination in time**
    - Simultaneous presence of gadolinium-enhancing and nonenhancing lesions at any time **or** by new T2-hyperintense or gadolinium-enhancing lesion on follow-up MR with reference to baseline scan, irrespective of timing of baseline MR
  - Unlike 2010 McDonald criteria, no distinction between symptomatic and asymptomatic MR lesions is required

Gross Pathologic & Surgical Features

- Acute: Poorly delineated, yellowish-white, periventricular plaques
- Chronic: Gray, granular, well-demarcated plaques ± generalized volume loss

CLINICAL ISSUES

Presentation

- Most common signs/symptoms
  - Variable; initially impaired/double vision of acute ON
    - ≈ 50% with positive MR develop MS
  - Weakness, numbness, tingling, gait disturbances
  - ↓ sphincter control, blindness, paralysis, dementia
  - Cranial nerve palsy; usually multiple, 1-5% isolated (CNV, CNVI most common)
  - Spinal cord symptoms in 80%
- Children may have similar clinical presentation to adults
  - Clinically distinct episodes of ON, brainstem or cerebellar syndrome, or transverse myelitis followed by at least partial resolution
- More likely (than adults) to present with isolated ON, brainstem syndrome, or encephalitic symptoms, such as headache, vomiting, seizure, or altered consciousness

Demographics

- Age
  - 20-40 years; peak onset: 30 years, 3-5% < 15 years, 9% > 50 years
- Sex
  - Adults: M:F = 1:2
  - Adolescents: M:F = 1:3
- Ethnicity
  - All groups, but White populations most common
  - Most often occurs in temperate zones
- Epidemiology
  - Rare disease; estimated frequency ~ 2.5 per 100,000 children
  - Most common disabling CNS disease of young adults; 1:1,000 in Western world

Natural History & Prognosis

- Prognostically, pediatric-onset MS (POMS) portends more inflammatory course and higher relapse rate compared with adult-onset MS (AOMS)
- Relapse recovery is faster and more complete compared to adults, disability progression is slower, and longer time elapses before transitioning to secondary progression
- Unfortunately, given younger age at diagnosis, POMS patients reach comparable level of handicap 10 years earlier than patients with AOMS

Treatment

- Immunomodulators &/or immunosuppressants
  - Emerging trend toward earlier use of disease modifying therapies to achieve prompt immunomodulatory disease control
- Newer, more specific and effective treatments rapidly entering clinical realm

DIAGNOSTIC CHECKLIST

Image Interpretation Pearls

- 95% with clinically definite MS have positive MR findings

SELECTED REFERENCES

1. Bower A et al: Radiologically isolated syndrome and the multiple sclerosis prodrome in pediatrics: early features of the spectrum of demyelination. Semin Pediatr Neurol. 46:101053, 2023
2. Kornbluh AB et al: Pediatric multiple sclerosis. Semin Pediatr Neurol. 46:101054, 2023
3. Teleanu RI et al: The state of the art of pediatric multiple sclerosis. Int J Mol Sci. 24(9), 2023
4. Thompson AJ et al: Diagnosis of multiple sclerosis: 2017 revisions of the McDonald criteria. Lancet Neurol. 17(2):162-73, 2018

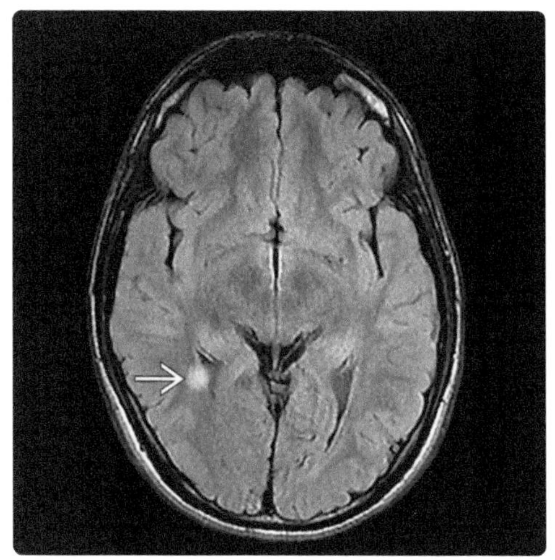

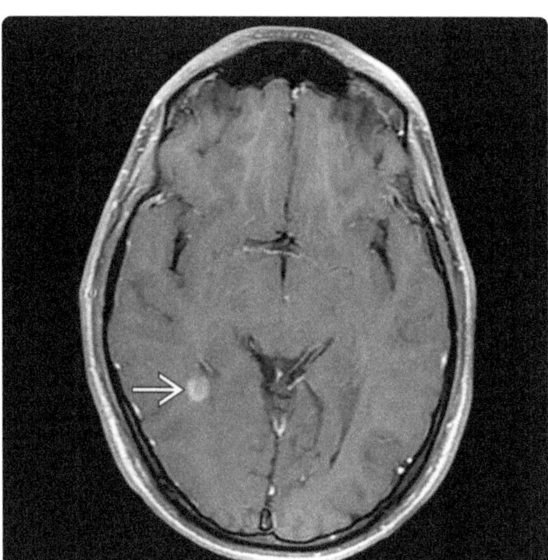

(Left) *Axial FLAIR MR in a teen patient with acute extremity sensory changes and visual disturbance shows a focal periventricular T2-hyperintense lesion ➡. Imaging also showed additional periventricular and callosal-septal lesions (not shown).* **(Right)** *Axial T1 C+ FS MR in the same patient confirms abnormal peripheral lesion enhancement with an incomplete ring pattern ➡.*

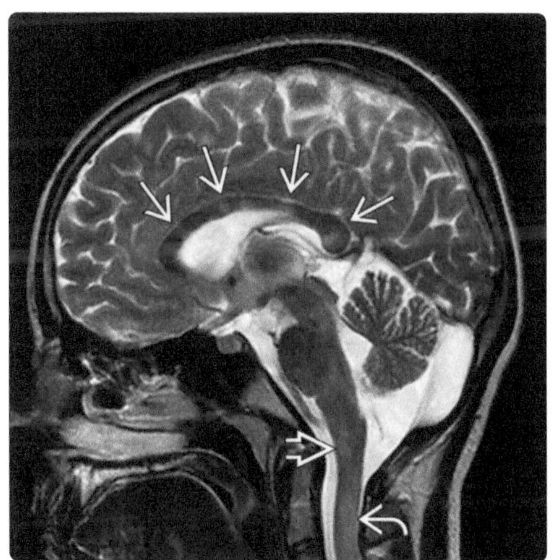

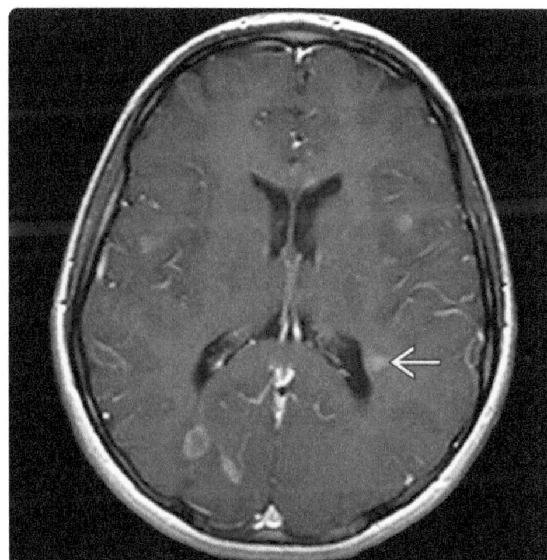

(Left) *Sagittal T2 MR in a teenager presenting with acute ataxia demonstrates numerous hyperintense corpus callosum lesions ➡ extending to the callosal-septal interface as well as brainstem, cervicomedullary ➡, and cord lesions ➡.* **(Right)** *Axial T1 C+ MR in the same patient confirms ring- and solid-enhancing demyelinating lesions, including a characteristic perpendicular periventricular lesion ➡.*

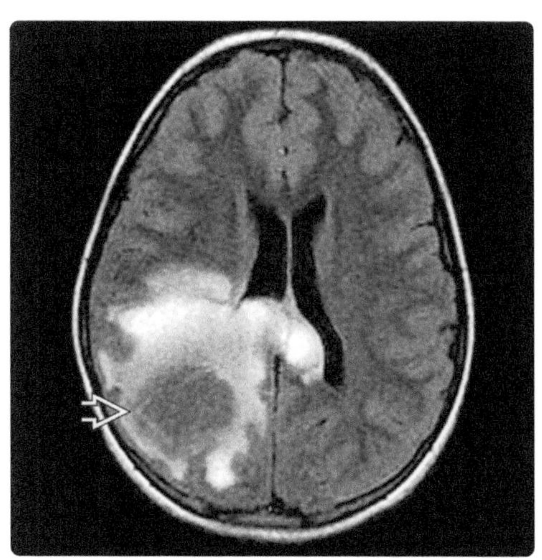

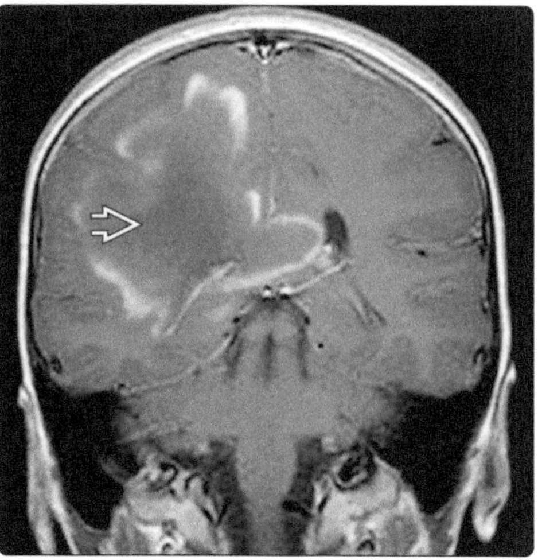

(Left) *Axial FLAIR MR in a teen patient with acute left body weakness and sensory disturbance shows a tumefactive lesion ➡ with surrounding T2 hyperintensity extending into the corpus callosum. Differential considerations include neoplasm and abscess in addition to demyelinating disease.* **(Right)** *Coronal T1 C+ MR in the same patient reveals an incomplete ring of enhancement surrounding the mildly hypointense lesion ➡, permitting a diagnosis of tumefactive MS.*

KEY FACTS

TERMINOLOGY

- Autoimmune-mediated white matter (WM) demyelination of brain &/or spinal cord, usually with remyelination

IMAGING

- Best diagnostic clue: Multifocal WM and deep gray lesions days to weeks following infection/vaccination
- May involve both brain and spinal cord; WM > gray matter, but usually both affected
- Multifocal punctate to large, flocculent FLAIR hyperintensities
  - Deep/juxtacortical WM > periventricular WM
  - Do not usually involve callososeptal interface
- Most lesions show increased signal on DWI (T2 shine-through)
- Punctate, ring, incomplete ring, peripheral enhancement
  - Absence of enhancement does not exclude diagnosis

TOP DIFFERENTIAL DIAGNOSES

- Multiple sclerosis (MS)
- Collagen-vascular disorders
- Neoplasms
- Hemophagocytic lymphohistiocytosis (HLH)
- Mitochondrial diseases
- Leukodystrophies
- Acute hypertensive encephalopathy, PRES

PATHOLOGY

- > 30 different infectious agents reported

CLINICAL ISSUES

- Mean age: 5-8 years but can occur at any age
- Usually monophasic, self-limited

DIAGNOSTIC CHECKLIST

- Imaging findings often lag behind symptom onset, resolution

(Left) *Axial FLAIR MR in a child with ADEM shows peripheral, confluent areas of hyperintensity predominantly involving subcortical white matter. Bilateral but asymmetric pattern is typical of ADEM.* **(Right)** *Axial T1 C+ MR in the same patient shows marked, irregular enhancement of nearly all lesions. As ADEM is a monophasic illness, enhancement of most lesions is typical; all lesions have a similar time course. Enhancement of multiple sclerosis lesions is more variable.*

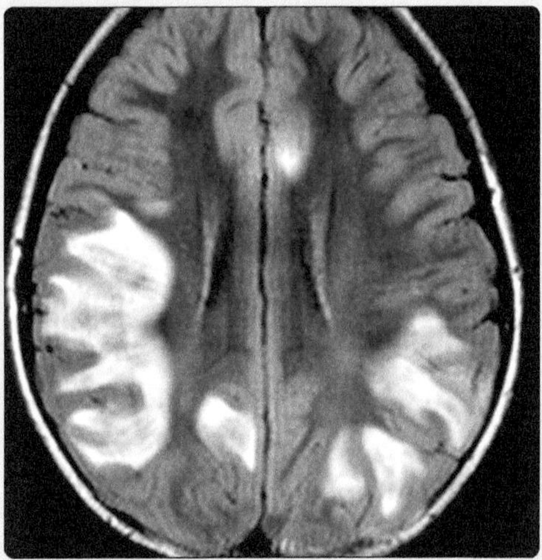

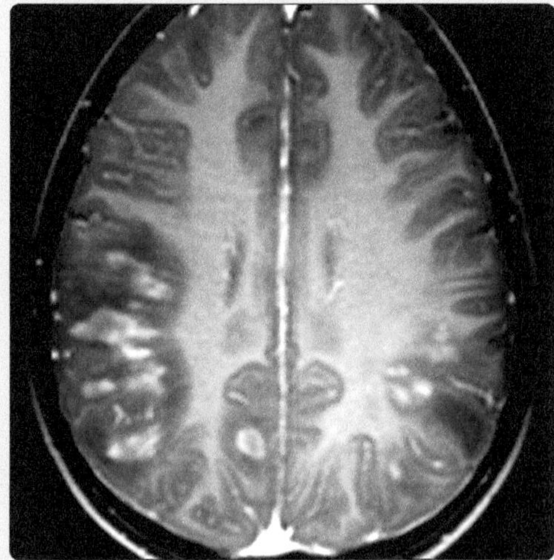

(Left) *Axial FLAIR MR in a 5-year-old with ADEM following an EBV infection demonstrates more subtle findings with abnormal hyperintensity in the left basal ganglia ➡ and right parietal cortex/subcortical white matter ➡.* **(Right)** *Axial T1 C+ MR in the same patient reveals no abnormal lesional contrast enhancement.*

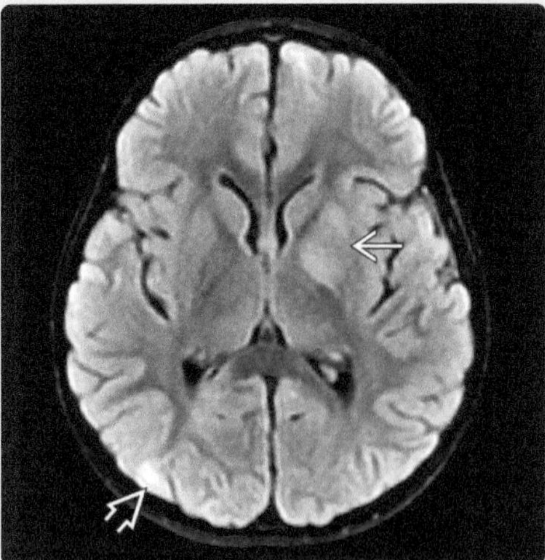

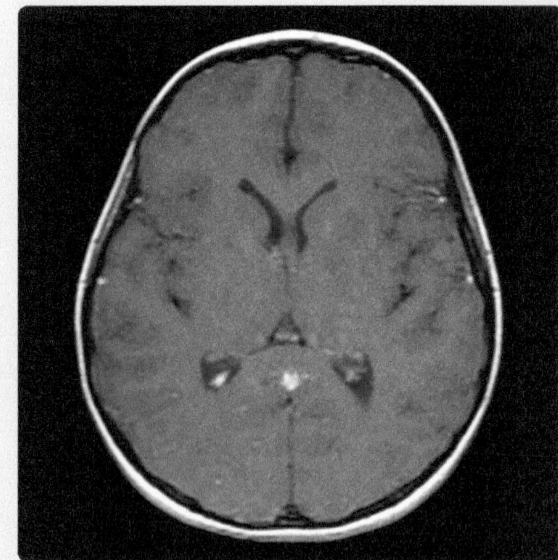

TERMINOLOGY

Abbreviations

- Acute disseminated encephalomyelitis (ADEM)

Definitions

- Autoimmune-mediated white matter (WM) demyelination of brain &/or spinal cord, usually with remyelination

IMAGING

General Features

- Best diagnostic clue
  - Multifocal WM/basal ganglia lesions days to weeks following preceding infection
    - 93% within 3 weeks of infection
- Location
  - Widespread WM and gray matter brain abnormalities
    - Both supratentorial and infratentorial lesions
  - May involve both brain and spinal cord; WM > gray matter, but usually both affected
  - Deep/juxtacortical WM > periventricular WM
- Size
  - Tumefactive lesions may be large but with less mass effect than expected from similar size tumor
- Morphology
  - Punctate to flocculent
  - Tumefactive, mass-like lesions possible

CT Findings

- NECT
  - Initial CT normal in 40% of patients
- CECT
  - Normal or multifocal punctate or ring-enhancing lesions

MR Findings

- T1WI
  - Hypointense "black holes" uncommon
- T2WI
  - Hyperintensities may be better visualized in brainstem and posterior fossa than on T2 FLAIR
- FLAIR
  - Widespread multifocal punctate to large, flocculent FLAIR hyperintensities
    - Bilateral, asymmetric, frequently poorly marginated
  - Involve peripheral WM-gray matter junction subcortical WM
  - Thalami and basal ganglia symmetrically involved, particularly in children
  - Can involve brainstem and posterior fossa
  - Usually do **not** involve callososeptal interface
- DWI
  - Variably hyperintense lesions on DWI (trace) images
  - ADC may be increased or decreased
    - Most lesions show increased signal (T2 shine-through)
    - Diffusion restriction uncommon, suggests worse prognosis
- T1WI C+
  - Punctate, ring, incomplete ring, peripheral enhancement
  - Cranial nerve(s) may enhance
  - Absence of enhancement does not exclude ADEM

Imaging Recommendations

- Best imaging tool
  - Contrast-enhanced brain MR, including FLAIR T2 imaging

DIFFERENTIAL DIAGNOSIS

Multiple Sclerosis

- Predilection for periventricular WM (callososeptal interface), subcortical U fibers, posterior fossa
- Relapsing-remitting course common

Collagen-Vascular Disorders

- e.g., systemic lupus erythematosus (SLE), Sjögren syndrome, and neuro-Behçet disease
- Can present with primarily CNS involvement in children
  - Imaging findings mimic ADEM
- Elevated markers of systemic inflammation help distinguish
- Behcet: Classic triad of oral and genital ulcerations with uveitis

Neoplasms

- Mimic features of pediatric demyelinating processes
- Optic pathway neoplasms, primary brain tumors, intramedullary spinal cord tumors
- Specific imaging features and clinical history can help distinguish from pediatric demyelinating disorders

Hemophagocytic Lymphohistiocytosis

- With primary CNS involvement can (rarely) precede systemic disease manifestations
- Mimics clinical presentation of ADEM
- Imaging manifestations are protean

Mitochondrial Diseases

- MELAS and MERRF may present in setting of intercurrent acute infection
- Typical brain MR features include abnormal T2-hyperintense signal in basal ganglia and nonvascular distribution hemispheric lesions
- DWI MR will show acute restriction reflecting "metabolic stroke"
- Elevation of serum, CSF lactate levels

Leukodystrophies

- Genetic WM diseases are typically symmetrical, sometimes with characteristic location or appearance
- e.g., metachromatic leukodystrophy, X-linked adrenoleukodystrophy, Alexander disease, globoid cell leukodystrophy (Krabbe disease)

Autoimmune-Mediated Vasculitis

- Multifocal gray matter-WM lesions
  - Bilateral, usually cortical/subcortical, basal ganglia/thalami
  - Ring-enhancing lesions may mimic infection

Acute Hypertensive Encephalopathy, PRES

- Typically posterior circulation in cortex/subcortical WM
- May affect deep gray nuclei

PATHOLOGY

General Features

- Etiology

- Autoimmune-mediated severe acute demyelination
- Pathogenesis incompletely understood, but thought to be triggered by environmental stimulus in genetically susceptible individuals
  - Myelin autoantigens, such as myelin basic protein (MBP), proteolipid protein (PLP), and myelin oligodendrocyte glycoprotein (MOG), share antigenic determinants with those of infecting pathogen
- Often follows antecedent nonspecific upper respiratory tract infection
  - > 30 different infectious agents and immunizations reported
  - Severe acute respiratory syndrome coronavirus 2 (SARS-CoV-2 or COVID) infection has been reported with ADEM, but overall incidence appears to be low
  - Some cases are spontaneous (no known cause)
- Neurologic symptoms typically appear 4-13 days after preceding infection
- Current studies show little or no association between ADEM and immunizations (postvaccinal ADEM)

- Acute hemorrhagic leukoencephalopathy variant associated with ulcerative colitis and asthma

Microscopic Features

- Acute myelin breakdown
- Perivenous inflammation; lymphocytic infiltrates
- Relative axonal preservation; atypical astrogliosis
- Virus particles generally not found, unlike viral encephalitides
- Similar to experimental allergic encephalomyelitis, supporting autoimmune-related etiology

CLINICAL ISSUES

Presentation

- Most common signs/symptoms
  - Usually preceded by prodromal phase: Fever, malaise, myalgia
  - Multifocal neurologic symptoms, 2 days to 4 weeks after viral illness
    - Initial symptoms: Headache, fever, drowsiness
    - Cranial nerve palsies, hemiparesis
    - Decreased consciousness (from lethargy to coma)
    - Behavioral changes
- Other signs/symptoms
  - Seizures in 10-35%
- Clinical profile
  - CSF normal in 60%
  - If abnormal (lymphocyte pleocytosis, elevated protein) usually lacks CSF oligoclonal bands

Demographics

- Age
  - Children > adults
  - Mean age: 5-8 years but can occur at any age
- Sex
  - Male predominance (M:F = 1.0:0.6-0.8), unlike MS
- Epidemiology
  - Pediatric ADEM is uncommon illness
    - Estimated annual incidence 0.2-0.5 per 100,000 children
  - Typically delay between symptom onset, imaging findings
  - Rare, yet most common para-/postinfectious disorder
  - Most common in winter and spring
  - Exact epidemiology unknown but increasingly reported

Natural History & Prognosis

- Usually monophasic and self-limited
- Variable prognosis
  - Complete recovery within 1 month (50-60%)
  - Neurologic sequelae (most commonly seizures) (20-30%)
  - Mortality (10-30%)
  - Relapses are rare
    - "Relapsing disseminated encephalomyelitis"
    - Many of these cases may actually be MOG antibody disease (MOGAD)
    - May be difficult to distinguish from relapsing-remitting MS
- Varicella and rubella ADEM have preferential patterns
  - Varicella ADEM characterized by cerebellar ataxia and mild pyramidal dysfunction
  - Rubella ADEM characterized by acute explosive onset, seizures, coma, and moderate pyramidal signs
- Rare manifestations of ADEM
  - Acute hemorrhagic leukoencephalopathy (2%)
    - Young patients with abrupt symptom onset and fulminant clinical course
    - Inflammatory hemorrhagic WM demyelination
    - Prognosis for survival or recovery of neurologic function is worse than for classic ADEM
  - Bilateral striatal necrosis (usually in infants, may be reversible)

Treatment

- Immunosuppressive/immunomodulatory therapy
  - MR may show prompt improvement after therapy
- Plasma exchange therapy
  - 40% of patients failing steroid treatment may show marked improvement

DIAGNOSTIC CHECKLIST

Image Interpretation Pearls

- Imaging findings often lag behind both symptom onset and resolution

SELECTED REFERENCES

1. Kalita IR et al: Acute abducens nerve palsy with acute disseminated encephalomyelitis-like presentation following COVID-19 vaccination. Indian J Ophthalmol. 71(5):2279-81, 2023
2. Chen LW et al: Prognostic factors for functional recovery in children with moderate to severe acute disseminated encephalomyelitis. Mult Scler Relat Disord. 66:104056, 2022
3. Wang Y et al: SARS-CoV-2-associated acute disseminated encephalomyelitis: a systematic review of the literature. J Neurol. 269(3):1071-92, 2022
4. Benallegue N et al: Neurological involvement in secondary hemophagocytic lymphohistiocytosis in children. Eur J Paediatr Neurol. 34:110-7, 2021
5. Pujari SS et al: Acute haemorrhagic leukoencephalitis (AHLE) - our experience and a short review. J Neuroimmunol. 361:577751, 2021

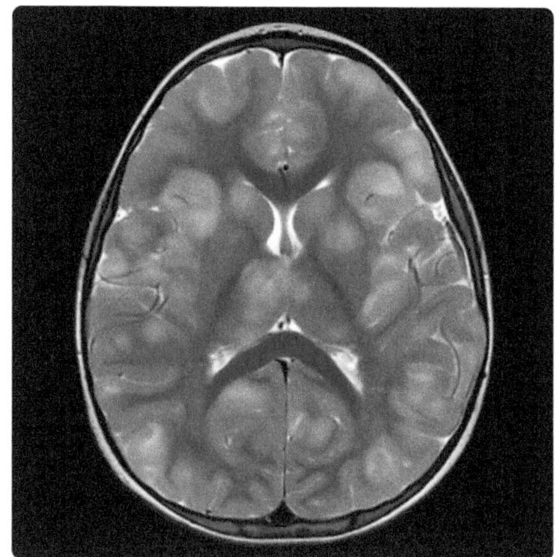

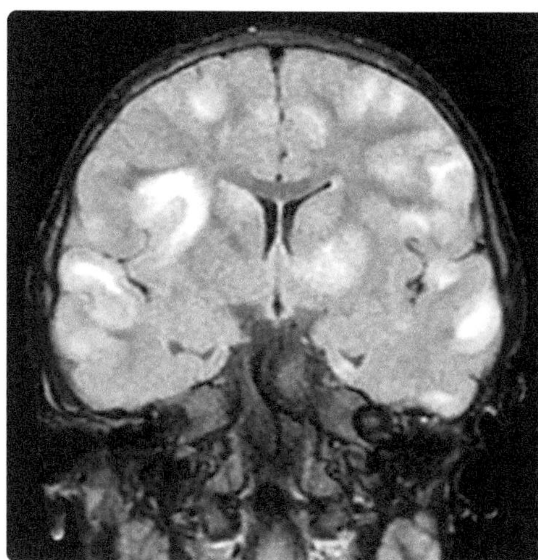

(Left) *Axial T2 MR in a 21-month-old who presented with seizures and encephalopathy demonstrates numerous lesions involving both subcortical white matter and gray matter (caudate nuclei, left basal ganglia, both thalami).* **(Right)** *Coronal FLAIR MR in the same patient confirms characteristic lesion distribution. Contrast-enhanced imaging (not shown) demonstrated no lesional enhancement.*

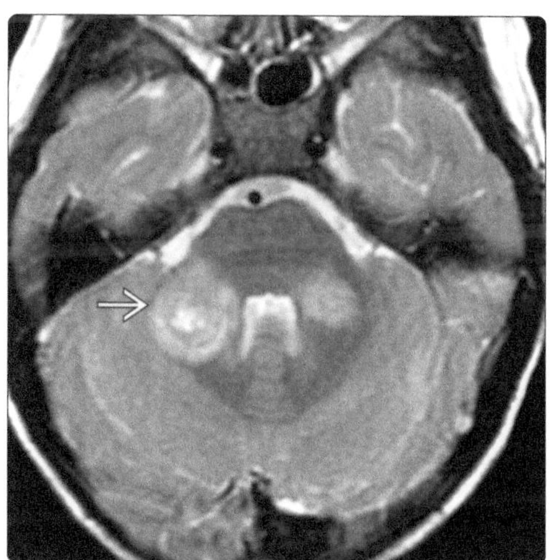

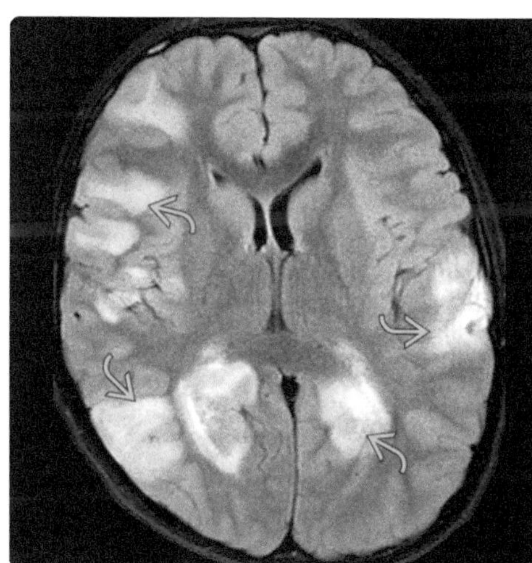

(Left) *Axial T2WI MR shows hyperintense lesions in the brachium pontis bilaterally, typical for demyelination. The right-sided lesion shows a targetoid ➔ appearance. Enhancement of several lesions was present on postcontrast T1 images (not shown).* **(Right)** *Axial FLAIR MR shows large, confluent regions of hyperintense signal ➔ in the periventricular and subcortical white matter in a 14-year-old who presented with neck stiffness, fatigue, and seizures.*

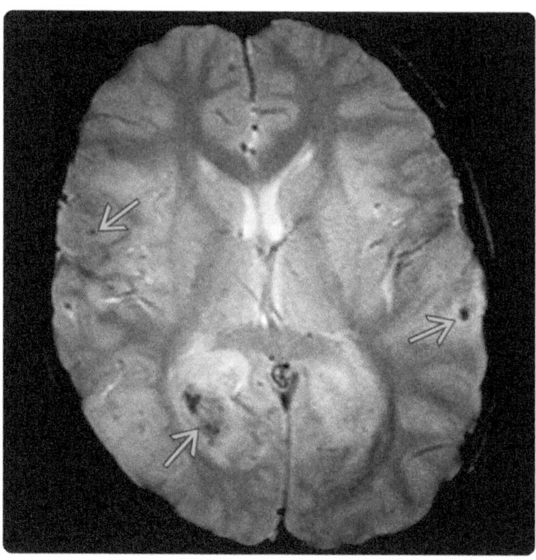

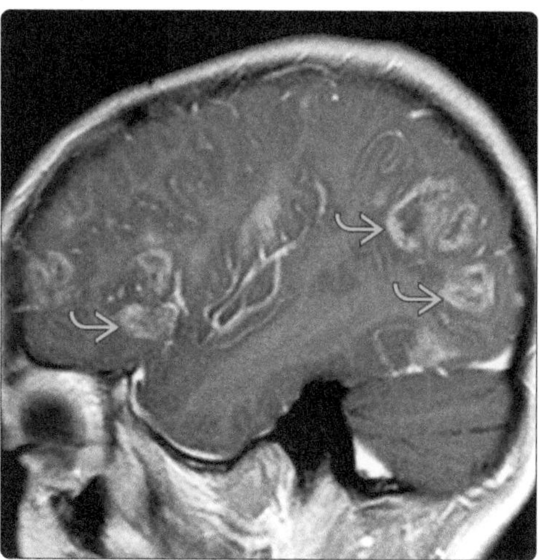

(Left) *Axial SWI MR in the same patient shows petechial hemorrhages ➔ in regions of FLAIR signal abnormality.* **(Right)** *Sagittal T1 C+ MR in same patient shows extensive irregular ring enhancement ➔ involving multiple subcortical white matter lesions. Acute hemorrhagic leukoencephalopathy (AHL) is a rare manifestation of ADEM, occurring in 2% of cases. AHL is associated with a very poor prognosis. Aggressive therapeutic management is a prerequisite to avoid usual disease course with fatal outcome.*

KEY FACTS

TERMINOLOGY

- Myelin oligodendrocyte glycoprotein (MOG), MOG antibody-associated disease (MOGAD)

IMAGING

- Orbits
  - Abnormal bilateral long-segment hyperintensity of optic nerve **anterior** segments
  - Usually spares optic chiasm, retrochiasmatic pathways
- Brain
  - T2-hyperintense, fluffy, poorly demarcated lesions
  - Bilateral, large brainstem and deep gray nuclei lesions more common in children

TOP DIFFERENTIAL DIAGNOSES

- Multiple sclerosis
- Acute disseminated encephalomyelitis (ADEM)
- Neuromyelitis optica spectrum disorder (NMOSD)
- Brain neoplasms

PATHOLOGY

- Cortical demyelination common, topographically adjacent meningeal inflammation

CLINICAL ISSUES

- Unilateral or bilateral optic neuritis (ON)
- Most common
  - Acute disseminated encephalomyelitis-like presentation with altered mental status, focal neurologic deficits
  - Transverse myelitis
- Less common: Cerebral cortical encephalitis
- Infectious prodrome precedes initial symptom onset ≤ 60% of patients

DIAGNOSTIC CHECKLIST

- Best diagnostic clue: Bilateral **anterior** ON + longitudinally extensive transverse myelitis (LETM)
- Evaluate optic nerves on brain imaging to identify concurrent ON

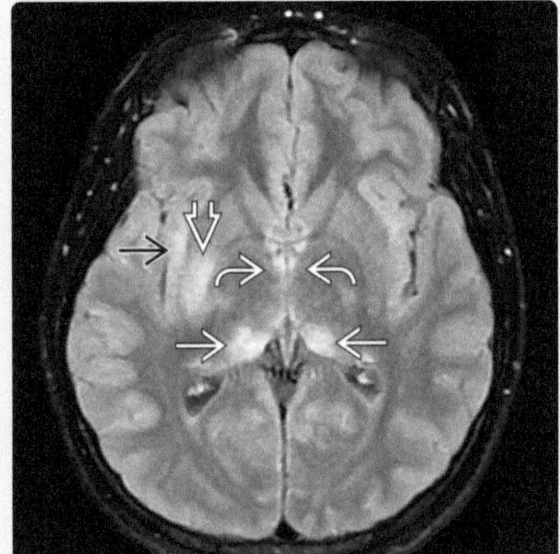

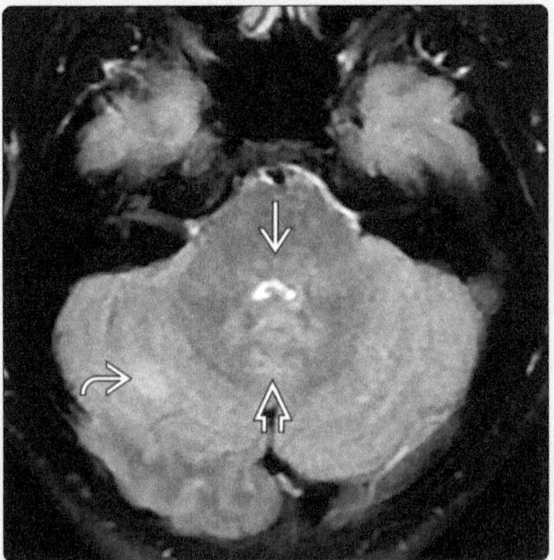

(Left) *Axial FLAIR MR in a 10-year-old with acute myelin oligodendrocyte glycoprotein antibody-associated disease (MOGAD) shows characteristic thalamic ➡, basal ganglia ➡, hypothalamic ➡, and insular cortex ➡ hyperintense lesions. The hypothalamic lesions are relatively subtle but correlated clinically with lethargy and hypothalamic symptoms and signs.* **(Right)** *Axial FLAIR MR in the same patient additionally reveals brainstem/cerebellar peduncle ➡, deep cerebellar white matter ➡, and cerebellar hemisphere ➡ lesions.*

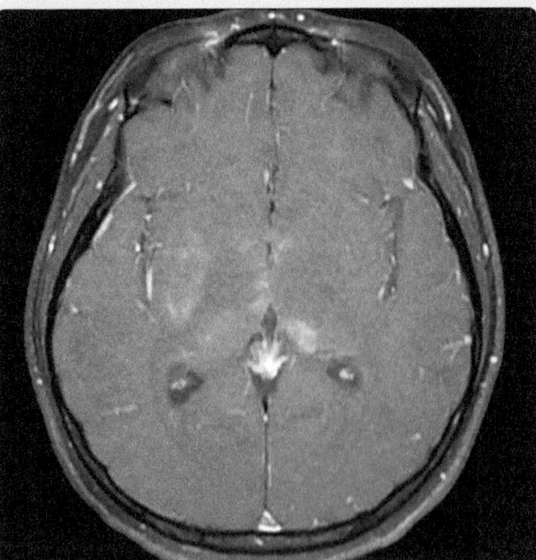

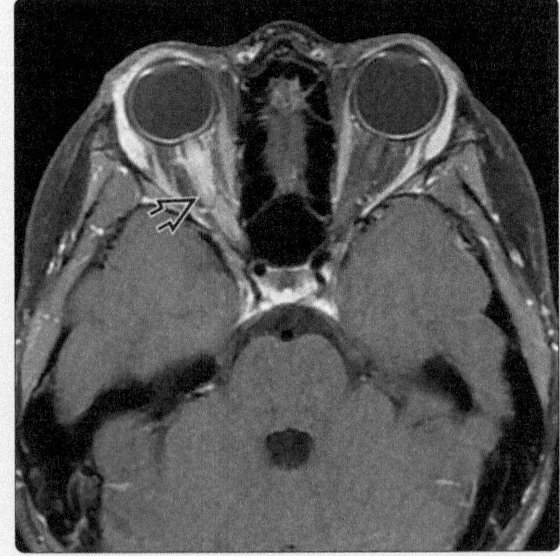

(Left) *Axial T1 C+ FS MR in the same patient shows patchy enhancement of the thalamic, basal ganglia, and hypothalamic lesions. In this patient, the hypothalamic lesions are conspicuous on contrast imaging but subtle on noncontrast FLAIR MR.* **(Right)** *Axial T1 C+ FS MR in the same patient 3 months prior reveals avid contrast enhancement of the left optic nerve (anterior segment) ➡. Laboratory assessment at that time confirmed MOG antibodies, but brain imaging was normal (not shown).*

TERMINOLOGY

Abbreviations

- Myelin oligodendrocyte glycoprotein (MOG), MOG antibody-associated disease (MOGAD)

Definitions

- Inflammatory process of CNS characterized by attacks of immune-mediated demyelination
- Clinically and laboratory distinguishable from multiple sclerosis (MS) and AQP4-IgG (+) neuromyelitis optica spectrum disorder (NMOSD)

IMAGING

General Features

- Best diagnostic clue
  - Bilateral **anterior** optic pathway neuritis + longitudinally extensive transverse myelitis (**LETM**)
    - Bilateral involvement during 1st optic neuritis (ON) presentation in 84% of MOGAD patients
- Location
  - Orbits, cerebral hemispheres, spinal cord
  - Cortical gray matter (GM)/paracortical white matter (WM) most common location for MOGAD lesions

CT Findings

- NECT
  - Hypodense lesions in areas of acute demyelination
- CECT
  - Variable enhancement pattern, similar to MR

MR Findings

- T1WI
  - ± hypointensity within brain lesions
- T2WI
  - Orbits
    - Abnormal bilateral long-segment hyperintensity of optic nerve **anterior** segments
      - □ Best seen on fat-saturated imaging
      - □ Usually spares optic chiasm, retrochiasmatic pathways
  - Brain
    - Hyperintensity in cortical GM, subcortical WM, deep WM, and deep GM
      - □ Perivenous confluent pattern around small veins, lacking radiologic central vein sign (as opposed to MS)
    - Bilateral hyperintense, fluffy, poorly demarcated lesions
      - □ Brain lesions present at onset < 1/2 of adults, more common in children
      - □ 1/3 infratentorial, predominantly in brainstem and cerebellar peduncles (children)
      - □ Ovoid periventricular (Dawson fingers) lesions **not** typical
    - Bilateral, large brainstem and deep gray nuclei lesions more common in children
- STIR
  - Orbits
    - Abnormal bilateral long-segment hyperintensity of anterior optic nerve segments
      - □ Spares optic chiasm, retrochiasmatic pathways
- FLAIR
  - Brain
    - Same as T2WI, lesions usually better seen
    - ± T2-hypointense subcortical WM lesions
- T1WI C+
  - Orbits
    - Avid optic nerve enhancement
    - Perioptic nerve sheath and surrounding orbital fat enhancement
  - Brain
    - Variable; absent, faint, or patchy
    - ± leptomeningeal enhancement, ± adjacent cortical lesions

Imaging Recommendations

- Protocol advice
  - MR ± contrast of orbits, brain, and spinal cord

DIFFERENTIAL DIAGNOSIS

Multiple Sclerosis

- Optic nerves: Typically unilateral, short-segment, less extensive enhancement than MOGAD, NMOSD
  - Bilateral ON during initial presentation ≈ 23% of patients with MS-associated ON
- Brain: Presence of perpendicular periventricular lesions (Dawson fingers), "black holes"
- (+) CSF oligoclonal bands, (-) MOG antibodies, (-) AQP4 antibodies

Acute Disseminated Encephalomyelitis

- Polyfocal neurologic deficits and encephalopathy not explainable by fever
- Diffuse T2 signal abnormality in cortical GM, subcortical WM, deep WM, deep GM (or combination)
- ± linear, patchy, nodular enhancement
- May clinically mimic NMOSD and MOGAD

Neuromyelitis Optica Spectrum Disorder

- Most patients (+) for AQP4-IgG antibodies (seropositive NMOSD)
- Optic nerves: Favors **posterior** optic pathway segments (optic chiasm, retrochiasmatic optic tract)
- Brain: Medulla oblongata (45.5%) and area postrema (31.8%) lesions most common

Brain Neoplasms

- Intracranial mass lesion
  - May mimic tumefactive MS on imaging
- Distinguish on clinical and imaging features

Collagen Vascular Disorders

- Systemic lupus erythematosus, Sjögren syndrome neuro-Behçet disease, neurosarcoidosis
- Look for elevated markers of systemic inflammation

Hemophagocytic Lymphohistiocytosis

- Primary involvement of CNS (rarely) precedes systemic manifestations of hemophagocytic lymphohistiocytosis (HLH)
- Pediatric CNS-isolated HLH can mimic acute disseminated encephalomyelitis (ADEM) clinically and on imaging

Mitochondrial Diseases

- Typical MR features include abnormal T2 hyperintensity in basal ganglia or parietooccipital regions
- (Mitochondrial) **m**yopathy, **e**ncephalopathy, **l**actic **a**cidosis, and **s**troke-like episodes syndrome (MELAS), Leigh disease, others
- Elevation of serum and CSF lactate levels

Leukodystrophies

- Metachromatic leukodystrophy (MLD), X-linked adrenoleukodystrophy (ALD), Alexander disease (AD), Krabbe disease (globoid cell leukodystrophy)
- Look for characteristic imaging or laboratory abnormalities

PATHOLOGY

General Features

- MOG is myelin protein expressed on outer surface of oligodendrocytes and myelin sheath
    - Function not known; may act as cell adhesion molecule, regulate microtubule stability, and modulate myelin immune interactions
- Cortical demyelination common, topographically associated with adjacent meningeal inflammation
- Intracortical > subcortical WM demyelinated lesions predominate (compared to MS)

Staging, Grading, & Classification

- **New diagnostic criteria for MOGAD (March 2023)**
    - 3 primary diagnostic criteria
        - 1 of 6 core clinical demyelinating events [i.e., ON, transverse myelitis (TM), ADEM-like encephalopathy, cerebral monofocal or polyfocal deficits, brainstem or cerebellar deficits, or cerebral cortical encephalitis]
        - MOG-immunoglobulin G (IgG) antibody test (+)
        - Exclusion of better diagnosis

Microscopic Features

- Initial peripheral T-cell activation of T cells → reactivation in subarachnoid/perivascular spaces by MOG-laden antigen-presenting cells and inflammatory CSF milieu
    - T cells, granulocytes cross blood brain barrier, infiltrate CNS parenchyma
    - Macrophages/microglia appear in lesions
- Anti-MOG antibodies opsonize MOG, activate complement- and antibody-dependent cellular cytotoxicity
- Extensive subpial cortical demyelination with microglial activation, inflammatory infiltrate
- Chronic active lesions absent

Laboratory Evaluation

- Serum MOG-IgG antibody testing by cell-based assay
- Serum AQP4-IgG testing to exclude NMOSD
- CSF testing for oligoclonal bands to evaluate for MS

CLINICAL ISSUES

Presentation

- Most common signs/symptoms
    - Unilateral or bilateral ON
        - Most common clinical MOGAD manifestation at onset
    - ADEM-like presentation with altered mental status, focal neurologic deficits
        - Up to 68% of cases at initial presentation
        - Recurrence of ADEM features after recovery suggests MOGAD
    - TM
        - Limb weakness, sensory loss, and bowel, bladder, or sexual dysfunction
    - Cerebral cortical encephalitis
        - Headache, seizures, stroke-like episodes, and focal neurologic deficits
- Other signs/symptoms
    - Rare: Progressive clinical decline with leukodystrophy-like MR pattern

Demographics

- Age
    - Predilection for children but can affect any age
        - Median age of MOGAD onset: 20-30 years
        - Children: ≈ 50% of MOGAD cases
- Sex
    - M = F

Natural History & Prognosis

- Infectious prodrome precedes initial symptom onset ≤ 60% of patients
- Monophasic or relapsing course (≈ 50/50)
    - ON is most common relapse manifestation (followed by TM)
- Most T2 lesions resolve completely over months to few years
    - Useful discriminator from MS and AQP4-IgG NMOSD, in which majority have residual T2-hyperintense lesions
- Visual outcomes after MOG-associated ON better than NMOSD
- Long-term disability rates lower than with NMOSD or MS

Treatment

- Glucocorticoid therapy 1st line

DIAGNOSTIC CHECKLIST

Consider

- Simultaneous bilateral ON involving anterior optic pathway with associated optic disc edema strongly implies MOGAD

Image Interpretation Pearls

- Evaluate optic apparatus carefully on brain imaging to identify concurrent ON

SELECTED REFERENCES

1. Banwell B et al: Diagnosis of myelin oligodendrocyte glycoprotein antibody-associated disease: International MOGAD Panel proposed criteria. Lancet Neurol. 22(3):268-82, 2023
2. Gadde JA et al: Rate of leptomeningeal enhancement in pediatric myelin oligodendrocyte glycoprotein antibody-associated encephalomyelitis. J Child Neurol. 36(11):1042-6, 2021
3. Shahriari M et al: MOGAD: How it differs from and resembles other neuroinflammatory disorders. AJR Am J Roentgenol. 216(4):1031-9, 2021
4. Höftberger R et al: The pathology of central nervous system inflammatory demyelinating disease accompanying myelin oligodendrocyte glycoprotein autoantibody. Acta Neuropathol. 139(5):875-92, 2020
5. Ogawa R et al: MOG antibody-positive, benign, unilateral, cerebral cortical encephalitis with epilepsy. Neurol Neuroimmunol Neuroinflamm. 4(2):e322, 2017

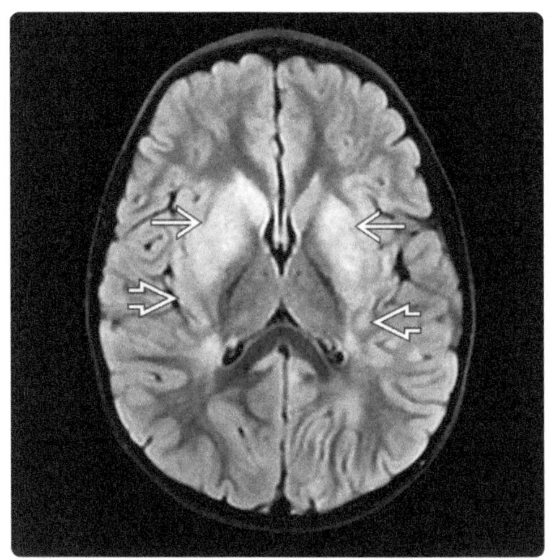

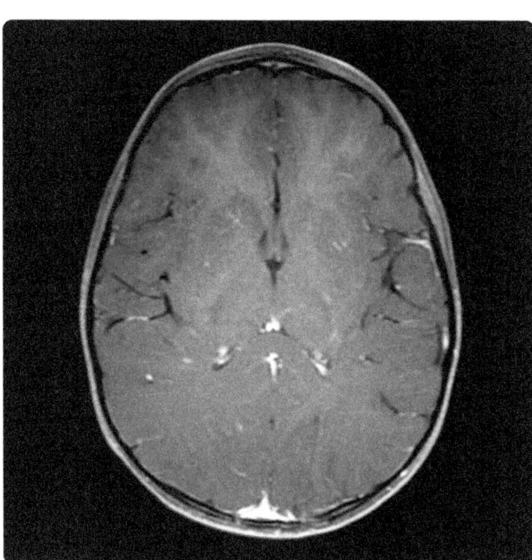

(Left) *Axial FLAIR MR in a 4-year-old with florid optic neuritis and encephalopathy with positive anti-MOG antibody titer reveals abnormal hyperintensity and swelling within the bilateral basal ganglia ➡, insular cortex ➡, perventricular white matter, and posterior thalami.* **(Right)** *Axial T1 C+ FS MR in the same patient reveals minimal, if any, enhancement within the same abnormal brain regions.*

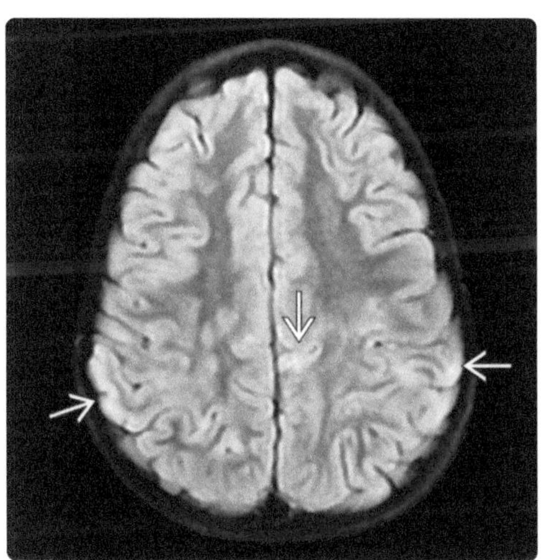

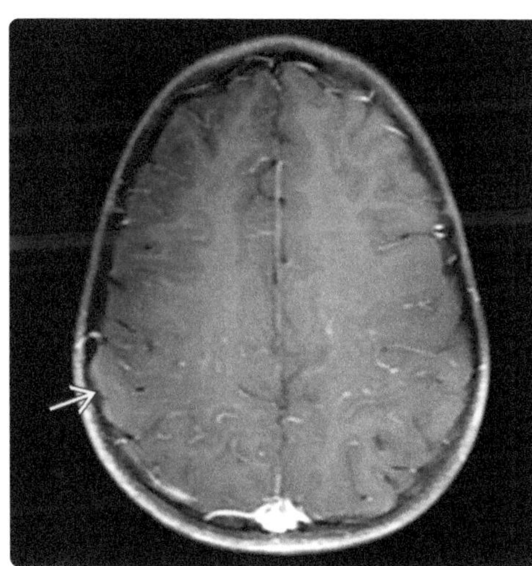

(Left) *Axial FLAIR MR in a 4-year-old with severe onset of encephalopathy with positive MOG antibody titer depicts several areas of abnormal cortical hyperintensity and edema ➡ as well as subcortical white matter signal abnormalities.* **(Right)** *Axial T1 C+ FS MR in the same patient reveals subtle leptomeningeal enhancement ➡ over the right parietal lobe. This constellation of findings represents cerebral cortical encephalitis, a finding unique to MOGAD and potentially predisposing to seizures.*

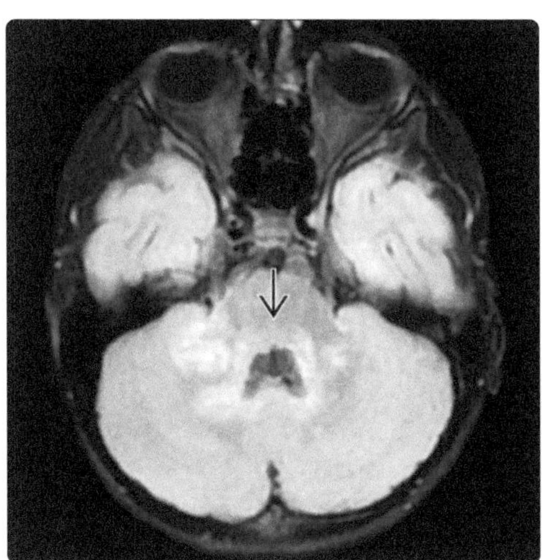

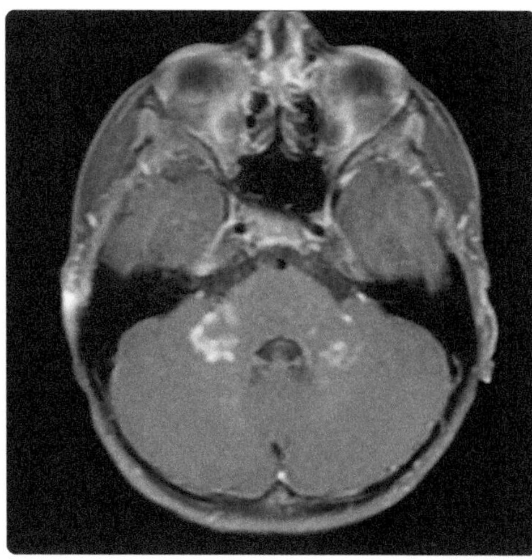

(Left) *Axial FLAIR MR in a 5-year-old patient with florid encephalopathy and emesis reveals multifocal T2-hyperintense lesions predominantly localizing to the brainstem and posterior fossa. Lesions are noted in the middle cerebellar peduncles, deep cerebellar white matter, and dorsal brainstem ➡ near the facial colliculus (area postrema, explaining vomiting).* **(Right)** *Axial T1 C+ FS MR in the same patient reveals patchy partial ring and nodular enhancement in these abnormal areas.*

Normal Brain Maturation

From the imaging perspective, normal brain maturation can be divided into 2 concurrent processes: Sulcation and myelination. Cerebral sulcation first starts in the early 2nd trimester with the formation of the sylvian fissures but really begins to accelerate in the middle-to-late 2nd trimester with formation of the callosal sulcus and the hippocampal and parietooccipital fissures by 23 weeks, the calcarine and cingulate sulci by 24 weeks, the collateral and central sulci by 26 weeks, and the superior temporal sulcus by 27 weeks, followed by the precentral, postcentral, and interparietal sulci by 28 weeks. The left superior temporal sulcus is usually several days advanced compared to the right. The superior and inferior frontal sulci are seen by 29 weeks. Afterward, multiple sulci are seen to form in rapid succession until birth with a few tertiary and quaternary sulci forming during the 1st year after birth.

Fetal imaging using single-shot half-Fourier techniques (HASTE, SSFSE) shows other signs of maturation with the presence of the "germinal matrices" and the subplate. The germinal matrices are actually multiple areas: The ganglionic eminences (caudal, medial, and lateral), the ventricular zone, and the inner and outer subventricular zones are the major supratentorial regions where neurons are generated, whereas the ventricular zone and the rhombic lips are the regions where most cerebellar neurons are generated. These zones are seen as areas of hypointensity lining the superior 3rd ventricle and the lateral ventricles of fetuses between the ages of 18-24 weeks. Just external to these areas is a region of intermediate intensity consisting of the so-called intermediate zone, composed mainly of the leading processes of the migrating neurons and axons from the neurons that are pathfinding through the developing hemispheres. External to the intermediate zone is the subplate, which is hyperintense on T2 images and consists of sparsely scattered neurons that form synapses with axons from neurons in the thalami and, likely, from other subplate neurons. Most peripheral is a layer with hypointensity similar to that of the germinal matrices: The developing cerebral cortex. By ~ 25-27 weeks, the germinal matrices disappear as the neurons complete their migratory path. The subplate fades at about the same time on SSPE images as the early subcortical synapses disappear and are replaced by more permanent synapses within the cortex itself. However, high-resolution, diffusion-weighted postnatal scans at the same adjusted age allow visualization of the subplate.

White matter maturation also begins in utero but is a later process than neuronal migration or sulcation. It is important to note in this regard that the imaging changes seen associated with white matter maturation [T1 and T2 shortening, reduced mean diffusivity, reduced radial diffusivity (RD), increased fractional anisotropy (FA), increased magnetization transfer, and increased bound water fraction] do not directly represent myelination. They represent the many changes associated with white matter and gray matter maturation, which can be most simply understood as increasingly complex intra- and extracellular structures that transiently bind water molecules and, thereby, alter their relaxation and diffusivity characteristics. Although some early myelination occurs in the dorsal brainstem in the early 3rd trimester (median longitudinal fasciculus, medial lemnisci, lateral lemnisci), the vast majority of maturational changes in both the supra- and infratentorial compartments take place in the late 3rd trimester and after birth. Myelination of the cerebrum and cerebellum begins just before birth along the corticospinal tracts; thus, T1 and T2 shortening is seen at term in normal neonates. It is important to note that the changes associated with white matter maturation are seen earlier on T1-weighted images than on T2-weighted images in all structures. Although this is often attributed to T1 imaging being "more sensitive to the changes of myelination," the reason for this is not known. On T1 images, the posterior portions of the posterior limbs of the internal capsules are hyperintense at birth with the entire posterior limb (PLIC) becoming hyperintense in the 2nd month and the anterior limb (ALIC) in the 3rd month. The callosal splenium is hyperintense by 6 months, the genu by 8 months, the frontal white matter by 9 months, and the entire brain by 12 months. On T2-weighted images, a focus of hypointensity is seen in the corticospinal tract portion of the PLIC at birth, the entire PLIC and the callosal splenium by 6 months, the ALIC and callosal genu by 8-9 months, the occipital white matter by 12 months, the deep frontal white matter by 14 months, and the subcortical superior frontal white matter by 20 months. The last areas to turn dark on T2-weighted images are the orbital regions of the frontal lobes and the most anterior temporal lobes, which may not be hypointense compared to cortex until 28-30 months.

Other imaging sequences can be used to quantify brain maturation (keep in mind that they do not quantify myelination per se). Of these, the easiest to use at this time are magnetization transfer, diffusion tensor imaging (in particular, RD and FA), and T1/T2 relaxometry. Standard values for these parameters at specific ages are published. The numbers can vary, however, with MR field strength and parameters used; therefore, the standard values should be used with caution. The "bound water fraction," a.k.a. the "myelin water fraction" imaging technique (which is still difficult to use on clinical scanners at the time of this writing), holds a great deal of promise for quantification of maturation.

Approach to Metabolic Diseases

The diagnosis of inborn errors of metabolism is extremely challenging unless a family history is present. The presenting signs and symptoms are typically nonspecific: Seizures, hypotonia, movement disorder, delayed achievement of milestones, or ataxia. Biochemical testing requires sending blood for a wide variety of chemical and genetic tests that may or may not be revealing. Imaging occasionally gives an answer or narrows the differential diagnosis, but the large majority of cases yield only nonspecific findings. As a result, > 60% of patients with presumed metabolic disorders never receive a specific diagnosis. Imaging can be a great help, however, if approached properly. The proper approach involves acquiring high-resolution images that maximize contrast between normal and abnormal tissue. All studies of children with suspected inborn errors of metabolism should include T1-weighted images ± contrast, T2-weighted images to assess for cortical malformations, T2 FLAIR images to assess for leukoencephalopathy, diffusion imaging to assess diffusivity and FA, and short- and long-echo proton MR spectroscopy to assess quantities of normal metabolites and to find abnormal metabolites.

Imaging Patterns

From an imaging perspective, it is best to look at inborn errors of metabolism by assessing the pattern of involvement of the brain: What parts of the brain are involved and what kind of involvement? For the parts of the brain, the primary differentiation is gray matter vs. white matter. Secondary differentiation points would be cortex vs. cerebral nuclei for gray matter disease with tertiary points being the location(s) of cortical involvement and the specific nuclei involved. For white matter involvement, differentiation of subcortical, deep, or periventricular white matter involvement and the presence of additional factors, such as cysts, cavitations, calcifications, inflammation (reduced diffusivity) or enhancement, are important points.

In children, the major disorders that cause diffuse cortical degeneration are neurodegenerative diseases, such as the neuronal ceroid lipofuscinoses (NCL), mucolipidoses, Rett syndrome, and Alpers-Huttenlocher syndrome. None of these have specific patterns (although the presence of diffuse mild cortical atrophy in a child presenting with ataxia and found to have early cerebellar atrophy should raise the question of late infantile onset NCL); therefore, the diagnosis has to be made by combining imaging findings with clinical exam results and laboratory or genetic testing.

A broader group of disorders causes deep gray nuclear involvement with the diagnosis being narrowed by the specific nuclei or combinations of nuclei involved. For example, isolated globus pallidus involvement generates a differential diagnosis of methylmalonic aciduria, succinate semialdehyde dehydrogenase deficiency, isovaleric acidemia, or toxins (carbon monoxide, cyanide, bilirubin). Striatal involvement suggests Leigh syndrome, 3-methylglutaconic aciduria, propionic acidemia, or ethylmalonic acidemia, among others.

Among white matter diseases, disorders that affect subcortical white matter early in the course of the disease include galactosemia, infantile Alexander disease (mainly frontal involvement), and megalencephaly with leukoencephalopathy and cysts (MLC), of which the latter 2 are associated with macrocephaly. MLC is unusual in that it presents as a leukodystrophy on imaging but has normal white matter; the appearance of leukodystrophy is actually the result of water leaking through volume-regulated ion channels into the interstitial space of the white matter. This is why the affected children are usually only mildly affected clinically despite a severe imaging appearance.

A larger group of white matter diseases spares the subcortical white matter in the early course of the disease. These include metachromatic leukodystrophy (MLD), Krabbe disease, GM2 gangliosidoses, X-linked adrenoleukodystrophy (X-ALD), phenylketonuria, and maple syrup urine disease (MSUD). All of these disorders have onset at different ages as well, while X-ALD has an inflammatory component, MSUD has markedly reduced diffusivity in affected areas, and GM2 has T1 hyperintensity/T2 hypointensity of the thalami.

A still larger group of disorders has involvement of both white matter and deep gray nuclei. The most common of these are the mitochondrial disorders, such as Leigh disease, but Canavan disease, urea cycle disorders, L-2 hydroxyglutaric aciduria, glutaric aciduria type I, Wilson disease, and many others belong in this group. These disorders can be further divided into white matter and gray matter diseases: Subcortical vs. deep vs. periventricular white matter involvement and the specific gray matter nuclei affected.

The final white matter disease category is composed of hypomyelinating disorders. These recently described disorders differ from other white matter disorders, which are associated with production of myelin that disappears, usually associated with edema or inflammation. In hypomyelinating disorders, myelin is never formed, or it is formed very slowly and deficiently, thus, the brain always looks like that of a young infant on T2-weighted images (in some cases, the white matter may appear to mature on T1 images). Due to the absence of edema/inflammation, it may be difficult to ascertain whether myelin is merely delayed as opposed to deficient. In such cases, a follow-up MR in 6 months is useful: Significant progress of myelination suggests earlier delay, while no or minimal progress suggest hypomyelination. Other features of the disorders, such as hypodontia, hypogonadotropic hypogonadism, or congenital cataracts, can help in the distinction as well. Some of the most common disorders in this group include Pelizaeus-Merzbacher disease, 4H syndrome (hypomyelination, hypodontia, and hypogonadotropic hypogonadism), hypomyelination with atrophy of the basal ganglia and cerebellum (HABC), and the 18q deletion syndrome.

Selected References

1. Ardissone A et al: Phenotyping mitochondrial DNA-related diseases in childhood: a cohort study of 150 patients. Eur J Neurol. 30(7):2079-91, 2023
2. Hong SY et al: Epilepsy in sulfite oxidase deficiency and related disorders: insights from neuroimaging and genetics. Epilepsy Behav. 143:109246, 2023
3. Huisman TAGM et al: Neuroimaging of primary mitochondrial disorders in children: a review. J Neuroimaging. 32(2):191-200, 2022
4. Servais A et al: Central nervous system complications in cystinosis: the role of neuroimaging. Cells. 11(4), 2022
5. Gonçalves FG et al: Primary mitochondrial disorders of the pediatric central nervous system: neuroimaging findings. Radiographics. 40(7):2042-67, 2020
6. Casanova MF et al: The modular organization of the cerebral cortex: evolutionary significance and possible links to neurodevelopmental conditions. J Comp Neurol. 1;527(10):1720-30, 2018
7. Mascalchi M et al: Neuroimaging in mitochondrial disorders. Essays Biochem. 62(3):409-21, 2018
8. Reddy N et al: Neuroimaging findings of organic acidemias and aminoacidopathies. Radiographics. 38(3):912-31, 2018
9. Tan AP et al: Clinical and neuroimaging spectrum of peroxisomal disorders. Top Magn Reson Imaging. 27(4):241-57, 2018
10. Longo MG et al: Brain imaging and genetic risk in the pediatric population, part 1: inherited metabolic diseases. Neuroimaging Clin N Am. 25(1):31-51, 2015
11. Deoni SC et al: One component? Two components? Three? The effect of including a nonexchanging "free" water component in multicomponent driven equilibrium single pulse observation of T1 and T2. Magn Reson Med. 70(1):147-54, 2013
12. Nossin-Manor R et al: Quantitative MRI in the very preterm brain: assessing tissue organization and myelination using magnetization transfer, diffusion tensor and T_1 imaging. Neuroimage. 64:505-16, 2013
13. Barkovich AJ et al: Metabolic, toxic and inflammatory brain disorders. In Barkovich AJ et al: Pediatric Neuroimaging. 5th ed. Wolters Kluwer, 2012
14. Deoni SC et al: Investigating white matter development in infancy and early childhood using myelin water faction and relaxation time mapping. Neuroimage. 63(3):1038-53, 2012
15. Dreha-Kulaczewski SF et al: Assessment of myelination in hypomyelinating disorders by quantitative MRI. J Magn Reson Imaging. 36(6):1329-38, 2012
16. Provenzale JM et al: Progression of corpus callosum diffusion-tensor imaging values during a period of signal changes consistent with myelination. AJR Am J Roentgenol. 198(6):1403-8, 2012
17. van der Knaap MS et al: Megalencephalic leukoencephalopathy with subcortical cysts: chronic white matter oedema due to a defect in brain ion and water homoeostasis. Lancet Neurol. 11(11):973-85, 2012
18. Deoni SC: Quantitative relaxometry of the brain. Top Magn Reson Imaging. 21(2):101-13, 2010
19. Steenweg ME et al: Magnetic resonance imaging pattern recognition in hypomyelinating disorders. Brain. 133(10):2971-82, 2010
20. van der Knaap MS et al: Defining and categorizing leukoencephalopathies of unknown origin: MR imaging approach. Radiology. 213(1):121-33, 1999

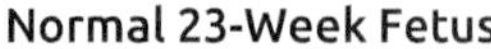

Normal 23-Week Fetus

Normal 27-Week Fetus

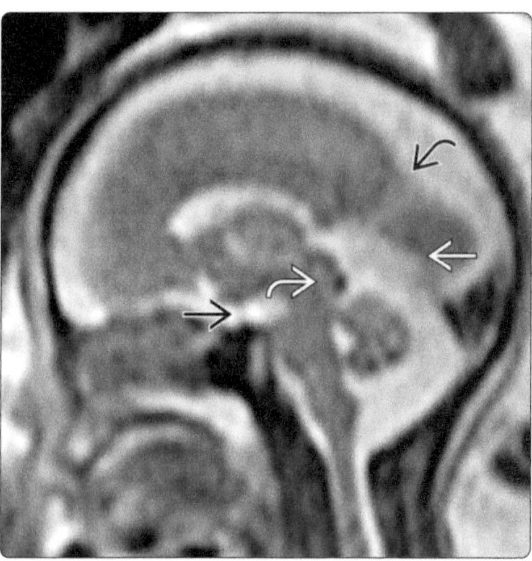

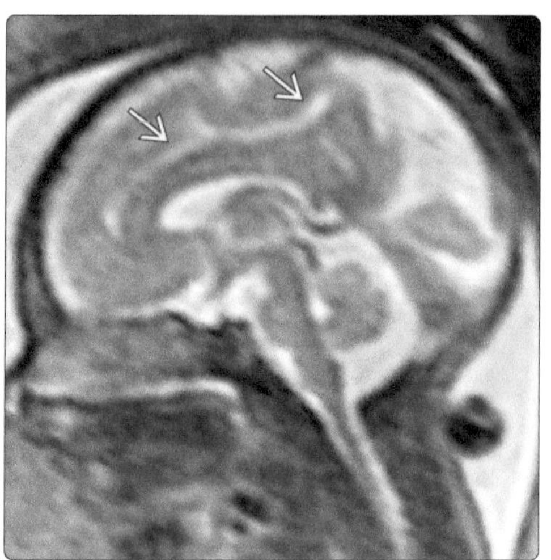

(Left) *Sagittal T2 MR SSFSE reformat in a 35-week fetus shows that the corpus callosum can already be confidently seen; the only sulci seen are the parietooccipital* ➩ *and calcarine* ➡*, and the cerebellum appears relatively small because it grows late. The cerebral aqueduct* ➡ *and pituitary stalk* ➩ *are seen at this age.* **(Right)** *Sagittal T2 MR SSFSE in a 27-week fetus shows significant sulcal development since 23 weeks. The cingulate and callosomarginal sulci* ➡ *are well seen on this image.*

Normal 35-Week Infant

Normal Term Infant

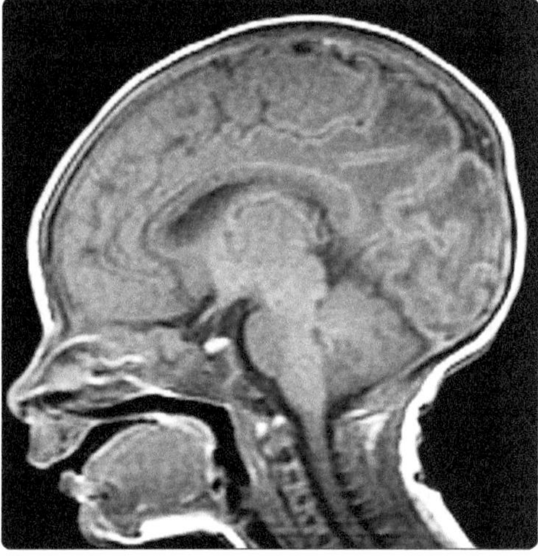

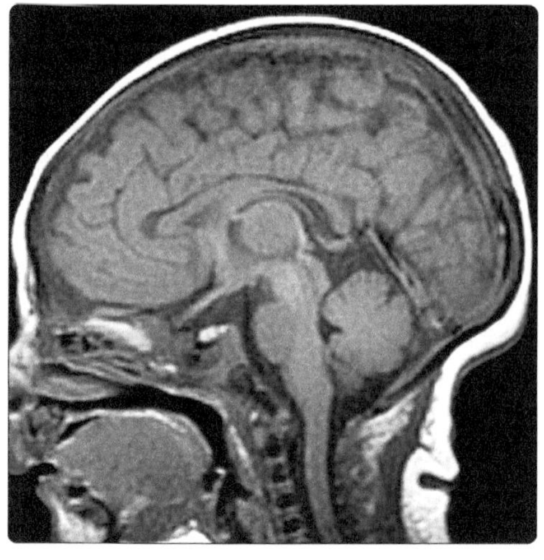

(Left) *Sagittal T1WI MR in a 35-week, adjusted-age infant shows a markedly more complex gyral pattern than at 27 weeks. The pituitary gland is always bright on T1 images in the 1st week after birth. Also note that the cerebellum is still relatively small at this age. Much cerebellar growth is postnatal.* **(Right)** *Sagittal T1WI MR in a term-born neonate shows more complex sulcation along the medial surface of the cerebral hemispheres. Posterior fossa and cerebellar size are increased.*

Normal 6-Month Infant

Normal 18-Month Child

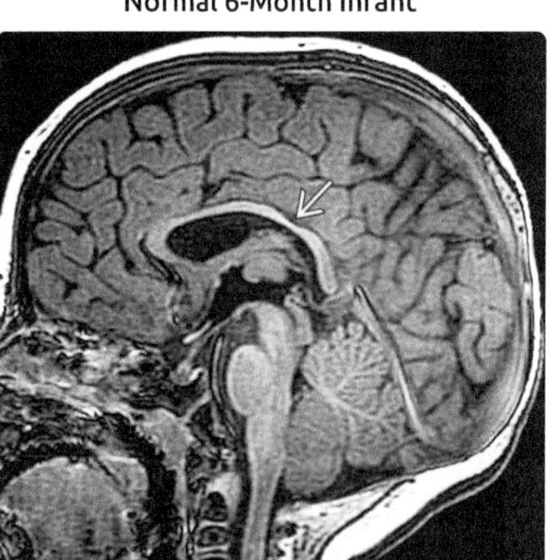

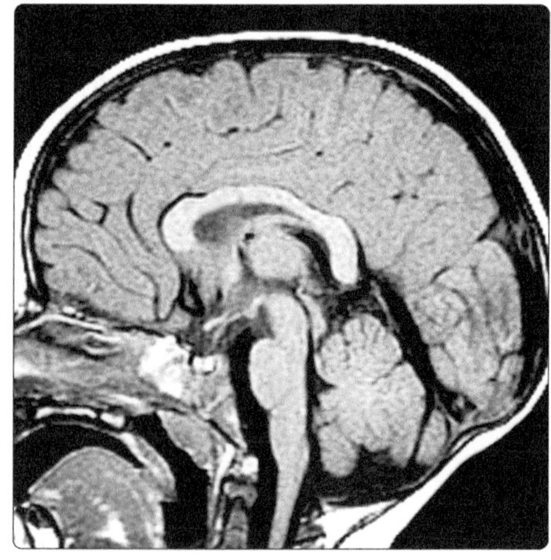

(Left) *Sagittal T1WI MR in a 6-month-old infant shows development of high signal in the posterior corpus callosum* ➡ *and some thickening of the genu and splenium. Complexity of sulcation of the medial hemisphere has further increased, as has cerebellar growth.* **(Right)** *Sagittal T1WI MR in an 18-month-old child shows a fully myelinated corpus callosum that has adult proportions and an adult-sized posterior fossa containing an adult-sized cerebellum.*

Normal 23-Week Fetus

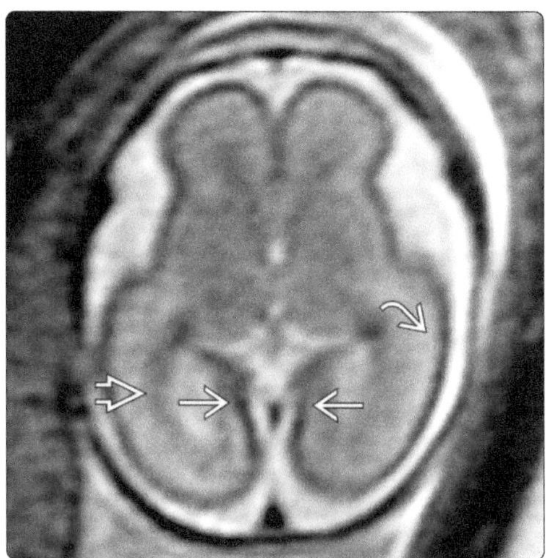

Normal 28-Week Fetus

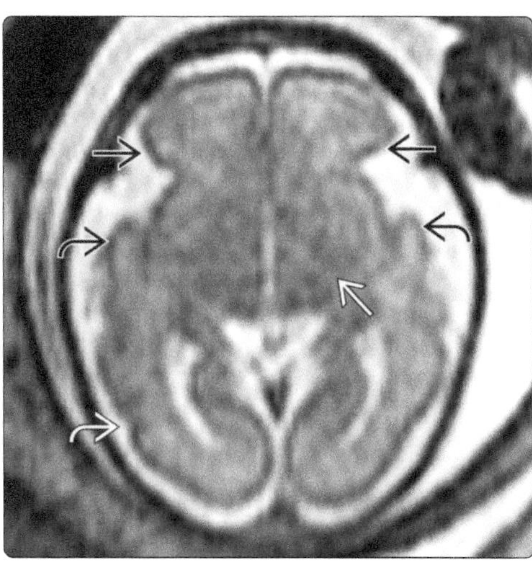

(Left) *Axial T2 MR SSFSE in a 23-week fetus shows sylvian fissures and very early calcarine fissures ➡. Hypointense germinal matrices ➡ line lateral ventricles. Hyperintense subplate ➡ is seen between the cortex and intermediate zone.* **(Right)** *Axial T2 MR SSFSE shows small parietal opercula ➡ and very small frontal opercula ➡ at the sylvian fissures at 28 weeks. The superior temporal sulcus ➡ is present on the right. The internal capsule ➡ helps localize basal ganglia.*

Normal 33-Week Infant

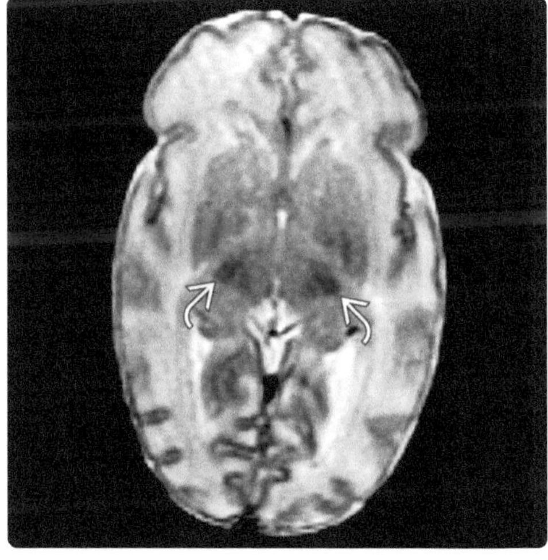

Normal Term Infant

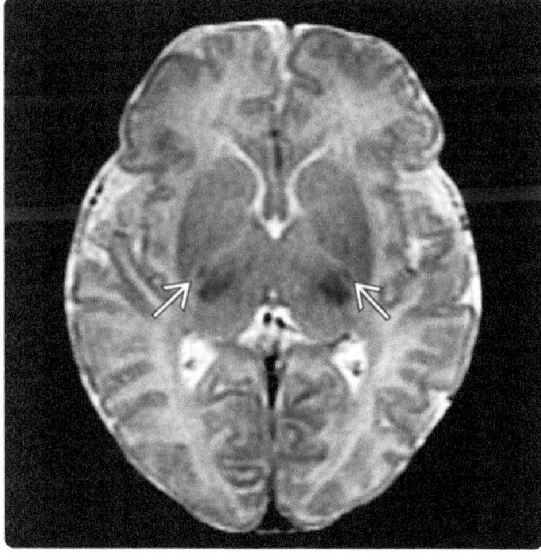

(Left) *Axial T2WI MR in a 33-week premature infant shows absence of any myelination. The ventrolateral thalamic nuclei ➡ are the most hypointense structures. Secondary sulci are present but still rather shallow. The insular sulci have just formed.* **(Right)** *Axial T2WI MR in a term-born neonate shows a much greater degree of sulcation with mature-appearing insular sulci, although the insula is not yet covered. Hypointensity is present in the posterior limbs of the internal capsules ➡.*

Normal 7-Month Infant

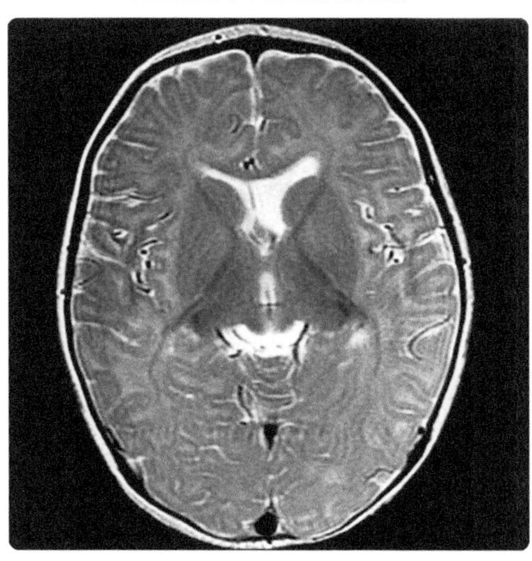

Normal 24-Month Child

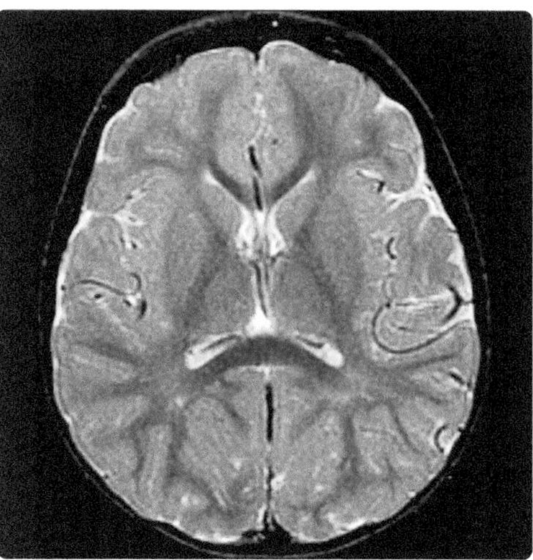

(Left) *Axial T2WI MR in a 7-month-old infant shows the insulae completely covered by opercula. The anterior and posterior limbs in the internal capsules are hypointense (a bit precociously). The hemispheric white matter, however, remains hyperintense. Sulcation appears nearly mature.* **(Right)** *Axial T2WI MR in a 24-month-old child shows nearly complete myelination; anterior temporal and orbitofrontal regions remain iso- to slightly hyperintense at this age.*

(Left) *Axial T2WI MR in a patient with late infantile neuronal ceroid lipofuscinosis (LI-NCL) shows gray matter involvement appearing as diffuse cortical atrophy with some sulcal and lateral ventricular enlargement.* **(Right)** *Axial T2WI MR through the cerebellum in the same patient with LI-NCL shows marked cerebellar atrophy, which was the cause of initial presentation, resulting in a prominent horizontal fissure and a significantly enlarged 4th ventricle.*

Late Infantile Neuronal Ceroid Lipofuscinosis

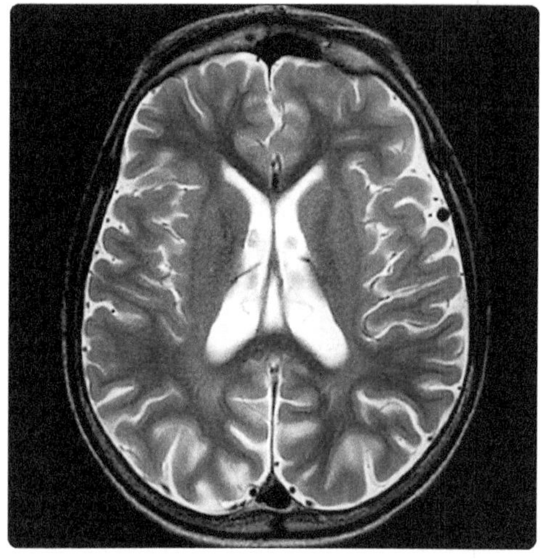

Late Infantile Neuronal Ceroid Lipofuscinosis

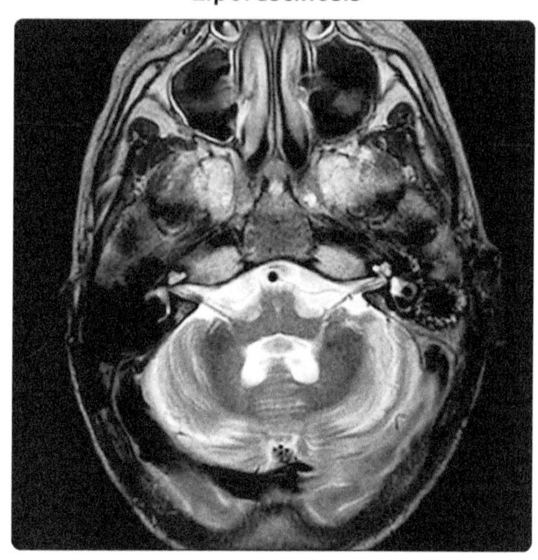

(Left) *Axial PDWI MR in a patient with methylmalonic aciduria shows deep gray matter involvement, appearing as abnormal hyperintensity of the globus pallidus ⇨ bilaterally.* **(Right)** *Axial T2WI MR in a patient with glutaric aciduria type 1 shows hypoplasia of the frontal and temporal insulae, resulting in open sylvian fissures. In addition, hyperintensity is seen in the posterior putamina ↷, another characteristic of this disorder.*

Methylmalonic Aciduria

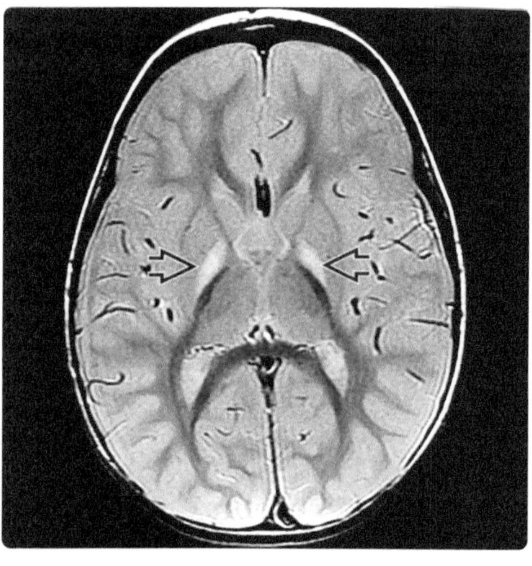

Glutaric Aciduria Type 1

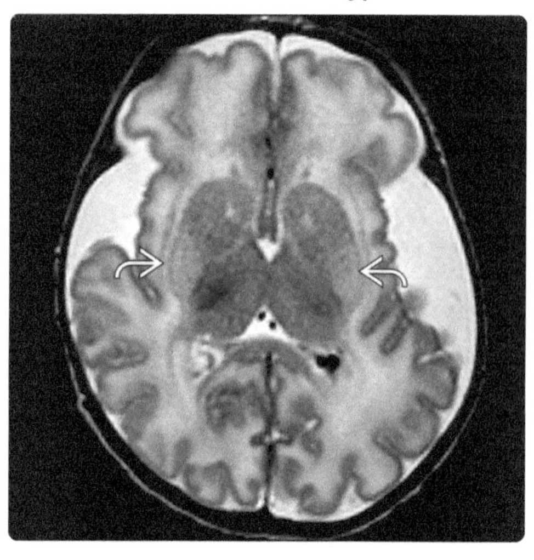

(Left) *Axial T1WI MR in a 7-month-old infant with GM2 gangliosidosis shows hypomyelination of the white matter, which should be hyperintense in much of the brain at this age, and abnormal hyperintensity of the thalami ➡.* **(Right)** *Axial T2WI MR in the same patient with GM2 gangliosidosis shows absence of hypointensity in the white matter (hypomyelination) and abnormally increased hypointensity of the bilateral thalami ➡.*

GM2 Gangliosidosis

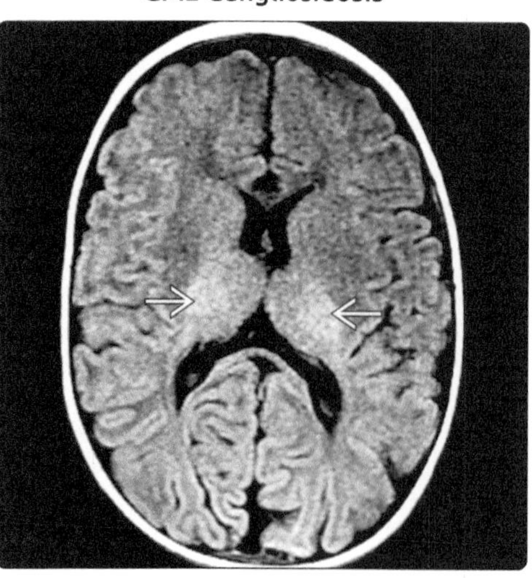

GM2 Gangliosidosis

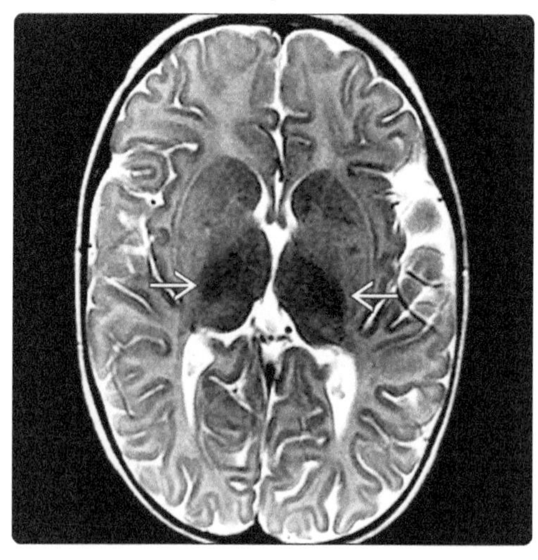

Pelizaeus-Merzbacher Disease

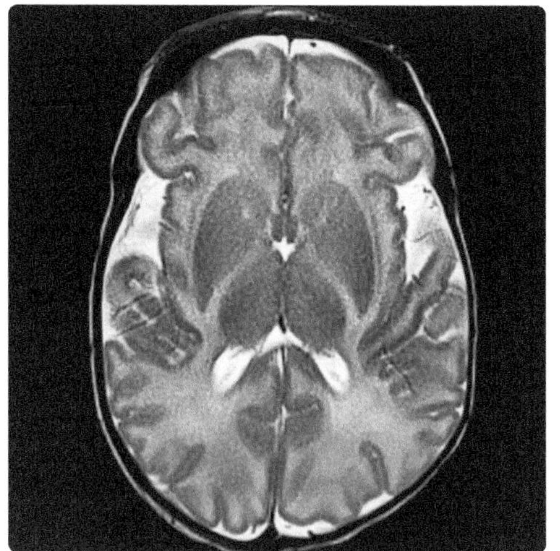

Vanishing White Matter Disease

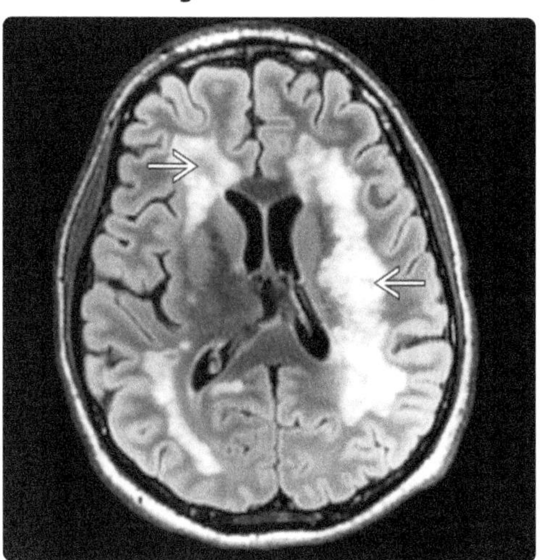

(Left) *Axial T2WI MR in a 3-year-old child with Pelizaeus-Merzbacher disease shows hypomyelination with diffuse abnormal hyperintensity of the white matter. This appearance would be more typical of a neonate, although a neonate would have some hypointensity in the posterior limb of the internal capsule.* **(Right)** *Axial T2WI MR in a 10-year-old patient with vanishing white matter disease shows abnormal hyperintensity in deep white matter, sparing of subcortical white matter, and areas of cavitation ➡.*

Infantile Alexander Disease

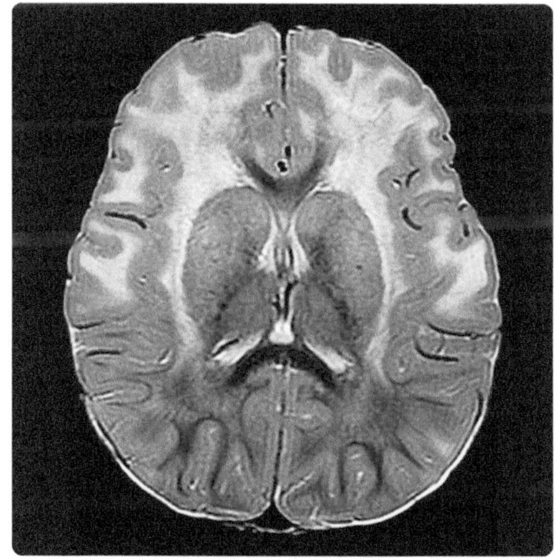

L2-Hydroxyglutaric Aciduria

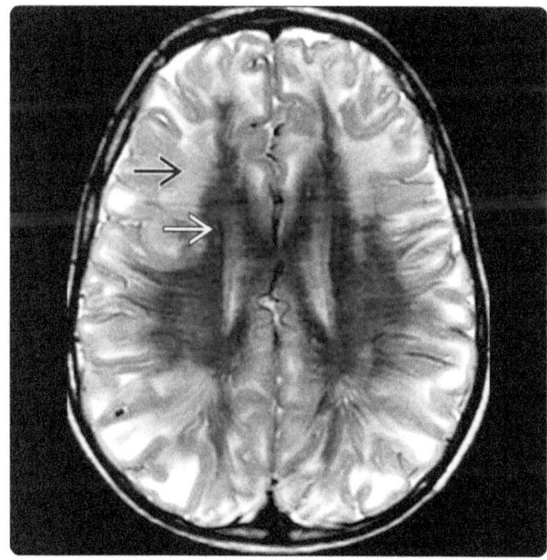

(Left) *Axial T2WI MR in a patient with infantile Alexander disease shows white matter hyperintensity in the frontal lobes that involves subcortical, deep, and periventricular white matter. Basal ganglia are slightly hyperintense.* **(Right)** *Axial T2WI MR in 7-year-old patient with L2-hydroxyglutaric aciduria shows abnormal hyperintensity ⇨ of the subcortical white matter but normal hypointensity ➡ of the deep and subcortical white matter.*

L2-Hydroxyglutaric Aciduria

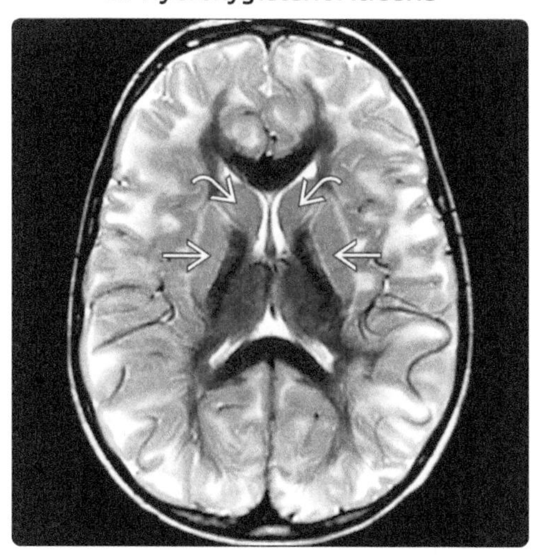

L2-Hydroxyglutaric Aciduria

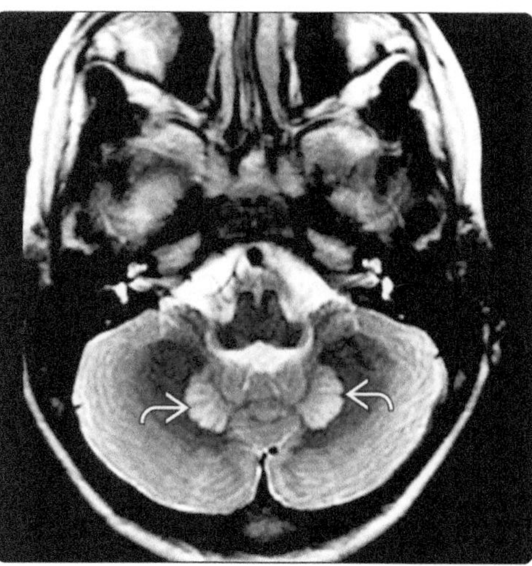

(Left) *Axial T2WI MR in same patient with L2-hydroxyglutaric aciduria shows combined white matter and deep gray matter involvement. Subcortical white matter is abnormally hyperintense. Bilateral caudates ➡ and putamina ➡ are also abnormally hyperintense.* **(Right)** *Axial T2WI MR in the same patient shows bilateral cerebellar nuclear hyperintensity ➡. The combination of subcortical white matter, basal ganglia, and cerebellar nuclei involvement is specific.*

Hypomyelination

KEY FACTS

TERMINOLOGY

- Primary hypomyelination = genetic defect resulting in diminished or absent myelin formation
- Delayed myelination = indicates ability to "catch up" with time

IMAGING

- Key areas to assess are internal capsule, pyramidal tracts, and peripheral frontal lobe white matter rami
  - Myelination on T1WI essentially complete by 1 year of age; T1 shortening reflects presence of mature oligodendrocytes with proteolipid protein (PLP)
  - Myelination on T2WI is complete by 3 years of age (usually by age 2 years)
    - T2 shortening reflects displacement of interstitial water by myelin wrapping on axons

TOP DIFFERENTIAL DIAGNOSES

- Pelizaeus-Merzbacher disease (PMD)
  - Classic hypomyelination syndrome caused by reduced production of PLP
- 18q-syndrome
  - Hemizygous deletion (1 copy of gene missing) of *MBP* gene
- *TUBB4A*-related hypomyelinating disorders
  - *TUBB4A* gene encodes for β-tubulin
  - Hypomyelination with atrophy of basal ganglia and cerebellum (H-ABC) is most severe phenotype
- POLR3-related leukodystrophies
  - 4H syndrome (hypomyelination, hypodontia, hypogonadotropic hypogonadism)

PATHOLOGY

- 87 different genes have been associated with hypomyelination

CLINICAL ISSUES

- Classic PMD is X-linked recessive and, thus, exclusive to males

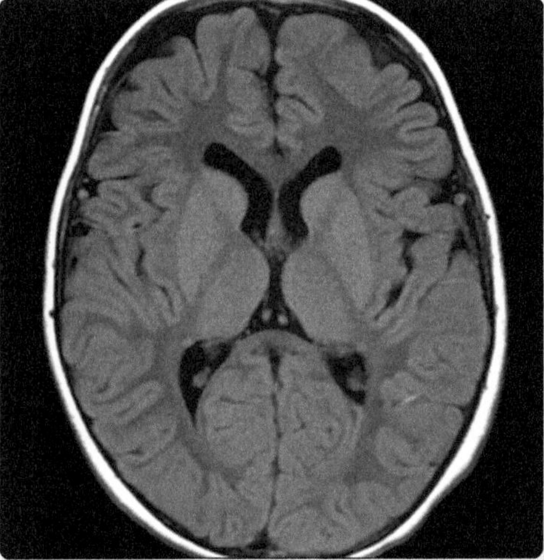

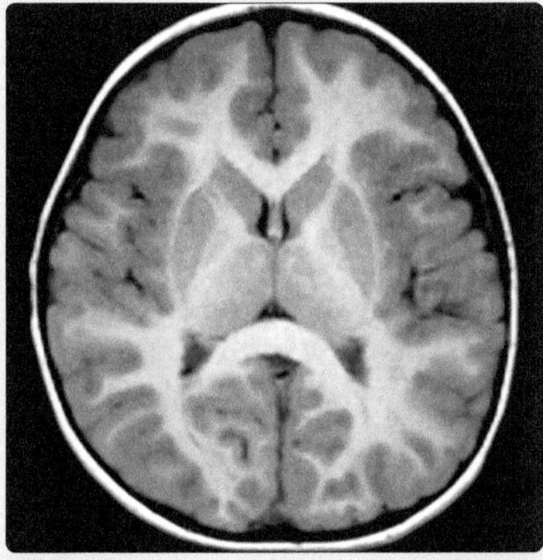

(Left) *Axial T1WI MR in a 2-year-old with Pelizaeus-Merzbacher disease looks like a normal FLAIR image due to the absence of expected T1 shortening caused by myelin. A 2-year-old's brain should look like an adult's on T1-weighted images.* **(Right)** *Conversely, there is bright signal throughout all of the normally myelinated white matter on this T1WI MR obtained at the same level of the brain from a normal 2-year-old.*

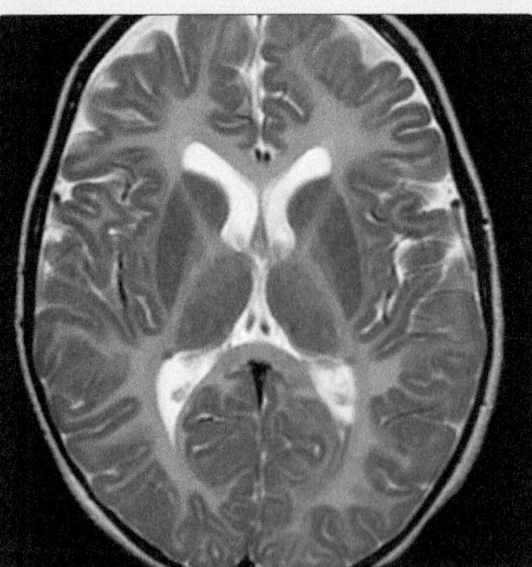

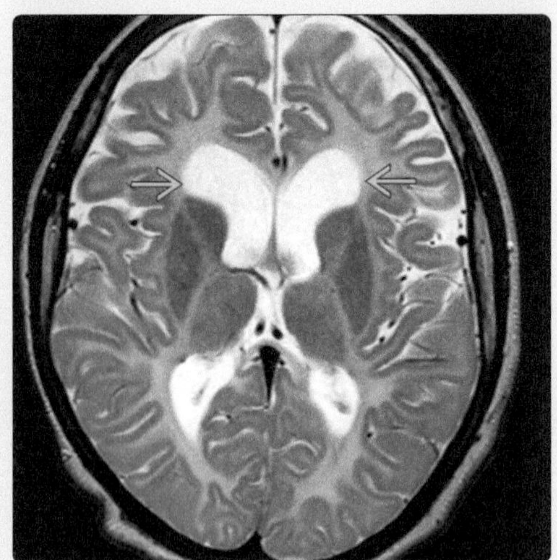

(Left) *Axial T2WI MR in the same child shows diffuse hyperintensity of white matter. At 2 years of age, normal thickening of myelin drives out interstitial fluid and makes most of the white matter hypointense relative to gray matter.* **(Right)** *Axial T2WI MR obtained in the same child 10 years later shows no progression of myelination and development of volume loss with enlargement of the frontal horns ➜ and peripheral sulci.*

TERMINOLOGY

Synonyms

- Delayed myelin maturation, undermyelination

Definitions

- Diminished or absent degree of white matter (WM) myelination expected for age
  - Myelin "milestones" not achieved
  - Stable on consecutive exams 6 months apart
- Primary hypomyelination = genetic defect resulting in diminished or absent myelin formation
  - Synonymous with dysmyelination
- Delayed myelination = indicates ability to "catch up" with time
  - Typically secondary to other pathology
- Demyelination = destruction of already present myelin

IMAGING

General Features

- Best diagnostic clue
  - Poor gray matter-WM differentiation on T1WI in children > 1 year of age
  - Poor gray matter- WM differentiation on T2WI in children > 2 years of age
- Location
  - Key areas to assess are internal capsule, pyramidal tracts, and peripheral frontal lobe WM rami

MR Findings

- T1WI
  - Myelinated WM is hyperintense
    - T1 shortening reflects presence of mature oligodendrocytes with proteolipid protein (PLP)
  - Myelination on T1WI appears complete by 1 year of age
- T2WI
  - Myelinated WM is hypointense
    - T2 shortening reflects displacement of interstitial water by myelin wrapping on axons
  - Hypointensity on T2WI lags hyperintensity on T1WI by 4-8 months
  - Myelination on T2WI appears complete by 3 years of age (usually by 2 years of age)
  - "Terminal zones"
    - Regions of persistent hyperintense signal on T2WI in otherwise normal brains
    - Typically around trigones of lateral ventricles
    - Greater concentration of interstitial fluid in these areas
      - Greater degree of myelin wrapping is required to displace excess interstitial fluid
    - Must be distinguished from periventricular leukomalacia or perivascular spaces
- PD/intermediate
  - Helpful in distinguishing gliosis from undermyelination
    - Gliosis is more hyperintense
- FLAIR
  - Not recommended in children < 2 years of age
    - Heterogeneous signal makes assessment of myelination and distinction of pathology more difficult
- DWI
  - ADC values predate T1- and T2-weighted signal changes
    - ADC, radial diffusivity decrease with maturation
  - Fractional anisotropy increases with brain maturation
    - More myelin wrapping = more resistance to water flow perpendicular to WM tracts
    - More directionality of water flow = greater anisotropy

Imaging Recommendations

- Best imaging tool
  - MR
- Protocol advice
  - T1WI most helpful in children < 10 months of age
  - T2WI most helpful in children > 10 months of age
  - Consider contrast administration if leukodystrophy (demyelination) is suspected

DIFFERENTIAL DIAGNOSIS

Primary Hypomyelination Syndromes

- Pelizaeus-Merzbacher disease (PMD)
  - Classic hypomyelination syndrome caused by reduced production of PLP
- PMD-like disease type 1
- Spastic paraplegia type 2 (SPG2)
- 18q-syndrome
- *TUBB4A*-related hypomyelinating disorders
  - Hypomyelination with atrophy of basal ganglia and cerebellum (H-ABC) is most severe phenotype
- POLR3-related leukodystrophies
  - 4H syndrome (hypomyelination, hypodontia, hypogonadotropic hypogonadism)
  - Hypomyelination with cerebellar atrophy and hypoplasia of corpus callosum
  - Leukodystrophy with oligodontia
- Hypomyelination with congenital cataracts
- 11q- syndrome
  - Delayed myelination rather than hypomyelination
- Trichothiodystrophy (photosensitive or nonphotosensitive)
- Sialic acid storage disease (Salla disease)
- Allan-Herndon-Dudley Syndrome

Prematurity

- Adjust chronologic age for degree of prematurity
- Use of normal milestones assumes full-term gestation

External Stresses

- Chronic debilitating conditions in infancy
  - Congenital vascular malformations (arteriovenous fistula); malnutrition
- Treatments for diseases in neonate
  - Organ transplantation, chemotherapy
- Myelination typically rebounds with treatment of primary illness

PATHOLOGY

General Features

- Etiology

- Normal myelination requires distribution/migration of mature oligodendrocytes
  - Seen on MR imaging as distribution of T1 shortening caused by presence of PLP
- After migration, process of myelin wrapping proceeds
  - Seen on MR imaging as progression of T2 hypointensity
- Hypomyelination may be caused by deficiency of oligodendrocytes &/or PLP
  - Absence of normal T1 shortening
- Less frequently, deficiency of myelin wrapping is cause
  - Near-normal appearance on T1WI with lack of progressive hypointensity on T2WI

- Genetics
  - 87 different genes have been associated with hypomyelination
  - PMD and SPG2 are both caused by mutations in *PLP1* gene, located on long (q) arm of X chromosome at position 22
    - Duplication of *PLP1* gene causes folded protein response, oligodendrocyte death
      - Result is nearly complete absence of myelin
  - PMD-like disease is caused by mutations in *GJC2* gene, located on long (q) arm of chromosome 1 at position 42.13
  - 18q-syndrome causes hemizygous deletion (1 copy of gene missing) of *MBP* gene
  - *TUBB4A* gene is located on short (p) arm of chromosome 19 at position 13.3
    - Encodes for β-tubulin
  - *POLR3A* gene is located on long (q) arm of chromosome 10 at position 22.3
  - *POLR3B* gene is located on long (q) arm of chromosome 12 at position 23.3
  - Trichothiodystrophy is associated with mutations involving 4 genes
    - *ERCC2* gene is located on long (q) arm of chromosome 19 at position 13.32
    - *ERCC3* gene is located on long (q) arm of chromosome 2 at position 14.3
    - *GTF2H5* gene is located on long (q) arm of chromosome 6 at position 25.3
    - *MPLKIP* (nonphotosensitive) gene is located on short (p) arm of chromosome 7 at position 14.1
  - Sialic acid storage diseases are caused by mutations in *SLC17A5* gene, located on long (q) arm of chromosome 6 at position 13
  - Hypomyelination and congenital cataract is caused by mutation in *FAM126A* gene

Microscopic Features

- PMD
  - Diffuse myelin deficiency: Looks like much less mature brain
  - Islands of persistent perivascular myelin result in classic tigroid appearance
  - Absent or deficient compact myelin sheaths, "redundant myelin balls"

CLINICAL ISSUES

Presentation

- Most common signs/symptoms
  - Developmental delay, hypotonia
- Other signs/symptoms
  - Classic PMD: Head titubation, hypotonia, only 50% able to sit
    - Optic nerve enlargement
  - 18q-syndrome: Developmental delays, short stature, delayed bone age, limb anomalies
  - Trichothiodystrophy: Short stature, osteosclerosis
  - POLR3 mutations: Oligodontia and abnormally placed or shaped teeth

Demographics

- Age
  - Primary hypomyelination syndromes typically present in infancy
- Sex
  - Classic PMD is X-linked recessive and, thus, exclusive to males

Natural History & Prognosis

- Late progression of symptoms may occur in some

Treatment

- No treatment yet for heritable disorders of hypomyelination

DIAGNOSTIC CHECKLIST

Consider

- Hypomyelination may be difficult to distinguish from dys- and demyelination
- Remember to adjust chronologic age for degree of prematurity when imaging infants

Image Interpretation Pearls

- Assess myelination prior to learning chronologic age of patient
  - Avoid predetermination bias

Reporting Tips

- Define degree of myelination by age at which it would be appropriate → "degree of myelination appropriate for x months of age"

SELECTED REFERENCES

1. Perrier S et al: Classifying hypomyelination: a critical (white) matter. Child Neurol Open. 7:2329048X20983761, 2020
2. Urbik VM et al: Expanded phenotypic definition identifies hundreds of potential causative genes for leukodystrophies and leukoencephalopathies. Child Neurol Open. 7:2329048X20939003, 2020
3. Nahhas N et al: Pelizaeus-Merzbacher-like disease 1. GeneReviews. University of Washington, 2017
4. Nahhas N et al: TUBB4A-related leukodystrophy. GeneReviews. University of Washington, 2016
5. Numata Y et al: Epidemiological, clinical, and genetic landscapes of hypomyelinating leukodystrophies. J Neurol. 261(4):752-8, 2014
6. Harreld JH et al: Trichothiodystrophy with dysmyelination and central osteosclerosis. AJNR Am J Neuroradiol. 31(1):129-30, 2010
7. Steenweg ME et al: Magnetic resonance imaging pattern recognition in hypomyelinating disorders. Brain. 133(10):2971-82, 2010

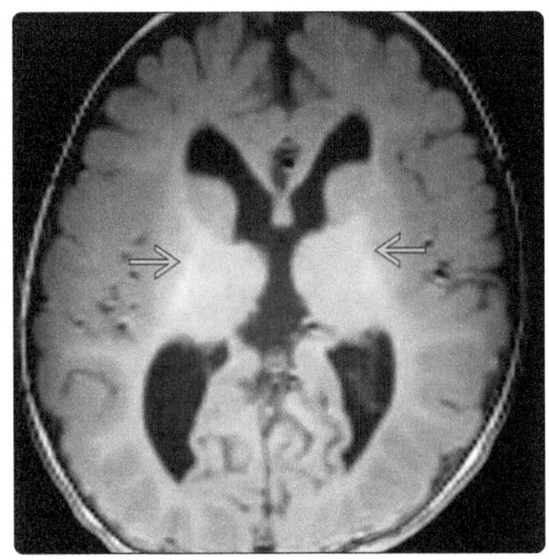

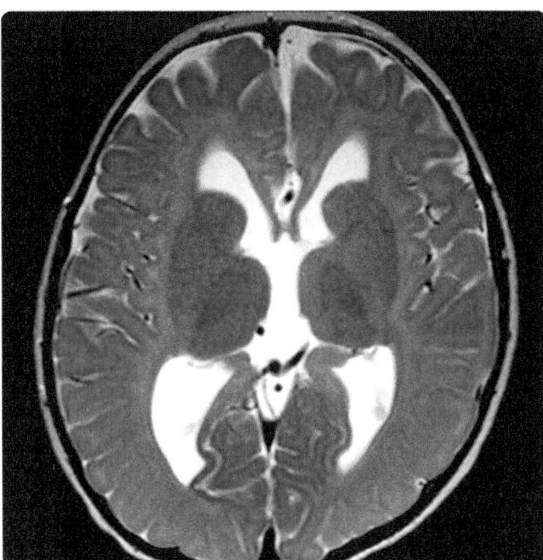

(Left) *Axial T1WI MR in an 18-month-old with 18q- syndrome shows faint T1 shortening in the internal capsules* ➙. *Myelination should appear essentially complete on T1-weighted images by 11 months of age.* **(Right)** *Axial T2WI MR in the same infant shows no evidence of myelin thickening. The gene for myelin basic protein is deleted in this condition, but there is some debate about whether the MR appearance is caused by gliosis or true hypomyelination.*

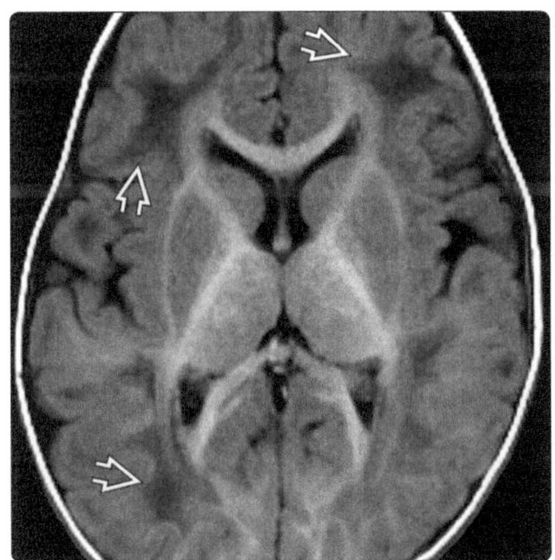

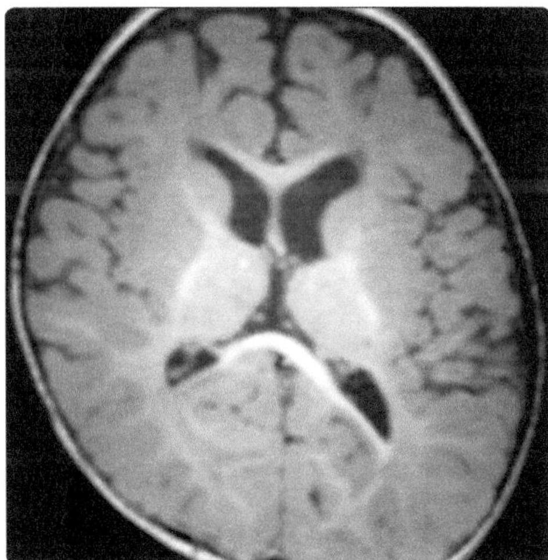

(Left) *Axial T1WI MR in a 12-year-old with 11q-syndrome (Jacobsen syndrome) shows that hypomyelination is limited to periventricular and subcortical white matter* ➙ *with normal T1-shortening in internal and external capsules.* **(Right)** *Axial T1WI MR shows that the degree of myelination in this 18-month-old would be more appropriate for 5 months of age. Herndon-Dudley syndrome is caused by a mutation that impairs delivery of thyroid hormone to the developing brain. Thyroid hormone is necessary for oligodendrocyte maturation.*

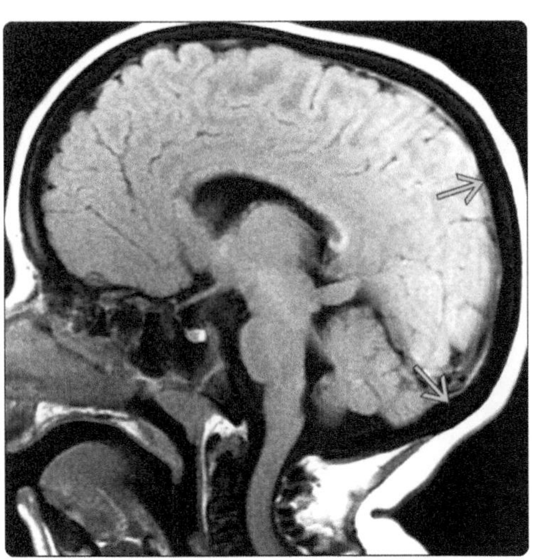

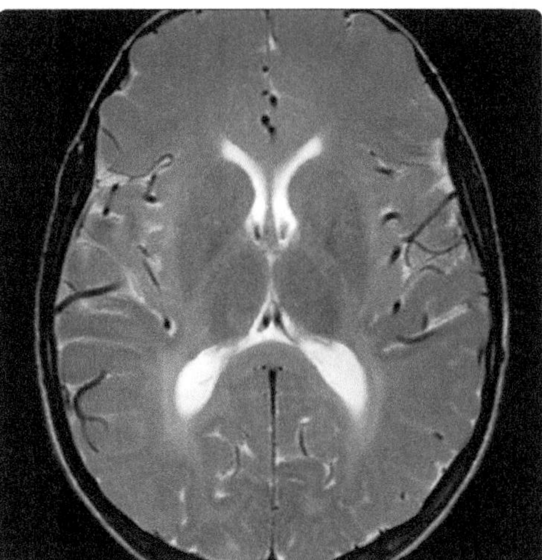

(Left) *The genetic mutations that cause trichothiodystrophy impact the general transcription factor 2H (TFIIH) complex, which is essential for DNA transcription and repair. In addition to hypomyelination, the syndrome causes brittle hair, developmental delay, and thickened bones* ➙*, as seen on this sagittal T1WI MR.* **(Right)** *Axial T2WI MR in a 9-year-old with spastic paraplegia type 2 shows near-complete absence of myelination in both central and peripheral white matter.*

KEY FACTS

TERMINOLOGY

- Mitochondrial myopathy, encephalopathy, lactic acidosis, and stroke-like episodes (MELAS)
- Inherited disorder of intracellular energy production caused by point mutation in mitochondrial DNA (mtDNA)

IMAGING

- Stroke-like cortical lesions crossing vascular territories
  - Posterior location most common
- "Shifting spread" (appearance, disappearance, reappearance elsewhere) is classic
- Lactate (Lac) "doublet" at 1.3 ppm in 60-65%
  - Elevated Lac in CSF, "normal" brain on MRS
- Basal ganglia lesions and Ca^{++}

PATHOLOGY

- mtDNA contribution to zygote exclusively maternal inheritance
- Caution: Relationship of phenotype to genotype complex, variable
- Mutations may present as MELAS but also as other mitochondrial phenotypes

CLINICAL ISSUES

- Classic MELAS triad: Lactic acidosis, seizures, stroke-like episodes
  - Onset of stroke-like episodes usually occurs in childhood/early adulthood
  - Sensorineural hearing loss, diabetes, short stature

DIAGNOSTIC CHECKLIST

- Think MELAS in patient with acute, stroke-like cortical lesion that crosses usual vascular territories
- Consider MELAS in adult presenting with unusual and recurrent stroke-like episodes

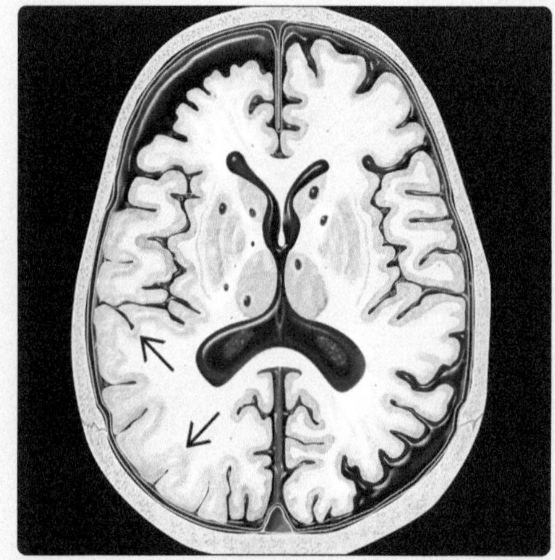

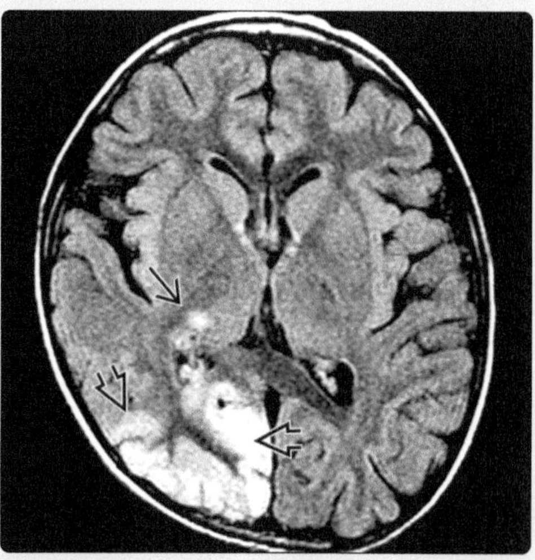

(Left) *Axial graphic shows pathology of MELAS. The acute onset of gyriform cortical swelling that crosses vascular territories* ➙ *is depicted. Note old lacunes, generalized/focal atrophy.* **(Right)** *Axial FLAIR MR in an 8-year-old girl with short stature and new-onset, stroke-like symptoms reveals a focus of abnormally increased signal intensity in the right thalamus* ➙ *and extensive hyperintensity and abnormal thickening of the cerebral cortex* ➙ *in the right occipital lobe. The underlying white matter (WM) is largely spared.*

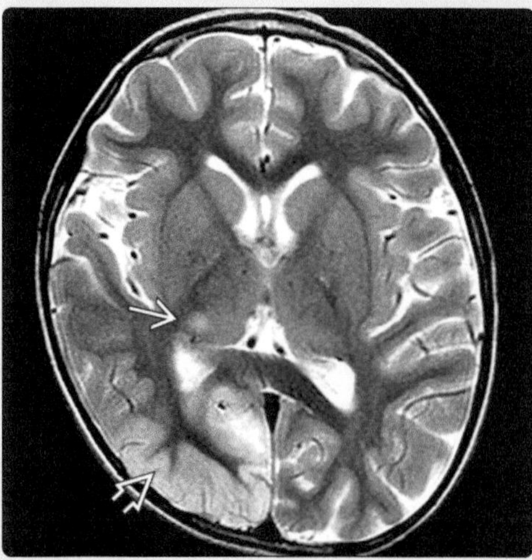

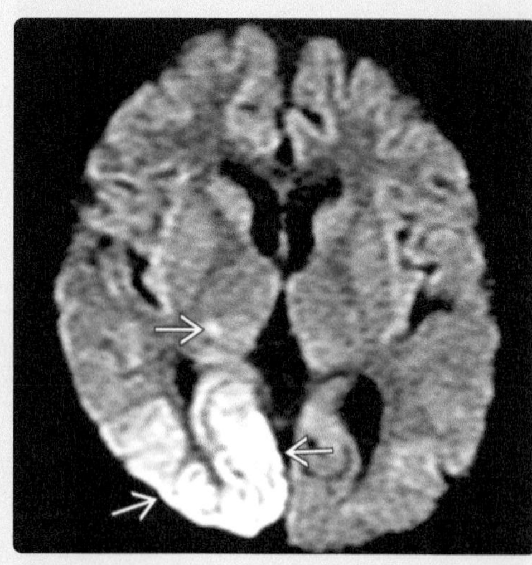

(Left) *Axial T2WI MR in the same patient shows similar abnormal signal hyperintensity lesions in the same thalamic focus of signal increase* ➙ *and in the edematous right occipital cortex* ➙*. Note the prominent subarachnoid spaces, which may result from malnutrition, medications, or the disease process itself.* **(Right)** *Axial DWI MR demonstrates reduced diffusion in the affected regions of the brain* ➙*, confirming the acuity of the lesion.*

TERMINOLOGY

Abbreviations

- Mitochondrial myopathy, encephalopathy, lactic acidosis, and stroke-like episodes (MELAS)

Definitions

- Inherited disorder of intracellular energy production caused by point mutations in mitochondrial DNA (mtDNA)

IMAGING

General Features

- Best diagnostic clue
  - Acute: Stroke-like cortical lesions
    - "Shifting spread" (appearance, disappearance, reappearance elsewhere) is classic
    - Lesions cross typical vascular territories
- Location
  - Stroke-like: Parietooccipital > temporoparietal
  - Ca^{++}: Basal ganglia (BG)
- Size
  - Variable, progressive, multifocal
- Morphology
  - Acute: Gyral swelling
  - Chronic: Supra- and infratentorial atrophy, deep white matter (WM), and BG lacunar infarcts

CT Findings

- NECT
  - Symmetric BG Ca^{++}
- CECT
  - Variable gyral enhancement

MR Findings

- T1WI
  - Acute: Swollen gyri, compressed sulci
  - Subacute: Band of cortical hyperintensity consistent with laminar necrosis
  - Chronic: Progressive atrophy of BG, temporal-parietal-occipital cortex with preservation of hippocampal, entorhinal structures
- T2WI
  - Acute: Hyperintense cortex/subcortical WM
  - Chronic: Multifocal BG, deep WM hyperintensities
- FLAIR
  - Infarct-like swelling and mass effect
- T2* GRE
  - No hemorrhage; SWI may show cortical hypointensity
- DWI
  - Acute: DWI positive, ADC variable
- T1WI C+
  - Acute: Gyral enhancement
- MRA
  - Often normal; may show cerebral artery vasodilatation, hyperperfusion in acute states
- MRS
  - Lactate (Lac) "doublet" at 1.3 ppm in 60-65%
  - Caution: Lac presence variable
    - Lac may be elevated in CSF but not brain (measure ventricular Lac)
    - Lac not always elevated and may precede imaging changes of brain
    - Other causes of elevated CNS Lac (e.g., hypoxia, ischemia, neoplasm, infection) must be excluded

Angiographic Findings

- Conventional
  - Acute: Dilated cortical arteries, prominent capillary blush without arterial occlusion

Nuclear Medicine Findings

- SPECT
  - Acute: Tc-99m HMPAO SPECT shows striking increase in tracer accumulation

Other Modality Findings

- Xenon CT shows focal hyperperfusion during acute, stroke-like episode, hypoperfusion later
- Electromyographic findings consistent with myopathy found in majority of cases
- EEG may show focal periodic epileptiform discharges

Imaging Recommendations

- Best imaging tool
  - MR with multivoxel MRS
- Protocol advice
  - Confirm Lac in normal appearing brain regions

DIFFERENTIAL DIAGNOSIS

Myoclonic Epilepsy With Ragged-Red Fibers

- Propensity for BG, caudate nuclei
- Watershed ischemia/infarcts common

Leigh Disease

- Mutations commonly involve electron transport chain complexes (COs) I-V
- Subacute necrotizing encephalomyopathy
- *SURF1* gene mutation
  - Involvement of subthalamic nuclei, lower brainstem characteristic

Kearns-Sayre Syndrome

- Ataxia, ophthalmoplegia, retinitis pigmentosa
- Diffuse symmetric Ca^{++} in BG, caudate nuclei, subcortical WM
- Hyperintense BG on T1 and T2; cerebellar WM, posterior columns of medulla often involved

Status Epilepticus

- May cause transient gyral swelling, enhancement
- No Lac elevation in normal unaffected brain, CSF

Maternally Inherited Diabetes and Deafness

- Also *A3243G* mutation of mitochondrial DNA
- Diabetes mellitus, sensorineural hearing loss, short stature, ± spontaneous abortion
- No stroke-like episodes
- NECT: Diffuse atrophy and BG Ca^{++}

PATHOLOGY

General Features

- Etiology

- Pathophysiology remains unclear
  - Impaired oxidative cerebral metabolism
  - Mitochondrial angiopathy of small cerebral arteries, arterioles, capillaries
- May also be hyperperfusion, vasogenic edema with blood-brain barrier disruption during acute, stroke-like episodes
- Genetics
  - mtDNA contribution to zygote exclusively maternal inheritance
  - Caution: Relationship of phenotype to genotype complex, variable
    - Mutations may present as MELAS but also as other phenotypes
      - *MTT1*: A-to-G translation at nucleotide 3243 of mtDNA most common
    - Polygenetic: *MTTQ, MTTL1, MTTH, MTTK, MTTC, MTTS1, MTND1, MTND5, MTND6, MTTS2*
    - MELAS overlap syndromes with Leigh syndrome, myoclonic epilepsy with ragged red fibers (MERRF), Kearns-Sayre syndrome (KSS), others
- Associated abnormalities
  - Some cortical malformations associated with *A3243G* mutations

Gross Pathologic & Surgical Features

- Diffuse generalized atrophy
- Multiple focal cortical, deep WM/BG infarcts
- Prominent mineralization of BG

Microscopic Features

- Trichrome stain shows increased numbers of ragged-red fibers in skeletal/cardiac muscle
- Perivascular Ca^{++} in both gray matter, WM may occur
- Immunohistochemistry: COX(+) ragged-red fibers (may help distinguish from MERRF)
- Electron microscopy: Swelling, increase in number of dysfunctional mitochondria in smooth muscle, endothelial cells of small arteries, and pial arterioles

CLINICAL ISSUES

Presentation

- Most common signs/symptoms
  - Triad: Lactic acidosis, seizures, stroke-like episodes
  - Common: Sensorineural hearing loss, diabetes, short stature
  - Cognitive deficits, depression, psychosis, dementia
  - Ataxia, muscle weakness (myopathy), peripheral neuropathy
  - Acute-onset headache, migraines, episodic vomiting, intermittent dystonia, alternating hemiplegia
- Other signs/symptoms
  - Heteroplasmy and random mitotic mtDNA segregation, tissue-to-tissue variability → phenotypic heterogeneity and "overlap" with other mitochondrial syndromes
    - Cardiac: Cardiomyopathy, cardiac conduction defects
    - Ocular findings: Scotomata, hemianopsia, ophthalmoplegia, maculopathy (progressive macular retinal pigment epithelial atrophy)
    - Renal dysfunction (including Fanconi syndrome and focal segmental glomerular sclerosis)
    - GI dysmotility, gastroparesis, intestinal pseudoobstruction
- Clinical profile
  - Older child or young adult with muscle weakness and epilepsy or acute, stroke-like syndrome

Demographics

- Age
  - Onset of stroke-like episodes usually occurs in childhood/early adulthood
    - Mean onset: 15 years
    - 90% symptomatic by 40 years
- Epidemiology
  - Uncommon but important cause of stroke in pediatric cases
  - Carrier prevalence of *m.3243A > G* mutation 0.6% or 60 per 100,000 individuals
  - Incidence (Finland): *3243A > G* = 18.4 per 100,000 individuals

Natural History & Prognosis

- Recurrent stroke-like events with either permanent or reversible neurologic deficits
- Progressive course with periodic acute exacerbation
  - May be triggered by relatively mild head injury or illness

Treatment

- Cofactor and supplement therapy
  - Intravenous arginine, CoQ10, L-carnitine, creatine

DIAGNOSTIC CHECKLIST

Consider

- Think MELAS in patient with acute, stroke-like cortical lesion that crosses usual vascular territories
- Consider MELAS in adult presenting with unusual and recurrent stroke-like episodes

Image Interpretation Pearls

- Obtain MRS in CSF, "uninvolved" brain

SELECTED REFERENCES

1. Yang X et al: Clinical features of epileptic seizures in patients with mitochondrial encephalomyopathy, lactic acidosis, and stroke-like episodes. Seizure. 106:110-6, 2023
2. Lopriore P et al: Mitochondrial epilepsy, a challenge for neurologists. Int J Mol Sci. 23(21), 2022
3. Zanotti S et al: Traumatic brain injury triggers neurodegeneration in a mildly symptomatic MELAS patient: implications on the detrimental role of damaged mitochondria in determining head trauma sequalae in the general population. Metabolites. 13(1), 2022
4. Zheng H et al: Mitochondrial encephalomyopathy with lactic acidosis and stroke-like episodes with an MT-TL1 m.3243A>G point mutation: enuroradiological features and their implications for underlying pathogenesis. Front Neurosci. 16:1028762, 2022
5. Finsterer J: Mitochondrial metabolic stroke: phenotype and genetics of stroke-like episodes. J Neurol Sci. 400:135-41, 2019
6. Miyahara H et al: Autopsied case with MERRF/MELAS overlap syndrome accompanied by stroke-like episodes localized to the precentral gyrus. Neuropathology. 39(3)-212-7, 2019
7. Li Y et al: Current insight into MELAS: clinical perspectives and multimodal MRI. J Magn Reson Imaging. 47(2):583-4, 2018
8. Minobe S et al: Vasodilatation of multiple cerebral arteries in early stage of stroke-like episode with MELAS. J Clin Neurosci. 22(2):407-8, 2015
9. Rodan LH et al: Cerebral hyperperfusion and decreased cerebrovascular reactivity correlate with neurologic disease severity in MELAS. Mitochondrion. 22:66-74, 2015

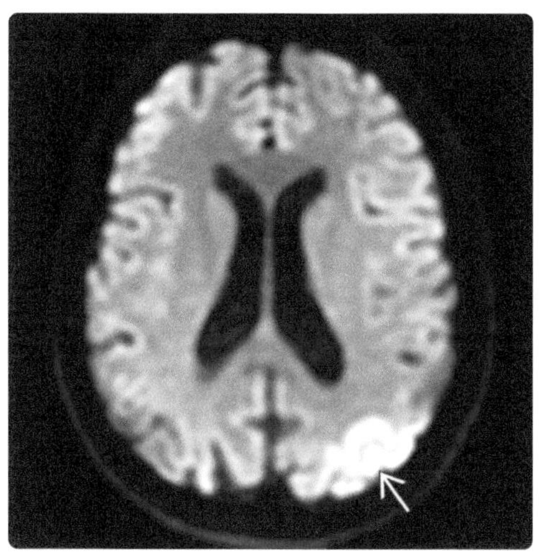

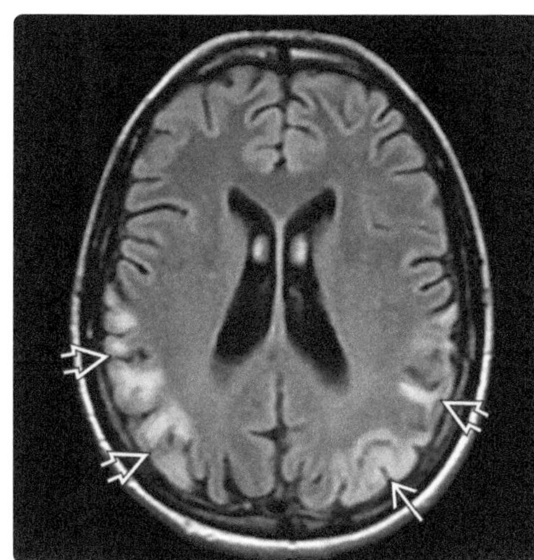

(Left) *Axial DWI MR in a young adult with severe MELAS reveals acute diffusion restriction → in the left parietal lobe. Note also sulcal prominence and chronic volume loss elsewhere in both hemispheres.* **(Right)** *Axial FLAIR MR in the same patient confirms cortical swelling in the left parietal lobe at the site of acute diffusion restriction → as well as chronic volume loss at prior injury sites →.*

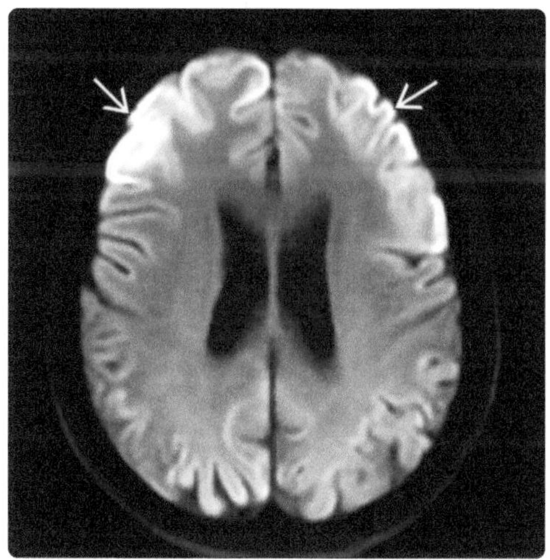

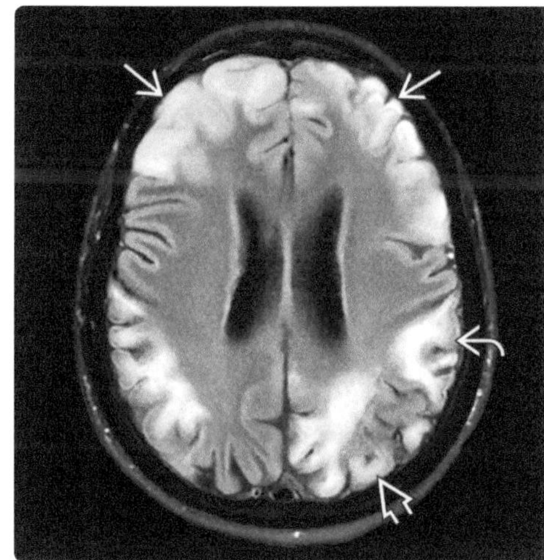

(Left) *Axial DWI MR in the same patient obtained 9 months later during an acute crisis shows new diffusion restriction → in both frontal lobes.* **(Right)** *Axial FLAIR MR in the same patient confirms gyral swelling and hyperintensity in both frontal lobes →, the right more swollen, suggesting a slightly different timeline of injury. More chronic changes are noted at prior site of acute injury →. Note also a new area of clinically unrecognized brain injury occurring between episodes →.*

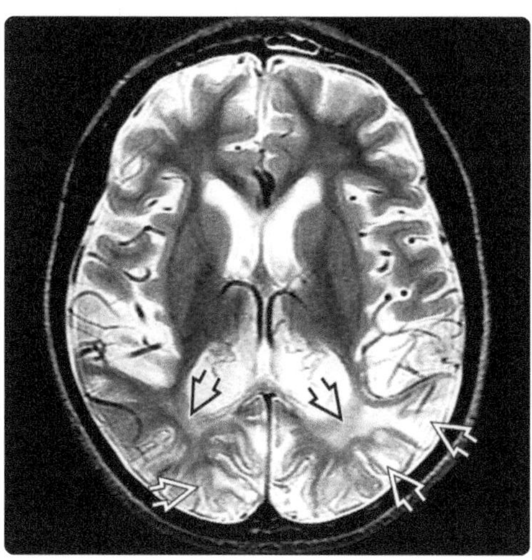

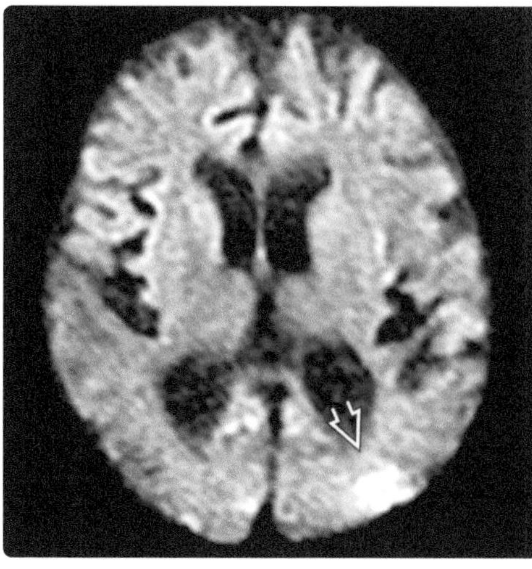

(Left) *Axial T2WI MR in a 12-year-old girl with longstanding MELAS reveals extensive volume loss in the cerebral cortex and subcortical white matter, in addition to increased signal intensity of peritrigonal white matter → and the parietooccipital subcortical WM/cortex →.* **(Right)** *Axial DWI MR in the same patient demonstrates reduced diffusivity → in the left occipital pole, indicating an acute exacerbation in superimposed upon chronic changes.*

KEY FACTS

TERMINOLOGY

- Genetically based disorders of mitochondrial function resulting in progressive or intermittent brain injury
    - Leigh syndrome (LS)
    - Myopathy, encephalopathy, lactic acidosis, and stroke-like episodes (MELAS)
    - Kearns-Sayre syndrome (KSS)
    - DNA polymerase γ-related disorders (POLG-RD)
    - Disorders of pyruvate metabolism
        - Pyruvate dehydrogenase (PDH) deficiency
    - Mitochondrial aminoacyl tRNA synthetase deficiencies
        - Leukoencephalopathy with brainstem and spinal cord involvement and high lactate (LBSL)
- Many other metabolic diseases primarily affect mitochondria but are not typically considered ME
    - Neurodegeneration with brain iron accumulation (NBIA), glutaric aciduria type 1, trichothiodystrophy are examples

IMAGING

- Broad range of imaging appearances, characterized by regions of edema, brain destruction, volume loss, &/or mineralization
- Typically hyperintense lesions on T2WI and FLAIR
    - LS typically causes speckled pattern in deep nuclei
- MRS can be helpful but is often nonspecific
    - ↑ lactate and restricted diffusion can be clue to true etiology
        - Especially if found in normal-appearing regions
- Cerebellar atrophy is common feature

PATHOLOGY

- LS → associated with mutations in > 75 genes, both mitochondrial (mtDNA) and nuclear (nDNA)
    - As specific mutations affecting specific metabolic pathways are determined, enzymatic deficiencies resulting in LS may now be diagnosed as separate entities

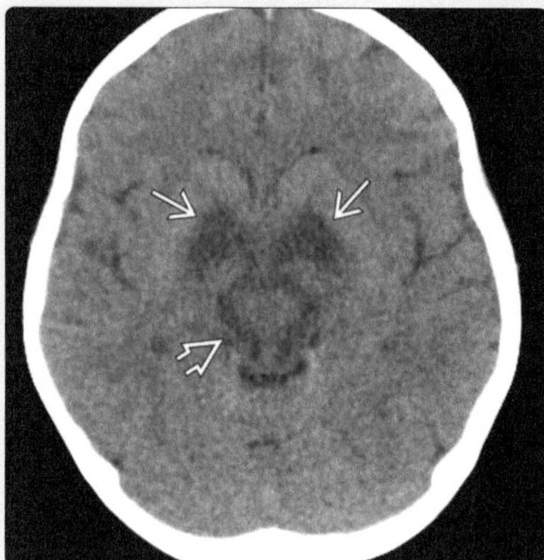

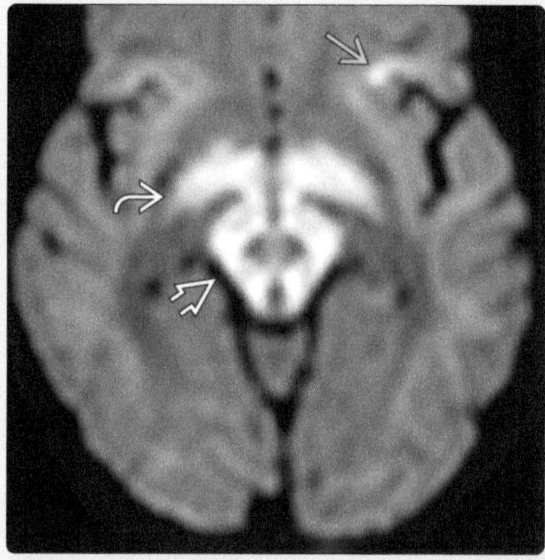

(Left) *Axial NECT in an 11-year-old found unresponsive after complaining of headache shows decreased brainstem and basal ganglia attenuation.* **(Right)** *Axial diffusion-weighted image from a subsequent MR in the same patient shows restricted diffusion in the upper brainstem and globus pallidus, bilateral and symmetric. Note subcortical diffusion restriction in the left frontal lobe. This is Kearns-Sayre syndrome.*

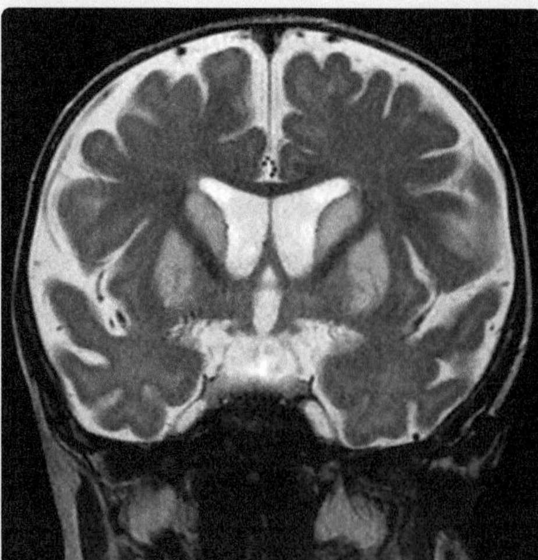

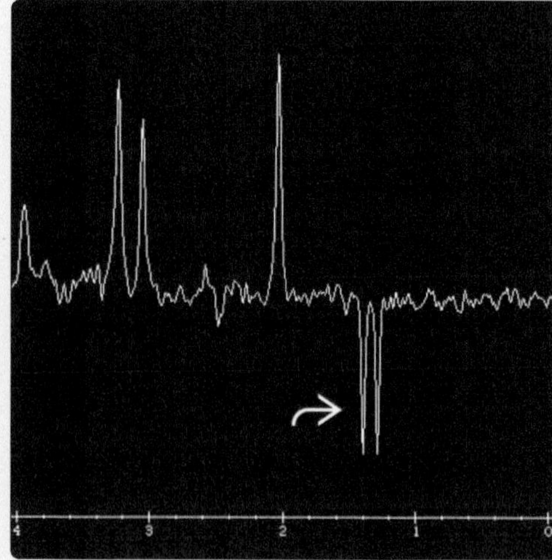

(Left) *Coronal T2WI MR in a 9-month-old presenting with hypotonia shows symmetric abnormal hyperintense signal in the putamen and caudate with visible perforating arteries. Subsequent genetic analysis confirmed the diagnosis of Leigh syndrome.* **(Right)** *Intermediate echo (144 msec) MRS in the left basal ganglia (same patient) shows a prominent inverted lactate doublet. Detection of lactate with MRS can lend credence to a suspected diagnosis of mitochondrial encephalopathy (ME), but a negative study is not exclusive.*

Mitochondrial Encephalopathies

TERMINOLOGY

Abbreviations

- Mitochondrial encephalopathies (MEs)

Definitions

- Genetically based disorders of mitochondrial function, resulting in progressive or intermittent brain injury
  - Leigh syndrome (LS)
    - a.k.a. subacute necrotizing encephalomyelopathy
    - Defined by its characteristic clinical and pathologic presentation rather than by specific enzymatic deficiency
      - Characteristic imaging appearance
  - Myopathy, encephalopathy, lactic acidosis, and stroke-like episodes (MELAS)
  - Kearns-Sayre syndrome (KSS)
  - DNA polymerase γ-related disorders (POLG-RD)
  - Disorders of pyruvate metabolism
    - Pyruvate dehydrogenase (PDH) deficiency
    - Pyruvate carboxylase (PC) deficiency
  - Mitochondrial aminoacyl tRNA synthetase deficiencies
    - Leukoencephalopathy with thalamus and brainstem involvement and high lactate (LTBL)
    - Leukoencephalopathy with brainstem and spinal cord involvement and high lactate (LBSL)
- Mitochondrial dysfunction has been associated with myriad clinical pathologies, ranging from autism to Alzheimer dementia to normal aging
  - This document addresses some of those primarily affecting brain, presenting in childhood, and not covered elsewhere
    - New mutations and phenotypes are constantly being discovered
- Many other metabolic diseases primarily affect mitochondria but are not typically considered ME
  - Neurodegeneration with brain iron accumulation (NBIA), glutaric aciduria type 1, trichothiodystrophy are examples

Classification

- Multiple classification schemes for metabolic diseases of mitochondria have been proposed
  - Clinical phenotype
    - Longest recognized syndromes are classified by their clinical/pathologic/radiologic presentation
      - LS is defined in this manner
  - Locale of genetic defect
    - Mutation in mitochondrial DNA (mtDNA) or nuclear DNA (nDNA)
  - Segment of metabolic pathway affected
    - Respiratory chain (RC) subunits: Complexes I-V
    - mtDNA transcription defects: POLG-RD
    - Pyruvate metabolism disorders: PDH and PC deficiency
- All these classifications have their strengths and weaknesses, reflecting complexity of structure and ubiquity of mitochondrial function in cellular metabolism

IMAGING

General Features

- Best diagnostic clue
  - Broad range of imaging appearances, characterized by regions of edema, brain destruction, volume loss, &/or mineralization
    - LS, PDH deficiency: Symmetric "speckled" lesions in basal ganglia (BG)
    - MELAS: Peripheral stroke-like lesions
    - KSS: Cerebellar atrophy, ↑ T2 in subcortical white matter (WM)
    - Leber hereditary optic neuropathy (LHON): Perivenular MS-like lesions
    - POLG-RD: Volume loss, asymmetric thalamic lesions with restricted diffusion
    - LBSL: ↑ T2 in WM, posterior limbs of internal capsules, dorsal columns of spinal cord
- Location
  - Variable
    - Most common in BG, brainstem, thalami, dentate nuclei
      - Often bilateral and symmetric
    - Less commonly diffuse WM, peripheral cortex, cerebellum
- Morphology
  - BG lesions often conform to original shape of nuclei
    - Edema/swelling characteristic of acute lesions; volume loss characteristic of late disease

MR Findings

- T1WI
  - Hypointense lesions
    - Foci of hyperintensity may reflect Ca^{++}, blood products, myelin breakdown (rare)
  - Cerebellar atrophy is common feature
- T2WI
  - Typically hyperintense lesions on T2WI and FLAIR
    - LS typically causes speckled pattern in deep nuclei
      - Sparing (islands of preserved signal) around vessels
- DWI
  - May or may not be associated with restricted diffusion
    - Likely reflecting acuteness of pathology
    - DWI not reliable for detection or exclusion of MEs
  - Strokes not matching known vascular territories may indicate MELAS
- MRS
  - Detection of lactate characteristic of MEs; however, absence of lactate does not exclude diagnosis
    - May only be elevated during acute crises
  - Chronic lesions typically have ↓ NAA

Imaging Recommendations

- Best imaging tool
  - MR is modality of choice in investigation of suspected metabolic disease of any sort
- Protocol advice
  - MRS can be helpful but is often nonspecific
  - ↑ lactate and restricted diffusion can be clue to true etiology
    - Especially if found in normal-appearing regions

DIFFERENTIAL DIAGNOSIS

Hypoxic-Ischemic Encephalopathy

- Central pattern of injury affects ventrolateral thalamus and BG
  - T2 signal abnormalities difficult to identify in unmyelinated brain
    - 1st echo (protein density) is very helpful
  - T1 hyperintensity seen acutely → posterior limb of internal capsular (PLIC) sign

Near Drowning

- History generally definitive
- High lactate implies poorer prognosis

Neurofibromatosis Type 1

- Signal abnormalities in globus pallidus (GP) most common brain manifestation in children

Kernicterus

- T2 prolongation in GP, subthalamic nuclei, hippocampi

Encephalitis

- Acute disseminated encephalomyelitis can affect BG, mimic MELAS/myoclonic epilepsy with ragged-red fibers (MERRF)

PATHOLOGY

General Features

- Etiology
  - Most pronounced effects on striated muscle and deep cerebral nuclei → presumed highest adenosine triphosphate (ATP) demand
- Genetics
  - Syndromes attributed to mutations in mtDNA
    - MELAS
    - KSS
    - LHON
    - MERRF
  - Syndromes attributed to mutations in nDNA
    - POLG-RD
      - Alpers-Huttenlocher syndrome
      - Myoclonic epilepsy, myopathy, sensory ataxia (MEMSA)
      - Ataxia neuropathy spectrum (ANS)
    - Coenzyme Q10 (CoQ10) deficiency
    - Mitochondrial DNA depletion syndromes (MDS)
      - Caused by mutations in nDNA genes necessary for mtDNA synthesis &/or replication
      - Encephalomyopathic MDS caused by defects in *SUCLG1* (chromosome 2), *SUCLA2* (chromosome 13), or *RRM2B* (chromosome 8) genes
      - Hepatocerebral MDS caused by defects in *DGUOK*, *MPV17*, *POLG*, or *TWNK* (*C10orf2*) genes
      - Mitochondrial neurogastrointestinal encephalomyopathy (MNGIE) caused by *TYMP* mutations
  - LS → associated with mutations in > 75 genes, both mtDNA and nDNA
    - Affecting functions of complexes I-V, mitochondrial transcription/translation, PDH, and thiamine metabolism
    - As specific mutations affecting specific metabolic pathways are determined, enzymatic deficiencies resulting in LS are now diagnosed as separate entities
      - Mitochondrial short-chain enoyl-coA hydratase deficiency (ECHS1D): Inborn error of valine and fatty acid metabolism
      - Holocarboxylase synthetase deficiency, multiple carboxylase deficiency
- Associated abnormalities
  - KSS → ophthalmoplegia, heart block, retinitis pigmentosa
  - Alpers → micronodular cirrhosis
- Broad phenotypic presentations due to varied distribution of mitochondria throughout various cell types

CLINICAL ISSUES

Presentation

- Most common signs/symptoms
  - Psychomotor delay/regression, hypotonia
  - Stroke-like episodes, episodic paresis
  - Metabolic stressors (e.g., infection) may unmask disease or cause deterioration
- Other signs/symptoms
  - Ataxia, ophthalmoplegia, ptosis, swallowing and respiratory difficulties, dystonia
  - Vomiting, diarrhea, cramping

Demographics

- Age
  - Majority have clinical symptoms in infancy
  - MELAS usually presents in teens
  - Age at onset and severity correlates with degree of enzyme deficit

Natural History & Prognosis

- Variable due to heterogeneity of clinical phenotype
  - Many have step-wise progression with periods of stability between episodes of decline
  - LS → progressive neurodegeneration leading to respiratory failure and death in childhood
  - MELAS → progressive course with episodic insults

DIAGNOSTIC CHECKLIST

Image Interpretation Pearls

- Consider MEs when encountering atypical presentation of stroke, severe encephalitis, or seizure
- Bilateral speckled hyperintense lesions on T2WI and FLAIR = LS or PDH deficiency
- Bilateral GP lesions = toxin exposure, hypoxic-ischemic encephalopathy (HIE)/injury, or mitochondrial dysfunction
  - These 3 are **not** exclusive diagnoses; toxins and HIE cause mitochondrial dysfunction
- Cerebellar atrophy is common feature in MEs

SELECTED REFERENCES

1. Distelmaier F et al: Neuroimaging in mitochondrial disease. Handb Clin Neurol. 194:173-85, 2023
2. Sofou K et al: Phenotype-genotype correlations in Leigh syndrome: new insights from a multicentre study of 96 patients. J Med Genet. 55(1):21-7, 2018
3. Baertling F et al: The many faces of paediatric mitochondrial disease on neuroimaging. Childs Nerv Syst. 32(11):2077-83, 2016

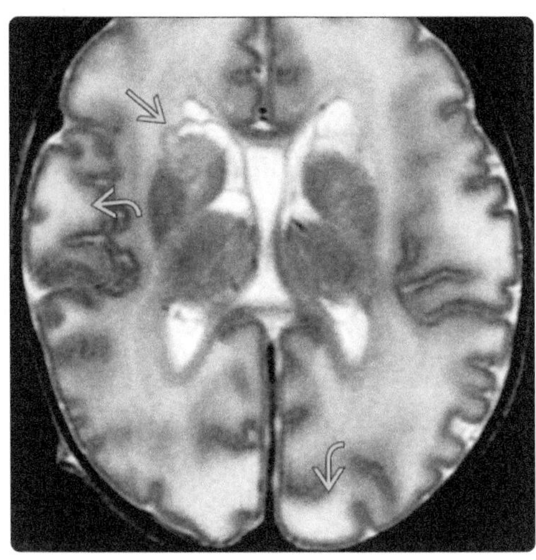

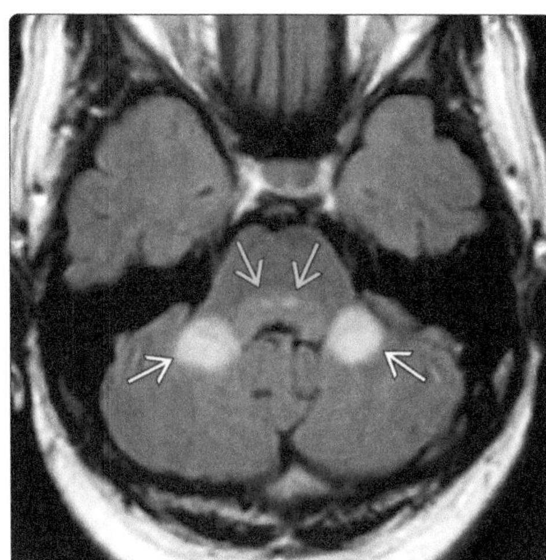

(Left) *Axial T2WI MR in a term neonate with metabolic acidosis and lethargy shows abnormal hyperintensity of the subcortical white matter (WM)* ↪ *and focal ischemic lesions in the right basal ganglia* →*. This is holocarboxylase synthetase deficiency.* **(Right)** *Axial FLAIR MR of the posterior fossa in an 18-year-old with holocarboxylase synthetase deficiency shows symmetric signal abnormalities* → *in the cerebellar peduncles and also in the central tegmental tracts* →*.*

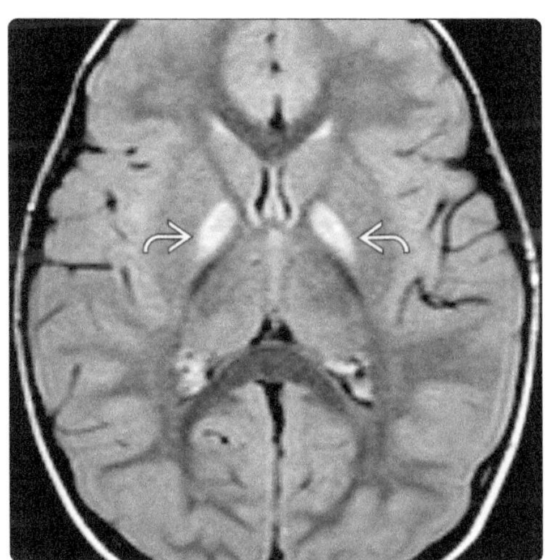

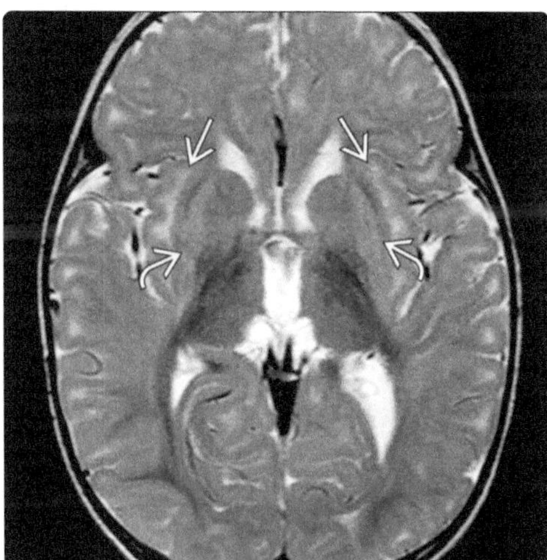

(Left) *Axial FLAIR MR shows there is symmetric abnormal hyperintense signal* ↪ *in each globus pallidus in this 3-year-old with dystonia, limp, and a diagnosis of mitochondrial short-chain enoyl-coA hydratase deficiency (ECHS1D).* **(Right)** *Axial T2WI MR in a 10-month-old with mitochondrial depletion syndrome caused by a SUCLG1 mutation shows abnormal hyperintense signal in the putamen* ↪ *and subinsular WM* →*.*

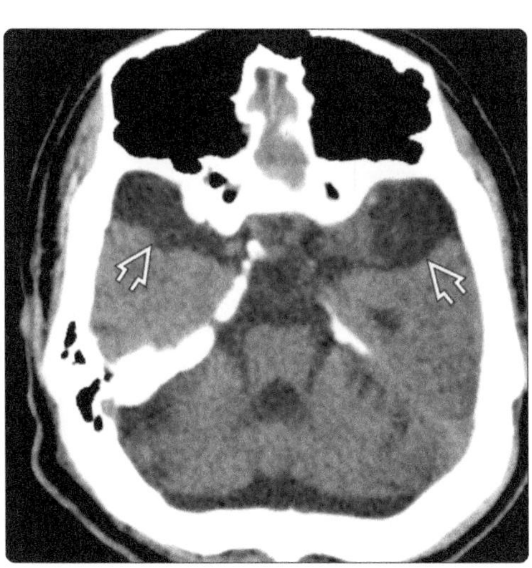

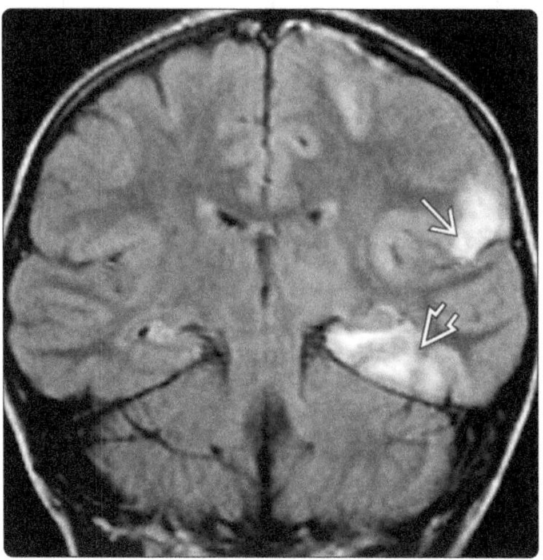

(Left) *Axial CT in a 19-year-old with pyruvate dehydrogenase (PDH) deficiency shows cerebellar volume loss and large subarachnoid spaces in the middle cranial fossae* ⇨*. This is a relatively common finding in MEs and can be mistaken for subdural collections secondary to abusive head injury in infants.* **(Right)** *Coronal FLAIR MR in a 9-year-old with a seizure and new-onset chorea shows scattered regions of abnormal hyperintensity in the cortical ribbon* → *and subcortical WM* ⇨*. Stroke-like lesions are the hallmark of MELAS.*

KEY FACTS

TERMINOLOGY

- Mucopolysaccharidoses (MPS): I-IX
- Group of lysosomal storage disorders
  - Characterized by inability to break down glycosaminoglycans (GAGs)
  - Undegraded GAGs toxic, accumulate in multiple organs
  - Each type of MPS causes accumulation of particular GAG in lysosomes, extracellular matrix
  - 11 known enzyme deficiencies, resulting in 7 distinct forms of MPS
    - Prototype MPS = MPS I-H (Hurler)

IMAGING

- Perivascular spaces (PVSs) dilated by accumulated GAGs
- Favored sites of dilated Virchow-Robin spaces (VRSs) in MPS: Corpus callosum, peritrigonal white matter (WM)
  - Can occur in other lobes
- Single to too many to count
- Dysostosis multiplex, broad ribs, trident hands
- Progressive odontoid dysplasia → risk atlantoaxial subluxation; some correction follows bone marrow transplant (BMT)

CLINICAL ISSUES

- Prognosis, deterioration rate depends upon specific enzyme deficiency
- Treatment: BMT or IV recombinant human enzyme (e.g., MPS I-H: α-L-iduronidase)
- Significant correlation exists between WM alterations and mental restrictions

DIAGNOSTIC CHECKLIST

- Always visualize foramen magnum on any CNS study to seek craniocervical junction (CVJ) compression
- Airway: Major sedation and anesthesia risk
- Not all MPS have typical facial features; dilated VRSs may still signal less common MPS
- Look at upper cervical spine on sagittal images; aids in making diagnosis

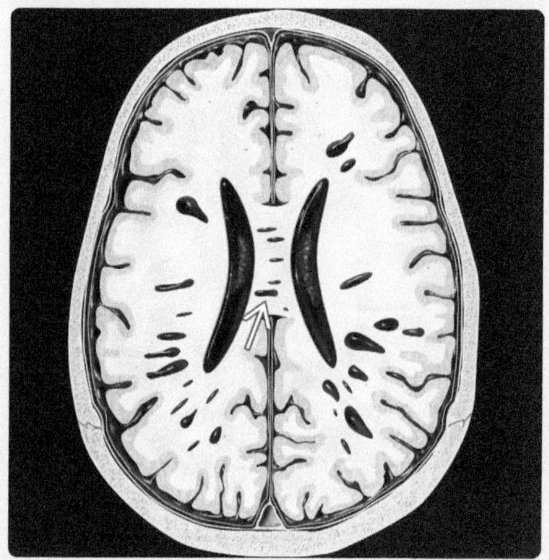

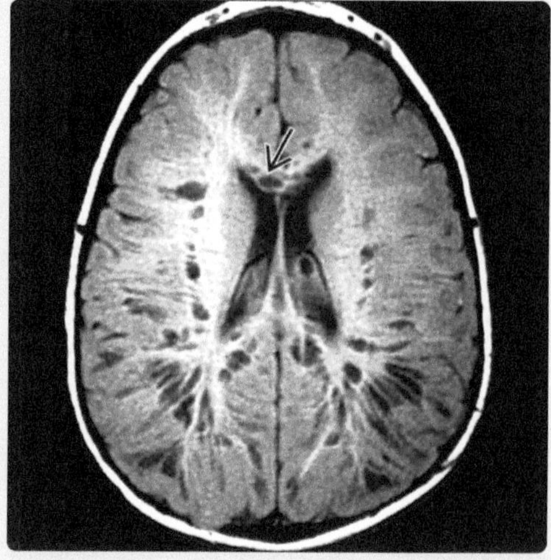

(Left) *Axial graphic of a prototype mucopolysaccharidosis (MPS) shows multiple dilated perivascular spaces that are radially oriented in the white matter (WM) of the brain. Note the posterior predominance and involvement of the corpus callosum ➡.* **(Right)** *Axial T1WI MR in a toddler with MPS I-H (Hurler) demonstrates prominent perivascular spaces involving the WM, including the corpus callosum ➡. Note the posterior predominance of involvement, which is typical in MPS.*

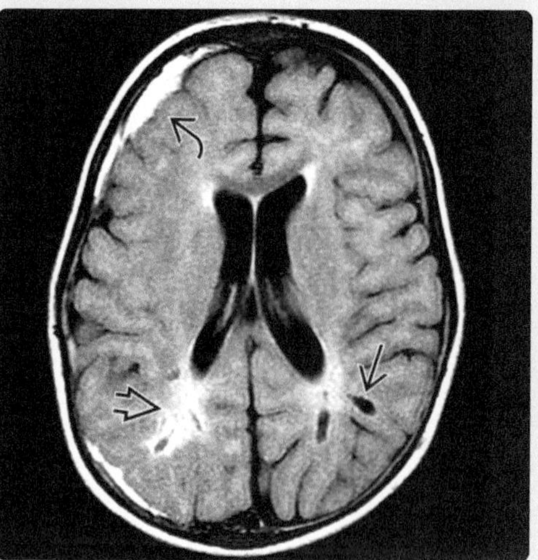

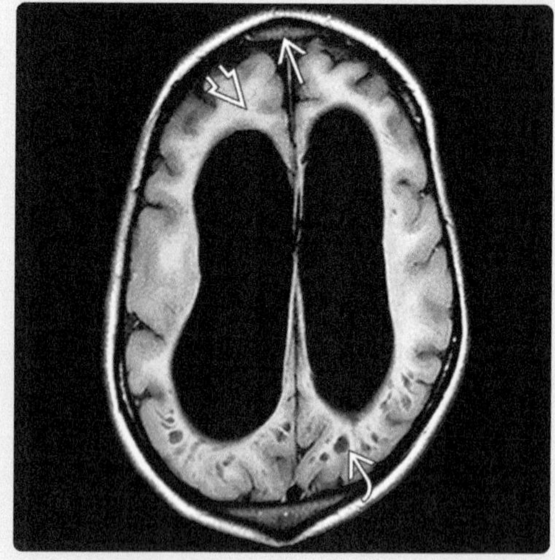

(Left) *Axial FLAIR MR in a male child with MPS II (Hunter) reveals a few dilated perivascular spaces ➡ surrounded by gliotic WM ➡. Note the unilateral subdural hematoma ➡. Extraaxial bleeds, while uncommon, have been reported in MPS with vasculopathy, trauma, or large subdural effusions.* **(Right)** *Axial FLAIR MR in a school-aged boy with MPS II (Hunter) demonstrates dilated perivascular spaces ➡, hyperintense WM ➡, and hydrocephalus. Note the typical anterior beaking ➡.*

TERMINOLOGY

Abbreviations

- Mucopolysaccharidoses (MPS)

Definitions

- Group of lysosomal storage disorders
  - Characterized by inability to break down glycosaminoglycans (GAGs)
  - Undegraded GAGs toxic, accumulate in multiple organs
  - Each type of MPS causes accumulation of particular GAG in lysosomes, extracellular matrix
  - 11 known enzyme deficiencies, resulting in 7 distinct forms of MPS
    - Prototype MPS = MPS I-H (Hurler)

IMAGING

General Features

- Best diagnostic clue
  - Perivascular spaces (PVSs), a.k.a. Virchow-Robin spaces (VRSs), dilated by accumulated GAGs
- Location
  - Favored sites of dilated VRSs in MPS: Corpus callosum (CC), peritrigonal white matter (WM)
    - Can occur in other lobes
- Size
  - Variably sized dilated VRSs, usually < 5 mm; occasional large obstructed VRS occur
  - Range: 1 to too many to count
- Morphology
  - Round, oval, spindle, parallel to veins

Radiographic Findings

- Radiography
  - Dysostosis multiplex, broad ribs, trident hands, J-shaped sella, rosette formation of multiple impacted teeth in single follicle

CT Findings

- NECT
  - Metopic beaking despite macrocrania
  - Macrocrania, ↓ density WM, dilated VRSs rarely visible on CT
  - Progressive hydrocephalus **and** atrophy
    - MPS I: Hydrocephalus is early finding in 25%
    - MPS IIIB: Severe atrophy
- CECT
  - Enhancing pannus associated with ligaments and dura at craniocervical junction (CVJ)

MR Findings

- T1WI
  - Cribriform appearance WM, CC, basal ganglia (BG)
    - Dilated VRS filled with GAG: "Hurler holes"
    - Especially in severe MPS (MPS IH, II > > other MPS types)
    - Except MPS IV (Morquio): CNS spared
  - Occasional arachnoid cysts (meningeal GAG deposition)
- T2WI
  - ↑ signal of WM surrounding dilated VRS: Gliosis, edema, de- or dysmyelination
  - ± additional patchy WM signal
- FLAIR
  - VRS isointense with CSF
  - ↑ signal surrounds VRSs
- T1WI C+
  - CVJ pannus enhances
- MRS
  - ↓ NAA, ↑ Cho:Cr ratio; ↑ peak at 3.7 ppm contains signals from MPS
    - Improvement in presumptive MPS peaks following bone marrow transplant (BMT)
- Spinal MR
  - Compression CVJ in majority of MPS
    - C2 meningeal hypertrophy
    - Progressive odontoid dysplasia → risk atlantoaxial subluxation; some correction reported following BMT
    - Short C1 posterior arch
  - ↑ T2 signal cord in 50% of CVJ compression
  - Upper lumbar gibbus
    - MPS IH (Hurler): Inferior beaking
    - MPS IV (Morquio): Middle beaking

Imaging Recommendations

- Best imaging tool
  - Multiplanar brain MR
- Protocol advice
  - Baseline MR/MRS
  - Follow-up: Complications (CVJ compression, hydrocephalus), therapeutic response to BMT
  - Always visualize foramen magnum on any CNS study to seek CVJ compression

DIFFERENTIAL DIAGNOSIS

Velocardiofacial Syndrome (22q11DS)

- Dilated VRSs and plaques, typical frontal predominance
- Deviated carotid arteries in pharynx is clue

Macrocephaly With Dilated Virchow-Robin Spaces

- Lacks typical beaked metopic suture and foramen magnum compression

Hypomelanosis of Ito

- Periventricular signal change (brighter and more persistent than MPS) with large VRS
- May also have hemimegalencephaly
- Typical whorled skin lesions
- Lack "beaked" metopic suture present in MPS

Perinatal Hypoxic-Ischemic Encephalopathy

- Transient phase of cystic change following hypoxic-ischemic encephalopathy → atrophy

Normal Virchow-Robin Spaces

- Vary in number and prominence

PATHOLOGY

General Features

- Etiology
  - Ganglioside accumulation (toxic to neurons)
- Genetics
  - Autosomal recessive (exception: X-linked MPS II)

- Associated abnormalities
  - Dermal melanocytosis (mongolian-like spots)
    - Extensive blue skin pigmentation differs from typical mongolian spots in persistence or progression
  - GAG accumulates in most organs/ligaments
    - Hepatosplenomegaly (HSM), umbilical hernia
    - Skeletal dysostosis multiplex, joint contractures
    - Arterial wall (midaortic stenosis) and cardiac valve thickening
    - Thick dura (cord compressed at foramen magnum)
    - Coarse facies (formerly "gargoylism")
    - Upper airway obstruction (38%): Submucosal deposition → small, abnormally shaped trachea (difficult intubation); abnormal configuration vocal cords
  - Embryology anatomy
    - Dilated VRSs may be seen in utero

Staging, Grading, & Classification

- Diagnosis depends on specific enzyme deficiency
  - MPS I-H, I-HS (Hurler/Hurler-Scheie): α-L-iduronidase (4p16.3)
  - MPS II (Hunter): Iduronate 2-sulfatase (Xq28)
  - MPS IIIA (Sanfilippo): Heparin N-sulfatase (17q25.3)
  - MPS IVA (Morquio): Galactose 6-sulfatase (16q24.3)
  - MPS VI (Maroteaux-Lamy): Arylsulfatase B (5q11-q13)
  - MPS VII (Sly): β-glucuronidase (7q11.21)

Gross Pathologic & Surgical Features

- Thick meninges
- Cribriform appearance to cut surface of brain

Microscopic Features

- MPS: GAGs accumulate in leptomeninges and VRSs

CLINICAL ISSUES

Presentation

- Most common signs/symptoms
  - Typical coarse facies develop (mild in MPS III, VI, VII)
    - Macroglossia, bushy eyebrows, flat nasal bridge
- Clinical profile
  - Prototype MPS I-H, appear normal at birth
    - Corneal clouding (except MPS II): Proteoglycans in keratocytes
    - Mental restrictions (except MPS IIb, IV, I-HS)
    - Joint contractures, dysostosis multiplex, short stubby fingers, carpal tunnel syndrome
    - Loss of walking skills: Spinal claudication/myelopathy C1-C2 and vascular claudication from midaortic stenosis
    - Recurrent upper respiratory infection, nasal discharge, ear infections, sleep apnea, sensorineural deafness
    - Middle ear effusions (73%); otolaryngologist notes this prediagnosis MPS
    - Cardiac valvular disease: Mitral > aortic
    - Skin blistering in MPS III
  - MPS VII may present with fetal nuchal translucency, hydrops fetalis, or isolated ascites

Demographics

- Age
  - MPS I-H presents in infancy
- Sex
  - MPS II (Hunter) is X-linked: Male
- Ethnicity
  - Geographic variability in prevalence of specific MPS disorders
- Epidemiology
  - 1:29,000 live births (series from Australia)
    - MPS I-H = 1:107,000 live births
    - MPS II = 1:165,000 male live births
    - MPS III = 1:58,000 live births
    - MPS IVA = 1:640,000 live births
    - MPS VI = 1:320,000 live births

Natural History & Prognosis

- Significant correlation exists between WM alterations and mental restrictions
- Rate of deterioration depends upon specific deficiency
  - MPS I-H death by 10 years without therapy
  - MPS IIA death in late teens (cardiac)
  - Others variable

Treatment

- Enzyme replacement therapy (e.g., α-L-iduronidase for MPS I-H), hematopoietic stem cell transplantation, substrate reduction therapy, gene therapy, antiinflammatory drugs
  - Goal: ↓ visceral accumulation MPS; ameliorate some manifestations

DIAGNOSTIC CHECKLIST

Consider

- Airway: Major sedation and anesthesia risk

Image Interpretation Pearls

- Not all MPS have typical facial features; dilated VRSs may still signal less common MPS
- Not all dilated VRSs are MPS
- Always look for CVJ compression
  - Treatable cause of morbidity in MPS
  - Lack of CVJ compression suggests there may be different etiology of dilated VRSs than MPS

SELECTED REFERENCES

1. Rossi A et al: Gene therapies for mucopolysaccharidoses. J Inherit Metab Dis. 47(1):135-44, 2024, 2023
2. Costanzo R et al: Burden of surgical treatment for the management of cervical myelopathy in mucopolysaccharidoses: a systematic review. Brain Sci. 13(1), 2022
3. Pontesilli S et al: Evidence of treatment benefits in patients with mucopolysaccharidosis type I-Hurler in long-term follow-up using a new magnetic resonance imaging scoring system. J Pediatr. 240:297-301.e5, 2022
4. Nicolas-Jilwan M et al: Mucopolysaccharidoses: overview of neuroimaging manifestations. Pediatr Radiol. 48(10):1503-20, 2018
5. Reichert R et al: Neuroimaging findings in patients with mucopolysaccharidosis: what you really need to know. Radiographics. 36(5):1448-62, 2016
6. Andrade F et al: Sanfilippo syndrome: overall review: Mucopolysaccharidosis type III. Pediatr Int. 57(3):331-8, 2015
7. Aronovich EL et al: Lysosomal storage disease: gene therapy on both sides of the blood-brain barrier. Mol Genet Metab. 114(2):83-93, 2015

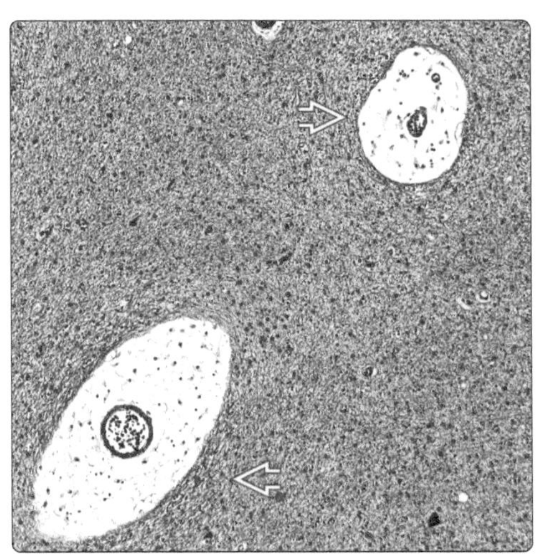

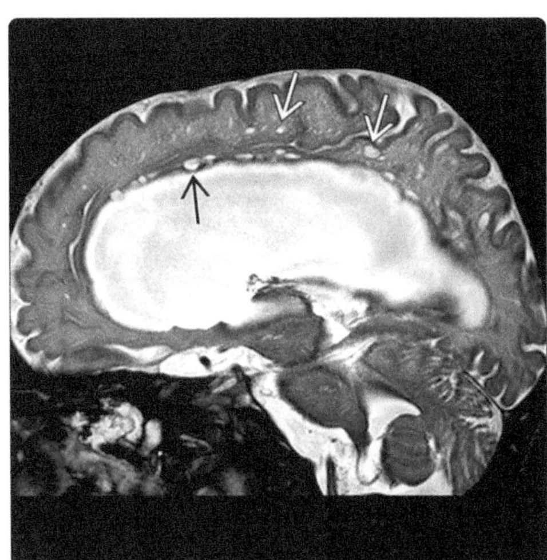

(Left) *Axial micropathology with Luxol fast blue stain in a teenager with MPS I-HS (Hurler-Scheie) reveals dilated perivascular spaces ➡ filled by mucopolysaccharide. (Courtesy P. Shannon, MD.)* **(Right)** *Sagittal T2WI MR in a 10-year-old boy with MPS II (Hunter) demonstrates ventriculomegaly due to hydrocephalus, scaphocephaly, and numerous dilated perivascular spaces ➡. Characteristic dilated perivascular spaces ➡ within the corpus callosum can be seen.*

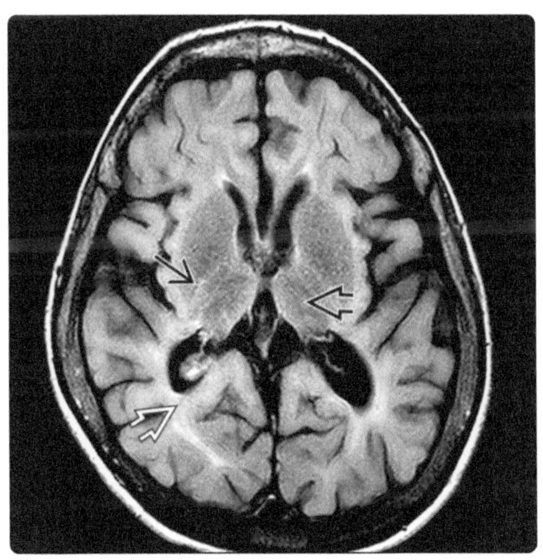

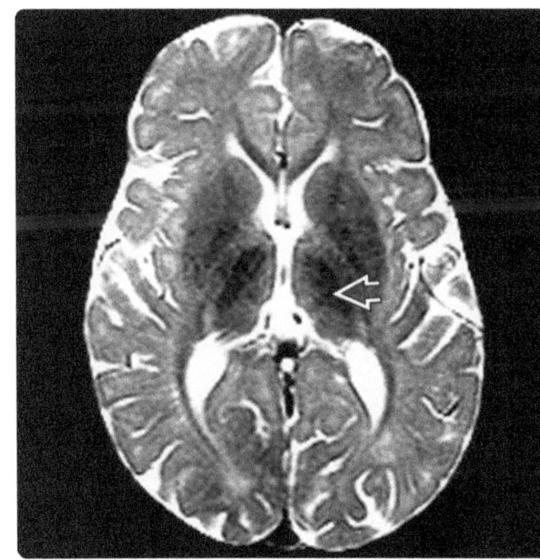

(Left) *Axial FLAIR MR in a child with MPS III reveals increased signal in the abnormal myelin of the peritrigonal WM ➡ and the internal capsules ➡. The thalami are dark and small ➡. Thalamic findings are uncommon in the other MPS disorders but can be seen in MPS III and other lysosomal disorders.* **(Right)** *Axial T2WI MR in a 2-year-old child with MPS III reveals similar thalamic hypointensity ➡. Notice the hypomyelination of the WM manifested as abnormal hyperintensity.*

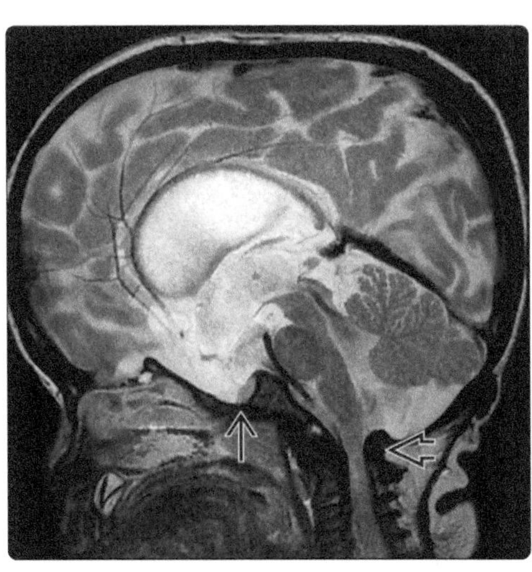

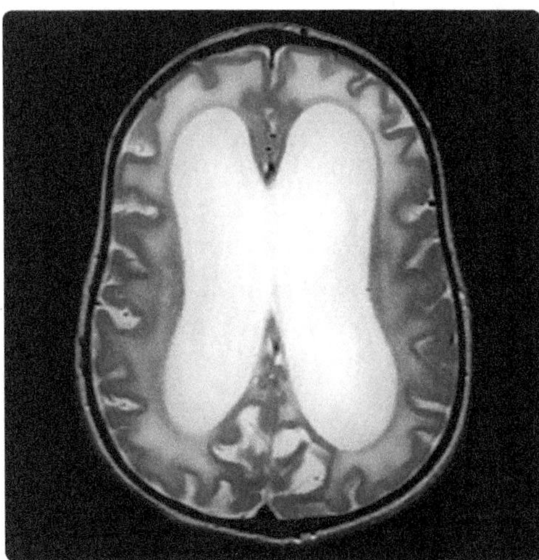

(Left) *Sagittal T2 MR (MPS I) demonstrates severe corpus callosum volume loss reflecting generalized brain atrophy. The sella ➡ shows a J-shape configuration typical of MPS. Additionally, there is severe foramen magnum stenosis ➡, reinforcing the importance of reviewing this area on sagittal images.* **(Right)** *Axial T2 MR in the same patient reveals ventriculomegaly (volume loss + foramen magnum obstruction). Rarely, MPS shows a leukoencephalopathy pattern, as in this patient with severe WM T2 hyperintensity.*

Gangliosidosis (GM2)

KEY FACTS

TERMINOLOGY

- Tay-Sachs disease (TS), Sandhoff disease (SD)
- Inherited lysosomal storage disorder characterized by gangliosidosis (GM2) ganglioside accumulation in brain
- TS and SD exist in infantile, juvenile, and adult forms

IMAGING

- Infantile: T2-hypointense, T1-hyperintense (CT-hyperdense) thalami
- Juvenile/adult: Cerebellar atrophy

TOP DIFFERENTIAL DIAGNOSES

- Krabbe disease
- Juvenile GM1, GM2
- Neuronal ceroid lipofuscinosis
- Status marmoratus

PATHOLOGY

- Autosomal recessive inheritance
- Accumulation of GM2 ganglioside in neuronal lysosomes causes neuronal degradation, apoptosis with secondary hypo-/demyelination

CLINICAL ISSUES

- TS: 1:30 carrier frequency in Ashkenazi Jewish and French Canadians
- SD, GM2 variant AB, juvenile/adult GM2 = panethnic (↑ in small gene pools)
- Presentation
    - Infant: Psychomotor restrictions/regression
    - Juvenile/adult: Atypical spinocerebellar ataxia
- Poor prognosis for infantile-onset GM2
    - Typically death by 4 years of age
- Treatment: Supportive, seizure control; promising new therapies on horizon

DIAGNOSTIC CHECKLIST

- Signal characteristics of abnormal thalami helps guide differential diagnosis

(Left) *Axial NECT shows classic hyperdense thalami ➡ in this developmentally delayed 1-year-old with infantile Tay-Sachs disease. The basal ganglia appear small and were hypodense on lower images (not shown).* **(Right)** *Axial T2WI MR in a patient with infantile Tay-Sachs disease shows thalamic hypointensity limited to the ventral nuclei ➡, findings in contrast to those in patients with Sandhoff disease. The dorsal thalamus (not shown) is often mildly hyperintense.*

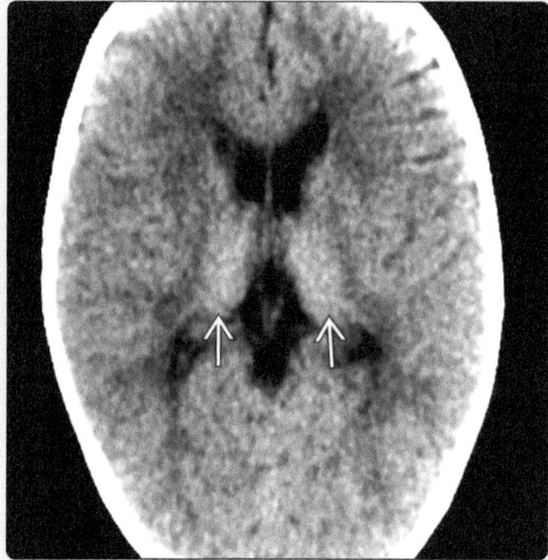

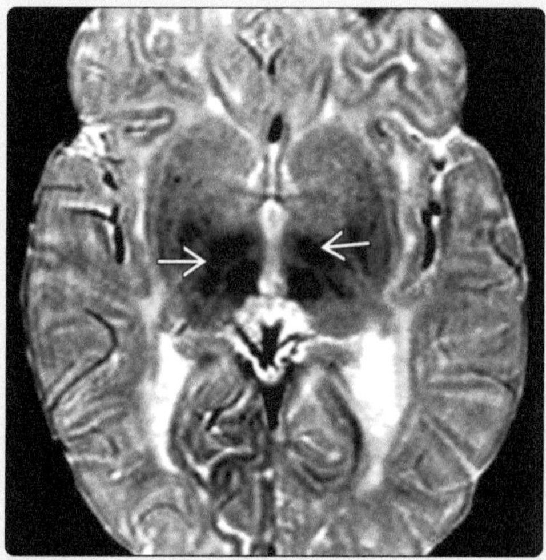

(Left) *Axial T2WI MR in a 3-month-old boy with seizures reveals bilateral abnormal T2 hypointensity within the thalami ➡. Axial T1 MR (not shown) showed corresponding T1 hyperintensity in the same regions.* **(Right)** *Axial T2WI MR in the same patient at 4 years of age performed for progressive loss of milestones and intractable seizures reveals marked diffuse brain atrophy, particularly involving the deep nuclear structures. Genetic testing revealed a homozygous HEXA genetic mutation, diagnostic of Tay-Sachs disease.*

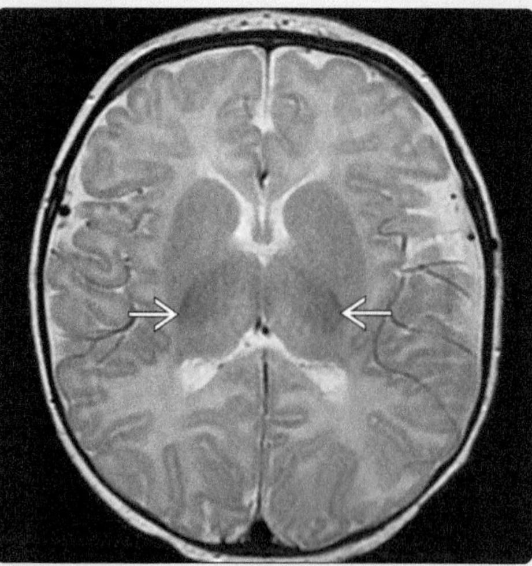

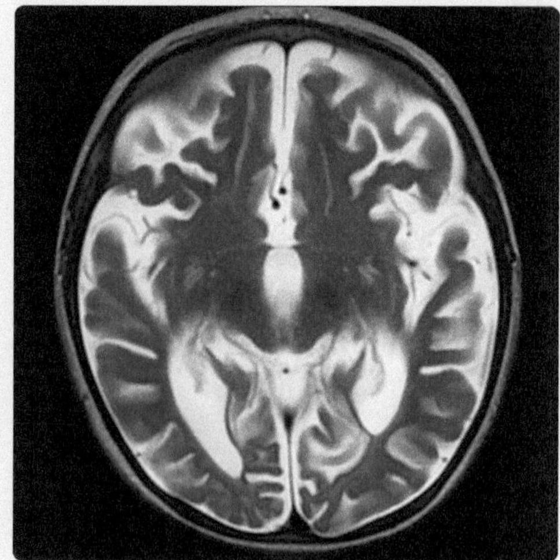

TERMINOLOGY

Abbreviations

- Gangliosidosis (GM2)

Synonyms

- Tay-Sachs (TS) disease, Sandhoff disease (SD)

Definitions

- Inherited lysosomal storage disorder
  - Characterized by GM2 ganglioside accumulation in brain
- 3 major biochemically distinct, but clinically indistinguishable types
  - TS disease
  - SD
  - GM2 variant AB (rare)
- TS and SD exist in infantile, juvenile, and adult forms
- GM2 variant AB exists in infantile form only

IMAGING

General Features

- Best diagnostic clue
  - Infantile
    - T2-hypointense, T1-hyperintense (CT-hyperdense) thalami
    - Mild T2-hyperintense striatum
  - Juvenile/adult
    - Cerebellar atrophy
- Location
  - Infantile: Thalami, striatum, cerebral > > cerebellar white matter (WM)
    - Corpus callosum (CC) spared
  - Juvenile/adult: Cerebellum, cerebral WM
    - Rare striatal and mass-like brainstem involvement
- Morphology
  - Symmetric involvement of deep gray structures
  - Late: Atrophy

CT Findings

- NECT
  - Infantile
    - Hyperdense thalami (classic but variable)
    - Hypodense striatum, WM
  - Juvenile/adult
    - Cerebellar atrophy
    - ± cerebral WM hypodensity
- CECT
  - No abnormal enhancement

MR Findings

- T1WI
  - Hyperintense thalami
  - Striatal intensity variable
  - Hypointense cerebral WM
- T2WI
  - TS: **Hypo**intense ventral thalami, **hyper**intense dorsal thalami
  - SD: Thalami diffusely hypointense
  - Mild striatal and cerebral WM hyperintensity
- DWI
  - Variably ↓ diffusivity ventral thalami (TS)
- T1WI C+
  - No abnormal enhancement
- MRS
  - Infantile: ↓ NAA, ↑ choline, ↑ myoinositol
  - Juvenile/adult: ↓ NAA; normal-appearing thalami, cerebral WM reported

Ultrasonographic Findings

- Infantile: Echogenic thalami

Imaging Recommendations

- Best imaging tool
  - Multiplanar MR (CT may confirm thalamic abnormality)

DIFFERENTIAL DIAGNOSIS

Krabbe Disease

- Hyperdense thalami, caudate and dentate nuclei
- T2-hyperintense cerebral, cerebellar WM
- CC involved

Juvenile GM1 Gangliosidosis

- Imaging findings identical to SD
- GM1 ganglioside accumulates in brain and viscera

Neuronal Ceroid Lipofuscinosis

- Thalami, globi pallidi hyperdense, T2 hypointense
- Cerebral, cerebellar atrophy

Status Marmoratus

- History of profound perinatal ischemia
- Hyperdense, atrophic thalami
- Atrophy putamina, perirolandic region

PATHOLOGY

General Features

- General pathology comments
  - Neuronal accumulation of GM2 ganglioside caused by deficient lysosomal enzyme, β-hexosaminidase A (HexA)
- Embryology anatomy
  - GM2 ganglioside resides in neuronal membranes; plays role in cell-cell recognition, synaptogenesis
  - β-HexA and GM2 activator protein (GMAP) required for lysosomal GM2 ganglioside catabolism
  - HexA is 1 of 3 isoenzymes of β-HexA formed by dimerization α and β subunits
    - HexA = αβ dimer, HexB = ββ, HexS = αα
  - HexA and HexB are major forms; HexS is minor form with unclear physiologic function
  - *HEXA*, Chr 15q23-24, encodes α subunit
  - *HEXB*, Chr 5q13, encodes β subunit
  - *GM2A*, Chr 5q31.3-q33.1, encodes GMAP
- Genetics
  - Autosomal recessive inheritance
  - > 100 different mutations of *HEXA* cause TS
  - > 30 different mutations of *HEXB* cause SD
  - ~ 4 mutations of *GM2A* cause GM2 variant AB
  - Mutations allowing residual HexA activity (0.5-4.0% normal activity) account for milder juvenile/adult phenotypes
- Etiology

- Accumulation of GM2 ganglioside in neuronal lysosomes causes neuronal degradation, apoptosis with secondary hypo-/demyelination
  - GM2 ganglioside accumulation in myelin membrane may also contribute to demyelination
- Exact mechanism by which GM2 ganglioside accumulation → neuronal apoptosis is unknown
  - Activation microglia, macrophages, and astrocytes suggest inflammatory component
  - Identification of autoantibodies in mouse models of SD suggests autoimmune component

Gross Pathologic & Surgical Features

- Infantile: Early megalencephaly, late atrophy
  - Gelatinous, hemispheric WM, ± cavitation
- Juvenile/adult: Cerebellar atrophy

Microscopic Features

- GM2 ganglioside accumulation in cerebral neurons
- Less severe GM2 ganglioside accumulation in glial, Purkinje, anterior horn, and retinal ganglion cells
- EM: GM2 ganglioside contained in membranous cytoplasmic bodies (MCBs) in neuronal cytoplasm, proximal nerve processes, axons
  - MCBs in cytoplasm cause distortion and ballooning
  - MCBs in proximal nerve processes form meganeurites
- Hypomyelination, demyelination, wallerian degeneration
- Juvenile/adult GM2: Ganglioside accumulation in anterior horn cells, cerebellar neurons, basal ganglia, brainstem
  - MCBs occasionally absent
- SD: Additional storage of GM2 (and globoside) in viscera

CLINICAL ISSUES

Presentation

- Most common signs/symptoms
  - Infantile
    - Psychomotor retardation/regression
  - Juvenile/adult
    - Atypical spinocerebellar ataxia
  - Other signs/symptoms
    - Infantile: Macrocranium, hypotonia, seizures, blindness (90% with cherry-red spot macula), exaggerated startle response to noise
    - Juvenile/adult: Dysarthria, extrapyramidal and pyramidal dysfunction, peripheral neuropathy, stuttering, psychosis/depression (late, 30%)
- Clinical profile
  - Diagnosis: Documentation HexA deficiency in serum leukocytes, cultured skin fibroblasts, amniotic fluid, or chorionic villus sample
  - Abnormal results should be followed by DNA analysis to detect mutation &/or exclude pseudodeficiency allele

Demographics

- Age
  - Infantile
    - Symptom onset in 1st year
  - Juvenile
    - Symptom onset by 2-6 years old
  - Adult
    - Symptom onset in 1st-3rd decades
- Sex
  - No predilection
- Epidemiology
  - TS
    - 1:30 carrier frequency in Ashkenazi Jewish and French Canadians
    - ↑ incidence in Cajuns, French Canadians
    - Normal carrier frequency in general population
  - SD, GM2 variant AB, juvenile/adult GM2 = panethnic (↑ in small gene pools)
    - 1:1,000 Jewish, 1:600 non-Jewish
    - 1:16-29 Creole population of Cordoba, Argentina
    - 1:7 Maronite Christian Cypriots
  - Incidence of TS in USA and Canada has ↓ by > 90% since 1970 due to carrier screening and prenatal diagnosis

Natural History & Prognosis

- Infantile: Rapidly progressive psychomotor regression culminating in paralysis, blindness, deafness; death typically by 4 years of age
- Juvenile: More slowly progressive with death between 5-15 years of age
  - Death often 2° to respiratory infection
  - Often several years of decerebrate rigidity in vegetative state precede death
- Adult: Prolonged survival to age 60-80 years can occur

Treatment

- Supportive therapy, seizure control
- Promising new therapies: Substrate deprivation, enzyme replacement, bone marrow transplantation, gene therapy, pharmacologic chaperone therapy

SELECTED REFERENCES

1. İnci A et al: Two patients from Turkey with a novel variant in the GM2A gene and review of the literature. J Pediatr Endocrinol Metab. 34(6):805-12, 2021
2. Yamamoto N et al: A case of infantile Tay-Sachs disease with late onset spasms. Brain Dev. 43(5):661-5, 2021
3. Masingue M et al: Natural history of adult patients with GM2 gangliosidosis. Ann Neurol. 87(4):609-17, 2020
4. Cachon-Gonzalez MB et al: Genetics and therapies for GM2 gangliosidosis. Curr Gene Ther. 18(2):68-89, 2018
5. Gupta L et al: Magnetic resonance imaging findings in Tay-Sachs disease. Neurol India. 66(4):1201-2, 2018
6. Jauhari P et al: Unusual neuroimaging finding in infantile Tay-Sach's disease. Indian J Pediatr. 85(2):158-9, 2018
7. Nestrasil I et al: Distinct progression patterns of brain disease in infantile and juvenile gangliosidoses: volumetric quantitative MRI study. Mol Genet Metab. 123(2):97-104, 2018
8. Mittal P et al: CT and MRI findings in a case of infantile form of GM2 gangliosidosis: Tay-Sachs disease. Neurol India. 64(6):1372-3, 2016
9. Pretegiani E et al: Pendular nystagmus, palatal tremor and progressive ataxia in GM2-gangliosidosis. Eur J Neurol. 22(6):e67-9, 2015
10. Bisel B et al: GM1 and GM2 gangliosides: recent developments. Biomol Concepts. 5(1):87-93, 2014
11. Cachón-González MB et al: Reversibility of neuropathology in Tay-Sachs-related diseases. Hum Mol Genet. 23(3):730-48, 2014
12. Deik A et al: Atypical presentation of late-onset Tay-Sachs disease. Muscle Nerve. 49(5):768-71, 2014
13. Hall P et al: Diagnosing lysosomal storage disorders: the GM2 gangliosidoses. Curr Protoc Hum Genet. 83:17.16.1-8, 2014
14. Harlalka GV et al: Mutations in B4GALNT1 (GM2 synthase) underlie a new disorder of ganglioside biosynthesis. Brain. 136(Pt 12):3618-24, 2013
15. Jamrozik Z et al: Late onset GM2 gangliosidosis mimicking spinal muscular atrophy. Gene. 527(2):679-82, 2013
16. Sandhoff K et al: Gangliosides and gangliosidoses: principles of molecular and metabolic pathogenesis. J Neurosci. 33(25):10195-208, 2013

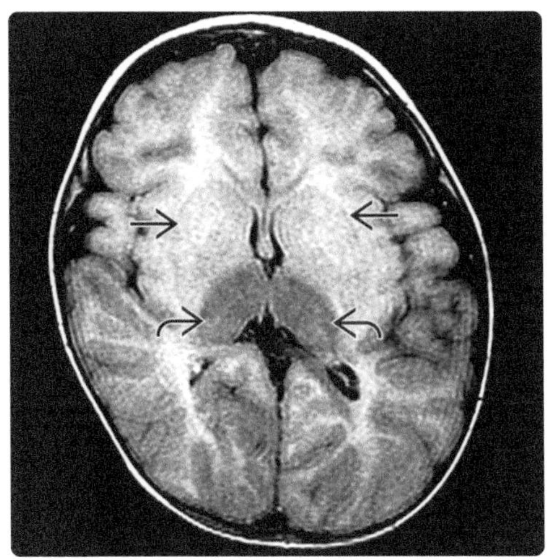

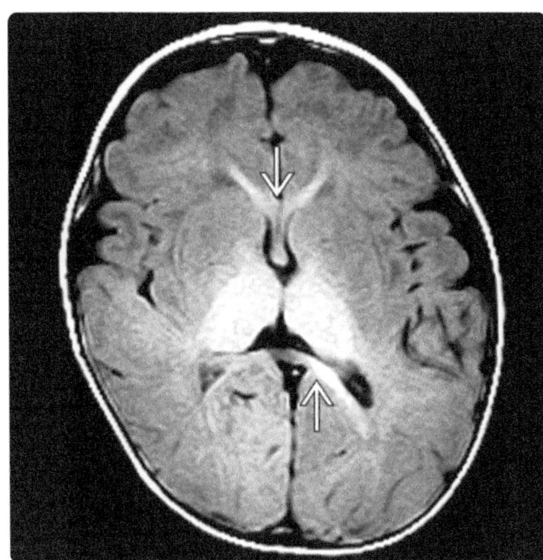

(Left) *Axial FLAIR MR in a 1-year-old with infantile Sandhoff disease shows diffusely hypointense thalami ➲. The striatum ➙ is diffusely hyperintense. Evaluation of the cerebral white matter on FLAIR MR is difficult at this age.* **(Right)** *Axial T1WI MR in the same patient shows symmetric thalamic hyperintensity and diffusely hypointense (hypo-/demyelinated) cerebral white matter. White matter should appear completely myelinated on T1WI at this age. Note the spared (hyperintense) corpus callosum ➡.*

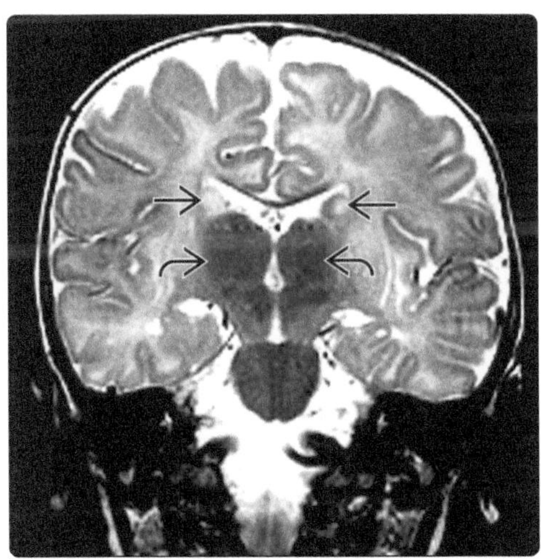

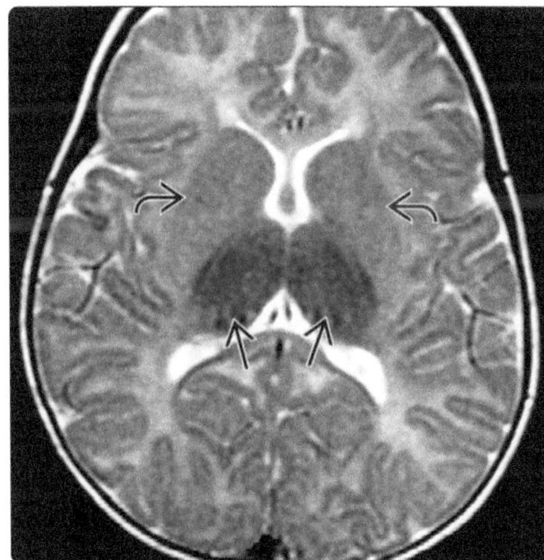

(Left) *Coronal T2WI MR in a 1-year-old with infantile Sandhoff disease shows diffusely hypointense thalami ➲. The striatum is abnormally hyperintense, particularly the caudate nuclei ➙. The cerebral white matter is also mildly hyperintense.* **(Right)** *Axial T2WI MR shows symmetric hypointense thalami ➙ in this 7-month-old with infantile Sandhoff disease. The putamina ➲ are mildly hyperintense, more so posteriorly than anteriorly. Myelination appears within a normal range.*

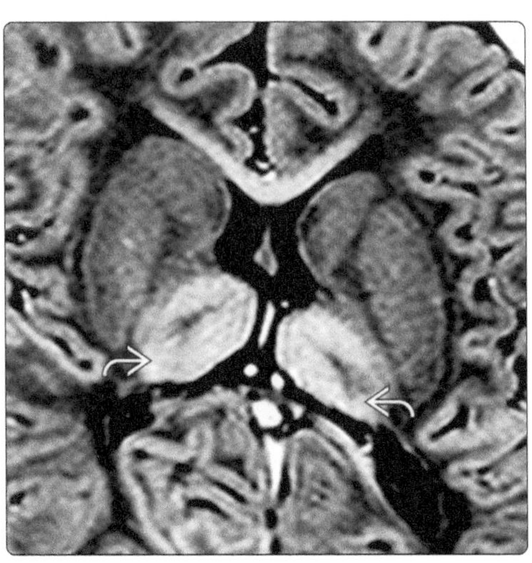

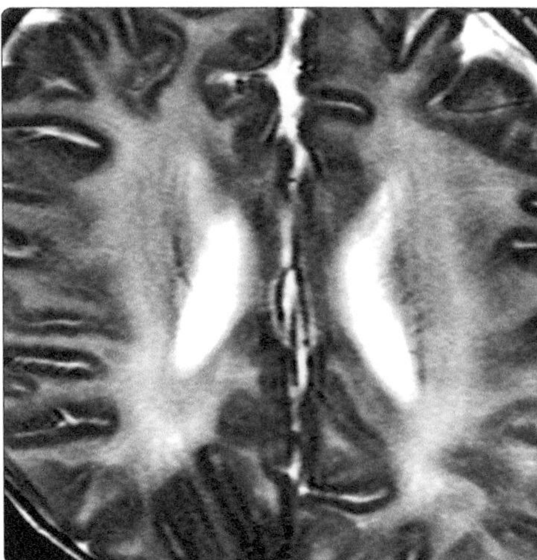

(Left) *Axial T1WI MR in a 2-year-old with infantile Sandhoff disease shows symmetric thalamic hyperintensity ➲. The central hypointense foci are atypical. The cerebral white matter is grossly hypointense with sparing of the corpus callosum.* **(Right)** *Axial T2WI MR in the same patient shows diffuse white matter hyperintensity, confirming extensive hypo-/demyelination. The cerebral cortex has a normal appearance.*

KEY FACTS

TERMINOLOGY

- Lysosomal storage disorder
  - Caused by ↓ arylsulfatase A (ARSA)
  - Results in CNS, peripheral nervous system (PNS) demyelination
- 3 clinical forms
  - Late infantile (most common), juvenile, adult

IMAGING

- Best diagnostic clue: Confluent butterfly-shaped ↑ T2 signal in deep cerebral hemispheric white matter (WM)
  - Early: Spares subcortical U fibers
    - Corpus callosum splenium, parietooccipital WM initially
    - Rapid centrifugal spread to frontal, temporal WM
  - Late: Involves subcortical U fibers
- Sparing of perivenular myelin = tigroid or leopard pattern
- No WM enhancement
  - Reports cranial nerve, cauda equina enhancement

TOP DIFFERENTIAL DIAGNOSES

- Pelizaeus-Merzbacher disease
- TORCH
- Pseudo-TORCH
- Periventricular leukomalacia
- Sneddon syndrome (ARSA pseudodeficiency)
- Krabbe disease
- Megalencephaly with leukoencephalopathy and cysts

CLINICAL ISSUES

- Clinical profile: Toddler with visuomotor impairment and abdominal pain

DIAGNOSTIC CHECKLIST

- Adult patients presenting with cryptic spasticity of legs should be screened for X-linked adrenoleukodystrophy/adrenomyeloneuropathy, lysosomal disorders (e.g., metachromatic leukodystrophy)

(Left) *Axial NECT in a 9-year-old with cognitive decline reveals bilateral symmetrical decreased attenuation in the deep white matter, sparing the U fibers. Gene testing revealed an arylsulfatase A (ARSA) gene mutation.* **(Right)** *Axial T1WI MR in the same patient confirms abnormal deep white matter hypointensity. There was no abnormal enhancement following intravenous contrast (not shown).*

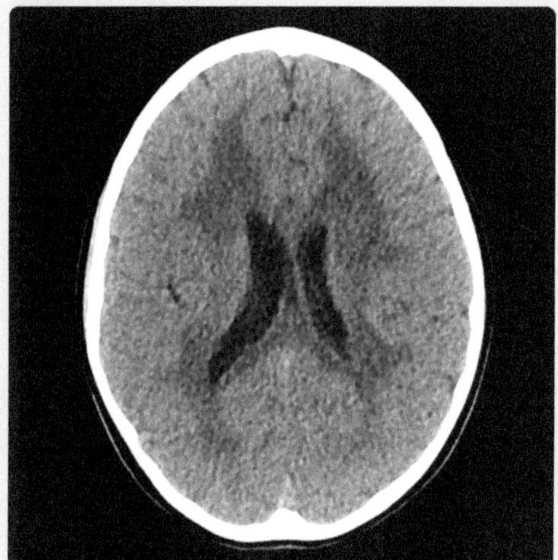

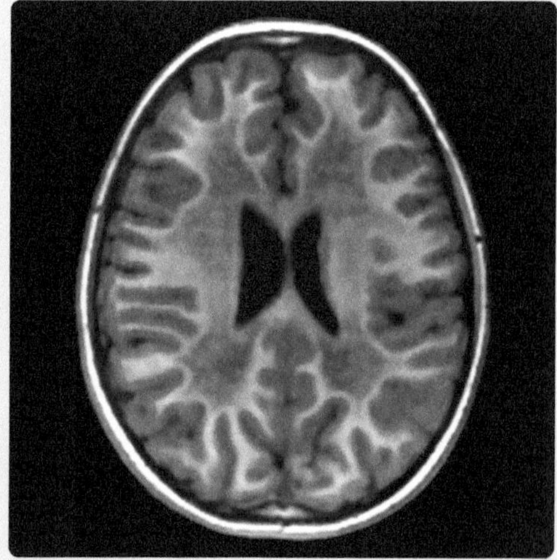

(Left) *Axial T2WI MR in the same patient shows abnormal hyperintensity in the deep white matter. The subcortical U fibers are spared in this patient. Note the faint tigroid striped pattern in the abnormal white matter.* **(Right)** *Axial FLAIR MR in the same patient better demonstrates the hypointense stripes (tigroid pattern) within the abnormally hyperintense white matter. This patient underwent bone marrow transplant with some stabilization of neurologic deterioration.*

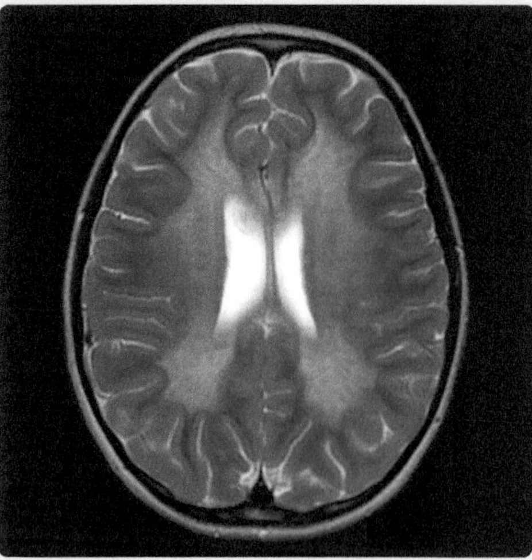

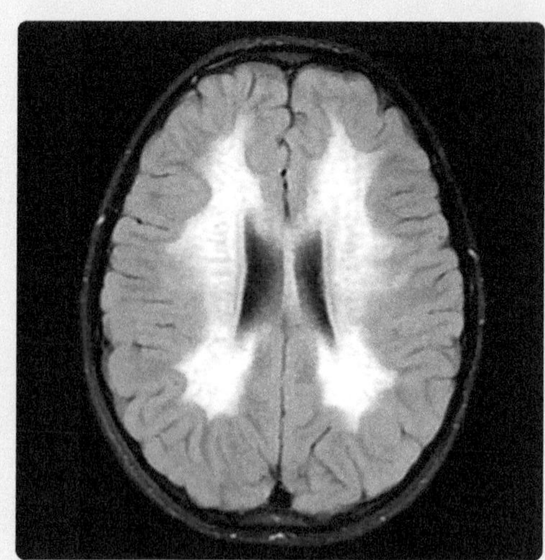

TERMINOLOGY

Abbreviations

- Metachromatic leukodystrophy (MLD)

Definitions

- Lysosomal storage disorder
  - Caused by ↓ arylsulfatase A (ARSA) enzyme
  - Results in CNS, peripheral nervous system (PNS) demyelination
- 3 clinical forms: Late infantile (most common), juvenile, adult

IMAGING

General Features

- Best diagnostic clue: Confluent butterfly-shaped ↑ T2 signal in deep cerebral hemispheric white matter (WM)
- Location: Deep cerebral hemispheric WM
  - Early: Spares subcortical U fibers
    - Initially, corpus callosum, parietooccipital WM
    - Rapid centrifugal spread to frontal, temporal WM
  - Late: Involves subcortical U fibers
- Morphology: Symmetric and confluent high T2 signal in periventricular (PV) and deep WM

CT Findings

- NECT
  - Symmetric ↓ attenuation of central cerebral hemispheric WM; late atrophy
- CECT
  - No enhancement (lacks inflammation)
- CT perfusion
  - ↓ perfusion in hemispheric WM

MR Findings

- T1WI
  - Early: ↓ T1 signal within PV/deep WM
  - Late: Atrophy
- T2WI
  - Early
    - Confluent PV hyperintensity (butterfly-shaped)
    - Sparing of perivenular myelin = tigroid or leopard pattern
    - Sparing of subcortical U fibers
  - Late
    - Progressive subcortical WM extension
    - Involvement of U fibers, corpus callosum, descending pyramidal tracts, internal capsules
    - Atrophy
- T1WI C+
  - No WM enhancement
  - ± cranial nerve, cauda equina enhancement
- FLAIR: Butterfly-shaped PV hyperintensity
- T2* GRE: No petechial hemorrhage
- DWI
  - ↑ diffusivity, ↓ fractional anisotropy in abnormal WM
  - May see reduced diffusivity (restriction) in areas of active demyelination
- MRS
  - ↑ choline, ± ↑ myoinositol, ↓ NAA later
  - Quantitative MRS may help stratify patients into good and poor predicted outcome after stem cell transplant

Imaging Recommendations

- Best imaging tool
  - Early MR and MRS in presymptomatic enzyme-deficient siblings
- Protocol advice
  - MR: Include FLAIR
  - MRS: Sample central hemispheric WM

DIFFERENTIAL DIAGNOSIS

Pelizaeus-Merzbacher Disease

- Usually manifests in neonates and infants
- Lack of myelination without myelin destruction
- Cerebellum may be markedly atrophic

TORCH

- Variable WM hyperintensity (demyelination and gliosis)
- Not progressive
- Varied patterns of Ca^{++} depending on etiology

Pseudo-TORCH

- Progressive cerebral and cerebellar demyelination
- Brainstem, basal ganglia, and PV Ca^{++}
- Elevated CSF neurotransmitters

Periventricular Leukomalacia

- Usually symmetric PV bright T2 signal
- PV volume loss (nonprogressive)
- Static spastic diplegia or quadriplegia

Sneddon Syndrome (Arylsulfatase A Pseudodeficiency)

- Demyelination
  - May be precipitated by hypoxic event
- PV WM bright T2 signal
- Confirmed by skin biopsy

Krabbe Disease

- Early involvement of cerebellar WM
- CT shows ↑ attenuation of thalami

Megalencephaly With Leukoencephalopathy and Cysts

- Slowly progressive, sparing of cognition, macrocephaly

PATHOLOGY

General Features

- General pathology comments
  - ↓ ARSA results in systemic storage of sulfatide
    - Symptomatic storage: CNS, PNS, gallbladder
    - Asymptomatic: Kidneys, adrenals, pancreas, liver
  - Diagnosis confirmed by
    - Excess urine sulfatide
    - Absent or deficient ARSA activity in fibroblasts &/or leukocytes
- Genetics: Autosomal recessive
  - *ARSA* gene located at 22q13.31-qter
  - > 110 different mutations

- Late infantile form caused by mutations, resulting in extremely low levels of ARSA
- Juvenile/adult forms associated with residual ARSA activity
- Etiology
  - Absent or ↓ ARSA → ↑ lysosomal storage sulfatide → lethal demyelination
- Associated abnormalities: Gallbladder disease, peripheral nerve enlargement

Gross Pathologic & Surgical Features

- Early
  - Enlarged brain and demyelination
  - Lack of inflammatory component to WM
- Late
  - Progressive cerebral hemispheric demyelination
  - Cerebral atrophy

Microscopic Features

- CNS
  - PAS (+) metachromatic material accumulates in glial cells, neurons, Schwann cells, macrophages
  - Sulfatide deposition within plasma membranes
  - Sulfatide membrane-bound inclusions at inner layer of myelin sheaths
  - Demyelination may be extensive, yet inflammatory component is lacking
  - Sulfatide content in WM is considerably higher in late infantile form

CLINICAL ISSUES

Presentation

- Most common signs/symptoms
  - Late infantile
    - Insidious onset in 2nd year of life
    - Strabismus, gait disturbance, ataxia, weakness, hypotonia
    - ± cherry-red macular spot
    - Bulbar signs → progressive hypotonia → decerebrate posturing → optic atrophy
    - Death frequently within 4 years of diagnosis
  - Juvenile
    - Appears between 5-10 years of age
    - Impaired school performance (nonverbal learning disability)
    - Spastic gait, ataxia, intellectual impairment
    - Brisk deep tendon reflexes
    - Progressive spasticity → progressive dementia → decerebrate posturing → seizures
    - Rare to survive longer than 20 years
  - Adult form
    - Can manifest as late as 6th decade
    - Presentation
      - May present as MS
      - Dementia, schizophrenia
      - Cryptic spasticity of legs
      - Progressive corticobulbar, corticospinal, and cerebellar changes
- Other signs/symptoms
  - Gallbladder disease common (polyps, hemobilia, rarely, cancer)
- Clinical profile: Toddler with visuomotor impairment and abdominal pain

Demographics

- Age: Variable depending on clinical form
- Sex: No predilection
- Epidemiology of all forms in USA: 1:100,000
  - ↑ in Habbanite Jewish patients (1:75 live births)
  - ↑ in Navajo Native American patients (1:2,500 live births)

Natural History & Prognosis

- Variable depending on clinical form and treatment efficacy

Treatment

- Hematopoietic stem cell, bone marrow, and umbilical cord blood transplant
  - May arrest motor and intellectual deterioration
  - Hematopoietic stem cell transplant shown to stabilize and even improve WM abnormalities
  - Mixed reports of effectiveness of bone marrow/cord blood transplants
    - Considered only in early phases of late infantile and juvenile/early adult forms
- Experimental: Lentivector-mediated *ARSA* gene transfer showing early promise

DIAGNOSTIC CHECKLIST

Consider

- If WM involvement appears as worst-case MLD, involving internal capsule and brainstem → MLD look-alike, consider
  - Pseudo-TORCH
  - Megalencephaly with leukoencephalopathy and cysts
- Adult patients presenting with cryptic spasticity of legs should be screened for X-linked adrenoleukodystrophy/adrenomyeloneuropathy, lysosomal disorders (e.g., MLD)

Image Interpretation Pearls

- Butterfly pattern of cerebral hemispheric WM
- Tigroid or leopard pattern on T2WI
- Early sparing of subcortical U fibers
- Lack of WM enhancement

SELECTED REFERENCES

1. Fumagalli F et al: Lentiviral haematopoietic stem-cell gene therapy for early-onset metachromatic leukodystrophy: long-term results from a non-randomised, open-label, phase 1/2 trial and expanded access. Lancet. 399(10322):372-83, 2022
2. Morton G et al: The importance of early diagnosis and views on newborn screening in metachromatic leukodystrophy: results of a caregiver survey in the UK and Republic of Ireland. Orphanet J Rare Dis. 17(1):403, 2022
3. Federico A et al: New disease modifying therapies for two genetic childhood-onset neurometabolic disorders (metachromatic leucodystrophy and adrenoleucodystrophy). Neurol Sci. 42(7):2603-6, 2021
4. Fumagalli F et al: Metachromatic leukodystrophy: a single-center longitudinal study of 45 patients. J Inherit Metab Dis. 44(5):1151-64, 2021
5. van Rappard DF et al: Quantitative MR spectroscopic imaging in metachromatic leukodystrophy: value for prognosis and treatment. J Neurol Neurosurg Psychiatry. 89(1):105-11, 2018
6. Grimm A et al: Thickening of the peripheral nerves in metachromatic leukodystrophy. J Neurol Sci. 368:399-401, 2016
7. van Rappard DF et al: Gallbladder and the risk of polyps and carcinoma in metachromatic leukodystrophy. Neurology. 87(1):103-11, 2016

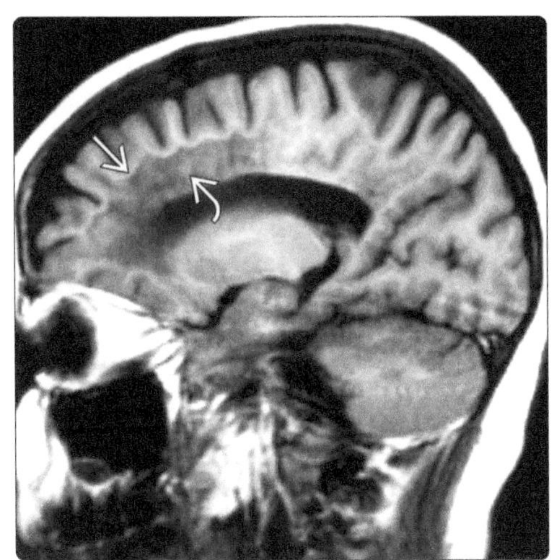

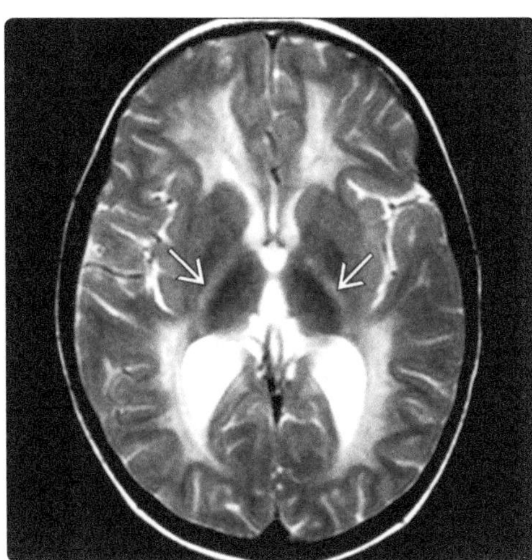

(Left) *Sagittal T1WI MR shows confluent hypointense signal in the periventricular and deep white matter with sparing of the subcortical U fibers ➡. Although less well evaluated in the sagittal plane, dot-like areas of spared perivenular myelin ➡ can be identified.* **(Right)** *Axial T2WI MR shows the butterfly-shaped pattern of white matter involvement, typical in more advanced metachromatic leukodystrophy (MLD). Although the subcortical U fibers remain spared, the posterior limbs of the internal capsules ➡ are involved.*

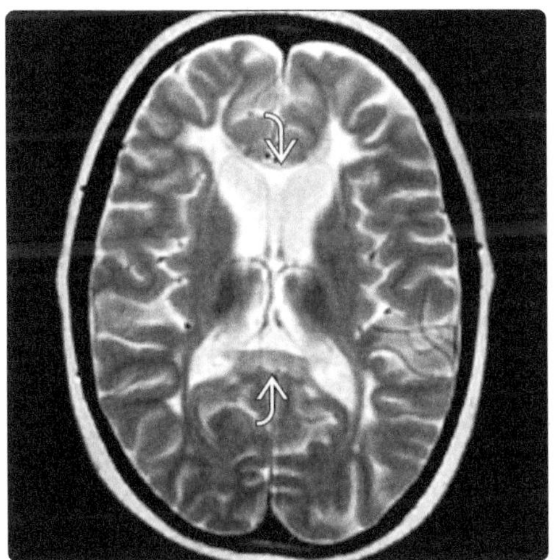

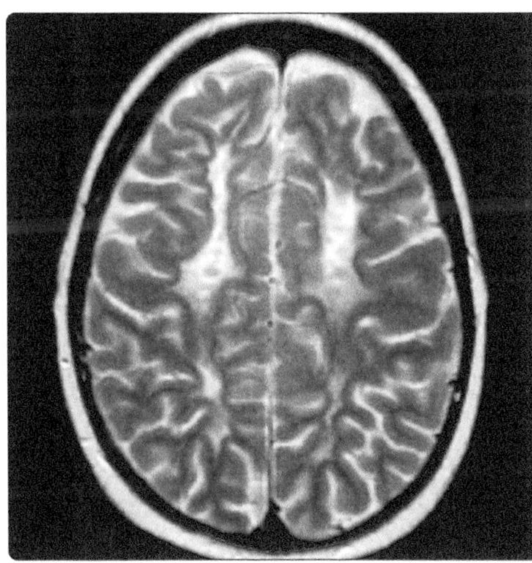

(Left) *In this axial T2WI MR of a patient with late MLD, the characteristic butterfly-shaped pattern of disease can be recognized despite severe loss of white matter volume. Lateral ventricles are enlarged (ex vacuo), and the basal ganglia are atrophic. Hyperintense signal is present in the corpus callosum ➡.* **(Right)** *Axial T2WI MR in the same patient shows confluent hyperintense signal and severe volume loss of the white matter. Although spared in this patient, the subcortical U fibers are often affected in late disease.*

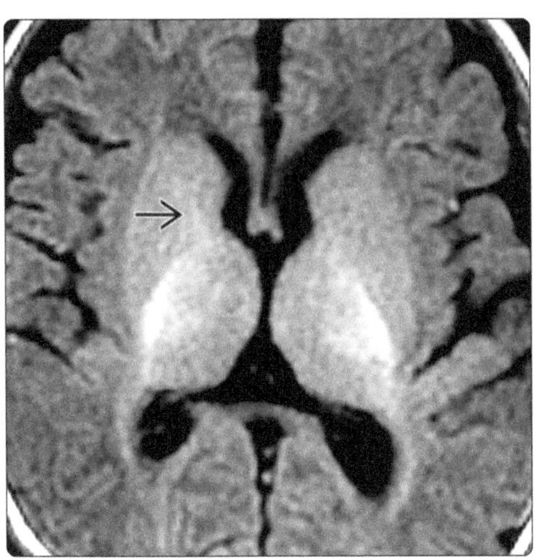

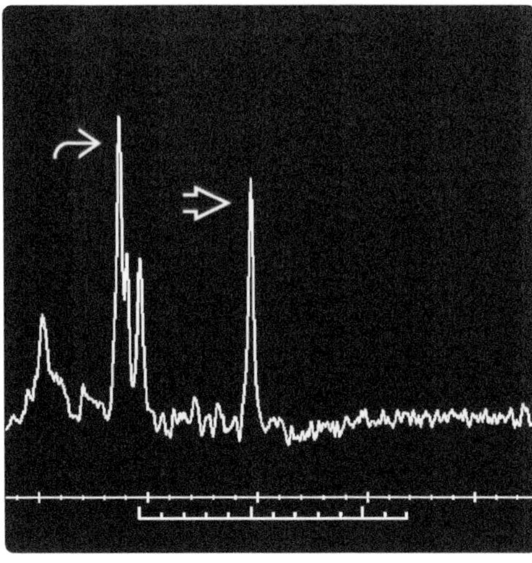

(Left) *Axial T1WI MR shows a 4-month-old infant with affected older siblings status post bone marrow transplant (BMT). Excepting mild myelin maturation delay in the anterior limbs of the internal capsule ➡, the conventional images were normal.* **(Right)** *Single-voxel MRS (TE = 288 msec) obtained from the periventricular white matter of the same patient shows increase in the choline peak ➡. The NAA peak ➡ should be the dominant peak at this age.*

KEY FACTS

TERMINOLOGY

- Krabbe disease
- Progressive autosomal recessive degenerative leukodystrophy of CNS and peripheral nervous system (PNS)

IMAGING

- Symmetric hyperdensity in thalami, basal ganglia (BG), corona radiata, cerebellum
  - Transient, sometimes seen in infants, but not older children
- Enlargement of optic nerves and cranial nerves
  - Enhancement of cranial nerves
- Enhancement and thickening of cauda equina nerve roots
- Confluent symmetric deep periventricular white matter (WM) hyperintensity on T2
  - Starts in corticospinal tracts, becomes diffuse over time
- Cerebellar WM hyperintense signal on T2
  - Concentric rings around dentate nuclei

PATHOLOGY

- Caused by homozygous or compound heterozygous mutations in *GALC* gene
  - Normally aids in cleavage of galactose from psychosine and galactosylceramide, leaving sphingosine and ceramide, respectively
- Autosomal recessive lysosomal disorder

CLINICAL ISSUES

- Early infantile (< 12 months); 85-90% of diagnoses
  - Hyperirritability
  - Seizures
  - Motor deterioration progressing to quadriparesis
  - Hypertonicity becomes flaccidity as PNS is involved

DIAGNOSTIC CHECKLIST

- Think of Krabbe when dealing with hyperirritable infant
- Use DTI for WM disease to enable fractional anisotropy analysis

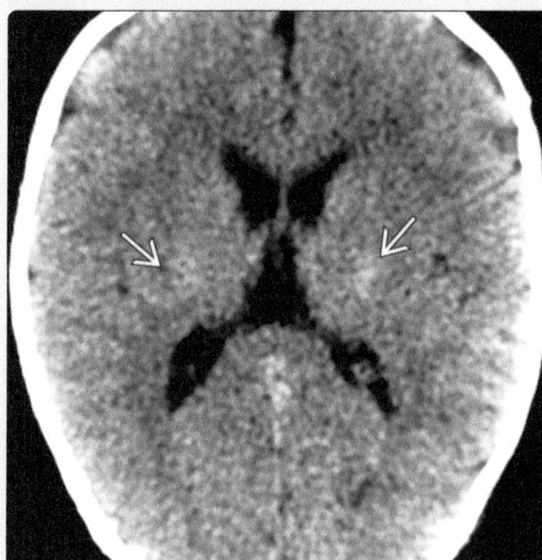

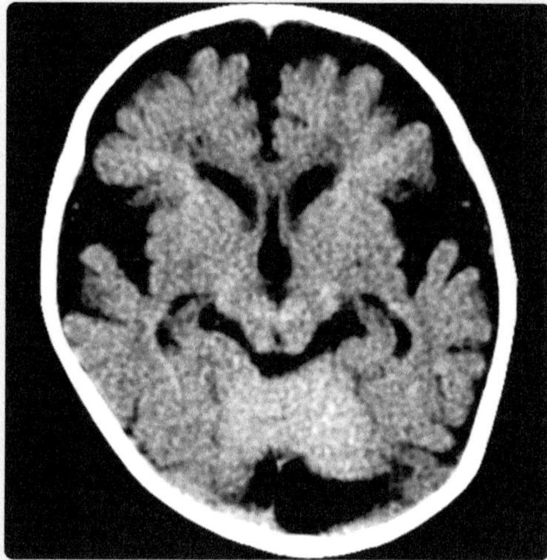

(Left) *Punctate hyperdensities* ➡ *are seen in this axial NECT from an 18-month-old with Krabbe disease. Infantile Krabbe is one of the few leukodystrophies in which CT features may be apparent before MR findings; however, DTI shows promise in detecting decreased fractional anisotropy in the corticospinal tracts in presymptomatic neonates.* **(Right)** *As the disease progresses, the hyperdensities fade and atrophy becomes the dominant imaging feature.*

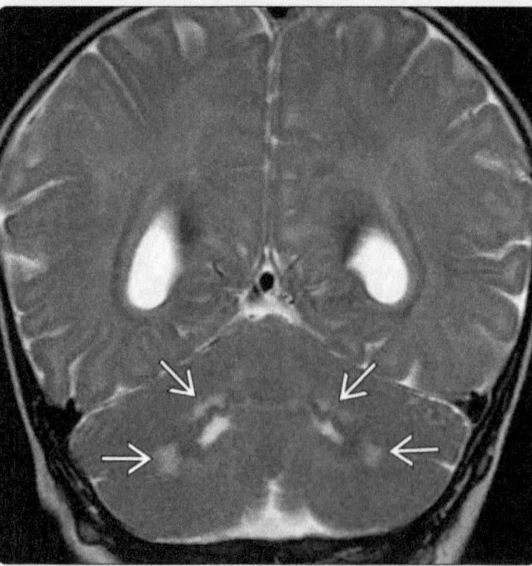

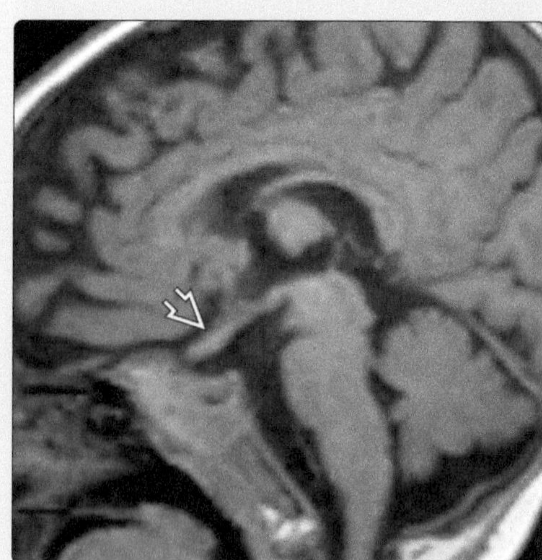

(Left) *Coronal T2WI MR in an 8-month-old boy with progressive spasticity and developmental regression due to globoid cell leukodystrophy (GLD) shows symmetric abnormal signal in the cerebellar white matter bordering the dentate nuclei* ➡. **(Right)** *Sagittal T1WI MR in a 10-month-old with failure to thrive and hypertonia shows marked thickening of the prechiasmatic optic nerve* ➡. *Optic nerve thickening was described by Krabbe in his original manuscript.*

TERMINOLOGY

Abbreviations

- Globoid cell leukodystrophy (GLD)

Synonyms

- Krabbe disease

Definitions

- Progressive autosomal recessive degenerative leukodystrophy of CNS and peripheral nervous system (PNS)

IMAGING

General Features

- Best diagnostic clue
  - Hyperintense signal in corticospinal tracts and bordering cerebellar dentate nuclei on T2-weighted imaging
- Location
  - Thalami, basal ganglia (BG), white matter (WM), corticospinal and pyramidal tracts, PNS

CT Findings

- NECT
  - Symmetric hyperdensity in thalami, BG, corona radiata, cerebellum
    - Globoid cell accumulation with Ca^{++}
    - Transient, sometimes seen in infants, but not older children
  - Deep, periventricular WM hypodensity
    - Demyelination, gliosis
  - Atrophy develops over time, leading to microcephaly

MR Findings

- T1WI
  - Deep, periventricular WM hypointensity
  - Faint hyperintensity in thalami and BG
  - Enlargement of optic nerves and cranial nerves
- T2WI
  - Confluent, symmetric, deep, periventricular WM hyperintensity
    - Starts in corticospinal tracts, becomes diffuse over time
    - Spares subcortical U fibers
    - May have tigroid appearance
  - Cerebellar WM hyperintense signal
    - Concentric rings around dentate nuclei
      - Prevalent in infantile phenotype
  - Corpus callosum frequently involved in adult-onset disease
- FLAIR
  - WM hyperintensities that parallel findings on T2WI
- DWI
  - Diffusion tensor imaging (DTI) can detect WM abnormalities prior to T2 signal abnormalities
    - Fractional anisotropy (FA) values in corticospinal tracts are lower in asymptomatic neonates with Krabbe disease than in age-matched controls
    - Differences are greater in symptomatic infants
    - Successful treatment with hematopoietic stem cell transplantation slows decline in FA values
- T1WI C+
  - Enhancement of cranial nerves
    - Infrequent finding
  - Enhancement and thickening of cauda equina nerve roots
    - Infrequent finding
- MRS
  - Infantile: Pronounced ↑ choline, myoinositol; moderate NAA reduction; mild lactate accumulation
  - Late infantile-juvenile: ↑ choline, myoinositol; mild NAA reduction
  - Adult: Mild ↑ choline and myoinositol, may be close to normal

Imaging Recommendations

- Best imaging tool
  - MR + contrast and DTI
- Protocol advice
  - Pay attention to cranial nerves
  - Include DTI with comparison of FA values to age-matched controls
  - Include lumbar spine imaging with contrast
  - Consider NECT to look for hyperdense thalami

DIFFERENTIAL DIAGNOSIS

Neuronal Ceroid Lipofuscinosis

- Batten disease
- Hyperdense thalami on CT
- Progressive cerebral atrophy

GM2 Gangliosidoses

- e.g., Tay-Sachs disease
- Lysosomal lipid storage disorders caused by mutations in ≥ 1 of 3 recessive genes: *HEXA, HEXB, GM2A*
- Hypointense/hyperdense thalami; patchy, hyperintense WM

Neurofibromatosis Type 1

- Optic nerve enlargement (optic nerve glioma)
- Patchy WM signal abnormalities
- Not progressive; does not present with irritability in infant

Metachromatic Leukodystrophy

- Progressive WM hyperintensity on T2WI
- Initial sparing of subcortical U fibers

PATHOLOGY

General Features

- Etiology
  - Caused by homozygous or compound heterozygous mutations in *GALC* gene
  - Gene defects result in deficiency of lysosomal galactocerebroside β-galactosidase (GALC)
    - Normally aids in cleavage of galactose from psychosine and galactosylceramide, leaving sphingosine and ceramide, respectively
      - Galactosylceramidase 2 and 3 can catalyze galactosylceramide but not psychosine
    - Results in accumulation of psychosine 100x normal concentrations

        - Psychosine is toxic to brain, especially oligodendroglia, leading to destruction of oligodendrocytes
      - Accumulation of psychosine causes
        - Upregulation of AP-1 (proapoptotic pathway)
        - Downregulation of NF-κB pathway (antiapoptotic pathway)
  - Sulfotransferase may also be deficient; suggests that galactosylceramide degradation may be complex
  - Accumulation of galactosylceramide leads to formation of globoid cells
- Genetics
  - Autosomal recessive lysosomal disorder
  - Gene mapped to chromosome 14 (14q24.3 to 14q32.1)
    - Different mutations may be associated with differing severity for both age of onset and progression
    - > 85 mutations and polymorphic changes have been identified

Staging, Grading, & Classification

- Infantile: Symptomatic < 12 months
  - 85-90% of diagnoses
  - Most severe
- Late infantile: 12 months to 16 years
- Adult: > 16 years
  - Corticospinal, pyramidal tract symptoms
  - Mimics peripheral neuropathy
  - May go undiagnosed for many years

Microscopic Features

- Myelin loss with gliosis and dysmyelination
  - Severe oligodendrocyte loss
- Perivascular large, multinucleated "globoid" and mononuclear epithelioid cells in demyelinated zones
  - "Globoid" cells = macrophages containing PAS (+) galactocerebrosides
- Demyelination is marked within cerebrum, cerebellum, brainstem, spinal cord with segmental involvement of peripheral nerves
- "Globoid" cells identified in enlarged optic nerves
- "Globoid" cell inclusions in sweat gland epithelial cells

CLINICAL ISSUES

Presentation

- Most common signs/symptoms
  - Early infantile (< 12 months)
    - Hyperirritability
    - Seizures
    - Abnormal protective reflexes
    - Axial hypotonia, appendicular hypertonia
    - Feeding difficulty, constipation
  - Late infantile-juvenile (12 months to 16 years)
    - Visual failure, cerebellar ataxia, spasticity, polyneuropathy, psychosis
  - Adult
    - Hemiparesis, spastic paraparesis, cerebellar ataxia, intellectual impairment, visual failure, peripheral polyneuropathy, talipes cavus
- Clinical profile
  - Diagnosis made from leukocyte or skin fibroblast β-galactosidase assay
  - Molecular assay available for genetic counseling, prenatal testing
  - Universal neonatal screening performed in Ohio, Kentucky, Missouri, and New York
    - Pending implementation in Pennsylvania, Illinois, Louisiana, New Mexico, New Jersey, and Tennessee

Demographics

- Sex
  - M = F
- Epidemiology
  - 1:100,000 in USA and Europe
  - 1:25-50,000 in Sweden
  - 6:1,000 in Druze community in Israel

Natural History & Prognosis

- Early infantile
  - Motor deterioration progressing to quadriparesis
  - Hypertonicity becomes flaccidity as PNS is involved
  - Blindness
- Infantile-juvenile: More protracted course, slower rate of progression
- Adult: Heterogeneous, progresses more slowly
  - MR may remain normal for many years, even in presence of symptoms

Treatment

- Hematopoietic stem cell transplantation
  - Effective in early infantile if instituted before symptoms develop
    - Halts or markedly slows disease progression
    - Both clinical and radiologic manifestations arrest
  - Less symptomatic at time of transplantation = better outcome
- Bone marrow transplant in combination with gene therapy, enzyme replacement therapy (ERT), and substrate reduction therapy (SRT) has shown some synergistic effect in animal models

DIAGNOSTIC CHECKLIST

Consider

- Think of Krabbe when dealing with hyperirritable infant
- Use contrast on MR when considering leukodystrophies
- Use DTI for WM disease to enable FA analysis
- Include lumbar spine imaging

Image Interpretation Pearls

- Look for faint hyperdensity on CT in deep cerebral nuclei

SELECTED REFERENCES

1. Maghazachi AA: Globoid cell leukodystrophy (Krabbe disease): an update. Immunotargets Ther. 12:105-11, 2023
2. Komatsuzaki S et al: Clinical characteristics of 248 patients with Krabbe disease: quantitative natural history modeling based on published cases. Genet Med. 21(10):2208-15, 2019
3. Bascou N et al: A prospective natural history study of Krabbe disease in a patient cohort with onset between 6 months and 3 years of life. Orphanet J Rare Dis. 13(1):126, 2018
4. Hwang M et al: Thickening of the cauda equina roots: a common finding in Krabbe disease. Eur Radiol. 26(10):3377-82, 2016
5. Jones BV et al: Optic nerve enlargement in Krabbe's disease. AJNR Am J Neuroradiol. 20(7):1228-31, 1999

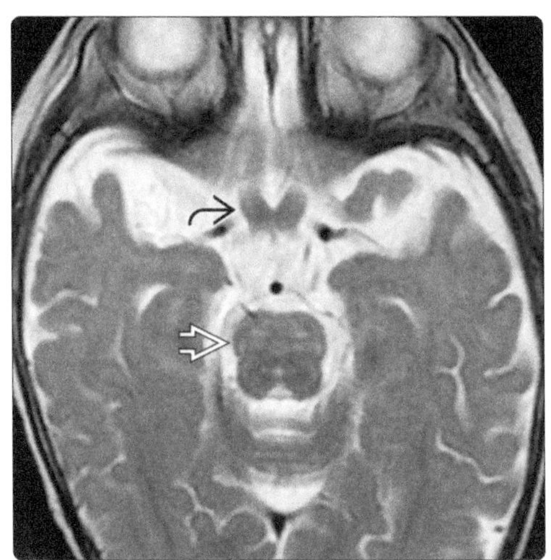

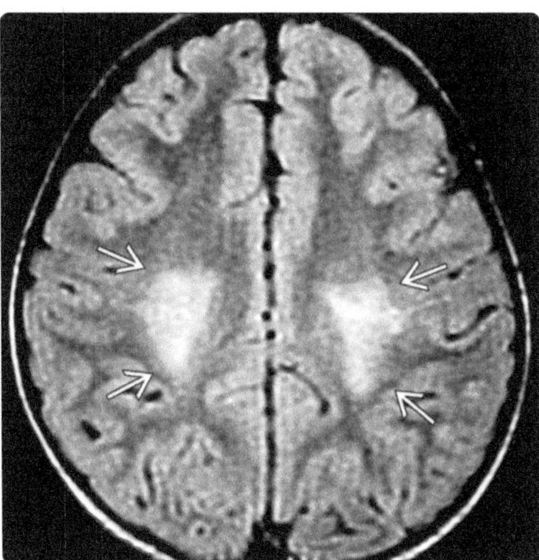

(Left) *Abnormal hyperintense signal ➡ is seen in the pons in this 6-month-old with progressive spasticity and vision loss due to Krabbe disease, reflecting demyelination in crossing corticospinal tract fibers. Note the thickened appearance of the optic nerves ➡.* **(Right)** *Axial FLAIR MR in a 30-year-old with juvenile-onset Krabbe disease demonstrates abnormal hyperintense signal ➡ in the corona radiata on each side. Symmetric corticospinal tract involvement is a hallmark of GLD.*

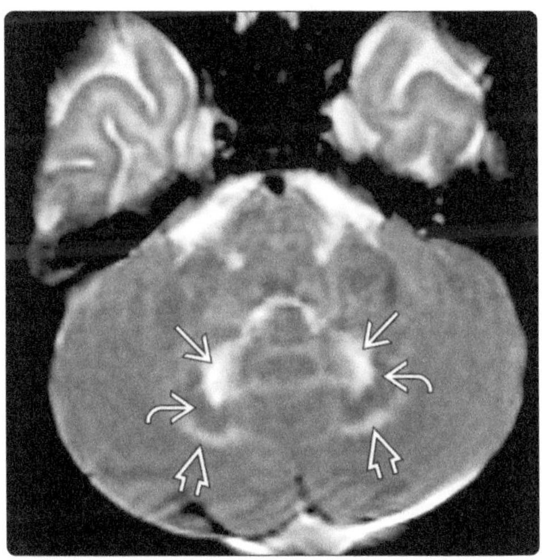

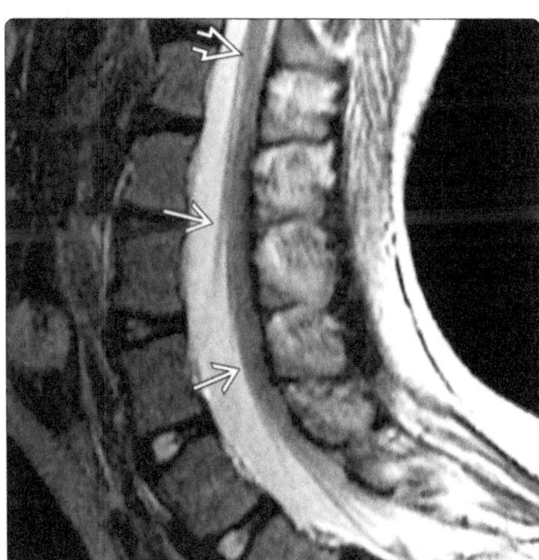

(Left) *Axial T2WI MR in an infant with GLD shows alternating hyper- ➡, hypo- ➡, and hyperintense ➡ signal around the cerebellar dentate nuclei. Krabbe is one of the few leukodystrophies that has early cerebellar imaging findings.* **(Right)** *Sagittal T2WI MR of the lumbar spine in a 12-year-old with Krabbe disease and severe scoliosis shows thickening and clumping of the nerve roots of the cauda equina ➡, which appear more solid and bulky than the distal spinal cord ➡.*

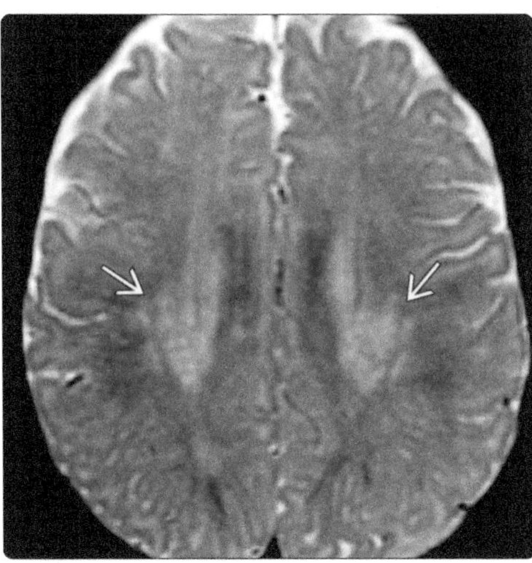

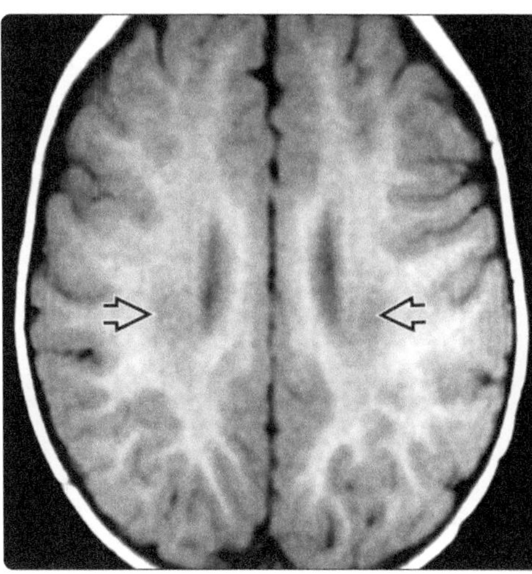

(Left) *Axial T2WI MR in a 4-year-old with Krabbe disease treated with stem cell transplantation shows confluent abnormal hyperintense signal in the periventricular white matter ➡, primarily affecting the descending corticospinal tracts.* **(Right)** *Axial T1WI MR in the same child shows subtle hypointense signal ➡ that appears less extensive but is in the same distribution. These findings did not progress after the stem cell transplant.*

Zellweger Syndrome and Peroxisomal Biogenesis Disorders

KEY FACTS

TERMINOLOGY

- Disorders of peroxisome biosynthesis, assembly, and biochemical functions
- Varying phenotypes reflect degree of dysfunction
  - Severe: Zellweger syndrome (ZS)
  - Moderate: Neonatal adrenoleukodystrophy (NALD)
  - Mild: Infantile Refsum disease (IRD), Heimler syndrome (HS)

IMAGING

- Polymicrogyria, pachygyria, hypomyelination, germinolytic cysts, heterotopic gray matter
- Leukoencephalopathy with abnormal myelin in corticospinal tracts and dentate nuclei
- Volume loss evident after 1 year
- Use short TE MRS: ↓ NAA; ↑ Cho
  - Lipid peaks at 0.9 and 1.33 ppm
- Polymicrogyria most severe in perisylvian region, especially posterior insula

TOP DIFFERENTIAL DIAGNOSES

- Congenital CMV
- Single peroxisomal enzyme deficiencies

PATHOLOGY

- Autosomal recessive
  - 70% associated with *PEX1* mutations
  - 15-20% associated with *PEX6* mutations
- Laboratory analysis demonstrates ↓ peroxisomal function

CLINICAL ISSUES

- Elevated liver enzymes, hepatomegaly
- Vision loss, hearing loss
- Severe deficiencies (ZS) manifest at birth
- Milder forms (IRD) may present later in childhood

DIAGNOSTIC CHECKLIST

- Polymicrogyria most severe in perisylvian region, especially posterior insula

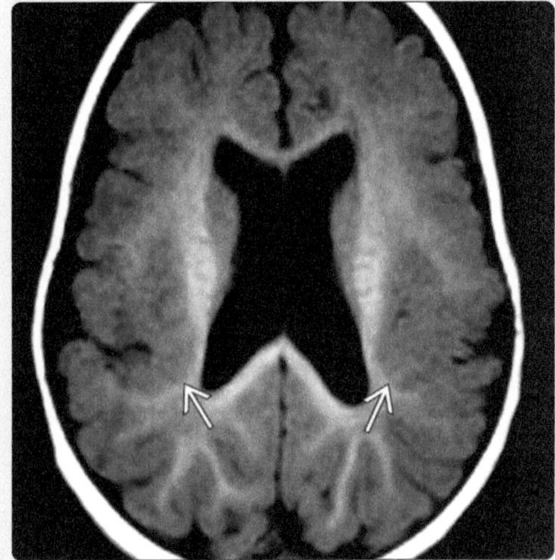
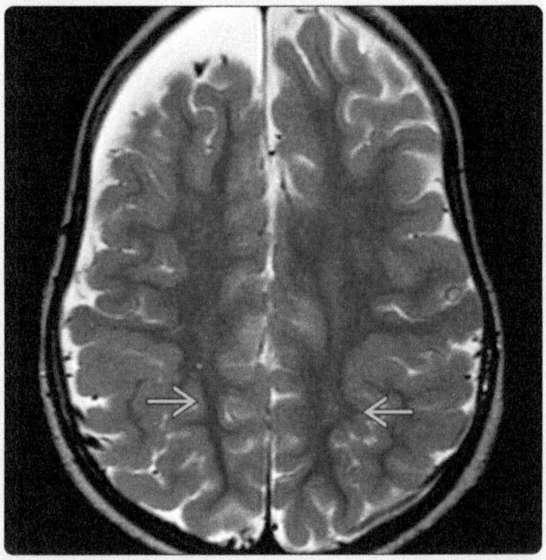

(Left) *Axial T1WI MR in an 8-month-old boy with Zellweger syndrome shows polymicrogyria ➔ at the apex of each sylvian fissure.* **(Right)** *Axial T2WI MR in the same patient at 3 years of age shows the thickening of the cortical ribbon on each side with an irregular gray matter-white matter interface. The complexity of white matter rami is diminished in the regions of polymicrogyria → when compared to the normal frontal white matter.*

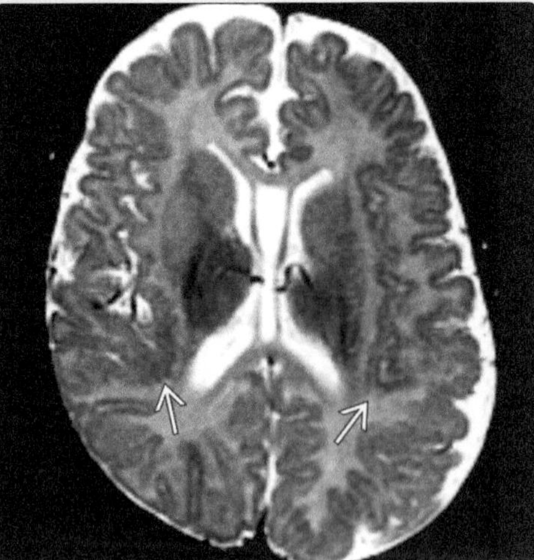
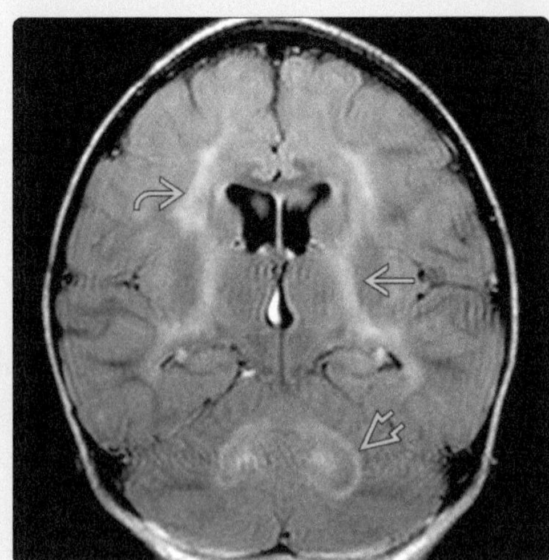

(Left) *Axial T2WI MR in a 5-month-old with neonatal adrenoleukodystrophy shows bilateral polymicrogyria ➔. Subtle areas of cortical malformation are best seen on T2WI in the neonatal period but can be more difficult to discern as myelination progresses.* **(Right)** *Dysmyelination in the periventricular white matter ↪, corticospinal tracts →, and dentate nuclei of the cerebellum ⇨ are evident in this 4-year-old with infantile Refsum disease.*

Zellweger Syndrome and Peroxisomal Biogenesis Disorders

TERMINOLOGY

Definitions

- Disorders of peroxisome biosynthesis, assembly, and biochemical functions
- Varying phenotypes reflect degree of dysfunction
  - Severe: Zellweger syndrome (ZS)
  - Moderate: Neonatal adrenoleukodystrophy (NALD)
  - Mild: Infantile Refsum disease (IRD), Heimler syndrome (HS)
- Related disorders
  - Multiple peroxisomal enzyme deficiencies (PEDs): Rhizomelic chondrodysplasia punctata (RCDP)
  - Single peroxisomal enzyme deficiency: Acyl-CoA oxidase deficiency, adrenoleukodystrophy protein deficiency (X-ALD), D-bifunctional protein deficiency (D-BP)

IMAGING

General Features

- Best diagnostic clue
  - Polymicrogyria, pachygyria, hypomyelination, germinolytic cysts, heterotopic gray matter
  - Leukoencephalopathy with abnormal myelin in corticospinal tracts and dentate nuclei
  - Volume loss evident after 1 year
- Location
  - Polymicrogyria most severe in perisylvian region, especially posterior insula
  - Diffuse hypomyelination; cerebellum and brainstem may be involved, especially if present > 1 year

MR Findings

- T1WI
  - Polymicrogyria, pachygyria
  - Germinolytic cysts (near foramina of Monro)
  - ± ↑ globus pallidus signal from hyperbilirubinemia
- T2WI
  - ↑ white matter (WM) signal in corticospinal tracts and dentate nuclei
- T1WI C+
  - May see enhancement of corticospinal tracts in brainstem
- MRS
  - Use short TE: ↓ NAA; ↑ Cho; lipid peaks at 0.9 and 1.33 ppm

Imaging Recommendations

- Best imaging tool
  - MR + MRS
- Protocol advice
  - Volumetric T1, high-resolution T2 for migrational abnormalities

DIFFERENTIAL DIAGNOSIS

Congenital CMV

- Ca^{++}, periventricular cysts usually not caudothalamic

Pseudo-TORCH

- Basal ganglia, thalamic, and periventricular Ca^{++}

Single Peroxisomal Enzyme Deficiencies

- Brain MR may be similar; biochemistry different

PATHOLOGY

General Features

- Etiology
  - Defect in biogenesis of peroxisomes
    - Defective transport of proteins into peroxisomal matrix → accumulation of very long chain fatty acids (VLCFA)
  - Laboratory analysis demonstrating ↓ peroxisomal function
    - Elevated plasma levels of sphingomyelin, VLCFA, pristanic acid, phytanic acid, pipecolic acid
- Genetics
  - Autosomal recessive
  - Caused by mutations in 1 of 14 known PEX genes
    - 70% associated with *PEX1* mutations
    - 15-20% associated with *PEX6* mutations
- Associated abnormalities
  - Characteristic facies in ZS: High forehead, broad nasal bridge, hypertelorism
  - Hepatomegaly, renal cortical cysts
  - Skeletal: Stippled chondral Ca^{++} in RCDP

CLINICAL ISSUES

Presentation

- Most common signs/symptoms
  - Severe hypotonia, seizures, poor sucking
  - Elevated liver enzymes, hepatomegaly
- Other signs/symptoms
  - Vision loss due to retinal dystrophy and abnormal optic nerves
  - Hearing loss

Demographics

- Age
  - Severe deficiencies (ZS) manifest at birth
  - Milder forms (IRD) may present later in childhood
- Epidemiology
  - 1:50,000 to 1:100,000
    - Incidence ↑ with detection of milder forms

Natural History & Prognosis

- Most severely affected die < 3 months, milder may live > 20 years

SELECTED REFERENCES

1. Bose M et al: Characterization of severity in Zellweger spectrum disorder by clinical findings: a scoping review, meta-analysis and medical chart review. Cells. 11(12):1891, 2022
2. Tan AP et al: Clinical and neuroimaging spectrum of peroxisomal disorders. Top Magn Reson Imaging. 27(4):241-57, 2018
3. Braverman NE et al: Peroxisome biogenesis disorders in the Zellweger spectrum: an overview of current diagnosis, clinical manifestations, and treatment guidelines. Mol Genet Metab. 117(3):313-21, 2016
4. Salpietro V et al: Zellweger syndrome and secondary mitochondrial myopathy. Eur J Pediatr. 174(4):557-63, 2015
5. Crane DI: Revisiting the neuropathogenesis of Zellweger syndrome. Neurochem Int. 69:1-8, 2014
6. van der Knaap MS et al: MRI as diagnostic tool in early-onset peroxisomal disorders. Neurology. 78(17):1304-8, 2012

KEY FACTS

TERMINOLOGY

- Abbreviations
  - X-linked adrenoleukodystrophy (X-ALD, ALD)
  - Classic childhood ALD (CCALD)
- Inherited peroxisomal disorder
  - *ABCD1* mutation → impaired β-oxidation (β-ox) of very long chain fatty acids (VLCFA)
  - Accumulation of VLCFAs in white matter (WM) causes severe inflammatory demyelination
- Several clinical forms of ALD and related disorders
  - Classic X-ALD
    - Severe form almost exclusively in boys 5-12 years
  - At least 6 variants other than classic childhood X-ALD
    - Presymptomatic X-ALD, adolescent (AdolCALD), adult (ACALD), adrenomyeloneuropathy (AMN), Addison only, symptomatic female carriers
  - AMN
    - "Mild" adult (spinocerebellar) form, cerebral involvement in up to 50%
    - X-ALD and AMN account for 80% of cases

IMAGING

- 3 zones of myelin loss in CCALD
  - Innermost: Necrotic astrogliotic core
  - Intermediate: Enhancing active demyelination, inflammation
  - Peripheral: Advancing demyelination without inflammation

DIAGNOSTIC CHECKLIST

- X-ALD presenting at atypical ages
  - Atypical appearances common
    - Lacks enhancement; may have frontal (rather than posterior) "gradient"
- Always enhance unknown leukodystrophy

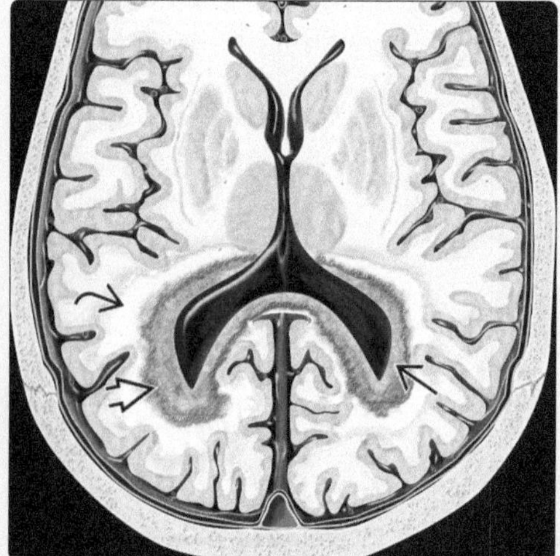

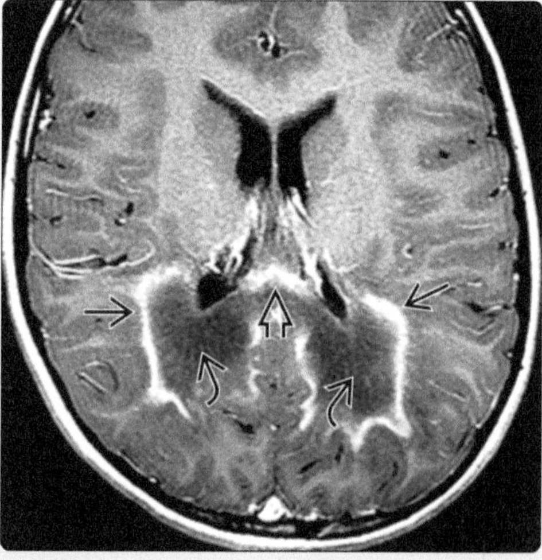

(Left) *Axial graphic shows multiple layers of demyelination, which correspond to 3 zones histopathologically. Outer layer ➙ consists of active destruction and middle layer ➙ of active inflammation. Note the central area ➙ is burned out.* **(Right)** *Axial T1WI C+ MR reveals marked rim enhancement ➙ surrounding the most severely damaged parietal white matter (WM) ➙ and the splenium of the corpus callosum ➙ in a preteen boy with typical classic childhood adrenoleukodystrophy (CCALD) (Loes pattern 1).*

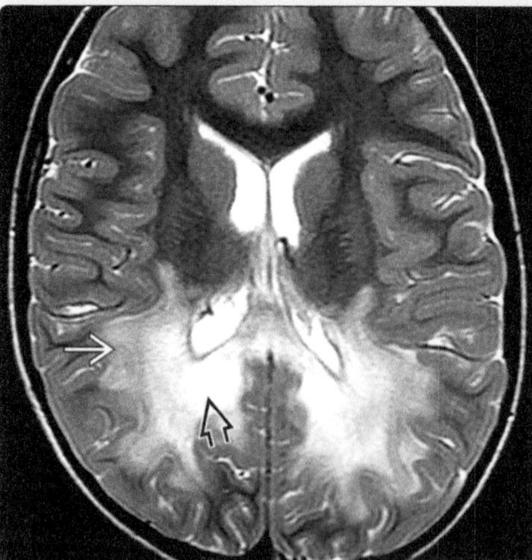

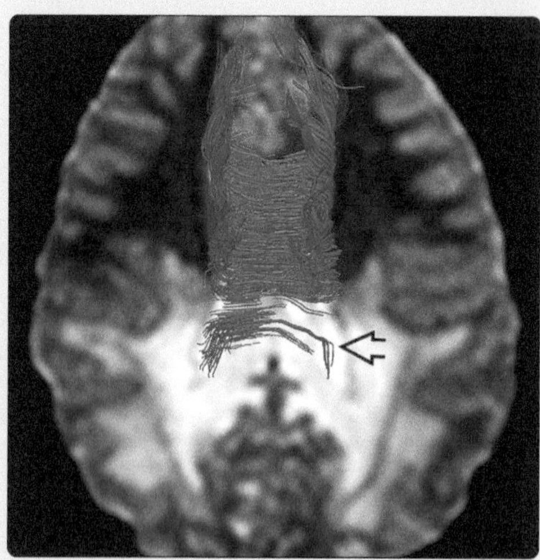

(Left) *Axial T2WI MR distinguishes the active inflammation of the outer zone ➙ from the innermost burned-out zone of WM destruction ➙ in this preteen boy who presented with well-developed brain involvement.* **(Right)** *Axial tractograph of the corpus callosum from a DTI sequence demonstrates significant loss of WM tracts crossing the splenium of the corpus callosum ➙ and forceps major in another preteen symptomatic boy with CCALD.*

TERMINOLOGY

Abbreviations

- X-linked adrenoleukodystrophy (X-ALD, ALD)
  - Classic childhood ALD (CCALD)

Definitions

- Inherited peroxisomal disorder
  - *ABCD1* mutation → impaired β-oxidation (β-ox) of very long chain fatty acids (VLCFA)
  - Accumulation of VLCFAs in white matter (WM) causes severe inflammatory demyelination
- Several clinical forms of ALD and related disorders
  - Classic X-ALD
    - Severe progressive form almost exclusively in boys 5-12 years
  - At least 6 variants other than classic childhood X-ALD exist: Presymptomatic X-ALD, adolescent (AdolCALD), adult (ACALD), adrenomyeloneuropathy (AMN), Addison only, symptomatic female carriers
    - AMN
      - "Mild" adult (spinocerebellar) form, cerebral involvement in up to 50%
  - X-ALD and AMN account for 80% of cases

IMAGING

General Features

- Best diagnostic clue
  - CCALD: Enhancing peritrigonal demyelination
- Location
  - Classic CCALD: Peritrigonal WM
    - Pattern: Splenium → peritrigonal WM → corticospinal tracts/fornix/commisural fibers/visual and auditory pathways
    - Typically spares subcortical U fibers
- Morphology
  - Usually symmetric, confluent, posterior involvement; rare frontal pattern occurs
  - Central (splenium) to peripheral gradient is usual

CT Findings

- NECT
  - ↓ density splenium/posterior WM
  - ± Ca^{++} of involved WM
- CECT
  - CCALD: Linear enhancement of intermediate zone

MR Findings

- T1WI
  - ↓ T1 signal of involved WM
- T2WI
  - ↑ T2 signal of involved WM
    - CCALD: Splenium → peritrigonal WM → corticospinal tracts/fornix/commisural fibers/visual and auditory pathways
    - AMN: Cerebellum, spinal cord; most common intracranial feature is corticospinal involvement but may resemble CCALD
- FLAIR
  - Same as T2WI
- DWI
  - Reduced diffusion in actively involved WM, ↑ in chronically involved WM
  - DTI: Reduced brain "connectivity," ↑ isotropic diffusion, and loss of fractional anisotropy in obvious WM change **and** in presymptomatic WM
- T1WI C+
  - Leading edge (intermediate zone) enhances
    - Enhancement strongly linked to progression
- MRS
  - Peaks between 0.9 and 1.4 ppm probably represent VLCFA macromolecules
  - X-ALD: ↓ NAA even in normal-appearing WM predicts progression; ↑ Cho, myoinositol, lactate
- Spinal MR: Spinal atrophy in AMN

Nuclear Medicine Findings

- PET
  - Hypometabolism of occipital lobes
- Tc-99m-HMPAO SPECT: ↑ regional cerebral blood flow (CBF) in enhancing zone (↓ elsewhere)

Imaging Recommendations

- Best imaging tool
  - MR + contrast
- Protocol advice
  - DWI/DTI and MRS may predict onset of presymptomatic disease

DIFFERENTIAL DIAGNOSIS

Neonatal Hypoglycemia (Acute and Follow-Up)

- May involve splenium, calcar avis, and posterior peritrigonal WM but does not enhance

White Matter Disease With Lactate

- WM disease with lactate (WML) involves splenium, peritrigonal WM, and corticospinal tracts but does not enhance

Alexander Disease

- Enhances, but frontal, not peritrigonal, WM

PATHOLOGY

General Features

- Etiology
  - Peroxisomes: Ubiquitous organelles involved in catabolic pathways
    - Involved with myelin formation/stabilization
    - Defect in VLCFA importer → impaired β-ox of VLCFA
    - VLCFA accumulate in WM → brittle myelin
- Genetics
  - X-ALD: X-linked recessive
    - Mutations of *ABCD1* gene at Xq28 (> 300 described)
    - ABCD1 is ATPase transporter protein: "Traffic" ATPase
    - Required for transport hydrophilic molecules across peroxisomal membrane
  - Phenotypic variability: CCALD, AMN, or presymptomatic presentations even within same family
  - Clinical heterogeneity attributed (in part) to specific mutations, modifying factors
    - Insertion allele of CBS c.844_845ins68 protects against CNS demyelination

- G allele of Tc2 c.776C > G more common in demyelinating forms (CCALD)
- Associated abnormalities
  - VLCFA accumulates in all tissues of body
  - Symptomatic accumulation: CNS myelin, adrenal cortex, Leydig cell testes
    - Adrenal failure: Skin bronzing
    - Testes: Early androgenetic alopecia in adults

Staging, Grading, & Classification

- Loes MR scoring system: Severity score based upon location, extent of disease, and atrophy
  - Pattern 1: Parietooccipital WM (rapid progression if contrast-enhancement present and very young)
  - Pattern 2: Frontal WM (same as pattern 1)
  - Pattern 3: Corticospinal tract (adults, slower progression)
  - Pattern 4: Corticospinal tract and cerebellar WM (adolescents, slower progression)
  - Pattern 5: Concomitant parietooccipital and frontal WM (mainly childhood, extremely rapid)

Gross Pathologic & Surgical Features

- Atrophy, WM softened

Microscopic Features

- Complete myelin loss (U fibers preserved), astrogliosis
- Zone-specific features
  - Innermost zone of necrosis, gliosis ± Ca^{++}
  - Intermediate zone of active demyelination and inflammation
  - Peripheral zone of demyelination without inflammation

CLINICAL ISSUES

Presentation

- Most common signs/symptoms
  - Incidental diagnosis on newborn screening
  - Skin bronzing, behavioral difficulties, hearing problems
- Clinical profile
  - Phenotypes unpredictable (even intrafamilial)
- Classic childhood cerebral X-ALD (CCALD): 35-50%, but percentage ↓ as new forms diagnosed
  - Preteen male (3-10 years): Behavioral, learning, gait, hearing, vision difficulties
  - Addison/adrenal insufficiency (skin bronzing, nausea and vomiting, fatigue) may predate X-ALD diagnosis
- AMN (25%)
  - 14-60 years
  - Spinal involvement > > brain involvement; peripheral nerve involvement
  - Brain inflammatory reaction eventually in 50%; variable demyelination/enhancement
- Presymptomatic ALD (12%)
  - Abnormal genetic testing (due to known symptomatic brother or maternal uncle)
- 20-50% female carriers develop AMN-like symptoms (milder, age related)
- Other presentations less common
  - AdolCALD: 10-20 years, symptoms and course similar to CCALD
  - ACALD: May be misdiagnosed as psychiatric disorder, very rapid progression, diffuse rather than posterior pattern

Demographics

- Age
  - CCALD: Preteen boys
- Sex
  - Male patients in classic X-ALD
  - Female carriers may show AMN-like symptoms
- Ethnicity
  - CCALD predominates in North America and France
  - AMN predominates in Netherlands
- Epidemiology
  - X-ALD and variants = 1:16,800 North American births

Natural History & Prognosis

- CCALD: Progresses to spastic quadriparesis, blindness, deafness, vegetative state
- AMN: Spastic, weak legs; sphincter/sexual dysfunction

Treatment

- CCALD: Vegetative state, death in 2-5 years without bone marrow transplant (BMT)
  - Lorenzo oil delays symptoms in presymptomatic ALD
  - Early BMT stabilizes demyelination: **Rare** reversal demyelination

DIAGNOSTIC CHECKLIST

Consider

- X-ALD presenting at atypical ages → atypical appearances (may lack enhancement or have frontal rather than posterior "gradient")
- Newborn screening test available, but not used in all USA states

Image Interpretation Pearls

- Always contrast enhance unknown leukodystrophy

Reporting Tips

- Loes scoring aids pattern analysis

SELECTED REFERENCES

1. Albersen M et al: Sex-specific newborn screening for X-linked adrenoleukodystrophy. J Inherit Metab Dis. 46(1):116-28, 2023
2. Pierpont EI et al: Neurocognitive and mental health impact of adrenoleukodystrophy across the lifespan: insights for the era of newborn screening. J Inherit Metab Dis. 46(2):174-93, 2023
3. Bonkowsky JL et al: Time to transplant in X-linked adrenoleukodystrophy. J Child Neurol. 37(5):397-400, 2022
4. Cebeci H et al: Contrast enhancement in cerebral adrenoleukodystrophy: a comparison of T1 TSE and MPRAGE sequences. Jpn J Radiol. 40(12):1241-5, 2022
5. Mao C et al: Typical and atypical phenotype and neuroimaging of X-linked adrenoleukodystrophy in a Chinese cohort. Neurol Sci. 43(5):3255-63, 2022
6. Liberato AP et al: MRI brain lesions in asymptomatic boys with X-linked adrenoleukodystrophy. Neurology. 92(15):e1698-708, 2019
7. de Beer M et al: Frequent occurrence of cerebral demyelination in adrenomyeloneuropathy. Neurology. 83(24):2227-31, 2014
8. McKinney AM et al: Childhood cerebral X-linked adrenoleukodystrophy: diffusion tensor imaging measurements for prediction of clinical outcome after hematopoietic stem cell transplantation. AJNR Am J Neuroradiol. 34(3):641-9, 2013
9. Santosh Rai PV et al: Childhood adrenoleukodystrophy - classic and variant - review of clinical manifestations and magnetic resonance imaging. J Pediatr Neurosci. 8(3):192-7, 2013

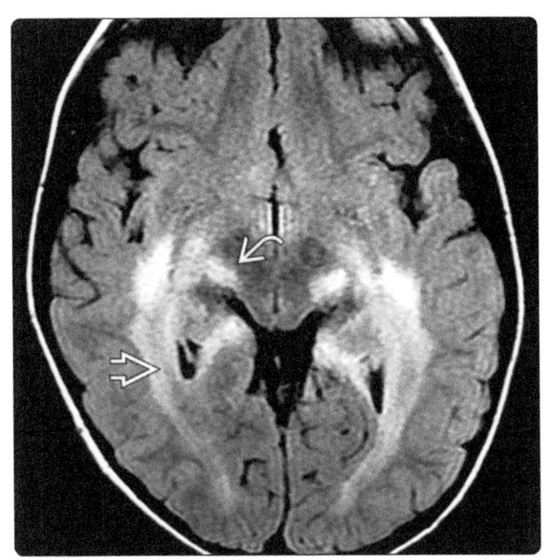

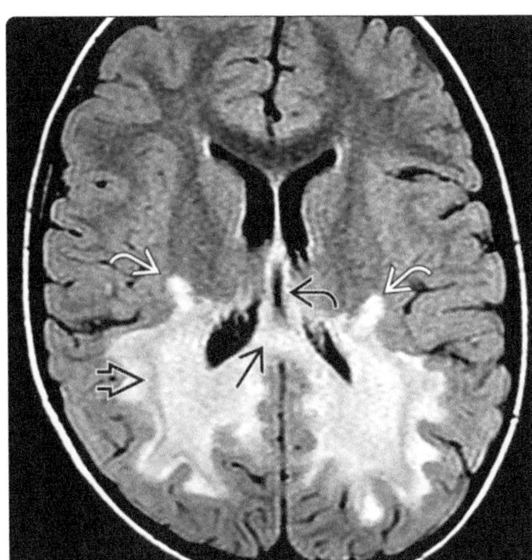

(Left) *Axial FLAIR MR in CCALD (ALD pattern 1) demonstrates hyperintensity of the medial geniculate body* ➡ *along with the periventricular and deep WM* ➡ *of the temporal and occipital lobes.* **(Right)** *Axial FLAIR MR in the same child with CCALD reveals hyperintensity of the posterior columns of the fornices* ➡*, the splenium of the corpus callosum* ➡*, and multilayered involvement in the peritrigonal WM* ➡ *and external/extreme capsules* ➡*.*

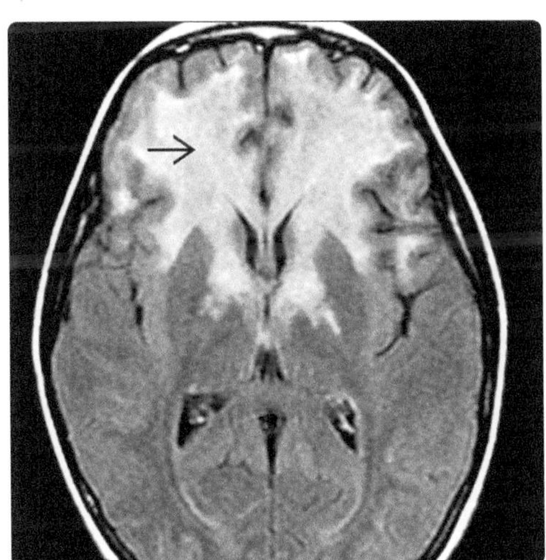

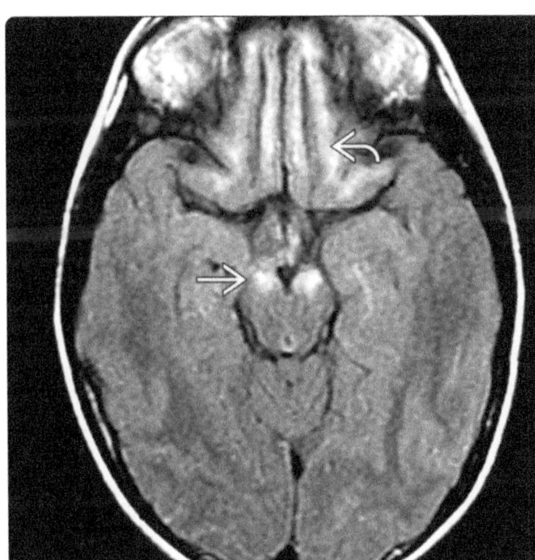

(Left) *Axial FLAIR MR shows confluent bifrontal WM hyperintensity* ➡*. Abnormal signal extends into the caudate heads, globi pallidi, and anterior limbs of internal capsules in this frontal variant case (Loes pattern 2) of proven X-linked ALD in a school-aged boy.* **(Right)** *Axial FLAIR MR in the same patient shows symmetric WM hyperintensities in the internal capsules as they extend into the cerebral peduncles* ➡ *and in the juxtacortical frontal WM* ➡*.*

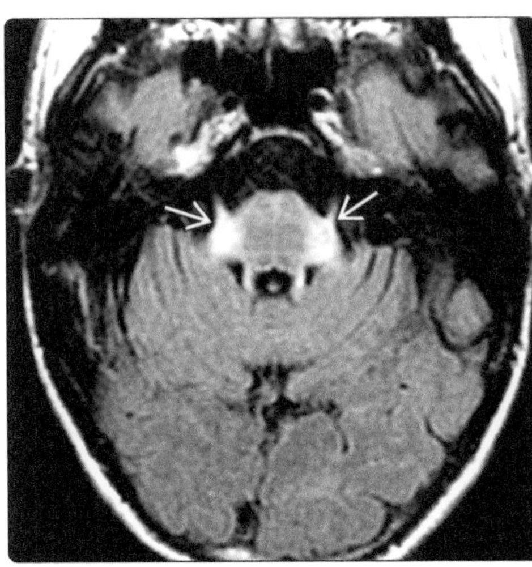

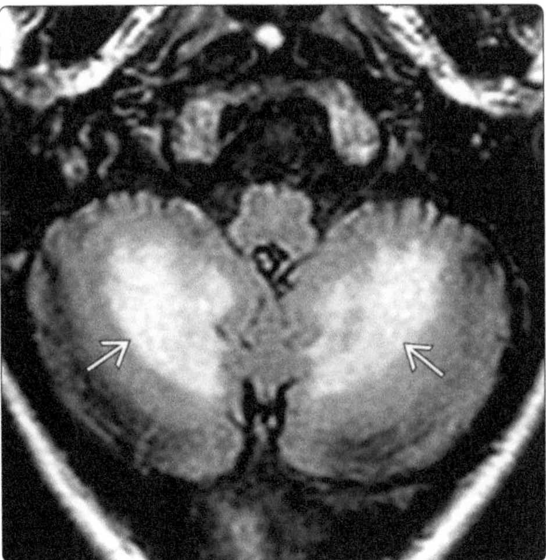

(Left) *Axial FLAIR MR through the midpons shows striking demyelination in the lateral pons/root entry zones and both CNVs* ➡ *in an adult with Loes pattern 4.* **(Right)** *Axial FLAIR MR at the level of the medulla and lower cerebellum in the same adult with trigeminal nerve involvement shows symmetric hyperintensity in the cerebellar WM* ➡ *(Loes pattern 4 of ALD).*

Maple Syrup Urine Disease

KEY FACTS

TERMINOLOGY

- Maple syrup urine disease (MSUD)
- Inherited disorder of branched-chain amino acid (BCAA) metabolism

IMAGING

- MR with DWI best, but CT can make diagnosis in critically ill infant
  - NECT (early): Diffuse edema **not** sparing brainstem and cerebellum
  - NECT (subacute): Rapid formation of typical (classic) MSUD edema pattern
- Classic MSUD edema/restriction pattern
  - Cerebellar white matter, dorsal brainstem, cerebral peduncles, thalami, globi pallidi
  - Pyramidal and tegmental tracts
  - Infratentorial > > > supratentorial edema
- MRS: Broad peak at chemical shift of 0.9 ppm

PATHOLOGY

- MSUD: ↓ activity branched-chain α-keto acid dehydrogenase complex (BCKD) → accumulation of branched-chain L-amino (BCAA) and metabolites (neuro- and leukotoxic)

CLINICAL ISSUES

- 1:850,000 in general population but as frequent as 1:170 in population isolates
- Initial symptoms of classic MSUD: Poor feeding, vomiting, poor weight gain, increasing lethargy, encephalopathy, seizures
- Patients in crisis often (but not always) smell like maple syrup (or burnt sugar)

DIAGNOSTIC CHECKLIST

- Typically presents at 4-10 days of age with neurologic deterioration, ketoacidosis, hyperammonemia

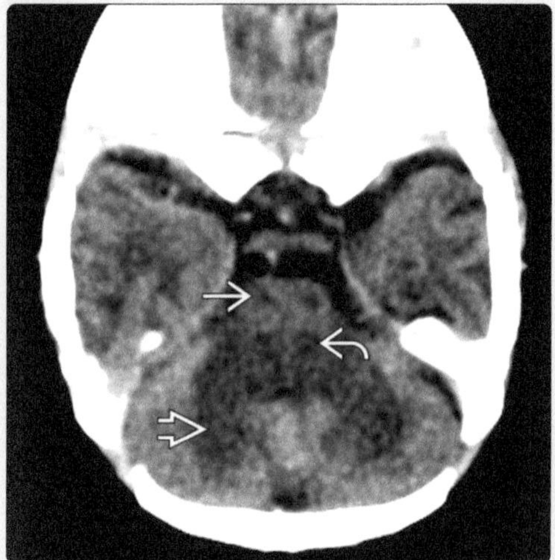

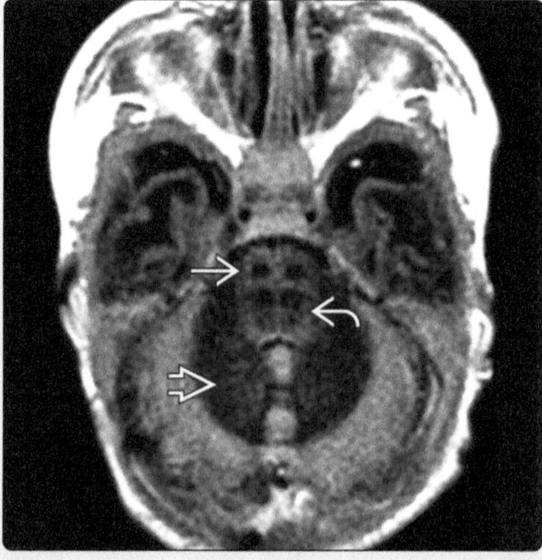

(Left) *Axial NECT in a seizing newborn who returned to the hospital at 10 days of age demonstrates the classic maple syrup urine disease (MSUD) edema pattern. Note hypodensity in cerebellar white matter ➡, dorsal pons, and 4 foci in the anterior and middle pons, which are paired pyramidal ➡ and tegmental ➡ tracts.* **(Right)** *Axial T1WI MR in an infant with lethargy and feeding difficulty shows the same MSUD pattern: Hypointensity in the cerebellar white matter ➡ and paired pyramidal ➡ and tegmental ➡ tracts.*

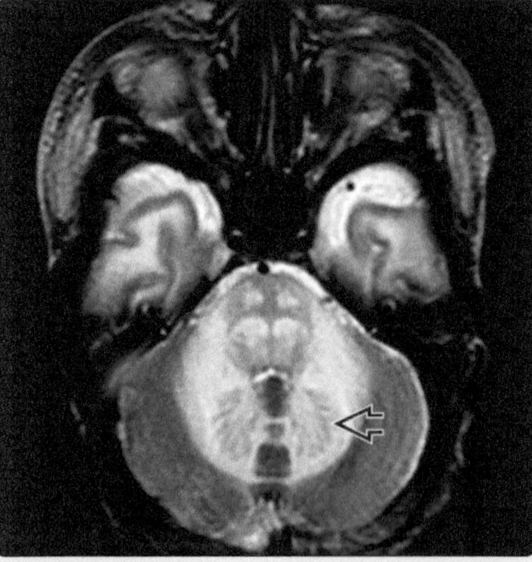

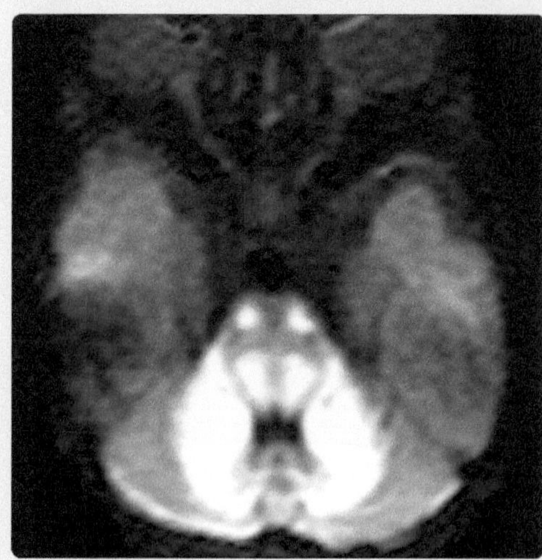

(Left) *Axial T2WI MR demonstrates crisp margins of signal abnormality of the cerebellar white matter. Again seen are the paired tracts (4 bright pontine foci) superimposed on signal abnormality in the pons. The dentate nuclei ➡ stand out against the abnormal MSUD edema.* **(Right)** *Axial DWI MR confirms intramyelinic edema in a MSUD pattern, showing reduced diffusivity (hyperintensity). DWI is extremely useful in the acute and subacute phases of MSUD.*

TERMINOLOGY

Abbreviations

- Maple syrup urine disease (MSUD)

Synonyms

- Leucine encephalopathy

Definitions

- Inherited disorder of branched-chain amino acid (BCAA) metabolism presenting in newborns with neurologic deterioration, ketoacidosis, and hyperammonemia
- Intermediate form presents later with developmental delay and failure to thrive
- Intermittent form presents in late infancy (or later) with episodic decompensation
  - Ataxia, disorientation, altered behavior

IMAGING

General Features

- Best diagnostic clue
  - Radiologist may be 1st to suggest diagnosis based on classic-appearing MSUD edema
    - Cerebellar white matter, brainstem, thalamus, globus pallidus
    - Pyramidal and tegmental tracts
- Location
  - Cerebellar and brainstem edema > > > supratentorial hemispheres
    - Most prominent in dorsal brainstem, cerebellar white matter
    - Edema of corticospinal tracts
    - These areas show reduced diffusivity on ADC maps

CT Findings

- NECT
  - Early: Diffuse edema **not** sparing brainstem and cerebellum
    - Recognize here for best neurocognitive outcome
  - Subacute: Rapid formation of typical (classic) MSUD edema pattern
    - Cerebellar white matter, dorsal brainstem, cerebral peduncles, thalami, pyramidal, and tegmental tracts > supratentorial hemispheres
    - Margins become sharp during subacute phase

MR Findings

- T1WI
  - ↓ signal intensity; margins may be sharp
- T2WI
  - Late: Generalized and MSUD edema disappear
    - Resolve to "pallor" and volume loss
- FLAIR
  - Insensitive to fluid shifts in newborns
- DWI
  - Marked restriction (↑ intensity) and ↓ ADC (MSUD edema = cytotoxic/intramyelinic)
  - DTI: ↓ anisotropy
- MRS
  - Broad peak at chemical shift of 0.9 ppm; this is present with both short-echo and long-echo spectra

Ultrasonographic Findings

- Grayscale ultrasound
  - ↑ echogenicity of globi pallidi, periventricular white matter, brainstem, cerebellar white matter

Imaging Recommendations

- Best imaging tool
  - DWI during hyperacute and acute phases
- Protocol advice
  - DWI MR best, but CT can make diagnosis in critically ill infant

DIFFERENTIAL DIAGNOSIS

Disorders Causing Brainstem and Cerebellar Swelling

- Mitochondrial *SURF1* mutations: Lactate may be seen in this **and** in MSUD during crisis
- Alexander disease: Abnormal signal and enhancement of brainstem and aqueduct
- Vanishing white matter: Findings are persistent

Hypoxic-Ischemic Encephalopathy

- No symptom-free interval, usually positive history
- Cerebellum, brainstem relatively spared (MSUD involves these areas)

Marchiafava-Bignami Disease

- Myelin-splitting disorder of adult red wine drinkers
- Splits corpus callosum

PATHOLOGY

General Features

- Etiology
  - MSUD: ↓ activity branched-chain α-keto acid dehydrogenase complex (BCKD) → accumulation of branched-chain L-amino (BCAA) and metabolites (neuro- and leukotoxic)
  - ↑ brain leucine displaces other essential amino → neurotransmitter depletion, disrupted brain growth and development
  - Branched-chain ketoacid accumulation → thought to disrupt Krebs cycle
- Genetics
  - > 50 different mutations in genes governing enzyme components of BCKD
    - e.g., E1α (33%), E1β (38%), E2 (19%)
  - Autosomal recessive
- Associated abnormalities
  - ↑ plasma isoleucine associated with maple syrup odor
  - Maternal ingestion of fenugreek during labor gives false impression of MSUD
    - Shares component and smell with MSUD urine

Staging, Grading, & Classification

- Classic, intermediate, and intermittent forms of MSUD; thiamine-responsive MSUD

Gross Pathologic & Surgical Features

- Brainstem edema
- Spongy degeneration: White matter, basal ganglia

Microscopic Features

- ↓ oligodendrocytes and astrocytes
- Alterations in neuronal migration, maturation
  - Aberrant orientation of neurons
  - Abnormal dendrites/dendritic spines

CLINICAL ISSUES

Presentation

- Most common signs/symptoms
  - Initial symptoms of classic MSUD: Poor feeding, vomiting, poor weight gain, increasing lethargy
    - In neonates, develops within 4-7 days
  - Patients in crisis often (but not always) smell like maple syrup (or burnt sugar)
    - Resuscitation with non-protein-containing oral or IV-hydrating fluids may "clear" odor
    - Maple syrup odor may be difficult to identify in 1st days of life unless urine-soaked diaper allowed to dry
    - Maple syrup odor of cerumen "more predictable"
  - Neonates in communities with known high MSUD risk diagnosed within hours of blood sampling
    - If tested **and** receive immediate results **and** therapy is instituted, then may have excellent outcome
    - Tandem mass spectrometry of whole blood filter paper shortens diagnosis time
    - Guthrie test insensitive before 24 hours, requires incubation period and has high false-positive rate
  - Classic MSUD, intermediate form, and E3 deficiency can usually be detected by screening in newborn period
    - Intermittent MSUD usually not detected, because patients' concentrations are normal when not in crisis
    - Thiamine-responsive MSUD may not be identified by newborn screening
- Clinical profile
  - Normal at birth
  - Presents after disease-free interval, usually within first 48 hours to 2 weeks of life
  - Mimic of sepsis: Acute encephalopathy, vomiting, seizures, neurologic distress, lethargy, coma, leukopenia/thrombopenia
    - Additionally, free water retention, renal salt wasting and hyponatremia, dehydration
  - Plasma detection of alloisoleucine diagnostic
    - May not appear until 6th day of life
  - Ketosis or ketoacidosis and hyperammonemia
  - Typical EEG: Comb-like rhythms
  - Prenatal diagnosis can be performed on cultured amniocytes or chorion villus cells

Demographics

- Age
  - May be diagnosed on day 1 of life if MSUD suspected
- Ethnicity
  - 1/170 live births in certain population isolates (founder effect in Old Order Mennonites)
  - High carrier rate in Middle East and Ashkenazi Jewish descendants
- Epidemiology
  - 1:850,000 in general population but as frequent as 1:170 in population isolates

Natural History & Prognosis

- Breastfeeding may delay onset of symptoms to 2nd week of life
- MSUD has potentially favorable outcome with strict dietary control and aggressive treatment of metabolic crises
  - Response to therapy, however, can be variable
  - Exposure to high levels, BCAAs and their metabolites neurotoxic
  - Uncontrolled BCAA levels → profound cognitive impairment/death
  - Pretreatment plasma leucine > 40 mg/100 mL **or** encephalopathy prolonged with poor cognitive outcome
- May survive to adulthood if well controlled
  - Metabolic "intoxication" **at any age** may be provoked by infection, injury, stress, fasting, or even pregnancy
- Reports of late (adulthood) development of peripheral neuropathy
- Exfoliative skin and corneal lesions from inadequate amino acid intake

Treatment

- Acute "metabolic rescue" to reverse cerebral edema
- May require hemodialysis during acute crisis to limit neurotoxicity/damage
- Metabolically appropriate diet (protein modified) minimizes severity
  - Inhibit endogenous protein catabolism while sustaining protein synthesis
  - Prevent deficiencies of essential amino acids
  - Maintain normal serum osmolarity
  - Commercially available formulas, foods are available without BCAAs or with reduced levels of BCAAs
  - Dietary therapy must be lifelong
- Neonatal screening (tandem mass spectrometry) can diagnose
- Orthotopic liver transplantation increases availability of BCKD (rarely used)
- Gene therapy experimental

DIAGNOSTIC CHECKLIST

Consider

- Neonatal testing for MSUD is **not** universal but part of US newborn screening
- Not all MSUD occurs in population isolates
- Even if testing performed, results may be available only after 1-2 weeks in nonendemic areas

Image Interpretation Pearls

- Neonatal brain edema that includes posterior fossa and brainstem is highly suggestive of MSUD

SELECTED REFERENCES

1. Kilgore MB et al: Development of a universal second-tier newborn screening LC-MS/MS method for amino acids, lysophosphatidylcholines, and organic acids. Anal Chem. 95(6):3187-94, 2023
2. Liu Q et al: Neonatal maple syrup urine disease case report and literature review. Medicine (Baltimore). 101(50):e32174, 2022
3. Sen K et al: In-hospital mortality from cerebral edema in MSUD during newborn screening era: what are we missing and what more can we do? Pediatr Neurol. 135:61-2, 2022
4. Unsal Y et al: Organic acidemias in the neonatal period: 30 years of experience in a referral center for inborn errors of metabolism. J Pediatr Endocrinol Metab. 35(11):1345-56, 2022

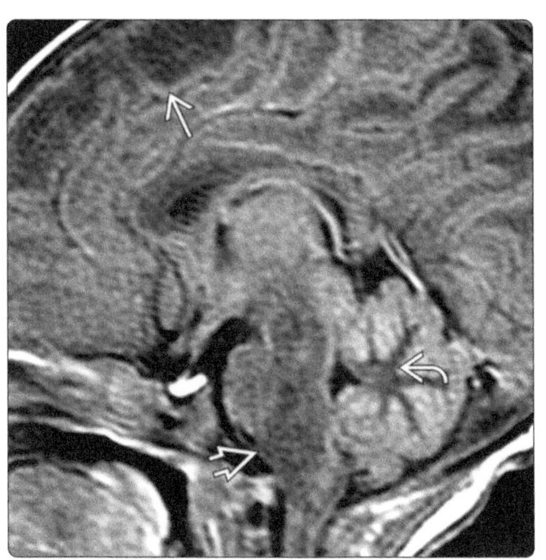

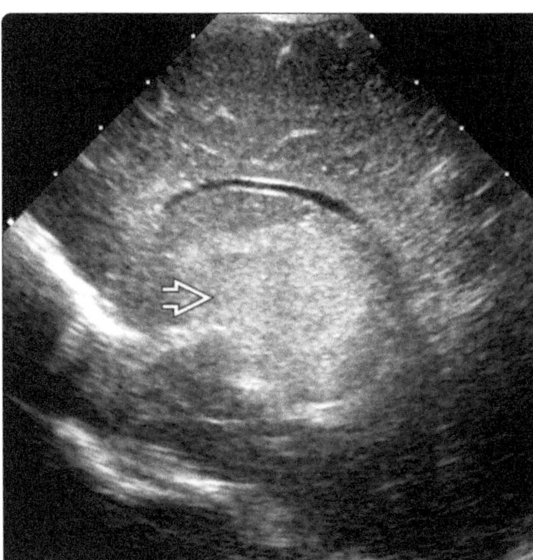

(Left) *Sagittal T1WI MR in an encephalopathic newborn reveals marked swelling of the entire brainstem. Low signal of the involved brainstem ➔, cerebellar white matter ➔, and subcortical cerebral white matter ➔ is also present.* **(Right)** *Parasagittal US in a symptomatic newborn with MSUD demonstrates markedly increased echogenicity ➔ of the thalami due to the severe edema.*

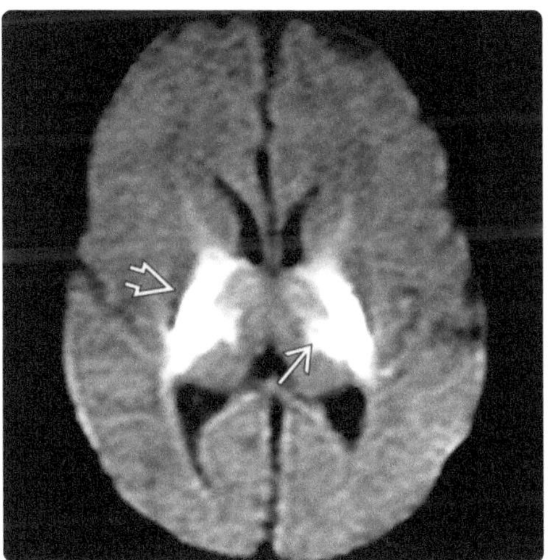

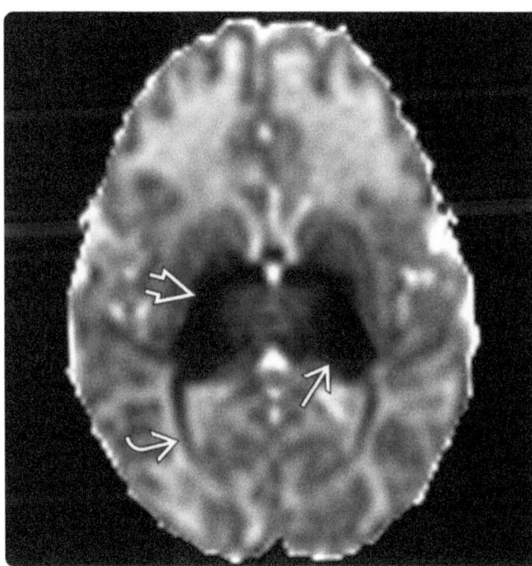

(Left) *Axial DWI MR shows markedly reduced diffusivity (hyperintensity) of the posterior limbs of the internal capsules ➔ and of the internal medullary lamina ➔ of the thalami during the acute phase of MSUD.* **(Right)** *Axial diffusivity (ADC) map in the same infant confirms reduced diffusivity of the posterior limbs of the internal capsules ➔ and of the internal medullary lamina ➔ of the thalami as well as the optic tracts ➔.*

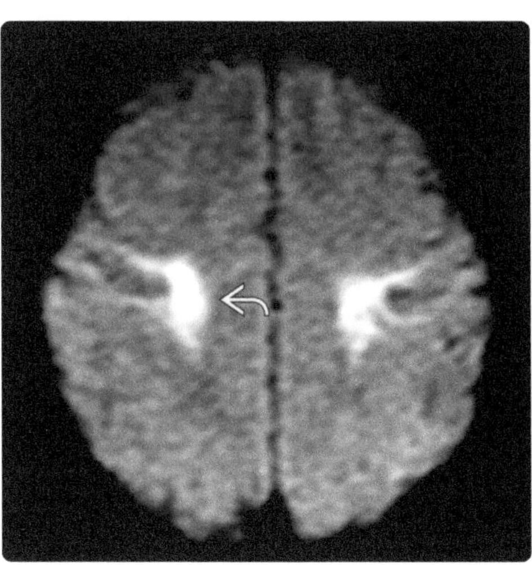

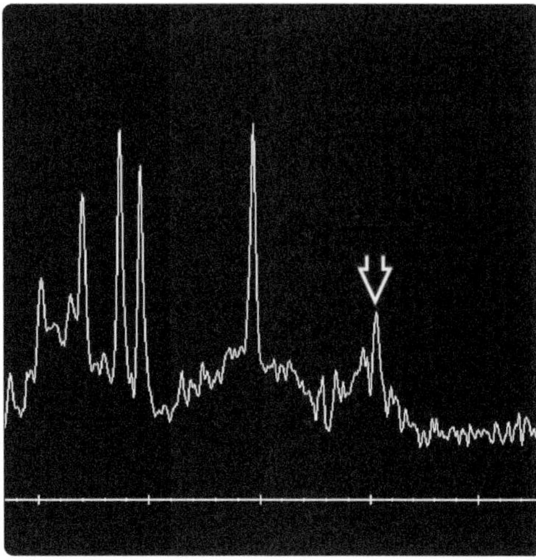

(Left) *Axial DWI MR demonstrates extension of intramyelinic edema (manifest as reduced diffusivity) in the corticospinal tracts as they extend upward to the perirolandic cortex ➔.* **(Right)** *Peaks at 0.9-1.0 ppm ➔ on MRS with an echo time of 30 ms represent branched-chain a-keto acid peaks, which can be seen during acute metabolic decompensation in MSUD. They are also seen at longer echo times, a finding that helps to confirm the diagnosis.*

Urea Cycle Disorders

KEY FACTS

TERMINOLOGY

- 6 disorders of urea cycle
  - Ornithine transcarbamylase deficiency (OTCD)
  - Carbamoyl phosphate synthetase 1 deficiency
  - Citrullinemia or argininosuccinate synthetase deficiency
  - Argininosuccinate aciduria or argininosuccinate lyase deficiency
  - Argininemia or arginase deficiency (AD)
  - N-acetylglutamate synthase deficiency

IMAGING

- Neonates: Deep gray nuclei, depths of sulci in frontal, parietal, and insular > temporal cortex
- Older: As above or asymmetric cortical/subcortical white matter mimicking stroke
- Posterior fossa spared
- T2WI: Acute/subacute: ↑ T2 signal, swelling areas involved
- DWI: Acute/subacute: Iso-/↑ DWI signal, iso-/↓ ADC
- MRS: Acute/subacute: ↓ myoinositol, ↑ glutamine-glutamate, ↑ lipids/lactate

TOP DIFFERENTIAL DIAGNOSES

- Hypoxic ischemic encephalopathy
- Arterial ischemic stroke
- Mitochondrial disorders
- Organic acidemias
- Nonketotic hyperglycinemia

PATHOLOGY

- Urea cycle incorporates nitrogen → urea → urine, prevents accumulation of toxic nitrogen products
- ↑ ammonia → ↑ glutamate → ↑ glutamine in astrocytes → swelling + dysfunction

CLINICAL ISSUES

- Triad of hyperammonemia, encephalopathy, respiratory alkalosis

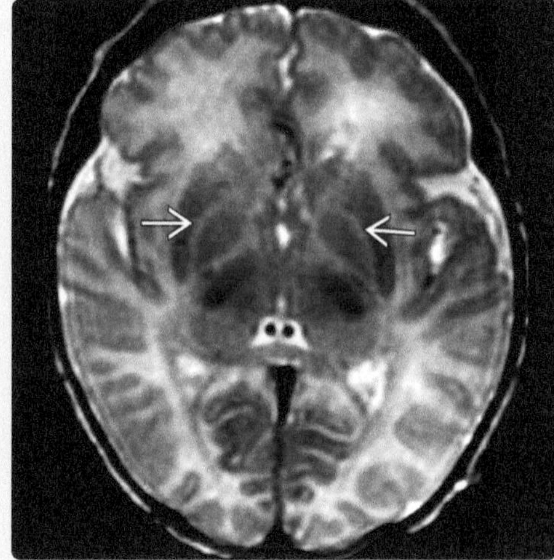

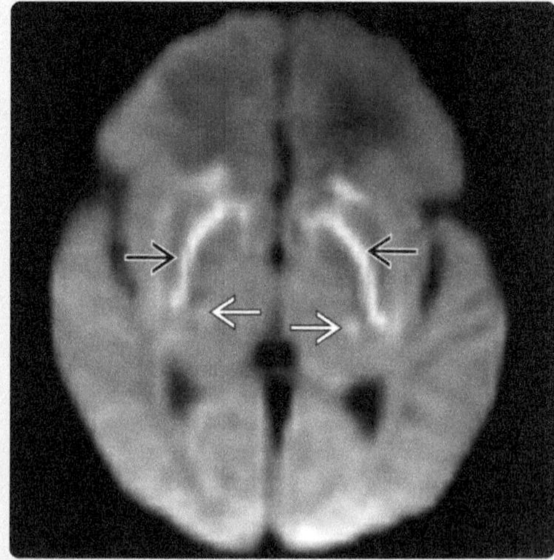

(Left) *Axial T2 MR shows abnormally increased signal ➡ between lateral nuclei of the globi pallidi and the putamina in a 2-day-old boy neonate presenting acutely with ornithine transcarbamylase deficiency (OTCD).* **(Right)** *Axial DWI MR in the same patient shows reduced diffusivity (abnormally increased signal ➡) in the same location between the globi pallidi and putamina, extending into the caudates; this corresponded to decreased ADC. More subtle thalamic hyperintensity ➡ (and low ADC) is also seen.*

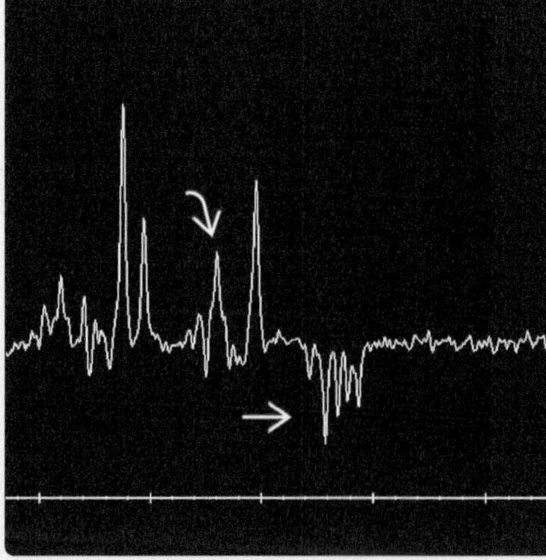

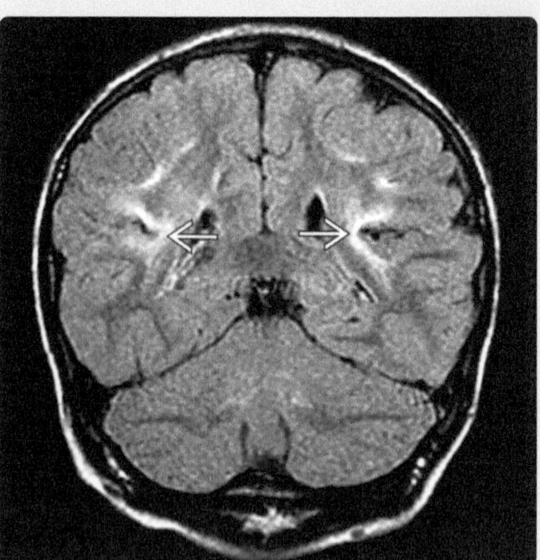

(Left) *Axial proton MRS (echo time = 144 ms) in a neonate presenting acutely demonstrates 2 inverted doublets ➡ of lactate (at 1.33 ppm) and 1,2-propene-diol (found in anticonvulsants, at 1.1 ppm). Also noted is a large glutamine-glutamate (glx) peak ➡ at 2.1-1.4 ppm.* **(Right)** *Coronal FLAIR MR in the chronic stage of a child with OTCD shows cortical and subcortical posterior insular and temporoparietal increased signal ➡ that is most marked at the depths of the sulci.*

TERMINOLOGY

Definitions

- 6 disorders of urea cycle
  - Ornithine transcarbamylase deficiency (OTCD)
  - Citrullinemia or argininosuccinate synthetase deficiency
  - Carbamoyl phosphate synthetase 1 deficiency
  - Argininosuccinate aciduria or argininosuccinate lyase deficiency
  - Argininemia or arginase deficiency (AD)
  - N-acetylglutamate synthase deficiency

IMAGING

General Features

- Best diagnostic clue
  - Neonate presenting 24-48 hours with basal ganglia (BG) and cortical ↑ DWI signal
- Location
  - Neonates: Deep gray nuclei, depths of sulci in frontal, parietal, and insular > temporal cortex
  - Older: As above or asymmetric cortical/subcortical white matter (WM) mimicking stroke
  - Posterior fossa spared

CT Findings

- NECT
  - ↓ attenuation deep gray nuclei, WM + cortex with swelling → atrophy when chronic

MR Findings

- T1WI
  - Subacute/chronic: ↑ signal in cortical, deep gray nuclei areas involved
- T2WI
  - Acute/subacute: ↑ signal, swelling areas involved
  - Chronic: Volume loss, gliosis ± cystic change
- DWI
  - Acute/subacute: Iso-/↑ DWI signal, iso-/↓ ADC
- MRS
  - Acute/subacute: ↓ myoinositol, ↑ glutamine-glutamate, ↑ lipids/lactate

Imaging Recommendations

- Best imaging tool: MR
- Protocol advice: T1WI, T2WI, DWI, MRS

DIFFERENTIAL DIAGNOSIS

Hypoxic Ischemic Encephalopathy

- Lateral putamen and ventrolateral thalamus involved; difficult to differentiate in chronic state

Arterial Ischemic Stroke

- Vascular distribution

Metabolic Disorders

- Mitochondrial disorders
- Organic acidemias: Globi pallidi but not cortex; metabolic acidosis/ketosis
- Nonketotic hyperglycinemia: No BG involvement

PATHOLOGY

General Features

- Etiology
  - Urea cycle incorporates nitrogen → urea → urine; prevents accumulation of toxic nitrogen products
  - ↑ ammonia → ↑ glutamate → ↑ glutamine in astrocytes → swelling + dysfunction
- Genetics
  - All autosomal recessive except OTCD (X-linked)

Gross Pathologic & Surgical Features

- Brain swelling in acute; atrophy + ulegyria in chronic

Microscopic Features

- Gray matter (GM) Alzheimer type 2 astrocytes; GM, WM spongiosis

CLINICAL ISSUES

Presentation

- Most common signs/symptoms
  - Triad of hyperammonemia, encephalopathy, respiratory alkalosis
  - Progressive lethargy, hypothermia, vomiting, apnea
  - Neonates develop encephalopathy > 24-48 hours
  - Episodic in older patients (often when ↑ protein intake or ↑ catabolism)
- Clinical profile
  - ↑ ammonium blood levels (except AD)
  - Diagnosis: Liver cell enzyme assessment/DNA

Demographics

- Age
  - Neonate if severe, older if less severe
- Epidemiology
  - Whites > Blacks; OTCD most common

Natural History & Prognosis

- Improved with treatment but most intellectually disabled
- Neonates: Worst prognosis with high mortality

Treatment

- Hemodialysis in acute crisis
- Liver transplant in severe cases
- ↓ protein intake, adequate caloric intake, supplements
- Sodium benzoate/phenylbutyrate/phenylacetate
- Valproate contraindicated; can cause death

SELECTED REFERENCES

1. Koç Yekedüz M et al: Early neuroimaging findings of infants diagnosed with inherited metabolic disorders in neonatal period: a case-control study. Clin Neurol Neurosurg. 222:107474, 2022
2. Ozturk K et al: Urea cycle disorders: a neuroimaging pattern approach using diffusion and flair MRI. J Neuroimaging. 31(1):144-50, 2021
3. Sen K et al: Review of multi-modal imaging in urea cycle disorders: the old, the new, the borrowed, and the blue. Front Neurol. 12:632307, 2021
4. Ninković D et al: The therapeutic hypothermia in treatment of hyperammonemic encephalopathy due to urea cycle disorders and organic acidemias. Klin Padiatr. 231(2):74-9, 2019
5. Jichlinski A et al: "Cerebral palsy" in a patient with arginase deficiency. Semin Pediatr Neurol. 26:110-4, 2018
6. Gropman AL: Patterns of brain injury in inborn errors of metabolism. Semin Pediatr Neurol. 19(4):203-10, 2012

KEY FACTS

TERMINOLOGY

- Glutaric acidemia type 1 (GA1), mitochondrial glutaryl-coenzyme A dehydrogenase (GCDH) deficiency
- Inborn error of metabolism characterized by encephalopathic crises and resultant severe dystonic-dyskinetic movement disorder

IMAGING

- Large sylvian fissures (from hypoplastic frontal/temporal opercula) and bright T2/FLAIR basal ganglia (BG)
  - Common: ↑ signal caudate/putamina > globus pallidus
  - Occasional: Pallidal and dentate signal change may occur, even in absence of crisis
  - Severe: White matter, thalami, dentate nuclei may be involved
  - Significant BG atrophy in late phases of disease
- Child abuse mimic: Easily torn bridging veins within enlarged CSF spaces → subdural hematomas

TOP DIFFERENTIAL DIAGNOSES

- Nonaccidental injury
- Disorders with bilateral middle fossa cyst-like spaces
  - Mucopolysaccharidoses
  - "Idiopathic" middle cranial fossae arachnoid cysts
- Other causes of macrocephaly
  - Hydrocephalus
  - Idiopathic enlargement of subarachnoid spaces (SASs) during 1st year of life
  - Benign familial macrocephaly

CLINICAL ISSUES

- Episodic crises follow trigger (infection, immunization, surgery)

DIAGNOSTIC CHECKLIST

- Consider GA1 in young children with bilateral enlargement of sylvian fissures and abnormal BG

(Left) *Axial graphic demonstrates the pattern of involvement in glutaric acidemia type 1 (GA1). The sylvian fissures are enlarged, and the basal ganglia are diffusely and symmetrically abnormal in signal.* **(Right)** *Axial T2WI MR in a 7-month-old reveals enlarged sylvian fissures ⇨. Note the swelling and abnormally increased signal intensity of the basal ganglia ➩, including the heads of caudate nuclei, the putamina, and the globi pallidi bilaterally. Myelination is delayed.*

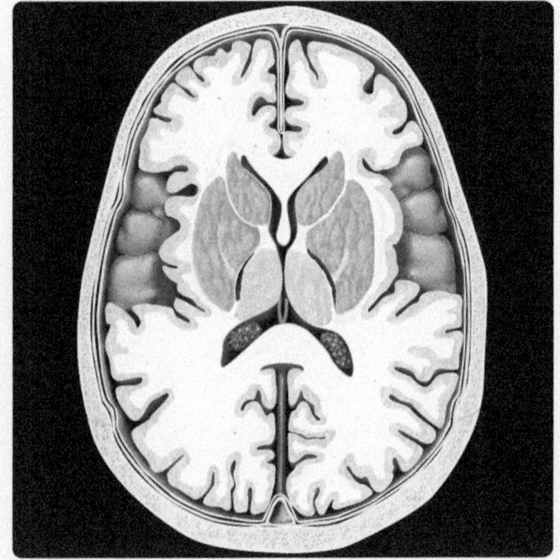

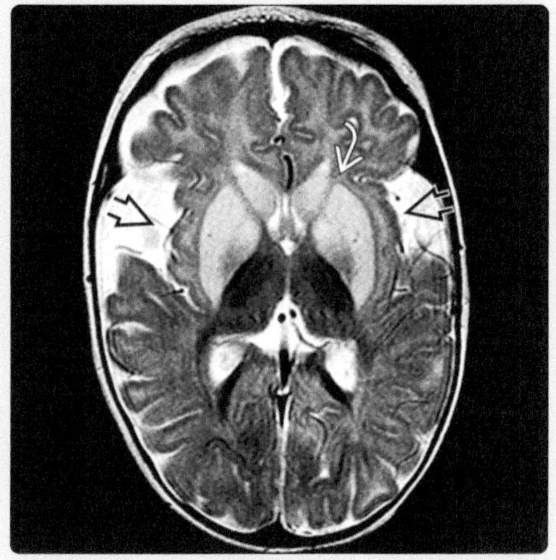

(Left) *Axial DWI MR in an infant in the midst of a severe metabolic crisis shows hyperintense signal resulting from reduced diffusion within the heads of the caudate nuclei ➩ and putamina ➡ bilaterally.* **(Right)** *ADC map shows hypointensity ➩ in the same areas, the caudates and putamina, confirming the presence of acute brain injury with resultant reduced diffusivity, rather than T2 shine-through.*

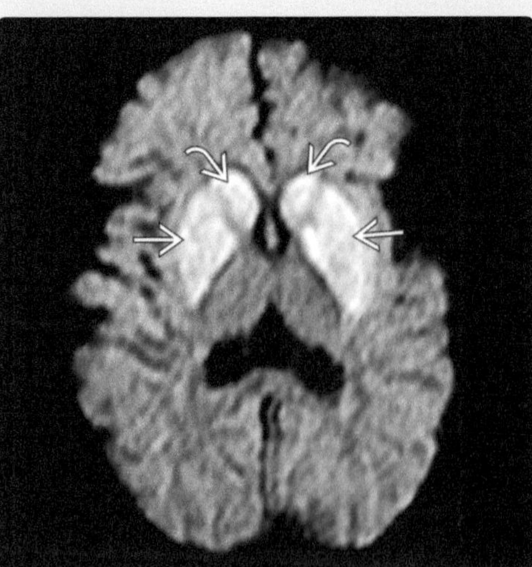

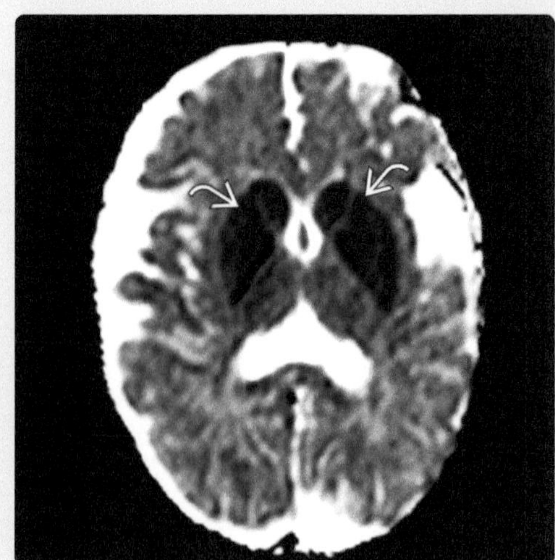

TERMINOLOGY

Abbreviations

- Glutaric acidemia type 1 (GA1)

Definitions

- Organic aciduria disorder
- Inborn error of metabolism characterized by encephalopathic crises and resultant severe dystonic-dyskinetic movement disorder

IMAGING

General Features

- Best diagnostic clue
  - Wide sylvian fissures and bright basal ganglia (BG)
- Location
  - Sylvian fissures, BG
- Size
  - Enlarged sylvian fissures
- Morphology
  - Small frontal and temporal opercula → bat wing dilatation of sylvian fissures

CT Findings

- NECT
  - > 95% have wide, cyst-like CSF spaces in middle cranial fossae
    - Sylvian fissure widening (93%), mesencephalic cistern widening (86%)
    - Frontal, temporal opercula, which normally cover insula, are hypoplastic
  - Striatal hypodensity
  - Early macrocephaly, late atrophy (mostly ventricular enlargement)
  - Subdural hematoma (SDH) with minimal trauma
- CECT
  - No enhancement

MR Findings

- T1WI
  - Sylvian fissure cyst-like spaces isointense to CSF
    - May ↓ in size over time
  - Subependymal pseudocysts (disappear by 6 months)
  - Frontotemporal hypoplasia
  - Delayed myelination
  - Occasional mild, immature-appearing gyral pattern
- T2WI
  - Common: ↑ signal caudate/putamina > globus pallidus
    - Frequently presents before 3 years of age
  - Occasional: Pallidal and dentate signal change may occur, even in absence of crisis
    - May predate involvement of caudate and putamina
  - Striatal atrophy over time
  - If severe: White matter (WM), thalami, dentate nuclei may be involved
- FLAIR
  - Same as T2WI
  - May show associated SDH better than T2WI
- DWI
  - Acute phase: Reduced diffusion in BG and selected WM tracts; may show more extensive disease than apparent on either CT or MR
- T1WI C+
  - No enhancement
- MRS
  - ↑ Cho:Cr ratio, ↓ NAA
  - During crisis: ± ↑ lactate

Imaging Recommendations

- Best imaging tool
  - Brain MR
- Protocol advice
  - Multiplanar brain MR ± MRS, DWI

DIFFERENTIAL DIAGNOSIS

Nonaccidental Injury

- Opercular hypoplasia may mimic atrophy
- GA1 does not cause fractures
- SDH in GA1 from torn bridging veins in presence of large CSF, atrophy
- SDH in GA1 does not occur without enlarged CSF spaces
- Head trauma = most common cause of death
  - SDH most common finding, often interhemispheric
  - Skull fracture subarachnoid, epidural hemorrhage
  - Cerebral edema, contusion(s), shear injuries

Other Disorders With Bilateral Middle Cranial Fossa Cyst-Like Spaces

- Mucopolysaccharidoses
  - Types 1-4: Hurler, Hunter, Sanfilippo, Scheie, Maroteaux-Lamy, Sly
  - CSF-like mucopolysaccharide pachymeningeal deposition in all but Morquio type 4
- "Idiopathic" middle cranial fossae arachnoid cysts
  - 5% may be bilateral, usually asymptomatic
  - CSF intensity; may be slightly different on FLAIR
  - No DWI restriction

Causes of Macrocephaly

- Hydrocephalus
  - Congenital, posttraumatic, or obstructive
  - Ventricular prominence out of proportion to sulci
  - Enlarged temporal horns, rounded frontal horns, transependymal CSF flow
- Idiopathic enlargement of subarachnoid spaces (SASs) during 1st year of life
- Benign familial macrocephaly
  - Family tendency toward large head size

PATHOLOGY

General Features

- Etiology
  - Mitochondrial glutaryl-coenzyme A dehydrogenase (GCDH) deficiency required for metabolism of lysine, hydroxylysine, and tryptophan
  - ↓ GCDH → accumulation glutaric, glutaconic, and 3-OH-glutaric acid
  - Accumulated substances toxic to striate cells and WM
- Genetics

- Autosomal recessive
- *GCDH* gene mutations (Chr 19p13.2) result in amino acid substitutions
- Multiple mutations govern varied clinical presentation
  - European variant (most common): Arg402-to-trp
  - Amish variant, riboflavin sensitive: Ala421-to-val
  - Severe, 1% residual enzyme, symptoms despite treatment: Glu365-to-lys
- Rare adult onset: Compound heterozygosity with deletion and novel missense mutation

- Associated abnormalities
  - Embryology: Toxic effects in utero impede operculization during 3rd trimester
  - Mild hepatocellular dysfunction during crisis

Staging, Grading, & Classification

- Symptomatic: Frontotemporal atrophy, BG signal changes
- Presymptomatic: Symptom free, lacks BG changes, but CSF spaces still enlarged

Gross Pathologic & Surgical Features

- Macrocrania, frontotemporal atrophy/hypoplasia; ↑ CSF spaces ± SDH
- Hypo- and demyelination

Microscopic Features

- Myelin vacuolation and splitting, excess intramyelinic fluid
- Spongiform changes, neuronal loss in BG

CLINICAL ISSUES

Presentation

- Most common signs/symptoms
  - Initially normal development
  - Acute encephalopathy, seizures, dystonia, choreoathetosis, intellectual disability
- Acute-onset group: Majority
  - Episodic crises follow trigger (infection, immunization, surgery)
    - Acute Reye-like encephalopathy, ketoacidosis, ↑ NH4, vomiting
    - Dystonia, opisthotonus, seizures, excessive sweating
    - Follow-up: Alert child (intellect preserved > > motor); rapid infantile head growth → frontal bossing; severe dystonia
- Insidious onset (25%): Dystonia without crisis
- Presymptomatic may remain asymptomatic: Diagnose, treat, avoid catabolic stress
- Rare asymptomatic without treatment: Still frontotemporal atrophy but normal BG
- Diagnosis: Frequent long interval between presentation and diagnosis
  - Tandem mass spectrometry of newborn filter paper blood specimens
    - Chromatography of mass; spectroscopy of urine
  - Deficient or absent GCDH activity in fibroblasts
  - Laboratory (may be relatively normal between crises)
    - Metabolic acidosis/ketosis, hypoglycemia, ↓ carnitine
    - Urinary organic acids: ↑ glutaric, glutaconic, and 3-OH-glutaric acid

Demographics

- Age
  - Generally manifests during 1st year of life
- Sex
  - No predilection
- Ethnicity
  - 10% carrier rate in Old Order Amish
- Epidemiology
  - 1:30,000 newborns

Natural History & Prognosis

- Symptomatic: Most severely handicapped; 20% die before 5 years of age
- Presymptomatic: Many (not all) remain asymptomatic with diagnosis and therapy
- Treat before 1st encephalopathic crisis; avoiding catabolic crises may improve outcome
- Prognosis poor if patient has already presented with encephalopathic crisis

Treatment

- Intrauterine diagnosis available
  - DNA analysis: Cultured amniotic fluid cells and chorionic villi biopsy
  - Fetal sonography and MR: Dilated perisylvian CSF in 3rd trimester
- Early treatment may prevent or ameliorate symptoms and imaging
  - Low-protein diet (reduced tryptophan and lysine), synthetic protein drink
  - Riboflavin (vitamin B2) to ensure cofactor supply for GCDH
  - Oral carnitine replacement; gamma aminobutyric acid (GABA), analog (baclofen)

DIAGNOSTIC CHECKLIST

Image Interpretation Pearls

- Consider GA1 in young children with bilateral enlargement of sylvian fissures and abnormal BG
- Pallidal and dentate signal change may occur, even in absence of crisis; may predate involvement of caudate and putamina

SELECTED REFERENCES

1. Boy N et al: Recommendations for diagnosing and managing individuals with glutaric aciduria type 1: third revision. J Inherit Metab Dis. 46(3):482-519, 2023
2. Forny P et al: How guideline development has informed clinical research for organic acidurias (et vice versa). J Inherit Metab Dis. 46(3):520-35, 2023
3. Healy L et al: Glutaric aciduria type 1: diagnosis, clinical features and long-term outcome in a large cohort of 34 Irish patients. JIMD Rep. 63(4):379-87, 2022
4. Biasucci G et al: Early neonatal glutaric aciduria type I hidden by perinatal asphyxia: a case report. Ital J Pediatr. 44(1):8, 2018
5. Thomas A et al: Favourable outcome in a child with symptomatic diagnosis of glutaric aciduria type 1 despite vertical HIV infection and minor head trauma. Metab Brain Dis. 33(2):537-44, 2018
6. Boy N et al: Extrastriatal changes in patients with late-onset glutaric aciduria type I highlight the risk of long-term neurotoxicity. Orphanet J Rare Dis. 12(1):77, 2017
7. Boy N et al: Proposed recommendations for diagnosing and managing individuals with glutaric aciduria type I: second revision. J Inherit Metab Dis. 40(1):75-101, 2017

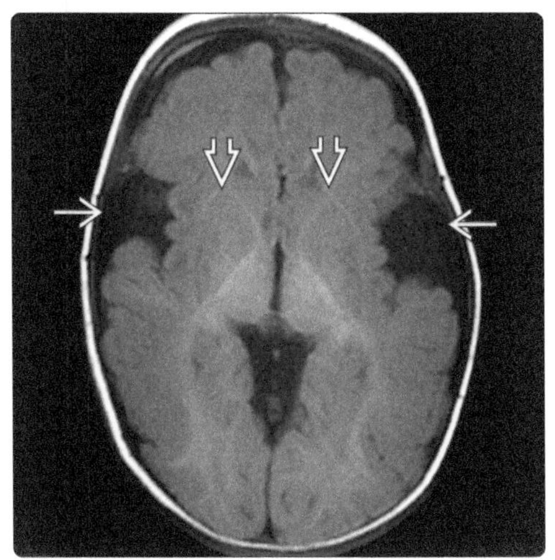

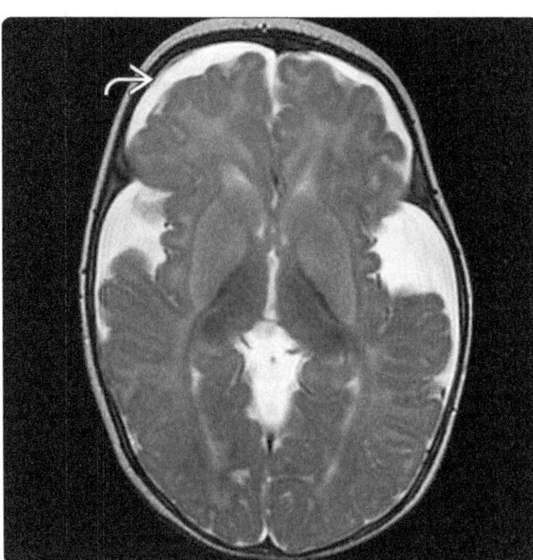

(Left) *Axial T1WI MR in a 12-month-old patient with GA1 presenting in metabolic crisis shows typical prominent sylvian fissures* ➡ *and hypointensity within the basal ganglia* ➡*. White matter is also undermyelinated for age, particularly in the frontal lobes.* **(Right)** *Axial T2WI MR in the same patient confirms abnormal T2 hyperintensity in both the putamina and globi pallidi. There is also a small right frontal subdural fluid collection* ➡*.*

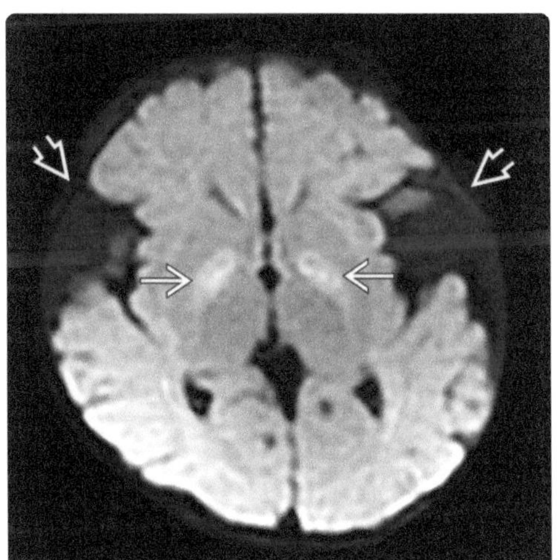

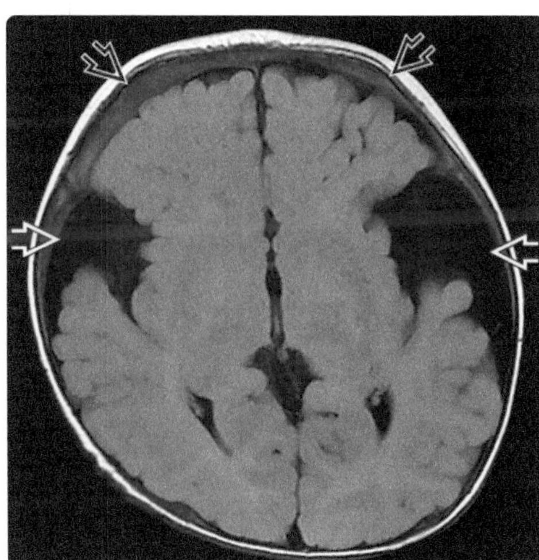

(Left) *Axial DWI MR in a 3-month-old reveals acute diffusion restriction within the bilateral globi pallidi* ➡*. Note also the wide sylvian fissures* ➡ *and small frontal and temporal opercula, compatible with GA1.* **(Right)** *Axial FLAIR MR in the same patient confirms typical classic widened sylvian fissures* ➡*. Note also bilateral chronic subdural hematoma* ➡*, an appearance that can mimic abusive head trauma.*

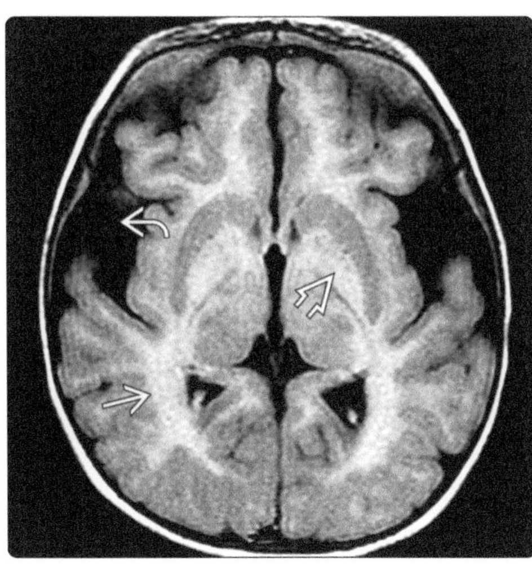

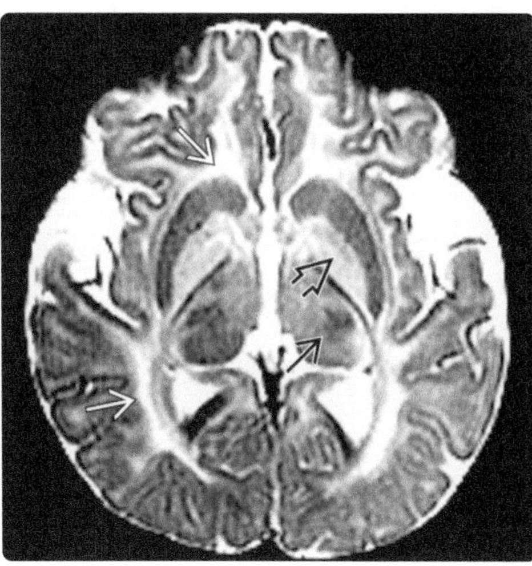

(Left) *Axial FLAIR MR demonstrates typical enlargement of the sylvian fissures* ➡ *in a 7-month-old child. Abnormal signal is identified within the globi pallidi* ➡*, as expected, and in cerebral white matter* ➡*. The latter finding is unusual and is thought to reflect the combination of GA1 and dihydropteridine reductase (DHPR) deficiency in this child.* **(Right)** *Axial T2WI MR in the same patient shows diffusely abnormal white matter* ➡ *and abnormal signal within the globi pallidi* ➡ *and thalami* ➡*.*

Canavan Disease

KEY FACTS

TERMINOLOGY

- Progressive autosomal-recessive spongiform leukodystrophy

IMAGING

- White matter (WM): Involves subcortical U fibers (may show small cysts), sparing internal capsule and corpus callosum
- Globi pallidi (GP) almost always involved, sparing putamen and often sparing caudate
- Thalami frequent, mainly in advanced cases, ± dentate nuclei, dorsal pons, midbrain, part of cerebellar peduncles
- ↑ T2 + DWI signal, normal to ↓ ADC in involved areas
- ↑ NAA/Cr, ↓ Ch/Cr
- US: Reversal of normal cortical and WM echogenicity

TOP DIFFERENTIAL DIAGNOSES

- Pelizaeus-Merzbacher disease
- Merosin-deficient congenital muscular dystrophy
- Alexander disease
- Sialuria (Salla disease): ↑ NAA

PATHOLOGY

- Deficiency of aspartoacylase → N-acetyl aspartic acid ↑ in brain and urine
- Spongiform degeneration of WM; GP and thalami with swollen astrocytes

CLINICAL ISSUES

- Early severe hypotonia and macrocephaly
- Evident by 4 months
- ↑ risk for Ashkenazi Jews (1 in 40 carriers)
- Relentless, progressive neurodegenerative disorder
- No proven treatment (gene therapy and acetate supplementation tried)

DIAGNOSTIC CHECKLIST

- **Macrocephaly** with ↑ T2, ↑ DWI signal in WM, involvement of GP and thalami and **↑ NAA** in MRS

(Left) *Axial T2WI MR in a 32-month-old child with Canavan disease shows hyperintense cerebral white matter ➡ and globus pallidus ➡ with relative sparing of T2 dark internal capsule ➡, corpus callosum ➡, caudate, and putamen ➡. Faint thalamic hyperintensity ➡ is also seen.* **(Right)** *Axial T1W MR in the same patient shows cerebellar dentate nucleus involvement with T1 hypointensity ➡. Also note slight T1 hypointensity of dorsal pons ➡ compared with normal bright middle cerebellar peduncles ➡ and ventral pons ➡.*

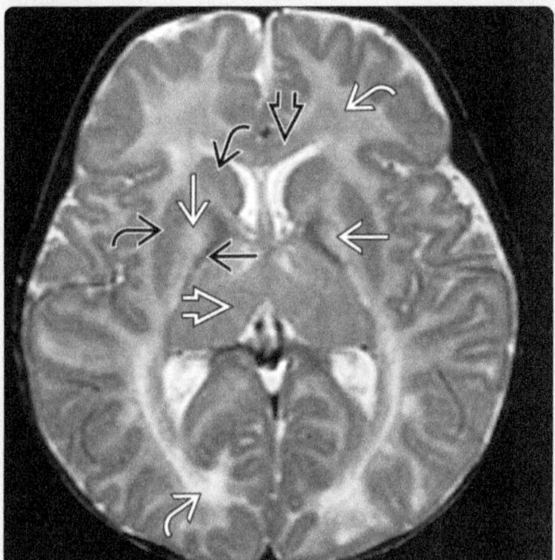

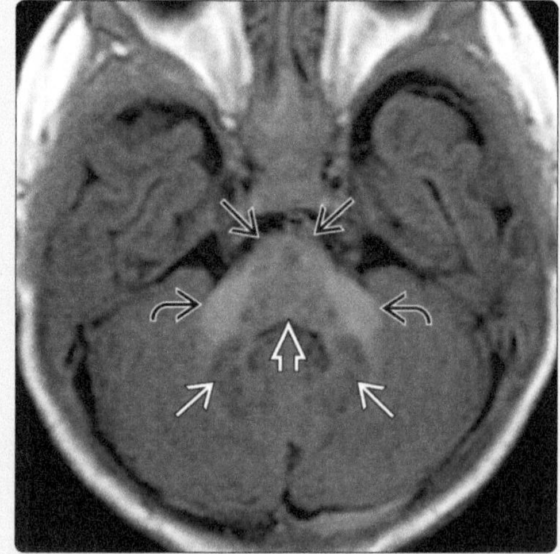

(Left) *Intermediate-echo (TE = 144 msec) proton MR spectroscopy acquired in the centrum semiovale at 1.5T shows a marked relative increase in NAA ➡ in the same patient.* **(Right)** *Axial DWI MR in a 6-month-old infant with Canavan disease shows diffusely ↑ signal (reduced diffusivity/diffusion restriction) in the cerebral white matter ➡, thalami ➡, and globi pallidi ➡. Normal diffusivity is seen in the myelinated internal capsule ➡ and corpus callosum ➡. Caudate nuclei and putamina ➡ also appear unaffected.*

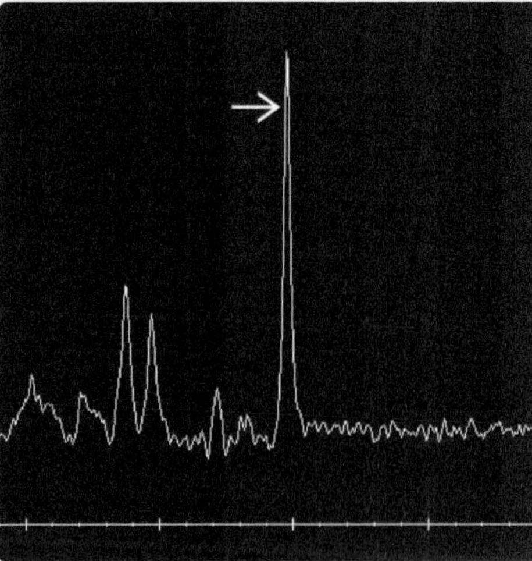

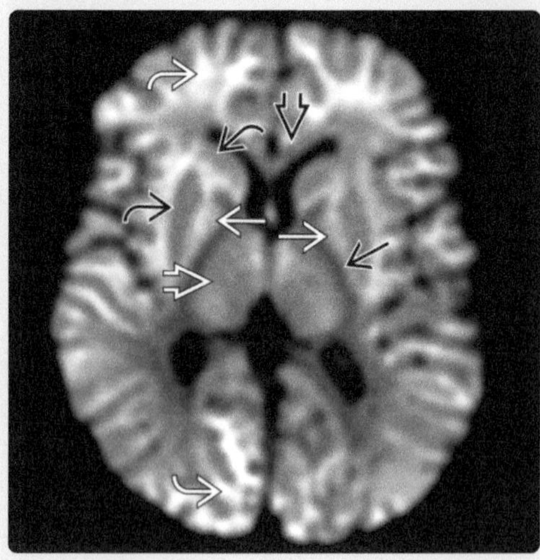

TERMINOLOGY

Abbreviations

- Canavan disease (CD)

Synonyms

- Spongiform leukodystrophy, aspartoacylase deficiency

IMAGING

General Features

- Best diagnostic clue
  - **Macrocephaly** with diffuse ↑ white matter (WM) T2 and DWI signal, and ↑ NAA in MRS
- Location
  - WM: Involves subcortical U fibers, sparing internal capsule, and corpus callosum
  - Globi pallidi (GP) almost always involved, sparing putamen and often sparing caudate
  - Thalami frequent, mainly in advanced cases
  - ± dentate nuclei, dorsal pons, midbrain, and part of cerebellar peduncles
  - Gradually diffuse WM atrophy and then cerebral cortex
  - Rare juvenile cases with absent WM changes but ↑ T2 in bilateral caudate, putamen, and medial thalami

CT Findings

- NECT
  - Diffuse ↓ attenuation in involved areas

MR Findings

- T1WI
  - Hypointense in involved areas
- T2WI
  - Hyperintense in involved areas
  - Multiple subcentimeter bilateral small round cysts may be seen within WM, mainly frontal and parietooccipital
- DWI
  - Bright DWI signal, normal to ↓ ADC in involved areas (due to myelin vacuolization)
  - DTI shows marked reduced fractional anisotropy (FA)
- T1WI C+
  - No enhancement
- MRS
  - ↑ NAA/Cr, ↓ Ch/Cr; **even without**/atypical **T2 findings**

Ultrasonographic Findings

- High-resolution ultrasound shows reversal of normal pattern of cortical and WM echogenicity
- Canavan: Cerebral cortex seen as hypoechoic ribbon covered on outside by thin hyperechoic pia mater and hyperechoic subcortical WM underneath
  - WM: Markedly hyperechoic homogeneous fine texture, may be interrupted by small multicystic changes
- Normal infant: Fine hyperechoic cortical ribbon and hypoechoic WM

DIFFERENTIAL DIAGNOSIS

Pelizaeus-Merzbacher Disease

- ↑ ADC; spares GP and thalami

Merosin-Deficient Congenital Muscular Dystrophy

- ↑ ADC; spares GP and thalami

Alexander Disease

- Predilection for frontal WM, enhances

Sialuria (Salla Disease)

- Unmyelinated subcortical WM; reduced volume of WM and corpus callosum
- Normal basal ganglia, and some myelination in posterior limb of internal capsule and peritrigonal WM
- **↑ NAA** (Acetyl protons of N-acetyl neuraminic [sialic] acid resonate at same frequency of NAA), ↓ Ch, ↑ Cr

PATHOLOGY

General Features

- Etiology
  - Deficiency of aspartoacylase (which metabolizes NAA) → ↑ ↑ NAA in brain and **urine (lab diagnosis)**
- Genetics
  - Autosomal recessive → *ASPA* gene = short arm chromosome 17

Staging, Grading, & Classification

- Earlier onset → more rapid progression

Gross Pathologic & Surgical Features

- Swollen brain

Microscopic Features

- Spongiform degeneration of WM; GP and thalami with swollen astrocytes

CLINICAL ISSUES

Presentation

- Most common signs/symptoms
  - 3 clinical variants (according to age at presentation)
    - Congenital (1st few days of life)
      - Hypotonia, rapid death
    - Infantile (3-6 months); most common form
      - Hypotonia, head lag, macrocephaly → seizures, spasticity, optic atrophy, visual loss
      - Death usually in 2nd year of life
    - Juvenile
      - Onset at 4-5 years; most slowly progressive form

Demographics

- Ethnicity
  - ↑ risk for Ashkenazi Jews (1 in 40 carriers)

Treatment

- No proven treatment

DIAGNOSTIC CHECKLIST

Image Interpretation Pearls

- Swollen brain, ↑ T2, ↑ DWI in WM, GP, and thalami

SELECTED REFERENCES

1. Rossler L et al: Canavan's spongiform leukodystrophy (aspartoacylase deficiency) with emphasis on sonographic features in infancy: description of a case report and review of the literature. J Ultrasound. 26(4):757-64, 2023

Alexander Disease

KEY FACTS

TERMINOLOGY

- Rare leukoencephalopathy characterized by **Rosenthal fibers** (RFs), intracytoplasmic astrocytic inclusions
- 3 clinical forms: Infantile (most common), juvenile, adult

IMAGING

- Infantile: Symmetric, ↑ T2-signal bifrontal white matter
- Juvenile/adult: ↑ T2-signal brainstem (especially medulla), cerebellum, cervical cord
  - Tectal plate enlargement (due to RF accumulation) can narrow aqueduct of Sylvius; mimic tectal plate glioma
- Other findings: ↓ T2, ↑ T1 **rabbit ear-like** enhancing nodular periventricular rim (**periventricular garland**) around lateral ventricles, especially frontal horns
  - 1 of few metabolic disorders that enhances
- Cavum septum pellucidum association

TOP DIFFERENTIAL DIAGNOSES

- Canavan disease
- Megaloencephalic leukoencephalopathy with subcortical cysts (MLC)

PATHOLOGY

- Dominant **mutations GFAP** (17q21) (> 95% of cases)
- **Glial fibrillary acidic protein (GFAP)** deficiency → astrocyte dysfunction, WM destruction, RF accumulation

CLINICAL ISSUES

- Clinical profile: Infant with macrocephaly, seizures
- Natural history: Variable rate of progression ultimately leading to death in all forms
- Treatment: Supportive

DIAGNOSTIC CHECKLIST

- Consider adult Alexander disease (AD) if ↑ T2 signal and atrophy in medulla (inferior olives and gracile nuclei) and cervical spinal cord
- Enhancing, symmetric bifrontal white matter disease in **macrocephalic** infant highly characteristic of AD

(Left) *Axial T2WI MR in infantile Alexander disease (AD) shows a nodular, hypointense periventricular rim with symmetric, mild hyperintensity in the striata and thalami. Cerebral white matter (WM) is diffusely hyperintense, greatest in frontal lobes where it extends from the ventricular margin to subcortical U-fibers.* **(Right)** *Axial T1WI MR shows diffusely hypointense, swollen WM with a frontal to occipital gradient. Only the occipital WM is myelinated. The nodular periventricular rim is hyperintense.*

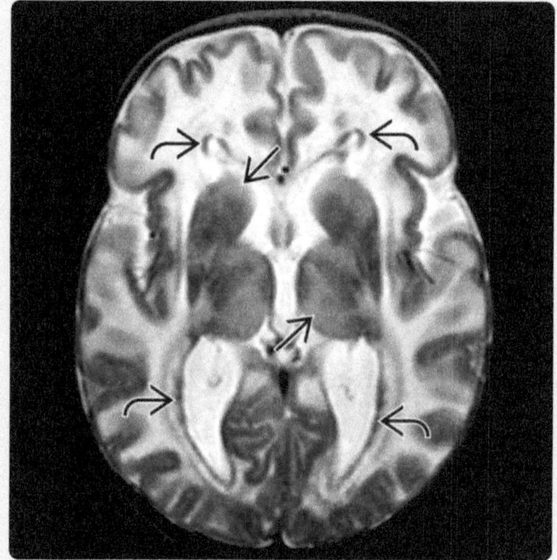

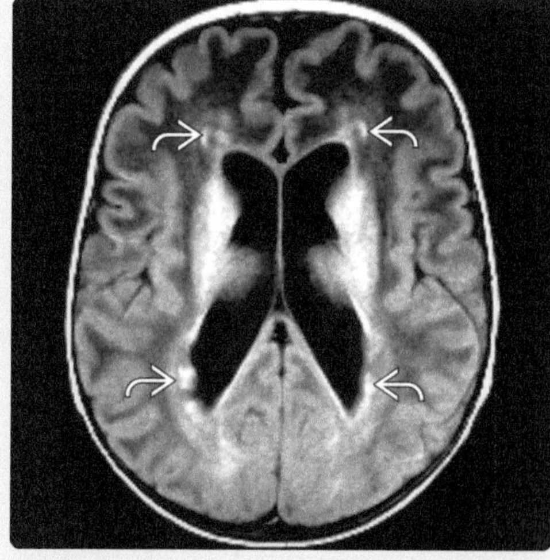

(Left) *Axial T1WI C+ MR shows enhancement of the anterior and posterior periventricular rim, caudate heads, putamina and faintly of the thalami bilaterally. The nodular, rabbit ear appearance of the frontal periventricular rim is typical of AD.* **(Right)** *Single-voxel MRS from WM in infantile AD shows typical ↑ myoinositol peak at 3.5 ppm, ↑ choline peak at 3.2 ppm, reduced NAA peak at 2 ppm, and ↑ inverted doublet peak of lactate at 1.3 ppm.*

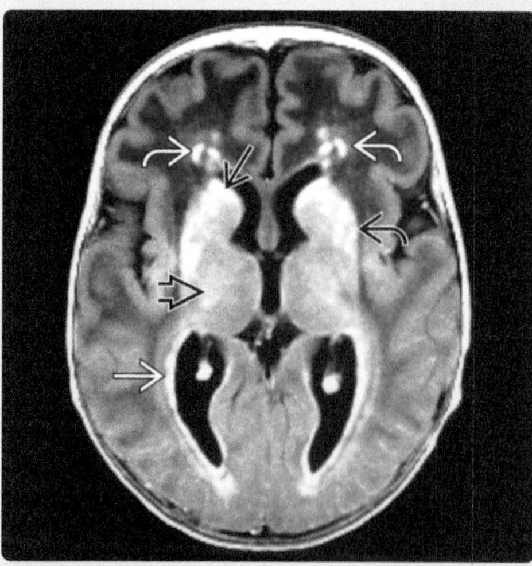

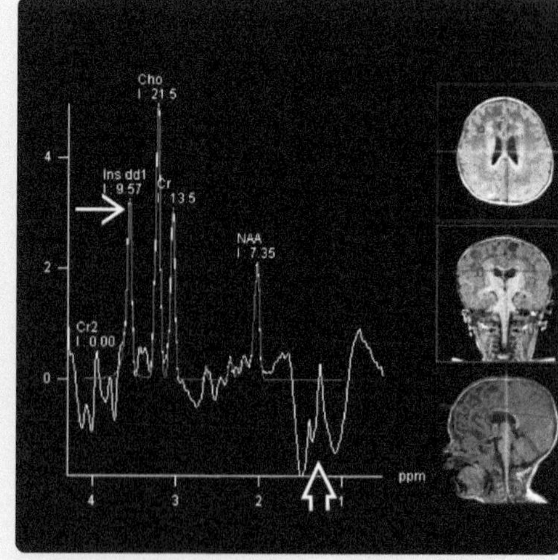

TERMINOLOGY

Abbreviations

- Alexander disease (AD)

Synonyms

- Fibrinoid leukodystrophy

Definitions

- Rare leukoencephalopathy characterized by **Rosenthal fibers (RFs)**, intracytoplasmic astrocytic inclusions
- 3 clinical forms: Infantile (most common), juvenile, adult
- Caused by dominant mutations in gene encoding GFAP

IMAGING

General Features

- Best diagnostic clue
  - **Infantile**: Macrocephalic infant with
    - Symmetric, ↑ T2-signal bifrontal white matter (WM)
    - ↓ T2, ↑ T1, enhancing nodular periventricular rim
  - **Juvenile**: Enhancing ↑ T2-signal brainstem, cerebellum
    - 1 of few metabolic disorders that enhances
  - **Adult**: ↑ T2 signal, atrophy medulla, cervical spinal cord
- Other findings
  - **Infantile**
    - ↑ T2 signal, enhancement striatum
    - Variable ↑ T2 signal, enhancement in brainstem (especially periaqueductal), dentate nuclei, optic chiasm, fornix, rarely hypothalamus, amygdala
    - ± hydrocephalus (periaqueductal disease)
  - **Juvenile/adult**
    - Characterized by brainstem, cerebellar, spinal cord (usually C1, C2) involvement
      - Inferior olives, gracile nuclei in medulla
      - Medial lemniscus, corticospinal tracts, deep cerebellar nuclei hila, cerebellar peduncles, midbrain tegmentum
      - Tectal plate enlargement (due to RF accumulation) may narrow aqueduct of Sylvius; mimic tectal plate glioma
    - Involvement of cerebral WM, periventricular rim, striatum variable (usually mild and developing few years later)
    - Subcortical WM may not be involved
  - Enhancement, swelling early in frontal WM, basal ganglia (BG) (infantile AD)
  - Atrophy, cystic encephalomalacia (infantile) late
  - Cavum septum pellucidum association often, significance uncertain
- Location
  - WM
    - Frontal: Periventricular → subcortical
    - External/extreme capsules, ± callosal genu
  - Periventricular rim
  - BG, thalami, brainstem, cerebellum, fornix, optic chiasm, spinal cord
- Morphology
  - Posterior extension WM changes frequent with disease progression
  - Rostral caudal gradient less pronounced in juvenile/adult disease

CT Findings

- NECT
  - Hypodense frontal WM typically extending into parietal WM and internal capsule
  - Dense periventricular rim, caudate heads
- CECT: Intense enhancement typical of early disease

MR Findings

- T1WI
  - Hypointense frontal WM
  - **Hyper**intense periventricular rim around lateral ventricles, especially frontal horns (**periventricular garland**)
  - Hyperintense ependyma of trigones of lateral ventricles
    - Relationship to garland uncertain
- T2WI
  - Hyperintense frontal WM extending into parietal WM and internal and external capsules
  - BG, especially caudate heads and anterior putamina (striatum) edematous early in disease
  - Globus pallidus and thalamic involvement less common
  - **Hypo**intense periventricular rim (**periventricular garland**)
  - Juvenile/adult: Hyperintense foci in brainstem, especially periaqueductal region, medulla, pons, middle cerebellar peduncles ± cervical cord
- FLAIR
  - **Cavities/cysts** in affected areas, frontal WM (late infantile)
- DWI: Normal to ↑ diffusivity (dark on DWI)
- T1WI C+: Intense enhancement typical of early disease
  - Infantile: Frontal periventricular WM (**rabbit ear** appearance), striatum, periventricular rim; rare in brainstem, fornix, optic chiasm
  - Juvenile/adult: Brainstem and cerebellar enhancement may mimic tumor
- MRS: ↓ NAA, ↑ myoinositol; ± ↑ choline, lactate
- Adult form may show ↑ myoinositol with other metabolite peaks normal

Nuclear Medicine Findings

- F-18 FDG PET
  - Hypometabolism in affected frontal WM
  - Preserved overlying normal glucose metabolism

Imaging Recommendations

- Best imaging tool: C+ MR/MRS
- Protocol advice: Enhance all "unknown" cases of hydrocephalus and abnormal WM

DIFFERENTIAL DIAGNOSIS

Canavan Disease

- Macrocephaly, WM: Diffuse; subcortical U fibers involved early, dorsal brainstem
- Deep gray matter: Globi pallidi, thalami, dentate nuclei
- No enhancement
- Characteristic ↑ ↑ NAA peak on MRS

Megalencephaly With Leukoencephalopathy and Cysts

- WM: Diffuse with subcortical U fiber involvement
- No involvement of deep gray matter structures
- No enhancement
- Characteristic temporal, frontoparietal, subcortical cysts

Glutaric Aciduria Type 1

- WM: Periventricular WM involved in severe disease
- Deep gray matter: Symmetric BG
- No enhancement
- Characteristic widened opercula

Mucopolysaccharidoses

- WM: Mild periventricular
- No involvement of deep gray matter structures
- Characteristic cribriform WM, corpus callosum

PATHOLOGY

General Features

- General pathology comments
  - AD characterized by accumulation of **RFs** in astrocytes and hypo-/demyelination
- Genetics
  - Dominant **mutations** *GFAP* (17q21) (> 95% of cases)
    - > 80 different mutations identified
    - Majority of mutations arise de novo; familial cases seen in adult AD
  - **Glial fibrillary acidic protein (GFAP)**: Major intermediate filament protein in astrocytes
  - GFAP deficiency → astrocyte dysfunction, WM destruction, RF accumulation
- Etiology
  - RF: Abnormal intracellular protein aggregates containing GFAP, αβ-crystalline, hsp27, and ubiquitin
  - Mechanism by which RF accumulation leads to hypo-/demyelination uncertain
    - Theory: RF accumulation causes cell dysfunction
      - Includes blood-brain barrier disruption and loss of normal cell-cell interaction with oligodendrocytes
  - **RFs** also seen in pilocytic astrocytomas, chronic glial scars, craniopharyngiomas
    - Rarely seen in astrocytes of cortical dysplasia and tuberous sclerosis

Gross Pathologic & Surgical Features

- Megaloencephalic, heavy brain with large ventricles
- Swollen, gelatinous WM with cortical thinning
- Frontal WM cavitation
- BG swelling early; atrophy and cystic change late

Microscopic Features

- RF: Eosinophilic, electron-dense, cytoplasmic inclusions in fibrous astrocytes
  - Greatest concentration in subependymal, subpial, and perivascular astrocytic end-feet areas of enhancement
- Hypomyelination/myelin loss frontal lobes > caudal brain, ± cerebellar WM, dentate nucleus, brainstem
- Generalized astrocytosis ± neuraxonal degeneration
- Abnormalities of muscle mitochondria reported

CLINICAL ISSUES

Presentation

- Most common signs/symptoms
  - **Infantile**: Macrocephaly, seizures, developmental delay/arrest, spasticity
  - **Juvenile**: Developmental regression, bulbar/pseudobulbar signs, ataxia, spasticity
  - **Adult**: Bulbar/pseudobulbar signs, ataxia
    - **Palatal myoclonus (40%)** highly suggestive
- Other signs/symptoms in juvenile/adult
  - Bowel/bladder dysfunction, sleep disturbance, dysautonomia
- Clinical profile: Infant with macrocephaly, seizures
- CSF: Variable ↑ protein, αβ-crystalline, hsp27, lactate
- Diagnosis: MR findings and *GFAP* gene blood analysis

Demographics

- Age
  - **Infantile**: Birth to 2 years
  - **Juvenile**: 2-12 years
  - **Adult**: > 12 years old
- Sex: Slight male predominance in infantile AD
- Epidemiology: Rare; incidence unknown
  - Adult AD more common than previously thought

Natural History & Prognosis

- Natural history
  - Variable rate of progression ultimately leading to death in all forms
    - Neonatal variant of infantile form most rapidly fatal; infantile form next most severe
    - Juvenile form more slowly progressive
    - Adult form mildest
- Prognosis
  - **Infantile**: Average survival 3 years after disease onset
  - **Juvenile**: Average survival 8 years after disease onset
  - **Adult**: Average survival 15 years after disease onset

Treatment

- Supportive; hydrocephalus may respond to shunting
- Potential future therapeutic role for agents causing downregulation of *GFAP* expression

DIAGNOSTIC CHECKLIST

Consider

- Infantile AD if macrocephaly with frontal predominant leukodystrophy
- Juvenile AD: Enhancing, ↑ T2-signal brainstem, cerebellum
- Adult AD if ↑ T2 signal, atrophy in medulla and cervical cord

Image Interpretation Pearls

- Enhancing symmetric bifrontal WM disease in macrocephalic infant highly characteristic of AD

SELECTED REFERENCES

1. Anderson NE et al: Alexander disease: the story behind an eponym. J Hist Neurosci. 1-24, 2023
2. Kang YR et al: Older adult-onset Alexander disease with atypical clinicoradiological features: a case report. Front Neurol. 14:1139047, 2023
3. Zampini L et al: Developmental profiles in children and young adults with Alexander disease. Dev Neurorehabil. 26(4):253-61, 2023

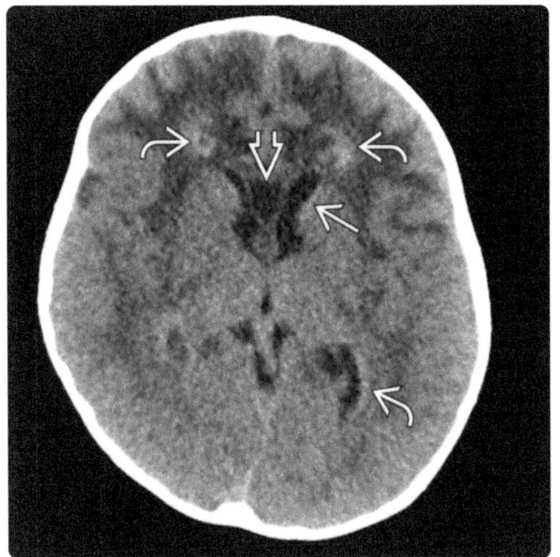

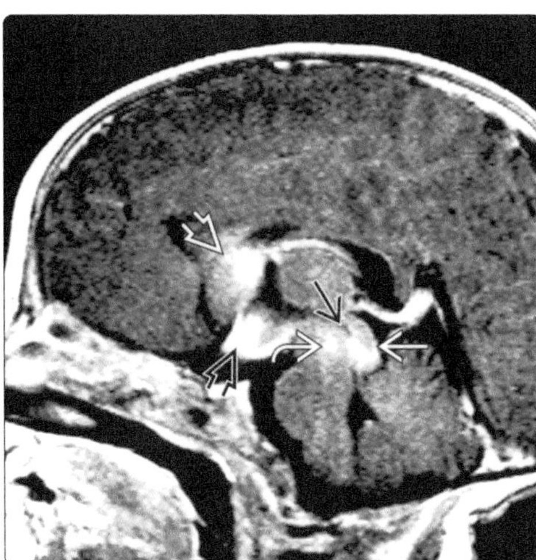

(Left) *Axial NECT in infantile AD shows hyperdense striatum ➡ and a periventricular rim ➦, which showed contrast enhancement on MR (not shown). Note the symmetric frontal predominant WM hypodensity. A cavum septum pellucidum ➡ is seen.* **(Right)** *Sagittal T1 C+ MR in an AD patient shows swelling and abnormal enhancement of the midbrain tegmentum ➦ and tectum ➡, compressing the cerebral aqueduct ➡. Note the abnormal hypothalamic enhancement ➡. Abnormal enhancement is also seen in the caudate head ➡.*

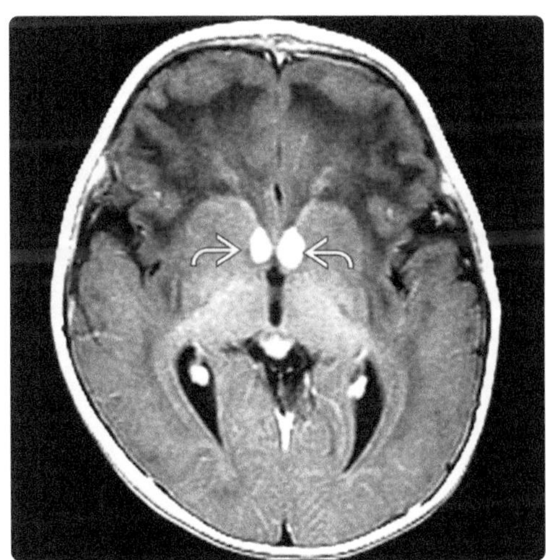

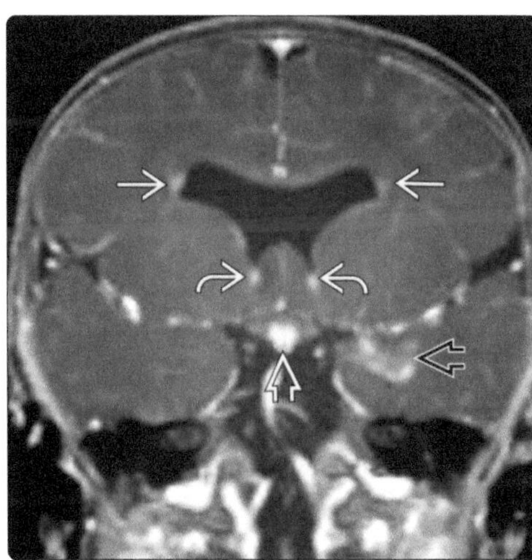

(Left) *Axial T1WI C+ MR in an AD patient shows intense enhancement of the columns of fornix ➦ bilaterally and mild enhancement over the surface of the caudate heads.* **(Right)** *Coronal T1WI C+ MR in an AD patient shows periventricular foci of enhancement surrounding the superolateral ➡ and inferior ➦ aspects of lateral ventricles. Also note the abnormal thickening and enhancement of hypothalamus ➡ and left amygdala ➡. (Courtesy T.J.E. Muttikkal, MD.)*

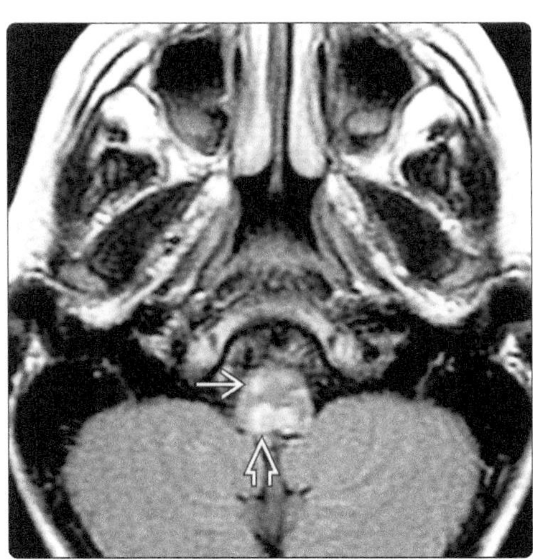

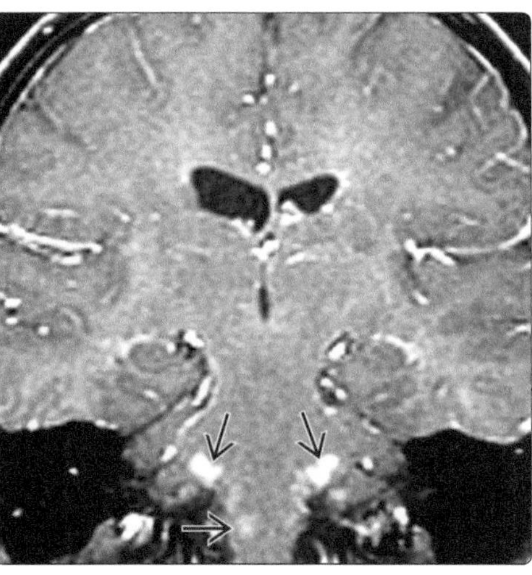

(Left) *Axial FLAIR MR in an older child with AD shows multiple foci of hyperintensity within the inferior olives ➡ and gracile nuclei ➡ in the medulla.* **(Right)** *Coronal T1WI C+ MR in the same patient shows focal enhancement in the medulla and middle cerebellar peduncles ➡. Note the normal cerebral WM. Juvenile and adult AD are characterized by involvement of the brainstem (especially medulla), cerebellum, and cervical cord (particularly adults) with little to no supratentorial involvement.*

Megalencephaly With Leukoencephalopathy and Cysts

KEY FACTS

TERMINOLOGY

- Megalencephaly with leukoencephalopathy (MLC)
- Inherited leukodystrophy

IMAGING

- Swollen white matter (WM)
  - Early WM swelling ↓ over time; atrophy ensues
- Subcortical temporal and frontoparietal cysts
- Cysts ↑ in size and number over time
- No contrast enhancement or reduced diffusion

PATHOLOGY

- Genetics
  - Autosomal recessive; mutations of *MLC1* or *GLIALCAM* gene
  - Mutations mostly private
  - Founder effect occurs in population subisolates

CLINICAL ISSUES

- Delayed onset of slow motor deterioration (despite very abnormal MR)
- Macrocephaly
- Seizures/deterioration after mild trauma
- Even slower cognitive decline
- Cerebellar ataxia
- Pyramidal tract involvement
- Rare disorder, but carrier rate in some communities with high levels of consanguinity as high as 1/40
- Prenatal diagnosis is option in families with known mutations

DIAGNOSTIC CHECKLIST

- Consider 1 of "new" leukodystrophies, such as MLC, when imaging features are more severe than metachromatic leukodystrophy

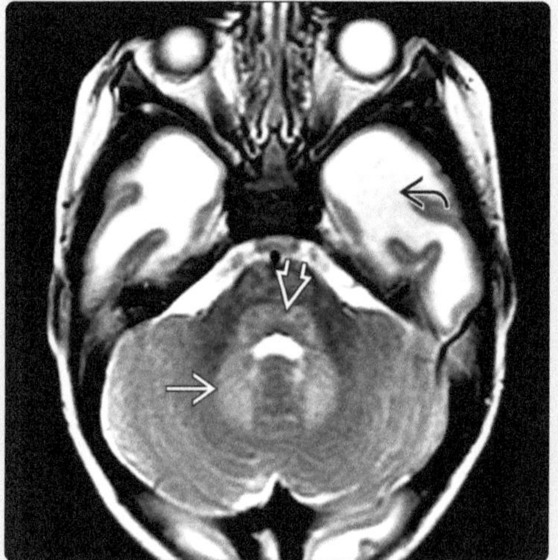

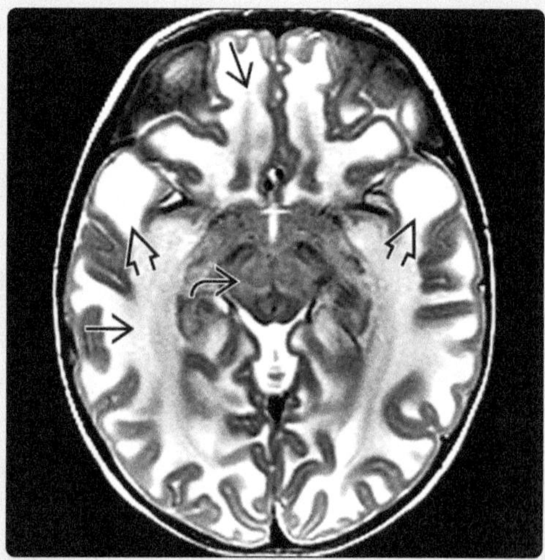

(Left) *Axial T2WI MR in a 10-month-old infant with increasing head circumference but normal development reveals abnormally increased signal intensity of the cerebellar white matter (WM) ➡, dorsal brainstem ➡, and anterior temporal lobes ➡.* **(Right)** *Axial T2WI MR in the same infant confirms extensive swelling and increased signal of WM of the cerebrum ➡ and the WM tracts ➡ surrounding the red nuclei in the midbrain. Note the anterior temporal lobe cysts ➡.*

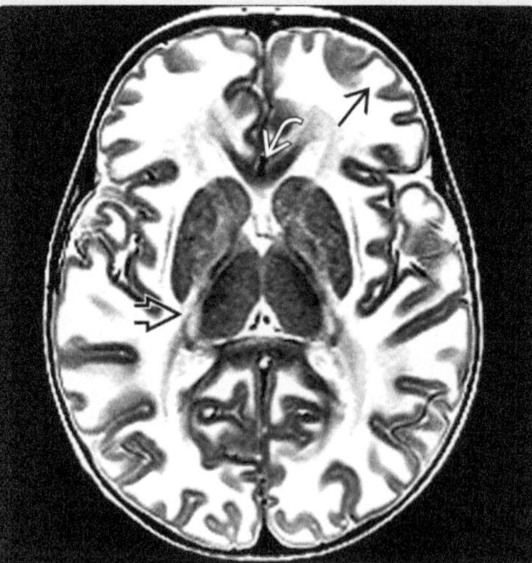

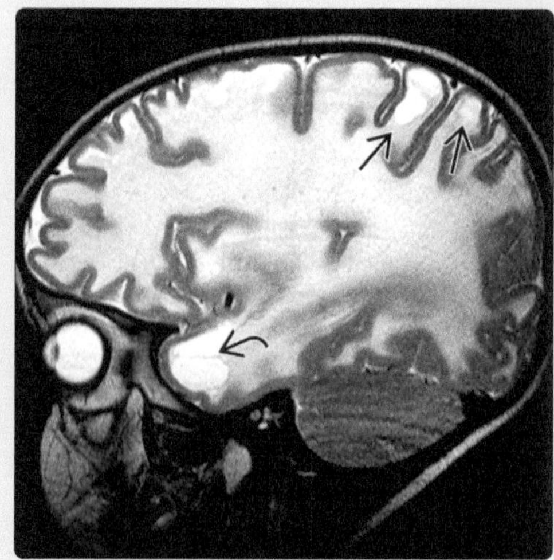

(Left) *Axial T2WI MR in the same 10-month-old infant reveals sparing (normal myelination) of the corpus callosum ➡, diminished myelination of portions of the posterior limb of the internal capsule ➡, and definitely impaired myelination of the subcortical U fibers throughout the cerebral hemispheres ➡.* **(Right)** *Sagittal T2WI MR in the same infant confirms the presence of temporal ➡ and frontoparietal ➡ cysts in addition to extensive hypomyelination.*

TERMINOLOGY

Abbreviations

- Megalencephaly with leukoencephalopathy (MLC)

Synonyms

- Formerly
  - Vacuolating megaloencephalic leukoencephalopathy with benign, slowly progressive course
  - Infantile-onset leukoencephalopathy with swelling and discrepantly mild course
  - van der Knaap disease
    - 1 of many disorders eponymously named after that author
  - Indian Agarwal megaloencephalic leukodystrophy

Definitions

- Autosomal recessive disorder of astrocytic, volume-regulated anion currents
  - Characterized by macrocephaly, motor/cognitive decline, ataxia, spasticity

IMAGING

General Features

- Best diagnostic clue
  - Diffusely abnormal, swollen hemispheric white matter (WM)
  - Subcortical cysts, predominantly anterotemporal, frontoparietal
- Location
  - Diffuse WM, includes subcortical U fibers
    - Subcortical cysts
      - Anterotemporal most common
      - Frontoparietal also common
    - ± involvement of posterior internal capsules
    - Cerebellar WM involvement subtle
- Size
  - Cysts ↑ in size and number over time

CT Findings

- NECT
  - Involved WM ↓ attenuation
- CECT
  - No contrast enhancement

MR Findings

- T1WI
  - Involved WM ↓ signal on T1WI
- T2WI
  - Involved WM ↑ signal on T2WI
    - Cerebral WM
      - Relative sparing of corpus callosum
    - Posterior 1/3 of posterior limb of internal capsule ± involvement
    - WM tracts of brainstem ± involvement in very young
- FLAIR
  - Involved WM ↑ signal on FLAIR
  - Subcortical cysts
    - Anterotemporal and frontoparietal most common
    - Cysts approximate CSF signal
- DWI
  - DTI shows ↓ anisotropy, ↑ ADC values
    - Results from ↑ water in interstitial space
- T1WI C+
  - No contrast enhancement
  - Probably not necessary
- MRS
  - All metabolites ↓ in cystic regions
  - ↓ NAA in WM
  - Normal myoinositol
  - ± lactate signal

Imaging Recommendations

- Best imaging tool
  - MR with MRS
    - ± contrast administration (to exclude enhancing leukodystrophies)

DIFFERENTIAL DIAGNOSIS

Other Leukodystrophies, Nonenhancing

- Metachromatic leukodystrophy (MLD)
  - Look for WM "stripes" on T2WI
- Hypomyelination
- Canavan
  - Subcortical U fibers involved early
  - Markedly elevated NAA on MRS
- Cree leukoencephalopathy
  - Involvement of WM
  - Deep structures
    - Involves globus pallidus, thalami, and medulla
    - Spares olives, red nuclei, and caudate nuclei

Other Leukodystrophies, Enhancing

- Alexander disease
  - Abnormal signal + enhancement of frontal WM and ependymal surfaces
  - Basal nuclei involved
- X-linked adrenoleukodystrophy
  - Abnormal signal and enhancement of peritrigonal WM and splenium

PATHOLOGY

General Features

- Etiology
  - Inborn genetic errors
  - Disturbed water homeostasis and osmotic balance to abnormal function of volume-regulated anion channels (VRACs)
    - VRACs in astrocytes respond to changes in extracellular osmolarity
    - Display prominent cell volume changes as part of osmoregulatory process
    - *MLC1* important in VRAC activity; *GlialCAM* is chaperone of *MLC1* in ion channels
- Genetics
  - Autosomal recessive; gene localized on Chr 22q(tel)
    - Many different mutations of *MLC1*, *HEPACAM*, and *GLIALCAM* genes
    - Mutations distributed along whole gene, types include
      - Splice-site mutations

- Nonsense mutations
- Missense mutations
- Deletions and insertions
- Mutations identified in 80%; 2nd locus suspected
- Mutations mostly private
- Founder effect occurs in population subisolates

- Associated abnormalities
  - *MLC1* in CNS expressed in astrocytic end-feet at blood-brain and CSF-brain barriers
    - GlialCAM is chaperone for MLC1 in ion channels of astrocytes
  - *MLC1* also expressed in peripheral WBCs, spleen
    - But no systemic or other organ involvement

Gross Pathologic & Surgical Features

- Spongiform leukoencephalopathy
  - Vacuolization in subcortical WM

Microscopic Features

- Myelin splitting at intraperiod line
- Vacuolization of outermost lamellae of myelin sheaths

CLINICAL ISSUES

Presentation

- Most common signs/symptoms
  - Macrocephaly at birth or within 1st year of life
  - Delayed onset of slow motor deterioration (even slower cognitive decline) despite very abnormal MR
    - Development during 1st year often normal
- Other signs/symptoms
  - Rare early presentation with developmental delay
  - Rare transient coma following minor head trauma
- Clinical profile
  - Macrocephaly
  - Very slow cognitive decline
    - Eventual learning problems in 50%
  - Cerebellar ataxia and pyramidal tract involvement
  - Motor deterioration
    - Late loss of ability to walk
    - Occasional delayed autonomous walking
  - Minor head trauma → seizures and temporary deterioration

Demographics

- Age
  - Macrocephaly before 1 year of age
- Ethnicity
  - ↑ in population isolates
    - Common *MLC* mutations in
      - Specific Indian community (Agarwal)
      - Libyan Jewish community
      - Turkish community
      - Some Japanese families due to founder effect
    - Agarwal community mutation
      - Insertion (c.135_136insC) usual, phenotypic variation occurs
- Epidemiology
  - Rare
  - Carrier rate in some communities with high levels of consanguinity as high as 1/40

Natural History & Prognosis

- Early WM swelling
  - Swelling ↓ over time
  - Atrophy ensues
- Clinical features progress slowly

Treatment

- Treat symptoms (seizures, spasticity)
- Prenatal diagnosis is option in families with known mutations

DIAGNOSTIC CHECKLIST

Consider

- 1 of "new" leukodystrophies when imaging involvement more severe than MLD

Image Interpretation Pearls

- Always enhance unknown leukoencephalopathy

Reporting Tips

- Differentiation from MLD
  - Involvement of subcortical U fibers
  - Subcortical cysts
- Differentiate from Canavan
  - No basal ganglia involvement in MLC
  - Normal NAA in MLC

SELECTED REFERENCES

1. Das S et al: The coexistence of two genetic astrocytopathies-megalencephalic leukoencephalopathy and vanishing white matter disease-in an Indian child. Neuropediatrics. 54(2):153-6, 2023
2. Kaushal H et al: Van Der Knaap disease: young male with megalencephalic leukoencephalopathy with subcortical cysts: a case report. Neurol India. 70(6):2437-9, 2022
3. Sadek AA et al: Clinicoradiologic correlation in 22 Egyptian children with megalencephalic leukoencephalopathy with subcortical cysts. J Child Neurol. 37(5):380-9, 2022
4. Ballesteros-Cogollos V et al: [Megalencephalic leukoencephalopathy with cysts -the clinical importance in the genetic era.] Rev Neurol. 71(10):373-6, 2020
5. Endrakanti M et al: Macrocephaly, epilepsy and intracranial cysts: an image to remember. BMJ Case Rep, 2018
6. Sun Y et al: Novel RNASET2 pathogenic variants in an East Asian child with delayed psychomotor development. Fetal Pediatr Pathol. 37(1):15-21, 2018
7. Abdel-Salam GM et al: Megalencephalic leukoencephalopathy with cysts in twelve Egyptian patients: novel mutations in MLC1 and HEPACAM and a founder effect. Metab Brain Dis. 31(5):1171-9, 2016
8. Dash PK et al: Megalencephalic leucoencephalopathy with subcortical cysts: subcortical diffuse leucoencephalopathy associated with white matter cystic degeneration. BMJ Case Rep, 2015
9. Kariminejad A et al: Eight novel mutations in MLC1 from 18 Iranian patients with megalencephalic leukoencephalopathy with subcortical cysts. Eur J Med Genet. 58(2):71-4, 2015
10. Koç K et al: Magnetic resonance imaging findings of two sisters with Van der Knaap leukoencephalopathy. Neuroradiol J. 28(5):519-22, 2015
11. Mahmoud IG et al: Clinical, neuroimaging, and genetic characteristics of megalencephalic leukoencephalopathy with subcortical cysts in Egyptian patients. Pediatr Neurol. 50(2):140-8, 2014
12. Capdevila-Nortes X et al: Insights into MLC pathogenesis: GlialCAM is an MLC1 chaperone required for proper activation of volume-regulated anion currents. Hum Mol Genet. 22(21):4405-16, 2013
13. van der Knaap MS et al: Megalencephalic leukoencephalopathy with subcortical cysts: chronic white matter oedema due to a defect in brain ion and water homoeostasis. Lancet Neurol. 11(11):973-85, 2012

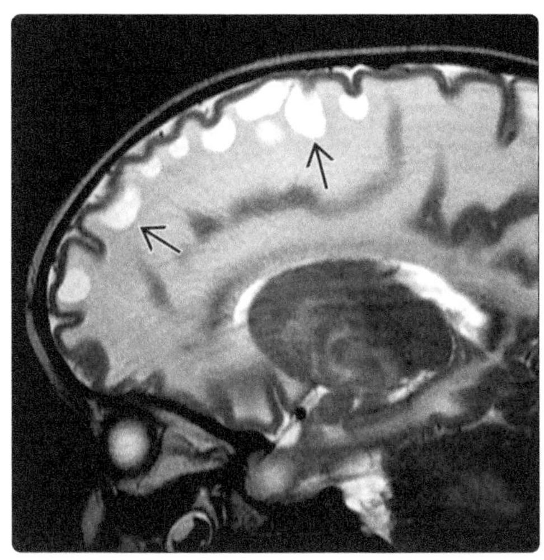

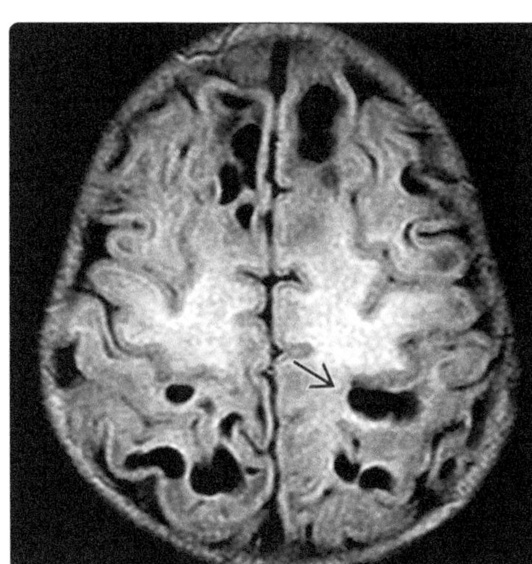

(Left) *Sagittal T2WI MR in a 2-year-old patient with megalencephaly and slowing of acquisition of developmental milestones shows swollen WM as well as fairly extensive subcortical cysts ➙ involving the frontal lobe.* **(Right)** *Axial FLAIR MR in the same patient shows WM with abnormally high signal intensity due to hypomyelination, in addition to extensive, bilateral, frontal, and frontoparietal subcortical cysts ➙.*

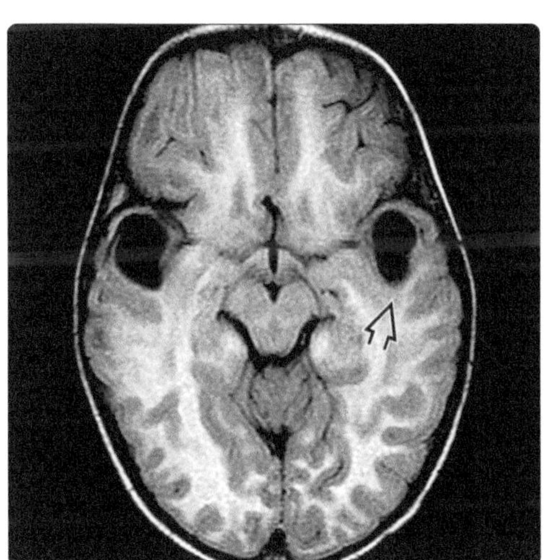

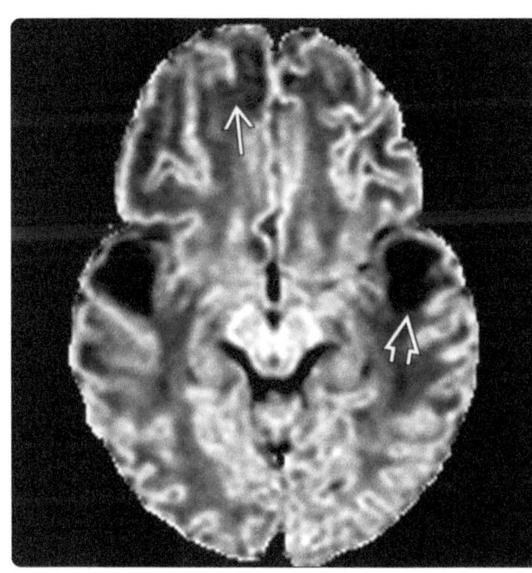

(Left) *Axial FLAIR MR in a 22-month-old child with macrocephaly and decreasing acquisition of developmental milestones shows large, bilateral temporal lobe cysts ➙, typical of megalencephaly with leukoencephalopathy and cysts (MLC) on a background of swollen, abnormally hyperintense WM.* **(Right)** *Axial DWI MR in the same 22-month-old infant confirms markedly increased diffusivity in the cysts ➙ and, less dramatically, in the subcortical WM ➙.*

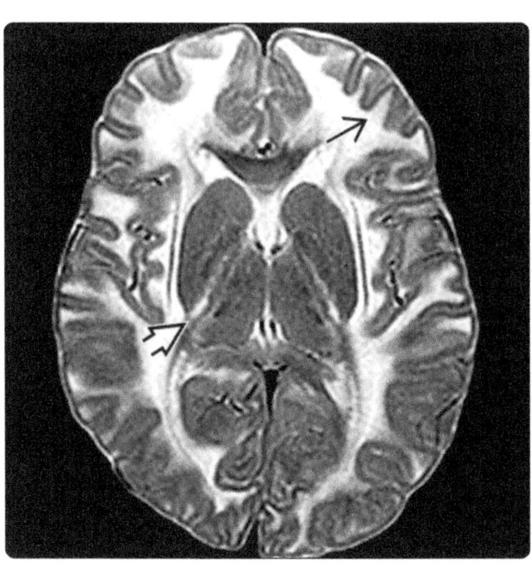

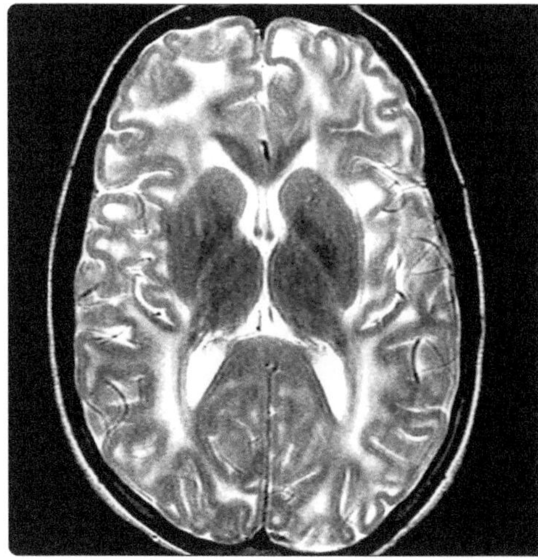

(Left) *Axial T2WI MR in a 6-year-old child with MLC shows less pronounced WM swelling, although the posterior limbs of the internal capsules ➙ and subcortical U fibers ➙ show persistence of abnormal signal hyperintensity.* **(Right)** *Axial T2WI MR in a 14-year-old patient with MLC demonstrates sulcal widening due to atrophy, a common finding as the disease progresses. Note the persistent hyperintensity of the cerebral WM with involvement of the subcortical U fibers.*

KEY FACTS

TERMINOLOGY

- Chronic, progressive white matter (WM) disorder featuring central WM loss + ataxia, spasticity

IMAGING

- Abnormal low T1 signal in affected WM approaching CSF signal, no abnormal enhancement
- High T2 signal intensity early within affected WM, continues to ↑ as cerebral WM is replaced by CSF
- FLAIR MR signal changes from high to low intensity as cerebral WM replaced by CSF
  - Radiating, stripe-like tigroid pattern within rarefied and cystic WM
- ± restricted diffusion early in relatively spared brain regions

TOP DIFFERENTIAL DIAGNOSES

- Megalencephalic leukoencephalopathy with subcortical cysts
- Multiple sclerosis
- Acute disseminated encephalomyelitis
- Infectious encephalitis
- Mitochondrial disorders
- Alexander disease
- Other leukodystrophies

PATHOLOGY

- Most patients have gene mutation encoding eukaryotic translation initiation factor eIF2B

CLINICAL ISSUES

- Early-childhood onset of chronic progressive neurologic deterioration dominated by cerebellar ataxia
- Spasticity, relatively mild mental decline

DIAGNOSTIC CHECKLIST

- Diffuse WM abnormality present **before** appearance of clinical signs/symptoms
- Absence of contrast enhancement helps distinguish from other leukodystrophies

(Left) *Axial T2 MR in a 19-month-old girl with ataxia who is losing milestones demonstrates diffuse abnormal white matter (WM) hyperintensity without volume loss or ventricular enlargement. In fact, the WM appears mildly "swollen."* **(Right)** *Axial T1 C+ MR in the same patient confirms abnormal hypointensity of the involved WM. The absence of abnormal enhancement helps distinguish from other differential diagnostic entities.*

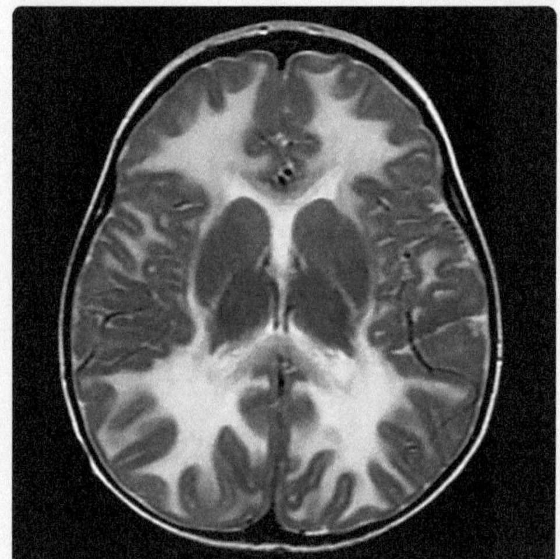

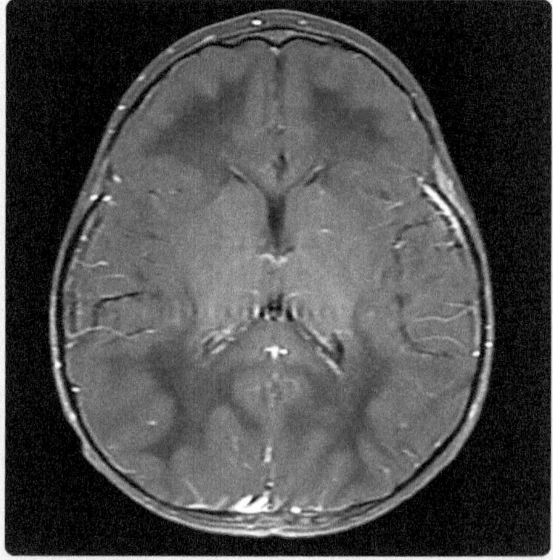

(Left) *Axial FLAIR MR in the same patient reveals abnormal (for this age) WM hypointensity with a characteristic striped or tigroid appearance. Subcortical U fibers are relatively spared.* **(Right)** *Axial DWI MR in the same patient depicts positive diffusion restriction (confirmed on ADC map, not shown) ➙ within the subcortical WM. This finding is seen within relatively unaffected WM early in disease course.*

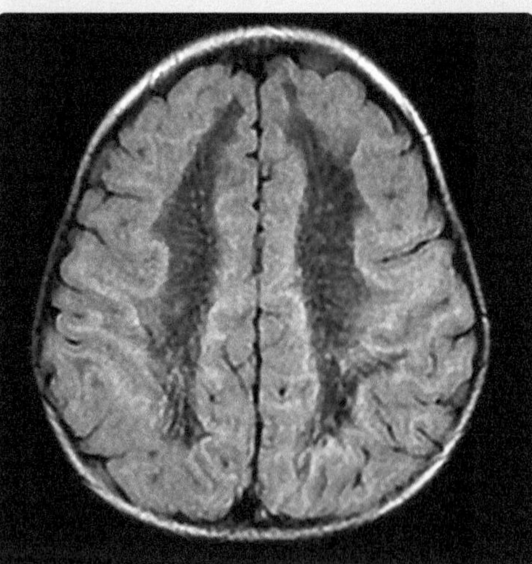

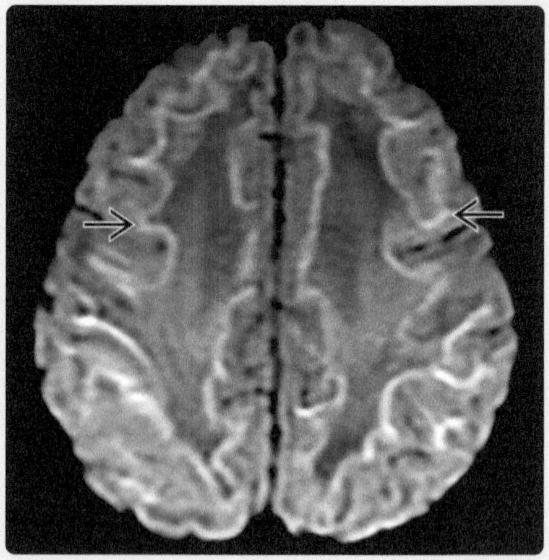

TERMINOLOGY

Abbreviations

- Vanishing white matter (VWM)

IMAGING

General Features

- Best diagnostic clue
  - "Tigroid stripes" on FLAIR MR within affected WM
- Location
  - Nearly all cerebral WM; relative sparing of U fibers, cerebellar WM, pyramidal tracts, corpus callosum, posterior limb of internal capsule
  - ± cerebellar atrophy (particularly vermis)
- Morphology
  - Antenatal/early infantile form
    - "Swollen" cerebral WM → gyral broadening
    - Subsequent cerebral WM rarefaction, cystic atrophy with disease progression (WM "vanishes")
    - Lateral ventricles remain normal in size until late in process despite WM loss
    - At end stage, all hemispheric WM is atrophic, leaving only ventricular walls and cortex with intervening CSF
  - Juvenile/adult form
    - WM better preserved; some cavitation but generally does not completely "vanish"
    - Progressive lateral ventricle dilation related to WM loss
  - Minimal cortical gray matter atrophy even at advanced stages

CT Findings

- NECT
  - Hypodense WM ± cystic change

MR Findings

- T1WI
  - Abnormal low signal in affected WM (both cystic and noncystic) approaching CSF signal
- T2WI
  - High signal intensity within affected WM early in process
  - Abnormal signal intensity continues to ↑ as cerebral WM is replaced by CSF
  - ± globus pallidus low signal 2° to mineralization
- FLAIR
  - High signal intensity within affected WM early in process
  - Signal changes from high to low intensity as cerebral WM "vanishes" 2° to replacement of WM by CSF
  - Radiating, stripe-like tigroid pattern within rarefied and cystic WM develops
    - Represents meshwork of residual tissue strands and vessels
- DWI
  - ± restricted diffusion in relatively spared brain regions early in process
    - Subcortical U fibers, cerebellar WM, middle cerebellar peduncles, pyramidal tracts, corpus callosum, posterior limb of internal capsule
    - Corresponds to relatively higher tissue cellular density
  - ↑ diffusivity within rarefied or cystic WM
- T1WI C+
  - No abnormal enhancement

DIFFERENTIAL DIAGNOSIS

Megalencephalic Leukoencephalopathy With Subcortical Cysts

- Presents with macrocephaly in 1st year of life
- Mild developmental delay, ataxia, spasticity, and seizures
- Supratentorial WM abnormality + cystic brain lesions (mostly frontoparietal border zone, anterior temporal subcortical WM)

Multiple Sclerosis

- Common WM demyelination disorder with generally focal, rather than large, confluent lesions
- Isolated juxtacortical lesions and lesions perpendicular to lateral ventricle are most discriminative for multiple sclerosis

Acute Disseminated Encephalomyelitis

- Asymmetric multifocal brain WM, spinal cord abnormalities ± contrast enhancement
  - Commonly involves centrum semiovale, basal ganglia
- Generally presents 1-2 weeks subsequent to febrile viral illness

Infectious Encephalitis

- Febrile illness with neurologic dysfunction ± altered state of consciousness
- Brain lesions typically involve both WM and gray matter ± contrast enhancement
- Laboratory testing may identify infectious agent

Mitochondrial Disorders

- e.g., pyruvate dehydrogenase deficiency, pyruvate carboxylase deficiency
- May cause leukoencephalopathy with diffuse rarefaction, cystic WM degeneration
- Unlike in VWM, MR typically shows well-delineated cysts, less diffuse WM abnormalities ± focal contrast enhancement, and areas of restricted diffusion

Alexander Disease

- Megalencephaly, psychomotor restrictions, pseudobulbar signs, spasticity, ataxia with progressive deterioration
- Initially frontal WM swelling, avid WM and basal ganglia enhancement → frontoparietal WM atrophy with cystic degeneration as disease evolves

Other Leukodystrophies

- e.g., adrenoleukodystrophy, metachromatic leukodystrophy, Krabbe disease, Pelizaeus-Merzbacher disease
- Not associated with diffuse cystic cerebral WM degeneration

PATHOLOGY

General Features

- Etiology
  - Astrocytic dysfunction produces 2° effects on oligodendroglia, axons → WM degeneration

- Oligodendrocytes receive conflicting proliferative, proapoptotic, and prosurvival signals during disease course
- Genetics
  - Autosomal recessive
  - Most patients have mutation in genes encoding eukaryotic translation initiation factor eIF2B
    - eIF2B essential for WM protein synthesis, regulation under cellular stress conditions
    - Oligodendrocytes, astrocytes predominantly affected
- Associated abnormalities
  - Ovarioleukodystrophy
    - Childhood ataxia with CNS hypomyelination (CACH)/VWM + 1° or 2° ovarian failure
    - Ovaries most frequently affected organ besides brain
  - Other organ involvement: Growth failure, cataracts, hepatosplenomegaly, pancreatitis, renal hypoplasia

Gross Pathologic & Surgical Features

- Extensive cystic, gelatinous, or cavitary degeneration of periventricular, immediate subcortical WM
- Gray matter volume generally preserved

Microscopic Features

- Myelin pallor and severe myelinolysis with atypical astrogliosis
  - Radiating stripes within rarefied WM on MR correlate with blood vessels accompanied by reactive astrocytes, tissue strands
- Complete axonal loss in cavitated areas, more variable axonal loss in less involved areas
- Abnormal vacuolated ("foamy") oligodendrocytes
- Absence of significant inflammatory response

Laboratory Testing

- Routine laboratory tests, standard CSF analysis generally normal

CLINICAL ISSUES

Presentation

- Most common signs/symptoms
  - Progressive neurologic deterioration featuring prominent ataxia, spasticity
  - Rapid neurologic deterioration or coma following febrile infection, minor head trauma, or acute fright
- Other signs/symptoms
  - Transient headache with hemiparesis or hemiparesthesia
    - Episodes may be triggered by stress
  - Asymptomatic patient identified incidentally
    - Otherwise healthy child or adult undergoes brain MR for other reasons
  - Seizures (relatively late in disease course)
- Clinical profile
  - Classic phenotype: Early childhood onset of chronic progressive neurologic deterioration dominated by cerebellar ataxia with less prominent spasticity, relatively mild mental decline

Demographics

- Age
  - Mostly affects children
- Ethnicity
  - More common in White populations
  - Phenotypic variant described in Cree Native American population
- Epidemiology
  - True incidence and prevalence unknown
    - Estimated incidence ≥ 1:80,000 live births (Netherlands)
    - May be one of most prevalent inherited childhood leukoencephalopathies
  - 1988 Canadian study described severe infantile leukodystrophy (Cree leukoencephalopathy) in 3 Cree Native American villages
    - Now recognized as phenotypic variant of CACH/VWM

Natural History & Prognosis

- High phenotypic variation: Ranges from antenatal onset, early demise → adult onset, slowly progressive disease
- Age at onset is important prognostic determinant
  - Earlier onset age (< 4 years) → more severe CACH/VWM with more rapid progression, higher severity, greater mortality
  - In contrast, presentation ≥ 4 years generally shows less progressive course, lower mortality
    - Wide severity variation in this group independent of onset age
- Febrile illness, minor head trauma, or severe fright may result in sudden neurologic deterioration, including coma, with incomplete recovery

Treatment

- Currently, there is no therapy for VWM, but various drugs are in clinical development or trials
- Liberal use of antibiotics, antipyretics, and vaccinations
- Avoidance of contact sports, stressful situations that may trigger deterioration
- Physical therapy, rehabilitation, and antispasmodic medications to improve gait and tone

DIAGNOSTIC CHECKLIST

Consider

- Chronic progressive WM disorder exacerbated by infection, head trauma, or severe fright
- Diagnosis supported by characteristic disease clinical and MR features
- Diffuse WM abnormality present **before** appearance of clinical signs/symptoms

Image Interpretation Pearls

- Absence of contrast enhancement helps distinguish from other leukodystrophies

SELECTED REFERENCES

1. Filareto I et al: EIF2B2 gene mutation causing early onset vanishing white matter disease: a case report. Ital J Pediatr. 48(1):128, 2022
2. Hanson FM et al: Regulation and function of eIF2B in neurological and metabolic disorders. Biosci Rep. 42(6):BSR20211699, 2022
3. Stellingwerff MD et al: MRI natural history of the leukodystrophy vanishing white matter. Radiology. 300(3):671-80, 2021
4. Bugiani M et al: Vanishing white matter: a leukodystrophy due to astrocytic dysfunction. Brain Pathol. 28(3):408-21, 2018
5. Hamilton EMC et al: Natural history of vanishing white matter. Ann Neurol. 84(2):274-88, 2018

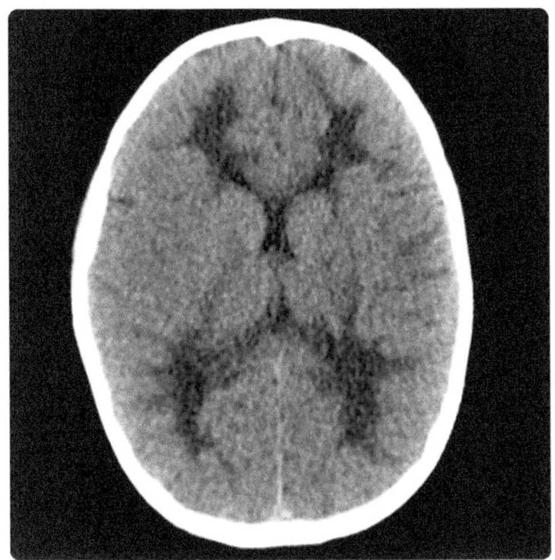

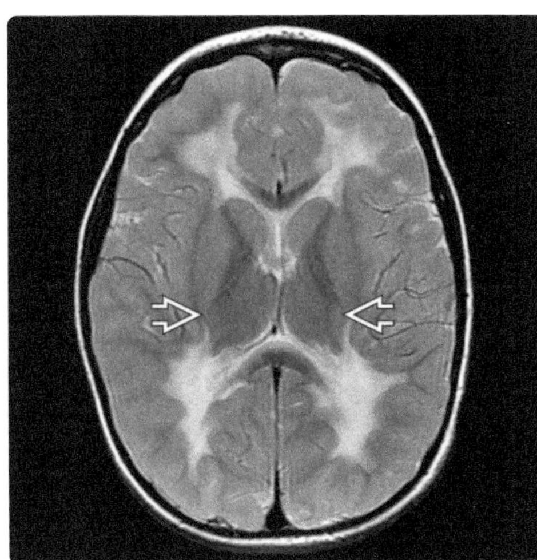

(Left) *Axial NECT in a 5-year-old boy reveals symmetric, bilateral, abnormal WM hypodensity within the centrum semiovale that spares subcortical WM, an incidental finding during imaging for a bicycle accident.* **(Right)** *Axial T2 MR in the same patient confirms abnormal central WM hyperintensity without volume loss. Note relative sparing of subcortical WM and the posterior limb internal capsule ➡ along with absence of cavitation.*

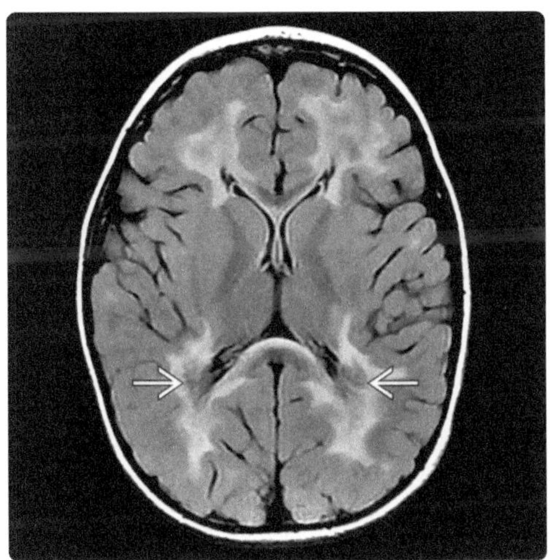

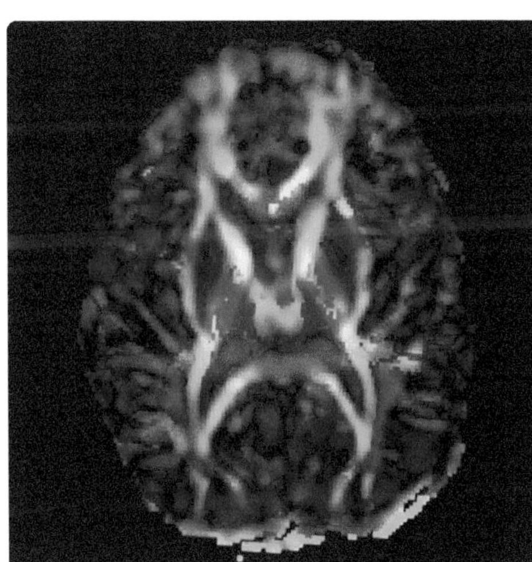

(Left) *Axial FLAIR MR in the same patient shows a mix of hyperintense and hypointense WM changes in the central WM and corpus callosum. The periventricular WM shows internal "stripes" ➡. No contrast enhancement was noted (not seen).* **(Right)** *Axial color FA map confirms preservation of underlying WM architecture and directional anisotropy within the areas of abnormal WM T1 and T2 signal abnormality.*

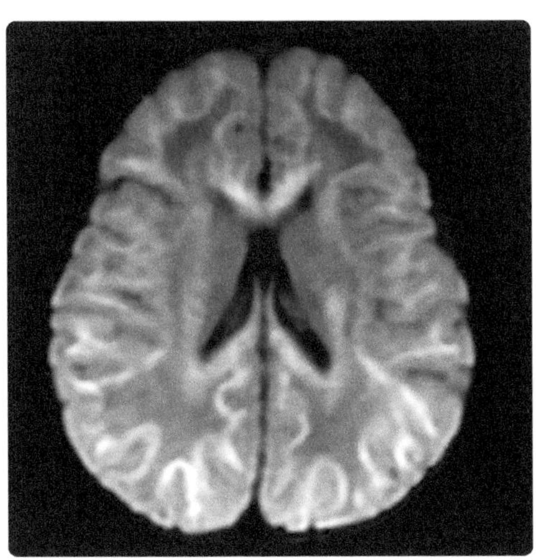

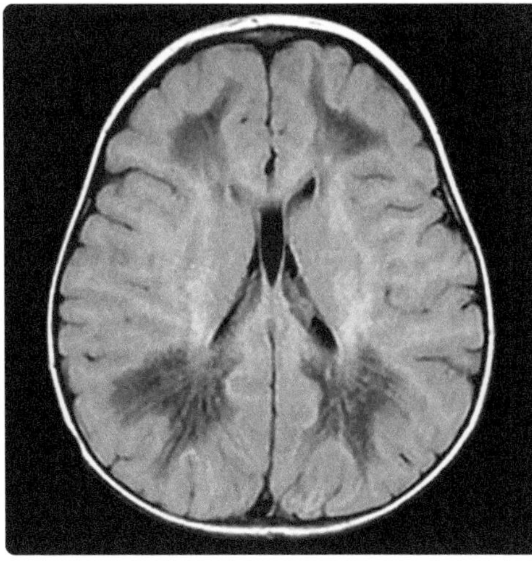

(Left) *Axial DWI MR in a 19-month-old child reveals extensive diffusion restriction in the subcortical regions, as well as corpus callosum. ADC map (not shown) showed concordant hypointensity. Clinical course was relatively indolent.* **(Right)** *Axial FLAIR MR in the same patient confirmed abnormally hypointense central WM and relatively hyperintense strands within the periventricular WM ("tiger stripes"), diagnostic of vanishing WM. This diagnosis was confirmed by genetic testing.*

X-Linked Charcot-Marie-Tooth

KEY FACTS

TERMINOLOGY

- X-linked hereditary peripheral sensory and motor neuropathy

IMAGING

- Initial presentation with confluent symmetric white matter T2-hyperintense lesions in posterior centrum semiovale, splenium
  - Acute lesions show diffusion restriction
  - Spares subcortical U fibers
  - No lesion enhancement
- White matter lesions transient; improvement or complete resolution common

TOP DIFFERENTIAL DIAGNOSES

- Acute disseminated encephalomyelitis (ADEM)
- Multiple sclerosis
- X-linked adrenoleukodystrophy (ALD)

PATHOLOGY

- X-linked
- Mutations in gap junction beta 1 gene (*GJB1*) on chromosome Xq13.1 coding for connexin-32

CLINICAL ISSUES

- Acute transient encephalopathy
- Transient motor weakness
- Chronic distal leg muscle wasting ± weakness of ankle flexion, absent lower extremity deep-tendon reflexes, pes cavus foot deformity

DIAGNOSTIC CHECKLIST

- Bilateral leg wasting and weakness + pes cavus foot deformity suggests Charcot-Marie-Tooth (CMT)
- Consider X-linked CMT (CMTX) in patients with peripheral neuropathy and CNS symptoms/signs ± recurrent white matter lesions
  - Lesion symmetry, posterior predilection suggest CMTX

(Left) *Axial DWI MR in a patient with acute onset of encephalopathy and a familial history of X-linked Charcot-Marie-Tooth (CMTX) demonstrates symmetric diffusion restriction ➡ within the posterior centrum semiovale.* **(Right)** *Axial FLAIR MR in the same patient confirms abnormal T2 hyperintensity ➡ within the posterior centrum semiovale conforming to areas of acute diffusion diffusion restriction. Brain imaging was otherwise normal.*

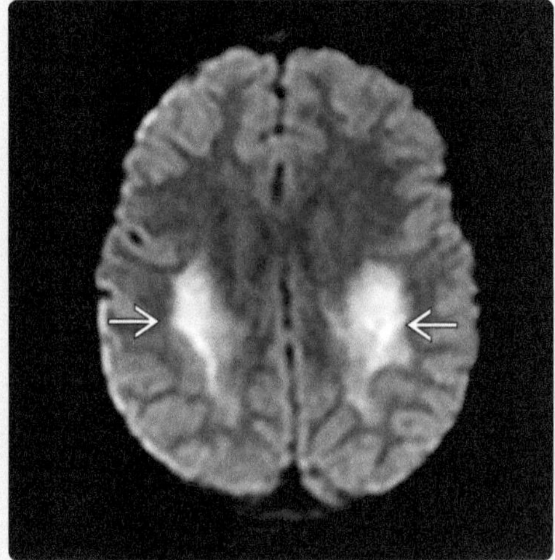

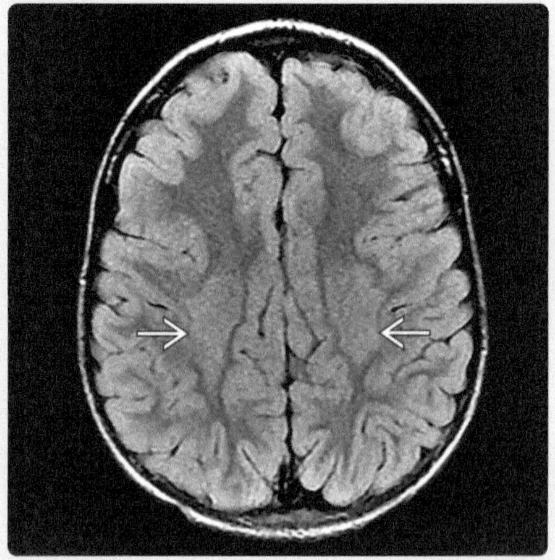

(Left) *Axial DWI MR 1 month later in the same patient shows resolution of acute diffusion restriction. Mild symmetric increased signal on ADC map (not shown) confirmed increased diffusivity.* **(Right)** *Axial FLAIR MR in the same patient for follow-up1 month later shows mild residua of abnormal T2 hyperintensity ➡ within the posterior centrum semiovale in clinical context of symptom resolution. Five years later, this patient presented with recurrent symptoms and imaging findings similar to the initial presentation.*

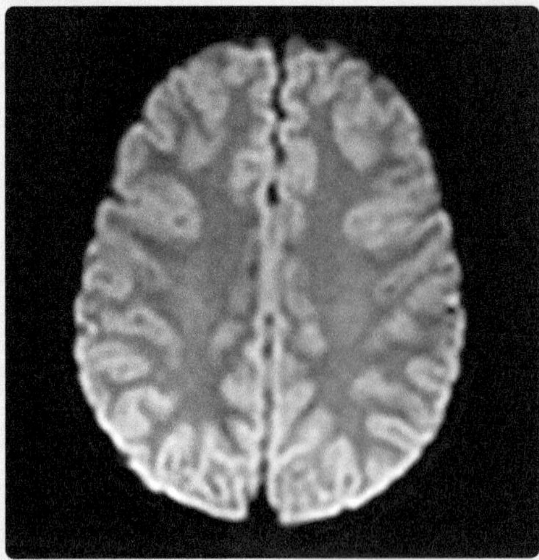

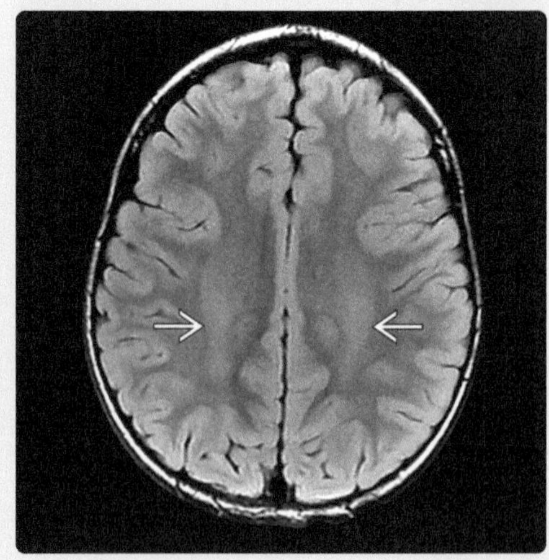

X-Linked Charcot-Marie-Tooth

TERMINOLOGY

Abbreviations

- X-linked Charcot-Marie-Tooth (CMTX)

Definitions

- X-linked hereditary peripheral sensory and motor neuropathy

IMAGING

General Features

- Best diagnostic clue
  - Initial presentation with symmetric posterior centrum semiovale T2-hyperintense lesions
  - Acute lesions show diffusion restriction
  - White matter lesions transient; improvement or complete resolution common
    - Subsequent lesion recurrence within same distribution highly suggestive of CMTX
- Location
  - Posterior centrum semiovale, corpus callosum splenium most common
  - Less commonly, may involve entire centrum semiovale

CT Findings

- NECT
  - Lesions normal (undetectable) to slightly hypodense

MR Findings

- T1WI
  - Lesions mildly hypointense or normal signal
- T2WI
  - Symmetric T2 hyperintensity in posterior centrum semiovale, splenium sparing subcortical U fibers
- DWI
  - Positive diffusion restriction during acute presentation
  - Restriction resolves with maturation of signal abnormality
- T1WI C+
  - No lesion enhancement

Imaging Recommendations

- Protocol advice
  - T2 MR and DWI MR essential for detection and characterization

DIFFERENTIAL DIAGNOSIS

Acute Disseminated Encephalomyelitis

- Monophasic clinical presentation (usually)
- Lesions multifocal, asymmetric, may involve U fibers, higher lesion load than CMT
- Frequent involvement of deep gray matter
- Variable peripheral enhancement

Multiple Sclerosis

- Polyphasic clinical presentation
- Asymmetric focal lesions with predilection for callosal-septal interface and posterior fossa
- Variable incomplete ring or peripheral enhancement

X-linked Adrenoleukodystrophy

- Rare metabolic disorder caused by peroxisomal enzyme failure → accumulation of very long chain fatty acid (VLCFA) in tissues and plasma
- X-linked, nearly always in boys
- Parietooccipital white matter lesions with edema, peripheral enhancement most common

PATHOLOGY

General Features

- Etiology
  - Most common type is CMTX type 1 (CMTX1), which arises from mutations in gap junction beta 1 gene (*GJB1*) on chromosome Xq13.1 coding for connexin-32
    - Gap junction protein expressed in Schwann cells and oligodendrocytes

CLINICAL ISSUES

Presentation

- Most common signs/symptoms
  - Acute transient encephalopathy
  - Transient motor weakness
  - Chronic distal extremity muscle weakness, atrophy
- Other signs/symptoms
  - Subclinical presentation with lesions detected on imaging
- Clinical profile
  - Chronic distal leg muscle wasting ± ankle flexion weakness, absent lower extremity deep-tendon reflexes, pes cavus foot deformity
  - Acute CNS symptoms/signs + peripheral neuropathy suggests CMTX

Natural History & Prognosis

- Gradual clinical progression, often into 2nd or 3rd decades
- Later presentation portends milder clinical course
- Brain lesions usually improve or resolve but may recur

Treatment

- Multidisciplinary supportive care to maintain mobility, prevent falls

DIAGNOSTIC CHECKLIST

Consider

- Consider CMTX in patients with characteristic peripheral neuropathy and CNS symptoms/signs ± recurrent white matter lesions

Image Interpretation Pearls

- Lesion symmetry and posterior centrum semiovale predilection suggest CMTX diagnosis

SELECTED REFERENCES

1. Karavasilis E et al: Structural and functional brain changes in X-linked Charcot-Marie-Tooth disease: insights from a multimodal neuroimaging study. Neuroradiology. 64(3):543-52, 2022
2. Liang Y et al: Recurrent episodes of reversible posterior leukoencephalopathy in three Chinese families with GJB1 mutations in X-linked Charcot-Marie-tooth type 1 disease: cases report. BMC Neurol. 19(1):325, 2019
3. Nishikura N et al: X-linked Charcot-Marie-Tooth disease type 5 with recurrent weakness after febrile illness. Brain Dev. 41(2):201-4, 2018

PKAN

KEY FACTS

TERMINOLOGY

- Pantothenate kinase-associated neurodegeneration (PKAN)
  - Pantothenate kinase 2 (*PANK2*) mutation
  - Most common form of neurodegeneration with brain iron accumulation (NBIA)

IMAGING

- Best diagnostic clue: Eye of tiger sign = diffuse pallidal T2 hypointensity with medial foci ↑ T2 signal
- Hyperintense "eye" may predate surrounding pallidal hypointensity

TOP DIFFERENTIAL DIAGNOSES

- Disorders with ↑ T2 signal globus pallidus
  - Metabolic: Methylmalonic acidemia, Kearns-Sayre, L-2-hydroxyglutaric aciduria, Canavan, neuroferritinopathy
  - Ischemic/toxic: Anoxic encephalopathy, carbon monoxide/cyanide poisoning, kernicterus

PATHOLOGY

- *PANK2* gene encodes mitochondrial-targeted pantothenate kinase 2, key enzyme in biosynthesis of coenzyme A (CoA)
- Progressive, physiologic brain iron accumulation occurs in globus pallidus, substantia nigra > red and dentate nuclei
- Basal ganglia and retina vulnerable to oxidative damage secondary to high metabolic demand
- Autosomal recessive (50% sporadic)

CLINICAL ISSUES

- Classic PKAN: Dystonia, dysarthria, rigidity, choreoathetosis in young child
- Atypical PKAN: Psychiatric, speech, pyramidal/extrapyramidal disturbances in older child/teenager

DIAGNOSTIC CHECKLIST

- Eye of tiger sign highly suggestive of PKAN

(Left) *Axial T2WI MR in a 5-year-old with a diagnosis of cerebral palsy demonstrates an eye of the tiger sign typical of PKAN: Symmetric areas of high T2 signal ➡ within the medial globus pallidus with surrounding pallidal hypointensity.* **(Right)** *Four years later, dystonia prompted repeat MR in the same patient. Axial T2WI MR shows that the "eyes" have diminished in size and intensity with greater surrounding pallidal hypointensity. Volume loss is now evident, particularly frontal.*

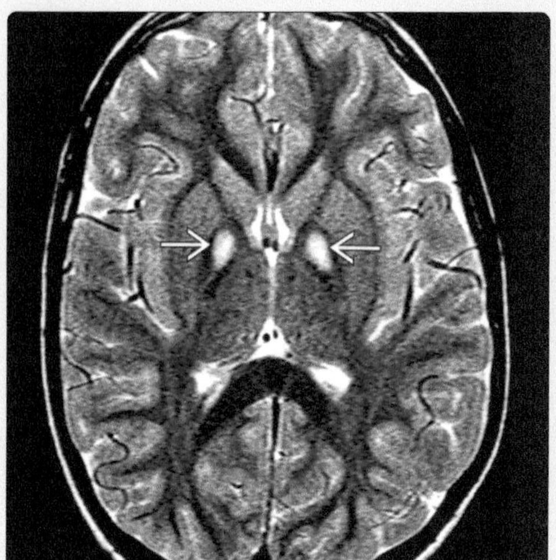

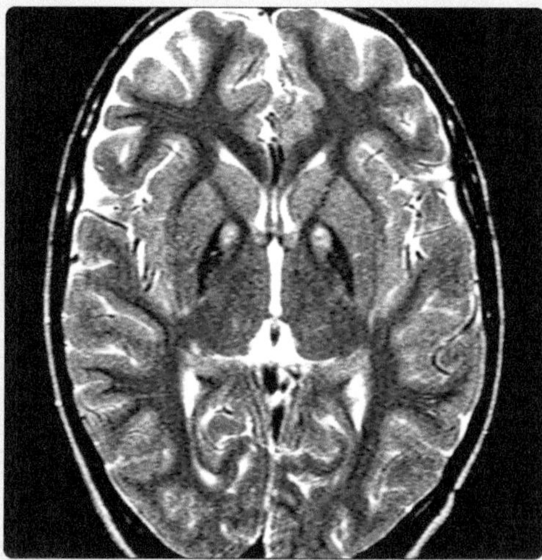

(Left) *Coronal T2WI MR of the same patient at 9 years of age shows abnormal hypointense signal in the globus pallidus ➡ and substantia nigra ⇨.* **(Right)** *Axial T2* GRE MR in the same patient at 9 years of age shows blooming of the hypointense signal in the globus pallidus secondary to the paramagnetic effect of iron. The findings in this patient are typical of the evolution of classic PKAN: Diminishing caliber of the "eye," increasing surrounding pallidal hypointensity, and progressive volume loss.*

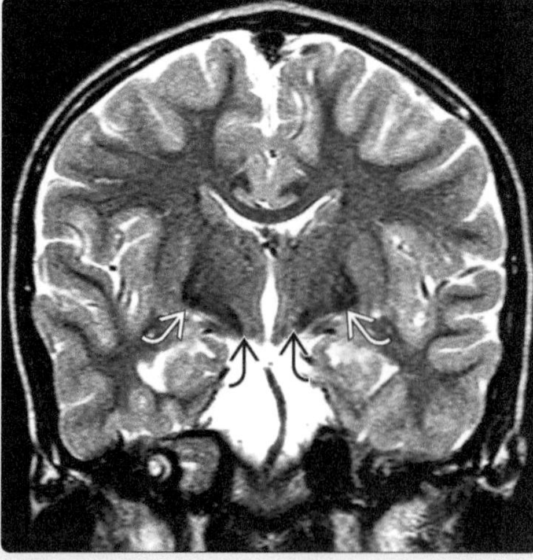

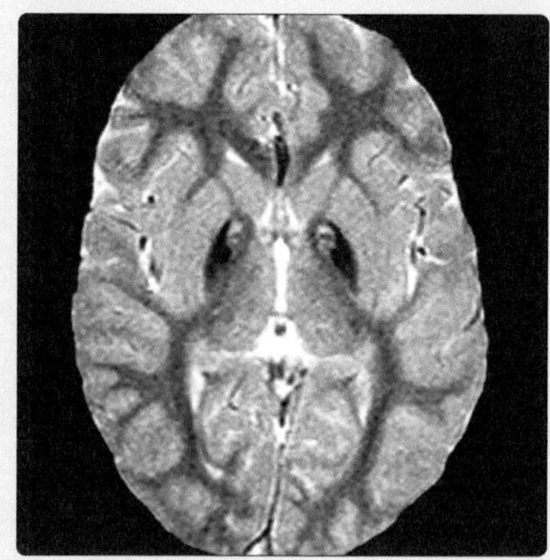

TERMINOLOGY

Abbreviations

- Pantothenate kinase-associated neurodegeneration (PKAN)

Synonyms

- Neurodegeneration with brain iron accumulation type 1 (NBIA-1)
- Hallervorden-Spatz syndrome (obsolete term)
  - PKAN and NBIA-1 = preferred terms

Definitions

- NBIA: Umbrella term for neurodegenerative disorders characterized by brain iron accumulation
  - Known causes include PKAN (most common), aceruloplasminemia, neuroferritinopathy, and infantile neuroaxonal dystrophy
- PKAN caused by mutation pantothenate kinase 2 gene (*PANK2*)

IMAGING

General Features

- Best diagnostic clue: Eye of tiger sign = diffuse pallidal T2 hypointensity with medial foci ↑ T2 signal
  - Highly suggestive of PKAN
  - Hyperintense "eye" may predate surrounding pallidal hypointensity
  - "Eye" caliber and intensity ↓ as disease progresses
  - Pallidal hypointensity increases as disease progresses
  - Eye of tiger sign has been described in neuroferritinopathy
- Variable ↓ T2 signal substantia nigra (SN) > > dentate nuclei (DN)
- Atrophy in advanced diseases
- Location: Globus pallidus (GP), SN, DN
- Morphology: Signal alteration of GP resembles tiger eyes
- Iron deposition (ferritin bound) responsible for T2-hypointense imaging appearance

CT Findings

- NECT: Variable; hypodense, hyperdense, normal GP
- CECT: No abnormal enhancement

MR Findings

- T1WI: Variable (ferritin bound iron has more T1 shortening than hemosiderin bound)
- T2WI
  - Eye of tiger sign = diffuse pallidal hypointensity with medial foci ↑ signal
  - Variable ↓ signal SN; more common in older patients
- FLAIR: "Eye" persists
- T2* GRE: ↓ T2 signal GP, SN "blooms" due to paramagnetic effect of iron
- SWI: Greater blooming artifact than T2* GRE
- T1WI C+: No abnormal enhancement
- MRS: ↓ NAA GP (neuronal loss)

Nuclear Medicine Findings

- Tc-99m SPECT: ↑ activity in medial GP
  - Possible chelation Tc-99m by pallidal cysteine

Imaging Recommendations

- Best imaging tool
  - Multiplanar MR with SWI
- Protocol advice
  - Consider SWI or T2* GRE sequence for mineralization
  - T2 hypointensity more conspicuous on spin-echo (vs. fast spin-echo) and high-field strength magnets

DIFFERENTIAL DIAGNOSIS

Disorders With ↑ T2 Signal Globus Pallidus

- Metabolic
  - Methylmalonic acidemia (MMA): ↑ T2 signal GP ± periventricular white matter (WM)
  - Kearns-Sayre/L-2-hydroxyglutaric aciduria: ↑ T2 GP (> other deep gray matter) and peripheral WM
  - Canavan: ↑ T2 GP (> other deep gray matter) and subcortical WM; macrocephaly; ↑ NAA
  - Neuroferritinopathy: Variable-sized foci ↑ T2 signal GP, putamen, caudate heads with ↓ T2 SN, DN; disease of adults
  - Guanidinoacetate methyltransferase deficiency (impairs creatine synthesis)
- Ischemic/toxic
  - Anoxic encephalopathy: ↑ T2 GP (and other deep gray matter) and cortex
  - Carbon monoxide poisoning: ↑ T2 GP (± other deep gray matter, cortex, WM)
  - Cyanide poisoning: ↑ T2 basal ganglia followed by hemorrhagic necrosis
  - Kernicterus: ↑ T2/T1 GP in neonate

PATHOLOGY

General Features

- Iron accumulation likely secondary phenomenon in PKAN
  - Serial MRs in patients with PKAN show hyperintense foci in GP predating surrounding hypointensity
- Embryology, anatomy
  - Progressive, physiologic brain iron accumulation occurs in GP, SN > red and DN
  - ↓ T2 signal GP identified in majority of normal patients by age 25 but < 10 years of age
- Genetics
  - Autosomal recessive (50% sporadic)
  - > 100 *PANK2* mutations Chr 20p12.3-p13 identified
    - Eye of tiger sign on MR highly correlative with *PANK2* mutation
    - *PANK2* gene encodes mitochondrial-targeted pantothenate kinase 2, key enzyme in biosynthesis of coenzyme A (CoA)
      - CoA essential to energy and fatty acid metabolism, among other functions
    - Null mutations are more common in early-onset, rapidly progressive disease
    - Missense mutations more common in late-onset, more slowly progressive disease
      - Suggests residual pantothenate kinase 2 activity in late-onset (less severe) disease
  - HARP: **H**ypoprebetalipoproteinemia, **a**canthocytosis, **r**etinitis pigmentosa, and **p**allidal degeneration

- Allelic with PKAN
- Prominent orofacial dystonia; early-onset parkinsonism
- Etiology
  - Leading theory
    - *PANK2* mutation → CoA deficiency → energy and lipid dyshomeostasis → production of oxygen-free radicals → phospholipid membrane destruction
    - Basal ganglia and retina vulnerable to oxidative damage secondary to high metabolic demand
  - Additional factors
    - Cysteine accumulation in GP secondary to ↓ phosphopantothenate causes iron chelation and peroxidative cell membrane damage
    - Axonal spheroids further compromise glial and neuronal function

Gross Pathologic & Surgical Features

- Symmetric, rust-brown pigmentation GP (interna > externa), and pars reticulata SN
  - In addition to iron, intra-/extraneuronal ceroid lipofuscin and melanin contribute to pigmentation
- Variable atrophy

Microscopic Features

- Classic features
  - ↑ iron GP interna and pars reticulata SN
    - Iron located in astrocytes, microglial cells, neurons, and around vessels
  - Neuronal loss, gliosis, and glial inclusions primarily involving GP interna and pars reticulata SN
  - Round or oval, nonnucleated, axonal swellings ("spheroids") in GP, SN, cortex, and brainstem
- Loose tissue (consisting of reactive astrocytes, dystrophic axons, and vacuoles in anteromedial GP) corresponds to "eye" in eye of tiger sign on MR
- Variably present acanthocytes (on blood smear)

CLINICAL ISSUES

Presentation

- Clinical classification into classic and atypical disease
  - Classic PKAN: Early-onset, more rapidly progressive disease, uniform phenotype
  - Atypical PKAN: Late-onset, more slowly progressive disease, heterogeneous phenotype
- Most common signs/symptoms
  - Classic PKAN: Dystonia
    - Other extrapyramidal signs/symptoms: Dysarthria, rigidity, choreoathetosis
    - Upper motor neuron signs/symptoms and cognitive decline are frequent
    - Pigmentary retinopathy (66%)
  - Atypical PKAN: Psychiatric and speech disturbances
    - Other signs/symptoms: Pyramidal/extrapyramidal disturbances (including freezing), dementia, seizures (10%)
- Clinical profile
  - Classic PKAN: Young child with gait, postural deficits
  - Atypical PKAN: Teenager with speech, psychiatric disturbance
- Normal serum and CSF iron levels
- Confirmatory *PANK2* mutation analysis should be performed in all suspected cases of PKAN

Demographics

- Age
  - Classic PKAN: Majority present < 6 years of age
  - Atypical PKAN: Mean age at presentation: 13 years
- Epidemiology: Rare; incidence unknown

Natural History & Prognosis

- Natural history
  - Classic PKAN: Rapid, nonuniform progression with periods of deterioration interspersed with stability, leading to early adulthood death
  - Atypical PKAN: More slowly progressive with loss of ambulation 15-40 years after disease onset
- Prognosis
  - Classic PKAN: Fatal; mean disease duration after symptom onset is 11 years
  - Atypical PKAN: Eventual severe impairment, ± death, adulthood

Treatment

- No curative treatment; iron chelation ineffective
- Palliative therapy
  - Baclofen, trihexyphenidyl frequently ineffective
  - Stereotactic pallidotomy
  - Subthalamic nucleus deep brain stimulation (STN-DBS)

DIAGNOSTIC CHECKLIST

Image Interpretation Pearls

- Eye of tiger sign highly suggestive of PKAN
- Physiologic GP hypointensity difficult to distinguish from pathologic hypointensity in teenager/adult

SELECTED REFERENCES

1. Emamikhah M et al: Seizure in neurodegeneration with brain iron accumulation: a systematic review. Can J Neurol Sci. 50(1):60-71, 2023
2. Kolarova H et al: Lifetime risk of autosomal recessive neurodegeneration with brain iron accumulation (NBIA) disorders calculated from genetic databases. EBioMedicine. 77:103869, 2022
3. Li H et al: Deep brain stimulation (DBS) with subthalamic nucleus (STN) as target for pediatric patients with PKAN. World Neurosurg. 163:e317-22, 2022
4. González Huerta LM et al: Psychiatric symptoms in an adolescent reveal a novel compound heterozygous mutation of the PANK2 gene in the atypical PKAN syndrome. Psychiatr Genet. 31(3):95-9, 2021
5. Chang X et al: Natural history and genotype-phenotype correlation of pantothenate kinase-associated neurodegeneration. CNS Neurosci Ther. 26(7):754-61, 2020
6. Zeng J et al: Magnetic resonance imaging, susceptibility weighted imaging and quantitative susceptibility mapping findings of pantothenate kinase-associated neurodegeneration. J Clin Neurosci. 59:20-8, 2019
7. Razmeh S et al: Pantothenate kinase-associated neurodegeneration: clinical aspects, diagnosis and treatments. Neurol Int. 10(1):7516, 2018
8. Sharma LK et al: A therapeutic approach to pantothenate kinase associated neurodegeneration. Nat Commun. 9(1):4399, 2018
9. Darling A et al: Clinical rating scale for pantothenate kinase-associated neurodegeneration: a pilot study. Mov Disord. 32(11):1620-30, 2017
10. Liu Z et al: Subthalamic nuclei stimulation in patients with pantothenate kinase-associated neurodegeneration (PKAN). Neuromodulation. 20(5):484-91, 2017
11. Arber C et al: Insights into molecular mechanisms of disease in neurodegeneration with brain iron accumulation; unifying theories. Neuropathol Appl Neurobiol. 42(3):220-41, 2016
12. Bosemani T et al: Susceptibility-weighted imaging in pantothenate kinase-associated neurodegeneration. J Pediatr. 164(1):212, 2014

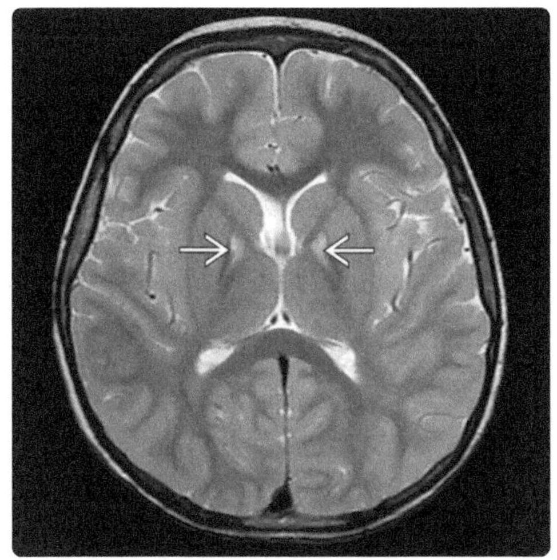

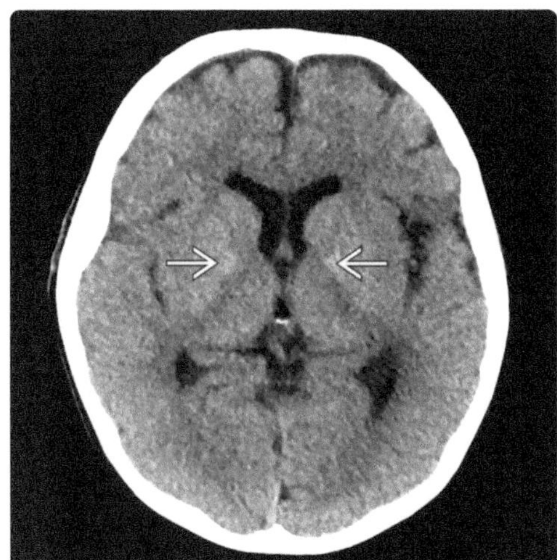

(Left) *Axial T2 MR in a 5-year-old patient with spastic gait reveals characteristic T2 hyperintensity surrounded by hypointense signal ➡ within the bilateral globi pallidi. This is the typical appearance of eye of the tiger in a younger patient. Genetic analysis confirmed PKAN.* **(Right)** *Axial NECT in the same PKAN patient confirms calcification with the bilateral globi pallidi ➡.*

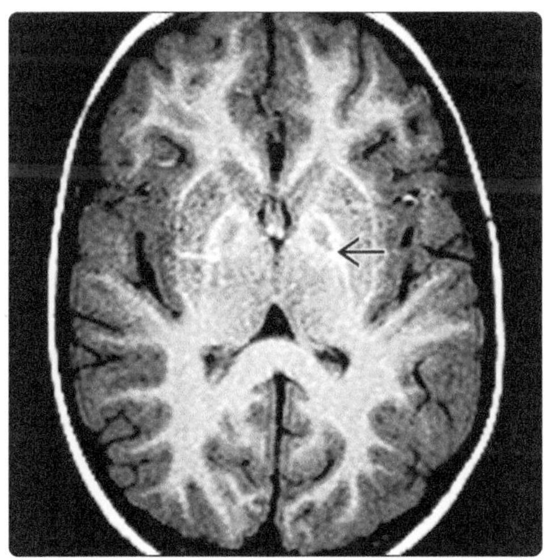

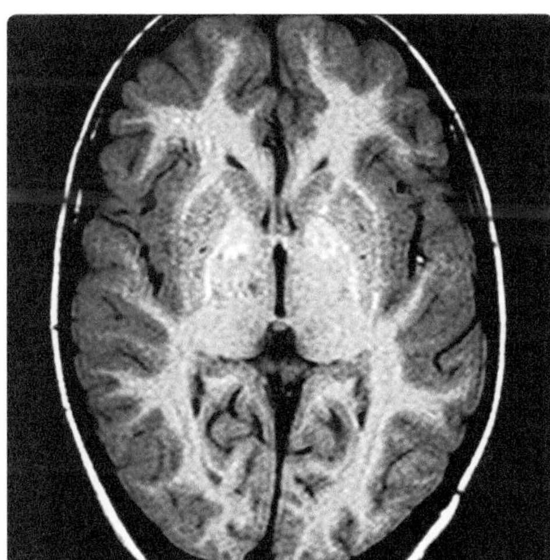

(Left) *Axial T1WI MR in a 5-year-old with classic PKAN shows that the "eye" in the eye of the tiger is hypointense with a few punctate areas of surrounding hyperintensity ➡.* **(Right)** *Axial T1WI MR in the same patient at 9 years of age shows the "eye" as mostly hyperintense. The appearance of the "eye" in eye of the tiger is variable depending on the stage of the disease. Progressive iron deposition within the globus pallidus likely accounts for greater T1 shortening seen in later disease.*

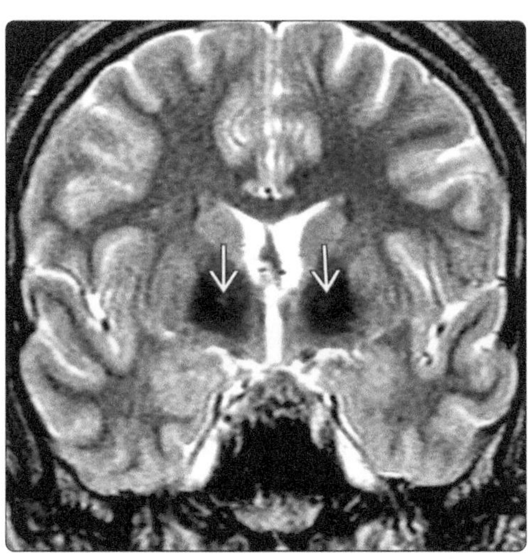

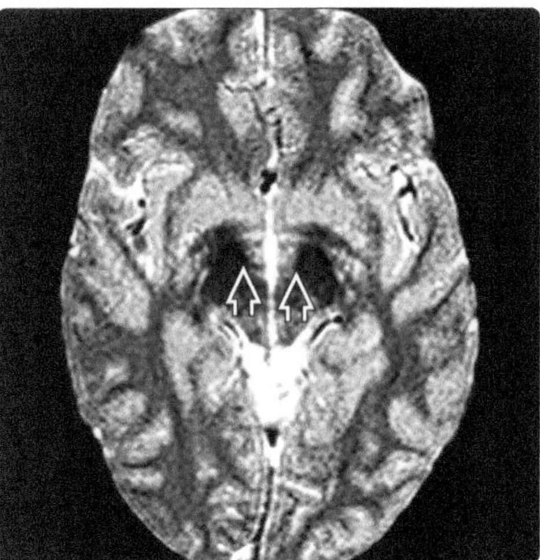

(Left) *Coronal T2WI MR in a patient with classic PKAN shows the classic eye of the tiger sign with small foci of increased T2 signal in the medial globi pallidi ➡ surrounded by abnormal pallidal hypointensity.* **(Right)** *Axial T2* GRE MR in a patient with classic PKAN shows blooming of hypointense signal in the inferior globus pallidus and substantia nigra ➡. Abnormal iron accumulation within the substantia nigra is more conspicuous on imaging as the disease progresses.*

KEY FACTS

TERMINOLOGY

- Huntington disease (HD): Autosomal dominant **CAG trinucleotide repeat** disease
  - Loss of GABAergic neurons of basal ganglia

IMAGING

- Diffuse cerebral atrophy
- Atrophy of caudate nucleus (CN) → frontal horns enlarged (**boxcar** appearance) → ↑ intercaudate distance (CC)
- **↑ CC:distance between inner tables of skull (IT) (bicaudate) ratio**: Most specific & sensitive for HD
- ↑ T2 signal in CN, putamina in juvenile HD
- SWI hypointensity suggesting striatal iron accumulation
  - Sometimes in midbrain red nucleus & substantia nigra pars reticularis & globus pallidus (GP) also
- ↓ FDG uptake in basal ganglia before any detectable atrophy ± frontal lobe hypometabolism
- Atrophy of CN, putamen, & (lesser degree) GP
- Diffuse cerebral atrophy, may be frontal predominant

TOP DIFFERENTIAL DIAGNOSES

- Neuroacanthocytosis; Leigh disease; Wilson disease
- Pantothenate kinase-associated neurodegeneration (formerly called Hallervorden-Spatz)
- Carbon monoxide poisoning
- Frontotemporal lobar degeneration with fused in sarcoma protein, multiple system atrophy (MSA), etc., in adults

PATHOLOGY

- Autosomal dominant with complete penetrance
- CAG trinucleotide repeat disease affecting HD gene on chromosome 4p16.3

CLINICAL ISSUES

- **Triad**: Early-onset dementia, choreoathetosis, psychosis

DIAGNOSTIC CHECKLIST

- Caudate atrophy main radiologic feature of HD
- Consider HD in child with ↑ T2 signal in CN/putamina

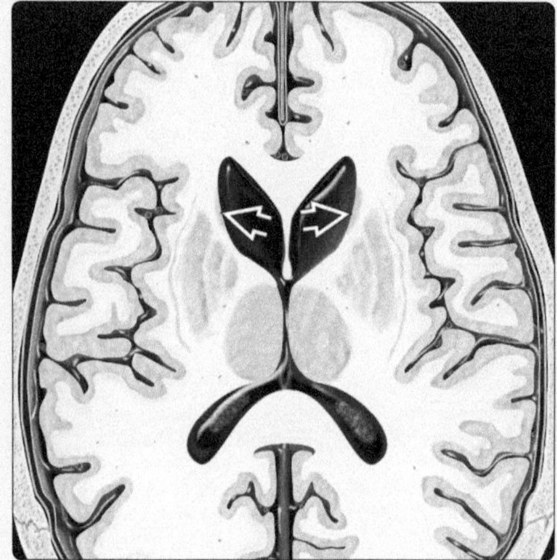

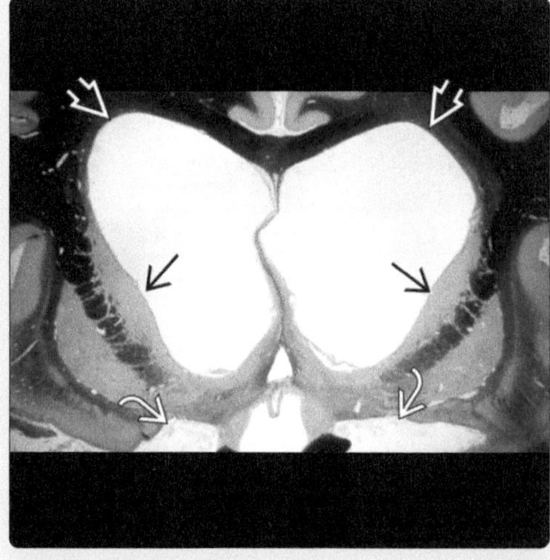

(Left) *Axial graphic shows the convex margins of the frontal horns ➡ (boxcar appearance) due to atrophy of the heads of the caudate nuclei in Huntington disease.* **(Right)** *Autopsy specimen sectioned in the coronal plane shows enlarged lateral ventricles ➡ and basal cisterns ➡. Both caudate nuclei ➡ appear thinned and atrophic. Note that the lateral borders of the frontal horns are straightened due to loss of normal convexity of the caudate heads.*

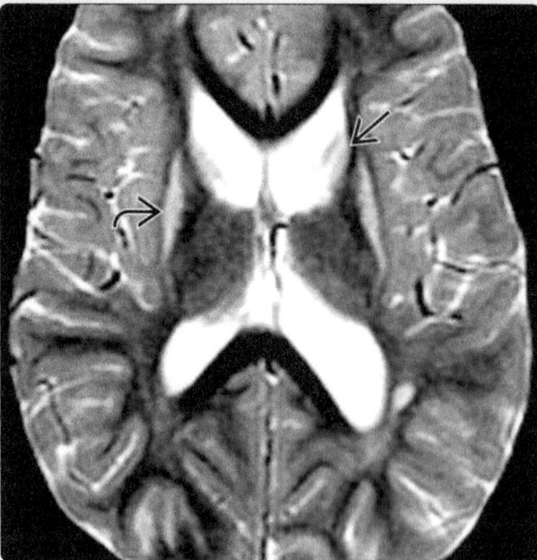

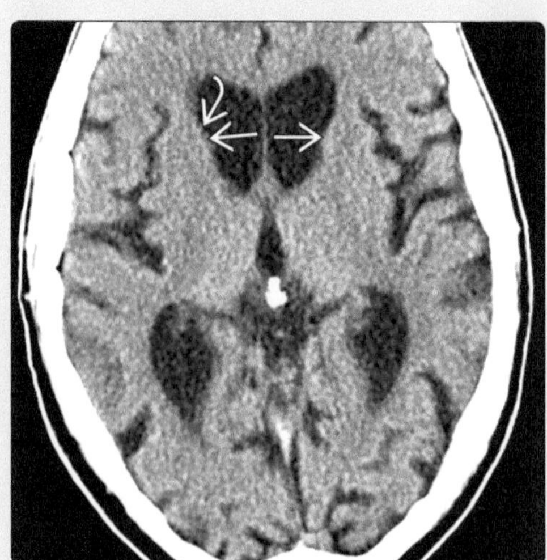

(Left) *Axial T2WI MR in a patient with juvenile Huntington disease shows generalized volume loss and striking atrophy and hyperintensity ➡ of both caudate heads. The frontal horns of the lateral ventricles are enlarged, and there is atrophy and hyperintensity in the putamina ➡.* **(Right)** *Axial NECT in Huntington disease shows generalized atrophy. The frontal horns are enlarged with a loss of normal concavity ➡ due to caudate head atrophy. Note the increased intercaudate distance ➡.*

TERMINOLOGY

Abbreviations

- Huntington disease (HD)

Synonyms

- Huntington chorea

Definitions

- Autosomal dominant neurodegenerative disease
  - Loss of GABAergic neurons of basal ganglia (BG)
- **Clinical triad**: Early-onset dementia, choreoathetosis, psychosis

IMAGING

General Features

- Best diagnostic clue
  - Atrophy of caudate nucleus (CN) → frontal horns (FH) enlarged (boxcar appearance)
- Location
  - Primarily striatum (especially CN, putamen)
  - Cerebral cortex, globus pallidus (GP), thalamus
  - Substantia nigra (SN), brainstem
  - Juvenile HD: GP, cerebellum may be involved
- Morphology
  - Loss of convex surface of caudate head

CT Findings

- NECT
  - Atrophy of CN, putamen, & (lesser degree) GP
  - Compensatory enlargement of FH of lateral ventricles
  - Diffuse cerebral atrophy (reported to be predominantly frontal in some studies)
  - CN atrophy is measured on axial images at level of 3rd ventricle
    - ↑ **intercaudate distance (CC)** between medial aspects of CN
    - CC can be compared with **distance between inner tables (IT)** of skull (CC:IT ratio)
    - In HD, CC is typically > 20 mm & often > 25 mm (compared to 10-14 mm in normal individuals)
    - **CC:IT (bicaudate) ratio** ↑ in HD; considered most specific & sensitive HD measurement
    - In HD, CC:IT ratio usually ranges from 0.175-0.185 compared to ~ 0.12 in normal individuals
    - CC compared with **distance across lateral margins of FH** provides FH:CC ratio
    - In HD, **FH:CC ratio** typically ranges from 1.3-1.8 compared to 2.3-2.8 in normal individuals
- CECT
  - No contrast enhancement of affected structures

MR Findings

- T1WI
  - Shrinkage of CN & ↑ CC
  - MR measurements: ↓ volume in all BG structures
    - Reported even in presymptomatic stage of HD
  - Diffuse cerebral atrophy
  - Selective hippocampal subfields perforant-pathway atrophy in presubiculum, subiculum, dentate gyrus, tail, right molecular layer
- T2WI
  - Hyperintense signal in CN & putamina in juvenile HD
    - Related to gliosis
  - Shrinkage of CN; ↑ CC
  - Striatum may have ↓ signal due to iron deposition
- T2* GRE
  - SWI hypointensity suggests striatal iron accumulation
    - Sometimes seen in midbrain red nucleus & SN pars reticularis & GP margins also
  - Predominantly rim hypointensities of BG may be seen
- MRS
  - ↑ lactate concentration in occipital cortex of symptomatic HD, also in BG in some patients
  - ↓ NAA:creatine ratio in BG (neuronal loss)
  - ↑ ↑ choline:creatine ratio in BG due to gliosis

Nuclear Medicine Findings

- PET
  - ↓ FDG uptake in BG precedes detectable atrophy
  - ± frontal lobe hypometabolism
- SPECT: Perfusion defects in motor cortex, prefrontal cortex, & BG correlate with clinical disease

Imaging Recommendations

- Best imaging tool
  - MR
- Protocol advice
  - T2WI

DIFFERENTIAL DIAGNOSIS

Neuroacanthocytosis

- Atrophy of CN heads with dilation of FH of lateral ventricles
- Chorea, orolingual dyskinesia, acanthocytosis in peripheral blood smear, ↑ serum creatine kinase

Leigh Disease

- Onset usually < 2 years old, but juvenile/adult forms exist
- Changes in putamen, CN, & tegmentum
  - T1 hypointensities, T2 hyperintensities (infarcts)
- Focal involvement of white matter, thalamus, brainstem, & cerebellum

Wilson Disease

- Rigidity, tremor, dystonia, gait difficulty, dysarthria
- Symmetrical T2 hyperintensity with irregular internal hypointense foci in putamina, CN
  - Putamen: ↑ T2 laminar appearance/peripheral rim
  - Rarely GP, thalami, asymmetrical frontal white matter
  - BG can be hypointense due to ↑ iron (rather than copper); better seen in SWI
- Atrophy of CN & brainstem on CT, MR
- Double panda sign: Axial T2 MR midbrain face of giant panda & midbrain-pons junction face of miniature panda

Pantothenate Kinase-Associated Neurodegeneration

- Type of neurodegeneration with brain iron accumulation (NBIA); formerly called Hallervorden-Spatz
- Involuntary movements (choreoathetosis), spasticity
- Progressive dementia in young adults
- Characteristic iron deposition in GP, red nuclei, SN

- Eye of tiger sign: Central high signal in T2-dark GP
- GP atrophy, ± cortical, CN atrophy

Carbon Monoxide Poisoning

- Bilateral CT hypodensity, T2 hyperintensity in GP

Other Neurodegenerative Disorders, Adults

- Multiple system atrophy
- Corticobasal degeneration
- **Frontotemporal lobar degeneration with fused in sarcoma protein (FTLD-FUS)**
  - Caudate head atrophy with enlarged FH
  - Caudate involvement more prominent in FTLD-FUS & FTLD-tau than in FTLD-TDP

PATHOLOGY

General Features

- Etiology
  - Polyglutamine expansion → huntingtin (HTT) fragments accumulate in nucleus; cytoplasm → aggregates in axonal terminals
- Genetics
  - Autosomal dominant with complete penetrance
  - CAG trinucleotide repeat disease affecting HD gene on chromosome 4p16.3
  - Genetic anticipation: ↑ severity or ↓ age of onset in successive generations
    - More commonly in paternal transmission of mutated allele
  - Homozygosity for HD mutation (very rare)
    - Associated with more severe clinical course

Staging, Grading, & Classification

- Based on gross striatal pathology, neuronal loss, gliosis
- Grade 0: Normal gross, histologic examination
- Grade 1: No gross striatal atrophy (only histologic changes)
- Grade 2: Striatal atrophy, convex CN
- Grade 3: More severe striatal atrophy, flat CN
- Grade 4: Most severe striatal atrophy, concave CN

Gross Pathologic & Surgical Features

- Diffuse cerebral atrophy (marked in CN, putamen)
- Juvenile HD: Involvement of GP, cerebellum (typically not involved in adults)

Microscopic Features

- Neuropathologic hallmarks of HD
  - Intranuclear inclusions containing huntingtin protein
  - Perinuclear aggregates in cortex, striatum
- Histochemistry may show ↑ iron in CN, putamen

CLINICAL ISSUES

Presentation

- Most common signs/symptoms
  - Classic triad: Choreoathetosis, dementia of subcortical type, & behavioral changes/psychosis
  - Memory impairment due to selective hippocampal subfields perforant-pathway atrophy
- Clinical profile
  - Pathognomonic feature of HD: Movement disorder
    - Chorea: Often facial twitching or writhing & twitching of distal extremities; ballism later on
    - Impaired gait ("dancing" gait)
    - Rigidity & dystonia in later stages (adult HD)
  - Juvenile HD: Rigidity > chorea
    - Rigidity & dystonia may occur as initial symptoms
    - Cerebellar signs, dyslalia, rapid cognitive decline
    - Seizures, parkinsonism, dystonia, long-tract signs

Demographics

- Age
  - Mean age at onset: 35-44 years in adult-onset HD
  - Juvenile HD (5-10% of cases): Onset at < 20 years
- Sex
  - M = F; sex-related factor affecting disease onset
    - Earlier onset, faster progression of HD in offspring of male patients
    - 70% of juvenile cases have affected father
- Ethnicity
  - Less common in African/Asian populations
- Epidemiology
  - Worldwide prevalence: 5-10/100,000 people
  - 3-7/100,000 in populations of Western European descent

Natural History & Prognosis

- Early symptoms: Personality changes & subtle movement disturbances
- Progression to choreoathetosis & dementia
- Behavioral disorganization, depression, suicidal behavior, psychotic features (visual hallucinations)
- Adult HD: Progressive deterioration until death 15-20 years after onset
- Higher degree of volume loss ↔ earlier age of onset
- Juvenile HD: More progressive clinical course
  - Average survival: 7-8 years after onset

Treatment

- Antidepressants, high-potency antipsychotics
- Tetrabenazine (dopamine depleters)
- Antiglutamatergic drugs (amantadine, memantine, riluzole)
- Ubiquinone (coenzyme Q10) → normalization of lactate levels in cortex & striatum
- Bilateral neural transplantation
- Experimental: Grafting of trophic factor-producing cell lines

DIAGNOSTIC CHECKLIST

Consider

- Reversible dementias & movement disorders

Image Interpretation Pearls

- Caudate atrophy main radiologic feature of HD
  - Bicaudate diameter: Sensitive for CN atrophy
- Decline in size of GP, putamen correlates with disease progression
- Consider HD in child with ↑ T2 signal in CN/putamina

SELECTED REFERENCES

1. Wibawa P et al: Selective perforant-pathway atrophy in Huntington disease: MRI analysis of hippocampal subfields. Eur J Neurol. 30(9):2650-60, 2023

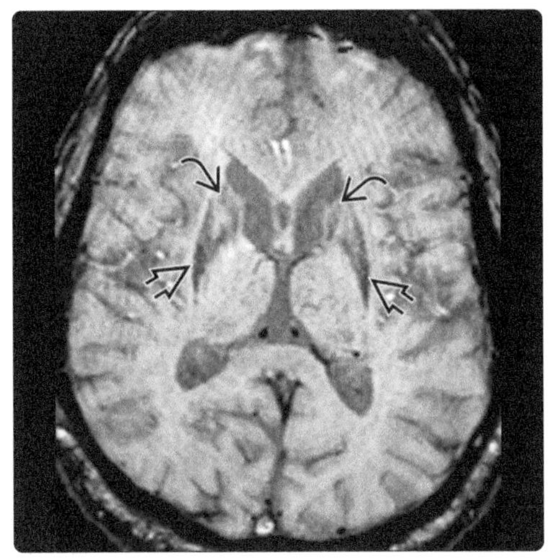

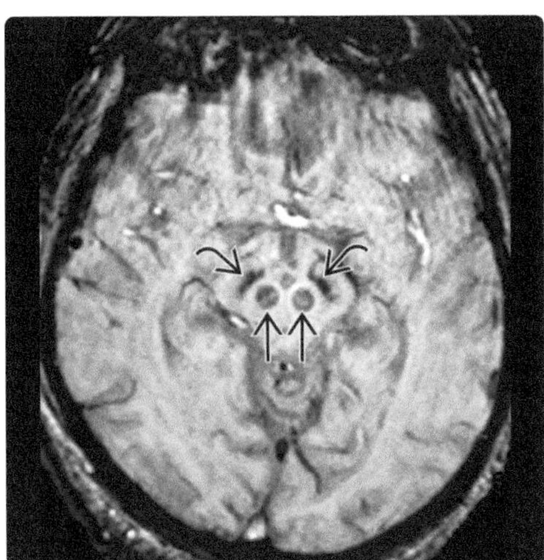

(Left) *Axial SWI MR in a patient with Huntington disease shows exaggerated hypointensities, suggesting excess iron deposition in the caudate heads ➲ and posterolateral putamina ➲. Note mild caudate atrophy.* **(Right)** *Axial SWI MR through the upper midbrain in the same patient shows increased iron deposition in the pars reticularis of the substantia nigra ➲ and red nuclei ➔ bilaterally. Neurodegeneration with brain iron accumulation (NBIA) is in the differential diagnosis with this MR pattern.*

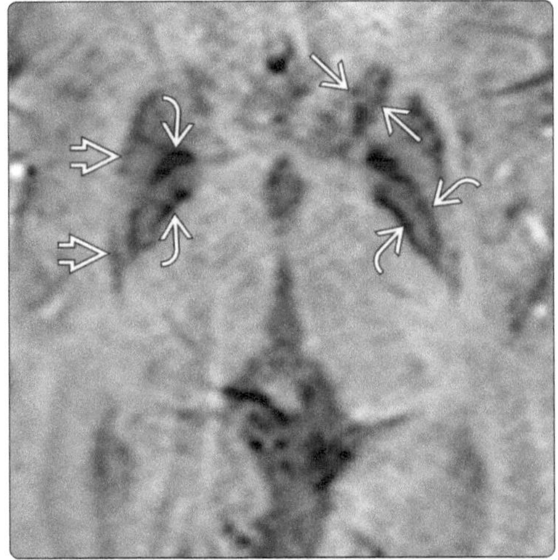

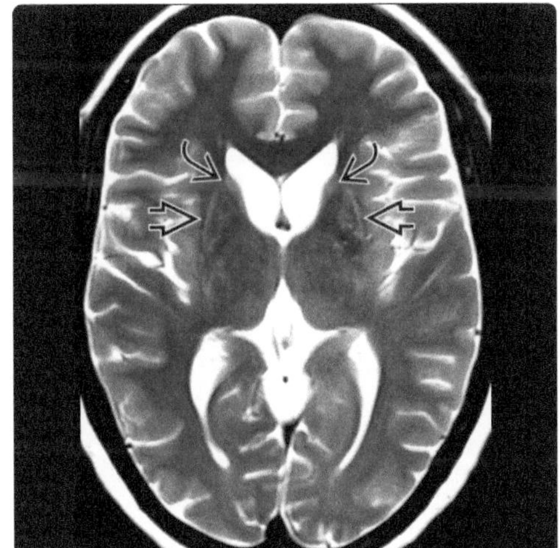

(Left) *Axial SWI MR in another patient with Huntington disease shows rim hypointensities around the globi pallidi ➲. Also note the marginal hypointensities surrounding caudate nuclei ➔ and putamina ➲. Pars reticularis of substantia nigra demonstrated solid hypointensity (not shown).* **(Right)** *Axial T2WI MR in a patient with Huntington disease shows bilateral mild caudate head and putaminal atrophy with T2-hyperintense abnormal signal in the caudate heads ➲ and lateral putamina ➲.*

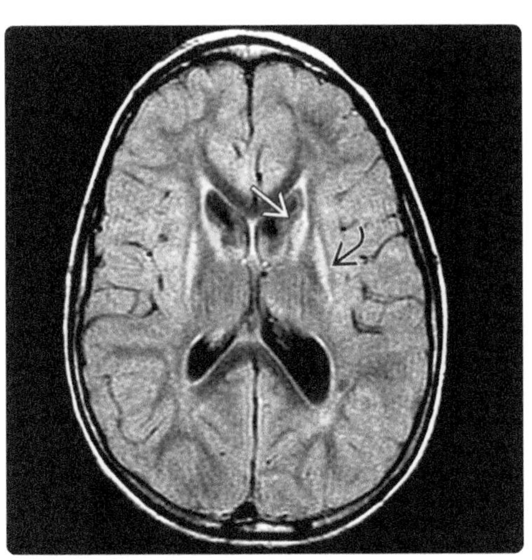

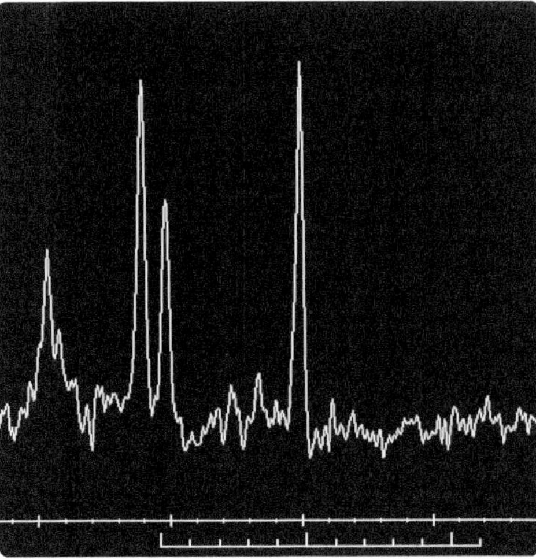

(Left) *Axial FLAIR MR in an 8-year-old with dysarthria, rigidity, and a family history of Huntington disease demonstrates a combination of volume loss and increased signal intensity of the caudate heads ➔ and putamina ➲.* **(Right)** *MRS (TR of 144) in the same patient demonstrates abnormal increased choline to creatine peak. Differential diagnosis would include mitochondrial disorders, such as Leigh syndrome. No lactate doublet and a positive family history of Huntington disease favors Huntington disease over Leigh syndrome.*

Wilson Disease

KEY FACTS

TERMINOLOGY

- Wilson disease (WD), hepatolenticular degeneration
- Autosomal recessive inherited copper (Cu) metabolism disorder characterized by
  - Abnormal accumulation of Cu in various tissues
  - Particularly in liver and brain [basal ganglia (BG)]

IMAGING

- Usually normal MR in presymptomatic patients
- Signal intensity improvement correlated with clinical response to Cu-chelating therapy
- Symmetric T2 hyper-/mixed intensity in putamina (with T2-hyperintense putaminal peripheral rim/laminar appearance), caudate nuclei, thalami, and globus pallidi (GP)
- **Double panda sign**: Axial T2 MR midbrain face of **giant** panda and midbrain-pons junction face of **miniature** panda

TOP DIFFERENTIAL DIAGNOSES

- Leigh disease
- Hypoxic-ischemic encephalopathy
- Creutzfeldt-Jakob disease
- Japanese encephalitis
- Organic aciduria

PATHOLOGY

- Brain lesions caused by accumulation of Cu, chronic ischemia, vasculopathy, or demyelination

CLINICAL ISSUES

- Kayser-Fleischer ring in cornea
- Neurologic: Asymmetric tremor, ataxia, dyskinesia, dysarthria, dystonia (mainly face), incoordination
  - Chelation therapy prevents progression

DIAGNOSTIC CHECKLIST

- T2 hyperintensity in striatum with neurologic dysfunction
- T1 hyperintensity in BG with hepatic dysfunction
- T1WI abnormal signal resolution correlated with clinical recovery post treatment, but T2WI signal changes variable

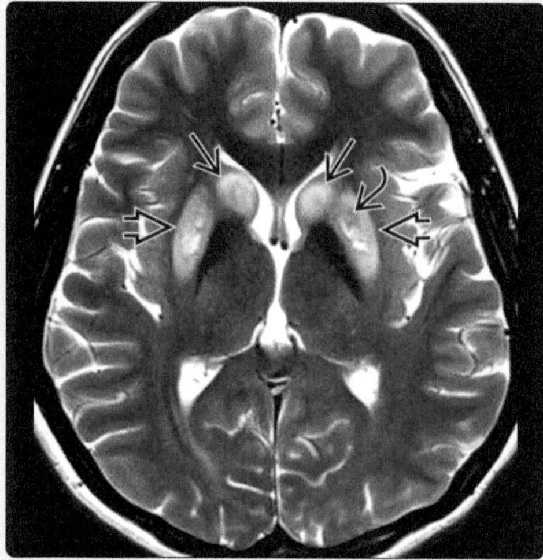
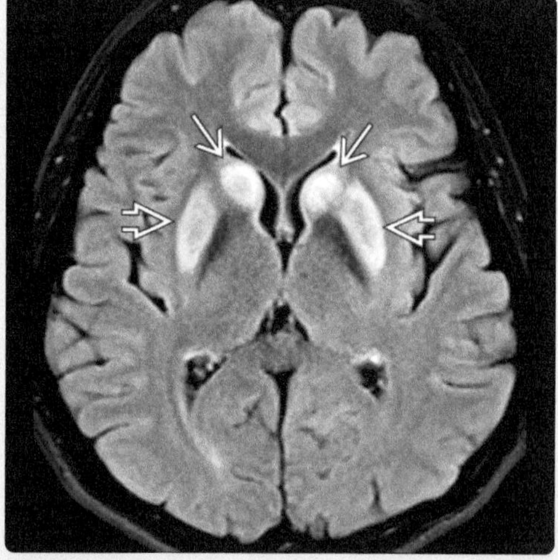

(Left) *Axial T2WI MR in a patient with Wilson disease shows hyperintensity in the bilateral caudate heads ➙ and putamina ➯ with areas of tiny hypointensities ➚. T2 hyperintensities could represent mineral deposition. Note that the globi pallidi and thalami are spared in this case.* **(Right)** *Axial FLAIR MR in the same patient also shows the bilateral caudate heads ➙ and putaminal ➯ hyperintensities.*

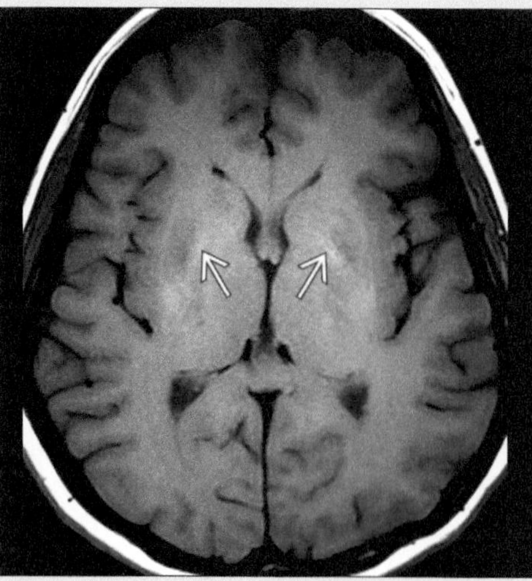
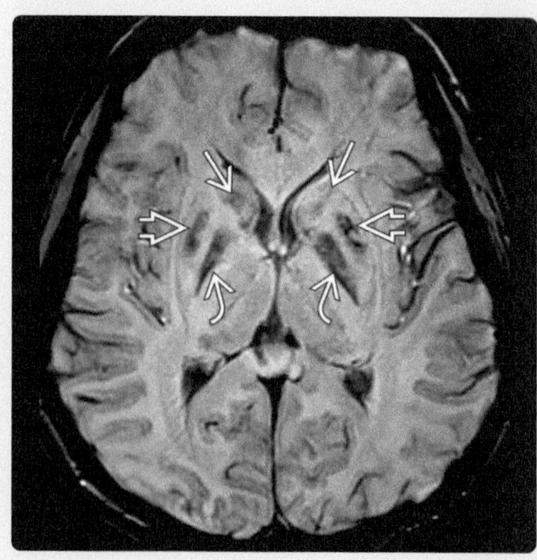

(Left) *Axial T1WI MR in the same patient shows subtle basal ganglia hyperintensities ➙, which could be due to paramagnetic effects of copper.* **(Right)** *Axial SWI MR in the same patient shows hypointensities in the caudate heads ➙ and putamina ➯. This suggests an effect of excess iron rather than copper deposition as based on evidence from SWI research studies. The globi pallidi ➚, which were unremarkable on T2/FLAIR MR, also show increased iron deposition on SWI.*

TERMINOLOGY

Abbreviations

- Wilson disease (WD)

Synonyms

- Progressive hepatolenticular degeneration

Definitions

- Autosomal recessive copper (Cu) metabolism disorder with abnormal accumulation of Cu in various tissues

IMAGING

General Features

- Best diagnostic clue
  - Symmetric T2 hyperintensity or mixed intensity in putamina, caudate nuclei, thalami, and globi pallidi (GP)
  - Clinical response to Cu-chelating therapy may correlate with improvement in signal abnormalities
  - Recent brain MR study with neurologic improvement after liver transplantation in pediatric WD
    - Resolution of T1 hyperintensities
    - Resolution, improvement, or stabilization of T2 signal
- Location
  - Most common: Putamen (predilection for outer rim)
  - Caudate nuclei, GP, thalami (ventrolateral nuclei)
  - Midbrain, pons, cerebellum (vermis and dentate nucleus)
  - Cortical and subcortical lesions (mostly frontal lobe)
- Size
  - Initially swelling, especially in basal ganglia (BG); later, widespread atrophy most pronounced in central structures
  - **Putaminal atrophy** negatively correlates with Unified WD Rating Scale score and can be used as surrogate imaging marker of neurologic clinical severity

CT Findings

- NECT
  - Widening of frontal horns of lateral ventricles; diffuse brain atrophy
  - ± hypodensity in lentiform nuclei and thalami
- CECT
  - Lesions do not contrast enhance

MR Findings

- T1WI
  - T1 signal generally reduced in BG
  - Signal intensity may ↑ in affected BG (paramagnetic effects of Cu)
- T2WI
  - Usually, normal MR in presymptomatic patients
  - Hyper-/hypo-/mixed intensity in putamen, GP, caudate, thalamus
    - Bilateral symmetric concentric-laminar T2 putaminal hyperintensity
    - BG can be hypointense due to ↑ iron (rather than Cu); better seen in SWI
  - **Upper midbrain**: Characteristic **face of giant panda sign**
    - Normal signal intensity in red nuclei and lateral portion of pars reticulata of substantia nigra
    - Against background of hyperintense signal in tegmentum and hypointensity of superior colliculus
  - **Midbrain-upper dorsal pons junction** (pontine tegmentum): **Face of miniature panda sign**
    - Hypointensity of medial longitudinal fasciculi and central tegmental tracts (eyes of miniature panda)
    - Against background of aqueductal CSF hyperintensity opening into 4th ventricle (nose and mouth)
      - Bordered inferiorly by superior medullary velum
    - Hyperintense superior cerebellar peduncles (cheeks)
  - **Double panda sign**: Midbrain giant panda and pontine miniature panda faces seen in same MR
  - **Central pons**: Central pontine myelinolysis-like T2 hyperintensities with 3 distinct patterns described
    - (1) Characteristic round central pontine hyperintensity
    - (2) Bisected hypointensity within it
    - (3) Trisected hypointensity within it (**trident sign** or **Mercedes-Benz sign)**
  - ± hyperintensity in callosal splenium, periaqueductal gray matter (GM), pontine tegmentum (dorsal pons)
  - ± medulla oblongata, **dentate nucleus**, and cerebral and cerebellar white matter (WM), especially **frontal lobe**
  - In adults, BG lesions may differ from those in children
    - Putaminal lesions may be absent; GP and substantia nigra may be hypointense on T2WI
- PD/intermediate
  - Symmetric high signal intensity in affected BG
- DWI
  - Diffusion restriction with abnormally low ADC values immediately after onset of neurologic symptoms
    - Subsequently high ADC values
- T1WI C+
  - No contrast enhancement typically
- MRS
  - ↓ N-acetylaspartate:creatine ratio (neuronal loss) in BG, parietooccipital cortex, frontal WM
  - ↓ myoinositol:creatine ratio in BG and ↓ choline:creatine ratio in GP
  - ↓ myoinositol:creatine ratio in WD with portosystemic shunting (pattern of hepatic encephalopathy)

Nuclear Medicine Findings

- PET
  - ↓ ↓ glucose metabolism in cerebellum, striatum, and, to lesser extent, in cortex and thalamus
  - ↓ ↓ dopa-decarboxylase activity (impaired nigrostriatal dopaminergic pathway)
- SPECT
  - (I-123)2β-carbomethoxy-3β-(4(I-123)iodophenyl)tropane binds to presynaptic striatal dopamine carriers
  - (I-123)iodobenzamide binds to postsynaptic striatal dopamine D2R
  - In symptomatic WD patients, ↓ ↓ striatal binding ratios of both tracers
  - In all WD cases, highly correlated binding ratios of both tracers corresponding to severity of neurologic features

Imaging Recommendations

- Best imaging tool: MR more sensitive than CT for detection of early lesions
- Protocol advice: T2WI, FLAIR, DWI

DIFFERENTIAL DIAGNOSIS

Leigh Disease

- Subacute necrotizing encephalomyelopathy
- Symmetric spongiform brain lesions with onset in infancy/early childhood
- Lesions predominantly bilateral and symmetric, in brainstem, BG (particularly putamen)

Hypoxic-Ischemic Encephalopathy

- Bilateral symmetric hyperintense lesions with restricted diffusion in putamen, caudate, thalamus, and cortex

Creutzfeldt-Jakob Disease

- Progressively hyperintense changes in BG, thalamus, and cerebral cortices on T2WI

Japanese Encephalitis

- Homogeneous T2 hyperintensities in BG and posteromedial thalami (usually ventrolateral nuclei in WD)

Organic Aciduria

- Symmetric diffuse WM changes, wide CSF spaces
- BG changes (↑ T2 signal ± volume loss in caudate &/or lentiform nuclei)

Methanol Poisoning

- Bilateral symmetric ↑ T2 signal in putamen, caudate ± WM

Osmotic Demyelination Syndrome

- Involvement of central pons, BG, and, rarely, midbrain

PATHOLOGY

General Features

- Etiology
  - Defective incorporation of Cu into ceruloplasmin and impaired biliary Cu excretion
  - Brain lesions caused by accumulation of Cu, chronic ischemia, vasculopathy, or demyelination
- Genetics
  - ATPase Cu transporting β-polypeptide (*ATP7B*) gene on chromosome 13q14.3-q21.1; autosomal recessive

Staging, Grading, & Classification

- Stage 1: Initial period of accumulation of Cu by hepatic binding sites
- Stage 2: Acute redistribution of Cu within liver and release into circulation
- Stage 3: Chronic accumulation of Cu in brain and other extrahepatic tissues

Gross Pathologic & Surgical Features

- Ventricular enlargement, sulcal widening

Microscopic Features

- Edema, necrosis, and spongiform degeneration of BG; gliosis and demyelination in WM
- Opalski cells = PAS (+) altered glial cells
- Deep pyramidal cell layers of cerebral cortex involved

CLINICAL ISSUES

Presentation

- Most common signs/symptoms
  - Neurologic: Asymmetric tremor, ataxia, incoordination, dyskinesia, dysarthria, dystonia (mainly facial)
    - Parkinsonian: Rigidity, bradykinesia
  - Psychiatric: Hyperkinetic, irritable, emotionally labile, mania, psychosis, depression, ↓ concentration
  - Seizures in patients with MR showing more subcortical and cortical lesions, severe dystonia, and higher serum-free Cu
  - Acute hepatitis
  - Kayser-Fleischer ring in cornea due to abnormal Cu accumulation in Descemet membrane
- Clinical profile
  - 40-50% of patients present with liver disease
  - 40-50% of patients present with neurologic or psychiatric symptoms (corneal rings almost always present)
  - ↓ ceruloplasmin and total serum Cu levels, ↑ 24-hour urinary Cu excretion, and ↑ ↑ hepatic Cu content

Demographics

- Age
  - Onset of liver disease usually at age 8-16 years
  - Neurologic symptoms often 1st recognized in 2nd-3rd decade (rarely, age < 12 years)
- Sex
  - Generally, M = F, but M:F = 1:4 for fulminant WD, i.e., liver failure, encephalopathy, coagulopathy
- Epidemiology
  - Prevalence: 1 in 30,000-40,000
  - Carrier frequency in USA: 1 in 90

Natural History & Prognosis

- Children: Liver disease most common presentation
- Older individuals: Neuropsychiatric symptoms
  - ↑ symptom severity with ↑ brain Cu deposition
- Once symptomatic, WD is fatal if untreated; 70% mortality for patients with fulminant liver failure
- Good prognosis with early chelation treatment
  - Prevents progression; may improve symptoms
- Best prognosis: Treated asymptomatic siblings

Treatment

- Restriction of food abundant in Cu (e.g., chocolate, liver, nuts, mushrooms, shellfish)
- Early administration of chelating therapy can ↓ brain damage
  - Penicillamine (side effect of initial neurologic deterioration in 20-50%)
  - Trientine (better alternative chelator), ammonium tetrathiomolybdate, zinc
- Liver transplant (for severe hepatic decompensation)

DIAGNOSTIC CHECKLIST

Image Interpretation Pearls

- T2 hyperintensity in striatum with neurologic dysfunction
- T1 hyperintensity in BG with hepatic dysfunction

SELECTED REFERENCES

1. Pinto C et al: Brain MRI in the decision for liver transplantation in pediatric neurological Wilson's disease. Mov Disord Clin Pract. 9(7):941-8, 2022
2. Dusek P et al: Associations of brain atrophy and cerebral iron accumulation at MRI with clinical severity in Wilson disease. Radiology. 299(3):662-72, 2021

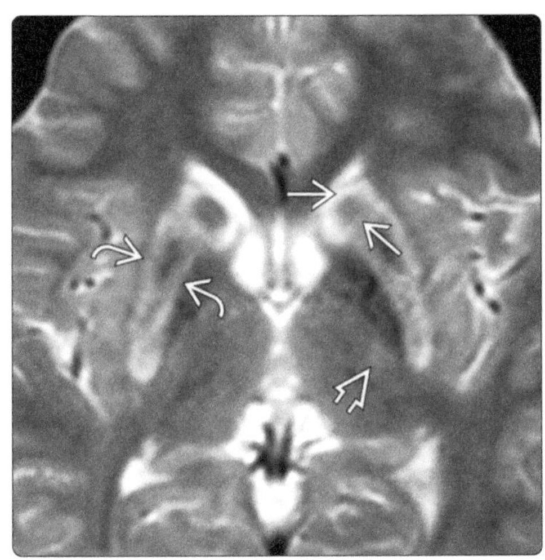

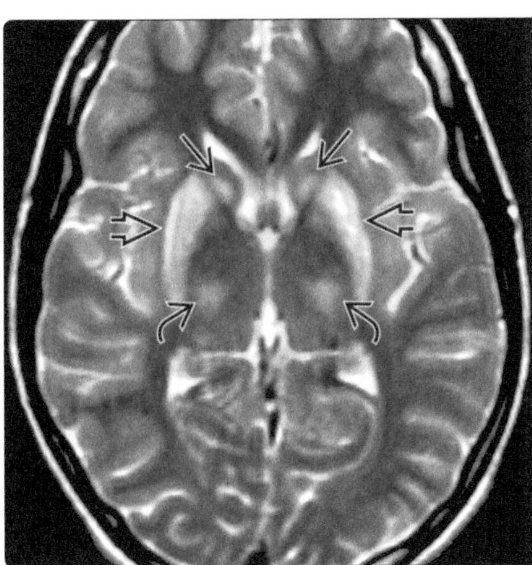

(Left) *Axial T2WI MR in a young patient with Wilson disease shows bilateral symmetric laminar outer rim hyperintensity in the bilateral caudate ➡ and putamina ➡ surrounding central hypointensity. Also note the faint hyperintense signal in the posterior limb of the internal capsule (more on the left) ➡.* **(Right)** *Axial T2WI MR in a 13-year-old boy with Wilson disease shows typical bilateral symmetric increased signal intensity in the caudate head ➡, putamen ➡, and ventrolateral thalamus ➡.*

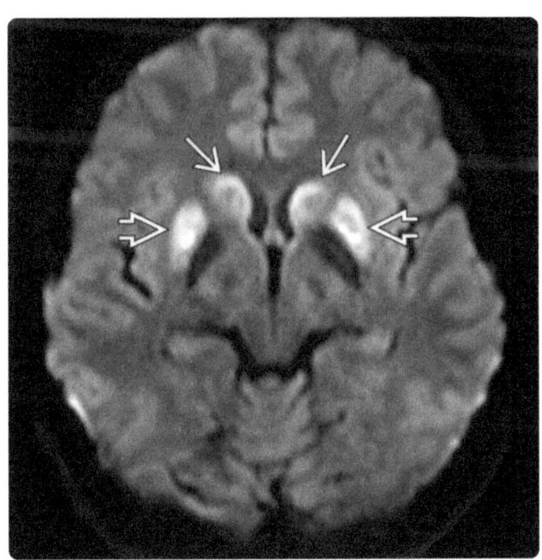

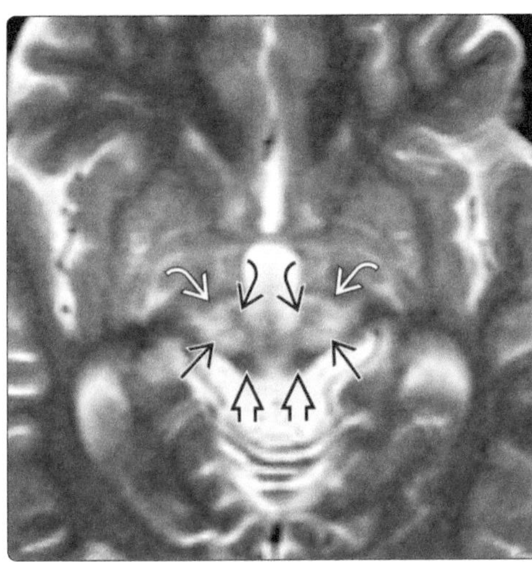

(Left) *Axial DWI MR in a patient with Wilson disease shows diffusion restriction in the bilateral caudate head ➡ and putamen ➡.* **(Right)** *Axial T2WI MR at the upper midbrain level in a patient with Wilson disease shows the face of giant panda sign with normally hypointense red nuclei ➡ and pars reticulata of substantia nigra ➡ against the background of abnormal high signal in midbrain tegmentum ➡ and the hypointensity of superior colliculi ➡.*

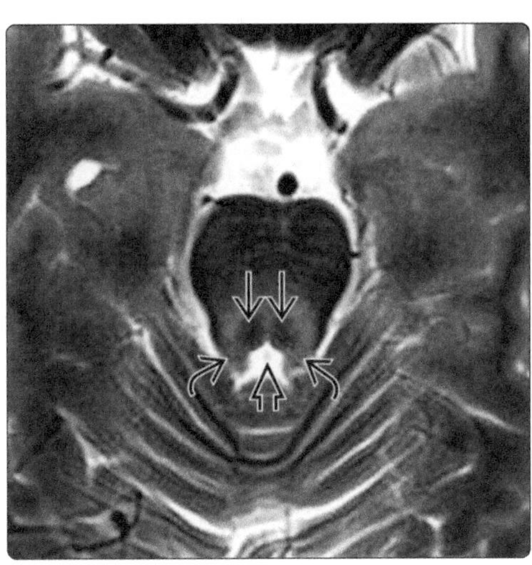

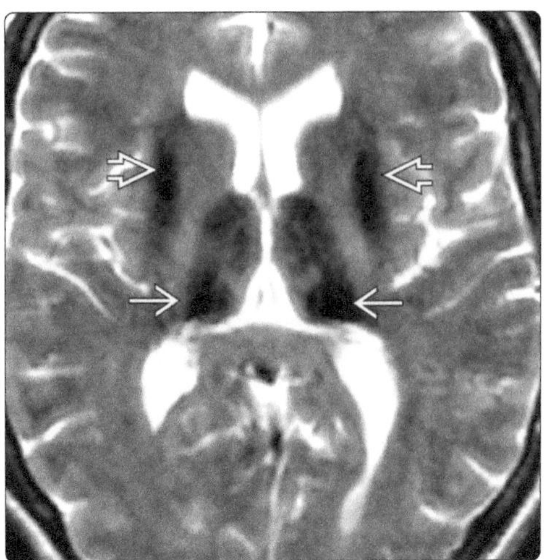

(Left) *Axial T2WI MR at the lower midbrain-upper pons junction in Wilson disease shows the face of miniature panda sign. Hypointensity of medial longitudinal fasciculi and central tegmental tracts (eyes of panda) ➡ are seen against the background of aqueductal CSF hyperintensity opening into the 4th ventricle (nose and mouth of panda) ➡. Note the hyperintense superior cerebellar peduncles (cheeks of miniature panda) ➡.* **(Right)** *Axial T2WI MR in a patient with Wilson disease shows hypointense thalami ➡ and basal ganglia ➡.*

Hypoglycemia

KEY FACTS

TERMINOLOGY

- Neonate with significant hypoglycemia

IMAGING

- Occipital > parietal > frontal, temporal lobe
- ± basal ganglia, thalamus, brainstem involvement
- White matter injury common, may be predominantly periventricular in premature
- ↑ DWI signal corresponds to normal to low ADC acutely, DWI normalizes after 1st week

TOP DIFFERENTIAL DIAGNOSES

- Term hypoxic-ischemic injury
- Preterm hypoxic-ischemic injury
- Mitochondrial encephalomyopathy, lactic acidosis, & stroke-like episodes
- Venous Infarct
- Acute hypertensive encephalopathy (posterior reversible encephalopathy syndrome)

PATHOLOGY

- Upper cortical layers involved, not intermediate & deep layers, as in hypoxic-ischemic injury
- No selective involvement of watershed areas

CLINICAL ISSUES

- Stupor, jitteriness, seizures, apnea, irritability, hypotonia
- Usually presents within first 3 days of life
- Threshold for injury unknown but likely factor of severity & duration as well as associated insults
- Prognosis depends on prompt recognition & treatment of hypoglycemia
- Long-term prognosis correlated with white matter damage on MR

DIAGNOSTIC CHECKLIST

- Consider if bilateral occipital/parietal bright DWI signal in neonate with seizures

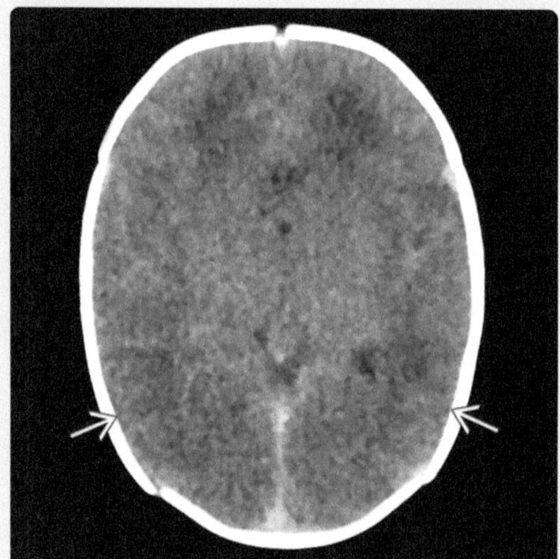

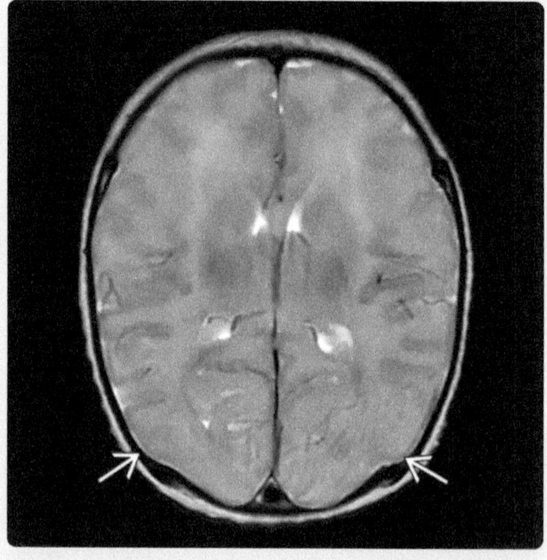

(Left) *Axial NECT in a 4-day-old infant who initially fed well and had no concerns for hypoxic-ischemic encephalopathy (HIE) at birth presents with seizures and poor oral intake. Note hypodensity and loss of gray matter (GM)-white matter (WM) differentiation ➡ in the bilateral occipital and parietal lobes.* **(Right)** *Axial T2 MR in the same patient confirms bilateral posterior cortical injury with loss of parietooccipital lobe GM-WM differentiation ➡.*

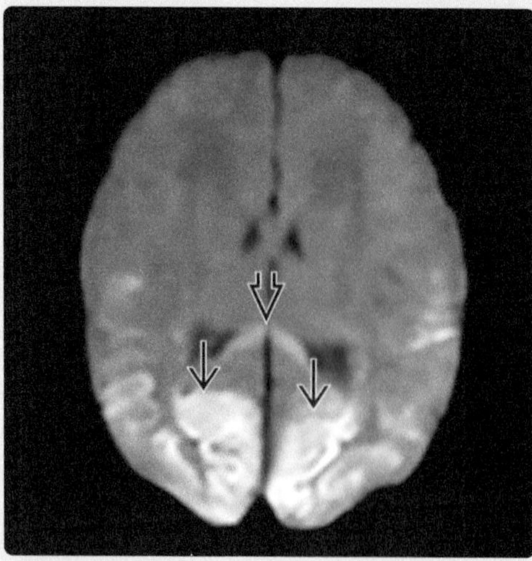

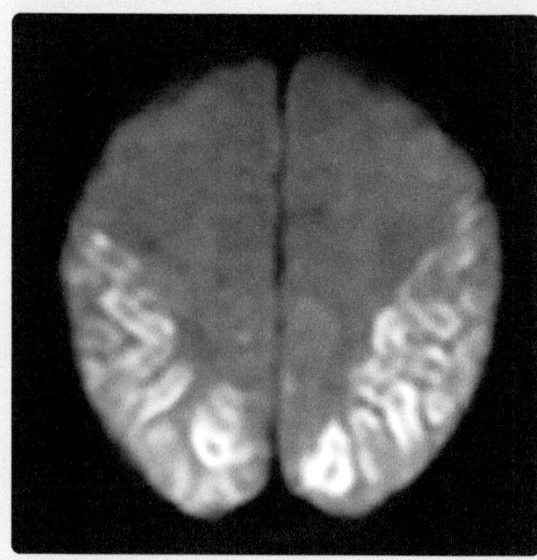

(Left) *Axial DWI MR in the same patient reveals avid diffusion restriction in the abnormal parietal and occipital lobes, including the calcarine cortex ➡ and corpus callosum splenium ➡. ADC map confirmed hypointense signal intensity in the abnormal areas (not shown).* **(Right)** *Axial DWI MR obtained more rostrally shows involvement of the posterior frontal lobes in a nonwatershed pattern. This infant recovered well neurologically without detectable atrophy on follow-up MR (not shown).*

TERMINOLOGY

Definitions

- Neonate with significant hypoglycemia
  - Plasma glucose level < 30-35 mg/dL in first 24 hours of life; < 40-45 mg/dL (after 24 hours)

IMAGING

General Features

- Best diagnostic clue
  - Bilateral occipital/parietal bright DWI in neonate with seizures
- Location
  - Occipital > parietal > frontal, temporal lobes
  - ± basal ganglia, thalamus, brainstem involvement
  - White matter (WM) injury common; may be predominantly periventricular in premature
  - Hypoglycemia that is less severe can accentuate watershed zone injuries in neonate hypoxic-ischemic injury (HII)

CT Findings

- NECT
  - ↓ attenuation with loss of gray matter (GM)-WM differentiation in acute & subacute phase
  - Cortical Ca^{++} in chronic phase

MR Findings

- T1WI
  - Cortical ± deep gray hyperintensity in subacute phase
  - ± foci of ↑ T1 signal in WM
- T2WI
  - ↑ signal in GM & WM with loss of GM-WM distinction in acute phase
  - ↑ signal in GM & WM with variable cortical low signal in subacute phase
  - Volume loss ± gliosis that may be subtle to cystic encephalomalacia in chronic phase
- DWI
  - ↑ DWI signal corresponds to low ADC acutely; normalizes after 1st week; most sensitive to identify parietal-occipital injury
- MRS
  - Normal to low NAA; ± lactate

Ultrasonographic Findings

- Grayscale ultrasound
  - ↑ echogenicity

Imaging Recommendations

- Best imaging tool
  - MR with DWI
- Protocol advice
  - Higher b values (b = 1,000-1,500 s/mm²) make areas of ↓ diffusion more conspicuous

DIFFERENTIAL DIAGNOSIS

Term Hypoxic-Ischemic Injury

- Hypoglycemia & HII often coexist & potentiate extent of brain injury
- HII causes hypoglycemia
- DWI in partial HII with hypoglycemia may be indistinguishable from posterior predominant normoglycemic partial HII

Preterm Hypoxic-Ischemic Injury

- Hypoglycemia potentiates periventricular leukomalacia

Mitochondrial Encephalomyopathy, Lactic Acidosis, & Stroke-Like Episodes

- Mitochondrial encephalopathy with lactic acidosis & stroke-like episodes
- Consider if marked elevation in lactate or if no history of hypoglycemia

Status Epilepticus

- Seizures are typical response of newborn brain to injury
  - DWI abnormalities in newborns more likely to be cause (not consequence) of seizures
- Vicious cycle may develop where cerebral injury is exacerbated by seizures

Venous Infarct

- Often associated hemorrhage & edema; MRV to rule out

Acute Hypertensive Encephalopathy (Posterior Reversible Encephalopathy Syndrome)

- Cortical & subcortical T2/FLAIR hyperintensity with predominant posterior distribution
- Predominantly ↑ ADC, older patients

PATHOLOGY

General Features

- Etiology
  - Inadequate energy substrate (oxygen, glucose, lactate) availability/reserve: Intrauterine growth restriction (IUGR), preeclampsia, maternal hypoglycemia, prolonged fasting, prematurity
  - ↑ glucose utilization: Hypoxia, stress
  - Hyperinsulinemia
    - Uncontrolled maternal diabetes
    - Hyperinsulinemic hypoglycemia, familial, 1 or 2 (HHF1 or HHF2)
  - Beckwith-Wiedemann syndrome (BWS)
    - Inherited disorder with macrosomia, macroglossia, visceromegaly, omphalocele, embryonal tumors, & renal abnormalities
    - BWS-associated hypoglycemia is mild & transient
  - Other endocrine abnormalities: Panhypopituitarism, hypothyroidism, adrenal insufficiency
  - Other: Polycythemia, congenital heart disease
  - Excitatory amino acids (glutamate) & oxidative stress are thought to play central role in neuronal death
- Glucose metabolism
  - Glucose primary metabolic fuel for brain
  - Brain is major determinant of hepatic glucose production
  - Neonates have disproportionally high glucose production relative to body size due to disproportionately large neonatal brain
  - Immature brain more resilient to hypoglycemia than adult
    - Lower absolute demand
    - ↑ ability to ↑ cerebral blood flow

- Utilization of other substrates (i.e., lactate)
- Resistance of neonatal heart to hypoglycemia
- Hypoglycemia potentiates hypoxic-induced damage

Staging, Grading, & Classification

- Clinical categories
  - Transitional adaptive hypoglycemia
    - Very early onset; mild, brief hypoglycemia
    - Responds rapidly to treatment
    - Diabetic mothers, erythroblastosis, difficulty transitioning to extrauterine life
  - Secondary associated hypoglycemia
    - Early 1st day; mild, short-duration hypoglycemia
    - Responds rapidly to treatment
    - Associated CNS disorder (HII, intracranial hemorrhage, sepsis)
  - Classic transient hypoglycemia
    - End of 1st day; moderate to severe, often prolonged hypoglycemia
    - Requires large amounts of glucose
    - IUGR, ↓ substrate/impaired gluconeogenesis
  - Severe recurrent hypoglycemia
    - Variable onset; severe, prolonged hypoglycemia
    - May persist despite treatment
    - Most have primary disorder of glucose metabolism
      - e.g., BWS, HHF1 or HHF2/persistent hyperinsulinemia hypoglycemia of infancy (PHHI)/nesidioblastosis, β-cell hyperplasia, endocrine deficiencies, inborn errors in metabolism

Gross Pathologic & Surgical Features

- Pale, edematous brain; blurred GM-WM junction

Microscopic Features

- Widespread injury to cerebral cortex, hippocampus, basal ganglia, thalamus, brainstem, spinal cord
- Upper cortical layers involved, not intermediate & deep layers as in HII
- No selective involvement of watershed areas
- Severe degeneration of glial cells
- Periventricular WM injury may be prominent

CLINICAL ISSUES

Presentation

- Most common signs/symptoms
  - Stupor, jitteriness, seizures, apnea, irritability, hypotonia
  - May have no symptoms
  - When associated with neonatal HIE, may present with neonatal encephalopathy
- Clinical profile
  - Small or large neonates

Demographics

- Age
  - Usually presents within first 3 days of life
- Sex
  - M > F

Natural History & Prognosis

- Cerebral glucose metabolism probably flow limited, thus, dependent on cerebral blood flow (CBF)
- Threshold for injury unknown but likely factor of severity & duration as well as associated insults
- < 45 mg/dL may have deleterious long-term effects even if no neonatal signs
- Epilepsy (may have intractable seizures), developmental delay, motor delay, learning & behavior problems, hyperactivity & attention difficulties, autistic features, microcephaly, cortical blindness
- DWI abnormalities associated with later deficits (occipital lobe low ADC associated with later cortical visual loss)
- Regions of bright DWI & minimal ADC ↓ may have minimal to no volume loss on follow-up
- Prognosis depends on prompt recognition & treatment of hypoglycemia
- Long-term prognosis correlated with WM damage on MR

Treatment

- Glucose level to treat controversial; consider if 40-45 mg/dL
- Glucose infusion to restore normal glucose levels, often even if asymptomatic
- Frequent feeds, ↑ caloric density, continuous NG feeds ± cornstarch, continuous IV dextrose, hydrocortisone, diazoxide, octreotide, glucagon, Ca^{++} channel blocker, partial pancreatectomy

Prevention

- Control maternal diabetes, preeclampsia/eclampsia, nutrition, prevention/rapid treatment of perinatal asphyxia
- Identify high-risk infant, temperature control, oral feeds in 1st hours of life, glucose test when indicated

DIAGNOSTIC CHECKLIST

Reporting Tips

- Do not equate DWI abnormalities with infarcts (pannecrosis), as acute DWI abnormalities may result in only mild volume loss, especially if ADC not ↓

SELECTED REFERENCES

1. Anderson Enni JB et al: Screening and diagnosis of neonatal hypoglycaemia in at-risk late preterm and term infants following AAP recommendations: a single centre retrospective study. BMJ Paediatr Open. 7(1):e001766, 2023
2. Zenker M et al: Syndromic forms of congenital hyperinsulinism. Front Endocrinol (Lausanne). 14:1013874, 2023
3. Misser SK et al: Thalamus L-sign: a potential biomarker of neonatal partial, prolonged hypoxic-ischemic brain injury or hypoglycemic encephalopathy? AJNR Am J Neuroradiol. 43(6):919-25, 2022
4. Smyczyńska J et al: Delayed diagnosis of congenital combined pituitary hormone deficiency including severe growth hormone deficiency in children with persistent neonatal hypoglycemia-case reports and review. Int J Mol Sci. 23(19), 2022
5. Zhang Y et al: Dynamic magnetic resonance imaging findings in the early stages of neonatal hypoglycemic brain injury. Eur J Pediatr. 181(12):4167-74, 2022
6. De Leon DD et al: Congenital hypoglycemia disorders: new aspects of etiology, diagnosis, treatment and outcomes: highlights of the proceedings of the congenital hypoglycemia disorders symposium, Philadelphia April 2016. Pediatr Diabetes. 18(1):3-9, 2017
7. Goode RH et al: Developmental outcomes of preterm infants with neonatal hypoglycemia. Pediatrics. 138(6), 2016
8. Bathla G et al: Neuroimaging in patients with abnormal blood glucose levels. AJNR Am J Neuroradiol. 35(5):833-40, 2014
9. Wong DS et al: Brain injury patterns in hypoglycemia in neonatal encephalopathy. AJNR Am J Neuroradiol. 34(7):1456-61, 2013
10. Burns CM et al: Patterns of cerebral injury and neurodevelopmental outcomes after symptomatic neonatal hypoglycemia. Pediatrics. 122(1):65-74, 2008
11. Barkovich AJ et al: Imaging patterns of neonatal hypoglycemia. AJNR Am J Neuroradiol. 19(3):523-8, 1998

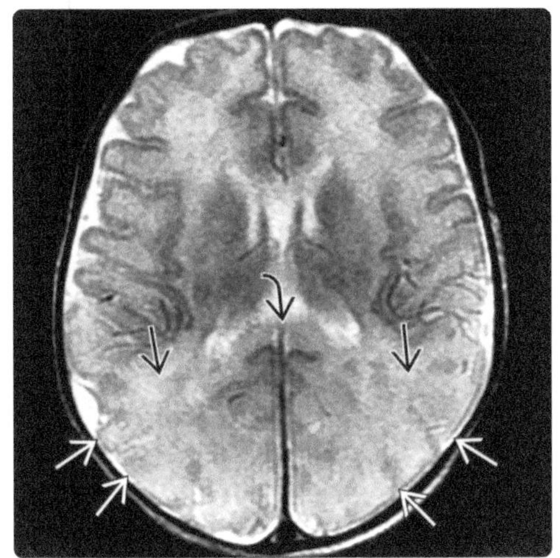
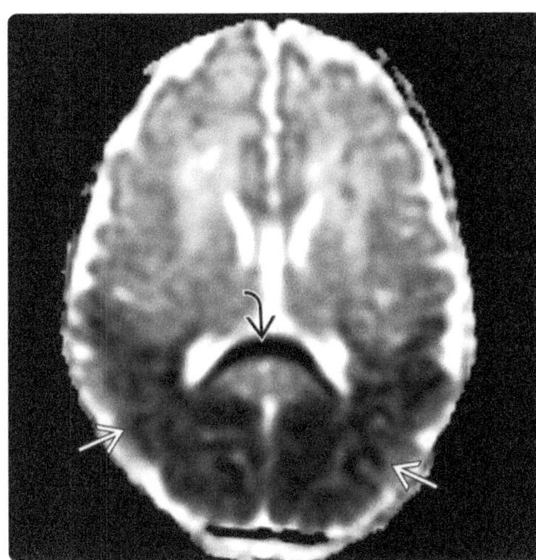

(Left) *Axial T2 MR in a 5-day-old hypoglycemic infant shows increased signal in the parietal cortex ➡ and underlying parietal WM ⇨ with loss of GM-WM distinction. Note the extension of hyperintensity ⇨, probably representing interstitial edema, into the splenium of the corpus callosum.* **(Right)** *Axial ADC in the same infant shows reduced diffusivity in the parietal cortex and WM ➡ as well as in the posterior corpus callosum ⇨.*

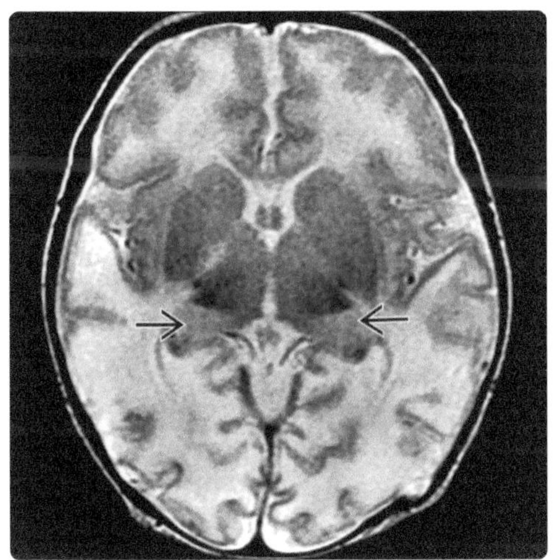
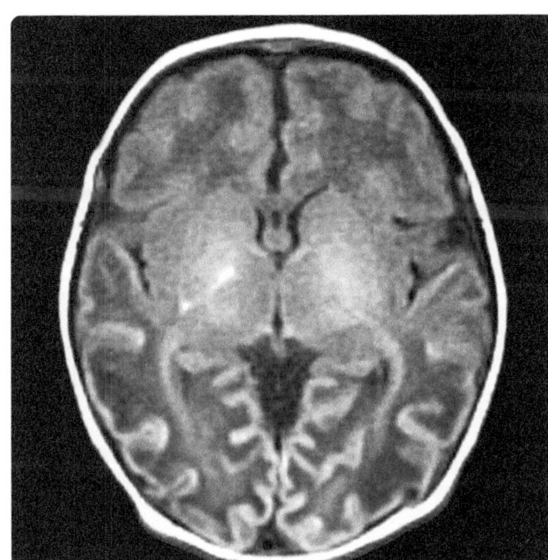

(Left) *Axial T2 MR in the same patient at 7 days of age shows the evolution of hypoglycemic injury with increased signal in the posterior WM, including posterior limb of the internal capsules and pulvinar thalamus ⇨. The overlying cortex shows patchy increased and decreased signal.* **(Right)** *Axial T1 MR in the same patient at 7 days of age shows evolving injury: Decreased signal in the posterior WM and pulvinar thalamus and increased signal in the overlying cortex and posterior limb internal capsule.*

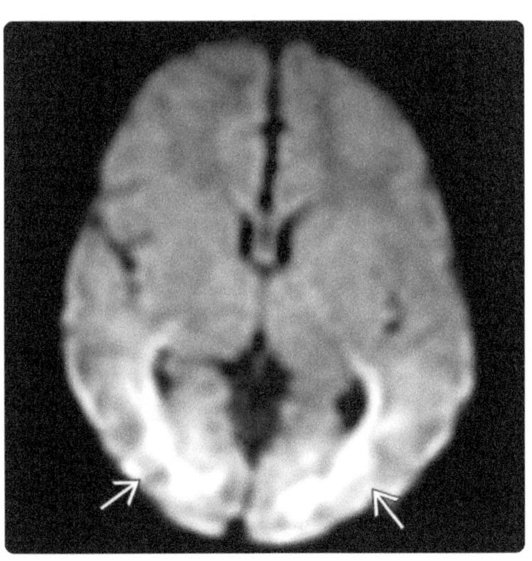
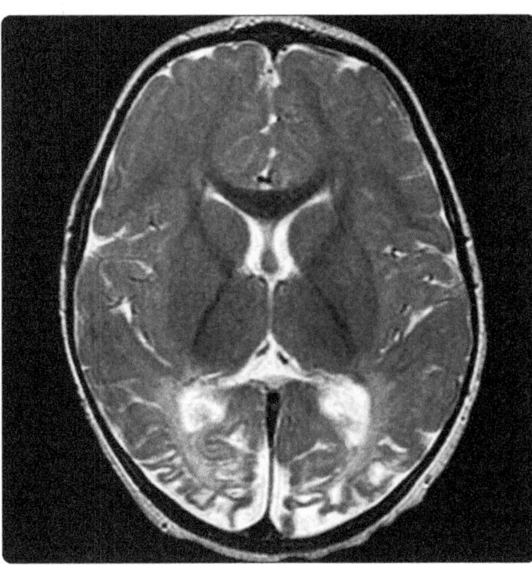

(Left) *Axial DWI MR at in the same patient with hypoglycemic injury at 7 days of age shows increased signal ➡ in the posterior WM and overlying cortex. At this stage, diffusivity is pseudonormalizing; therefore, the increased signal is likely a result of T2 shine-through.* **(Right)** *Axial T2 MR in the same patient at 1 year of age shows chronic injury with marked volume loss and gliosis involving the cortex and WM of the posterior temporal lobes, parietal lobes (not shown), and occipital lobes.*

Kernicterus

KEY FACTS

TERMINOLOGY

- Kernicterus or bilirubin encephalopathy: Pathologic bilirubin staining of basal ganglia, brainstem, & hippocampi associated with hyperbilirubinemia

IMAGING

- Acute: ↑ T1 signal in globus pallidus (GP), subthalamic nuclei (STN), hippocampi, substantia nigra (SN)
- Chronic: ↑ T2 signal in GP, hippocampi
- MRS: ↑ Tau/Cr, ↑ Glx/Cr, ↑ mI/Cr, ↓ Cho/Cr

TOP DIFFERENTIAL DIAGNOSES

- Hyperalimentation, liver failure: ↑ T1 signal GP, SN
- Toxic: CO poisoning
- Metabolic: Methylmalonic acidemia, creatine deficiency, succinic semialdehyde dehydrogenase deficiency, L2-hydroxyglutaric aciduria
- Term hypoxic-ischemic injury

PATHOLOGY

- Encephalopathy due to ↑ unconjugated bilirubin crossing immature blood-brain barrier (BBB)
- Neurons > glia, neuropil spongiosis
- Yellow staining > MR abnormality

CLINICAL ISSUES

- Stupor, hypotonia, poor suckling, high-pitched cry
- Incidence ↑ with early discharge, ↑ breastfeeding
- Specific damage to brainstem auditory nuclei, ± deafness or abnormal auditory processing (most common)
- Athetosis, gaze abnormal in most; intellectual deficits in few

DIAGNOSTIC CHECKLIST

- Normal MR does not rule out long-term sequelae
- ↑ T1 signal in GP can be normal in neonates; look for other areas of involvement
- Findings may resolve with therapy

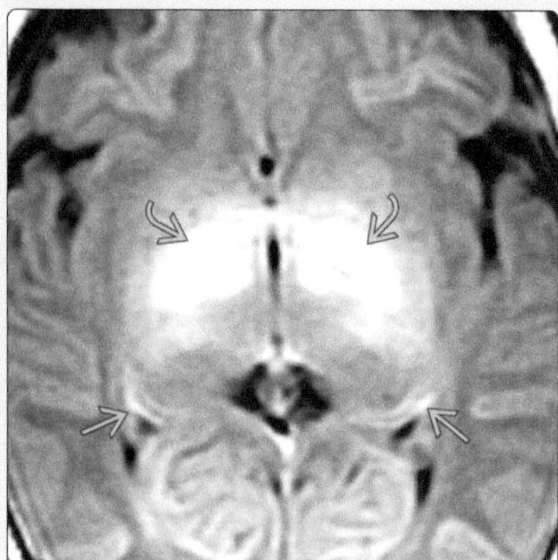

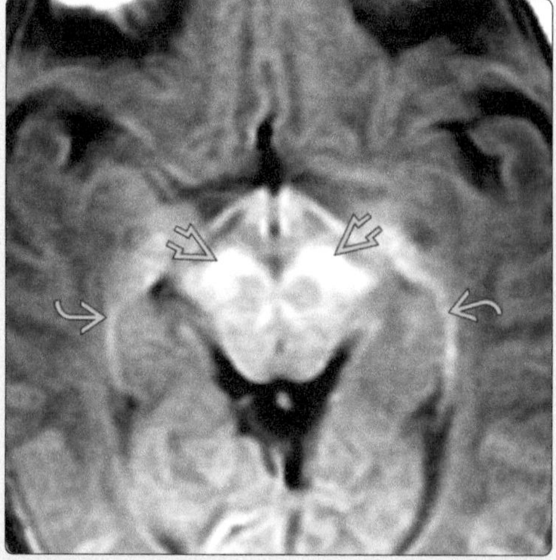

(Left) *Axial T1 MR in a neonate with hyperbilirubinemia, stupor, hypotonia, and increased irritability shows increased signal with the globi pallidi ➢ and hippocampal tails ➢.* **(Right)** *Axial T1 MR in the same neonate shows abnormally increased signal within the substantia nigra ➢ and hippocampus bilaterally ➢. The cerebral cortex and the underlying white matter have a normal appearance.*

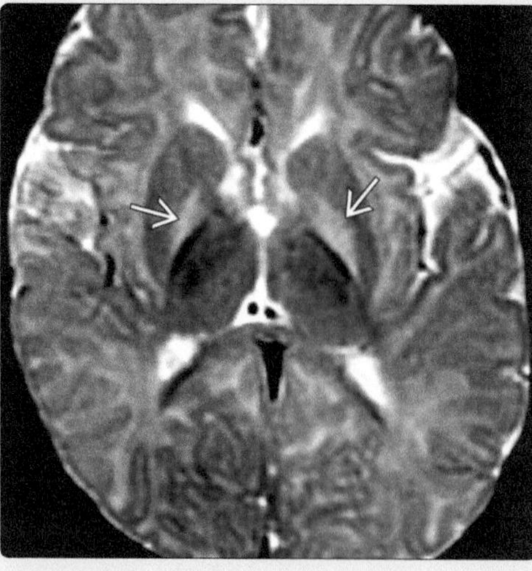

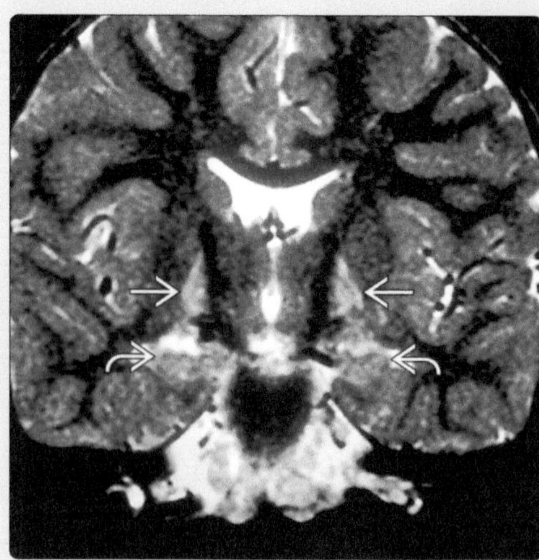

(Left) *Axial T2 MR in the same infant at 6 months of age shows high T2 signal intensity and volume loss in the globus pallidus bilaterally ➡. The volume of the cerebral white matter is somewhat diminished.* **(Right)** *Coronal T2 MR in a young child who had severe neonatal hyperbilirubinemia shows increased T2 signal and volume loss in the bilateral globi pallidi ➡ as well as in the hippocampal heads ➡ bilaterally.*

TERMINOLOGY

Synonyms

- Bilirubin (BR) or posticteric encephalopathy

Definitions

- Kernicterus or BR encephalopathy: Pathologic BR staining of basal ganglia, brainstem, & hippocampi associated with hyperbilirubinemia

IMAGING

General Features

- Best diagnostic clue
  - Acute: ↑ T1 signal in globus pallidus (GP), subthalamic nuclei (STN), hippocampi, substantia nigra (SN)
  - Chronic: ↑ T2 signal in GP, hippocampi

MR Findings

- T1WI
  - Acute: ↑ T1 signal in GP > STN > hippocampi > SN
    - Deposition of unconjugated BR (UBR) or ↑ manganese (Mn)
- T2WI
  - Subacute & chronic: ↑ T2 signal/volume loss in GP, hippocampi, ± SN
- MRS
  - ↑ Tau/Cr, Glx/Cr, mI/Cr, ↓ NAA/Cho,NAA/Cr, Cho/Cr

Imaging Recommendations

- Best imaging tool
  - Multiplanar MR

DIFFERENTIAL DIAGNOSIS

T1-Hyperintense Globus Pallidus

- Hyperalimentation, liver failure, asphyxia, neurofibromatosis, gadolinium accumulation

T2-Hyperintense Globus Pallidus

- Toxic: CO poisoning
- Metabolic: Methylmalonic acidemia, creatine deficiency, succinic semialdehyde dehydrogenase deficiency, L2-hydroxyglutaric aciduria
- Normotensive hypoxia

Term Hypoxic Ischemic Injury

- Acute: ↑ T2 signal; subacute/chronic: ↑ T1 signal in ventrolateral thalamus, corticospinal tract

PATHOLOGY

General Features

- Etiology
  - Encephalopathy due to ↑ UBR crossing immature blood-brain barrier (BBB)
  - Risk factors for ↑ BR
    - Hemolytic disorders (especially erythroblastosis fetalis), breastfeeding, > 10% loss of birth weight, polycythemia, dehydration
  - Risk factors for ↑ susceptibility to brain damage at ~ normal BR levels
    - Drugs compete for albumin binding of BR
    - Sulphonamides, ceftriaxone, salicylates, Na benzoate, hormones
    - Renal hypoalbuminemia, hepatic failure, ↓ thyroidism
    - Prematurity, asphyxia, sepsis
    - ↑ cerebral blood flow; abnormal BBB
- Genetics
  - Some 2q37 (Crigler-Najjar syndrome, etc.)

Gross Pathologic & Surgical Features

- Yellow staining > MR abnormality
  - GP, SN, STN, hippocampi > thalamus, striatum, cranial nerve nuclei (3, 8), dentate nuclei, reticular formation, spinal cord
  - Also Purkinje cells (premature infants)

Microscopic Features

- Neurons > glia, neuropil spongiosis

CLINICAL ISSUES

Presentation

- Most common signs/symptoms
  - Stupor, hypotonia, poor suckling, high-pitched cry
  - Over days, may develop stupor, irritability, ↑ tone
  - May have no or equivocal neurologic signs

Demographics

- Age
  - Preterm > term; 1st days of life
- Sex
  - M > F
- Ethnicity
  - More prevalent in Asians, Hispanics
- Epidemiology
  - Incidence ↑ with early discharge, ↑ breastfeeding

Natural History & Prognosis

- Specific damage to brainstem auditory nuclei → ± deafness or abnormal auditory processing (common)
- Athetosis, gaze abnormality; intellectual deficits in few

Treatment

- Maternal screen, anti-Rh; fetal blood transfusion
- Hydration, phototherapy for moderate + exchange transfusion for severe
- Other, e.g., heme oxygenase inhibitors

DIAGNOSTIC CHECKLIST

Consider

- Normal MR does not rule out long-term sequelae

Image Interpretation Pearls

- ↑ T1 signal in GP can be normal in neonates; look for other areas; findings may resolve with therapy

SELECTED REFERENCES

1. Qattea I et al: Neonatal hyperbilirubinemia and bilirubin neurotoxicity in hospitalized neonates: analysis of the US Database. Pediatr Res. 91(7):1662-8, 2022
2. Sarı S et al: Brain magnetic resonance imaging and magnetic resonance spectroscopy findings of children with kernicterus. Pol J Radiol. 80:72-80, 2015

KEY FACTS

TERMINOLOGY

- Cerebrovascular autoregulatory disorder
- Many etiologies with HTN as common component
  - Glomerulonephritis, lupus nephritis, sepsis
  - Drug toxicity (e.g., chemotherapy, cyclosporine)

IMAGING

- General
  - Patchy parietooccipital cortical/subcortical edema in patient with severe acute/subacute HTN
- CT
  - Bilateral, nonconfluent, hypodense foci
  - ± symmetric lesions in basal ganglia
- MR
  - Parietooccipital T2/FLAIR hyperintensities in 95%
  - ± basal ganglia, pontine, cerebellar involvement
  - 3 patterns of hemorrhage: Focal parenchymal hemorrhage, microhemorrhages, convexity SAH
  - Generally no restriction on DWI
  - Variable patchy enhancement
  - However, atypical imaging patterns common

TOP DIFFERENTIAL DIAGNOSES

- Acute cerebral ischemia-infarction
- Encephalitis
- Acute disseminated encephalomyelitis
- Status epilepticus
- Hypoglycemia
- Thrombotic microangiopathies (DIC, TTP, mHTN)

PATHOLOGY

- Acute HTN damages vascular endothelium
- Failed autoregulation causes blood-brain barrier disruption
- Result = vasogenic (not cytotoxic) edema

CLINICAL ISSUES

- Headache, seizure, ↓ mental status, visual symptoms
- Caution: Some patients may be normotensive or have only minimally elevated BP

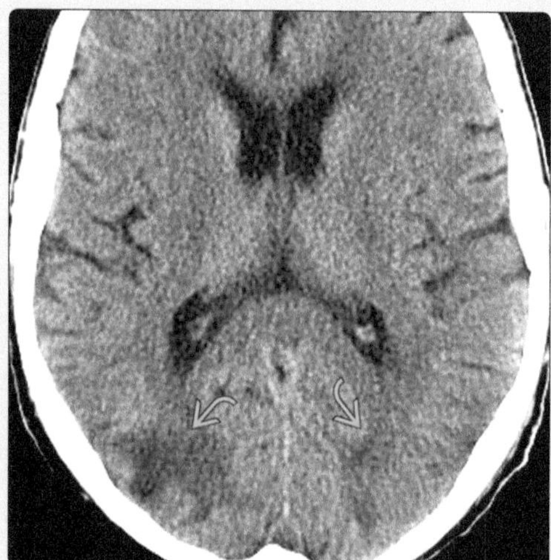

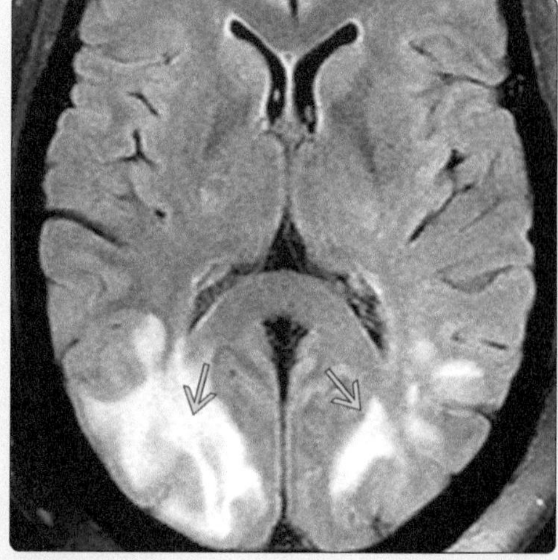

(Left) *Axial NECT in a 54-year-old with liver transplant on Tacrolimus FK 506 who presented with seizures demonstrates asymmetric subcortical edema in the occipital lobes bilaterally ➢. Findings are typical of posterior reversible encephalopathy syndrome (PRES).* **(Right)** *Axial FLAIR MR in a 20-year-old eclamptic woman who presented with severe hypertension, seizures, and altered sensorium shows classic findings of PRES with occipital cortical/subcortical edema ➢. Her BP at presentation was 210/140.*

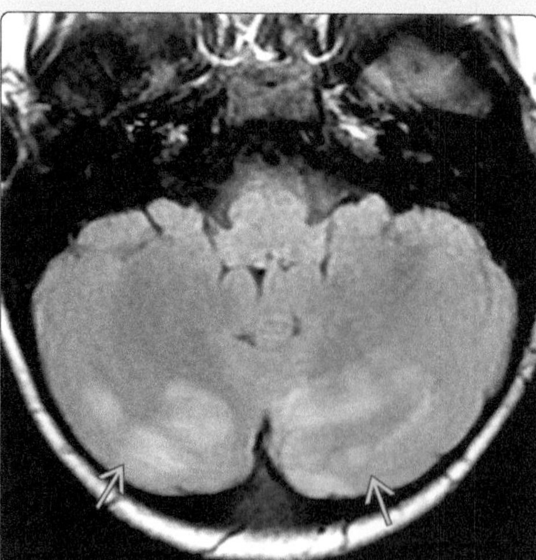

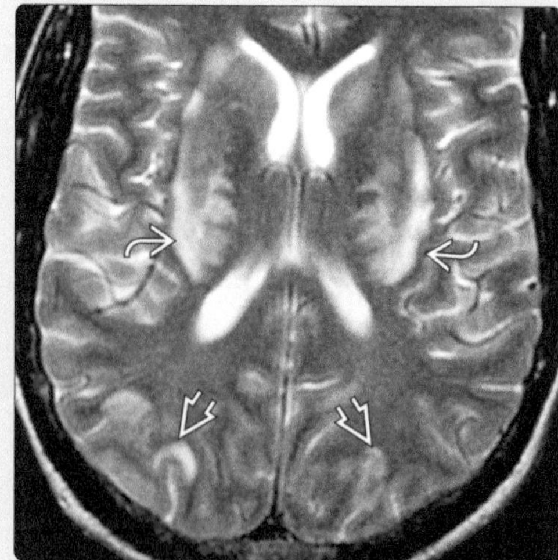

(Left) *Axial FLAIR MR in a 5-year-old with neuroblastoma and new onset of seizures shows bilateral signal abnormalities ➢ within the posterior periphery of the cerebellar hemispheres. Cerebellar involvement occurs in ~ 50% of cases.* **(Right)** *Axial T2WI MR shows symmetric hyperintensity in both basal ganglia ➢ with relatively subtle findings in the occipital poles ➢. Basal ganglia involvement occurs in a minority of cases (~ 30%).*

TERMINOLOGY

Abbreviations

- Posterior reversible encephalopathy syndrome (PRES)

Synonyms

- Hypertensive encephalopathy
- Reversible posterior leukoencephalopathy syndrome (RPLS)

Definitions

- Cerebrovascular autoregulatory disorder
  - Multiple etiologies
  - Most cases associated with acute HTN
  - Symptoms: Headache, visual disturbances, altered mental function, & seizures

IMAGING

General Features

- Best diagnostic clue
  - Patchy parietooccipital cortical/subcortical edema in patient with severe acute/subacute HTN
- Location
  - Most common: Cortex & subcortical white matter (WM)
    - Arterial territory junctions (watershed territory)
    - Usually bilateral, often somewhat asymmetric
    - Parietooccipital lobes (> 90%)
    - Frontal lobes (> 70%)
    - Temporal lobes (> 60%)
  - Less common: Cerebellum, deep gray nuclei, brainstem, periventricular WM
    - Cerebellum (> 50%)
    - Deep gray nuclei (> 30%)
    - Brainstem (< 30%)
    - Periventricular WM (< 25%)
- Size
  - Extent of abnormalities highly variable
- Morphology
  - Patchy > confluent; atypical patterns common

CT Findings

- NECT
  - Insensitive exam: May be normal or subtly abnormal
    - If PRES suspected, MR is much more sensitive
  - Common: Bilateral nonconfluent hypodense foci
    - Posterior parietal, occipital lobes
    - Cortical watershed zones
  - Less common: Petechial cortical/subcortical or basal ganglionic hemorrhages
- CECT
  - Usually no enhancement
  - Occasionally mild patchy/punctate enhancement
- CTA
  - Major vessels usually normal
  - Distal vessels may show diffuse vasoconstriction, focal irregularity, & beaded appearance

MR Findings

- T1WI
  - Hypointense cortical/subcortical lesions
- T2WI
  - Subtle cases may be inconspicuous
  - More advanced cases show obvious gyral signal abnormality & swelling
- FLAIR
  - Most sensitive sequence for detection of PRES
  - Common: Cortical/subcortical ↑ signal with swelling
  - Uncommon: ↑ signal in deep gray nuclei, cerebellum
  - Rare: ↑ signal in brainstem
  - "Leaky" blood-brain barrier may cause gadolinium accumulation in CSF, FLAIR hyperintensity
- T2* GRE
  - 3 patterns of hemorrhage
    - Focal parenchymal hemorrhage evident on conventional imaging (usually ↑ T1/↓ T2)
    - Parenchymal microhemorrhage usually evident only on SWI/GRE
    - Subarachnoid hemorrhage most conspicuous on FLAIR & SWI
- DWI
  - Most common: No restriction (usually ↑ ADC)
  - Less common: Small areas of diffusion restriction (much smaller than FLAIR abnormality)
- PWI
  - May show variable perfusion findings depending on phase
    - Acute vasoconstrictive phase: ↓ cerebral blood volume (CBV), ↓ cerebral blood flow (CBF)
    - Acute vasodilatory phase: ↑ CBV, ↑ CBF
    - Over time, perfusion abnormalities normalize but often lag behind FLAIR reversal
- T1WI C+
  - Variable patchy enhancement
    - Most common: No enhancement
    - Less common: Leptomeningeal enhancement
    - Uncommon: Patchy cortical enhancement
- MRS
  - May show widespread metabolic abnormalities
    - ↑ Cho, Cr, mildly ↓ NAA
    - Usually return to normal within 2 months

Nuclear Medicine Findings

- SPECT: Variable findings reported; more common hypoperfusion in affected areas

Imaging Recommendations

- Best imaging tool
  - MR ± contrast
- Protocol advice
  - If question of diagnosis, repeat scan after symptom resolution to confirm resolution

DIFFERENTIAL DIAGNOSIS

Acute Cerebral Ischemia-Infarction

- MCA distribution > > PCA
- Infarcts restrict on DWI; PRES usually does not

Encephalitis

- May involve deep gray nuclei & cortical/subcortical regions similar to PRES
- Typically do not selectively affect watershed regions, as PRES does

Acute Disseminated Encephalomyelitis

- May involve deep & cortical gray matter similar to PRES
- Predominantly affects WM, often asymmetrically
- Enhancement is more common than in PRES

Status Epilepticus

- May cause transient gyral edema, enhancement
- Can mimic PRES, stroke, infiltrating neoplasm
- Unilateral (PRES often bilateral), often involves hippocampi

Hypoglycemia

- Severe parietooccipital edema
- Can resemble PRES; thus, history is important

Thrombotic Microangiopathies

- Malignant HTN, disseminated intravascular coagulation DIC, HUS, TTP
- Significant overlap as PRES common imaging manifestation

Gliomatosis Cerebri

- Entire lobe(s) involved
- Can mimic brainstem PRES

PATHOLOGY

General Features

- Etiology
  - Diverse causes with acute HTN as frequent component
  - Acute HTN, inflammation, & drug toxicity damage vascular endothelium
  - Failed autoregulation → blood-brain barrier disruption
  - Result = predominantly vasogenic edema
    - Hydrostatic leakage (extravasation, transudation of fluid/macromolecules through arteriolar walls)
    - Interstitial fluid accumulates in cortex, subcortical WM
- Associated abnormalities
  - Acute/subacute systemic HTN
  - Drug toxicity ± tumor lysis syndrome
    - Chemotherapeutic agents
      - □ e.g., cisplatin
    - Posttransplant immunosuppressants
      - □ (e.g., cyclosporine, tacrolimus)
  - Thrombotic microangiopathies (DIC, TTP, malignant HTN)
  - Uremic encephalopathies
    - Acute glomerulonephritis (GN), lupus nephropathy, etc.
  - Severe infection
    - 25% of septic patients in shock develop PRES
    - BP can be normal or elevated

Microscopic Features

- Autopsy in severe cases shows microvascular fibrinoid necrosis, ischemic microinfarcts, variable hemorrhage
- Chronic: Demyelination, laminar necrosis, older hemorrhage

CLINICAL ISSUES

Presentation

- Most common signs/symptoms
  - Headache, seizure, ↓ mental status, visual disturbances
  - Caution: Some patients, especially children, may be normotensive or have only minimally elevated BP
- Clinical profile
  - Child s/p transplant on immunosuppressant (e.g., cyclosporine, tacrolimus)
  - Child with acute renal disease (e.g., GN) & HTN
  - Child with tumor on chemotherapy ± HTN

Demographics

- Age
  - Any, but young > old
- Sex
  - F > M
- Epidemiology
  - In children, underlying disease is almost always present
    - Cancer, posttransplant, systemic inflammatory disorders
  - Differences in children vs. adults
    - Multiorgan failure: 84% in children, 50% in adults
    - Temporal lobe involvement: 63% vs. 39%
    - Cerebellar involvement: 21% vs. 57%
    - Restricted diffusion: 42% vs. 18%

Natural History & Prognosis

- Usually no residual abnormalities after HTN corrected
  - Reversibility related to BP normalization
  - Brainstem, deep WM lesions less reversible than cortical/subcortical
  - Diffusion restriction & hemorrhage more likely to result in permanent sequelae
  - Recent study (Pringle et al) suggests permanent injury may be more likely in children compared to adults
- PRES itself is typically not life threatening but most often occurs in serious multiorgan illness with high mortality
- 4% of patients develop recurrent PRES

Treatment

- Control BP, remove precipitating factors
- Delayed diagnosis/therapy can result in chronic neurologic sequelae

DIAGNOSTIC CHECKLIST

Consider

- Patchy bilateral parietooccipital hypodensities may be earliest NECT manifestation of PRES

Image Interpretation Pearls

- Major DDx of PRES is cerebral ischemia; DWI is positive in latter, usually negative in former
  - Ischemia is usually within vascular territory & unilateral; PRES crosses vascular territories & is usually bilateral

SELECTED REFERENCES

1. Pringle C et al: Imaging findings in neonatal and pediatric posterior reversible encephalopathy syndrome (PRES) differ from adults. Pediatr Neurol. 135:6-11, 2022
2. Triplett JD et al: Posterior reversible encephalopathy syndrome (PRES): diagnosis and management. Pract Neurol. 22(3):183-9, 2022
3. Anderson RC et al: Posterior reversible encephalopathy syndrome (PRES): pathophysiology and neuro-imaging. Front Neurol. 11:463, 2020
4. Li K et al: Clinical and MRI Features of posterior reversible encephalopathy syndrome with atypical regions: a descriptive study with a large sample size. Front Neurol. 11:194, 2020

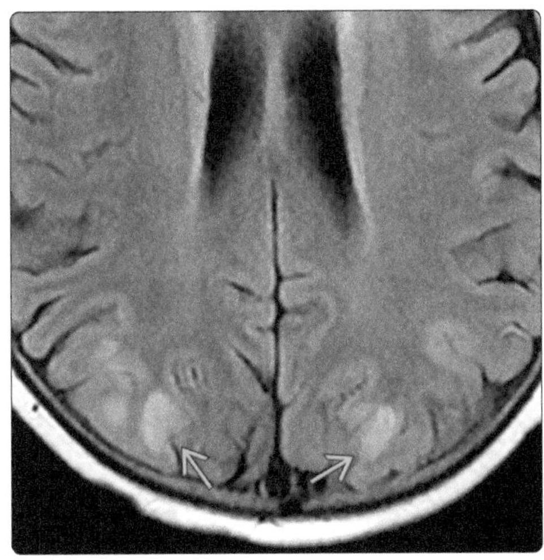

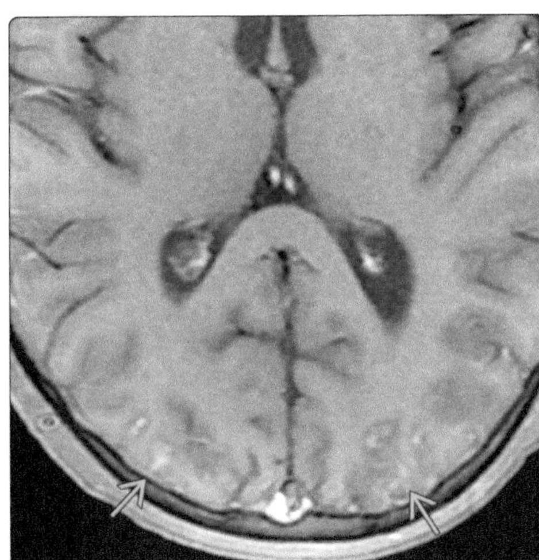

(Left) *Axial FLAIR MR in an 8-year-old with leukemia on chemotherapy, now with new-onset seizures, shows symmetric parietooccipital signal abnormality ➡. This is the most typical anatomic distribution and extent of PRES.* **(Right)** *Axial T1 C+ MR in the same patient shows leptomeningeal enhancement ➡ adjacent to the areas of signal abnormality. Enhancement is uncommon in PRES, but when it is present, a leptomeningeal pattern is most common.*

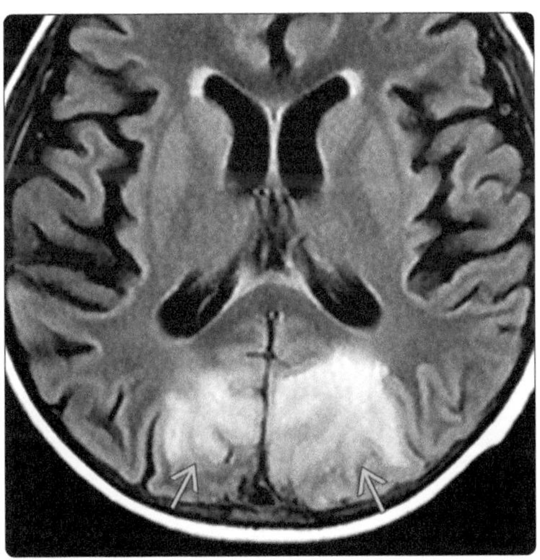

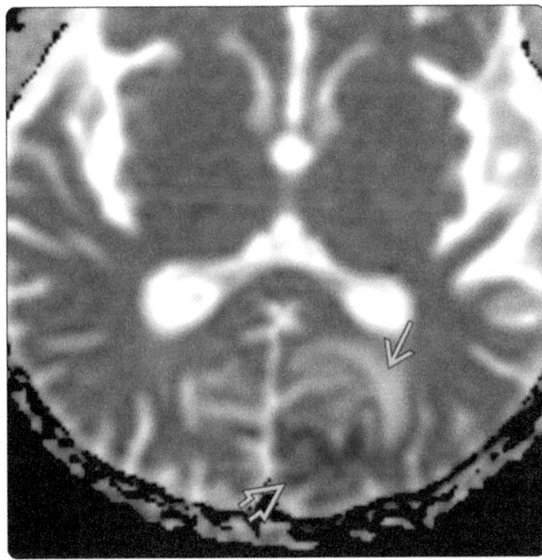

(Left) *Axial FLAIR MR in a 10-year-old with ALL shows nearly symmetric extensive signal abnormality ➡ in the bilateral parietooccipital region, the most common location of PRES.* **(Right)** *Axial ADC shows ↑ signal in the left deep occipital white matter (WM) ➡, consistent with vasogenic edema. More posteriorly within the cortex and subcortical WM ➡, there is ↓ signal consistent with diffusion restriction. Such findings are typically much smaller than the extent of FLAIR abnormality and may be irreversible.*

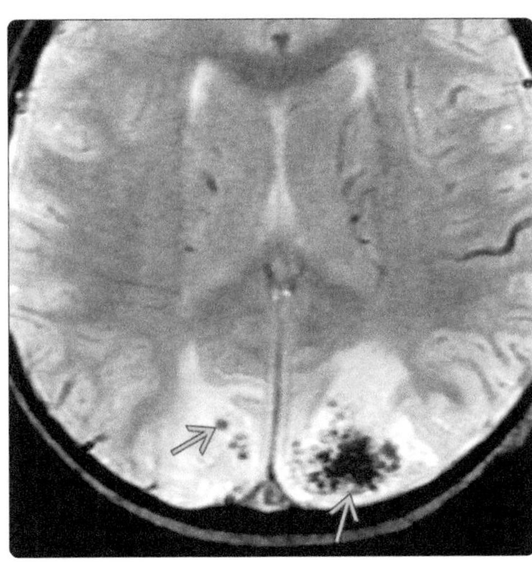

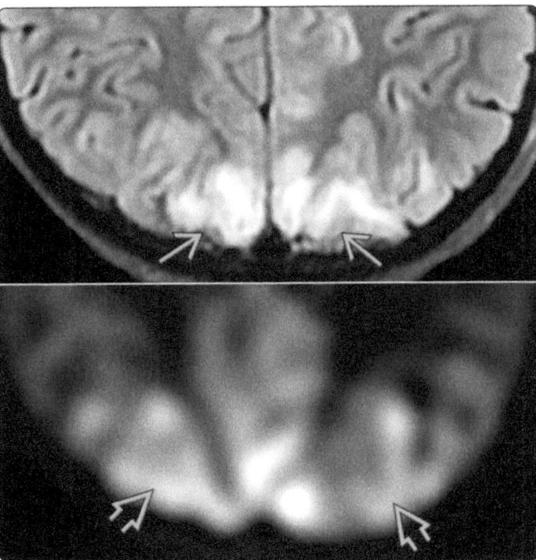

(Left) *Axial SWI MR in the same patient shows signal loss ➡ in bilateral (L > R) parietooccipital regions, consistent with microhemorrhage. Hemorrhage is seen in a small minority of cases, often resulting in permanent brain injury.* **(Right)** *Axial FLAIR (top) and ASL perfusion (bottom) MR in a 9-year-old girl with IgA nephropathy and HTN is shown. Note ↑ perfusion signal ➡ corresponding to areas of ↑ FLAIR signal ➡. Perfusion in areas of PRES involvement varies depending on disease phase.*

Mesial Temporal Sclerosis

KEY FACTS

TERMINOLOGY

- Mesial temporal sclerosis (MTS)
- Seizure-associated neuronal loss and gliosis in hippocampus and adjacent structures

IMAGING

- Primary features: Abnormal T2 hyperintensity, hippocampal volume loss/atrophy, obscuration of internal architecture
- Secondary signs: Ipsilateral fornix and mammillary body atrophy; enlarged ipsilateral temporal horn and choroidal fissure
- ↑ hyperintensity on DWI (T2 shine-through)
- ↓ NAA in hippocampus, temporal lobe

TOP DIFFERENTIAL DIAGNOSES

- Status epilepticus
- Low-grade astrocytoma
- Choroidal fissure cyst
- Hippocampal sulcus remnant

PATHOLOGY

- Prolonged febrile seizures may produce acute hippocampal injury → subsequent atrophy
- Coexistent 2nd developmental lesion in 15% of patients with MTS

CLINICAL ISSUES

- Partial complex seizures
- Often history of childhood febrile or medically intractable seizures
- Surgical temporal lobectomy reserved for medically intractable seizures, intolerable drug side effects

DIAGNOSTIC CHECKLIST

- Most common cause of partial complex epilepsy in adult age group
- Low-grade neoplasms and cortical dysplasia more common causes of partial complex epilepsy than MTS in pediatric age group

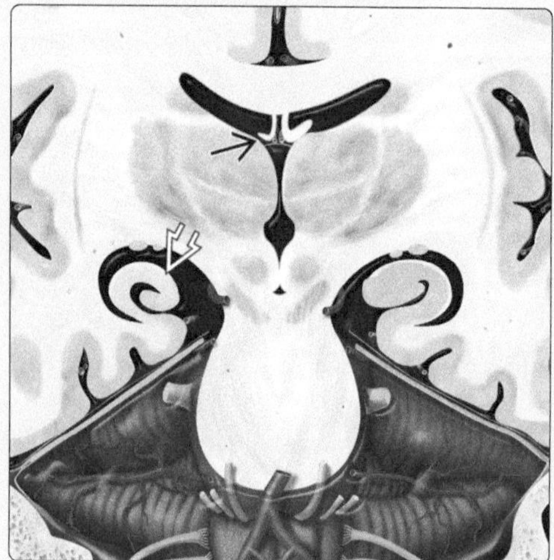

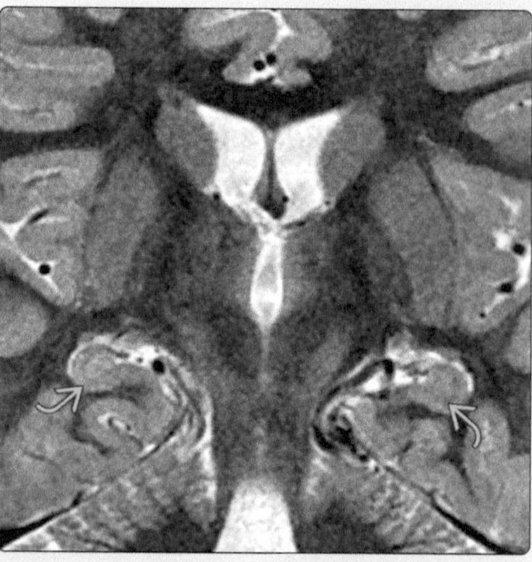

(Left) *Coronal graphic depicts the characteristic appearance of mesial temporal sclerosis (MTS). The right hippocampus ➔ is small (atrophic) with loss of normal internal architecture reflecting neuronal loss and gliosis. Note concordant atrophy of the ipsilateral fornix ➔ and widening of the ipsilateral temporal horn and choroidal fissure.* **(Right)** *Coronal STIR MR at 3T in a normal nonepileptic patient imaged for headaches demonstrates normal bilateral hippocampal anatomy ➔, size, and signal intensity.*

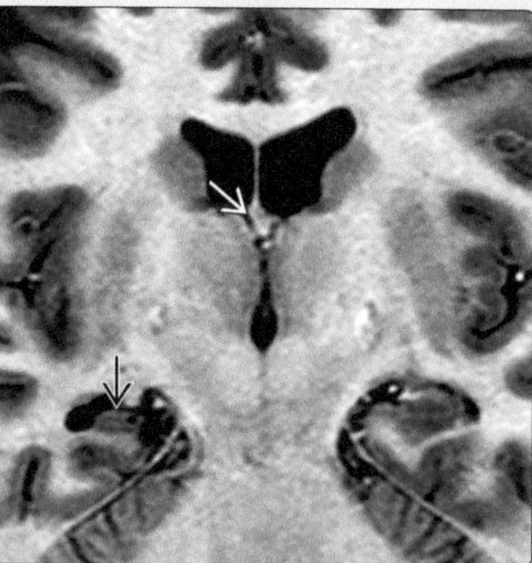

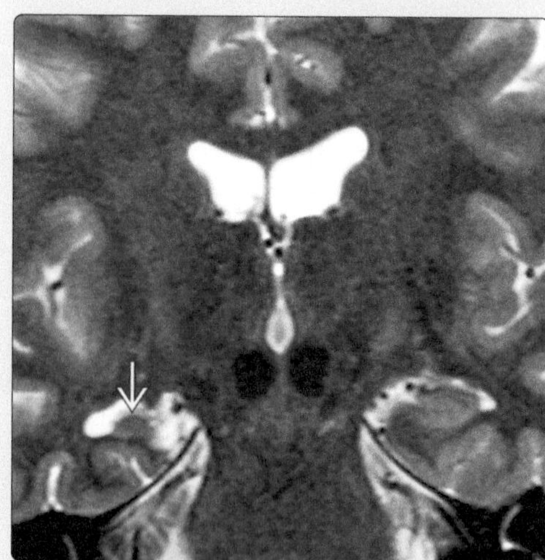

(Left) *Coronal T1 true inversion recovery MR at 3T shows asymmetric right hippocampal volume loss ➔ and obscuration of normal internal gray matter-white matter differentiation. The ipsilateral fornix ➔ is smaller than the normal left fornix.* **(Right)** *Coronal T2 MR at 3T in the same patient with right hippocampal sclerosis (HS) ➔ shows hippocampal volume loss and obscuration of normal internal architecture but normal T2 signal intensity. FLAIR MR better shows the increase in signal intensity.*

TERMINOLOGY

Abbreviations

- Mesial temporal sclerosis (MTS)

Synonyms

- Ammons horn sclerosis, hippocampal sclerosis (HS)

Definitions

- Seizure-associated neuronal loss and gliosis in hippocampus and adjacent structures

IMAGING

General Features

- Best diagnostic clue
  - Primary features: Abnormal T2 hyperintensity, hippocampal volume loss/atrophy, obscuration of internal architecture
  - Secondary signs: Ipsilateral fornix and mammillary body atrophy; enlarged ipsilateral temporal horn and choroidal fissure
  - Additional findings: Loss of ipsilateral hippocampal head (pes) digitations, parahippocampal gyrus white matter atrophy, ↑ T2 signal in anterior temporal white matter
- Location
  - Mesial temporal lobe(s), 10-20% bilateral
  - Hippocampus > amygdala > fornix > mammillary bodies
- Size
  - Slight to marked ↓ in hippocampal volume
- Morphology
  - Abnormal shape, size of affected hippocampus

CT Findings

- NECT
  - Usually normal; CT insensitive to MTS

MR Findings

- T1WI
  - ↓ hippocampal size
  - Loss of normal hippocampal gray matter-white matter differentiation
  - ± ipsilateral fornix, mammillary body atrophy
  - Quantitative hippocampal volumetry: ↑ sensitivity of MTS detection (particularly bilateral MTS)
- T2WI
  - Hippocampal atrophy
  - Obscuration of normal internal architecture
  - ↑ hippocampal signal intensity
  - ± ipsilateral fornix, mammillary body atrophy, dilatation of ipsilateral temporal horn
  - ± abnormal hyperintensity, volume loss in ipsilateral anterior temporal lobe
- FLAIR
  - Hyperintense signal in abnormal hippocampus
- DWI
  - ↑ hyperintensity on DWI (T2 shine-through)
  - ↑ diffusivity on ADC
- T1WI C+
  - No enhancement
- MRS
  - ↓ NAA in hippocampus, temporal lobe
  - ↓ NAA/Cho and ↓ NAA/Cho+Cr suggests MTS
  - ± lactate/lipid peaks after 24 hours of continual seizure

Angiographic Findings

- Presurgical Wada testing: Neuropsychologic testing after intracarotid amobarbital (Amytal) injection
  - Lateralize memory and language functions
  - Predict postoperative memory loss, feasibility of surgery
  - May help lateralize seizure onset
- fMRI mapping replacing Wada testing

Nuclear Medicine Findings

- FDG PET: Hypometabolism in abnormal mesial temporal lobe
- SPECT: Hypoperfusion (interictal) or hyperperfusion (ictal) in epileptogenic zone
  - Sensitivity of ictal > interictal

Imaging Recommendations

- Best imaging tool
  - High-resolution MR
  - MRS, quantitative volumetry may help lateralize MTS in difficult cases
- Protocol advice
  - Thin-section coronal T2WI and FLAIR (3 mm), angled perpendicular to long axis of hippocampus
  - Thin-section coronal 3D SPGR (1-2 mm), angled perpendicular to long axis of hippocampus

DIFFERENTIAL DIAGNOSIS

Status Epilepticus

- Clinical history of multiple seizures or status epilepticus
- Temporary T2 hyperintensity ± gyriform enhancement in affected cortex, hippocampus

Low-Grade Astrocytoma

- Hyperintense temporal lobe white matter mass (usually nonenhancing)
- ± seizures, young adults typical

Choroidal Fissure Cyst

- Asymptomatic CSF signal cyst in choroidal fissure distorts normal hippocampus
  - Round on axial, coronal images
  - Oval, parallels temporal lobe long axis on sagittal imaging
- No abnormal T2 hyperintensity in mesial temporal lobe

Hippocampal Sulcus Remnant

- Failure of normal hippocampal sulcus involution → asymptomatic cyst between dentate gyrus, cornu ammonis (CA)
- Common normal variant (10-15%)

Cavernous Malformation

- Heterogeneous hyperintense "popcorn" lesion with dark complete hemosiderin rim
- ± seizures

Dysembryoplastic Neuroepithelial Tumor

- Demarcated "bubbly," variably enhancing cortical mass ± regional cortical dysplasia
- Partial complex seizures

Cortical Dysplasia

- Most common dual pathology associated with MTS
- T2 hyperintensity in anterior temporal white matter

PATHOLOGY

General Features

- Etiology
  - Controversial whether acquired or developmental
    - Acquired: Follows complicated febrile seizures (FSs), status epilepticus, encephalitis
    - Developmental: 2nd developmental lesion identified in 15%
    - 2-hit hypothesis: 1st, initial precipitating injury (like complicated seizures); 2nd, ↑ vulnerability (such as genetic predisposition or developmental anomaly)
    - Most likely MTS represents common outcome of both acquired and developmental processes
  - FSs most common childhood seizure disorder (2-5%)
    - Prolonged FSs may produce acute hippocampal injury → subsequent atrophy
- Genetics
  - Familial cases of mesial temporal lobe epilepsy (TLE), FSs reported
  - Recent studies suggest relationship between FSs and later epilepsy development may be genetic
  - Syndrome-specific genes for FSs (channelopathies) account for small proportion of FS cases
- Associated abnormalities
  - Coexistent 2nd developmental lesion (15%)

Gross Pathologic & Surgical Features

- Normal hippocampus divided anatomically into head (pes), body, tail
  - Subdivision into Ammons horn, dentate gyrus, hippocampal sulcus, fimbria, alveus, subiculum, parahippocampal gyrus, collateral sulcus
- Mesial temporal lobe atrophy: Hippocampal body (88%), tail (61%), head (51%), amygdala (12%)
- Absence of hemorrhage or necrosis

Microscopic Features

- Chronic astrogliosis with fine fibrillary background of bland astrocytic nuclei and ↓ residual neurons
- Ammons horn, CA, contains 4 zones of granular cells: CA1, CA2, CA3, CA4
  - CA1, CA4 pyramidal cell layers most susceptible to ischemia
  - All hippocampal regions may show varying neuronal cell loss

CLINICAL ISSUES

Presentation

- Most common signs/symptoms
  - Partial complex seizures, automatisms
    - Simple at younger ages and increasingly complex and discrete with age
- Other signs/symptoms
  - May progress to generalized tonic-clonic seizures
- Clinical profile
  - Often history of childhood febrile or medically intractable seizures
    - History of complex or prolonged FSs ↑ risk for development of hippocampal injury, MTS
  - Surface electro- (EEG) or magneto- (MEG) encephalogram helpful for localization (60-90%)
  - Intracranial EEG (subdural or depth electrodes) may be indicated if noninvasive studies discordant

Demographics

- Age
  - Disease of older children, young adults
- Sex
  - No predominance
- Epidemiology
  - MTS accounts for majority of epilepsy patients undergoing temporal lobe seizure surgery

Natural History & Prognosis

- Anterior temporal lobectomy 70-95% successful if MR findings are of MTS
- Success of anterior temporal lobectomy 40-55% if MR normal
- ↓ surgical success when amygdala involved

Treatment

- Clinical management based on phenotypic features of initial febrile and subsequent seizures
- Medical treatment initial approach
- Surgical temporal lobectomy reserved for medically intractable seizures, intolerable drug side effects
  - Resection includes anterior temporal lobe, majority of hippocampus, variable portions of amygdala
- Stereotactic laser amygdalohippocampectomy (LiTT) less invasive option in early phases of use

DIAGNOSTIC CHECKLIST

Consider

- Most common cause of partial complex epilepsy in adults
- Bilateral in 10-20%; difficult to detect without quantitative volumetry unless severe

Image Interpretation Pearls

- Coronal high-resolution T2WI, FLAIR MR most sensitive for MTS
- Dual pathology in 15%
- In pediatric age group, low-grade neoplasms (epilepsy associated tumors) and cortical dysplasia more common causes of partial complex epilepsy than MTS

SELECTED REFERENCES

1. Jayalakshmi S et al: Long-term seizure freedom, resolution of epilepsy and perceived life changes in drug resistant temporal lobe epilepsy with hippocampal sclerosis: comparison of surgical versus medical management. Neurosurgery. 92(6):1249-58, 2023
2. Jesus-Ribeiro J et al: Resective epilepsy surgery and respective histopathological diagnoses: a retrospective cohort study. Acta Med Port. 36(4):229-35, 2023
3. Kanner AM et al: Long-term seizure and psychiatric outcomes following laser ablation of mesial temporal structures. Epilepsia. 63(4):812-23, 2022
4. Fayed I et al: MR-guided laser interstitial thermal therapy for medically refractory lesional epilepsy in pediatric patients: experience and outcomes. Pediatr Neurosurg. 53(5):322-9, 2018

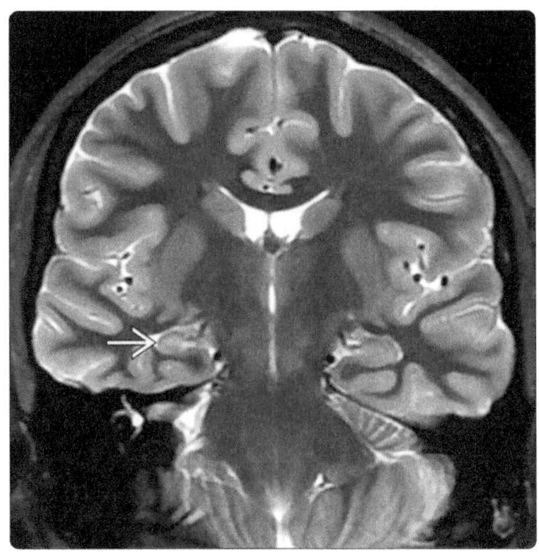

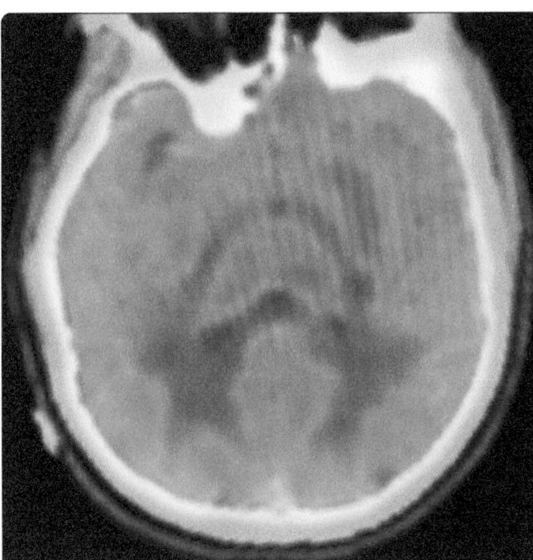

(Left) *Coronal STIR MR in an adolescent patient with complex partial epilepsy shows right hippocampal volume loss ➡, internal T2 hyperintensity, and obscuration of internal architecture compatible with MTS. FLAIR MR (not shown) confirmed abnormal hyperintensity.* **(Right)** *Axial PET/CT in the same patient reveals hypometabolic uptake of radiotracer in the right temporal lobe compared to normal left side. Semiology and EEG correlated with right MTS.*

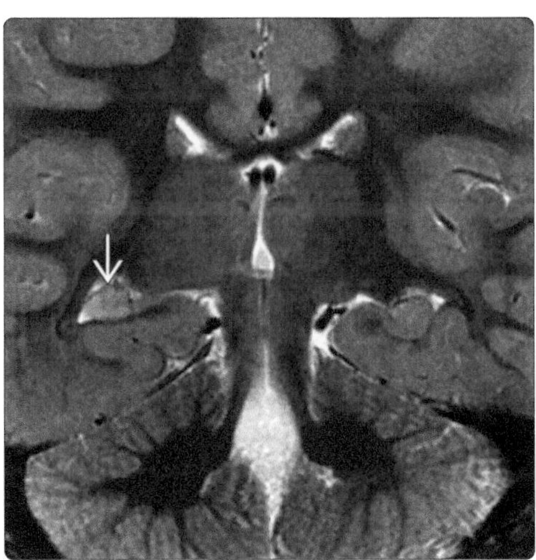

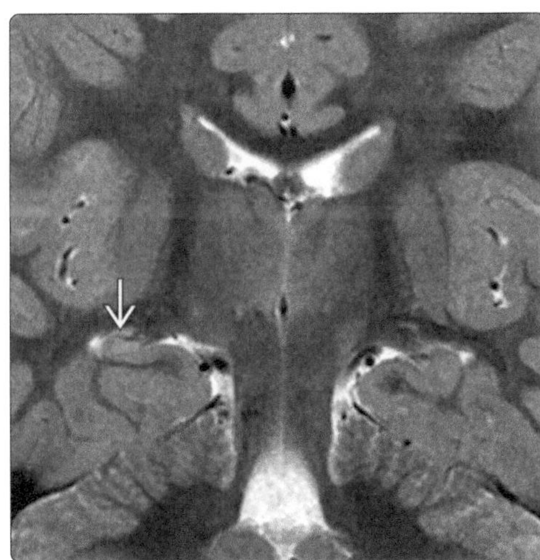

(Left) *Coronal STIR MR in a 2-year-old with acute febrile complex partial seizures demonstrates abnormal T2 hyperintensity (and diffusion restriction, not shown) within the right hippocampal formation ➡ compared to the normal left hippocampus.* **(Right)** *Coronal STIR MR in the same patient performed during follow-up 9 months later for persistent seizures shows T2 hyperintensity as well as volume loss within the right hippocampal formation ➡ compatible with evolving HS.*

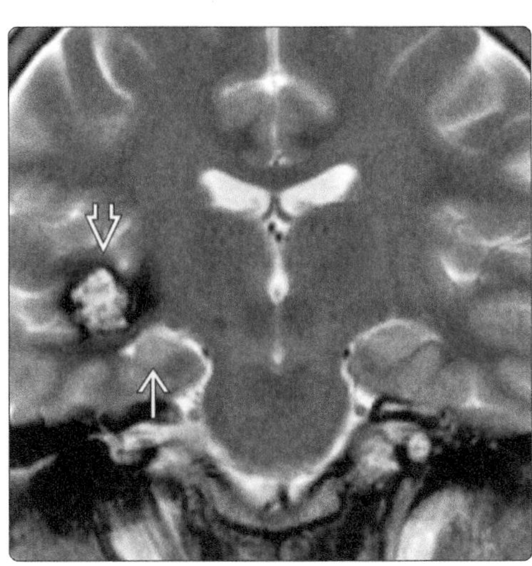

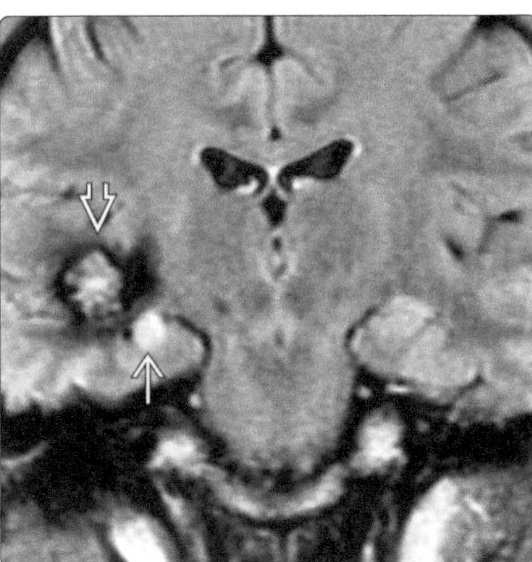

(Left) *Coronal T2 MR in a chronic seizure patient with a large right temporal lobe cavernous malformation ➡ demonstrates all 3 primary determinants of right HS ➡ (volume loss, T2 hyperintensity, and loss of internal architecture).* **(Right)** *Coronal FLAIR MR in the same patient with right temporal lobe cavernous malformation ➡ better shows HS ➡. Hyperintensity is usually more conspicuous on FLAIR MR, while T2 is better for depicting internal structure.*

Cerebellitis

KEY FACTS

TERMINOLOGY
- Acute cerebellitis

IMAGING
- Bilateral cerebellar hemispheric gray matter & white matter low attenuation (NECT), T2/FLAIR hyperintensity (MR); unilateral involvement less common
- Confluent regions of T2 prolongation, affecting gray matter & white matter
- ± pial or subtle parenchymal enhancement
- DWI/ADC → affected regions typically show ↑ diffusivity

TOP DIFFERENTIAL DIAGNOSES
- Demyelinating disease (multiple sclerosis or acute disseminated encephalomyelitis)
- Cerebellar infarct
- Infiltrating cerebellar neoplasm

PATHOLOGY
- Reported in association with COVID-19, varicella, EBV, enterovirus, rotavirus, human herpesvirus 7 (HHV-7), mumps, measles, influenza, & mycoplasma pneumoniae
- Difficult to distinguish infectious vs. immune etiologies
- Moderate to severe cerebellar swelling → vascular compression, upward transtentorial herniation, tonsillar herniation, brainstem compression, obstructive hydrocephalus

CLINICAL ISSUES
- Truncal ataxia, dysmetria, & headache
- Symptoms of ↑ intracranial pressure: Irritability, occipital headache & vomiting may overshadow manifestations of cerebellar dysfunction
- Most symptoms & signs resolve completely over weeks to months
- Surgery rarely necessary to decompress herniating cerebellum; ventricular drain for hydrocephalus

(Left) *Axial NECT in an 8-year-old with subtle low attenuation in the right cerebellar hemisphere ➡ with effacement of 4th ventricle ➡ & posterior fossa cisterns ➡ is shown. CT attenuation changes are often very subtle in cerebellitis, so it's important to look for loss of CSF spaces to suggest the diagnosis.* **(Right)** *Axial FLAIR MR in a 5-year-old with acute cerebellitis shows nearly symmetric swelling & signal abnormality within the cerebellar hemispheres. The majority of cerebellitis cases involve both cerebellar hemispheres.*

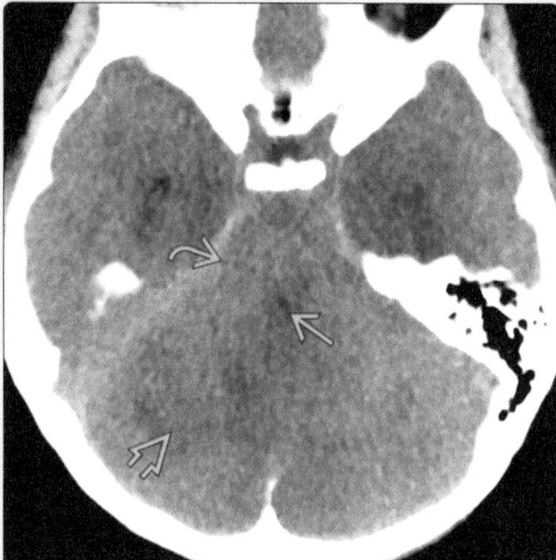

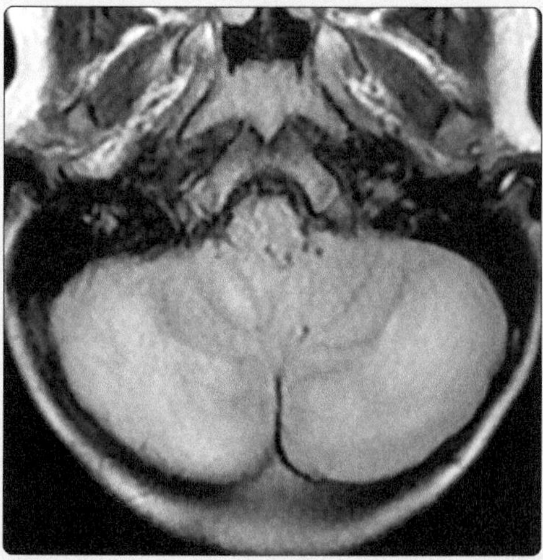

(Left) *Axial FLAIR MR in a 2-year-old with lethargy & imbalance shows diffusely increased signal ➡ throughout the bilateral cerebellar hemispheres, suggesting acute cerebellitis. Note the marked increase in signal compared to normal occipital lobes ➡.* **(Right)** *Axial T1 C+ MR in the same patient shows increased leptomeningeal enhancement ➡ in the affected cerebellar hemispheres. Enhancement is often subtle & most often affects the leptomeningeal spaces with parenchymal enhancement less common.*

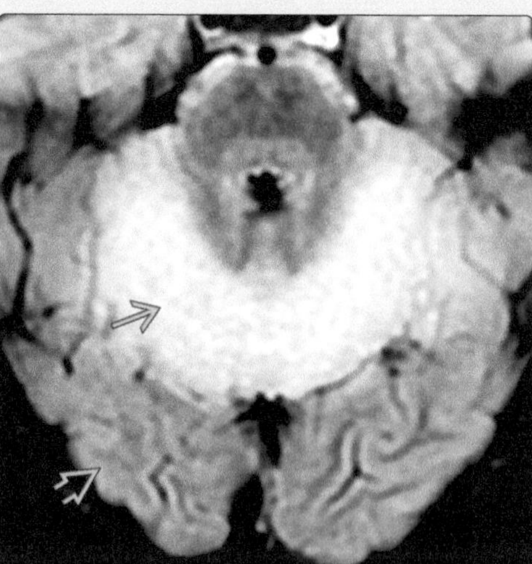

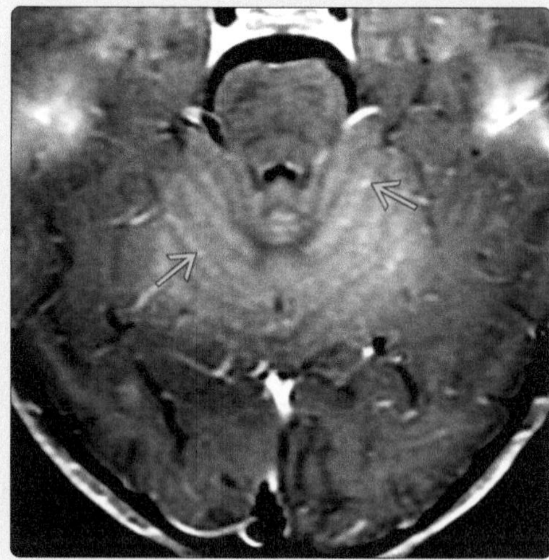

TERMINOLOGY

Synonyms

- Acute cerebellitis

Definitions

- Infectious, postinfectious, or postvaccination cerebellar inflammation

IMAGING

General Features

- Best diagnostic clue
  - Bilateral cerebellar hemispheric gray matter & white matter low attenuation (NECT), T2/FLAIR hyperintensity (MR); unilateral involvement less common
- Location
  - Cerebellar gray matter & white matter, typically bilateral
- Morphology
  - Often associated with upward transtentorial & downward tonsillar herniation

Imaging Recommendations

- Best imaging tool
  - MR, including C+, DWI, MRS

CT Findings

- NECT
  - Bilateral or, less commonly, unilateral low attenuation involving gray matter & white matter of cerebellar hemispheres

MR Findings

- T1WI
  - Regions of T1 hypointensity in cerebellum
- T2WI
  - T2 hyperintensity affecting gray matter & white matter of cerebellum
- DWI
  - Typically shows ↑ diffusivity
- T1WI C+
  - ± pial or subtle parenchymal enhancement
- MRS
  - Acutely: ↑ excitatory neurotransmitters, ↑ choline, ± lactate & lipid, NL to ↓ NAA

DIFFERENTIAL DIAGNOSIS

Demyelinating Disease (Multiple Sclerosis or Acute Disseminated Encephalomyelitis)

- Look for supratentorial peripheral white matter, basal ganglia (BG), & brainstem lesions

Cerebellar Infarct

- Typical vascular distribution, DWI positive

Infiltrating Cerebellar Neoplasm

- Typical bilateral involvement of gray matter & white matter in cases of cerebellitis is helpful
- Use MRS as adjunct when tumor is considered (↓ NAA, ± ↓ creatine, ↑ choline, myoinositol, ± lactate & lipid)

PATHOLOGY

General Features

- Etiology
  - Reported in association with COVID-19, varicella, EBV, enterovirus, rotavirus, human herpesvirus 7 (HHV-7), mumps, measles, influenza, & mycoplasma pneumoniae
  - Difficult to distinguish infectious vs. immune etiology
  - In most cases, definite etiology remains unknown
- Associated abnormalities
  - Moderate to severe cerebellar swelling → upward transtentorial herniation, tonsillar herniation, brainstem compression, obstructive hydrocephalus

Gross Pathologic & Surgical Features

- Acutely, cerebellar edema, nonhemorrhagic involving gray matter & white matter

Microscopic Features

- Acute: Edema with lymphocytic & eosinophilic infiltrates
- Chronic: ± cerebellar atrophy

CLINICAL ISSUES

Presentation

- Most common signs/symptoms
  - Truncal ataxia, dysmetria, & headache
  - Symptoms of ↑ intracranial pressure: Irritability, occipital headache, & vomiting may overshadow manifestations of cerebellar dysfunction

Demographics

- Age
  - Usually in younger children
- Epidemiology
  - Typically follows viral infection

Natural History & Prognosis

- Most symptoms resolve completely over weeks to months
- Severe cases with herniation & hydrocephalus: Variable outcome from full recovery to death

Treatment

- Typically supportive, ± steroids, ± antivirals if specific diagnosis is confirmed
- Surgery rarely necessary to decompress herniating cerebellum; ventricular drain for hydrocephalus

DIAGNOSTIC CHECKLIST

Consider

- Acute cerebellitis when bihemispheric gray matter & white matter cerebellar involvement

Image Interpretation Pearls

- Bilateral cerebellar hemispheric gray matter & white matter edema; unilateral involvement less common

SELECTED REFERENCES

1. Orman G et al: Can MRI Differentiate between infectious and immune-related acute cerebellitis? A retrospective imaging study. AJNR Am J Neuroradiol. 42(12):2231-7, 2021
2. Yildirim M et al: Acute cerebellitis or postinfectious cerebellar ataxia? Clinical and imaging features in acute cerebellitis. J Child Neurol. 35(6):380-8, 2020

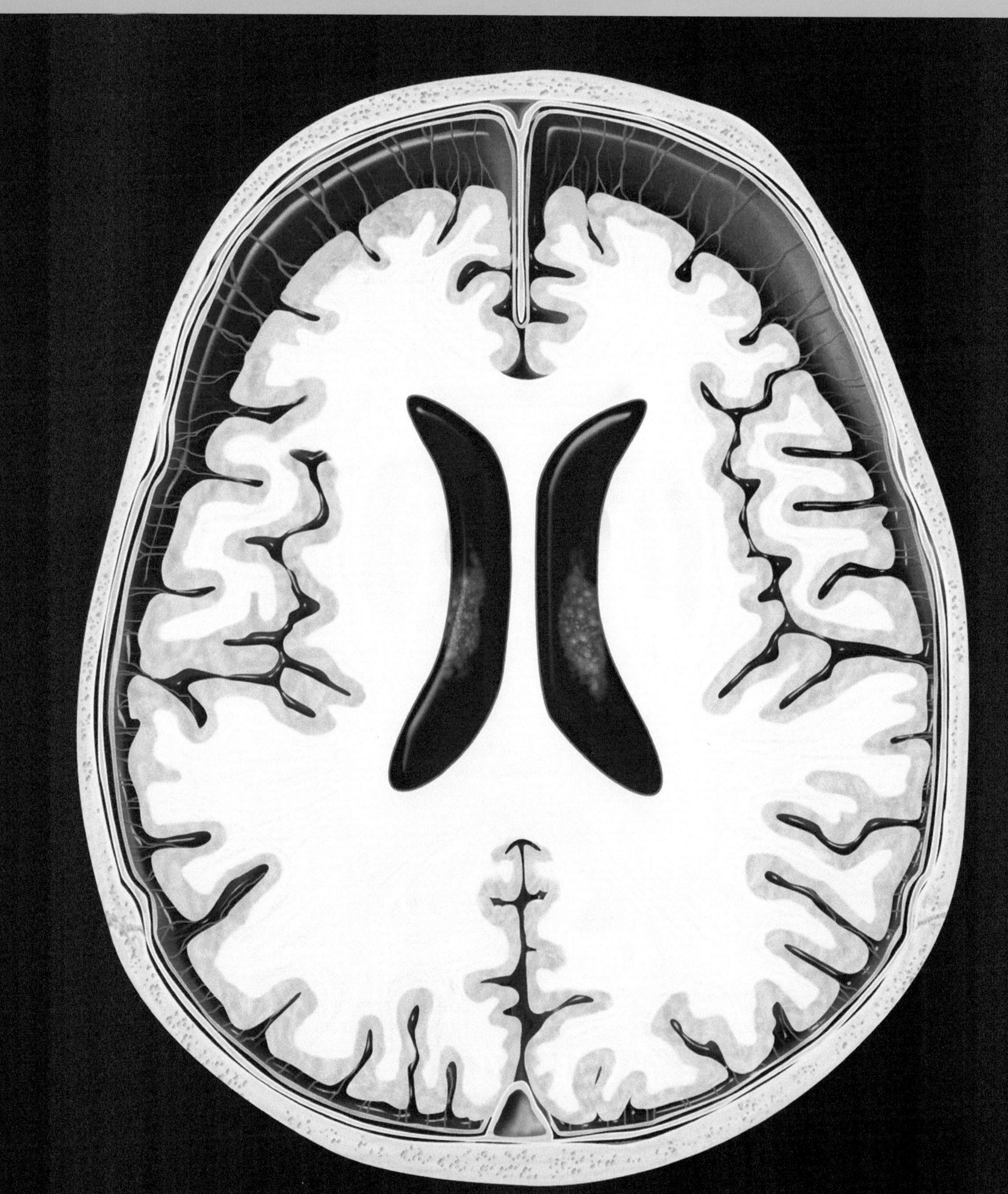

PART I
SECTION 2

Anatomy-Based Diagnoses

Ventricles and Cisterns

Sella and Pituitary

Skull, Scalp, and Meninges

Embryology

Ventricular development starts with the closing of the neural tube, which occurs in humans at ~ 28 postconceptual days with the closure of the posterior neuropore. Subsequently, the central lumen of the neural tube enlarges to form the forebrain, midbrain, and hindbrain vesicles, which will become the lateral, 3rd, and 4th ventricles. At ~ the 2nd gestational month, neuroependyma and some mesenchyme from the developing leptomeninges invaginates into the lumen of the 4th ventricle to form the epithelium (from the neuroependyma), stroma, and vasculature (from the leptomeninges) of the choroid plexus, soon followed by similar invaginations into the 3rd and lateral ventricles. These structures secrete the early CSF that helps the ventricles expand. In addition, the choroid plexuses secrete multiple proteins that are postulated to stimulate proliferation of the neuroependymal cells, stimulating mitosis to generate the cells that will be the building blocks of the developing cerebral hemispheres. Although the choroid plexuses initially occupy > 70% of the ventricular lumen, their relative sizes diminish with growth of the brain and ventricular system.

The production, circulation, and resorption of CSF are key functions of the ventricular system. CSF is found in the brain prior to development of intrinsic brain vasculature, and it is believed to initially form from degeneration of gel-like meninx primitiva that surrounds the developing brain. Later, CSF production begins, primarily in the choroid plexuses, but it is likely that some is produced by ependymal cells and possible that some is produced in the parenchyma, perhaps via filtration through capillary walls. Flow of CSF is primarily from the lateral ventricles to the 3rd ventricle and then through the cerebral aqueduct and the 4th ventricle and its outflow foramina (of Magendie and Luschka) into the cisterna magna and cisterns around the brainstem. From these locations, CSF pulsations result in mixing of this CSF with that already present in the subarachnoid spaces, probably by a combination of diffusion and laminar flow propelled by CSF exiting the ventricular system. Eventually, this CSF is resorbed either into the circulating blood via capillaries or venous structures. In adults, CSF is produced at a rate of ~ 500 mL/day, completely replacing existing CSF (volume ~ 300-400 mL in adults) at least daily.

In addition to cell proliferation and CSF production, the walls of the ventricles contain the **circumventricular organs**, 7 structures that (1) permit polypeptide hypothalamic hormones to leave the brain without disrupting the blood-brain barrier (BBB), and (2) permit substances that do not cross the BBB to trigger changes in brain function, particularly the regulation of endocrine and autonomic function. These include the area postrema, the organum vasculosum of the lamina terminalis, and the subfornical organ, which are sensory organs, in addition to the subcommissural organ, the neurohypophysis and median eminence of the hypothalamus, and the pineal gland, which are secretory organs. All allow the brain to sense noxious stimuli or disrupted body regulation (osmoregulation, electrolyte regulation, polypeptide regulation, cardiovascular regulation), circadian oscillations, patency of the sylvian aqueduct, and other functions under investigation. As the CSF enters the ventricles without having to cross the BBB, it brings clues of extra-CNS disruptions of homeostasis and allows CNS-mediated responses without exposing the brain to noxious materials.

Imaging Anatomy

The normal anatomy of the cerebral ventricles in children is quite consistent. The lateral ventricles are composed of the frontal horns, bodies (in the posterior frontal and parietal regions), occipital horns, temporal horns, and trigones (also called atria, where the bodies, occipital, and temporal horns intersect). CSF from the lateral ventricles flows through the paired foramina of Monro (between the upper forniceal columns and the anterior thalami) into the 3rd ventricle, and then through the cerebral aqueduct into the 4th ventricle (lying between the cerebellar vermis and the dorsal surface of the brainstem), exiting dorsally into the cisterna magna via the midline foramen of Magendie and ventrally into the prepontine/premedullary spaces via the paired foramina of Luschka.

Several features of the anatomy of the normal pediatric cerebral ventricles are important. The medial and lateral walls of the frontal horns and bodies are parallel and straight, not rounded. The temporal horns are quite narrow, and their anteromedial borders (in front of the hippocampi) form a sharp point. The occipital horns initially extend very far posteriorly; portions of the walls of the posterior occipital horns may fuse, leaving an (apparently) isolated, CSF-containing structure of variable size in the posterior occipital lobe; this is an "isolated" occipital horn, not a cyst or tumor. On T2 FLAIR images, the fused ventricular walls between this structure and the main portion of the occipital horn can be seen as a small streak of hyperintensity. Other important features of ventricular anatomy are the 3rd ventricular recesses: The chiasmatic recess between the inferior border of the lamina terminalis and the optic chiasm, the infundibular recess extending into the proximal pituitary stalk, and the suprapineal recess. When normal, these are sharply pointed; rounding or expansion suggests hydrocephalus.

Another important feature of the ventricular system is the cerebral aqueduct, the narrowest portion of the ventricular system. Due to its narrow diameter, the aqueduct is the section with most rapid CSF flow, leading to a characteristic signal hypointensity (the so-called flow void) on T2WI acquired using 2D spin-echo acquisition. Also, because of its narrow diameter, the aqueduct is the section of the ventricular system most commonly narrowed or obstructed by intrinsic and extrinsic processes.

Blockage in the ventricles results in "intraventricular obstructive hydrocephalus." The appearance of the ventricles in these cases depends on the location of the blockage and the severity. Narrowing or obstruction of a single foramen of Monro causes enlargement of the ipsilateral lateral ventricle: The frontal and temporal horns and ventricular body become enlarged and rounded, and the trigones and occipital horns enlarge. The anterior temporal horns become round in their anteromedial portion, which is normally sharply pointed. Typically, both foramina are narrowed or obstructed, and both lateral ventricles enlarge, usually commensurately, although small lesions like colloid cysts or bilateral subependymal nodules/giant cell tumors from tuberous sclerosis may result in asymmetrical enlargement. Narrowing of the distal 3rd ventricle or aqueduct causes enlargement of the lateral ventricles and 3rd ventricle. Early or mild 3rd ventricular enlargement is characterized by dilated chiasmal, infundibular, and, occasionally, suprapineal, recesses, and flattening or inferior convexity/rounding (rather than the normal inferior concavity) of the ventricle. Obstruction of the 4th ventricle or its outflow foramina results in tetraventricular hydrocephalus, in which all 4 ventricles are enlarged. Typically, however, the 4th ventricle is less severely enlarged than the 3rd ventricle or lateral ventricle in these situations, possibly because the supratentorial compartment is larger than the infratentorial compartment, allowing more room for expansion. If the 4th ventricle is disproportionately enlarged compared to the lateral and 3rd ventricles, stenosis of both the aqueduct and the 4th ventricular outflow foramina should be considered. CSF flow within the ventricular system can also result from septations within the ventricles. This is most often the result of bacterial infections of the CNS in which frank pus accumulates within the ventricles and subarachnoid spaces. CSF obstruction occurs at multiple sites; this condition is discussed below.

Blockage of CSF flow in the subarachnoid spaces (most commonly in the basilar cisterns) or at the sites of CSF absorption into the venous system results in "extraventricular obstructive hydrocephalus." The imaging appearance of the ventricles differs slightly in this condition. Massive dilation of the lateral ventricles, as is sometimes seen in 3rd ventricular or aqueductal narrowing/obstruction, is not seen in this scenario, nor is the disproportional enlargement of the anterior and pineal recesses of the 3rd ventricle. The reason for this is likely the lack of large pressure differential between the intraventricular and cisternal CSF when CSF freely communicates between the 2 spaces. A final imaging appearance is what is sometimes (incorrectly) called "pentaventricular hydrocephalus." In this condition, scarring and flow obstruction occurs in the 4th ventricular outflow foramina and the basilar cisterns. In this situation, the 4th ventricle massively enlarges and herniates through the foramen of Magendie (occasionally through the Luschka foramina as well), pushing the cerebellar vermis posteriorly and upward. The appearance on sagittal images appears to be enlargement of both ventricles and cisterna magna (but is in fact a very severe case of tetraventricular hydrocephalus).

Hydrocephalus becomes complex when flow is obstructed at multiple sites, particularly when the sites are both intra- and extraventricular. The most common cause for this is infection, particularly ventriculitis secondary to meningitis or large intraventricular hemorrhages (IVHs). In bacterial ventriculitis, the inflammatory response may result in multiple fluid loculations separated by septations of various thickness. Some of the loculations are in the parenchyma, while others are intraventricular; the pattern of loculations, therefore, obscures the location of the ventricular lumen. IVH rarely causes multiple loculations, most often narrowing the aqueduct and, less commonly, the outflow foramina of the lateral and 4th ventricles. In these situations, the imaging appearance after ventriculoperitoneal shunting or 3rd ventriculostomy is often that of an enlarged 4th ventricle with decompressed lateral and 3rd ventricles, the "trapped" or "isolated" 4th ventricle.

Imaging Protocols

In the assessment of the cerebral ventricles and processes that alter normal CSF flow dynamics, one should always start with good anatomic imaging sequences. Sagittal images will show enlargement of the lateral ventricles and the recesses of the 3rd ventricle, inferior convexity, rather than the normal concavity, of the 3rd ventricular floor (resulting in decrease of the mamillopontine distance), patency or narrowing of the aqueduct and the presence of periaqueductal masses, and size/shape of the 4th ventricle. Coronal images show enlargement of the temporal horns with rounding of the medial aspect (above the hippocampus) along with enlargement of the anterior recesses of the 3rd ventricle (with the thin hypothalamus forming the lateral walls) greater than the superior 3rd ventricle (with the thicker thalami forming the lateral walls).

Steady-state free precession studies (FIESTA, CISS) can be very useful to demonstrate intraventricular cysts of membranes and should always be obtained if the precise cause or location of the obstruction of CSF flow is uncertain. Cysts, membranes, and small organisms (such as cysticerci) within the ventricles or thickened membranes at the outflow foramina can be very difficult to see on T1 or T2/FLAIR images, and the use of steady-state imaging techniques often allows a diagnosis to be made without intraventricular contrast injections. An additional use of Steady-State-free precession techniques is to accurately locate the course and tip of an intraventricular catheter in complicated hydrocephalus. The sagittal plane is generally the most useful, but axial and coronal planes may detect septations and other abnormalities not conspicuous on sagittal imaging.

If steady-state imaging does not give an answer, CSF flow studies may be helpful. These are performed most commonly using cardiac-gated, phase-contrast MR imaging, taking advantage of the CSF pulsations induced by expansion of intracranial vessels after each cardiac systole. Because the cranium contains a fixed volume, the entrance of blood into intracranial vessels with each cardiac systole requires the same amount of fluid to exit the brain (Monro-Kellie doctrine). The expansion of cerebral capillaries causes contraction of the ventricles and pulsations in the subarachnoid space that drive CSF out of the ventricles into the cisterns and out of the intracranial cisterns into the spinal subarachnoid space. This movement and its direction of flow can be evaluated by the phase encoding of the protons at the time of each ventricular contraction via cardiac gating. Although this technique is used primarily at the foramen magnum, it can also be used to measure flow at the cerebral aqueduct.

Selected References

1. Gallo P et al: Trapped fourth ventricle: pathophysiology, history and treatment strategies. Adv Tech Stand Neurosurg. 46:205-20, 2023
2. Robinson S et al: Pathogenesis of posthemorrhagic hydrocephalus of prematurity: new horizons. Semin Perinatol. 46(5):151596, 2022
3. Spennato P et al: The effect of image-guided ventricular catheter placement on shunt failure: a systematic review and meta-analysis. Childs Nerv Syst. 38(6):1069-76, 2022
4. Abdelhamed Z et al: A mutation in Ccdc39 causes neonatal hydrocephalus with abnormal motile cilia development in mice. Development. 145(1), 2018
5. Korzh V: Development of brain ventricular system. Cell Mol Life Sci. 75(3):375-83, 2018
6. Bueno D et al: Evolutionary development of embryonic cerebrospinal fluid composition and regulation: an open research field with implications for brain development and function. Fluids Barriers CNS. 13:5, 2016
7. Gandhoke GS et al: Role of magnetic resonance ventriculography in multiloculated hydrocephalus. J Neurosurg Pediatr. 11(6):697-703, 2013
8. Bateman GA et al: The measurement of CSF flow through the aqueduct in normal and hydrocephalic children: from where does it come, to where does it go? Childs Nerv Syst. 28(1):55-63, 2012
9. Vinchon M et al: Pediatric hydrocephalus outcomes: a review. Fluids Barriers CNS. 9(1):18, 2012
10. Rekate HL: A consensus on the classification of hydrocephalus: its utility in the assessment of abnormalities of cerebrospinal fluid dynamics. Childs Nerv Syst. 27(10):1535-41, 2011

(Left) *Midline sagittal T1WI MR of the 3rd and 4th ventricles shows the chiasmal, infundibular, and suprapineal recesses of the 3rd ventricles at their normal sizes. Note that the aqueduct is normally narrower proximally than distally. The fastigium of the 4th ventricle and the foramen of Magendie are well seen.* **(Right)** *Axial T1WI MR at the level of the frontal horns and trigones shows normal ventricular size in a child, including slender occipital horns.*

Normal 3rd and 4th Ventricles

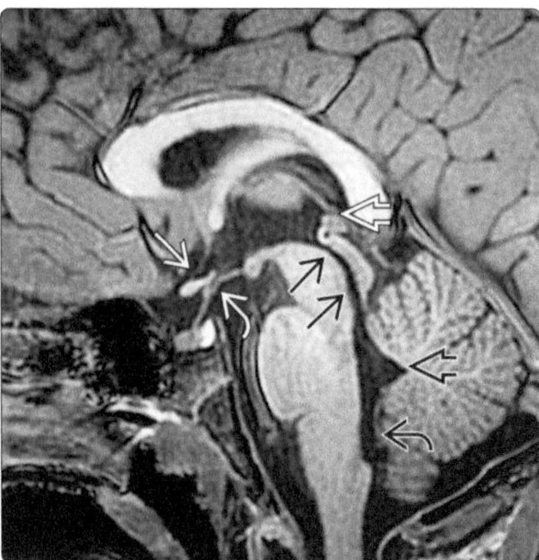

Normal Lateral Ventricles

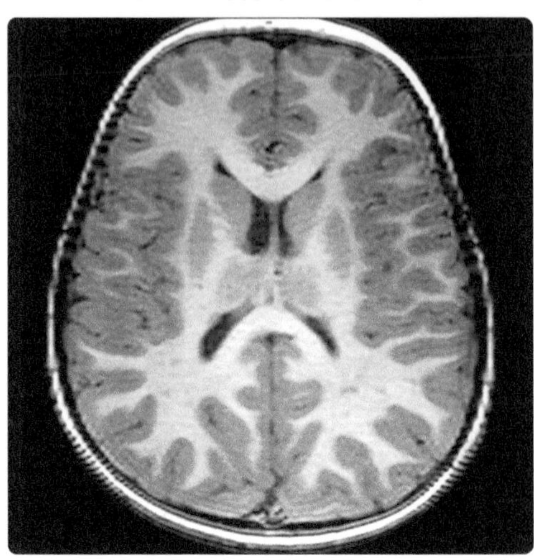

(Left) *Axial FLAIR MR shows the normal slit-like anterior recesses of the 3rd ventricle. In addition, note the high signal intensity in the medial occipital lobes, where the curvilinear coapted left occipital horn and the small, cyst-like residuum of the left occipital horn are seen.* **(Right)** *Coronal FLAIR MR through the occipital lobes shows small hyperintensities representing the coapted occipital horns. These should not be mistaken for dysplasias or injuries.*

Normal Lateral and 3rd Ventricles

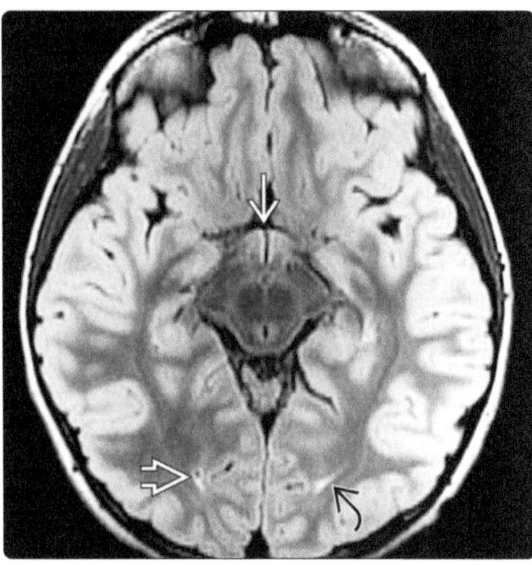

Normal Occipital Horns

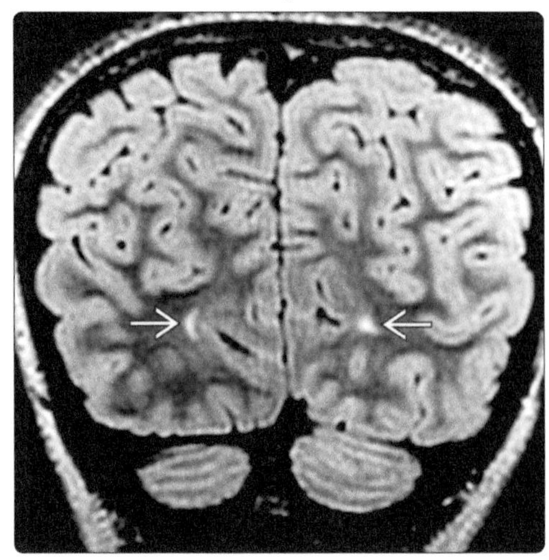

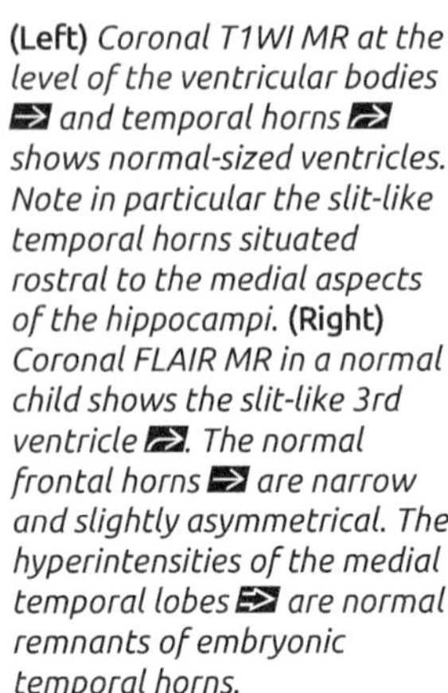

(Left) *Coronal T1WI MR at the level of the ventricular bodies and temporal horns shows normal-sized ventricles. Note in particular the slit-like temporal horns situated rostral to the medial aspects of the hippocampi.* **(Right)** *Coronal FLAIR MR in a normal child shows the slit-like 3rd ventricle. The normal frontal horns are narrow and slightly asymmetrical. The hyperintensities of the medial temporal lobes are normal remnants of embryonic temporal horns.*

Normal Lateral Ventricles

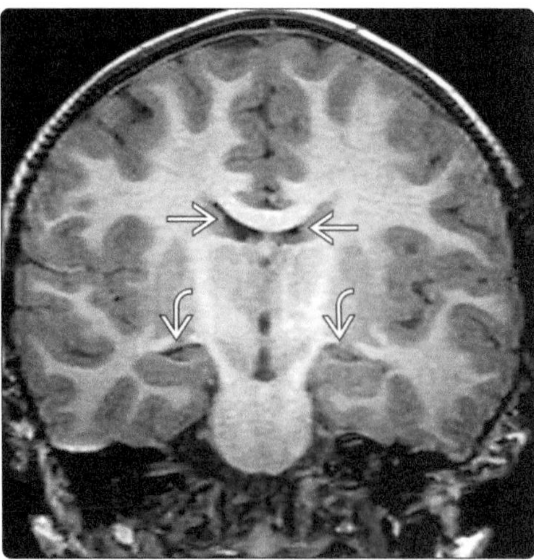

Normal Lateral and 3rd Ventricles

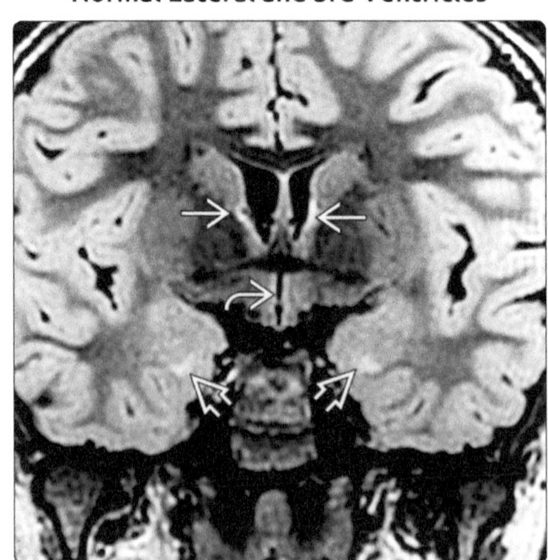

Intraventricular Cyst

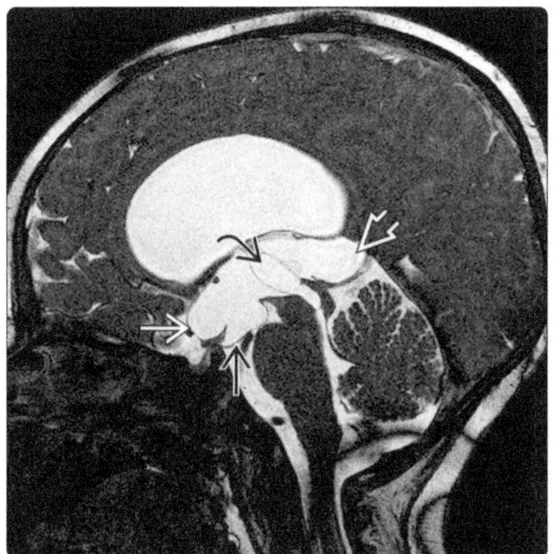

Entrapped 4th Ventricle

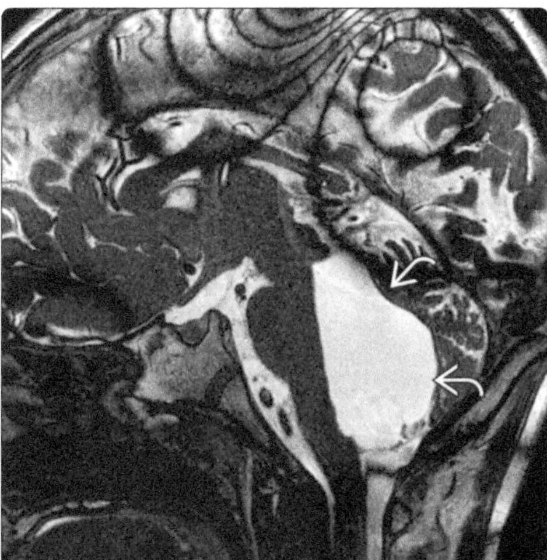

(Left) *Sagittal FIESTA MR shows markedly expanded lateral and 3rd ventricles due to blocking of the aqueduct by an intraventricular cyst. Note the widely expanded chiasmatic recess, depressed inferiorly convex 3rd ventricular floor, and suprapineal recess.* **(Right)** *Sagittal FIESTA MR shows disproportion between the markedly dilated 4th ventricle and the decompressed 3rd and lateral ventricles caused by aqueductal narrowing.*

Hydrocephalus

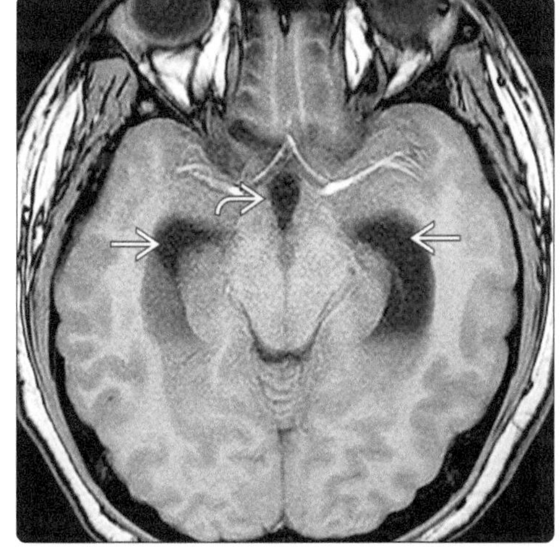

Hydrocephalus

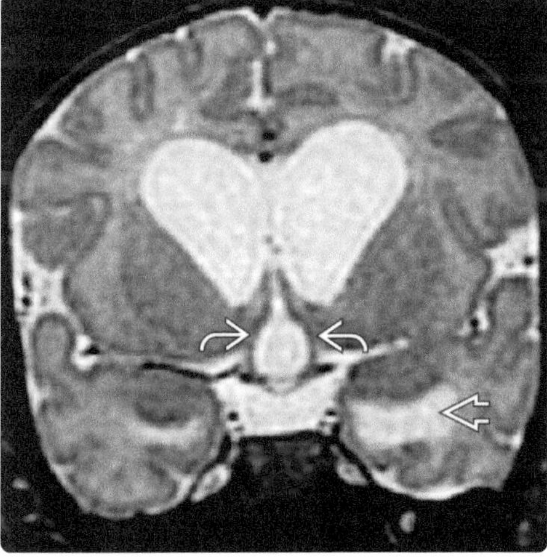

(Left) *Axial T1WI MR in a patient with aqueductal narrowing shows marked enlargement on the temporal horns of the lateral ventricles and anterior recesses of the 3rd ventricle.* **(Right)** *Coronal T2WI MR shows marked lateral ventricular enlargement, including the temporal horns (seen better on the left, expanding below the amygdala). Note how the anterior recess of the 3rd ventricle balloons inferiorly where the wall is thinner.*

Hydrocephalus

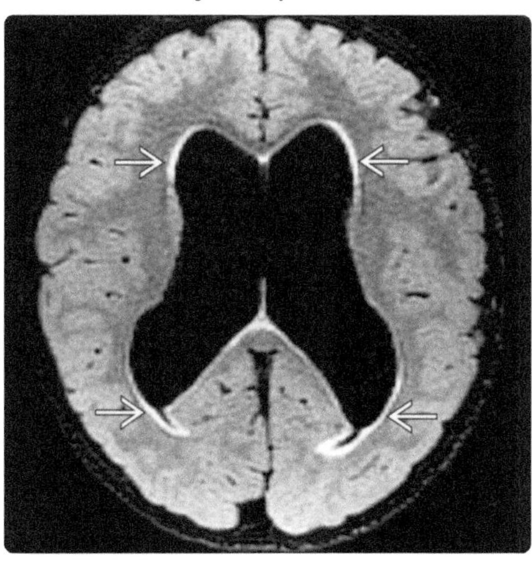

Posthemorrhagic Hydrocephalus

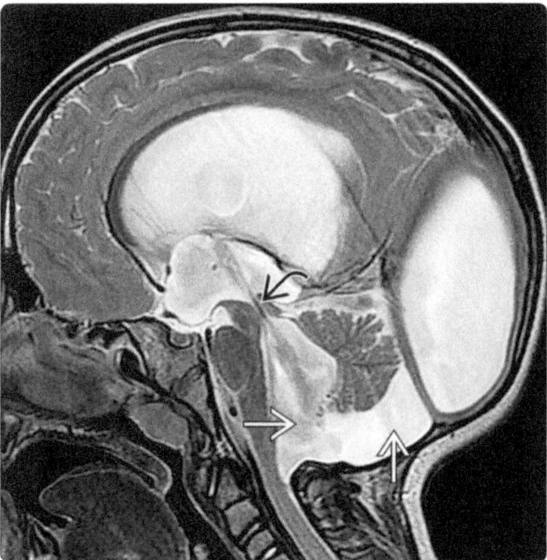

(Left) *Axial FLAIR MR shows dilated lateral ventricles with surrounding interstitial edema.* **(Right)** *Sagittal T2WI MR shows severe hydrocephalus from scarring of the 4th ventricular outflow foramina and basilar cisterns (large intraventricular hemorrhage in a preterm baby). Lateral ventricles are massively enlarged, stretching the corpus callosum. Third ventricular recesses are dilated, narrow aqueduct creates massive flow void, and 4th ventricle herniates through foramen of Magendie and beneath the vermis.*

Cavum Septi Pellucidi

KEY FACTS

TERMINOLOGY

- Cystic CSF cavity of septum pellucidum (SP)
  - Occurs ± cavum vergae (CV)

IMAGING

- Elongated, finger-shaped CSF collection between lateral ventricles
  - Cavum septi pellucidi (CSP): Between frontal horns of lateral ventricles
  - CV: Posterior extension between fornices
- Size varies from slit-like to several mm, occasionally > 1 cm
- SP invariably cystic in fetus
  - Width of fetal CSP increases between 19-27 weeks
  - Plateaus at 28 weeks
  - Gradually closes in rostral direction between 28 weeks and term
  - CSP present in 100% of premature, 85% of term infants
- CSP seen in up to 15-20% of adults

TOP DIFFERENTIAL DIAGNOSES

- Asymmetric lateral ventricles
- Cavum velum interpositum
- Ependymal cyst
- Absent SP

PATHOLOGY

- CSP forms if fetal SP fails to obliterate
- CSP is not "5th ventricle"
- CV is not "6th ventricle"

CLINICAL ISSUES

- Usually asymptomatic, incidental
- CSP frequent among athletes with history of repeated traumatic brain injury, such as boxers

DIAGNOSTIC CHECKLIST

- Absence of CSP in fetus or newborn prompts evaluation for possible congenital brain malformation

(Left) *Coronal graphic with axial insert shows classic cavum septi pellucidi (CSP) with cavum vergae (CV) ⇨. Note the finger-like CSF collection between the lateral ventricles.* **(Right)** *Axial T2WI MR shows CSP as a CSF collection between the leaves of the septum pellucidum ⇨. Although seen incidentally, some studies have reported that CSP is frequent among athletes with a history of repeated traumatic brain injury (TBI), such as boxers and American professional football players.*

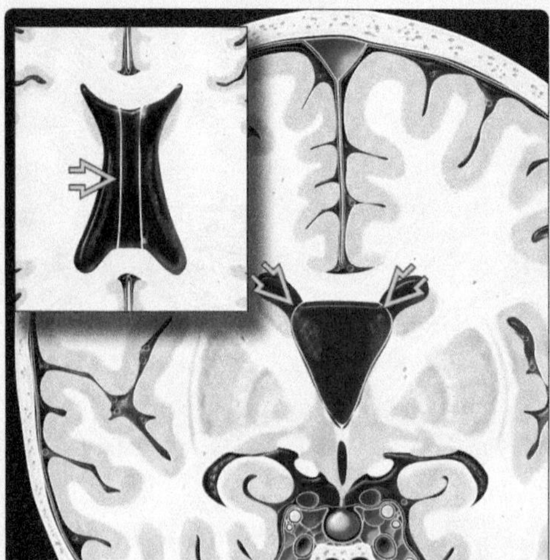

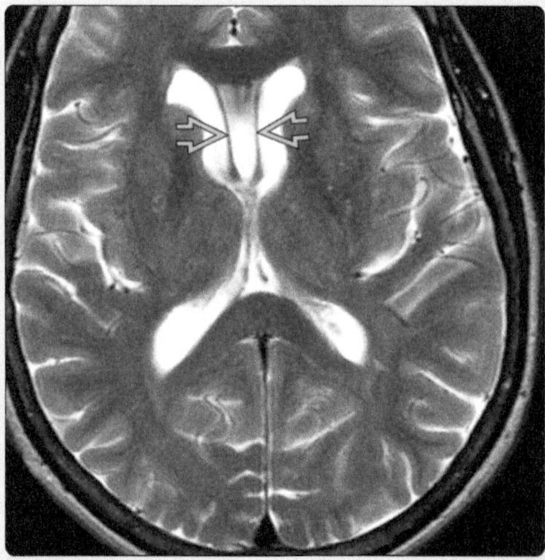

(Left) *Coronal T1WI MR shows a classic large CSP between the frontal horns ⇨ bowing the leaves of the septum pellucidum laterally ⇨.* **(Right)** *Axial FLAIR MR shows a large CSP with CV as a large CSF collection between the leaves of the septum pellucidum ⇨ continuing directly posteriorly with the CSF collection, splaying the fornices laterally ⇨.*

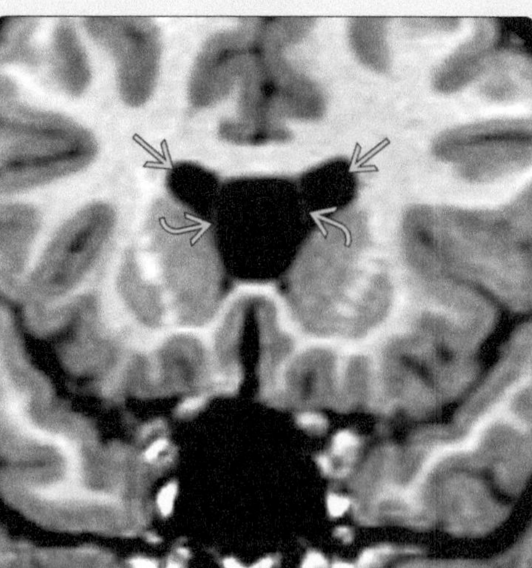

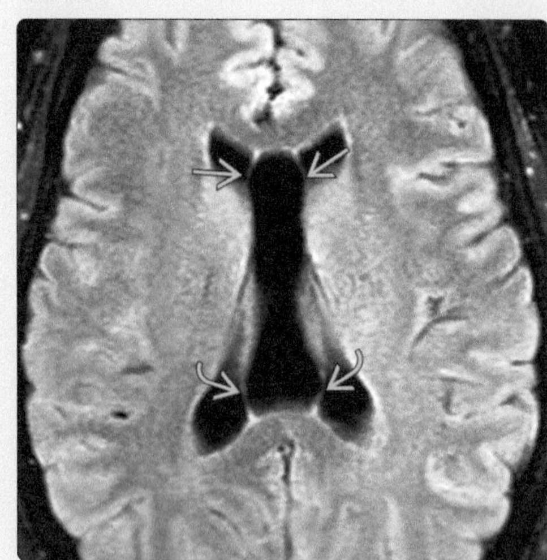

Cavum Velum Interpositum

KEY FACTS

TERMINOLOGY

- Cavum velum interpositum (CVI), cyst of velum interpositum (VI)

IMAGING

- Triangular CSF space
  - Between lateral ventricles, over thalami
  - Apex points toward foramen of Monro
  - Elevates, splays fornices
  - Flattens, displaces internal cerebral veins inferiorly
- Size varies from slit-like linear to triangular to round/ovoid CSF collection
- Isodense/isointense with CSF
  - Suppresses completely on FLAIR
  - Does not restrict on DWI
  - Does not enhance
- US shows hypoechoic midline interhemispheric cyst

TOP DIFFERENTIAL DIAGNOSES

- Normal cistern of VI
- Cavum septi pellucidi, cavum vergae
- Arachnoid cyst
- Epidermoid cyst

CLINICAL ISSUES

- Can be found at any age
  - Common in infants, rare in adults
- Symptoms
  - Usually asymptomatic, found incidentally
  - Headache (relationship to cyst unclear)
  - Large CVI can obstruct normal CSF flow; treated by endoscopic fenestration

DIAGNOSTIC CHECKLIST

- May be normal fetal or infant finding
- Include FLAIR and DWI to distinguish between CVI, epidermoid cyst

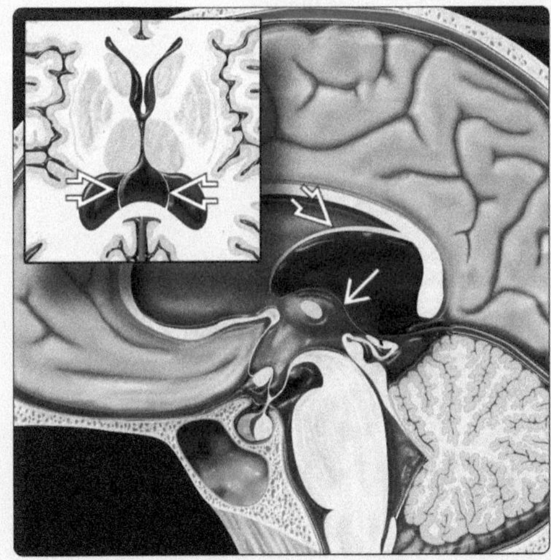

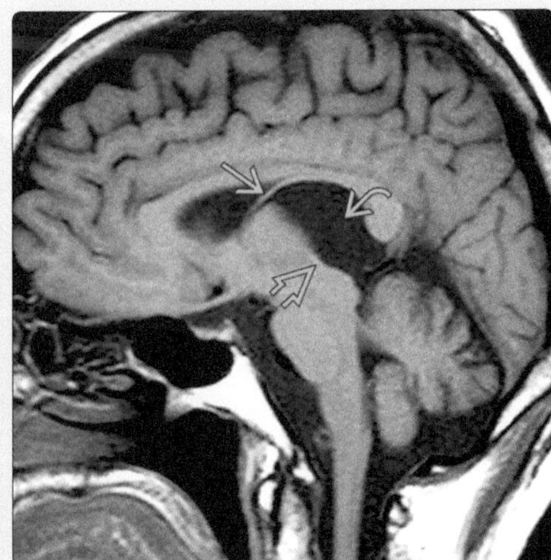

(Left) *Sagittal graphic with axial insert shows a cavum velum interpositum (CVI). Note the elevation and splaying of the fornices ➡. Also noted is the inferior displacement of the internal cerebral veins and 3rd ventricle ➡.* **(Right)** *Sagittal T1WI MR shows a classic CVI ➡ as a CSF-like enlargement that elevates the fornix ➡ and flattens and displaces the internal cerebral vein ➡ inferiorly. These are usually asymptomatic; however, large ones can cause CSF obstruction and can be treated by fenestration.*

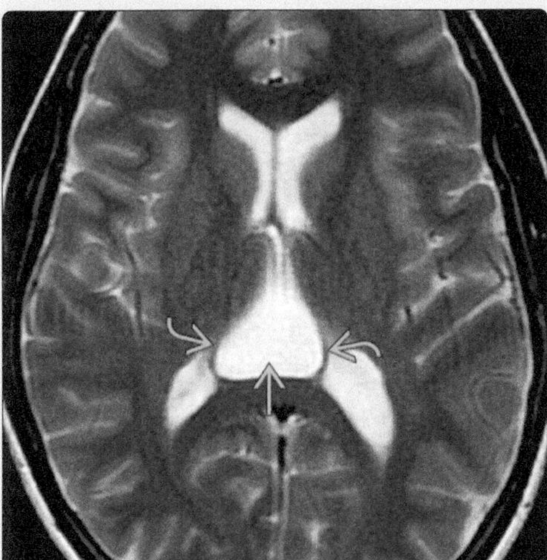

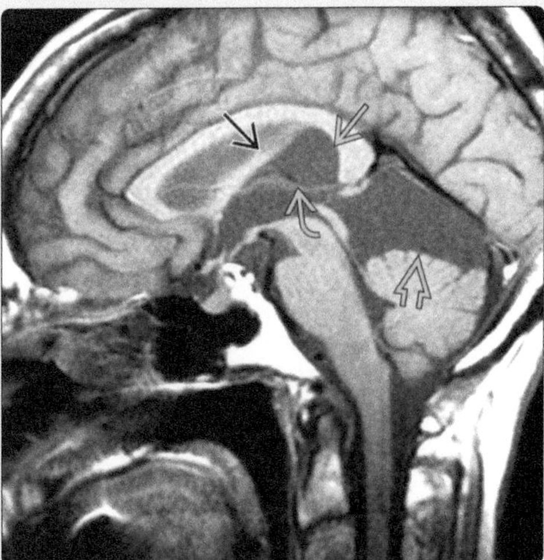

(Left) *Axial T2WI MR in a 37-year-old man with headaches shows a classic CVI with a triangular-shaped CSF collection ➡ between the lateral ventricles spreading the fornices laterally ➡.* **(Right)** *Sagittal T1WI MR shows a variant CVI ➡ that elevates the fornix ➡, flattens the internal cerebral vein ➡, and extends into the quadrigeminal and suprasellar cisterns ➡. This case probably represents an arachnoid cyst of the CVI.*

Benign Enlarged Subarachnoid Spaces

KEY FACTS

TERMINOLOGY

- Idiopathic enlargement of subarachnoid spaces (SASs) during infancy

IMAGING

- Primary imaging modality: US
- Best clue: Enlarged SASs & ↑ orbitofrontal circumference (> 95th percentile)
  - Ventricles may be mildly enlarged
- Symmetric bifrontal & bitemporal SASs
- All modalities show veins coursing through SASs
- SASs follow CSF appearance on all modalities
- No compression of veins or gyri
- No inward displacement of arachnoid membrane by subdural fluid; small, nonhemorrhagic subdural collections seen in ~ 4% of patients with enlarged SAS

TOP DIFFERENTIAL DIAGNOSES

- Atrophy
- Acquired progressive communicating hydrocephalus
- Nonaccidental trauma (NAT)

PATHOLOGY

- Etiology uncertain: Immature CSF drainage pathways likely
- Family history of macrocephaly > 80%

CLINICAL ISSUES

- Mild developmental delay alone should not prompt further imaging or subspecialty evaluation
  - Further evaluation required only in setting of focal neurologic signs &/or developmental regression
- Consider NAT if enlarged extraaxial spaces atypical
- SAS enlargement & developmental delay typically resolve without therapy by 2 years of age

DIAGNOSTIC CHECKLIST

- Even small/simple subdural collections should be discussed with referring clinician to identify any concerns for NAT that merit further work-up

(Left) *Axial graphic shows classic enlarged subarachnoid spaces (SASs) in a macrocephalic infant (head circumference > 95%). Note the symmetric enlargement with idiopathic enlargement of SASs during the 1st year of life.* **(Right)** *Axial T2 MR in a 7-month-old with macrocephaly & normal development shows enlargement of the bifrontal ➙ & interhemispheric ➙ SASs, consistent with benign enlargement of SASs of infancy (BESSI). Also note mild ventriculomegaly ➙, a common associated finding in BESSI.*

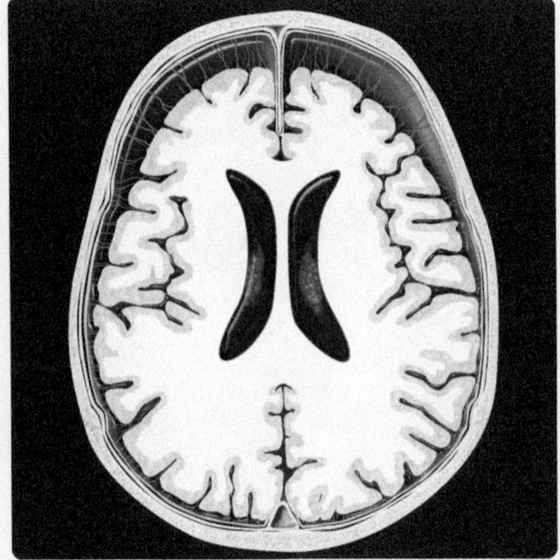

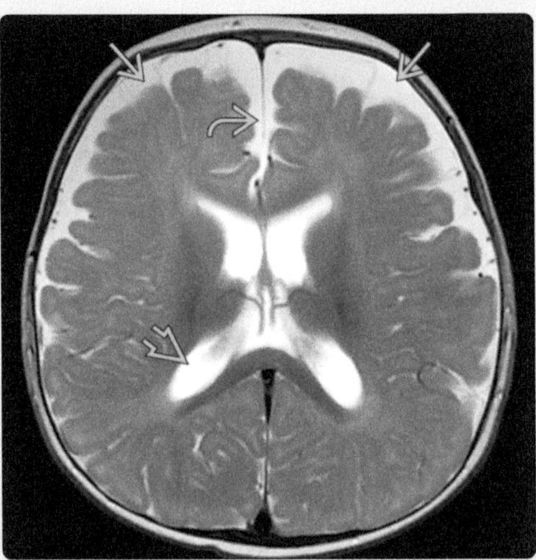

(Left) *Coronal US in a 7-month-old boy with macrocrania shows enlarged SASs ➙ & normal ventricular ➙ size. Note the normal size of the sulci. This is the typical clinical history & imaging appearance for benign enlargement of SASs.* **(Right)** *Coronal color Doppler US in a 4-month-old girl shows vessels ➙ traversing the enlarged SASs ➙. Doppler US can be helpful to exclude subdural collections by demonstrating normal veins in the SASs.*

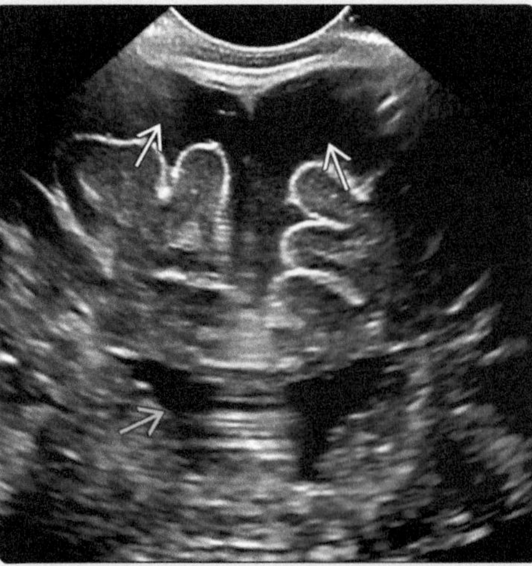

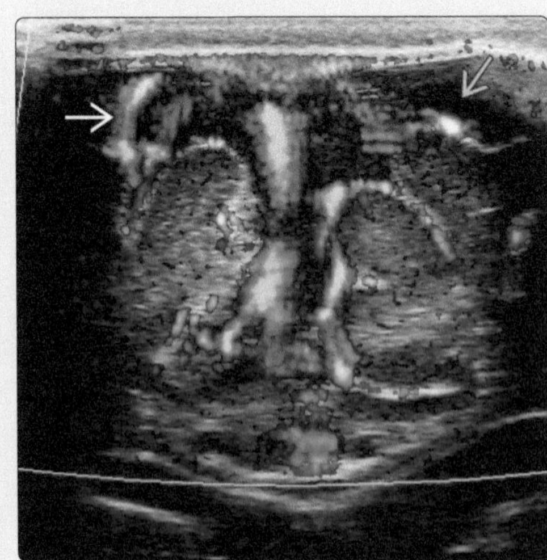

Benign Enlarged Subarachnoid Spaces

TERMINOLOGY

Abbreviations

- Subarachnoid spaces (SASs)

Synonyms

- Benign enlargement of SASs of infancy (BESSI)
- Benign external hydrocephalus
- Benign extracerebral fluid collections of infancy
- Benign communicating hydrocephalus
- Physiologic extraventricular obstructive hydrocephalus
- Benign macrocephaly of infancy

Definitions

- Enlarged SASs in patient < 1 year of age with macrocrania [head circumference (HC) > 95%]

IMAGING

General Features

- Best diagnostic clue
  - Symmetric bilateral SAS enlargement ± mild ventriculomegaly
    - Patient with normal or mildly delayed development
- Location
  - Enlarged SASs in infant with macrocrania
    - Symmetric at bifrontal & bitemporal SASs
- Size
  - Normal SAS values differ significantly between studies
    - Normal maximum width peaks at 28 postnatal weeks (7 months of age)
    - Interhemispheric width: 95th percentile: ~ 8 mm
      - Widest distance between hemispheres
    - Craniocortical width: 95th percentile: ~ 10 mm
      - Widest vertical distance between brain & inner table of calvarium
    - Sinocortical width: 95th percentile: ~ 7 mm
      - Widest distance between cortex & superior sagittal sinus
- Morphology
  - CSF space follows (not flattens) gyral contour

Radiographic Findings

- Radiography
  - ↑ craniofacial ratio

CT Findings

- NECT
  - Enlarged SASs with normal sulci; no hemorrhage
  - Enlarged cisterns (especially suprasellar/chiasmatic)
  - Associated subdural collections often not visible
- CECT
  - Demonstrates veins traversing SASs
  - No abnormal meningeal enhancement

MR Findings

- T1WI
  - Normal brain parenchyma without edema
  - Small subdural collections sometimes visible on T1
- T2WI
  - Arachnoid membranes
  - Small, nonhemorrhagic subdural collections ~ 4%
- FLAIR
  - SAS fluid follows CSF signal on all sequences
  - Incomplete signal suppression in subdural collections
- DWI
  - ↑ fractional anisotropy & mean diffusivity in brain of patients with enlarged SASs compared to controls
    - Normalizes over time with resolution of SAS enlargement
- T1WI C+
  - Demonstrates veins traversing SASs
- SSFSE
  - May be used for follow-up to avoid sedation in children

Ultrasonographic Findings

- Grayscale ultrasound
  - Primary modality used whenever possible
  - Symmetric enlargement of bifrontal SASs
  - ± mild ventricular enlargement
- Color Doppler
  - Cortical veins seen within subarachnoid fluid space
    - No mass effect displacing veins against pia
    - No inward displacement of arachnoid membrane by subdural fluid
  - Subdural collections lack traversing veins

Imaging Recommendations

- Best imaging tool
  - US if acoustic window available
  - CT/MR if no acoustic window available
- Protocol advice
  - Doppler sonography: Documents veins traversing SASs
  - Linear high-resolution US most sensitive for detection of associated subdural fluid
  - After diagnosis, best follow-up: Clinical monitoring of HC & development of any neurologic findings
  - Follow-up with MR/CT typically not necessary, unless
    - Focal neurologic signs/symptoms
    - Suspicion for subdural collection on US

DIFFERENTIAL DIAGNOSIS

Associated Subdural Fluid Collections

- Subdural fluid not normally visualized
  - Small, nonhemorrhagic subdural collections seen in 4% of benign macrocrania patients
  - ↑ incidence of subdural collections with ↑ size of SASs
  - Characterized by crescentic fluid collection separating dura from arachnoid
    - Discrete arachnoid membrane displaced toward cortex; may be compressing SAS veins
    - May have different signal intensity on PD & other MR sequences compared to CSF
  - Discuss need for further work-up with referring clinician
    - Management remains controversial
      - Some authors recommend universal diagnostic work-up for nonaccidental trauma (NAT)
      - Others recommend more nuanced approach

Nonaccidental Trauma

- Moderate/large or hemorrhagic subdurals or unusual clinical findings should raise concern

Atrophy

- Small HC; sulcal prominence out of proportion

Glutaric Aciduria Type 1

- Enlarged sylvian fissures with delayed myelination
- Subdural collections may be present
- T2-hyperintense basal ganglia

Elevated Venous Pressures

- Causes: Cardiac disease, internal jugular vein sacrifice for ECMO, arteriovenous fistula, or sinus venous thrombosis

Communicating Hydrocephalus

- Often posthemorrhagic/postinflammatory/neoplastic
  - Density of extraaxial collection does not = CSF
- Achondroplasia & other skull base anomalies
  - Coarctation of foramen magnum (narrow)

PATHOLOGY

General Features

- Etiology
  - Remains incompletely understood
  - Immature CSF drainage pathways: Most accepted theory
    - CSF primarily drained via extracellular space → capillaries
    - Pacchionian granulations (PGs) do not mature until 18 months
    - PGs then displaced into veins (as Starling-type resistors)
    - PGs regulate venous drainage of CSF when fontanels close
    - Benign SAS enlargement usually resolves at that time
  - Disproportionate growth of skull & brain
    - Faster growth of skull results in ↑ SASs ± ↑ ventricles
    - This theory helps to explain frequent identification of subdural fluid collections
  - Family history of macrocephaly > 80%
- Associated abnormalities
  - Subdural collections (typically small & incidental) in ~ 4%
  - Predisposition to bleed with minor trauma: Controversial
    - Possibility of ↑ risk for bridging vein injury & subdural collection/hematoma in absence of major trauma
    - Venous "stretching" implicated
  - May ↑ risk of arachnoid cyst development compared to normal population

Gross Pathologic & Surgical Features

- Deep/prominent but otherwise normal-appearing SASs
- No pathologic membranes

Microscopic Features

- Ependymal damage not seen in benign SAS enlargement

CLINICAL ISSUES

Presentation

- Most common signs/symptoms
  - Macrocrania: HC > 95th percentile
  - Frontal bossing
  - No signs of elevated intracranial pressure (ICP); normal pressure on lumbar puncture
  - Danger signs
    - Elevated ICP
    - Persistent or rapid deviation of HC from normal curve
    - Developmental regression, focal neurologic signs, vomiting, bruising
- Other signs/symptoms
  - Mild developmental delay common (20-50%) & usually resolves over time
    - Mild developmental delay should not necessarily prompt further evaluation
- Clinical profile
  - Family history of benign macrocephaly common
  - Male infants, ± late to walk

Demographics

- Most common imaging diagnosis for macrocrania < 1 year
  - Usually presents at 3-9 months
- Sex: M:F = 2:1

Natural History & Prognosis

- Enlarged SASs → ↑ suture/calvarial malleability/compliance → predisposes to posterior plagiocephaly
- Self-limited; resolves without therapy by 12-24 months
  - Spontaneous resolution of spaces & symptoms
- Macrocephaly may persist

Treatment

- No treatment necessary
- Normal outcome (developmental delay usually resolves as prominent SAS resolves)

DIAGNOSTIC CHECKLIST

Image Interpretation Pearls

- Crucial to know HC
- Further evaluation with brain MR or CT if US atypical
  - Moderate/large/complex subdural collection → NAT work-up
  - Even small/simple subdural collections should be discussed with referring clinician to identify any concerns for NAT that merit further work-up

SELECTED REFERENCES

1. Huang J et al: Systematic approach to pediatric macrocephaly. Radiographics. 43(5):e220159, 2023
2. Raissaki M et al: Benign enlargement of the subarachnoid spaces and subdural collections-when to evaluate for abuse. Pediatr Radiol. 53(4):752-67, 2023
3. Alshareef M et al: Prevalence of visible subdural spaces in benign enlargement of subarachnoid spaces in infancy: a retrospective analysis utilizing magnetic resonance imaging. World Neurosurg. 164:e973-9, 2022
4. Caré MM: Macrocephaly and subdural collections. Pediatr Radiol. 51(6):891-7, 2021
5. Zahl SM et al: Clinical, radiological, and demographic details of benign external hydrocephalus: a population-based study. Pediatr Neurol. 96:53-7, 2019
6. Zahl SM et al: Quality of life and physician-reported developmental, cognitive, and social problems in children with benign external hydrocephalus-long-term follow-up. Childs Nerv Syst. 35(2):245-50, 2019
7. Haws ME et al: A retrospective analysis of the utility of head computed tomography and/or magnetic resonance imaging in the management of benign macrocrania. J Pediatr. 182:283-9.e1, 2017

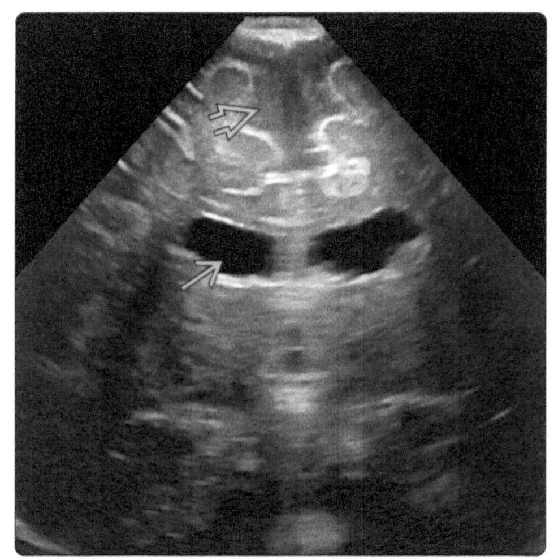

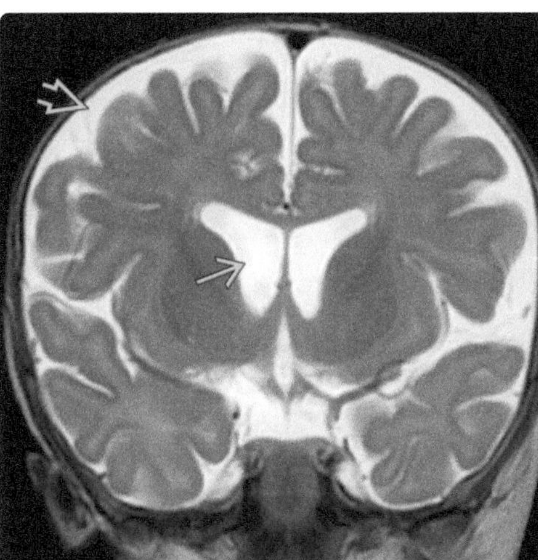

(Left) *Coronal US in a 3-month-old with macrocephaly shows prominent SASs* ⇨ *as well as mild enlargement of the lateral ventricles* →*. Mild lateral ventricular enlargement is common in BESSI.* **(Right)** *Coronal T2 MR in a 6-month-old with macrocephaly shows symmetrically prominent bifrontal SASs* ⇨ *with mild enlargement of the lateral ventricles* →*. Mild enlargement of the lateral ventricles should not dissuade one from suggesting BESSI.*

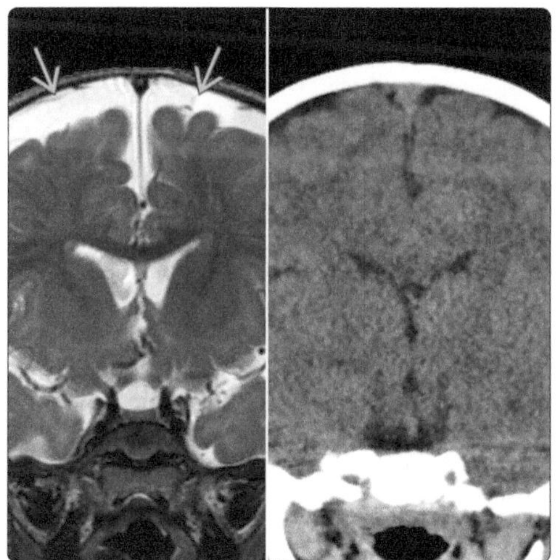

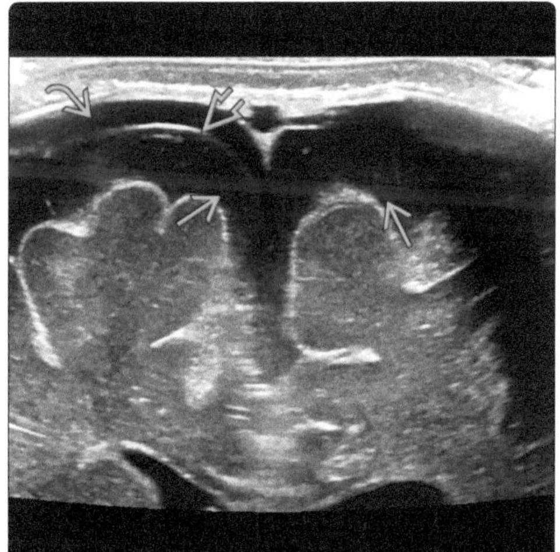

(Left) *Coronal T2 MR at 13 months (left) & NECT at 5 years (right) of age show expected resolution of the enlarged SASs* → *over a 4-year period. Enlarged SASs typically resolve by 24 months of age.* **(Right)** *Coronal high-resolution US in a 2-month-old with macrocrania shows bilateral enlargement of the SASs* →*. Also present is a small subdural collection* ↷ *on the right, which is anechoic compared to the SASs. Note the separation of the arachnoid membrane* ⇨*.*

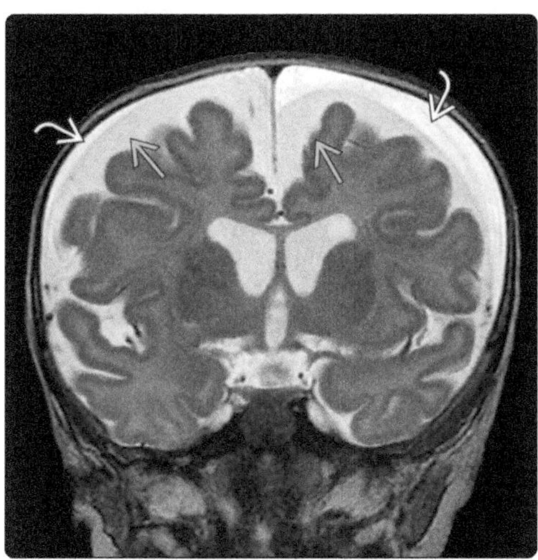

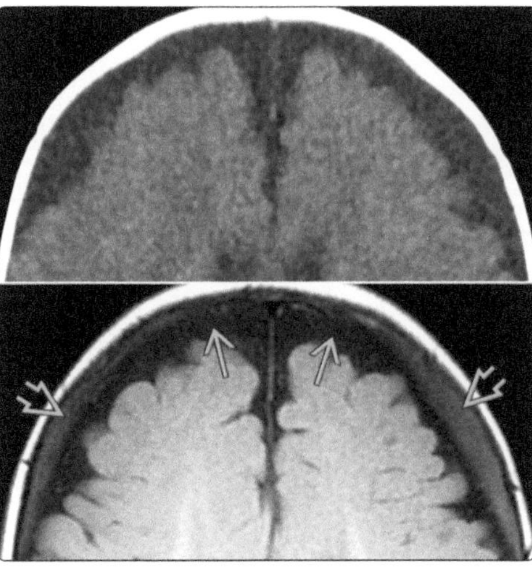

(Left) *Coronal T2 MR in a BESSI patient shows symmetrically enlarged SASs* → *as well as small, bilateral, nonhemorrhagic subdural fluid collections* ↷*. Small subdural fluid collections are seen in ~ 4% of patients with enlarged SASs.* **(Right)** *Axial NECT (top) and T2 FLAIR MR (bottom) in a 5-month-old with BESSI is shown. It is not possible to delineate the low attenuation subdural fluid collections from the SASs on CT. In contrast, the subdural collections* ⇨ *are very pronounced compared to the SASs* → *on the FLAIR sequence.*

KEY FACTS

TERMINOLOGY

- Ventriculomegaly caused by
  - Obstruction of CSF egress from ventricles: Intraventricular obstructive hydrocephalus
  - Decreased CSF resorption from subarachnoid space: Extraventricular obstructive hydrocephalus
  - Increased CSF production
- Use FOHR to track ventricle size over time
  - (Transverse diameter of frontal horns + transverse diameter of occipital horns) ÷ 2x transverse diameter of cranium

IMAGING

- 3D FIESTA/CISS
  - Acquire in sagittal plane to outline aqueduct
- Limited shunt MR protocol
  - 30-second acquisition in each plane
  - Useful substitute for CT
  - Insensitive for parenchymal abnormalities

PATHOLOGY

- Extracellular, extravascular fluid in brain is managed by glymphatic system
  - CSF circulates from within ventricles → subarachnoid space → perivascular spaces ↔ interstitium ↔ perivenular spaces → subarachnoid space
  - CSF is resorbed from subarachnoid space at multiple sites
    - Along sheaths of cranial nerves (especially olfactory bulb) into head and neck lymphatics
    - Along sheaths of spinal nerves into perispinal lymphatics
    - Into meningeal (dural) lymphatics
    - Into dural sinuses via arachnoid granulations
      - Previously thought to be major site of resorption
- Hydrocephalus results from obstruction of CSF egress from ventricular system or reduced resorption from subarachnoid space

(Left) *Depiction of normal CSF flow through the glymphatic system. CSF descends along periarterial perivascular spaces (PVS) and through the interstitium before exiting along perivenular PVS, clearing macromolecules (black particles). The exchange between interstitium and PVS is modulated by astrocytic endfeet expressing AQP4 (pink channels).* **(Right)** *An isoattenuating colloid cyst ➔ obstructs the foramina of Monro in this 7-year-old, causing obstructive hydrocephalus.*

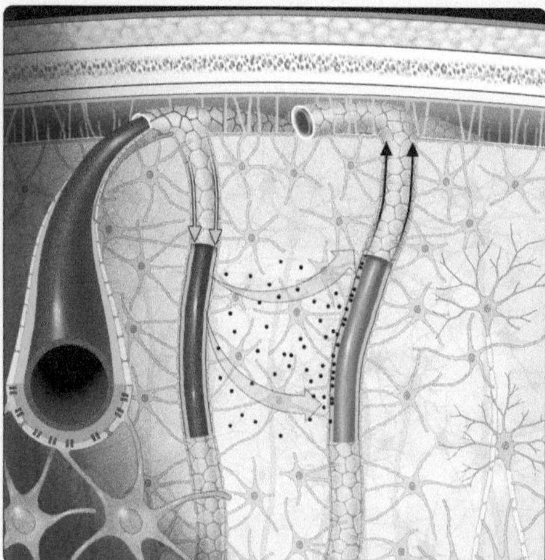

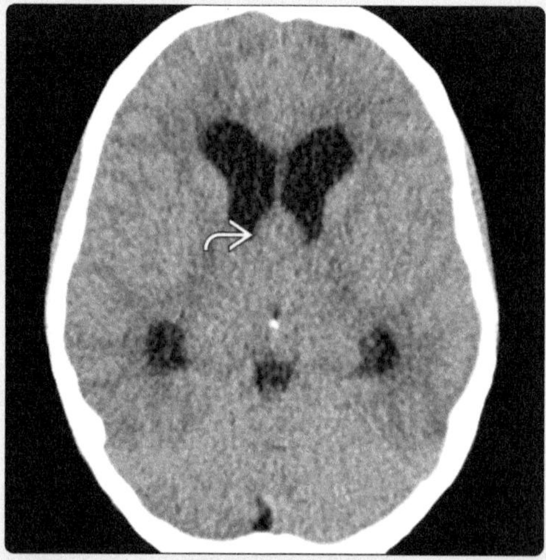

(Left) *A large suprasellar arachnoid cyst balloons upward ➔ and obstructs the foramina of Monro in this 1-year-old with macrocrania.* **(Right)** *This 3-month-old with hydrocephalus has a Blake pouch cyst obstructing outflow of CSF from the 4th ventricle. Note the membrane across the posterior foramen magnum ➔ and the uplifting of the vermis ➔.*

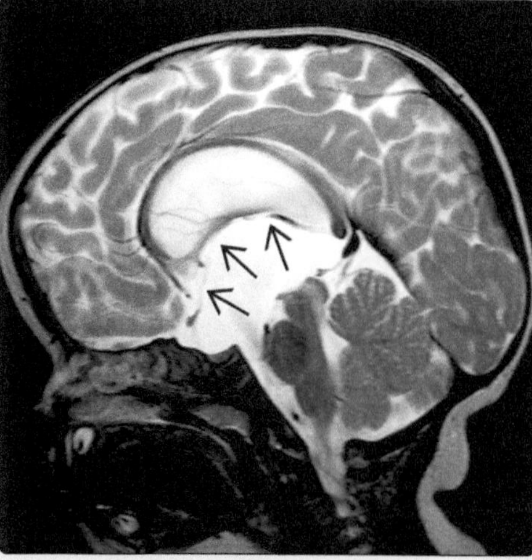

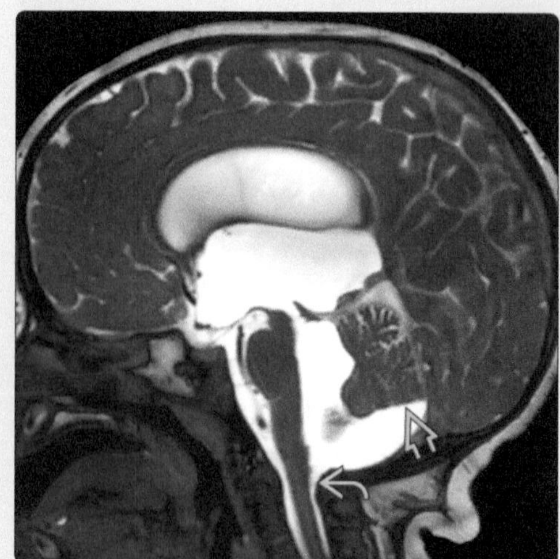

TERMINOLOGY

Abbreviations

- Intraventricular obstructive hydrocephalus (IVOH)
- Extraventricular obstructive hydrocephalus (EVOH)
- Frontal occipital horn ratio (FOHR)
  - (Transverse diameter of frontal horns + transverse diameter of occipital horns) ÷ 2x transverse diameter of cranium
- Subarachnoid lymphatic-like membrane (SLYM)
  - Recently discovered 4th meningeal membrane that divides subarachnoid space into inner and outer compartments

Definitions

- Ventriculomegaly caused by
  - Obstruction of CSF egress from ventricles: IVOH
  - Decreased CSF resorption from subarachnoid space: EVOH
  - Increased CSF production
- Ventriculomegaly secondary to loss of parenchyma, a.k.a. ex vacuo dilation, is **not** hydrocephalus

IMAGING

General Features

- Best diagnostic clue
  - Enlarged ventricles
    - With decreased extraaxial spaces (EAS): IVOH
    - With periventricular (transependymal) edema: Acute IVOH
    - With enlarged EAS: EVOH
- Size
  - FOHR > 0.33
- Morphology
  - Ventricles proximal to obstruction enlarge, appear more rounded
  - Trigones and occipital horns typically enlarge most
    - Wall pressure is proportional to diameter: Laplace law
    - Optic and infundibular recesses of 3rd ventricle may preferentially enlarge
    - Optic nerve sheaths may enlarge → papilledema

CT Findings

- NECT
  - Large ventricles proximal to obstruction
  - Basal cisterns, sulci compressed/obliterated

MR Findings

- T1WI
  - Lateral ventricles enlarged
  - Corpus callosum (CC) thinned, stretched upward
    - May be impinged against falx
  - Enlarged 3rd ventricle often herniated into expanded sella
  - Funnel-shaped aqueduct of Sylvius in aqueductal stenosis
- T2WI
  - Acute obstruction
    - Transependymal edema extends into periventricular white matter (WM)
      - Accentuated around frontal and occipital horns
  - Chronic obstruction
    - Large ventricles without transependymal edema
    - CC may show hyperintensity after decompression (15% of shunted IVOH cases)
- T1WI C+
  - Diffuse leptomeningeal disease can cause EVOH
    - May only be apparent on postcontrast imaging
- MRS
  - Small lactate resonances can be detected in up to 20% of CSF spaces, even if no hydrocephalus

Other Modality Findings

- Contrast-enhanced ventriculography
  - MR can be used for assessing CSF flow
- Cardiac-gated phase-contrast MR
  - May show loss of CSF flow through aqueduct
  - Useful for assessing status of endoscopic 3rd ventriculostomy (ETV)

Imaging Recommendations

- Best imaging tool
  - Sagittal T2WI MR
  - Administer contrast if pattern suggests EVOH and no etiology is apparent
- Protocol advice
  - 3D FIESTA/CISS
    - Acquire in sagittal plane to outline aqueduct
    - Decreases CSF flow artifact
    - Allows better delineation of ventricular contour, septa
  - SWI to assess for superficial siderosis in posthemorrhagic hydrocephalus
  - Limited shunt MR protocol
    - Single-shot rapid technique with heavy T2 weighting
    - 30-second acquisition in each plane
    - Useful substitute for CT
      - Reduce radiation exposure in frequently imaged population
      - Rapid aquisition reduces need for sedation
    - Insensitive for parenchymal abnormalities
  - Use FOHR to track ventricle size over time
    - Especially in younger children with open sutures
    - Accounts for increase in head circumference with increase in ventricular size

DIFFERENTIAL DIAGNOSIS

Ventricular Enlargement Secondary to Parenchymal Loss

- a.k.a. ex vacuo ventriculomegaly
- Associated enlargement of sulci, cisterns
- Normal lateral ventricles can be asymmetric

Benign Enlargement of Subarachnoid Spaces and Ventricles

- a.k.a. benign macrocrania
- Seen in association with macrocephaly in infants
- Transient and self-limited
  - Not associated with developmental delay
  - Does not require CSF diversion
- Likely reflects relative immaturity of glymphatic system

- Diminished ability to resorb CSF as interstitial fluid compartment is shrunk by progressive myelination

PATHOLOGY

General Features

- Etiology
  - Extracellular, extravascular fluid in brain is managed by glymphatic system
    - Maintains homeostatic balance between interstitial fluid compartment, cellular compartment, and intravascular compartment
    - Analogous to lymphatic system in other organs
  - While brain parenchyma does not have lymphatic vessels, they are present in dura mater and along sheaths of cranial nerves
  - CSF circulates from within ventricles → subarachnoid space → perivascular spaces ↔ interstitium ↔ perivenular spaces → subarachnoid space
  - CSF is resorbed from subarachnoid space at multiple sites
    - Along sheaths of cranial nerves (especially olfactory bulb) into head and neck lymphatics
    - Along sheaths of spinal nerves into perispinal lymphatics
    - Into meningeal (dural) lymphatics
    - Into dural sinuses via arachnoid granulations
      - Previously thought to be major site of resorption
  - SLYM is thought to facilitate CSF flow
    - Disruption after trauma may explain reduced glymphatic flow and posttraumatic cerebral edema
  - Hydrocephalus results from obstruction of CSF egress from ventricular system or reduced resorption from subarachnoid space
  - Obstruction within ventricular system results in IVOH
    - Ventricles expand, compress adjacent parenchyma; stretching may rupture/open ependymal cell junctions
    - Periventricular interstitial fluid increases → myelin destruction
  - Etiology depends on site
    - Foramen of Monro
      - Colloid cyst
      - Subependymal giant cell astrocytoma in tuberous sclerosis
    - 3rd ventricle
      - Craniopharyngioma, hypothalamic glioma, arachnoid cyst
    - Aqueduct of Sylvius
      - Aqueductal stenosis, tectal glioma, pineal region tumor
      - Obstruction by hemorrhage or inflammatory debris
      - Enlarged vein of Galen due to arteriovenous fistula
    - 4th ventricle
      - Medulloblastoma, ependymoma, pilocytic astrocytoma
      - Chiari, Dandy-Walker malformation, Blake pouch cyst
    - Metastasis, neurocysticercosis, or meningioma can occur at multiple intraventricular locations
  - Reduced resorption from subarachnoid space results in EVOH
    - Subarachnoid pathology may reduce absorptive capacity
      - Hemorrhage or inflammation (acute or chronic)
    - Metabolic disorders may reduce resorptive capacity
  - Overproduction of CSF may overwhelm ability of glymphatic system to manage and resorb CSF
    - Choroid plexus papilloma or carcinoma
      - Focally enlarged and hyperenhancing choroidal mass
    - Choroid plexus villous hyperplasia
      - Diffusely enlarged choroid
- Genetics
  - Cell adhesion molecule L1 (*L1CAM*) recognized as cause of X-linked aqueductal stenosis
    - Located on X chromosome (Xq28)

CLINICAL ISSUES

Presentation

- Most common signs/symptoms
  - Headache, papilledema (aIVOH)
  - Nausea, vomiting
  - Diplopia
    - 6th nerve palsy caused by compression of cisternal segment

Treatment

- Obstructive hydrocephalus is managed surgically
  - CSF diversion (shunt or ETV)
  - Resection of obstructing or hypersecreting lesion
- Most common neurosurgical procedure in children = CSF shunting for hydrocephalus
- CSF diversion is typically delayed in EVOH
  - Tendency to be much more shunt dependent
    - Less tolerant of minor pressure changes
  - Lesser degree of ventriculomegaly increases difficulty of surgery

DIAGNOSTIC CHECKLIST

Consider

- Longstanding aqueductal stenosis can be caused by slow-growing tectal tumor
  - Compensated IVOH
- CSF function and homeostasis are far more complex than previously thought
  - Free communication among anatomic/functional compartments is necessary for proper brain health

Image Interpretation Pearls

- Size of ventricles generally correlates poorly with intracranial pressure
- Pulsatile CSF may create confusing signal intensity, even mimic intraventricular mass

SELECTED REFERENCES

1. Møllgård K et al: A mesothelium divides the subarachnoid space into functional compartments. Science. 379(6627):84-8, 2023
2. Krishnan P et al: Neuroimaging in pediatric hydrocephalus. Indian J Pediatr. 86(10):952-60, 2019
3. Jessen NA et al: The glymphatic system: a beginner's guide. Neurochem Res. 40(12):2583-99, 2015

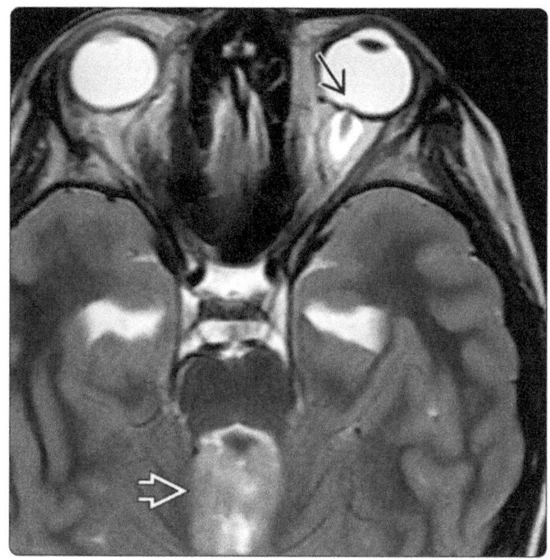

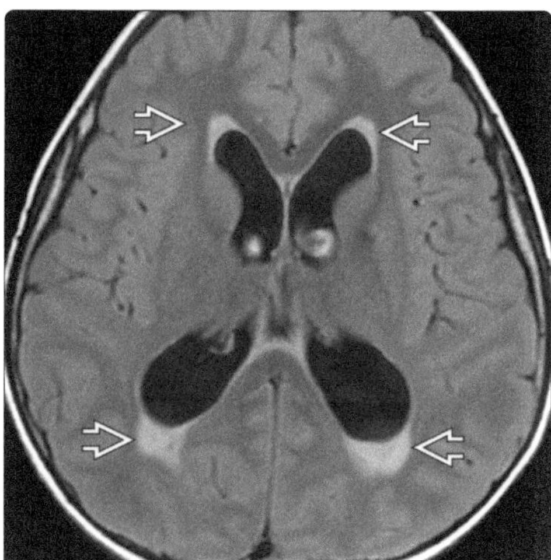

(Left) *A medulloblastoma* ➡ *fills and obstructs the 4th ventricle in this 10-year-old, leading to supratentorial ventriculomegaly and papilledema* ➡*. Papilledema visible on MR typically correlates to grade 3 on the Frisen scale (moderate edema).* **(Right)** *Axial FLAIR MR through the lateral ventricles in the same child shows transependymal edema capping the frontal and occipital horns* ➡*, reflecting the increased pressure in the ventricular system.*

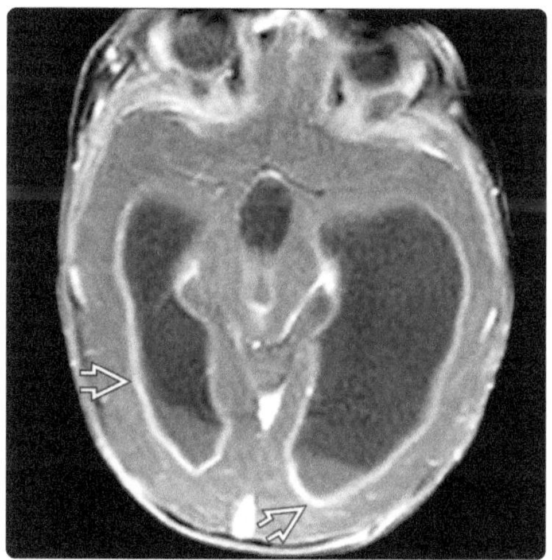

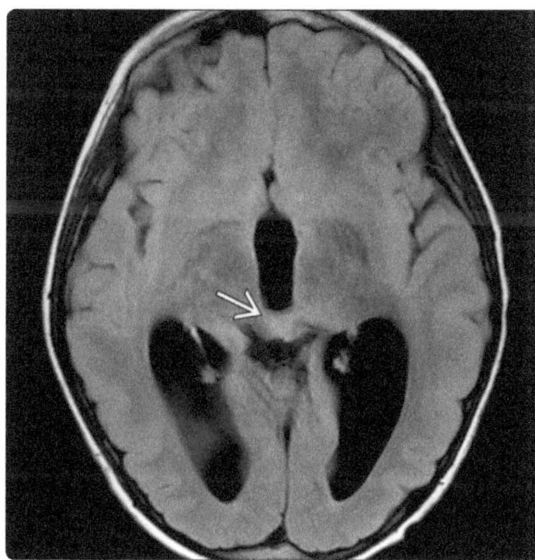

(Left) *Bacterial meningitis (group A Streptococcus in this example) can restrict resorption of CSF but can also obstruct at the cerebral aqueduct and 4th ventricular outlets when complicated by ventriculitis, evident on this image by abnormal enhancement of the ependyma* ➡*.* **(Right)** *An infiltrating tectal glioma* ➡ *obstructs the cerebral aqueduct in this 10-year-old. Absence of transependymal edema suggests a compensated hydrocephalus.*

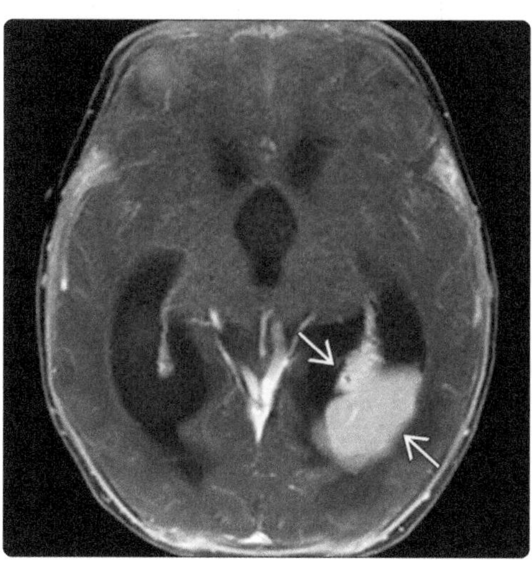

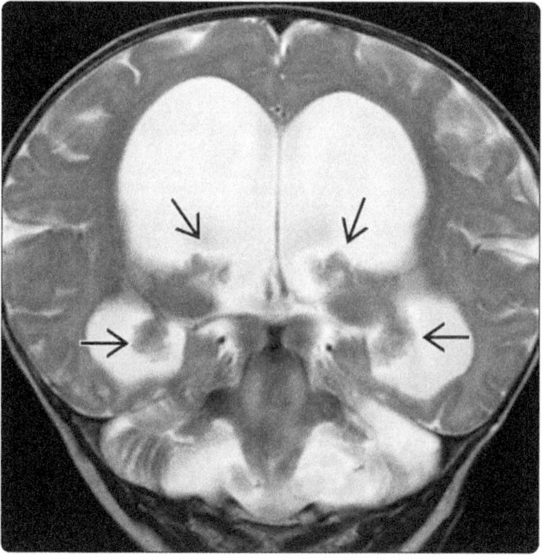

(Left) *A papilloma of the choroid plexus in the occipital horn of the left lateral ventricle* ➡ *causes moderate hydrocephalus by excessive CSF production in this 2-month-old.* **(Right)** *CSF overproduction can rarely be nonneoplastic in nature, as in this 6-month-old with villous hyperplasia of the choroid plexus in each lateral ventricle* ➡*. Note the preservation of peripheral sulci, as the unfused sutures of the infant can widen in response to increased intracranial volume.*

Aqueductal Stenosis

KEY FACTS

TERMINOLOGY

- Aqueductal stenosis (AS)

IMAGING

- Ventriculomegaly of lateral and 3rd ventricles with normal-sized 4th ventricle
- Obstruction of cerebral aqueduct ± tectal thickening
- Macrocephaly in fetus and infant
- Multiplanar MR with sagittal 3D TrueFISP/bFFE sequence to evaluate aqueduct

TOP DIFFERENTIAL DIAGNOSES

- Supratentorial volume loss
- Benign enlargement of subarachnoid fluid spaces of infancy
- Communicating hydrocephalus
- Secondary obstructive hydrocephalus

PATHOLOGY

- Congenital AS is common cause of fetal hydrocephalus
- Can be acquired (isolated) or associated with genetic disorder
- Subsets include stenosis from tectal thickening, obstructing web/gliotic tissue, or forking

CLINICAL ISSUES

- Though may present at any time from birth to adulthood, bimodal distribution in 1st year of life and adolescence
- Headache, papilledema, 6th nerve palsy, macrocephaly, bulging fontanelle
- C-section may be required for prenatally diagnosed cases due to macrocephaly

DIAGNOSTIC CHECKLIST

- Look for coexisting brain anomalies, such as rhombencephalosynapsis or diencephalic-mesencephalic dysplasia

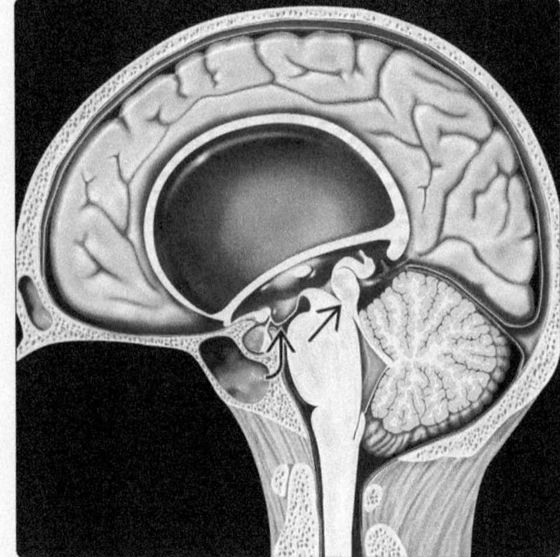

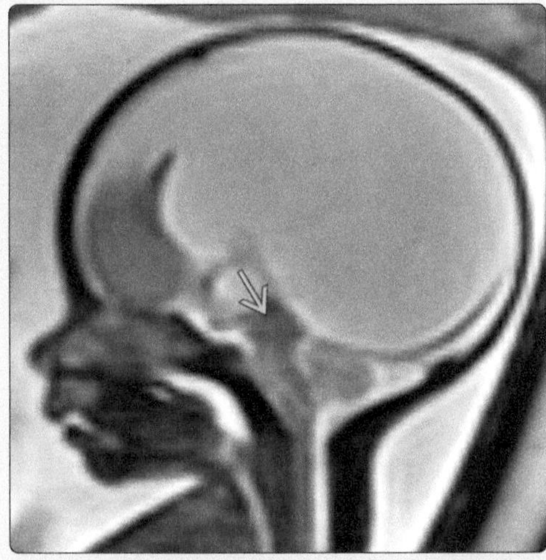

(Left) *Sagittal graphic shows obstructive hydrocephalus with markedly enlarged lateral and 3rd ventricles, a stretched (thinned) corpus callosum, and a funnel-shaped cerebral aqueduct ➔ related to distal obstruction. Note the normal size of the 4th ventricle and depression of the floor of the 3rd ventricle ➢ from the hydrocephalus.* **(Right)** *Sagittal T2WI from a fetal MR at 25-weeks gestational age with aqueductal stenosis shows macrocephaly, lateral and 3rd ventriculomegaly, and no CSF in the cerebral aqueduct ➔.*

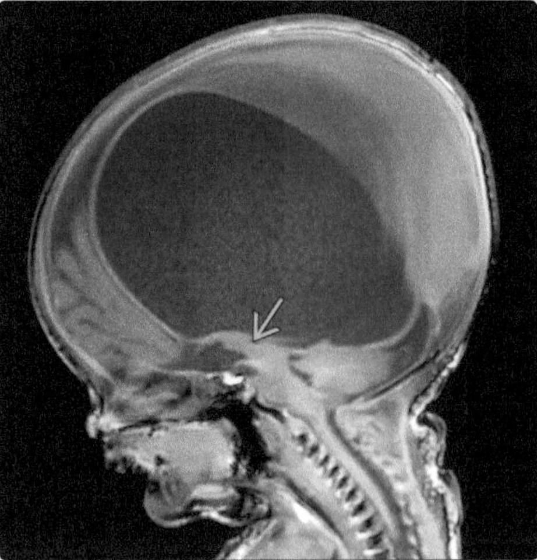

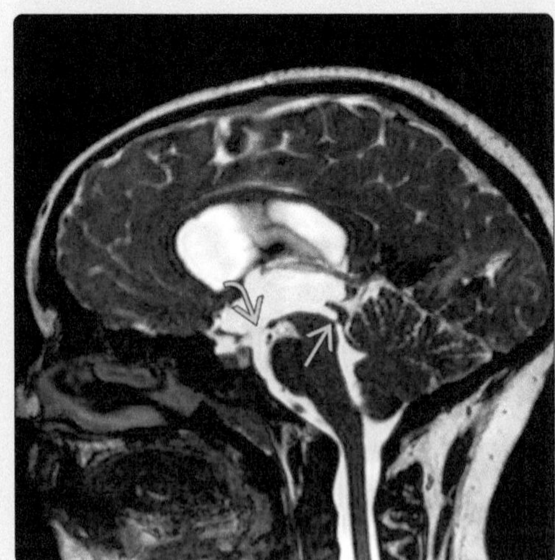

(Left) *Sagittal T1WI MR in a 1-day-old boy with prenatal diagnosis of aqueductal stenosis demonstrates incomplete separation ➔ of the massa intermedia from the thick midbrain tectum compatible with diencephalic-mesencephalic junction dysplasia.* **(Right)** *Sagittal FIESTA in a 5-year-old with aqueductal stenosis secondary to a small obstructing web ➔ is shown. This patient underwent a 3rd ventriculostomy ➢ and is doing well. There are no other brain anomalies.*

TERMINOLOGY

Abbreviations

- Aqueductal stenosis (AS)

Definitions

- Ventriculomegaly involving lateral and 3rd ventricles as result of complete or partial obstruction to CSF flow within cerebral aqueduct
- AS diagnosis generally refers to congenital form characterized by varying degree of obstruction at level of cerebral aqueduct
  - However, tumors, germinal matrix hemorrhage, or vascular lesions can obstruct aqueduct as well

IMAGING

General Features

- Best diagnostic clue
  - Ventriculomegaly of lateral and 3rd ventricles with normal-sized 4th ventricle
- Location
  - Cerebral aqueduct

CT Findings

- NECT
  - Ventriculomegaly of lateral and 3rd ventricles, normal-sized 4th ventricle

MR Findings

- T1WI
  - Ventriculomegaly of lateral and 3rd ventricles
    - Corpus callosum (CC) thinned, stretched upward
      - Often limits evaluation for coexisting callosal dysgenesis
    - ± lateral ventricular diverticulum (a.k.a. ventricular rupture or dehiscence)
    - Extraaxial CSF effacement
      - Limits ability to evaluate gyral-sulcal pattern
  - Normal size of 4th ventricle
  - Aqueductal web: Thin tissue membrane separating dilated aqueduct from normal-sized 4th ventricle
  - ± coexisting anomalies: Rhombencephalosynapsis, diencephalosynapsis (large massa intermedia/incomplete thalamic separation) or diencephalic-mesencephalic dysplasia (incomplete segmentation between diencephalon and mesencephalon)
- T2WI
  - Presence of dephasing jet or flow void through aqueduct may suggest that AS is less likely, though does not exclude diagnosis
  - ± periventricular interstitial edema
  - Tectal plate thickening
    - Loss of differentiation between superior and inferior colliculi
    - May be difficult to differentiate from tectal plate glioma in certain cases
      - AS should **not** have T2-/FLAIR-hyperintense signal or enhancement in tectal plate (tectum should be isointense to rest of midbrain on all pulse sequences)
      - Unlikely to be tectal plate glioma < 3 years of age
  - Septum pellucidum often absent or partially absent secondary to perforation
- T2* GRE
  - May have trace amounts of blood products in aqueduct and ventricular system, but no frank germinal matrix hemorrhage or other cause for bleeding
- MR cine
  - Phase-contrast imaging may demonstrate absent or diminished CSF flow in aqueduct
- 3D FIESTA/CISS/TrueFISP/bFFE
  - Higher spatial resolution allows evaluation of degree of aqueductal occlusion and anatomy of 3rd ventricle floor for endoscopic 3rd ventriculostomy (ETV) assessment

Ultrasonographic Findings

- Grayscale ultrasound
  - Ventriculomegaly of lateral and 3rd ventricles with normal-sized 4th ventricle in newborn with macrocephaly is highly suggestive of AS
  - Obstetrical ultrasound may permit prenatal diagnosis
    - Usually severe lateral ventriculomegaly (> 15 mm)
    - Decreased transverse cerebellar diameter with coexisting rhombencephalosynapsis; fetal MR can help confirm
    - Adducted thumbs in male fetus raise possibility of X-linked hydrocephalus/*L1CAM* mutation

Imaging Recommendations

- Best imaging tool
  - Multiplanar MR with sagittal 3D TrueFISP/bFFE sequence to evaluate aqueduct

DIFFERENTIAL DIAGNOSIS

Supratentorial Volume Loss

- Should have normal or decreased head circumference (HC)

Benign Enlargement of Subarachnoid Spaces in Infancy

- a.k.a. benign macrocrania, thought to be mild form of communicating hydrocephalus from immaturity of CSF absorption mechanisms
- Patients have normal neurologic exam
- Ventricles are normal in size or mildly enlarged

Communicating Hydrocephalus

- Secondary to impaired absorption of CSF in subarachnoid spaces rather than anatomic obstruction
- Causes include meningitis, leptomeningeal metastatic disease, venous hypertension

Secondary Obstructive Hydrocephalus

- Cause of obstruction is extrinsic to aqueduct: Tumor, germinal matrix hemorrhage, vascular lesion, etc.

PATHOLOGY

General Features

- Etiology
  - AS
    - AS pathologically obstructs CSF flow into 4th ventricle

- CSF production in choroid plexus continues → lateral/3rd ventricular fluid increased pressure, ventriculomegaly
- Ventricles expand, compress adjacent parenchyma, stretch CC
  - May rupture/open ependymal cell junctions → periventricular edema, ventricular diverticulum/dehiscence
- May be acquired or genetic
  - Isolated acquired forms from prior injury/insult, such as trace hemorrhage or infection, which results in webs or gliotic tissue obstructing aqueduct
  - Genetic forms often have other associated anomalies
- Genetics
  - *L1CAM* mutation (a.k.a. X-linked AS)
    - Most common genetic cause of AS
    - Caused by mutation of *L1CAM* gene
    - Associated syndromes
      - MASA: Intellectual disability (**m**ental restrictions), **a**phasia, **s**huffling gait, and **a**dducted thumbs
      - CRASH: **C**allosal hypoplasia, intellectual disability (mental **r**etardation), **a**dducted thumbs, **s**pastic paraplegia, and X-linked **h**ydrocephalus
  - α-dystroglycanopathy
    - Genes: *POMT1, POMT2, POMGNT1, FKTN, FKRP, LARGE1, CRPPA*
    - Congenital muscular dystrophies: Walker-Warburg, muscle-eye-brain disease, Fukuyama
    - Brain findings: Cobblestone cortex, Z-shaped brainstem, cerebellar cysts, vermian hypoplasia, pontine cleft, cephalocele
  - Tubulinopathy
    - Genes: *TUBA1A, TUBA8, TUBB2B, TUBB2A, TUBB3, TUBB, TUBG1*
    - Dysmorphic basal ganglia, lissencephaly/dysgyria, dysgenesis of CC, hypoplastic/Z-shaped brainstem
  - VACTERL-H association
    - Usually sporadic, some genetic mutations identified (*FANCB, ZIC3*)
    - ± rhombencephalosynapsis
- Associated abnormalities
  - Rhombencephalosynapsis
    - Up to 65% of patients with rhombencephalosynapsis have coexisting AS
  - Diencephalic-mesencephalic junction dysplasia
    - Associated with *L1CAM* mutation
    - Usually with diencephalosynapsis
    - ± pontine hypoplasia, vermian hypoplasia, and cerebellar hypoplasia
  - Chiari 2
    - Not well described, but coexisting AS suspected in cases with increased HC (majority of Chiari 2 patients have decreased HC)

CLINICAL ISSUES

Presentation

- Most common signs/symptoms
  - Symptoms depend upon patient age at time of diagnosis
  - Onset can be insidious, may occur from birth to adulthood but typically bimodal distribution
- Other signs/symptoms
  - Headache, papilledema, 6th nerve palsy, bulging fontanelles
  - Macrocrania, especially if sutures open
  - Parinaud syndrome

Demographics

- Age
  - Presentation, 2 peaks of distribution: One in 1st year of life (more common), other in adolescence
- Sex
  - M:F = 2:1
- Epidemiology
  - 0.5-1 per 1,000 births, recurrence rate of 1-4.5% in siblings
  - AS responsible for ~ 20% of congenital hydrocephalus
    - Most common cause of prenatal obstructive hydrocephalus

Natural History & Prognosis

- Hydrocephalus usually progressive unless treated
  - May stabilize as "arrested" or compensated hydrocephalus
- While isolated congenital AS has much better prognosis than AS with genetic disorder or other brain anomalies, only ~ 1/3 of patients with isolated AS have normal neurodevelopmental outcomes

Treatment

- CSF shunt diversion
- ETV
- Cerebral aqueductoplasty for membranous and short-segment aqueductal stenoses (selected cases)
- Prenatally diagnosed cases may require C-section due to macrocephaly

DIAGNOSTIC CHECKLIST

Consider

- Look for coexisting brain anomalies as they make difference in prognosis

Image Interpretation Pearls

- Use thin-section 3D TrueFISP/bFFE to better delineate aqueduct

SELECTED REFERENCES

1. Accogli A et al: L1CAM variants cause two distinct imaging phenotypes on fetal MRI. Ann Clin Transl Neurol. 8(10):2004-12, 2021
2. Heaphy-Henault KJ et al: Congenital aqueductal stenosis: findings at fetal mri that accurately predict a postnatal diagnosis. AJNR Am J Neuroradiol. 39(5):942-8, 2018
3. Kline-Fath BM et al: Congenital aqueduct stenosis: progressive brain findings in utero to birth in the presence of severe hydrocephalus. Prenat Diagn. 38(9):706-12, 2018
4. Tonetti DA et al: Clinical outcomes of isolated congenital aqueductal stenosis. World Neurosurg. 114:e976-81, 2018
5. Yamada S et al: Current and emerging MR imaging techniques for the diagnosis and management of CSF flow disorders: a review of phase-contrast and time-spatial labeling inversion pulse. AJNR Am J Neuroradiol. 36(4):623-30, 2015

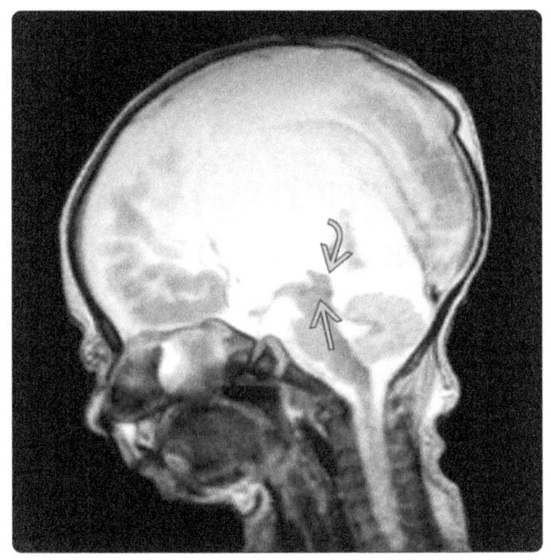

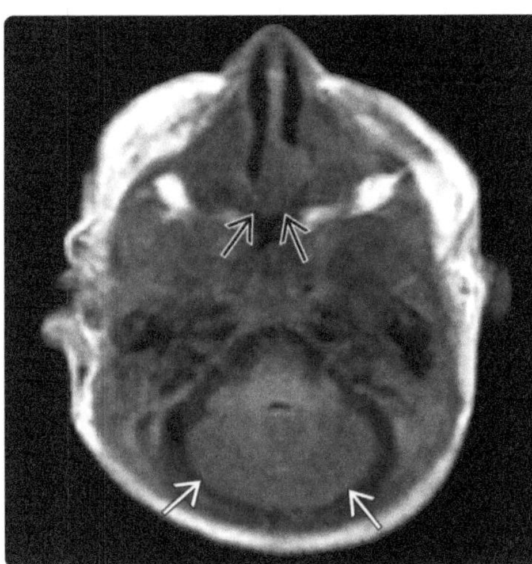

(Left) *Sagittal T2WI MR in a 5-day-old with prenatal diagnosis of aqueductal stenosis demonstrates effacement of the cerebral aqueduct ⇨ with thickening of the tectum ⇨.* **(Right)** *Axial T1WI MR in the same patient demonstrates rhombencephalosynapsis ➡ and bilateral choanal atresia ⇨. Other anomalies in this patient included bilateral microphthalmia and tracheoesophageal fistula. This patient had a partial deletion of chromosome 3q and SOX2 gene mutation.*

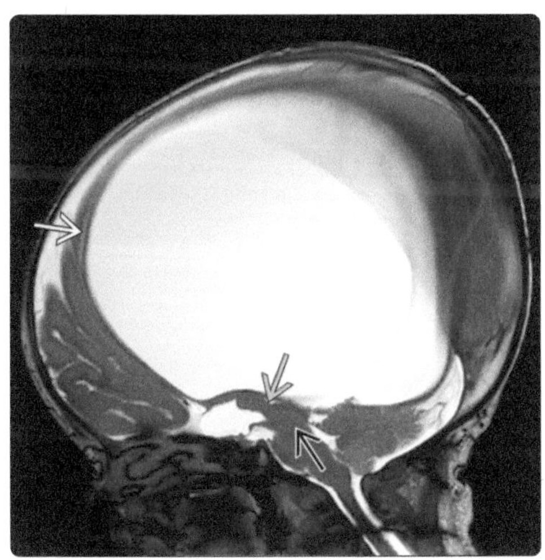

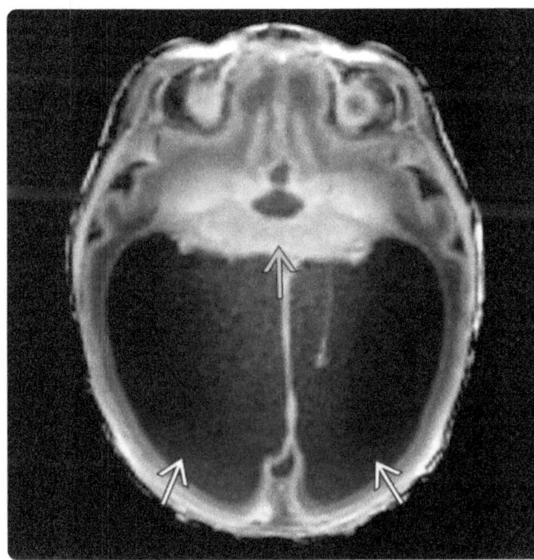

(Left) *Sagittal 3D FIESTA in a 1-day-old boy with prenatal diagnosis of aqueductal stenosis demonstrates thinning of the corpus callosum ➡, diencephalic-mesencephalic junction dysplasia ⇨, and effacement of the aqueduct ⇨.* **(Right)** *Axial T1WI MR in the same patient shows severe ventriculomegaly of the lateral ventricles ➡ and thickening of the massa intermedia/ diencephalosynapsis ⇨. This patient was negative for L1CAM mutation.*

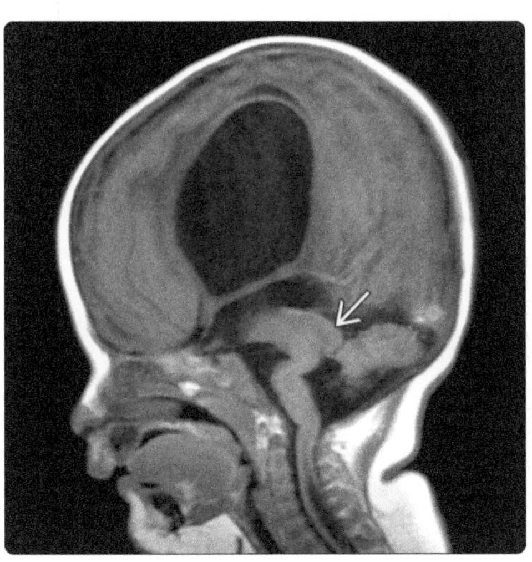

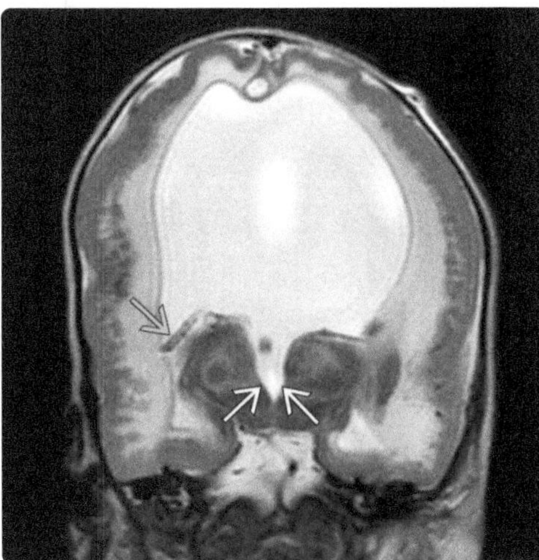

(Left) *Sagittal T1WI MR in a patient with Walker-Warburg syndrome shows rounded thickened tectal plate ➡ with aqueductal occlusion. Marked enlargement of the lateral and 3rd ventricles is present. A Z-shaped brainstem and very small cerebellum are characteristic of this syndrome.* **(Right)** *Coronal T2WI MR in the same patient with Walker-Warburg syndrome confirms marked ventriculomegaly, funnel-shaped 3rd ventricle above aqueduct ➡, and classic cobblestone cortex. Shunt ⇨ is partially imaged.*

KEY FACTS

TERMINOLOGY

- Hydrocephalus (HCP)
  - Enlargement of cerebral ventricles secondary to abnormal CSF formation, flow, or absorption resulting in ↑ CSF volume

IMAGING

- Shunt failure → dilated ventricles + edema around ventricles, along catheter and reservoir
- Use CT or MR to evaluate ventricle size, plain radiograph shunt series to identify mechanical shunt failure
- Baseline CT/MR following shunt insertion, follow-up at 1 year and as clinically needed
- Shunt radionuclide studies: Used to confirm distal obstruction

TOP DIFFERENTIAL DIAGNOSES

- Shunt failure with normal ventricle size or lack of interstitial edema
- Noncompliant (slit) ventricle syndrome
- Acquired Chiari 1/tonsillar ectopia

PATHOLOGY

- Obstructive HCP: Secondary to physical blockage by tumor, adhesions, cyst
- Communicating HCP: Secondary to ↓ CSF absorption across arachnoid granulations

CLINICAL ISSUES

- Older children/adults: Headache, vomiting, lethargy, seizure, neurocognitive symptoms
- Infants: Bulging fontanelle, ↑ head circumference, irritability, lethargy

DIAGNOSTIC CHECKLIST

- Shunt + headache not always shunt failure
- Confirm programmable shunt valve setting after MR
- Compare current CT with prior studies to detect subtle changes in ventricle size

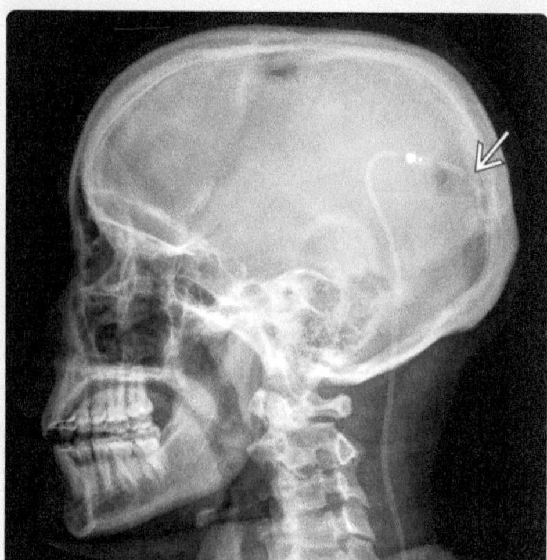

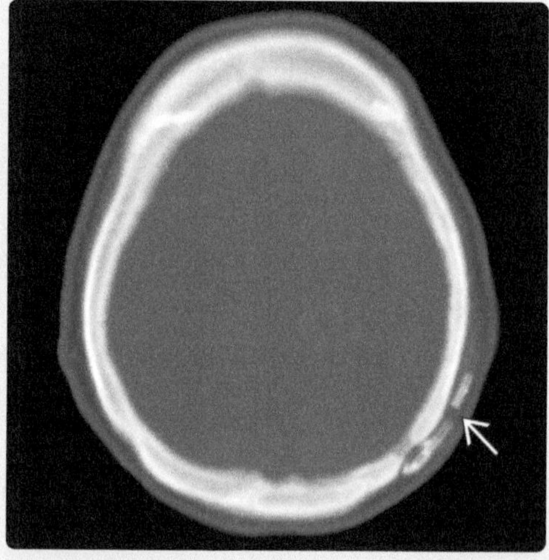

(Left) *Lateral skull radiograph of acute ventriculoperitoneal (VP) shunt failure from a plain radiograph shunt series demonstrates a mechanical shunt catheter disconnection ➡ between the programmable valve and the reservoir.* **(Right)** *Axial bone CT in the same patient reveals the mechanical catheter disconnection ➡ between the reservoir and the programmable shunt valve. This finding had not appeared on the most recent comparison CT scan (not shown).*

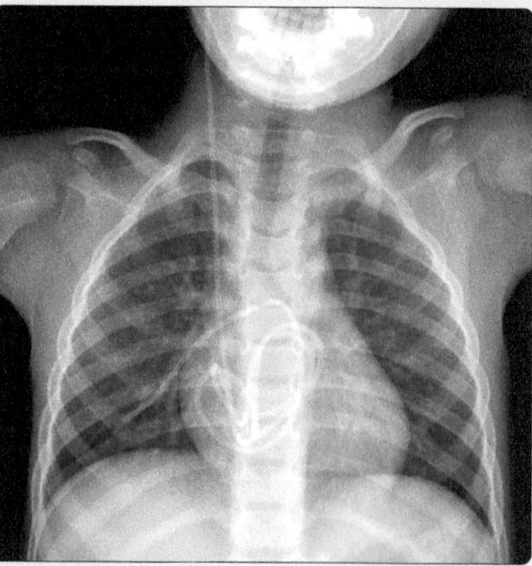

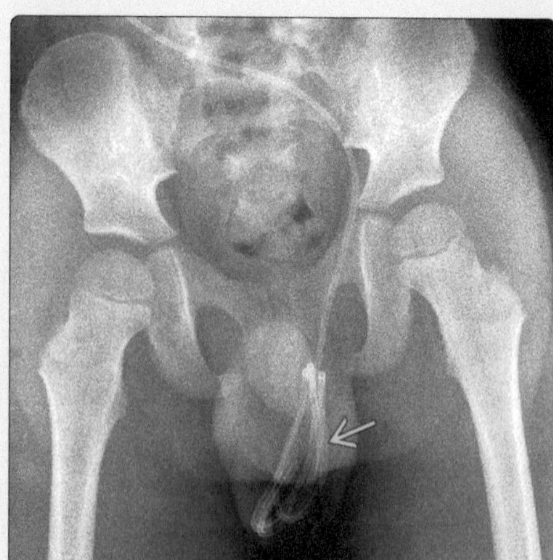

(Left) *AP radiograph from a shunt series demonstrates intracardiac migration of the VP shunt catheter with the tip residing in the right interlobar pulmonary artery.* **(Right)** *AP radiograph of the pelvis in a 4-year-old with a VP shunt who presented with left scrotal swelling demonstrates a coiled distal shunt catheter ➡ in the left scrotum. The migration of the catheter to the scrotum is due to a patent processus vaginalis.*

TERMINOLOGY

Abbreviations

- Shunt types: Ventriculoperitoneal (VP), ventriculoatrial (VA), ventriculopleural (VPL), lumboperitoneal (LP)

Definitions

- Ventriculomegaly
  - General term for enlargement of cerebral ventricles
- Hydrocephalus (HCP)
  - Enlargement of cerebral ventricles secondary to abnormal CSF formation, flow, or absorption resulting in ↑ CSF volume
    - Subset of ventriculomegaly
    - Onset over days (acute), weeks (subacute), or months to years (chronic)

IMAGING

General Features

- Best diagnostic clue
  - Shunt failure: Dilated ventricles + edema ("blurring") around ventricles and along catheter, reservoir
- Location
  - VP shunt common; VA and VPL used rarely unless VP contraindicated
- Size
  - Ventricular size is relative; ventriculomegaly may indicate shunt failure in one patient and be stable finding in another
    - Change in ventricular size in individual patient probably significant
    - Conversely, some patients manifest shunt failure with minimal to no change in ventricular size
  - Distal catheter must be sized long enough to permit somatic growth, prevent retraction out of abdomen or chest
- Morphology
  - Shunt system components
    - Proximal catheter in ventricles, subarachnoid space, syrinx cavity, or thecal sac
    - Unidirectional valve prevents reflux into ventricles
    - Reservoir used to sample CSF, acutely relieve pressure
    - Distal catheter tunneled through subcutaneous tissues → tip in peritoneal cavity, cardiac atrium, or pleural cavity

Radiographic Findings

- Radiography
  - Evaluate shunt catheter system integrity
    - Shunt fracture, separation, migration
    - Distal catheter may retract out of abdomen if significant somatic growth since shunt placement

CT Findings

- NECT
  - Ventricular dilatation (diffuse or loculated)
    - Isolated ventricle after infection, hemorrhage → interventricular synechia
    - Periventricular interstitial edema ("blurred" ventricle margins) → acute HCP
  - Small, slit ventricles → noncompliant ventricle syndrome, chronic overdrainage
  - ± subdural hematoma (CSF overdrainage)

MR Findings

- T1WI
  - Assess ventricular size, characterize brain anatomy
- T2WI
  - ± interstitial parenchymal edema (transependymal CSF flow) → acute shunt failure
- FLAIR
  - Interstitial edema more conspicuous than on T1WI or T2WI
- T1WI C+
  - ± enhancement with ventriculitis, abscess, neoplasm
  - Pachymeningeal enhancement due to low intracranial pressure (ICP)
- MRA
  - Stretched, displaced arteries around dilated ventricles secondary to ventriculomegaly
- MRV
  - Venous thrombosis may precede HCP or follow shunting
    - Leads to ↑ intraventricular/ICP
- MR cine
  - Evaluate patency of normal CSF pathways, 3rd ventriculostomy

Ultrasonographic Findings

- Grayscale ultrasound
  - Useful in neonates for serial assessment of ventricular size (requires open fontanelle)

Nonvascular Interventions

- Interventricular contrast injection through shunt + NECT → detect ventricular isolation needing additional catheter

Nuclear Medicine Findings

- Shunt radionuclide studies
  - Radiotracer injected into shunt reservoir, serial imaging to document timing of radiotracer egress from distal catheter tip
  - Used to confirm distal obstruction

Imaging Recommendations

- Best imaging tool
  - Brain NECT to assess for acute ventricular size change
  - Fast MR protocols (HASTE, SSFSE) used in many centers to avoid cumulative radiation exposure
    - Can be successfully performed without sedation in many patients
- Protocol advice
  - Brain CT or "fast" MR to evaluate ventricle size
  - Plain film shunt series to identify mechanical shunt fracture or disconnection

DIFFERENTIAL DIAGNOSIS

Shunt Failure With Normal Ventricle Size or Lack of Interstitial Edema

- Look for fluid along shunt catheter or reservoir as only sign of malfunction
- May require diagnosis on clinical grounds

Noncompliant (Slit) Ventricle Syndrome

- Usually older child (shunted in infancy)
- Small ventricles + intermittent signs of shunt obstruction
- Ventricles normal/small, even if shunt malfunctioning

Acquired Cerebellar Tonsillar Ectopia

- Functioning LP shunt produces tonsillar descent through foramen magnum
- More common with valveless systems
- Do **not** call this "acquired Chiari 1"!

PATHOLOGY

General Features

- Etiology
  - Impairment of CSF circulation
    - Obstructive
      - Usually at narrowest points in CSF circulation (aqueduct, foramina of Monro)
      - Tumor, web/synechia, congenital aqueductal stenosis
    - Inadequate reabsorption across arachnoid granulations into venous sinuses
      - Arachnoid granulations "clogged" after hemorrhage, inflammation
      - Diminished pressure gradient from subarachnoid space to venous sinuses secondary to venous hypertension
      - Impaired CSF absorption → CSF accumulation, ↑ ICP
  - CSF shunt establishes accessory drainage pathway to bypass obstructed natural CSF flow pathways
    - Restores or maintains normal ICP
  - Each shunt, valve, device carries its own set of complications
    - All types → material degradation/fatigue, mechanical stress (especially craniocervical junction, inferior ribs)
    - VP → abdominal complications (CSF pseudocyst, ascites, bowel perforation)
    - VPL → symptomatic pleural effusion
    - VA → shunt nephritis, cor pulmonale, pulmonary embolus
    - LP → arachnoiditis, cerebellar tonsillar herniation, high catheter migration rate
    - Programmable shunt → unintentional reprogram during MR
- Associated abnormalities
  - Shunts placed with CSF blood/protein > 1 g/dL prone to early blockage, failure
  - Shunt infection
  - Ventricular loculation or isolation
  - Overshunting

Gross Pathologic & Surgical Features

- Ventricular ependymal adhesions (scar)
- Extracranial shunt tubing calcification

Microscopic Features

- Gliosis along intracranial shunt tract

CLINICAL ISSUES

Presentation

- Most common signs/symptoms
  - Children, adults
    - Headache, vomiting, lethargy, seizure
    - Neuropsychologic, cognitive, or behavioral
  - Infants
    - Bulging fontanelle, ↑ head circumference, irritability, lethargy

Natural History & Prognosis

- Acute shunt obstruction in shunt-dependent patients may lead to death
- Majority of shunts eventually fail; complication rate: 25-37%
  - ≤ 40% of shunts fail in 1st year, 80% fail by 10 years
  - 50% of patients need multiple revisions, progressively shorter time interval to next failure

Treatment

- Shunt revision
  - Replace intraventricular component/valve for proximal obstruction
  - Alter valve pressure setting/type if over- or underdraining
    - Programmable shunt valves permit transcutaneous adjustment of pressure setting
  - Lengthen distal shunt as child grows
- 3rd ventriculostomy to avoid indwelling shunt if blockage is distal to 3rd ventricle
  - Becoming commonly used in pediatric hospitals to avoid shunt placement
- Laparoscopic or open abdominal procedure for distal obstruction related to CSF pseudocyst

DIAGNOSTIC CHECKLIST

Consider

- Shunt + headache does not always mean shunt failure
  - Consider sinusitis, trauma, sinovenous thrombosis, viral infection
- Confirm programmable shunt valve setting after MR
- Plain film shunt series has extremely low yield in absence of clinical evidence for mechanical shunt failure

Image Interpretation Pearls

- Compare with prior studies to detect subtle ventricular size changes
- Fluid tracking along shunt may be only sign of failure; possibly even if ventricles normal or unchanged size

SELECTED REFERENCES

1. Pedersen SH et al: How to define CSF overdrainage: a systematic literature review. Acta Neurochir (Wien). 165(2):429-41, 2023
2. Simsek O et al: Acquired hump of the corpus callosum: a rare morphologic complication after CSF shunting. Childs Nerv Syst. 39(5):1253-9, 2023
3. McAlpine A et al: Cerebrospinal fluid shunt infections: a multicenter pediatric study. Pediatr Infect Dis J. 41(6):449-54, 2022
4. Kraemer MR et al: Overdrainage-related ependymal bands: a postulated cause of proximal shunt obstruction. J Neurosurg Pediatr. 1-11, 2018
5. Hanak BW et al: Cerebrospinal fluid shunting complications in children. Pediatr Neurosurg. 52(6):381-400, 2017
6. Sivaganesan A et al: Neuroimaging of ventriculoperitoneal shunt complications in children. Pediatr Radiol. 42(9):1029-46, 2012

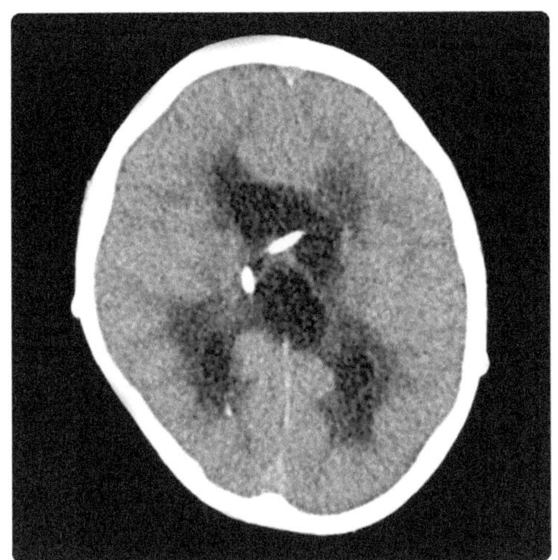

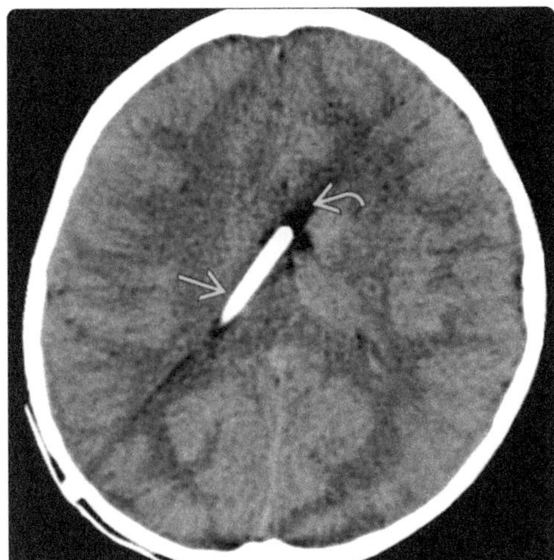

(Left) *Axial NECT depicts symmetric interstitial edema within the periventricular white matter. Ventricular size is significantly larger than demonstrated on a prior CT (not shown), supporting the diagnosis of acute shunt failure.* **(Right)** *Axial NECT in a patient with VP shunt ➔ who presented with severe headaches shows collapsed lateral ventricles ➔. Slit ventricle syndrome presents as severe headaches due to noncompliant ventricles and should not be confused with radiologic slit ventricles.*

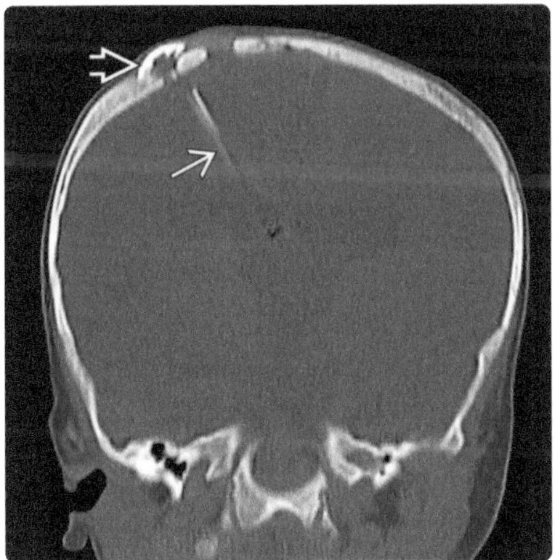

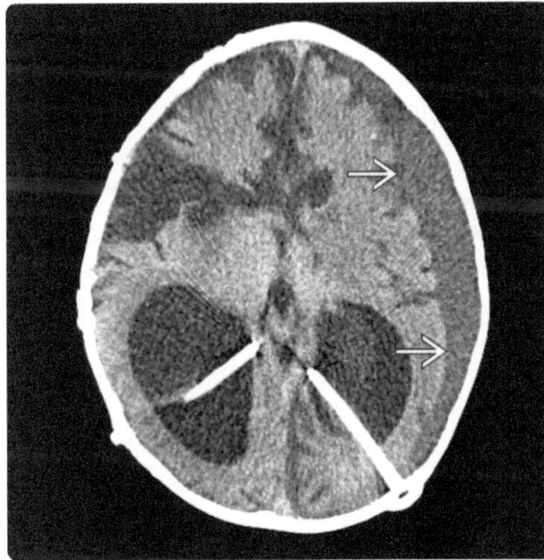

(Left) *Coronal bone CT demonstrates fracture or disconnection of the ventricular catheter ➔ from the reservoir ➔, resulting in clinical shunt failure (larger ventricles on NECT).* **(Right)** *Axial NECT following bilateral ventricular catheter placement in a patient with severe hydrocephalus and brain atrophy reveals development of a large left subdural hematoma ➔ following VP shunting.*

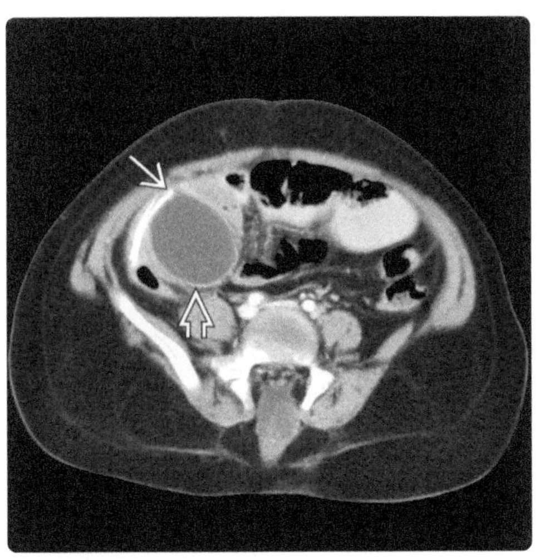

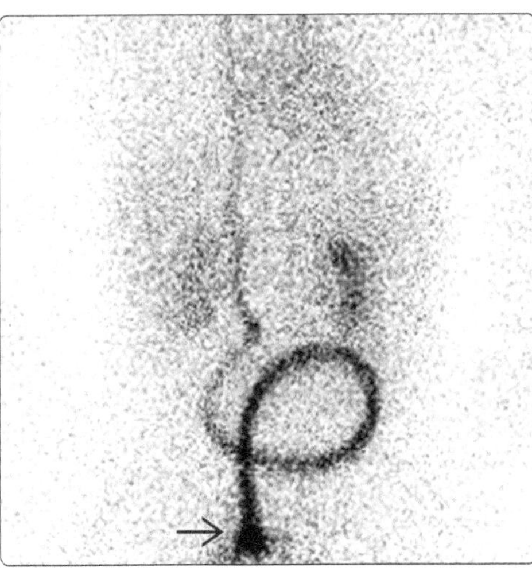

(Left) *Axial NECT in a hydrocephalic patient presenting with distal VP shunt failure shows the peritoneal catheter tip ➔ within a loculated pelvic fluid collection (CSF pseudocyst ➔).* **(Right)** *Frontal cisternogram-radionuclide shuntogram examination performed after injecting the shunt valve reservoir reveals no spillage from the distal catheter ➔ after 10 minutes. Further delayed imaging (not shown) confirmed absence of spillage from the catheter, substantiating distal shunt obstruction.*

Embryology

The pituitary gland is composed of 3 lobes, which are derived from dual-embryonic ectodermal origins. The endocrine hormone-producing anterior and intermediate lobes originate from the ectoderm of the oral cavity, whereas the posterior lobe develops from overlying neuroectoderm. A persistent apposition, with resultant interactions between these ectodermal layers, is essential for normal pituitary development. The location of the pituitary and hypothalamus in the midline, and their close developmental associations with other structures of the ventral forebrain and eyes, results in frequent association of congenital hypopituitarism with heterogeneous midline defects, most commonly optic nerve hypoplasia and septo-optic dysplasia. Less common associated conditions include holoprosencephaly (HPE), Kallmann syndrome, and cleft palate.

During the 5th week of embryonic life, a thickening appears in the oral ectoderm of the foregut, rostral to the notochord. This structure invaginates to form a vesicle, the rudimentary **Rathke pouch** (a.k.a. Rathke cleft). As this vesicle extends anteriorly, it becomes positioned rostral to a ventral extension of the embryonic hypothalamus, which develops into the **neurohypophysis**, or the posterior pituitary lobe. The connection of Rathke cleft with the buccal cavity disappears shortly after contacting the neurohypophysis; at this time, it becomes known as the **adenohypophysis** or anterior pituitary lobe. Portions of the anterior lobe may remain as nests of pituitary tissue in the nasopharynx, sphenoid sinus, or in remnants of the craniopharyngeal canal.

During the 6th week of embryonic life, the anterior pituitary lobe develops lateral processes called the tuberal processes, which will differentiate into the pars tuberalis. Soon after, the tuberal processes surround the entire infundibulum and anterior lobe laterally, and the posterior midline adenohypophysial cells differentiate into the primordium of the pars intermedia. By the end of the 7th gestational week, all of the components of the mature hypothalamus and pituitary axis are present. These will slowly evolve into the mature hypothalamic-pituitary axis.

The various transcription factors involved in these processes have been determined over the past decade. Maturation of the oral ectoderm occurs under the influence of zinc finger factors, such as GLI1, GLI2, and GLI3. Incorporation of Rathke cleft into the pituitary seems to be dependent upon the activation of several extrinsic signaling pathways; these include sonic hedgehog (SHH), fibroblast growth factors (FGF8, FGF10), bone morphogenetic proteins (BMP2, BMP4), and wingless (WNT) pathways. Mutations affecting certain transcription factors in these pathways are specifically associated with abnormal hypothalamic or pituitary development. These include *GLI2* (hypopituitarism), *LHX3* (pituitary hormone deficiencies associated with cervical abnormalities), *LHX4* [hypoplastic anterior pituitary ± ectopic posterior pituitary (EEP)], *HESX* (anterior pituitary deficiency with septo-optic dysplasia phenotypes), and *SOX3* (hypopituitarism or infundibular hypoplasia). The details of these pathways are beyond the scope of this book but are important in that they are also involved in the induction of other transcription factors that are important in development of the ventral forebrain and midline structures. Therefore, it is not surprising that **other brain anomalies are commonly found in patients with hypothalamic-pituitary anomalies.** After assessing the basal forebrain for the presence of a complete interhemispheric fissure (and thereby exclude HPE), the optic nerves, olfactory nerves, septum pellucidum, and corpus callosum should be particularly scrutinized.

Imaging Anatomy

The key to interpreting abnormalities of hypothalamic and pituitary development is an understanding of the normal anatomy of the structures. This anatomy is closely tied in with the anatomy of the 3rd ventricle. The hypothalamus forms the floor and the anterolateral walls of the 3rd ventricle, and the infundibulum descends from the floor of the ventricle into the sella turcica, where it ends in the neurohypophysis (posterior pituitary lobe). Anterior to the neurohypophysis is the much smaller pars intermedia (intermediate lobe), which is situated posterior to the adenohypophysis (anterior pituitary lobe). The neurohypophysis is easy to identify on noncontrast T1-weighted images, as it is usually hyperintense, whereas the adenohypophysis is isointense to brain on noncontrast images (except in the newborn). In the newborn, the adenohypophysis is hyperintense on T1, often equal to the neurohypophysis. This T1 hyperintensity of the neonatal adenohypophysis decreases over the first few months of life. The pars intermedia is difficult to see unless a mass (or, more commonly, a cyst) is present. The neurohypophysis is a direct extension of the hypothalamus, receiving vasopressin and oxytocin that are synthesized in hypothalamic nuclei, transported along axons of the tuberohypophyseal tract (from the tuber cinereum) and the supraopticohypophyseal tract (from the supraoptic nucleus) through the infundibulum, and stored in neurohypophysial vesicles to be released into the blood stream after reception of signals from outside the nervous system by way of the circumventricular organs.

Although the specific hypothalamic nuclei cannot (yet) be seen on routine diagnostic imaging, several hypothalamic structures and other structures adjacent to or within the hypothalamus can be identified. On sagittal images, the optic chiasm and lamina terminalis define the rostral (anterior) borders of the hypothalamus, while the mammillary bodies define the caudal (posterior) borders. On sagittal T2-weighted images, the columns of the fornices can often be seen ascending obliquely dorsally from the mammillary bodies toward the foramina of Monro. The forniceal columns can also be identified on coronal images as thin bands of dorsoventral white matter intensity in the medial aspect of the gray matter intensity hypothalamic nuclei. Directly rostral to the mammillary bodies, the floor of the hypothalamus arches slightly upward to the pituitary stalk (infundibulum). This section of the hypothalamus is known as the **tuber cinereum**. Along with the infundibulum, it can be seen to enhance after administration of paramagnetic contrast material. The dorsal-most aspect of the infundibulum (at the 3rd ventricle) will often be seen as slightly widened and containing some fluid. This should not be mistaken for a mass, as it is almost always the infundibular recess of the 3rd ventricle and is seen to communicate with the ventricle on thin-section sagittal or coronal images. Immediately rostral to the infundibulum is the chiasmal recess of the 3rd ventricle and its ventrorostral border, the optic chiasm, from which the optic nerves can be seen to course obliquely toward the optic canals. In close proximity to the optic nerves, the olfactory tracts divide into olfactory stria, which may be seen on very high-resolution imaging entering the entorhinal cortex, amygdala, anterior perforated substance, and uncus.

Pathologic anatomy of the hypothalamus and pituitary in children is typically developmental or neoplastic. The most common developmental abnormality is the ectopic neurohypophysis, more commonly called the **EPP**. In this condition, the neurohypophysis is located within the infundibulum or at the median eminence (the junction of the infundibulum and the tuber cinereum, appearing as a focus of hyperintensity on T1-weighted images). If the neurohypophysis is of normal size, it often functions normally in its ectopic location and is detected incidentally. If the ectopic neurohypophysis is small or absent, the patient will likely have diabetes insipidus. The posterior pituitary bright spot can be seen in almost all normal patients (especially with high-spatial-resolution 3D imaging) but can occasionally not be confidently visualized. In the absence of a clinical history of diabetes insipidus, this is likely within limits of normal variation. However, if there is diabetes insipidus, a careful evaluation for an infundibular mass should be performed. Even in the absence of an infundibular mass, index of suspicion should be high, and a follow-up examination should be recommended to evaluate for development of an infiltrative infundibular mass (usually germinoma).

Another anomaly of the hypothalamic-pituitary region is the **hypothalamic hamartoma** (a.k.a. **hamartoma of the tuber cinereum**): A nodular mass of predominantly neurons that may be located in the walls or floor of the 3rd ventricle, between the infundibulum and the mammillary bodies, or as a pedunculated mass situated in the suprasellar or interpeduncular cistern with a narrow waist between the mass and the tuber cinereum. The hamartoma is isointense to gray matter on T1-weighted images, is iso- to slightly hyperintense on T2/FLAIR images, has gray matter diffusivity and perfusion, and does not enhance. Patients typically present with precocious puberty or gelastic ("laughing") seizures. The morphology of the hypothalamic hamartoma is somewhat predictive of clinical presentation with sessile masses being associated with seizures and pedunculated masses being more likely associated with precocious puberty.

The tuber cinereum is a common location for lipomas, which are presumed to result from abnormal development of the primitive leptomeninges (which normally evolve into the CSF of the subarachnoid space). They are ovoid, T1-hyperintense masses that are almost always an incidental finding. Differentiation from an ectopic neurohypophysis is made by location. Lipomas are found attached to the ventral surface of the tuber cinereum, between the infundibulum and the mammillary bodies, whereas the ectopic neurohypophysis is seen within the infundibulum or at its junction with the floor of the 3rd ventricle. Diagnosis is confirmed by acquiring a sequence with the use of a fat-suppression pulse; the hyperintense signal of the lipoma disappears, but that of the EEP does not.

The most common brain anomalies associated with pituitary dysgenesis or hypogenesis are optic nerve hypoplasia and septo-optic dysplasia, usually associated with EPP and hypoplastic adenohypophysis. However, the most bizarre pituitary anomalies are usually associated with HPEs and sphenoethmoidal cephaloceles. In HPE, the basal forebrain is improperly formed because the transcription factors that guide the development of the region are incompletely or improperly expressed. The result is hypoplasia or aplasia of structures that normally develop in the basal midline. Patients with the more severe forms of HPE, therefore, typically have severe hypopituitarism; the hypothalamus and pituitary should always be evaluated in patients with HPE. In sphenoidal cephaloceles, portions of the pituitary gland, hypothalamus, optic chiasm/nerves, anterior cerebral arteries, and inferior frontal lobe may herniate through defects in the sphenoid bones, often through the craniopharyngeal canal. These patients may present with endocrinologic or visual deficiencies. Less commonly, they may be discovered because of a soft tissue mass in the roof of their mouth; such masses should never be biopsied without prior neuroimaging, as neurologic damage, CSF leak, or meningitis may result.

Although the brain abnormalities in hypopituitarism may be isolated to the hypothalamus and pituitary gland, the observation that genes and transcription factors involved in pituitary and hypothalamic development are also expressed in other areas of the developing forebrain suggests that imaging should not be restricted to the hypothalamic-pituitary axis. The entire brain should be imaged with particular attention to the ventral and rostral forebrain. In addition to EPP, malformations associated with hypopituitarism include olfactory bulb hypoplasia with hypoplastic olfactory sulci (Kallmann syndrome), optic nerve hypoplasia ± absent septum pellucidum or schizencephaly (septo-optic dysplasia), and periodic hypothermia with absent corpus callosum (Shapiro syndrome).

Imaging Protocols

In general, anomalies of the hypothalamus and pituitary gland do not require special imaging protocols. Standard T1- and T2-weighted images of the entire brain should be acquired, preferably with additional smaller field of view, thin-section (< 3-mm) sequences through the basal forebrain and pituitary fossa. Contrast enhancement is useful when evaluating masses. Fat suppression may be useful to differentiate EPP from hypothalamic lipoma (although differences in location are diagnostic). Thin-section (2- to 3-mm) coronal FSE T2-weighted images are essential to assess the olfactory bulbs, nerves, and sulci. Thin-section steady-state sequences (e.g., FIESTA) provide unparalleled spatial resolution and resolve any CSF flow artifact in the suprasellar cistern. Optic nerves can be assessed simultaneously, as can the interhemispheric fissures, septum pellucidum, and the basal ganglia, all of which will be abnormal in the vast majority of HPEs. The optic nerves and septum will be abnormal in most patients with septo-optic dysplasia. Intravenous contrast is useful to rule out hypothalamic glioma (usually bright on T2/FLAIR sequences, however) or germinoma.

A slightly different protocol is necessary if sphenoidal or sphenoethmoidal encephalocele is suspected. These patients require very high-resolution, thin-section studies through the entire brain. Particular attention should be given to the anterior cerebral arteries, optic nerves/chiasm, and pituitary gland, which may extend ventrally into the cephalocele. Therefore, MRA and thin-section, steady-state images (CISS, FIESTA) should be added and scrutinized.

Selected References

1. Serrallach BL et al: Duplication of the pituitary gland: CT, MRI and DTI findings and updated review of the literature. Brain Sci. 12(5):574, 2022
2. Chapman PR et al: Neuroimaging of the pituitary gland: practical anatomy and pathology. Radiol Clin North Am. 58(6):1115-33, 2020
3. Boruah DK et al: Extra-pituitary cerebral anomalies in pediatric patients of ectopic neurohypophysis: an uncommon association. J Clin Imaging Sci. 7:19, 2017

(Left) *Sagittal illustration at ~ 30 days of embryonic life shows thickening of the roof of the stomodeum, immediately rostral to the notochord. The cleft is associated with a downward bowing of the diencephalon.* **(Right)** *Sagittal illustration 1 day later shows that the infolding has ↑ and established contact with the diencephalon, which is extending ventrally behind the pouch to eventually form a rudimentary neurohypophysis.*

Pituitary Embryology

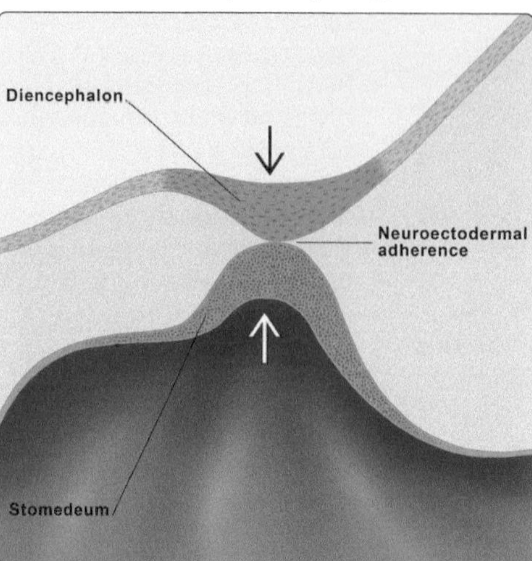

Pituitary Embryology

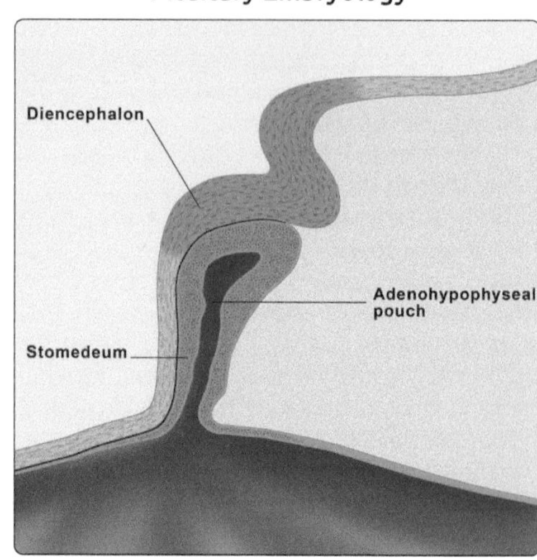

(Left) *Sagittal illustration at ~ 40 days shows narrowing of the connection of rudimentary pouch to buccal cavity; it may remain as a persistent craniopharyngeal (CP) canal. The definitive Rathke pouch is formed when its connection to oral ectoderm is lost and neurohypophysis fully evaginates. Progenitors of hormone-producing cells then proliferate.* **(Right)** *Sagittal illustration shows mature pituitary: Stalk, anterior and posterior gland, and location of the CP canal, when persistent.*

Pituitary Embryology

Pituitary Embryology

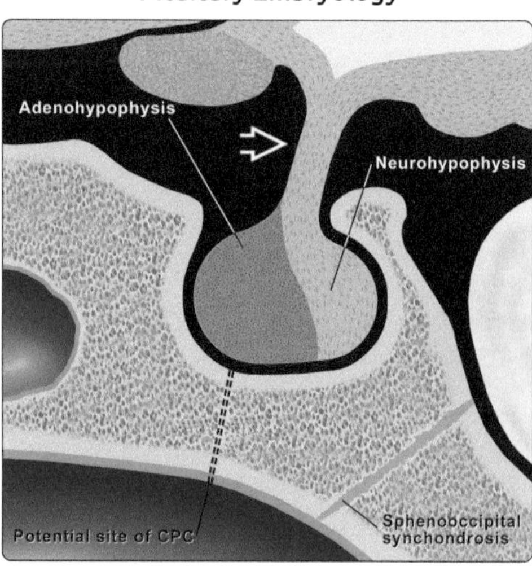

(Left) *Sagittal T1WI MR in a normal teenage male patient shows a normal pituitary with a bright posterior pituitary (neurohypophysis) and anterior pituitary (adenohypophysis), which is isointense to the pons.* **(Right)** *Midline sagittal FIESTA in a normal 4-year-old shows the normal hypothalamic-pituitary axis. Note the optic and infundibular recesses of the 3rd ventricle. Also note the thin membrane of Liliequist, which lies just posterior to the pituitary infundibulum.*

Normal Pituitary

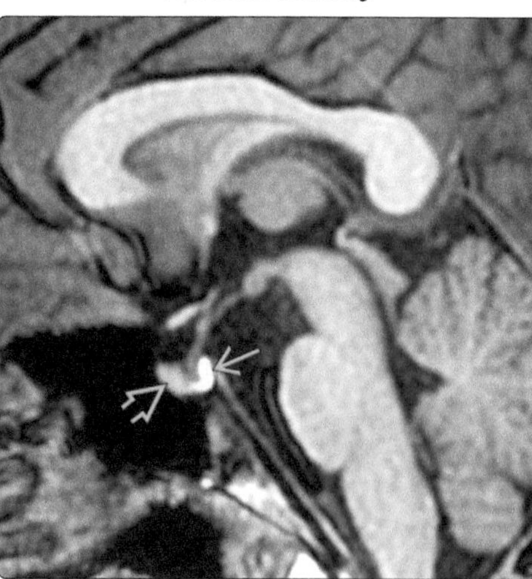

Normal Pituitary

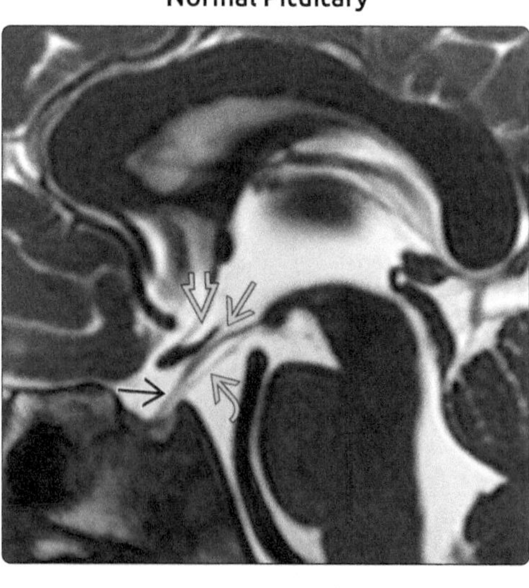

Normal Newborn Pituitary

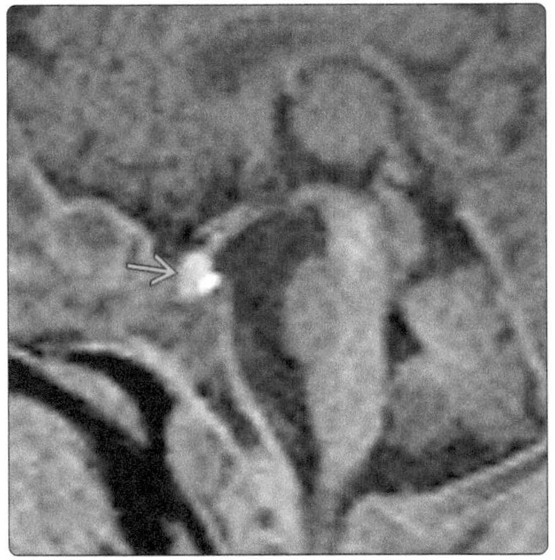

Normal Pubertal Female Pituitary

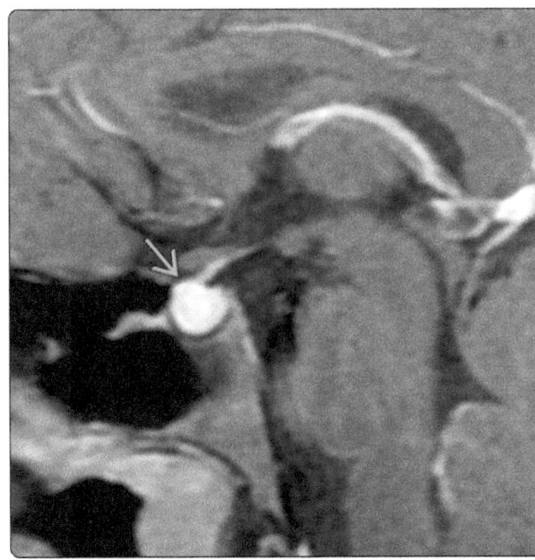

(Left) *Midline sagittal T1WI MR in a 4-day-old shows a hyperintense adenohypophysis ➔, which is a normal appearance for a neonate. Over the 1st few weeks of life, the T1 signal intensity will slowly decrease to become isointense to myelinated white matter.* **(Right)** *Midline sagittal T1WI C+ FS MR in a 13-year-old girl shows convex prominence of the superior margin ➔ of the pituitary gland. The superior margin of the pituitary is often convex in teenage girls and should not be mistaken for a pituitary mass.*

Pars Intermedia Cyst

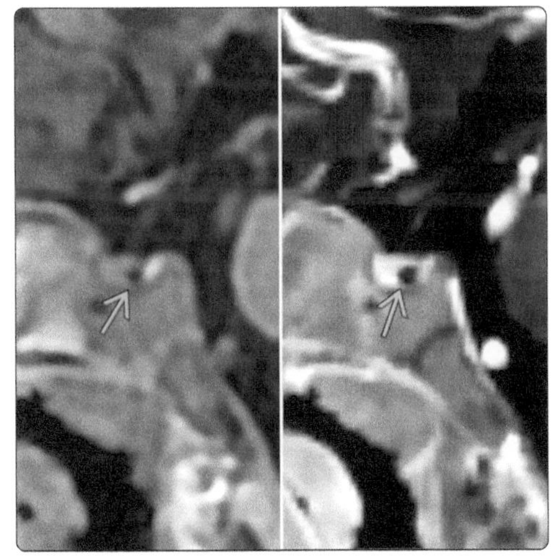

Pars Intermedia Cyst

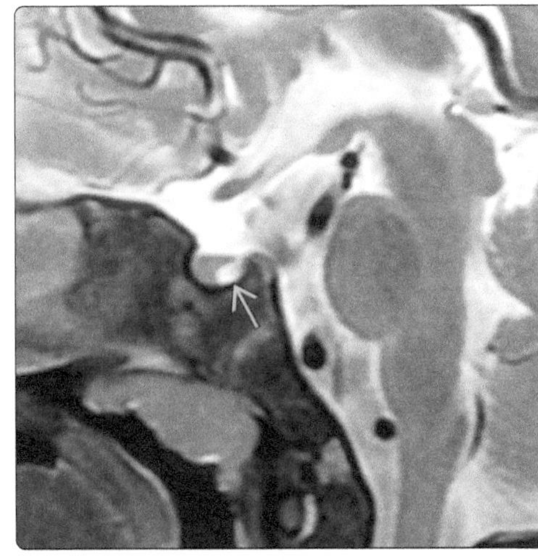

(Left) *Sagittal T1WI (L) and T1WI C+ (R) MRs in a 7-month-old with developmental delay show hypointense nonenhancing focus ➔ between anterior and posterior pituitary glands, consistent with pars intermedia cyst.* **(Right)** *Sagittal T2WI MR in 7-month-old with developmental delay shows hyperintense focus ➔ between anterior and posterior pituitary glands, consistent with pars intermedia cyst. This is an incidental finding and does not require clinical or imaging follow-up.*

Rathke Cleft Cyst

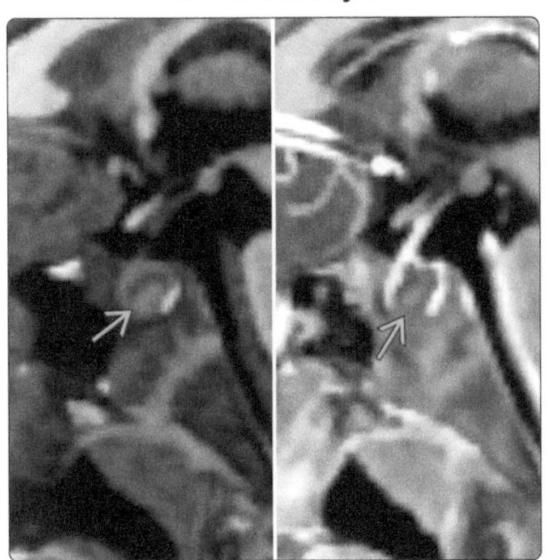

Rathke Cleft Cyst

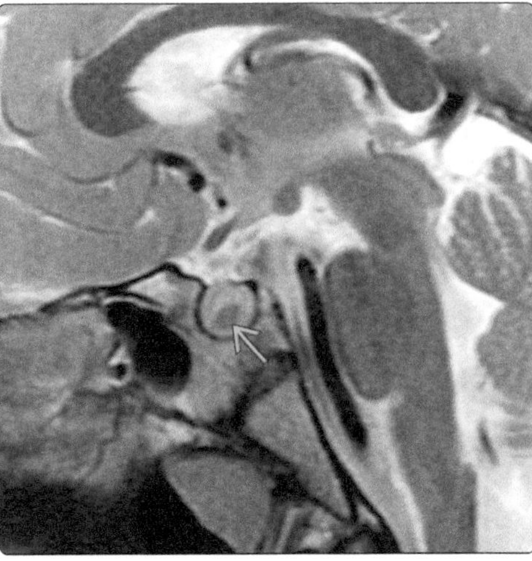

(Left) *Midline sagittal T1WI (L) and T1WI C+ (R) MR images in an 8-year-old shows an incidentally identified Rathke cleft cyst ➔. Cyst contains T1-hyperintense nodule, is nonenhancing, and is located between neurohypophysis and adenohypophysis. T1 signal intensity of Rathke cleft cysts is highly variable.* **(Right)** *Midline sagittal T2WI MR (same patient) with Rathke cleft cyst shows a characteristic T2-hypointense nodule ➔ in the inferior aspect of the cyst, a characteristic imaging feature of Rathke cleft cysts.*

(Left) *Sagittal T1WI MR in an 11-year-old with pituitary dysfunction and ectopic posterior pituitary shows a globular focus of ↑ signal* → *in the pituitary infundibulum. Ectopic neurohypophysis can occur anywhere from along the infundibulum to the base of the hypothalamus.* **(Right)** *Sagittal T1WI MR in a 3-week-old with septo-optic dysplasia (SOD) shows absence of normal signal along posterior pituitary. Neurohypophysis* → *is located ectopically at the base of the hypothalamus. Pituitary anomalies are common in SOD.*

Ectopic Neurohypophysis

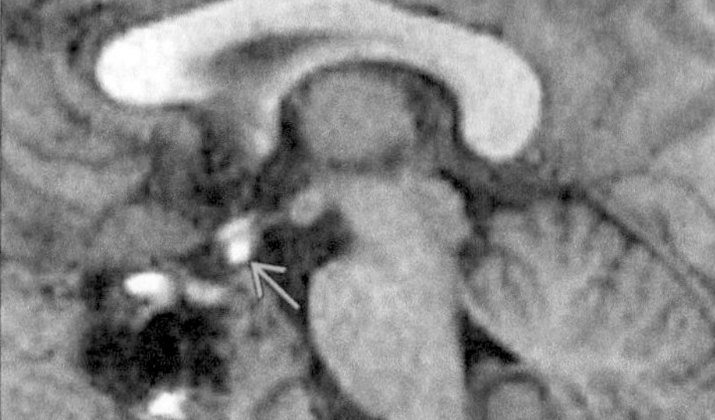

Ectopic Neurohypophysis in Septo-Optic Dysplasia

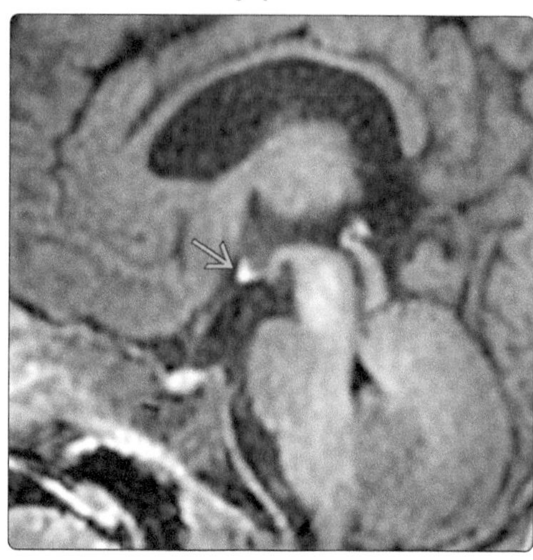

(Left) *Midline sagittal FIESTA in a 15-year-old with SOD plus shows a hypoplastic optic chiasm* → *and absence of the pituitary infundibulum in its expected location* ⇨. **(Right)** *Sagittal T1WI MR in a 12-year-old with SOD plus shows that an ectopic neurohypophysis* → *is located at the base of the hypothalamus and small anterior pituitary* ⇨. *Identification of an ectopic neurohypophysis should prompt a search for findings of SOD, such as optic nerve/chiasm hypoplasia* ↷, *as in this case.*

Absent Infundibulum and Ectopic Neurohypophysis in Septo-Optic Dysplasia

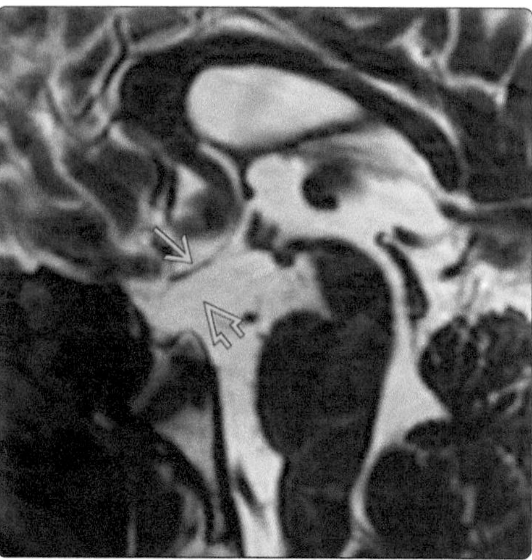

Pituitary Malformation in Septo-Optic Dysplasia

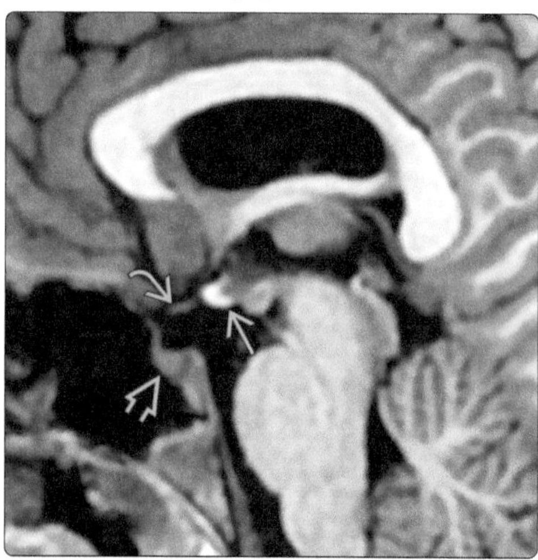

(Left) *Sagittal FIESTA in a neonate with persistent CP canal containing a duplicated pituitary* → *shows the persistent fetal osseus CP canal* ↷ *with anterior tethering of the 3rd ventricle* ⇨. **(Right)** *T1WI MR in the same neonate with duplicated pituitary shows 2 separate pituitary infundibula* → *and incomplete separation of the pituitary gland* ⇨ *itself. Coronal images are key to making this diagnosis, as they allow confident identification of 2 separate infundibula.*

Persistent Craniopharyngeal Canal and Pituitary Duplication

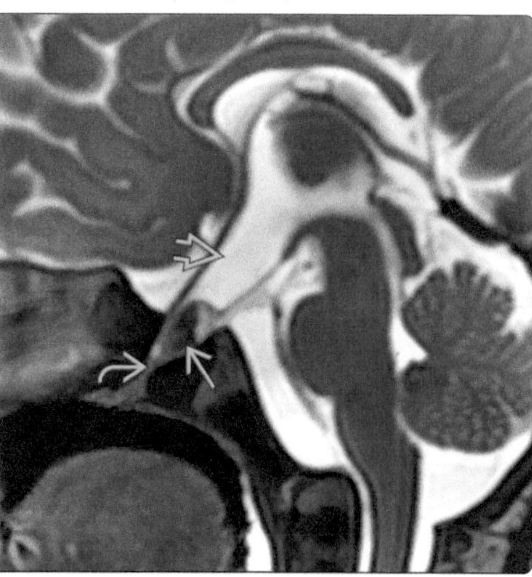

Persistent Craniopharyngeal Canal and Pituitary Duplication

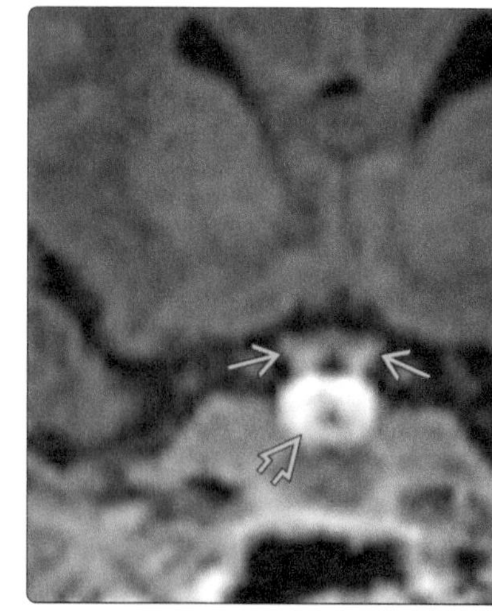

Pituitary Duplication

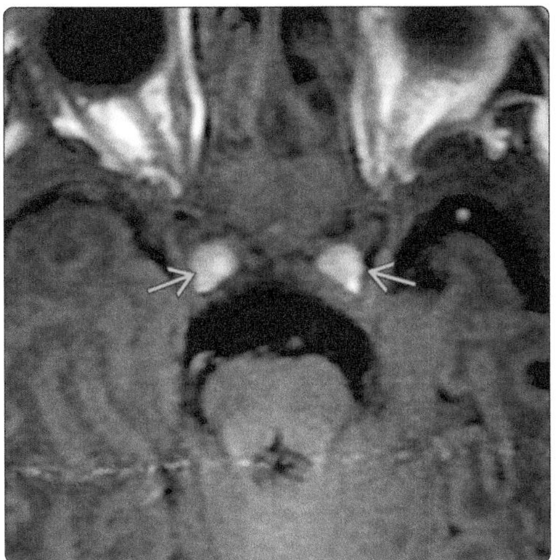

Pituitary Duplication

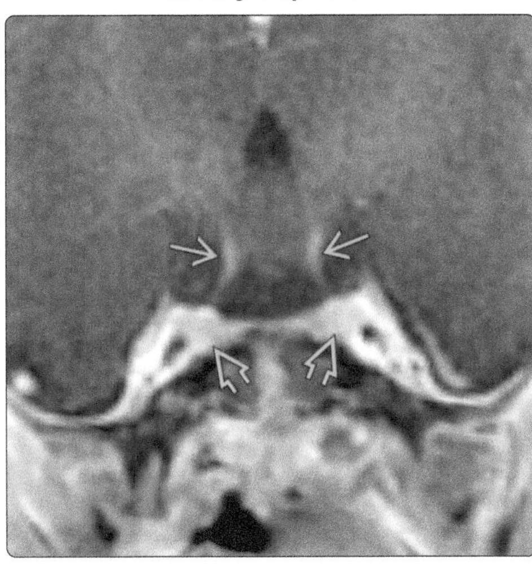

(Left) *Axial T1WI MR in a 2-day-old with pituitary duplication shows 2 separate hyperintense pituitary glands ➔ at the level of the sella turcica. Note that the adenohypophysis is T1 hyperintense in neonates, so this finding is most conspicuous on precontrast images.* **(Right)** *Coronal T1WI C+ FS MR in the same patient shows enhancement of the separate pituitary infundibula ➔. The pituitary glands ➔ are less conspicuous after contrast due to the adjacent cavernous sinus.*

Germinoma

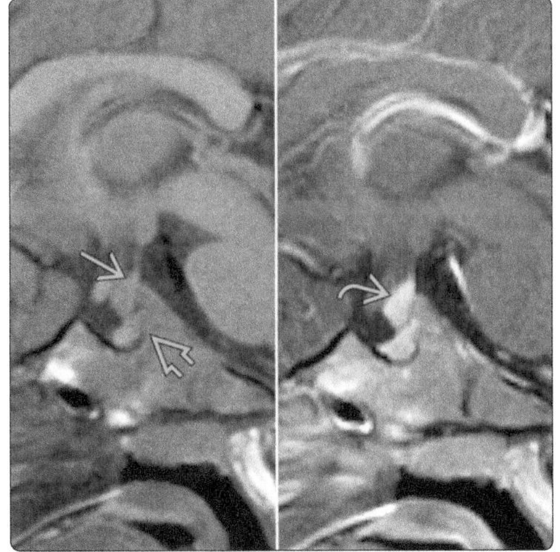

Germinoma

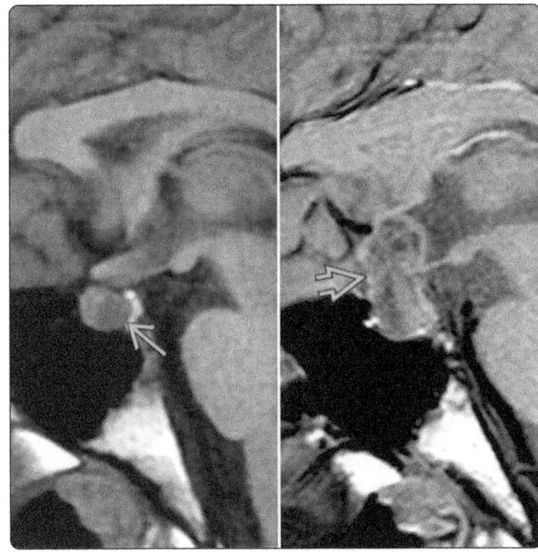

(Left) *Sagittal T1WI C+ MR (L) in a 4-year-old boy with central diabetes insipidus (DI) shows an infundibular mass ➔ and absence of posterior pituitary bright spot ➔. After contrast (R), the mass enhances homogeneously ➔.* **(Right)** *Sagittal T1WI MR in a 17-year-old boy with DI show initial absence of the posterior pituitary bright spot ➔ (L) with interval development of a large sellar and suprasellar mass ➔ 2 months later (R). Patients with DI and absent posterior pituitary bright spot require follow-up imaging to detect occult germinoma.*

Hypothalamic Hamartoma

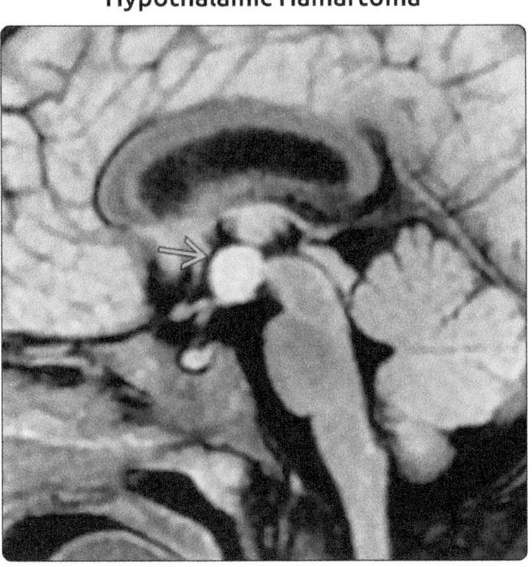

Hypothalamic Hamartoma

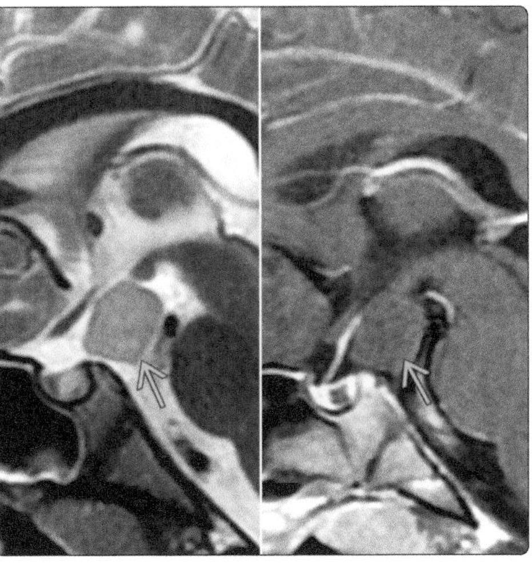

(Left) *Sagittal FLAIR MR in a 2-year-old with gelastic seizures shows a sessile well-defined mass ➔ arising from the hypothalamus, extending into the 3rd ventricle. Patients with sessile lesions are more likely to present with gelastic seizures.* **(Right)** *Midline sagittal T2 (L) and T1 C+ (R) MRs in a 5-year-old girl with precocious puberty show a pedunculated mass ➔ in the suprasellar cistern arising from the hypothalamus with signal intensity equal to gray matter and lack of enhancement, consistent with a hypothalamic hamartoma.*

Pituitary Anomalies

KEY FACTS

TERMINOLOGY

- Congenital anomalies of pituitary stalk → potential hypothalamic/pituitary axis malfunction

IMAGING

- Posterior pituitary ectopia (PPE): No (or tiny) pituitary stalk, ectopic posterior pituitary (EPP) on midline sagittal T1WI MR
  - Look for associated anomalies: Heterotopia, optic nerve hypoplasia, corpus callosum anomalies
- Duplicated pituitary gland/stalk (DP): 2 pituitary stalks on coronal view, thick tuber cinereum on midline sagittal view

TOP DIFFERENTIAL DIAGNOSES

- PPE
  - Surgical or traumatic stalk transection
  - Central diabetes insipidus
  - Hypothalamic lipoma (in tuber cinereum)
- DP
  - Dilated infundibular recess of 3rd ventricle (pseudoduplication)
  - Tuber cinereum hamartoma

PATHOLOGY

- PPE: Genetic mutation → defective neuronal migration during embryogenesis
- DP: Genetic mutation unknown; may constitute polytopic field defect due to splitting of notochord

CLINICAL ISSUES

- PPE: Short stature
- DP: Unsuspected finding on craniofacial imaging for other indications

DIAGNOSTIC CHECKLIST

- PPE: Assess optic and olfactory nerves, frontal cortex
- DP: Oral tumors compromise airway patency

(Left) *Sagittal graphic demonstrates ectopia of the posterior pituitary gland ➡ located at the distal end of a truncated pituitary stalk along the median eminence of the hypothalamus. The sella turcica and adenohypophysis ➡ are both small.* **(Right)** *Sagittal T1WI MR in an 11-year-old with pituitary dysfunction and ectopic posterior pituitary shows a globular focus of ↑ signal ➡ in the pituitary infundibulum. An ectopic neurohypophysis can occur anywhere from along the infundibulum to the base of the hypothalamus.*

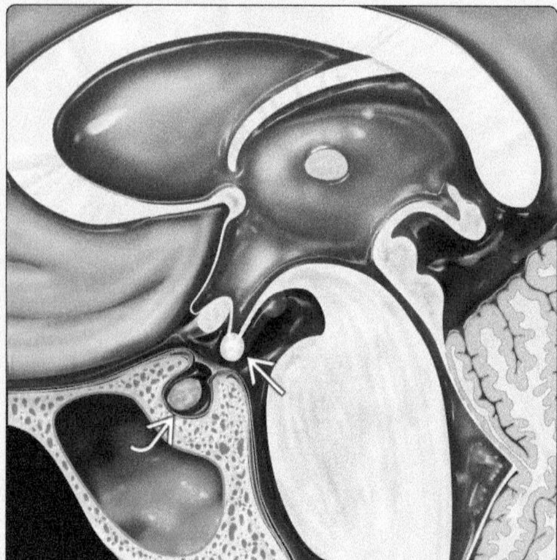

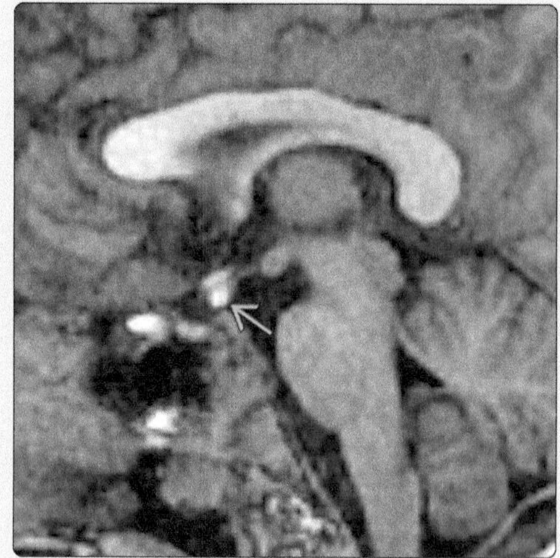

(Left) *Sagittal T1WI MR in a 15-year-old with septo-optic dysplasia (SOD) plus shows that the ectopic neurohypophysis ➡ is ectopically located at the hypothalamus, and the adenohypophysis ➡ is very small.* **(Right)** *Midline sagittal FIESTA MR in the same patient shows a hypoplastic optic chiasm ➡ and absence of the pituitary infundibulum in its expected location ➡. The spectrum of pituitary anomalies in SOD is broad. Correlation with pituitary function is critical in SOD, regardless of MR findings.*

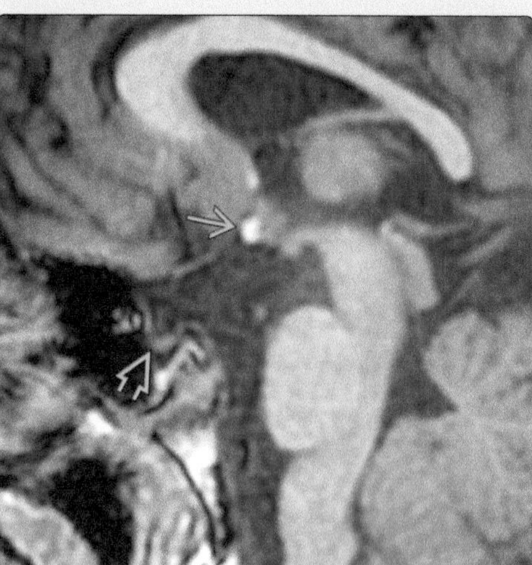

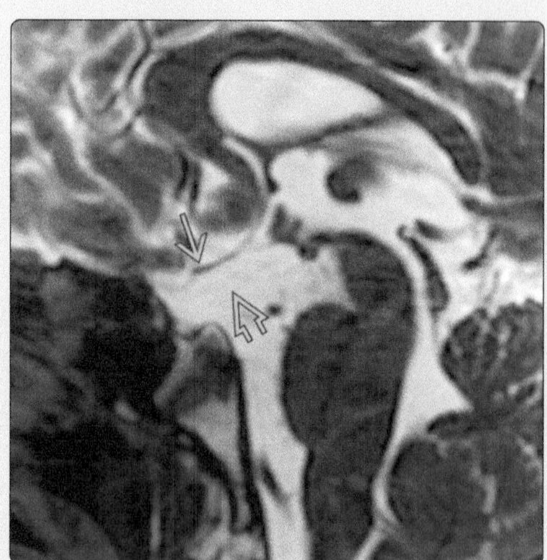

TERMINOLOGY

Definitions

- Congenital anomalies of pituitary stalk → potential hypothalamic/pituitary axis malfunction

IMAGING

General Features

- Best diagnostic clue
  - Posterior pituitary ectopia (PPE): No (or tiny) pituitary stalk, ectopic posterior pituitary (EPP) on midline sagittal T1WI MR
  - Duplicated pituitary gland/stalk (DP): 2 pituitary stalks on coronal view, thick tuber cinereum on midline sagittal view
    - Tuberomammillary fusion: Tuber cinereum/mammillary bodies fused into single mass
  - Pituitary hypoplasia: Small sella turcica and adenohypophysis
- Location
  - PPE: EPP located along median eminence of tuber cinereum or truncated pituitary stalk
  - DP: Paired lateral stalks, pituitary glands, bony fossae
- Size
  - PPE: Anterior pituitary (adenohypophysis) is small
  - DP: Each pituitary gland is normal in size
- Morphology
  - PPE: Small adenohypophysis and osseous sella
  - DP: Each pituitary gland and osseous sella is normal in morphology but laterally located

Radiographic Findings

- Radiography
  - PPE: Small sella turcica on lateral radiography
  - DP: Craniofacial/craniocervical anomalies common; may observe 2 fossae on AP view

CT Findings

- NECT
  - PPE: Narrow pituitary fossa and skull base structures and clivus ± persistent sphenopharyngeal foramen
  - DP: 2 widely separated pituitary fossae ± midline basisphenoid cleft or frontonasal dysplasia
- CTA
  - PPE: Medial deviation of juxtasellar/supraclinoid carotid arteries ("kissing" carotids)
  - DP: Duplicated basilar artery (BA) ± widely separated juxtasellar/supraclinoid carotid arteries

MR Findings

- T1WI
  - PPE: Absent, truncated, or thread-like pituitary stalk; small adenohypophysis
    - EPP located along truncated stalk or median eminence of tuber cinereum
      - Usually ↑ signal on T1WI (phospholipids/secretory granules)
      - Posterior pituitary may "dim" as patient outgrows available hormone levels
  - DP: Mass-like thickening of tuber cinereum on sagittal view portends duplicated pituitary axis
    - Mammillary bodies fused with tuber cinereum into thickened 3rd ventricle floor
    - 2 lateralized but otherwise normal pituitary glands/stalks
- T2WI
  - PPE: Variable signal of posterior pituitary
  - DP: Normal signal of glands, stalk, tuberomammillary fusion mass
- T1WI C+
  - PPE and DP: Stalks and remnants enhance (absent blood-brain barrier)
  - PPE: Hyperintensity absent if multiple endocrine anomalies/diabetes insipidus; contrast enhancement helps find neurohypophysis
- MRA
  - PPE: Supraclinoid carotid arteries medially deviated, "kiss" in midline; rare absent carotid artery/canal
  - DP: Fenestration (common) or total duplication (rare) of BA; widely separated juxtasellar carotid arteries

Imaging Recommendations

- Best imaging tool
  - Multiplanar MR
- Protocol advice
  - PPE and DP: Sagittal and coronal T1WI of hypothalamic/pituitary axis
  - PPE: Assess olfactory nerves, anterior frontal lobes with coronal T2WI FSE
    - 3D T1WI SPGR can identify small posterior pituitaries, occult on conventional 2D sagittal T1WI
    - bSSFP (FIESTA/CISS/TrueFISP) to evaluate pituitary stalk
    - Recent studies suggest gadolinium contrast is not necessary
  - DP: 3D CT of skull base and face in selected patients
    - Gadolinium contrast and bSSFP helpful to identify 2 pituitary stalks

DIFFERENTIAL DIAGNOSIS

Posterior Pituitary Ectopia

- Central diabetes insipidus
  - Hyperintensity of posterior pituitary lobe is absent but normal location of stalk and gland
- Surgical or traumatic stalk transection
  - Permits build-up of neurosecretory granules along stump
- Hypothalamic lipoma (located at tuber cinereum)
  - Posterior pituitary is not suppressed by fat saturation; lipoma is suppressed

Duplicated Pituitary Gland/Stalk

- Dilated infundibular recess of 3rd ventricle (pseudoduplication)
  - Simulates duplicated stalk but only 1 gland and 1 pituitary fossa
- Tuber cinereum hamartoma
  - Round mass of 3rd ventricle floor but 1 midline pituitary stalk/gland

PATHOLOGY

General Features

- Etiology
  - PPE: Genetic mutation → defective neuronal migration during embryogenesis
    - Adenohypophysis (anterior pituitary) grows up from stomodeal ectoderm (Rathke pouch)
      - Hypothalamic releasing hormones reach adenohypophysis via infundibular portal system
      - Anterior pituitary dysfunction thought to be related to absent infundibulum
    - Neurohypophysis (posterior pituitary) grows down from diencephalon, remains attached by stalk
      - ADH and oxytocin transported to neurohypophysis via neurosecretory cells along infundibulum
  - DP: Congenital anomaly, presumed genetic duplication of stomodeal origin structures 2° to aberrant ventral induction
    - Theory: Duplication prechordal plate and tip of rostral notochord leads to duplicated pituitary primordium
- Genetics
  - PPE: Mutations in genes encoding developmental transcription factors allow maldevelopment
    - *HESX1* (homeobox gene), *PIT1*, *PITX2*, *LHX3*, *LHX4*, *PROP1*, *SF1*, and *TBX19* (TPIT)
  - DP: Gene mutation unknown; may constitute polytopic field defect due to splitting of notochord
- Associated abnormalities
  - DP
    - Midline tumors in oral, nasopharyngeal, palate
      - Epignathus, teratomas, hypothalamic hamartoma, dermoids, lipomas
    - Spinal anomalies include segmentation/fusion anomalies, schisms, hydromyelia, enteric cysts
  - PPE and DP: Common midline CNS anomalies
    - Posterior pituitary ectopia
      - ± anomalies of structures formed at same time (anterior pituitary, forebrain, eyes, olfactory bulbs)
      - ± septo-optic dysplasia (most common)
      - ± lobar holoprosencephaly, Joubert syndrome (less common)
    - DP
      - Callosal dysgenesis, Dandy-Walker spectrum, frontonasal dysplasia
      - Craniofacial clefting and duplication anomalies: Frontonasal dysplasia; clefts/duplication of skull base, face, mandible, nose, palate

Gross Pathologic & Surgical Features

- PPE: Hypoplastic anterior lobe, stalk truncation or aplasia
  - Sella may be covered over with dura
- DP: Tuberomammillary fusion, 2 normal glands/stalks

CLINICAL ISSUES

Presentation

- Most common signs/symptoms
  - PPE: Short stature
  - DP: Unsuspected finding on craniofacial imaging for other indications
- Other signs/symptoms
  - PPE: Multiple pituitary hormone deficiencies common
  - DP: Rarely symptomatic from pituitary causes
- Clinical profile
  - PPE: Short stature (growth hormone deficiency) ± multiple endocrine deficiencies
    - Peak growth hormone levels < 3 g/L more likely to have abnormal MR
    - ± anosmia, poor vision, seizures (cortical malformations)
    - Neonatal hypoglycemia or jaundice, micropenis, single central incisor
  - DP: ± facial midline anomalies, oral or nasal mass (hamartoma or teratoma)
    - Face: ± hypertelorism or frontonasal dysplasia
    - Craniocervical segmentation and fusion anomalies
    - Airway or oral obstruction from pharyngeal tumor

Demographics

- Age
  - PPE: Early growth failure apparent in childhood
  - DP: Usually discovered in early infancy during imaging for complicated facial anomalies
- Sex
  - PPE: M > F
  - DP: M < F
- Epidemiology
  - PPE: Prevalence of 1:4,000 to 1:20,000 births
  - DP: Extremely rare (20+ reported cases)

Natural History & Prognosis

- PPE: Stable if no pituitary/hypothalamic crises; growth may be normal for a while
  - Severity and number of hormone deficiencies predicted by degree of stalk and gland hypoplasia
- DP: Usually significant intracranial, upper airway, or craniocervical malformations (some lethal)
  - Clinical outcome unrelated to pituitary function

Treatment

- Assess/treat endocrine malfunction

DIAGNOSTIC CHECKLIST

Consider

- PPE: Assess optic and olfactory nerves, frontal cortex
- DP: Oral tumors compromise airway patency

Image Interpretation Pearls

- PPE and DP: Can miss findings/diagnosis if thick sections (MR) are used or osseous structures (bone CT) not evaluated

SELECTED REFERENCES

1. Jakobsen LK et al: Diagnosis and incidence of congenital combined pituitary hormone deficiency in Denmark-a national observational study. J Clin Endocrinol Metab. 108(10):2475-85, 2023
2. Serrallach BL et al: Duplication of the pituitary gland: CT, MRI and DTI findings and updated review of the literature. Brain Sci. 12(5):574, 2022
3. Almaghraby A et al: Is gadolinium contrast necessary for pituitary MRI in the evaluation of pediatric short stature and growth hormone deficiency? Horm Res Paediatr. 94(5-6):201-10, 2021

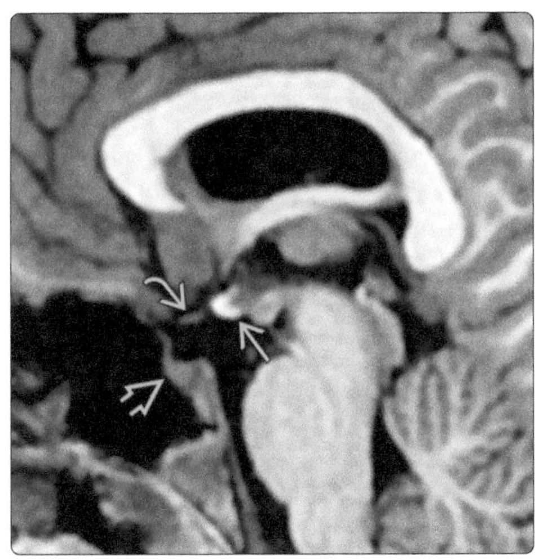

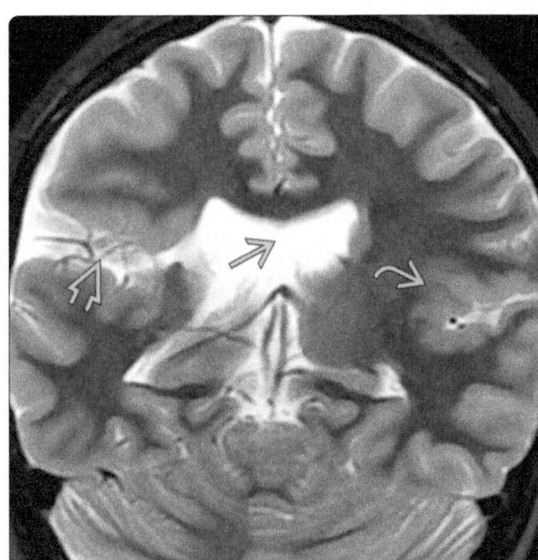

(Left) *Sagittal T1WI MR in a 12-year-old with SOD plus shows an ectopic neurohypophysis located at the base of the hypothalamus and small anterior pituitary. Ectopic neurohypophysis should prompt a search for findings of SOD, such as optic nerve/chiasm hypoplasia.* **(Right)** *Coronal T2WI MR in the same patient shows absent septum pellucidum (SP), dysplastic gray matter cleft in the right insula (closed-lip schizencephaly), and left perisylvian polymicrogyria (PMG), consistent with SOD plus.*

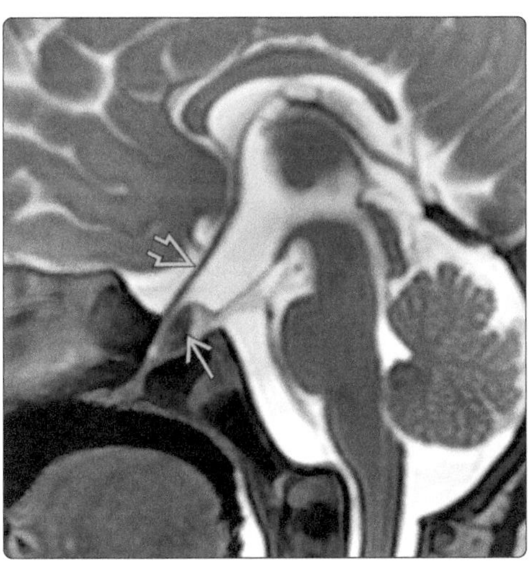

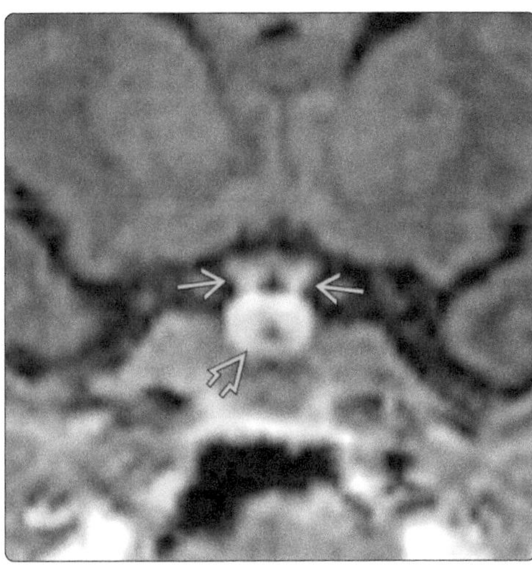

(Left) *Sagittal FIESTA MR shows a neonate with persistent craniopharyngeal canal containing the pituitary with inferior tethering of the optic chiasm. Not evident on sagittal imaging is the associated pituitary duplication.* **(Right)** *Coronal T1WI MR in the same patient shows duplicated pituitary infundibulae and incompletely duplicated pituitary gland. Note that the adenohypophysis is T1 hyperintense in neonates, making the entire pituitary very conspicuous.*

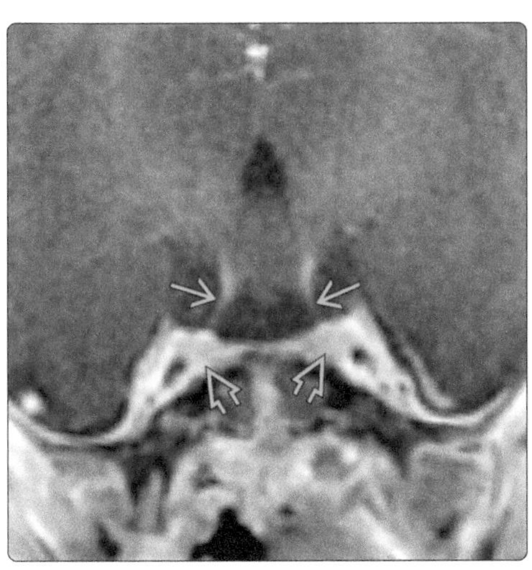

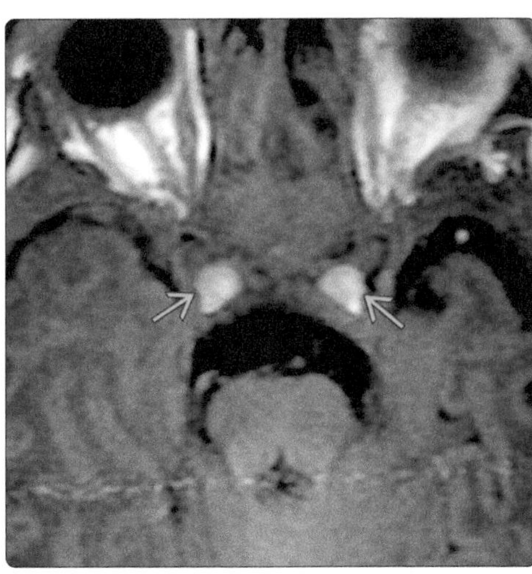

(Left) *Coronal T1WI C+ MR in a 2-year-old with duplicated pituitary shows 2 separate pituitary infundibulae and pituitary glands. High-resolution coronal imaging is very helpful in identifying duplicated pituitary infundibulae.* **(Right)** *Axial T1WI MR in the same patient shows 2 separate pituitary glands in 2 separate sellae turcica. Because the neonatal pituitary is intrinsically bright on T1WI, this finding is typically most conspicuous on precontrast images.*

Craniopharyngioma

KEY FACTS

IMAGING

- Best clue: Complex suprasellar cystic mass with Ca^{++} & wall enhancement
- Location: Sellar + suprasellar ~ 2/3; suprasellar ~ 1/3
  - Larger tumors can extend into multiple cranial fossae
- "90% rule"
  - 90% cystic: MR signal intensity highly variable
    - Cystic components frequently T1 hyperintense
  - 90% calcified: SWI/T2* GRE MR helpful to identify Ca^{++}
  - 90% enhance (wall & solid portions)
- Often develop obstructive hydrocephalus
- Optic chiasm, hypothalamus, & vessels often involved
  - Thin sagittal T2 or SSFP MR sequences help assess

TOP DIFFERENTIAL DIAGNOSES

- Rathke cleft cyst
- Pituitary adenoma
- Germinoma
- Hypothalamic-chiasmatic glioma

PATHOLOGY

- 2 clinically & pathologically distinct subtypes
  - Adamantinomatous: Cystic & solid, mostly in children
  - Squamous-papillary: Mostly solid tumor found in adults

CLINICAL ISSUES

- Most common nonglial pediatric intracranial tumor
- Symptoms: Visual changes, endocrine symptoms, academic decline, headache/vomiting (obstructive hydrocephalus)
  - ~ 1/3 of patients with endocrine symptoms (↓ growth hormone, ↓ thyroid function, diabetes insipidus)
- Benign tumor with high rate of recurrence
  - 88% overall 20-year survival
- Poor prognostic factors: Hypothalamic involvement, ↑ tumor size

DIAGNOSTIC CHECKLIST

- Must identify relationship of tumor to optic chiasm, hypothalamus, & vessels

(Left) *Sagittal graphic shows typical features of a mixed intra- & suprasellar craniopharyngioma with a nodule of solid tissue ➔ in the wall of a complex cyst that projects into the sella. Note the fluid level ⇨ within the cystic component.* **(Right)** *Sagittal T1WI MR in a teen with craniopharyngioma shows a very heterogeneous suprasellar mass ⇨ with multiple cystic spaces containing T1-hyperintense material ⇨. T1-hyperintense cysts not corresponding to fat are essentially pathognomonic for craniopharyngioma.*

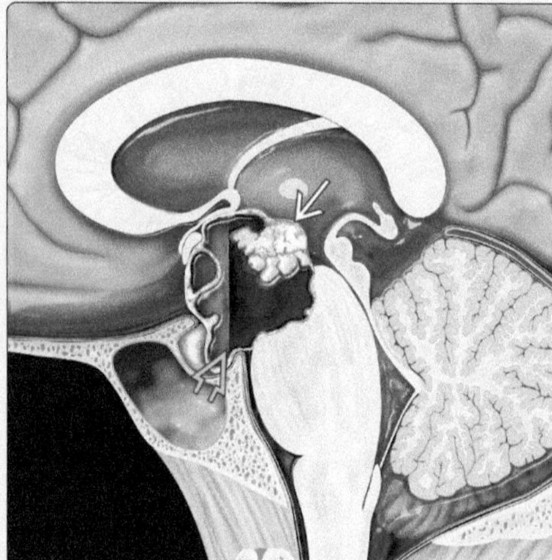

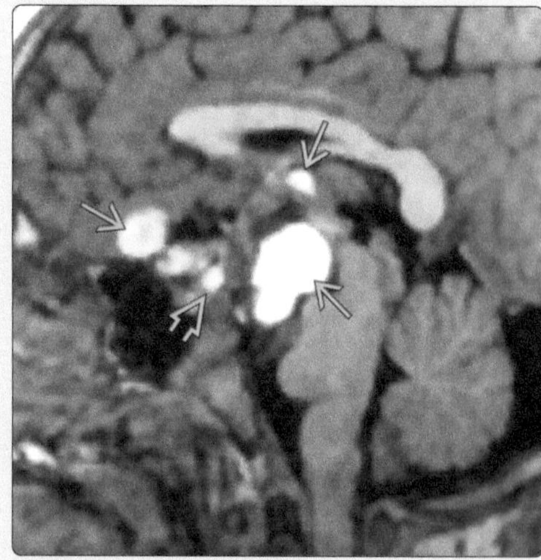

(Left) *CT scout view in a 10-year-old boy with increasing headaches shows enlargement of the bony sella ⇨, suggesting a sellar mass. Craniopharyngioma frequently remodels the sella turcica.* **(Right)** *Sagittal T1WI C+ MR in the same patient confirms a predominantly cystic mass with a very thin rim of enhancement ➔. The majority of craniopharyngiomas have some solid component, but not all. Cystic contents often show intrinsic T1 shortening ⇨ before contrast, as in this case.*

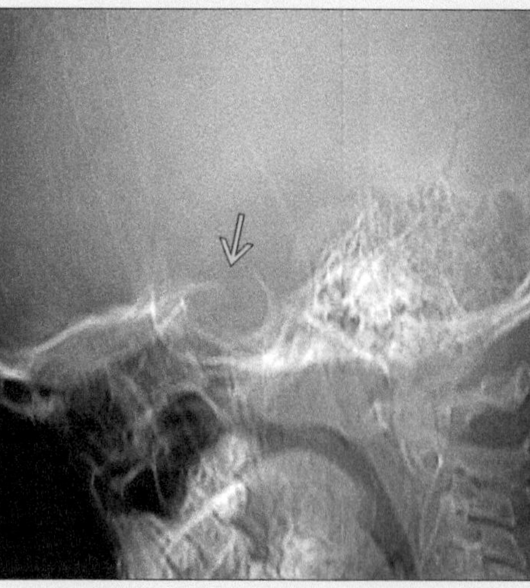

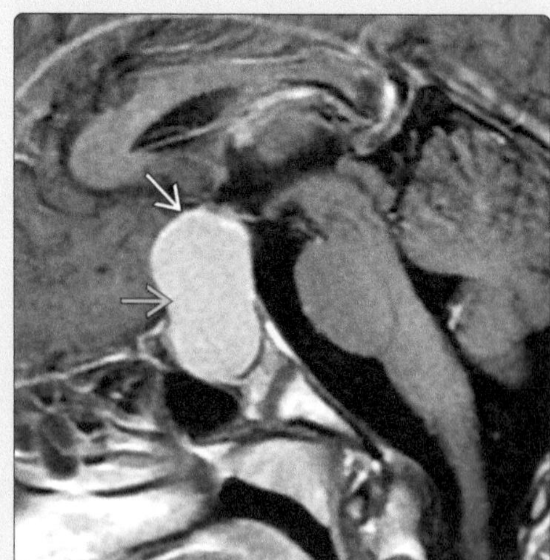

TERMINOLOGY

Abbreviations

- Craniopharyngioma (CP)

Synonyms

- Craniopharyngeal duct tumor, Rathke pouch tumor, adamantinoma

Definitions

- Histologically benign epithelial tumor arising from squamous rests along involuted hypophyseal-Rathke duct

IMAGING

General Features

- Best diagnostic clue
  - Cystic suprasellar mass with Ca^{++} & enhancing wall or mural nodule
- Location
  - Sellar + suprasellar: ~ 2/3; suprasellar: ~ 1/3; isolated sellar: Uncommon
    - Rare ectopic locations: 3rd ventricle, nasopharynx, sphenoid sinus
  - Retrochiasmatic vs. prechiasmatic configuration key determinant for surgical approach
    - Prechiasmatic often grow into anterior cranial fossa
    - Retrochiasmatic often grow into retroclival space & cerebellopontine angle cisterns
  - Larger tumors can extend into multiple cranial fossae
- Often large at presentation (> 5 cm)
  - Cyst typically largest component

Radiographic Findings

- Skull radiographs
  - Sellar enlargement, erosion of clinoids
  - Suprasellar Ca^{++}

CT Findings

- "90% rule": 90% cystic, 90% calcified, 90% enhance (wall & solid portions)
- May present with obstructive hydrocephalus from compression on 3rd ventricle & foramen of Monro

MR Findings

- T1WI
  - T1 signal within cysts is highly variable from near CSF to very hyperintense
  - ↑ T1 signal is one of most characteristic MR findings
    - ↑ T1 signal reflects protein, cholesterol, &/or blood products in fluid
    - Most characteristic of adamantinomatous subtype
- T2WI
  - Hypointense foci of Ca^{++}
  - Variable signal intensity of cysts
- FLAIR
  - Cysts typically do not suppress like CSF
    - ± hyperintense signal in adjacent brain
- T2* GRE
  - Areas of signal loss correspond to Ca^{++}
- DWI
  - Variable cystic signal, typically closer to CSF than brain
- MRA
  - Vessels often displaced, but large lesions may encase vessels; important for preoperative planning
    - Look for moyamoya arteriopathy following XRT
- MRS
  - Cyst contents show broad lipid spectrum at 0.9-1.5 ppm

Imaging Recommendations

- Best imaging tool
  - Contrast-enhanced MR with thin-section, postcontrast sagittal & coronal imaging
- Protocol advice
  - Volumetric T1 ± contrast; SWI/GRE for Ca^{++}
  - Thin-section sagittal T2 or SSFP sequences help define relationship of tumor to adjacent structures
  - MRA helpful in preoperative identification of arterial involvement
  - Consider including CT in long-term postoperative follow-up
    - May detect small calcified recurrences before detectable on MR

DIFFERENTIAL DIAGNOSIS

Rathke Cleft Cyst

- Ca^{++} uncommon; no nodular/solid component
- Cyst more homogeneous, although small T2-hypointense intracystic nodules may be present
- No/minimal enhancement of cyst wall on T2 FLAIR C+

Germinoma

- Predominantly solid & lobular
- Ca^{++} very rare in suprasellar germinoma
- Strong association with diabetes insipidus

Pituitary Adenoma

- Solid tumor arising from adenohypophysis
- Diffuse & homogeneous enhancement
- Rare in young children

Hypothalamic-Chiasmatic Glioma

- More solid & homogeneous
- Extension into prechiasmatic optic nerves/tracts
- Infiltrate/enlarge chiasm instead of displacing it

Arachnoid Cyst

- Thin/imperceptible, nonenhancing wall
- Cyst contents follow CSF

Dermoid & Epidermoid Cysts

- Epidermoids solid but mimic cysts
- Suprasellar locations uncommon in children
- Minimal enhancement; marked diffusion restriction

Aneurysm

- "Onion-skin" layers of aging blood products
- Bright enhancement of residual lumen

Meningioma

- Planum sphenoidale & dorsal clival meningiomas may mimic CP
- Cystic component unusual
- Uncommon in children

PATHOLOGY

General Features

- Arise from rests of epithelial cells
- 2 proposed sites of origin
  - In pars tuberalis at distal aspect of infundibulum
  - Along tract of involuted craniopharyngeal duct
- Overactivation of WNT/β-catenin signaling pathway
- 2 clinically & pathologically distinct subtypes
  - Adamantinomatous (~ 90%): Classic calcified cyst with mural nodule seen in children
    - Cyst walls of simple stratified squamous epithelium with collagenous basement membrane
    - Peripheral cellular palisading & stellate reticulum with dystrophic Ca^{++}
  - Papillary (~ 10%): Mostly solid tumor almost exclusively found in adults
    - Formation of papillae with rare Ca^{++} or necrosis
  - 15% of tumors have mixed histology but behave like adamantinomatous form
  - Adamantinomatous & papillary: WHO grade 1
- Genetics
  - Targetable mutations are present in subset of tumors
    - *BRAF* V600 & *CTNNB1* mutations present in many CPs
      - V600 mutations in most papillary CPs (rare in children)
      - *CTNNB1* mutations very common in adamantinomatous CPs

Gross Pathologic & Surgical Features

- Cyst fluid usually straw colored & thick ("crankcase oil")
- Adamantinomatous
  - Mixed cystic & solid tumor
  - Cysts > > solid components
- Papillary
  - Solid > > cysts

CLINICAL ISSUES

Presentation

- Headache, vomiting, hydrocephalus, papilledema
- Visual disturbance, decline in school performance
- Endocrine symptoms in at least 1/3 of cases
  - Growth hormone deficiency, hypothyroidism, diabetes insipidus
  - Due to mass effect on pituitary/hypothalamus

Demographics

- Age
  - Peak at 8-12 years
    - Peak for papillary type at 40-60 years
- Sex
  - M = F
- Epidemiology
  - Most common nonglial pediatric intracranial tumor
    - > 50% of all pediatric suprasellar region tumors
    - 6-9% of all pediatric intracranial tumors
  - 0.5-2.5 new cases per 1,000,000 per year

Natural History & Prognosis

- Slow-growing benign tumor
- 88% overall survival at 20 years
- Hypothalamic involvement: ↓ overall survival, quality of life
  - Obesity, physical fatigue, reduced motivation, dyspnea, diarrhea, & poor psychosocial development
- Factors affecting recurrence
  - Gross total vs. partial resection
    - Gross total resection: 23% recurrence
    - Subtotal resection: 63% recurrence
  - Radiation therapy (for residual tumor) ↓ recurrence
    - XRT reduces recurrence risk from 63% to 20%
  - Tumor size (↑ recurrence in larger tumors)
    - 30% short-term (18 months) recurrence if > 4 cm
    - 7% short-term (18 months) recurrence if < 4 cm
    - Larger tumors more likely to have hypothalamic involvement & less likely to have complete resection
  - Late recurrences (decades later) reported
  - Occasional ectopic sites of recurrence, often along surgical tract

Treatment

- Surgical: Complete resection ideal but must be weighed against high morbidity associated with extensive resection
  - Gross total resection
    - Limited by tumor size, adherence to vessels & hypothalamus
- Radiation therapy for incomplete resection
  - Patients at ↑ risk for moyamoya arteriopathy & stroke after XRT
- Treatment associated with high rate of morbidity
  - Perioperative hyperthermia
  - Vascular injury & pseudoaneurysm
  - Hypopituitarism
  - Long-term hypothalamic syndrome
    - Morbid obesity from compulsive eating
- Targeted biologic therapies
  - Targeted therapies may become important pre- & postsurgical adjuvant
    - Case reports of BRAF inhibitors used in V600 mutants is promising
    - Control with targeted therapies may support less aggressive surgical resection

DIAGNOSTIC CHECKLIST

Consider

- Rathke cleft cyst can be identical to small CP
  - Rathke cleft cyst unlikely to have Ca^{++}, more homogeneous
  - Use NECT & SWI/GRE to identify Ca^{++} in CP
- Relationship of tumor to optic chiasm & other adjacent structures important for surgical planning

SELECTED REFERENCES

1. Huang ZS et al: Machine learning-based multiparametric magnetic resonance imaging radiomic model for discrimination of pathological subtypes of craniopharyngioma. J Magn Reson Imaging. 54(5):1541-50, 2021
2. Azuma M et al: Usefulness of contrast-enhanced 3D-FLAIR MR imaging for differentiating rathke cleft cyst from cystic craniopharyngioma. AJNR Am J Neuroradiol. 41(1):106-10, 2020

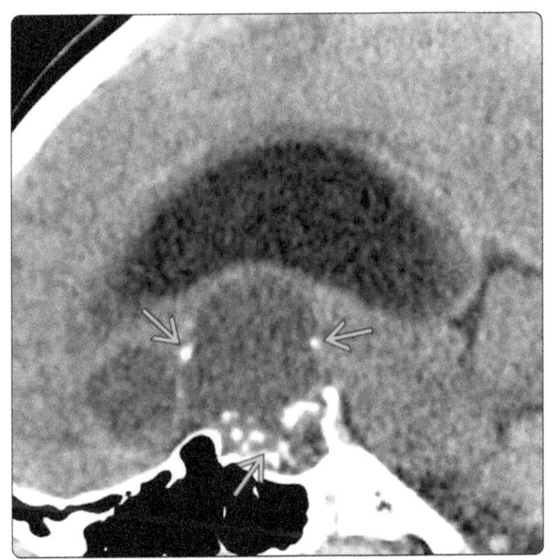

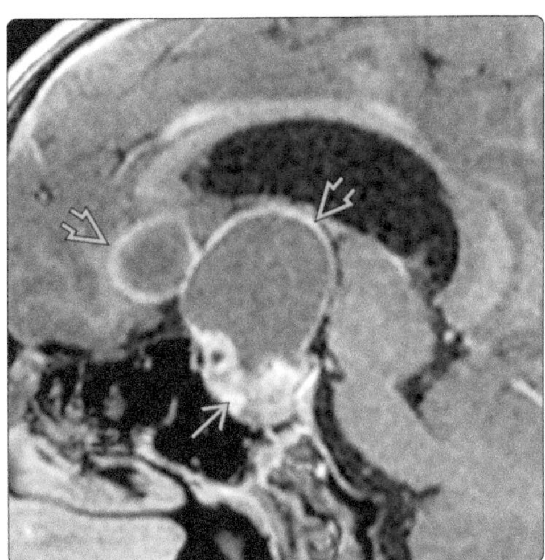

(Left) *Sagittal NECT in a 9-year-old boy shows a mixed solid & cystic sellar/suprasellar mass with Ca^{++} within the solid component as well as along the margins of the cystic component. Ca^{++} are seen in ~ 90% of craniopharyngiomas & are the most important CT finding to discriminate from other DDxs.* **(Right)** *Sagittal T1WI C+ MR in the same patient shows avid enhancement within the inferior solid components as well as linear enhancement along the margins of the cystic components.*

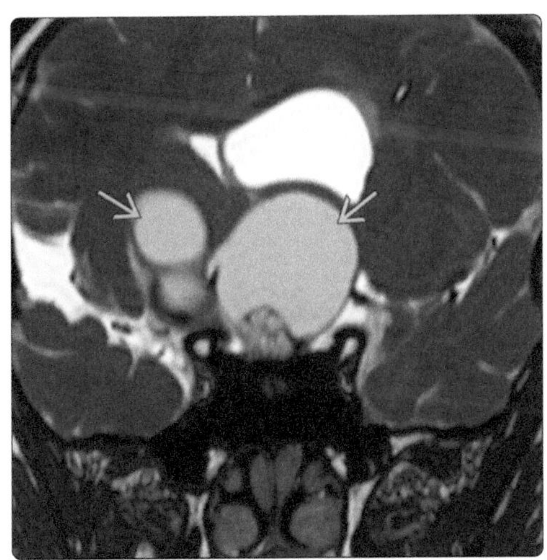

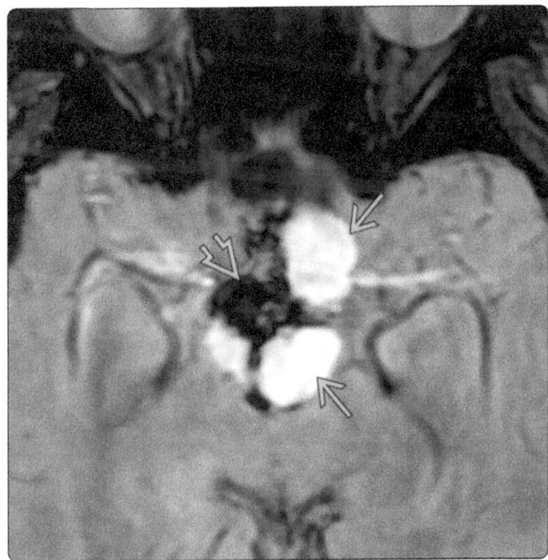

(Left) *Coronal FIESTA in the same patient shows the often multicystic nature of craniopharyngioma with cystic components extending into spaces adjacent to the suprasellar cistern.* **(Right)** *Axial SWI MR in a 13-year-old boy with craniopharyngioma shows areas of signal loss corresponding to Ca^{++} amongst the cystic spaces. Without a comparison CT, SWI is an extremely helpful sequence to identify Ca^{++} in the setting of a suprasellar mass to aid the radiologist in narrowing the DDx.*

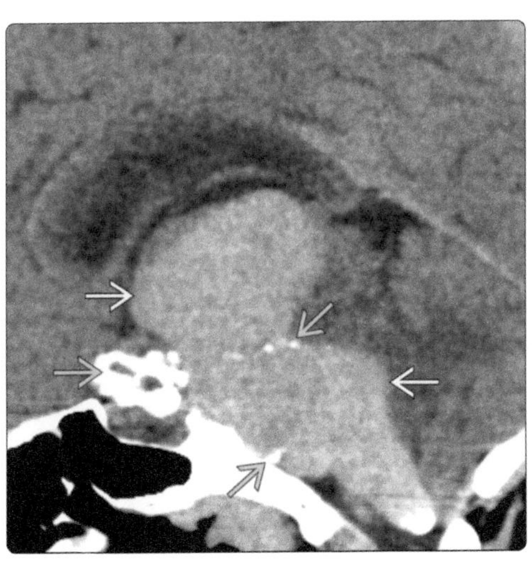

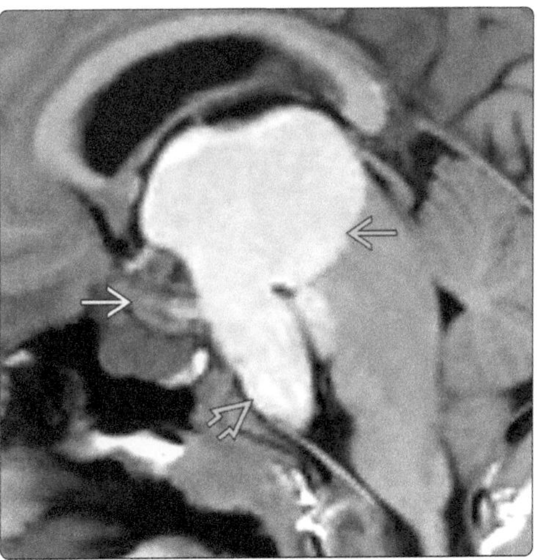

(Left) *Sagittal NECT in a 10-year-old boy with left vision loss shows a mixed solid & cystic mass in the suprasellar & retroclival regions with multiple foci of Ca^{++} as well as high-density cystic contents.* **(Right)** *Sagittal T1WI MR in the same patient shows predominantly low signal in the solid component with high signal in the dorsal cystic component. High T1 signal often (but not always) corresponds to high CT density. Retroclival extension is common in retrochiasmatic masses when they become large.*

Hypothalamic Hamartoma

KEY FACTS

TERMINOLOGY

- Hypothalamic hamartoma (HH)
- Nonneoplastic; congenital gray matter heterotopia

IMAGING

- Hypothalamic mass contiguous with tuber cinereum
  - Located between mammillary bodies and infundibulum
  - Can be sessile or pedunculated ("collar button")
  - Size ranges from few mm to several cm
- Isointense with gray matter on T1WI MR
  - Can be slightly hyperintense on T2/FLAIR MR
  - Large lesions can be heterogeneous, contain cysts
  - No enhancement on T1WI C+ MR

TOP DIFFERENTIAL DIAGNOSES

- Craniopharyngioma
- Chiasmatic/hypothalamic astrocytoma
- Ectopic posterior pituitary
- Germinoma
- Langerhans cell histiocytosis
- Lipoma

PATHOLOGY

- Mature but dysplastic neuronal ganglionic tissue

CLINICAL ISSUES

- Infant with epilepsy or precocious puberty
  - Cognitive, neuropsychiatric comorbidities common
- Older children with precocious puberty
  - Often tall and overweight with advanced bone age
- Shape, size of hamartoma often predicts symptoms, presentation
  - Large, sessile lesions → seizures
  - Small, pedunculated lesions → central precocious puberty

DIAGNOSTIC CHECKLIST

- If hypothalamic mass in imaging for seizure or precocious puberty → HH

(Left) *Sagittal graphic shows a classic pedunculated tuber cinereum hamartoma ➔ interposed between the infundibulum anteriorly & mammillary bodies posteriorly. The mass resembles gray matter (GM).* **(Right)** *Sagittal T1WI MR in an 8-year-old girl with precocious puberty shows a classic pedunculated "collar button" hypothalamic hamartoma (HH) ➔. The lesion is interposed between the infundibular stalk ➔ anteriorly & mammillary bodies ➔ posteriorly. HHs are classically isointense with GM.*

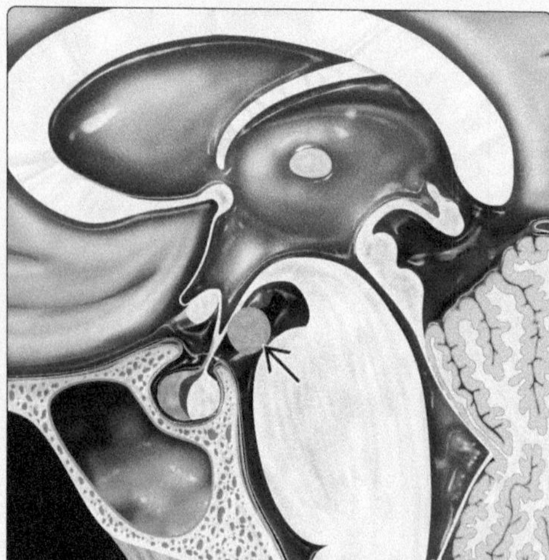

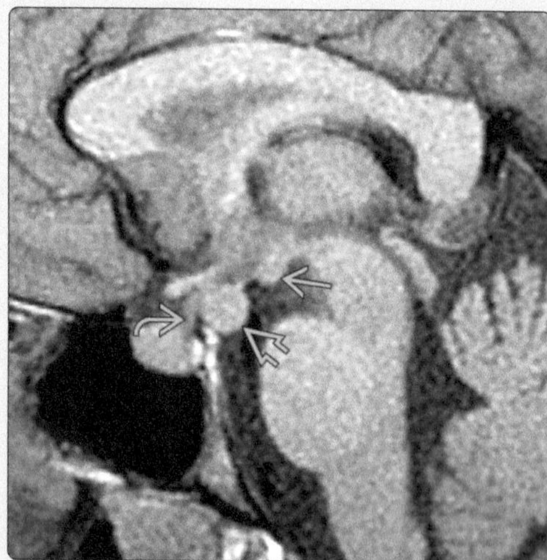

(Left) *Midline sagittal T2WI (left) & T1WI C+ (right) MR in a 5-year-old girl with precocious puberty shows a pedunculated mass ➔ in the suprasellar cistern arising from the hypothalamus with signal intensity equal to GM & lack of enhancement, consistent with an HH.* **(Right)** *Sagittal T2WI MR in the same patient 5 years later following laser ablation therapy for intractable seizures shows a cystic defect ➔ at the site of laser ablation. Laser ablation therapy has been found to be effective with relatively few complications.*

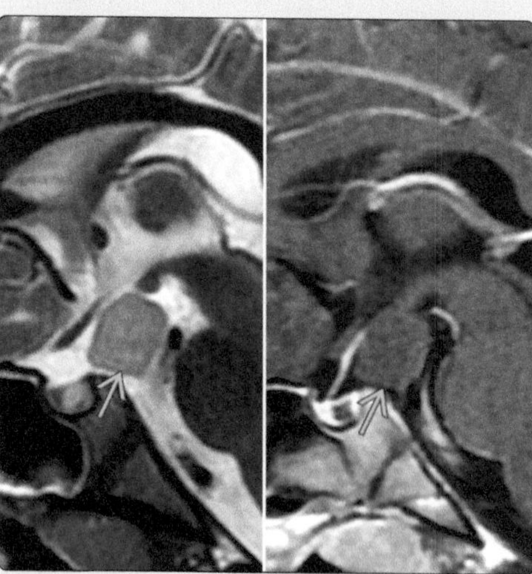

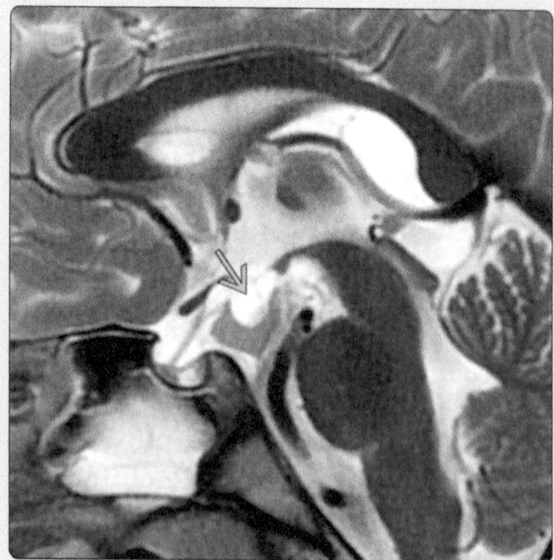

TERMINOLOGY

Abbreviations

- Hypothalamic hamartoma (HH)

Synonyms

- Tuber cinereum hamartoma, diencephalic hamartoma

Definitions

- Nonneoplastic congenital gray matter heterotopia in region of tuber cinereum

IMAGING

General Features

- Best diagnostic clue
  - Nonenhancing hypothalamic mass contiguous with tuber cinereum
- Location
  - Tuber cinereum of hypothalamus
  - Located between pons/mammillary bodies and hypothalamic infundibulum
- Size
  - Variable, few mm to giant (3-5 cm)
- Morphology
  - Sessile or pedunculated mass
  - Similar in density/intensity to gray matter

Radiographic Findings

- Radiography
  - ± suprasellar calcifications, eroded dorsum, enlarged sella (rare)

CT Findings

- NECT
  - Homogeneous suprasellar mass
    - Isodense → slightly hypodense
    - Cysts and calcification are uncommon
    - ± patent craniopharyngeal canal (very rare)
- CECT
  - No pathologic enhancement

MR Findings

- T1WI
  - Mass located between mammillary bodies and infundibulum
  - Isointense → slightly hypointense to gray matter
- T2WI
  - Isointense → slightly hyperintense (secondary to fibrillary gliosis)
- PD/intermediate
  - Hyperintense to CSF, slightly hyperintense to gray matter
- FLAIR
  - Isointense → slightly hyperintense to gray matter
- T1WI C+
  - Nonenhancing; if enhances, consider other diagnosis
- MRS
  - ↓ NAA and NAA:Cr, mild ↑ Cho and Cho:Cr, ↑ myoinositol (mI) and mI:Cr
    - ↓ NAA and ↑ Cho indicate reduced neuronal density and relative gliosis, respectively, compared to normal gray matter
    - ↑ mI:Cr correlates with ↑ glial component and lesion T2 hyperintensity

Imaging Recommendations

- Best imaging tool
  - Multiplanar MR with contrast
- Protocol advice
  - Thin-section sagittal and coronal T2, T1WI C+ MR

DIFFERENTIAL DIAGNOSIS

Craniopharyngioma

- Most common suprasellar mass in children
- Variable signal intensity cysts (90%), calcifications (90%), and enhancement (90%)
- Longstanding lesion, frequently with short stature and pituitary abnormalities

Chiasmatic/Hypothalamic Astrocytoma

- 2nd most common pediatric suprasellar mass (± neurofibromatosis type 1)
- Hyperintense on T2WI MR ± contrast enhancement (heterogeneous, often vigorous)
- Optic pathway or hypothalamus ± optic tract extension

Ectopic Posterior Pituitary

- Ectopic hyperintense focus on T1WI MR
- No normal orthotopic posterior pituitary hyperintensity

Germinoma

- Thickening, abnormal enhancement of pituitary stalk rather than tuber cinereum
- Diabetes insipidus common
- ± multicentric: Suprasellar, pineal, thalamus, basal ganglia
- Early leptomeningeal metastatic dissemination

Langerhans Cell Histiocytosis

- Thickening, abnormal enhancement of pituitary stalk rather than tuber cinereum
- Diabetes insipidus common
- Look for lytic bone lesions in typical locations

Lipoma

- Hyperintense fat signal on T1WI MR
- Hypointense on STIR or fat-saturated sequences

PATHOLOGY

General Features

- Etiology
  - Neuronal migration anomaly (occurs between gestational days 33-41)
  - Affects normal hypothalamic regulation of autonomic, endocrine, neurologic, behavioral functions
  - Pathogenesis of precocious puberty-induced sexual precocity
    - ± luteinizing hormone-releasing hormone (LHRH) granules in hamartoma/connecting axons in some
    - Activating astroglial-derived factors in tumors may stimulate endogenous LHRH secretion if no intratumoral LHRH granules

- Shape and size of hamartoma postulated to predict symptoms
  - Large, sessile lesions → seizures
  - Small, pedunculated lesions → central precocious puberty (CPP)
  - Presentation with both seizures and CPP common
- Genetics
  - *GLI3* mutation
    - Pallister-Hall syndrome (PHS)
      - Hamartoma or hamartoblastoma of tuber cinereum; often large mass
      - Digital malformations (short metacarpals, syndactyly, polydactyly)
      - Other midline (epiglottis/larynx) and cardiac/renal/anal anomalies
    - Greig cephalopolysyndactyly syndrome (GCPS)

Staging, Grading, & Classification

- Valdueza classification
  - Pedunculated, CPP, or asymptomatic
    - Originates in tuber cinereum
    - Originates in mammillary bodies
  - Sessile, hypothalamus displaced, seizures
    - More hypothalamic dysfunction and abnormal behavior

Gross Pathologic & Surgical Features

- Mature neuronal ganglionic tissue projecting from hypothalamus, tuber cinereum, or mammillary bodies
- Pedunculated or sessile, rounded or nodular

Microscopic Features

- Well-differentiated neurons interspersed with glial cells, myelinated/unmyelinated axons, variable amounts of fibrillary gliosis
  - Hamartoblastomas include primitive undifferentiated cells

CLINICAL ISSUES

Presentation

- Most common signs/symptoms
  - LHRH-dependent CPP presenting at very young age
  - Refractory symptomatic mixed seizure types, including gelastic seizures
    - Gelastic seizures are recurrent automatic bursts of laughter without mirth
    - Presentation usually encompasses both epileptic seizures and encephalopathy with behavioral cognitive impairment
    - May progress to partial epilepsy, partial complex seizures, generalized tonic clonic seizures
    - Rarely occur in conjunction with focal cortical dysplasia or hypothalamic astrocytoma
  - Other seizure types frequent with HH; always look for HH in child with epilepsy
- Other signs/symptoms
  - Depression, anxiety common in adult HH patients
- Clinical profile
  - Infant with gelastic seizures or precocious puberty
  - Older children with precocious puberty; tall, overweight, and advanced bone age

Demographics

- Age
  - Usually present between 1-3 years of age
- Sex
  - No predilection; some reports M > F
- Ethnicity
  - No predilection
- Epidemiology
  - Of histologically verified lesions, 3/4 have precocious puberty and 1/2 have seizures
  - Up to 33% of patients with CPP have HH

Natural History & Prognosis

- Size should remain stable; if growth is detected, surgery/biopsy is indicated
  - Postsurgical hypothalamic complications include headache, mental slowing, and weight gain
- Symptomatic lesions: Sessile > > pedunculated
  - Sessile lesions nearly always symptomatic
- Syndromic patients generally do poorly

Treatment

- Medical: Hormone-suppressive therapy, treat seizures
- Surgical: If medical therapy failure or rapid lesion growth
  - Endoscopic or transcallosal surgical resection
  - Many studies have shown stereotactic laser ablation to have equivalent efficacy to open surgery with fewer complications
  - Laser ablation therapy results in > 90% freedom from gelastic seizures at 1 year

DIAGNOSTIC CHECKLIST

Consider

- If hypothalamic mass identified in seizure imaging, think HH

Image Interpretation Pearls

- Classic = nonenhancing hypothalamic mass
  - Isointense to gray matter on T1WI, slightly ↑ signal on T2WI/FLAIR
  - Hypothalamic astrocytoma, Langerhans cell histiocytosis (LCH), and germ cell tumor all show some contrast enhancement

SELECTED REFERENCES

1. Lombardi S et al: Intraoperative MRI assessment of the tissue damage during laser ablation of hypothalamic hamartoma. Diagnostics (Basel). 13(14):2331, 2023
2. Lu D et al: Advances in hypothalamic hamartoma research over the past 30 years (1992-2021): a bibliometric analysis. Front Neurol. 14:1176459, 2023
3. Candela-Cantó S et al: Robot-assisted, real-time, MRI-guided laser interstitial thermal therapy for pediatric patients with hypothalamic hamartoma: surgical technique, pitfalls, and initial results. J Neurosurg Pediatr. 29(6):681-92, 2022
4. Curry DJ et al: MR-guided laser ablation for the treatment of hypothalamic hamartomas. Epilepsy Res. 142:131-4, 2018
5. Du VX et al: Laser interstitial thermal therapy: a first line treatment for seizures due to hypothalamic hamartoma? Epilepsia. 58 Suppl 2:77-84, 2017
6. Harrison VS et al: Hypothalamic hamartoma with epilepsy: review of endocrine comorbidity. Epilepsia. 58 Suppl 2:50-9, 2017
7. Scholly J et al: Hypothalamic hamartoma: epileptogenesis beyond the lesion? Epilepsia. 58 Suppl 2:32-40, 2017
8. Mittal S et al: Hypothalamic hamartomas. Part 1. Clinical, neuroimaging, and neurophysiological characteristics. Neurosurg Focus. 34(6):E6, 2013

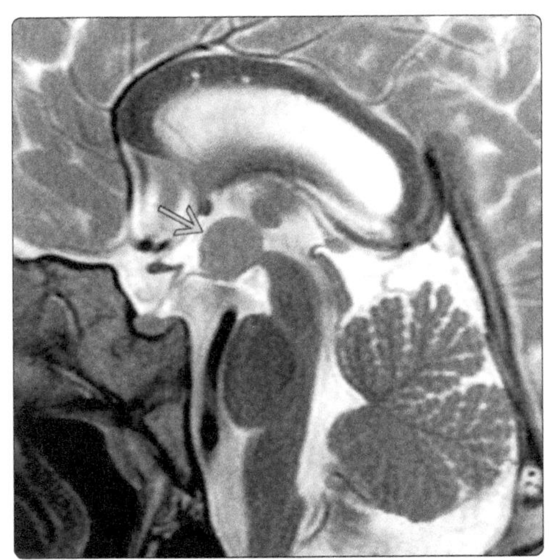

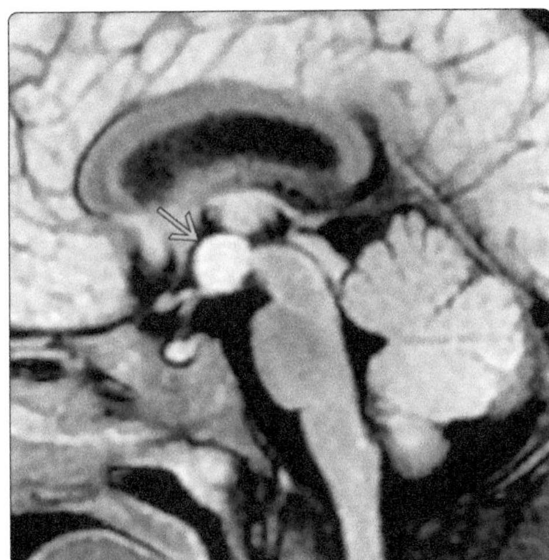

(Left) *Sagittal T2WI MR in a 2-year-old with gelastic seizures shows a sessile, well-defined mass ⇒ arising from the hypothalamus extending into the 3rd ventricle. HHs may protrude into the suprasellar cistern, 3rd ventricle, or both. Patients with sessile lesions are more likely to present with gelastic seizures, whereas pedunculated HHs more often present with precocious puberty.* **(Right)** *Sagittal FLAIR MR in the same patient shows the HH ⇒ to be isointense to GM, a typical appearance.*

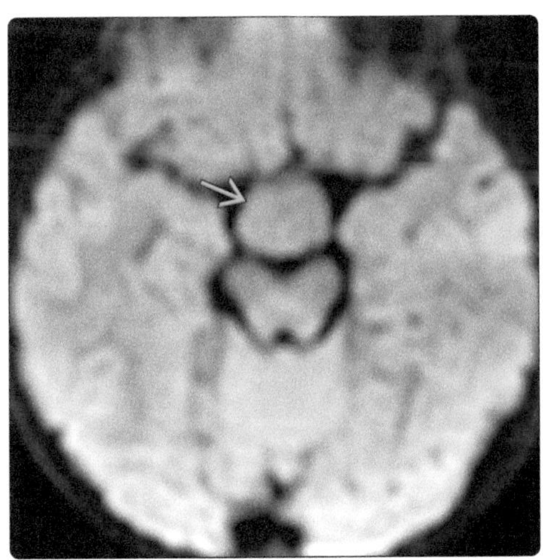

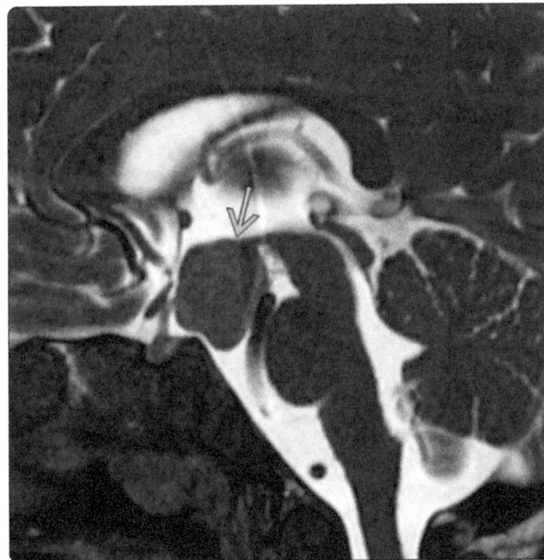

(Left) *Axial DWI MR in a 2-year-old with a tuber cinereum hamartoma shows a large suprasellar mass ⇒ that is isointense to the brain parenchyma. DWI helps for evaluating suprasellar masses. Pilocytic astrocytoma usually shows ↑ ADC signal, & germinoma typically shows ↓ ADC signal.* **(Right)** *Sagittal FIESTA MR in the same patient shows the relationship of the mass ⇒ with adjacent structures. FIESTA eliminates CSF flow artifact & provides high spatial resolution evaluation of suprasellar lesions with a CSF interface.*

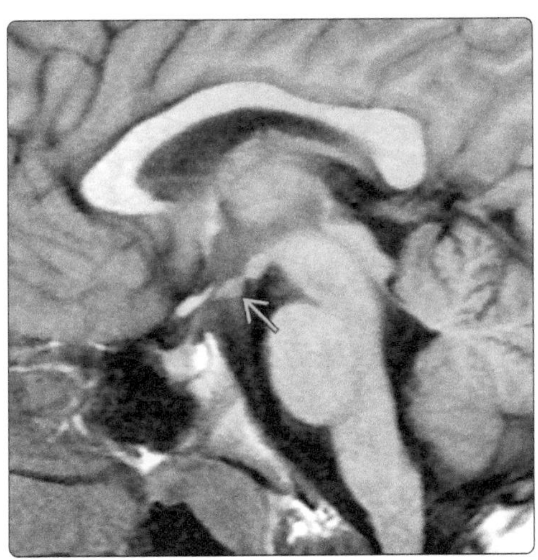

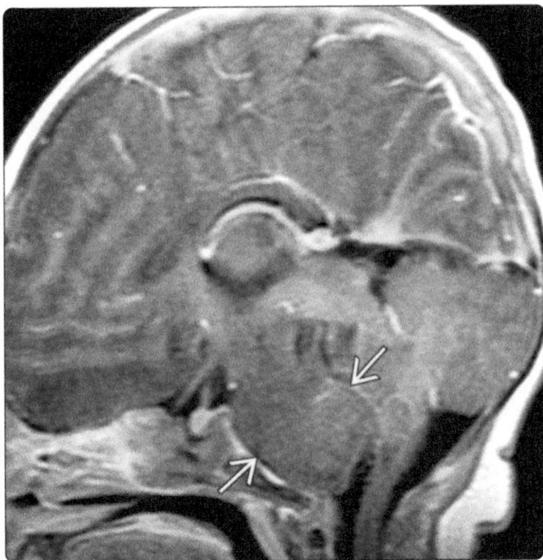

(Left) *Sagittal T2WI MR in an 8-year-old girl with precocious puberty shows a small, sessile lesion ⇒ in the tuber cinereum. While most hamartomas are quite large at presentation, one must be diligent in searching for small lesions that may only be evident on careful inspection.* **(Right)** *Sagittal T1WI C+ MR of an infant reveals a giant, pedunculated HH ➡ that posteriorly displaces the cerebellum & brainstem. No incremental enhancement of the mass is identified.*

Congenital Calvarial Defects

KEY FACTS

TERMINOLOGY

- Parietal foramina
  - Nonossification of medial parietal bone embryonal rest
- Sinus pericranii
  - Abnormal communication between intracranial and extracranial venous systems through calvarial defect
- Aplasia cutis congenita
  - Congenital skin malformation; may have underlying skull defect
- Cleidocranial dysplasia
  - Defective membranous and endochondral bone formation → delayed skull ossification
- Amniotic band syndrome
  - Strands of amniotic sac (bands) from ruptured amnion entangle digits, limbs, or other fetal parts
- Cranium bifidum occultum

IMAGING

- Symmetry, location best clues for diagnosis
- CT for calvarium, MR for underlying brain

TOP DIFFERENTIAL DIAGNOSES

- Epidermoid/dermoid
- Hemangioma
- Langerhans cell histiocytosis
- Metastasis
- Lacunar skull (Lückenschädel)

CLINICAL ISSUES

- Incidental finding on imaging or palpable scalp/calvarial mass that may protrude with crying, ↑ intracranial pressure

DIAGNOSTIC CHECKLIST

- Patients with enlarged parietal foramen (> 5 mm) warrant imaging of brain parenchyma and vasculature
- Use MR to differentiate sinus pericranii from arteriovenous malformation, hemangioma, dermoid cyst, encephalocele, abscess

(Left) *Lateral skull radiograph in a patient with cleidocranial dysplasia depicts large anterior/posterior fontanelles and a wide sagittal suture ➔. Note the numerous wormian bones ➔ characteristically distributed along the lambdoid sutures.* **(Right)** *Axial bone CT of the calvarium in a young patient with cleidocranial dysplasia demonstrates diminished midline bone structures with abnormally large anterior and posterior fontanelles ➔ and wide sagittal suture.*

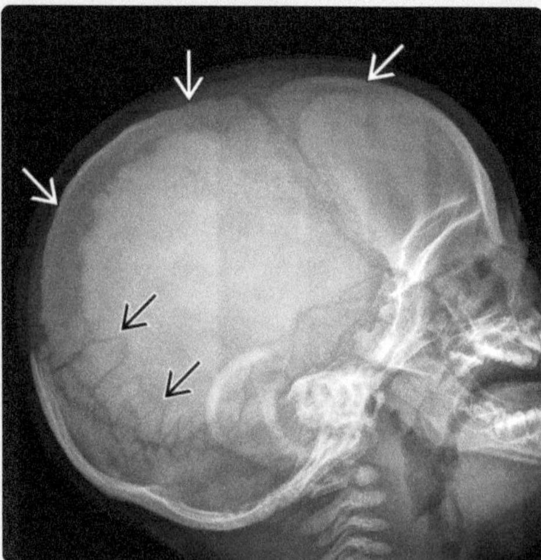

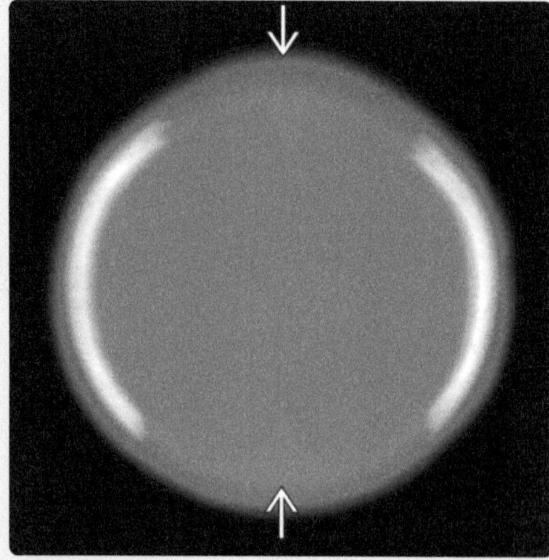

(Left) *Sagittal T2WI MR in a patient with a large calvarial defect secondary to amniotic band syndrome reveals a markedly abnormal head shape with encephalomalacia and gliotic brain extending through the large calvarial defect ➔.* **(Right)** *Sagittal oblique 3D bone CT reconstruction (same patient) nicely demonstrates the large calvarial defect resulting from amniotic band syndrome. Note the absence of the superior portions of the bilateral frontal and parietal bones, resulting in an open superior cranial vault.*

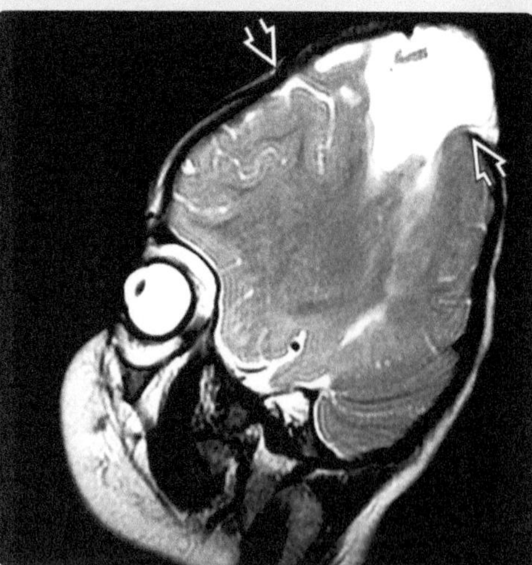

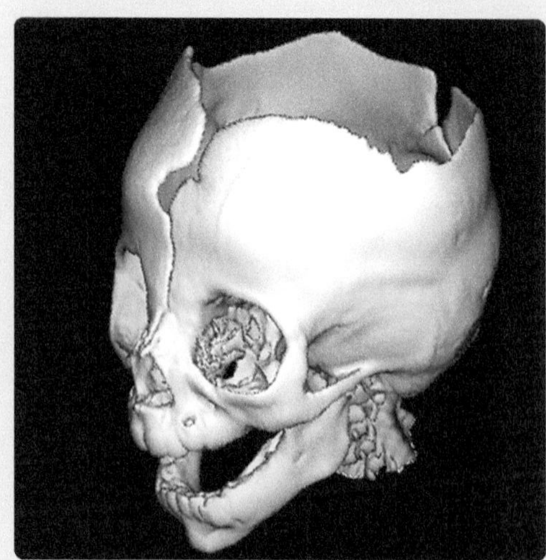

TERMINOLOGY

Definitions

- Parietal fissure (common)
  - Small, residual, incomplete medial parietal bone suture
- Parietal foramina (common; 60-70% of normal skulls)
  - Nonossification of medial parietal bone embryonal rest
  - Emissary vein portal between superior sagittal sinus and extracranial scalp veins
- Enlarged parietal foramina (EPF) (rare; prevalence 1:15,000-25,000)
  - Delayed/incomplete ossification of membranous parietal bone → round or oval parietal bone defects
  - Calvarial defect may be large, palpable
- Sinus pericranii
  - Abnormal communication between intracranial, extracranial venous systems through calvarial defect
  - Soft (often red or blue) scalp mass near superior sagittal or transverse dural sinuses
  - ↑ size with ↑ intracranial pressure (ICP) (Valsalva, dependent positioning)
- Craniolacunia (venous lakes)
  - Patulous calvarial diploic veins
  - Irregular, geographic, well-demarcated contour
  - Variable size and number
- Arachnoid (pacchionian) granulations
  - Located within 3 cm of superior sagittal sinus
  - Often multiple; irregular contour
- Abnormally large fontanelle
  - Secondary to ↑ ICP (suture spreading) or skeletal dysplasia
  - Search for ventriculomegaly, skeletal anomalies
- Cleidocranial dysplasia (uncommon)
  - Defective membranous and endochondral bone formation → delayed skull ossification
  - Enlarged sagittal and metopic sutures, wide anterior and posterior fontanelles, broad cranial diameter, multiple wormian bones along lambdoid sutures
- Cranium bifidum occultum (cleft skull)
  - Delayed ossification of parietal bones → large midline skull defects
  - Progressive parietal bone ossification fills defects; may persist as parietal foramina
    - Persistence in adulthood rare (< 1%)
  - Brain covered by dura, intact scalp
- Amniotic band syndrome
  - Occurs when inner amnion membrane ruptures or tears without disruption of outer chorion
  - Strands of amniotic sac (bands) from ruptured amnion entangle digits, limbs, or other fetal parts
- Aplasia cutis congenita (uncommon)
  - Congenital skin malformation; may have underlying skull defect
  - Skin defects most frequent on midline scalp > trunk, face, limbs
- Acalvaria (rare)
  - Absent superior osseous cranial vault, dura mater
  - Normal skull base, facial bones, brain (usually)
- Acrania (rare)
  - Partial or complete absence of cranial vault bones, abnormal cerebral hemisphere development

IMAGING

General Features

- Best diagnostic clue
  - Symmetry, location best clues for diagnosis
- Size
  - Variable; small → large

CT Findings

- NECT
  - Variable soft tissue component
  - Intracranial extent may not be well demonstrated
- Bone CT
  - Characterize osseous margins as sharp or destructive, sclerotic or nonsclerotic, inner or outer table

MR Findings

- Variable; depends on composition of soft tissue component, size and etiology of calvarial defect

Imaging Recommendations

- Best imaging tool
  - Bone CT with 3D shaded surface reformats best demonstrates calvarial defect, bone margins
  - MR best demonstrates soft tissue component composition, intracranial extension, brain anomalies

DIFFERENTIAL DIAGNOSIS

Epidermoid/Dermoid

- Most common childhood benign calvarial tumor
- Sharp, slightly sclerotic osseous margins
- Most common along frontal, parietal bone sutures or adjacent to fontanelles

Hemangioma

- Honeycomb or sunburst pattern of bony spicules, avid enhancement
- Outer > inner table, nonsclerotic, nonbeveled margins
- ± prominent vascular grooves

Langerhans Cell Histiocytosis

- Lytic lesion(s) with nonsclerotic rim
- Beveled (outer > inner table)
- Predilection for calvarium, temporal bone

Metastasis

- Multiple poorly defined destructive osteolytic lesions
- Advanced leukemia, neuroblastoma most common
  - Neuroblastoma ± hair-on-end appearance
- Look for additional appendicular skeletal lesions, hepatosplenomegaly (leukemia)

Lacunar Skull (Lückenschädel) of Newborn

- Membranous bone dysplasia present at birth
- Well-defined calvarial lucencies = nonossified fibrous bone surrounded by normally ossified bone
- Resolve spontaneously by ~ 6 months, unrelated to hydrocephalus severity
- Associated with myelomeningocele or encephalocele, Chiari 2 malformation

Leptomeningeal Cyst

- Growing fracture with adjacent encephalomalacia
- 0.6% of skull fractures (usually in child < 3 years)

Convolutional Markings

- True convolutional markings occur after sutural closure → differentiate from Lückenschädel

Osteomyelitis

- Lytic, poorly defined infiltrating margins, overlying soft tissue edema, fever or ↑ serum inflammatory markers

Cephalocele

- Osseous defect in characteristic location
- Brain anomalies, soft tissue component often clinically obvious

PATHOLOGY

General Features

- Etiology
  - Variable; many are developmental and present early in life
  - Fortunately, majority of pediatric skull masses are histologically and clinically benign
- Genetics
  - Enlarged parietal foramina
    - Isolated autosomal dominant or syndromal
      - Chromosome 11p deletion with *ALX4* gene mutation
    - No causative mutation identified in nonsyndromic cases
  - Cleidocranial dysplasia
    - Autosomal dominant, locus on chromosome 6p21
      - Mutation in *RUNX2* (a.k.a. CBFA1) gene coding for transcription factor activating osteoblastic differentiation
    - Variable expression, high penetrance
  - Cranium bifidum
    - Autosomal dominant, strong genetic heterogenicity
- Associated abnormalities
  - Enlarged parietal foramina
    - Scalp defects, cleft lip/palate, structural brain malformations
    - Vascular anomalies, including persistent falcine venous sinus ± adjacent focal encephalomalacia, occipital cortical infolding variations, atretic occipital encephalocele
  - Abnormally large fontanelles
    - Variable; depends on etiology or syndrome
  - Cleidocranial dysplasia
    - Absent/hypoplastic clavicles, small bell-shaped thorax, widened pubic symphysis, spinal anomalies, hypoplastic middle and distal phalanges, delayed deciduous dentition, hearing loss (38%)
  - Cranium bifidum
    - Midline neural tube malformations (myelomeningocele, meningoencephalocele, dermal sinus)
  - Amniotic band syndrome
    - ± constriction bands around limbs, congenital amputations, abdominal wall defects, and facial clefting
  - Acrania
    - Amniotic bands, anencephaly

CLINICAL ISSUES

Presentation

- Most common signs/symptoms
  - Palpable scalp or calvarial mass may bulge with crying, ↑ ICP
  - Incidental finding detected during imaging for other reasons
- Other signs/symptoms
  - Abnormally large anterior fontanelle (seen in osteogenesis imperfecta, cleidocranial dysplasia)

Natural History & Prognosis

- Dependent on severity of associated anomalies (especially orthopedic, neurologic)

Treatment

- Surgical closure of calvarial defect with autologous bone or alloplastic material
- Multidisciplinary supportive care

DIAGNOSTIC CHECKLIST

Consider

- Patients with EPF (> 5 mm) warrant imaging of brain parenchyma and vasculature

Image Interpretation Pearls

- Confirm presence or absence of skull base, vascular, skeletal anomalies

SELECTED REFERENCES

1. Fiaschi P et al: Peculiar bony involvement of sinus pericranii in children: extensive diploic erosion in three "karstic" variants. Clin Neurol Neurosurg. 219:107334, 2022
2. Scotti A et al: A case of large aplasia cutis congenita with underlying skull defect: effective surgical treatment with Integra® dermal regeneration template. Pediatr Neurosurg. 56(3):268-73, 2021
3. Walters ME et al: Vertical transmission of a large calvarial ossification defect due to heterozygous variants of ALX4 and TWIST1. Am J Med Genet A. 185(3):916-22, 2021
4. Tyrell R et al: Sinus pericranii in posterior cranial vault distraction. J Craniofac Surg. 31(7):e715-7, 2020
5. Alalade AF et al: Fossa navicularis in a pediatric patient: anatomical skull base variant with clinical implications. J Neurosurg Pediatr. 1-5, 2018
6. Sanders FH et al: Extremely large sinus pericranii with involvement of the torcular and associated with Crouzon's syndrome. Childs Nerv Syst. 33(9):1445-9, 2017
7. Singh I et al: Growing skull fractures: guidelines for early diagnosis and surgical management. Childs Nerv Syst. 32(6):1117-22, 2016
8. Pavanello M et al: Sinus pericranii: diagnosis and management in 21 pediatric patients. J Neurosurg Pediatr. 15(1):60-70, 2015
9. Ramdurg SR et al: Pediatric encephaloceles: a series of 20 cases over a period of 3 years. J Pediatr Neurosci. 10(4):317-20, 2015
10. Hawasli AH et al: Acalvaria. J Neurosurg Pediatr. 14(2):200-2, 2014
11. Singh S et al: Cleidocranial dysplasia: a case report illustrating diagnostic clinical and radiological findings. J Clin Diagn Res. 8(6):ZD19-20, 2014
12. Griessenauer CJ et al: Enlarged parietal foramina: a review of genetics, prognosis, radiology, and treatment. Childs Nerv Syst. 29(4):543-7, 2013
13. Vij R et al: Cleidocranial dysplasia: complete clinical, radiological and histological profiles. BMJ Case Rep. 2013
14. Glass RB et al: The infant skull: a vault of information. Radiographics. 24(2):507-22, 2004

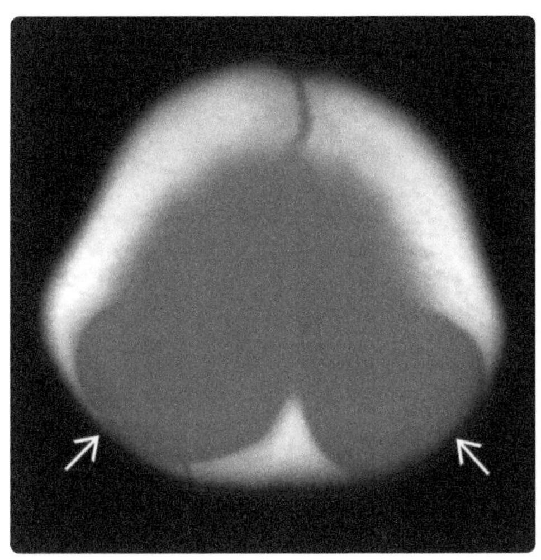

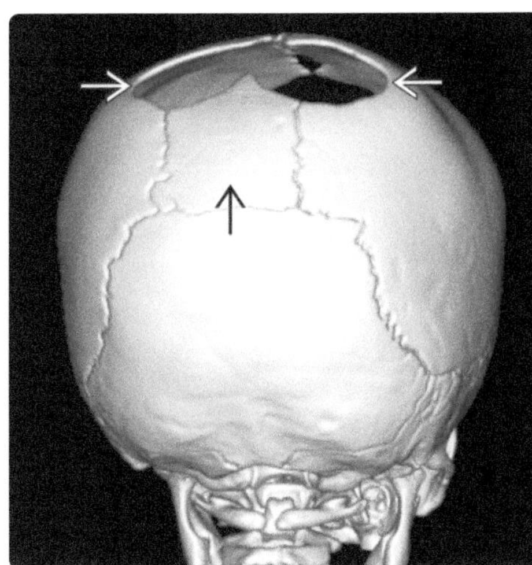

(Left) *Axial bone CT from a study ordered in an infant for "prominent posterior fontanelle" shows there are large bilateral parietal foramina ➡ communicating with the posterior fontanelle. The underlying brain (not shown) was normal.* **(Right)** *3D surface-rendered image of the skull (same patient) demonstrates the large parietal foramina ➡. There is also a large intrasutural bone ➡ at the lambda. Follow-up CT at 15 months (not shown) demonstrated smaller size of the foramina.*

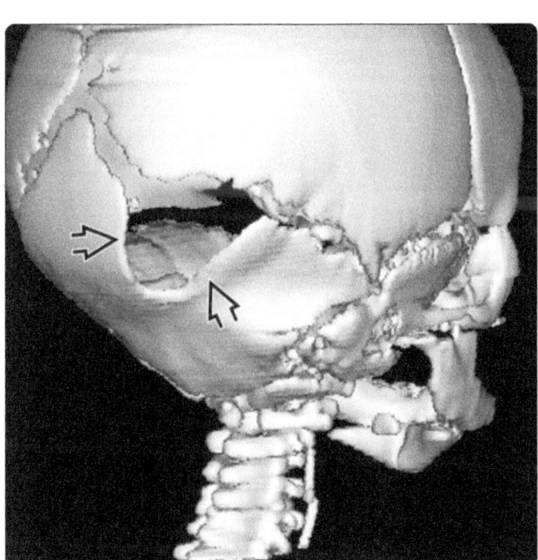

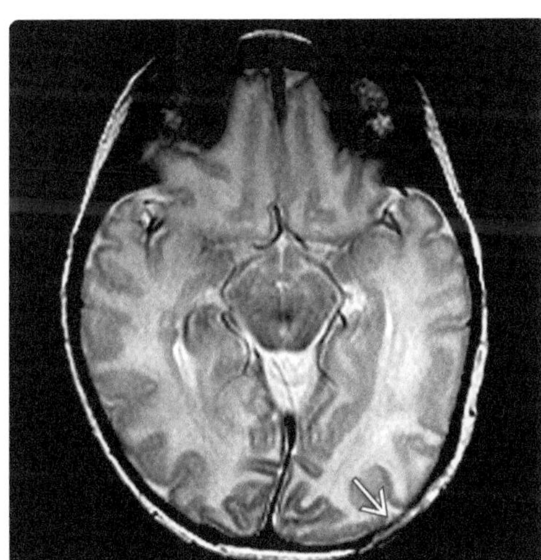

(Left) *Coronal oblique 3D bone CT reconstruction of the calvarium in a patient with focal cutis aplasia congenita of the scalp depicts a large calvarial defect ➡ subjacent to the region of cutis aplasia abutting the lambdoid suture.* **(Right)** *Axial T2WI MR in the same patient with focal cutis aplasia congenita and a left occipital calvarial defect demonstrates thinning of subcutaneous fat but intact dura ➡ in the region immediately beneath the area of cutis aplasia.*

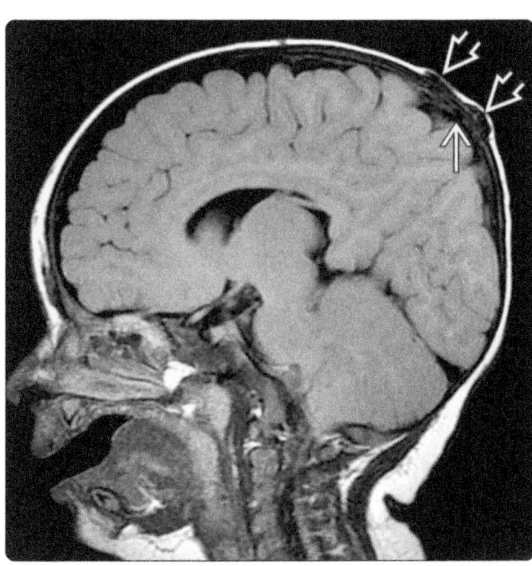

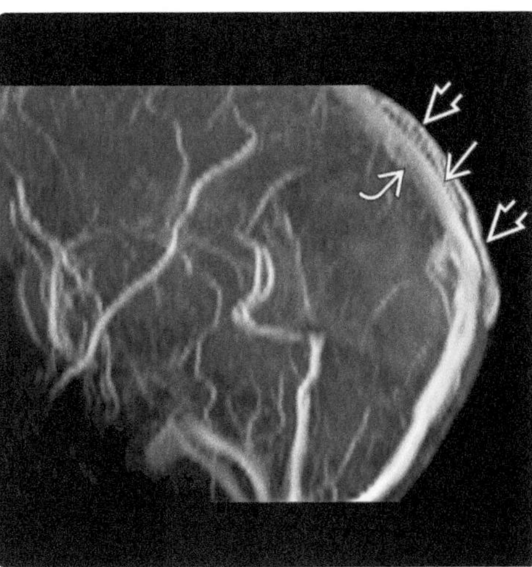

(Left) *Sagittal T1WI MR in a patient with sinus pericranii shows dilated parietal scalp veins ➡ in contiguity with the superior sagittal sinus through a small calvarial defect ➡.* **(Right)** *Sagittal MRV MIP reconstruction in the same patient confirms the presence of large parietal scalp veins ➡ in contiguity with the superior sagittal sinus ➡ via a small transcalvarial vein ➡. These are the classic imaging findings of sinus pericranii.*

KEY FACTS

TERMINOLOGY

- Synonyms: Craniosynostosis, sutural synostosis, cranial dysostosis, craniofacial dysostosis
- Heterogeneous group with abnormal head shape, premature sutural closure and fusion

IMAGING

- Calvarial (and facial) distortion predictable based on suture(s) involved
- Fibrous or bony "bridging" ± "beaking" along suture

TOP DIFFERENTIAL DIAGNOSES

- Postural flattening or positional molding
- Secondary craniosynostosis

PATHOLOGY

- Premature upregulation of growth factors signaling sutural fusion → craniosynostosis
- Head shape may be abnormal before osseous sutural changes detectable on imaging
- Some single sutural and nonsyndromic synostoses are genetic
- Syndromic synostoses usually autosomal dominant

CLINICAL ISSUES

- Asymmetric face/cranium, ↓ head growth, extremity anomalies, developmental delay
- Patients with more severe anomalies often present at time of birth
- Treatment with surgical cranial vault reconstruction or cranial vault distraction osteogenesis

DIAGNOSTIC CHECKLIST

- Nonsyndromic does not necessarily mean nongenetic; single sutural synostoses also governed by genes
  - Gene expression often suture specific
- Look for venous drainage anomalies or occlusion (particularly with multisutural synostosis)

(Left) *Sagittal bone CT 3D shaded surface reformat of the calvarium in a 1-day-old with Carpenter syndrome shows an abnormal head shape and frontal bossing with facial hypoplasia and premature closure of the squamosal, coronal, lambdoid, and sagittal sutures.* **(Right)** *Anterior coronal bone CT 3D shaded surface reformat in the same patient shows a very wide metopic suture* ➚ *and anterior fontanelle with harlequin eyes and a small face due to premature closure of the facial sutures.*

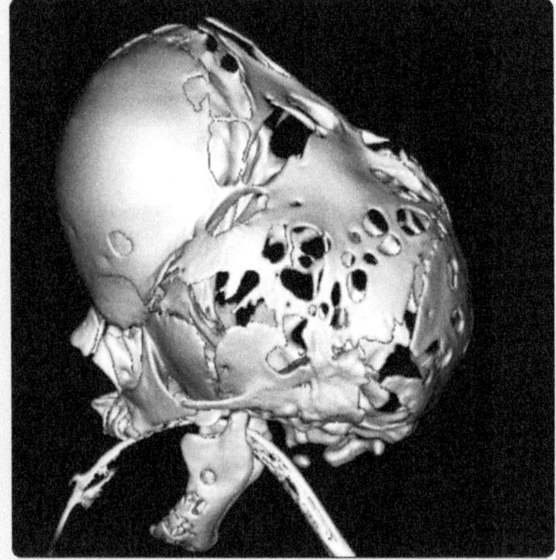

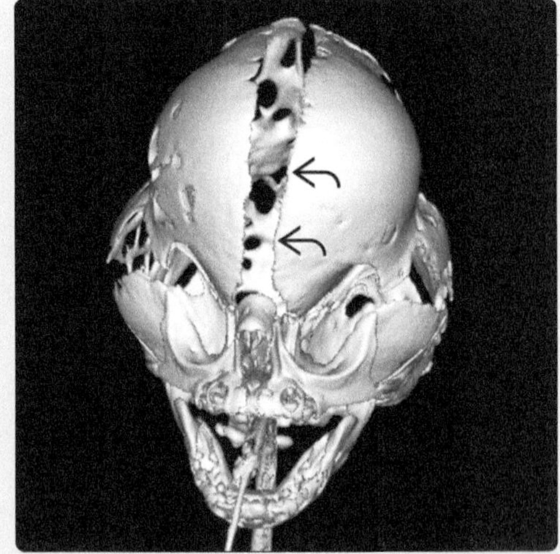

(Left) *Posterior coronal bone CT 3D shaded surface reformat in the same patient shows an abnormal head shape with occiput flattening, partial or complete closure of the lambdoid, sagittal sutures, and apparent holes* ➚ *due to focal calvarial thinning.* **(Right)** *Axial NECT in the same patient reveals marked irregularity of the calvarium. The intracranial compartment is small, producing brain compression with posterior effacement of the convexity sulci.*

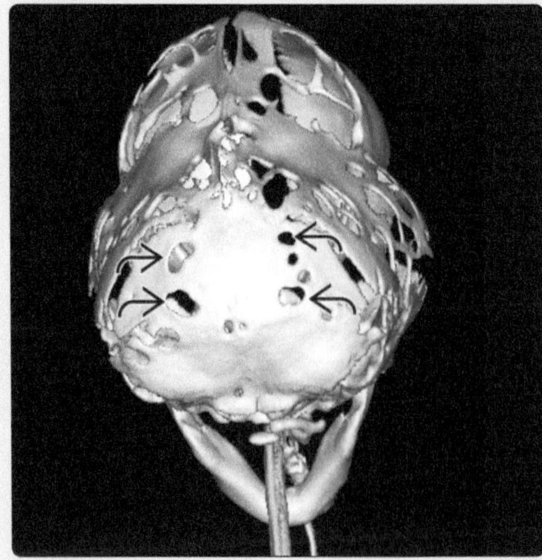

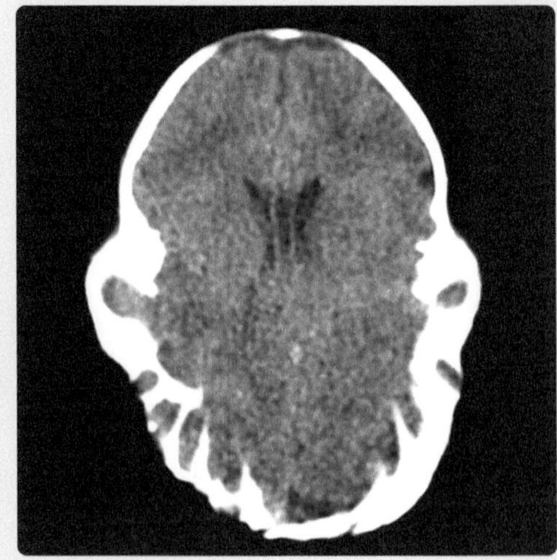

TERMINOLOGY

Synonyms

- Craniosynostosis, sutural synostosis, cranial dysostosis, craniofacial dysostosis

Definitions

- Heterogeneous group with abnormal head shape, premature sutural closure and fusion
  - Nonsyndromic (85%); isolated, classified according to involved suture(s)
    - Simple (single) suture (75-80%)
      - Abnormal head shape, (usually) normal intelligence
      - Sagittal > coronal > metopic > lambdoid
      - Usually sporadic, operated for cosmetic reasons
    - Multiple sutures (20-25%)
      - Oxycephaly (40-50%), brachycephaly (30-40%), unclassified (20%)
  - Syndromic [> 180 syndromes (15%)]; multiple anomalies with (frequent) developmental delay
    - Association with craniofacial, skeletal, nervous system, other anomalies
    - Syndrome description based on clinical features
      - Acrocephalosyndactyly type 1 (Apert)
      - Acrocephalosyndactyly type 2 (Apert-Crouzon)
      - Acrocephalosyndactyly type 3 (Saethre-Chotzen)
      - Acrocephalosyndactyly type 4 (Waardenburg)
      - Acrocephalosyndactyly type 5 (Pfeiffer)
      - Acrocephalopolysyndactyly type 2 (Carpenter)

IMAGING

General Features

- Best diagnostic clue
  - Head shape predicts abnormal suture(s)
- Size
  - Part or all of abnormal suture may be fused
- Morphology
  - Classic imaging appearance: Calvarial (and facial) distortion predictable based on suture(s) involved
    - Scaphocephaly (dolichocephaly): ↓ transverse, ↑ AP, forehead bossing → sagittal synostosis
    - Trigonocephaly: Wedge-shaped forehead, hypotelorism → metopic synostosis
    - Plagiocephaly: Asymmetry → unilateral single or asymmetric multiple sutures
      - Unilateral coronal synostosis: Unilateral harlequin orbit, hemicalvarium shortened and pointed
      - Lambdoid synostosis: Trapezoid skull, ipsilateral posterior ear displacement, occipital flattening
    - Brachycephaly: ↑ transverse, ↓ AP → bicoronal or bilambdoid synostosis
      - Bilateral coronal synostosis: Bilateral harlequin orbit, brachycephaly, skull base and craniofacial aberrations
    - Turricephaly: "Towering skull" → bicoronal or bilambdoid synostosis
    - Oxycephaly: Coronal, sagittal, lambdoid sutures
    - Kleeblattschädel: "Cloverleaf skull," bulging temporal bone, shallow orbits → bicoronal and bilambdoid synostosis
    - Unclassified: Multiple assorted sutural synostoses

CT Findings

- Bone CT
  - Fibrous or bony "bridging" ± "beaking" along suture
  - Head shape determined by involved suture(s)

MR Findings

- T1WI
  - Syndromic: Abnormal head shape ± cerebellar tonsillar ectopia, hydrocephalus, agenesis corpus callosum
  - Nonsyndromic: Abnormal head shape, brain (usually) normal
- T2WI
  - Same as T1WI
- MRV
  - ± congenital venous drainage anomalies
  - Postoperative dural venous occlusion

Imaging Recommendations

- Best imaging tool
  - Low-dose 3D bone CT reconstruction for sutural status
  - MR for brain abnormalities

DIFFERENTIAL DIAGNOSIS

Postural Flattening or Positional Molding

- Sutures normal
- Normal infants: Marked ↑ in incidence after 1994 pediatric "back to sleep" campaign
  - Parallelogram skull, ipsilateral anterior ear displacement
- Hypotonic infant: Lies on back → posterior flattening
- Premature infant: Lies on side → dolichocephaly

Secondary Craniosynostosis

- Brain growth arrest (myriad causes) → premature sutural fusion (especially metopic or universal craniosynostosis)

PATHOLOGY

General Features

- Etiology
  - Normal sutures permit skull growth perpendicular to long axis; close when brain growth slows
    - Order of closure: Metopic > coronal > lambdoid > sagittal
  - Premature upregulation of growth factors signaling sutural fusion → anomalous skull base development, craniostenosis
    - Transforming growth factor (TGF), fibroblast growth factor/receptor (FGF/FGFR) mutations expressed in face, skull base, limb buds
  - Abnormal head shape before osseous sutural changes apparent
    - Identifiable as early as 13-weeks gestation
    - Only part of suture needs to close → craniosynostosis
  - ↓ growth of 1 suture compensated by ↑ growth of other sutures
    - Skull growth ↓ perpendicular, ↑ parallel to fused suture → abnormal head shape
- Genetics
  - Some single sutural and nonsyndromic synostoses are genetic

- High-throughput DNA sequencing techniques have identified gene mutations in both syndromic and nonsyndromic cases
- Gene expression often suture specific
  - Syndromic synostoses usually autosomal dominant
    - *FGFR1* (Pfeiffer syndrome)
    - *FGFR2* (Apert, Pfeiffer, Crouzon, Jackson-Weiss)
    - *FGFR3* (thanatophoric dysplasia types 1 and 2, Crouzon)
    - *TWIST1* (Saethre-Chotzen syndrome)
    - *MSX2* (Boston-type craniosynostosis)
- Associated abnormalities
  - Limb anomalies [syndactyly and polysyndactyly (30%), deficiencies (22%)]
  - Neurologic abnormalities/complications
    - ↑ intracranial pressure (ICP): Mechanical brain distortion, hydrocephalus, dural and collateral venous outflow obstruction at skull base leading to venous hypertension
    - Tonsillar herniation ± syringohydromyelia
    - Exophthalmos, visual loss, intellectual disabilities (secondary to ↑ ICP)

Gross Pathologic & Surgical Features

- Fibrous or osseous "bridging," "beaking" along suture

Microscopic Features

- ↑ osteoblastic cell differentiation/maturation

CLINICAL ISSUES

Presentation

- Most common signs/symptoms
  - Asymmetric face/cranium, ↓ head growth
  - Affected patients with more severe abnormalities often present at birth
- Other signs/symptoms
  - Extremity anomalies, developmental delay
- Clinical profile
  - Craniofacial asymmetry ± extremity anomalies
  - More common in twins, perhaps related to mechanical forces

Demographics

- Age
  - Usually present at birth or in infancy
- Sex
  - Overall: M:F = 4:1
  - Scaphocephaly: M:F = 3.5:1
  - Trigonocephaly: M:F = 3:1
  - Coronal synostosis: M:F = 1:2
  - Apert: M:F = 1:1
- Epidemiology
  - Overall: 1:2,500
  - Sagittal (55-60%), coronal (20-30%), metopic (1-2%)

Natural History & Prognosis

- Single suture → cosmetic only or secondary mandibular/maxillary deformities (suture dependent)
- Multiple suture → cosmetic with secondary mandibular/maxillary deformities, ↑ ICP, ↓ cerebral blood flow (CBF); airway/aural/visual compromise
  - Craniofacial deformity socially stigmatizing
- Nonsyndromic → normal cognitive and motor development (debated)
- Syndromic ± midline brain anomalies → developmental delay

Treatment

- Mild deformity or positional molding
  - Aggressive physiotherapy, head repositioning, orthotic headband/helmet therapy
- Moderate to severe deformity
  - Surgical cranial vault reconstruction or cranial vault distraction osteogenesis
- Postoperative CT important
  - Establishes baseline
  - Rate of reossification assessed in regions where dura left uncovered
  - Focal or generalized copper-beaten appearance and sclerotic hyperdense bands represent recurrence
  - As skull grows, evaluate for migration of fixation screws, plates, and wires
    - May end up buried within skull or even intracranially
    - Development of absorbable hardware may eradicate this problem

DIAGNOSTIC CHECKLIST

Consider

- Nonsyndromic does not mean nongenetic; single sutural synostoses also governed by genes
- Venous drainage anomalies (multisutural synostosis)

Image Interpretation Pearls

- Positional lambdoid flattening: Long axis of skull is oblique (forehead to contralateral occiput)
- Unilateral lambdoid synostosis: Long axis of skull remains unilateral AP (forehead to ipsilateral occiput)

SELECTED REFERENCES

1. Santiago GS et al: Positional plagiocephaly and craniosynostosis. Pediatr Ann. 52(1):e10-7, 2023
2. Blessing M et al: Epidemiology, genetics, and pathophysiology of craniosynostosis. Oral Maxillofac Surg Clin North Am. 34(3):341-52, 2022
3. Dempsey RF et al: Nonsyndromic craniosynostosis. Clin Plast Surg. 46(2):123-39, 2019
4. Wu X et al: Signaling mechanisms underlying genetic pathophysiology of craniosynostosis. Int J Biol Sci. 15(2):298-311, 2019
5. Cyprus GN et al: Spatial regulation of gene expression in nonsyndromic sagittal craniosynostosis. J Neurosurg Pediatr. 1-7, 2018
6. Dalle Ore CL et al: Endoscopic surgery for nonsyndromic craniosynostosis: a 16-year single-center experience. J Neurosurg Pediatr. 22(4):335-43, 2018
7. Ghali GZ et al: Intracranial venous hypertension in craniosynostosis: mechanistic underpinnings and therapeutic implications. World Neurosurg. S1878-8750(18)31740-6, 2018
8. Ginat DT et al: CT imaging findings after craniosynostosis reconstructive surgery. Pediatr Neurosurg. 53(4):215-21, 2018
9. Isaac KV et al: Analysis of clinical outcomes for treatment of sagittal craniosynostosis: a comparison of endoscopic suturectomy and cranial vault remodeling. J Neurosurg Pediatr. 1-8, 2018
10. Kestle JRW et al: Variation in the management of isolated craniosynostosis: a survey of the Synostosis Research Group. J Neurosurg Pediatr. 1-5, 2018
11. Moosa S et al: Altered FGF signalling in congenital craniofacial and skeletal disorders. Semin Cell Dev Biol. 53:115-25, 2016
12. Blaser SI et al: Skull base development and craniosynostosis. Pediatr Radiol. 45 Suppl 3:S485-96, 2015
13. Calandrelli R et al: Identification of skull base sutures and craniofacial anomalies in children with craniosynostosis: utility of multidetector CT. Radiol Med. 119(9):694-704, 2014

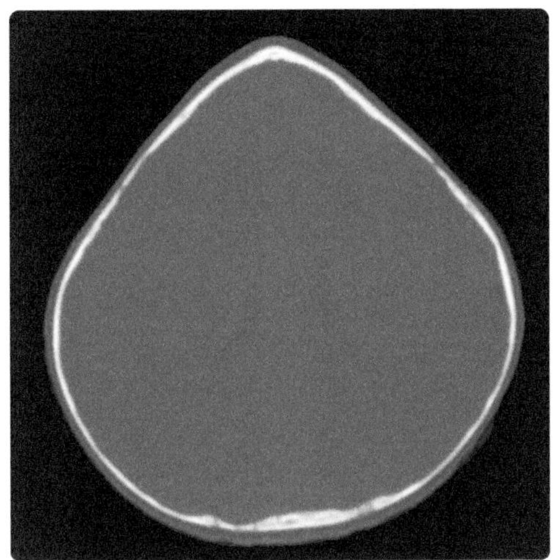

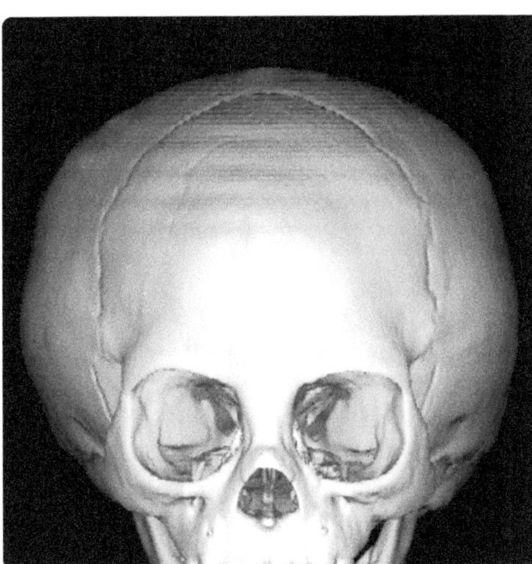

(Left) *Axial bone CT in a patient with metopic synostosis demonstrates a prominent pointed forehead with the wedge shape characteristic of trigonocephaly.* **(Right)** *Coronal bone CT 3D shaded surface reformat of the skull in a patient with metopic synostosis depicts premature fusion of the metopic suture, producing hypotelorism and trigonocephaly. The sagittal and coronal sutures are open.*

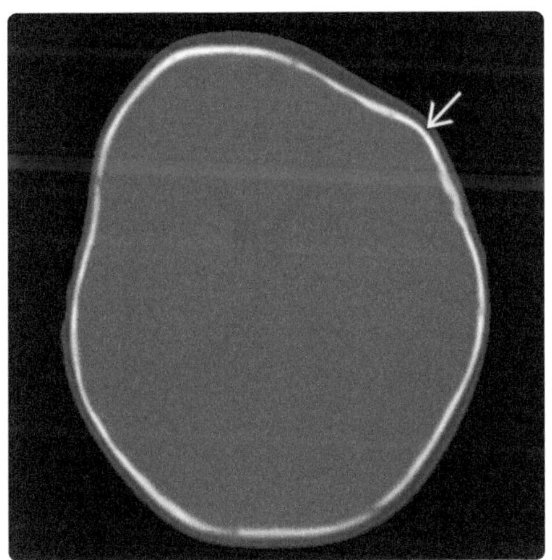

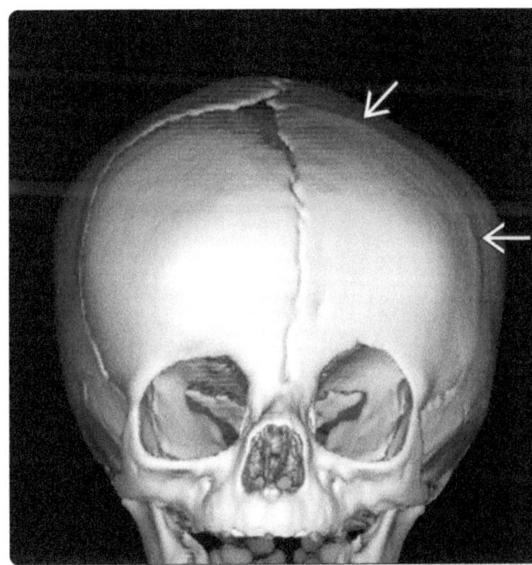

(Left) *Axial bone CT of the calvarium in a patient with plagiocephaly reveals abnormal flattening of the left forehead and pointed configuration ➔ at the left coronal suture from premature closure and fusion of the suture. The right coronal and lambdoid sutures are open.* **(Right)** *Coronal 3D bone CT reformat of the skull in the same patient confirms closure of left coronal suture ➔ with characteristic flattening of the ipsilateral forehead and retrusion of lateral superior orbit ("harlequin eye").*

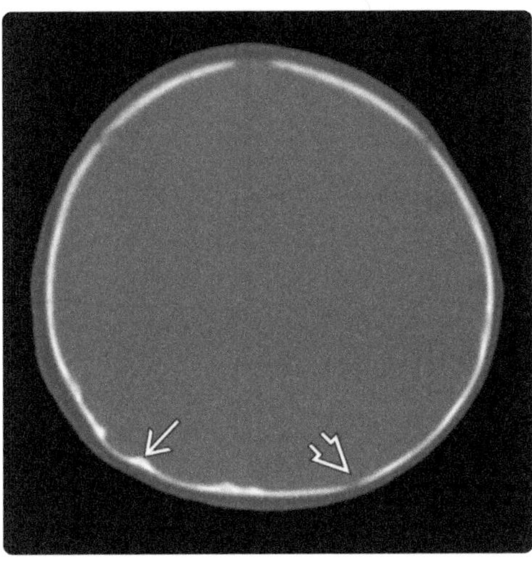

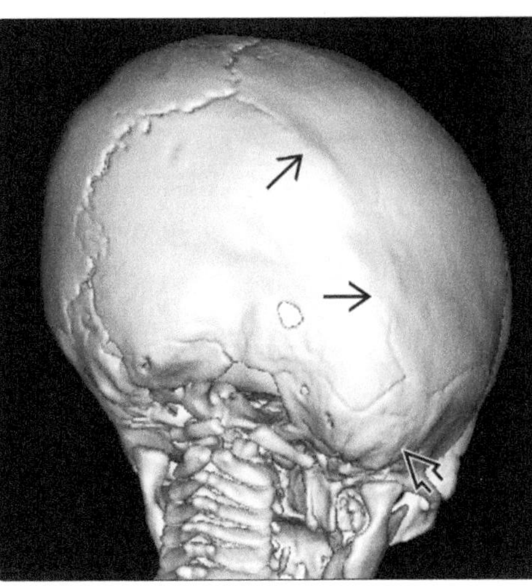

(Left) *Axial bone CT of the skull in a patient with unilateral lambdoid synostosis demonstrates a fused right lambdoid suture ➔ producing asymmetric occipital flattening. The left lambdoid ➔ suture is normal.* **(Right)** *Coronal oblique 3D bone CT shaded surface reformat in the same patient confirms obliteration of the right lambdoid suture ⇨, producing occipital flattening and protrusion of the right mastoid bone ("mastoid bump") ⇨. The left lambdoid and sagittal sutures are open.*

Cephalocele

KEY FACTS

TERMINOLOGY

- Extracranial extension of intracranial contents through defect in skull
  - Contents
    - Meningocele: Meninges & CSF
    - Encephalocele: Brain tissue, meninges, CSF
  - Locations
    - Occipital (most common)
    - Frontoethmoidal
    - Parietal (usually atretic)/cranial vault
    - Basal/nasopharyngeal

IMAGING

- Meninges & CSF ± brain tissue protrude through defect
  - Herniated brain tissue is often dysplastic
- MR + MRV to assess cephalocele contents & abnormal venous sinuses; CT to assess bone defect

TOP DIFFERENTIAL DIAGNOSES

- Dermoid/epidermoid cyst
- Nasal glial heterotopia ("nasal glioma")
- Sinus pericranii
- Assorted vascular anomalies (neoplasms & malformations)

CLINICAL ISSUES

- Congenital is more common than acquired
- Most cephaloceles (occipital) are clinically obvious at birth
- Basal/nasopharyngeal cephaloceles may not manifest until end of 1st decade
- Prognosis & surgical options depend on cephalocele size, location, contents, & associated anomalies

DIAGNOSTIC CHECKLIST

- Normal cartilaginous nasofrontal region in infants can mimic defect on CT; correlate with MR

(Left) *Sagittal T1 MR in a 2-day-old girl shows a large occipital cephalocele containing brain & a thin-walled ventricle → (encephalocystocele). The posterior fossa structures are herniated into the sac ➡ (a.k.a. Chiari 3). Microcephaly ➡ is also noted.* **(Right)** *Sagittal T2 MR in a 5-day-old patient shows a parietal cephalocele containing CSF & fibrous tissue →. Note the persistent falcine sinus →. Special attention to vascular involvement is critical in cephalocele evaluation.*

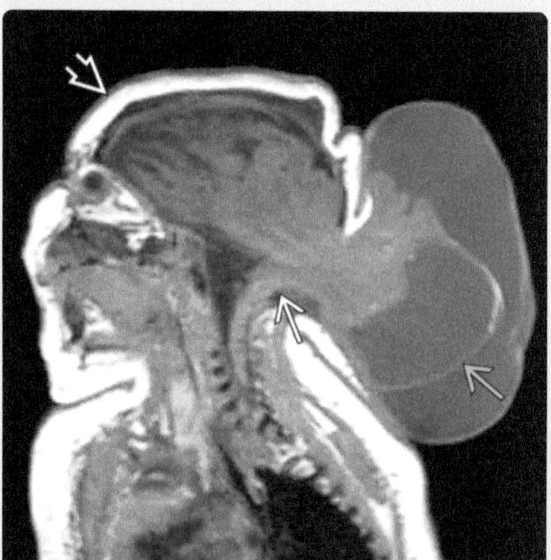

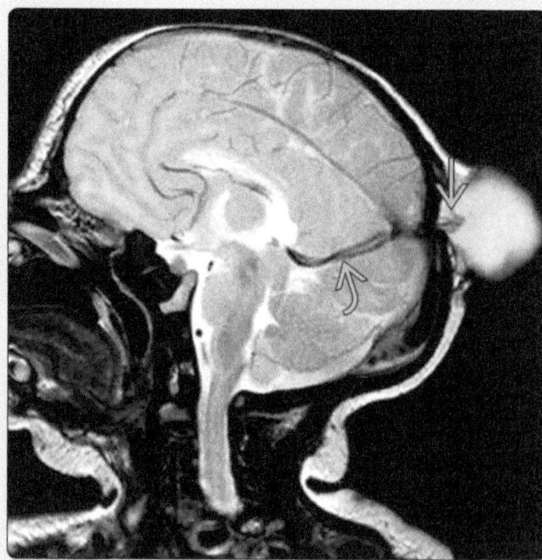

(Left) *Sagittal T2 MR in a 1-month-old shows a frontonasal encephalocele →. There is associated microcephaly & lateral ventriculomegaly →.* **(Right)** *Sagittal T2 MR in a 6-day-old girl shows a large sphenoethmoidal cephalocele →. Prenatal diagnosis prompted EXIT to airway so a tracheostomy could be placed while on placental support ➡. There is also agenesis of the corpus callosum ➡ & eye anomalies (not shown) consistent with Sakoda complex.*

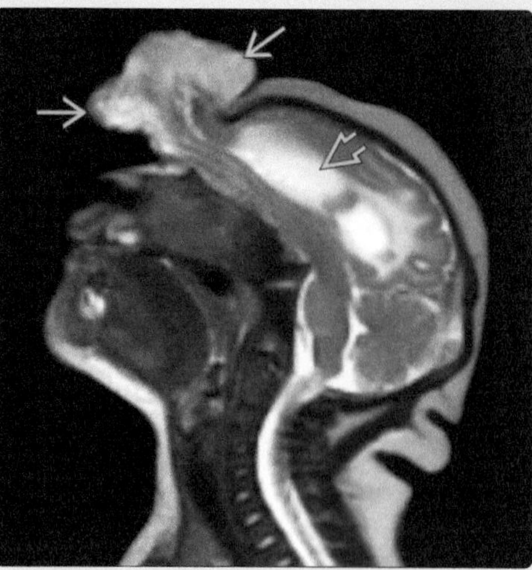

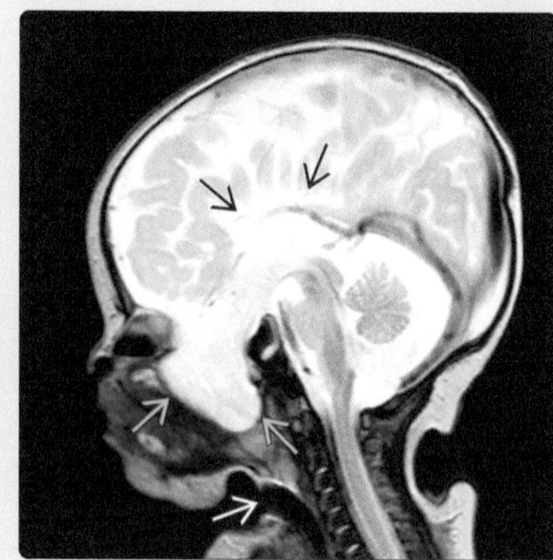

TERMINOLOGY

Definitions

- Extracranial extension of intracranial contents through defect in skull; categorized by contents & location
  - Congenital is more common than acquired
  - Associated anomalies in up to 50%
    - Brain: Neuronal migrational anomalies, dural venous sinus anomalies, callosal agenesis/dysgenesis, Dandy-Walker continuum, Chiari 3, vermian hypoplasia, holoprosencephaly spectrum, interhemispheric cysts, hydrocephalus
    - Craniofacial: Microcephaly, hypertelorism, cleft lip/palate, eye anomalies
- Contents
  - Cephalocele: Broad term for any focal extracranial extension of intracranial contents
  - Meningocele: Meninges & CSF only
  - Encephalocele: Brain, meninges, CSF
    - a.k.a. meningoencephalocele
  - Meningoencephalocystocele: Ventricle, brain, meninges, CSF
  - Atretic cephalocele: Meningeal & neuroglial elements retain fibrous connection to intracranial compartment, often without significant protrusion through defect
- Locations
  - Occipital: Most common location, up to 80% of cases
    - Supra- &/or infratentorial structures in cephalocele, including tentorium cerebelli & dural venous sinuses
  - Frontoethmoidal (a.k.a. sincipital): 15% (↑ in Southeast Asia)
    - 3 subtypes: Nasoethmoidal, nasofrontal, & nasoorbital
  - Parietal/cranial vault: 10-20%
    - Atretic parietal cephalocele most common
  - Basal/nasopharyngeal: Up to 10% of cases

IMAGING

General Features

- Best diagnostic clue
  - Meninges & CSF ± brain tissue protruding through skull defect

CT Findings

- Best for delineation of osseous defect

MR Findings

- T1, T2, FLAIR
  - Heterogeneous signal intensity of cephalocele contents reflecting brain parenchyma & CSF
    - Neural tissue may be dysplastic/gliotic/hemorrhagic
- MRV
  - Helps to characterize venous relationships to cephaloceles, particularly occipital
    - ± herniation of dural venous sinuses into cephalocele
- CISS/FIESTA
  - Helpful for delineating dermal sinus tract in frontoethmoidal cephaloceles

Ultrasonographic Findings

- Prenatal: Cephaloceles (mainly occipital) can be detected in utero
- Postnatal: Small superficial bumps over calvarium may receive ultrasound request first (particularly atretic parietal cephaloceles)

DIFFERENTIAL DIAGNOSIS

Dermoid/Epidermoid Cyst

- ± T1-hyperintense fat, diffusion restriction

Nasal Glial Heterotopia

- Dysplastic neural tissue

Sinus Pericranii

- Anomalous connection of intracranial & extracranial veins

Vascular Anomaly

- Variety of solid & cystic lesions found in neonatal period

PATHOLOGY

General Features

- Associated abnormalities
  - Meckel-Gruber syndrome: Occipital encephalocele + cystic renal disease + postaxial polydactyly
  - Frontoethmoidal: ± skin dimple/dermal sinus tract, dermoid/epidermoid cysts, nasal glial heterotopia (a.k.a. "nasal glioma")
    - Association with midline craniofacial dysraphism (a.k.a. frontonasal dysplasia), such as hypertelorism, telecanthus, microcephaly, micro-/anophthalmia
  - Atretic parietal cephalocele: ± superior sagittal sinus fenestration/duplication, persistent falcine sinus, absence of vein of Galen, & straight sinus

CLINICAL ISSUES

Presentation

- Most common signs/symptoms
  - Majority (occipital) are clinically obvious
  - Smaller lesions: Soft & bluish mass if skin covered (majority) or moist & red if lacking skin covering (rare)
- Other signs/symptoms
  - Occipital: Microcephaly, hydrocephalus
  - Basal/nasopharyngeal: Occult mass in oro-/nasopharynx → changes in size with Valsalva + upper airway obstruction, nasal stuffiness/mouth breathing
  - Seizures, developmental delay

Treatment

- Depends on cephalocele location, contents, size, & associated anomalies
- Goals of surgery: Prevent CSF leak & meningitis, improve functional & cosmetic deformities

DIAGNOSTIC CHECKLIST

Image Interpretation Pearls

- Always consider cephalocele when encountering cystic skull base lesion

SELECTED REFERENCES

1. Khodarahmi I et al: Imaging spectrum of calvarial abnormalities. Radiographics. 41(4):1144-63, 2021
2. Pejic M et al: Pediatric cephaloceles: a multimodality review. Appl Radiol. 49(5):26-32, 2020

Atretic Cephalocele

KEY FACTS

TERMINOLOGY

- Atretic parietal cephalocele (APC)
- Cephalocele "forme fruste" consisting of dura, fibrous tissue, and dysplastic brain tissue

IMAGING

- Heterogeneous subcutaneous scalp mass with intracranial extension
- Focal fenestration of superior sagittal sinus at APC
- CSF tract and vertical falcine vein point to subcutaneous scalp mass
- Cephalocele itself may be very small

TOP DIFFERENTIAL DIAGNOSES

- Dermoid or epidermoid cyst
- Proliferating (infantile) hemangioma
- Sinus pericranii
    - Often associated with APC
- Cephalohematoma or subgaleal hematoma
- Sebaceous cyst
- Metastasis

PATHOLOGY

- Considered involuted true cephalocele (meningocele or encephalocele) connected to dura mater via fibrous stalk
- Syndromic patients have increased incidence of associated intracranial anomalies

CLINICAL ISSUES

- Soft palpable interparietal subgaleal mass
- Usually identified in infants and young children
    - M ≤ F

DIAGNOSTIC CHECKLIST

- Consider APC in differential diagnosis for child with midline parietal skin-covered subgaleal mass
- Prognosis depends more on associated "occult" brain anomalies than existence of cephalocele itself

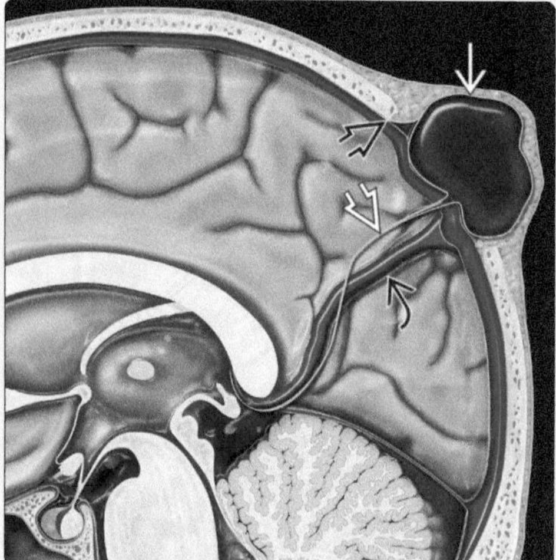

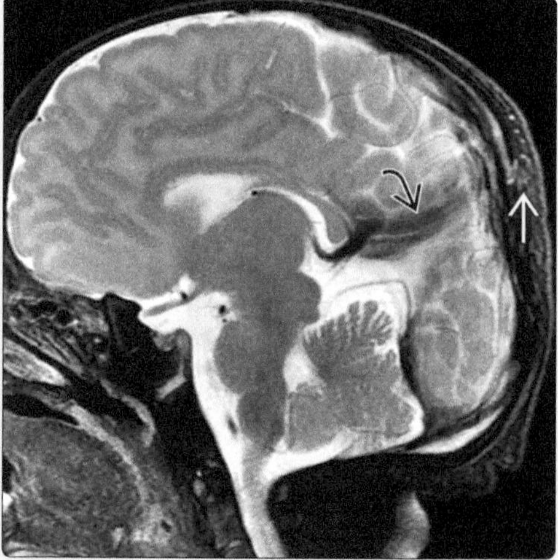

(Left) *Sagittal graphic shows a skin-covered midline atretic parietal cephalocele ➡ protruding through a sharply demarcated skull defect ⇨. The atretic cephalocele is associated with a dura-lined sinus tract ➡ and a persistent falcine venous sinus ↷.* **(Right)** *Sagittal T2 FS MR in an infant with a palpable parietal mass demonstrates the persistent falcine venous sinus ↷ and a tiny atretic parietal cephalocele ➡.*

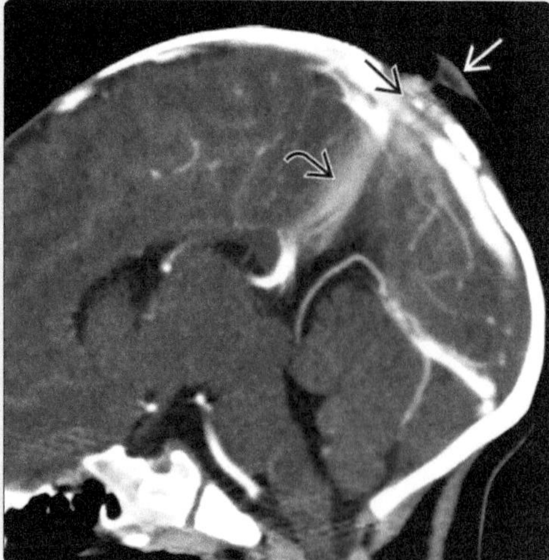

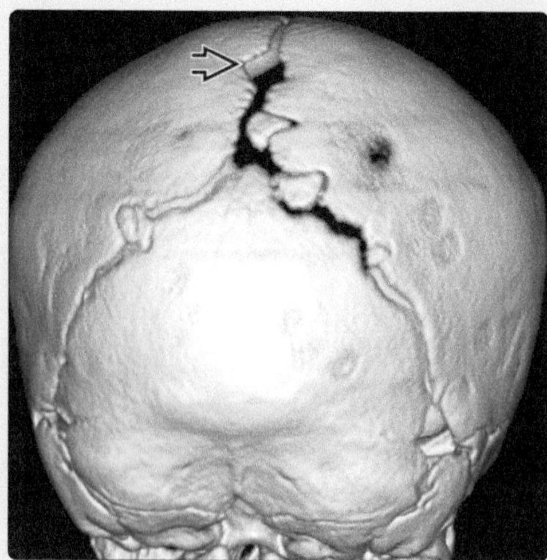

(Left) *Sagittal CTA in the same patient confirms the persistent falcine venous sinus ↷, atretic cephalocele ➡ passing between a split superior sagittal sinus ⇨.* **(Right)** *3D-rendered bone CT in the same child with an atretic parietal cephalocele reveals a small, sharply delineated midline skull defect ⇨ through which the dural-lined tract and cephalocele would pass.*

TERMINOLOGY

Abbreviations

- Atretic parietal cephalocele (APC)

Definitions

- Cephalocele "forme fruste" consisting of dura, fibrous tissue, and dysplastic brain tissue

IMAGING

General Features

- Best diagnostic clue
  - Fibrous tract and vertical falcine vein point to subcutaneous scalp mass (APC)
- Location
  - Midline interparietal most common
  - Occasionally occipital
- Size
  - Usually small (5-15 mm)
- Morphology
  - Skin-covered subgaleal mass with sharply marginated calvarial defect

Radiographic Findings

- Radiography
  - Cranium bifidum at obelion
    - May be difficult to appreciate

CT Findings

- NECT
  - Subgaleal soft tissue mass
  - Small cranium bifidum superior to lambda
  - Spinning top configuration of tentorial incisura (axial)
- CECT
  - Extension of subcutaneous scalp mass through dura delineated by enhancing veins
  - Fenestration of superior sagittal sinus, vertically oriented primitive falcine vein
- CTA
  - Vertical embryonic positioning of straight sinus equivalent (falcine sinus)
  - Fenestration of superior sagittal sinus

MR Findings

- T1WI
  - Heterogeneous subcutaneous scalp mass with intracranial extension
  - ± cigar-shaped CSF tract within interhemispheric fissure
  - Prominent superior cerebellar cistern and suprapineal recess
  - Characteristic appearance of tentorial incisura
    - Spinning top (axial) and peaked (coronal) configuration
  - Tissues are stretched in direction of defect and may point to lesion
- T2WI
  - Subcutaneous scalp mass representing APC is usually hyperintense
  - Other findings similar to T1WI
- STIR
  - Fat suppression better delineates subgaleal hyperintense cephalocele
- T1WI C+
  - Subcutaneous scalp mass usually shows heterogeneous enhancement
  - APC fibrous tract delineated by adjacent enhancing veins
- MRV
  - Vertically positioned straight sinus equivalent (persistent falcine vein)
  - Focal fenestration or lateral displacement of superior sagittal sinus at APC

Ultrasonographic Findings

- Grayscale ultrasound
  - Scalp mass with heterogeneous echotexture
  - Cranium bifidum osseous defect usually too small to identify

Imaging Recommendations

- Best imaging tool
  - Multiplanar MR with intravenous contrast + MRV
- Protocol advice
  - MR: Thin section, small field of view, sagittal T1 and T2 with fat saturation
  - Intravenous contrast with fat saturation to define sagittal sinus and falcine vein; exclude sinus pericranii

DIFFERENTIAL DIAGNOSIS

Dermoid or Epidermoid Cyst

- Often located near sutures
- Scallops outer table of calvarium
- + marginal enhancement, no internal enhancement

Proliferating (Infantile) Hemangioma

- Lobulated soft tissue mass with internal flow voids
- + avid contrast enhancement

Sinus Pericranii

- Often associated with APC
- Abnormal communication between intracranial and extracranial venous systems through osseous calvarial defect
- Soft red or blue scalp mass adjacent to superior sagittal or transverse dural sinuses
- ↑ size with ↑ intracranial pressure (Valsalva, dependent positioning)
- Internal venous flow, robust enhancement

Cephalohematoma or Subgaleal Hematoma

- Fluid in subgaleal space adjacent to intact calvarium
- Consider in newborn post trauma or following vaginal delivery

Sebaceous Cyst

- Dermal inclusion in scalp
- No calvarial defect or venous anomalies

Metastasis

- Destructive calvarial lesion + soft tissue mass
- Consider neuroblastoma in infant or toddler

Heterotopic Scalp Nodule

- Neuroectodermal malformation containing heterotopic leptomeningeal or glial tissue
- Focal alopecia surrounded by ring of long coarse hair (hair collar sign) ± surrounding capillary stain
  - May have rudimentary stalk with intracranial communication
- Clinically resembles dermoid cyst

PATHOLOGY

General Features

- Etiology
  - Considered involuted true cephalocele (meningocele or encephalocele)
  - Originates from overdistended rhombencephalic vesicle at 7-10 weeks of fetal life
    - Presence of persistent midline neural crest cells may prevent mutual induction of ectoderm and mesoderm
  - Postulated link to folate deficiency, valproic acid exposure
- Genetics
  - Typically sporadic, some cases syndromic
  - Syndromic more likely to have associated intracranial anomalies
- Associated abnormalities
  - Variable incidence
    - Most APC are incidentally identified without additional intracranial anomalies
    - Holoprosencephaly, callosal agenesis, eye anomalies, and interhemispheric cyst most common

Gross Pathologic & Surgical Features

- Hamartomatous subgaleal mass with adjacent focal cranium bifidum
- Connects to dura mater via fibrous stalk terminating in falx or tentorium
- CSF tract to supracerebellar, suprapineal, and quadrigeminal cisterns

Microscopic Features

- Meningeal and vestigial neural tissue rests
- CSF tract ependymal lined

CLINICAL ISSUES

Presentation

- Most common signs/symptoms
  - Soft palpable interparietal subgaleal mass
  - Overlying skin may be abnormally thin (cutis aplasia) and hairless (alopecia)
- Other signs/symptoms
  - APC may enlarge with crying
- Clinical profile
  - Subgaleal mass identified incidentally or during imaging evaluation for other anomalies

Demographics

- Age
  - Infants and young children
  - Occasionally described in adults
- Sex
  - M ≤ F
- Epidemiology
  - APC 10x more common than large parietal cephalocele
  - More common in Western hemisphere

Natural History & Prognosis

- Outcome determined more by associated anomalies than presence of APC
  - Children with no associated intracranial anomalies usually have normal clinical outcome
  - Additional intracranial anomalies (more common in syndromic patients) → worse outcome

Treatment

- Surgical resection of cephalocele with dural repair

DIAGNOSTIC CHECKLIST

Consider

- APC in differential diagnosis for child with midline parietal skin-covered subgaleal mass
- Prognosis depends more on associated occult brain anomalies than existence of cephalocele itself

Image Interpretation Pearls

- Persistent falcine sinus points to cephalocele
- Lack of abnormally dilated scalp veins, absence of falcine vein, and characteristic fibrous tract distinguish from sinus pericranii

SELECTED REFERENCES

1. Rousslang LK et al: Persistent falcine sinus in the newborn: 3 case reports of associated anomalies. Radiol Case Rep. 18(3):886-94, 2023
2. Khodarahmi I et al: Imaging spectrum of calvarial abnormalities. Radiographics. 41(4):1144-63, 2021
3. Sencer S et al: The spectrum of venous anomalies associated with atretic parietal cephaloceles: a literature review. Surg Neurol Int. 12:326, 2021
4. Ertuğrul Ö et al: Recurrence of atretic parietal cephalocele in adult: report a case and review of literature. Folia Morphol (Warsz). 77(3):591-6, 2018
5. Demir MK et al: Atretic cephaloceles: a comprehensive analysis of historical cohort. Childs Nerv Syst. 32(12):2327-37, 2016
6. Ramdurg SR et al: Pediatric encephaloceles: a series of 20 cases over a period of 3 years. J Pediatr Neurosci. 10(4):317-20, 2015
7. Siverino RO et al: Parietal atretic cephalocele: associated cerebral anomalies identified by CT and MR imaging. Neuroradiol J. 28(2):217-21, 2015
8. Leykamm S et al: Atretic cephalocele and associated anomalies in a newborn child. Clin Neuroradiol. 23(1):37-40, 2013
9. Hsu SW et al: Atretic parietal cephalocele associated with sinus pericranii: embryological consideration. Brain Dev. 34(4):325-8, 2012
10. Şengöz A et al: Atretic cephalocele in adults. Acta Neurochir (Wien). 153(11):2275-7, 2011
11. Morioka T et al: Detailed anatomy of intracranial venous anomalies associated with atretic parietal cephaloceles revealed by high-resolution 3D-CISS and high-field T2-weighted reversed MR images. Childs Nerv Syst. 25(3):309-15, 2009
12. Güzel A et al: Atretic parietal cephalocele. Pediatr Neurosurg. 43(1):72-3, 2007
13. Yamazaki T et al: Atretic cephalocele--report of two cases with special reference to embryology. Childs Nerv Syst. 17(11):674-8, 2001
14. Brunelle F et al: Intracranial venous anomalies associated with atretic cephalocoeles. Pediatr Radiol. 30(11):743-7, 2000
15. Gulati K et al: Atretic cephalocele: contribution of magnetic resonance imaging in preoperative diagnosis. Pediatr Neurosurg. 33(4):208-10, 2000
16. Reddy AT et al: Enlarged parietal foramina: association with cerebral venous and cortical anomalies. Neurology. 54(5):1175-8, 2000
17. Patterson RJ, et al: Atretic parietal cephaloceles revisited: an enlarging clinical and imaging spectrum? AJNR 19:791-5, 1998

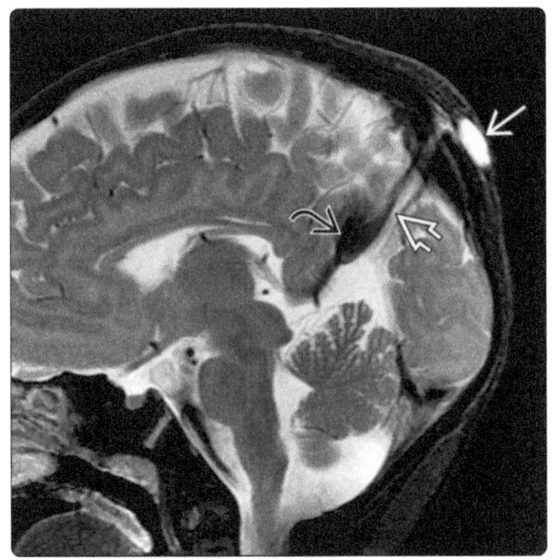

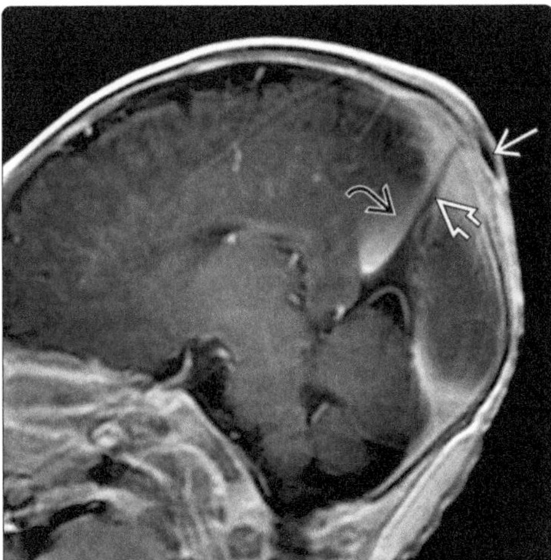

(Left) *Sagittal T1 FS MR shows a classic atretic parietal cephalocele with falcine vein and fluid collection. The fibrous stalk connecting the cephalocele through the calvarial defect is difficult to distinguish from the falcine vein flow void.* **(Right)** *Sagittal T1 C+ MR in the same patient shows a persistent falcine vein and the fluid-filled, skin-covered cephalocele. The fibrous stalk connecting to the cephalocele through the calvarial defect is clearly visible next to the enhancing falcine vein.*

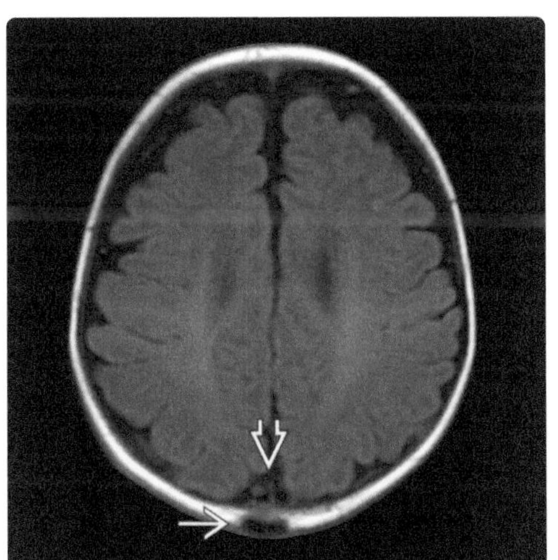

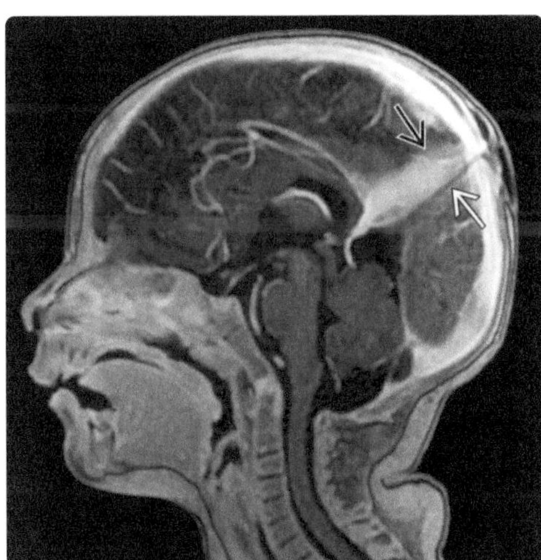

(Left) *Axial T1 MR in a 3-month-old infant with a palpable scalp mass reveals intrinsic fluid signal and a faint mildly hyperintense stalk extending intracranial, splitting the superior sagittal sinus. Finding represents a subtle atretic parietal cephalocele.* **(Right)** *Sagittal T1 C+ MR in the same patient confirms hypointense stalk connected to the palpable cephalocele with adjacent aberrant falcine vein.*

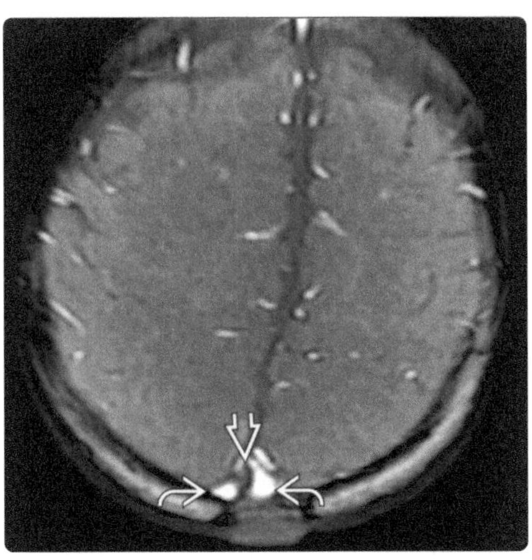

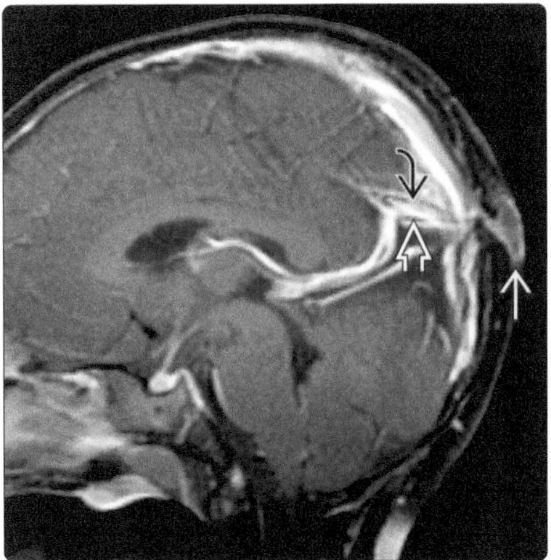

(Left) *Axial 2D time-of-flight MRV source image clearly demonstrates a focal split of the superior sagittal sinus surrounding the hypointense atretic cephalocele fibrous stalk.* **(Right)** *Sagittal T1 C+ FS MR demonstrates the uncommon occipital variant of atretic cephalocele. As in the parietal variant, there is an aberrant vein and fibrous tract pointing to the atretic cephalocele.*

Calvarial Fracture

KEY FACTS

TERMINOLOGY

- Synonyms: Calvarial, skull, skull base, basilar skull fracture

IMAGING

- Best diagnostic clue: Linear calvarial lucency
- Morphology: Linear, depressed, elevated; also comminuted, overriding, and closed or open
- Middle cranial fossa weakest with thin bones and foramina → look for epidermal hematoma at pterion
- Bone CT: Sharply delineated lucent line
  - Depressed fracture: Fragment(s) displaced inward
  - Skull base fracture → pneumocephalus common
  - Air in TMJ glenoid fossa may be only CT sign of inconspicuous skull base fracture
- CTA quickly and easily evaluates for vascular injury
- Best imaging tool: CT; add MR if complicated

TOP DIFFERENTIAL DIAGNOSES

- Suture line
- Calvarial fissure
- Vascular groove
- Arachnoid granulation
- Venous lake

PATHOLOGY

- Skull fracture extends through entire thickness of bone

CLINICAL ISSUES

- Linear fracture: Usually asymptomatic without LOC
- Symptoms often referable to epidural hematoma
- "Raccoon eyes" = periorbital ecchymosis
- Battle sign = mastoid ecchymosis
- Sequelae: CSF leak, delayed CN deficit(s), infarct
- Most skull fracture, even depressed, do not require surgery

DIAGNOSTIC CHECKLIST

- Sutures curvilinear, symmetric; fractures linear, asymmetric
- Raised suspicion of child abuse if multiple, complex, bilateral, depressed, or unexplained without trauma

(Left) *Coronal NECT (newborn infant, vaginal delivery) demonstrates a mildly elevated right parietal bone fracture ➡ with adjacent epidural hematoma ➡ and a large scalp hematoma.* **(Right)** *Axial composite of an NECT and bone CT in an infant with abusive head trauma (AHT) and multiple ages of acute ➡ and chronic ➡ subdural blood reveals a small, nondisplaced frontal bone fracture ➡. Evaluate AHT cases carefully for skull fracture, remembering that they do not heal with a callus.*

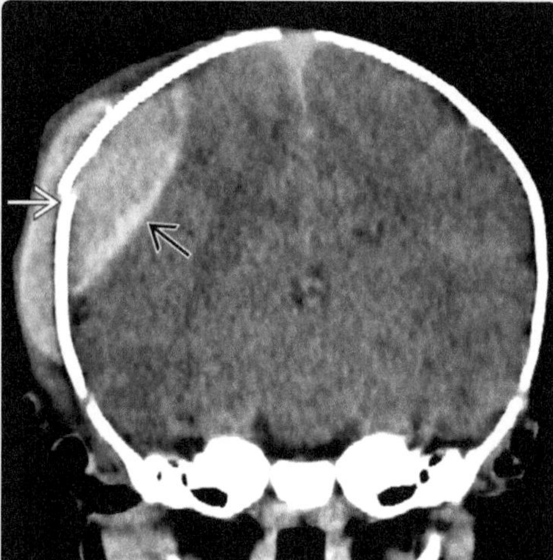

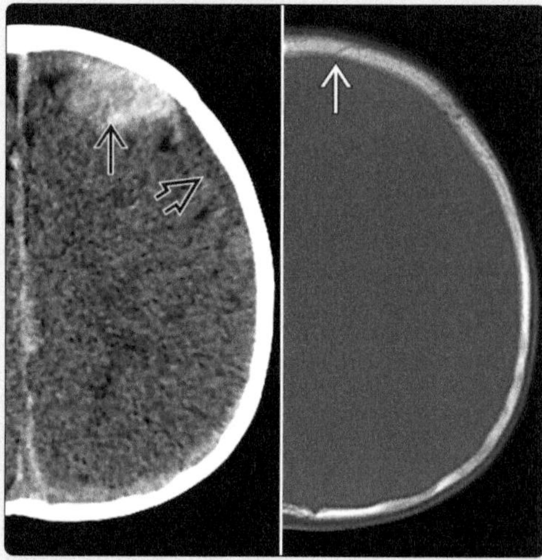

(Left) *Axial bone CT in a 13-year-old boy with closed head injury after helmet-less bicycle injury shows wide diastasis of the sagittal suture ➡ and circumferential scalp soft tissue swelling.* **(Right)** *3D shaded surface rendering in the same patient shows diastasis of both the previously closed sagittal ➡ and left coronal ➡ sutures. This implies a significant force directly to the calvarium.*

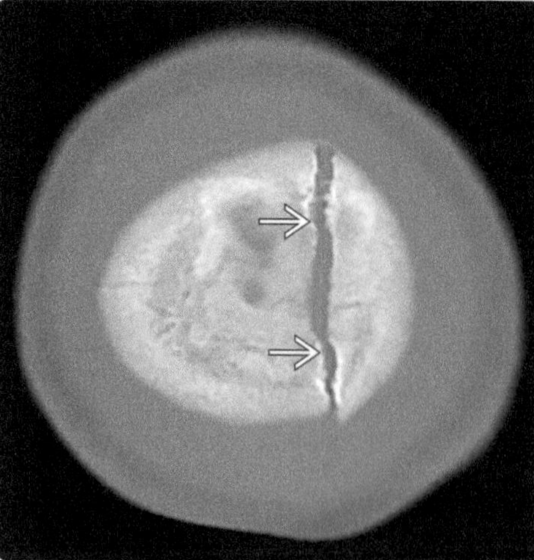

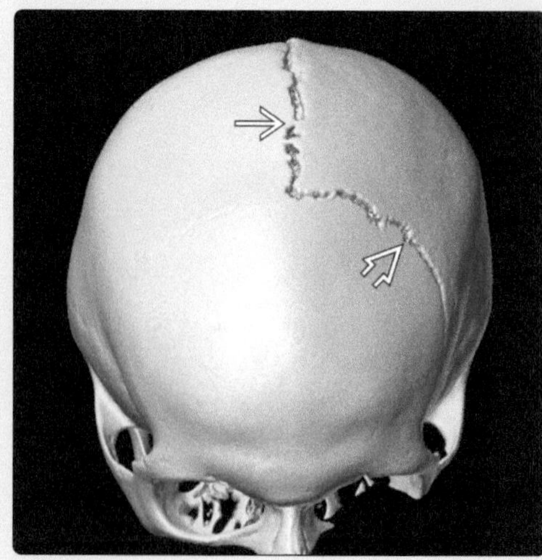

TERMINOLOGY

Synonyms

- Calvarial, skull, skull base, basilar skull fracture

IMAGING

General Features

- Best diagnostic clue
  - Linear calvarial lucency
- Morphology
  - Linear, depressed, elevated
  - Comminuted, overriding, closed or open

Radiographic Findings

- Radiography
  - Linear fracture: Sharply defined linear lucent line
  - Growing skull fracture (GSFx): Widening fracture line over time
    - Associated with leptomeningeal cyst/brain parenchymal injury

CT Findings

- Bone CT
  - Linear fracture: Sharply delineated lucent line
  - Depressed fracture: Fragment(s) displaced inward
  - Elevated fracture: Fragment(s) displaced outward
  - Skull base fracture
    - Pneumocephalus common (fracture through pneumatized skull)
    - Air-fluid level within adjacent air cell(s)
    - Nasal cavity fluid → CSF rhinorrhea
    - Ear cavity fluid from CSF otorrhea or blood density from hemotympanum
    - Air in TMJ glenoid fossa may be only CT sign of inconspicuous skull base fracture
  - Temporal bone fracture: Longitudinal or transverse
  - Ping pong-type depressed fracture
    - Pediatric specific (younger children)
    - Analogous to buckle fractures that occur in appendicular skeleton (i.e., incomplete fractures)
    - Usually no significant underlying hemorrhage or brain injury
  - Occipital condyle fracture
  - GSFx: Herniation of CSF and perhaps brain tissue through widened fracture defect with rounded margins
    - Intradiploic GSFx: Intact outer table, CSF-filled cyst, with defect of inner table and dura

MR Findings

- T2WI
  - Best to delineate dural injury, adjacent brain parenchyma
- FLAIR
  - Hyperintense cerebral contusion
- T2* GRE
  - Foci of hemorrhage susceptibility

Imaging Recommendations

- Trauma screen recommendations
  - Plain films have no role
  - CT scan for any clinical suspicion
  - Evaluate for vascular injury if carotid canal involved
    - CTA better than MRA
  - CTA or DSA if suspected traumatic carotid cavernous fistula

DIFFERENTIAL DIAGNOSIS

Suture Line

- < 2-mm width, same width throughout length
- At specific anatomic sites
- Not straight line, appears curvilinear or serrated ("zig-zag")
- Less distinct than fracture, has dense sclerotic borders

Calvarial Fissure

- Residual cartilage "fissure"
- Linear, often parietal, connects to sagittal suture

Vascular Groove

- Corticated margins, nonlinear (branches like tree)
- Frequently typical location (i.e., middle meningeal artery) but can be variable

Arachnoid Granulation

- Corticated margins; typical location (i.e., parasagittal, transverse sinus)

Venous Lake

- Corticated margins; typical location (i.e., parasagittal)

PATHOLOGY

General Features

- Etiology
  - Linear fracture: Low-energy blunt trauma over wide surface area of skull
  - Depressed fracture: High-energy direct blow to small surface area with blunt object (e.g., baseball bat)
  - Elevated fracture: Long, sharp wounding object elevates fragments (lateral pull, head rotation)
  - Occipital condylar fracture: High-energy trauma with axial load, lateral bending, or rotational injury
- Associated abnormalities
  - Linear fracture: Associated with epi-/subdural hematoma
  - Depressed fracture: Lacerated dura/arachnoid + parenchymal injury
  - Skull base fracture: Cranial nerve (CN) injury, CSF leak
    - CN palsies may be immediate or delayed
  - Raised suspicion of child abuse if multiple, complex, bilateral, depressed, and unexplained without trauma
  - Delayed intracranial hypertension from disturbance of superior sagittal sinus by depressed fracture
  - Traumatic carotid cavernous fistula may accompany basilar skull fracture

Gross Pathologic & Surgical Features

- Open fractures
  - Skin laceration over fracture
  - Fracture results in communication between external environment, intracranial cavity
  - May be clean or contaminated/dirty
- Depressed fracture
  - Comminution of fragments starts at point of maximum impact and spreads centrifugally
  - May compromise venous sinuses

- Elevated fracture: Always compound
- CN deficits: Transection by bone fragments, arterial ischemia, nerve stretching, or nerve root avulsion
- GSFx: Progressively enlarging diastatic fracture with underlying dural laceration, encephalomalacia
  - Herniation of CSF, brain, or vessels through defect

CLINICAL ISSUES

Presentation

- Most common signs/symptoms
  - Linear fracture: Often asymptomatic without LOC
  - Depressed fracture: LOC (25% none, 25% < 1 hour)
    - Often symptoms referable to epidural hematoma
  - Skull base fracture: Vernet/jugular foramen syndrome
    - Foraminal involvement → CNIX, X, and XI deficits
    - Difficulty in phonation, aspiration
    - Ipsilateral paralysis: Vocal cord, soft palate, superior pharyngeal constrictor, sternocleidomastoid, and trapezius
  - Longitudinal temporal bone fracture
    - **Conductive** hearing loss
    - 10-20% CNVII palsy from facial canal involvement
  - Transverse temporal bone fracture
    - **Neurosensory** hearing loss, vertigo
    - 50% CNVII palsy from internal auditory canal fracture
  - Mixed temporal bone fracture: Signs/symptoms of both longitudinal and transverse fracture
  - Occipital condylar fracture
    - Coma, associated cervical spinal injuries, lower CN deficits, hemiplegia, quadriplegia
    - Collet-Sicard syndrome: CNIX, X, XI, XII deficits
  - Traumatic carotid cavernous fistula: Vision impairment, limitation of ocular movements
- Clinical profile
  - Fracture present in majority of severe head injury cases
  - Linear fracture: Most common skull fracture; swelling at impact site, skin often intact
  - Depressed fracture: Often palpable abnormality
  - Skull base fracture
    - "Raccoon eyes" = periorbital ecchymosis
    - Battle sign = mastoid ecchymosis
  - Sphenoid bone fracture
    - CSF rhinorrhea/otorrhea, hemotympanum
  - Traumatic carotid cavernous fistula: Exophthalmos, bruit, chemosis

Demographics

- Age
  - GSFx: > 50% before 12 months, 90% before 3 years
  - "Ping pong" fractures occur in infants
- Epidemiology
  - Skull fracture present in 80% of fatal injuries at autopsy
  - Skull base fracture = 19-21% of all skull fractures
    - Sphenoid fracture accounts for 15% of skull base fractures
  - 75-90% of depressed fractures are open fractures
  - GSFx: 0.05-1.60% of pediatric skull fractures
  - Traumatic carotid cavernous fistula in 3.8% of basilar skull fractures
    - Incidence with fracture of anterior fossa (2.4%), middle fossa (8.3%), and posterior fossa (1.7%)

Natural History & Prognosis

- Sequelae: CSF leak, delayed CN deficit(s), infarct
- Healing process
  - Infants: Usually heals in 3-6 months without trace
  - Children: Heals within 12 months
  - Adults: Heals within 2-3 years, often residual lucency
- Transverse temporal bone fracture
  - Permanent neurosensory hearing loss
  - Persistent vertigo, unrelenting CNVII palsy
- Growing fracture (posttraumatic encephalocele) can be late complication
  - Infants < 3 months with head injury and scalp hematoma are at high risk
  - Herniated brain matter may be damaged by fracture edge
- Immediate CN palsies have lower rate of recovery than delayed deficits
- Traumatic carotid cavernous fistula: Untreated can lead to blindness

Treatment

- Most skull fractures, even depressed, do not require surgery
- Contaminated open fractures: Broad spectrum of antibiotics and tetanus vaccination
- Indications for surgery
  - Depressed segment > 8-10 mm or > thickness of skull; cosmesis
  - Gross contamination, dural tear with pneumocephalus, underlying hematoma
  - Brain function difficulties related to pressure or injury of underlying brain
  - Correction of ossicle disarticulation
  - Occipital condylar type 3 fracture (unstable) with atlantoaxial arthrodesis
  - Persistent CSF leak
  - Persistent intracranial hypertension secondary to superior sagittal sinus involvement and conservative treatment not effective
- Traumatic carotid cavernous fistula: Endovascular therapy

DIAGNOSTIC CHECKLIST

Consider

- Raised suspicion of child abuse if multiple, complex, bilateral, depressed, or unexplained without trauma

Image Interpretation Pearls

- Sutures curvilinear, symmetric; fractures linear, asymmetric

SELECTED REFERENCES

1. Hodges H et al: Pitfalls in the interpretation of pediatric head CTs: what the emergency radiologist needs to know. Emerg Radiol. 29(4):729-42, 2022
2. Purushothaman R et al: Utility of three-dimensional and reformatted head computed tomography images in the evaluation of pediatric abusive head trauma. Pediatr Radiol. 51(6):927-38, 2021
3. Sidpra J et al: Skull fractures in abusive head trauma: a single centre experience and review of the literature. Childs Nerv Syst. 37(3):919-29, 2021

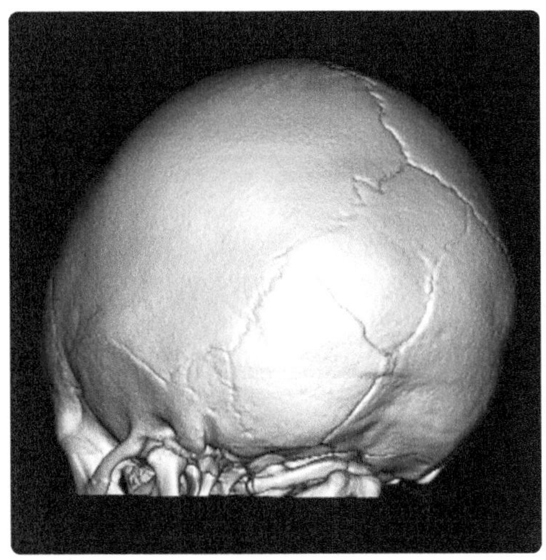

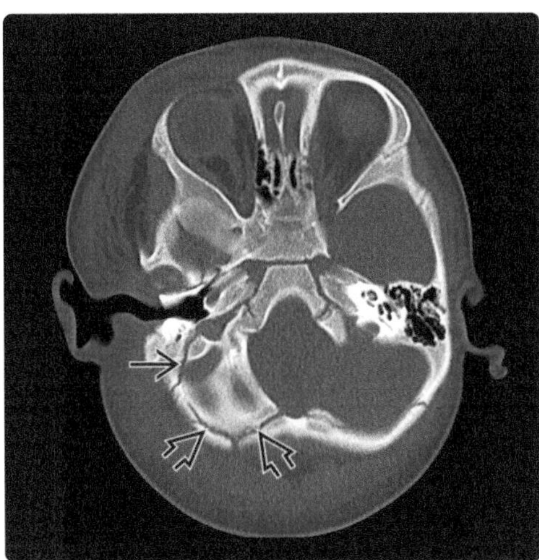

(Left) *3D shaded surface CT reformat of a comminuted stellate fracture of the occipital bone in an infant with confirmed AHT was associated with scalp soft tissue swelling and intracranial hemorrhage (not shown).* **(Right)** *Axial bone CT in the same patient confirms fracture extension into the posterior skull base with diastasis of the occipito-mastoid ➔ and intraoccipital ➔ sutures.*

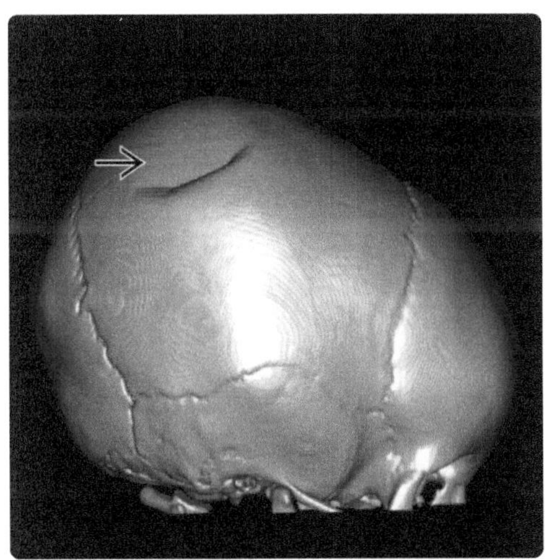

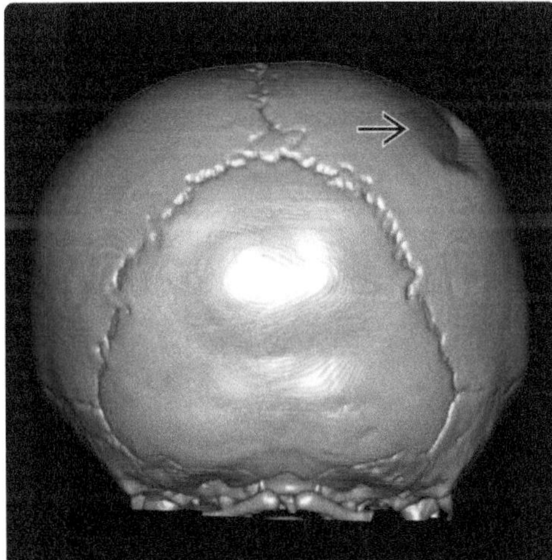

(Left) *3D shaded surface reconstruction from a brain CT demonstrates a depressed, incomplete fracture of the right parietal bone ➔, often referred to as a ping pong ball-type fracture. This occurs because the calvarium is quite soft in young children and is analogous to buckle fractures that occur in the appendicular skeleton.* **(Right)** *Sequential 3D reconstruction from a brain CT confirms depression of the right parietal bone fracture ➔.*

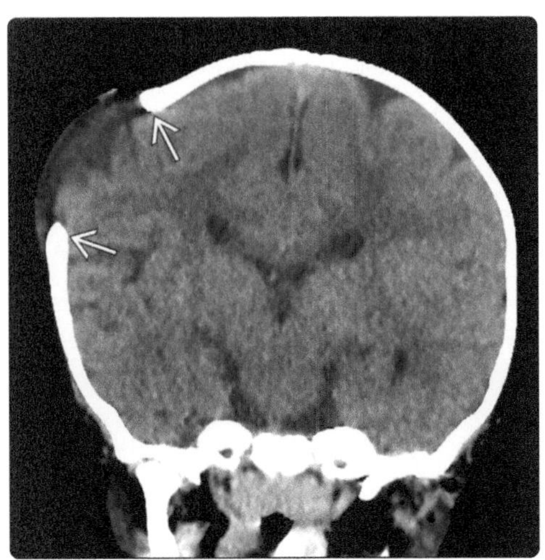

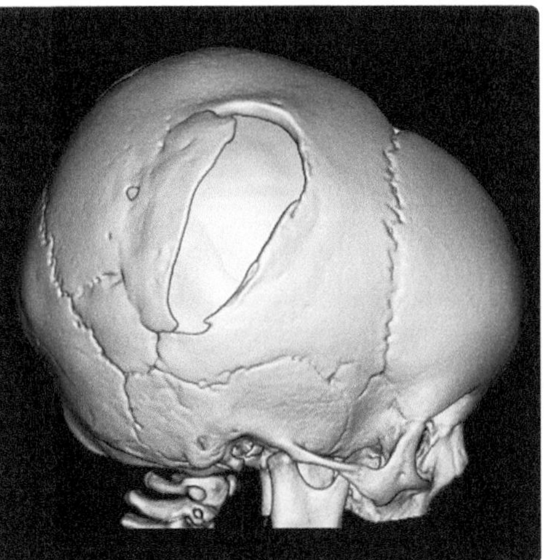

(Left) *Coronal NECT in a patient with prior head trauma and persistent soft palpable right parietal abnormality demonstrates extension of encephalomalacic brain through a parietal bone defect ➔. Note the rounded bone margins. This likely reflects sequelae of "growing fracture."* **(Right)** *3D shaded surface rendering in the same patient best depicts a large parietal bone defect. Note the rounded margins of the defect, reflecting chronic remodeling.*

KEY FACTS

TERMINOLOGY

- intracranial hypotension (IH): Headache caused by ↓ intracranial CSF pressure

IMAGING

- Classic imaging
  - Diffuse dural thickening/enhancement
    - Smooth, not nodular or "lumpy-bumpy"
  - Downward displacement of brain through incisura ("slumping" midbrain)
  - Veins, dural sinuses distended
  - ± subdural hygromas/hematomas
- Lack of ≥ 1 of 4 classic findings does not preclude diagnosis

TOP DIFFERENTIAL DIAGNOSES

- Meningitis
- Meningeal metastases
- Chronic subdural hematoma
- Dural sinus thrombosis
- Postsurgical dural thickening
- Idiopathic hypertrophic cranial pachymeningitis

CLINICAL ISSUES

- Severe headache (orthostatic, persistent, pulsatile, or even associated with nuchal rigidity)
- Uncommon: cranial nerve palsy (e.g., abducens), visual disturbances
- Profile: Young/middle-aged adult with orthostatic headache

DIAGNOSTIC CHECKLIST

- Frequently misdiagnosed clinically; imaging is key to diagnosis
  - Do not misdiagnose IH as Chiari 1
- Only rarely are **all** classic findings of IH present in same patient
- Recent LP or shunted hydrocephalus most common predisposing conditions in children

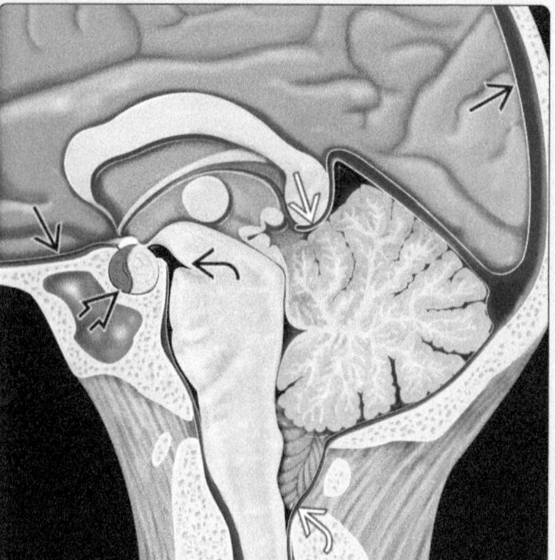

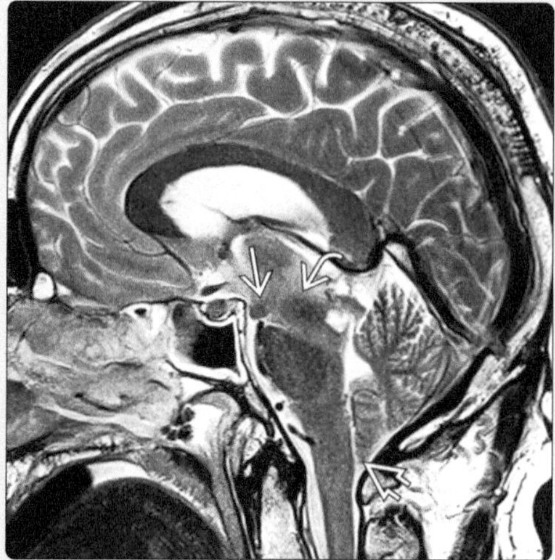

(Left) *Graphic shows intracranial hypotension (IH) with distended dural sinuses ➙, enlarged pituitary ➙, & herniated tonsils ➙. Central brain descent → midbrain slumping, inferiorly displaced pons, closed pons-midbrain angle ➙, & splenium depressing ICV/vein of Galen junction ➙.* **(Right)** *Sagittal T2 MR in a patient treated for "migraine" shows midbrain slumping ➙, downwardly displaced cerebellar tonsils ➙, & draping of hypothalamus over dorsum sellae with mammillary bodies ➙ below dorsum.*

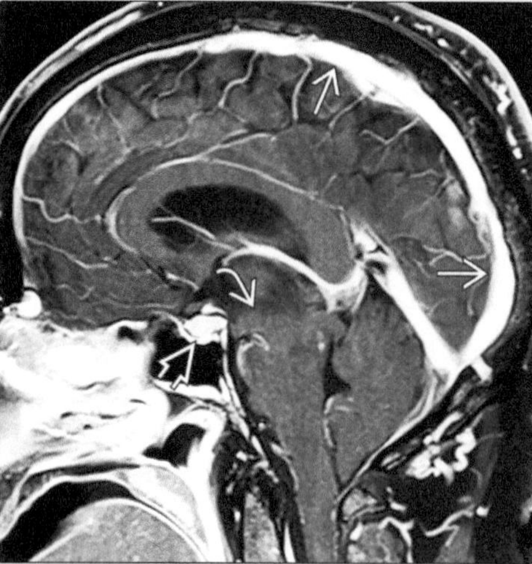

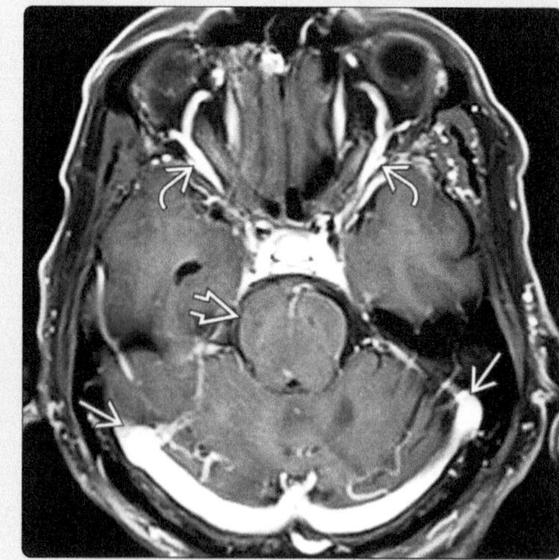

(Left) *Sagittal T1 C+ FS MR in the same patient shows the severe midbrain slumping ➙ and inferiorly displaced tonsils. In addition, the pituitary gland appears "fat" ➙, and the dural venous sinuses are engorged ➙.* **(Right)** *Axial T1 C+ FS in the same patient demonstrates a "fat" midbrain/pons ➙, prominent superior ophthalmic veins ➙, and engorged, outwardly convex transverse/sigmoid sinuses ➙. Severe IH was treated successfully with blood patch.*

TERMINOLOGY

Abbreviations

- Intracranial hypotension (IH)

Definitions

- Headache caused by ↓ intracranial CSF pressure

IMAGING

General Features

- Best diagnostic clue
  - Classic imaging quartet
    - Downward displacement of brain through incisura ("slumping" midbrain)
    - Diffuse dural thickening/enhancement
    - Veins, dural sinuses distended
    - Subdural hygromas/hematomas
  - Lack of 1 or more of 4 classic findings does **not** preclude diagnosis
- Location
  - Pachymeninges (dura)
    - Both supra- and infratentorial
    - May extend into internal auditory canals
    - Spinal dura, epidural venous plexuses may be involved
- Morphology
  - Dural enhancement is smooth, not nodular or "lumpy-bumpy"

CT Findings

- NECT
  - Relatively insensitive; may appear normal
  - Look for effaced suprasellar/basilar cisterns, "fat" midbrain/pons
  - ± thick dura
  - ± subdural fluid collections
    - Usually bilateral
    - CSF (hygroma) or blood (hematoma)
  - Atria of lateral ventricles may appear deviated medially, abnormally close ("tethered") to midline
- CECT
  - Diffuse dural thickening, enhancement

MR Findings

- T1WI
  - Sagittal view shows brain descent in 40-50% of cases
    - "Sagging" midbrain
      - Midbrain displaced inferiorly below level of dorsum sellae
      - Pons may be compressed against clivus
    - Decreased angle between peduncles, pons
    - Caudal displacement of tonsils in 25-75%
    - Optic chiasm, hypothalamus draped over sella
    - Pituitary enlarged above sella in 50%
    - Veins/dural sinuses distended (convex margins)
    - Decreased angle between internal cerebral veins (ICVs), vein of Galen
  - Axial
    - Suprasellar cistern crowded/effaced
    - Midbrain, pons appear elongated ("fat" midbrain)
    - Temporal lobes herniated over tentorium, into incisura
    - Lateral ventricles small, often distorted
      - Atria pulled medially by downward displacement of midbrain
  - Coronal
    - Severe cases show decreased venous angle (< 120°) between roofs of lateral ventricles
  - Bilateral subdural fluid collections in 15%
    - 70% hygromas (clear fluid collects within dural border cell layer)
    - 10% hematomas (blood of variable signal intensity)
- T2WI
  - Thickened dura usually hyperintense
  - Subdural fluid (variable signal)
- FLAIR
  - Hyperintense dura, subdural fluid
- T2* GRE
  - May bloom if hemorrhage present
- T1WI C+
  - Diffuse, intense dural enhancement in 85%
  - Often extends into CPAs

Nonvascular Interventions

- Myelography
  - May demonstrate epidural contrast accumulation at site of CSF leak
    - Dynamic CT myelogram may show "fast" high-flow leaks
  - Caution: Myelography may facilitate CSF leak, worsen symptoms

Nuclear Medicine Findings

- Radionuclide cisternography (RNC)
  - Direct findings: Focal accumulation of radioactivity outside of subarachnoid space at leakage site
  - Indirect findings
    - Rapid washout from CSF space
    - Early appearance of activity in kidneys, urinary bladder
    - Poor migration of isotope over convexities

Imaging Recommendations

- Best imaging tool
  - Contrast-enhanced cranial MR for diagnosis
  - RNC or dynamic myelography if localization required
- Protocol advice
  - Search for actual leakage site only if
    - 2 technically adequate blood patches fail
    - Posttraumatic leak is suspected

DIFFERENTIAL DIAGNOSIS

Meningitis

- Pia-subarachnoid enhancement > dura-arachnoid

Meningeal Metastases

- Enhancement usually thicker, irregular ("bumpy")

Chronic Subdural Hematoma

- Look for enhancing membranes with blood products

Dural Sinus Thrombosis

- Look for thrombosed sinus (empty delta sign, etc.)

Postsurgical Dural Thickening

- Look for other postoperative findings (e.g., burr holes)
- May occur almost immediately after surgery, persist for months/years

Idiopathic Hypertrophic Cranial Pachymeningitis

- Headache usually not orthostatic
- May cause bone invasion

PATHOLOGY

General Features

- Etiology
  - Dural thickening, enhancement due to venous engorgement
  - Common cause of IH = spontaneous spinal CSF leak
    - Weak dura ± arachnoid diverticula common
    - Aberrant extracellular matrix with abnormalities of fibrillin-containing microfibrils
  - Most (but not all) cases caused by reduced CSF pressure precipitated by
    - Diagnostic lumbar puncture
    - Surgery (CSF overshunting) or trauma (including trivial fall)
    - Vigorous exercise or violent coughing
    - Spontaneous dural tear, ruptured arachnoid diverticulum
    - Severe dehydration
    - Disc herniation or osteophyte (rare)
    - Spinal CSF-venous fistula
  - Pathophysiology = Monro-Kellie doctrine
    - CSF, intracranial blood volume vary inversely
    - In face of low CSF pressure, dural venous plexuses dilate
- Associated abnormalities
  - Dilated cervical epidural venous plexus, spinal hygromas, retrospinal fluid collections
  - Typical
    - Low opening pressure (OP), < 6 cm H_2O
    - CSF frequently shows pleocytosis, ↑ protein
  - Variant
    - OP occasionally normal (CSF hypovolemia rather than hypotension)
  - Stigmata of systemic connective tissue disorder found in up to 2/3 of patients
    - Marfan, Ehlers-Danlos type 2
    - Clinical findings = minor skeletal features, small joint hypermobility, etc.; may be subtle

Gross Pathologic & Surgical Features

- Surgical specimen generally unremarkable with grossly normal-appearing dura
- Spinal meningeal diverticula (often multiple), dural holes/rents common
- No specific leakage site identified at surgery in at least 50%

Microscopic Features

- Meningeal surface normal
  - No evidence for inflammation or neoplasia
- Inner surface
  - Layer of numerous delicate, thin-walled, dilated vessels often attached to inner surface
  - Nests of meningothelial cells may be prominent, should not be misinterpreted as meningioma
  - May show marked arachnoidal, dural fibrosis if longstanding

CLINICAL ISSUES

Presentation

- Most common signs/symptoms
  - Severe headache (orthostatic, persistent, pulsatile, or even associated with nuchal rigidity)
  - Uncommon: cranial nerve palsy (e.g., abducens), visual disturbances
  - Rare: Severe encephalopathy with disturbances of consciousness
- Clinical profile
  - Young/middle-aged adult with orthostatic headache
  - Recent LP or shunted hydrocephalus by far most common predisposing conditions in children

Demographics

- Age
  - Peak in 3rd, 4th decades

Natural History & Prognosis

- Most IH cases resolve spontaneously
  - Dural thickening, enhancement disappears; midline structures return (ascend) to normal position
- Rare: Coma, death from severe intracranial herniation

Treatment

- Epidural blood patching
- Surgery if blood patch fails (usually large dural tear) or subdural hematomas with acute clinical deterioration

DIAGNOSTIC CHECKLIST

Consider

- Frequently misdiagnosed clinically; imaging is key to diagnosis
  - Do not misdiagnose IH as Chiari 1
    - Surgery can exacerbate symptoms; in rare cases can be fatal

Image Interpretation Pearls

- Only rarely are **all** classic findings of IH present in same patient
- Look for enlarged spinal epidural venous plexuses

SELECTED REFERENCES

1. Amrhein TJ et al: Efficacy of epidural blood patching or surgery in spontaneous intracranial hypotension: a systematic review and evidence Map. AJNR Am J Neuroradiol. 44(6):730-9, 2023
2. Baram A et al: Intracranial hypotension syndrome after lumbar drainage in skull base surgery: diagnosis and correct management. J Neurol Surg A Cent Eur Neurosurg. 84(6):578-83, 2023
3. Bin Wan Hassan WMN et al: Overview of spontaneous intracranial hypotension and differential diagnosis with Chiari I malformation. J Clin Med. 12(9), 2023
4. Ballmann L et al: Subdural hygroma in an infant with Marfan's syndrome. Neuropediatrics. 52(6):423-30, 2021
5. Peterson EE et al: Pediatric intracranial hypotension and post-dural puncture headache. Semin Pediatr Neurol. 40:100927, 2021
6. Shah LM et al: Intracranial hypotension: improved MRI detection with diagnostic intracranial angles. AJR Am J Roentgenol. 200(2):400-7, 2013

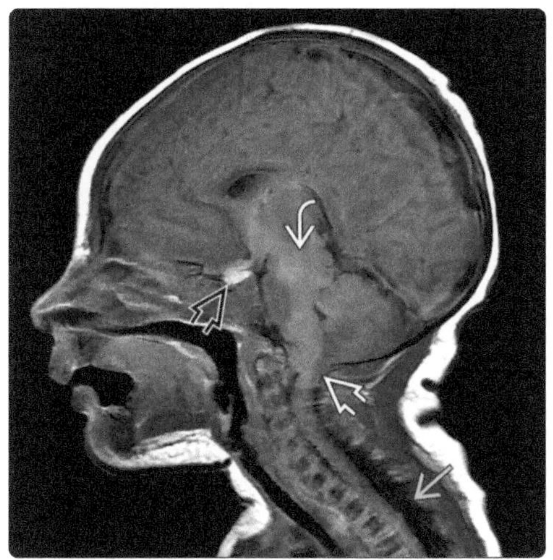

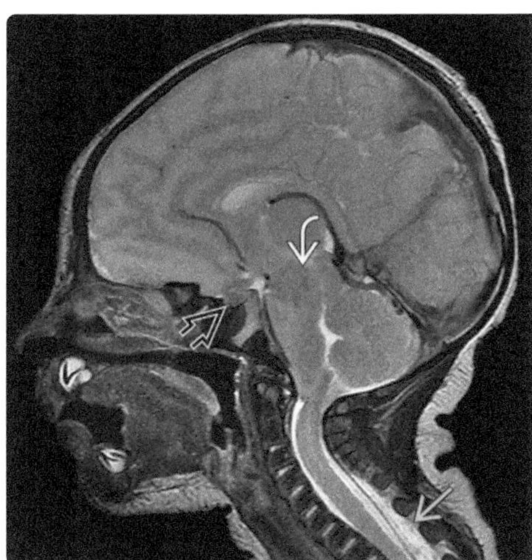

(Left) *Sagittal T1 MR in an 11-day-old infant with CSF leak after an LP reveals engorgement of the pituitary gland →, tonsillar ectopia →, and downward brainstem "slumping" →. Prominent CSF is also noted behind the cervical spinal cord →.* **(Right)** *Sagittal T2 MR in the same patient confirms brainstem "slumping" → and effacement of the suprasellar cistern with pituitary engorgement → as well. T2 imaging depicts prominent extradural CSF collection → reflecting post lumbar puncture CSF leak.*

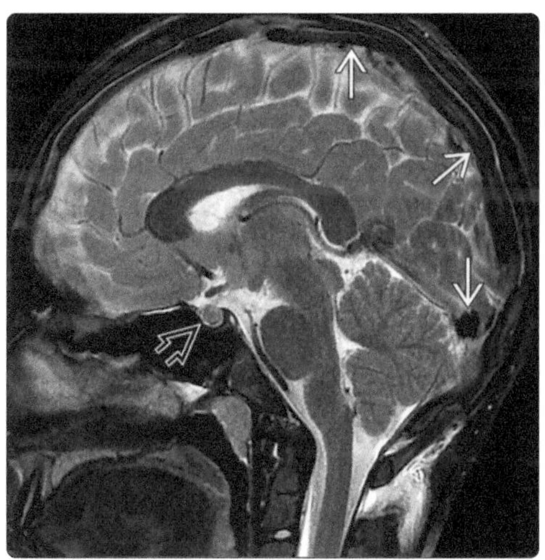

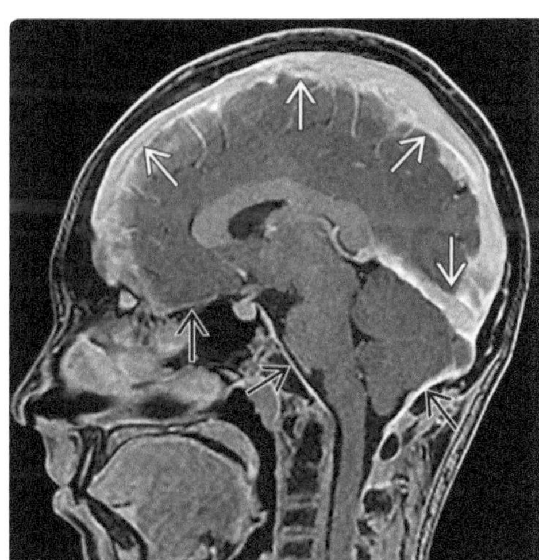

(Left) *Sagittal T2 MR in an 11-year-old patient with back trauma and postural headache reveals engorgement of the dural venous sinuses → and pituitary engorgement → as well as ligamentum nuchae injury, but no brainstem "slumping" or tonsillar ectopia is present.* **(Right)** *Sagittal T1 C+ MR in the same patient confirms marked dural venous engorgement → and demonstrates smooth dural thickening and enhancement →.*

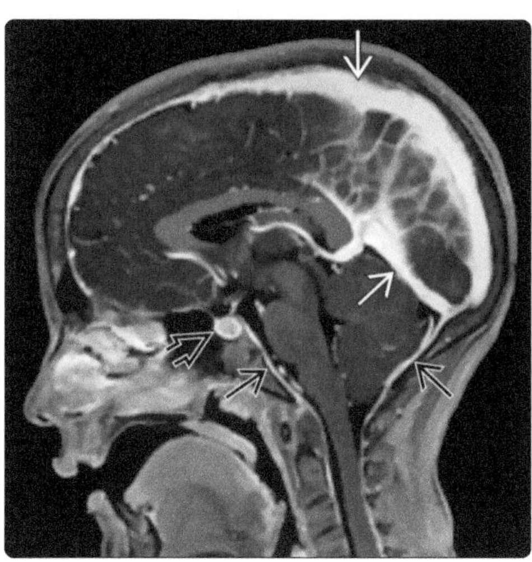

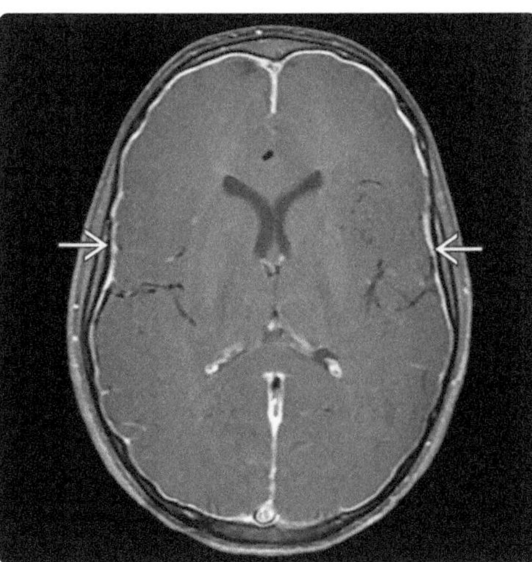

(Left) *Sagittal T1 C+ FS MR in a 6-year-old patient with back injury and significant postural headache reveals mildly reduced pontomesencephalic angle, plump pituitary (unusual for age) →, dural venous engorgement →, and dural thickening and enhancement →.* **(Right)** *Axial T1 C+ FS MR in the same patient confirms smooth symmetrical dural thickening and enhancement →. Spinal imaging (not shown) demonstrated longitudinally extensive extradural CSF collection.*

Fibrous Dysplasia

KEY FACTS

TERMINOLOGY

- Fibrous dysplasia (FD)
  - Synonyms: Craniofacial fibrous dysplasia (CFD), osteitis fibrosa, osteodystrophy fibrosa
- McCune-Albright syndrome (MAS)
- Congenital disorder characterized by expanding lesion(s)
  - Defect in osteoblastic differentiation, maturation
  - Contains mixture of fibrous tissue, woven bone

IMAGING

- Best diagnostic clue: Ground-glass matrix in bone lesion on CT
- CFD: Majority have > 1 bone involved
- MR: ↓ T2WI signal throughout (if solid) or in rim (if cystic)
  - Variable enhancement
  - Rim, diffuse, or none

TOP DIFFERENTIAL DIAGNOSES

- Paget disease
- Garré sclerosing osteomyelitis
- Meningioma

CLINICAL ISSUES

- Most common signs/symptoms: Painless swelling or deformity
- Demographics
  - < 6 years (39%), 6-10 years (27%), > 10 years (39%)
  - MAS usually (but not exclusively) female patients
  - Calvarial involvement differs: Polyostotic FD (50%) > monostotic FD (25%)
- **Rare** progression to fibro-, osteo-, chondro-, and mesenchymal sarcoma

DIAGNOSTIC CHECKLIST

- Ground-glass appearance on plain films or CT, homogeneously decreased signal on T2WI characteristic
- MR enhancement characteristics may look aggressive; low signal on both T1 and T2 reassuring for FD

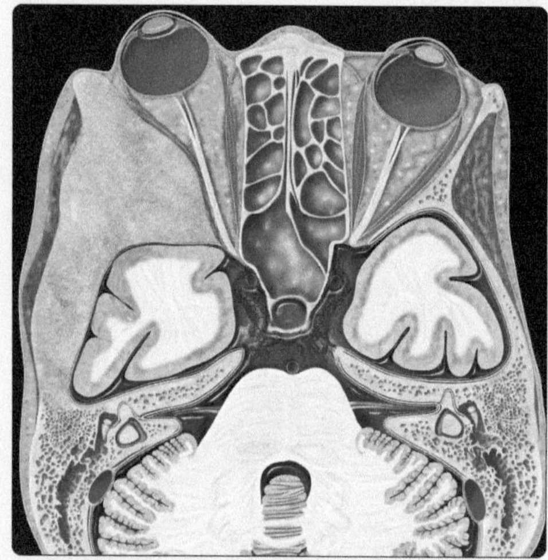

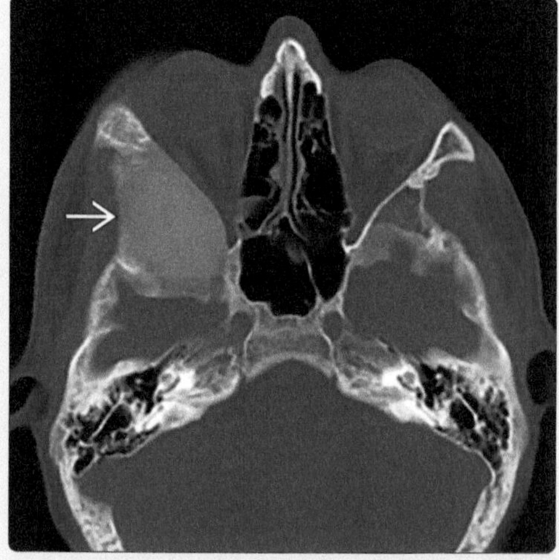

(Left) *Axial graphic shows expansion of the lateral orbital rim, sphenoid wing, and temporal squamosa by fibrous dysplasia. Note the exophthalmos and stretching of the optic nerve on the ipsilateral side.* **(Right)** *Axial bone CT in a patient presenting with facial asymmetry demonstrates classic smooth ground-glass expansion of the right greater wing of sphenoid bone ➡, mildly encroaching on the right orbit.*

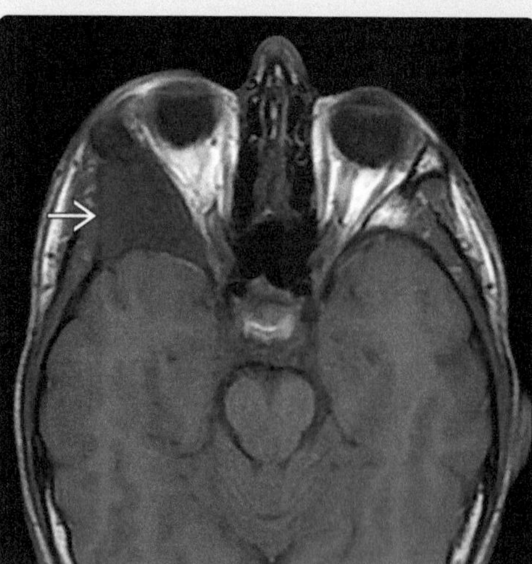

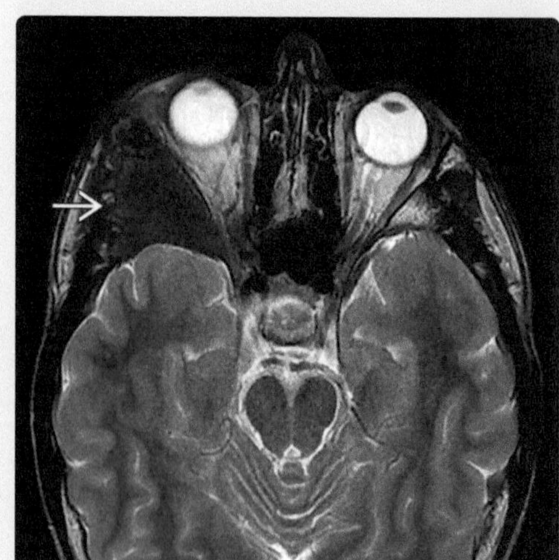

(Left) *Axial T1 MR in the same patient reveals smooth hypointense expansion of the sphenoid bone ➡. Note the mass effect on the right globe. Contrast images (not shown) revealed heterogeneous enhancement.* **(Right)** *Axial T2 MR in the same patient confirms homogeneous low signal intensity within the area of fibrous dysplasia ➡. Hypointensity on both T1 and T2 MR is characteristic of typical fibrous dysplasia.*

TERMINOLOGY

Abbreviations

- Fibrous dysplasia (FD)

Synonyms

- Craniofacial fibrous dysplasia (CFD), osteitis fibrosa, osteodystrophy fibrosa
- McCune-Albright syndrome (MAS): One of most common FD syndromes
- Jaffe-Lichtenstein dysplasia (monostotic FD)

Definitions

- Congenital disorder characterized by expanding lesions with mixture of fibrous tissue and woven bone
- Defect in osteoblastic differentiation and maturation
- One of most common fibroosseous lesions

IMAGING

General Features

- Best diagnostic clue
  - Ground-glass matrix in bone lesion on CT
- Location
  - May involve any aspect of skull
  - CFD: Majority have > 1 bone involved
    - Maxilla, orbit, and frontal bones most common in one series; ethmoids and sphenoids in another

Radiographic Findings

- Radiography
  - Expanded bone with ground-glass appearance
  - CFD: Dental malocclusions in 20%

CT Findings

- NECT
  - Imaging patterns relate to relative content of fibrous and osseous tissue
  - Expansile bone lesion, widened diploic space
  - Ground-glass, sclerotic, cystic, or mixed bone changes
    - If cystic, may have thick sclerotic rind

MR Findings

- T1WI
  - Usual: ↓ signal
- T2WI
  - Usual: ↓ signal (if solid) or in rind (if cystic)
  - ↑ clinical-pathologic activity leads to ↑ signal
- T1WI C+
  - Variable enhancement depends on lesion pattern (rim, diffuse, or none)

Nuclear Medicine Findings

- Bone scan
  - Variable radionuclide uptake: Perfusion/delayed phases
  - Nonspecific; sensitive to extent of skeletal lesions in polyostotic FD
- PET
  - Accumulation of 11C-MET
  - Can be variably hot on FDG PET
    - Should not be mistaken for metastasis
    - Correlation with radiograph, CT helps

Imaging Recommendations

- Best imaging tool
  - Bone CT
- Protocol advice
  - CT or MR to define local extent
  - Bone scan to search for additional lesions

DIFFERENTIAL DIAGNOSIS

Paget Disease

- Pagetoid ground-glass FD mimics Paget disease
- Paget: Calvarium, not craniofacial; "cotton wool" CT

Garré Sclerosing Osteomyelitis

- Bony expansion but inhomogeneous sclerotic pattern; ± dehiscent bone cortex; ± periosteal reaction

Jaffe-Campanacci Syndrome

- Nonossifying fibromas, axillary freckling, and café au lait (lacks neurofibromas)
- Mimics polyostotic forms of FD
  - Jaffe-Campanacci café au lait: Coast of California (like neurofibromatosis type 1)
  - McCune-Albright café au lait: Coast of Maine

Craniometaphyseal Dysplasia

- Hyperostosis and sclerosis of craniofacial bones → facial distortion, cranial nerve compression
- Abnormal modeling of long bone metaphyses; paranasal "bossing"

Meningioma

- Resulting hyperostosis mimics FD
- MR spectroscopy: Characteristic alanine peak

Other Disorders With Expanded Bone and Abnormal Bony Density

- Thalassemia: Maxillary sinus involvement typical; "hair on end" skull
- Osteopetrosis: Involvement of all bones
- Neurocutaneous disorders: Osteitis fibrosa cystica in
  - Tuberous sclerosis
  - Neurofibromatosis type 1
- Chronic renal failure: Renal osteodystrophy may simulate leontiasis ossea
- Morgagni syndrome of hyperostosis frontalis interna
  - Postmenopausal women, limited to frontal bone

PATHOLOGY

General Features

- Etiology
  - Mutation of Gsα protein in osteoblastic progenitor cells leads to ↑ proliferation; abnormal differentiation
- Genetics
  - Numerous up-/downregulated genes described
    - Mutations in regulatory Gsα protein (encoded by *GNAS1* gene) common to monostotic, polyostotic, and MAS
    - *ADAMTS2* significantly overexpressed in FD tissues

Staging, Grading, & Classification

- Monostotic vs. polyostotic

- Specific lesion type (pagetoid, sclerotic, cystic) relates to disease activity
  - Cystic, pagetoid, and sclerotic FD believed to represent (in order) most to least active
    - Cystic FD (11-21%): Hypodense (CT) except rind
    - Pagetoid mixed FD (56%): Ground glass plus cystic change
    - Homogeneous sclerotic FD (23-34%)

Gross Pathologic & Surgical Features

- Fibrous, tan to gray gritty tissue
- Variable consistency depends upon fibrous vs. osseous components
- Woven bone immature, structurally weak, prone to fractures
- Hemorrhage, cystic change may be present

Microscopic Features

- Fibrous stroma, usually avascular, low cellularity
- Osseous metaplasia: Bone trabeculae made up of immature, woven bone seen as peculiar shapes floating in fibrous stroma ("alphabet soup")

CLINICAL ISSUES

Presentation

- Most common signs/symptoms
  - Swelling &/or deformity, pain
- Clinical profile
  - Proptosis, cranial neuropathy (diplopia, hearing loss, blindness), atypical facial pain or numbness, headache
  - Multiple endocrine disorders typically with severe polyostotic FD
- Presentations: Monostotic, polyostotic, craniofacial (CFD), syndromic (many known syndromes)
  - Monostotic FD
    - 70% of all FD cases; single osseous site affected
      - Skull, face involved in 27%
      - Most common: Maxilla (especially zygomatic process), mandible (molar area)
      - Less common: Frontal > ethmoid, sphenoid > temporal > occipital bones
    - Older children/young adults (75% present < 30 years)
  - Polyostotic FD
    - 30% of all FD cases; involves ≥ 2 separate sites
    - Skull, face involved in 50%
    - Younger group, 67% have symptoms by age 10
  - CFD
    - Autosomal dominant, stabilizes with skeletal maturity
  - MAS
    - Subtype of unilateral polyostotic FD: Clinical triad of polyostotic FD, hyperfunctioning endocrinopathies, café au lait spots
    - 5% of FD cases; appears earlier; affects more bones more severely
    - Renal phosphate wasting (50%) associated with elevation of circulating factor FGF-23; may result in rickets and osteomalacia
  - Mazabraud syndrome
    - Polyostotic FD, intramuscular myxoma
  - Cherubism: Familial bilateral FD of jaw
  - Mulibrey nanism: Severe, progressive growth failure; pericardial constriction; primarily in Finland
    - **Mu**scle, **li**ver, **br**ain, **ey**e = triangular face, yellow ocular fundi pigment, hypoplastic tongue, peculiar high voice, nevi flammei (65%)
    - FD of long bones in 25%

Demographics

- Age
  - < 6 years (39%), 6-10 years (27%), > 10 years (39%)
- Sex
  - MAS usually (but not exclusively) female patients
- Epidemiology
  - Actual incidence unknown
    - Monostotic FD is 6x more common than polyostotic FD
    - Calvarial involvement differs: Polyostotic FD (50%) > monostotic FD (25%)
    - Monostotic FD (75%): 25% found in skull, face
    - Polyostotic FD (25%): 50% found in skull, face

Natural History & Prognosis

- **Rare** progression to osteo-, fibrous-, chondro-, and mesenchymal sarcoma
  - Usually polyostotic/syndromic forms
  - Nearly 50% arise following irradiation (marked increase in malignant potential)
- Monostotic craniofacial FD has excellent prognosis
- Most spontaneously "burn out" in teens, 20s

Treatment

- Aggressive resection reserved for visual loss, severe deformity ("vault" more accessible than skull base)
- No radiation therapy → malignant progression
- Alendronate treatment does not change pain scores, skeletal disease burden scores, or functional parameters

DIAGNOSTIC CHECKLIST

Consider

- Monostotic and polyostotic FD likely on same spectrum of phenotypic expression; consider checking for gene to predict complications
- Chiari 1 common due to reduction of posterior fossa volume from skull thickening

Image Interpretation Pearls

- Ground-glass appearance on plain films or CT, homogeneously decreased signal on T2WI characteristic

SELECTED REFERENCES

1. Behbahani M et al: Endoscopic endonasal optic nerve decompression: treatment of fibrous dysplasia in a pediatric population. J Neurosurg Pediatr. 31(2):179-85, 2023
2. Sato K et al: Long-term imaging course of Chiari malformation type I due to fibrous dysplasia/McCune-Albright syndrome. Childs Nerv Syst. 38(9):1817-20, 2022
3. Mierzwiński J et al: Different clinical presentation and management of temporal bone fibrous dysplasia in children. World J Surg Oncol. 16(1):5, 2018
4. Wilson M et al: Fibro-osseous lesions of the skull base in the pediatric population. J Neurol Surg B Skull Base. 79(1):31-6, 2018
5. Frisch CD et al: Fibrous dysplasia of the temporal bone: a review of 66 cases. Laryngoscope. 125(6):1438-43, 2015

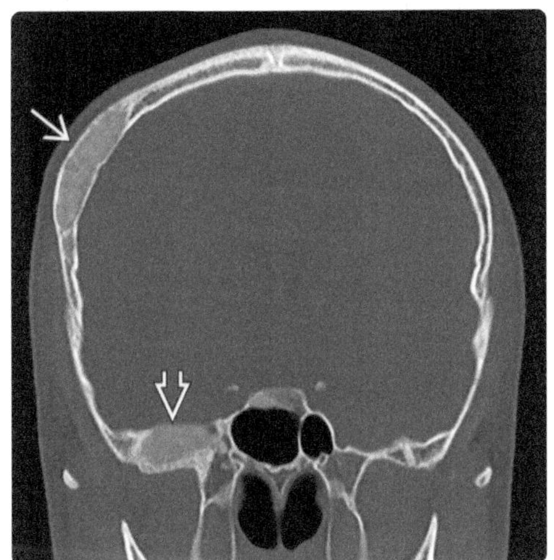

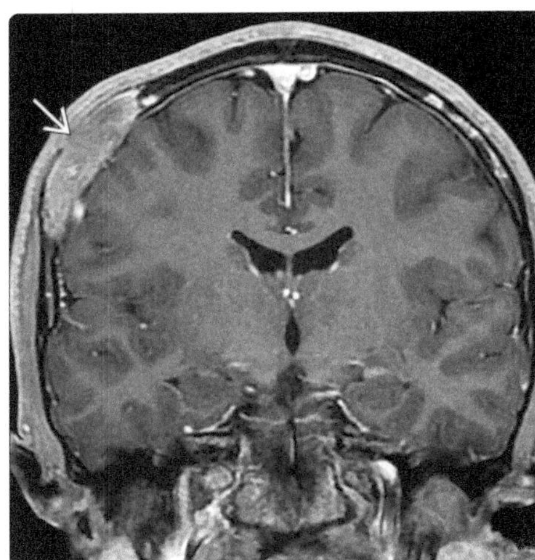

(Left) *Coronal bone CT in a patient with a palpable hard mass of the right parietal bone* ➡ *shows mildly heterogeneous bone expansion with ground-glass attenuation. Note the 2nd focus of fibrous dysplasia* ➡ *in the right sphenoid bone.* **(Right)** *Coronal T1 C+ FS MR in the same patient demonstrates mildly heterogeneous enhancement of the fibrous dysplasia* ➡*. Note that the lesion is more aggressive-appearing on MR than CT.*

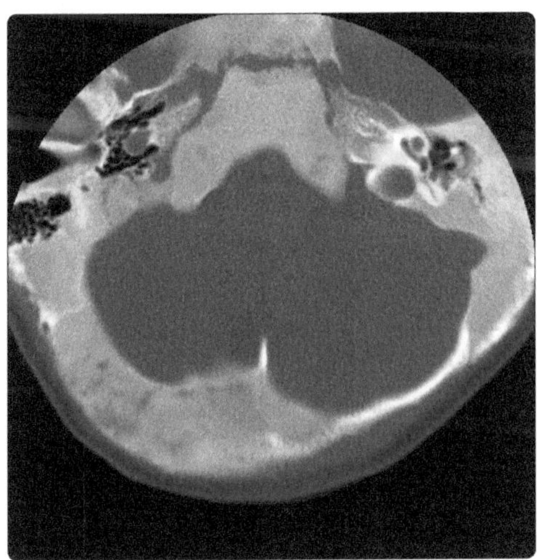

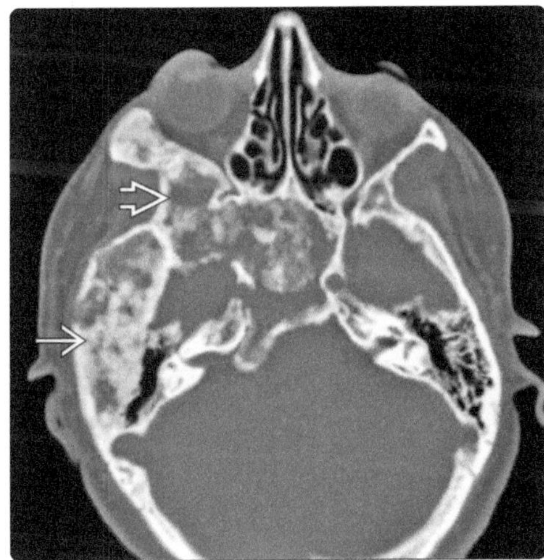

(Left) *Axial bone CT of the temporal and occipital bones in a patient with conductive hearing loss reveals extensive fibrous dysplasia with bone expansion and ground-glass matrix within the diploic spaces.* **(Right)** *Axial bone CT demonstrates the pagetoid mixed fibrous dysplasia variant with a ground-glass matrix* ➡ *and cystic changes* ➡ *involving the sphenoid, zygomatic, and temporal bones.*

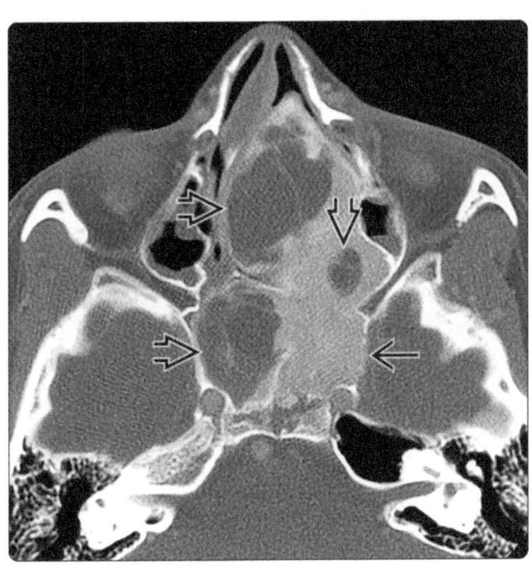

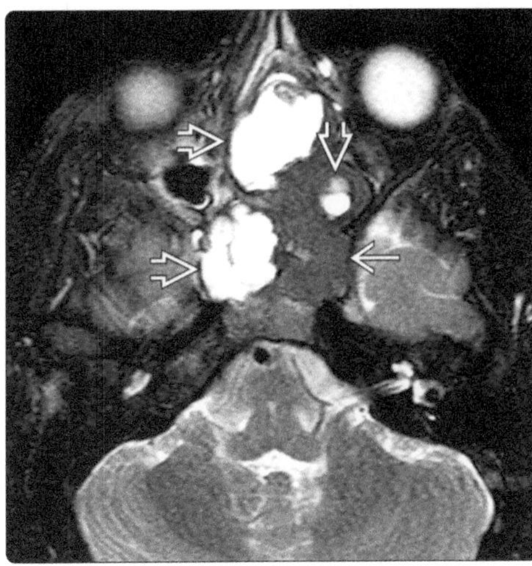

(Left) *Axial bone CT in a 9-year-old girl demonstrates the cystic variant of fibrous dysplasia. Note the areas of frank cystic formation* ➡ *within and adjacent to more characteristic ground-glass appearance* ➡*.* **(Right)** *Axial T2 FS MR confirms the complex nature of this lesion. The ground-glass components* ➡ *show a quite low signal while the cystic areas* ➡ *show high (fluid) signal intensity. The cystic variant of fibrous dysplasia is the least common and is felt to represent the most active phase of the disease.*

Extramedullary Hematopoiesis

KEY FACTS

TERMINOLOGY

- Extramedullary compensatory formation of blood elements due to decreased medullary hematopoiesis

IMAGING

- Skull (epidural, dura matter, sinuses), spine (paraspinal, epidural)
  - Too thick or dense skull
  - May show findings of underlying disease
- Contrast-enhanced MR
  - Smooth, juxtaspinal or cranial homogeneous masses in patients with chronic anemias or marrow depletion
- Look for local complication
  - Cranial foramina, nerves
  - Spinal nerve involvement
  - Cord compression

TOP DIFFERENTIAL DIAGNOSES

- Meningioma
- Metastases
- Subdural collections
- Intracranial hypotension

PATHOLOGY

- Trilineage hyperplasia: Erythroid, myeloid, and megakaryocytic elements
- Primarily patients with congenital hemoglobinopathies
  - Thalassemia, sickle cell disease
- May be secondary to any depleted, infiltrated, or hyperactive bone marrow
  - Myelofibrosis/myelodysplastic syndromes
  - Leukemia

DIAGNOSTIC CHECKLIST

- EMH is dural &/or subdural hematoma mimic
- Think of EMH in unexplained extraaxial "collections" or perivertebral masses in child with congenital anemia or other hematologic disorder

(Left) *Graphic depicts cranial manifestations of extramedullary hematopoiesis (EMH). The diploic space converts from fatty to hematopoietic ("red") marrow ➡. Multiple lobulated, extraaxial masses ➡, usually subdural, can occur in severe cases.* **(Right)** *Axial NECT in a patient with myelofibrosis shows a well-delineated, lobulated, hyperdense mass ➡ adjacent to the falx cerebri.*

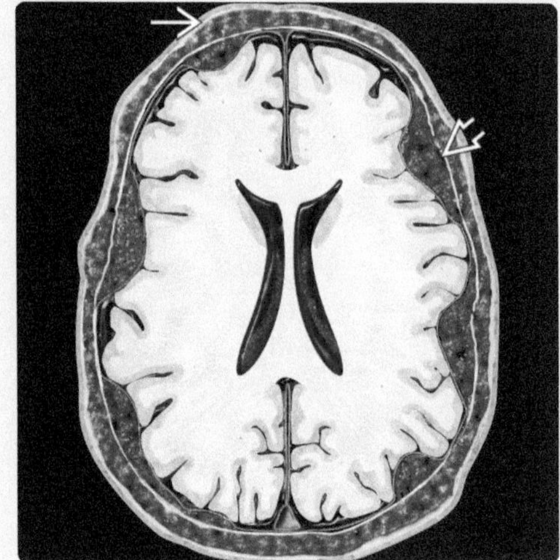

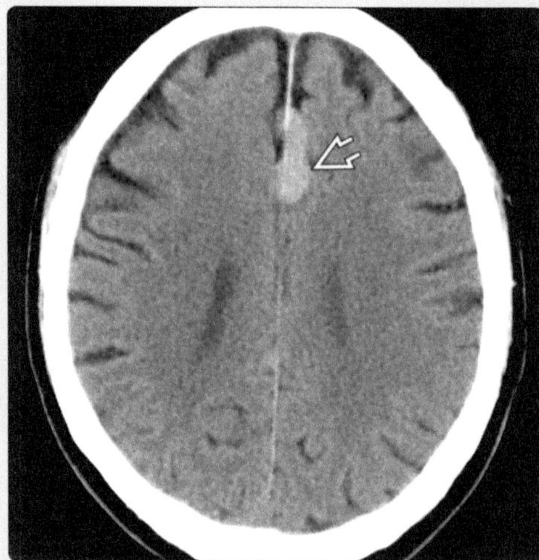

(Left) *Axial T2WI FS MR in the same patient shows multiple extraaxial, dural-based, hypointense masses ➡ along the falx.* **(Right)** *Axial T1WI C+ FS MR in the same patient shows the masses enhance intensely and uniformly ➡. Myelofibrosis/myelodysplastic syndromes are 2nd only to anemia as the most common underlying cause of EMH.*

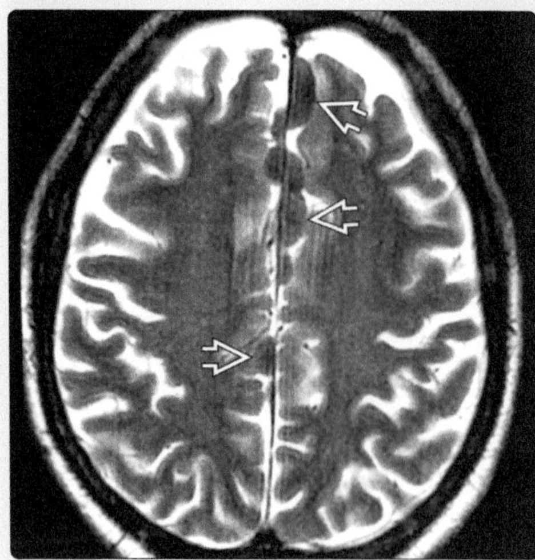

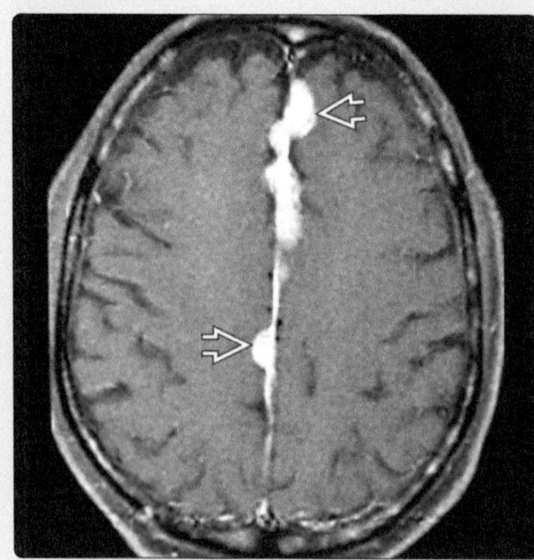

TERMINOLOGY

Abbreviations

- Extramedullary hematopoiesis (EMH)

Synonyms

- Extramedullary erythropoiesis

Definitions

- Extramedullary compensatory formation of blood elements due to decreased medullary hematopoiesis

IMAGING

General Features

- Best diagnostic clue
  - Smooth, juxtaspinal or cranial homogeneous masses in patients with chronic anemia or marrow depletion
- Location
  - Skull (epidural, dura matter, sinuses), spine (paraspinal, epidural)
  - May be seen in multiple other organs: Kidneys, adrenals, thyroid, liver, spleen, lymph nodes, peritoneum
- Size
  - Variable, sometimes huge
- Morphology
  - Smooth, juxtaosseous circumscribed masses
  - Hypercellular tissue

Radiographic Findings

- Radiography
  - May show findings of underlying disease
    - Thalassemia → "hair on end" skull
    - Osteopetrosis → dense bone obliterating medullary space

CT Findings

- NECT
  - Smooth, homogeneous, isodense masses
    - May mimic subdural hematoma, lymphoma
    - Also simulates en plaque meningioma
  - May show osseous findings of underlying disease
    - Too thick or dense skull
    - Enlarged diploë
    - Changes of vertebral structure
  - Soft tissue filling paranasal sinus(es), orbits, juxtasellar regions
- CECT
  - Homogeneous enhancement

MR Findings

- T1WI
  - Isointense to slightly hyperintense to cortex
- T2WI
  - Slightly hypointense to cortex
- FLAIR
  - Hyperintense
  - No underlying parenchymal edema
- T1WI C+
  - Homogeneous enhancement
  - Simulates en plaque meningioma

Nuclear Medicine Findings

- Uptake by Tc-99m sulfur colloid

Imaging Recommendations

- Best imaging tool
  - Contrast-enhanced multiplanar MR
- Protocol advice
  - Investigate bone as well as soft tissue masses
    - Etiologic context usually known
    - CT: Thickening of diploë, erosions, paranasal sinus disease
    - MR: Bone marrow changes in vertebral bodies
  - Look for local complication
    - Cranial foramina, nerves
    - Spinal nerve involvement
    - Cord compression

DIFFERENTIAL DIAGNOSIS

Meningioma

- Different context, different bony findings
- MRS (often impossible in masses adjacent to bone): Characteristic alanine peak

Metastases

- Often multifocal, infiltrative, skull invasion

Subdural Collections

- Trauma history
- Enhancement of limiting membranes, not diffuse

Intracranial Hypotension

- Thick skull, thick enhancing dura
- May have associated subdural hematomas
- Enlarged dural venous sinuses
- Tonsillar descent, bulging pituitary
- ± history of CSF diversion or leak

Neurosarcoid

- Abnormal chest radiograph, labs

Other Paraspinal Masses

- Spondylitis, abscesses: Bone, disk involved, peripheral abscesses
- Lymphoma

PATHOLOGY

General Features

- Etiology
  - Hematogenous stem cell spread to different organs
    - Liver and spleen
    - Kidneys
    - Lungs
    - Peritoneum
    - Juxtaosseous also common
      - Face
      - Skull
      - Spine
  - Primarily patients with congenital hemoglobinopathies
    - Thalassemia
    - Sickle cell disease

- Hereditary spherocytosis
- Hemorrhagic thrombocytopenia
- Leukemia
- Lymphoma
- Myeloid metaplasia

o Others
- May be secondary to any depleted, infiltrated, or hyperactive bone marrow
  - Can be seen after granulocyte colony-stimulating factor therapy
- May be seen in any myelofibrosis/myelodysplastic syndrome
  - Hematologic disorders (e.g., polycythemia vera)
  - Bone diseases
  - Exposure to ionizing radiation, benzene

o Occasionally, no etiology found

- Genetics
  - Causal disease
    - Congenital hemoglobinopathies
    - Genetic hemopathies
    - Myelosclerosis of genetic causes
- Associated abnormalities
  - Secondary subdural hemorrhage from EMH involvement of dura reported

Gross Pathologic & Surgical Features

- Periosseous soft tissue masses
- Epidural EMH may compress underlying neural tissue
- Associated bony changes

Microscopic Features

- Trilineage hyperplasia
  - Erythroid elements
  - Myeloid elements
  - Megakaryocytic elements

CLINICAL ISSUES

Presentation

- Most common signs/symptoms
  - Asymptomatic
  - Seizures
  - Cranial nerve deficit(s) at skull base
  - Increased intracranial pressure, if compressing dural sinuses
  - Myelopathy, if compressing spinal cord
- Clinical profile
  - Generally older adults with myelofibrosis
  - Younger patients with congenital hemolytic anemias

Demographics

- Age
  - Generally in older patients, but EMH has its own specific pediatric causes
- Sex
  - Equal
- Epidemiology
  - Rare

Natural History & Prognosis

- Evolution dependent on primary underlying disease
- Compensatory for bone marrow failure
- Uncommonly, local complications related to compression

Treatment

- Treat primary disease
- Low-dose radiotherapy is treatment of choice
  - Remember that hematopoietic tissue is extremely sensitive to irradiation
- Surgical resection

DIAGNOSTIC CHECKLIST

Consider

- Think of EMH in unexplained extraaxial "collections" or perivertebral masses in child with congenital anemia or other hematologic disorder

Image Interpretation Pearls

- EMH is dural &/or subdural hematoma mimic

SELECTED REFERENCES

1. Nichols NM et al: Intracranial extramedullary hematopoiesis in a patient with beta-thalassemia presenting with head trauma. Surg Neurol Int. 13:542, 2022
2. Woodward Z et al: Intracranial sclerosing extramedullary haematopoietic tumour mimicking meningioma in a patient with myelofibrosis: case report. J Clin Neurosci. 88:268-70, 2021
3. Xue JY et al: Expanding the phenotypic spectrum of TNFRSF11A-associated dysosteosclerosis: a case with intracranial extramedullary hematopoiesis. J Hum Genet. 66(6):607-11, 2021
4. Merchant R et al: Intracranial hematopoiesis in beta thalassemia: a case series. Indian J Pediatr. 85(8):679-81, 2018
5. Reddy R: Intracranial extramedullary hematopoiesis in primary myelofibrosis. Neurol India. 65(4):913-4, 2017
6. Mehta S et al: Intracranial extramedullary haematopoiesis: a case report. Br J Neurosurg. 1-3, 2015
7. Mughal TI et al: Myelofibrosis-associated complications: pathogenesis, clinical manifestations, and effects on outcomes. Int J Gen Med. 7:89-101, 2014
8. Singer A et al: Intracranial extramedullary hematopoiesis: a rare cause of headaches. J Neuroimaging. 24(5):524-7, 2014
9. Ghieda U et al: Progressive spinal cord compression due to epidural extramedullary hematopoiesis in thalassemia intermedia. A case report and literature review. Neuroradiol J. 26(1):111-7, 2013
10. Palma JA et al: Intracranial extramedullary hematopoiesis associated with multiple myeloma. Neurology. 80(17):1620, 2013
11. Tefferi A: Primary myelofibrosis: 2013 update on diagnosis, risk-stratification, and management. Am J Hematol. 88(2):141-50, 2013
12. Eskazan AE et al: Intracranial extramedullary hematopoiesis in patients with thalassemia: a case report and review of the literature. Transfusion. 52(8):1715-20, 2012
13. Sohawon D et al: Extra-medullary haematopoiesis: a pictorial review of its typical and atypical locations. J Med Imaging Radiat Oncol. 56(5):538-44, 2012
14. Jiang WX et al: 37-year-old woman with multiple intracranial masses. Brain Pathol. 21(5):607-10, 2011
15. Zherebitskiy V et al: Extramedullary hematopoiesis involving the central nervous system and surrounding structures. Hum Pathol. 42(10):1524-30, 2011
16. Debard A et al: Dural localization of extramedullary hematopoiesis. Report of a case. J Neurol. 256(5):837-8, 2009
17. Tun K et al: Meningeal extramedullary haematopoiesis mimicking subdural hematoma. J Clin Neurosci. 15(2):208-10, 2008
18. Collins WO et al: Extramedullary hematopoiesis of the paranasal sinuses in sickle cell disease. Otolaryngol Head Neck Surg. 132(6):954-6, 2005
19. Haidar S et al: Intracranial involvement in extramedullary hematopoiesis: case report and review of the literature. Pediatr Radiol. 35(6):630-4, 2005
20. Koch CA et al: Nonhepatosplenic extramedullary hematopoiesis: associated diseases, pathology, clinical course, and treatment. Mayo Clin Proc. 78(10):1223-33, 2003

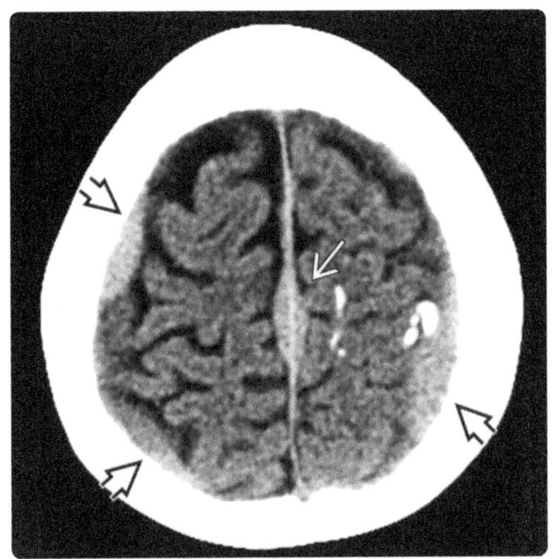

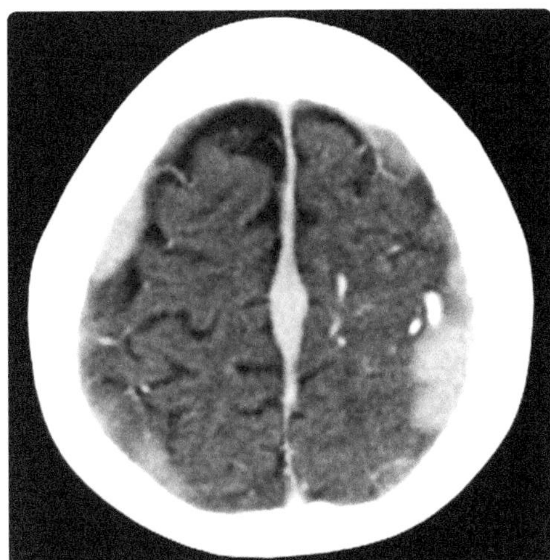

(Left) *Axial NECT in an 8-year-old girl with myelofibrosis shows multiple extraaxial masses ⇨, most likely due to dural, epidural, &/or subdural intramedullary hematopoiesis. Note the falx ➡, where the mass is shown on both sides of the dural layer. The masses are slightly denser than the brain with (probably) dural calcifications, consistent with EMH.* **(Right)** *Axial CECT in the same patient demonstrates diffuse, rather homogeneous enhancement of the lesions, again in keeping with EMH. EMH was confirmed by surgical biopsy.*

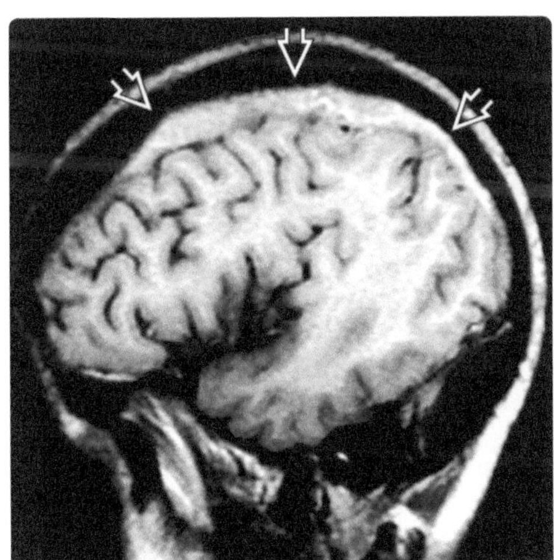

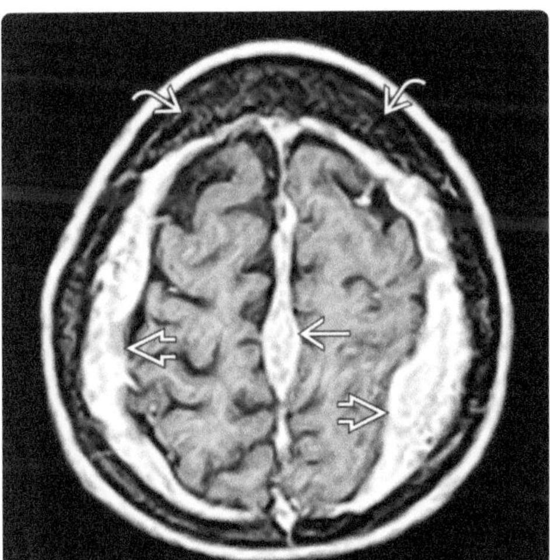

(Left) *Sagittal T1WI MR in an 8-year-old girl with myelosclerosis of an unknown cause reveals slightly T1-hyperintense extradural tissue ➡ overlying the hemisphere. Note that the adjacent bone appears normal.* **(Right)** *Axial T1WI C+ MR demonstrates avid enhancement in bilateral dural/epidural lesions over the cerebral convexities ➡ and along the falx cerebri ➡. The diagnosis of EMH was confirmed by a dural biopsy. Note also the marked overlying calvarial thickening ➡.*

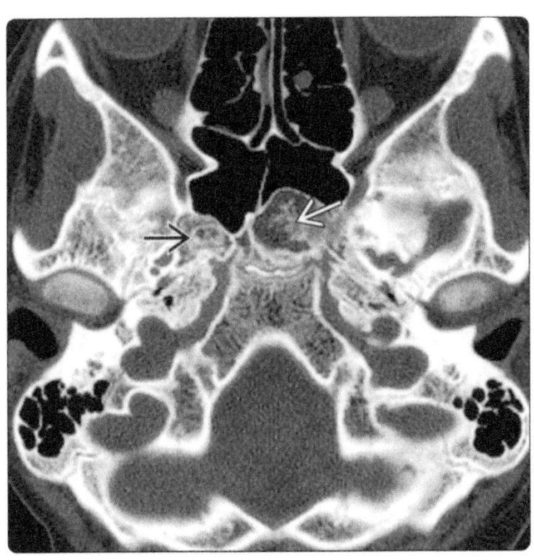

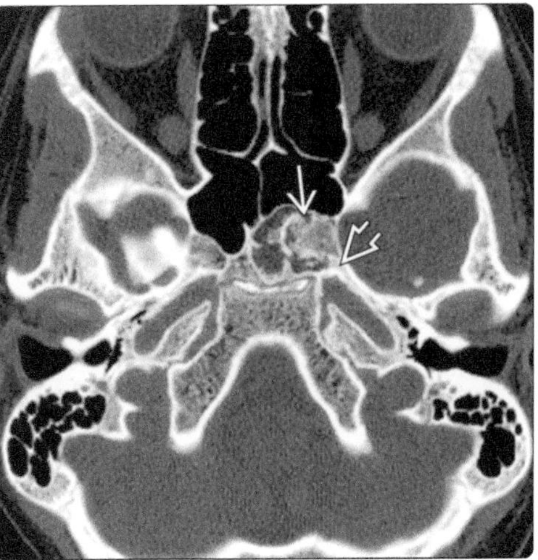

(Left) *Axial bone CT in a 13-year-old with thalassemia shows asymptomatic masses within the body of the sphenoid ➡ and the base of the right pterygoid plate ⇨ with bone expansion but preservation of the cortex, suggestive of, but not specific for, EMH.* **(Right)** *Axial bone CT at a higher level shows the proximity of the sphenoid body lesion ➡ to the carotid canal ➡. This patient had multiple sites of proven EMH in other locations; therefore, this is the most likely diagnosis.*

Thick Skull

KEY FACTS

TERMINOLOGY

- Skull thickening (ST)
  - Diploic space expanded ± thickened cortex

IMAGING

- Widened calvarium (skull width)
  - Can be diffuse or focal
- NECT best for most causes of ST
  - Thin-section MDCT for detailed skull base evaluation
- MR C+: Look for adjacent dural involvement

TOP DIFFERENTIAL DIAGNOSES

- Normal variation (most common cause)
- Shunted hydrocephalus or infantile brain injury
  - Neonatal meningitis or cerebritis
  - Hypoxia/ischemia/hypoglycemia in neonatal period
  - Metabolic/genetic disease with infantile brain atrophy
  - ± phenytoin
- Metastases (diffuse sclerotic)
- Microcephaly
- Chronic anemias

CLINICAL ISSUES

- Often asymptomatic
- Patients with skull base ST
  - Look for foraminal/canal overgrowth/encroachment
  - May cause cranial neuropathy
- In many cases, evaluation of underlying brain can help to establish diagnosis
- Many tests can help discriminate among etiologies
- Skull findings often harbinger of underlying disease
- Therapy aimed at treating underlying etiology

DIAGNOSTIC CHECKLIST

- What is underlying cause of ST?
  - Keep in mind: Most often it is normal variant
- Consider focal vs. diffuse, other involved bones, intracranial findings

(Left) *Sagittal T1 MR in a patient with seizures on chronic phenytoin therapy reveals characteristic diffuse skull hyperostosis with expansion of the diploic space. Note also cerebellar vermian atrophy.* **(Right)** *Axial T2 MR in a pediatric patient with bilateral Sturge-Weber syndrome reveals bilateral brain atrophy (worse on the right) with chronic subdural fluid collections as well as compensatory diffuse skull thickening favoring the frontal bones.*

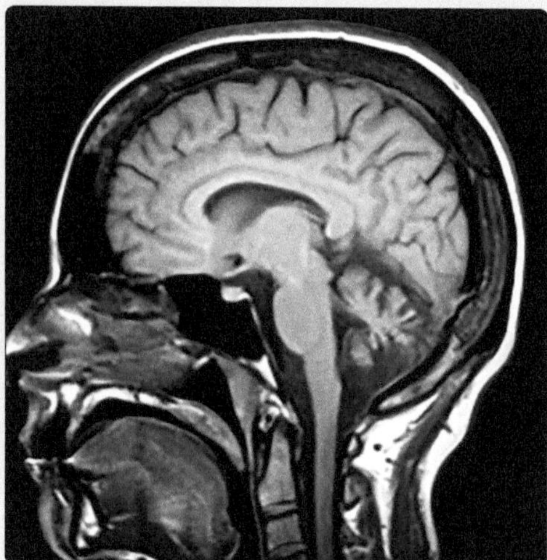

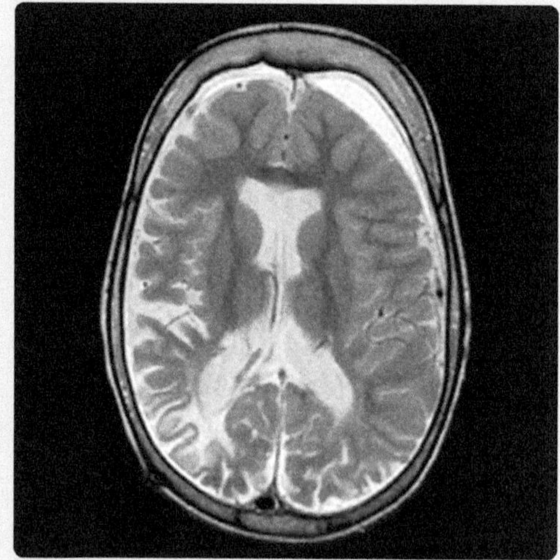

(Left) *Coronal bone CT in a case of severe polyostotic fibrous dysplasia shows extensive calvarial and skull base thickening with ground-glass attenuation. Note curious sparing of the left squamous temporal bone* ➙. **(Right)** *Coronal bone CT in an infant with development of a hard left parietal mass prompting imaging shows a characteristic appearance for ossifying cephalohematoma* ➙. *Recognizing an intact inner table and eliciting pertinent neonatal history assists in the diagnosis.*

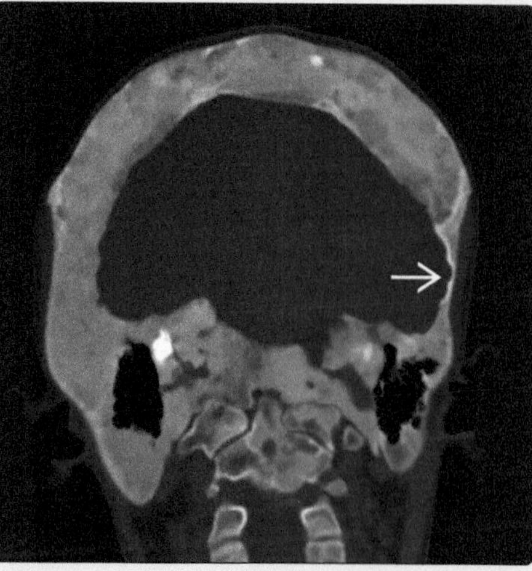

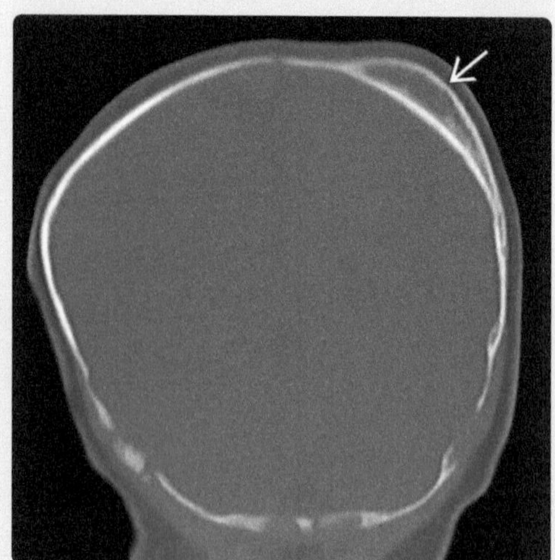

TERMINOLOGY

Synonyms

- Skull thickening (ST), calvarial thickening

Definitions

- Diploic space expansion ± adjacent cortical thickening

IMAGING

General Features

- Best diagnostic clue
  - Diffuse/focal increased skull width; variable size
- Location
  - Any bone can be involved; calvarium > skull base > occipital squamae
- Morphology
  - Generalized, regional or focal, depending on etiology

Radiographic Findings

- Radiography
  - Not useful for diffuse unless thickening is striking
  - Focal thickening more easily appreciated

CT Findings

- NECT
  - Thick skull: Findings may be classic/pathognomic
    - Local brain atrophy: Ipsilateral compensatory osseous hypertrophy/hyperpneumatization of paranasal sinuses
    - β-thalassemia: Hair-on-end skull appearance
    - Shunted hydrocephalus: Thick skull + shunt + chronic collapsed ventricles
    - Fibrous dysplasia: Medullary expansion with ground-glass appearance

MR Findings

- T1, T2 may show diploic widening; depends on etiology
- Any sequence: Dural sinus displacement in focal thickening

Nuclear Medicine Findings

- Bone scan
  - Variable, dependent on cause of ST
- PET
  - Rarely useful in children

Imaging Recommendations

- Best imaging tool
  - NECT for most causes of ST
  - MR for brain assessment
- Protocol advice
  - Thin-section, high-resolution MDCT
    - Coronal and sagittal reformats
    - Goal: Thoroughly evaluate foramina and canals

DIFFERENTIAL DIAGNOSIS

Normal Anatomic Variation

- Normal skulls may have symmetric areas of thickening

Microcephaly

- Skull overgrowth occurs secondary to decreasing brain size in child

Many Others

- Shunted hydrocephalus
- Localized atrophy (e.g., Sturge-Weber disease)
- Chronic anemias

PATHOLOGY

General Features

- Etiology
  - Generalized ST: Drugs (phenytoin), microcephaly, hyperparathyroidism, osteopetrosis
  - Regional ST: Calcified cephalohematoma, localized cerebral atrophy, epidermal nevus syndrome, fibrous dysplasia
- Associated anomalies vary with genetic involvement/predisposition and systemic causes

Microscopic Features

- Specific histopathology varies greatly, dependent on underlying cause

CLINICAL ISSUES

Presentation

- Most common signs/symptoms
  - Most often asymptomatic; varies with etiology
  - Without skull base disease: Most symptoms referable to disease affecting systems outside skull
  - Patients with skull base ST may be symptomatic from foraminal or canal encroachment
    - Manifests as cranial nerve (CN) deficit(s)
    - Sinoorbital and auditory complications

Natural History & Prognosis

- Aggressive lesions, especially those involving skull base, have associated morbidity; usually CN deficit(s)

Treatment

- Usually no treatment required

DIAGNOSTIC CHECKLIST

Consider

- What is underlying cause of ST?

Reporting Tips

- Focal vs. diffuse, other bones, intracranial findings

SELECTED REFERENCES

1. Sato K et al: Long-term imaging course of Chiari malformation type I due to fibrous dysplasia/McCune-Albright syndrome. Childs Nerv Syst. 38(9):1817-20, 2022
2. Guzik A et al: Abnormal cranium development in children and adolescents affected by syndromes or diseases associated with neurodysfunction. Sci Rep. 11(1):2908, 2021
3. Wang Y et al: Whether cranial expansion is indicated in selected cases with microcephaly? Clin Neurol Neurosurg. 207:106748, 2021
4. Kandemirli SG et al: Temporal evolution of imaging findings in ossified cephalohematoma. J Craniofac Surg. 31(4):e375-8, 2020
5. Warne RR et al: The bone does not predict the brain in Sturge-Weber syndrome. AJNR Am J Neuroradiol. 39(8):1543-9, 2018
6. Wilson M et al: Fibro-osseous lesions of the skull base in the pediatric population. J Neurol Surg B Skull Base. 79(1):31-6, 2018
7. Tomlinson AR et al: Pediatric calvarial bone thickness in patients with and without aural atresia. Otol Neurotol. 38(10):1470-5, 2017
8. Sharma B et al: Dyke-Davidoff-Masson syndrome: a clinicoradiological amalgam. BMJ Case Rep. 2014, 2014

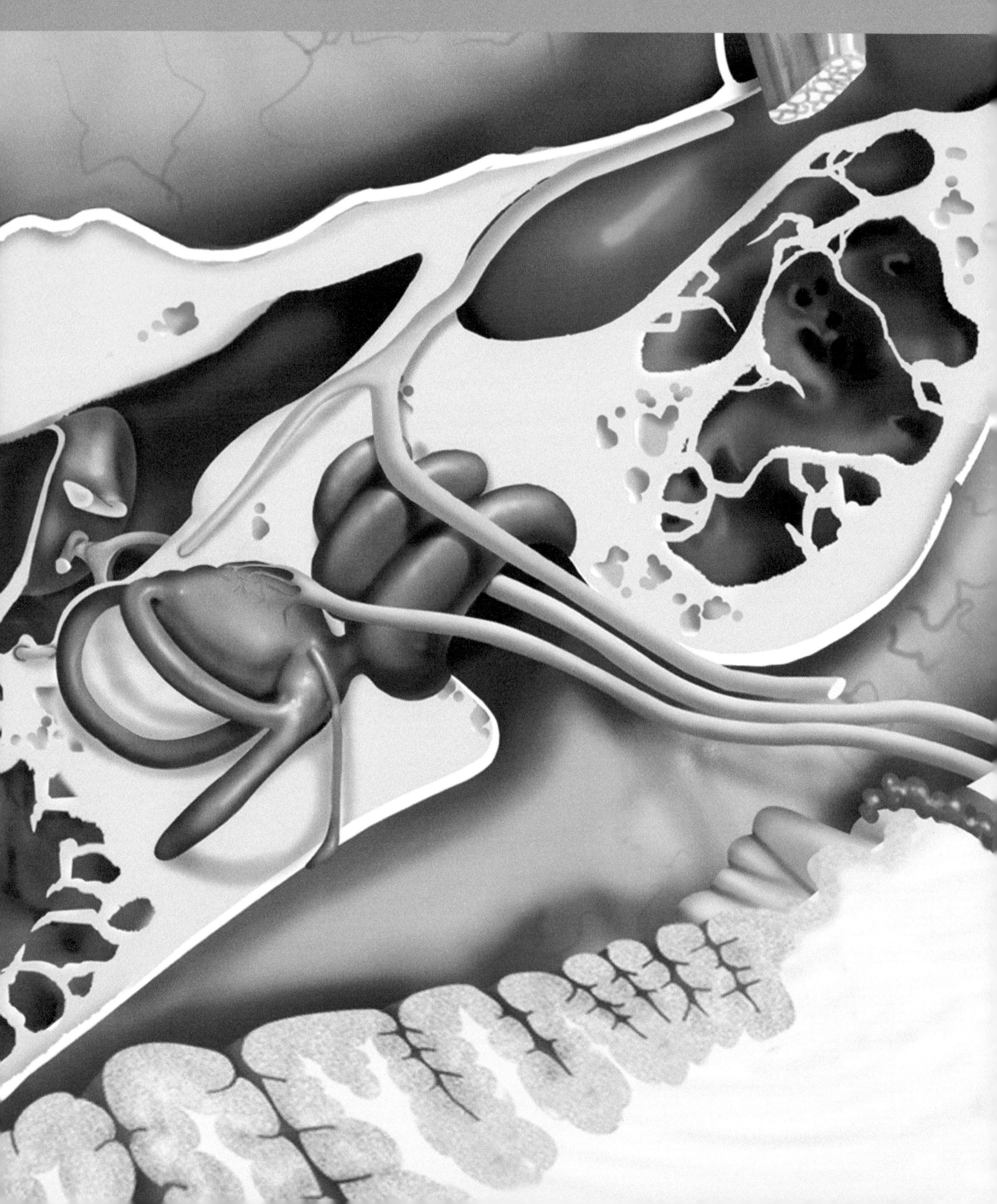

Part II

SECTION 1

Temporal Bone and Skull Base

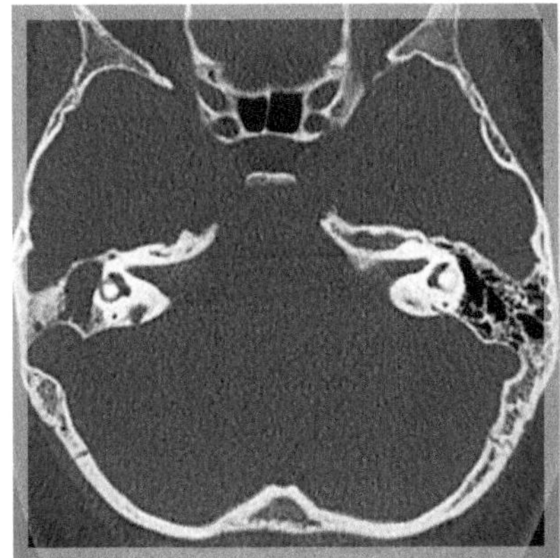
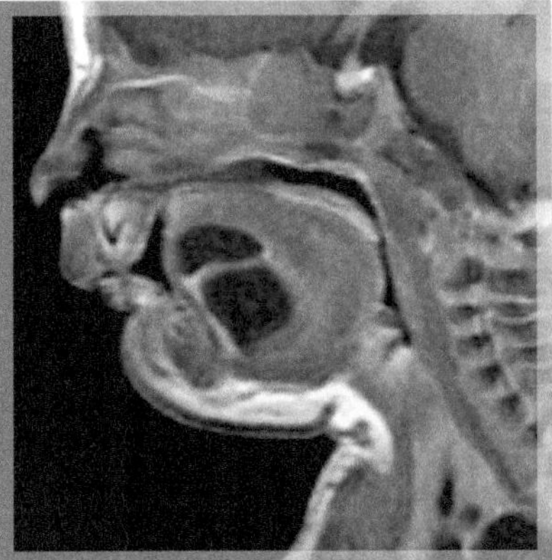
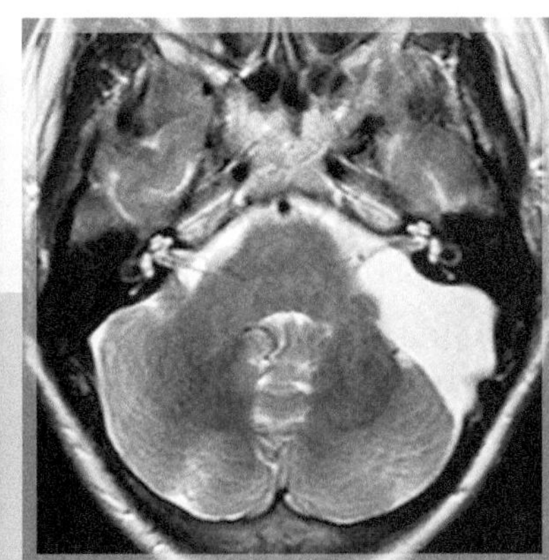

Introduction

Membranous malformations with pathology involving inner ear hair cells cause **80%** of congenital hearing loss in which high-res CT and heavily T2-weighted 3D MRs appear normal; **20%** have inner ear malformations (IEMs) involving the bony labyrinth with findings that are **seen on CT/MR.**

Jackler et al. (1987) classified IEMs into 5 groups based on embryogenesis and developmental arrest: Complete labyrinthine aplasia (CLA) (Michel deformity), cochlear aplasia, common cavity (CC), cochlear hypoplasia (CH), and incomplete partition (IP). **Sennaroglu and Saatci (2002)** revised the IEM classification, including IP types I and II. In 2006, X-linked deafness was recognized as IP type III, and Sennaroglu et al. later made updates in the IEM classification.

The current classification includes **8 distinct IEM groups. Similar-appearing cochlear anomalies are grouped together**, and they have similar clinical findings and treatment options. However, a functional outcome with cochlear implantation (CI) also depends on cochlear nerve status.

Treatment, including CI or auditory brainstem implantation (ABI) choice, is based on 3 factors: Classification of IEM, cochlear nerve status, and preoperative audiologic findings.

A stapes footplate fistula is seen in 3.6% of all IEMs. It is most commonly in the CC (18%), followed by IP-I (15%), and, rarely, in cochlear aplasia (5.2%), CH-I (5.6%), CH-II (4.4%), and IP-II (0.85%).

Radiologic signs of a stapes footplate fistula with recurrent meningitis necessitating middle ear exploration and the above IEM subgroups include an oval window area, round soft tissue density on CT/cystic structure on MR, and middle ear effusion continuous with and similar to the signal of the CSF-containing inner ear on MR, which may extend through the eustachian tube into the nasopharynx.

1. Complete Labyrinthine (Michel) Aplasia

Complete absence of inner ear structures, such as the cochlea, vestibule, and semicircular canals (SCCs) has 3 subgroups. Embryologically, it is due to arrest of **otic placode** development **before** the **3rd** gestational **week**. The treatment is **ABI**.

(1) CLA with hypoplastic or aplastic petrous bone: Middle ear could be adjacent to posterior fossa.

(2) CLA without otic capsule: Hypo/aplastic otic capsule but normal petrous bone.

(3) CLA with otic capsule: Normal otic capsule and petrous bone. Labyrinthine segment of the facial canal is in the normal location only for this subgroup. Otic capsule development is essential for normal facial canal location.

2. Rudimentary Otocyst

This is a round or ovoid, tiny (a few mm in size) otocyst **without an inner auditory canal (IAC)**. It may have accompanying small, rudimentary parts of SCCs.

Do not mistake this for a CC malformation, which has an IAC with a cochleovestibular nerve (CVN) connecting the brainstem to the CC.

3. Cochlear Aplasia

The cochlea is absent, but the vestibule, SCCs, and IAC are present in some form. The facial nerve canal is anteriorly displaced, occupying the normal cochlea location, and the anterior genu may have an obtuse angle. Embryologically, it is due to arrest of **otic placode** development at the **late 3rd** gestational **week**. The treatment is **ABI**.

Two subgroups, defined by the size of the vestibular system, are as follows.

(1) Cochlear aplasia with normal labyrinth: Normally developed vestibule and SCCs.

(2) Cochlear aplasia with dilated vestibule (CADV): Dilated vestibule and normal or dilated SCCs. It is extremely important to **distinguish CADV from a CC malformation**. CI is contraindicated in cochlear aplasia and requires ABI, whereas CI can be done in the CC if the CVN is present.

In CADV, the **IAC fundus opens into the anteromedial aspect of the dilated vestibule**, whereas, in the CC, the IAC fundus opens into the center of the cavity medially. If differentiation of a CADV (ABI) from a CC malformation (CI) is difficult at imaging, audiology should be critically analyzed preoperatively. Audiologically, CADV demonstrates no hearing compared to a CC malformation, which demonstrates profound hearing loss.

4. Common Cavity Malformation

The CC is a cystic space representing an undifferentiated cochlea and vestibule. Embryologically, a CC malformation is due to developmental arrest after differentiation of the otic placode into the **otocyst** in the **4th** gestational **week**.

Normally, cochlear and vestibular nerves originate from the brainstem as a single common **CVN** and separate in the IAC into the cochlear, superior, and inferior vestibular nerves. In the CC, **the IAC fundus usually opens into the cavity's center, and** an unbranched **CVN enters the CC**. Cochlear nerve fiber content in the CVN is impossible to assess with current clinical MR, but it can be considered normal if its **size** is similar to the contralateral normal CVN or it is **1.5-2x** that of the ipsilateral **facial nerve**.

The treatment is **CI** if the CVN has enough cochlear nerve fibers (determined by the size on MR or by a hearing aid trial). An **ABI** should be done if the cochlear fibers are questionable, as in nondemonstrated or a small CVN on MR.

5. Cochlear Hypoplasia

CH and incomplete partition anomalies have clear differentiation into the cochlea and vestibule. CH has an underdeveloped cochlea with smaller external dimensions than a normal cochlea and shows variable internal architectural deformities. The term cochlea with 1.5 turns is used to define CH (especially CH type III) but should be avoided for cochlear IP-II. Also, note that a miniature cochlea (dwarf cochlea) is not synonymous with CH and is used to denote a normal-appearing cochlea with a normal number of turns but with reduced diameter. Embryologically, CH results from arrested development at the **6th** gestational **week** and has 4 different types. **Treatment is variable** and includes hearing aids, stapes surgery, CI, and ABI.

(1) CH type I (bud-like cochlea): Small, ovoid/round, bud-shaped cochlea arising from the IAC. The internal architecture is severely deformed with no modiolus and interscalar septa (ISS).

(2) CH type II (cystic hypoplastic cochlea): Small cochlea with a defective modiolus and ISS but a normal external outline.

The modiolus may be totally absent with large communication with the IAC, leading to a **CSF gusher at surgery** and the potential for **CI electrode misplacement into the IAC**. The vestibular aqueduct (VA) may enlarge, and vestibule dilation may occur. The **stapes footplate** may be **defective** due to an **endosteal** development defect [such as IP-I, cystic cochleovestibular malformation (CCVM)], leading to **spontaneous CSF fistula** and **recurrent meningitis**.

(3) CH type III (cochlea with < 2 turns): Small cochlea with a short modiolus and reduced overall length of ISS. The vestibule and SCCs are usually hypoplastic, and the cochlear aperture (CA) may be hypoplastic or aplastic.

(4) CH type IV (cochlea with hypoplastic middle and apical turns): Small cochlear middle and apical turns **located anteromedially** (instead of centrally) over a **normal basal turn**. The facial nerve labyrinthine segment is usually located anterior to the cochlea.

6. Incomplete Partition of Cochlea

Like CH, IP anomalies have clear differentiation into the cochlea and vestibule and various internal architecture defects. However, unlike CH, the **cochlear external dimensions are normal**.

6a. IP-I (Cystic Cochleovestibular Malformation)

CCVM: Cochlea lacks ISS, modiolus (IP-I), and a dilated vestibule and lateral (horizontal) SCC. The cystic, featureless cochlea and vestibule have the appearance of a **figure 8** or **sloping snowman** on axial CT/MR. The defect between the IAC fundus and cochlea results from a CA defect, and an absent modiolus may cause CSF to completely fill the cochlea. Embryologically, IP-I/CCVM is due to arrested **otocyst** development at the **5th** gestational **week**.

A stapes footplate may be **defective** due to an **endosteal** developmental anomaly (as in CH-I, CH-II, and CC) with CSF filling the cochlea and a **cystic** structure at the stapes footplate. It can be easily infected during an otitis media attack with a **spontaneous stapes footplate CSF fistula** and **recurrent meningitis**.

The treatment is CI, the risks being a CSF gusher (deficient IAC fundus) and facial nerve damage (dehiscent CN VII). An **ABI** should be done if the cochlear nerve is aplastic. Patients with IP-I who have recurrent meningitis and normal tympanic membranes, but fluid filling the middle ear and mastoid, should undergo a middle ear exploration to excise the stapes footplate cyst and repair the oval window defect.

6b. IP-II

A deficient modiolus and ISS **between the middle and apical cochlear turns** (IP-II) is often seen associated with a **large VA (LVA)**. Enlarged **scala vestibuli** and scala communis may be seen in the cochlea with an increased 2nd interscalar ridge notch angle and reduced depth. Embryologically, IP-II is due to arrested development at the **7th** gestational **week**.

Modiolar defects in IP-II may result from transmission of high CSF pressure into the inner ear due to LVA. *SLC26A4* gene mutations are seen in ~ 50% of LVA patients. LVA may be associated with **Pendred** syndrome [sensorineural hearing loss (SNHL) and goiter]. **Mondini** deformity is LVA + minimally dilated vestibule + IP-II.

Hearing is normal at birth. Progressive/fluctuating SNHL is apparently from high pulsating CSF pressure or head trauma. **Contact sports should be avoided** and head trauma prevented. A hearing aid should be used before CI. All IP-II have a cochlear nerve; ABI is not indicated.

6c. IP-III

X-linked deafness with a **stapes gusher** shows a bulbous IAC and cochlear IP-III. In IP-III, cochlear ISS is present, but the modiolus and cochlear base are absent, giving rise to a **corkscrew** appearance of the **cochlea**. This always leads to a severe CSF gusher during CI and stapes surgery and a very high chance of electrode misplacement into the IAC during CI. The cochlea lies directly at the lateral end of the IA instead of in its usual anterolateral location.

The vestibule is enlarged in most IP-III, and SCCs are dilated in the majority. **Cystic/diverticular lesions** are contiguous with a vestibule (in 1/3) &/or SCCs (in 1/6). The VA has a more medial origin than usual with varying degrees of dilatation. The **facial nerve** canal **labyrinthine segment** is located almost **above the cochlea** (due to a thin otic capsule) and forms the **superior-most structure** seen on axial temporal bone CT.

A spontaneous CSF fistula through a stapes footplate and recurrent **meningitis** happens **very rarely** in IP-III, although a CSF gusher at surgery is very severe. This is because the **defect** in IP-III is in the **outer periosteal and enchondral layers** with a **normal/thick** endosteal layer and a **stapes footplate** (unlike in IP-I, CC, CH-I, and CH-II, in which the defect is endosteal and stapes footplate, CSF fistula and recurrent meningitis are very common). Oval window atresia/hypoplasia can be associated.

The treatment is **CI**. All IP-III (like IP-II) have a cochlear nerve, so ABI is not indicated. **Stapes surgery is contraindicated** in IP-III, as it may lead to a severe gusher and further increased SNHL.

7. Enlarged Vestibular Aqueduct

This is an enlarged VA with a vertical and axial VA width > 1.5 mm at the midpoint of the labyrinth and operculum, along with a normal cochlea, vestibule, and SCCs.

8. Cochlear Aperture Abnormalities

CA abnormalities, a.k.a. cochlear fossette or bony cochlear nerve canal, include stenosis **(width < 1.4 mm)** or atresia. Cochlear nerve deficiency, which is cochlear nerve hypoplasia or absence (aplasia), should always be evaluated with MR.

In MR, the **normal cochlear nerve is usually larger than** either the superior or inferior **vestibular** nerves. Also, the normal cochlear nerve is almost similar in size to the **facial** nerve or larger than it in 2/3 of cases.

Audiologic evaluation shows severe to profound SNHL. The newborn may pass a hearing screening test if automated auditory brainstem response is not obtained because otoacoustic emissions may be present, as the cochlea is normal. The treatment is CI and ABI if CI fails. ABI is the 1st-line therapy for cochlear nerve canal (CA) aplasia. Simultaneous CI and ABI can be done if the cochlear nerve is barely visible on MR in children between 2-3 years of age to avoid losing valuable time for language development.

Selected References

1. Parlak S et al: X-linked deafness/incomplete partition type 3: radiological evaluation of temporal bone and intracranial findings. Diagn Interv Radiol. 28(1):50-7, 2022
2. Sennaroğlu L et al: Classification and current management of inner ear malformations. Balkan Med J. 34(5):397-411, 2017

Labyrinthine Aplasia

KEY FACTS

TERMINOLOGY

- Synonyms: Complete labyrinthine aplasia (CLA); Michel anomaly (old synonym)

IMAGING

- Bilateral or unilateral anomaly
- Temporal bone CT findings
  - Otic capsule bone: Aplasia/hypoplasia
  - Absent cochlea, vestibule, semicircular canals, & vestibular aqueduct
  - Cochlear promontory: Absent/flattened
  - Ossicles: Normal, or malformed stapes
  - Tegmen tympani: Normal, low, or defective
  - Facial nerve canal: Aberrant course
  - Petrous apex: Hypoplasia
  - Internal auditory canal: Aplasia/hypoplasia
  - Carotid canal: Normal or absent
- MR: Absent vestibular & cochlear nerves

TOP DIFFERENTIAL DIAGNOSES

- Cochlear aplasia
- Common cavity
- Labyrinthine ossificans, obliterative type

PATHOLOGY

- Genetic mutation: *FGF3* mutations [LAMM (C**LA**, **m**icrotia, **m**icrodontia) syndrome], *HOXA1* mutations, thalidomide exposure, or unknown etiology
- **Otic placode** development arrest **before 3rd week**

CLINICAL ISSUES

- Congenital sensorineural hearing loss
- **Horizontal gaze palsy** (*HOXA1*) or **abnormal teeth** (LAMM) suggest underlying syndrome
- Auditory brainstem implantation (ABI) treatment

DIAGNOSTIC CHECKLIST

- Often asymmetric: Contralateral common cavity, inner ear hypoplasia, or cochlear IP-I anomaly

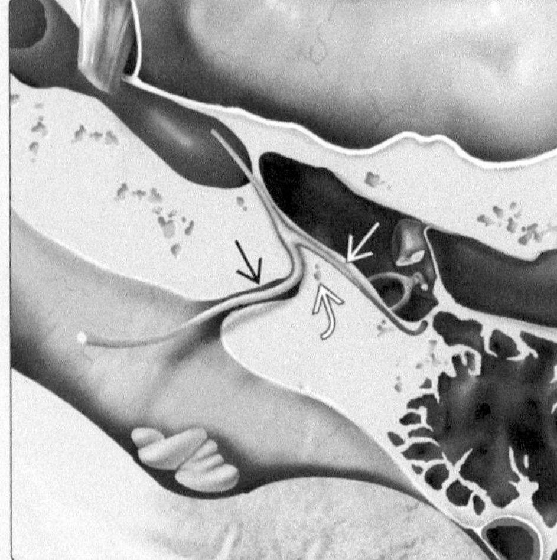

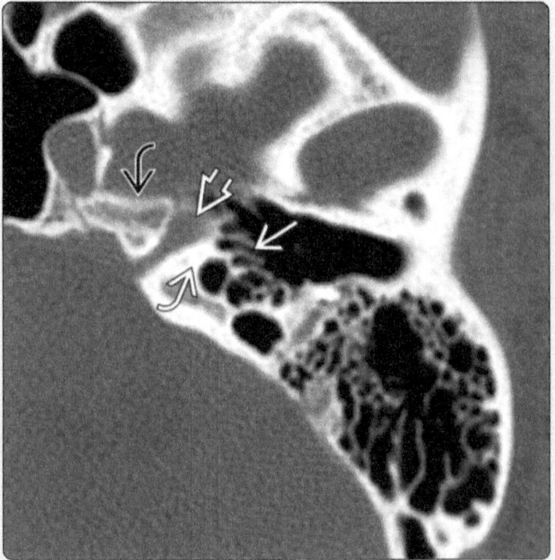

(Left) *Axial graphic depicts labyrinthine aplasia. Note complete absence of all inner ear structures ➡ with the exception of a small IAC with only CNVII ➡. The lateral wall of the inner ear (promontory) is flattened ➡.* **(Right)** *Axial bone CT in 21-year-old woman with SNHL shows severe hypoplasia of the otic capsule bone with air cells in expected location of the promontory ➡. The inner ear structures are absent ➡. CNVII canal is present with a broadened anterior genu ➡. Note the petrous apex is hypoplastic ➡, narrow in width.*

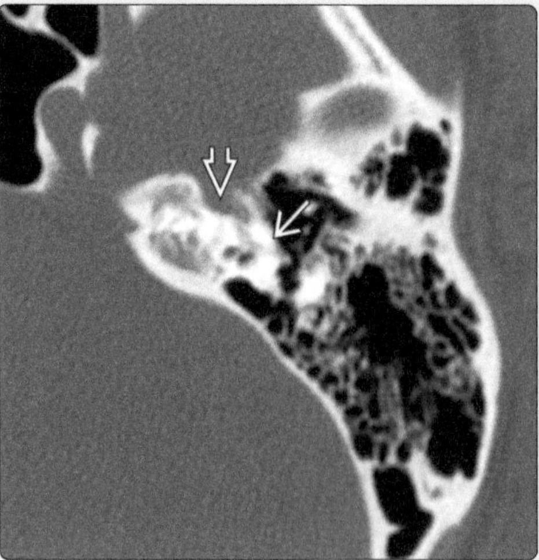

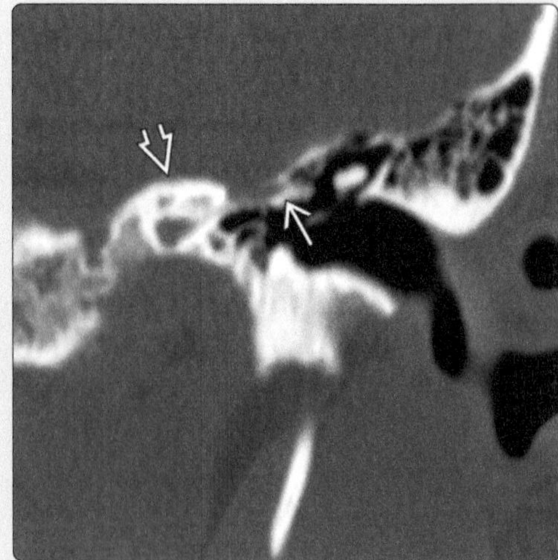

(Left) *Axial bone CT in the same patient at a more cephalad level shows hypoplastic otic capsule bone ➡. The anterior genu & proximal tympanic segment of the anomalous CNVII canal are visible ➡.* **(Right)** *Coronal bone CT in the same patient reveals complete absence of inner ear structures & severe hypoplasia of the otic capsule bone ➡ & petrous apex ➡. Note the normal middle ear & ossicles despite complete inner ear aplasia.*

TERMINOLOGY

Synonyms

- **Complete labyrinthine aplasia** (CLA)
- Old synonym: Michel anomaly

Definitions

- **Absent cochlea, vestibule, & semicircular canals** (SCCs)

IMAGING

General Features

- Best diagnostic clue
  - Complete absence of inner ear structures
- Morphology
  - **3 subgroups** based on radiologic findings
  - **CLA with hypoplastic or aplastic petrous bone**
    - Middle ear could be adjacent to posterior fossa
  - **CLA without otic capsule**
    - Hypo/aplastic otic capsule but normal petrous bone
  - **CLA with otic capsule**
    - Normal otic capsule and petrous bone
    - Labyrinthine segment of facial canal in normal location only in this subgroup
    - Otic capsule essential for normal facial canal location

CT Findings

- Bone CT
  - Otic capsule bone: Aplasia/hypoplasia
  - Absent cochlea, vestibule, SCC, vestibular aqueduct
  - Cochlear promontory: Absent/flattened
  - Ossicles: Normal usually, or malformed stapes
  - Tegmen tympani: Normal, low, or defective (look for associated cephalocele)
  - Middle ear & mastoid: Normal or hypoplastic
  - Facial nerve canal: Aberrant course
  - Petrous apex: Hypoplasia
  - Internal auditory canal (IAC): Aplasia/hypoplasia
  - Jugular bulb/vein: Normal, dehiscent or stenotic + large emissary veins
  - Carotid canal: Normal or absent
  - Clivus: Normal or narrowed
  - Cervical spine: Normal or + anomalies

MR Findings

- T2WI
  - Absent membranous labyrinth
  - Absent vestibular & cochlear nerves
    - IAC contains only facial nerve
  - Large cerebellopontine angle cistern/arachnoid cyst
  - Pontine anomaly

Imaging Recommendations

- Best imaging tool
  - High-resolution temporal bone CT
  - Heavily T2WI 3D (CISS, FIESTA) MR IAC/temporal bones

DIFFERENTIAL DIAGNOSIS

Cochlear Aplasia

- **Late 3rd-week arrest**: Absent cochlea, dysmorphic vestibule, & SCC

Common Cavity

- **4th-week arrest**: Ovoid globular sac of cochlea + vestibule

Labyrinthine Ossificans

- Postmeningitic ossification, promontory well formed

PATHOLOGY

General Features

- Etiology
  - Genetic mutation, thalidomide exposure, or unknown
- Genetics
  - *FGF3* mutations: LAMM (C**LA**, **m**icrotia, **m**icrodontia) syndrome
  - *HOXA1* mutations: Bosley-Salih-Alorainy syndrome (BSAS) & Athabaskan brainstem dysgenesis (ABDS)
- Associated abnormalities
  - BSAS & ABDS: Congenital heart disease, horizontal gaze palsy, absent internal carotid arteries
- Embryology
  - Arrest of **otic placode** development **before 3rd** gestational **week**

Gross Pathologic & Surgical Features

- Failure of bony & membranous labyrinth formation

CLINICAL ISSUES

Presentation

- Most common signs/symptoms
  - Congenital sensorineural hearing loss (SNHL)
- Other signs/symptoms
  - *FGF3* mutations: Microtia, **microdontia**
  - *HOXA1* mutations: Central hypoventilation, cardiac failure, **horizontal gaze restriction**, stroke
- **Audiologic evaluation findings**
  - No response
  - May show findings of profound SNHL on low frequencies
    - Actually vibrotactile stimulation

Treatment

- Unilateral CLA: Assess contralateral side for cochlear implantation if bilateral SNHL
- Bilateral CLA: Auditory brainstem implantation (ABI)

DIAGNOSTIC CHECKLIST

Consider

- CLA if cochlea, vestibule, & SCC are absent

Image Interpretation Pearls

- Often asymmetric: Contralateral common cavity, inner ear hypoplasia, or cochlear IP-I anomaly

Reporting Tips

- Variable pathognomonic flattening of cochlear promontory: Subtle to marked
- Evaluate tegmen tympani integrity on coronal reformats

SELECTED REFERENCES

1. Jamshidi F et al: Identification of a homozygous frameshift mutation in the FGF3 gene in a consanguineous Iranian family: first report of labyrinthine aplasia, microtia, and microdontia syndrome in Iran and literature review. Mol Genet Genomic Med. 11(5):e2168, 2023

Oval Window Atresia

KEY FACTS

TERMINOLOGY

- Oval window atresia (OWA): Absent space between lateral semicircular canal above & cochlear promontory below
- Associated with anomalous stapes & malpositioned CNVII

IMAGING

- Temporal bone CT findings
  - Normal OW replaced by ossific "web" or plate
  - **Inferomedially positioned** tympanic segment **CNVII**
    - May completely overlie OW
    - May reside on superior or inferior OW margin
- Key surgical finding on CT = facial nerve location prevents safe surgical correction
- Best imaging tool: Multiplanar temporal bone CT
  - OW niche best seen in coronal plane
  - CNVII location relative to OW best seen in coronal plane
  - Stapes crura best seen in axial plane
- Bony plate over OW + inferomedially displaced tympanic segment of facial nerve = OWA

TOP DIFFERENTIAL DIAGNOSES

- Tympanosclerosis
- Fenestral otosclerosis

PATHOLOGY

- Best hypothesis for OWA etiology
  - Primitive stapes fails to fuse with primitive vestibule during 7th week of gestation
- **Deformed stapes** & **lenticular process of incus** (both develop from 2nd branchial arch) can be associated, especially in **CHARGE** syndrome

CLINICAL ISSUES

- Clinical presentation
  - Nonprogressive conductive hearing deficit from birth
  - Lack of history of otomastoiditis; normal EAC

DIAGNOSTIC CHECKLIST

- Thickened bone over OW + inferomedially displaced tympanic of facial nerve (CNVII) = OWA

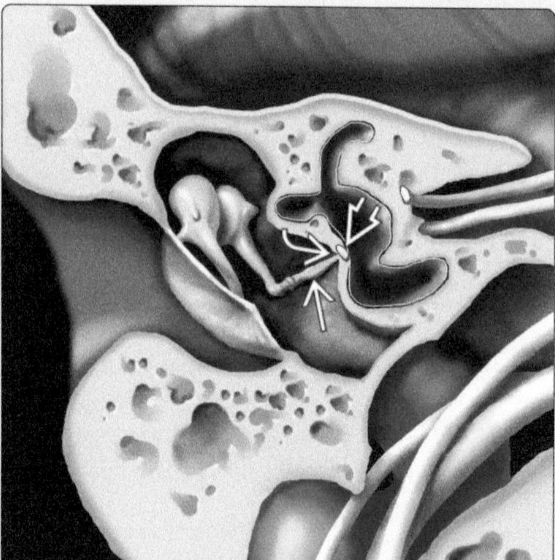

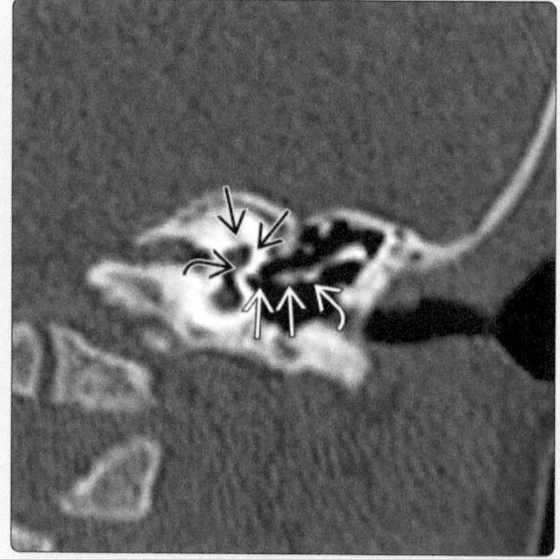

(Left) *Coronal graphic illustrates features of oval window atresia ➡, including malformation of the stapes crura & footplate ➡ & the tympanic segment of the facial nerve in an abnormal location ➡.* **(Right)** *Coronal bone CT in a 6-month-old girl with CHARGE syndrome shows left oval window atresia with thick bony plate in the location of oval window ➡. Note the deformed lenticular process of incus ➡ & stapes ➡ (both develop from 2nd branchial arch). Semicircular canals are absent ➡.*

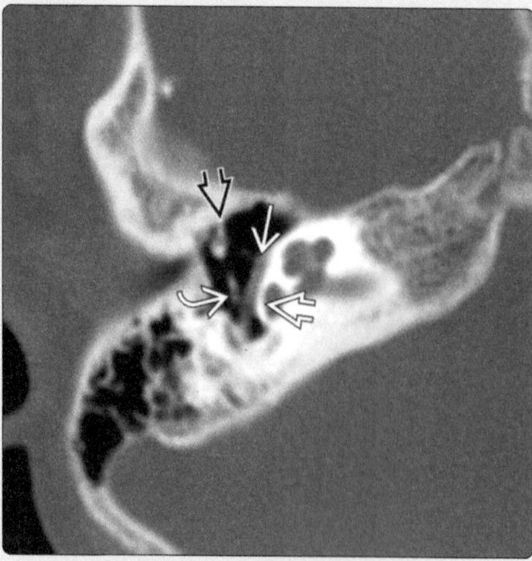

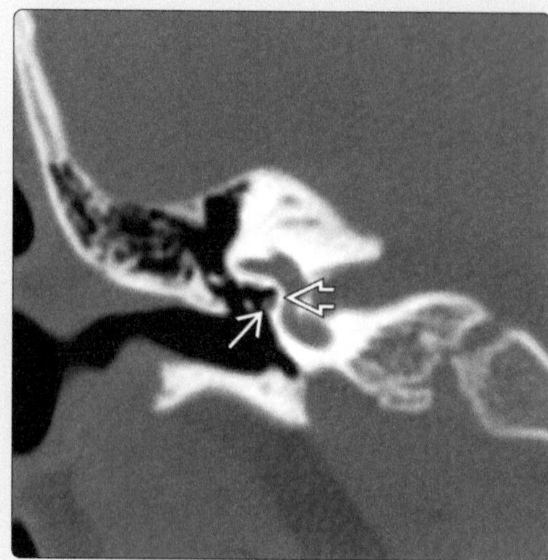

(Left) *Axial bone CT in an adolescent patient with conductive hearing loss shows deformed ossicles with angulation of the incus ➡ and anterior malleolar ligament calcification ➡. The oval window is bone covered ➡ with the tympanic segment of CNVII traversing its margin ➡.* **(Right)** *Coronal bone CT in the same patient reveals the bony plate within the oval window ➡. Notice that the tympanic segment is present along the inferior margin of the oval window niche ➡.*

TERMINOLOGY

Abbreviations

- Oval window atresia (OWA)

Definitions

- Absent space between lateral semicircular canal above & cochlear promontory below
- Associated with anomalous stapes & malpositioned CNVII

IMAGING

Normal OW Shape

- OW oval-shaped in > 1/2 (53%)
- Kidney (18%), D (17%), rectangle (7%), trapezoid (5%)

Normal OW Size

- **Age**: **Height** (mm) x **width** (mm) → **area** (mm^2)
- **Fetal/infant**: 1.36 ± 0.18 x 2.53 ± 0.36 → 2.69 ± 0.60
- **Child**: 1.40 ± 0.20 x 2.61 ± 0.20 → 2.87 ± 0.62
- **Adult**: 1.50 ± 0.19 x 2.63 ± 0.23 → 3.05 ± 0.57

General Features

- Best diagnostic clue
  - Absence of OW lucency with bony plate at its location between vestibule & middle ear (ME)

CT Findings

- Bone CT
  - Normal OW replaced by ossific web
  - Malformed stapes superstructure (absence of normal paired crura) & distal incus
  - **Inferomedially positioned** tympanic segment **CNVII**
    - May reside on superior or inferior margin of OW
    - May completely overlie expected location of OW
      - **Critical surgical importance** (associated in > 60%)
      - OW drill-out may be contraindicated if present
  - External auditory canal (EAC) usually normal but may be malformed rarely
    - Most congenital ME anomalies are associated with congenital external ear dysplasia

Imaging Recommendations

- Best imaging tool
  - Multiplanar high-resolution temporal bone CT
    - OW niche best seen in coronal plane
    - Stapes crura best seen in axial plane

DIFFERENTIAL DIAGNOSIS

Tympanosclerosis

- Clinical: Chronic otomastoiditis
- Imaging: Stapes may be thickened, including footplate
  - Ossific deposits on ossicle surface may be seen
  - ME debris/sclerotic mastoid = chronic otomastoiditis
  - Facial nerve normal

Fenestral Otosclerosis

- Clinical: Rare in childhood
- Imaging: Lucent lesions anterior to OW
  - Obliterative variety (< 10%) results in similar appearance to OWA, but stapes & facial nerve normal

Congenital External Ear Malformation

- Clinical: Microtia, EAC malformation
- Imaging: Variable EAC narrowing or absence
  - Ossicle fusion, rotation; CNVII anomalous course
  - OWA may be associated

PATHOLOGY

General Features

- Etiology
  - Best hypothesis: Primitive stapes fails to fuse with primitive vestibule during 7th week of gestation
  - Alternate hypothesis: Developing facial nerve displaced & interposed between primitive stapes & otic capsule
  - If stapes forms but annular ligament does not, stapes footplate gets ankylosed (**congenital stapes fixation**)
    - Caution: This may result in congenital conductive hearing loss in absence of imaging findings

Gross Pathologic & Surgical Features

- Tympanic segment of CNVII abnormal in many cases
  - Inferomedially positioned
- **Abnormal incus lenticular process** associated
  - Expected since **distal incus & stapes** superstructure both formed from 2nd branchial arch
  - Especially in **CHARGE** syndrome
- OWA rarely associated with **persistent stapedial artery**
- OWA seen in 1/3 of cases & severe OW hypoplasia in < 1/3 cases of **X-linked stapes gusher** (DFNX2) syndrome

CLINICAL ISSUES

Presentation

- Most common signs/symptoms
  - Profound conductive hearing deficit in child
    - Nonprogressive; air-bone gap > 40 dB

Demographics

- Epidemiology
  - OWA **bilateral** in ~ **40%**

Natural History & Prognosis

- Surgical correction results modest over long term

Treatment

- Vestibulotomy with ossiculoplasty
  - Difficult, as landmarks for vestibule are few; risk of ectopic facial nerve injury
- Fenestration above OWA & piston prosthesis placement
- Alternative treatment (**round** window vibroplasty)
  - Version of active ME implants (vibrant sound bridge)

DIAGNOSTIC CHECKLIST

Image Interpretation Pearls

- Thickened bone over OW + inferomedially displaced tympanic CNVII = OWA

SELECTED REFERENCES

1. Gheorghe DC et al: Persistent stapedial artery, oval window atresia and congenital stapes agenesis-case report. Medicina (Kaunas). 59(3), 2023
2. Singal A et al: Anatomic variability of oval window as pertaining to stapes surgery. Surg Radiol Anat. 42(3):329-35, 2020

Cochlear Aplasia

KEY FACTS

TERMINOLOGY

- Absent cochlea, but vestibule, semicircular canals (SCC), & internal auditory canal (IAC) present in some form

IMAGING

- Cochlea: **Absent** bilaterally or unilaterally
- Cochlear nerve canal & cochlear nerve: **Absent**
- Cochlear **promontory**: Hypoplastic, **flattened**
- Vestibule & SCC: Dilated **[cochlear aplasia with dilated vestibule (CADV)]** or hypoplastic or normal
- Vestibular aqueduct: **Normal**
- Facial nerve canal: **Anomalous**, obtuse angle anterior genu
- IAC: Hypoplastic; **IAC fundus opens** into **anteromedial** aspect of dilated vestibule in **CADV**
- Middle ear: Normal size; normal or malformed stapes
- Oval window: Normal or stenotic/atretic
- Rare stapes footplate endosteal developmental anomaly → spontaneous CSF fistula/recurrent meningitis

TOP DIFFERENTIAL DIAGNOSES

- Complete labyrinthine (Michel) aplasia
- Common cavity (CC) deformity
  - Dilated cochlea & vestibule form common cavity
  - **IAC fundus opens** at **center** of CC medially
- Cochlear hypoplasia: 4 types
- Cystic cochleovestibular anomaly
  - **Figure 8** or **sloping snowman** appearance
- Labyrinthine ossificans
  - Acquired SNHL, postmeningitic, **normal promontory**

PATHOLOGY

- Arrested **otic placode** at **late 3rd** gestational **week**

CLINICAL ISSUES

- Extremely rare, congenital SNHL, usually bilateral

DIAGNOSTIC CHECKLIST

- **CADV (ABI)** vs. **common cavity (cochlear implant)**

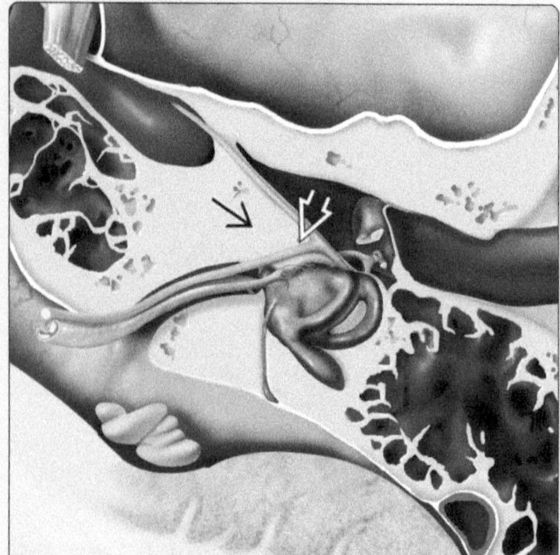

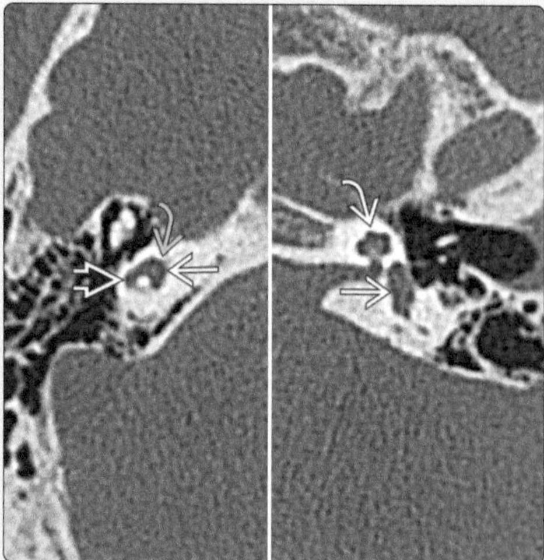

(Left) *Axial graphic shows cochlear aplasia, including a small IAC with absence of the cochlear nerve, an absent cochlea ➔, vestibular & semicircular canal (SCC) malformation, & flattening of CNVII anterior genu ➔. The facial nerve canal occupies the normal cochlear location.* **(Right)** *Axial bone CT shows absence of right cochlea ➔ with visualization of vestibule ➔ & lateral semicircular canal ➔ in a girl with right cochlear aplasia. Note the presence of cochlea on the left side ➔. (Courtesy R. H. Ramakrishnaiah, MD.)*

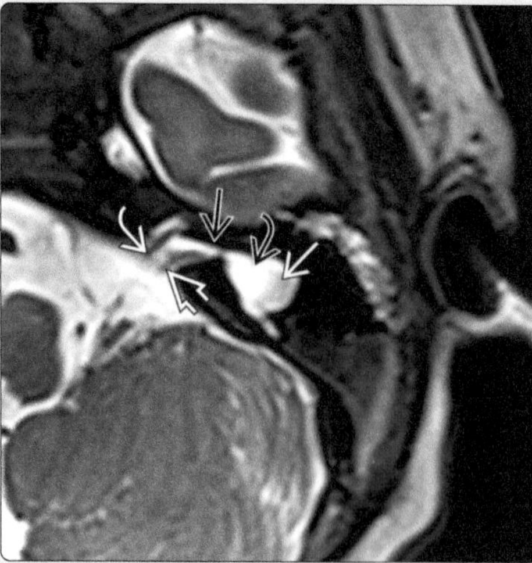

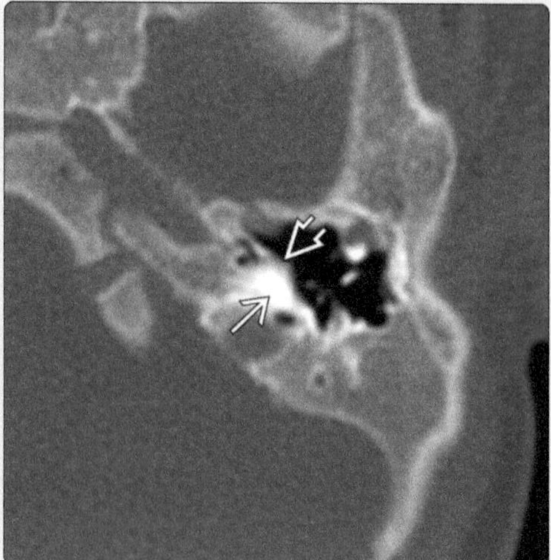

(Left) *Axial T2 SPACE MR in a 4-month-old girl shows cochlear aplasia with dilated vestibule (CADV). IAC fundus ➔ opens into anteromedial aspect of dilated vestibule ➔, whereas IAC fundus opens at the center of cavity medially in common cavity malformation. Note globular vestibule-horizontal SCC anomaly ➔. Narrow IAC contains vestibular ➔ & facial ➔ nerves, without cochlear nerve.* **(Right)** *Axial bone CT in the same patient demonstrates absence of cochlea ➔ & mild flattening of cochlear promontory ➔.*

TERMINOLOGY

Definitions

- Absent cochlea, but vestibule, semicircular canals (SCCs), & internal auditory canal (IAC) present in some form

IMAGING

General Features

- Morphology
  - **2 subgroups** according to vestibular system
  - **Cochlear aplasia (CA) with normal labyrinth**
    - Normally developed vestibule & SCCs
  - **CA with dilated vestibule (CADV)**
    - Dilated vestibule and normal or dilated SCCs
  - Extremely important to **distinguish CADV from common cavity (CC)** malformation
    - Cochlear implant (CI) contraindicated in CA/CADV
    - CI done in CC if cochleovestibular nerve present
    - In CADV, **IAC fundus** opens into anteromedial aspect of dilated vestibule
    - In CC, IAC fundus opens into center of cavity medially

CT Findings

- Bone CT
  - Cochlea: **Absent**, bilaterally or unilaterally
  - Cochlear nerve canal: **Absent**
  - **Cochlear promontory**: Hypoplastic, **flattened**
    - In contrast with normal cochlear promontory in labyrinthine ossificans
  - Vestibule & SCC: Often **malformed**, globular, & dilated, or hypoplastic or normal
  - **Vestibular aqueduct: Usually normal**
  - **Facial nerve** canal: Anteriorly displaced **occupying normal location of cochlea**; obtuse angle anterior genu
  - IAC: Usually **hypoplastic; IAC fundus opens** into **anteromedial** aspect of dilated vestibule in **CADV**
    - In contrast with IAC fundus opening into center of cavity medially in CC
  - Middle ear: **Normal size**
  - Ossicles: Normal or malformed stapes
  - Oval window: Normal or stenotic/atretic
  - Round window: Atretic

MR Findings

- T2WI
  - Cochlea & cochlear nerve: Absent
  - Vestibule & SCC: Variable abnormality

Imaging Recommendations

- Best imaging tool
  - T-bone CT or heavily T2W 3D (CISS, FIESTA) MR

DIFFERENTIAL DIAGNOSIS

Complete Labyrinthine (Michel) Aplasia

- Developmental arrest **before** 3rd gestational week

Common Cavity Malformation

- **Dilated cochlea & vestibule form common cavity (CC)**
- Developmental arrest in 4th gestational week
- **IAC fundus opens** at **center** of CC medially

Cochlear Hypoplasia: 4 Types

- Cochlear hypoplasia (CH)-I (bud-like cochlea)
- CH-II (cystic hypoplastic cochlea): Recurrent meningitis due to defective stapes foot plate
- CH-III (cochlea with < 2 turns)
- CH-IV (cochlea with hypoplastic middle and apical turns)

Cystic Cochleovestibular Anomaly

- Cochlea & vestibule cystic with no internal architecture; **figure 8 or snowman appearance**
- Developmental arrest in 5th gestational week

Labyrinthine Ossificans

- **Acquired sensorineural hearing loss (SNHL)**, usually following meningitis
- Ossified membranous labyrinth, **normal promontory**

PATHOLOGY

General Features

- Associated abnormalities
  - Vestibule & SCC may be normal or dilated
- Embryology: Arrest of **otic placode** development at **late 3rd** gestational **week**

Gross Pathologic & Surgical Features

- Absent cochlea; remaining inner ear present but abnormal
- Rare **stapes footplate endosteal** developmental anomaly **→ spontaneous CSF fistula/recurrent meningitis**
  - CSF fills cochlea & cystic structure may be seen at stapes footplate on CT/MR
  - Most commonly in CC malformation (18%), followed by IP-I (15%), and rarely in CA (5.2%), CH-I (5.6%), CH-II (4.4%), & IP-II (0.85%)

CLINICAL ISSUES

Presentation

- Most common signs/symptoms
  - Congenital SNHL, usually bilateral
- **Audiologic evaluation findings**
  - No hearing level; only stimulation vibrotactile

Treatment

- Auditory brainstem implantation (ABI)
- Satisfactory short-term outcomes of cochlear implantation (CI) for cochlear aplasia anecdotally reported

DIAGNOSTIC CHECKLIST

Consider

- CA diagnosed if **no** cochlea is seen on CT or T2 MR but rest of membranous labyrinth present
  - Distinguish **CA (flat promontory)** from **labyrinthine ossificans (normal promontory)**
- If differentiation of **CADV (ABI)** from **CC (CI)** difficult
  - Audiologically no hearing in CADV; profound hearing loss in CC malformation

SELECTED REFERENCES

1. Kim BJ et al: How to maximize the outcomes of cochlear implantation in common cavity and cochlear aplasia with dilated vestibule, the most severe inner ear anomalies? Clin Exp Otorhinolaryngol. 15(1):3-4, 2022

Cochlear Hypoplasia

KEY FACTS

TERMINOLOGY

- Small, underdeveloped cochlea; 4 types

IMAGING

- Cochlear hypoplasia (CH) of variable severity
  - **CH-I** (bud-like cochlea)
  - **CH-II** (cystic hypoplastic cochlea)
  - **CH-III** (cochlea with < 2 turns)
  - **CH-IV** (cochlea with hypoplastic middle & apical turns)
- Cochlear nerve canal: Absent, narrow, normal, wide
- Cochlear nerve: Often absent or hypoplastic
- Facial nerve canal: Aberrant course ± dehiscence
- Internal auditory canal: Normal or narrow/anomalous
- Vestibule: Normal, dilated, or hypoplastic
- Vestibular aqueduct: Normal or large

TOP DIFFERENTIAL DIAGNOSES

- **Dwarf cochlea (miniature cochlea)**
  - Normal number but smaller diameter of turns
- **Cochlear incomplete partition type-III (IP-III)**
- **Cochlear incomplete partition type-II (IP-II)**
- **Branchiootorenal syndrome**
  - Hypoplastic offset middle & apical turns, ± funnel-shaped large vestibular aqueduct
- **CHARGE syndrome**

PATHOLOGY

- Arrested development at **6th** gestational **week**

CLINICAL ISSUES

- Congenital sensorineural or sometimes mixed hearing loss
- Rare stapes footplate endosteal developmental anomaly → spontaneous CSF fistula/recurrent meningitis in CH-I & CH-II
- Treatment variable, including hearing aids, stapes surgery, cochlear implant, & auditory brainstem implant

DIAGNOSTIC CHECKLIST

- Consider CHARGE & branchiootorenal syndromes if other associated findings present

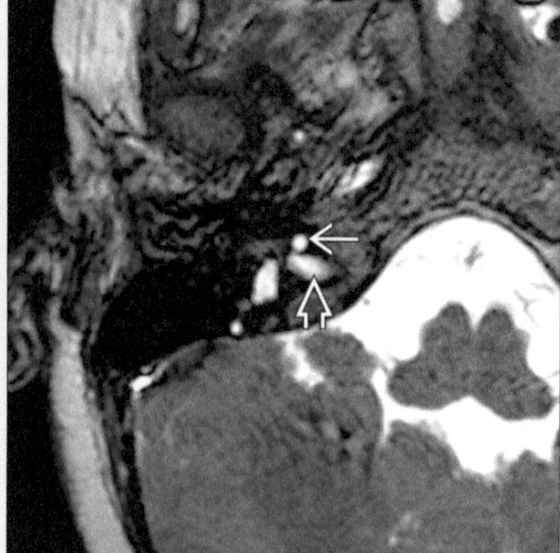

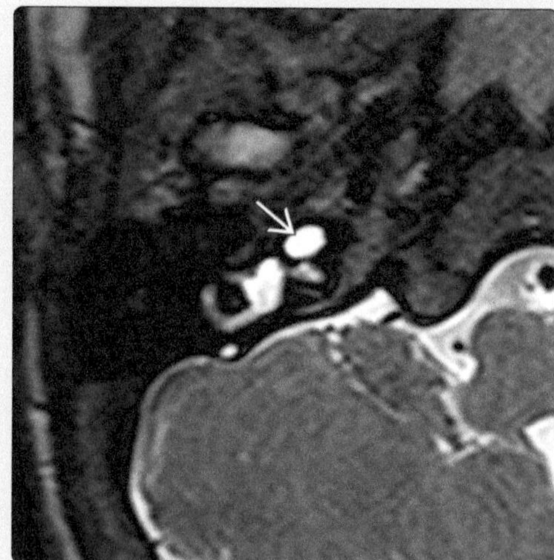

(Left) *Axial T2 MR shows a small, bud-like structure consistent with cochlear hypoplasia type I (CH-I, bud-like cochlea) ➡ arising from the internal auditory canal ➡.* **(Right)** *Axial 3D T2 SPACE MR in an infant boy with bilateral profound sensorineural hearing loss (SNHL) shows CH-II (cystic hypoplastic cochlea) with a single rounded cochlear turn ➡ without modiolus and interscalar septa. Note that the cochlea has smaller dimensions but with a normal external outline. CSF gusher and recurrent meningitis may occur in CH-II.*

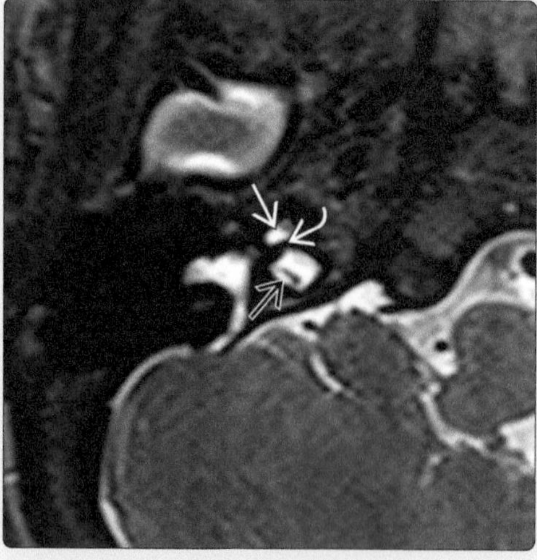

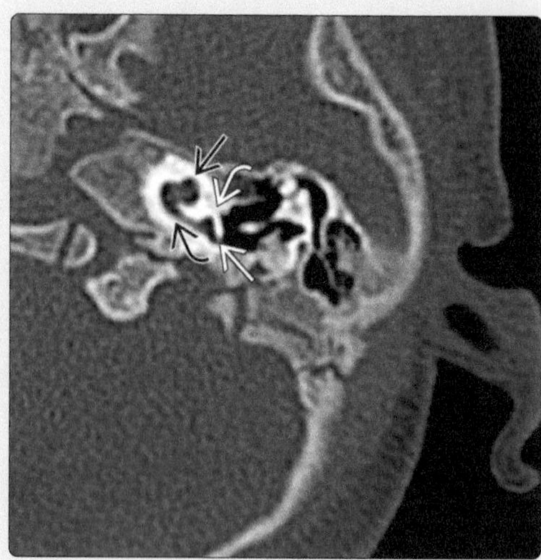

(Left) *Axial T2 MR in an infant shows CH-III (cochlea with < 2 turns) ➡. Inferior vestibular nerve ➡ appears normal. The cochlear nerve is not seen, and the cochlear nerve canal is absent ➡.* **(Right)** *Axial bone CT in an infant with CHARGE syndrome shows CH-IV (cochlea with hypoplastic middle and apical turns). The middle and apical turns ➡ are severely hypoplastic and located anteromedially over the normal basal turn ➡ (instead of their normal central position). Note oval window atresia ➡ and round window hypoplasia ➡.*

TERMINOLOGY

Abbreviations

- Cochlear hypoplasia (CH)

Definitions

- Cochlear underdevelopment: External dimensions < normal cochlea with internal architecture deformities

IMAGING

General Features

- Best diagnostic clue
  - Small cochlea; CH classified into 4 types

CT Findings

- Bone CT
  - **CH-I (bud-like cochlea)**: Small ovoid/round, bud-shaped cochlea arising from internal auditory canal (IAC)
    - Severely deformed internal architecture with no modiolus & interscalar septa (ISS)
  - **CH-II (cystic hypoplastic cochlea)**: Small cochlea with defective modiolus & ISS but normal external outline
    - Modiolus may be totally absent with large communication with IAC → **CSF gusher** at surgery
    - Cochlear implant **electrode misplacement** into IAC
    - Vestibular aqueduct may enlarge & vestibule dilate
  - **CH-III (cochlea with < 2 turns)**: Small cochlea, short modiolus, & reduced overall length of ISS
    - Vestibule & semicircular canals (SCCs) usually hypoplastic
    - Cochlear aperture (CA) may be hypoplastic or aplastic
  - **CH-IV (cochlea with hypoplastic middle & apical turns)**: Small cochlear middle & apical turns
    - Located **anteromedially** (instead of normal central position) over **normal basal turn**
    - Facial nerve labyrinthine segment usually located anterior to cochlea
  - Round window: Absent or present
  - Cochlear nerve canal (CNC): Absent, narrow, or wide
  - IAC: Normal or narrow/anomalous
  - Vestibule: Normal, dilated, or hypoplastic
  - SCCs: Normal, dilated, hypoplastic, or absent
  - Vestibular aqueduct: Normal or large
  - **Facial nerve canal**: **Aberrant course**, associated SCC (especially lateral SCC) abnormalities ± dehiscence
  - Middle ear space & contents: Usually normal, but **stapedial fixation** may occur, especially in CH-III & CH-IV
  - **Cochlear promontory may lack normal protuberance**

MR Findings

- Cochlea: Small internal structure present or absent
- **Cochlear nerve (CN)**: **Often absent or hypoplastic**, especially in CA hypoplasia/aplasia

DIFFERENTIAL DIAGNOSIS

Dwarf Cochlea (Miniature Cochlea)

- **Small**, morphologically normal-appearing cochlea with **normal number** of turns but **reduced diameter of turns**

Cochlear Incomplete Partition Type III (IP-III)

- Corkscrew cochlea, normal to large in size

Cochlear Incomplete Partition Type II (IP-II)

- Cochlear modiolus deficient ± plump apical & middle turns

Branchiootorenal Syndrome

- Tapered cochlear basal turn
- Hypoplastic, offset middle & apical cochlear turns

CHARGE Syndrome

- CH, most commonly with basal turn relatively preserved & upper turns underdeveloped

PATHOLOGY

General Features

- Embryology
  - Arrested development at **6th** gestational **week**

Microscopic Features

- **CH-III & CH-IV**: Genetically predetermined earlier stoppage of membranous labyrinth development
- **CH-I & CH-II**: Arrested development of internal architecture, severely defective vascular supply from IAC
- **Stapes footplate** may be **defective** due to **endosteal** developmental **anomaly**
  - CSF fills cochlea, & cystic structure may be seen at stapes footplate
  - Can be infected during otitis media attack with **stapes footplate CSF fistula** & **recurrent meningitis**
  - Most commonly in **common cavity** malformation (18%), followed by **IP-I** (15%) &, rarely, in **cochlear aplasia** (5.2%), **CH-I** (5.6%), **CH-II** (4.4%), & **IP-II** (0.85%)

CLINICAL ISSUES

Presentation

- Most common signs/symptoms
  - Congenital sensorineural hearing loss (SNHL)
  - Stapedial fixation may produce conductive hearing loss (CHL), especially in CH-III & CH-IV
- **Audiologic evaluation findings**
  - Full spectrum of hearing loss from normal to profound

Treatment

- Hearing aids only: Mild or moderate SNHL; stapes surgery: Pure CHL; both: Mixed hearing loss
- Cochlear implantation (CI): Profound SNHL if CN present
- Auditory brainstem implantation (ABI): Profound SNHL if CN deficient (frequent)
- CI on side with better developed CN/better audiologic findings
- Contralateral ABI if limited language development with CI
- Simultaneous CI & ABI if 2-3 years age & barely visible CN
  - To avoid losing valuable time for language development

DIAGNOSTIC CHECKLIST

Image Interpretation Pearls

- 3D T2WI MR (inner ear) with sagittal oblique reformats (CN)

SELECTED REFERENCES

1. Lewis MA et al: The spectrum of cochlear malformations in CHARGE syndrome and insights into the role of the CHD7 gene during embryogenesis of the inner ear. Neuroradiology. 65(4):819-34, 2023

Cochlear Nerve and Cochlear Nerve Canal Aplasia-Hypoplasia

KEY FACTS

TERMINOLOGY

- Stenosis or atresia of cochlear nerve canal (CNC)
- Cochlear nerve deficiency (CND): Cochlear nerve (CN) hypoplasia/aplasia

IMAGING

- CNC or cochlear aperture (CA) extends from internal auditory canal (IAC) fundus to modiolus
  - **Diameter** measured **at narrowest point**
  - **CNC (CA) stenosis**: < **1.4 mm**
- Cochlea (spectrum of findings)
  - Normal
  - Normal modiolus + mildly stenotic CNC
  - Thickened modiolus + stenotic/atretic CNC
  - Cochlear anomaly + stenotic/atretic CNC
- IAC: Normal, small, absent or "duplicated" (separate CNVII canal)
- CND: **CN smaller than** normal **ipsilateral facial nerve (hypoplasia)** or absent (aplasia)
- **Normal CN** almost similar size of facial nerve or slightly larger, & larger than vestibular nerves

TOP DIFFERENTIAL DIAGNOSES

- CHARGE syndrome
- Cochlear aplasia or hypoplasia

PATHOLOGY

- CN size correlates with spiral ganglion cell population, but thin cochlear nerve may still transmit impulses for hearing

CLINICAL ISSUES

- Presents with congenital sensorineural hearing loss
- 2% of congenital profound deafness due to CND
- Treat with cochlear implantation (CI), ABI if CI fails

DIAGNOSTIC CHECKLIST

- Most cases of CND have normal cochlea ± modiolar thickening ± CNC stenosis or atresia
- Assess CNs on axial & **oblique sagittal** heavily T2WI 3D MR

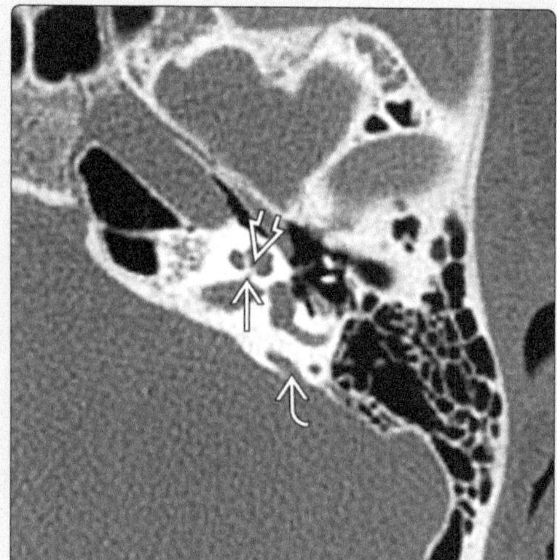
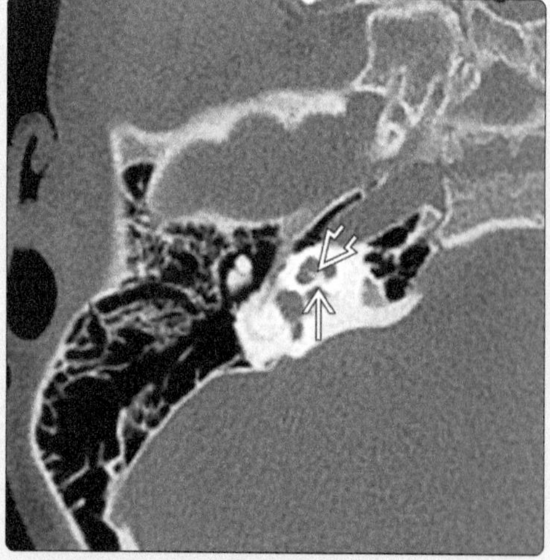

(Left) *Axial bone CT in an 11-year-old girl with profound bilateral sensorineural hearing loss (SNHL) is shown. There is severe stenosis of the cochlear nerve canal (CNC) ➡. The modiolus ➡ is thickened. This patient also has a mildly enlarged vestibular aqueduct ➡.* **(Right)** *Axial bone CT in a 4-year-old girl with profound right SNHL is shown. There is absence of the CNC ➡ (trapped isolated cochlea) & marked thickening of the modiolus ➡.*

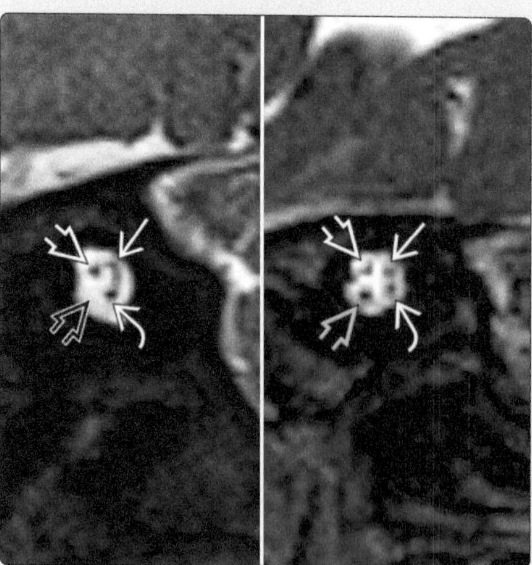
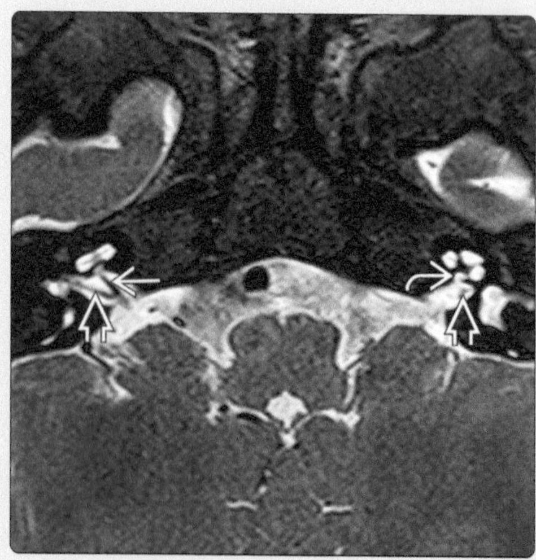

(Left) *Sagittal oblique 3D T2 (SPACE) MR of IAC shows cochlear nerve (CN) aplasia ➡, with intact facial & superior/inferior vestibular nerves. Right side of image in another patient shows the normal 4 nerves in IAC. Note that the anteroinferior CN ➡ should be larger than facial nerve ➡ above it & superior ➡ /inferior ➡ vestibular nerves posterior to it.* **(Right)** *Axial T2 SPACE MR in a 1-year-old boy with profound left SNHL shows absent left CN & mildly stenotic CNC ➡. Note normal right CN ➡ & bilateral vestibular nerves ➡.*

Cochlear Nerve and Cochlear Nerve Canal Aplasia-Hypoplasia

TERMINOLOGY

Abbreviations

- **Cochlear nerve canal (CNC)**

Synonyms

- **Cochlear aperture (CA)** (a.k.a. **cochlear fossette** or **bony CNC**) stenosis or atresia
- **Trapped (isolated) cochlea**: CNC absent; filled with bone

Definitions

- CNC hypoplasia-aplasia: Narrowing or absence of CNC
- **CN deficiency (CND)**: CN hypoplasia or absence (aplasia)

IMAGING

General Features

- Best diagnostic clue
  - **Normal CN larger than** either superior **vestibular nerves** (SVN) or inferior **vestibular nerves** (IVNs) in 90%
  - Normal CN almost **similar size of facial nerve or larger** than CNVII in 64%
  - **CND**: **CN smaller than normal CNVII (hypoplasia)** or absent (aplasia) on MR
  - **CNC (CA) width**: At **narrowest point** between internal auditory canal (IAC) fundus & modiolus on axial images
  - **CNC (CA) hypoplasia**: CNC **width < 1.4 mm**
- Location
  - CNC extends from IAC fundus to modiolus
  - CNVII anterosuperior; **CN anteroinferior** (7UP, Coke down); SVN posterosuperior; IVN posteroinferior **in IAC**

Imaging Recommendations

- Protocol advice
  - Sagittal oblique 3D T2 MR perpendicular to plane of CN

CT Findings

- Bone CT
  - **CNC (CA)**: Seen on axial mid modiolar section
    - Normal: In some cases of CND on MR
    - Stenosis: Severity varies
    - Atresia: Complete absence of CNC
  - **Cochlea**
    - Normal turns & modiolus with normal or mildly stenotic CNC
    - Normal turns & **thickened modiolus** with moderate to severe stenosis of CNC
    - Abnormal cochlea with stenotic/atretic CNC (less common) (e.g., cochlear hypoplasia)
  - Vestibule & semicircular canal (SCC): Normal (most); less commonly abnormal (e.g., syndromic etiology)
  - IAC: Normal or small, rarely separate CNVII canal ("duplicated IAC")
    - **Narrow IAC**: **< 2.5 mm** at midpoint of IAC
  - CNVII canal: Normal (most) or anomalous (rare)

MR Findings

- **CN**: Hypoplasia or aplasia
  - CNC (CA) normal: Occasional CND
  - CNC (CA) mildly stenotic: CN normal or CND
  - CNC (CA) stenotic < 1.4 mm ± thickened modiolus: CND
  - CNC (CA) stenosis + IAC narrowing: CND difficult to see on MR because of ↓ CSF around CNVIII & CNVII
  - CNC (CA) aplasia: CN aplastic
- VNs
  - Normal IAC: VN usually normal
  - Narrow IAC: VN normal or deficient

DIFFERENTIAL DIAGNOSIS

CHARGE Syndrome

- CNC stenosis/atresia, CNVIII deficiency, hypoplastic vestibule, absent/hypoplastic SCC

Cochlear Aplasia

- Cochlea absent

Cochlear Hypoplasia

- Small cochlea, 4 subtypes

PATHOLOGY

Microscopic Features

- CN size correlates with spiral ganglion cell population, but thin CN may still transmit impulses for hearing

CLINICAL ISSUES

Presentation

- Most common signs/symptoms
  - Congenital sensorineural hearing loss (SNHL)
    - Unilateral > > bilateral SNHL; usually static
- **Audiologic evaluation findings**
- Neural-type SNHL typical of isolated CND
  - Otoacoustic emissions or cochlear microphonics present (intact cochlea with outer hair cell function)
  - Absent auditory brainstem response (ABR)

Treatment

- Hearing aids do not provide enough amplification in CNC (CA) hypoplasia/aplasia
- Bilateral hypoplastic CNC (CA) with hypoplastic CN, hearing aid trial necessary
  - If no functional hearing after trial, perform **cochlear implantation (CI)**
- MR differentiation of CN hypoplasia from aplasia difficult, especially if IAC is narrow
- Perform full audiometric test battery even if MR CN aplasia
  - Evidence of hearing sometimes detected, then CI
- **Auditory brainstem implantation (ABI)** when CI contraindicated or fails
- **ABI 1st-line** therapy for CNC (CA) **aplasia**
- **Simultaneous CI & ABI** if barely visible CN in children between 2-3 years age
  - To avoid losing valuable time for language development

DIAGNOSTIC CHECKLIST

Image Interpretation Pearls

- CND: CNC stenosis ± modiolar thickening

SELECTED REFERENCES

1. Liang W et al: Heterozygous MYH9 mutations in 2 children with cochlear nerve canal stenosis. Ear Nose Throat J. 1455613221135644, 2022

X-Linked Stapes Gusher (DFNX2)

KEY FACTS

TERMINOLOGY

- **X-linked mixed hearing loss (bilateral)**
- Cochlear **incomplete partition type III (IP-III)**

IMAGING

- Cochlea: **Interscalar septa present** but **absent modiolus** & cochlear base → **corkscrew cochlea**
- **Cochlea directly at lateral end of IAC**
- ↓ otic capsule thickness; ↓ transverse cochlear dimension
- **IAC**: **Bulbous** dilation + deficient lamina cribrosa
- **Cysts/diverticuli** contiguous with vestibule &/or SCCs
- **SCC dehiscence** (mainly posterior SCC); ± SCC ossification
- **Vestibular aqueduct**: More **medial origin** ± large
- **CNVII**: **Labyrinthine** segment located **above cochlea**
- **Hypothalamus** thickened/lobular ± hamartoma-like

TOP DIFFERENTIAL DIAGNOSES

- Cochlear incomplete partition types I & II (IP-I & IP-II)
- Cochlear hypoplasia type II (CH-II)

PATHOLOGY

- X-linked recessive: **Males** affected, female carriers
- Molecular cause: *POU3F4* gene mutation
- Absent lamina cribrosa → communication between CSF & cochlear perilymph → perilymph hydrops
- **Outer** periosteal & enchondral **layers defective**
  - Predispose to very severe CSF gusher at surgery
- **Normal/thick** inner **endosteal** layer & stapes foot plate
  - Spontaneous CSF fistula through stapes footplate & recurrent meningitis very rare

CLINICAL ISSUES

- Bilateral profound SNHL (treat by **cochlear implant**) ± CHL
- **Severe gusher** at cochlear implantation surgery & very high chance of **electrode misplacement into IAC**
- IP-III: **Stapes surgery contraindicated** → gusher & ↑ SNHL

DIAGNOSTIC CHECKLIST

- CT/MR: Widened IAC & IP-III (corkscrew cochlea)

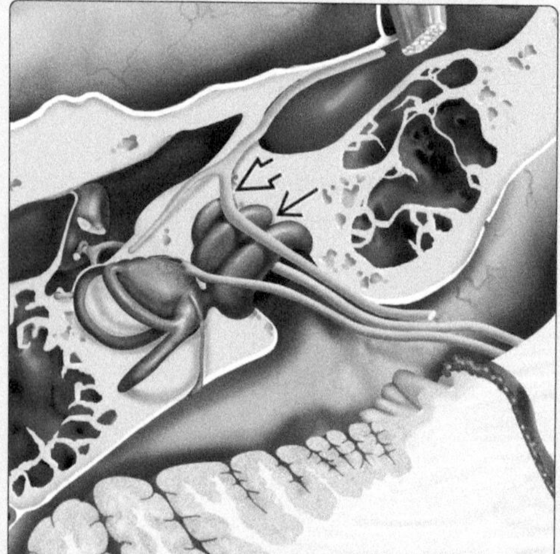

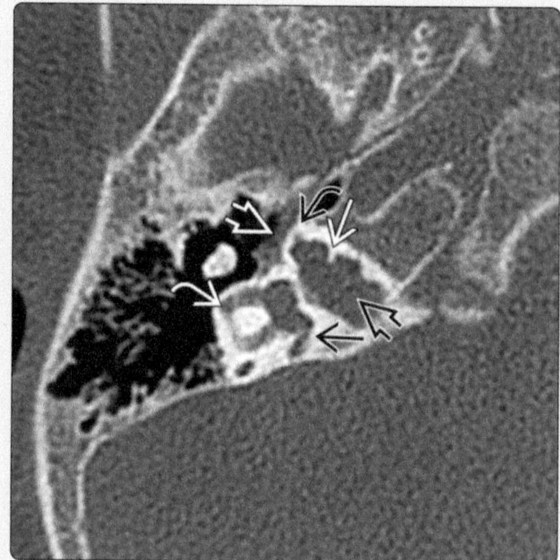

(Left) *Axial graphic of X-linked stapes gusher reveals a corkscrew cochlea (IP-III) ⇒ with no modiolus. IAC is small and wide. CNVII labyrinthine segment ⇒ is the superior-most structure in temporal bone located above cochlea.* **(Right)** *Axial bone CT in a 2-year-old boy shows a corkscrew cochlea with interscalar septa ➡, but absent modiolus, and thin otic capsule ⇗. IAC ⇒ is wide and merges with cochlea. Note mildly dilated tympanic CNVII canal ➡, lateral SCC ➡, and vestibular aqueduct (VA) ⇒. VA has more medial origin.*

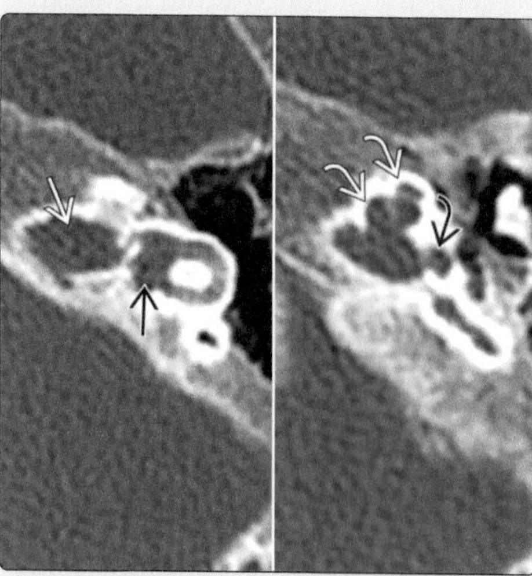

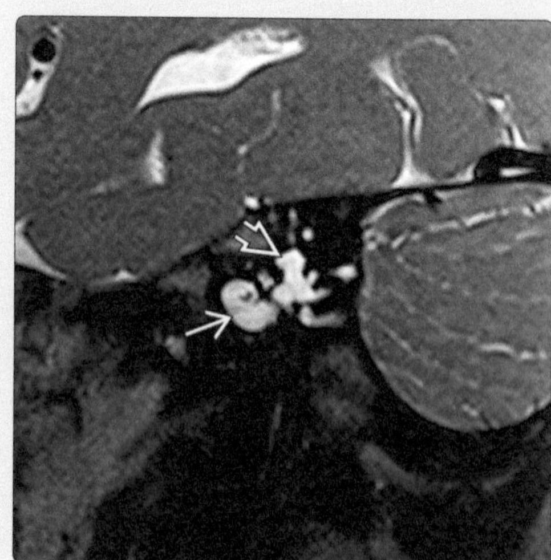

(Left) *Axial bone CT images in a patient with DFNX2 show bulbous IAC ➡ leading laterally directly to a corkscrew cochlea (IP-III) ➡ (unlike normal anterolateral cochlear location). Note a small cystic/diverticular lesion ⇗ contiguous with a mildly enlarged vestibule ⇒. (Courtesy T. J. E. Muttikkal, MD.)* **(Right)** *Sagittal oblique T2 SPACE MR in a 2-year-old boy with DFNX2 shows the deficient internal structure of cochlea ➡, which is dilated. Note globular cystic protrusion off the superior aspect of vestibule ➡.*

X-Linked Stapes Gusher (DFNX2)

TERMINOLOGY

Abbreviations

- Deafness X-linked 2 (DFNX2);X-linked mixed hearing loss (XLMHL)

Synonyms

- **Bilateral** X-linked deafness with **stapes gusher**
- Deafness 3, conductive, with stapes fixation (DFN3)
- Nance deafness
- Cochlear **incomplete partition type III (IP-III)**

IMAGING

General Features

- Best diagnostic clue
    - **Bulbous** internal auditory canal (**IAC**) & cochlear **IP-III**

CT Findings

- Bone CT
    - ↓ otic capsule (OC) thickness & ↓ **transverse** & slightly ↑ **vertical** dimensions of **cochlea** on axial CT frequent
        - Could affect selection of **cochlear implant type**
        - **OC thickness** measured anterior to cochlea, from anterior cochlear apex to anterior cortical margin
    - **Cystic/diverticular lesions** contiguous with vestibule (in 1/3) &/or semicircular canals (SCCs) (in 1/6)
    - ± **superior bulge protruding from vestibule**
    - **Dilated vestibule** in most & **SCC** in majority
    - **SCC dehiscence** in most, mainly posterior SCC
    - ± **SCC ossification**
    - **Cochlea**: **Interscalar septum (ISS) present,** but absent modiolus & cochlear base → **corkscrew** cochlea (**IP-III**)
    - Cochlea directly **at lateral end of IAC** instead of usual anterolateral location
    - Cochlear nerve canal: Widened
    - **IAC**: **Bulbous dilatation laterally**, absent lamina cribrosa
    - **Vestibular aqueduct** (VA): More **medial origin** than usual with varying degrees of dilatation
    - **Facial nerve** canal: **Labyrinthine segment** located almost above cochlea (**due to thin OC**)
        - **Superior-most structure in axial** temporal bone **CT**
        - Wide labyrinthine & proximal tympanic segments
        - Distal tympanic & mastoid segments normal
    - Oval window: Atresia in 1/3 & severe hypoplasia in < 1/3
    - Stapes footplate: Thick in 3/4; rarely, stapes dislocation

MR Findings

- T2WI
    - Inner ear findings similar to CT
    - **Hypothalamus** thickened/lobular, with hamartoma-like appearance in 1/2 of cases

DIFFERENTIAL DIAGNOSIS

Cochlear Incomplete Partition Type I (IP-I)

- Absent internal cochlear structure; figure 8 or snowman

Large Vestibular Aqueduct (IP-II)

- Large VA ± absent apical septation & deficient modiolus

Cochlear Hypoplasia Type II

- CH-II: Defective cochlear modiolus & ISS

PATHOLOGY

General Features

- Genetics
    - Inheritance: **X-linked recessive**
    - Chromosomal locus: **Xq21**; *POU3F4* **gene** mutation

Gross Pathologic & Surgical Features

- Absent lamina cribrosa → subarachnoid space & cochlear perilymph communication → perilymphatic hydrops
- Stapes fixation → perilymph/CSF gusher at stapedectomy
- **IP-III: Defective vascular supply from middle ear**
    - **Outer periosteal & enchondral layers defective**
    - Predispose to very **severe CSF gusher at surgery**
- **Normal/thick** inner **endosteal** layer & **stapes foot plate**
    - Hence, **spontaneous CSF fistula** through stapes footplate & recurrent meningitis **very rare**
- In IP-III, cochlear base defective & modiolus totally absent
    - **Cochlear base** consists of middle enchondral (main bulk) & inner endosteal layers
    - When enchondral layer absent, inner endosteal layer not enough to form thick base to support modiolus
        - Modiolus cannot form attachment points
    - **Defective cochlear base** & **absent modiolus**, even with normal vascularization of modiolus from IAC

CLINICAL ISSUES

Presentation

- Most common signs/symptoms
    - Males affected; female carriers normal (most) or mild-/delayed-onset hearing loss
        - **Bilateral profound** sensorineural hearing loss (**SNHL)** (may be progressive)
- **Audiologic evaluation findings**
    - IP-III may have profound SNHL or mixed hearing loss
    - **Conductive hearing loss** may be due to thin OC, stapes fixation, or perilymphatic pressure on stapes foot plate

Treatment

- Profound SNHL: **Cochlear implantation**
- All IP-III have **severe gusher** at cochlear implant surgery & very high chance of **electrode misplacement into IAC**
    - Due to absent modiolus & large cochlear base defect
- All IP-III (like IP-II) have cochlear nerve; auditory brainstem implant (ABI) not indicated
- IP-III: **Stapes surgery contraindicated** → gusher & ↑ SNHL

DIAGNOSTIC CHECKLIST

Image Interpretation Pearls

- Key features: **Bulbous IAC** + cochlear **IP-III**

SELECTED REFERENCES

1. Parlak S et al: X-linked deafness/incomplete partition type 3: radiological evaluation of temporal bone and intracranial findings. Diagn Interv Radiol. 28(1):50-7, 2022
2. Sennaroğlu L: Radiological features and pathognomonic sign of stapes footplate fistula in inner ear malformations. Turk Arch Otorhinolaryngol. 59(2):95-102, 2021
3. Sennaroğlu L et al: Incomplete partition type III: a rare and difficult cochlear implant surgical indication. Auris Nasus Larynx. 45(1):26-32, 2018

Common Cavity Malformation

KEY FACTS

TERMINOLOGY

- Common cavity (CC): Cystic space representing undifferentiated cochlea & vestibule

IMAGING

- **Cochlea, vestibule, & horizontal semicircular canal (SCC)**: CC, variable size
- Posterior & superior SCC: Usually absent or malformed
- IAC: Variable size, anomalous course, deficient fundus
  - **Small CC**: Stenotic IAC; **large CC**: Widened IAC
- CNVIII: Small or absent components
- Facial nerve canal: Anomalous course

TOP DIFFERENTIAL DIAGNOSES

- **Rudimentary otocyst**: Not connected to IAC
- Cochlear aplasia with dilated vestibule (CADV): **IAC fundus opens into anteromedial aspect of vestibule**
- Cystic cochleovestibular malformation (CCVM)/incomplete partition type I (IP-I): **Figure 8 or sloping snowman**

PATHOLOGY

- Arrested **otocyst** development at **4th** gestational **week**
- *HOXA1* mutations: Bosley-Salih-Alorainy syndrome

CLINICAL ISSUES

- Congenital sensorineural hearing loss
- Cochlear implantation if cochleovestibular nerve (CVN) with enough cochlear nerve fibers (size/hearing aid trial)
- Auditory brainstem implantation if cochlear fibers questionable, as in nondemonstrated or small CVN in MR
- Potential risk of **spontaneous CSF fistula/recurrent meningitis** for large CC & large IAC

DIAGNOSTIC CHECKLIST

- **CC** if cochlea & vestibule form undifferentiated single cavity
- **CCVM (IP-I)** if differentiated into partially separate but featureless cochlea & vestibule
- **CC**: IAC fundus usually opens into **center** of cavity medially
- **CADV**: IAC fundus opens into its **anteromedial** aspect

(Left) *Axial graphic shows features of a common cavity (CC) malformation. Note that the cochlea and vestibule are merged into a common cyst. Semicircular canals are not distinct from cystic vestibular component.* **(Right)** *Axial bone CT in a 6-month-old boy with unilateral sensorineural hearing loss reveals a CC anomaly of the inner ear with a cystic structure representing the rudimentary cochlea bud, vestibule, and horizontal semicircular canal ➔. A dilated posterior semicircular canal ➔ is seen.*

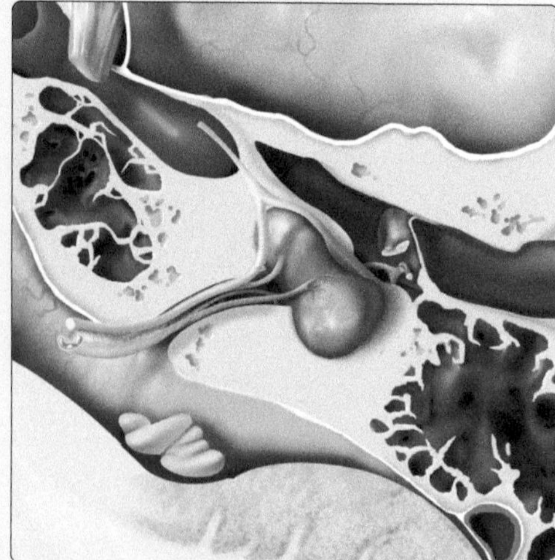

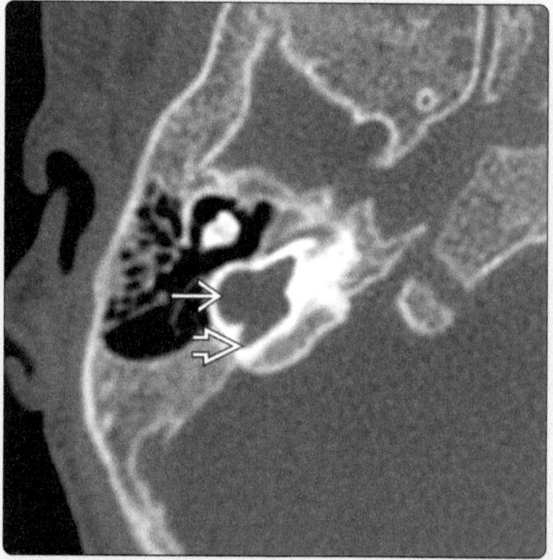

(Left) *Axial 3D FIESTA in an 18-month-old child with bilateral congenital sensorineural hearing loss demonstrates a CC anomaly with a cystic structure representing the vestibule, rudimentary cochlear bud, and horizontal semicircular canal ➔. There is a small posterior semicircular canal ➔. Middle ear cavity is fluid filled ➔.* **(Right)** *Axial 3D T2 MR shows a small rudimentary otocyst ➔ without an IAC. Do not mistake this for a CC malformation (usually has an IAC). Note small facial nerve in cerebellopontine angle ➔.*

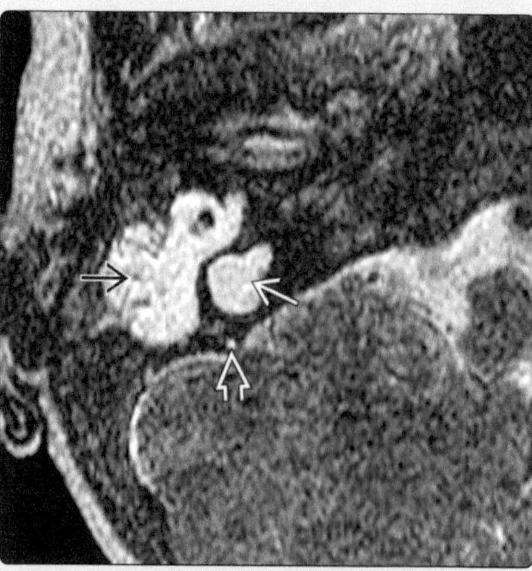

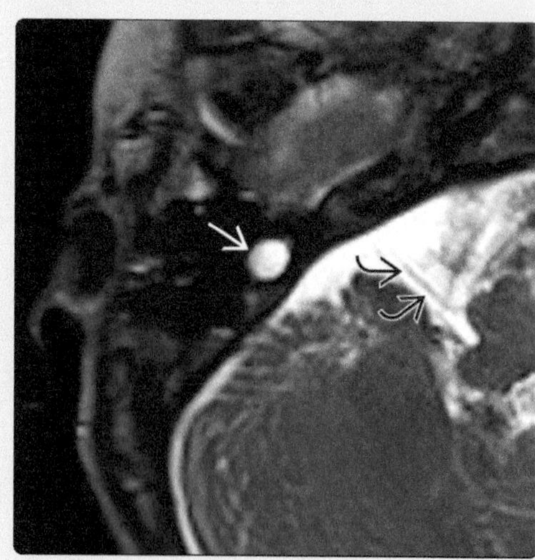

TERMINOLOGY

Definitions

- Common cavity (CC): Cystic space representing **undifferentiated cochlea & vestibule**

IMAGING

General Features

- Best diagnostic clue
  - Featureless CC represents rudimentary cochlea, vestibule, & semicircular canals (SCCs)

CT Findings

- Bone CT
  - Unilateral or bilateral & often asymmetric
  - **Cochlea, vestibule, & horizontal SCC**: CC, variable size
  - Posterior & superior SCC: Usually absent or malformed
  - Internal auditory canal (IAC)
    - **Small CC**: Stenotic IAC; **large CC**: Widened IAC
    - Defective fundus
    - **IAC fundus** may **enter center of CC medially**
    - If open at anterior aspect, more likely to be cochlear aplasia with dilated vestibule (CADV) than CC
  - Facial nerve canal: Anomalous labyrinthine segment & anterior genu
  - Middle ear space & ossicles: Normal or anomalous stapes & stenotic oval window
  - Vestibular aqueduct: Not dilated, may be absent

MR Findings

- T2WI
  - High signal intensity fluid within CC
  - Posterior & superior SCC: Usually absent or malformed
  - IAC: Single common **cochleovestibular nerve (CVN)** ± anomalous course of CNVII
  - Normally cochlear & vestibular nerves originate from brainstem as CVN & separates in IAC
    - Into cochlear, superior, & inferior vestibular nerves
    - In **CC, unbranched CVN** enters CC
  - **Cochlear nerve fiber content in CVN** impossible to assess with current imaging; considered normal if
    - Size similar to contralateral normal CVN or 1.5-2x that of ipsilateral facial nerve

DIFFERENTIAL DIAGNOSIS

Cochlear Aplasia

- Imaging: Absent cochlea, normal or dilated vestibule
- **CADV: IAC fundus opens at its anteromedial aspect**

Rudimentary Otocyst

- Anomaly between labyrinthine aplasia & CC
- **No IAC connection** (unlike CC); needs auditory brainstem implantation (ABI), cochlear implant (CI) contraindicated
  - Anecdotal case reports of CI with some benefit

Cystic Cochleovestibular Malformation (CCVM)/Incomplete Partition Type I (IP-I)

- Imaging: Cochlea & vestibule are usually enlarged & cystic without internal architecture; figure 8 or sloping snowman

Incomplete Partition Type III (IP-III)

- Modiolus absent but interscalar septa present, giving corkscrew appearance of cochlea
- Contiguous with bulbous IAC

PATHOLOGY

General Features

- Etiology
  - Unknown or genetic mutation
  - *HOXA1* mutations: Bosley-Salih-Alorainy syndrome
  - May have associated **endosteal/stapes footplate** developmental anomaly → **spontaneous CSF fistula/recurrent meningitis**
    - CSF fills cochlea, & cystic structure may be seen at stapes footplate on CT/MR
    - Most commonly in **CC malformation (18%)**, followed by IP-I (15%), &, rarely, in cochlear aplasia (5.2%), CH-I (5.6%), CH-II (4.4%), & IP-II (0.85%)
- Embryology
  - Developmental arrest in **4th** gestational **week**, after differentiation of otic placode into **otocyst**

CLINICAL ISSUES

Presentation

- Most common signs/symptoms
  - Congenital sensorineural hearing loss (SNHL)
  - Potential risk of **spontaneous CSF fistula/recurrent meningitis** for large CC & large IAC
- **Audiologic evaluation findings**
  - Profound hearing loss

Treatment

- **CI** if **CVN with enough cochlear nerve fibers**
- **Hearing aid trial**: If behavioral audiometric response or language development occurs with hearing aid use
  - Enough cochlear fibers possibly exist in CVN
- **ABI** if cochlear fibers questionable, as in nondemonstrated or small CVN in MR
- Contralateral ABI if limited language development with CI

DIAGNOSTIC CHECKLIST

Consider

- **CC** if cochlea & vestibule form undifferentiated single cavity
- **CCVM (IP-I)** if differentiated into partially separate but featureless cochlea & vestibule
- **CC**: IAC fundus usually opens into **center** of cavity medially
- **CADV:** IAC fundus opens into its **anteromedial** aspect
- Profound hearing loss in CC; no hearing in CADV
- **Rudimentary otocyst**: No IAC connection

Image Interpretation Pearls

- Oblique sagittal IAC 3D T2 MR to determine presence & size (cochlear fiber content) of CNV

SELECTED REFERENCES

1. Lu S et al: Cochlear implantation for rudimentary otocysts: two case reports. Otol Neurotol. 44(5):e295-9, 2023
2. Al-Mahboob A et al: Cochlear implantation in common cavity deformity: a systematic review. Eur Arch Otorhinolaryngol. 279(1):37-48, 2022

KEY FACTS

TERMINOLOGY

- Cochlear **incomplete partition type I (IP-I)** + dilated vestibule & horizontal semicircular canal (SCC)

IMAGING

- Cochlea: Absent internal septation & modiolus (IP-I)
- Vestibule & SCC: Dilated vestibule & lateral (horizontal) SCC form single cavity, wide communication with cochlea
- CNVII canal: Normal or mildly obtuse anterior genu angle; normal or dehiscent tympanic segment
- Internal auditory canal (IAC): Small or dilated, fundus defect
- IAC fundus opens **in between** vestibule & cochlea medially
- CNVIII: Nerves hypoplastic or absent
- Oval window: Normal or stenotic + stapedial anomaly

TOP DIFFERENTIAL DIAGNOSES

- Cochlear aplasia (CA), especially CA with dilated vestibule
    - IAC fundus opens at its anteromedial aspect
- Common cavity: IAC fundus enter center of cavity medially
- Cochlear hypoplasia type II (cystic hypoplastic cochlea)
- IP-III

PATHOLOGY

- Arrested **otocyst** development at **5th** gestational **week**

CLINICAL ISSUES

- Congenital sensorineural hearing loss
- Cochlear implant (CI) or auditory brainstem implant (ABI) (if deficient cochlear nerve)
- Contralateral ABI if limited language development with CI
- Recurrent meningitis: Middle ear exploration to excise & repair stapes footplate/oval window cyst & defect

DIAGNOSTIC CHECKLIST

- **Cystic cochleovestibular malformation (IP-I)**
    - **Figure 8/sloping snowman** cochlea & vestibule
    - Defective IAC fundus: Risk of CSF gusher at surgery
    - **Stapes foot plate defect**: Spontaneous **CSF fistula** & **recurrent meningitis**

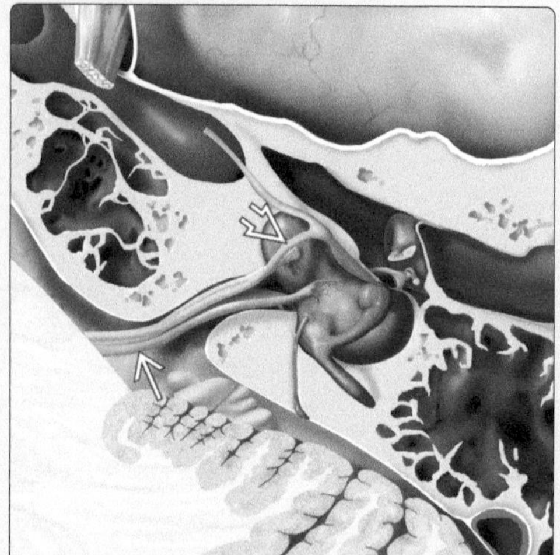

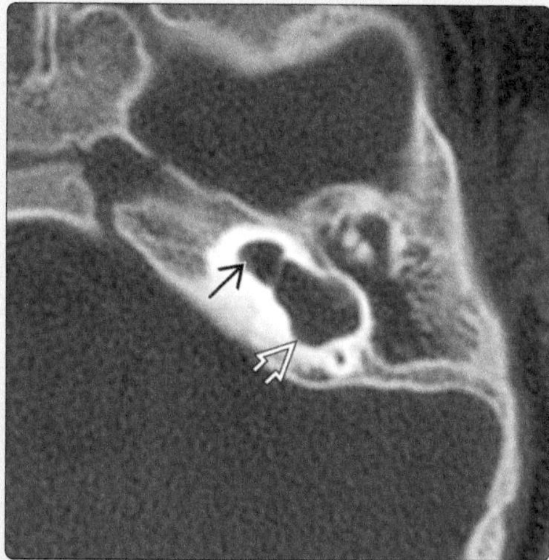

(Left) *Axial graphic shows cystic cochleovestibular malformation (CCVM) with featureless cochlea & vestibule. Cochlear interscalar septum & modiolus are absent (incomplete partition type I [IP-I]). CNVIII is hypoplastic ➡. IAC is narrow and shortened. CNVII labyrinthine segment has lost its anteriorly curving shape & appears straightened ➡.* **(Right)** *CT in an 18-month-old boy with CCVM shows a cochlea that lacks internal architecture (IP-I) ➡. Vestibule & horizontal semicircular canal form a single globular cavity ➡.*

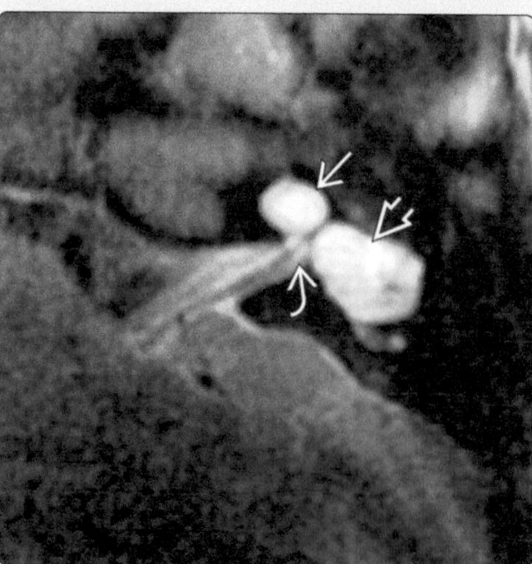

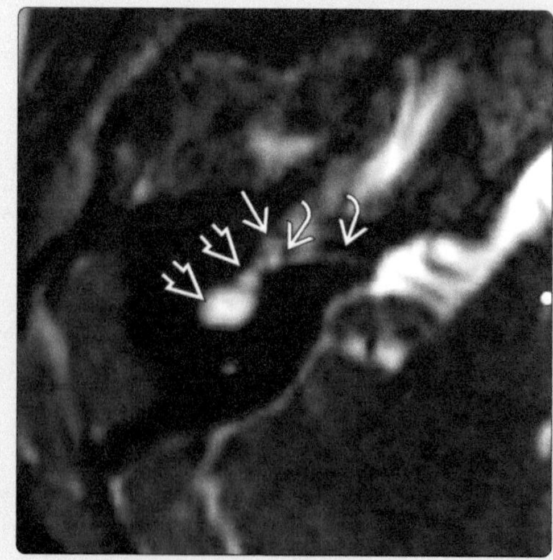

(Left) *Axial T2WI MR shows classic figure 8/sloping snowman-like CCVM with dilated, featureless cochlea (IP-I) ➡ & vestibule ➡. IAC fundus ➡ opens in between the medial aspects of vestibule & cochlea.* **(Right)** *Axial 3D T2 MR shows CCVM with hypoplastic IAC fundus ➡ opening between a tiny cochlea ➡ & a posterior gradually enlarging vestibular cavity ➡. In contrast, IAC opens at anteromedial aspect of vestibule in cochlear aplasia with dilated vestibule (CADV) & at center of cavity medially in common cavity (CC).*

Cystic Cochleovestibular Malformation

TERMINOLOGY

Abbreviations

- Cystic cochleovestibular malformation (CCVM)

Synonyms

- Cystic cochleovestibular anomaly
- Cochlear **incomplete partition type I (IP-I)**

Definitions

- Cochlea lacks interscalar septum & modiolus (IP-I) + dilated vestibule & lateral (horizontal) semicircular canal (SCC)

IMAGING

General Features

- Best diagnostic clue
  - Cystic, featureless cochlea + dilated vestibule/lateral SCC
- Morphology
  - Cochlea & vestibule: **Figure 8** or **sloping snowman**

CT Findings

- Bone CT
  - Cochlea: **Absent internal septation & modiolus (IP-I)**, variable size
  - Vestibule: **Dilated, large cochlear communication**
  - SCC: **Dilated, lateral SCC** forms common cavity (CC) with vestibule, anterior limb superior SCC ± dilated
  - Internal auditory canal (IAC): Small or dilated
    - **Defect between IAC fundus** & cochlea due to cochlear aperture defect & absent modiolus
      - CSF may completely fill cochlea
  - IAC fundus opens **in between** vestibule & cochlea
  - CNVII canal: Normal or mildly obtuse anterior genu angle; normal or dehiscent tympanic segment
  - Vestibular aqueduct: Usually normal
  - Oval window: Normal or stenotic + stapedial anomaly
  - **Stapes footplate defect** & CSF filling cochlea with **cystic structure** in stapes footplate
    - **Endosteal** developmental anomaly
    - Easily infected during otitis media attack
    - **Spontaneous CSF fistula & recurrent meningitis**
  - Cerebellar flocculus herniation into IAC reported
    - Due to predisposition to IAC fundus CSF leak & ↑ intracranial pressure because of meningitis

MR Findings

- T2WI
  - Cochlea + vestibule: Figure 8 contour
  - Cochlea: Lacks internal septation & modiolus
  - Vestibule & horizontal SCC: Dilated
  - CNVIII: Nerves hypoplastic or absent

Imaging Recommendations

- Best imaging tool
  - MR for CNVIII components, mainly cochlear nerve (**CN**)
- Protocol advice
  - 3D T2 (CISS, FIESTA): Axial & oblique sagittal

DIFFERENTIAL DIAGNOSIS

Cochlear Aplasia

- **Absent cochlea**; vestibule & SCC variable
- Cochlear aplasia (CA) with dilated vestibule: IAC fundus opens at **anteromedial aspect** of dilated vestibule

Common Cavity Malformation

- **Cystic cochlea & vestibule** form undifferentiated or minimally differentiated CC
- IAC fundus opens at **center of cavity medially**

Cochlear Hypoplasia Type II

- Defective cochlear modiolus & interscalar septa
- **Endosteal** developmental anomaly with **defective stapes footplate** development & **recurrent meningitis**: CC (18%), IP-I (15%), CA (5.2%), cochlear hypoplasia type 1 (CH-I) (5.6%), CH-II (4.4%), & IP-II (0.85%)

Incomplete Partition Type III

- Modiolus absent, but interscalar septa present, giving corkscrew appearance of cochlea
- Contiguous with bulbous IAC; predisposes to high-volume CSF **gusher** during cochlear implant (CI) surgery
- **Outer** periosteal & enchondral **layers defective** but with thick endosteal layer & **normal stapes foot plate**
  - Meningitis rare (unlike others with endosteal defect)

PATHOLOGY

General Features

- Embryology
  - Arrested **otocyst** development: ~ **5th** gestational **week**

CLINICAL ISSUES

Presentation

- Most common signs/symptoms
  - Congenital sensorineural hearing loss (SNHL)
  - CSF leak & meningitis from translabyrinthine fistula
  - Risk of labyrinthine ossification from meningitis
- **Audiologic evaluation findings**
  - Severe to profound SNHL in majority

Treatment

- CI: Risks in CCVM: CSF gusher (deficient IAC fundus), facial nerve damage (dehiscent)
  - CSF leakage from cochleostomy should be sealed; then, only subtotal petrosectomy to seal middle ear from nose
- Auditory brainstem implantation (ABI) if aplastic CN
- Contralateral ABI if limited language development with CI
- IP-I with recurrent meningitis & normal tympanic membranes, & fluid filling middle ear & mastoid
  - Middle ear exploration to excise & repair stapes footplate/oval window cyst & defect

DIAGNOSTIC CHECKLIST

Image Interpretation Pearls

- CCVM: **Figure 8** or **sloping snowman** cochlea & vestibule
- Look for IAC fundus opening **in between** vestibule & cochlea in CCVM, to differentiate from CADV & CC
- MR to detect hypoplasia/aplasia of CNVIII components

SELECTED REFERENCES

1. Parlak Ş et al: Flocculus herniation into the internal acoustic canal in incomplete partition type I: a case report. J Int Adv Otol. 19(3):266-8, 2023

Large Vestibular Aqueduct

KEY FACTS

TERMINOLOGY

- Large vestibular aqueduct (LVA)
- **Incomplete partition type II (IP-II)** between middle & apical cochlear turns; **often seen with LVA**
- IP-II + LVA + minimally dilated vestibule: **Mondini** deformity

IMAGING

- Axial CT: **Midpoint of vestibular aqueduct** between posterior labyrinth & operculum **> 1.5 mm**
- MR: Enlarged endolymphatic sac & duct
- Cochlea: Abnormal in ~ 75% of LVA cases
    - Absent septation & modiolus between middle & apical turns (**IP-II**); enlarged **scala vestibuli > 1.2 mm**
- 2nd interscalar ridge notch **angle** > **114°**, **depth ≤ 0.31 mm**
- Vestibule & semicircular canal: Normal or mildly enlarged

TOP DIFFERENTIAL DIAGNOSES

- Cystic cochleovestibular malformation (IP-I)
- Cochlear hypoplasia
- CHARGE syndrome (funnel-shaped LVA)
- Branchiootorenal syndrome (funnel-shaped LVA)

PATHOLOGY

- *SLC26A4* mutations in ~ 50% of LVA patients
- **IP-II**: Arrested development at **7th** gestational **week**
- Modiolar defects in IP-II may be from **transmission of high CSF pressure** into inner ear **due to LVA**

CLINICAL ISSUES

- Most common imaging abnormality in pediatric SNHL
- Bilateral anomaly (most); **initially normal hearing**
- **Progressive/fluctuating SNHL** due to high pulsating CSF pressure or head trauma
- Avoid contact sports & try to prevent head trauma
- **Hearing aid** first, **cochlear implantation** later
- All IP-II have cochlear nerve, ABI not indicated

DIAGNOSTIC CHECKLIST

- LVA diagnosis: Look for associated cochlear IP-II anomaly

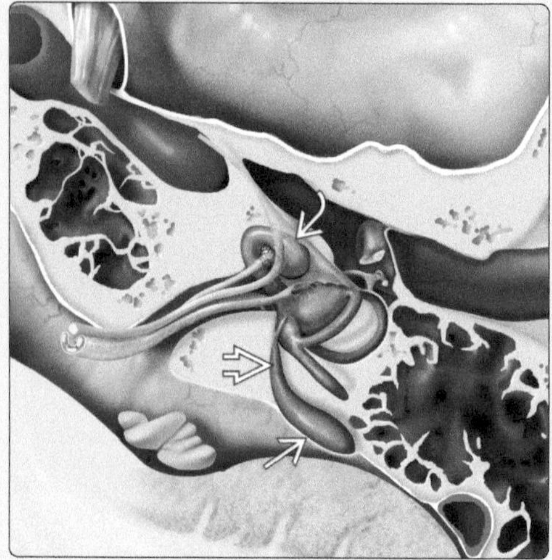

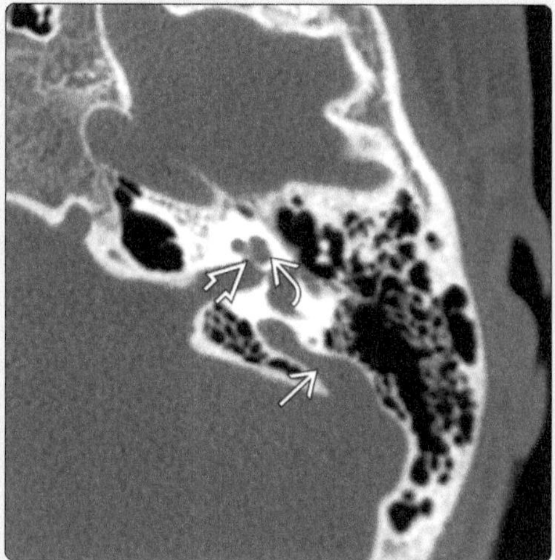

(Left) *In the left inner ear, large endolymphatic sac (ES) epidural ➡ & intraosseous ➡ components are shown. Cochlea is malformed with absent septation between middle & apical turns, which appear bulbous ➡.* **(Right)** *Axial temporal bone CT in a 15-year-old boy with sensorineural hearing loss (SNHL) shows a large vestibular aqueduct (LVA) ➡. The modiolus is defective toward apex & present at base ➡. Note that the scalar chambers are asymmetric (anterior scala vestibuli > posterior scala tympani) ➡.*

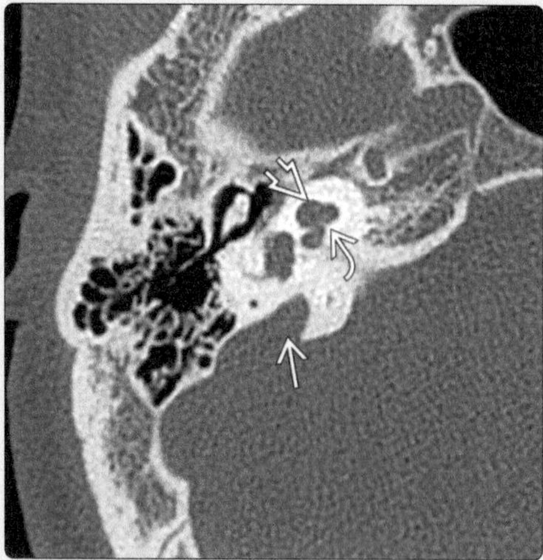

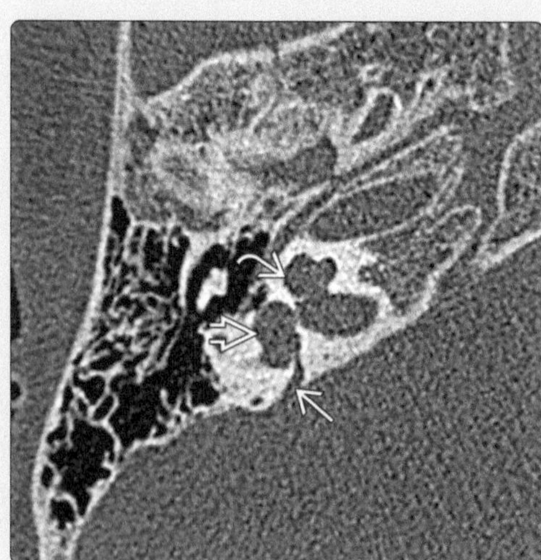

(Left) *Axial temporal bone CT in a 17-year-old girl with Pendred syndrome shows an LVA ➡ & absent septation between the middle & apical cochlear turns ➡ with a deficient modiolus ➡. This is typical of incomplete partition type II (IP-II), which results in a baseball cap-shaped cochlea.* **(Right)** *Axial bone CT in a 3-year-old boy with SNHL shows Mondini deformity with LVA ➡, typical IP-II cochlear anomaly ➡ with plump cochlear middle & apical turns, absent modiolus, & no apical septation, and the vestibule is mildly enlarged ➡.*

TERMINOLOGY

Abbreviations

- Large vestibular aqueduct (LVA)

Synonyms

- Large endolymphatic sac anomaly (**LESA**): T2 MR term
- Enlarged vestibular aqueduct (**EVA**): CT term
- **Mondini** deformity (historic terminology): LVA + minimally dilated vestibule + incomplete partition type II (IP-II)

Definitions

- LVA: Enlarged bony vestibular aqueduct (VA) houses large endolymphatic sac (ES) & duct
  - Associated with variable cochlear malformation
- **IP-II**: Deficient modiolus & interscalar septum (ISS) between **middle & apical** cochlear turns; often seen with LVA
- IP-II: Normal cochlear external dimensions
  - Not correct to classify IP-II as cochlea with 1.5 turns
  - Term cochlea with 1.5 turns should be used only for cochlear hypoplasia (CH) (especially CH-III)

IMAGING

General Features

- Best diagnostic clue
  - CT: EVA ± IP-II; 3D T2 MR: LESA ± IP-II
- Location
  - **Endolymphatic duct (ELD) & sac (ELS)** located within bony **VA**
  - Connects crus communis [meeting point of posterior & superior semicircular canals (SCCs)] to fovea
    - **Fovea**: Cup-shaped area at posterior T-bone margin; **operculum**: Opening of VA into fovea
  - ELD: Short, proximal part connected to crus communis
  - ELS: Longer, distal part with both intraosseous & intradural (fovea area) components
  - ELD transition to ELS defined by change in wall cell architecture (not seen at imaging)
  - Normal ELS & ELD barely visible on heavily T2WI 3D MR
- Size
  - **Cincinnati** criteria: Axial T-bone CT: **LVA ≥ 1 mm at midpoint**, ± ≥ 2 mm at opercular margin perpendicular to long axis of VA
  - Literature variable for LVA; vertical & axial VA width **> 1.5 mm at midpoint** of labyrinth & operculum (classic **Valvassori** criteria)
  - Transverse oblique reformat (**Pöschl view**) parallel to plane of superior SCC: LVA **≥ 0.8-0.9 mm at midpoint**
- Morphology
  - Axial bone CT: V-shaped, enlarged bony VA
  - Axial T2 MR: Large ELS along posterior wall of petrous bone, lateral to dural reflection

CT Findings

- Bone CT
  - LVA: May scallop posterior margin of petrous bone
  - Cochlea: Abnormal on CT in ~ 75% of LVA cases
    - Normal or **deficient septation** between **plump apical & middle turns** (IP-II); normal basal turn
    - **Asymmetric scalar chambers**: Anterior > posterior
    - **Deficient** (typical), absent, or normal **modiolus**
  - Vestibule: Normal or mildly enlarged
  - SCC: Normal or mildly dilated
    - Reduced size of lateral SCC bone island with enlargement of lateral SCC may be seen in IP-II
  - Middle ear space & ossicles: Normal

MR Findings

- 3D T2 SPACE, FIESTA, CISS or equivalent
  - ELS & ELD: Enlarged, variable hyperintense signal
  - Cochlea: **Deficient septation** between **plump apical & middle turns (IP-II)** or normal in LVA only
  - **Asymmetric perilymphatic scalar chambers**: Anterior **scala vestibuli larger** than posterior scala tympani
    - Intervening scala media (endolymph) not seen on MR
    - Scala media has anterior vestibular (Reissner) & posterior basilar membranes with organ of Corti
    - **Spiral lamina**: Thin, bony plate tapers laterally connecting to medial aspect of basilar membrane
      - □ Separates scala media from posterior scala tympani (osseous spiral lamina-basilar membrane complex)
    - Cochlear nerve fibers traverse modiolus, branching onto spiral lamina-basal membrane & organ of Corti
    - In 3D T2 MR, **spiral lamina-basilar membrane complex** seen as **thin, hypointense**, transverse **line**
      - □ **Between scala vestibuli** anteriorly **& scala tympani** posteriorly in each cochlear turn
  - **ISS**: Membranous bony struts extending toward modiolus: **Thin, hypointense lines** in MR; **separates** basal, middle, & apical **turns of cochlea**
  - ISS continuous, has 3 parts, & forms 3 interscalar ridges or notches (R1, R2, R3) along outer margin of cochlea
  - 1st part (enchondral ossification) divides lower basal turn & lower middle turn (posterior medial)
  - 2nd/3rd parts (membranous ossification) faulty in IP-II
  - 2nd divides upper basal & upper middle turns (lateral)
  - 3rd part divides lower middle & apical turns (medial)
  - **R2 notch** formed by 2nd part located along **lateral margin of cochlea**; best seen on 3D T2 **MR**
  - R2 notch **angle > 114°** & **depth ≤ 0.31** mm suggest **IP-II & scala communis**
  - **Scala communis**: Due to defect of osseous ISS, which separates cochlear turns
  - In IP-II, 2nd part of **ISS bulges anteriorly** due to **enlarged scala vestibuli** in 3D T2 MR
    - **> 1.2 mm** between **spiral lamina-basilar membrane complex** of upper basal turn **&** 2nd part of **ISS**
    - **Spiral lamina-basilar membrane thin line** denotes apparent posterior margin of its scala vestibuli
    - 1st signal void anteriorly represents 2nd part of **ISS**; denotes anterior margin of scala vestibuli
  - **Deficient**/absent (IP-II), or normal **modiolus**

Imaging Recommendations

- Protocol advice
  - T-bone CT or heavily T2WI 3D (CISS, FIESTA) MR

DIFFERENTIAL DIAGNOSIS

Cystic Cochleovestibular Malformation (IP-I)

- Cystic cochlea & vestibule without internal structure

Cochlear Hypoplasia

- Small cochlea; usually < 2 turns

CHARGE Syndrome

- Funnel-shaped LVA, small vestibule, & small/absent SCC
- Cochlear nerve canal stenosis/atresia & thickened modiolus; occasional cochlear hypoplasia

Branchiootorenal Syndrome

- Funnel-shaped LVA, tapered basal turn, & small, offset middle & apical turns

High-Riding Jugular Bulb

- Communicates with jugular foramen, not vestibule

PATHOLOGY

General Features

- Etiology
  - LVA + large ELS/ELD occur during embryogenesis
  - **IP-II** may be from **transmission of high CSF pressure** into inner ear **due to LVA**
  - Mild: May be EVA only, or EVA & mild vestibule dilation
  - Transmission of CSF pressure into cochlea → spectrum of anomalies: Dilated scala vestibuli, scala communis, &
    - **Modiolar defects**: Superior (cystic apex), partial, subtotal, or rarely complete
  - **ISS bulging** upward due to high **pressure in scala vestibuli** constant finding in IP-II
  - **Cochlea "fragile"** & susceptible to injury from mild trauma due to microscopic infrastructure deficiencies
  - **Conductive** component of mixed hearing loss (MHL) due to **"3rd window" effect of EVA** on sound transmission
- Genetics
  - *SLC26A4* mutations (chromosome 7)
    - ~ **50%** of **LVA** patients have *SLC26A4* mutations
    - Autosomal recessive inheritance
  - *SLC26A4* gene encodes **pendrin protein** (chloride/bicarbonate anion exchanger)
    - ↑ endolymphatic pH by bicarbonate secretion
  - ↓ or **absent pendrin** expression → **acidification** & **abnormal expansion** of developing inner ear
  - Acidification → ↓ **endolymphatic potassium** concentration with loss of endocochlear potential
  - Acidification → ↑ **endolymphatic calcium** concentration, which is toxic to stria vascularis & organ of Corti; *FOXI1* mutations (less common): *SLC26A4* transcriptional **activator gene**
  - **Syndromic deafness: Pendred syndrome**
    - Sensorineural hearing loss (**SNHL**) + thyroid organification defect ± **goiter**
    - Autosomal recessive; biallelic *SLC26A4* mutation; ~ 10% of hereditary deafness
  - **Nonsyndromic deafness (Nsd)**: Deafness autosomal recessive 4 **(DFNB4)**
    - Isolated familial SNHL; ~ 4% of Nsd; 2nd most common cause of Nsd after *GJB2* mutation
- Associated abnormalities
  - **Pendred syndrome**: Goiter (2nd decade)
  - Distal renal tubular acidosis (rare)
- Embryology: **IP-II**: Arrested development at **7th** gestational **week**
- Mondini deformity described in association with thalidomide, rubella, Pendred syndrome, CHARGE syndrome, Klippel-Feil syndrome, DiGeorge syndrome, & Wildervanck syndrome (cervico-ocular-acoustic dysplasia)

Gross Pathologic & Surgical Features

- Enlarged VA houses large ES found in dural sleeve in fovea in posterior wall of T-bone

CLINICAL ISSUES

Presentation

- Most common signs/symptoms
  - SNHL (or MHL due to "3rd window" effect)
    - Fluctuating or **progressive course** ± linear relationship between VA width & progressive SNHL; SNHL precipitated by minor head trauma
- Other signs/symptoms
  - Tinnitus, vertigo, dizziness
  - Pendred syndrome: Hypothyroidism in ~ 50%, ± goiter in adolescence
- **Audiologic evaluation findings**
  - Varies from normal to profound hearing loss
  - Air bone gap due to "3rd window" effect from EVA; may resemble superior SCC dehiscence syndrome

Demographics

- Epidemiology
  - LVA: Most common CT/MR abnormality in pediatric SNHL; bilateral (most) or unilateral anomaly

Treatment

- Avoid contact sports & try to prevent head trauma
- **Hearing aid** first, **cochlear implantation** later
- All IP-II have cochlear nerve, auditory brainstem implant (ABI) not indicated
- **CSF oozing/gusher** occasionally at cochlear implant (CI) surgery in IP-II: Due to modiolar defects from high CSF pressure transmission
- **Pulsating round window** at CI surgery in IP-II: "3rd window" effect of EVA transmitting CSF pressure into cochlea

DIAGNOSTIC CHECKLIST

Consider

- Known *SLC26A4* mutation/Pendred syndrome: Look for EVA/LESA
- EVA/LESA: Recommend *SLC26A4* testing, US thyroid, thyroid function tests, ± perchlorate discharge test
- Obtain MR if borderline VA measurements on CT

Image Interpretation Pearls

- LVA diagnosis: Look for associated cochlear anomaly

Reporting Tips

- Reformatted coronal CT or transverse oblique view differentiates LVA from high-riding jugular bulb

SELECTED REFERENCES

1. Yu K et al: The correlation between deafness progression and SLC26A4 mutations in enlarged vestibular aqueduct patients. Eur Arch Otorhinolaryngol. 281(2): 649-54, 2024
2. Connor SEJ et al: Is CT or MRI the optimal imaging investigation for the diagnosis of large vestibular aqueduct syndrome and large endolymphatic sac anomaly? Eur Arch Otorhinolaryngol. 276(3):693-702, 2019

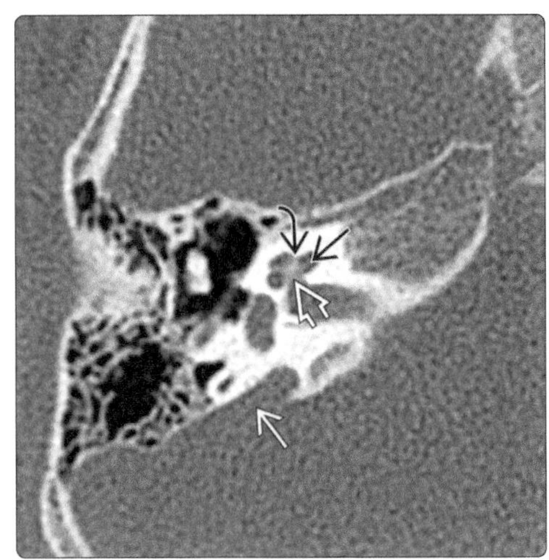

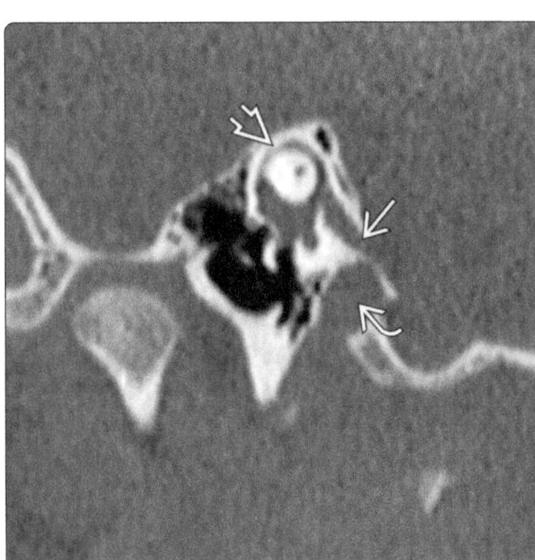

(Left) *Axial temporal bone CT in a 3-year old girl with SNHL shows LVA ➡. Cochlea is normal with interscalar septum (R2) ➡ separating the cochlear turns, spiral lamina ➡ separating scala vestibuli from scala tympani inside a turn, & normal modiolus ➡.* **(Right)** *Reformatted short-axis oblique (Pöschl view) temporal bone CT in a 3-year-old girl with SNHL demonstrates the right LVA ➡ in its entirety. The reconstructed image is parallel to the plane of the superior semicircular canal ➡. The jugular bulb ➡ lies inferior to the LVA.*

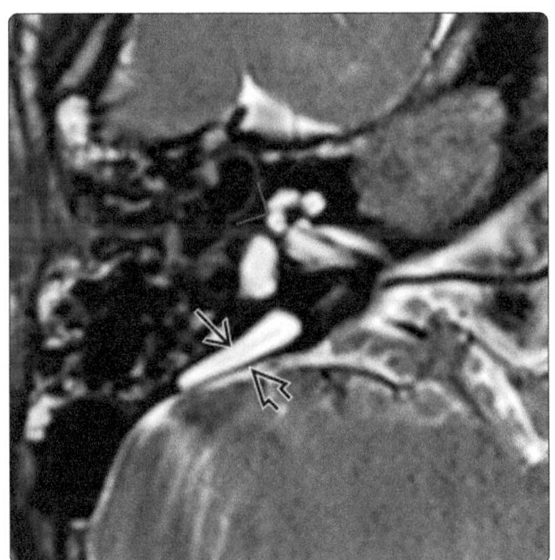

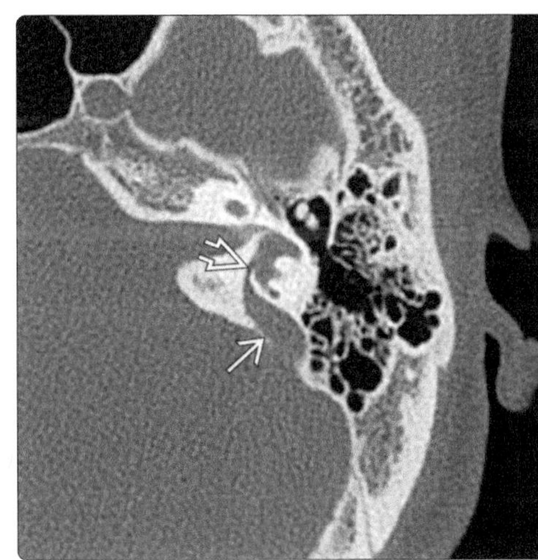

(Left) *Axial T2 MR shows hyperintense LESA ➡ lying anterolateral to hypointense dura ➡. Note normal lateral R2 notch angle (red) & depth (from lateral tangential line along cochlear turns to angle vertex) associated with the 2nd part of interscalar septum between upper basal & upper middle cochlear turns.* **(Right)** *Axial temporal bone CT in 17-year-old girl with Pendred syndrome reveals the entirety of the left LVA ➡ extending from the crus communis ➡ of the vestibule to the operculum at posterior aspect of the petrous bone.*

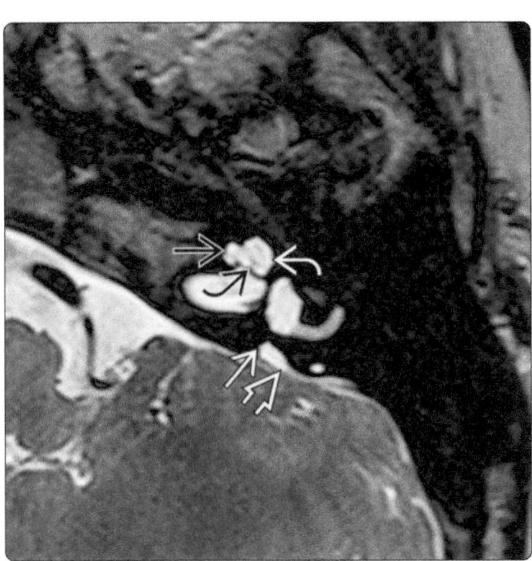

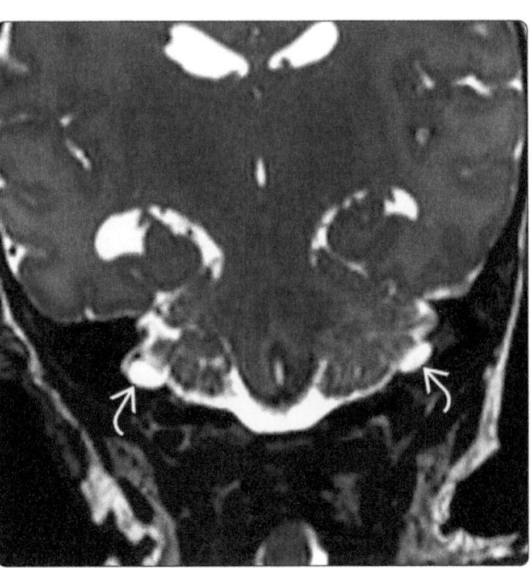

(Left) *Axial 3D FIESTA MR in a 3-year-old boy with SNHL shows a large ES ➡ lateral to hypointense dura ➡. There is a deficient 2nd part of ISS, & the lateral R2 notch angle between the distal cochlear turns is abnormally wide with narrowed depth ➡. Note the modiolar deficiency ➡. The hypointense line in the center of each cochlear turn is the normal osseous spiral lamina-basilar membrane complex ➡.* **(Right)** *Coronal 3D T2 MR through posterior petrous bone margins in another child shows bilateral large ESs ➡.*

Semicircular Canal Hypoplasia-Aplasia

KEY FACTS

TERMINOLOGY

- Definition: Hypoplasia/aplasia of 1 or multiple semicircular canals (SCCs) ± hypoplastic vestibule

IMAGING

- Hypoplastic vestibule + hypoplasia/aplasia of all SCCs in **CHARGE** syndrome
- Hypoplasia of single SCC + normal (or large) vestibule
  - Posterior SCC (PSCC) + normal or flattened cochlear apical turn: **Waardenburg (WS)** & **Alagille** syndromes
  - PSCC + hypoplastic, offset middle & apical cochlear turns: **Branchiootorenal (BOR)** syndrome
  - Lateral SCC (LSCC) + dense stapes superstructure, IP-II: 22q11.2 deletion (**DiGeorge** syndrome)
- Central lucency of LSCC bony island significantly associated with congenital severe-to-profound SNHL

TOP DIFFERENTIAL DIAGNOSES

- **Down syndrome**
  - Small or absent LSCC bone island; globular SCC-vestibule
- **Labyrinthine ossificans**: Prior meningitis or surgery

PATHOLOGY

- Superior SCC (SSCC) forms 1st, followed by PSCC, & then LSCC; isolated LSCC anomalies therefore most common

CLINICAL ISSUES

- Hearing loss, vestibular symptoms

DIAGNOSTIC CHECKLIST

- **CHARGE** if hypoplasia vestibule + SCC
- Consider **BOR** for hypoplastic, offset middle & apical turns cochlea; look for PSCC anomaly
- Consider WS for PSCC anomaly & Hirschsprung disease
- Consider Alagille syndrome for PSCC anomaly, peripheral pulmonary artery stenosis, & cholestatic liver disease
- Consider sporadic, 22q11.2 deletion or Down syndrome for LSCC anomalies

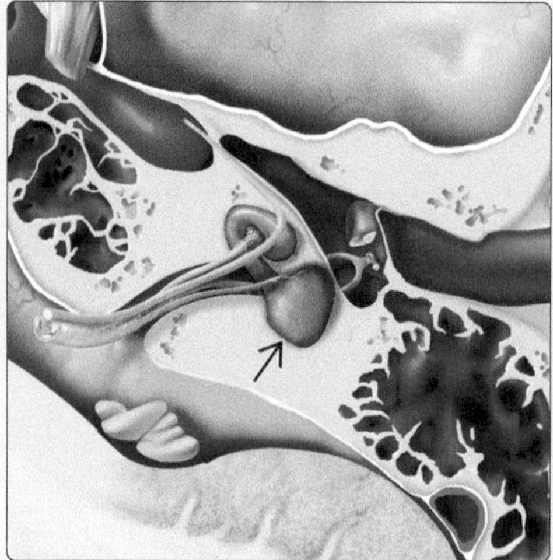

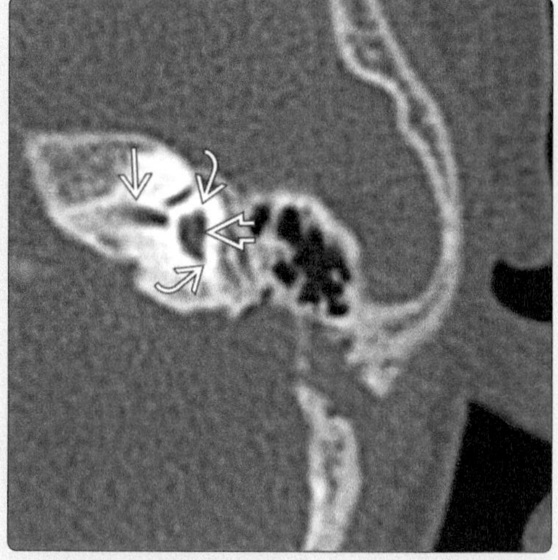

(Left) *Axial graphic depicts severe, syndromic type of semicircular canal (SCC) anomaly with complete absence of all SCCs, cochlear malformation, and dysmorphic small vestibule ➡.* **(Right)** *Axial CT in a patient with CHARGE syndrome shows near-aplasia of the horizontal (lateral) SCC with only minute nibbles at its origin ➡ from the hypoplastic vestibule ➡. The posterior SCC is aplastic and not visualized along the posterior petrous temporal bone. Also note the hypoplastic internal auditory canal (IAC) ➡.*

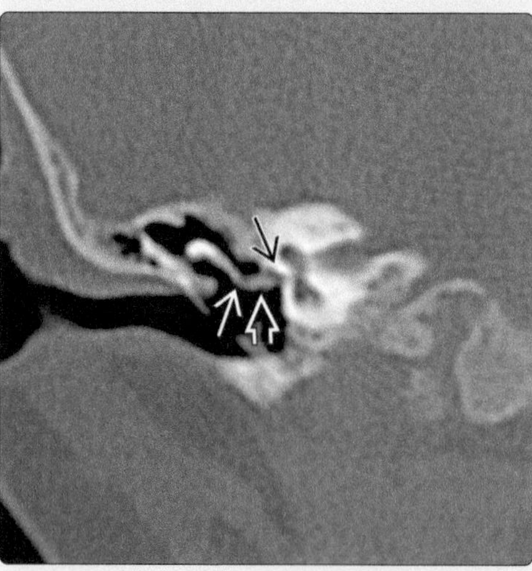

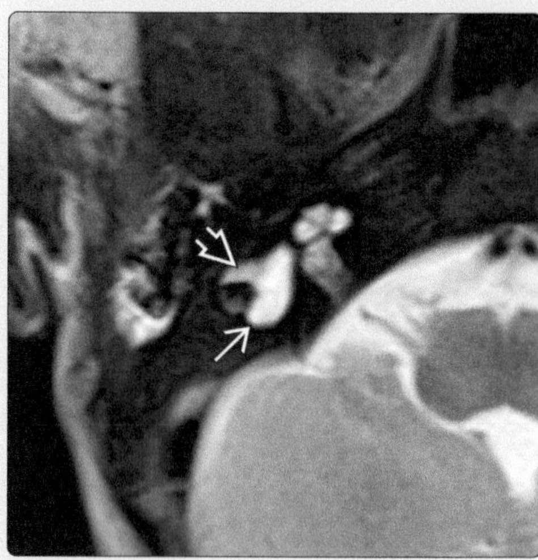

(Left) *Coronal T-bone CT in another patient shows absence of SCCs and bone covering the oval window ➡. Note the characteristic lack of lenticular process of incus ➡ and thick stapes ➡ in this patient with CHARGE syndrome.* **(Right)** *Axial T2WI MR in a 1-day-old girl with Waardenburg syndrome shows a rudimentary posterior SCC bud along the posterior aspect of the vestibule ➡. A normal horizontal SCC ➡ is seen.*

TERMINOLOGY

Synonyms

- Semicircular canal (SCC)-vestibule malformation

IMAGING

General Features

- Best diagnostic clue
  - Hypoplasia/aplasia of 1 or multiple SCCs ± hypoplasia vestibule
- Location
  - Posterior membranous labyrinth
- Size
  - Varies from aplasia of all SCCs + hypoplasia vestibule to hypoplasia of 1 SCC & normal vestibule
- Morphology
  - SCCs short or aplastic; small bone island
  - Vestibule normal or small

CT Findings

- Bone CT
  - Hypoplasia vestibule + hypoplasia/aplasia of **all SCCs**
    - Oval window stenosis/atresia
    - Anomalous ± dehiscent tympanic segment CNVII
    - Cochlea: Thickened modiolus, flattened apical ± middle turns, deficient cochlear septation [incomplete partition type I (IP-I)], cochlear hypoplasia
    - Cochlear nerve canal (CNC): Stenosis or atresia
    - Vestibular aqueduct (VA): Dilated, funnel-shaped
    - Associated findings of **CHARGE syndrome** (**c**oloboma, **h**eart disease, **a**tresia choanae, intellectual disability or growth **r**estriction, **g**enital hypoplasia, **e**ar anomalies)
  - Hypoplasia **single SCC** + normal or large vestibule
    - Posterior SCC (PSCC) hypoplasia (uncommon)
      - □ Small bone island with small, globular or rudimentary/absent PSCC
      - □ Anomalous origin PSCC from horizontal SCC (HSCC) & superior SCC (SSCC)
      - □ Syndromic etiology: Waardenburg (WS), Alagille, & **branchiootorenal (BOR) syndromes**
      - □ Anomaly often overlooked on CT
      - □ Cochlea: Flattened apical turn (WS) or hypoplastic, offset middle & apical turns (BOR)
    - HSCC or lateral SCC (LSCC) hypoplasia/aplasia
      - □ Hypoplasia: Small bone island with small or globular LSCC: **Trisomy 21, 22q11.2 deletion (DiGeorge)**
      - □ Aplasia: Absent part/all LSCC (rare) + oval window stenosis/atresia
      - □ Anomalous ± dehiscent tympanic segment CNVII
      - □ Cochlea: Typically normal depending on syndromic etiology
  - **Central lucency of LSCC bony island** significantly associated with congenital severe-to-profound sensorineural hearing loss (SNHL)
    - Central lucency may be manifestation of overlooked SCC malformation or inner ear hypoplasia
    - Prevalence of central lucency in congenital severe-to-profound SNHL ≈ 47%
      - □ ≈ 52% among patients without inner ear malformations
      - □ ≈ 41% among patients with inner ear malformations

MR Findings

- T2WI
  - Hypoplasia or absent SCC fluid signal
  - Normal or small vestibule
  - Cochlea: Normal or abnormal (e.g., CHARGE, BOR)

Imaging Recommendations

- Best imaging tool
  - Temporal bone CT or MR
- Protocol advice
  - Axial & reconstructed coronal images

DIFFERENTIAL DIAGNOSIS

Sporadic Semicircular Canal Dysplasia

- Dilated vestibule & dysmorphic LSCC forming confluent common sac
- Normal or mildly dysplastic PSCC & SSCC

CHARGE Syndrome

- Small vestibule + hypoplasia/aplasia of all SCC
- Variable cochlea: Normal to extreme hypoplasia
  - Flattened apical turn; normal middle & basal turns
  - Flattened middle & apical turns
  - Single globular cochlear turn, absent internal structure
  - Cochlear hypoplasia, most commonly with basal turn relatively preserved & upper turns underdeveloped
- Funnel-shaped large VA (LVA)
- Ossicular malformation

Branchiootorenal Syndrome

- Hypoplasia/absence of PSCC, normal vestibule
- Characteristic cochlear anomaly: Hypoplastic, unwound middle & apical turns
- Funnel-shaped LVA
- Ossicular malformation

Down Syndrome

- Small LSCC bone island, small or globular LSCC, CNC ± internal auditory canal (IAC) stenosis, ± LVA

Labyrinthine Ossificans

- Fibrosis & ossification of membranous labyrinth
- When affects SCCs, may mimic hypoplasia

Waardenburg Syndrome

- Characterized by deafness & pigmentation abnormalities
- 4 distinct subtypes involving several genes
- All showing deafness & pigmentary disturbance
- SNHL due to absent melanocyte-derived intermediate cells of stria vascularis
  - Endolymphatic collapse & secondary agenesis of organ of Corti (cochleosaccular degeneration)
- PSCC agenesis most frequent, followed by SSCC & LSCC anomalies
- Normal or large vestibule
- Normal or flattened cochlear apical turn
- Normal, hypoplastic or absent CN
- Normal VA or LVA

Alagille Syndrome (Arteriohepatic Dysplasia)

- PSCC anomaly/hypoplasia
- Peripheral pulmonary artery stenosis
- Paucity or stenosis of intrahepatic bile ducts → cholestatic liver disease, cirrhosis, hepatic failure

22q11.2 Deletion Syndrome (DiGeorge/Velocardiofacial Syndrome)

- Malformed LSCC with small bony island (33%)
- LSCC & vestibule fused to be single cavity (29%)
- Dense stapes superstructure (36%); IP-II (23%)

Goldenhar Syndrome (Oculoauriculovertebral Dysplasia)

- Rare, unilateral aplasia of all SCCs reported

PATHOLOGY

General Features

- Etiology
  - SCC begins to develop from utricle segment of otocyst at 6-8 gestational weeks
  - Development completed between 19th & 22nd weeks
  - Otic vesicle ventral pars inferior develops into vestibular sacculus & cochlear canal, fully formed by week 9
  - Otic vesicle dorsal pars superior develops into utricle & then SCC by week 8
  - SSCC forms 1st, followed by PSCC, & then LSCC
    - Isolated LSCC anomalies are therefore most common
  - Cochlear & vestibular development may be dependent on independent mechanisms
- Genetics
  - SCC aplasia or hypoplasia usually **syndromic**, rarely isolated
    - **CHARGE syndrome**: *CHD7* mutation
    - **BOR syndrome** (ear malformations, branchial & renal anomalies): *EYA1* mutations
    - **WS**: Several genes *PAX3, MITF, EDN3, EDNRB, SOX10*
      - *SOX10* mutations cause 15% of type 2 WS & 50% of type 4 WS (WS2 + Hirschsprung disease)
      - *SOX10* mutation patients may also show impaired myelination of CNS & PNS
      - Peripheral/central dysmyelinating leukodystrophy, WS, Hirschsprung disease (PCWH)
    - **AS** (arteriohepatic dysplasia): *JAG1* (90%) or *NOTCH2* (1-2%) mutations
    - **22q11.2 deletion syndrome** (DiGeorge/velocardiofacial syndrome): Most common chromosomal microdeletion disorder
      - De novo nonhomologous meiotic recombination events
- Associated abnormalities
  - Common & varies with syndromic etiology

Gross Pathologic & Surgical Features

- SCC atresia, hypoplasia ± anomalous origin
- HSCC hypoplasia/atresia: Oval window hypoplasia/atresia common
- Tympanic segment CNVII anomalous course ± dehiscent
- Cochlea, endolymphatic duct & sac anomaly varies with syndrome

CLINICAL ISSUES

Presentation

- Most common signs/symptoms
  - SNHL
    - Common even when cochlea appears normal on imaging
  - Conductive hearing loss from oval window atresia & ossicular anomalies
  - Vestibular symptoms
    - Vestibular function variable, even with SCC aplasia
    - Caloric responses may be absent
    - Positional vertigo
  - Facial nerve weakness/palsy

Demographics

- Age
  - Congenital
- Epidemiology
  - Uncommon inner ear anomaly
  - Typically syndromic etiology: CHARGE & BOR most common syndromes

DIAGNOSTIC CHECKLIST

Consider

- CHARGE syndrome: Hypoplasia vestibule + SCC
- BOR: Hypoplastic, offset middle & apical cochlear turns; look for PSCC anomaly
- WS type IV (rare): Constipation & SNHL; look for PSCC anomaly
- Alagille syndromes (rare): Liver disease & pulmonary stenosis; look for PSCC anomaly

Image Interpretation Pearls

- Axial & coronal temporal bone to assess oval window & CNVII tympanic segment

SELECTED REFERENCES

1. Lewis MA et al: The spectrum of cochlear malformations in CHARGE syndrome and insights into the role of the CHD7 gene during embryogenesis of the inner ear. Neuroradiology. 65(4):819-34, 2023
2. Wang Q et al: Research on congenital severe-to-profound sensorineural hearing loss associated with central lucency of the bony island of the lateral semicircular canal. Acta Otolaryngol. 143(2):134-40, 2023
3. Verheij E et al: Anatomic malformations of the middle and inner ear in 22q11.2 deletion syndrome: case series and literature review. AJNR Am J Neuroradiol. 39(5):928-34, 2018
4. Green GE et al: CHD7 mutations and CHARGE syndrome in semicircular canal dysplasia. Otol Neurotol. 35(8):1466-70, 2014
5. Saliba I et al: Down syndrome: an electrophysiological and radiological profile. Laryngoscope. 124(4):E141-7, 2014
6. Breheret R et al: Bilateral semicircular canal aplasia. Eur Ann Otorhinolaryngol Head Neck Dis. 130(4):225-8, 2013
7. Elmaleh-Bergès M et al: Spectrum of temporal bone abnormalities in patients with Waardenburg syndrome and SOX10 mutations. AJNR Am J Neuroradiol. 34(6):1257-63, 2013
8. Intrapiromkul J et al: Inner ear anomalies seen on CT images in people with Down syndrome. Pediatr Radiol. 42(12):1449-55, 2012
9. Blaser S et al: Inner ear dysplasia is common in children with Down syndrome (trisomy 21). Laryngoscope. 116(12):2113-9, 2006
10. Jongmans MC et al: CHARGE syndrome: the phenotypic spectrum of mutations in the CHD7 gene. J Med Genet. 43(4):306-14, 2006
11. Koch B et al: Partial absence of the posterior semicircular canal in Alagille syndrome: CT findings. Pediatr Radiol. 36(9):977-9, 2006

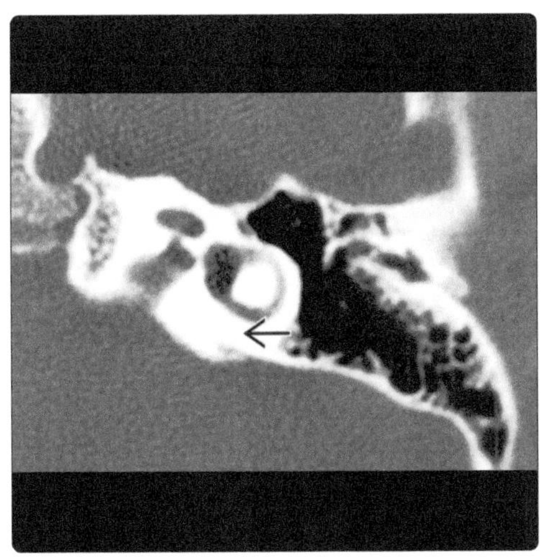

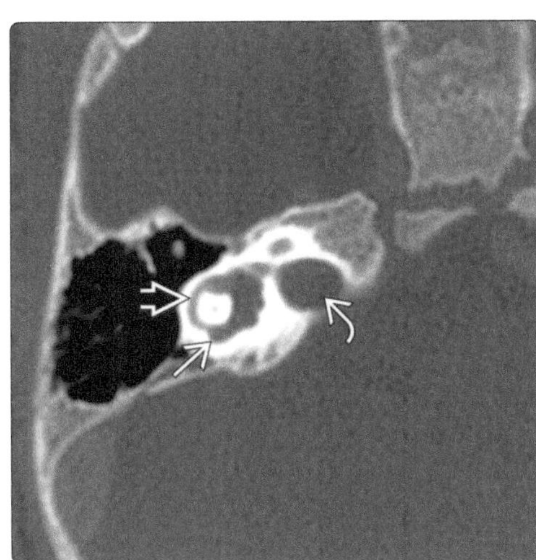

(Left) *Axial bone CT shows absence of the normally seen left posterior SCC ➡ in this child with Alagille syndrome.* **(Right)** *Axial bone CT in a 19-month-old boy with branchiootorenal (BOR) syndrome shows an underdeveloped and anomalous posterior SCC ➡ alongside a normal horizontal SCC ➡. Note the bulbous IAC ➡.*

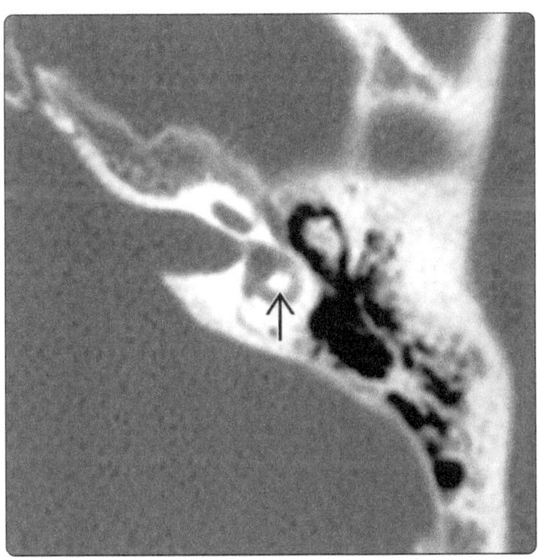

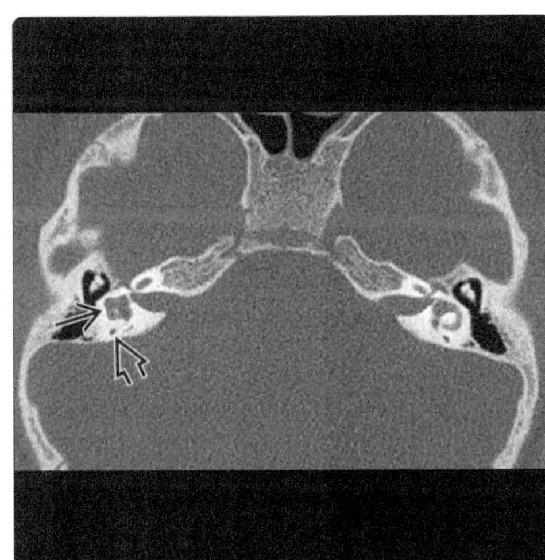

(Left) *Axial bone CT in an 11-year-old boy with Down syndrome (trisomy 21) shows a mildly underdeveloped bone island ➡ between the lateral SCC and vestibule. This anomaly is usually bilateral, often symmetric, and frequently overlooked when mild.* **(Right)** *Axial bone HRCT of temporal bones shows "nonsyndromic" right lateral SCC hypoplasia with shorter radius of its semicircle ➡ and underdeveloped tiny bone island between it and the vestibule. The right posterior SCC is intact ➡. The left SCCs are normal.*

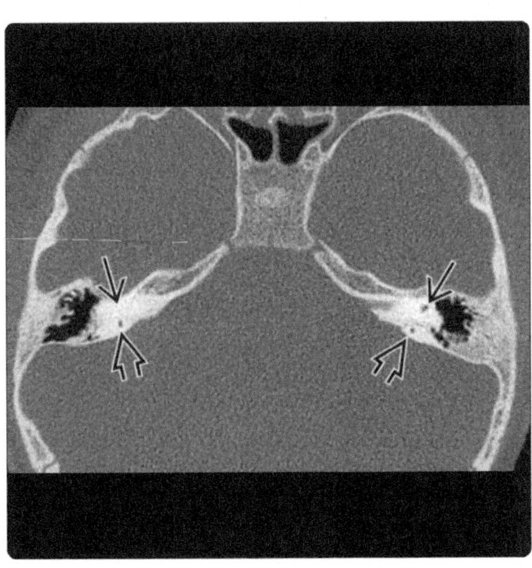

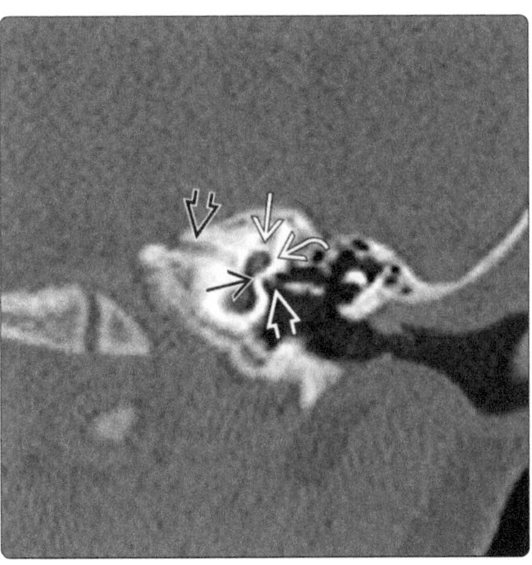

(Left) *Axial bone HRCT at a higher level in the same nonsyndromic patient shows hypoplasia of the anterior limb/apex ➡ of the right superior SCC, but its posterior limb ➡ is intact. Note normal counterparts of the left superior SCC.* **(Right)** *Coronal bone CT in a patient with CHARGE syndrome shows superior ➡ & lateral ➡ SCC aplasia (with their expected origin locations from vestibule marked). Also note oval window atresia ➡ with stapes ➡ attaching to the upper margin of oval window atresia plate. The IAC ➡ is small.*

Endolymphatic Sac Tumor

KEY FACTS

TERMINOLOGY

- Endolymphatic sac tumor (ELST)
- Synonyms: Adenomatous tumor of ELS, Heffner tumor
- Papillary cystadenomatous tumor of ELS
  - Originates from epithelium of ELS

IMAGING

- CT findings
  - **Permeative-destructive** retrolabyrinthine mass
  - Central spiculated tumor **Ca**$^{++}$ (100%)
  - Thin, **calcified rim** at posterior tumor margin
- MR findings
  - T1-hyperintense foci in 80%; inhomogeneous T2 signal
  - Heterogeneous enhancement
- Angiographic findings
  - Tumors < 3 cm supply from external carotid artery
  - Tumors > 3 cm internal carotid artery branches also

TOP DIFFERENTIAL DIAGNOSES

- Glomus jugulotympanicum paraganglioma
- Bony lesions, such as metastasis, osteosarcoma or hemangioma (bony spicules), aneurysmal bone cyst (fluid/blood levels)

PATHOLOGY

- Sporadic occurrence more common than von Hippel-Lindau disease (VHL)-associated ELST
  - **15% of VHL patients** develop **ELST**, 30% bilateral
- VHL: Cerebellar & spinal cord hemangioblastoma, renal cell carcinoma, pheochromocytoma, kidney & pancreas cysts

CLINICAL ISSUES

- Sensorineural hearing loss = most common symptom
- Treatment: Complete surgical resection
- If sporadic ELST, check patient & family for VHL

DIAGNOSTIC CHECKLIST

- Posterior wall T-bone **tumor with ↑ T1 foci** = **ELST**

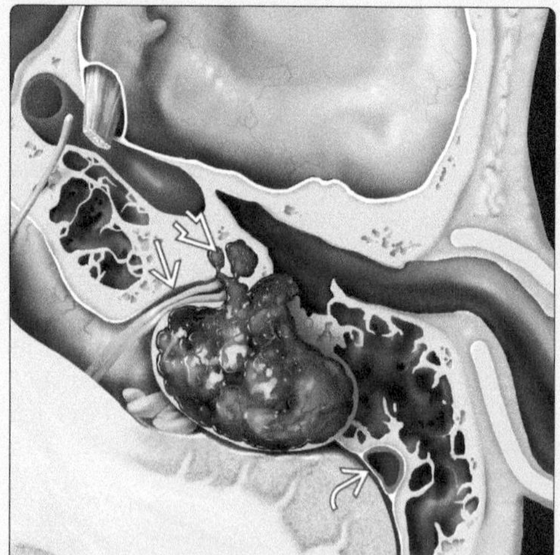

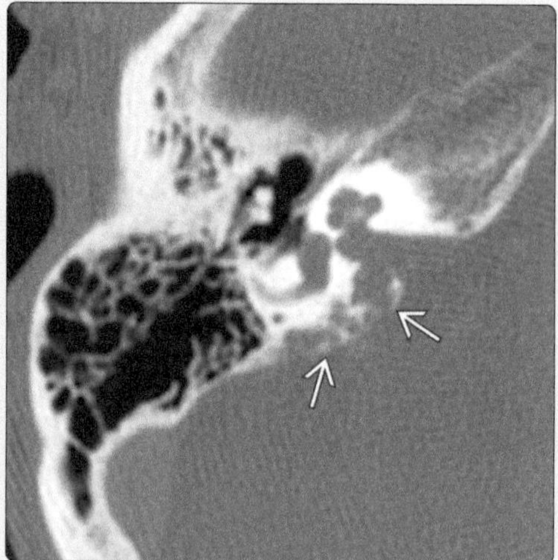

(Left) *Axial graphic of temporal bone illustrates the typical appearance of an endolymphatic sac tumor (ELST). Important features include its vascular nature, tendency to fistulize in inner ear ➡, & bone fragments within tumor matrix. Note the classic retrolabyrinthine location between the IAC ➡ & sigmoid sinus ➡.* **(Right)** *Axial bone CT shows a medium-sized ELST. Note the classic retrolabyrinthine location, permeative changes, & thin, "eggshell" rim of residual cortex posteriorly ➡, all classic features of an ELST.*

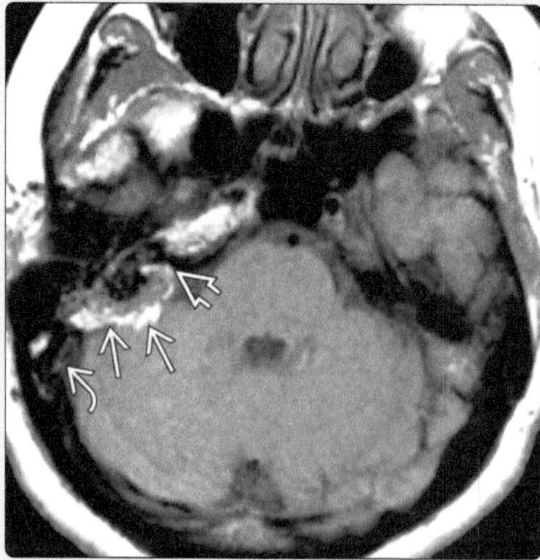

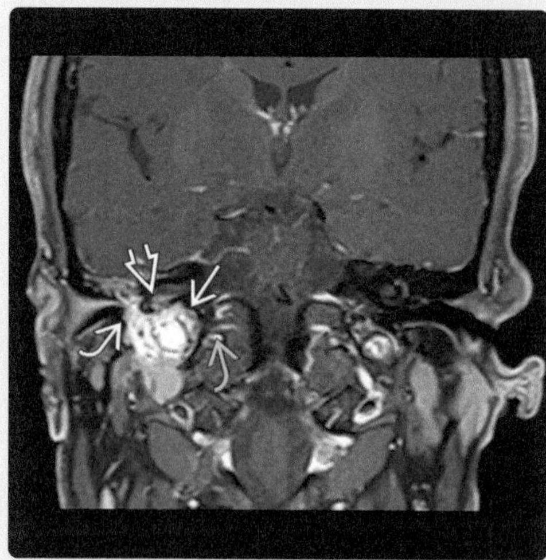

(Left) *Axial T1 MR reveals the classic posterior petrous ridge location between the IAC medially ➡ & sigmoid sinus posterolaterally ➡. Note the high-signal foci in an ELST matrix ➡. IAC is involved by the ELST.* **(Right)** *Coronal T1 C+ MR shows an intensely enhancing right ELST with IAC erosion ➡ & inferior extension along the mastoid eroding the skull base ➡ & reaching the jugular foramen ➡. Note that the bony jugular tubercle ➡ is spared (eroded early in glomus jugulotympanicum).*

TERMINOLOGY

Abbreviations

- Endolymphatic sac tumor (ELST)

Definitions

- Papillary cystadenomatous tumor of ELS
  - Originates from epithelium of endolymphatic sac

IMAGING

General Features

- Best diagnostic clue
  - Bone CT: Central intratumoral **bone spicules** & **posterior rim Ca^{++}**
  - MR: **High-signal** foci on **unenhanced T1**
- Location
  - **Retrolabyrinthine**: Posteromedial T-bone
  - Centered in **fovea of ELS** in presigmoid, posterior surface petrous T-bone
  - Large lesions (> 3 cm) involve cerebellopontine angle (CPA) cistern, middle ear/mastoid, & jugular foramen
- Morphology
  - Infiltrative, poorly circumscribed lesion

CT Findings

- Bone CT
  - **Permeative-destructive** retrolabyrinthine mass
    - Central spiculated tumor **Ca^{++}** (**100%**)
    - Thin, **calcified rim**, posterior margin tumor

MR Findings

- T1WI
  - **Hyperintense foci** in **80%** (hemorrhage, cholesterol)
  - Tumors > 2 cm may have **flow voids**
- T2WI
  - Inhomogeneous signal from bone fragments & cysts
  - Fluid (blood) levels
- T1WI C+
  - Heterogeneous enhancement

Angiographic Findings

- Tumors < 3 cm supplied by external carotid artery (ECA) branches
  - **Ascending pharyngeal** > stylomastoid & petrosal branch middle meningeal arteries & occipital artery branches
- Tumors > 3 cm also recruit internal carotid artery (ICA) branches
- Hypervascular tumor blush without early venous return

Imaging Recommendations

- Best imaging tool
  - Bone CT & T1 C+ MR (both necessary)

DIFFERENTIAL DIAGNOSIS

Glomus Jugulotympanicum Paraganglioma

- Jugular tubercle & spine erosion (spared in ELST)
- MR: ↑ T1 foci rare; T2 flow voids very common

Bony Lesions

- Metastasis: Renal cell or papillary thyroid carcinoma
- Osteosarcoma or hemangioma: Bony spiculation mimics
- Aneurysmal bone cyst: Fluid (blood) level mimics, especially if larger mastoid or skull base involvement

Petrous Apex Cholesterol Granuloma

- Smooth expansile margins
- MR: Entire lesion has ↑ signal on T1 & T2

Petrous Apex Meningioma

- Hyperostosis ± permeative sclerotic bones, no spicules
- MR: T1 C+ homogeneous enhancement; dural tail

PATHOLOGY

General Features

- Genetics
  - Sporadic > von Hippel-Lindau disease (VHL) ELST
  - *VHL* tumor suppressor gene mutated in both
- Associated abnormalities
  - 15% of VHL patients develop ELST, 30% bilateral

Staging, Grading, & Classification

- Grade 1: Confined to T-bone, middle ear, ± EAC
- Grade 2: Posterior cranial fossa extension
- Grade 3: Posterior & middle fossa extension
- Grade 4: Clival ± sphenoid wing extension

Gross Pathologic & Surgical Features

- Heaped up tumor on posterior wall of T-bone

CLINICAL ISSUES

Presentation

- Most common signs/symptoms
  - Sensorineural hearing loss
- Other signs/symptoms
  - Tinnitus, vertigo (mimics Ménière disease)
  - Facial nerve palsy

Demographics

- Age
  - Sporadic: 40-50 years; VHL: 30 years

Natural History & Prognosis

- Prognosis excellent with complete surgical resection
  - VHL ELST found earlier (annual MR screening)
- Late recurrence possible; perform follow-up imaging

Treatment

- Complete surgical resection
  - Preoperative embolization for larger lesions
- Radiation therapy if unresectable or nonsurgical candidate

DIAGNOSTIC CHECKLIST

Consider

- Bilateral ELST = VHL diagnosis

Image Interpretation Pearls

- Posterior wall T-bone **tumor with ↑ T1 foci** = **ELST**

SELECTED REFERENCES

1. Wu N et al: Surgical management of endolymphatic sac tumor: classification, outcomes and strategy. A single institution's experience. Eur Arch Otorhinolaryngol. 280(1):69-76, 2023

KEY FACTS

TERMINOLOGY

- Definition: Cystic mass resulting from congenital epithelial inclusion or rest
  - Epidermoid: Epithelial elements only
  - Dermoid: Epithelial elements + dermal substructure, including dermal appendages

IMAGING

- Epidermoid: Cystic, well-demarcated mass with fluid contents only
- Dermoid: Cystic, well-demarcated mass ± fatty, fluid, or mixed contents
- Location
  - Oral cavity: Submandibular space, sublingual space, or root of tongue
  - Anterior neck, usually midline
  - Orbit: Adjacent to frontozygomatic suture > frontolacrimal suture
  - Nasal cyst in association with nasal dermal sinus (NDS) ± intracranial extension
- Scalloping or remodeling of bone common
- Subtle rim enhancement of wall sometimes seen
- Restricted diffusion: Epidermoid > dermoid cysts
- Protocol advice
  - Routine CECT of cervical soft tissues
  - MR: T1 precontrast, & use fat-saturation post contrast for orbit, neck, & oral cavity lesions
  - High-resolution anterior skull base MR in NDS; image from tip of nose to posterior to crista galli
  - Sagittal to define tract: Nose → anterior skull base

DIAGNOSTIC CHECKLIST

- If complex lesion with fat, consider dermoid cyst
- Simple lesion (may be proteinaceous fluid) = epidermoid or dermoid cyst

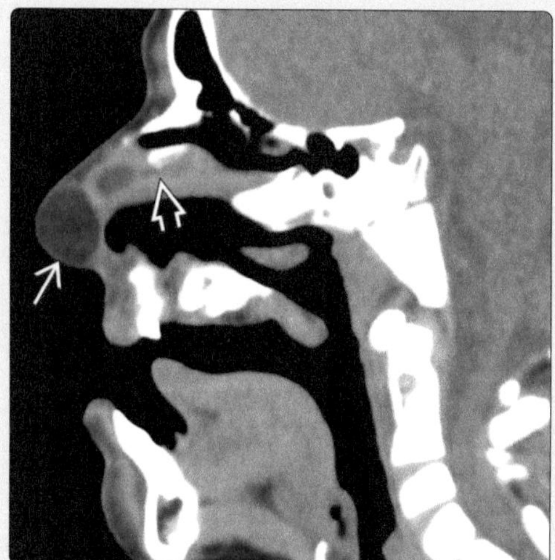

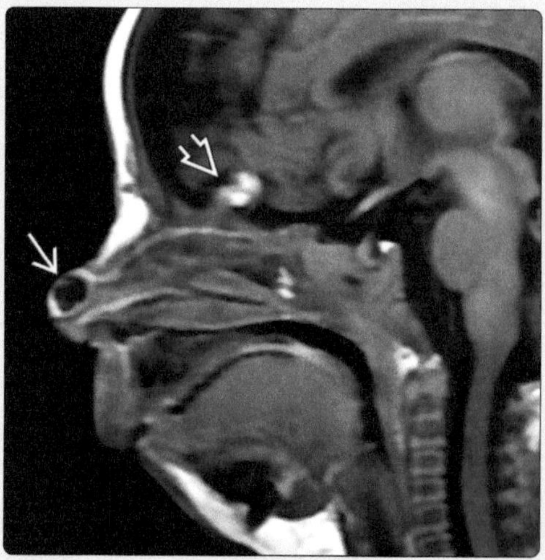

(Left) *Sagittal CT reconstruction in a 10-year-old child following cleft palate repair shows a large nasal dermoid ➡ with nasal dermal sinus tract ➡ extending toward the cribriform plate without intracranial extension.* **(Right)** *Sagittal T1 MR in a 1-year-old girl with micrognathia shows a fluid signal intensity mass at the tip of the nose ➡ and a fat signal intensity intracranial, extradural mass ➡ superior to the foramen cecum. These were connected via a linear tract, and both histologically proved to be dermoid cysts.*

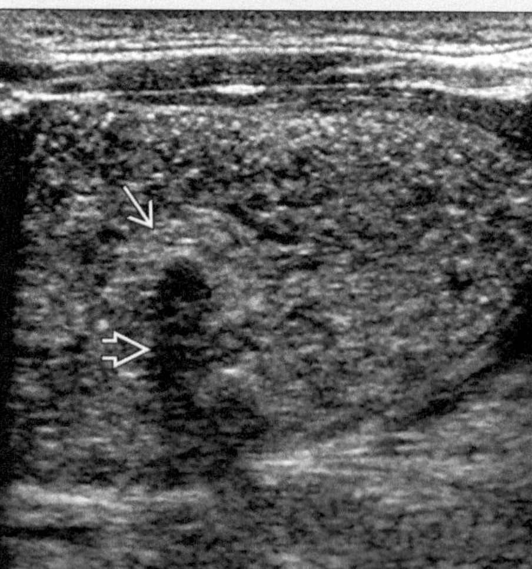

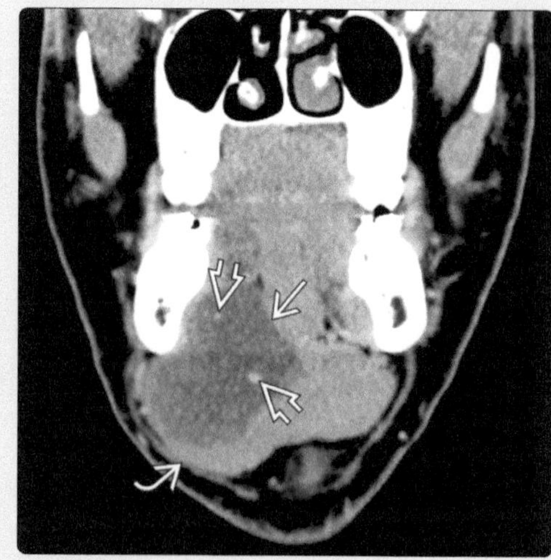

(Left) *Longitudinal ultrasound in a 14-year-old boy shows a oral cavity mass with heterogeneous echotexture and minimal increased through-transmission. One hyperechoic focus ➡ has posterior acoustical shadowing ➡, consistent with Ca^{++}, in this dermoid cyst.* **(Right)** *Coronal CECT in the same patient shows a low-density oral cavity mass ➡ with a few Ca^{++} ➡. Inferior displacement of the mylohyoid muscle ➡ indicates this dermoid cyst is in the sublingual space.*

TERMINOLOGY

Synonyms

- Developmental cyst, ectodermal inclusion cyst, dermoid cyst

Definitions

- Congenital epithelial inclusion or rest → cystic mass
  - Epidermoid: Epithelial elements only
  - Dermoid: Epithelial elements + dermal substructure, including dermal appendages

IMAGING

General Features

- Best diagnostic clue
  - Epidermoid: Cystic, well-demarcated mass with fluid contents only
  - Dermoid: Cystic, well-demarcated mass ± fatty, fluid, or mixed contents
- Location
  - Epidermoid & dermoid lesions
    - Oral cavity (OC): Submandibular space (SMS), sublingual space (SLS), or root of tongue
    - Anterior neck, usually midline
    - Orbit: Adjacent to frontozygomatic suture > frontolacrimal suture
    - Nasal cyst + nasal dermal sinus (NDS) ± intracranial extension
      - Tract or cyst nasal bridge to crista galli
      - Large foramen cecum with bifid or deformed crista galli or cribriform plate clue to intracranial extension
      - Classification by location: Superficial, intraosseous, intracranial extradural, intracranial intradural
- Morphology
  - Ovoid or tubular

CT Findings

- Low-density, well-circumscribed cystic mass
  - Epidermoid: Fluid-density material inside lesion without complex features
  - Dermoid: Fatty internal material, mixed density fluid, Ca^{++} (< 50%) all possible
    - When fluid density without complex features, indistinguishable from epidermoid
  - Scalloping or remodeling of bone common
  - Lesion wall may be imperceptible
  - Subtle rim enhancement of wall sometimes seen

MR Findings

- T1WI
  - Epidermoid: Well-circumscribed mass with homogeneous fluid signal
    - Diffuse ↑ signal if high protein fluid
  - Dermoid: Well-circumscribed mass with complex fluid signal
    - If fatty elements, focal or diffuse ↑ signal
- T2WI
  - Epidermoid: Homogeneous high signal
  - Dermoid: Heterogeneous high signal
    - Intermediate signal if fat
    - Focal areas of low signal if Ca^{++}
- DWI
  - Restricted diffusion epidermoid > dermoid cysts
- T1WI C+
  - Thin rim enhancement or no enhancement
  - If fat saturation used, fat will be low signal in dermoid

Ultrasonographic Findings

- Epidermoid: Pseudosolid appearance + uniform internal echoes
  - Cellular material in cyst → pseudosolid appearance
  - Posterior wall acoustic enhancement = cystic lesion
- Dermoid: Mixed internal echoes from fat with echogenic foci & dense shadowing if Ca^{++}

Imaging Recommendations

- Best imaging tool
  - CECT is best imaging tool for OC lesions (unless obscured by dental amalgam, then MR best)
  - MR or CECT for neck lesions
  - MR for orbit lesions
  - MR for NDS to better evaluate intracranial extent
    - CT to evaluate skull base & crista galli deformity
- Protocol advice
  - Routine CECT or MR with contrast for cervical soft tissues
  - MR: Include T1 precontrast, & use fat-saturation techniques post contrast for orbit, neck, & OC lesions
  - High-resolution anterior skull base MR in NDS; image from tip of nose to posterior to crista galli
    - Sagittal to define tract: Nose → anterior skull base
    - DWI hyperintensity may diagnose epidermoid

DIFFERENTIAL DIAGNOSIS

Pediatric Sublingual Space, Submandibular Space, or Neck Lesions

- Thyroglossal duct cyst
  - Midline unilocular cystic mass between hyoid bone & foramen cecum
  - No fat or Ca^{++}
- Lymphatic malformation
  - Unilocular or multilocular, transspatial common
  - Fluid-fluid levels common
- Ranula
  - Simple: Unilateral low-density/-signal mass in SLS with thin, nonenhancing wall
  - Diving: Comet-shaped unilocular mass with tail in collapsed SLS (tail sign) & head in posterior SMS
- Abscess
  - Clinical: Fever, erythema, elevated WBC count
  - Imaging: Rim-enhancing cyst often with soft tissue cellulitis, edema, & adenopathy

Pediatric Orbital Lesions

- Orbital Langerhans cell histiocytosis
  - Enhancing soft tissue mass with smoothly marginated lytic bone lesion
- Rhabdomyosarcoma
  - Moderately enhancing mass frequently inseparable from extraocular muscle
  - Frequently without bone erosion when in orbit

- Orbital infantile hemangioma
  - Significant contrast enhancement, no bone erosion, & presents in infancy
- Orbital lymphatic malformation
  - Intraconal, extraconal, or both
  - Nonenhancing; fluid-fluid levels common
- Orbital venous malformation
  - Moderate enhancement
  - Ca^{++}/phleboliths common
  - Positional proptosis may be present
- Orbital venolymphatic malformation
- Orbital idiopathic inflammatory pseudotumor
  - Painful proptosis common
  - Moderately enhancing mass, any area of orbit

Pediatric Nasal Lesions

- Normal fatty marrow in crista galli
  - No mass or pit on nose
- Nonossified foramen cecum
  - Ossifies postnatally in first 5 years of life
  - Normal crista galli
- Frontoethmoidal cephalocele
  - Direct extension of meninges, subarachnoid space, &, sometimes, brain through bone defect in cribriform plate or frontal bone
- Nasal glioma (nasal glial heterotopia is preferred term)
  - Most commonly projects extranasally onto paramedian bridge of nose
  - Less commonly, along anterior nasal septum

PATHOLOGY

General Features

- Etiology
  - Congenital inclusion of dermal elements at site of embryonic fusion
    - Sequestration of trapped surface ectoderm

Gross Pathologic & Surgical Features

- Oily or cheesy material; tan, yellow, or white
- Cyst wall = fibrous capsule; 2-6 mm in thickness

Microscopic Features

- Epidermoid
  - Simple squamous cell epithelium with fibrous wall
- Dermoid
  - Contains dermal structures, including sebaceous glands, hair follicles, blood vessels, fat ± collagen
    - Sweat glands in minority (20%)
    - Lined by keratinizing squamous epithelium
- Teratoid cysts (rare lesion)
  - Contain elements from all 3 germ cell layers

CLINICAL ISSUES

Presentation

- Most common signs/symptoms
  - Painless mass in floor of mouth (FOM), anterior neck, orbit, or nasoglabellar region
- Other signs/symptoms
  - OC lesions: Dysphagia, globus oral sensation, airway encroachment when large
  - Orbit lesions: Proptosis, diplopia
  - Nasal lesions: Pit on skin of nasal bridge ± protruding hair, recurrent meningitis, intermittent sebaceous material discharged from pit

Demographics

- Age
  - OC lesions: Mean age: Late teens to 20s
    - Most dermoid cysts of FOM present at 5-50 years
    - Average age: 30 years
  - Orbit lesions: Children or early adulthood
  - Nasal lesions: Newborn to 5 years
    - Mean age: 32 months
- Epidemiology
  - Present from birth; spontaneous occurrence
  - Dermoid/epidermoid are least common of all congenital neck lesions
  - Orbit most common dermoid of H&N
  - OC dermoids account for < 25% of all H&N dermoids

Natural History & Prognosis

- Benign lesion, very slow growth
  - Present during childhood but small & dormant
  - Symptomatic during rapid growth phase in young adult
- Sudden growth or change following rupture
  - Significant inflammation & ↑ size (rare complication)

Treatment

- Surgical resection is curative
  - Entire cyst must be removed to prevent recurrence
  - OC lesions: Surgical approach may be decided by lesion position relative to mylohyoid muscle
    - SLS: Intraoral approach
    - SMS: Submandibular approach

DIAGNOSTIC CHECKLIST

Image Interpretation Pearls

- If complex lesion with fat density or signal intensity, consider dermoid cyst
- Simple lesion (may be proteinaceous fluid) = epidermoid or dermoid cyst
- If dermal sinus tract reaches dura anterior cranial fossa, crista galli may be bifid & foramen cecum large
- Foramen cecum normally unossified up to 5 years

SELECTED REFERENCES

1. Booth TN: Congenital cystic neck masses. Neuroimaging Clin N Am. 33(4):591-605, 2023
2. Naina P et al: Pediatric nasal dermoid- a decade's experience from a South Indian tertiary care centre. Int J Pediatr Otorhinolaryngol. 139:110418, 2020
3. Rodriguez DP et al: Masses of the nose, nasal cavity, and nasopharynx in children. Radiographics. 37(6):1704-30, 2017
4. Hartley BE et al: Nasal dermoids in children: a proposal for a new classification based on 103 cases at Great Ormond Street Hospital. Int J Pediatr Otorhinolaryngol. 79(1):18-22, 2015
5. LaPlante JK et al: Common pediatric head and neck congenital/developmental anomalies. Radiol Clin North Am. 53(1):181-96, 2015
6. Hughes DC et al: Dimensions and ossification of the normal anterior cranial fossa in children. AJNR Am J Neuroradiol. 31(7):1268-72, 2010
7. Hedlund G: Congenital frontonasal masses: developmental anatomy, malformations, and MR imaging. Pediatr Radiol. 36(7):647-62; quiz 726-7, 2006

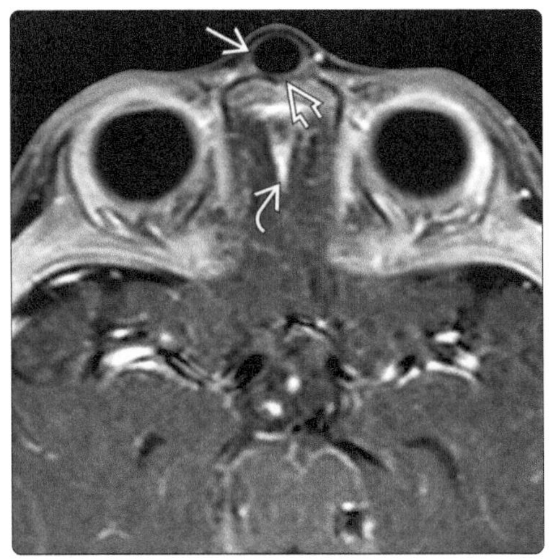

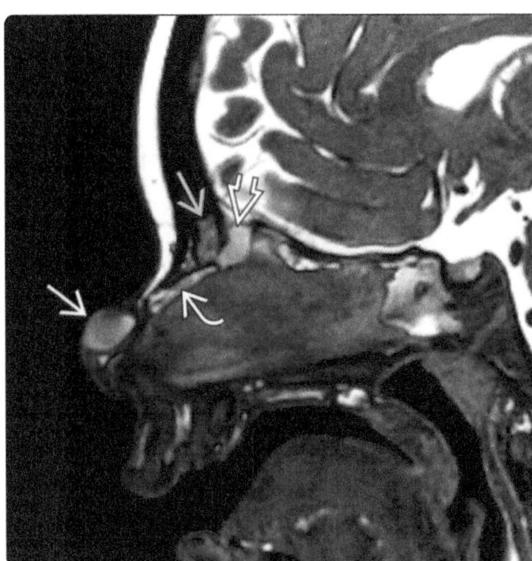

(Left) *Axial T1 C+ FS MR in a 6-month-old infant shows a typical nasal glabella dermoid cyst ➔, well defined and nonenhancing, with adjacent smooth osseous remodeling ➔. Notice the normal appearance of the crista galli ➔.* **(Right)** *Sagittal FIESTA MR in a 1-year-old girl shows a complex dermoid cyst with a nasal component ➔ and a component extending into the foramen cecum ➔, the 2 connected by a linear tract ➔. In addition, there is another component ➔ that remodels the dorsal aspect of the nasal bone.*

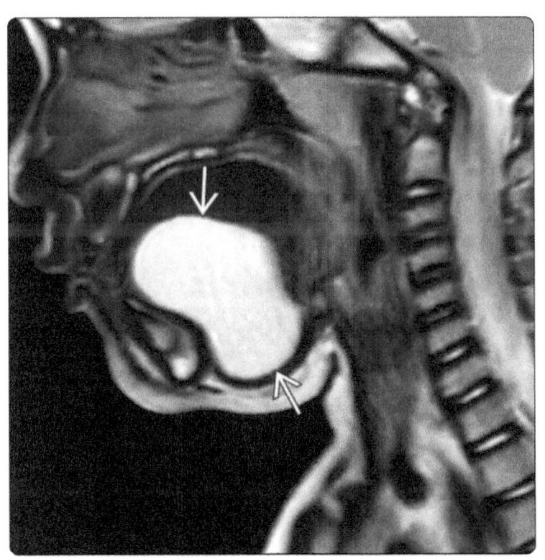

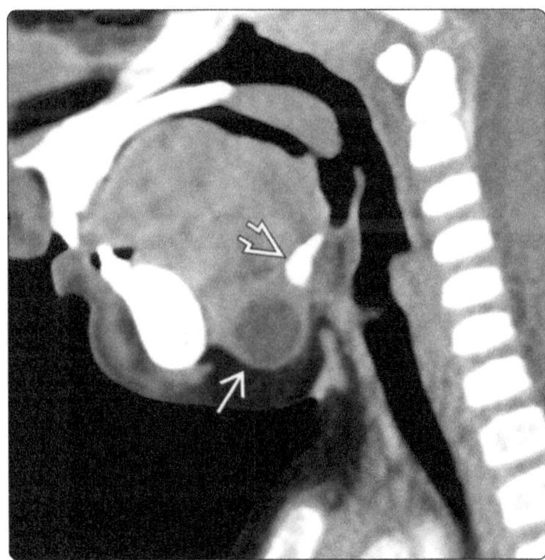

(Left) *Sagittal T2 MR in 5-year-old with recent increase in oral cavity mass shows well-defined, homogeneously hyperintense midline floor of mouth mass ➔, which showed diffusion restriction without contrast enhancement.* **(Right)** *Sagittal CECT in 20-month-old with midline anterior upper neck mass shows well-defined, round, nonenhancing dermoid cyst ➔ with thin, smooth wall just anterior to the midline hyoid bone ➔. Differential diagnosis at imaging was thyroglossal duct cyst vs. dermoid/epidermoid cyst.*

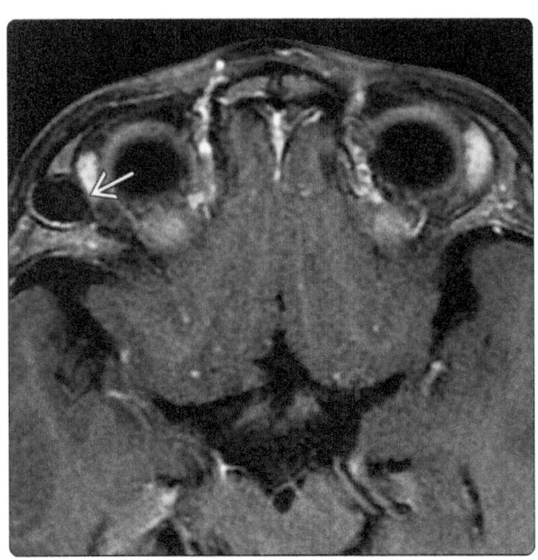

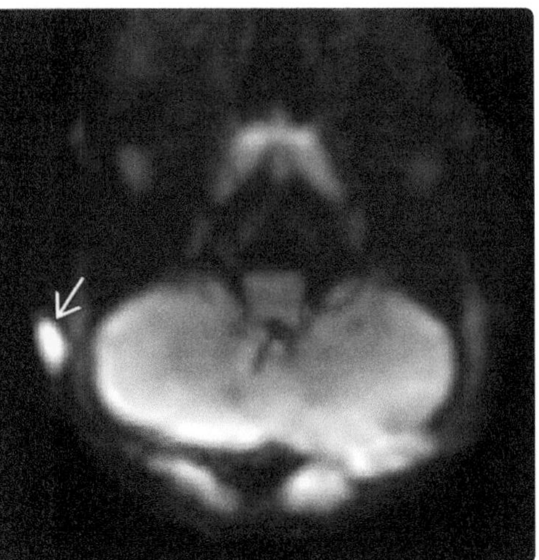

(Left) *Axial T1 C+ FS MR in a 3-year-old shows the typical location and appearance of an orbital dermoid cyst ➔ extending into the zygomaticofrontal suture: Well-defined, cystic-appearing lesion without enhancement and with diffusion restriction (not shown).* **(Right)** *Axial DWI MR in a young child with a longstanding right retroauricular lesion ➔ demonstrates a well-defined lesion with diffusion restriction. Lesion was fluid signal on other sequences and histologically proven to be epidermoid cyst.*

KEY FACTS

TERMINOLOGY

- Arachnoid cyst (AC): Developmental arachnoid duplication anomaly creating CSF-filled sac

IMAGING

- Sharply demarcated ovoid extraaxial cisternal cyst with imperceptible walls & CSF density (CT) or intensity (MR)
- AC signal closer to CSF intensity on **all** MR sequences
- Remember: T2 signal may be higher than CSF (due to lack of CSF pulsation, choroid plexus, or blood vessels)
- Complete fluid attenuation on FLAIR MR
- **No** diffusion restriction on DWI MR

TOP DIFFERENTIAL DIAGNOSES

- Epidermoid cyst in cerebellopontine angle (CPA)
- Cystic vestibular schwannoma
- Neurenteric cyst
- Cerebellar pilocytic astrocytoma
- Racemose neurocysticercosis

PATHOLOGY

- Embryonic meninges fail to merge, remain separate as duplicated arachnoid with CSF content

CLINICAL ISSUES

- Clinical presentation
  - Small AC: Asymptomatic, incidental finding (MR)
  - Large AC: Mostly asymptomatic
    - Symptoms may arise from direct compression ± ↑ intracranial pressure
  - Extremely rare intracystic/subdural hemorrhage
- Natural history
  - Vast majority of ACs **do not** enlarge over time
- Treatment options
  - Most cases require **no** treatment

DIAGNOSTIC CHECKLIST

- Differentiate AC from epidermoid cyst
- AC: No restriction on DWI = best clue

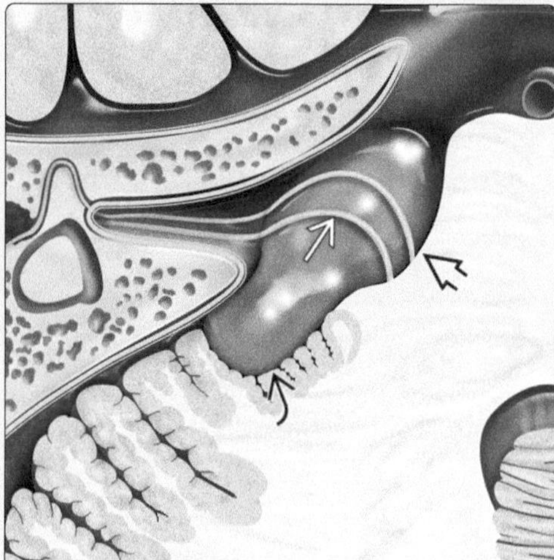

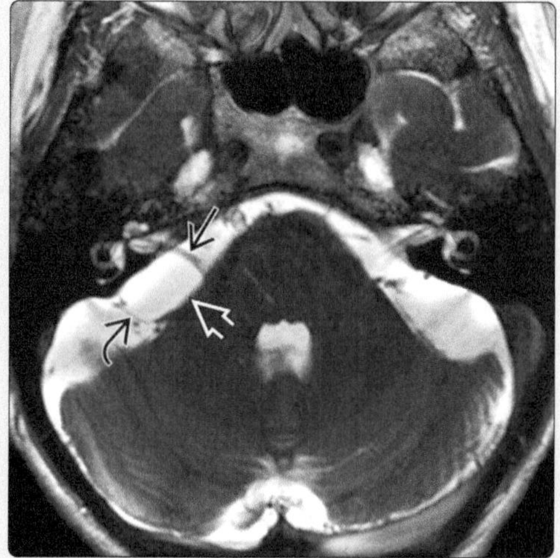

(Left) *Axial graphic of an arachnoid cyst in the cerebellopontine angle (CPA) shows a thin, translucent wall. Notice the cyst bowing CNVII and CNVIII anteriorly ➡ as well as effacing the brainstem ⇨ and cerebellum ⇨.* **(Right)** *Axial T2WI MR reveals a right CPA arachnoid cyst causing bowing of the facial and vestibulocochlear nerves anteriorly ⇨, small bridging veins posteriorly ⇨, and flattening of the lateral margin of the brachium pontis (middle cerebellar peduncle) ➡.*

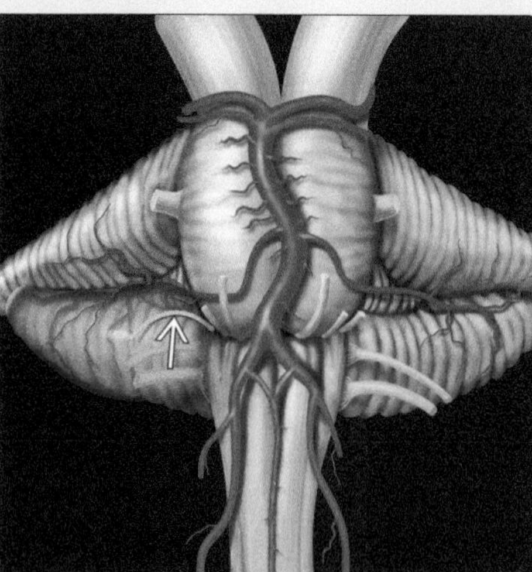

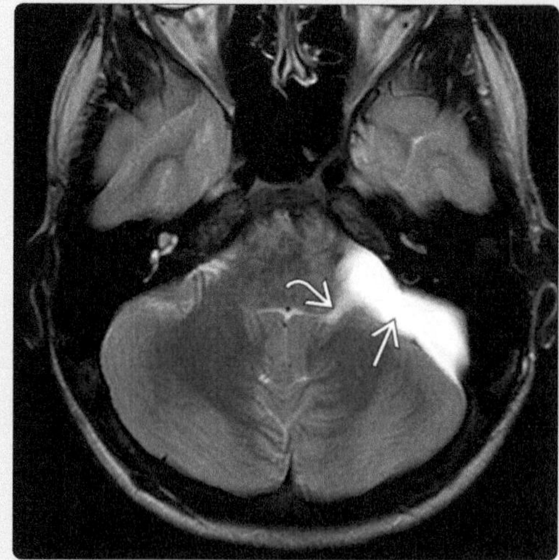

(Left) *Coronal graphic of a CPA arachnoid cyst depicts a typical translucent cyst wall. CNVII and CNVIII are pushed by the cyst ➡ without being engulfed by it. Cranial nerves are usually engulfed in an epidermoid cyst.* **(Right)** *Axial T2WI MR shows a fluid-signal hyperintense left CPA arachnoid cyst ➡. Notice that its signal is slightly brighter than the CSF in foramen of Luschka ➡, as the cyst lacks CSF pulsations, choroid plexus, or blood vessels within it.*

TERMINOLOGY

Abbreviations

- Arachnoid cyst (AC)

Synonyms

- Primary or congenital AC, subarachnoid cyst

Definitions

- Developmental arachnoid duplication anomaly creating **intraarachnoid** CSF-filled sac

IMAGING

General Features

- Best diagnostic clue
  - Sharply demarcated ovoid or lentiform extraaxial cisternal cyst with imperceptible walls
  - **No blood vessels** pass through cyst
    - If blood vessels seen within postcontrast CT/MR or heavily T2-weighted MR → just prominent subarachnoid space
  - AC signal parallels CSF signal on all MR sequences
    - **Complete fluid attenuation** on FLAIR MR
    - **No diffusion restriction** on DWI MR
- Location
  - 10-20% of all ACs occur in posterior fossa
    - Cerebellopontine angle (CPA) = most common infratentorial site
    - **10%** found in CPA
  - Spread patterns
    - Most remain confined to CPA (60%)
    - May spread dorsally along brainstem (25%)
    - Rarely spread into internal auditory canal (IAC)
- Size
  - Broad range: 1 cm to giant (> 8 cm)
  - In posterior fossa: When very large, may be symptomatic
  - When large, will exert mass effect on vestibulocochlear & facial nerves, adjacent brainstem, & cerebellum
- Morphology
  - Sharply demarcated with broad-arching margins
  - Displaces, does not engulf, surrounding structures
  - Pushes cisternal structures but does not insinuate
    - Epidermoid cyst insinuates adjacent structures

CT Findings

- NECT
  - Density same as CSF
  - Rare high density from hemorrhage or proteinaceous fluid
- CECT
  - No enhancement of cavity or wall
- Bone CT
  - Rarely causes expansile remodeling of bone
    - Seen mostly in children
- CT (and MR) cisternography
  - 3 types of communication with subarachnoid space
    - Complete (cyst filling time at 1 hour)
    - Incomplete (filling time beginning at 3 hours)
    - Noncommunicating (no or slight filling after 24 hours)

MR Findings

- T1WI
  - Low-signal cyst isointense to CSF
- T2WI
  - High-signal cyst isointense to CSF
    - May have brighter signal than CSF
      - Cyst fluid lacks CSF pulsations
  - Well-circumscribed lesion: Compresses adjacent CNVII-VIII bundle, brainstem, & cerebellum when large
- FLAIR
  - Suppresses cyst fluid completely
- DWI
  - No diffusion restriction
- T1WI C+
  - No enhancement
- High-resolution, thin-section 3D heavily T2-weighted MR (CISS, FIESTA, T2 SPACE)
  - Help define cyst wall, relationship to adjacent structures (CNVII, CNVIII, anterior inferior cerebellar artery, etc.)
- Phase-contrast cine CSF flow study MR
  - Flow quantification may distinguish AC from subarachnoid space
  - May rarely show connection between AC & cistern

Ultrasonographic Findings

- Grayscale ultrasound
  - Shows hypoechoic AC in infants < 1 year of age
  - Larger AC diagnosed in utero

Imaging Recommendations

- Best imaging tool
  - MR ± contrast
- Protocol advice
  - Add FLAIR (suppresses); add DWI (no restricted diffusion)

DIFFERENTIAL DIAGNOSIS

Epidermoid Cyst in CPA

- Major lesion of differential concern in setting of AC
- FLAIR: Incomplete fluid attenuation
- DWI: Restricted diffusion (high signal)
- Morphology: Insinuates into adjacent CSF spaces

Cystic Vestibular Schwannoma in CPA-IAC

- Intramural or marginal cysts seen in larger lesions
- Foci of enhancing tumor always present on T1 C+ MR
- Rarely, larger lesions have associated AC

Cystic Meningioma in CPA-IAC

- Rare meningioma variant
- Dural tails, asymmetry to IAC still present with mixed enhancement on T1 C+ MR

Neurenteric Cyst

- Rare prepontine cistern near midline
- Often contains proteinaceous fluid (↑ on T1 MR)

Cystic Infratentorial Ependymoma

- Ependymoma pedunculates from 4th ventricle
  - Via foramen of Luschka
- 50% calcified
- Cystic & solid enhancing components

Cerebellar Pilocytic Astrocytoma

- Cystic tumor in cerebellar hemisphere
- Enhancing mural nodule

Racemose Neurocysticercosis in CPA

- Cysts with multiple thin membranes
- No diffusion restriction (mimicking AC)
  - But FLAIR heterogeneous (mimicking epidermoid)

PATHOLOGY

General Features

- Etiology
  - Embryonic meninges fail to merge
    - Remain separate as **duplicated** arachnoid
    - Split arachnoid contains CSF
  - 2 types
    - Noncommunicating; most common type
    - Communicating with subarachnoid space/cistern
- Genetics
  - Usually sporadic; rarely familial
  - Inherited disorders of metabolism
    - "Sticky" leptomeninges: Mucopolysaccharidoses
- Associated abnormalities
  - Vestibular schwannoma has AC associated in 0.5%

Gross Pathologic & Surgical Features

- Fluid-containing cyst with translucent membrane
- Displaces adjacent vessels or cranial nerves

Microscopic Features

- Thin wall of flattened but normal arachnoid cells

CLINICAL ISSUES

Presentation

- Most common signs/symptoms
  - Small AC: **Asymptomatic, incidental** finding (MR)
  - Large AC: Symptoms from direct compression ± ↑ intracranial pressure
  - Pediatric AC associated with higher symptom rate
- Other signs/symptoms
  - Defined by location & size
    - Headache
    - Dizziness, tinnitus ± sensorineural hearing loss
      - Rarely facial nerve symptoms
    - Hemifacial spasm or trigeminal neuralgia
  - Extremely rare subdural hemorrhage **(SDH)** & intracystic hemorrhage with ↑ intracranial pressure
    - After minor head injury (delayed hemorrhage usually) or spontaneously

Demographics

- Age
  - May be initially seen at any age
    - 75% of AC identified in childhood
- Sex
  - M:F = 3:1
- Epidemiology
  - Most common congenital intracranial cystic lesion
  - Accounts for 1% of intracranial masses

Natural History & Prognosis

- Most ACs **do not enlarge** over time
  - Infrequently enlarge via CSF pulsation through ball-valve opening into AC
  - Hemorrhage with subsequent ↓ in size or resolution reported
- If surgery, limited to AC where symptoms clearly related, prognosis excellent
- Radical cyst removal may result in cranial neuropathy ± vascular compromise

Treatment

- Most cases require **no treatment**
  - Pediatric AC more commonly treated than adult AC
- Surgical intervention highly selective process
  - Reserved for cases where clear symptoms can be directly linked to AC anatomic location
  - Complicated AC in children should be more aggressively treated than adults
  - Endoscopic cyst fenestration
  - Open microsurgical cyst resection or fenestration
  - Cystoperitoneal shunt

DIAGNOSTIC CHECKLIST

Consider

- Differentiate AC from epidermoid cyst
  - AC: No restriction on DWI = best clue
- Determine if symptoms match location of AC before considering surgical treatment

Image Interpretation Pearls

- AC signal follows CSF on all MR sequences
  - Remember: AC **T2 signal may be higher than CSF**
    - Due to lack of CSF pulsation, choroid plexus, or blood vessels within cyst
- **DWI** sequence shows AC as **low signal**
- **FLAIR** sequence shows AC as **low signal**
- **No** enhancement of AC, including wall expected
  - Nodular enhancement suggests alternative diagnosis

Reporting Tips

- Since AC usually not treated surgically, avoid offering any differential diagnosis when imaging findings diagnose AC

SELECTED REFERENCES

1. Makhchoune M et al: Reversible hearing loss after 3D video-assisted marsupialization of several posterior fossa arachnoid cysts: a case report. Ann Med Surg (Lond). 3:75:103468, 2022
2. Olsson SE et al: Tinnitus triggered by a cerebellopontine arachnoid cyst in an adolescent. Am J Case Rep. 28:23:e938294, 2022
3. Nadi M et al: Resolution of middle fossa arachnoid cyst after minor head trauma - stages of resolution on MRI: case report and literature review. Pediatr Neurosurg. 52(5):346-50, 2017
4. Tan Z et al: Children with intracranial arachnoid cysts: classification and treatment. Medicine (Baltimore). 94(44):e1749, 2015
5. Karegowda LH et al: A rare case of racemose neurocysticercosis of the posterior fossa. BMJ Case Rep, 2014
6. Liu Z et al: Arachnoid cysts with subdural hematoma or intracystic hemorrhage in children. Pediatr Emerg Care. 30(5):345-51, 2014
7. Wang X et al: CT cisternography in intracranial symptomatic arachnoid cysts: classification and treatment. J Neurol Sci. 318(1-2):125-30, 2012
8. Gangemi M et al: Endoscopy versus microsurgical cyst excision and shunting for treating intracranial arachnoid cysts. J Neurosurg Pediatr. 8(2):158-64, 2011

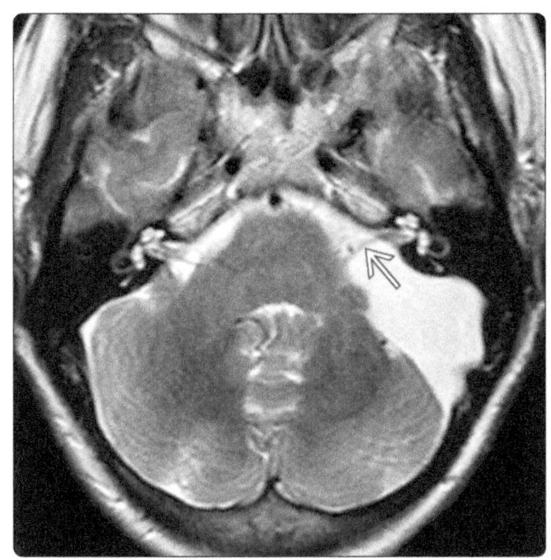

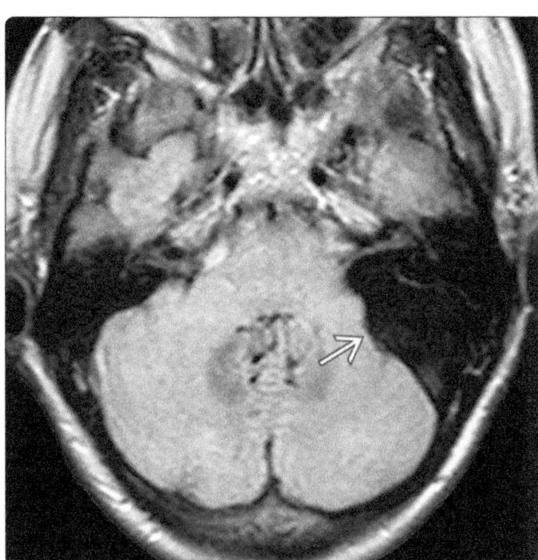

(Left) *Axial T2WI MR shows a high-signal, large arachnoid cyst enlarging the left CPA cistern. The facial and vestibulocochlear nerves are visibly bowing over the anteromedial surface of the arachnoid cyst ➡.* **(Right)** *Axial FLAIR MR in the same patient shows the low-signal arachnoid cyst ➡ and complete fluid attenuation. FLAIR suppression is expected, as the arachnoid cyst is essentially CSF collecting between arachnoid layers.*

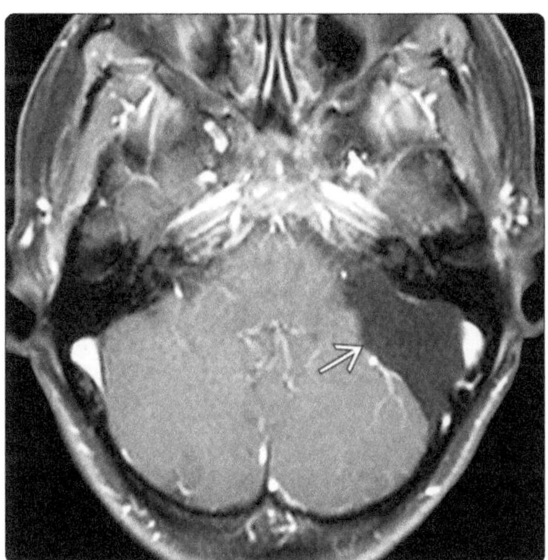

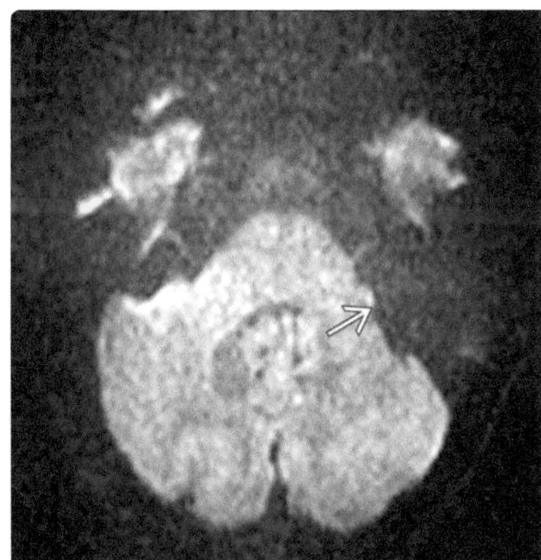

(Left) *Axial T1 C+ FS MR in the same patient demonstrates that the CPA arachnoid cyst ➡ does not enhance.* **(Right)** *Axial DWI MR in the same patient shows that the arachnoid cyst ➡ has no associated signal (no restricted diffusion). If this were an epidermoid cyst, high signal on DWI (restricted diffusion) would be present. DWI is the best way to differentiate an arachnoid cyst from an epidermoid cyst.*

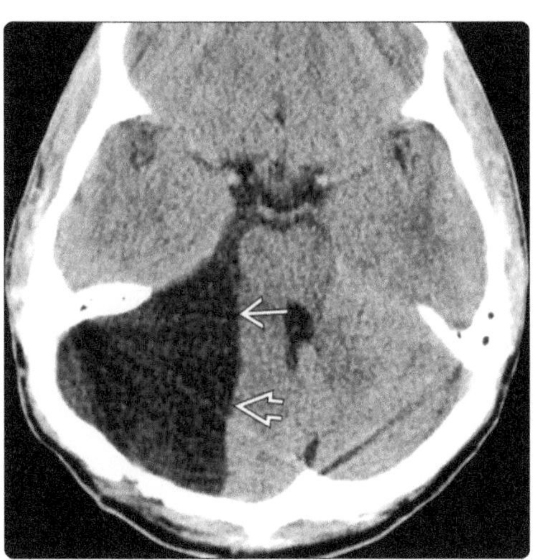

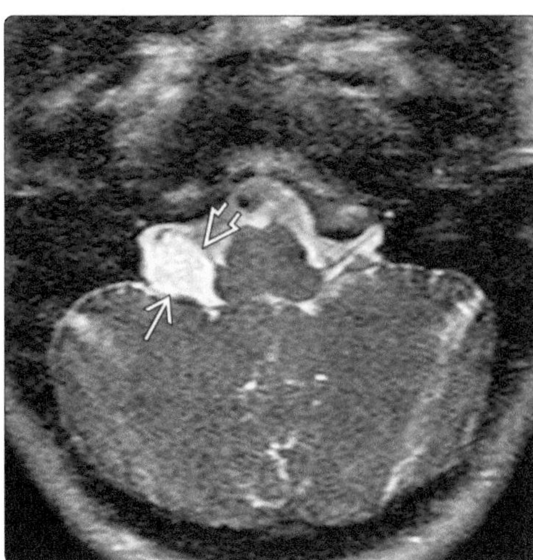

(Left) *Axial NECT through the upper CPA cistern shows a large low-density arachnoid cyst causing flattening of the lateral brachium pontis ➡ and cerebellar hemisphere ➡.* **(Right)** *Axial T2 FS MR demonstrates an incidental hyperintense CPA arachnoid cyst ➡ found at the time of imaging for headache. This lenticular-shaped lesion displaces the glossopharyngeal nerve (CNIX) anteriorly ➡. These small lesions require no additional imaging or treatment.*

KEY FACTS

TERMINOLOGY

- Congenital cholesteatoma (CCh): Benign mass secondary to epithelial rests of embryonal origin
- CCh most commonly occurs in middle ear (ME), behind intact tympanic membrane (TM) in patient without history of surgery, chronic otitis media (COM), or otorrhea

IMAGING

- Majority are in ME (CCh-ME)
  - Anterosuperior tympanic cavity near eustachian tube or stapes is most common
  - Posterior epitympanum at tympanic isthmus
  - Other sites include EAC, petrous apex, & mastoid
- Temporal bone CT findings
  - Small, well-circumscribed ME lesion medial to ossicles
  - Large mass may erode ossicles, ME wall, lateral semicircular canal, or tegmen tympani
- MR findings: Peripherally enhancing ME mass with diffusion restriction in larger lesions

TOP DIFFERENTIAL DIAGNOSES

- Acquired cholesteatoma
- Rhabdomyosarcoma
- Langerhans cell histiocytosis
- Glomus tympanicum paraganglioma
- ME cholesterol granuloma

CLINICAL ISSUES

- Avascular, pearly white ME mass behind intact TM without prior history of inflammation or trauma
- Unilateral conductive hearing loss in 30%
- Large ME lesions can obstruct eustachian tube → ME effusion & infection
- Complete surgical extirpation = treatment of choice

DIAGNOSTIC CHECKLIST

- Child with ME mass medial to ossicles, normal mastoid aeration, & no history of COM = CCh-ME

(Left) *Coronal graphic shows a congenital cholesteatoma (CCh) involving the middle ear (ME) cavity. The lesion has extended medial to the ossicles ➡ as it engulfs the entire ossicular chain. The tympanic membrane (TM) is intact, a typical finding in congenital lesions, as opposed to acquired cholesteatomas, which are associated with TM perforation.* **(Right)** *Axial DWI in a 4-year-old shows typical diffusion restriction ➡ in a well-defined ME cholesteatoma, lateral to the facial nerve canal.*

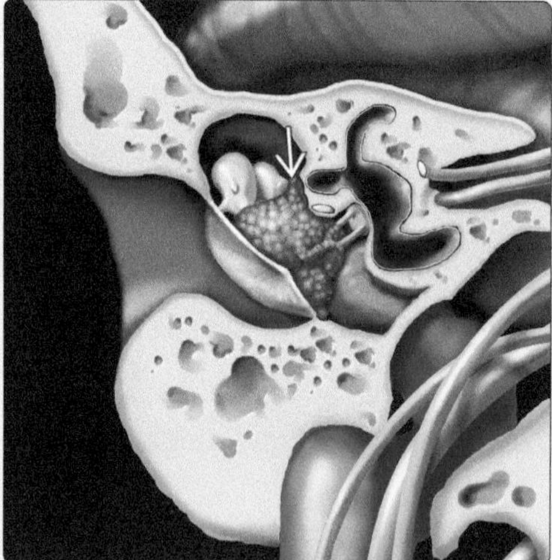

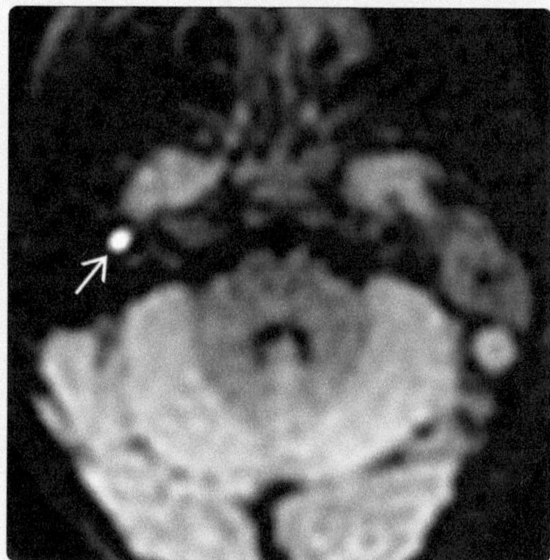

(Left) *Axial bone CT in a 3-year-old child without a history of chronic otitis media shows a typical round, well-circumscribed CCh ⇨ anteromedial to the malleus manubrium.* **(Right)** *Axial T1 C+ FS MR in the same patient shows the centrally nonenhancing CCh with a thin rim of peripheral enhancement ➡ adjacent to the cochlea ➡. This is a typical appearance & location for a CCh.*

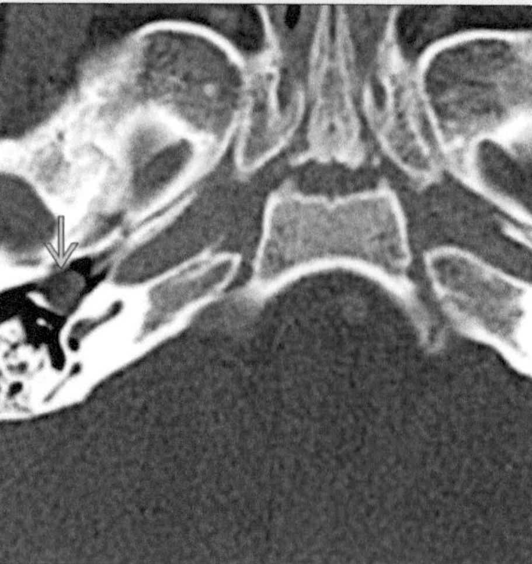

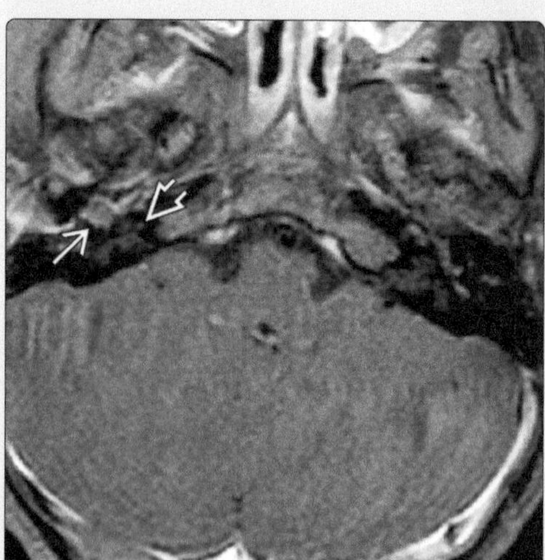

TERMINOLOGY

Synonyms

- Primary cholesteatoma, epidermoid

Definitions

- Congenital cholesteatoma (CCh): Benign mass secondary to epithelial rests of embryonal origin
- Most commonly occurs in middle ear (ME), behind intact tympanic membrane (TM) in patient without history of surgery, chronic otitis media, or otorrhea

IMAGING

General Features

- Best diagnostic clue
  - Smooth, well-circumscribed ME mass ± ossicular erosions
- Location
  - Majority in ME (CCh-ME)
  - Other locations: External auditory canal (EAC), mastoid, petrous apex, cerebellopontine angle, facial nerve canal, incudostapedial joint

CT Findings

- Bone CT
  - Appearance depends on size of lesion & location
  - Small CCh-ME: Well-circumscribed lesion
  - Large CCh-ME: Mass may erode ossicles, ME wall, lateral semicircular canal, or tegmen tympani [similar to acquired cholesteatoma (ACh)]
    - Bone erosion < ACh; occurs late in disease
    - Long process of incus & stapes superstructure are most commonly destroyed ossicles
    - If aditus ad antrum is occluded, mastoid air cells opacify with retained secretions
  - Petrous apex CCh: Expansile mass with smooth bone remodeling/erosion
    - May become very large before discovered
  - Mastoid CCh: Expansile mass with smooth bone erosion; may exit mastoid into EAC, parotid space, carotid space
  - EAC CCh: Rare; ↑ with EAC malformations

MR Findings

- T1: Iso- to hypointense mass
- T2: Intermediate signal intensity mass
  - Larger ME lesions → aditus ad antrum obstruction → high-signal retained secretions in mastoid air cells
- DWI: Larger lesions demonstrate diffusion restriction
- T1 C+: Peripherally enhancing ME mass
  - CCh-ME shows nonenhancing material surrounded by thin, subtle rim enhancement

DIFFERENTIAL DIAGNOSIS

Acquired Cholesteatoma

- Pars flaccida-ACh
- Pars tensa-ACh

Rhabdomyosarcoma

- Destructive mass in petrous apex, ME, or mastoid

Langerhans Cell Histiocytosis

- Enhancing soft tissue mass with bone destruction

Glomus Tympanicum Paraganglioma

- Pulsatile, vascular mass behind TM
- Enhancing mass on cochlear promontory; no bone erosion
- Unusual in pediatric & adolescent patients

Middle Ear Cholesterol Granuloma

- ME mass with high signal intensity on T1 MR

Facial Nerve Schwannoma

- Enlarged bony facial nerve canal

PATHOLOGY

General Features

- Etiology
  - 2 principal theories of CCh-ME
    - Congenital ectodermal rest in ME cavity left behind at time of neural tube closure
    - Lack of regression of epidermoid formation
      - Epidermoid formation: Point of epithelial transformation between tympanic cavity & eustachian tube
- Associated abnormalities
  - EAC atresia may have associated CCh of ME or EAC

Staging, Grading, & Classification

- CCh-ME staging system
  - Stage 1: Single quadrant; no ossicular involvement or mastoid extension
  - Stage 2: Multiple quadrants; no ossicular involvement or mastoid extension
  - Stage 3: Ossicular involvement; no mastoid extension
  - Stage 4: Mastoid extension

CLINICAL ISSUES

Presentation

- Most common signs/symptoms
  - Avascular, pearly white ME mass behind intact TM without prior history of inflammation or trauma

Demographics

- Age
  - Average age of presentation or detection
    - Anterior or anterosuperior: 4 years
    - Posterosuperior & mesotympanum: 12 years
    - Attic & mastoid antrum: 20 years or older
- Epidemiology
  - 2-5% of temporal bone cholesteatomas are congenital

Natural History & Prognosis

- CCh-ME: Smaller anterior lesions have better outcome with complete surgical resection
- Large lesions or posterior epitympanic CCh have recurrence rates as high as 20%

SELECTED REFERENCES

1. Wei B et al: Congenital cholesteatoma clinical and surgical management. Int J Pediatr Otorhinolaryngol. 164:111401, 2023
2. Hao J et al: The significance of staging in the treatment of congenital cholesteatoma in children. Ear Nose Throat J. 100(10_suppl):1125S-1131S, 2021
3. McCabe R et al: The endoscopic management of congenital cholesteatoma. Otolaryngol Clin North Am. 54(1):111-23, 2021

KEY FACTS

TERMINOLOGY

- Secondary or acquired cholesteatoma (ACh)
  - Tympanic membrane (TM) retraction or perforation → accumulation of stratified squamous epithelial cells in middle ear (ME) → mass-like keratin ball
- Pars flaccida cholesteatoma (PFC) (80%)
- Pars tensa cholesteatoma (PTC) (15%)
- Sinus cholesteatoma = PTC in sinus tympani
- EAC cholesteatoma (EACC)

IMAGING

- Best modalities
  - Noncontrast bone CT: Axial & coronal
    - Ossicular & adjacent bone evaluation
  - Coronal T1 C+ FS MR
    - Suspected intracranial extension/infection
- Nonenhancing ME soft tissue mass + ossicular erosion
  - PFC: In Prussak space with scutum erosion
    - ± tegmen tympani, lateral semicircular canal, facial nerve canal, or sigmoid sinus plate dehiscence
  - PTC: In posterior mesotympanum medial to ossicles
    - ± ossicular erosion, involvement of sinus tympani, facial recess, aditus ad antrum, or mastoid
- Restricts diffusion on DWI MR
- Associated granulation tissue or scar may enhance

TOP DIFFERENTIAL DIAGNOSES

- Congenital cholesteatoma
- Chronic otitis media with ossicular erosion
- Acute coalescent otomastoiditis with abscess
- Langerhans cell histiocytosis
- Rhabdomyosarcoma

CLINICAL ISSUES

- Recurrent or chronic ME infections with TM perforation or retraction pocket
- Conductive hearing loss (CHL)

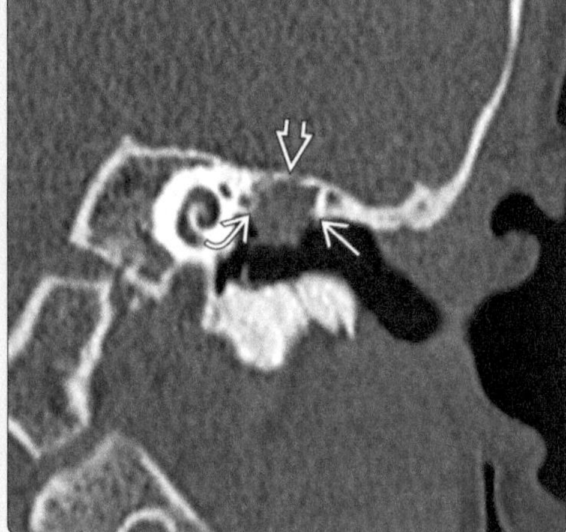

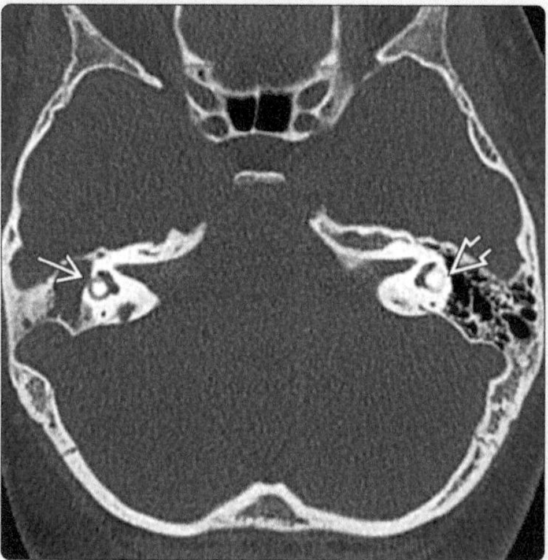

(Left) *Coronal bone CT in a teenager with recurrent otitis media shows opacity in the left middle ear cavity, truncated scutum ➡, and absence of the incus body and malleus neck (should be seen at this location). The tegmen tympani ➡ and facial nerve canal ➡ are intact.* **(Right)** *Axial bone CT in a child demonstrates focal dehiscence of the right lateral SCC ➡ compared to the normal covering of the left lateral SCC ➡. Also note underdevelopment of the right mastoid air cells, common in chronic inflammatory disease.*

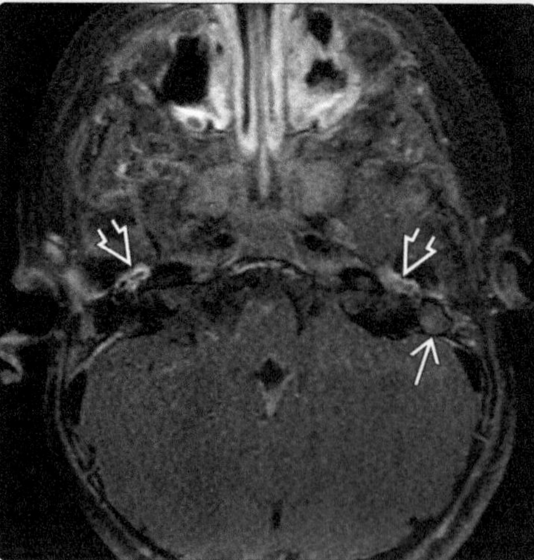

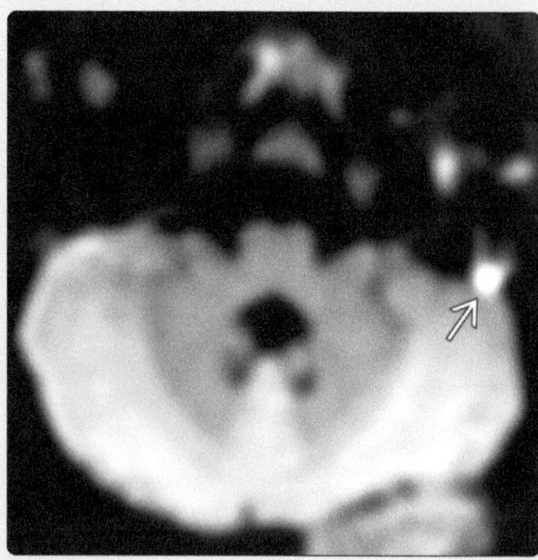

(Left) *Axial T1 C+ FS MR in a child with recurrent otitis media demonstrates a nonenhancing opacity in the left mastoid antrum ➡, mildly enhancing bilateral middle ear disease ➡, and bilateral maxillary sinus mucosal thickening.* **(Right)** *Axial DWI-B0 MR in the same child shows marked hyperintense signal corresponding to the nonenhancing lesion in the left mastoid antrum ➡. There was similar hypointense signal on ADC map, typical of cholesteatoma, which was proven at surgery.*

TERMINOLOGY

Abbreviations

- Secondary or acquired cholesteatoma (ACh)

Definitions

- Stratified squamous epithelium-lined sac filled with exfoliated keratin debris in middle ear (ME)
  - "Attic" or Prussak space cholesteatoma = pars flaccida cholesteatoma (PFC)
  - Pars tensa cholesteatoma (PTC) in posterior mesotympanum, medial to ossicles
- Abnormal migration of ectoderm in EAC cholesteatoma (EACC): secondary to surgery or trauma

IMAGING

General Features

- Best diagnostic clue
  - PFC: Nonenhancing soft tissue mass in Prussak space with scutum erosion
    - ± tegmen tympani, lateral semicircular canal, facial nerve canal, or sigmoid sinus plate dehiscence
  - PTC: Nonenhancing erosive mass in posterior mesotympanum, medial to ossicles
    - ± ossicular erosion, involvement of sinus tympani, facial recess, aditus ad antrum, or mastoid
  - EACC: Soft tissue mass + scalloping EAC + bony flecks
- Location
  - PFC: 80% of all cholesteatomas
    - 2° to tympanic membrane (TM) perforation or retraction pocket in anterior superior pars flaccida portion of TM (a.k.a. Shrapnell membrane)
  - PTC: 15% of all cholesteatomas
    - Secondary to TM perforation or retraction pocket in inferior pars tensa portion of TM
  - External auditory canal (EAC)

CT Findings

- Bone CT
  - PFC: Soft tissue mass in Prussak space, lateral to malleus head; scutum erosion characteristic
    - Ossicular erosion in 70%: Most commonly involves incus long process
    - ± posterolateral extension to aditus ad antrum & mastoid antrum or inferiorly to posterior ME recesses
    - ± erosion involving lateral semicircular canal, facial nerve canal, tegmen tympani, &/or sigmoid sinus plate
  - PTC: Erosive mass in posterior mesotympanum, medial to ossicles
    - ± sinus tympani, facial recess, aditus ad antrum, &/or mastoid involvement
    - Ossicular erosion common (90%): Especially medial aspect of incus long process, stapes suprastructure, & malleus manubrium
  - EACC: Soft tissue mass → scalloping EAC ± bone flecks

MR Findings

- ↓ T1, mildly ↑ T2 (< trapped secretions) ME mass
- PFC & PTC do not enhance; EACC ± rim-enhancement
- Associated granulation tissue or scar may enhance
- If tegmen tympani dehiscent, coronal may show dural enhancement adjacent to bony defect
- Restricted diffusion on DWI

Imaging Recommendations

- Noncontrast bone CT: Axial & coronal
- Coronal T1 C+ MR useful adjunct when cephalocele, intracranial extension, or intracranial infection suspected

DIFFERENTIAL DIAGNOSIS

Congenital Cholesteatoma

- Well-defined ME mass behind intact TM, medial to ossicles

Chronic Otitis Media With Ossicular Erosion

- Noncholesteatomatous ossicular erosion

Acute Coalescent Otomastoiditis With Abscess

- Rim-enhancing fluid collection adjacent to opacified mastoid air cells = intracranial or extracranial abscess

Langerhans Cell Histiocytosis

- Enhancing soft tissue mass with smooth bone destruction

Rhabdomyosarcoma

- Soft tissue mass with variable contrast enhancement & permeative bone destruction

PATHOLOGY

General Features

- Etiology
  - TM retraction or perforation → accumulation of stratified squamous epithelial cells in ME → mass-like keratin ball
  - Gradually increasing, ± erosion of adjacent bone
  - Inflammation may cause further bone erosion

CLINICAL ISSUES

Presentation

- Most common signs/symptoms
  - Recurrent or chronic ME infections with TM perforation or retraction pocket
  - Conductive hearing loss (CHL)
  - ME mass with TM perforation on otoscopy

Treatment

- Surgical excision, mastoidectomy, & ossicular chain reconstruction if needed

DIAGNOSTIC CHECKLIST

Image Interpretation Pearls

- When ME & mastoid opacified, difficult to differentiate effusion from ACh
- Presence of ossicular erosion favors ACh (but may also occur in noncholesteatomatous chronic otitis media)

SELECTED REFERENCES

1. Lourençone LFM et al: Management of acquired cholesteatoma in patients with craniofacial anomalies: an institutional experience. Am J Otolaryngol. 41(6):102591, 2020
2. Norris CD et al: Diffusion MR imaging in the head and neck: principles and applications. Neuroimaging Clin N Am. 30(3):261-82, 2020
3. He G et al: Clinical analysis of pediatric primary external auditory canal cholesteatoma. Int J Pediatr Otorhinolaryngol. 118:25-30, 2019

Skull Base Chondrosarcoma

KEY FACTS

TERMINOLOGY

- Skull base chondrosarcoma (CSA-SB): Chondroid malignancy of SB

IMAGING

- Typically **off-midline**, centered on **petrooccipital fissure**
- CT: Characteristic **arc or ring-like chondroid tumor matrix calcification** in **50%**
  - Sharp, narrow, nonsclerotic transition zone to adjacent normal bone
- MR: **High T2** signal & scattered hypointense calcifications
  - Heterogeneously enhancing
  - Whorls of enhancing lines within tumor matrix common
  - **ADC** of CSA **higher** than in chordoma & metastasis
  - Dynamic contrast enhanced (DCE) perfusion MR: Ve, Vp, Ktrans useful to differentiate tumor types

TOP DIFFERENTIAL DIAGNOSES

- Most common: Clival chordoma & SB metastasis
- Plasmacytoma
- Nasopharyngeal carcinoma (invasive)
- Meningioma
- Benign petrous apex lesions
- Cavernous sinus hemangioma

PATHOLOGY

- From remnants of embryonal cartilage, endochondral bone, or from primitive mesenchymal cells in meninges

CLINICAL ISSUES

- Typically middle-aged patient with insidious onset of headache & cranial nerve palsies (especially CNVI)

DIAGNOSTIC CHECKLIST

- Location: Off-midline (CSA) or midline (chordoma)
- Calcifications: **Arc-whorl intralesional calcifications** (CSA) or fragmented destroyed bone (chordoma)
- Consider MR angiography or CTA for preoperative characterization of vessel involvement

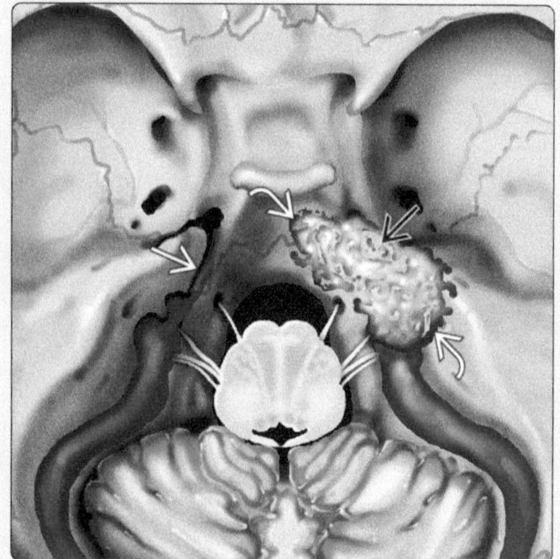

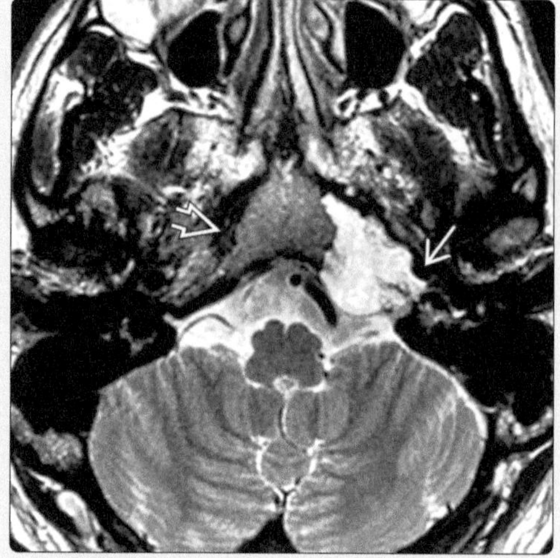

(Left) *Axial graphic depicts the classic location of a chondrosarcoma (CSA) of the skull base centered in the left petrooccipital fissure ➡. Note the normal right petrooccipital fissure with inferior petrosal sinus (blue) along its margins ➡. Chondroid calcifications, depicted in yellow, are seen within the lesion ➡.* **(Right)** *Axial T2 MR reveals a large, high-signal CSA of the left petrooccipital fissure. Note that the vertical segment of the petrous internal carotid artery (ICA) is compressed ➡. Note the normal right petrooccipital fissure ➡.*

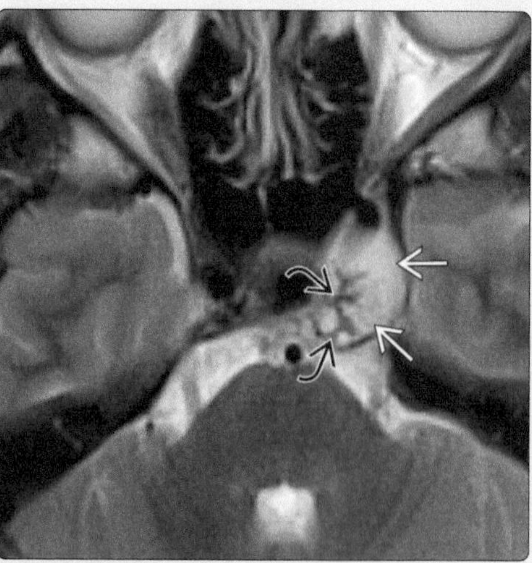

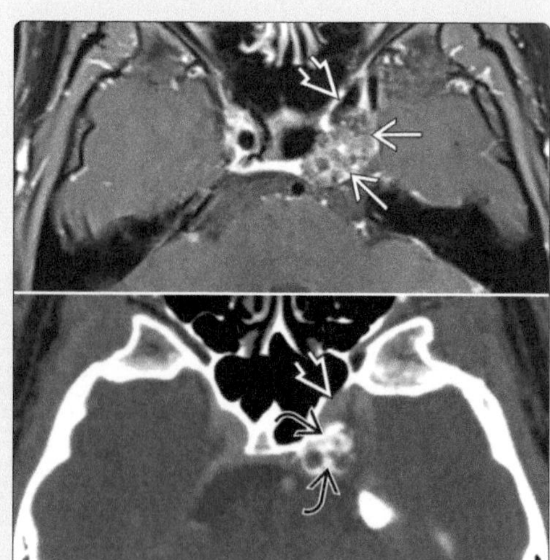

(Left) *Axial T2 MR in a 17-year-old boy shows a hyperintense expansile mass lesion filling the left cavernous sinus ➡, proven to be a CSA on surgical excision. Posteromedial hypointense areas are from chondroid calcifications ➡.* **(Right)** *Axial T1 C+ FS MR (top) in the same patient shows heterogeneous contrast enhancement ➡ of the CSA. Axial CECT (bottom) shows chondroid calcifications along its posteromedial aspect ➡. Left cavernous ICA is displaced anteromedially but is patent ➡. (Courtesy R. H. Ramakrishnaiah, MD.)*

TERMINOLOGY

Abbreviations

- Chondrosarcoma-skull base (CSA-SB)

Definitions

- Chondroid malignancy of SB

IMAGING

General Features

- Best diagnostic clue
  - Solitary, enhancing osteolytic soft tissue mass, centered at **petrooccipital fissure (POF)/petroclival fissure** ± chondroid matrix
  - Difficult to distinguish benign chondroma from CSA-SB
- Location
  - Off-midline at **POF** (2/3): POF occupied by cartilaginous plate
    - POF margins grooved for inferior petrosal sinus
    - Continuous posteriorly with jugular foramen
  - Anterior basisphenoid (1/3)
    - Lesion can extend across posterior to middle cranial fossa with dumbbell appearance
    - Frequently located extradurally in parasellar middle cranial fossa SB
  - Rarely multiple
- Size
  - Variable, usually > 3 cm at time of diagnosis
- Morphology
  - Well-circumscribed, lobulated margins
  - Lobulated growth in 3 dimensions results in cauliflower shape

CT Findings

- NECT
  - Soft tissue component relatively dense
- CECT
  - Variable, heterogeneous enhancement
- Bone CT
  - Expansile mass at POF producing erosive or destructive bone changes in clivus & petrous apex
  - ~ **50%** have radiographically classic chondroid matrix with **rings & arcs calcification**
  - Sharp, narrow, nonsclerotic transition zone to adjacent normal bone

MR Findings

- T1WI
  - Low to intermediate signal intensity relative to gray matter
    - ↓ signal foci within tumor may suggest coarse matrix mineralization or fibrocartilaginous elements
- T2WI
  - Variable, usually **high signal**
    - CSA-SB may be homogeneously hyperintense on T2WI or simply contain localized zones of hyperintensity
    - Degree of T2 hyperintensity inversely related to degree of calcified matrix
    - Steady-state free precession T2 images may be low signal (even if bright on T2 spin-echo)
  - Hypointense foci (calcifications) less conspicuous than CT
- DWI
  - Normalized mean **ADC** significantly **higher in CSA** (2.4) than in chordoma (1.3) & metastasis (1.39)
- PWI
  - **Dynamic contrast enhanced (DCE) perfusion MR**
  - Fractional plasma volume (**Vp**): **Differentiates all 3** common SB tumors from each other
    - CSA (0.015), chordoma (0.045), metastasis (0.12)
  - Fractional volume of extracellular space (**Ve**): **Differentiates CSA** (0.25) **from metastasis** (0.48)
    - Ve difference of chordoma (0.35) & metastasis (0.48) statistically insignificant
    - Ve difference of CSA (0.25) & chordoma (0.35) statistically insignificant
  - Forward volume transfer constant (**Ktrans**): **Differentiates CSA** (0.08) **from metastasis** (0.39)
    - **Also differentiates chordoma** (0.16) **from metastasis** (0.39)
    - Ktrans difference of CSA (0.08) & chordoma (0.16) statistically insignificant
- T1WI C+
  - Heterogeneous enhancement
    - Whorls of enhancing lines within tumor matrix common

Angiographic Findings

- Avascular or hypovascular mass
- Internal carotid artery displacement ± encasement

Imaging Recommendations

- Best imaging tool
  - Combination of multiplanar, gadolinium-enhanced MR & high-resolution bone CT
- Protocol advice
  - High-resolution axial bone CT for evaluation of chondroid matrix & pattern of bone destruction
  - MR of SB to include T2WI & multiplanar T1WI, followed by T1 C+ FS in same planes for direct comparison
  - MRA & MRV or CTA helpful to assess vascular involvement preoperatively
  - Preoperative angiography with test occlusion if vessel sacrifice necessary

DIFFERENTIAL DIAGNOSIS

Chordoma

- Destructive clival lesion; bone fragments within matrix
- Midline > lateral location
- Low T1 & markedly **high T2** signal; enhancing mass
- Chondroid chordomas more aggressive & worse prognosis
- SB chordomas have **lower ADC values than CSA-SB**

Skull Base Metastasis

- Bone CT: Destructive mass, can be anywhere in SB
- MR: Often multiple enhancing, invasive lesions
- Typically **low** to intermediate **T2** signal
- Known primary tumor

Plasmacytoma & Multiple Myeloma

- Usually more midline, within clivus
- **T2 signal low** to intermediate
- > 50% have concurrent multiple myeloma

Nasopharyngeal Carcinoma

- Primary mass in nasopharyngeal mucosal space
- Tumor invades superiorly to clivus, foramen lacerum, POF
- **Low** to intermediate **T2**, DWI restriction if highly cellular

Meningioma

- Calcification in meningioma can mimic chondroid matrix
- Hyperostosis possible; not typically destructive in absence of invasion
- **Low** to intermediate **T2** signal; enhancing with dural tails

Non-Hodgkin Lymphoma

- Lymphoproliferative neoplasm with focal or multifocal, osseous, &/or extraosseous involvement of SB
- **Low** to intermediate **T2** signal, may restrict on DWI

Nonneoplastic Lesion of Petrous Apex

- Includes benign expansile lesions: Cholesteatoma, mucocele, cholesterol granuloma
  - Should be nonenhancing, smoothly marginated without calcified matrix
- High signal from asymmetric petrous apex marrow can mimic enhancing tumor
- Petrous apicitis shows inflammatory enhancement of petrous apex with permeative bone changes
  - Expect acute clinical syndrome with fever, leukocytosis, Gradenigo syndrome

Chondromyxoid Fibroma

- Rare, expansile, noninfiltrating SB mass
- Areas of ground-glass density may be seen
- Appearance may overlap with CSA-SB
- **High T2** signal, similar to any chondroid tumor

Cavernous Sinus Hemangioma

- Lesion with **intensely high T2** signal (light bulb-like) & enhancement
- May mimic paracavernous CSA

PATHOLOGY

General Features

- Etiology
  - From remnants of embryonal cartilage, endochondral bone, or from primitive mesenchymal cells in meninges
    - May arise from metaplasia of meningeal fibroblasts
- Genetics
  - May complicate **Ollier** disease & **Maffucci** syndromes

Staging, Grading, & Classification

- Classification
  - Conventional [hyaline (7%), myxoid (30%), or mixed (63%)], clear cell, mesenchymal, dedifferentiated
- Grading from low to high grade
  - Based on degree of cellularity, pleomorphism, mitoses, & multinucleated cells

Microscopic Features

- Histology may overlap with/confused with chordoma
  - Particularly in chondroid chordoma & myxoid CSA
  - Differentiation by immunohistochemical staining
- Histopathologic differentiation between low-grade CSA & benign chondroma may be difficult

CLINICAL ISSUES

Presentation

- Most common signs/symptoms
  - **Abducens (CNVI) palsy** due to proximity of Dorello canal
  - **Headache**
  - Mean duration of symptoms at diagnosis: 27 months
- Other signs/symptoms
  - Other cranial nerve palsies (CNIII, CNV, CNVII, CNVIII)
- Clinical profile
  - Middle-aged patient with insidious onset of headaches & cranial nerve palsies

Demographics

- Age
  - Range: 10-80 years
    - Mean: 40 years
- Epidemiology
  - 6% of all SB tumors
  - 75% of all cranial CSA occur in SB

Natural History & Prognosis

- Prognosis depends on extent at diagnosis, histologic grade, & completeness of surgical resection
  - Disease-specific 10-year survival rates of 99% reported
  - Most central CSA-SBs well to moderately differentiated
  - High-grade CSA can metastasize to bones & lung
- Conventional CSA: Indolent growth pattern
  - Slow growing, locally invasive but rarely metastasize
- Mesenchymal & dedifferentiated forms: Aggressive behavior; poor prognosis

Treatment

- Aggressive resection associated with significant morbidity & low likelihood of complete resection
- Combined radical resection & postoperative high-dose fractionated precision conformal radiation therapy
  - Charged particle radiotherapy (proton beam or carbon ions) alone or combined with subtotal resection

DIAGNOSTIC CHECKLIST

Consider

- Location: Off-midline (CSA) or midline (chordoma)
- Calcifications: **Arc-whorl intralesional calcifications** (CSA) or fragmented destroyed bone (chordoma)
- Look for known primary neoplasm (metastasis), myeloma (plasmacytoma), or nasopharyngeal carcinoma

Image Interpretation Pearls

- Classic appearance: Heterogeneously enhancing tumor located at **POF** with hyperintense signal on T2 MR
  - CT shows chondroid mineralization & bone destruction
- Any SB chondroid tumor [including chondroma, CSA, & chondromyxoid fibroma (CMF)] & chordoma show **high T2** signal
  - Other common SB tumors usually low T2 signal

SELECTED REFERENCES

1. Ota Y et al: Differentiation of skull base chondrosarcomas, chordomas, and metastases: utility of DWI and dynamic contrast-enhanced perfusion MR imaging. AJNR Am J Neuroradiol. 43(9):1325-32, 2022

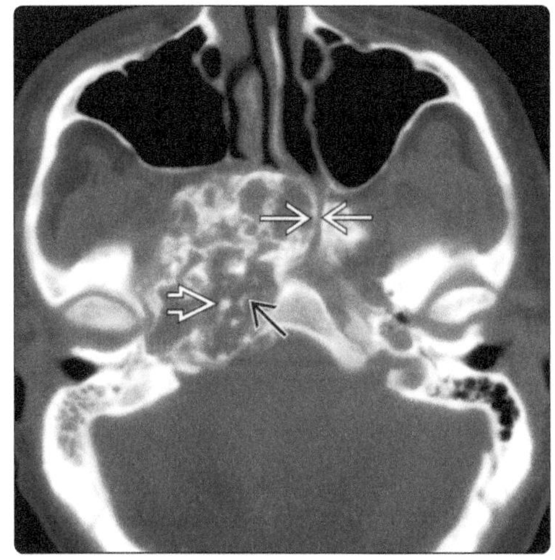

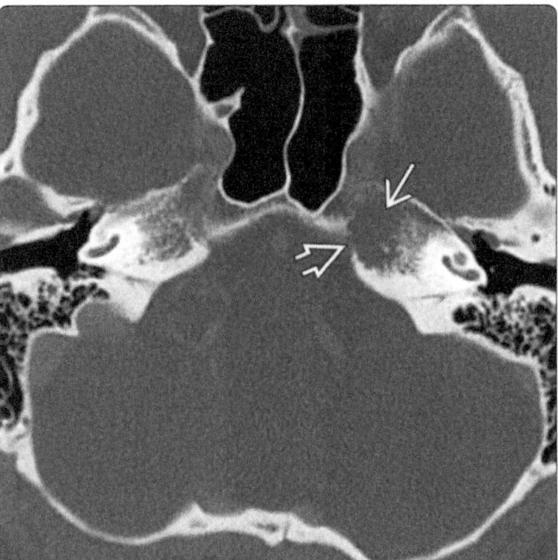

(Left) *Axial bone CT shows rounded ➡ and arc-like ➡ calcified foci in this large CSA centered at the right petrooccipital fissure. Up to 50% of CSAs demonstrate matrix calcification. Note slight narrowing of the left vidian canal ➡.* **(Right)** *Axial bone window CT shows subtle bone destruction ➡ with cortical erosion ➡ in this small left petrous apex CSA. No calcified matrix is seen. MR showed a corresponding T2-hyperintense and enhancing mass in this location.*

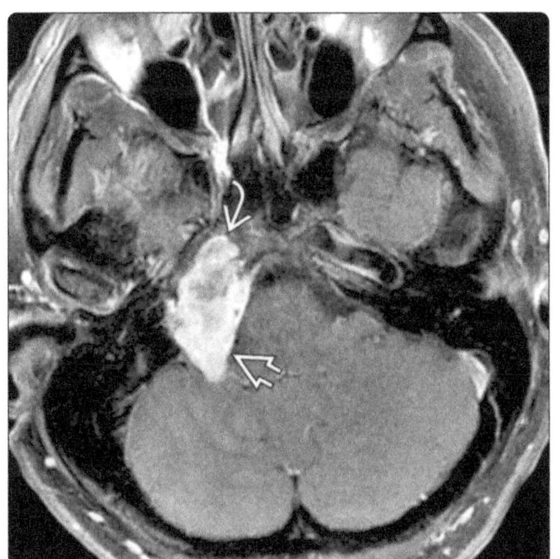

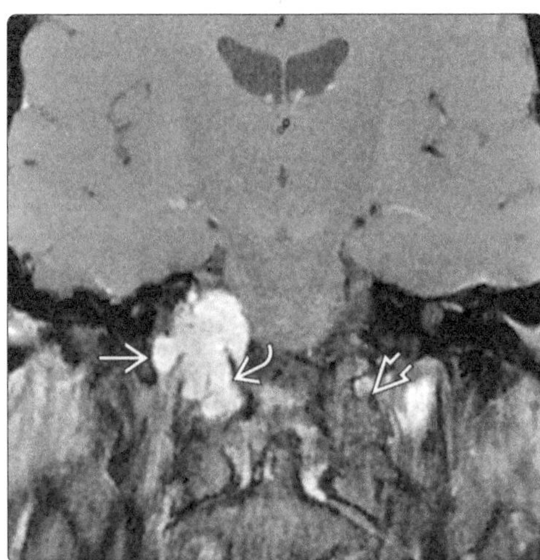

(Left) *Axial T1 C+ FS MR demonstrates avid enhancement in a CSA. Note petrous apex ➡ and CPA cistern ➡ involvement. Most skull base CSAs emanate from the petrooccipital fissure. However, when they become large, it may be hard to see the point of origin.* **(Right)** *Coronal T1 C+ FS MR delineates tumor invasion into the jugular foramen ➡ and occipital condyle ➡. Note the normal left occipital condyle ➡.*

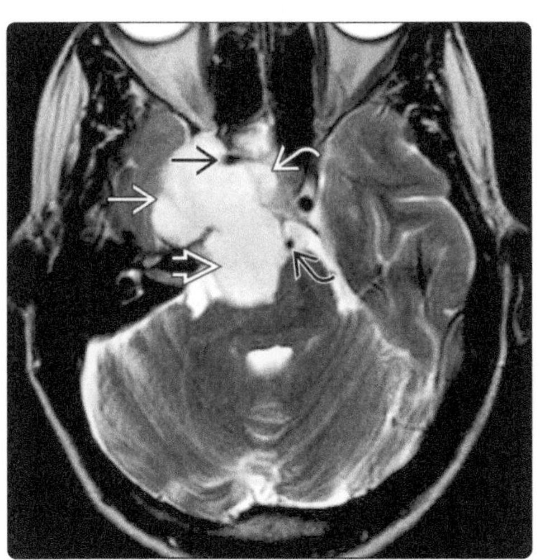

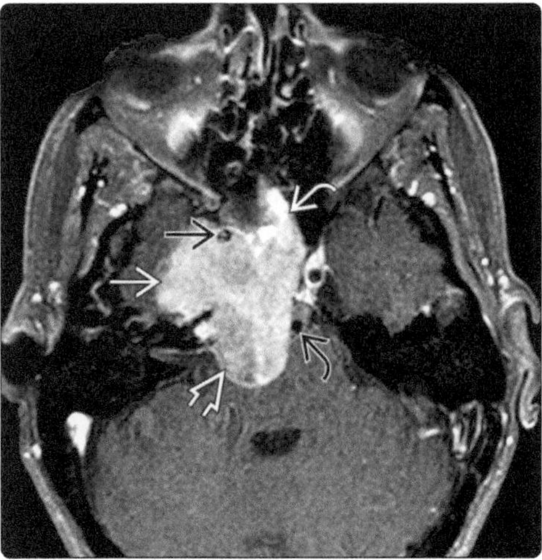

(Left) *Axial T2 MR shows a hyperintense right parasellar CSA ➡ that extends into the prepontine cistern ➡ and sphenoid sinus ➡. Note internal carotid ➡ and basilar ➡ arterial displacement by the mass. Differential diagnosis includes cavernous sinus hemangioma (light bulb-like high T2 signal).* **(Right)** *Axial T1 C+ FS MR shows moderate enhancement within a right parasellar CSA ➡. Tumor invades prepontine cistern ➡ and sphenoid sinus ➡, partly encases the right ICA ➡, and displaces the basilar artery ➡.*

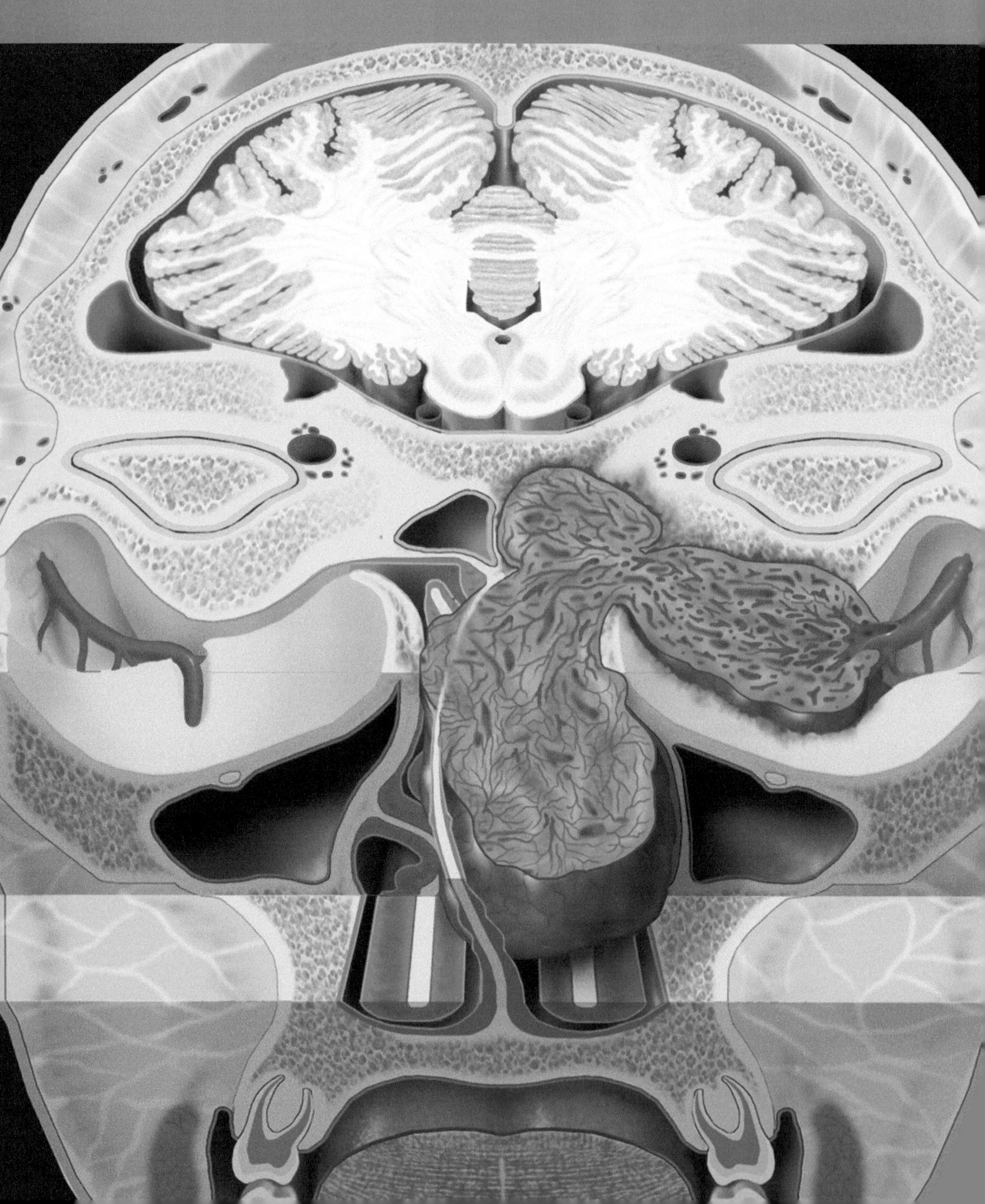

PART II
SECTION 2
Orbit, Nose, and Sinuses

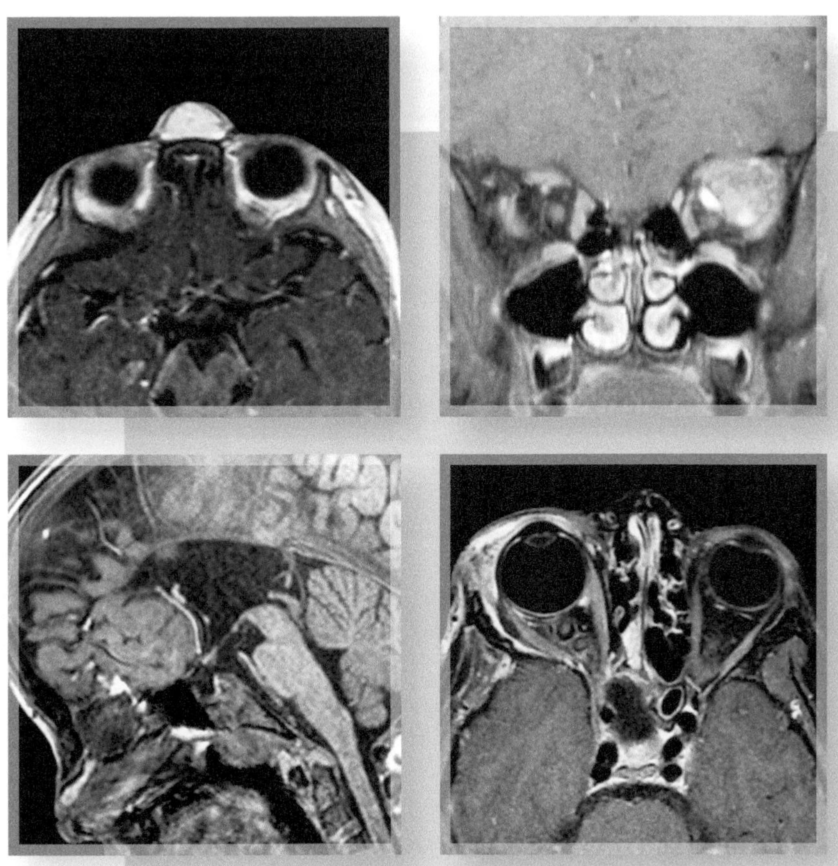

Nasal Glioma

KEY FACTS

TERMINOLOGY

- Synonym: **Nasal cerebral heterotopia**; glial heterotopia
- Developmental mass of dysplastic neurogenic tissue sequestered & isolated from subarachnoid space
  - **Glioma misnomer**; tissue nonneoplastic
  - Extranasal glioma (ENG), intranasal glioma (ING)

IMAGING

- Well-circumscribed soft tissue mass at superior nasal dorsum (ENG) or within nasal cavity (ING)
  - With no intracranial CSF or brain continuity
- Wide foramen cecum alone not strong indicator of intracranial extension; correlate with MR
- Multiplanar MR
  - May show pedicle of fibrous tissue (not brain parenchyma) between ING & intracranial cavity
  - Better than CT to differentiate from cephalocele or dermoid
  - Gyral structure of gray matter rarely visible
  - Commonly shows hyperintensity related to gliosis

TOP DIFFERENTIAL DIAGNOSES

- Frontoethmoidal cephalocele
- Nasal dermal sinus
- Sinonasal solitary polyp

PATHOLOGY

- Similar spectrum of congenital anomalies as frontoethmoidal cephaloceles
  - Does **not** contain CSF nor brain contiguous intracranially
- Rarely associated with other brain or systemic anomalies

CLINICAL ISSUES

- Usually identified at birth
- Treatment of choice: Complete surgical resection

DIAGNOSTIC CHECKLIST

- Caution: Anterior skull base **ossification widely variable** in 1st few years of life; do not overcall bony defects

(Left) *Sagittal graphic of a nasal glioma [better term is nasal glial (or cerebral) heterotopia; glioma is a misnomer] shows a mass of dysplastic glial tissue ➡ along the nasal dorsum. Notice the absence of a connection to the intracranial contents.* **(Right)** *Sagittal T2W MR demonstrates an extranasal glioma ➡ as a mass along the nasal dorsum near the glabella, mildly hyperintense to the brain. Extranasal gliomas may be rarely found at the medial canthus of eye or, extremely rarely, at other sites.*

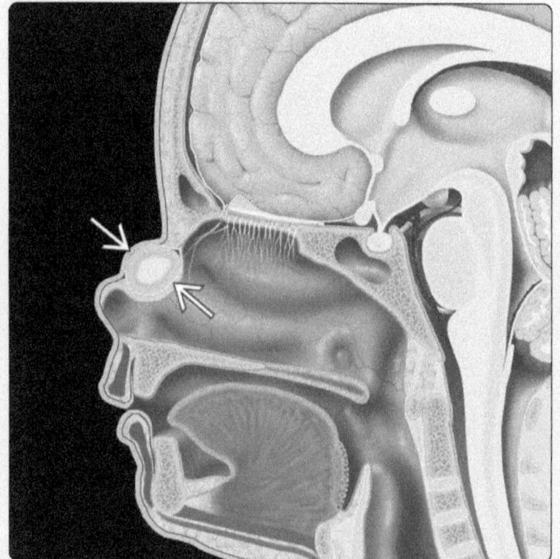

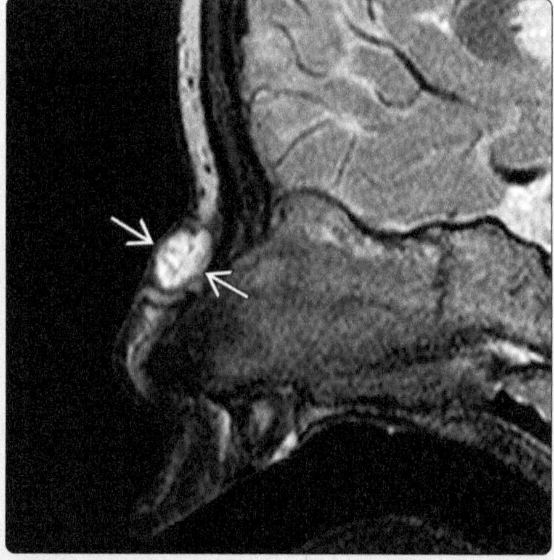

(Left) *Sagittal T2 MR in a 3-day-old with a nasal mass demonstrates an intermediate signal intensity intranasal glioma ➡ without intracranial extension.* **(Right)** *Axial T1 C+ MR shows central enhancement ➡ within a large extranasal glioma ➡. The lesion is located slightly off the midline. Enhancement is uncommon in these lesions. Dysplastic tissue of nasal glial (cerebral) heterotopia typically does not enhance but may rarely have focal or diffuse enhancement.*

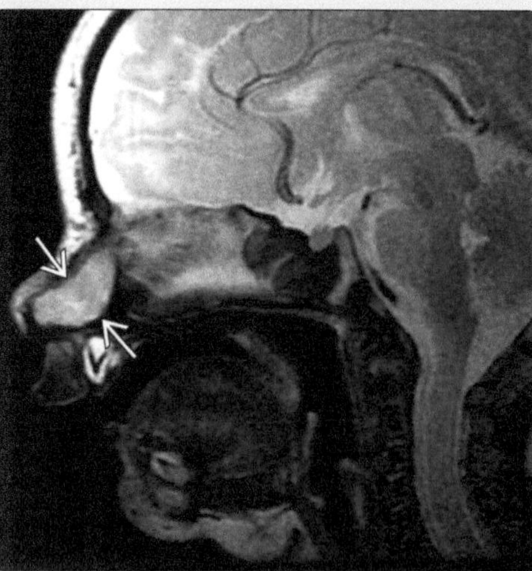

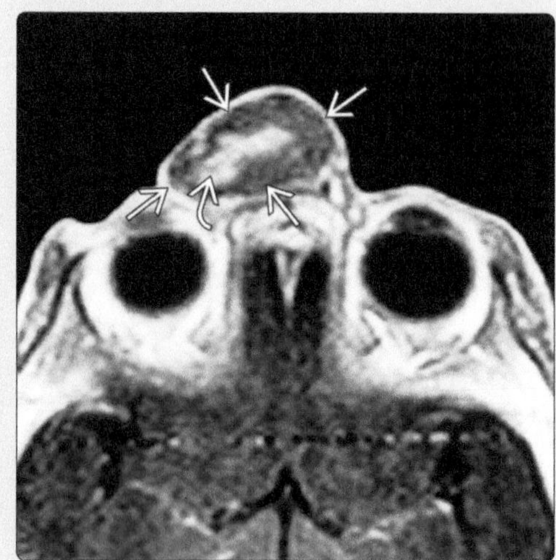

TERMINOLOGY

Abbreviations

- Nasal glioma (NG)
  - Extranasal glioma (ENG), intranasal glioma (ING)

Synonyms

- Nasal glial heterotopia; nasal cerebral **heterotopia**

Definitions

- Developmental mass of **dysplastic neurogenic tissue** sequestered & isolated from subarachnoid space
  - **Glioma misnomer**; tissue nonneoplastic
  - Best thought of as cephalocele without intracranial connection to brain

IMAGING

General Features

- Best diagnostic clue
  - Well-circumscribed soft tissue mass at superior nasal dorsum (ENG) or within nasal cavity (ING)
    - **No** connection to brain
- Location
  - Most occur at bridge of nose or in & around nasal cavity
  - Most commonly around glabella & nasomaxillary suture
  - Usually off-midline; right > left side
  - ENG: Mass along nasal dorsum
    - Glabella most frequent location
    - ENG may also be found at medial canthus
  - Other sites of ENG
    - Ethmoid sinus, sphenoid sinus, palate, middle ear, tonsil, nasopharynx, mouth, pterygopalatine fossa (very rare)
  - ING: Nasal cavity mass
    - May be attached to middle turbinate, nasal septum, or lateral nasal wall
- Size
  - 1-3 cm in diameter
- Morphology
  - Well-circumscribed, round, ovoid, or polypoid mass

CT Findings

- NECT
  - ENG: Well-circumscribed soft tissue attenuation/isodense to brain mass at glabella
    - Superficial to point of fusion of frontal & nasal bones (fonticulus frontalis); nasal bones may be thinned
  - ING: Soft tissue attenuation mass within nasal cavity
    - Typically high in nasal vault
    - Fibrous pedicle may extend toward skull base but not intracranially
    - Defect in cribriform plate (10-30%)
    - Caution: Anterior skull base **ossification widely variable** in 1st few years of life
      - ◻ Complete ossification by 3 year 10 months (earliest by 14 months)
      - ◻ Foramen cecum (anterior to crista galli) may still persist further later
      - ◻ Wide foramen cecum alone not strong indicator of intracranial extension; correlate with MR
  - Calcification rare
- CECT
  - Typically no significant enhancement
  - If intrathecal contrast used
    - Fails to document connection of lesion to subarachnoid space

MR Findings

- T1WI
  - Predominantly mixed to low signal intensity mass
  - Gyral structure of gray matter rarely visible
- T2WI
  - Commonly shows hyperintensity related to gliosis
  - No CSF around lesion connecting to subarachnoid space
- T1WI C+
  - Dysplastic tissue typically does not enhance
    - "Perceived" enhancement at periphery of intranasal lesions may actually represent adjacent nasal mucosa
    - Internal enhancement may occur rarely

Imaging Recommendations

- Best imaging tool
  - Multiplanar MR
    - May show pedicle of fibrous tissue (not brain parenchyma) between ING & intracranial cavity
    - MR better than CT for differentiating NG from cephalocele or dermoid
    - Avoids radiation to radiosensitive eye lenses in young patients
- Protocol advice
  - Thin-section sagittal T1 & T2 MR important sequences
  - Heavily T2W 3D sequences, such as CISS, FIESTA, or SPACE
    - Better demonstrate lack of brain parenchymal or CSF continuity intracranially
  - Preoperative thin-section axial bone CT with coronal reformatted images may also help in surgical planning
    - Bone only without IV contrast

DIFFERENTIAL DIAGNOSIS

Frontoethmoidal Cephalocele

- Frontonasal (FN) & nasoethmoidal (NE) cephaloceles
- Clinical: Congenital mass on anterior forehead at glabella-dorsum of nose (FN), or in superomedial nasal cavity (NE)
- Imaging: MR shows connection to intracranial brain parenchyma or CSF
  - Through unobliterated fonticulus frontalis (FN)
  - Through foramen cecum (NE)

Nasal Dermal Sinus

- Clinical: Pit on tip or bridge of nose
- Imaging
  - Dermoid or epidermoid along course from tip of nose to skull base at foramen cecum, anterior to crista galli
    - Single or multiple; within nasal septum
  - T2: Fluid-signal tract in septum from nasal dorsum to skull base (sinus)

Sinonasal Solitary Polyps

- Clinical: Polyp less firm, more translucent than ING
  - Unusual < 5 years
- Imaging

- Typically inferolateral to middle turbinate (ING medial)
- Homogeneous ↑ T2 MR signal with thin enhancement of peripheral mucosa

Orbital Dermoid & Epidermoid

- Clinical: Focal mass in medial orbit near nasolacrimal suture
- Imaging
  - Dermoid: Fluid or fat density/signal intensity
  - Epidermoid: Fluid density/signal intensity

PATHOLOGY

General Features

- Etiology
  - Dysplastic, heterotopic neuroglial & fibrous tissue separated from brain
    - During development of anterior skull/skull base
  - Similar spectrum of congenital anomalies as frontoethmoidal cephaloceles but does not contain CSF
    - Not contiguous with subarachnoid spaces or ventricles
  - Premature fusion of potential anterior skull base spaces prior to regression of dural diverticulum
  - **ENG**: Premature fusion of **fonticulus frontalis** (potential space prior to fusion of frontal & nasal bones)
    - Dysplastic parenchyma sequestered over nasal bones/nasofrontal suture
  - **ING**: Premature fusion of **prenasal space** (potential space between nasal bones & cartilaginous nasal capsule)
    - Dysplastic parenchyma sequestered in nasal cavity
- Associated abnormalities
  - Rarely associated with other brain or systemic anomalies

Gross Pathologic & Surgical Features

- Firm, smooth mass
- Rarely recognized as brain tissue at surgery
- Mixed extraintranasal lesions connect through defect in nasal bone
- 10-30% attached to brain by stalk of fibrous tissue through defect in or near cribriform plate
- Cribriform plate ossification begins near vertical attachments of superior & middle turbinates & spreads to reach crista galli at by ~ 2 months age
- Only 4% have complete anterior skull base ossification by 2 years of age
- Anterior skull base fully ossified at 3 years 10 months of age (foramen cecum may persist later)

Microscopic Features

- Fibrous or gemistocytic astrocytes & neuroglial fibers
- Fibrous, vascularized connective tissue & sparse neurons
- GFAP & S100 protein positive
- No mitotic features or bizarre nuclear forms

CLINICAL ISSUES

Presentation

- Most common signs/symptoms
  - **ENG**
    - Congenital subcutaneous blue or red mass along nasal dorsum (glabella)
    - Usually nonprogressive midfacial swelling
  - **ING**
    - Firm, polypoid submucosal nasal cavity mass
    - Nasal obstruction & septal deviation may be present
    - May be confused clinically with nasal polyp
    - Nasal congestion main symptom
- Other signs/symptoms
  - No change in size with crying, Valsalva, or pressure on jugular vein (size ↑ in frontoethmoidal cephalocele)
  - **ENG**: Capillary telangiectasia may cover
  - **ING**: Respiratory distress; epiphora; may protrude through nostril
  - Rhinorrhea, epistaxis, meningitis, chronic rhinosinusitis, strabismus
- Clinical profile
  - Firm mass at glabella (**ENG**) or within nasal cavity (**ING**) in newborn

Demographics

- Age
  - Identified at birth or within 1st few years of life
  - May be detected in antenatal ultrasound & fetal MR
- Epidemiology
  - Very rare lesion; male:female ratio = 3:2
  - **ENG: 36%**; **ING: 45%**; mixed: 19%
  - 66% diagnosed & treated before 1 year of age
  - 8% occur in adults; always ING
  - ING diagnosis delayed usually

Natural History & Prognosis

- Grows slowly in proportion to adjacent tissue or brain if attached by pedicle
  - May deform nasal skeleton, maxilla, or orbit
- May become infected, resulting in meningitis
- Complete resection curative
  - 10% recurrence rate with incomplete resection

Treatment

- Treatment of choice is complete surgical resection
  - **ENG** without intracranial connection removed via external incision with stalk dissection
  - **ING** without intracranial connection may be removed endoscopically
    - Less postoperative deformity than with craniotomy
  - Stalk removal imperative to decrease recurrence rate & minimize CSF leak & subsequent meningitis

DIAGNOSTIC CHECKLIST

Consider

- Most important to **differentiate** NG **from cephalocele**
- Document lack of connecting brain tissue &/or contiguous CSF space

Image Interpretation Pearls

- Must evaluate images for connection to intracranial cavity through skull base defect (cephalocele)
- Combined use of thin-section MR & bone CT accomplishes this task: Focus imaging to frontoethmoid area

SELECTED REFERENCES

1. Gallego Compte M et al: Nasal glial heterotopia: a systematic review of the literature and case report. Acta Otorhinolaryngol Ital. 42(4):317-24, 2022

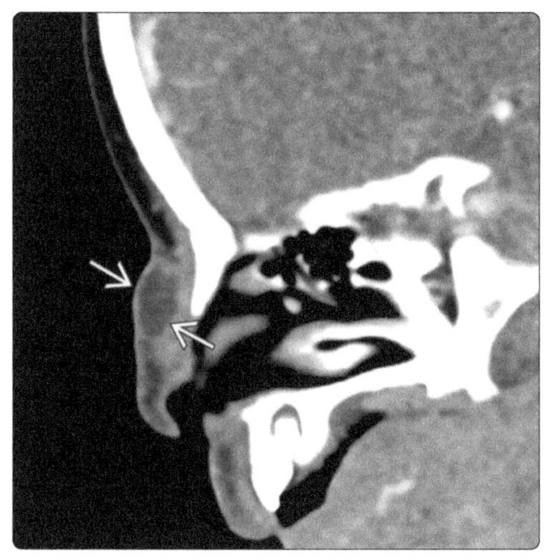

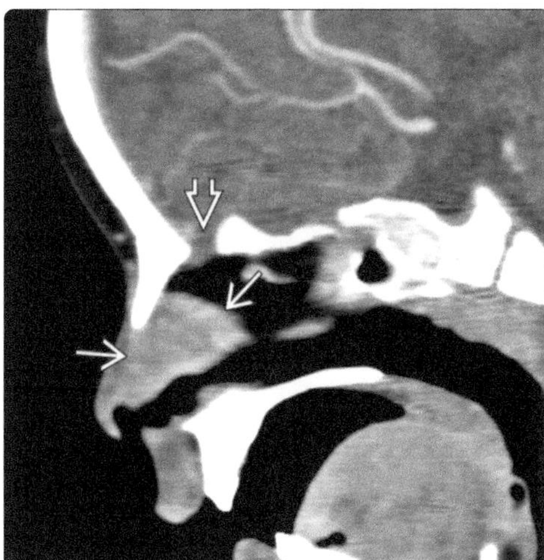

(Left) *Sagittal CECT shows nonenhancing soft tissue mass along the nasal dorsum near the glabella without any intracranial connection, consistent with an extranasal glioma ➡.* **(Right)** *Sagittal CECT demonstrates a mildly enhancing nasal cavity soft tissue mass, consistent with intranasal glioma ➡. Nasal gliomas rarely enhance. "Perceived" enhancement at the periphery of intranasal glioma may actually represent adjacent nasal mucosa. No connection is seen with a normally prominent foramen cecum ➡ in this child.*

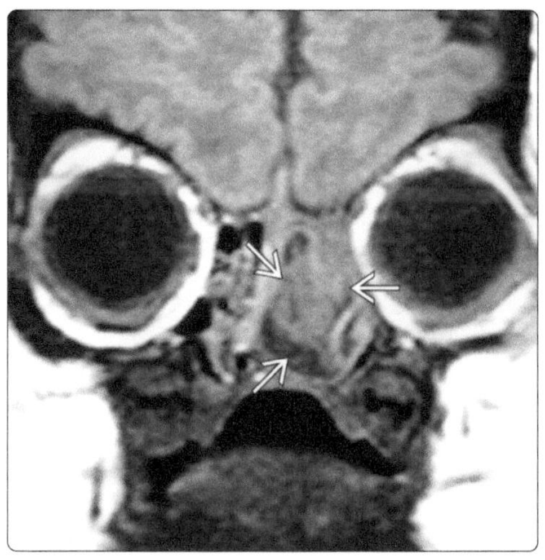

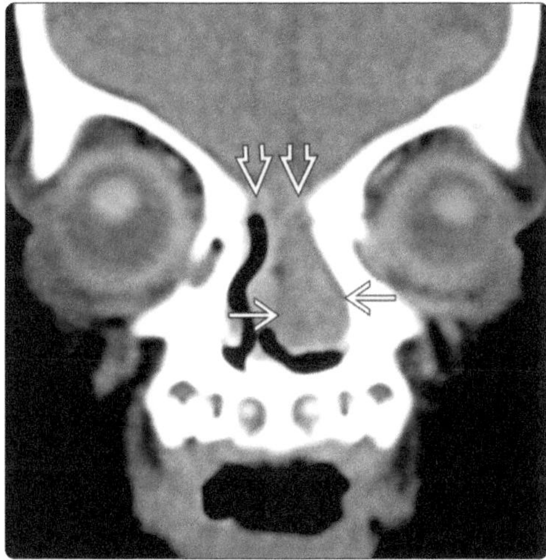

(Left) *Coronal FLAIR MR shows mixed signal intensity within an intranasal glioma ➡. There is no connection to the left frontal lobe to suggest a cephalocele.* **(Right)** *Coronal NECT shows a well-defined, polypoid soft tissue mass in the left nasal cavity ➡ without definite connection to brain, consistent with an intranasal glioma. Nasal septum is slightly deviated toward the right. Anterior skull base defects in a child should be interpreted with caution; there is wide variation in unossified areas ➡ in the 1st few years of life.*

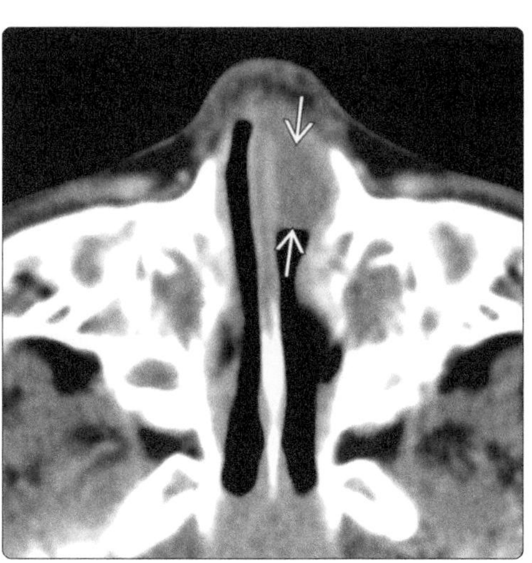

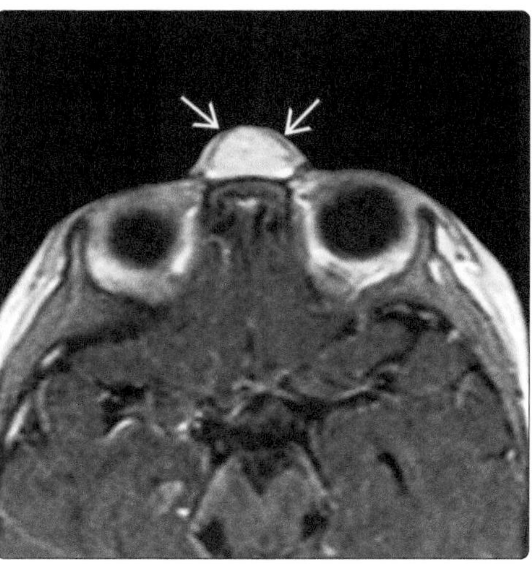

(Left) *Axial CECT shows a left-sided intranasal glioma ➡ widening the anterior nasal vault. These develop in relation to premature fusion of the prenasal space (potential space between nasal bones and cartilaginous nasal capsule).* **(Right)** *Axial T1 C+ MR shows a well-defined extranasal glioma ➡ along the dorsum of the nose in the midline with rare intense diffuse enhancement in this nasal glial heterotopia. These develop in relation to premature fusion of fonticulus frontalis (between frontal and nasal bones).*

Frontoethmoidal Cephalocele

KEY FACTS

TERMINOLOGY

- Congenital herniation of meninges, CSF ± brain tissue through mesodermal defect in anterior skull/skull base
- Synonym: **Sincipital** cephalocele
  - Do not confuse term for basal cephalocele, which occur through cribriform plate or sphenoid defects

IMAGING

- Heterogeneous, mixed density mass (variable amounts of CSF & parenchyma) extending through bony defect
  - Midline frontal: **Frontonasal** type (FNCeph)
  - Intranasal: **Nasoethmoidal** type (NECeph)
  - Inferomedial orbital: **Nasoorbital** type (NOCeph)

TOP DIFFERENTIAL DIAGNOSES

- Nasal glioma
- Orbital dermoid & epidermoid
- Nasal dermal sinus
- Nasolacrimal duct mucocele

PATHOLOGY

- **Frontonasal**
  - Protrudes through unobliterated **fonticulus frontalis**
- **Nasoethmoidal**
  - Protrudes through **foramen cecum** into **prenasal space**
- **Nasoorbital**
  - Protrudes into inferomedial orbit through defect in **lacrimal bone/frontal process of maxilla**

CLINICAL ISSUES

- Intracranial abnormalities in **~ 80%**
- F = 67%, M = 33%
- Most common in Southeast Asians

DIAGNOSTIC CHECKLIST

- Sagittal & coronal T1 MR & T2 MR optimal for showing contiguity of mass with intracranial contents
- Bone CT used to evaluate size & location of bony defect prior to surgical repair

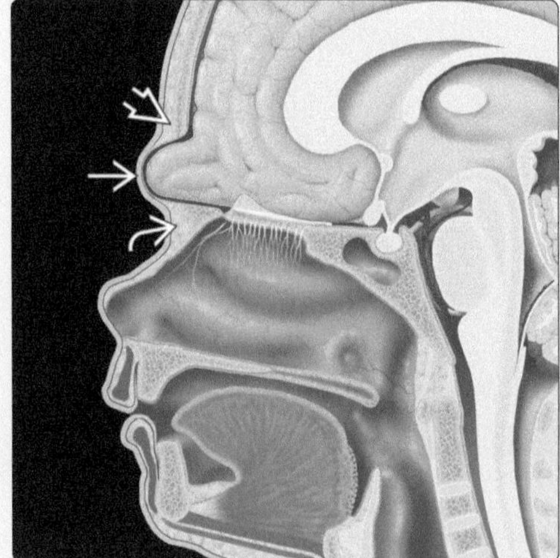

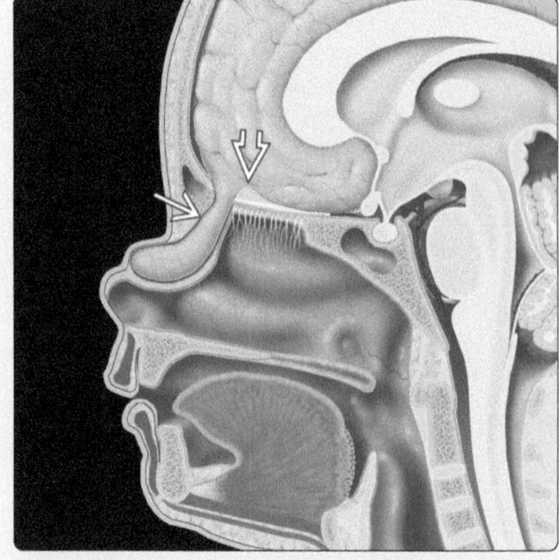

(Left) *Sagittal graphic of a frontonasal cephalocele shows herniation of the brain through a patent fonticulus frontalis ➡ between the frontal bone above ➡ and nasal bones below ➡.* **(Right)** *A nasoethmoidal cephalocele is depicted in this sagittal graphic. Notice the herniation of brain tissue ➡ into the nasal cavity through a patent foramen cecum. Also note that the crista galli is positioned posterior to the skull base defect ➡.*

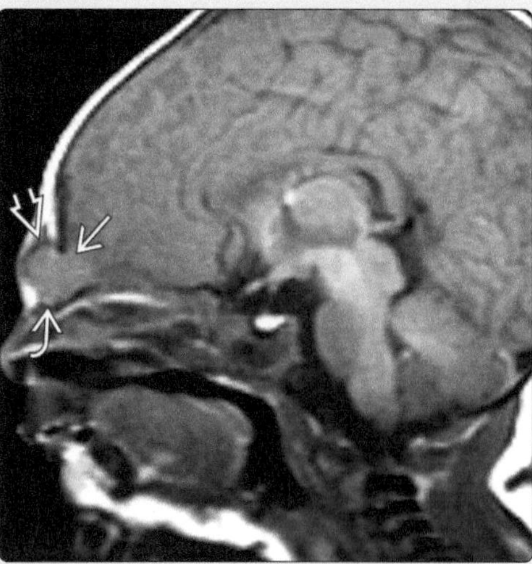

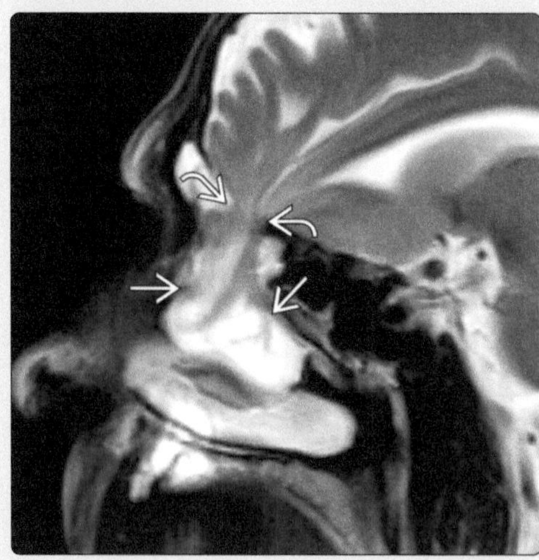

(Left) *Sagittal T1 MR in a 1-week-old shows a frontonasal cephalocele ➡ with protrusion of the dysplastic-appearing inferior left frontal lobe through a patent fonticulus frontalis. The frontal bone ➡ is above and the nasal bone ➡ is below the cephalocele.* **(Right)** *Sagittal T2 FS MR shows a nasoethmoidal cephalocele with herniation of brain parenchyma and meninges ➡ through a defect in the foramen cecum region of the anterior skull base ➡.*

TERMINOLOGY

Abbreviations

- Frontoethmoidal cephalocele (FECeph)
  - Fronto**nasal** cephalocele (FNCeph)
  - **Naso**ethmoidal cephalocele (NECeph)
  - **Naso**orbital cephalocele (NOCeph)

Synonyms

- **Sincipital** cephalocele

Definitions

- Cephalocele: Outward herniation of CNS contents through defect in cranium
  - Term includes meningocele & meningoencephalocele
- Congenital herniation of meninges & CSF (meningocele) + brain tissue (meningoencephalocele)
- Through mesodermal defect in anterior skull/skull base presenting as extranasal, intranasal, or medial orbital mass
- **Do not confuse for basal cephalocele**, which occur through cribriform plate or sphenoid defects
  - Basal cephaloceles: Transsphenoidal, sphenoethmoidal, transethmoidal, sphenoorbital

IMAGING

General Features

- Best diagnostic clue
  - Midline frontal (FNCeph), intranasal (NECeph), or medial orbital (NOCeph) soft tissue mass
  - Contiguous with intracranial brain parenchyma extending through bony defect
- Location
  - FNCeph: Anterior forehead at glabella-dorsum of nose
  - NECeph: Superomedial nasal cavity
    - Intracranially, 90% terminate at single midline defect at foramen cecum
    - 10% terminate at paired openings at anterior cribriform plates separated by midline bony bridge
  - NOCeph: Inferomedial orbit
- Size
  - Variable; 1-2 cm to larger than infant head
- Morphology
  - Well circumscribed, round, globular

CT Findings

- NECT
  - Heterogeneous, mixed-density mass (variable amounts CSF & parenchyma) extending through bony defect
- Bone CT
  - FNCeph: Frontal bone displaced superiorly while nasal bones, frontal processes of maxillae pushed inferiorly
  - NECeph: Nasal bone bowed anteriorly with tract through anterior ethmoid area
    - Crista galli may be bifid or absent
    - Deficient or absent cribriform plate
- CT myelogram
  - Intrathecal contrast: Fills subarachnoid space & surrounds soft tissue extending through bony defect

MR Findings

- T1WI
  - Soft tissue mass isointense to gray matter contiguous with intracranial parenchyma through bony defect
- T2WI
  - Hyperintense CSF surrounds herniated soft tissue parenchyma
  - Tissue may show ↑ signal due to gliosis
- T1WI C+
  - No abnormal enhancement noted within soft tissue
  - Meninges may enhance if infected/inflamed

Ultrasonographic Findings

- OB US: Frontal (FNCeph), intranasal (NECeph), or medial periorbital (NOCeph) soft tissue mass
  - Widened interorbital distance

Imaging Recommendations

- Best imaging tool
  - MR superior to CT for cephalocele evaluation
    - Differentiates CSF-filled meningocele & parenchymal components
    - Superior for showing other associated brain anomalies
- Protocol advice
  - Thin (3-mm) multiplanar T1 MR & T2 MR
    - Sagittal & coronal planes optimal for visualizing parenchymal herniation through defects
  - Heavily T2WI 3D sequences (like CISS, FIESTA, or SPACE)
    - Demonstrates intra- & extracranial continuity of CSF & brain better
  - Bone CT can provide important information about skull defects for surgical planning
    - CT or MR with intrathecal contrast used only when full MR & bone CT still leave unanswered questions

DIFFERENTIAL DIAGNOSIS

Nasal Glioma (Nasal Cerebral Heterotopia, Glial Heterotopia)

- Clinical: Soft tissue mass along dorsum of nose (extranasal type) or under nasal bones (intranasal type)
- Imaging: MR shows no connection between mass in intracranial contents

Orbital Dermoid & Epidermoid

- Clinical: Focal mass in medial orbit without associated tract
- Imaging: Fat density/intensity if dermoid; fluid density/intensity if epidermoid

Nasal Dermal Sinus

- Clinical: Pit on tip or bridge of nose
- Imaging: Midline sinus from tip of nose to skull base
  - Dermoid or epidermoid may be seen anywhere along tract
  - Possible intracranial connection via sinus tract; does not contain brain parenchyma

Nasolacrimal Duct Mucocele

- Clinical: Small, round, bluish, medial canthal mass seen at birth with submucosal nasal cavity mass at inferior meatus
- Imaging: Nasolacrimal duct dilatation may be present to inferior meatus
  - No connection to skull base or brain parenchyma

PATHOLOGY

General Features

- Etiology
  - Prior to 8th week of gestation, 2 potential spaces
  - **Fonticulus frontalis**: Fontanelle between developing frontal bone superiorly & nasal bones inferiorly
  - Fonticulus frontalis closes when chondrocranium begins to ossify; failure of closure → **FNCeph**
  - **Prenasal space**: Dura-filled space between developing nasal bones anteriorly & nasal capsule posteriorly
  - Chondrocranium of anterior skull base ossifies from posterior to anterior
    - Except small cartilage in front for nasal capsule
  - Nasal bones also ossify further
  - Prenasal space lying in between these becomes encased in bone & obliterates
    - Leaves small dural diverticulum, called **foramen cecum**, just anterior to future crista galli
  - Foramen cecum transiently communicates with nasal skin anteroinferiorly
    - Through dura-lined stalk called **anterior neuropore**
  - Anterior neuropore regression failure → **NECeph** via foramen cecum into prenasal space & nasal cavity
  - Defect in **lacrimal bone/frontal process of maxilla → NOCeph** protruding into inferomedial orbit
- Genetics
  - Sporadic occurrence
  - Not linked to neural tube defects, such as occipital cephaloceles
  - Siblings have 6% incidence of congenital CNS abnormalities
- Associated abnormalities
  - **Intracranial abnormalities (~ 80%)**
    - Callosal hypogenesis & interhemispheric lipomas
    - Neuronal migration anomalies
    - Microcephaly
    - Aqueductal stenosis & hydrocephalus
    - Colloid or arachnoid cysts
  - Midline craniofacial dysraphisms & hypertelorism
  - Microphthalmos
  - Morning glory disc anomaly with basal encephaloceles (cribriform plate or sphenoid defects); not FECeph

Gross Pathologic & Surgical Features

- Meningeal-lined mass containing CSF ± brain tissue

Microscopic Features

- **Meningoencephalocele**: CSF, brain tissue, & meninges
- **Meningocele**: Meninges & CSF only
- **Atretic cephalocele**: Forme fruste of cephalocele with dura, fibrous tissue, & degenerated brain tissue
- **Gliocele**: Glial-lined CSF-filled cyst

CLINICAL ISSUES

Presentation

- Most common signs/symptoms
  - Externally visible, firm midline forehead (FNCeph), intranasal (NECeph), or medial orbital (NOCeph) mass
- Other signs/symptoms
  - Hypertelorism & orbital dystopia
  - Hyperpigmentation of overlying skin
  - Change in size with crying, Valsalva, jugular compression
  - Seizures & intellectual disability < 50%
  - Occasionally cause recurrent meningitis

Demographics

- Age
  - Congenital lesion detected on prenatal US or presenting at birth
- Sex
  - F = 67%, M = 33%
- Ethnicity
  - FECeph most common in Southeast Asians
- Epidemiology
  - Less common in Western countries
  - 1 in 4,000-5,000 live births in Southeast Asia
  - FECeph account for 15% of all cephaloceles
  - FNCeph (50-61%), NECeph (30-33%), NOCeph (6-10%)

Natural History & Prognosis

- Present at birth; require surgical repair
- If untreated, may grow with child
- If thin skin covering or no skin, prone to rupture, CSF leak, & infection
- When CSF filled, may ↑ rapidly in size
- Hydrocephalus & presence of intracranial abnormalities predictors of developmental delay/poor outcome

Treatment

- Biopsy contraindicated: CSF leak, seizures, meningitis
- Complete surgical resection
  - Combined plastic surgery & neurosurgery
  - Herniated brain tissue dysfunctional (usually no neurologic deficits result)
- Meningeal & skull base defect repaired; otherwise CSF leak, meningitis, or recurrent herniation may result

DIAGNOSTIC CHECKLIST

Consider

- Sagittal & coronal T1 MR & T2 MR optimal for showing contiguity of mass with intracranial contents
- Bone CT used to evaluate size & location of bony defect prior to surgical repair

Image Interpretation Pearls

- Determine location of lesion relative to nasal bones
  - Above: FNCeph
  - Below: NECeph
- Evaluate brain for associated anomalies

SELECTED REFERENCES

1. Deniz M et al: Frontoethmoidal encephalocele as a cause of recurrent meningitis. Rev Soc Bras Med Trop. 56:e02362023, 2023
2. Oley MC et al: Evaluation of long-term results following surgical correction of frontoethmoidal encephalomeningocele. Int J Surg Case Rep. 107:108278, 2023
3. Keshri AK et al: Transnasal endoscopic repair of pediatric meningoencephalocele. J Pediatr Neurosci. 11(1):42-5, 2016
4. Vattoth S et al: Anterior skull base. In Watanabe K, et al: Anatomy for Plastic Surgery of the Face, Head, and Neck. 1st ed. Thieme Medical Publishers. 13-9, 2016

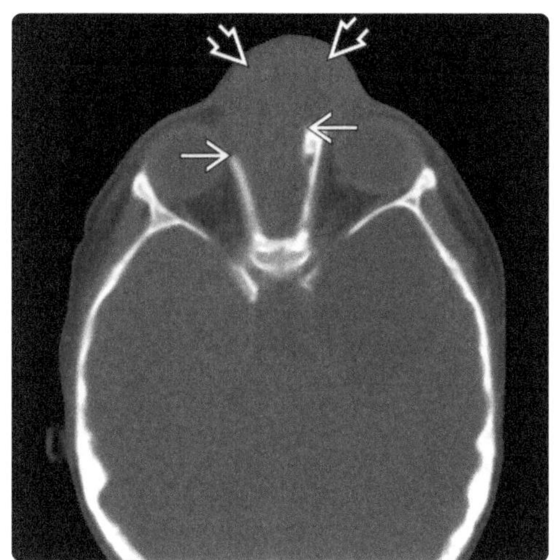

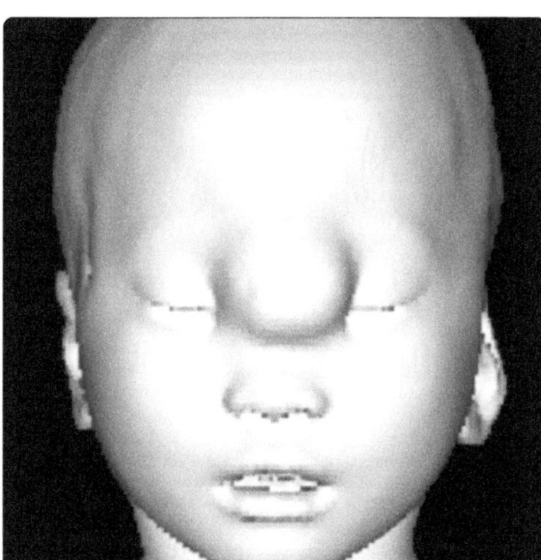

(Left) *Axial bone CT in a newborn with a soft tissue mass in the midline of the forehead shows a large anterior skull defect* ➔ *through which a large "frontonasal" cephalocele protrudes* ➔. **(Right)** *Frontal projection 3D surface-rendered CT in the same patient shows the clinical appearance of the large cephalocele between the eyes. This frontonasal cephalocele protrudes through a patent fonticulus frontalis.*

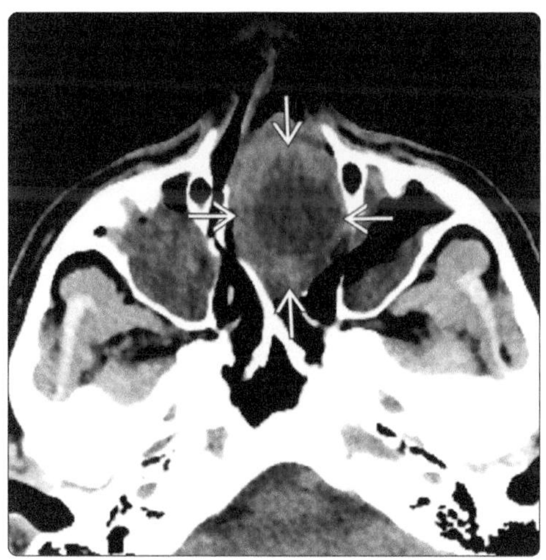

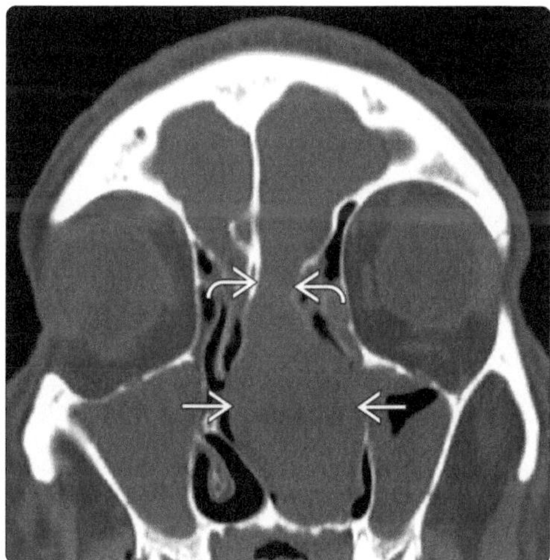

(Left) *Axial NECT in a child shows a heterogeneous left nasal cavity soft tissue mass* ➔ *deviating the nasal septum toward the right side.* **(Right)** *Coronal bone CT in the same patient shows anterior skull base defect/widened foramen cecum* ➔ *continuous with the nasal cavity soft tissue mass* ➔.

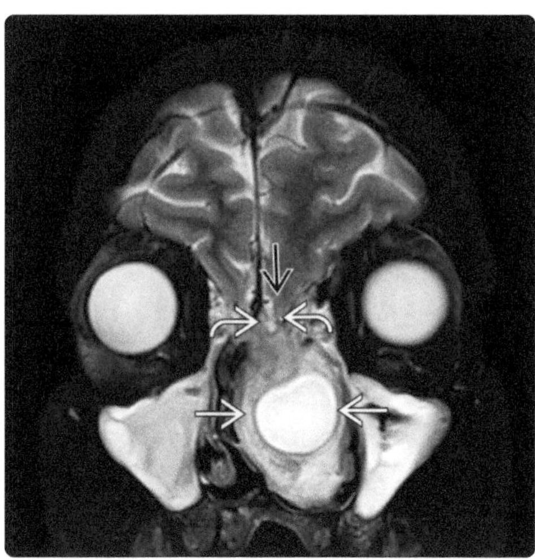

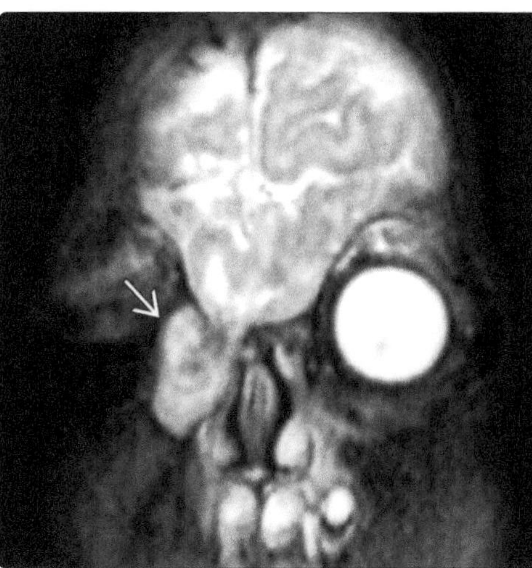

(Left) *Coronal T2 FS MR in the same patient shows that the heterogeneous nasal cavity soft tissue* ➔ *is continuous intracranially across the skull base defect/widened foramen cecum* ➔ *with the left frontal lobe* ➔. *Findings are consistent with a nasoethmoidal cephalocele.* **(Right)** *Coronal T2 MR shows the rarest type of frontoethmoidal cephalocele, the "nasoorbital" cephalocele* ➔ *herniating through a defect between the nasal and lacrimal bones on right.*

Nasal Dermal Sinus

KEY FACTS

TERMINOLOGY

- Defective embryogenesis of anterior neuropore
- Resulting in any mixture of dermoid cyst, epidermoid cyst, &/or sinus tract in frontonasal region

IMAGING

- Midline location anywhere from nasal tip to anterior skull base at foramen cecum
- MR
    - T2: Fluid signal tract in septum from nasal dorsum to skull base (sinus)
    - T1: Focal low-signal (epidermoid) or high-signal (dermoid) mass between tip of nose & apex of crista galli
- CT
    - Bifid crista galli with large foramen cecum
    - Fluid-attenuation tract (sinus)/cyst (epidermoid) or fat-containing mass (dermoid)
        - From nasal dorsum to skull base **within nasal septum**

TOP DIFFERENTIAL DIAGNOSES

- Fatty marrow in crista galli
- Nonossified foramen cecum
- Frontoethmoidal cephalocele
- Nasal glioma (nasal cerebral heterotopia)

PATHOLOGY

- Intracranial extension of nasal dermal sinus (NDS) in 20%
    - May rarely lead to meningitis
- Associated craniofacial anomalies in 15%

CLINICAL ISSUES

- Nasoglabellar mass (30%)
- Pit (± protruding hair) on skin of nasal bridge at osteocartilaginous nasal junction

DIAGNOSTIC CHECKLIST

- Nasoglabellar mass or pit on nose sends clinician in search of NDS with intracranial extension

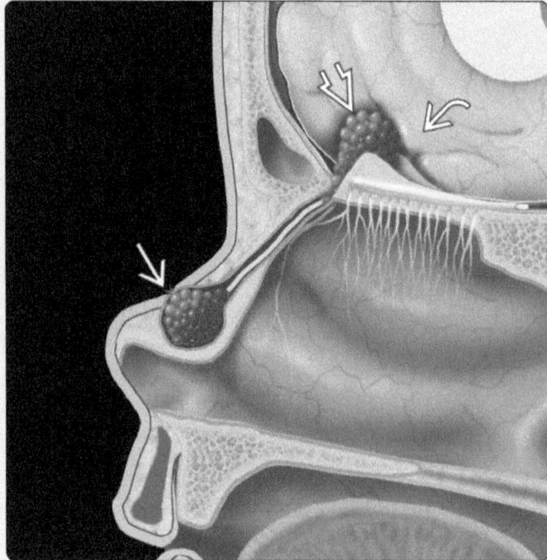

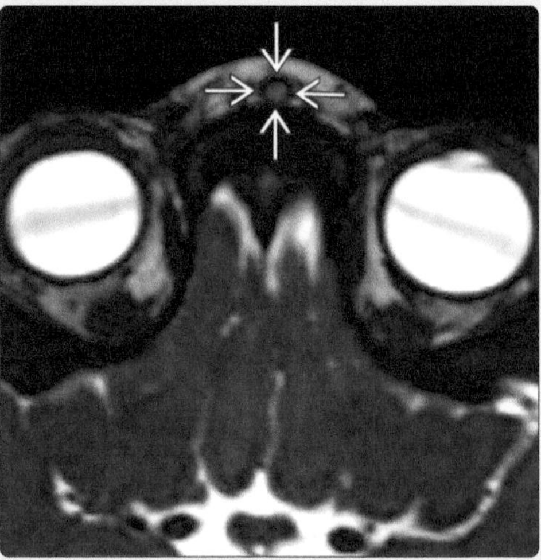

(Left) *Lateral graphic depicts a nasal dermal sinus with 2 dermoids. An extracranial dermoid is present just deep to a cutaneous nasal pit ➔. An intracranial dermoid ➔ splits a bifid crista galli ➔.* **(Right)** *Axial high-resolution 3D T2WI MR shows a nasal dermal sinus ➔ at the root of the nose, just below the glabella. This was an isolated nasal dermal sinus tract without associated dermoid/epidermoid.*

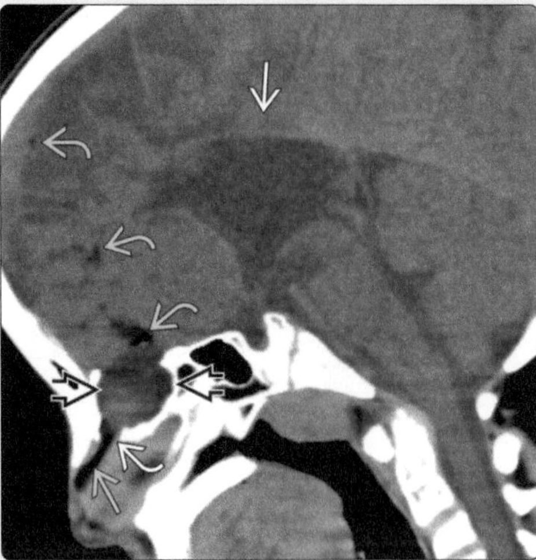

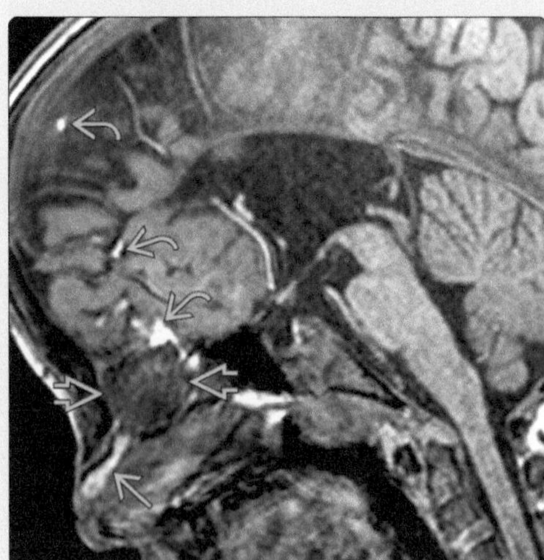

(Left) *Sagittal NECT in an 8-year-old with known midline anomalies shows a fat-lined nasal dermal sinus ➔ deep to the nasal bones. The sinus leads to a large fat & fluid attenuation dermoid ➔. There is a wide foramen cecum ➔ with fatty foci ➔ extending along the falx. Agenesis of the corpus callosum ➔ is also noted.* **(Right)** *Sagittal T1WI MR in the same patient shows fat-lined nasal dermal sinus ➔, mixed signal intensity dermoid ➔, & falcine foci of fat ➔ (consistent with intracranial extension & rupture).*

TERMINOLOGY

Abbreviations

- Nasal dermal sinus (NDS)

Synonyms

- Nasal dermoid, nasal dermal cyst, anterior neuropore anomaly

Definitions

- Defective embryogenesis of anterior neuropore
- Resulting in any mixture of dermoid cyst, epidermoid cyst, &/or sinus tract in frontonasal region

IMAGING

General Features

- Best diagnostic clue
  - CT
    - Bifid crista galli with large foramen cecum
    - Fluid-attenuation tract (sinus)/cyst (epidermoid) or fat-containing mass (dermoid)
      - From nasal dorsum to skull base **within nasal septum**
  - MR
    - Fluid signal tract in septum from nasal dorsum to skull base (sinus)
    - Focal T1 low signal (epidermoid) or high signal (dermoid) between tip of nose & apex of crista galli
- Location
  - Midline lesion anywhere from nasal tip to anterior skull base at foramen cecum
- Size
  - 5 mm to 2 cm for dermoid/epidermoid
- Morphology
  - Ovoid mass ± tubular sinus tract

CT Findings

- Bone CT
  - Focal tract (sinus) or mass (dermoid or epidermoid) anywhere from nasal bridge to crista galli
    - Fluid density tract = sinus
    - Fluid density mass = epidermoid
    - Fat-density mass = dermoid
  - Signs of intracranial extension
    - Large foramen cecum with bifid or deformed crista galli or, sometimes, cribriform plate
    - Caution: Anterior skull base ossification widely variable in 1st few years of life
    - Wide foramen cecum alone not strong indicator of intracranial extension; correlate with MR

MR Findings

- T1WI
  - ↓ signal tract = sinus
  - ↑ signal mass = dermoid (fat becomes ↓ on fat-suppressed images)
  - ↓ signal mass = epidermoid
- T2WI
  - ↑ signal in sinus, epidermoid, or dermoid
  - Coronal plane shows septal lesions to best advantage
- DWI
  - ↑ signal = epidermoid usually; dermoid rarely
  - Susceptibility artifacts at skull base may obscure signal from epidermoid

Imaging Recommendations

- Best imaging tool
  - MR more sensitive for delineating sinus tract, detecting intracranial extension
    - MR characterizes epidermoid/dermoid lesions better
  - Bone CT optimal for identifying skull base defect & crista galli deformity
- Protocol advice
  - Imaging "sweet spot" small & anterior
    - Focus imaging from tip of nose to back of crista galli
    - Inferior end of axial imaging: Hard palate
    - Contrast helps with infectious complications or consideration of other differential diagnoses
      - Not for primary dermoid/epidermoid diagnosis
  - CT
    - Thin-section (1-2 mm) bone & soft tissue axial & coronal images
  - MR
    - Sagittal plane displays course of sinus tract from nasal dorsum to skull base
    - Fat-suppressed T1 images confirm presence of fat in dermoids
    - DWI important additional sequence
    - Heavily T2 3D sequences like CISS, FIESTA, or SPACE
      - Demonstrates sinus tract, intracranial continuity, & associated tiny epidermoid/dermoid better

DIFFERENTIAL DIAGNOSIS

Fatty Marrow in Crista Galli

- No nasoglabellar mass or pit on nose
- CT & MR otherwise normal

Nonossified Foramen Cecum

- Small midline pit lying between frontal & ethmoid bones, just anterior to crista galli of ethmoid
- ~ 4-mm diameter at birth
- Foramen cecum ossification usually completes by 2 years
  - Sometimes delayed until 5 years
- Crista galli not deformed or bifid

Frontoethmoidal Cephalocele

- Bone dehiscence typically larger, involving broader area of midline cribriform plate or frontal bone
- Direct extension of meninges, subarachnoid space ± brain can be seen projecting into cephalocele on sagittal MR

Nasal Glioma

- Solid mass of dysplastic glial tissue separated from brain by subarachnoid space & meninges
- Preferred terms: Nasal cerebral heterotopia, glial heterotopia
- Most commonly projects extranasally onto paramedian bridge of nose
- Less commonly intranasal & along anterior nasal septum, off-midline

Nasoseptal Tuberculosis Mimicking Dermoid

- Extremely rare

PATHOLOGY

General Features

- Etiology
  - **Anterior neuropore anomaly**: General term for anomalous anterior neuropore regression; 3 main types
    - **NDS**
    - **Nasal glioma** (nasal cerebral heterotopia)
    - **Frontoethmoidal (sincipital) cephalocele**
  - Embryology-anatomy: Development of anterior neuropore in 4th gestational week
    - Dural stalk passes from area of future foramen cecum to area of osteocartilaginous nasal junction
      - □ Later regresses completely
    - Failure of involution may leave neuroectodermal remnants along tract of dural stalk
    - Results in **dermoid** or **epidermoid** alone or in association with NDS tract
    - Intracranial **neurenteric cyst** instead of typical epidermoid/dermoid with NDS recently reported
- Genetics
  - Familial clustering
- Associated abnormalities
  - Intracranial extension of NDS seen in 20%
  - Craniofacial anomalies (15%)

Gross Pathologic & Surgical Features

- Sinus = tube of tissue can be followed through bones
- Epidermoid = well-defined cyst; dermoid = lobular, well-defined mass

Microscopic Features

- Sinus = midline epithelial-lined tract
- Epidermoid cyst contains desquamated epithelium
- Dermoid cyst contains epithelium, keratin debris, skin adnexa

CLINICAL ISSUES

Presentation

- Most common signs/symptoms
  - Nasoglabellar mass (30%)
  - Pit on skin of nasal bridge at osteocartilaginous nasal junction
    - ± protruding hair
- Other signs/symptoms
  - Intermittent sebaceous material discharge from pit
  - < 50% have broadening nasal root & bridge
  - If nasal sinus tract present, recurrent meningitis may occur (rare)
  - Infected dermoid or epidermoid usual cause of neonatal nasal septal abscess
    - Nasal obstruction most common presenting symptom
- Clinical profile
  - Child (mean age: 32 months) with nasal pit ± nasoglabellar mass
  - Rarely presents in adult population
    - Episode of meningitis may be 1st problem leading to diagnosis

Demographics

- Age
  - Newborn to 5 years old
- Sex
  - Male patients with dermal sinus more likely to have intracranial extension
- Epidemiology
  - Congenital midline nasal lesions rare (1 in 20,000-40,000 births)
    - Nasal dermoids most common

Natural History & Prognosis

- Isolated problem when surgical correction successful
- Untreated patients have nasal bridge broadening ± recurrent meningitis

Treatment

- 80% require extracranial excision only
  - Local procedure to remove pit
  - Any associated dermoid or epidermoid also simultaneously removed from nasal bridge
    - Open rhinoplasty vs. transnasal endoscopic excision
- 20% undergo combined extracranial & intracranial resection
  - Biorbitofrontal nasal craniotomy approach
    - Dermoid or epidermoid along with involved dura & crista galli removed
    - Primary closure of surgical margins of dura

DIAGNOSTIC CHECKLIST

Consider

- Nasoglabellar mass or pit on nose sends clinician in search of NDS with intracranial extension
- Focused thin-section MR key to radiologic diagnosis
  - Axial coverage from cephalad margin of crista galli to hard palate
  - Coronal coverage from tip of nose to crista galli
- Add bone CT if NDS with intracranial extension found on MR

Image Interpretation Pearls

- If dermal sinus tract reaches dura of anterior cranial fossa → crista galli will be bifid with large foramen cecum
- If foramen cecum large but crista galli not bifid & tract not seen → foramen cecum normal & not yet closed
  - Foramen cecum may not close before age of 5 years
  - Do not overcall "large foramen cecum" or unnecessary craniotomy may result
  - Repeat imaging in 6-12 months to confirm foramen cecum closure acceptable approach in difficult cases

Reporting Tips

- Consider NDS if **mass or tract** seen in relation to **nasal septum/nasoglabellar region**

SELECTED REFERENCES

1. Shimizu R et al: The necessity of dural resection for nasal dermal sinus cyst with intracranial extension. J Craniofac Surg. 34(6):e589-90, 2023
2. Yang X et al: [Clinical analysis of 59 cases of pediatric nasal dermal sinus cysts with midfacial infection as the first symptom.] Lin Chuang Er Bi Yan Hou Tou Jing Wai Ke Za Zhi. 36(11):849-54, 2022
3. Sagar P et al: Naso-septal tuberculosis mimicking dermoid in a 3-year old child. Iran J Otorhinolaryngol. 30(99):231-5, 2018

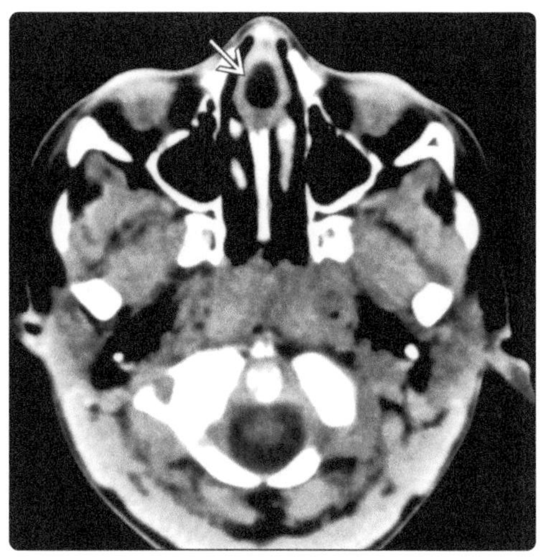

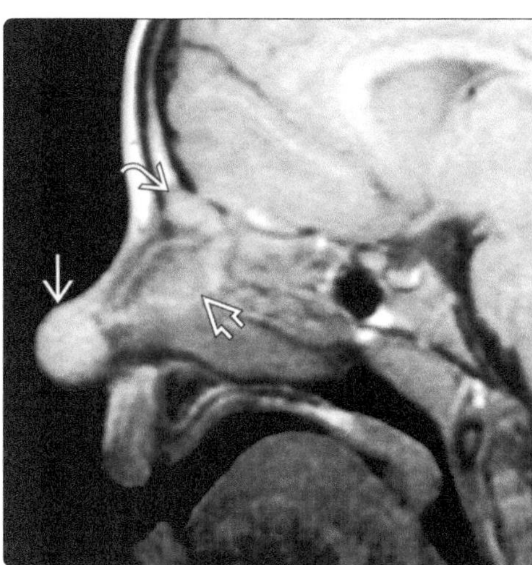

(Left) *Axial NECT demonstrates a characteristic low-attenuation dermoid centered in the cartilaginous portion of the nasal septum. The mass is slightly higher in attenuation than adjacent fat.* **(Right)** *Sagittal T1WI MR in another patient shows a hyperintense dermoid at the nasal tip. Additional dermoids are noted in the nasal septum & at the skull base.*

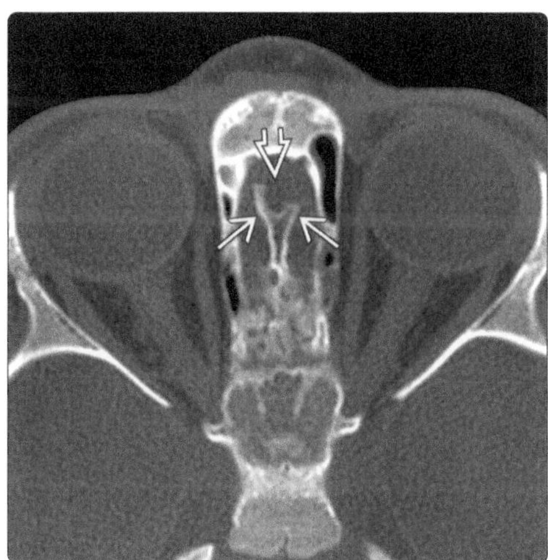

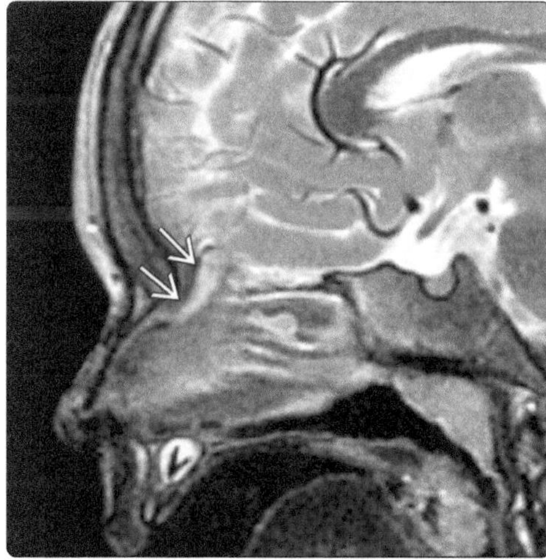

(Left) *Axial bone CT demonstrates a bifid crista galli surrounding an intracranial dermoid along a persistently large foramen cecum.* **(Right)** *Sagittal T2WI MR in a 3-year-old boy with a bump on the tip of his nose shows a hyperintense sinus tract extending from the anterior skull base into the nasal septum. These features are characteristic of a dermal sinus.*

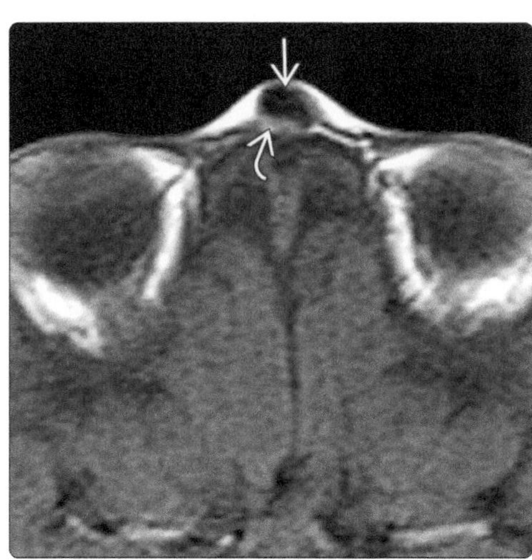

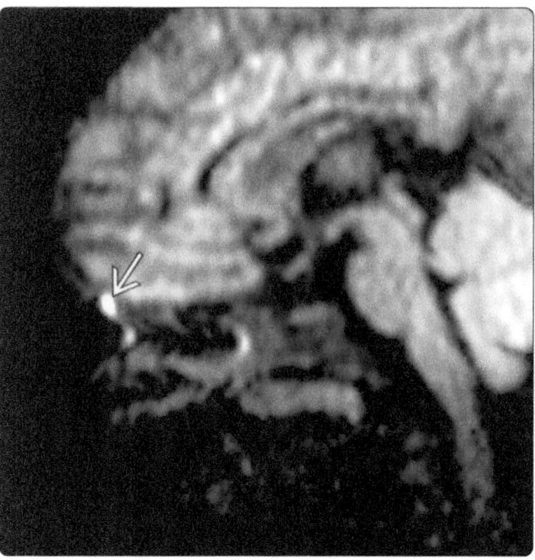

(Left) *Axial T1WI MR in a young child shows a hypointense cystic lesion with a small focal area of T1-hyperintense fat posteriorly, located anterior to the root of the nose, consistent with a dermoid cyst.* **(Right)** *Sagittal DWI MR reveals an epidermoid in the region of the foramen cecum as a high-signal focus of restricted diffusion. A 2nd (extracranial) lesion is not visible due to air-bone susceptibility artifact.*

KEY FACTS

TERMINOLOGY

- Congenital obstruction of posterior nasal aperture(s)

IMAGING

- Unilateral or bilateral osseous narrowing of posterior nasal cavity with complete obstruction by associated membrane or bony plate
  - Thickening of vomer
  - Medial bowing of posterior maxilla(e)
  - ± air-fluid level in obstructed nasal cavity
- Unilateral in up to 75% (right > left)
- Bilateral in up to 25%
  - 75% of bilateral cases have other anomalies

TOP DIFFERENTIAL DIAGNOSES

- Choanal stenosis
- Pyriform aperture stenosis
- Nasolacrimal duct mucocele

PATHOLOGY

- Most common congenital abnormality of nasal cavity
- Choanal atresia types
  - Mixed bony & membranous atresia in up to 70%
  - Purely bony atresia in up to 30%

CLINICAL ISSUES

- **Inability to pass nasogastric tube** through nasal cavity beyond 3-4 cm despite **aerated lungs** on radiograph
  - Bilateral choanal atresia: Newborn respiratory distress
    - Due to their physiologic obligate nasal breather status
  - Unilateral choanal atresia: Chronic, purulent, unilateral rhinorrhea & mild airway obstruction in older child
  - Diagnosed in newborns, rarely in adolescence/adulthood
  - May very rarely develop rhinolith in missed cases

DIAGNOSTIC CHECKLIST

- Respiratory distress & suspected nasal obstruction in newborn should be evaluated with thin-section bone CT

(Left) *Axial bone CT shows right bony choanal atresia ➡ with thickened posteroinferior bony nasal septum (vomer) ➡. Note posteromedial angulation of the medial wall of right maxillary sinus (lateral nasal wall) ➡. Left posterior choana ➡ is patent, & the left medial maxillary sinus (lateral nasal) wall ➡ is relatively straight.* **(Right)** *Axial bone CT in a respiratory distress infant shows bilateral membranous choanal atresia ➡. Posterior maxillae are medialized ➡ without bony fusion to a normal vomer ➡. Note air-fluid level in nasal cavities ➡.*

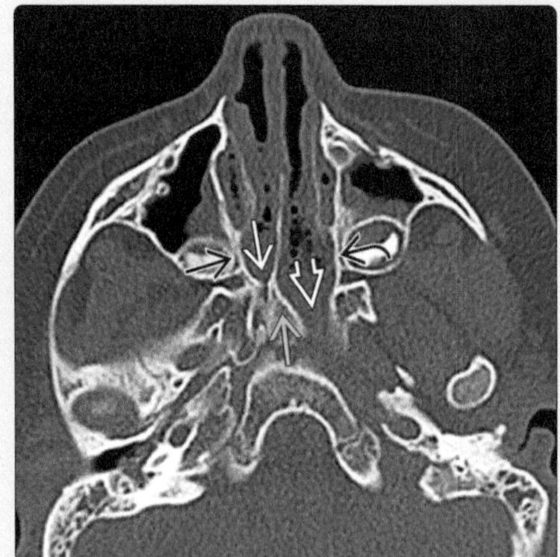

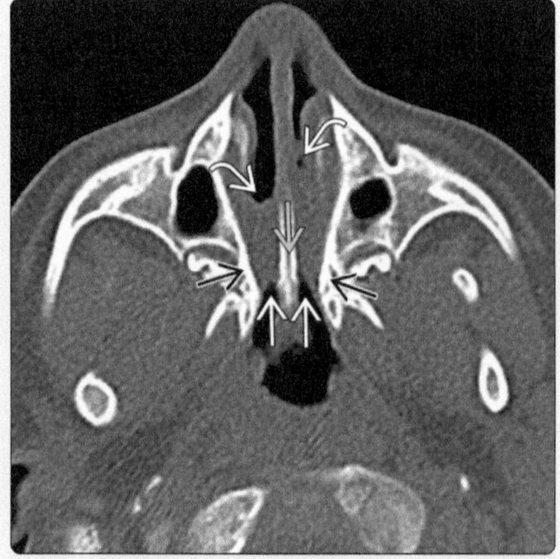

(Left) *Axial bone CT in another patient shows a membranous atresia ➡ at the narrowed inferior aspect of the choana. Note also the retained right nasal cavity secretions with air-fluid level ➡ secondary to choanal obstruction. Left posterior choana is patent ➡ with clear nasal cavity.* **(Right)** *Axial bone CT in another patient shows mixed left choanal atresia with severe bony stenosis ➡ of the left posterior choana, along with membranous component of obstruction ➡. Note air-fluid level in the left nasal cavity more anteriorly ➡.*

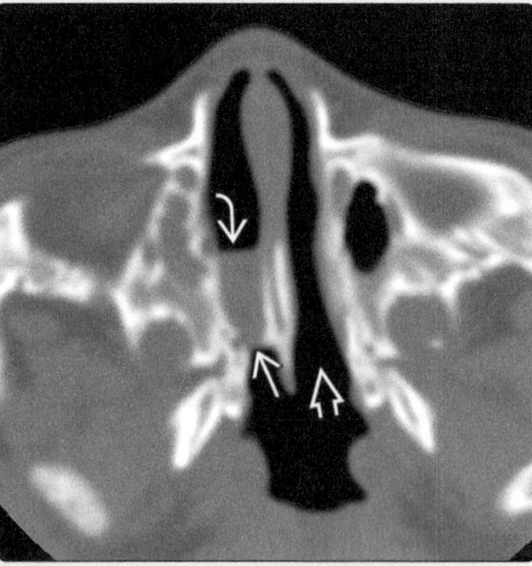

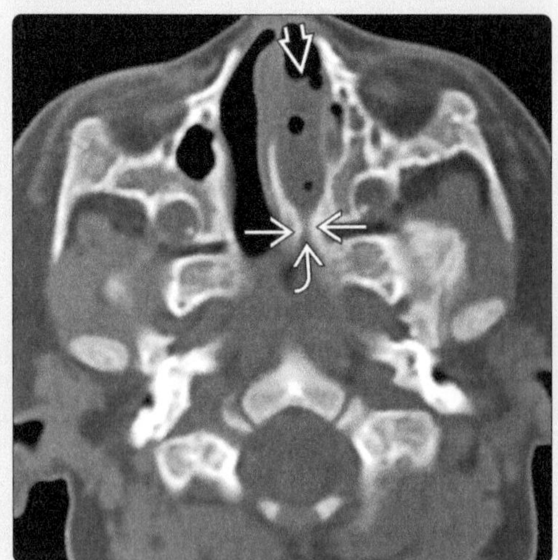

TERMINOLOGY

Definitions

- Congenital obstruction of posterior nasal apertures
  - Choana: Junction of posterior nasal cavity & nasopharynx
  - Choanal atresia: Lack of communication between nasal cavity & nasopharynx

IMAGING

General Features

- Best diagnostic clue
  - Bony narrowing of posterior nasal cavity with membranous &/or osseous obstruction of choana
- Location
  - Unilateral in ~ 75% (right > left), bilateral in ~ 25%
- Size
  - Newborn **choanal opening** abnormal if **< 0.34 cm** wide
  - Newborn **vomer** (posteroinferior part of bony nasal septum) abnormal if **> 0.23 cm** thick
- Morphology
  - Medial bowing of posterior maxilla (lateral nasal wall) & pterygoid plate
  - Large/thickened vomer
  - Bony narrowing ± soft tissue membrane/plug or bony plate obstructing choana
    - Mixed bony & membranous atresia in up to 70%
    - Purely bony atresia in up to 30%

CT Findings

- Bone CT
  - Choanal narrowing by medially bowed posterior maxilla/pterygoid & thickened vomer
  - Narrow gap between maxilla & vomer bridged by continuous bony plate or membrane
    - Membranous atresia may be thin/strand-like or thick/plug-like
  - Air-fluid level frequent in obstructed nasal passage
    - Nasal cavity may also be filled with soft tissue, hypertrophied inferior turbinates

Imaging Recommendations

- Best imaging tool
  - High-resolution unenhanced bone CT
- Protocol advice
  - Suction secretions from nasal cavity prior to scanning
  - Axial images angled 5° cephalad to palate
    - If angulated too much, region of choanae at level of skull base creates false appearance of choanal atresia
  - Edge enhancement bone kernel helps delineate bone margins in partially ossified skull base
  - Multiplanar reformations as needed
    - Sagittal usually best plane for this entity
  - 3D reconstructions may be helpful for clinical decision making & surgical planning

DIFFERENTIAL DIAGNOSIS

Choanal Stenosis

- Posterior nasal airway narrowed (not completely occluded)

Pyriform Aperture Stenosis

- Pyriform aperture (PA) of nose: Pear-shaped anterior aperture at mucocutaneous junction (limen nasi) level
- PA: Anterior bony margin of nasal skeleton
- Superior margin: Nasal bone lower margin
- Inferolateral margin: Maxillary bone thin sharp margins separating anterior from nasal surfaces of maxilla
- Narrowed anterior inferior nasal passage(s)
- Thickened anteromedial maxilla(e)
- Abnormal fusion (synostosis) of midline palatal suture with lateral growth restriction of midface
- ± **solitary** central **megaincisor tooth**
- Must evaluate brain for **holoprosencephaly**

Nasolacrimal Duct Mucocele

- Bilobed cystic mass extending from medial orbital nasolacrimal fossa to inferior meatus

PATHOLOGY

General Features

- Associated abnormalities
  - Syndromes common in bilateral atresia (up to 75%)
  - CHARGE syndrome: **C**oloboma, **h**eart defect, choanal **a**tresia, **r**estricted growth, **g**enitourinary & **e**ar defects
  - Unilateral choanal atresia more likely to be isolated

CLINICAL ISSUES

Presentation

- Most common signs/symptoms
  - Bilateral choanal atresia: Respiratory distress in newborn
    - Infants breathe through nose (obligate nasal breathers) up to 6 months of age
    - Aggravated by feeding, relieved by crying
  - Unilateral choanal atresia or stenosis: Chronic, purulent, unilateral rhinorrhea in older child
  - **Inability to pass nasogastric (NG) tube** through nose beyond 3-4 cm despite **aerated lungs** on radiograph

Treatment

- Establish oral airway immediately for proper breathing
- Membranous atresia may perforate on passage of NG tube
- Surgical treatment as needed

DIAGNOSTIC CHECKLIST

Reporting Tips

- Describe choanal atresia as unilateral or bilateral
  - Mixed membranous/bony or purely bony
- Comment on thickness of atretic bone plate & vomer, medial bowing of posterior maxilla(e), & air-fluid level in obstructed nasal cavity
- Associated syndromes like CHARGE & rare rhinoliths

SELECTED REFERENCES

1. Abraham ZS et al: Unilateral choanal atresia and a co-existent long-standing medium-sized ipsilateral rhinolith in a 15-year old boy: Case report and literature review. Int J Surg Case Rep. 105:107999, 2023
2. Legesse TK et al: Bilateral choanal atresia in an adolescent female: a rare case report. Int Med Case Rep J. 16:103-7, 2023
3. Wine TM et al: Congenital nasal pyriform aperture stenosis: evidence of premature fusion of the midline palatal suture. AJNR Am J Neuroradiol. 42(6):1163-6, 2021

Congenital Nasal Pyriform Aperture Stenosis

KEY FACTS

TERMINOLOGY

- Congenital nasal pyriform aperture stenosis (CNPAS): Congenital narrowing of anterior bony nasal passageway

IMAGING

- Best tool: Bone CT in axial & coronal planes
  - Medial deviation of anterior maxillae ± thickening of nasal processes
  - Abnormal maxillary dentition: **Solitary median maxillary central incisor (SMMCI)** (in up to 75%)
  - Triangle-shaped palate

TOP DIFFERENTIAL DIAGNOSES

- Nasolacrimal duct mucoceles
  - Intranasal component narrows anterior nasal cavity
- Nasal choanal stenosis/atresia
  - Narrow posterior nasal passage by membrane or bone

PATHOLOGY

- CNPAS without SMMCI is almost always isolated anomaly
- Solitary maxillary central incisor in 75% of cases
  - Associated with **holoprosencephaly**

CLINICAL ISSUES

- Respiratory distress in newborn/infant
  - Can mimic choanal atresia/stenosis
  - Breathing problems may be triggered by upper respiratory infection
  - Symptoms may be more pronounced with feeding
- Narrow nasal inlet on clinical exam
- CNPAS 1/5 to 1/3 as common as choanal atresia

DIAGNOSTIC CHECKLIST

- Bone CT recommended for diagnosis or bony narrowing & dental abnormalities
- Brain MR recommended in cases of SMMCI to exclude midline brain anomalies

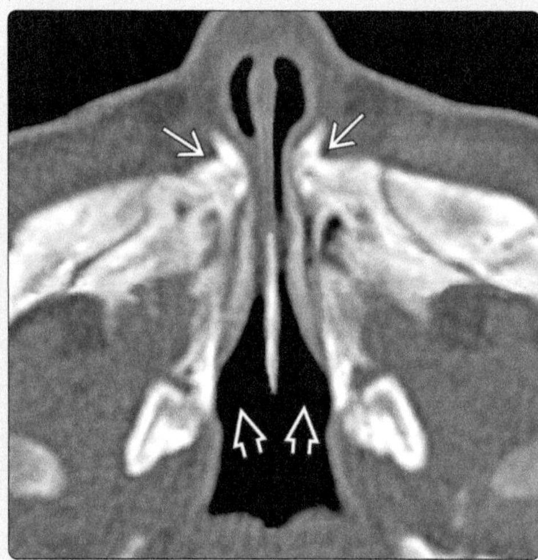

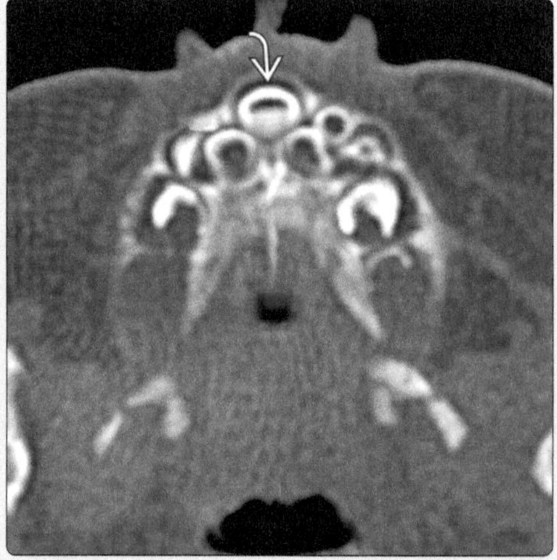

(Left) *Axial bone CT in a newborn shows the typical features of congenital nasal pyriform aperture stenosis. There is overgrowth of the anterior maxillae ➡ with marked narrowing of the anterior nasal passages. There is no associated choanal atresia ⇨.* **(Right)** *Axial bone CT at the level of the palate in the same patient shows a classic associated finding in patients with pyriform aperture stenosis: A solitary median maxillary central incisor, or megaincisor ➡.*

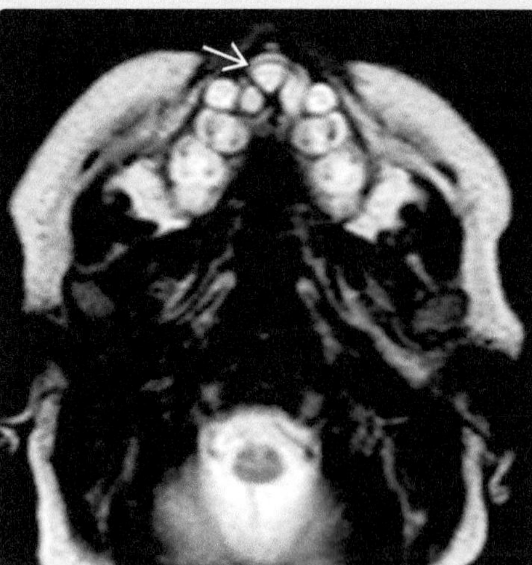

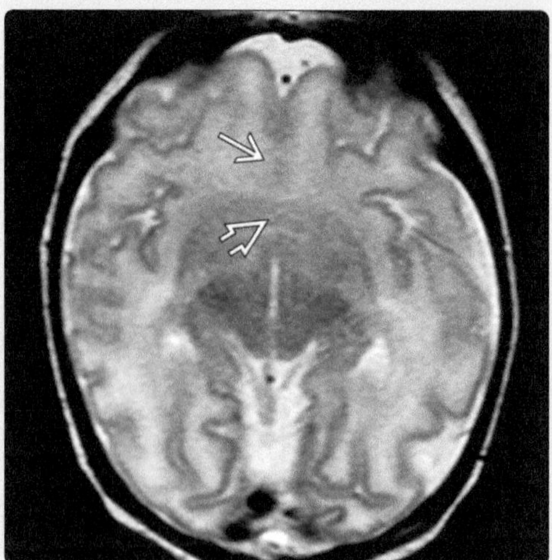

(Left) *Axial T2 MR in a 3-day-old infant with congenital nasal pyriform aperture stenosis demonstrates associated solitary median maxillary central incisor ➡.* **(Right)** *Axial T2 MR in the same infant with congenital nasal pyriform aperture stenosis and solitary central maxillary incisor shows midline fusion of the inferior frontal lobes ➡ and hypothalamus and inferior basal ganglia ⇨, consistent with semilobar holoprosencephaly.*

TERMINOLOGY

Abbreviations

- Congenital nasal pyriform aperture stenosis (CNPAS)

Definitions

- Congenital narrowing of anterior bony nasal passageway/nasal aperture

IMAGING

General Features

- Best diagnostic clue
  - Medialization & thickening of anterior maxillae with narrowing of nasal airway
- Size
  - Pyriform aperture (PA) size in CNPAS
    - PA width < 11 mm in term infant is diagnostic (normal = 13.4-15.6 mm)

Imaging Recommendations

- Best imaging tool
  - Bone CT in axial & coronal planes

CT Findings

- Narrowed bony nasal inlet
  - Medial deviation of lateral wall of PA (anterior maxillae) ± thickening of nasal processes
- Triangle-shaped hard palate
  - Bony ridge along oral surface of hard palate on coronal images
- Abnormal maxillary dentition may occur
  - Fused or malaligned central & lateral incisors
  - Solitary median maxillary central incisor (SMMCI) syndrome (in up to 75%)
- Decreased width of nasal cavity, midface, & palate
- Thinning of anterior nasal septum
- Posterior choanae normal in caliber

DIFFERENTIAL DIAGNOSIS

Nasolacrimal Duct Mucocele

- Obstruction of distal nasolacrimal ducts → cysts at bilateral inferior meatus → narrow anterior nasal cavity
- Bony aperture is normal

Nasal Choanal Stenosis/Atresia

- Narrow or occluded posterior nasal passage: Membranous, osseous, or mixed
- Anterior nasal passage normal in caliber

PATHOLOGY

General Features

- Etiology
  - 3 theories of pathogenesis
    - Deficiency of primary palate derived from midline mesodermal tissue
      - Embryologically, medial maxillary swelling forms structures of primary palate, including 4 incisors
      - Mesoderm thought to have inductive effect on forebrain, hence association of SMMCI syndrome with holoprosencephaly
    - Overgrowth or dysplasia of nasal processes of maxilla
    - Premature ossification of midline palatal suture (recently proposed theory)
- Associated abnormalities
  - CNPAS without SMMCI is almost always isolated anomaly
  - Upper teeth anomalies
    - **SMMCI syndrome** (75% of CNPAS cases)
  - Semilobar or alobar **holoprosencephaly**
  - Endocrine dysfunction: Pituitary-adrenal axis

CLINICAL ISSUES

Presentation

- Most common signs/symptoms
  - Symptoms may be more pronounced with feeding
  - Respiratory distress, especially with feeding, as infants are obligate nasal breathers
    - Can mimic choanal atresia/stenosis
    - Breathing problems may be triggered by upper respiratory infection further compromising airway
  - Cyanosis
  - Nasogastric tube difficult to pass

Demographics

- Age
  - Newborns or infants in 1st few months of life
- Epidemiology
  - Congenital airway obstruction affects 1 in 5,000 infants
    - Majority are choanal atresia
    - CNPAS 1/5 to 1/3 as common as choanal atresia
      - 1 in 25,000 live births

Treatment

- Conservative with special feeding techniques
  - Nasal cavity eventually grows, & mild obstruction is relieved
- Surgical intervention in patients with persistent respiratory difficulty & poor weight gain
  - Resection of anteromedial maxilla ± anterior aspect inferior turbinates & reconstruction of anterior nasal orifice
  - PA width < 5.7 mm in neonate may correlate with need for surgical intervention

DIAGNOSTIC CHECKLIST

Image Interpretation Pearls

- Brain MR recommended in cases of solitary maxillary central incisor to exclude midline brain anomalies

SELECTED REFERENCES

1. Galluzzi F et al: Congenital bony nasal cavity stenosis: a review of current trends in diagnosis and treatment. Int J Pediatr Otorhinolaryngol. 144:110670, 2021
2. Wine TM et al: Congenital nasal pyriform aperture stenosis: evidence of premature fusion of the midline palatal suture. AJNR Am J Neuroradiol. 42(6):1163-6, 2021
3. Ruda J et al: Radiologic, genetic, and endocrine findings in isolated congenital nasal pyriform aperture stenosis patients. Int J Pediatr Otorhinolaryngol. 128:109705, 2020
4. Shah GB et al: Congenital nasal pyriform aperture stenosis: analysis of twenty cases at a single institution. Int J Pediatr Otorhinolaryngol. 126:109608, 2019

Juvenile Angiofibroma

KEY FACTS

TERMINOLOGY

- Benign, vascular, nonencapsulated, locally invasive mass originating in nasal cavity

IMAGING

- Centered in posterior nasal cavity arising at sphenopalatine foramen; extends into nasopharynx, sphenoid sinus, pterygopalatine fossa, masticator space, orbit, skull base
- CT findings
  - Heterogeneous vs. diffuse, avid enhancement
  - Bone remodeling and destruction
    - Posterior wall of maxillary sinus bowed anteriorly
    - ± skull base invasion, intracranial extension
- MR findings
  - Tubular signal voids on spin-echo-based sequences due to fast flow in enlarged vessels
  - Intense enhancement, diffuse or heterogeneous
- Angiography typically performed at time of preoperative embolization; shows tumor blush
  - Most common feeding artery: Internal maxillary branch of external carotid artery

TOP DIFFERENTIAL DIAGNOSES

- Rhabdomyosarcoma
- Childhood nasopharyngeal carcinoma
- Antrochoanal polyp
- Esthesioneuroblastoma

CLINICAL ISSUES

- Unilateral nasal obstruction (90%), epistaxis (60%)
  - Occurs almost exclusively in adolescent males
- Preferred treatment: Complete surgical resection using preoperative embolization to ↓ blood loss
  - ± adjuvant radiation therapy after surgery or as primary treatment in some cases

DIAGNOSTIC CHECKLIST

- Look for extension into surrounding structures
- Consider other diagnoses (or genetic testing) in females

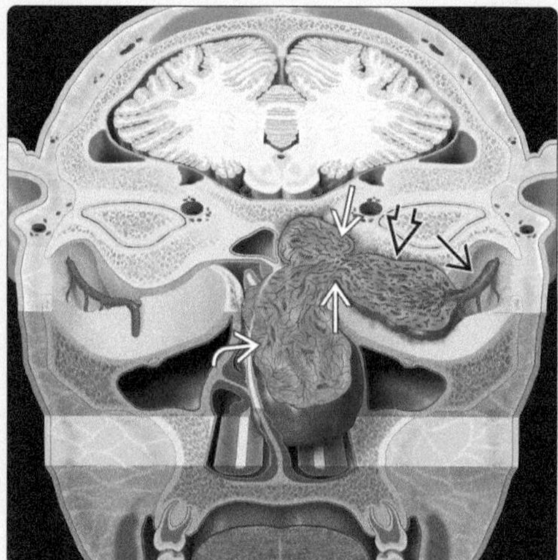

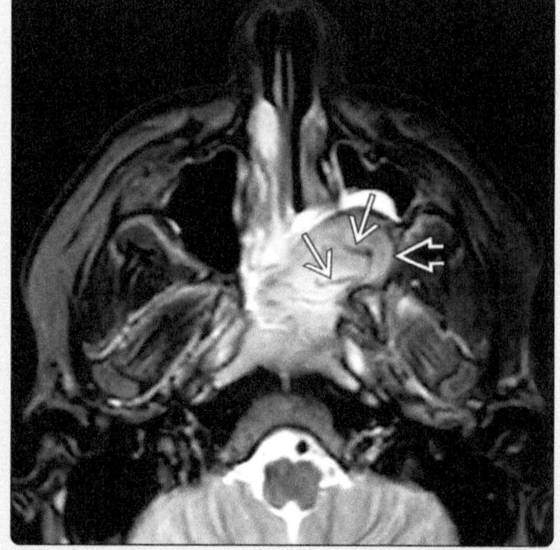

(Left) *Graphic shows the classic features and location of juvenile angiofibroma (JAF). The site of origin is the sphenopalatine foramen (SPF) ➡ with tumoral extension into the pterygopalatine fossa (PPF) ⇨ and nasal cavity ➡. The internal maxillary artery ⇨ is the dominant feeding vessel.* **(Right)** *Axial STIR MR in a teenage patient shows a well-defined mass with intralesional flow voids ➡ widening the left PPF, deviating the posterior wall of the maxillary sinus forward and extending into the left infratemporal fossa ➡.*

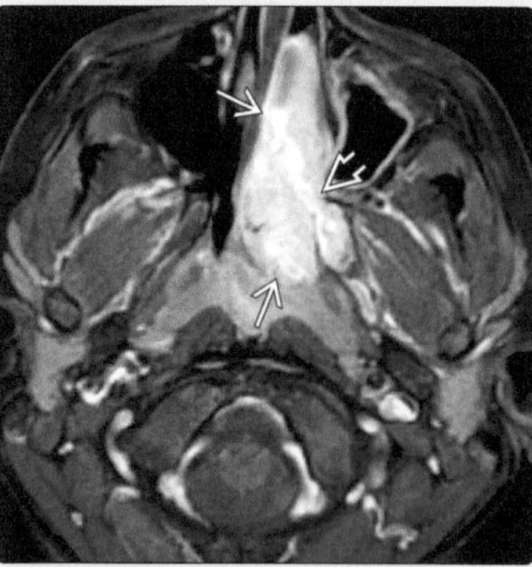

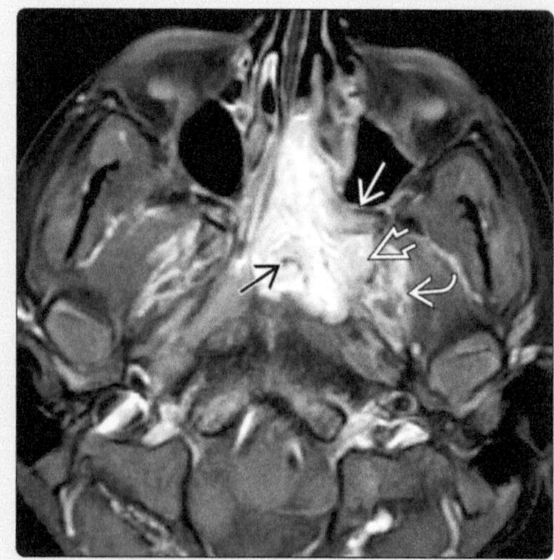

(Left) *Axial T1 C+ FS MR in a 15-year-old patient with nasal obstruction shows an enhancing JAF ➡ filling the left nasal cavity and extending into the nasopharynx. The presumed site of origin is the SPF ➡.* **(Right)** *Axial T1 C+ FS MR in the same patient shows a few intralesional high-flow vessels ⇨ with extension of the JAF into the widened PPF ➡. There is destruction of the left pterygoid ➡ with extension of the mass into the masticator space ➡.*

TERMINOLOGY

Abbreviations

- Juvenile angiofibroma (JAF)

Synonyms

- Juvenile nasopharyngeal angiofibroma (JNA); fibromatous or angiofibromatous hamartoma
  - JAF of nasal cavity more correct terminology
  - JNA commonly used term, but tumor begins in nasal cavity, not in nasopharynx

Definitions

- Benign, vascular, nonencapsulated, locally invasive nasal cavity mass

IMAGING

General Features

- Best diagnostic clue
  - Intensely enhancing soft tissue mass originating at sphenopalatine foramen (SPF) in adolescent male
- Location
  - Centered in posterior wall of nasal cavity off-midline, at margin of SPF
    - SPF is medial opening of pterygopalatine fossa (PPF) into superior meatus of nose
    - Extends anteriorly into nasal cavity, posteriorly into nasopharynx, and laterally into PPF
      - Penetrates PPF early (90%) with involvement of upper medial pterygoid lamina
    - Sphenoid sinus extension (60%)
    - May extend into maxillary (43%) and ethmoid sinuses (35%), masticator space, and inferior orbital fissure
    - 5-20% extend into middle cranial fossa via vidian canal or foramen rotundum
  - Extranasopharyngeal angiofibroma, entity showing pathologic findings of JAF but with other differences
    - Located at nasal septum, turbinate, etc.
    - M:F = 2.1:1; mean age: 28.7 years
    - Mainly nasal obstruction; epistaxis only 25%
    - Female sex or normal vascularity does not exclude
- Size
  - Usually 2-6 cm but may become massive
- Morphology
  - Lobular, usually well-circumscribed mass
    - Large lesions have infiltrating margins

Radiographic Findings

- Lateral skull radiograph shows anterior displacement of posterior wall of maxillary antrum
  - Called antral sign, bow sign, or Holman-Miller sign
  - Nonspecific sign, denotes any slow-growing mass
- Associated with nasal cavity opacification
- ± nasal cavity/nasopharyngeal soft tissue mass

CT Findings

- CECT
  - Heterogeneous vs. diffuse, avid enhancement of soft tissue mass in nasal cavity originating near SPF
  - Frequent extension into adjacent nasopharynx and PPF
  - ± opacified sphenoid sinus (obstructed nonenhancing secretions vs. enhancing tumor infiltration)
  - ± intracranial or orbital extension
- Bone CT
  - Bone remodeling ± destruction
    - Antral sign; nonspecific
    - Ipsilateral nasal cavity and PPF enlarged
    - ± skull base invasion; pterygoid lamina erosion specific
- CTA
  - Enlarged ipsilateral external carotid artery (ECA) and internal maxillary (IMAX) artery

MR Findings

- T1WI: Heterogeneous, intermediate signal
  - Signal voids represent flow in enlarged vessels
- T2WI: Heterogeneous, intermediate to high signal
  - Punctate and serpentine flow voids within tumor
- T1WI C+ FS: Intense enhancement ± flow voids
  - Coronal plane shows cavernous sinus, sphenoid sinus, or skull base extension
- MRA: Enlarged ipsilateral ECA and IMAX artery
  - Lesional vessels may be too small to evaluate with MRA

Angiographic Findings

- Conventional angiography typically performed at time of preoperative embolization
- Intense capillary tumor blush is fed by enlarged feeding vessels from ECA
  - Most common feeding vessels: IMAX and ascending pharyngeal arteries from ECA
  - If skull base or cavernous sinus extension, then internal carotid artery (ICA) supply common
  - ± supply from contralateral ECA branches

Imaging Recommendations

- Best imaging tool
  - Maxillofacial bone-only NECT in axial and coronal planes for evaluating bone remodeling vs. destruction
  - Postcontrast MR optimal for mapping lesion extent and determining vascularity
  - Catheter angiography of both ECA and ICA
    - Often in conjunction with embolization therapy
    - Helps plan surgery and ↓ intraoperative blood loss
- Protocol advice
  - Maxillofacial MR with T1 C+ FS in axial and coronal planes
    - Multiplanar imaging for evaluating extension into sphenoid sinus, orbit, skull base
  - Precontrast non-fat-suppressed T1 vital in evaluating infiltration of normal fat in PPF and adjacent bone
  - CECT may be helpful for evaluating residual disease in postoperative period

DIFFERENTIAL DIAGNOSIS

Rhabdomyosarcoma

- Intermediate- to mildly high-signal mass with variable enhancement (often mild to moderate) ± bone destruction
- Can arise in many locations (not necessarily nasal cavity)
- Rarely penetrates SPF into PPF

Childhood Nasopharyngeal Carcinoma

- Mostly EBV-related, undifferentiated carcinoma

- Invasive mass of lateral nasopharynx
- Mild to moderate enhancement
- 90% + nodal metastases, diagnosed at advanced stage

Antrochoanal Polyp

- Maxillary antrum opacified
- Homogeneous mass herniates into anterior nasal cavity, then nasopharynx; PPF not involved
- Peripheral enhancement only

Encephalocele

- Nasoethmoidal type presents as intranasal mass
- Connection to intracranial cavity seen on imaging
- No enhancement
- Usually more anterior in position

Esthesioneuroblastoma

- 1st incidence peaks in 2nd decade; F > M
- Presenting symptoms same as JAF
- Nasal cavity mass near cribriform plate
- Cystic intracranial components characteristic

PATHOLOGY

General Features

- Etiology
  - Unknown: Recent consideration as vasoproliferative tumor, positive staining for markers that may promote angiogenesis and proliferation

Staging, Grading, & Classification

- Staging systems based on tumor size (< or > 6 cm), invasion to PPF anterior &/or posterior to pterygoid plates, and skull base/intracranial invasion

Microscopic Features

- Unencapsulated, highly vascular polypoid mass of angiomatous tissue in fibrous stroma
- Myofibroblast thought to be cell of origin
- ± estrogen, testosterone, or progesterone receptors

CLINICAL ISSUES

Presentation

- Most common signs/symptoms
  - Unilateral nasal obstruction (90%), epistaxis (60%)
- Other signs/symptoms
  - Nasal voice, nasal discharge, anosmia, pain or swelling in cheek, proptosis, serous otitis media
- Clinical profile
  - Adolescent male with nasal obstruction and epistaxis
  - Nasal endoscopy: Vascular-appearing nasal cavity mass
    - Biopsy in outpatient setting should be avoided due to risk of hemorrhage

Demographics

- Age
  - 10-25 years; average age at onset: 15 years
- Sex
  - Almost exclusively occurs in male patients
    - If found in female, may have genetic mosaicism
- Epidemiology
  - 0.5% of all H&N neoplasms

Natural History & Prognosis

- May rarely spontaneously regress
- Local recurrence rate with surgery: 6-24%
  - Local recurrence more common with large lesions (> 6 cm), intracranial spread, previous treatment

Treatment

- Preferred: Complete surgical resection using preoperative embolization to ↓ blood loss
  - Transarterial embolization most often, direct puncture embolization in some centers
- Multiple surgical approaches
  - Open resection (midface degloving) vs. endoscopic or endoscopic-assisted removal ± laser assistance
  - Endoscopic resection associated with ↓ bleeding and shorter hospital stay
- Radiation therapy (RT)
  - Adjuvant to surgery for unresectable intracranial disease and cavernous sinus involvement
    - 78% control rates reported
  - Used with caution in young patients due to potential to induce malignancies
- Hormonal therapy (estrogen) controversial
  - Not routine; complete tumor regression not achieved
  - Feminization side effects undesirable in adolescent male
- Recent reports of some success with sirolimus

DIAGNOSTIC CHECKLIST

Consider

- JAF in adolescent male patient with epistaxis and enhancing posterior nasal cavity mass
- Consider other diagnoses (or genetic testing) in female patients

Image Interpretation Pearls

- Evaluate JAF extension into surrounding structures
  - Orbit, infratemporal fossa, sphenoid sinus, and skull base
  - Failure to identify subtle deep growth will result in incomplete surgical resection

SELECTED REFERENCES

1. Baba A et al: MRI features of sinonasal tract angiofibroma/juvenile nasopharyngeal angiofibroma: case series and systematic review. J Neuroimaging. 33(5):675-87, 2023
2. Diaz A et al: Embolization in Juvenile nasopharyngeal angiofibroma surgery: a systematic review and meta-analysis. Laryngoscope. 133(7):1529-39, 2023
3. Jurlina M et al: Endoscopic, endoscopic-assisted and open approaches in the treatment of juvenile angiofibroma: what has been new in the past decade (and 1586 cases)? Eur Arch Otorhinolaryngol. 280(5):2081-9, 2023
4. Kothari DS et al: Preoperative embolization techniques in the treatment of juvenile nasopharyngeal angiofibroma: a systematic review. Otolaryngol Head Neck Surg. 169(3):454-66, 2023
5. Mamlouk MD: Solid and vascular neck masses in children. Neuroimaging Clin N Am. 33(4):607-21, 2023
6. Scholfield DW et al: Midfacial degloving for juvenile angiofibroma: a case-series of 21 adult males: an alternative to the endoscopic approach and when it should be considered. Clin Otolaryngol. 46(3):659-64, 2021
7. Schreiber A et al: Early postoperative magnetic resonance in the diagnosis of persistent juvenile angiofibroma. Laryngoscope. 131(8):E2436-41, 2021
8. Fernández KS et al: Sirolimus for the treatment of juvenile nasopharyngeal angiofibroma. Pediatr Blood Cancer. 67(4):e28162, 2020
9. Bertazzoni G et al: Contemporary management of juvenile angiofibroma. Curr Opin Otolaryngol Head Neck Surg. 27(1):47-53, 2019
10. Rodriguez DP et al: Masses of the nose, nasal cavity, and nasopharynx in children. Radiographics. 37(6):1704-30, 2017

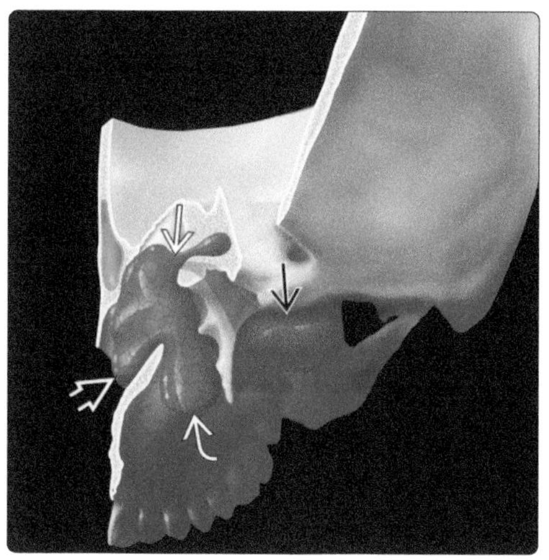

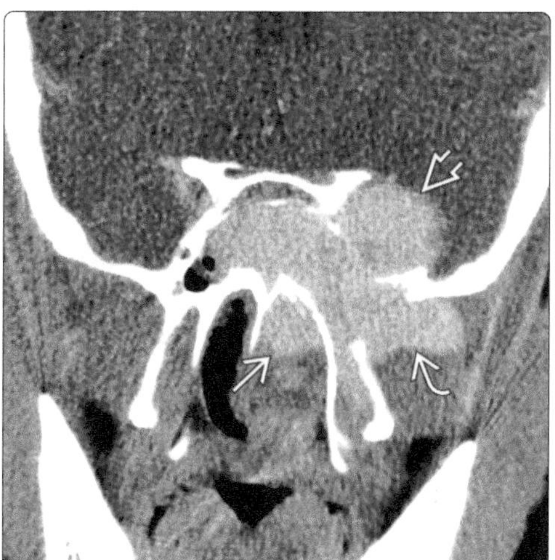

(Left) *Posterior oblique sagittal graphic shows the spread patterns of JAF. The lesion originates at the SPF ➡ and extends into the nasal cavity ➡, nasopharynx/oropharynx ➡, and infratemporal fossa ⇨.* **(Right)** *Coronal CECT shows a large JAF extending into the nasopharynx ➡, infratemporal fossa ➡, and middle cranial fossa ➡. The sphenoid sinus is replaced by the tumor. As seen in this case, JAF classically shows avid enhancement.*

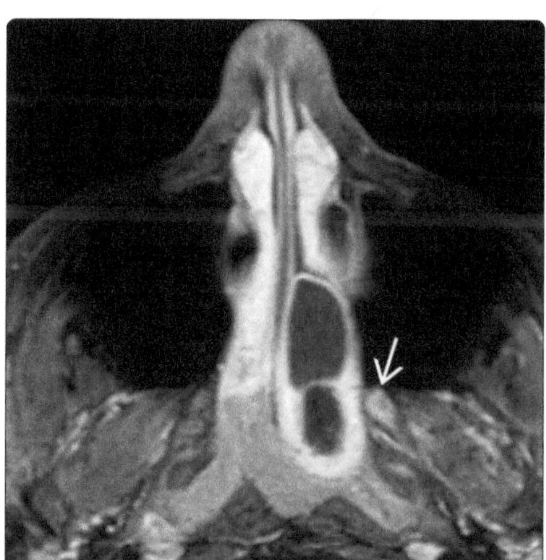

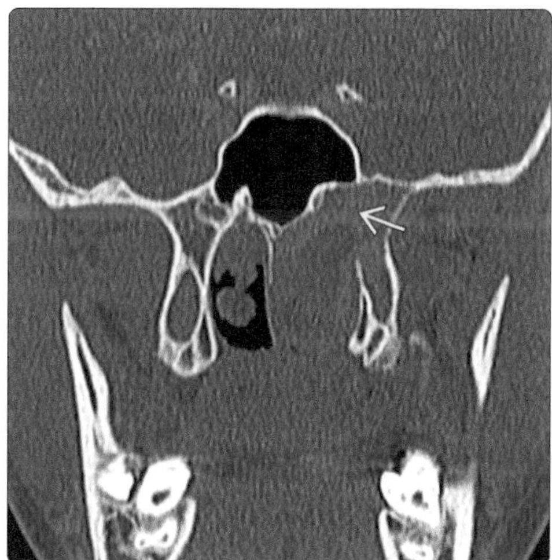

(Left) *Axial T1 C+ FS MR in a 13-year-old boy with epistaxis shows an enhancing mass obstructing the left nasal cavity, extending into the left nasopharynx, compressing the adenoids, with minimal enhancement in the left pterygoid ➡. Cystic areas are uncommon in JAF, but the location is typical.* **(Right)** *Coronal bone CT in the same patient shows an intact but thin floor of the left sphenoid sinus and floor of the middle cranial fossa, but destruction and infiltration of the left pterygoid plate ➡, typical of JAF.*

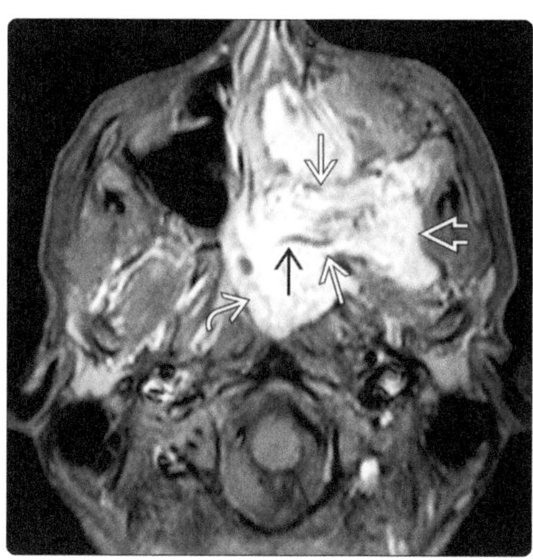

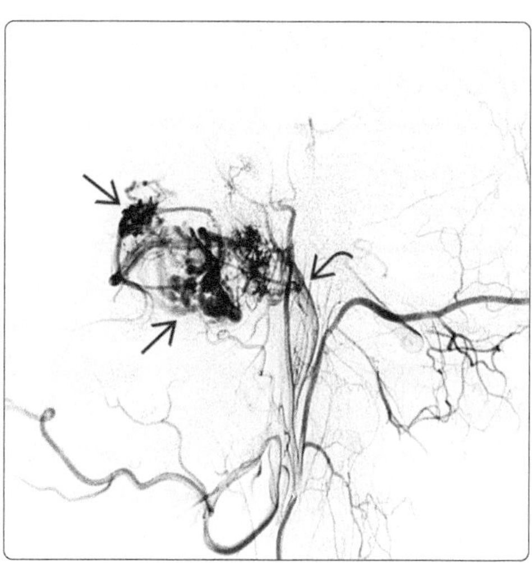

(Left) *Axial T1 C+ FS MR shows avid enhancement throughout JAF. The mass enlarges the PPF ➡ and extends laterally into the masticator space ➡ and medially into the nasopharynx ➡. Several serpiginous flow voids ⇨ are noted, consistent with enlarged feeding vessels.* **(Right)** *Lateral DSA from an external carotid artery injection shows areas of dense tumor blush ⇨ within JAF prior to embolization. As is typical, the main arterial feeding vessel for this JAF is the internal maxillary artery ⇨.*

Anophthalmia/Microphthalmia

KEY FACTS

TERMINOLOGY

- Anophthalmia: Complete absence of globe in presence of ocular adnexa
- Microphthalmia: Globe with total axial length (TAL) < 2 standard deviations below mean for age
  - < 19 mm in 1 year old or < 21 mm in adult

IMAGING

- Absent or small globe ± persistent hyperplastic primary vitreous (PHPV), colobomatous cyst, or intracranial anomalies

TOP DIFFERENTIAL DIAGNOSES

- Enophthalmos
  - Globe normal in size but sunken
- Phthisis bulbi
  - End stage, small/calcified globe remnant
- Surgical enucleation
- Large contralateral globe

PATHOLOGY

- Anophthalmia
  - Primary anophthalmia very rare: Failure of optic vesicle development (during weeks 1-3 of gestation)
  - Secondary as part of general abnormality of forebrain development
- Congenital microphthalmia
  - ± PHPV or large posterior colobomatous cyst
- Acquired microphthalmia
  - Trauma
  - Retinopathy of prematurity (ROP)
  - Congenital infection: Congenital rubella (also cataracts), CMV, syphilis
  - Postnatal infection: Ocular toxocariasis (sclerosing endophthalmitis)
  - Coats disease

DIAGNOSTIC CHECKLIST

- Consider genetic counseling

(Left) *Axial NECT in a 5-week-old with congenital anophthalmia demonstrates complete absence of the globes. Structures not derived from neuroectoderm (extraocular muscles, eyelids, conjunctiva, lacrimal apparatus) are present but small.* **(Right)** *Axial CECT demonstrates a large colobomatous cyst ➡ posterior to a microphthalmic left globe ➡ and a smaller right posterior coloboma ➡. Notice mild malposition of the left lens as well.*

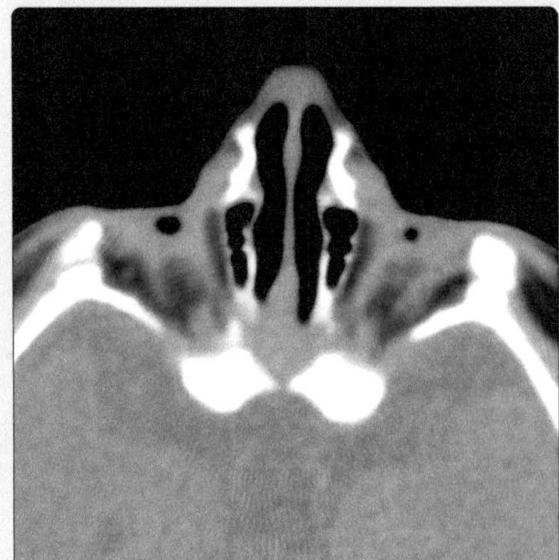

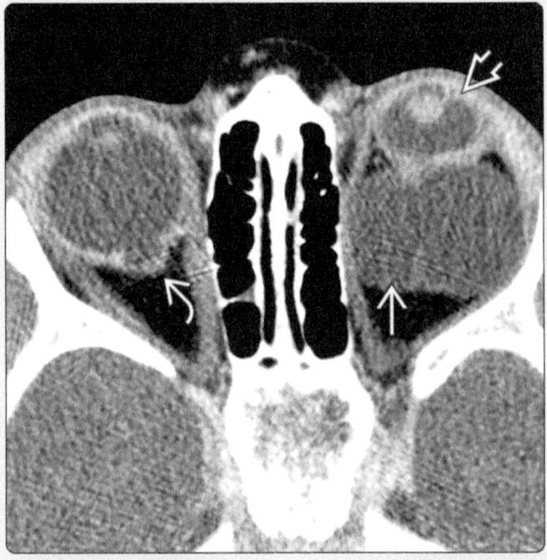

(Left) *Axial NECT in a 9-year-old boy with Lenz microphthalmia syndrome shows bilateral microphthalmia with small intraocular Ca^{++}. In the absence of known trauma, prematurity, or infection, these findings should raise the question of a genetic etiology.* **(Right)** *Axial T1WI MR in a former premature infant with retinopathy of prematurity shows right > left microphthalmia with complex intraocular signal abnormality, consistent with varying stages of hemorrhagic ocular detachments ➡.*

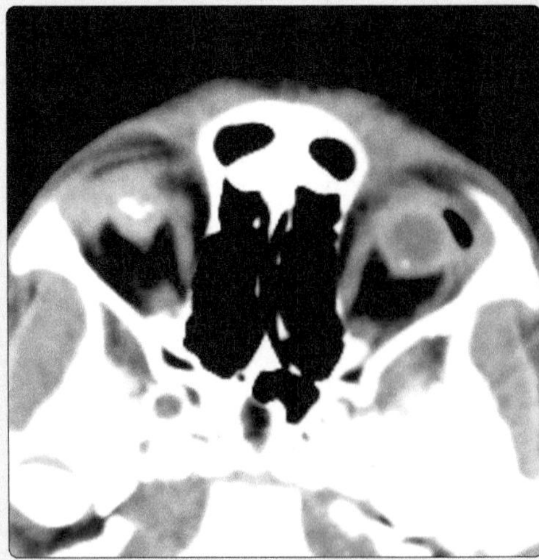

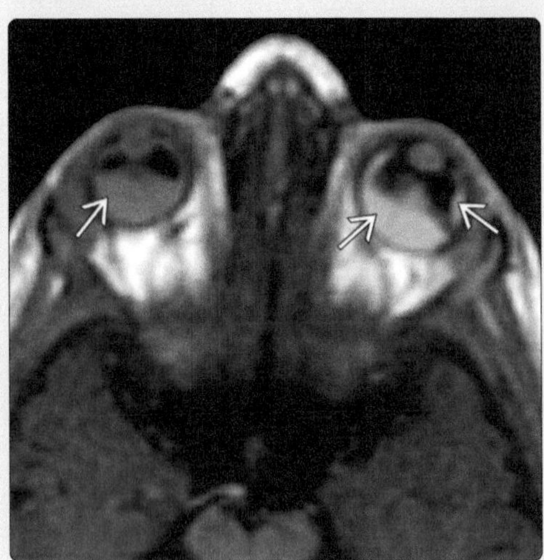

TERMINOLOGY

Synonyms

- Anophthalmos = anophthalmia
- Microphthalmos = microphthalmia

Definitions

- Anophthalmia: Complete absence of globe in presence of ocular adnexa
- Microphthalmia: Globe with total axial length (TAL) < 2 standard deviations below mean for age
  - < 19 mm in 1 year old or < 21 mm in adult
    - Normal neonatal eye is 17 mm, achieves adult-sized globe by 3 years of age
- Nanophthalmos: Type of simple microphthalmia + microcornea, bilateral TAL < 18 mm and hyperopia

IMAGING

General Features

- Location
  - Unilateral or bilateral
- Morphology
  - Absent or small globe ± persistent hyperplastic primary vitreous (PHPV), colobomatous cyst, or intracranial anomalies
- Embryology
  - 4th week of gestation: Optic vesicle begins to invaginate and form optic cup
    - Failure of optic vesicle development results in primary anophthalmos
  - 5th week of gestation: Mesenchyme invades open choroidal fissure, contributing to formation of hyaloid artery
  - 6th week of gestation: Closure of optic vesicle (globe)
  - At 36 weeks, hyaloid artery within globe has regressed
    - Incomplete regression of hyaloid artery → remnant vessels in persistent primary vitreous of posterior chamber
  - Between 4th and 8th weeks, face develops
    - Anlage of corpus callosum also forms around same time (between 3rd and ~ 8th weeks)
  - Therefore, congenital abnormalities involving closure of midface (medial cleft syndromes) or corpus callosum formation may be accompanied by coloboma, microphthalmia, or anophthalmia

Imaging Recommendations

- Best imaging tool
  - MR for internal structure of globe, ocular contents, and associated brain abnormalities

DIFFERENTIAL DIAGNOSIS

Enophthalmos

- Globe normal in size but sunken

Phthisis Bulbi

- End stage, small/calcified globe remnant secondary end-stage damage to globe from any cause

Surgical Enucleation

- If prior to 20 years of age, may lead to decreased orbital volume

Large Contralateral Globe

- Macrophthalmia

Microcornea With Normal Globe

- TAL within normal limits

PATHOLOGY

General Features

- Etiology
  - Anophthalmia
    - Primary anophthalmia very rare: Failure of optic vesicle development (during weeks 1-3 of gestation)
    - Secondary as part of general abnormality of forebrain development
    - Degenerative due to regression or involution of previously formed optic vesicle
    - Unilateral + severe craniofacial anomalies
    - Bilateral associated with absence of optic chiasm, diminished posterior optic pathways, agenesis/dysgenesis corpus callosum
  - Congenital microphthalmia
    - Congenital underdevelopment of globe
      - Sporadic, autosomal dominant, recessive and X-linked forms
      - ± fetal vasculature (previously called PHPV), cataracts, large posterior colobomatous cyst, or anterior segment dysgenesis
      - Microphthalmia secondary to small initial optic vesicle associated with small palpebral fissure
      - Microphthalmia caused by delayed or incomplete closure of optic fissure associated with normal palpebral fissure
    - More common than true anophthalmia
    - Less common than acquired microphthalmia
  - Acquired microphthalmia
    - More common than congenital microphthalmia
    - Trauma
      - Globe trauma may → small globe ± ocular hemorrhage, detachment
      - Flattened with flat tire or mushroom shape
    - Retinopathy of prematurity (ROP)
      - Vasculoproliferative disorder in low birth weight, premature infants
      - Small, noncalcified globes, frequently bilateral (Ca^{++} may be seen as late finding)
    - Congenital infection: Rubella (also cataracts), CMV, syphilis
    - Postnatal infection: Primarily ocular toxocariasis (sclerosing endophthalmitis)
      - Anterior segment may be uninvolved; retinal detachment, normal-sized globe early, no Ca^{++}
      - Other infections: Viral (herpes simplex, herpes zoster, rubeola, mumps, EBV), bacterial (Lyme, brucellosis, cat-scratch disease, *Escherichia coli*), and other fungal disease, such as candidiasis

 - Maternal exposure to alcohol (fetal alcohol syndrome) and toxins, such as benomyl (fungicide), thalidomide, retinoic acid, LSD, hydantoin
 - Coats disease
 - Exudate and retinal detachment with normal-sized globe and no Ca^{++}
 - Any cause may lead to phthisis bulbi = end stage, small/calcified globe
 - When extreme, may mimic anophthalmos
 - Growth of globe influences size of osseous orbit; therefore, anophthalmia and microphthalmia are frequently associated with small bony orbit
- Genetics
 - Many chromosomal abnormalities, syndromic and nonsyndromic single gene disorders
 - Genetic basis now identifiable in up to 30% of congenital microphthalmia
 - Anophthalmia/microphthalmia (A/M)
 - Isolated: Anophthalmos most autosomal recessive (AR), microphthalmos ~ 10% AR
 - Aneuploidy: Trisomy 13 (Patau syndrome), mosaic trisomy 19
 - Deletions (involving chromosomes 4, 7, 14, or X)
 - Chromosomal rearrangements
 - *SOX2*-related eye disorders, including anophthalmia-esophageal-genital (AEG) syndrome
 - *PAX6* (paired box gene) mutations
 - Waardenburg anophthalmia syndrome (distal limb anomalies, missense mutation *SMOC1* gene)
 - Oculocerebrocutaneous syndrome (Delleman syndrome)
 - Anophthalmia plus syndrome (multiple congenital malformations)
 - Microphthalmia with linear skin defects (MLS) or microphthalmia, dermal aplasia, and sclerocornea (MIDAS) (X-linked male-lethal disorder, *HCCS* or *COX7B* mutations)
 - Cerebro-oculo-facio-skeletal (COFS) (*ERCC6* gene)
 - Nance-Horan syndrome (X-linked with congenital cataracts, dental anomalies, ± intellectual disability)
 - Micro syndrome (AR *RAB3GAP1* gene mutation, intellectual disability, microcephaly, congenital cataract, microcornea, microphthalmia, agenesis/hypoplasia corpus callosum, hypogenitalism)
 - CHARGE syndrome (**c**oloboma, **h**eart detects, choanal **a**tresia, **r**estricted growth and development &/or CNS abnormalities, **g**enital anomalies in males, and **e**ar anomalies/deafness) (*CHD7* mutations)
 - Lenz microphthalmia syndrome [X-linked recessive, *ANOP1* and ANOP2 (*BCOR*)]
 - Branchiooculofacial (BOF) syndrome (*TFAP2A* gene)
 - Focal dermal hypoplasia (FDH) (Goltz syndrome, X-linked, *PORCN* gene)
 - Aicardi syndrome (infantile spasm, corpus callosum agenesis, chorioretinal lacunae)
 - X-linked dominant
 - Walker-Warburg (WWS), muscle-eye-brain (MEB) syndromes
 - Meckel-Gruber syndrome (AR)
 - Norrie disease (X-linked recessive)
 - Incontinentia pigmenti (IP) (X-linked dominant, *IKBKG*)
 - *SIX6* gene mutation (SIX homeobox 6)
 - *RAX* gene mutation (retina and anterior neural fold homeobox)
 - Lowe syndrome (oculocerebral renal disease); also cerebral white matter lesions, glaucoma, and cataracts
 - Hemifacial microsomia (oculo-auriculo-vertebral spectrum, Goldenhar syndrome)
 - Associated with CNS anomalies, such as encephaloceles, heterotopia, agenesis corpus callosum, midface abnormalities

Staging, Grading, & Classification

- Severe: Globe with corneal diameter < 4 mm and TAL < 10 mm at birth or < 12 mm after 1 year
- Simple: Globe intact but typically mild decrease in TAL
- Complex: Globe with anterior &/or posterior segment dysgenesis and mild, moderate, or severe decrease in TAL
 - Anterior segment dysgenesis: Developmental abnormalities of cornea, iris, iridocorneal angle, ciliary body
 - Posterior segment dysgenesis: Developmental abnormalities of globe posterior to lens

Gross Pathologic & Surgical Features

- Anophthalmos: Structures not derived from neuroectoderm (extraocular muscles, eyelids, conjunctiva, lacrimal apparatus) remain

CLINICAL ISSUES

Presentation

- Most common signs/symptoms
 - Small globe, decreased vision
- Other signs/symptoms
 - Depends on whether isolated or part of syndrome

Natural History & Prognosis

- Variable, depending on severity and associated abnormalities

Treatment

- Oculoplastic surgeon: Prosthesis, surgery
- Early intervention and therapy
- If residual sight, good eye patched to strengthen vision in microphthalmic eye
- Surveillance by geneticist to detect emerging features of syndromic causes

DIAGNOSTIC CHECKLIST

Consider

- Genetic counseling
- Chromosomal studies to look for evidence of aneuploidy, chromosomal duplication, deletion or rearrangement as well as TORCH titers for congenital infection

SELECTED REFERENCES

1. Fahnehjelm C et al: Anophthalmia and microphthalmia in children: associated ocular, somatic and genetic morbidities and quality of life. Ophthalmic Genet. 43(2):172-83, 2022
2. Monticelli M et al: Lenz microphthalmia syndrome in neurosurgical practice: a case report and review of the literature. Childs Nerv Syst. 37(8):2713-8, 2021

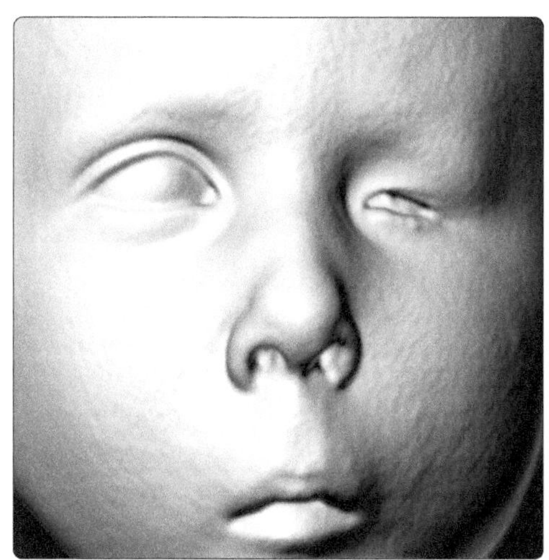

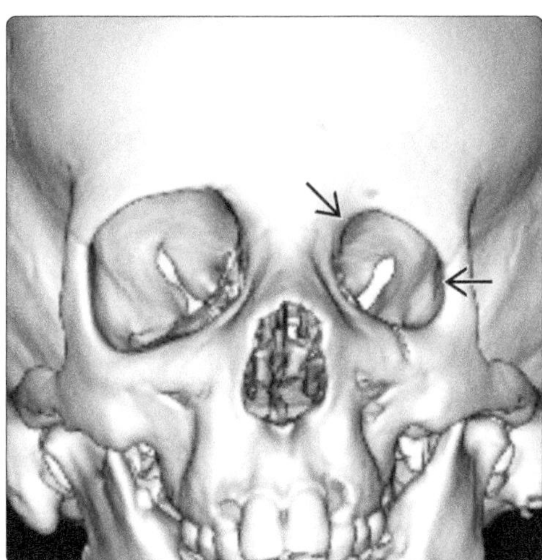

(Left) *AP soft tissue surface-rendered 3D reformation shows severely underdeveloped left eyelids in a child with multiple congenital anomalies, including congenital anophthalmia.* **(Right)** *AP 3D CT in the same child shows significant asymmetry in the orbital size, much smaller on the left ➔, secondary to congenital anophthalmia. Growth of the globe influences size of the osseous orbit; therefore, anophthalmia and microphthalmia are frequently associated with small bony orbits.*

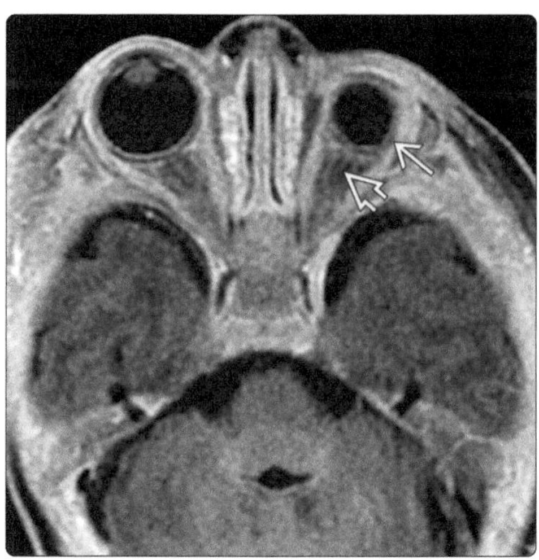

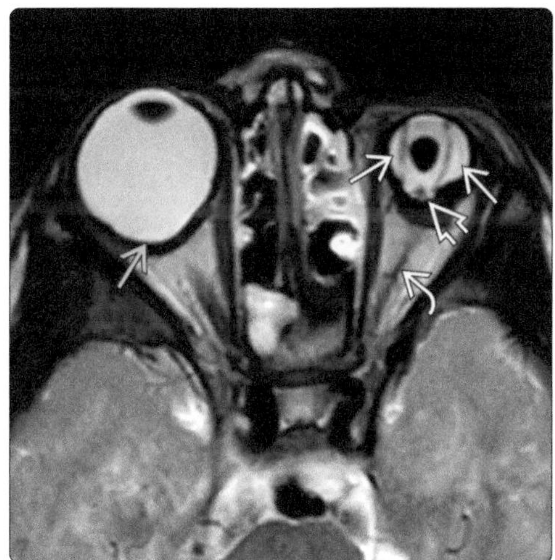

(Left) *Axial T1WI C+ FS MR in a 3-month-old with congenital microphthalmia, without genetic cause, shows a very small left globe ➔ that lacks a lens and ciliary body. Note mild left optic nerve hypoplasia ➔.* **(Right)** *Axial T2WI MR in CHARGE syndrome shows bilateral orbital abnormalities. There is severe left-sided microphthalmia with subluxed/rotated lens, choroidal detachments ➔, small posterior coloboma ➔, and optic nerve hypoplasia ➔. The right globe is enlarged with a broad-based posterior coloboma ➔.*

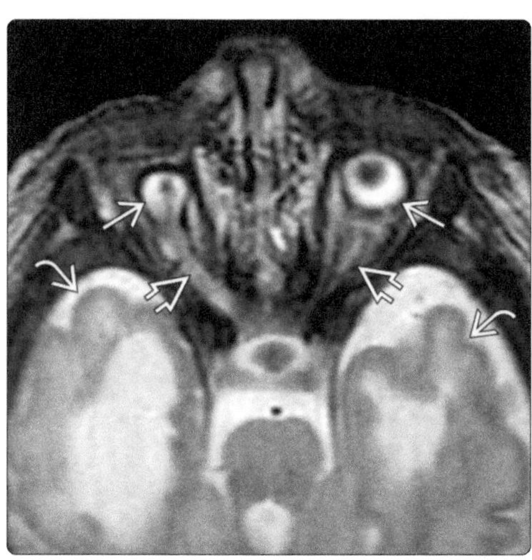

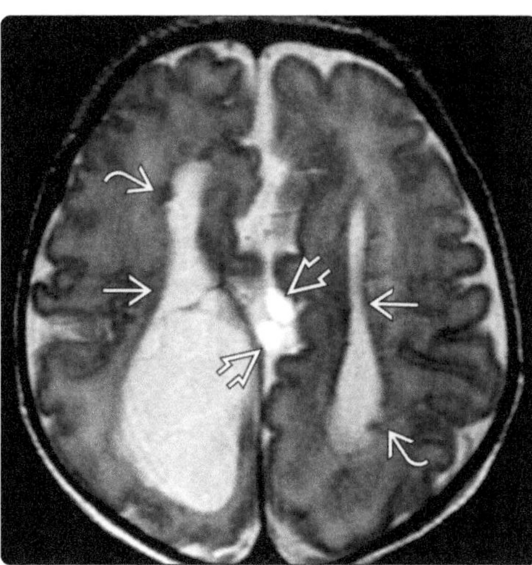

(Left) *Axial T2WI MR in an infant with Aicardi syndrome shows serve bilateral microphthalmia, right greater than left ➔, bilateral optic nerve hypoplasia ➔, enlarged temporal horns with abnormal cortical/gyral formation involving the temporal lobes ➔.* **(Right)** *Axial T2WI MR of the brain in the same child shows typical parallel configuration of the lateral ventricles ➔ related to absent corpus callosum, small posterior interhemispheric cysts ➔, diffusely abnormal cortex, and bilateral foci of gray matter heterotopia ➔.*

Macrophthalmia

KEY FACTS

TERMINOLOGY

- Enlarged globe: AP or both AP and transverse dimension
  - AP dimension secondary to myopia, staphyloma, or coloboma
  - AP and transverse dimension = buphthalmos secondary to increase in intraocular pressure in young patients

IMAGING

- Generalized enlargement of globe + increased depth of anterior chamber in primary congenital glaucoma (PCG) and early childhood glaucoma
  - Adult sclera is more rigid; glaucoma usually not associated with increase in ocular size
- Progressive myopia → AP elongation of globe/staphyloma

TOP DIFFERENTIAL DIAGNOSES

- Proptosis
  - Intraorbital extraocular mass, coloboma + retroocular cyst, thyroid ophthalmopathy, idiopathic orbital inflammatory disease
- Small contralateral eye

PATHOLOGY

- Etiology
  - PCG, neurofibromatosis type 1 (NF1), Sturge-Weber syndrome, staphyloma, collagen disorder, congenital myopia
  - Secondary to intraocular mass or trauma
- Associated abnormalities
  - Optic nerve atrophy and subluxated lens in PCG
  - Intraocular mass if secondary to ocular lesion
  - Enhancing choroidal angioma and leptomeningeal enhancement of pial angiomatosis in Sturge-Weber syndrome
  - Plexiform neurofibroma, sphenoid wing bony dysplasia, pulsatile exophthalmos in NF1

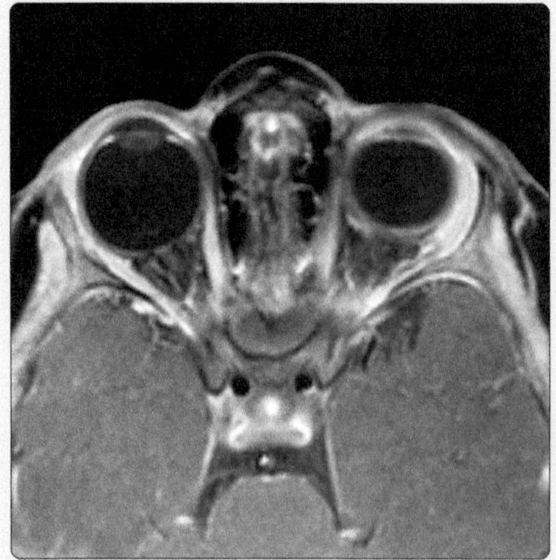

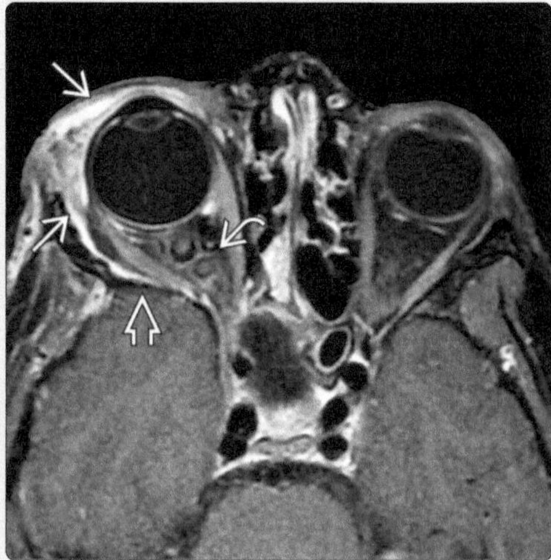

(Left) *Axial T1 C+ FS MR in a 1-year-old demonstrates diffuse right globe enlargement secondary to glaucoma.* **(Right)** *Axial T1 C+ FS MR in a 4-year-old with neurofibromatosis type 1 demonstrates an enhancing right orbital plexiform neurofibroma ➡, partial absence of the right sphenoid wing ⇨, an enlarged right globe, and incomplete visualization of a right optic nerve glioma ↪.*

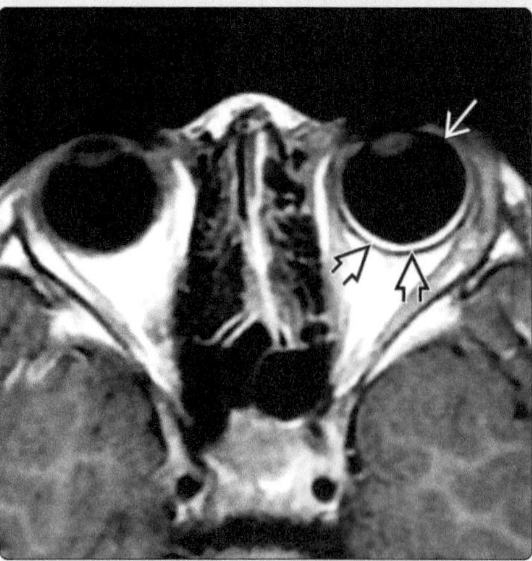

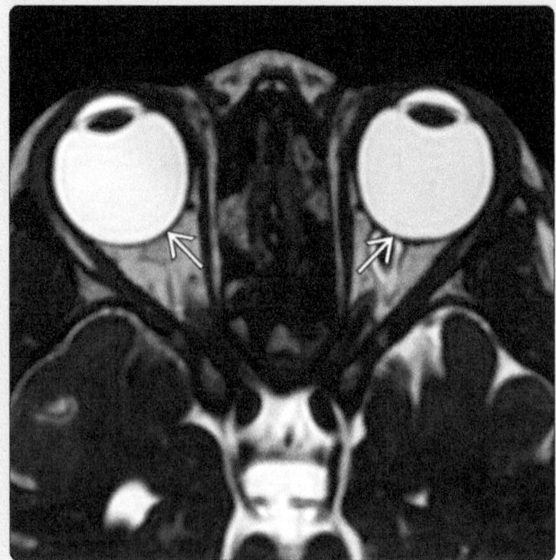

(Left) *Axial T1 C+ MR in a 5-year-old girl with Sturge-Weber syndrome shows a large left globe ➡ and smooth, intense enhancement of posterior choroidal angioma ⇨. Brain MR also demonstrated ipsilateral leptomeningeal enhancement and choroid plexus enlargement (not shown).* **(Right)** *Axial FIESTA MR in a 4-year-old girl with congenital myopia shows bilateral AP elongation of the globes ➡, typical of myopia, which leads to convergence of light anterior to the retina and subsequent nearsightedness.*

TERMINOLOGY

Definitions

- Enlarged globe: AP or both AP and transverse dimension
  - AP secondary to myopia, staphyloma, or coloboma
  - AP and transverse = buphthalmos ("ox eye" or "cow eye")
    - Secondary to increased intraocular pressure (IOP) when sclera is still pliable, as in primary congenital glaucoma (PCG) or glaucoma in children up to 4 years

IMAGING

General Features

- Best diagnostic clue
  - Enlarged globe
- Size
  - Globe larger than normal for age
    - Normal mature globe is 24 mm AP, 23 mm superior-inferior, 23.5 mm horizontal
    - Normal infant globe is 10-10.5 mm; > 12 mm is concerning for macrophthalmia
  - PCG mean anterior chamber depth: 6.3 mm (normal: 3 mm)
- Morphology
  - Generalized in PCG and early childhood glaucoma
    - Adult sclera is more rigid; adult-onset glaucoma not associated with increase in ocular size, unless associated with connective tissue disorder
  - Adults: Pathologic axial myopia → posterior segment elongated, depth of anterior chamber normal

Imaging Recommendations

- Best imaging tool
  - US is best initial modality for intraocular evaluation, usually performed by ophthalmologist, including US biomicroscopy
  - MR best evaluates intraocular masses and associated intracranial abnormalities

DIFFERENTIAL DIAGNOSIS

Proptosis

- Intraorbital extraocular masses
  - Subperiosteal abscess
  - Infantile hemangioma
  - Vascular malformations
  - Neoplasms: Rhabdomyosarcoma, optic nerve glioma, Langerhans cell histiocytosis, metastasis
- Coloboma with large retroocular cyst
- Thyroid ophthalmopathy
  - Painless enlargement of extraocular muscles (EOMs); bilateral in 90%, symmetric in 70%
- Idiopathic orbital inflammatory disease
  - Painful enlargement of EOMs, usually unilateral

Small Contralateral Eye

- Contralateral microphthalmia: Congenital or secondary to prior trauma, infection, &/or retinal detachment

PATHOLOGY

General Features

- Etiology
  - PCG
    - Obstruction to flow of aqueous humor from anterior chamber → elevated IOP and enlargement of globe and deep anterior chamber
  - Neurofibromatosis type 1 (NF1)
    - Possibly due to neurofibroma infiltrating angle or involving ciliary body; occurs in up to 50% of patients with facial and eyelid involvement
  - Sturge-Weber syndrome (SWS)
    - Glaucoma in 30-70%
  - Staphyloma
    - Focal enlargement secondary to posterior scleral wall thinning
    - Progressive myopia → posterior staphyloma
      - Glaucoma, connective tissue disorders, scleritis, necrotizing infection, or trauma
  - Collagen disorder
  - Congenital myopia
    - – Idiopathic globe enlargement in AP dimension → convergence of light anterior to retina → nearsightedness
  - Secondary to intraocular mass or trauma
    - Large intraocular mass may → enlarged globe
    - Smaller intraocular mass or trauma may → glaucoma → enlarged globe
- Genetics
  - PCG: Sporadic > autosomal recessive
    - *CYP1B1* and *LTBP2* biallelic pathogenic variants; *GLC3B* on 1p36 and *GLC3C* on 14q24.3 loci implicated, but gene is not known
- Associated abnormalities
  - Optic nerve atrophy &/or subluxated lens in PCG
  - Intraocular mass if secondary to primary ocular lesion
  - Enhancing choroidal angioma and leptomeningeal enhancement of pial angiomatosis in SWS
  - Plexiform neurofibroma, sphenoid wing bony dysplasia, pulsatile exophthalmos in NF1
    - May see buphthalmos in absence of elevated IOP in NF1 (etiology unknown)

CLINICAL ISSUES

Presentation

- Most common signs/symptoms
  - Classic triad in PCG: Photophobia, excessive tearing, blepharospasm
  - Corneal clouding

Natural History & Prognosis

- Vision prognosis fair with early treatment
- Blindness invariable, if untreated

SELECTED REFERENCES

1. Janssens R et al: Ultrasound biomicroscopy of the anterior segment in patients with primary congenital glaucoma: a review of the literature. Acta Ophthalmol. 100(6):605-13, 2022
2. Vachha BA et al: Imaging of pediatric orbital diseases. Neuroimaging Clin N Am. 25(3):477-501, 2015

Coloboma

KEY FACTS

TERMINOLOGY

- Coloboma: Gap or defect of ocular tissue
- May involve any or all structures of embryonic cleft
- Types of posterior coloboma
  - Optic disc coloboma
  - Choroidoretinal coloboma
- Related but distinct anomalies
  - Morning glory disc anomaly (MGDA)
  - Peripapillary staphyloma

IMAGING

- Focal defect at posterior pole of globe
- Outpouching contiguous with vitreous
- Microphthalmos & retrobulbar cysts often present
- Isodense/isointense to vitreous on CT/MR
- Bulging of posterior globe on prenatal MR
- MGDA on MR: Uveoscleral discontinuity, funnel-shaped optic disc, adjacent focal retinal surface elevation with ↑ T1
  - Less commonly, fat within adjacent optic nerve sheath
- MGDA on MR: Abnormal ↓ T2-hypointense tissue associated with adjacent optic nerve showing occasional Gd (+) enhancement with focal perioptic CSF effacement

TOP DIFFERENTIAL DIAGNOSES

- Congenital microphthalmos, neurofibromatosis type 1, congenital glaucoma, degenerative staphyloma

PATHOLOGY

- Failure of embryonic fissure fusion
- Isolated, sporadic, & syndromic genetic etiologies
- Bilateral when syndromic

CLINICAL ISSUES

- ↓ visual acuity; leukocoria
- Treatment to address refractive errors, strabismus, amblyopia, retinal detachment

DIAGNOSTIC CHECKLIST

- Look for syndromic & systemic associations

(Left) *Axial graphic of classic optic disc coloboma shows a focal defect in the posterior globe at the site of the optic nerve head insertion ⇨.* **(Right)** *Axial CECT demonstrates a broad colobomatous defect ➡ centered on the upper margin of the optic disc. Note the vitreous appears contiguous with retrobulbar outpouching. Apart from the retrobulbar outpouching, the globe is small.*

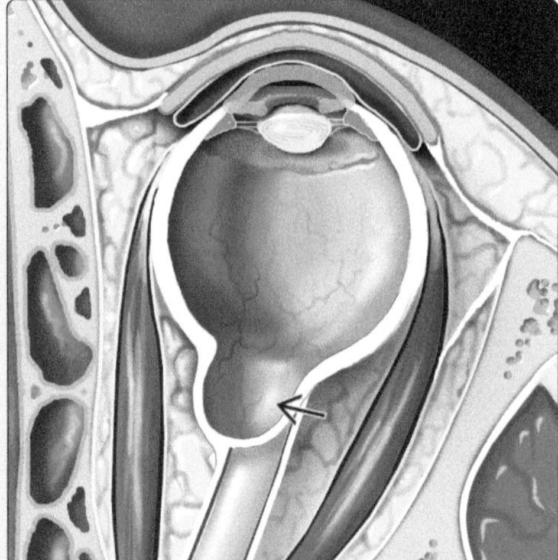

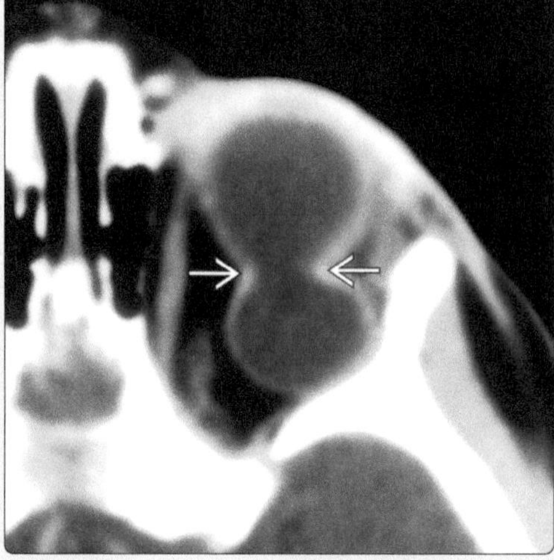

(Left) *Funduscopy shows a large posterior coloboma centered at the optic nerve head ⇨. Associated marginal pigmentation ⇨ suggests chorioretinal involvement.* **(Right)** *Sagittal reformatted 3D T2 CISS MR shows optic disc coloboma ➡ situated just inferior to the optic nerve insertion site ➡ at the posterior eye globe. Note that the fluid signal within the outpouching of coloboma is identical to that of vitreous.*

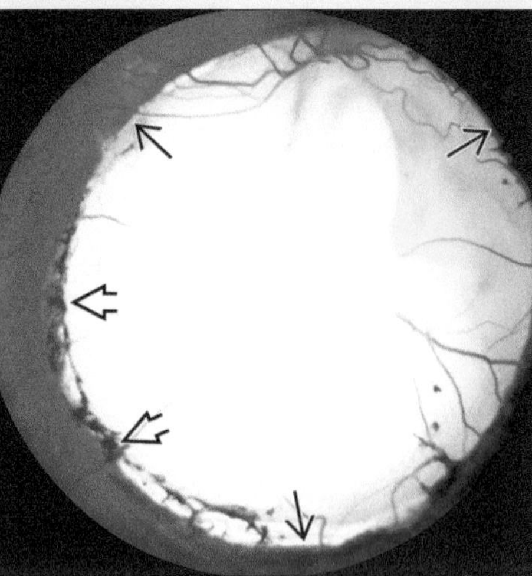

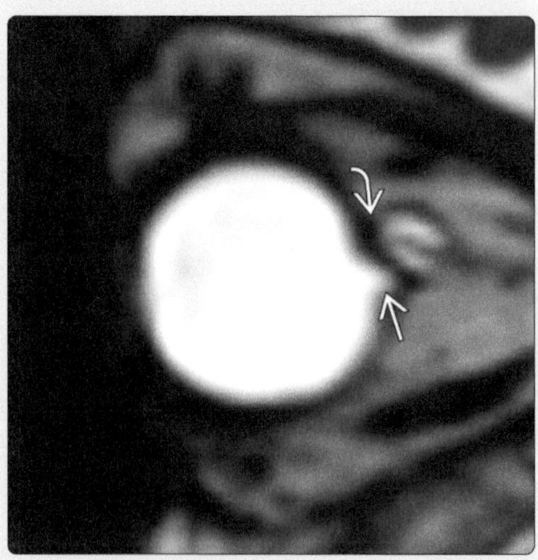

TERMINOLOGY

Abbreviations

- Optic disc coloboma (ODC)
- Choroidoretinal coloboma (CRC)

Definitions

- Coloboma: **Gap** or defect of ocular tissue
- Types of **posterior** coloboma
  - **ODC**: Excavation confined to **optic disc**
  - **CRC**: Defect separate from or extends **beyond disc**
- Related anomalies
  - Morning glory disc anomaly (**MGDA**): Defect with glial tissue & pigmented rim
  - Peripapillary staphyloma (**PPS**): Congenital scleral excavation at optic nerve head
- Other colobomatous lesions
  - May involve any or all structures of **embryonic cleft**
    - Iris, ciliary body, lens, or eyelid
  - Fuchs coloboma
    - Inferiorly tilted disc with crescent-shaped defect along inferonasal margin

IMAGING

General Features

- Best diagnostic clue
  - Focal defect with outpouching at posterior pole of globe; vitreous contiguous with defect
  - **Microphthalmos** & retrobulbar **cysts** often present
- Location
  - Posterior globe (usually inferomedial) at optic **nerve head** insertion
- Size
  - Usually small (few to several mm)
  - MGDA & PPS larger than simple coloboma
- Morphology
  - **Crater-shaped** excavation, contiguous with vitreous
  - Oriented posteriorly with **long axis** of globe
  - MGDA defect funnel-shaped with focal retinal elevation
  - PPS excavation encircles optic disc
- Laterality
  - Unilateral when sporadic, bilateral when syndromic
  - MGDA almost always unilateral, R > L
  - PPS usually unilateral

CT Findings

- NECT
  - Fluid in defect ± retrobulbar cyst **isodense to vitreous**
  - Subretinal hyperdensity if hemorrhage
- Bone CT
  - Ca^{++} may develop at margins of chronic defects

MR Findings

- T1WI & T2WI
  - **Isointense to vitreous**
  - Complex signal if retinal detachment, including hemorrhagic or proteinaceous fluid (T1 hyperintense)
- Prenatal MR
  - Bulging of posterior globe profile
- **MR findings in MGDA**
  - **Primary abnormality** in MGDA: **Uveoscleral coat discontinuity** at optic nerve insertion
    - Normal uveoscleral coat continuous across lamina cribrosa: Curvilinear T2 hypointensity & Gd (+) enhancement of inner choroid (with hypointense nonenhancing outer sclera)
  - **Funnel-shaped optic disc** with adjacent T2 hypointense **retinal surface elevation**
  - **T1 hyperintensity** within **elevated** region of **retina**
  - Less commonly, T1 hyperintense **fat** within adjacent distal **optic nerve sheath**
  - **Abnormal T2 hypointense tissue** associated with adjacent distal intraorbital segment of **optic nerve,** with perioptic CSF **subarachnoid space effacement** here
    - Abnormal tissue: Choroid & peripapillary retina evaginating into perineural space
    - Less commonly, focal **Gd (+) enhancement** of distal **optic nerve region** here thought to represent displaced choroidal tissue along with glial, fibrous, & pigment epithelial proliferation
  - **Variable** developmental irregular **optic nerve thickness**, hypertrophy, & hypoplasia, from orbit to optic chiasm
    - MGDA has rare association with **optic nerve glioma** reported; follow up to exclude this being just developmental thickening
  - Less commonly, **small size of eye globe**
  - Rarely, **retinal detachment**

Ultrasonographic Findings

- Outpouching of posterior globe at optic nerve head
- Hypoechoic retrobulbar mass if cyst present

Imaging Recommendations

- Best imaging tool
  - MR or CT shows globe & extraocular features, especially if defects prevent direct visualization
  - CT provides reasonable depiction without sedation
  - MR of brain helpful if **syndromic** to evaluate for associated **intracranial abnormalities**

DIFFERENTIAL DIAGNOSIS

Congenital Microphthalmos

- Congenital severe ocular derangement
- Deformed small globe with adjacent cyst

Congenital Glaucoma

- Present at birth, usually bilateral
- Enlarged globe

Neurofibromatosis Type 1

- Globe enlargement = buphthalmos
- May have associated optic glioma, sphenoid wing dysplasia, plexiform neurofibroma

Degenerative Staphyloma

- Thinning of posterior sclera-uveal rim
- Enlarged globe, associated with myopia
- Usually off center, temporal to disc (coloboma usually at optic nerve head)

Axial Myopia

- Elongated anteroposterior dimension

PATHOLOGY

General Features

- Etiology
  - Embryologic considerations
    - Embryonic fissure extends along **inferonasal** aspect of optic cup & stalk
    - Fissure fusion (**5th-7th weeks**) required for normal globe & nerve formation
  - Coloboma (ODC/CRC)
    - Failure of embryonic fissure fusion superiorly
  - MGDA
    - Faulty scleral closure (4th week)
    - Mesoectodermal dysgenesis of optic nerve head
  - PPS
    - Incomplete differentiation of sclera
    - Diminished peripapillary structural support
- Genetics
  - **Sporadic** coloboma
    - Noninherited
    - Unilateral; especially isolated ODC
    - Possible maternal environmental factors
  - **Nonsyndromic** coloboma
    - Typically **autosomal dominant**
    - Identified with many specific mutations
      - *PAX2*, *PAX6*, *SHH*, *VSX2* (CHX10), *MAF*, *SOX2*, others
  - **Syndromic** coloboma
    - Usually **autosomal recessive**
    - Typically bilateral, especially CRC
    - Associated with trisomies
    - Dozens of syndromes (CHARGE, Aicardi, papillorenal, COACH, Meckel, Warburg, Lenz)
  - **MGDA**
    - Typically sporadic; rare familial cases
    - Unilateral, except when familial
  - **PPS**
    - Typically sporadic
    - Unilateral, usually isolated anomaly
- Associated abnormalities
  - Triad of major congenital globe anomalies
    - Microphthalmos, anophthalmos, & coloboma (**MAC**)
  - Orbital
    - Microphthalmia; optic tract & chiasm atrophy
    - Retrobulbar **colobomatous cyst**, may be multiple
      - Typically retrobulbar but may project anteriorly
      - May be separate or communicate with globe
    - Retinal detachment (25-40%) (ODC, MGDA)
    - Congenital optic pit (ODC, MGDA)
    - Cataract; hyaloid artery (ODC, MGDA)
    - Iris coloboma (ODC)
    - Persistent hyperplastic primary vitreous, aniridia (MGDA)
  - Systemic
    - Renal, CNS, & many other systemic associations, particularly when bilateral
    - MGDA: **Basal cephaloceles**, moyamoya, callosal agenesis, **craniopharyngeal canal**, hypopituitarism
    - PPS: Usually isolated; rare associated facial lesions, **frontonasal dysplasia**, facial capillary hemangioma

CLINICAL ISSUES

Presentation

- Most common signs/symptoms
  - ↓ **visual acuity** (VA)
- Other signs/symptoms
  - **Leukocoria**
  - Iris involvement causes typical keyhole defect
  - Microphthalmia or anophthalmia in severe cases
  - Associated **syndromic** features
- Clinical profile
  - Vision depends on extent of optic disc involvement & retinal detachment
    - Strabismus & nystagmus secondary to poor VA
    - Reduced visual evoked potentials
- Funduscopic examination
  - ODC
    - Enlarged disc with excavation
    - May resemble glaucomatous cupping
  - CRC
    - White with pigmented margins
    - Extends inferiorly from or inferior to disc
  - MGDA
    - Enlarged, excavated disc; central core of tissue
    - Central tuft of tissue with surrounding ring of pigment; resembles morning glory blossom
  - PPS
    - Central crater with recessed optic nerve
    - Optic disc sunken, otherwise normal; atrophy of surrounding pigment epithelium

Demographics

- Sex
  - No predilection
    - Except MGDA: M < F = 1:2
- Epidemiology
  - Coloboma (nonsyndromic): 1:12,000
  - MGDA & PPS: Rare

Natural History & Prognosis

- VA correlates with retinal status
  - Detachment leads to precipitous vision loss
  - Nerve atrophy & cataracts may lead to more insidious vision loss

Treatment

- Address refractive errors, strabismus, amblyopia
- Retinal detachment management

DIAGNOSTIC CHECKLIST

Consider

- Coloboma is ophthalmoscopic diagnosis
- Imaging confirms ocular features, identifies retrobulbar findings, such as cyst, & evaluates coexistent anomalies

Image Interpretation Pearls

- Look for **syndromic** & systemic associations

SELECTED REFERENCES

1. Nguyen DT et al: Optic nerve abnormalities in morning glory disc anomaly: an MRI study. J Neuroophthalmol. 42(2):199-202, 2022

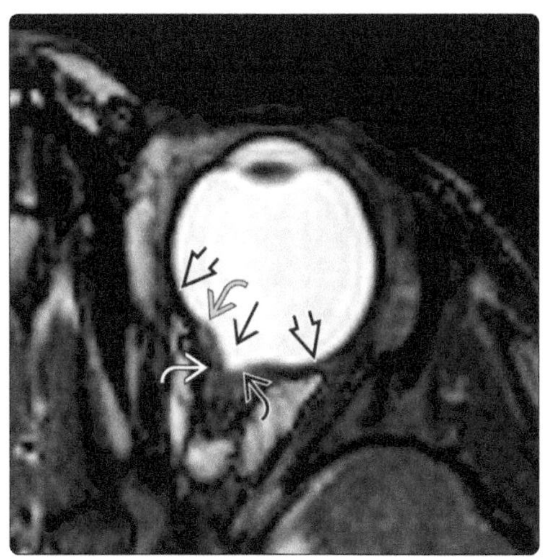

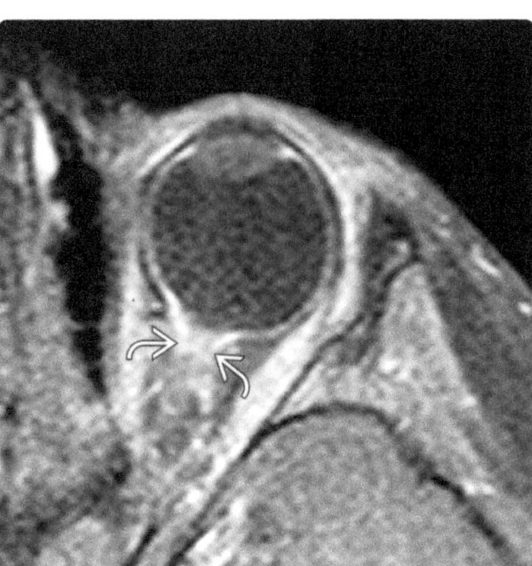

(Left) *Axial T2WI MR of morning glory disc anomaly (MGDA) shows funnel-shaped left optic disc* ➔ *with uveoscleral coat* ➔ *discontinuity at optic nerve insertion site* ➔*. Note the elevated adjacent retinal surface* ➔ *& abnormal tissue* ➔ *along adjacent optic nerve causing focal effacement of perioptic CSF.* **(Right)** *Axial T1 C+ FS MR shows enhancing distal optic nerve region tissue* ➔ *(displaced choroidal tissue/glial, fibrous & pigment epithelial proliferation). (Courtesy Raghu H. Ramakrishnaiah, MD.)*

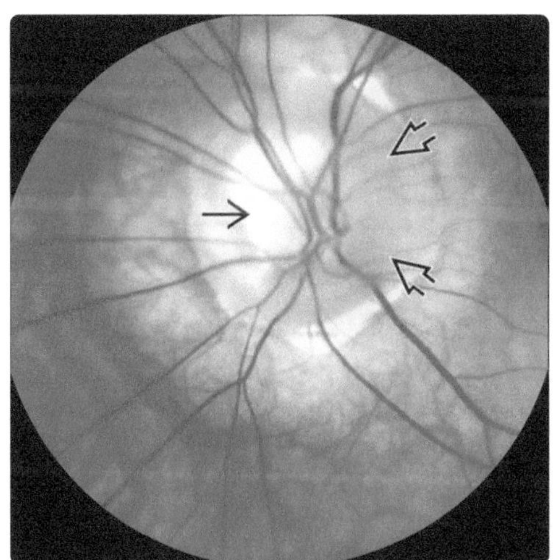

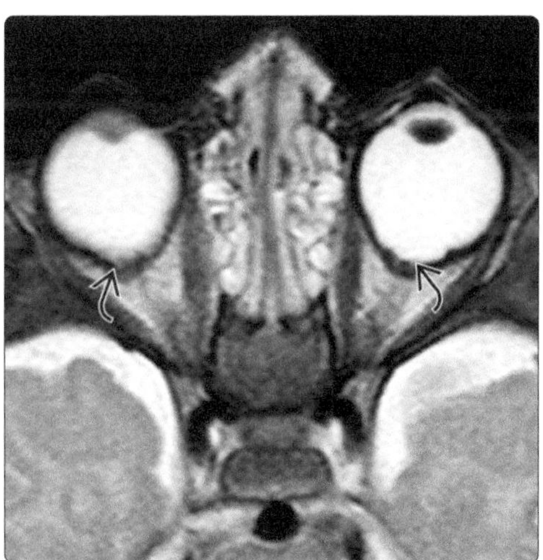

(Left) *Funduscopy in a patient with MGDA shows an enlarged, funnel-shaped optic disc* ➔ *with central glial tissue as well as annular pigmentation* ➔*, resulting in an appearance resembling a morning glory flower.* **(Right)** *Axial T2WI MR in another patient shows bilateral optic nerve head colobomas* ➔*. Do not confuse this with staphyloma, which occurs due to stretching & ectasia of uveoscleral coats & can be seen in glaucoma & high axial myopia. Staphylomas are located off center, typically temporal to the optic disc.*

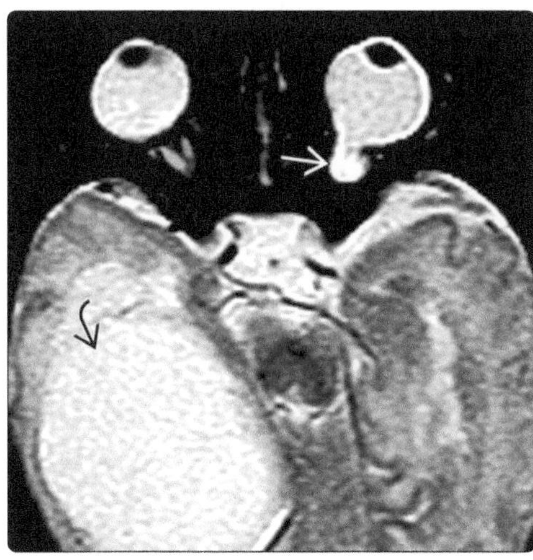

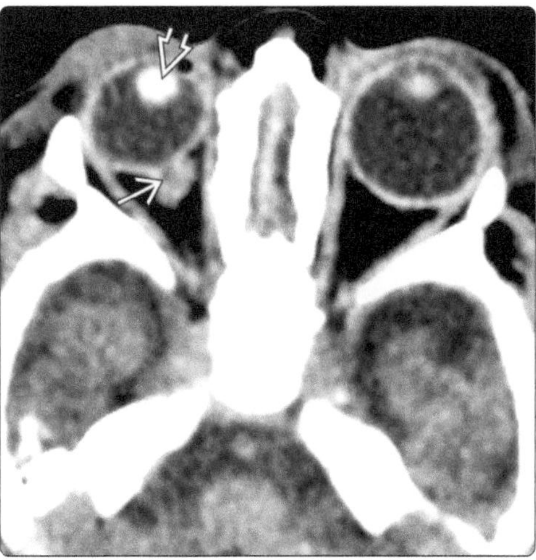

(Left) *Axial STIR MR in a patient with Aicardi syndrome demonstrates a moderate-sized left coloboma* ➔ *at the optic nerve insertion. A large choroid plexus cyst is present* ➔*, a common finding in patients with this X-linked syndrome.* **(Right)** *Axial CECT in a patient with CHARGE syndrome shows a small defect at the posterior pole of the right eye with focal vitreal herniation* ➔*. The right eye is microphthalmic with an abnormal appearance of the lens* ➔*.*

KEY FACTS

TERMINOLOGY

- Synonym: Congenital dacryocystocele

IMAGING

- Well-defined, cystic, medial canthal mass in continuity with enlarged lacrimal sac & nasolacrimal duct (NLD) in newborn
  - Unilateral or bilateral
- Absent or minimal wall enhancement (unless infected)
- Coronal/sagittal reformatted images show continuity of proximal cyst at lacrimal sac with distal inferior meatus cyst through dilated NLD

TOP DIFFERENTIAL DIAGNOSES

- Orbital dermoid & epidermoid
  - Lateral > medial canthus
- Frontoethmoidal (nasoorbital) cephalocele
  - Swelling at inferomedial orbit connected to brain/meninges on imaging
- Acquired dacryocystocele
  - Typically posttraumatic, usually adults

PATHOLOGY

- Tears & mucus accumulate in NLD with imperforate Hasner membrane (i.e., distal duct obstruction)
- Most common abnormality of infant lacrimal apparatus

CLINICAL ISSUES

- Proximal cyst: Small, round, bluish, medial canthal mass identified at birth or shortly after; ± **preseptal** cellulitis
- Distal cyst: Nasal airway obstruction with respiratory distress if bilateral (especially during feeding)

DIAGNOSTIC CHECKLIST

- CT or MR evaluates lacrimal apparatus lesion extent
  - Excludes other sinonasal causes of respiratory distress in newborn
- Comment on full extent of lesion from medial canthus to inferior meatus
- Exclude contralateral lesion

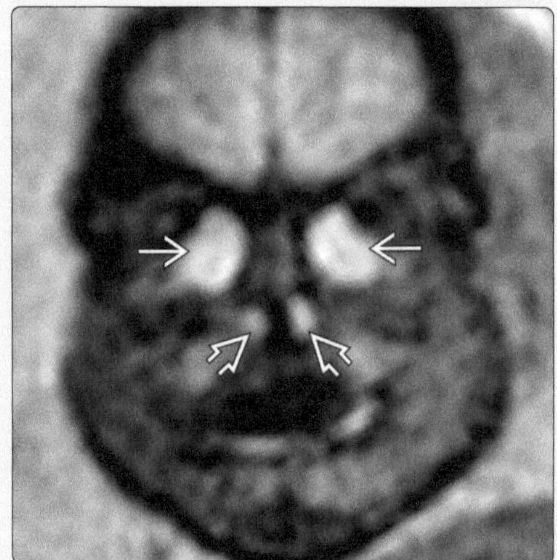

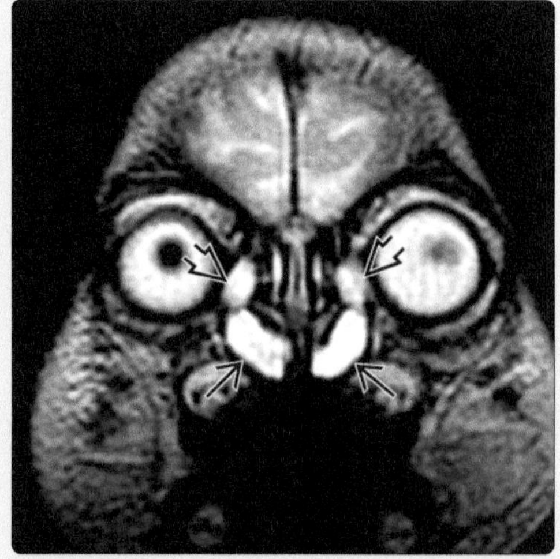

(Left) *Coronal T2 MR SSFSE in a 2nd-trimester fetus demonstrates bilateral lacrimal sac enlargement ➔ with distal extension into each inferior meatus ➔, a typical appearance of nasolacrimal duct mucoceles.* **(Right)** *Coronal T2 MR in an infant shows hyperintense nasolacrimal duct mucoceles extending from the dilated lacrimal sacs ➔ proximally along the nasolacrimal ducts ➔ to project into the inferior meatuses of bilateral nasal cavities.*

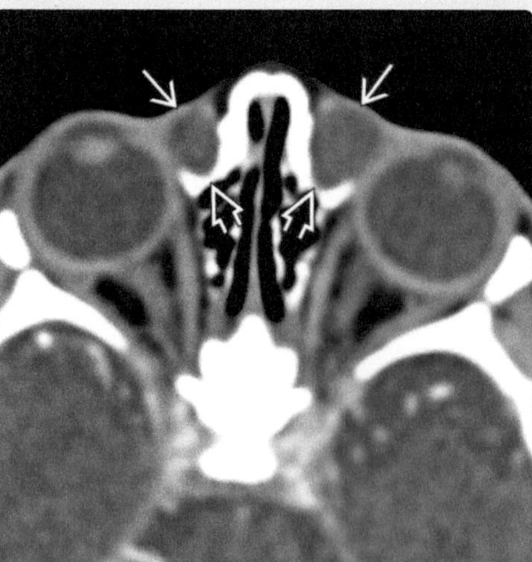

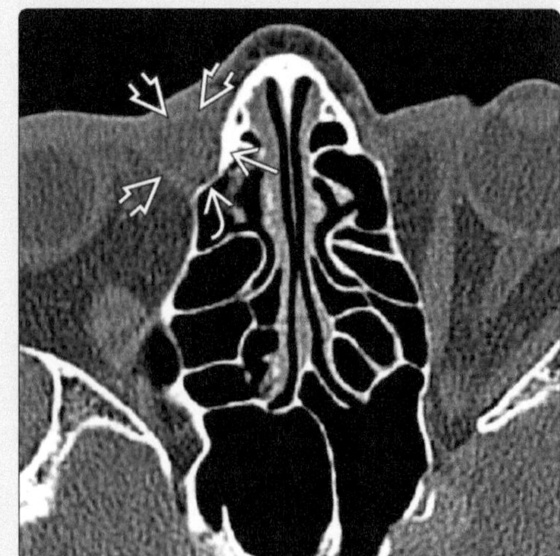

(Left) *Axial CECT in a 4-day-old with bluish, bilateral, medial orbital swelling shows bilateral lacrimal sac enlargement ➔ with splaying of the lacrimal fossae ➔.* **(Right)** *Axial bone CT in an adult with dacryocystocele shows dilated lacrimal sac ➔ in the lacrimal fossa. Lacrimal fossa is formed by thick anterior lacrimal crest (ALC) of frontal process of maxilla ➔ & thin posterior lacrimal crest (PLC) of lacrimal bone ➔. Medial orbital septum attach just posterior to PLC, making the lacrimal fossa & lacrimal sac preseptal structures.*

TERMINOLOGY

Synonyms

- Congenital dacryocystocele

Definitions

- Cystic dilation of nasolacrimal apparatus secondary to obstruction of nasolacrimal duct (NLD)
- Canthus: Corner of eye where eyelids meet

IMAGING

General Features

- Best diagnostic clue
  - Well-defined, cystic, medial canthal mass in continuity with enlarged NLD in newborn
- Location
  - Unilateral or bilateral
  - From lacrimal sac in lacrimal fossa at medial canthus of eye to distal aspect of NLD at inferior meatus
  - Lacrimal fossa formed by thick anterior lacrimal crest (ALC) of frontal process of maxilla & thin posterior lacrimal crest (PLC) of lacrimal bone
  - Medial orbital septum (& check ligament of medial rectus muscle) attach just posterior to PLC
    - Lacrimal fossa & lacrimal sac **preseptal** structures
  - Lacrimal sac lies within lacrimal fossa & is invested by superficial & deep parts of orbicularis oculi muscle
  - Lacrimal sac below medial canthal tendon not covered by orbicularis oculi muscle, hence potential weakness site for intraorbital spread of infection

CT Findings

- Hypodense, thin-walled cyst at medial canthus ± bulging cystic component at inferior meatus
  - Cysts communicate through enlarged NLD
- Minimal wall enhancement normally; thick rim enhancement ± fluid/debris level if infected

MR Findings

- T1-hypo-/T2-hyperintense, well-circumscribed mass(es)
- Signal intensity varies with protein content &/or infection
- Minimal wall enhancement normally
- If inflamed/infected → thick rim of enhancement with surrounding poorly defined soft tissue stranding

Imaging Recommendations

- Best imaging tool
  - Thin-section bone CT
  - ± contrast (for better soft tissue characterization)

DIFFERENTIAL DIAGNOSIS

Orbital Dermoid & Epidermoid

- Lateral > medial canthus
- Near suture: Frontozygomatic > frontonasal/nasolacrimal
- 50% show fat density/intensity with thin rim enhancement

Frontoethmoidal (Nasoorbital) Cephalocele

- Swelling at inferomedial orbit connected to brain/meninges

Acquired Dacryocystocele

- Typically in adults with history of prior regional trauma

PATHOLOGY

General Features

- Etiology
  - Tears & mucus accumulate in NLD due to distal **imperforate Hasner membrane** at distal duct
  - Distended lacrimal sac may compress lacrimal canaliculi, which bend on themselves → trapdoor obstruction
    - Massage cannot decompress lacrimal sac
    - Indicates dual obstruction of proximal canalicular-punctal system & distal inferior lacrimal system

CLINICAL ISSUES

Presentation

- Most common signs/symptoms
  - Small, round, bluish, medial canthal mass identified at or shortly after birth = distended lacrimal sac
  - Nasal airway obstruction & respiratory distress (especially during feeding) with bilateral nasal components
    - Obligate nose breathers during infancy
- Other signs/symptoms
  - Tearing & crusting at medial canthus, preseptal cellulitis, dacryocystitis

Demographics

- Age
  - Infancy: Typically 4 days to 10 weeks
- Sex
  - M < F (1:3)
- Epidemiology
  - 3rd most common etiology in neonatal nasal obstruction
    - 1st = mucosal edema, 2nd = choanal atresia

Natural History & Prognosis

- 90% of simple distal NLD obstructions (or congenital dacryostenosis) resolve spontaneously by age 1

Treatment

- Lacrimal fossa & sac **preseptal** in location; antibiotics for acute dacryocystitis with preseptal cellulitis
- Postseptal orbital cellulitis from dacryocystitis requiring surgical debridement rare
- Daily manual massage ± prophylactic antibiotics
  - Manual massage inappropriate if NLD mucocele infected or causing airway obstruction
- 10% require probing with irrigation ± silastic stent
- If endonasal component & no response to above → endoscopic resection with marsupialization
- Theoretical risk of nasolacrimal apparatus scarring, amblyopia, & permanent canthal asymmetry if untreated

DIAGNOSTIC CHECKLIST

Image Interpretation Pearls

- Comment on full extent of lesion from medial canthus to inferior meatus, bilaterality, & signs of infection

SELECTED REFERENCES

1. Pur DR et al: Management of congenital dacryocystocele: a case series and literature review. J Pediatr Ophthalmol Strabismus. 60(3):e31-4, 2023

Orbital Dermoid and Epidermoid

KEY FACTS

TERMINOLOGY

- Congenital orbital ectodermal inclusion lesion resulting in choristomatous cyst
- Dermoid: Includes dermal appendages
- Epidermoid: Dermal adnexal structures absent

IMAGING

- Cystic, well-demarcated, extraconal mass with lipid, fluid, or mixed contents
- Adjacent to orbital periosteum, near suture lines
- Superolateral at frontozygomatic suture most common
- May contain debris or fluid levels
- Osseous remodeling in majority of lesions with smooth, scalloped margins and thinning or dehiscence
- Distinguishing features
  - Dermoid: Typically but not exclusively contains fat; more heterogeneous, complex signal on MR, DWI variable
  - Epidermoid: Density and intensity similar to fluid; more homogeneous; diffusion restriction on MR

TOP DIFFERENTIAL DIAGNOSES

- Dermolipoma
- Frontal or ethmoid sinus mucocele
- Lacrimal gland cyst

PATHOLOGY

- Congenital inclusion of trapped ectoderm at suture site
- Fibrous capsule lined by squamous epithelium

CLINICAL ISSUES

- Firm, nontender mass, fixed to underling bone
- Slowly progressive; may rupture with acute inflammation
- Presentation typically in childhood; deeper lesions in adults
- Surgical resection curative

DIAGNOSTIC CHECKLIST

- Features distinctive, but deep or inflamed lesions may present diagnostic challenge
- Fat presence essentially pathognomonic for dermoid cyst

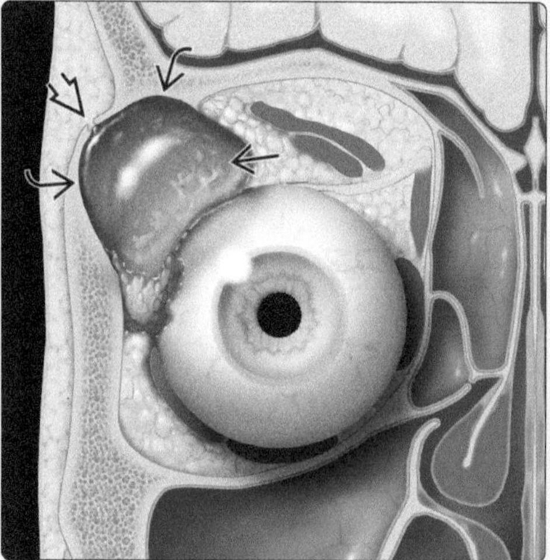

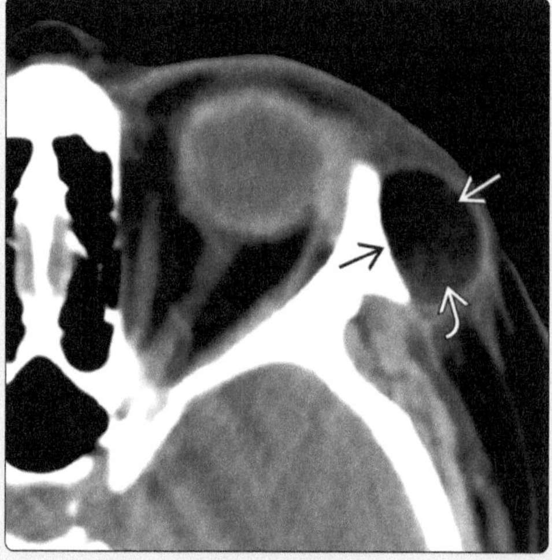

(Left) *Coronal graphic depicts a superotemporal dermoid cyst → located adjacent to the frontozygomatic suture of the right orbit →. There is resultant mass effect on the globe with remodeling of the bony orbit →.* **(Right)** *Axial NECT shows an ovoid mass in the temporal fossa adjacent to the lateral orbit near the "frontozygomatic" suture →. This dermoid cyst shows fat density with slightly more dense debris layering dependently →. Note the broad, scalloped remodeling of the adjacent bone →.*

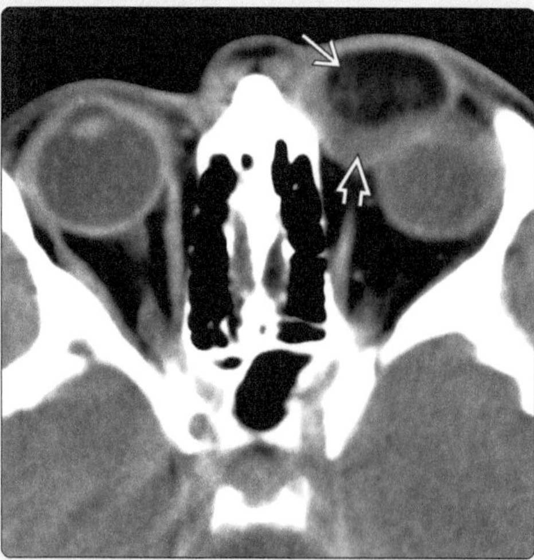

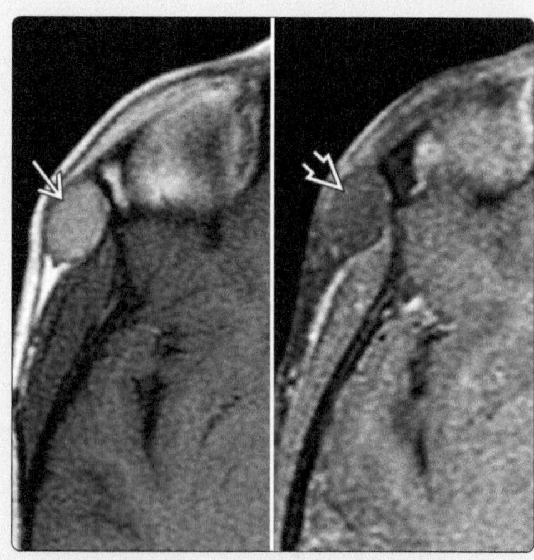

(Left) *Axial NECT shows a dermoid cyst → located medially in the orbit, near the location of the "frontolacrimal" suture. The cyst has fat-density contents as well as dependent soft tissue density debris →.* **(Right)** *Axial MR shows a right "pterional" dermoid cyst lateral to the orbit in the temporal fossa on T1 noncontrast → and T1 fat-saturated postcontrast → MR. Signal suppression with fat saturation indicates lipid content.*

TERMINOLOGY

Synonyms

- Congenital orbital **ectodermal inclusion cyst**

Definitions

- Cystic, **choristomatous** mass lesion of orbit resulting from congenital epithelial **inclusion**
- Dermoid lesions
  - Epithelial elements + dermal substructure, including **dermal appendages**
- Epidermoid lesions
  - Epithelial elements **without adnexal structures**

IMAGING

General Features

- Best diagnostic clue
  - Cystic, well-demarcated, anterosuperior extraconal mass with **lipid, fluid,** or **mixed contents**
- Location
  - Adjacent to orbital periosteum, near **suture lines**
  - Majority extraconal in **superolateral** aspect of anterior orbit, at **frontozygomatic** suture (65-75%)
  - Remainder mostly in **superonasal** aspect, at frontolacrimal suture, but can occur anywhere
- Size
  - Typically < 1-2 cm in superficial lesions
  - Larger in deep, complicated lesions
- Morphology
  - Ovoid, **well-demarcated** cystic mass
  - Most show thin, definable wall (75%)
  - No nodular soft tissue outside cyst (80%)
- Subtypes
  - **Superficial** (simple, exophytic)
    - Typically smaller, discrete, rounded
    - Present in early childhood
  - **Deep** (complicated, endophytic)
    - More insidious, extensive bony changes
    - Rarely intradiploic
- Contents
  - Lipid components evident in 40-50% of lesions
  - May contain mixed **fluid** or **debris**
  - **Fluid-fluid levels** in 5-10% of lesions
- Distinguishing features
  - Dermoid: Typically but not exclusively contains **fat**; more heterogeneous
  - Epidermoid: Density and intensity similar to **fluid**; more homogeneous

Radiographic Findings

- Radiography
  - Scalloped bony lucency with sclerotic margins

CT Findings

- NECT
  - **Hypodense fat** in ~ 1/2
    - Density -30 to -80 HU
  - **Calcification** in 15%
    - Fine or punctate, in cyst wall
- CECT
  - Mild, thin rim enhancement
  - Irregular margins and enhancement indicate rupture with inflammatory reaction
- Bone CT
  - **Osseous remodeling** in majority of lesions (85%)
    - Pressure excavation; smooth, **scalloped** margins
    - **Thinning** of bone, may cause focal dehiscence
    - Bony tunnel, cleft, or pit in up to 1/3, leading to dumbbell appearance

MR Findings

- T1WI
  - Strongly **hyperintense** if **fatty** contents
  - Isointense or slightly hyperintense otherwise
- T2WI
  - Isointense or mildly hypointense
  - Heterogeneous **debris**
  - May show fluid-fluid levels
- DWI
  - Epidermoid shows diffusion restriction
    - Spatial restriction of diffusion of water molecules between keratin layers within cyst
  - Dermoid cysts DWI variable depending upon contents; may or may not restrict diffusion
    - Ectodermal components, such as fat and hair, may cause decreased water diffusion within cyst
- T1WI C+
  - Thin **rim enhancement**
  - More extensive **inflammation if ruptured**
- Fat-saturation techniques
  - Dermoid shows **suppression** of lipid signal

Ultrasonographic Findings

- Grayscale ultrasound
  - Adequate for evaluation of simple superficial lesions without posterior extension
  - High internal **reflectivity**, variable attenuation
  - Debris may impair determination of cystic nature

Imaging Recommendations

- Best imaging tool
  - CT without contrast often adequate for diagnosis
- Protocol advice
  - Pursue MR with contrast if features not characteristic, particularly with lesion growth

DIFFERENTIAL DIAGNOSIS

Orbital Dermolipoma

- Clinical: Soft, solid, lateral canthus mass
- Imaging: Homogeneous episcleral fat

Frontal or Ethmoid Sinus Mucocele

- Clinical: Chronic obstructive sinusitis
- Imaging: Expansile, obstructed sinus space

Lacrimal Gland Cyst

- Clinical: Lacrimal swelling and inflammation
- Imaging: Fluid density and intensity within gland

Orbital Cellulitis

- Clinical: May mimic ruptured dermoid

- Imaging: Preseptal or intraorbital infiltration

Orbital Rhabdomyosarcoma

- Clinical: Enlarging orbital mass in child
- Imaging: Variably enhancing, aggressive orbital mass

Lacrimal Gland Neoplasm

- Clinical: Minor salivary tumors
  - Pleomorphic adenoma; adenoid cystic carcinoma
- Imaging: Benign or invasive lacrimal mass with **enhancing solid components**

PATHOLOGY

General Features

- Etiology
  - **Congenital inclusion** of dermal elements
  - Sequestration of trapped surface **ectoderm**
  - Typically at site of embryonic **suture** closure
  - Acquired epidermoid may occur after remote surgery or trauma (**implantation** cyst)

Gross Pathologic & Surgical Features

- Tethered to orbital **periosteum** by fibrovascular tissue
- Oily or cheesy tan, yellow, or white material

Microscopic Features

- Dermoid
  - **Sebaceous** glands and hair **follicles**, blood vessels, **fat**, and collagen; sweat glands in minority (20%)
  - Contains keratin, sebaceous secretions, lipid metabolites, and hair
- Epidermoid
  - **No adnexal** structures
  - Filled with **keratinaceous** debris and cholesterol

CLINICAL ISSUES

Presentation

- Most common signs/symptoms
  - Firm, rounded mass at **lateral eyebrow**
  - **Nontender**, slowly progressive
- Other signs/symptoms
  - Painless in 90% but **inflamed if ruptured**
    - May rarely present as orbital cellulitis
  - Relatively **fixed** to underlying bone
- Clinical profile
  - Childhood presentation
    - More common than adult
    - **Subcutaneous** nodule near orbital rim
    - Smaller, little globe displacement
  - May present with **rupture** (10-15%)
    - Secondary to **trauma** or **spontaneous**
    - Acute inflammation **mimics cellulitis** or inflammatory tumor
    - Can result in entrapment, neuropathy
  - Mass effect if very large
    - Diplopia due to restricted movement
    - Compromise of globe or optic nerve

Demographics

- Age
  - Usually presents in **childhood** and teenage years
  - Simple, superficial lesions often present in infancy
  - May present or **grow at any age**
  - Occasionally will appear in adult and grow significantly over several months
- Sex
  - Equal or slight male predominance
- Epidemiology
  - Most common noninflammatory, nonneoplastic, space-occupying lesion of orbit
    - 1/2 of childhood orbital lesions
    - 90% of cystic orbital lesions
  - 10% of head and neck dermoid and epidermoid cysts periorbital in location

Natural History & Prognosis

- Benign lesion, usually cosmetic considerations
- Very **slow growth**, usually dormant for years
  - Present during childhood but small and dormant
  - May become symptomatic during **rapid growth** phase in **young adult**
- Sudden growth or change following **rupture**
  - Significant **inflammation** and increased size
- Dermoid cysts along scalp midline have higher potential of intracranial extension
- Dermoid cysts in more lateral areas of skull/scalp rarely associated with intracranial extension
  - But temporal dermoid cysts have higher rate of intracranial extension

Treatment

- **Surgical resection** curative
  - Entire cyst must be removed to prevent recurrence
    - Including growth center at periosteal interface
  - **Brow** or **eyelid crease** incision most common
    - Approach depends on location in orbit
  - Lesions evident in early childhood should be removed to avoid traumatic rupture
- Steroids or nonsteroidal drugs to calm inflammation in ruptured lesions
- Asymptomatic small lesions may be observed expectantly
  - Particularly small epidermoid with less inflammatory response in event of rupture

DIAGNOSTIC CHECKLIST

Consider

- Features of typical lesions distinctive, but deep or inflamed lesions may present diagnostic challenge
- Dermoid cyst distinct from dermolipoma

Image Interpretation Pearls

- Presence of fat essentially **pathognomonic**
- Posterior extent of **complex lesions** may not be clinically apparent; therefore, imaging is warranted

SELECTED REFERENCES

1. Menousek JP et al: A unique case of frontotemporal dermoid cyst presenting as orbital cellulitis. Cureus. 15(4):e37050, 2023
2. Oh HJ et al: Craniofacial epidermoid and dermoid cysts. J Craniofac Surg. ePub, 2023
3. Lee BG et al: Intradiploic epidermoid cyst of the orbital roof: a case report. Orbit. 1-3, 2018

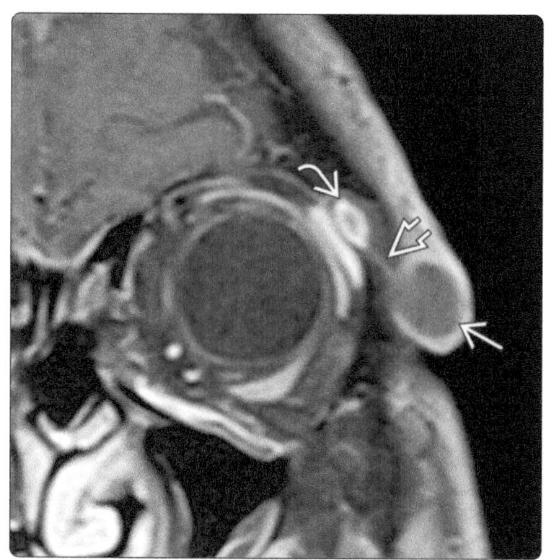

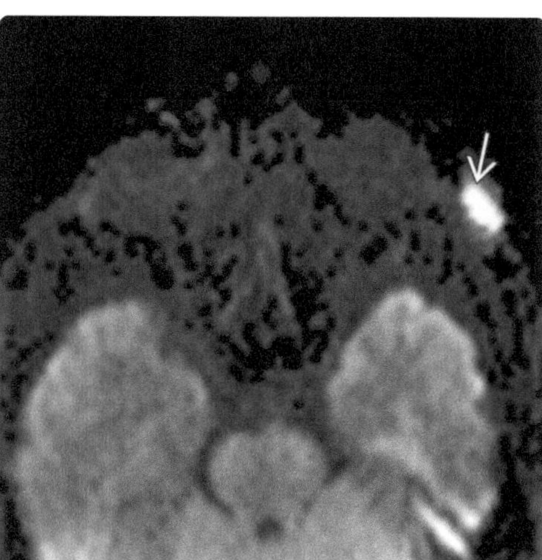

(Left) *Coronal T1 postcontrast MR shows an epidermoid cyst with thin marginal enhancement ➡ lateral to the left orbital rim. A smaller intraorbital component is seen along the inner margin of the orbital wall ➡ with scalloping of the bone at the lacrimal fossa. A small connecting stalk is visible near the frontozygomatic suture ➡.* **(Right)** *Axial DWI MR shows diffusion restriction in the same lesion at the left lateral orbital rim ➡, suggesting an epidermoid cyst. Note that dermoid cysts may sometimes restrict diffusion.*

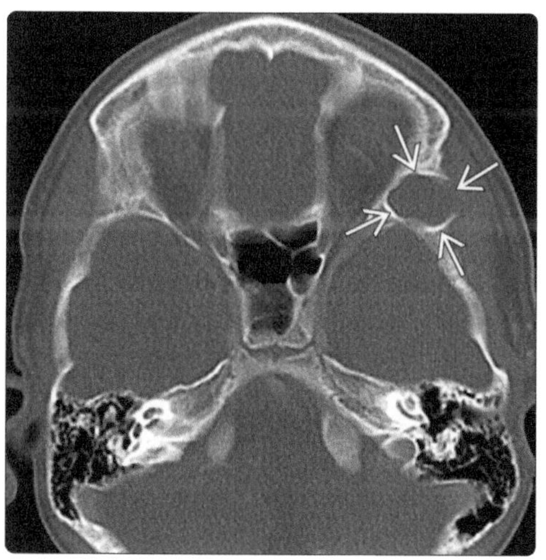

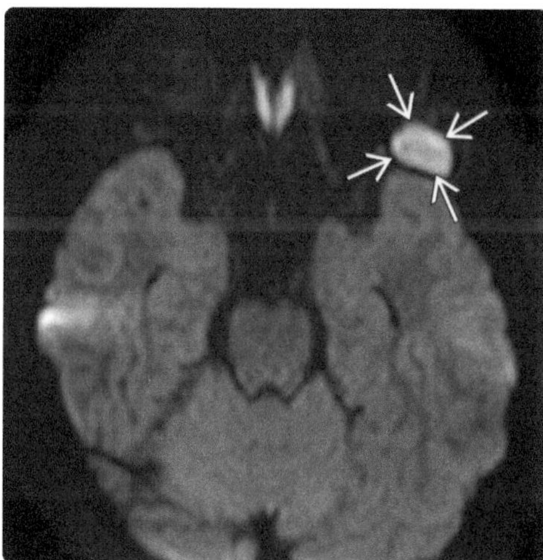

(Left) *Axial NECT bone window shows a left pterional expansile intradiploic dermoid cyst ➡ lateral to the orbit, projecting toward the temporal fossa. No definite fatty contents are detected on imaging.* **(Right)** *Axial DWI MR in the same patient shows diffusion restriction ➡ of the cyst contents. Even though the presence of diffusion restriction and the absence of fatty contents should favor epidermoid, this lesion was proven to be a dermoid cyst. Remember, dermoid cysts may also restrict diffusion.*

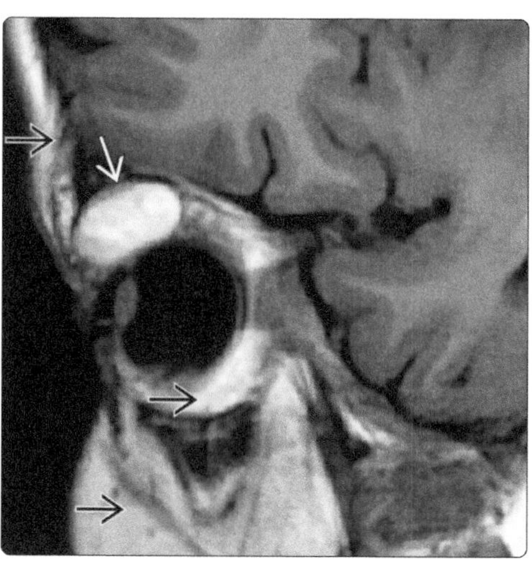

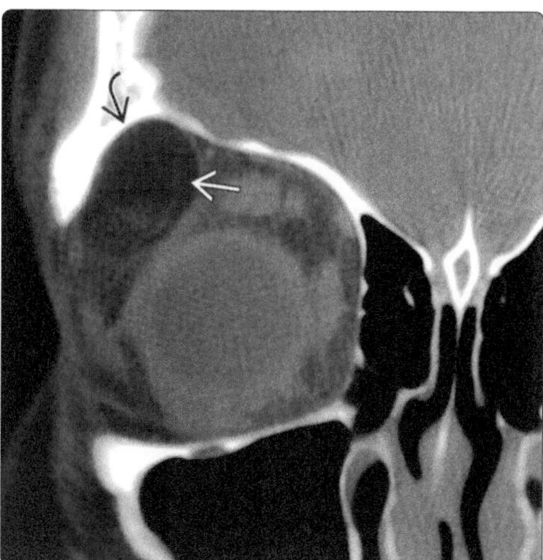

(Left) *Sagittal oblique unenhanced T1 MR without fat suppression shows a hyperintense superior orbital dermoid cyst ➡ due to fatty contents. Note similar signal intensity of normal fat in the scalp, orbit, and face ➡. If T1 hyperintensity is due to proteinaceous or hemorrhagic contents, it will not suppress in fat-saturated sequences.* **(Right)** *Coronal CT shows a lipid-containing dermoid cyst in superotemporal quadrant of the right orbit ➡. Smooth scalloping of the adjacent bony orbit ➡ suggests a longstanding benign lesion.*

KEY FACTS

TERMINOLOGY

- Preseptal cellulitis: Infection anterior to orbital septum
- Postseptal cellulitis: Infection posterior to orbital septum
- Orbital septum: Periosteal reflection of bony orbit → upper lid levator aponeurosis & lower lid tarsal plate

IMAGING

- Thickening & edema of orbital/periorbital soft tissues
- Preseptal cellulitis: Limited to anterior tissues
- Postseptal cellulitis
  - Low-attenuation, rim-enhancing collection
    - Drainable subperiosteal abscess (SPA) in majority
    - 20% without drainable abscess (phlegmon)
  - Associated myositis is common with swollen extraocular muscles, ± abnormal enhancement
  - ± thrombosed superior ophthalmic vein
- ± extraorbital complications of sinusitis
  - Frontal osteomyelitis, meningitis, subdural/epidural effusion or empyema, cerebritis, parenchymal abscess

TOP DIFFERENTIAL DIAGNOSES

- Idiopathic orbital inflammation
- Langerhans cell histiocytosis
- Orbital soft tissue or osseous neoplasm
  - Rhabdomyosarcoma
  - Metastatic neuroblastoma
- Orbital vascular anomaly
  - Infantile hemangioma
  - Venous malformation

PATHOLOGY

- Preseptal/periorbital cellulitis: Typically due to trauma (skin infection, insect bites, etc.)
- Postseptal cellulitis: Most common cause is sinusitis

CLINICAL ISSUES

- Treatment: Intravenous antibiotics ± sinus drainage procedures, SPA drainage

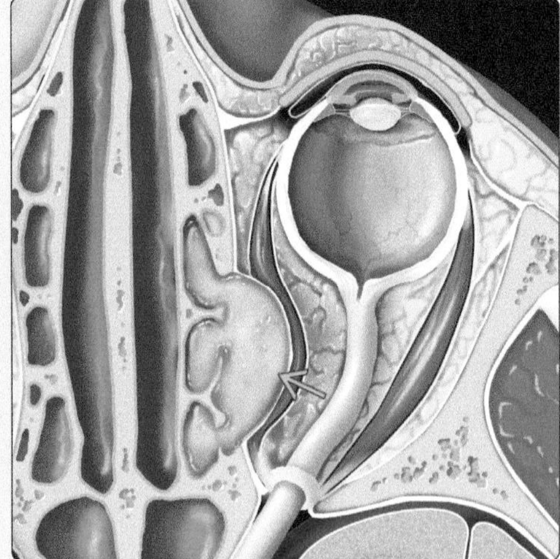

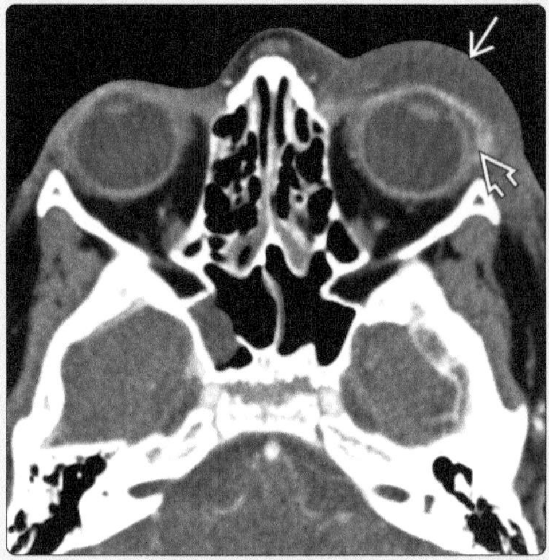

(Left) *Axial graphic shows the spread of infection from the ethmoid sinuses through the lamina papyracea into the medial orbit, resulting in a subperiosteal abscess (SPA) ⇨ that places the optic nerve at risk.* **(Right)** *Axial CECT in a 7-year-old with neutropenia & left eyelid swelling demonstrates marked preseptal periorbital soft tissue edema ➡. There is a low-attenuation crescent with rim enhancement marginating the anterolateral globe ➡, consistent with chemosis. The postseptal orbit is normal.*

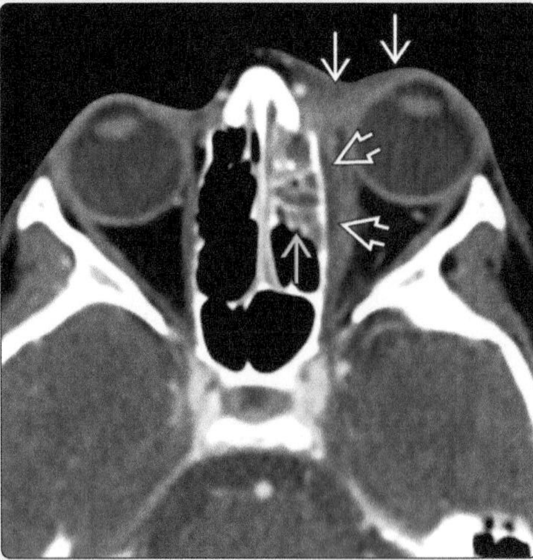

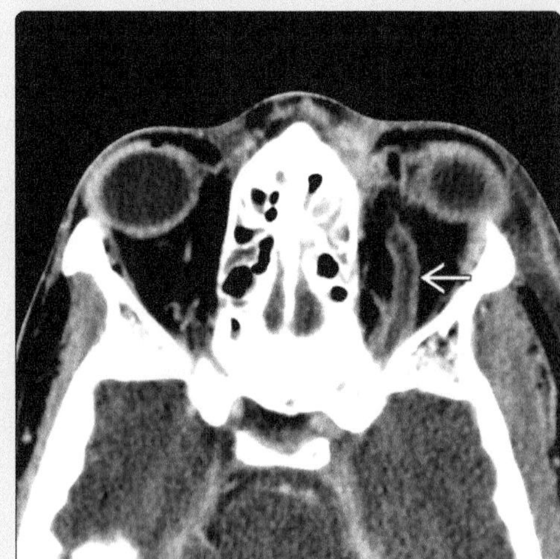

(Left) *Axial CECT in a 6-year-old boy demonstrates moderate preseptal cellulitis ➡, a medial subperiosteal fluid collection ➡ deviating the left medial rectus muscle, & ipsilateral left ethmoid sinus disease ⇨, which is the typical cause of postseptal inflammation. There is also mild associated proptosis.* **(Right)** *Axial CECT shows diffuse enlargement & lack of central enhancement in a thrombosed left superior ophthalmic vein ➡. There is associated ethmoid sinus disease with preseptal & postseptal orbital cellulitis.*

TERMINOLOGY

Definitions

- Preseptal cellulitis: Inflammation anterior to orbital septum
- Postseptal cellulitis: Inflammation posterior to orbital septum
- Orbital septum: Periosteal reflection bony orbit → upper lid levator aponeurosis & lower lid tarsal plate

IMAGING

General Features

- Best diagnostic clue
  - Thickening & edema of periorbital &/or orbital soft tissues = cellulitis
  - Low-attenuation, rim-enhancing subperiosteal collection in medial or superior orbit
    - Drainable subperiosteal abscess (SPA) in majority
    - Phlegmon in 20% without drainable abscess
- Location
  - Preseptal: Disease limited to periorbital soft tissues, anterior to orbital septum
  - Postseptal: Disease posterior to orbital septum
    - Intraconal: Within cone formed by extraocular muscles (EOMs)
    - Extraconal: Between bony orbit & EOMs
    - Subperiosteal: Between bony orbit & orbital periosteum
    - Associated myositis is common
      - ▫ Swollen EOMs ± abnormal enhancement
  - ± extraorbital complications of sinusitis
    - Frontal osteomyelitis, meningitis, subdural/epidural effusion or empyema, cerebritis, parenchymal abscess

CT Findings

- CECT
  - Infiltration of periorbital &/or intraorbital fat with poorly defined diffuse mild enhancement
  - ± focal elongated/lentiform rim-enhancing SPA or intraorbital abscess
    - Medial > > superior orbit
    - ± foci of gas in abscess
  - ± EOM enlargement due to myositis; EOM deviation by inflammatory collections
  - ± enlarged, centrally nonenhancing superior ophthalmic vein due to thrombosis
  - Careful review of anterior & middle cranial fossae for fluid collection or findings of parenchymal edema

MR Findings

- T1: Hypointense infiltration of normal fat
- T2 FS: Heterogeneous hyperintensity of fat ± fluid in focal collection
- DWI: Restricted diffusion suggests abscess
- T1 C+ FS: Heterogeneous enhancement of inflamed tissues ± rim-enhancing SPA

Imaging Recommendations

- Best imaging tool
  - CECT: Axial & coronal reformatted images
  - MR with contrast: Best for evaluation of intracranial complications of sinusitis

DIFFERENTIAL DIAGNOSIS

Idiopathic Orbital Inflammation

- Acute to subacute orbital pain, swelling, restricted motion, diplopia, proptosis, & impaired vision
- Poorly marginated, mass-like, enhancing soft tissue involving any region of orbit
  - Unilateral or bilateral

Langerhans Cell Histiocytosis

- Classic punched-out round or geographic lytic bone lesion
- Bone lesion is often filled with homogeneously enhancing soft tissue mass ± intra- & extracranial extension

Orbital Neoplasm

- Variably enhancing mass originating in bone or soft tissues
- Bone-centered lesions (primary or metastatic) show aggressive permeative destruction & periosteal reaction, particularly in superolateral orbit
  - Metastatic neuroblastoma: Perpendicular radiating spicules of new bone; may show mild osseous expansion
- Soft tissue neoplasms are often well defined without surrounding edema

Orbital Vascular Anomaly

- Infantile hemangioma
  - Well-circumscribed, lobular, diffusely enhancing mass
  - Superficial lesions typically show characteristic cutaneous features (raised red "strawberry mark")
    - Appear in 1st days-weeks of life with rapid growth prior to gradual involution
- Venous malformation
  - Infiltrative pre- &/or postseptal fluid signal lesion with septated mass-like components &/or tubular channels
  - ± fluid-fluid levels, low-signal thrombi, patchy gradual enhancement
  - ± bluish skin discoloration that bulges with Valsalva
    - Present at birth
    - May ↑ at puberty/pregnancy or with thrombosis

PATHOLOGY

General Features

- Etiology
  - Most common causes of preseptal or periorbital cellulitis
    - Trauma (skin infection, insect bites, foreign body), sinusitis, & primary bacteremia (< 36 months of age)
  - Most common cause of postseptal cellulitis: Sinusitis
    - Up to 3% of sinusitis patients develop cellulitis (most common complication)
      - ▫ May precede signs & symptoms of sinusitis
      - ▫ Usually secondary to ethmoiditis
    - Spread of sinus infection to orbit
      - ▫ Direct extension via thin bone with acquired dehiscence &/or normal foramina in lamina papyracea
      - ▫ Valveless venous system (diploic veins of Breschet) connects orbital circulation with ethmoid, frontal, & maxillary sinus circulation
    - Occasional underlying cause of sinusitis
      - ▫ Antrochoanal polyp
      - ▫ Sinonasal foreign body

- Odontogenic sinusitis
  - Other causes: Nasolacrimal duct mucocele or dacryocystocele may lead to periorbital cellulitis; retinoblastoma rarely presents as periorbital cellulitis
- Associated abnormalities
  - Superior ophthalmic vein &/or cavernous sinus thrombosis
    - Expanded with central heterogeneous or nonenhancing thrombus
  - Frontal osteomyelitis (Pott puffy tumor)
    - Forehead cellulitis, phlegmon ± subgaleal abscess
    - Frontal bone lytic lesion may be difficult to detect
  - Meningitis
    - ± abnormal meningeal contrast enhancement
      - Absence of enhancement does not exclude meningitis with clinical suspicion
  - Effusions
    - Epidural (lenticular) or subdural (crescentic) fluid collections without rim enhancement or restricted diffusion
  - Empyema
    - Epidural (lenticular) or subdural (crescentic) collection of pus
    - Usually shows peripheral dural enhancement
    - Restricted diffusion on MR (↑ signal on DWI with ↓ signal on ADC map)
  - Cerebritis
    - Amorphous parenchymal edema without rim-enhancing collection
  - Brain abscess
    - Round or ovoid collection of pus within brain
    - Ring-enhancing wall may be thicker superficially; ± low T2 signal rim on MR
    - Hyperintense DWI, hypointense ADC on MR

Staging, Grading, & Classification

- Chandler classification: Orbital complications of sinusitis
  - Preseptal cellulitis
    - Inflammation anterior to orbital septum
    - Eyelid edema
    - No tenderness, visual loss, or impaired EOM motility (ophthalmoplegia)
  - Orbital cellulitis without abscess
    - Diffuse postseptal edema of orbital fat
  - Orbital cellulitis with SPA
    - ± proptosis, impaired vision, or ophthalmoplegia
  - Orbital cellulitis with abscess in orbital fat
    - Usually severe proptosis, ↓ vision, & ophthalmoplegia
  - Cavernous sinus thrombosis secondary to orbital phlebitis: Unilateral or bilateral

CLINICAL ISSUES

Presentation

- Most common signs/symptoms
  - Depends on degree of inflammation
    - Fever, eyelid swelling, erythema, tenderness, chemosis, proptosis, ophthalmoplegia resulting in diplopia, ↓ visual acuity
- Other signs/symptoms
  - Cranial nerve palsies (III-VI) with cavernous sinus thrombosis
  - Seizures, mental status changes with intracranial complications

Demographics

- 50% of affected children < 4 years of age

Natural History & Prognosis

- Excellent with appropriate treatment
- Rare cause of blindness if untreated

Treatment

- Medical management: Intravenous antibiotics
- Surgical management
  - Chandler classification + imaging characteristics ↑ ability to predict surgical need
  - SPA: Not absolute surgical indication
    - Younger children may only require antibiotics with more aggressive surgical drainage in older children
    - Emergent surgery if visual disturbance develops from optic nerve or retinal compromise
  - Drainage of orbital fat abscess
  - Sinus drainage procedures
  - Intracranial empyema is classically considered surgical emergency, particularly with neurologic signs/symptoms
    - Collection may resolve with antibiotics

DIAGNOSTIC CHECKLIST

Consider

- Imaging indications: CECT
  - Impairment in visual acuity or ophthalmoplegia
  - No improvement or worsening of symptoms on appropriate antibiotics
  - Severe eyelid edema prohibiting evaluation of vision & EOM motility
- Imaging indications: MR with contrast
  - Suspected intracranial complications
    - Fluid collection is presumed infected if neurologic symptoms (seizure, altered mental status) are present
    - Clinical & CT findings may dictate operative intervention before MR

Image Interpretation Pearls

- Distinguishing SPA from phlegmon may be difficult
- Cavernous sinus thrombosis may be subtle
- Look for underlying cause of sinusitis & extraorbital complications

SELECTED REFERENCES

1. Winegar BA: Imaging of painful ophthalmologic disorders. Neurol Clin. 40(3):641-60, 2022
2. Nagaraj UD et al: Imaging of orbital infectious and inflammatory disease in children. Pediatr Radiol. 51(7):1149-61, 2021
3. Santos JC et al: Pediatric preseptal and orbital cellulitis: a 10-year experience. Int J Pediatr Otorhinolaryngol. 120:82-8, 2019
4. Jabarin B et al: Indicators for imaging in periorbital cellulitis secondary to rhinosinusitis. Eur Arch Otorhinolaryngol. 275(4):943-8, 2018
5. Wong SJ et al: Management of pediatric orbital cellulitis: a systematic review. Int J Pediatr Otorhinolaryngol. 110:123-9, 2018
6. Le TD et al: The effect of adding orbital computed tomography findings to the Chandler criteria for classifying pediatric orbital cellulitis in predicting which patients will require surgical intervention. J AAPOS. 18(3):271-7, 2014

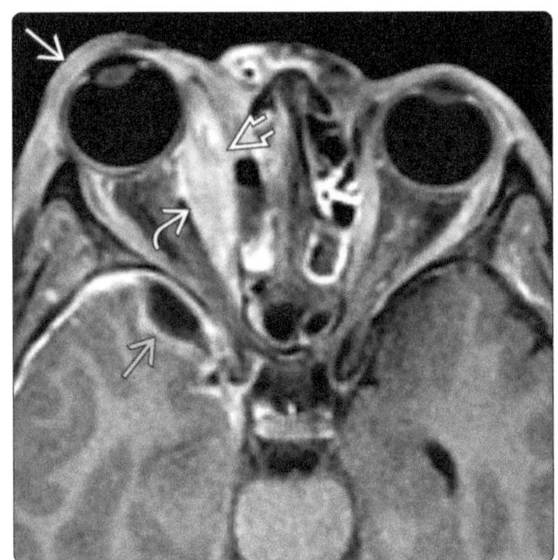

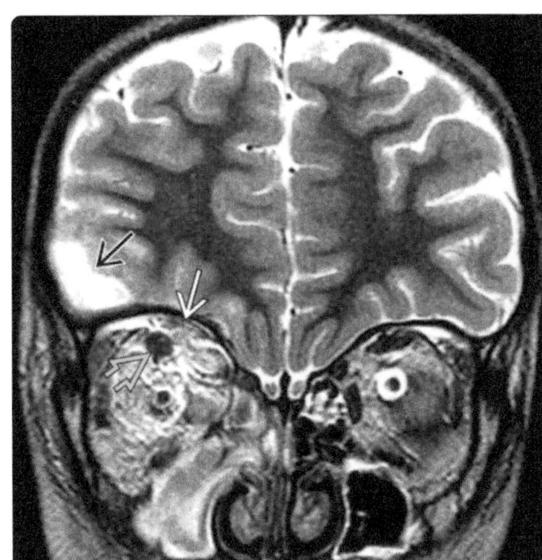

(Left) *Axial T1WI C+ FS MR in a 5-year-old with right proptosis & seizures shows ethmoid sinus disease, preseptal orbital cellulitis ➡, medial extraconal postseptal phlegmon ➡ with an enlarged medial rectus muscle ➡, & a middle cranial fossa epidural abscess ➡.* **(Right)** *Coronal T2WI MR in the same patient shows additional extraconal disease in the superior right orbit ➡ with inferior displacement of the superior rectus muscle complex ➡. There is an extraaxial fluid collection in the right anterior cranial fossa ➡.*

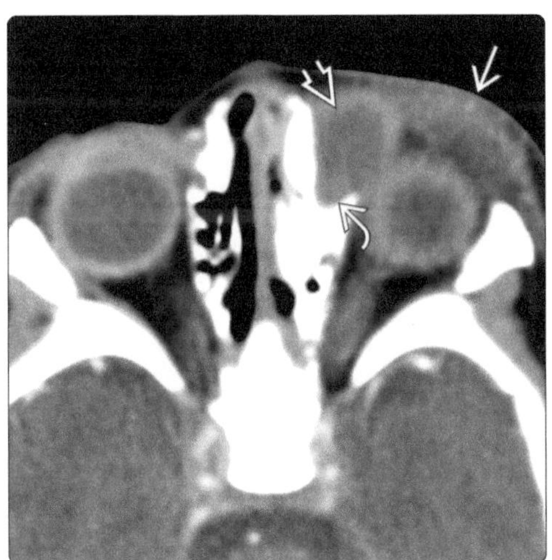

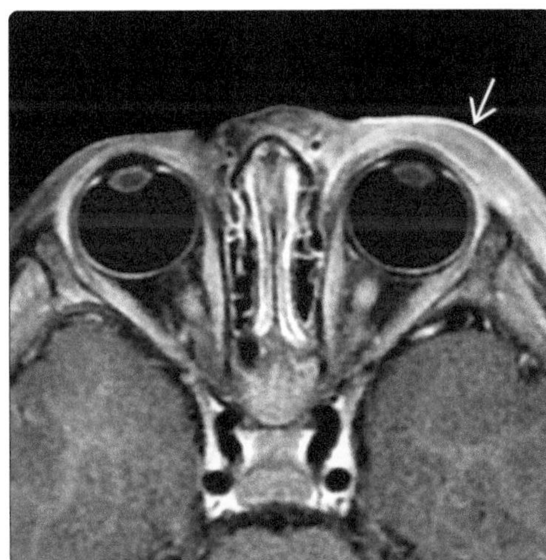

(Left) *Axial CECT in a 9-day-old presenting with eye swelling shows left preseptal orbital edema ➡ in the setting of a nasolacrimal duct mucocele. The lacrimal sac ➡ & lacrimal fossa/proximal canal ➡ are enlarged. There was an associated distal intranasal component to the mucocele (not shown).* **(Right)** *Axial T1WI C+ FS MR in a 7-year-old imaged for follow-up of an intracranial abnormality demonstrates new, unsuspected left preseptal cellulitis ➡. In this case, the cellulitis was secondary to a bee sting 1 day prior.*

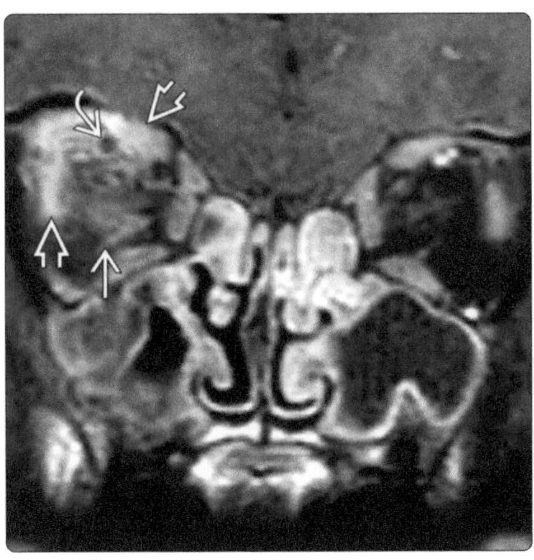

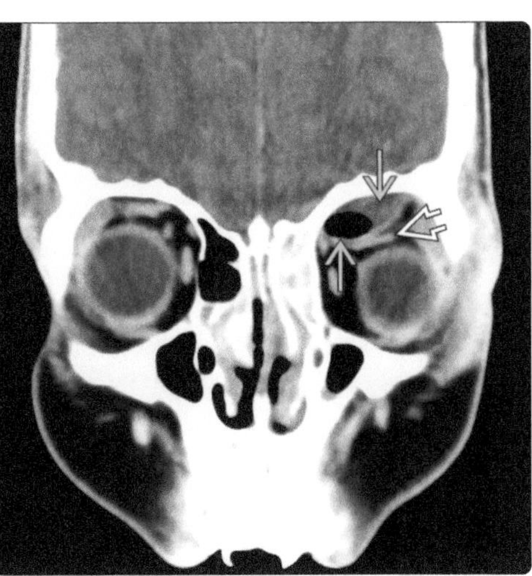

(Left) *Coronal T1WI C+ FS MR in a child with extensive sinusitis shows hazy ↑ enhancement of the right intraconal fat ➡, thickening of the superior & lateral rectus muscles ➡ (consistent with myositis), & enlargement of a nonenhancing superior ophthalmic vein ➡, consistent with thrombosis.* **(Right)** *Coronal CECT in a child with left ethmoid sinusitis shows an ipsilateral superior orbital gas-containing SPA ➡. The left superior rectus muscle complex ➡ & globe are deviated inferiorly.*

Orbital Vascular Malformations

KEY FACTS

TERMINOLOGY

- Congenital vascular malformation with variable lymphatic & venous vascular elements **(venolymphatic malformation)**

IMAGING

- Poorly marginated, lobulated, **transspatial** mass
- Multiloculated cystic features with **fluid-fluid levels**, blood products, & variable irregular enhancement
- Variants: Superficial vs. deep, macrocystic vs. microcystic
- CT: Irregular, cystic, hypodense mass with mixed hyperdense blood products
- MR: Variable signal resulting from mixed-age hemorrhagic, lymphatic, or proteinaceous fluid
- Variable enhancement, typically at margins, more pronounced if prominent venous components
- Look for associated developmental venous anomalies in cerebrofacial venous metameric syndromes (CVMS)
- US: Hypoechoic with heterogeneous internal echoes
- Dedicated fat-suppressed T2 & enhanced orbital MR

TOP DIFFERENTIAL DIAGNOSES

- Orbital varix
- Orbital cavernous hemangioma
- Infantile capillary hemangioma
- Plexiform neurofibroma

PATHOLOGY

- Congenital nonneoplastic vascular malformation
- Dilated dysplastic lymphatic ± venous channels

CLINICAL ISSUES

- Mass effect with proptosis in pediatric patient
- May rapidly ↑ in size due to acute hemorrhage
- Conservative therapy preferred due to surgical risk
- Percutaneous sclerotherapy for suitable lesions
- Surgical resection difficult; recurrence common

DIAGNOSTIC CHECKLIST

- Blood products & fluid-fluid levels highly suggestive

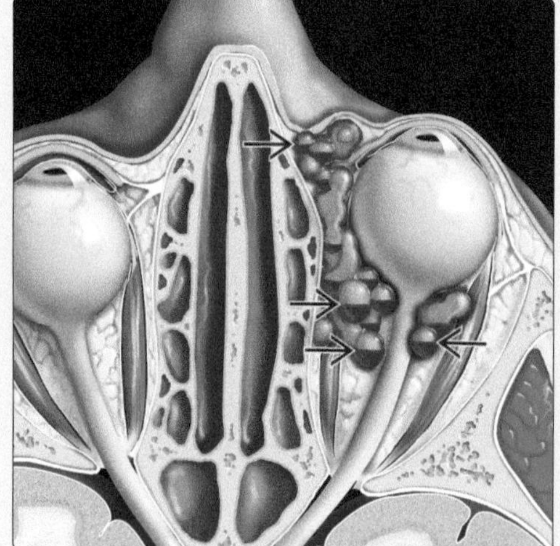

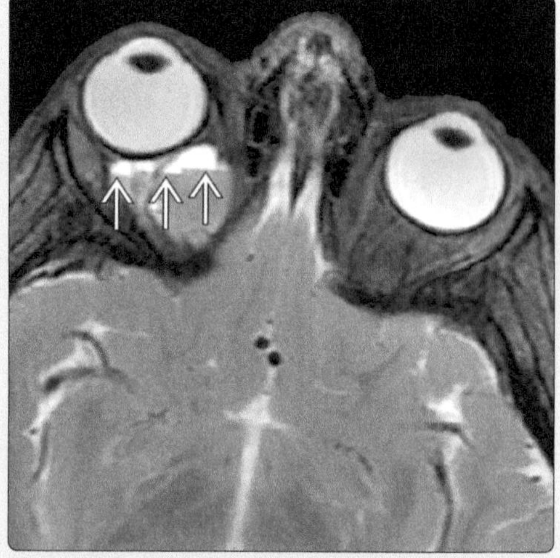

(Left) *Axial graphic depicts typical features of orbital venolymphatic malformation, including transspatial extension and characteristic fluid-fluid levels within loculations ➙.* **(Right)** *Axial T2WI FS MR in an older child with acute worsening of right proptosis shows a large, lobulated retrobulbar mass with characteristic fluid-fluid levels ➙. The differing heights of levels are indicative of the multilocular nature of the lesion.*

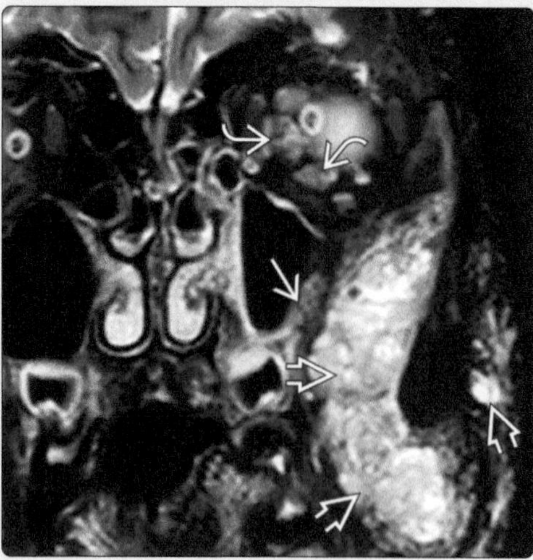

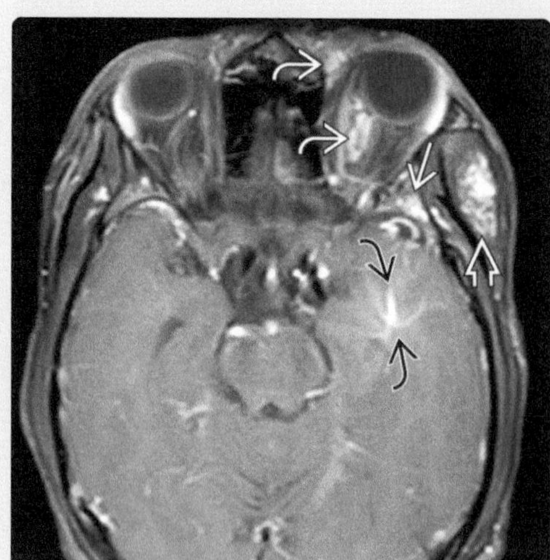

(Left) *Coronal T2WI FS MR in cerebrofacial venous metameric syndrome type 2 shows extensive hyperintense venous malformations in the left face ➙, maxilla ➙, and orbit ➙.* **(Right)** *Axial T1WI C+ FS MR (same patient) shows contrast enhancement of the orbital venous malformation ➙. Also note enhancing venous malformations in the left temporalis muscle ➙ and greater wing of sphenoid bone ➙. Brain shows a left temporal lobe developmental venous anomaly (DVA) ➙. (Courtesy R. H. Ramakrishnaiah, MD.)*

TERMINOLOGY

Abbreviations

- Orbital venolymphatic malformation (VLM or OVLM
- Orbital lymphatic-venous malformation (LVM or OLVM)
- Orbital lymphatic malformation (LM or OLM)

Synonyms

- Outdated terms: Lymphangioma, cystic hygroma

Definitions

- Congenital vascular malformation with variable **lymphatic** & **venous** vascular elements

IMAGING

General Features

- Best diagnostic clue
  - **Poorly marginated**, lobulated, **transspatial** mass
  - Multiloculated cystic features with **fluid-fluid levels**, **blood products**, & variable **irregular enhancement**
- Location
  - **Superficial**: Often confined to conjunctiva
    - Relatively common type of VLM
  - **Deep**: Extending into orbit
    - Extraconal > intraconal but often transspatial
- Morphology
  - **Irregular** margins, **multilocular cysts** with fluid levels
  - Macrocystic (> 1 cm), microcystic (< 1 cm), or mixed
  - Posterior venous lesions with more well-defined margins may mimic orbital cavernous hemangioma

CT Findings

- NECT
  - Irregular, multicystic, hypodense mass
  - Hemorrhage with mixed hyperdense blood products
  - Punctate calcification or **phleboliths**; uncommon
- CECT
  - Cystic structures with mild **rim enhancement**
  - More diffuse enhancement of **venous components**
- Bone CT
  - **Remodeling** of bony orbit with large lesions

MR Findings

- T1WI
  - Fluid-fluid levels with variable signal due to mixed-age hemorrhagic, lymphatic, or proteinaceous fluid in multilocular cystic spaces
  - Different ages of **blood products**; subacute blood characteristically **hyperintense**
- T2WI FS
  - Lobulated, **very hyperintense** fluid signal
  - **Fluid-fluid levels** show signal corresponding to age of blood products
  - No flow voids (unlike infantile capillary hemangioma)
- T1WI C+ FS
  - Variable enhancement, typically rim-enhancing cysts
  - More pronounced irregular enhancement if prominent venous components present
  - Nonenhancing **thrombus** in acute exacerbation
- MRA
  - Low-flow isolated vessels; may not be visible on MRA

Ultrasonographic Findings

- Grayscale ultrasound
  - **Hypoechoic** blood & lymph-filled cystic spaces
  - **Heterogeneous** internal echoes
  - Echogenic spikes at endothelial walls

Imaging Recommendations

- Best imaging tool
  - Dedicated enhanced orbital MR with fat suppression

DIFFERENTIAL DIAGNOSIS

Orbital Varix

- Clinical: **Intermittent** pain & **proptosis**
- Imaging: Similar to VLM, but **dynamic expansion** demonstrated with **Valsalva**; typically **extraconal**
- Pathology: Often considered part of **VLM spectrum** but with **distensible** venous component

Orbital Cavernous Hemangioma

- Clinical: Slowly growing, **painless** mass, most **common** benign orbital mass in **adults**
- Imaging: Circumscribed, ovoid, solid mass with **dynamic** fill-in enhancement; typically **intraconal**
- Pathology: **Pseudoencapsulated** venous malformation

Infantile Capillary Hemangioma

- Clinical: Highly vascular tumor of **infancy**; frequently **regresses** spontaneously
- Imaging: Poorly marginated, intensely enhancing orbitofacial mass with **flow voids**
- Pathology: True vascular **neoplasm**

Plexiform Neurofibroma

- Clinical: Associated with **neurofibromatosis** type 1
- Imaging: Infiltrative, transspatial masses, associated with **sphenoid dysplasia** & orbitofacial deformity
- Pathology: Nerve sheath tumor

Rhabdomyosarcoma

- Clinical: **Most common pediatric primary** orbital malignancy
- Imaging: Infiltrative, **destructive** orbital mass
- Pathology: **Embryonal** & **alveolar** subtypes usually

Lymphoproliferative Lesions

- Clinical: Lymphoid **proliferation** with mass primary to orbit; may be associated with systemic disease
- Imaging: Pliable mass, commonly involving **lacrimal** gland, or **multifocal** or diffuse in orbit
- Pathology: **Spectrum** ranging from benign reactive hyperplasia to malignant non-Hodgkin lymphoma

Idiopathic Inflammatory Pseudotumor

- Clinical: Inflammatory changes with **painful** proptosis & ophthalmoplegia
- Imaging: Asymmetric **mass-like inflammation** of muscles, lacrimal gland, & other orbital structures
- Pathology: **Unknown**; some cases associated with **IgG4**

PATHOLOGY

General Features

- Etiology

- Congenital **nonneoplastic vascular malformation** with low or no venous flow
- Arise from pluripotent venous anlage
- Lymphatic tissue not normally found in orbit
- Associated abnormalities
  - Malformations in other regions of head & neck
  - Generalized lymphangiomatosis
  - Noncontiguous **intracranial** vascular malformations, especially in **cerebrofacial venous metameric syndrome (CVMS)**
    - Include developmental venous anomaly (DVA), dural arteriovenous malformation (AVM), absent/occluded dural sinuses & jugular veins, cavernomas & pial AVMs
  - **CVMS: 3 types** based on concept of segmental organization of neural tube into 34 somites
    - 3 somites for brain & 31 for spinal cord with later metameric distribution migration of neural crest cells
    - Blood vessel endothelium derived from mesoderm & media derived from neural crest
    - Neural crest cells & mesoderm at any segmental level occupy same facial vascular territory due to segmental distribution → metameric vascular malformations
    - Complex venous vascular malformations that may affect soft tissues, bone, dura, orbit, & brain
    - **CVMS I**: Medial prosencephalic (**olfactory**): Involvement of nose, forehead, corpus callosum, hypothalamus, & pituitary
    - **CVMS II**: Lateral prosencephalic (**optic**): Involvement of orbit, eye, face/cheek, maxilla, optic nerve, chiasm, tract, thalamus, & temporoparietooccipital lobes
    - **CVMS III**: Rhombencephalic/mesencephalic (**otic**): Involvement of lower face, mandible, petrous bone, brainstem, & cerebellum
  - Concomitant **spontaneous orbital arteriovenous (AV) fistula** reported
    - Postulated to be due to mechanical erosion of ophthalmic artery by masses of orbital VLM

Staging, Grading, & Classification

- General classification of orbital vascular malformations
  - **Type 1**: No flow (LM)
  - **Type 2**: Venous flow (VLM)
    - Nondistensible vs. distensible (associated with varix)
  - **Type 3**: Arterial flow (low flow: Cavernous hemangioma; high flow: AVM)

Microscopic Features

- **Unencapsulated** mass of irregularly shaped sinuses; infiltrates into adjacent stroma
- Dilated **dysplastic** venous ± lymphatic channels lined with flattened endothelial cells
- **Cystic** spaces with lymphatic fluid or chronic blood
- Positive **lymphatic** immunohistochemical **markers**

CLINICAL ISSUES

Demographics

- Age
  - Younger patients: **Infants to young adults**
    - May be seen at birth (unlike infantile hemangioma)
  - 40% present by age 6; 60% present by age 16

Natural History & Prognosis

- **Progressive slow growth** during childhood, through puberty, & into early adulthood
  - **Episodic acute enlargement** due to hemorrhage
  - Lesions may intermittently ↑ & ↓ in size in conjunction with upper respiratory infection (lymphatic tissue)
- Infiltrating nature results in frequent **recurrence**
- Refractory visual problems & disfigurement common
- Poor visual acuity associated with multiple surgeries
- Optic nerve compromise with recurrent large lesions

Treatment

- Options, risks, complications
  - Conservative therapy
    - **Observation** preferred if vision not threatened
    - Systemic **steroids** may ↓ pain, swelling, & proptosis, especially in younger patients
    - 45% of smaller lesions show **regression**
    - CO2 laser, beta irradiation, & adjunctive systemic corticosteroids other options
    - Oral sildenafil for microcystic lesions has been tried
  - Image-guided sclerotherapy
    - Percutaneous **intralesional** injection of sclerosing agent, particularly for macrocystic lesions
    - Bleomycin, doxycycline, ethanol, picibanil (OK-432), sodium tetradecyl sulfate
  - Surgery
    - Difficult resection due to complex **insinuation** with normal orbital structures
    - **Recurrence** after surgery common (~ 50%)
    - Acute mass effect due to hemorrhage may require emergent **decompression**
    - Indications include optic nerve dysfunction, corneal compromise, & intractable amblyopia
  - Endovascular treatment
    - Orbital VLM may not have any accessible vascular channel for endovascular treatment
    - Concomitant orbital ophthalmic AV fistula treated with transvenous coil & glue embolization reported
  - Transcaruncular approach direct puncture of orbital venous malformation with angiography/embolization with Onyx, followed by safe surgical resection reported

DIAGNOSTIC CHECKLIST

Consider

- Deep circumscribed lesions in adults may mimic orbital cavernous hemangioma
- VLM & orbital varix-related lesions
  - VLM hemodynamically isolated
  - Varix possesses systemic drainage, which accounts for pressure-dependent distensibility

Image Interpretation Pearls

- Presence of blood products with **fluid-fluid levels** highly suggestive of VLM

SELECTED REFERENCES

1. Peer S et al: Cerebrofacial venous metameric syndrome type 2+3: face is the index of brain. Radiol Case Rep. 18(1):126-30, 2023
2. Wier GP et al: Orbital venous malformation excision after transcaruncular embolization with Onyx. Case Rep Ophthalmol. 14(1):121-6, 2023

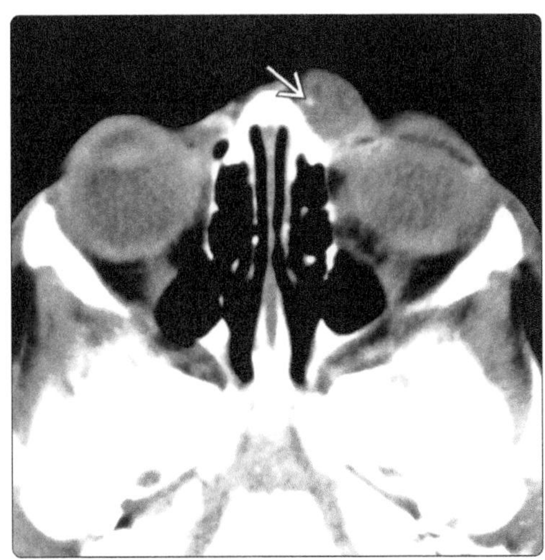

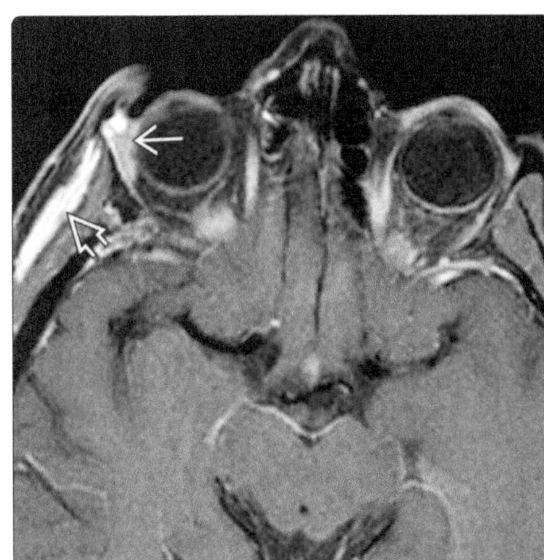

(Left) *Axial NECT shows a preseptal superficial hypodense mass in a 2-year-old child. A punctate Ca^{++} is present ➡, a relatively uncommon finding in venolymphatic malformation.* **(Right)** *Axial T1WI C+ FS MR shows a small, irregular, extraconal venolymphatic malformation in the lateral right orbit ➡ with mixed hyperintense signal and heterogeneous enhancement. Enhancing component is also seen extending into the adjacent temporal fossa ➡.*

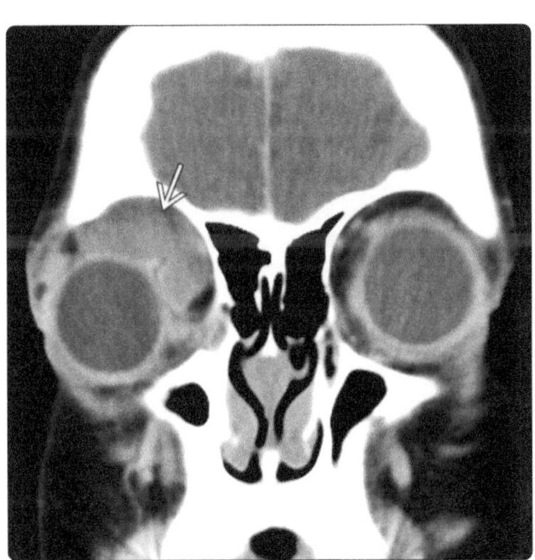

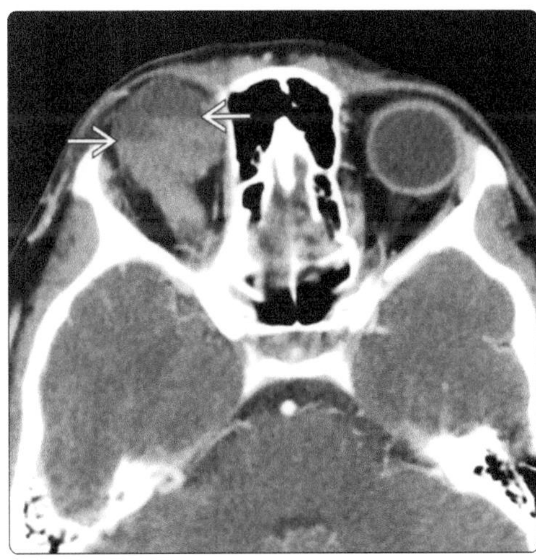

(Left) *Coronal CECT in a child with intermittently progressive proptosis shows a lobulated, intermediate- to low-density mass in the superomedial anterior orbit ➡, which causes displacement of the globe.* **(Right)** *Axial CECT in the same patient shows multiple loculations within the mass and demonstrates fluids of varying density with discrete levels ➡. The more dense chronic hemorrhagic products are seen layering dependently.*

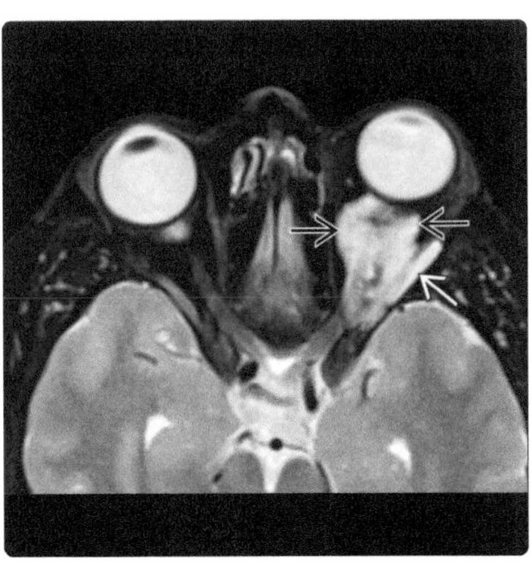

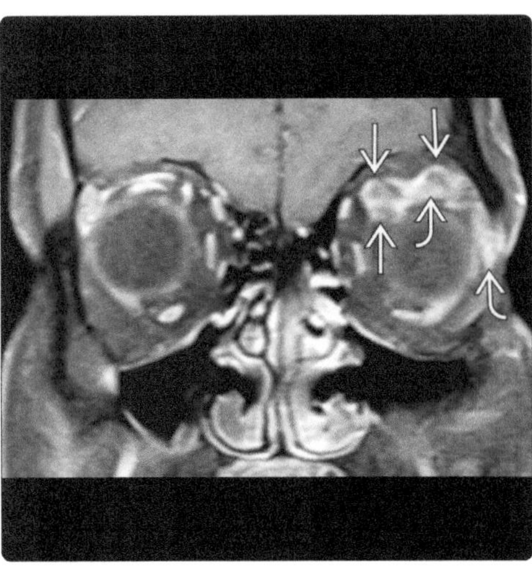

(Left) *Axial T2WI FS MR shows a very hyperintense transspatial venolymphatic malformation in the left postseptal orbit, involving the intraconal ➡ and extraconal ➡ compartments.* **(Right)** *Coronal T1WI C+ FS MR in the same patient shows rim enhancement of lymphatic components ➡ and more solid enhancement of venous components ➡.*

Orbital Infantile Hemangioma

KEY FACTS

TERMINOLOGY

- Synonyms: Orbital **capillary hemangioma**, infantile periocular hemangioma
- Definition: **Benign vascular tumor** of infancy

IMAGING

- Location: Preseptal &/or postseptal orbit
- CT findings
  - Lobular, slightly hyperdense, homogeneous
  - Intense enhancement
- MR findings
  - T1 intermediate; prominent internal **flow voids**
  - Moderate ↑ **T2**, ↑ blood flow on **perfusion MR**
- US: High vessel density, absent arteriovenous shunting, high peak arterial Doppler shift

TOP DIFFERENTIAL DIAGNOSES

- Rhabdomyosarcoma
- Metastatic neuroblastoma
- Orbital Langerhans cell histiocytosis
- Orbital venolymphatic malformation
- Plexiform neurofibroma
- Orbital non-Hodgkin lymphoma

PATHOLOGY

- **Proliferation** of vascular endothelium; cellular hyperplasia
- Immunohistochemical marker **GLUT1 positive**

CLINICAL ISSUES

- **Not present at birth**; has 3 distinct phases
  - **Proliferative phase**: Appears **few weeks after birth** and grows rapidly for year 1 or 2
  - **Involuting phase**: Regression over 3-5 years
  - **Involuted phase**: Complete regression by late childhood
- Distinguish from vascular malformations (VMs)
  - VM present at birth; grows in monophasic fashion

DIAGNOSTIC CHECKLIST

- T2-hyperintense enhancing mass with flow voids in infant

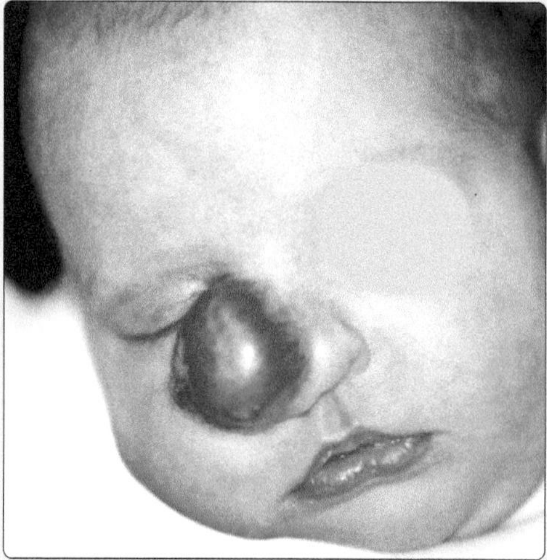

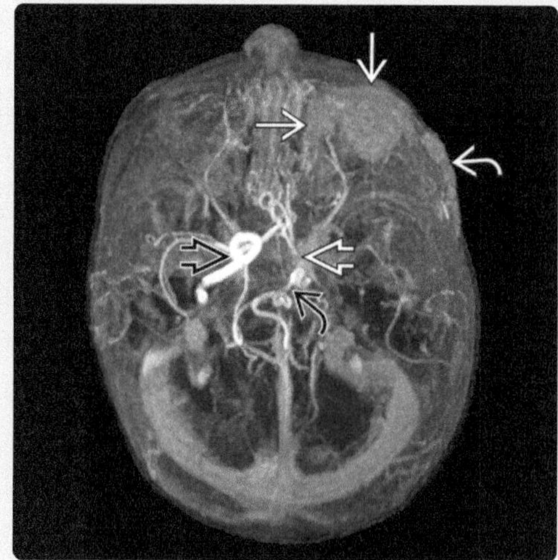

(Left) *Clinical photograph shows a superficial vascular mass centered at the medial orbit & nose with typical violaceous discoloration seen in infantile hemangioma.* **(Right)** *Axial MIP reformat of postcontrast MRA in a child with PHACE(S) syndrome shows left periorbital ➡ & zygomaticotemporal soft tissue ➡ capillary hemangiomas. There is severe hypoplasia of the left distal ICA ➡ compared with normal right ICA ➡. Note a persistent trigeminal artery ➡ connecting cavernous ICA to basilar artery on the left side.*

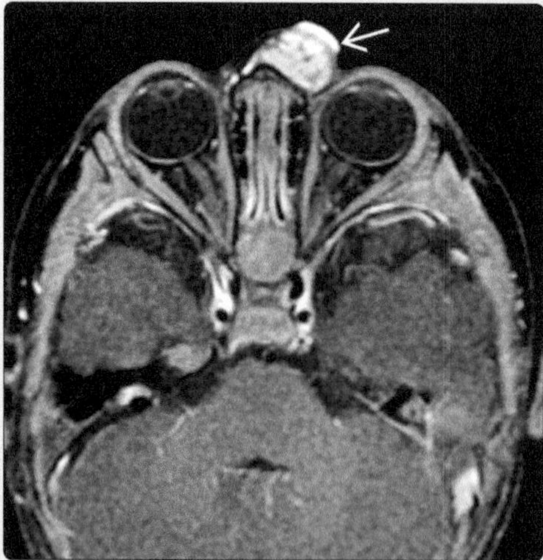

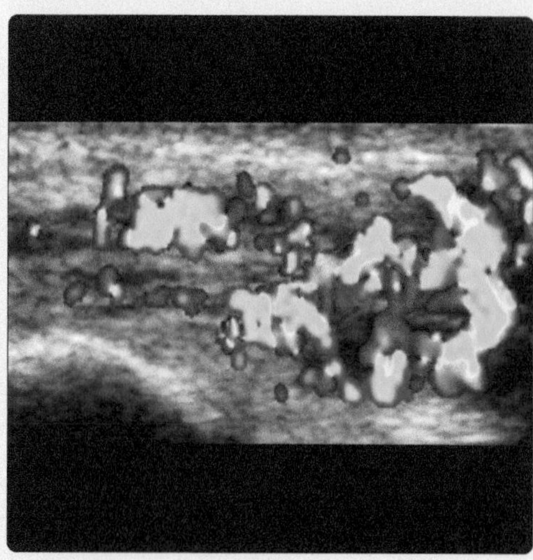

(Left) *Axial enhanced T1WI MR depicts a well-delineated, intensely enhancing infantile hemangioma ➡ with internal septations &/or flow voids in a typical periorbital location. Once again, postseptal extension is absent.* **(Right)** *Doppler US in the same patient shows striking internal flow, typical for phase I (proliferating) infantile hemangioma.*

TERMINOLOGY

Synonyms

- Orbital **capillary hemangioma**, infantile periocular hemangioma

Definitions

- **Benign vascular tumor** of infancy
- Distinct lesion from vascular malformation

IMAGING

General Features

- Best diagnostic clue
  - Lobular or infiltrative, **hypervascular, intensely enhancing** mass in infant
- Location
  - May involve multiple contiguous areas
  - Predilection for eyelids, supranasal periorbita
  - Sites of orbital involvement
    - Most commonly superficial superomedial extraconal location
    - May extend postseptal into superior orbital fissure or intraconal space
    - Exclusively retrobulbar in 10%
- Size
  - Variable, small superficial lesions rarely imaged
- Morphology
  - Ranges from lobular to infiltrative
    - Infiltrative pattern typical in postseptal component

CT Findings

- CECT
  - Intense enhancement, usually homogeneous
    - ↓ with involution
  - Prominent vessels during proliferative phase
  - ↑ fat content and septations with involution
  - No Ca^{++}

MR Findings

- T1WI
  - Slightly hyperintense to muscle
  - Internal flow voids
- T2WI
  - Moderate **hyperintensity** reflects high cellularity
  - **Flow voids** frequently visible
- PWI
  - Noncontrast arterial spin-labeling (ASL) perfusion MR shows ↑ blood flow on cerebral blood flow (CBF) images of brain perfusion MR (light-bulb appearance)
    - Excellent tool to identify tiny infantile hemangiomas, which may be difficult to identify on T1/T2/routine contrast-enhanced MR
    - Especially in **PHACE(S)** syndrome (**p**osterior fossa anomalies, **h**emangioma, **a**rterial, **c**ardiac, **e**ye and **s**ternal anomalies) where it can show small hemangiomas in unusual places
  - Perfusion ↑ in hemodynamically active high-flow lesions
    - Infantile hemangioma
    - Congenital hemangiomas (CHs) like rapidly involuting and partially involuting CH (RICH & NICH)
    - Arteriovenous malformation/fistula (AVM/AVF)
  - No measurable ↑ of perfusion in low-flow vascular malformations, such as venous, lymphatic, or venolymphatic malformations, and also hamartoma
  - Infantile hemangioma and CH: Marked hyperperfusion (median flow: 436 mL/min/100 g; range: 212.5-603 mL/min/100 g)
  - AVMs and AVFs: Marked hyperperfusion (median: 779 and 451 mL/min/100 g, respectively)
  - Lymphatic malformations: Low flow (median: 22.5 mL/min/100 g; range: 16-60 mL/min/100 g)
  - Venous malformations: Low flow (median: 25 mL/min/100 g; range: 15-66.5 mL/min/100 g)
  - IV contrast-enhanced perfusion MR, such as dynamic contrast enhancement (DCE) techniques, also demonstrate similar findings to ASL
- T1WI C+
  - Diffuse, **intense enhancement**
  - Enhancement may appear heterogeneous, particularly in involuting phase
- MRA
  - Generally not necessary for diagnosis but helpful in assessing associated arterial abnormalities in **PHACE(S)**

Ultrasonographic Findings

- Lobular soft tissue mass with high vessel density, high peak arterial Doppler shift, absent arteriovenous (AV) shunting

Angiographic Findings

- Enlarged feeding branches from external carotid, ophthalmic arteries
- Dense parenchymal stain, **no AV shunting**

Imaging Recommendations

- Best imaging tool
  - When small and superficial, US may be sufficient to confirm clinical diagnosis
  - MR for mapping larger, deeper, more complex lesions
  - Perfusion MR for tiny lesion, especially in PHACE(S)

DIFFERENTIAL DIAGNOSIS

Rhabdomyosarcoma

- Rapidly progressive invasive orbital mass
- Bone destruction present when large
- Mean ADC value of rhabdomyosarcomas significantly lower compared with infantile hemangiomas
  - ADC threshold of < 1159 × 10-6 mm^2/s and lesion:medulla ADC ratio of < 1.38

Metastatic Neuroblastoma

- Rapidly progressive osseous metastatic mass
- Predilection for greater sphenoid wing

Orbital Cellulitis

- Inflammatory changes ± abscess formation

Orbital Langerhans Cell Histiocytosis

- Well-defined, lytic bone lesion with enhancing soft tissue

Orbital Venolymphatic Malformation

- Hypointense T1, hyperintense T2, diffuse contrast enhancement of venous elements, ± phleboliths
- Nonenhancing lymphatic components
- Blood and fluid levels

Plexiform Neurofibroma

- Infiltrative + sphenoid dysplasia

Orbital Non-Hodgkin Lymphoma

- Multicompartmental infiltrating mass

Orbital Leukemia

- Homogeneous masses that mold to orbital walls ± periosteal reaction, usually without frank bone destruction

PATHOLOGY

General Features

- Etiology
  - **Proliferation** of vascular endothelium
    - Grows by **endothelial cellular hyperplasia**
  - **Distinguish from vascular malformation**: Localized defect of vascular morphogenesis
    - With quiescent endothelium
- Genetics
  - Most cases sporadic
  - Some associated with pleiotropic genetic syndromes
  - Small percent autosomal dominant
    - Gene map locus 5q35.3, 5q31-q33
- Associated abnormalities
  - Large lesions may involve ectodermal structures of face, neck, and airway; parotid involvement common
  - **PHACE(S)** syndrome

Staging, Grading, & Classification

- Classification by location
  - Deep: Within deep tissues of lid and anterior orbit, or entirely retrobulbar
  - Superficial: Confined to dermis
  - Combined: Both dermal and deep components

Microscopic Features

- Unencapsulated lobulated **cellular neoplasm**
- Thin-walled, **capillary-sized vascular spaces** in lobules with thin fibrous septa
  - Venous malformation has larger vascular spaces
- ↑ numbers of endothelial and mast cells during proliferative phase
- ↓ cellularity during involutional phase
- Immunohistochemical marker **GLUT1 positive in all phases**

CLINICAL ISSUES

Presentation

- Most common signs/symptoms
  - Unilateral eyelid, brow, or nasal vascular lesion
  - Ophthalmologic symptoms common: Amblyopia, astigmatism, proptosis, and ↓ visual acuity
    - Risk of amblyopia highest when diffuse, > 1 cm in size, and associated with PHACE(S) syndrome
- Clinical profile
  - Rubbery, soft mass
  - **Bluish discoloration of skin** or conjunctiva (80%)
    - **Blanche with pressure** unlike port-wine stain
  - Enlarges with Valsalva or crying in 50%
  - Occasional periorbital fat excess following involution
- Distinguish from **vascular malformations**: Present at birth and grow in monophasic fashion with age
- Distinguish from **CHs:** Present at or before birth, more commonly on trunk; **GLUT1 negative**
  - Noninvoluting CH (**NICH**)
  - Partially involuting CH (**PICH**)
  - Rapidly involuting CH (**RICH**)

Demographics

- Age
  - Typically not present at birth; most **appear within 1st few weeks**
    - Vascular malformations present at birth; deep lesions may not become apparent until later in life
- Sex
  - M:F = 1:2-3
  - Even higher female predominance in genetic syndromes
- Epidemiology: Affects ~ 1% of neonates

Natural History & Prognosis

- 3 distinct phases
  - **Proliferative phase**: Appears few weeks after birth and grows rapidly for year 1 or 2
  - **Involuting phase**: Regression over 3-5 years
  - **Involuted phase**: Usually complete regression by late childhood

Treatment

- Expectant observation unless complications
- Indications for treatment
  - Ophthalmologic: Visual disturbance, nerve compromise, proptosis
  - Dermatologic: Ulceration, infection, cosmesis
- Propranolol now recognized as very effective treatment
- Corticosteroids: Intralesional, systemic, or topical administration
- Intratumoral laser therapy in larger lesions
- Interferon, vincristine, surgical resection, or laser ablation for recalcitrant lesions
- Intravascular embolization contraindicated for intraorbital lesions

DIAGNOSTIC CHECKLIST

Consider

- Remember, differential diagnosis for rapidly growing mass in infant includes malignancy

Image Interpretation Pearls

- In appropriate age group, T2-hyperintense, enhancing mass with prominent flow voids and ↑ blood flow on perfusion MR

SELECTED REFERENCES

1. Melgosa Ramos FJ et al: Congenital and infantile hemangiomas: epidemiological, clinical, and treatment characteristics based on 3 years' experience at a tertiary care hospital - a retrospective case comparison and review of the literature. Actas Dermosifiliogr. 114(7):T631-5, 2023
2. Tanaka F et al: Pseudocontinuous arterial spin labeling: clinical applications and usefulness in head and neck entities. Cancers (Basel). 14(16):3872, 2022
3. Boulouis G et al: Arterial spin-labeling to discriminate pediatric cervicofacial soft-tissue vascular anomalies. AJNR Am J Neuroradiol. 38(3):633-8, 2017
4. Mamlouk MD et al: Arterial spin-labeled perfusion for vascular anomalies in the pediatric head and neck. Clin Imaging. 40(5):1040-6, 2016

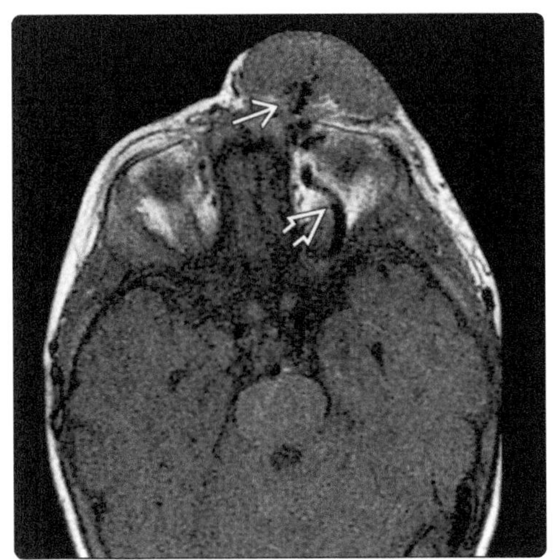

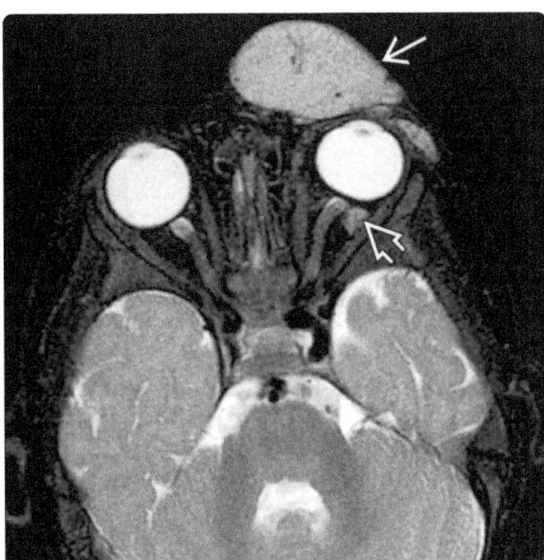

(Left) *Axial T1WI MR in a large, supraorbital infantile hemangioma reveals prominent internal flow voids* ➡ *& enlargement of the superior ophthalmic vein* ⇨*, which serves as the primary venous drainage pathway.* **(Right)** *Axial T2WI MR of a large, infantile hemangioma in a similar location* ➡ *demonstrates a small lobular retrobulbar component* ⇨*. Careful inspection of the postseptal soft tissues is critical when reviewing imaging studies in periorbital hemangioma.*

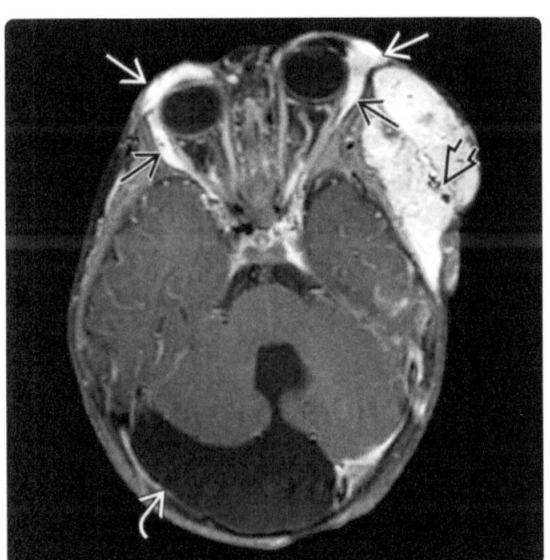

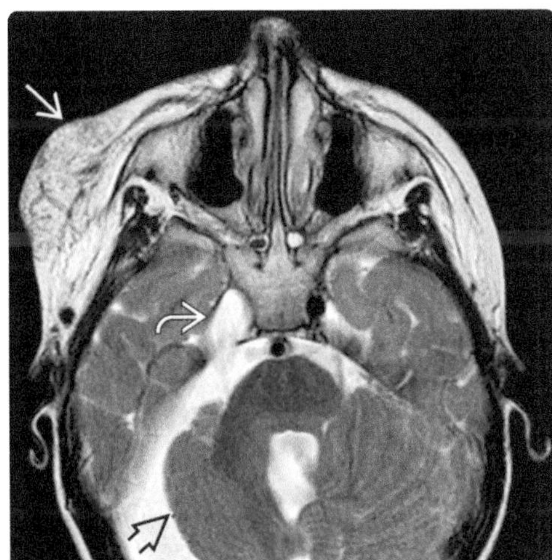

(Left) *Axial T1WI C+ FS MR shows a child with PHACE(S) syndrome. Bilateral orbital infantile hemangiomas have preseptal* ➡ *& postseptal* ➡ *components. The component in the masticator space has flow voids* ⇨*. Note cerebellar asymmetry* ↪*.* **(Right)** *Axial T2WI MR in a child with right orbitofacial hemangioma* ➡ *& PHACE(S) syndrome shows right cerebellar hypoplasia* ⇨ *& absence of the expected flow void for the right cavernous ICA* ↪*.*

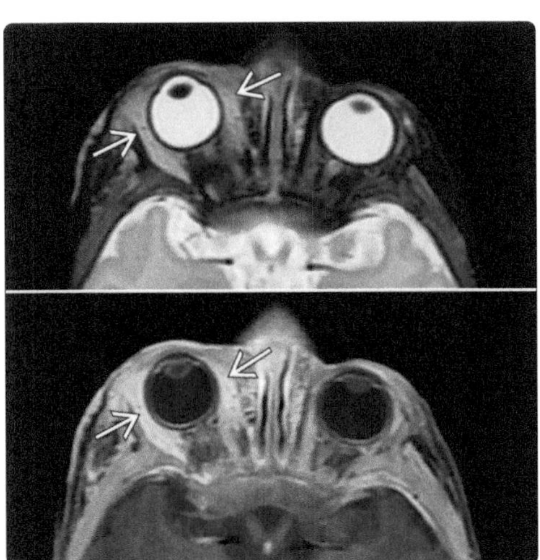

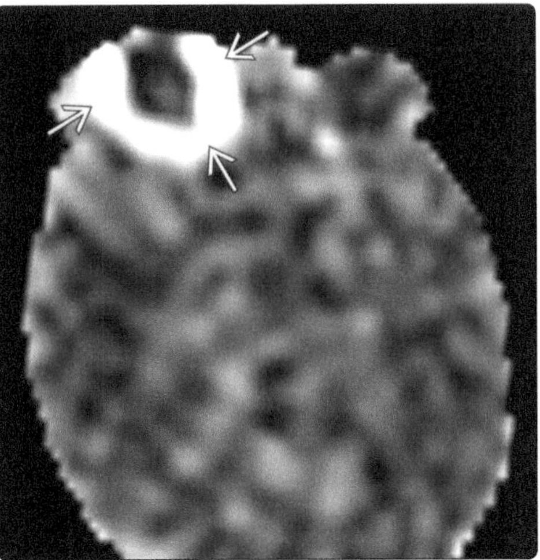

(Left) *Axial T2WI FS (top) & T1WI C+ FS (bottom) brain MRs in a 5-week-old show a right orbital T2-hyperintense & enhancing infantile hemangioma* ➡*.* **(Right)** *Axial cerebral blood flow (CBF) grayscale image of brain arterial spin-labeling (ASL) perfusion MR shows light-bulb appearance of this infantile hemangioma* ➡*. Other high-flow lesions like congenital hemangiomas & arteriovenous malformations/fistulae also show significantly ↑ CBF. Venolymphatic malformations show no detectable perfusion ↑.*

KEY FACTS

TERMINOLOGY

- Retinoblastoma (RB)
- Malignant primary retinal neoplasm
- Trilateral/quadrilateral RB: Bilateral ocular RB + pineal ± suprasellar tumors

IMAGING

- Unilateral in 60%; bilateral in 40%
- Trilateral or quadrilateral disease rare
- **Extraocular extension** in **< 10%**
  - Indicates poor prognosis
- CT: **Ca⁺⁺** in **> 90%**
- MR: Assess extent of intraocular tumor and presence of optic nerve, orbital, or intracranial involvement
  - T1: Mild hyperintensity
  - T2: Moderate to marked hypointensity
  - Moderate to marked heterogeneous enhancement

TOP DIFFERENTIAL DIAGNOSES

- Persistent hyperplastic primary vitreous
- Coats disease
- Retinopathy of prematurity
- Orbital toxocariasis

PATHOLOGY

- **Primitive neuroectodermal tumor**
- Inherited (germline): Multilateral > unilateral

CLINICAL ISSUES

- Most common intraocular tumor of childhood
- **Leukocoria** in 50-60%
- 90-95% diagnosed by 5 years of age

DIAGNOSTIC CHECKLIST

- Calcified intraocular mass in child is RB until proven otherwise

(Left) *Axial graphic depicts retinoblastoma (RB) with lobulated tumor extending through the limiting membrane into the vitreous. Punctate Ca⁺⁺ ➡ are characteristic.* **(Right)** *Axial T1 C+ FS MR in a 19-month-old with leukocoria and rubeosis iridis shows a heterogeneously enhancing intraocular mass ➡ with anterior segment enhancement ⇨, which carries a worse prognosis. In addition, there is another focal plaque-like mass along the nasal margin ↪.*

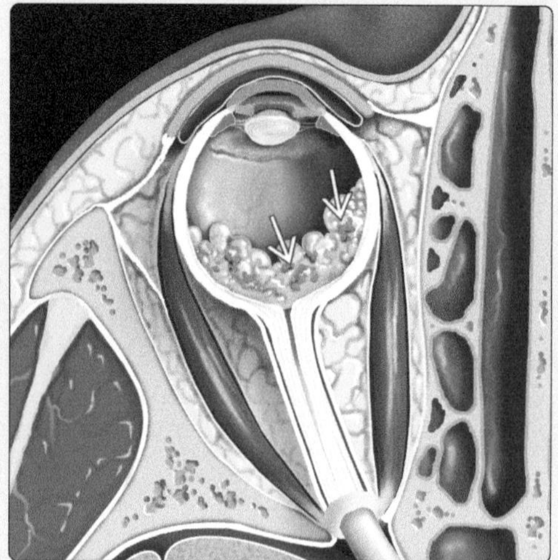

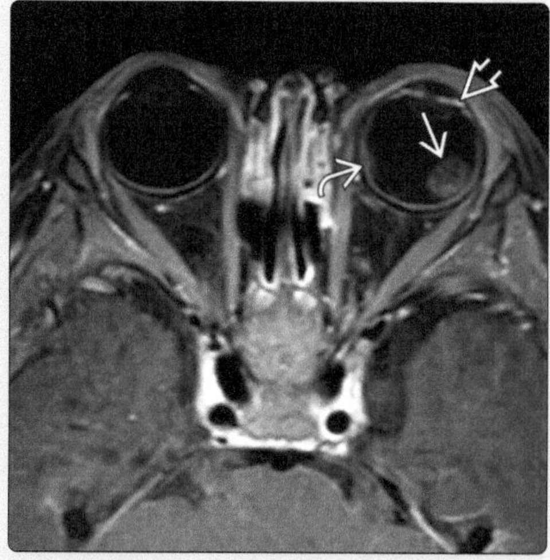

(Left) *Axial b-FFE MR in the same child shows the enhancing masses as hypointense ➡, consistent with CA⁺⁺ as well as associated retinal detachment ↪ and vitreous seeding ⇨.* **(Right)** *Axial ADC map (top) and DWI (bottom) images demonstrate classic diffusion restriction within the primary left ocular RB. Overall disease is endophytic, and on exam, under anesthesia, the patient had extensive vitreous seeding and neovascular glaucoma and was therefore treated with enucleation.*

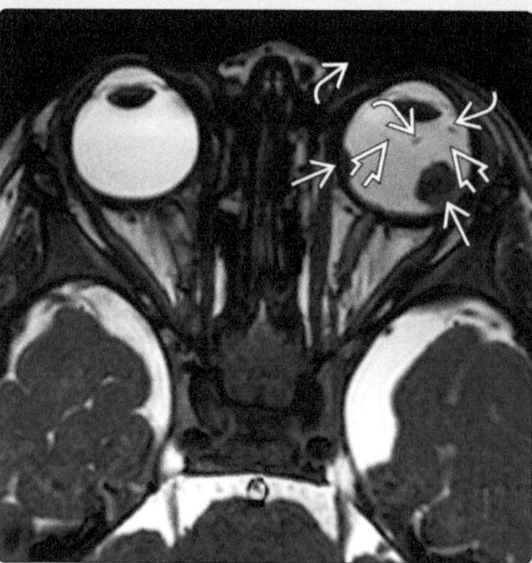

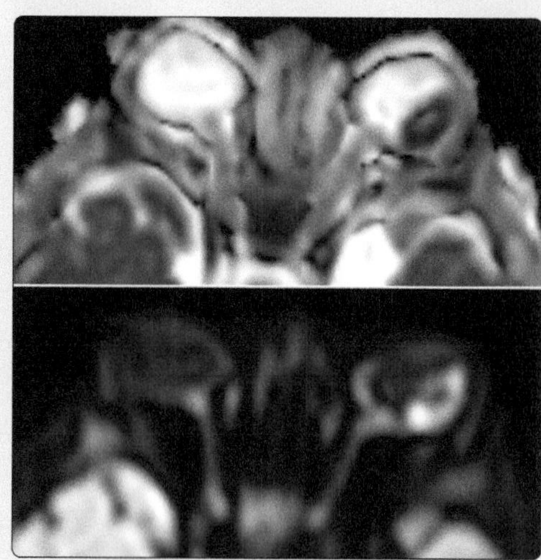

TERMINOLOGY

Abbreviations

- Retinoblastoma (RB)

Definitions

- Malignant primary retinal neoplasm
- **Trilateral** RB: Bilateral ocular tumors + midline intracranial neuroblastic tumor, typically pineal
- **Quadrilateral** (tetralateral) RB: Bilateral disease + pineal and suprasellar tumors

IMAGING

General Features

- Best diagnostic clue
  - Intraocular **calcified** mass in child
- Location
  - Diagnosis typically with ophthalmoscopy and ultrasound
    - MR for tumor mapping and prognostication
  - Unilateral in 60%; **bilateral in 40%**
  - Trilateral or quadrilateral disease rare
    - 5-15% of familial lesions
  - Extraocular extension in < 10%
    - Spreads along scleral vessels into orbit and along optic nerve to subarachnoid space
  - Predictors for metastatic disease: Involvement of optic nerve, choroid, anterior chamber, or orbit
    - Anterior chamber enhancement reflects neoangiogenesis and is associated with more aggressive tumor behavior
  - Role of MR
    - Exclude pseudoneoplastic lesions
    - Intraocular (choroid, sclera, prelaminar optic nerve), extraocular (postlaminar optic nerve, orbital), intracranial (pineal, parasellar, metastatic) involvement
- Growth patterns
  - **Endophytic** form (45%)
    - Inward protrusion into vitreous chamber
    - Associated with vitreous seeding
  - **Exophytic** form (45%)
    - Outward growth into subretinal space (between sensory retina and retinal pigment epithelium), typically with hemispherical configuration
    - Associated with retinal detachment and subretinal exudate
  - **Mixed** endophytic and exophytic (10%)
  - **Diffuse infiltrating** form (rare, older children)
    - Plaque-like growth along retina; often no Ca^{++}
    - Simulates inflammatory or other conditions

CT Findings

- Punctate or finely speckled **Ca^{++}** (> 90-95%)
- Moderate to marked heterogeneous enhancement
- CT not recommended for initial diagnosis or work-up
  - Potential ↑ risk for 2nd cancers with ionizing radiation, especially in patients with germline mutations

MR Findings

- T1WI: Variable, mildly hyperintense (vs. vitreous)
- T2WI: Moderate to markedly hypointense (vs. vitreous)
  - Helps distinguish from other hyperintense lesions (persistent hyperplastic primary vitreous, Coats disease)
  - Best sequence for subretinal fluid ± vitreous hemorrhage
  - Best to assess extent of intraocular disease and presence of optic nerve or extraocular invasion
    - **Choroidal invasion**: Localized thickening and heterogeneous contrast enhancement of choroid near tumor
    - **Scleral invasion**: Interruption in normal thin, hypointense T1/T2 sclera surrounding enhancing choroid
    - **Optic nerve invasion**: Thickening of optic disc (prelaminar), enhancement of nerve (postlaminar)
      - MR low sensitivity and specificity
- T1WI C+: Moderate to marked heterogeneous enhancement
- Imaging of orbital prosthesis
  - Fibrovascularization (indicated by heterogeneous enhancement) secures prosthesis and provides surface for muscular attachment

Ultrasonographic Findings

- A scan: Highly reflective spikes at Ca^{++}
- B scan: Echodense, irregular mass with focal shadows

Imaging Recommendations

- Best imaging tool
  - Enhanced MR with fat-saturated T1WI and T2WI best for tumor mapping
  - Ca^{++} on CT relatively specific
- Protocol advice
  - Include whole brain to assess for trilateral disease

DIFFERENTIAL DIAGNOSIS

Persistent Hyperplastic Primary Vitreous

- Small globe, hyperdense; no Ca^{++}
- Hyperintense on T2WI; retrolental tissue stalk

Coats Disease

- Normal-sized globe, hyperdense; no Ca^{++}
- Hyperintense on T1WI and T2WI

Retinopathy of Prematurity

- Retrolental fibroplasia; associated with excess oxygen and premature retinal vessels
- Small globe, hyperdense, bilateral; Ca^{++} if advanced

Retinal Astrocytoma

- Rare lesion, associated with tuberous sclerosis; ± Ca^{++}

Toxocariasis, Orbit

- Uveoscleral enhancement; no Ca^{++} acutely
- Moderately enhancing retinal nodule
- Intravitreal membranes and retinal detachment

Other Causes of Leukocoria

- Retinal detachment
  - Subretinal hemorrhage, retinal folds
- Choroidal osteoma
- Choroidal hamartoma
- Retinal dysplasia

PATHOLOGY

General Features

- Etiology
  - Primitive neuroectodermal tumor
  - **Sporadic** (nongermline): **60%** of RBs
    - Majority (85%) of unilateral disease
  - **Inherited** (germline): **40%** of RBs
    - Essentially all bilateral and multilateral disease
      - Minority (15%) of unilateral disease
    - Autosomal dominant with 90% penetrance
    - Positive family history in 5-10%
    - New germline mutations in 30-35%
- Genetics
  - *RB1*: Chromosome 13, q14 band
  - Somatic mosaicism in 10-20% of RB patients
- Associated abnormalities
  - Risk of 2nd malignancy ↑ in germline disease
    - Sarcoma, melanoma, CNS tumors, epithelial tumors (lung, bladder, breast)
    - 20-30% in nonirradiated patients
    - 50-60% in irradiated patients
    - Occur within 30 years; average: 10-13 years
  - 13q deletion syndrome: RB, multiple organ anomalies

Staging, Grading, & Classification

- Reese-Ellsworth classification: Groups 1-5
  - Based on size, location, and multifocality
  - More useful in radiation therapy management
- International (Murphree) classification of RB (ICRB); newer
  - Groups A-E
  - Based on size, retinal location, subretinal or vitreous seeding, and several specific prognostic features
  - More useful in chemotherapy management

Gross Pathologic & Surgical Features

- Yellowish-white irregular pedunculated retinal mass

Microscopic Features

- Small round cells, scant cytoplasm, and large nuclei
- Flexner-Wintersteiner rosettes and fleurettes

CLINICAL ISSUES

Presentation

- Most common signs/symptoms
  - **Leukocoria** (50-60%)
- Other signs/symptoms
  - Severe vision loss
  - Strabismus if macular involvement or retinal detachment
  - Proptosis if significant orbital disease
  - Rubeosis iridis (redness of iris secondary to neovascularization) correlates with anterior chamber enhancement on MR
  - Inflammatory signs in 10%
  - Less common: Anisocoria, heterochromia, glaucoma, cataract, nystagmus

Demographics

- Age
  - RB is congenital but usually not apparent at birth
  - Average age at diagnosis: 18 months
    - Unilateral: 24 months; bilateral: 13 months
    - Earlier with family history and routine screening
  - 90-95% diagnosed by 5 years of age
- Epidemiology
  - Most common intraocular tumor of childhood
  - Incidence 1:17,000 live births, ↑ in past 60 years
  - 3% of cancers in children < 15 years of age
  - 1% of cancer deaths; 5% of childhood blindness

Natural History & Prognosis

- Degree of nerve involvement correlates with survival
  - Superficial or no invasion: 90%
  - Invasion to lamina cribrosa (prelaminar): 70%
  - Invasion beyond lamina cribrosa (postlaminar): 60%
  - Involvement at surgical margin: 20%
- Poor prognosis for extraocular disease: < 10% 5-year disease-free survival
- Poor prognosis for trilateral disease or CSF spread
  - < 24-month survival

Treatment

- > 95% of children with RB in USA cured with modern techniques; challenge is maintaining eye and vision
- Based on tumor volume and localization, intraocular tumor extension, and extraocular stage of disease
- Intraarterial chemotherapy (IAC): Now standard of care 1st-line therapy for advanced unilateral tumors
- Systemic IV chemotherapy ("chemoreduction")
- Intraocular chemotherapy + IAC to treat vitreous seeding
- Plaque radiotherapy: Locally directed, I-125 or other isotope
  - Selected solitary or small tumors that are chemoresistant
- Cryotherapy: Small peripheral tumors
- Photocoagulation: Primary local treatment of small posterior tumors
- Enucleation: Advanced disease without chance to preserve useful vision
- External beam radiation therapy: Historically for bulky tumors with seeding, now avoided
  - Unfavorable complications: Radiation-induced 2nd primary malignancies and arrested bone growth

DIAGNOSTIC CHECKLIST

Consider

- Assess for intraocular and extraocular spread, including optic nerve
  - Check for intracranial trilateral or quadrilateral disease in pineal and suprasellar regions

Image Interpretation Pearls

- Calcified intraocular mass in child is RB until proven otherwise

SELECTED REFERENCES

1. Silvera VM et al: Retinoblastoma: what the neuroradiologist needs to know. AJNR Am J Neuroradiol. 42(4):618-26, 2021
2. Li Z et al: Diagnosis of postlaminar optic nerve invasion in retinoblastoma with MRI features. J Magn Reson Imaging. 51(4):1045-52, 2020
3. Nadiarnykh O et al: Optical coherence tomography (OCT) to image active and inactive retinoblastomas as well as retinomas. Acta Ophthalmol. 98(2):158-65, 2020

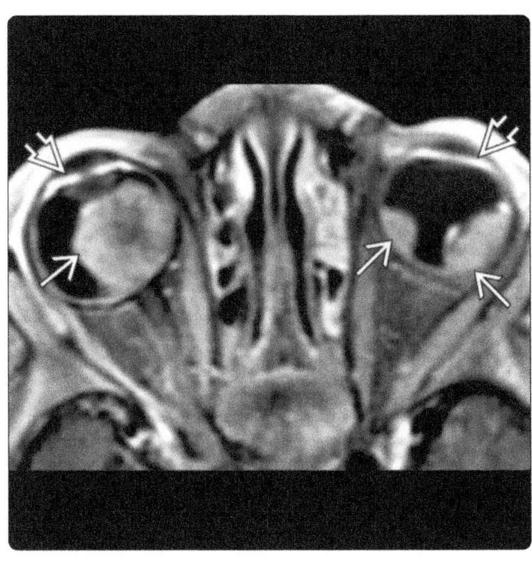

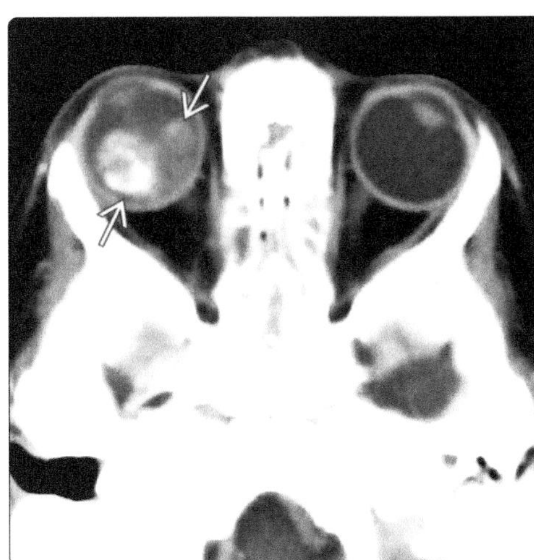

(Left) *Axial T1 C+ FS MR shows bulky, enhancing intraocular masses compatible with bilateral RBs. Note the prominent enhancement of each iris; anterior segment enhancement is associated with more aggressive tumor behavior.* **(Right)** *Axial CECT in a 15-month-old boy with leukocoria shows a partially calcified right ocular mass. CT is no longer a 1st-line imaging modality, but it is important to recognize the typical finding.*

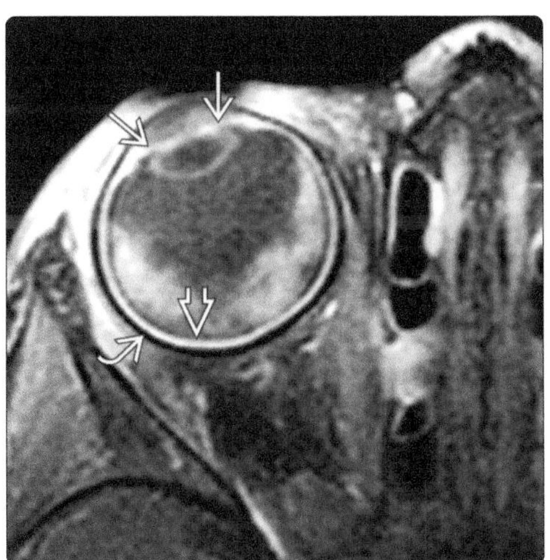

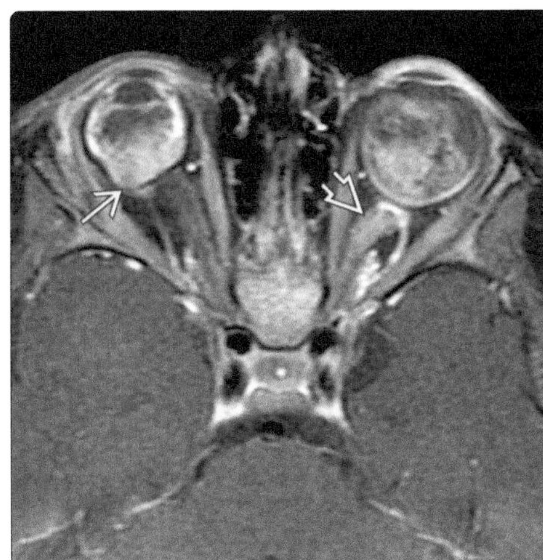

(Left) *Axial T1 C+ MR shows moderately enhancing RB associated with anterior segment enhancement. Note intact thin lines of enhancing choroid and hypointense sclera, indicating absence of invasion.* **(Right)** *Axial T1 C+ FS MR in a child with bilateral RB shows interruption of linear hypodensity with a focal contour abnormality, indicating scleral invasion of RB on the right. The left postlaminar optic nerve demonstrates asymmetric enlargement and enhancement.*

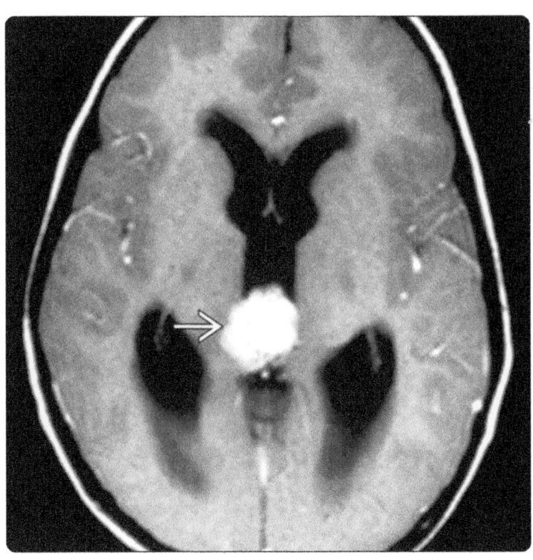

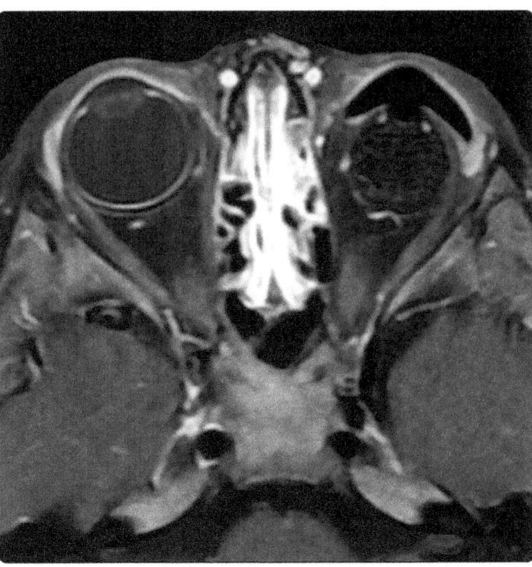

(Left) *Axial T1 MR in a patient with bilateral RB shows an intensely enhancing pineal region primitive neuroectodermal tumor, representing trilateral disease.* **(Right)** *Axial T1 C+ FS MR in a child after enucleation of the left globe for treatment of RB shows a typical ocular prosthesis with mild heterogeneous enhancement of the hydroxyapatite intraorbital spherical portion of the prosthesis.*

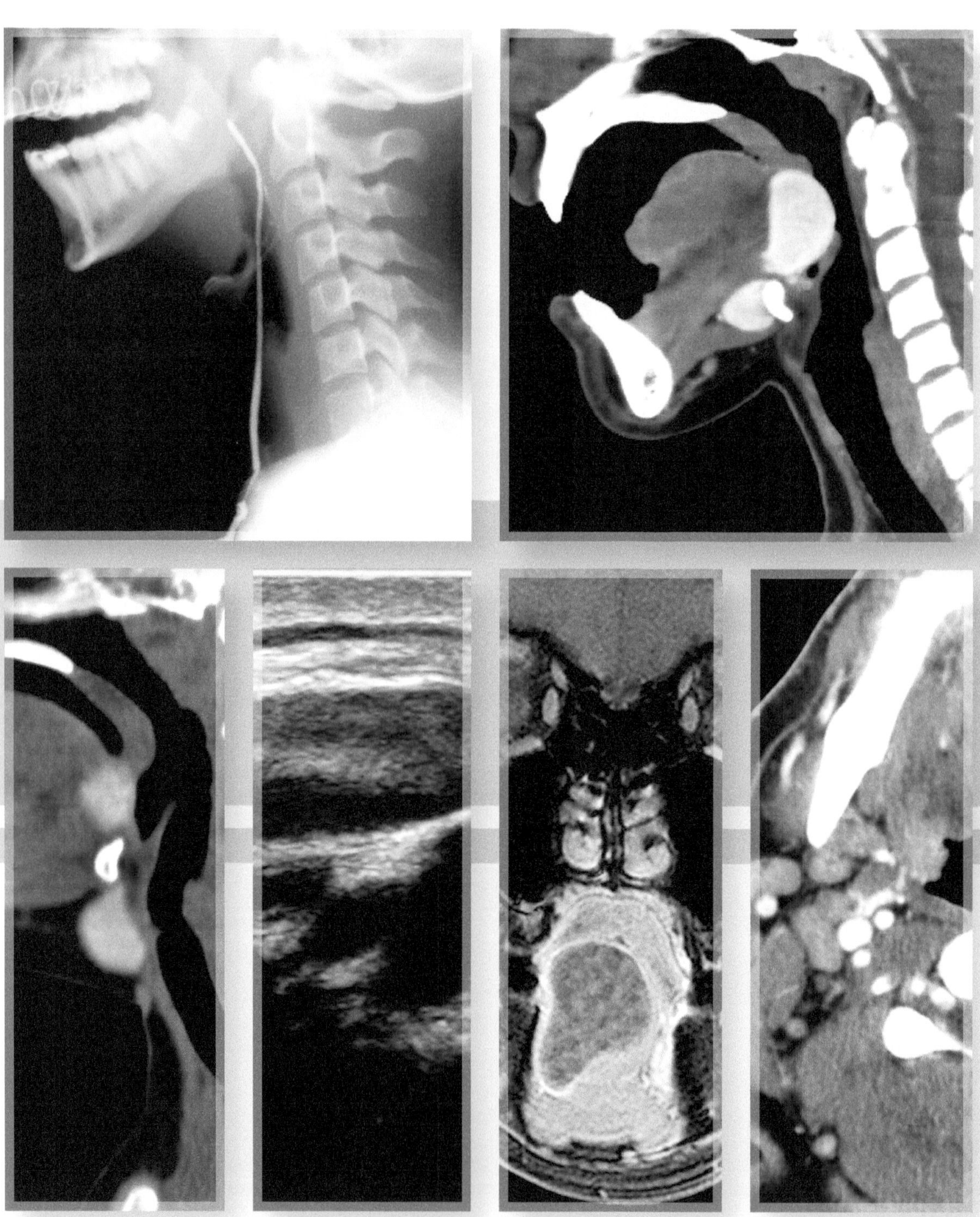

PART II
SECTION 3

Suprahyoid and Infrahyoid Neck

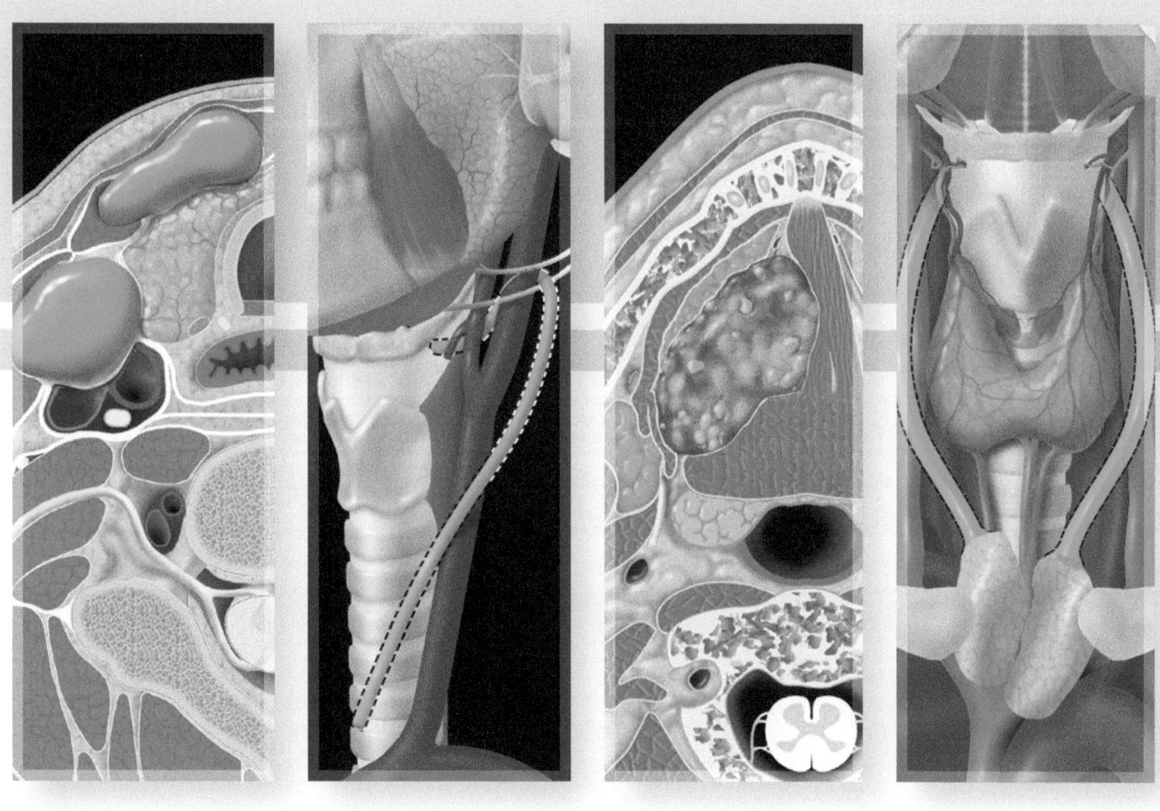

Summary Thoughts: Congenital Cystic Neck Masses

Palpable masses are a common indication for imaging the pediatric head & neck (H&N). Most are congenital or inflammatory in children; only 5% of childhood neoplasms occur in the H&N (excluding the brain). The most common extrathyroid, nonneoplastic **solid** neck masses in children are related to inflammatory disease & do not require imaging at all, unless there is concern for deep neck infection or abscess. The most common **cystic** masses in the pediatric H&N are congenital lesions secondary to abnormal embryogenesis involving the thyroglossal duct (TGD), the branchial apparatus, or the vascular endothelium. TGD cysts (TGDCs) account for 70-90% of all congenital neck abnormalities in children. The most common branchial apparatus lesion is the 2nd branchial cleft or apparatus cyst (BCC/BAC), & lymphatic malformations are the most common vascular malformations in the H&N.

Whenever a cystic neck mass is encountered on a pediatric imaging study, a very reasonable differential diagnosis can be made based on its **location** (midline, paramidline, or lateral as well as location relative to carotid sheath), **imaging appearance** (simple cyst, complicated cyst, enhancement, ± solid component), & **clinical presentation** (present since birth or acute onset ± clinical evidence of infection).

Terminology

A **TGDC** or tract is an anomalous remnant of the TGD that, under normal circumstances, completely involutes. Failure of involution may result in cysts (or solid foci of thyroid tissue) along the tract, anywhere from the midline posterior tongue at the foramen cecum, to the thyroid bed in the lower neck.

Branchial apparatus anomalies can be cysts, sinus tracts, or fistulae. **Cysts** are fluid filled with well-defined walls secondary to the failure of obliteration of a branchial cleft or pouch. **Sinus tracts** are congenital tracts with 1 opening, either externally to the skin surface (or external auditory canal) or internally to the pharynx (2nd branchial cleft), superolateral hypopharynx (3rd branchial cleft), or pyriform sinus (4th or 3rd branchial pouch). **Fistulae** are congenital tracts with 2 openings (1 internal & 1 external) secondary to failure of normal obliteration of the branchial cleft & pouch.

Imaging Techniques & Indications

US, CT, & MR are all reasonable options for imaging of neck masses in children. Modality choice depends on the clinical presentation, the referring clinical service, & the modalities available at the time. For instance, if there is concern that a child with cellulitis & cervical adenitis has a drainable abscess deep to a palpable neck mass, US is ideal for determining the presence of underlying drainable fluid. Likewise, if a child is thought to have a TGDC, US is the imaging modality of choice to evaluate the suspected TGDC & identify the presence of a normal-appearing thyroid gland in the lower neck. US is also the modality of choice in patients with suspected infantile hemangioma, as color Doppler findings can be quite characteristic. However, CECT is the initial imaging modality of choice to evaluate the total extent of disease in children with suspected deep neck infection & to assess for a possible underlying pyriform sinus tract in children with left-sided neck abscesses that involve the left thyroid lobe.

In children not presenting with signs & symptoms of infection, MR imaging is the preferred modality in many other settings, but frequently requires sedation in children less than 4-6 years of age. MR is also the preferred imaging modality for children with suspected vascular malformations due to its excellent soft tissue contrast resolution, variety of methods of interrogation, lack of limitations regarding depth, & lack of exposure to ionizing radiation.

Embryology

The thyroid gland migrates from the foramen cecum at the midline posterior tongue to the paramidline location in the lower neck via the path of the **TGD**. The TGD normally involutes during the 5th or 6th week of gestation. However, remnant epithelium anywhere along the tract may persist & form a TGDC. As the TGD diverticulum descends caudally, it passes along the anterior surface of the developing hyoid bone; therefore, remnants may be found anterior to the preepiglottic space of the larynx.

Branchial apparatus structures develop between the 4th & 6th week of gestation & consist of 6 pairs of mesodermal arches separated by 5 paired endodermal pouches internally & 5 paired ectodermal clefts externally. During the 6th week of gestation, the 2nd branchial arch overgrows the 3rd & 4th branchial arches, resulting in a combined 2nd, 3rd, & 4th branchial cleft, termed the "cervical sinus of His." Anomalies of the branchial apparatus include cysts, sinus tracts, & fistulae. The most common lesions for which imaging is indicated are BCCs/BACs, & most of these are related to anomalous development of a branchial cleft. However, a few are related to anomalous development of a branchial pouch.

The location of the lesion is the best clue to the origin of a branchial apparatus anomaly. **First BCCs** account for ~ 8% of all branchial anomalies. They are located in or around the external auditory canal, ear lobe, or parotid gland & may extend inferiorly to the angle of the mandible. **Second BCCs** account for up to 95% of all branchial apparatus anomalies & are subclassified by location using the Bailey system: Type I cysts are located deep to the platysma muscle/anterior to the sternocleidomastoid (SCM) muscle; type II cysts are posterior to the submandibular gland/anterior to the SCM (& are the most common); type III cysts protrude between the external & internal carotid arteries; & type IV cysts are directly adjacent to the pharyngeal wall (thought to be a remnant of the 2nd pouch). Fistulas are rare; however, a 2nd branchial apparatus fistula is occasionally identified with an internal opening at the level of the pharynx & an external skin opening anterior to the lower aspect of the SCM.

Third BCCs are rare & located in the posterior compartment of the upper neck or anterior compartment of the lower neck. Third pharyngeal pouch remnants are more common than cleft remnants & are related to descent of the thymic primordium from the lateral margins of the pharynx to the upper anterior mediastinum (via the thymopharyngeal duct) during the 6th-9th weeks of gestation. If the duct does not undergo normal involution, a cervical thymic cyst may form that is in close association with the anterior margin of the carotid sheath. The cyst formation is from interactions between the endodermal primordia & neural crest cells during normal thymic development & migration. Histologically, Hassall corpuscles will be identifiable within the cyst wall. Ectopic foci of solid thymic tissue may also be deposited along the remnant duct.

Pyriform sinus tracts, or rarely fistulae, represent a unique congenital anomaly of the **4th (or 3rd) pharyngeal pouch**.

Types of Congenital Cystic Neck Masses

Types of Congenital Cystic Neck Masses
Thyroglossal Duct Lesions
Thyroglossal duct cyst: Tongue base to thyroid bed; embedded in strap muscles when infrahyoid
Ectopic thyroid tissue: Lingual location is most common
Branchial Apparatus Lesions
1st branchial cleft cyst (type I): Located anterior, inferior, or posterior to external auditory canal
1st branchial cleft cyst (type II): Located in or adjacent to parotid gland; may extend inferiorly to angle of mandible
2nd branchial cleft cyst: Most common location is posterior to submandibular gland, lateral to carotid space, & anteromedial to SCM muscle
3rd branchial cleft cyst: Posterior cervical space in upper neck or anterior to SCM in lower neck
3rd branchial pouch remnant → thymopharyngeal duct cyst or ectopic thymus: Along course from pharynx to upper mediastinum
4th branchial pouch remnant → pyriform sinus tract: Patients present with left-sided abscess involving thyroid gland
Vascular Malformations
Venous malformation: Patchy, gradual enhancement; phleboliths are common; ± fluid-fluid levels
Lymphatic malformation: Multilocular cyst ± fluid-fluid levels; rim/septal enhancement
Venolymphatic malformation: Mixed enhancing venous & nonenhancing lymphatic components
SCM = sternocleidomastoid.

This lesion should be suspected in any child presenting with neck infection involving the left thyroid lobe. The inflammation can frequently be traced superiorly to an asymmetric pyriform sinus apex. A postbarium swallow CT study is helpful to define the barium-filled tract extending from the pyriform sinus to the anterior lower neck.

Vascular malformations are congenital malformations of endothelial development that can be divided into simple or combined lesions with combined lesions containing 2 or more vessel types in 1 lesion. Simple lesions can be divided based on the predominant endothelial characteristics of the lesion into capillary malformations, lymphatic malformations, venous malformations, arteriovenous malformations, & arteriovenous fistulae. The most common vascular malformations identified in the H&N are lymphatic, venous, & combined venolymphatic lesions.

Imaging Anatomy

Recognizing the defined **location** of a congenital abnormality, particularly congenital cysts, is key to arriving at the correct diagnosis or differential diagnosis. **TGD** remnants may be in the form of cysts or solid ectopic thyroid tissue anywhere from the midline tongue base to the infrahyoid paramidline thyroid bed. **First BCCs** are in or around the external auditory canal or parotid gland. **Second BCCs** are most commonly posteromedial to the submandibular gland & anteromedial to the SCM. Cysts in the posterior triangle of the upper neck may be 3rd BCCs or lymphatic malformations. Cysts along the lower anterior margin of the SCM may be from the 2nd or 3rd branchial cleft or may be lymphatic malformations. Cysts or solid masses in close association with the carotid sheath along the tract of the thymopharyngeal duct (from the angle of the mandible to the upper mediastinum) should raise the question of cervical thymic cyst or ectopic thymus (**3rd pouch** remnants), & left-sided neck abscesses involving the thyroid gland should raise the question of a pyriform sinus sinus tract as a cause, a **4th (or 3rd) pharyngeal pouch** remnant.

Differential Diagnosis

Thyroglossal Duct Lesions

- TGDC: Tongue base to thyroid bed
- Ectopic thyroid: Lingual thyroid is most common

Branchial Apparatus Lesions

- 1st BCC: Type I cysts lie anterior, inferior, or posterior to external auditory canal; type II cysts in superficial, parotid, or parapharyngeal space may extend as low as posterior submandibular space
- 2nd BCC: Most common posterolateral to submandibular gland, lateral to carotid space, & anteromedial to SCM
- 3rd BCC: Posterior cervical space upper neck, along anterior border of SCM in mid- & lower neck
- 3rd branchial pouch remnant: Thymopharyngeal duct cyst or ectopic thymus
- 4th branchial pouch remnant: Pyriform sinus tract → recurrent thyroiditis or thyroid abscess, usually left sided; some literature suggests this may be 3rd pouch remnant

Vascular Malformations

- Venous malformations: Patchy, gradual enhancement; ± fluid-fluid levels & phleboliths
- Lymphatic malformations: Classically multilocular & transspatial with fluid-fluid levels & minimal rim/septal enhancement
- Venolymphatic malformations: Nonenhancing lymphatic & enhancing venous elements ± phleboliths

Selected References

1. Booth TN: Congenital cystic neck masses. Neuroimaging Clin N Am. 33(4):591-605, 2023
2. Mamlouk MD: Solid and vascular neck masses in children. Neuroimaging Clin N Am. 33(4):607-21, 2023
3. Tokarz E et al: Proposed ultrasound algorithm to differentiate thyroglossal duct and dermoid cysts. Int J Pediatr Otorhinolaryngol. 142:110624, 2021
4. Corvino A et al: Thyroglossal duct cysts and site-specific differential diagnoses: imaging findings with emphasis on ultrasound assessment. J Ultrasound. 23(2):139-49, 2020
5. Merrow AC et al: 2014 revised classification of vascular lesions from the International Society for the Study of Vascular Anomalies: radiologic-pathologic update. Radiographics. 36(5):1494-516, 2016
6. Thomas B et al: Revisiting imaging features and the embryologic basis of third and fourth branchial anomalies. AJNR Am J Neuroradiol. 31(4):755-60, 2010

6-Week Embryo

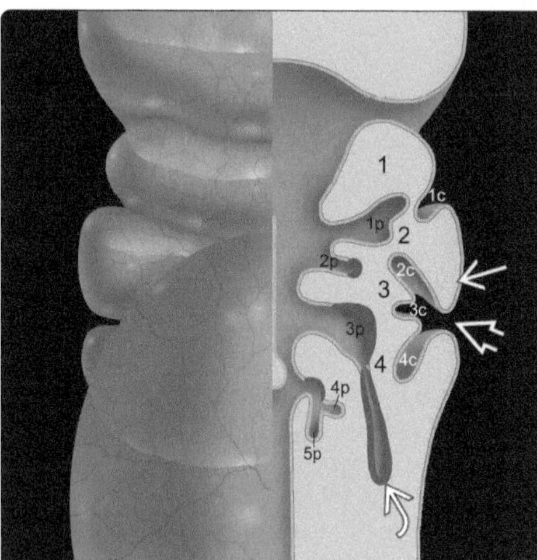

1st Branchial Cleft Anomaly

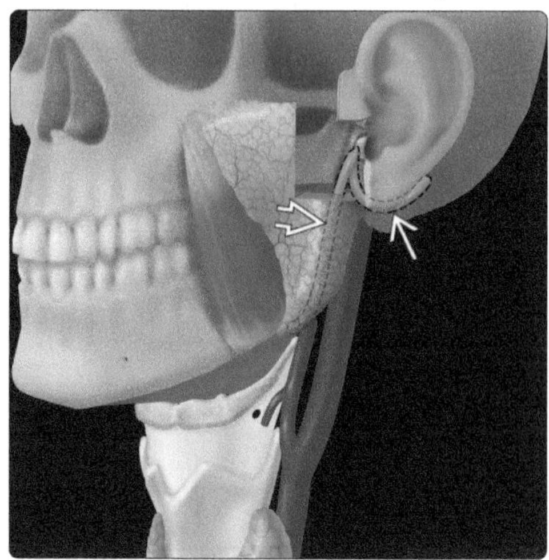

(Left) *Anterior graphic of a 6-week embryo shows the 2nd branchial arch growing inferiorly over the 3rd & 4th arches, resulting in the cervical sinus of His that combines the 2nd, 3rd, & 4th branchial clefts (BCs). Note that the thymopharyngeal duct is a remnant of the 3rd branchial pouch.* **(Right)** *Oblique graphic shows the tract of a type I 1st BC anomaly from the medial bony external auditory canal (EAC) toward the retroauricular area. The tract of a type II 1st BC anomaly connects the EAC to the angle of the mandible.*

2nd Branchial Cleft Anomaly

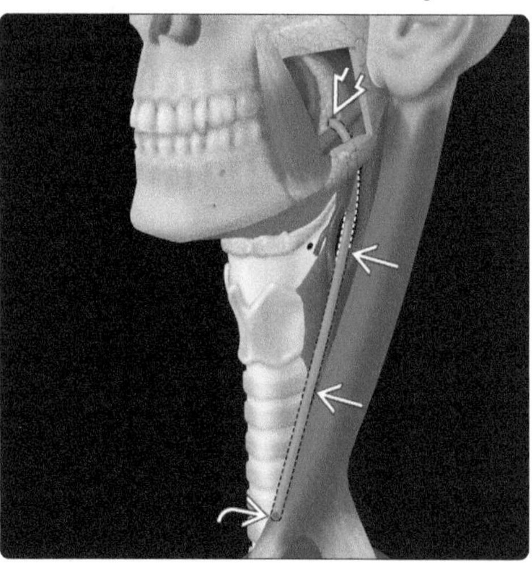

3rd Branchial Cleft Anomaly

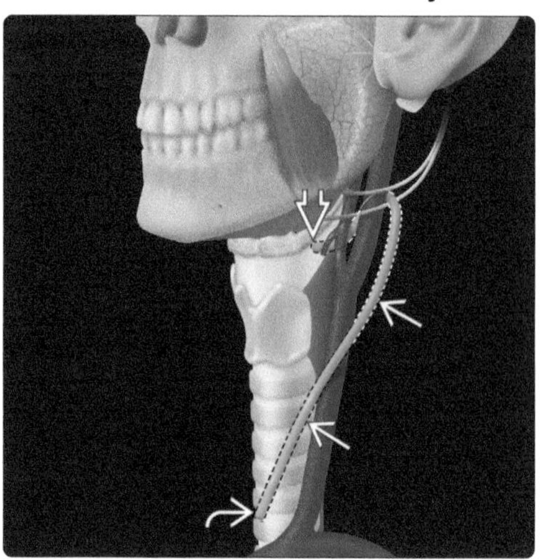

(Left) *Oblique graphic of the tract of a 2nd BC fistula shows a proximal opening in the faucial tonsil & a distal opening in the anterior supraclavicular neck. Second BC cysts (BCCs) may occur anywhere along this tract & are the most common of the BCCs.* **(Right)** *Oblique graphic illustrates the tract of a 3rd BC anomaly extending from the cephalad aspect of the lateral hypopharynx to the supraclavicular anterior neck skin. Notice cysts would lie in the posterior upper neck or the anterior lower neck.*

Thymopharyngeal Duct

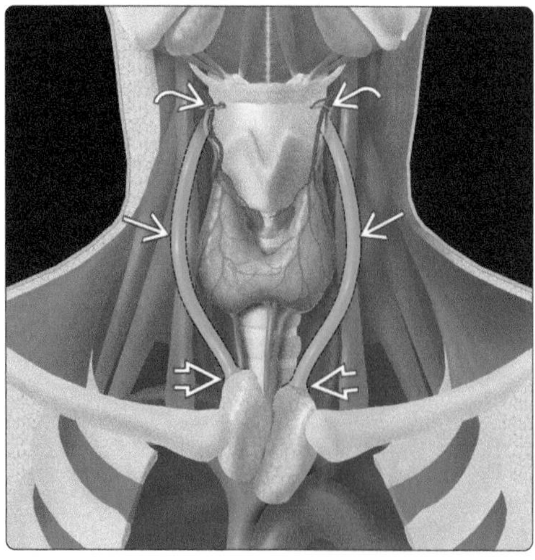

4th Branchial Cleft Anomaly

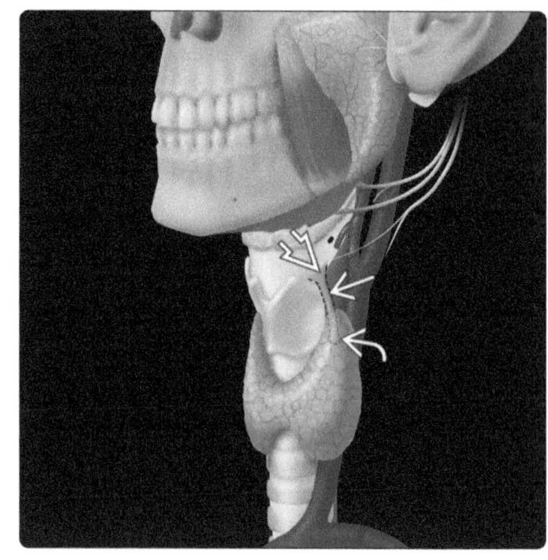

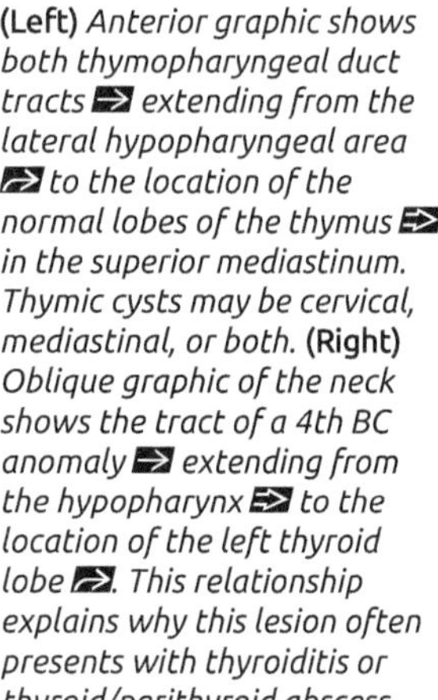

(Left) *Anterior graphic shows both thymopharyngeal duct tracts extending from the lateral hypopharyngeal area to the location of the normal lobes of the thymus in the superior mediastinum. Thymic cysts may be cervical, mediastinal, or both.* **(Right)** *Oblique graphic of the neck shows the tract of a 4th BC anomaly extending from the hypopharynx to the location of the left thyroid lobe. This relationship explains why this lesion often presents with thyroiditis or thyroid/perithyroid abscess.*

Thyroglossal Duct

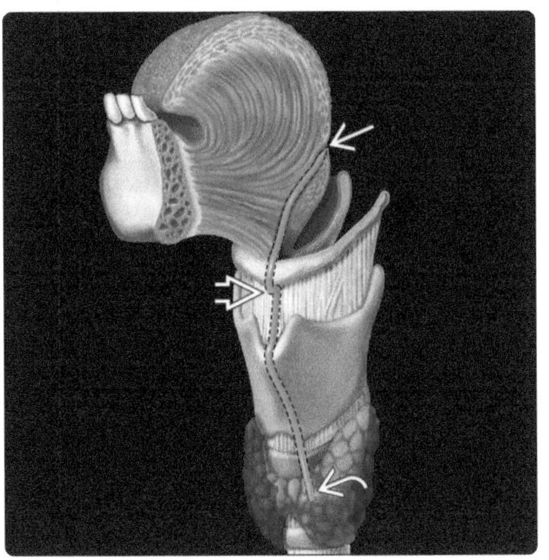

Localization of Major Congenital Cystic Neck Lesions

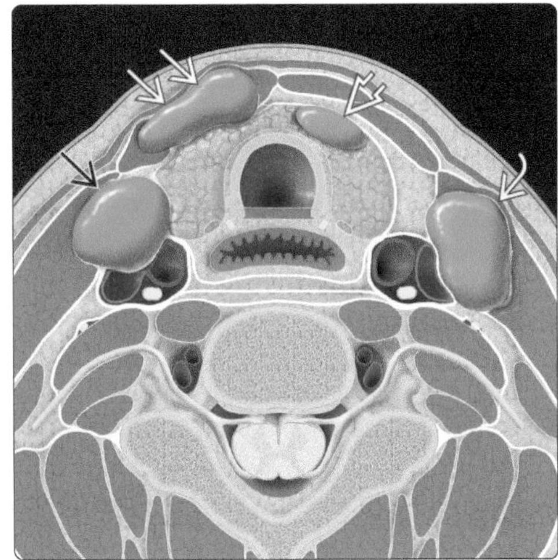

(Left) *Oblique graphic illustrates the tract of the thyroglossal duct descending from the foramen cecum ➡ (at the midline tongue base) to the midline hyoid bone ➡ before tracking off-midline to the thyroid lobe ➡.* **(Right)** *Axial graphic demonstrates the locations of 4 major congenital cystic lesions of the neck. Shown here are the location of infrahyoid 2nd & 3rd BCCs ➡, infrahyoid thyroglossal duct cysts ➡ (embedded in strap muscle), cervical thymic cysts ➡, & 4th branchial apparatus sinus tracts ➡.*

1st Branchial Cleft Anomaly

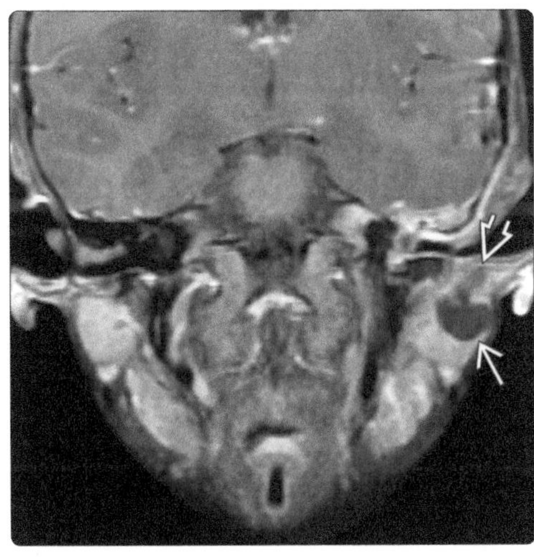

2nd Branchial Cleft Anomaly

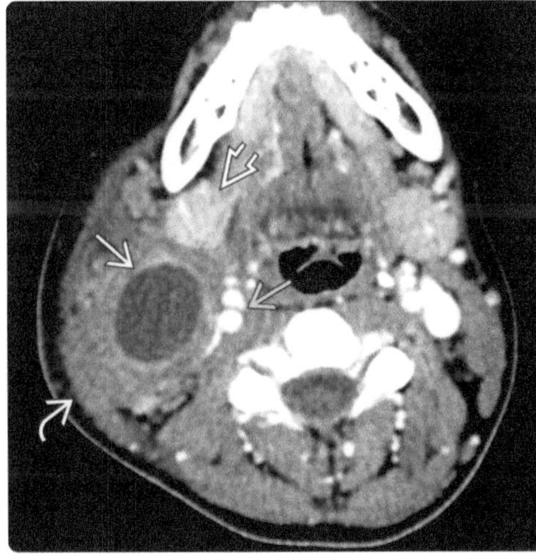

(Left) *Coronal T1 C+ FS MR in a 3-year-old patient with a 1st BAC shows a lobulated, nonenhancing periparotid cyst ➡ extending toward the junction of the cartilaginous & bony EAC ➡.* **(Right)** *Axial CECT in a teenager with an enlarging mass shows a cystic-appearing lesion ➡ in the typical location of a 2nd BCC: Dorsal to submandibular gland ➡, anterior to sternocleidomastoid (SCM) muscle ➡ & lateral to carotid sheath vessels ➡.*

Thymic Cyst

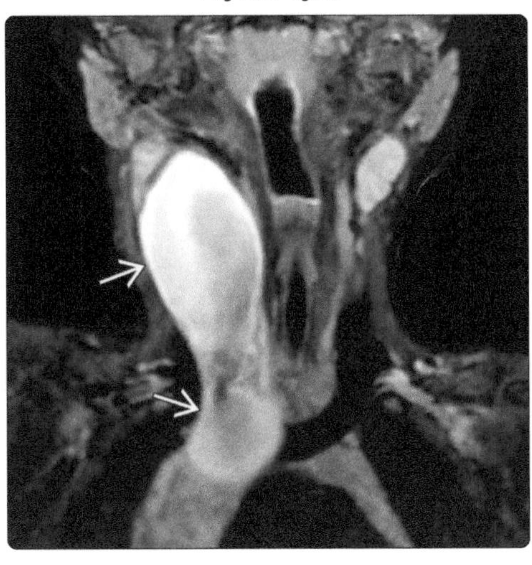

4th Branchial Cleft Anomaly

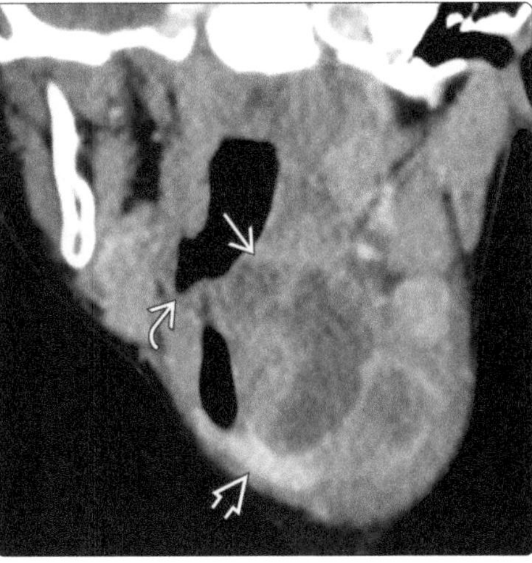

(Left) *Coronal FSEIR in a child with a right-sided neck mass shows a bilobed hyperintense cystic mass ➡ extending from the upper neck to the upper mediastinum, the location typical of a thymic cyst.* **(Right)** *Coronal CECT in a 2-year-old with a heterogeneously enhancing left neck mass that extends from the region of the effaced left pyriform sinus ➡ to the upper left thyroid lobe ➡, typical of an abscess secondary to congenital 4th (or 3rd) pharyngeal pouch sinus tract, is shown. Notice the air-filled normal right pyriform sinus ➡.*

KEY FACTS

TERMINOLOGY

- Thyroid tissue in abnormal ectopic location in base of tongue (BOT) or floor of mouth [root of tongue (ROT)/sublingual space]

IMAGING

- Well-circumscribed, rounded midline BOT mass
  - Usually at site of foramen cecum
- Less commonly in sublingual space or ROT
- Imaging features similar to normal thyroid tissue
- High density on NECT due to iodine content
- Usually avid homogeneous enhancement
- Tc-99m pertechnetate, radioiodine scan or early phase of 99mTc-sestamibi confirms diagnosis and determines other sites of thyroid tissue

TOP DIFFERENTIAL DIAGNOSES

- Venous malformation
- Hemangioma, upper airway
- Tonsillar tissue, prominent/asymmetric
- Non-Hodgkin lymphoma, lingual tonsil

PATHOLOGY

- Arrest of thyroid precursor descent in 1st trimester

CLINICAL ISSUES

- Most common location of ectopic thyroid (90%)
  - In 75%, lingual thyroid is only functioning thyroid tissue
- Thyroid hormone production may be insufficient, resulting in ectopic thyroid gland enlargement
- Lingual thyroid may expand rapidly during puberty
- Goiter in ectopic gland rarely with obstructive symptoms
- Differentiated thyroid carcinoma in lingual thyroid extremely rare, but serious potential complication

DIAGNOSTIC CHECKLIST

- Well-defined, ovoid or round mass in BOT or floor of mouth
- Intrinsic high density on CT characteristic
- Must check for additional cervical thyroid tissue

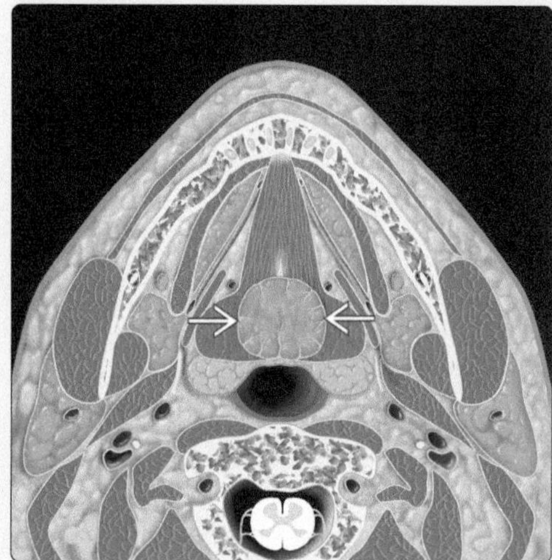

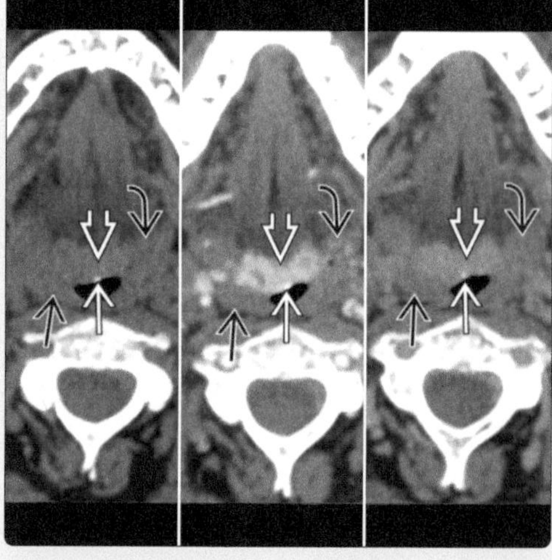

(Left) *Axial graphic depicts lingual thyroid ➡ in posterior midline of tongue, just deep to location of foramen cecum. Sharply defined contour and midline location in floor of mouth or tongue base are typical of lingual thyroid.* **(Right)** *Axial 3-phase (precontrast, 30-sec arterial & 90-sec venous phases) side-by-side CT scans show a lingual thyroid ➡ with density higher than that of lingual ⇨ & palatine ⇨ tonsils on all phases. Note a tiny Ca^{++} in the lingual thyroid posteriorly ➡.*

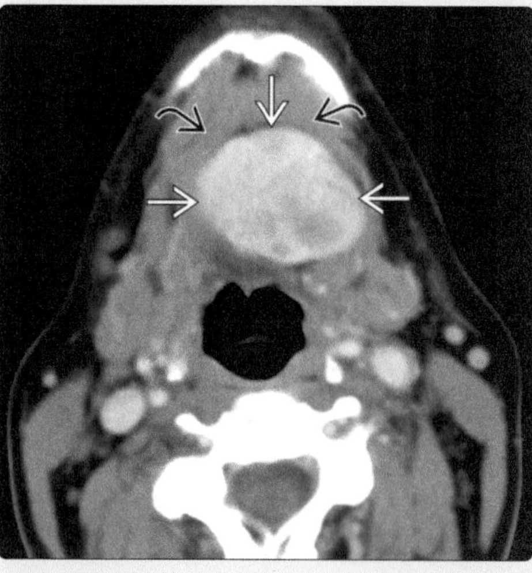

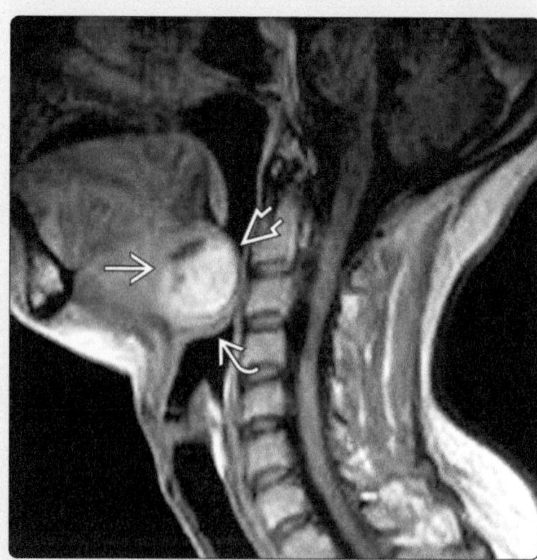

(Left) *Axial CECT demonstrates a sharply defined submucosal mass ➡ in the midline floor of the mouth involving the root of the tongue (ROT). Note the lateral splaying of ROT genioglossus muscles ⇨. Heterogeneous density suggests development of a goiter.* **(Right)** *Sagittal T1WI MR shows a heterogeneous hyperintense mass ➡ in the midline base of the tongue. Note the narrowing of the oropharyngeal airway ➡ and posterior and inferior displacement of the epiglottis ⇨.*

TERMINOLOGY

Definitions

- Thyroid tissue in abnormal ectopic location in base of tongue (BOT) or floor of mouth [root of tongue (ROT)/sublingual space]

IMAGING

General Features

- Best diagnostic clue
  - Imaging characteristics similar to normal thyroid
- Location
  - Midline BOT at level of foramen cecum
  - Less commonly in sublingual space or ROT
- Morphology
  - Well circumscribed, round or ovoid, 1-3 cm

CT Findings

- NECT
  - Sharply marginated, rounded mass
  - High density secondary to iodine accumulation
- CECT
  - Avid homogeneous enhancement

MR Findings

- T1WI
  - Isointense to mildly hyperintense relative to tongue
- T2WI
  - Mildly to strikingly hyperintense relative to tongue
- T1WI C+
  - Variable; most often homogeneous enhancement greater than tongue

Nuclear Medicine Findings

- **Tc-99m pertechnetate** or radioiodine scan to confirm
  - **I-123** scan for diagnosis
  - **I-131** scan for diagnosis/radioablation
- Parathyroid dual-phase **99mTc-sestamibi** scintigraphy shows normal or ectopic thyroid gland on **early images (15 min)** only and wash-out on delayed images
  - Parathyroid adenoma: Persistent focus of uptake on both early (15 min) and delayed (2 hr) phase images

Imaging Recommendations

- Protocol advice
  - Image through infrahyoid neck to determine if orthotopic thyroid tissue present in normal thyroid bed

DIFFERENTIAL DIAGNOSIS

Venous Malformation

- Vasoformative anomaly demonstrates prominent T2 hyperintensity and contrast enhancement

Infantile Hemangioma, Upper Airway

- Cavernous more common than capillary (infantile)

Tonsillar Tissue, Prominent/Asymmetric

- Prominent lingual lymphoid tonsils at entire width of BOT

Non-Hodgkin Lymphoma, Lingual Tonsil

- Isolated or in association with nodal or tonsillar lymphoma

PATHOLOGY

General Features

- Associated abnormalities
  - Thyroid migration anomalies (e.g., thyroglossal duct cyst)

Embryology

- Around 24th day of gestation, thyroid develops from endodermal diverticulum (called medial anlage)
  - Arising from paramedian aspect of 1st and 2nd branchial pouches (foramen cecum of tongue area)
- Lower end of diverticulum enlarges to form thyroid gland
  - Rest remains narrow (called thyroglossal duct), begins to involute by 7-10 gestational weeks
- Descends through BOT, floor of mouth, around and in front of hyoid bone, and through area of infrahyoid strap muscles
  - Final position in cervical thyroid bed of visceral space
- Lingual thyroid when arrest of thyroid anlage migration within BOT between 3rd and 7th gestational week
  - Complete arrest: No cervical thyroid in thyroid bed (75%)
  - Partial arrest: High cervical thyroid (25%)

CLINICAL ISSUES

Presentation

- Most common signs/symptoms
  - Dysphagia, dysphonia, dyspnea, obstructive sleep apnea
  - Most patients hypothyroid (60%) or euthyroid

Demographics

- Lingual most common site of ectopic thyroid (90%)
- Extremely rare; incidence (1:10,000 to 1:100,000)
- Female patients more often than male patients (M:F = 1:4)
- 25% of infants with congenital hypothyroidism have ectopic gland

Natural History & Prognosis

- Lingual thyroid may expand rapidly during puberty
- Goiter in ectopic gland rarely with obstructive symptoms
- Carcinoma of lingual thyroid extremely rare
  - Most often follicular thyroid carcinoma (unlike orthotopic cervical thyroid gland)
- Synchronous ectopic lingual thyroid and mediastinal ectopic parathyroid adenoma rarely occur

Treatment

- Thyroid hormone replacement 1st to shrink gland at BOT
- Surgical resection if obstructive symptoms
- Look for thyroid tissue in other locations before excision to prevent extreme postoperative hypothyroidism
- Some advocate radioiodine ablation

DIAGNOSTIC CHECKLIST

Consider

- Comment on infrahyoid thyroid tissue in thyroid bed
  - Lingual thyroid only functioning thyroid tissue in 75%

SELECTED REFERENCES

1. Palot Manzil FF et al: Synchronous ectopic thyroid gland and ectopic parathyroid adenoma on (99m)Tc-sestamibi scintigraphy and correlative imaging. J Nucl Med Technol. 51(3):263-4, 2023

Oral Cavity Dermoid and Epidermoid

KEY FACTS

TERMINOLOGY

- Cystic oral cavity (OC) lesion resulting from congenital epithelial inclusion or rest

IMAGING

- Dermoid, epidermoid appear as well-demarcated OC cysts
- Both dermoid and epidermoid may have restricted diffusion on DWI
- Dermoid: Complex cystic mass, often with fat &/or calcification (sack of marbles appearance pathognomonic)
  - More often midline
  - Fat bright on T1WI, low signal with fat saturation + chemical shift artifact
- Epidermoid: Fluid contents only

TOP DIFFERENTIAL DIAGNOSES

- Ranula
- Lymphatic malformation of OC
- Heterotopic gastrointestinal cyst of OC
- Submandibular cystic metastatic squamous cell carcinoma lymph node
- Thyroglossal duct cyst
- OC abscess

PATHOLOGY

- Dermoid: Epithelial elements plus dermal adnexa
- Epidermoid: Epithelial elements only

CLINICAL ISSUES

- Painless subcutaneous or submucosal mass (85-90%)
- Often grows rapidly during puberty when sebaceous glands activated
- Surgical resection curative

DIAGNOSTIC CHECKLIST

- OC dermoid, epidermoid, ranula, and lymphatic malformation may appear indistinguishable
- Only abscess and metastatic nodes solid components may restrict diffusion among top differential diagnoses

(Left) *Axial graphic depicts a dermoid ➡ within the sublingual space (SLS) that appears well defined and distorts only adjacent anatomy. The mass is complex, containing a mixture of fluid, fat globules (sack of marbles appearance), and calcifications.* **(Right)** *Axial T1 MR through the floor of the mouth shows an ovoid, well-circumscribed mass ➡. There are internal hyperintense globules (sack of marbles appearance) with chemical shift artifact ⮫, indicating fatty content, consistent with a dermoid cyst.*

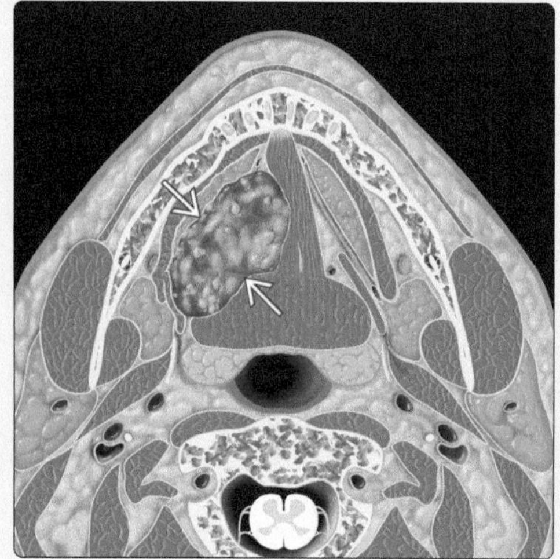

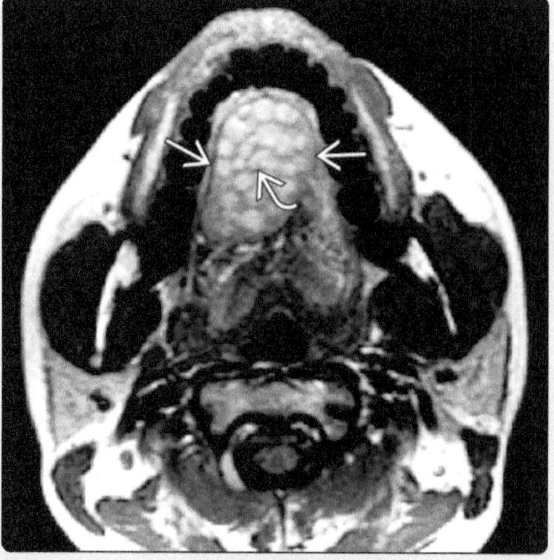

(Left) *Sagittal T2 FS MR in a child shows multiseptated fluid intensity cystic lesion in the tongue/SLS ➡. No definite fatty contents are detected on imaging.* **(Right)** *Axial DWI MR in the same patient shows diffusion restriction of the cyst contents ➡. Even though the presence of diffusion restriction and absence of fatty contents should favor epidermoid, this lesion was proven to be a lingual dermoid cyst extending to the SLS. Remember, dermoid cysts may also restrict diffusion.*

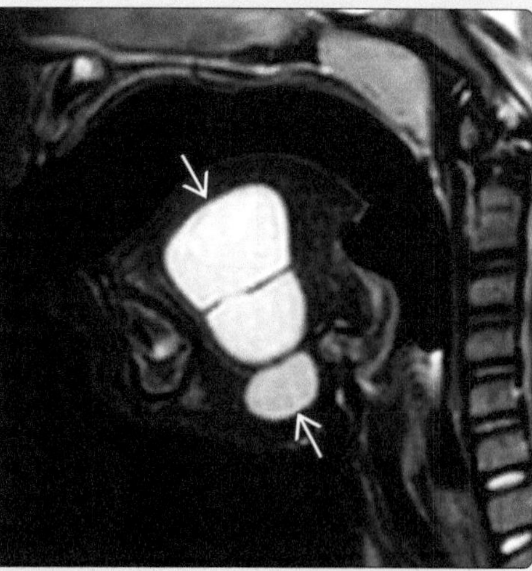

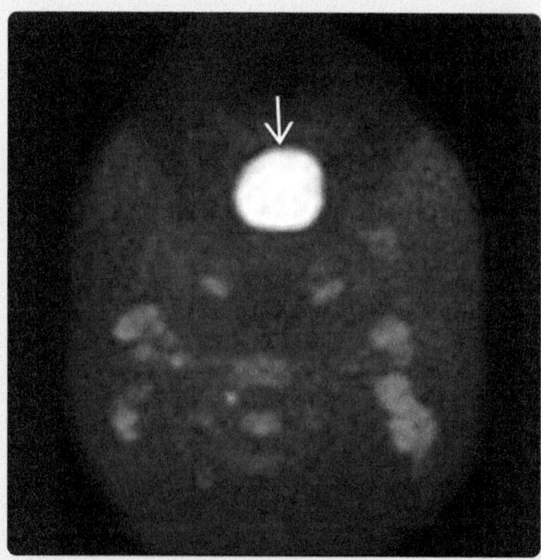

TERMINOLOGY

Synonyms

- Developmental oral cavity (OC) cyst, ectodermal inclusion cyst, dermoid cyst

Definitions

- Cystic OC lesion resulting from congenital epithelial inclusion or rest
  - **Dermoid**: Epithelial elements + dermal adnexa
  - **Epidermoid**: Epithelial elements only
- **Teratoid** cyst: Rarer; epithelial elements + other tissue, such as bone, cartilage, or muscle

IMAGING

General Features

- Best diagnostic clue
  - Dermoid and epidermoid appear as well-demarcated cysts in OC
  - Dermoid: Fatty, fluid, or mixed contents
    - Pathognomonic sack of marbles appearance from coalescence of fat into small nodules within fluid matrix
      - Sometimes even calcifications (< 50%)
  - Epidermoid: Fluid only
- Location
  - Submandibular space (SMS), sublingual space (SLS), or root of tongue (ROT)
  - Dermoid cyst more frequently midline
- Size
  - Typically < 4 cm
- Morphology
  - Ovoid or tubular
    - Most show thin, definable wall (75%)
    - 20% have nodular soft tissue in wall or on periphery of cyst

CT Findings

- NECT
  - Low-density, unilocular, well-circumscribed mass
    - Dermoid: Fatty internal material, mixed-density fluid, calcification (< 50%)
    - Epidermoid: Fluid density without complex features
- CECT
  - May see subtle enhancement of wall
  - If dermoid has only minimal complex elements, can be indistinguishable from epidermoid

MR Findings

- T1WI
  - Well-circumscribed mass in OC
  - Dermoid: Complex fluid signal characteristic
    - Focal or diffuse high signal suggests fat
      - Fat proven by chemical shift artifact or fat-saturation techniques
  - Epidermoid: Homogeneous fluid signal
    - Diffuse high signal may reflect protein content
- T2WI
  - Dermoid: Heterogeneous high signal
    - Intermediate signal if fat
    - Focal areas of low signal if calcifications
  - Epidermoid: Homogeneous high signal
- DWI
  - Dermoid or epidermoid may show restricted diffusion
    - Feature of epidermoid characteristically
  - ADC values only moderately low compared with intracranial epidermoids
- T1WI C+
  - Thin rim enhancement often evident

Ultrasonographic Findings

- May be useful for evaluation of superficial lesions
- Dermoid: Mixed internal echoes from fat; echogenic foci with dense shadowing if calcifications
- Epidermoid: Pseudosolid appearance with uniform internal echoes
  - Cellular material within cyst creates pseudosolid appearance
  - Posterior wall echo enhancement clue to cystic nature

Imaging Recommendations

- Best imaging tool
  - CECT or MR for localization
  - MR best for distinguishing dermoid and epidermoid
    - If complex signal, then lesion most likely represents dermoid
- Protocol advice
  - CT: Thin section with multiplanar reconstructions aids in specific OC localization
  - MR: Include fat-suppression sequences to prove presence of fat

DIFFERENTIAL DIAGNOSIS

Ranula

- Simple ranula may exactly mimic SLS epidermoid
  - Unilateral, thin-walled SLS cystic mass
- Diving ranula may also mimic SLS-SMS epidermoid
  - Comet-shaped, unilocular mass with "tail" in collapsed SLS and "head" in posterior SMS

Oral Cavity Lymphatic Malformation

- Transspatial cystic mass
- May hemorrhage, resulting in fluid levels
- Infected lymphatic malformation may have complex proteinaceous contents

Heterotopic Gastrointestinal Cyst of Oral Cavity

- Extremely rare; may coexist with sublingual dermoid cyst

Squamous Cell Carcinoma Nodes

- Cystic metastatic node; usually from OC 1°, including lip
- Submandibular nodes (level IB)
- Solid components if any, may restrict diffusion

Thyroglossal Duct Cyst

- Midline cystic neck mass between hyoid and foramen cecum
- In posterior tongue root, mimics epidermoid
- Important distinction for surgical excision technique
  - Sistrunk procedure for thyroglossal duct (TGD) cyst
  - Simple excision for epidermoid cyst

Oral Cavity Abscess

- Clinical setting of septic patient with painful OC mass distinctive
- Rim-enhancing, cystic mass, often with extensive tongue and soft tissue cellulitis-edema
- Pyogenic abscess restricts diffusion

PATHOLOGY

General Features

- Etiology
  - 2 theories: Congenital and acquired
    - Congenital inclusion of dermal elements at site of embryonic 1st and 2nd branchial arches
      - Sequestration of trapped surface ectoderm during midline fusion in 3rd-4th embryonic weeks
    - Acquired traumatic implantation of epithelial elements within OC mucosa

Staging, Grading, & Classification

- Meyer classification (pathologic)
  - Dermoid: Epithelium-lined cyst containing skin appendages, such as sebaceous and sweat glands, and hair follicles in cyst wall
  - Epidermoid: Lined with simple squamous epithelium and surrounding connective tissue
  - Teratoid: Epithelium-lined cyst containing mesodermal or endodermal elements, such as muscle, bones, teeth, and mucous membranes

Gross Pathologic & Surgical Features

- Oily or cheesy material; tan, yellow, or white
- May contain blood or chronic blood products
- Cyst wall 2-6 mm thick with fibrous capsule

Microscopic Features

- Dermoid
  - Contains dermal structures, including sebaceous glands, hair follicles, blood vessels, **fat** ± collagen
    - Sweat glands in minority (20%)
    - Lined by keratinizing squamous epithelium
  - Dermoid diagnosis can be difficult for pathologist if full cyst lining not available
- Epidermoid
  - Simple squamous cell epithelium with fibrous wall
- Teratoid cyst
  - Contains elements from all 3 germ cell layers
    - Dermoid features + other contents, such as bone, muscle, and cartilage

CLINICAL ISSUES

Presentation

- Most common signs/symptoms
  - Painless subcutaneous or submucosal mass (85-90%)
  - Other signs/symptoms
    - Dysphagia, globus oral sensation
    - Airway encroachment when large
    - Uncommonly acute presentation with cyst rupture and inflammation
- Clinical profile
  - Young adult with painless SMS/SLS mass

Demographics

- Age
  - Most often in late teens to 20s; much earlier with epidermoids, including infants
- Sex
  - No predilection
- Epidemiology
  - Dermoid and epidermoid least common of congenital neck lesions
  - < 25% of head and neck dermoids occur in OC, dermoids more commonly than epidermoids
  - 90% of OC/oropharynx masses squamous cell carcinoma

Natural History & Prognosis

- Benign lesion with slow growth; malignant transformation rare
- Present during childhood but small and dormant
- May enlarge, become symptomatic when sebaceous glands activated during adolescence
- Rapid growth due to cyst rupture, sudden increase in desquamation, during pregnancy, or association with sinus tract

Treatment

- Surgical resection curative
  - Entire cyst must be removed to prevent recurrence
- Extracapsular excision can be performed by intraoral or external approach
- Surgical approach may be decided by lesion position relative to mylohyoid muscle
  - SLS: Superomedial to mylohyoid muscle
    - Intraoral approach with good cosmetic and functional results
  - SMS: Inferolateral to mylohyoid
    - Submandibular approach
- Postoperative complications rare
- Steroids or nonsteroidal drugs calm inflammation in ruptured lesions

DIAGNOSTIC CHECKLIST

Consider

- OC dermoid, epidermoid, ranula, and lymphatic malformation often seem indistinguishable

Image Interpretation Pearls

- Presence of fat ± calcium characterizes dermoid
- When hemorrhagic fluid levels are present, consider lymphatic malformation
- Comet shape with components in SLS and SMS supports diving ranula

SELECTED REFERENCES

1. Oh HJ et al: Craniofacial epidermoid and dermoid cysts. J Craniofac Surg. 34(8):2405-9, 2023
2. Godinho GV et al: Epidermoid cyst mimicking a thyroglossal duct cyst in a pediatric patient: a case report. Gen Dent. 70(1):61-4, 2022
3. Giarraputo L et al: Dermoid cyst of the floor of the mouth: diagnostic imaging findings. Cureus. 10(4):e2403, 2018
4. Ginat DT et al: Heterotopic gastrointestinal cyst of the oral cavity radiology-pathology correlation. Head Neck Pathol. 13(4):668-70, 2018
5. Tsai A et al: Occipital intraosseous dermoid cyst with restricted diffusion on magnetic resonance imaging in a child. Radiol Case Rep. 13(1):248-53, 2018

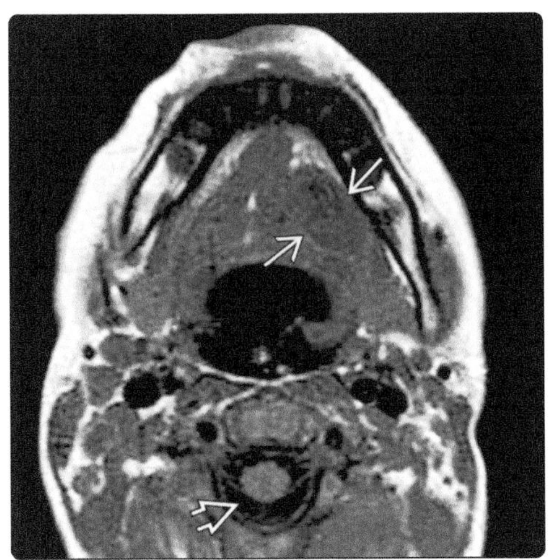

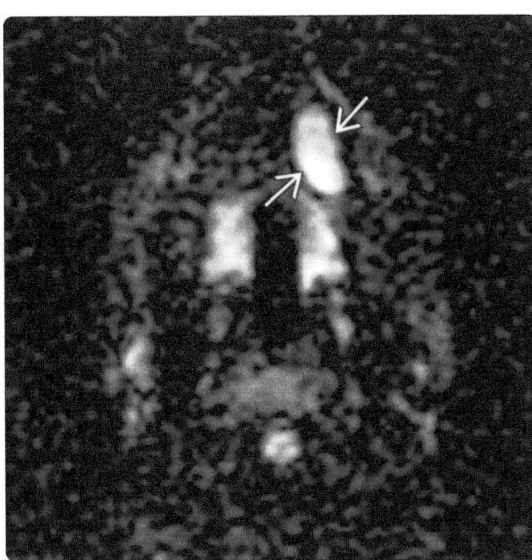

(Left) *Axial T1 MR reveals an SLS epidermoid →. Lesion signal is only minimally hypointense relative to the skeletal muscle and considerably hyperintense to CSF ⇨. This appearance is consistent with increased protein content and suggests prior infection or possibly hemorrhage.* **(Right)** *Axial DWI MR shows restricted diffusion → within the same sublingual lesion. Both dermoids and epidermoids may exhibit diffusion restriction, and it is difficult to differentiate from a fluid-like dermoid without visible complex elements.*

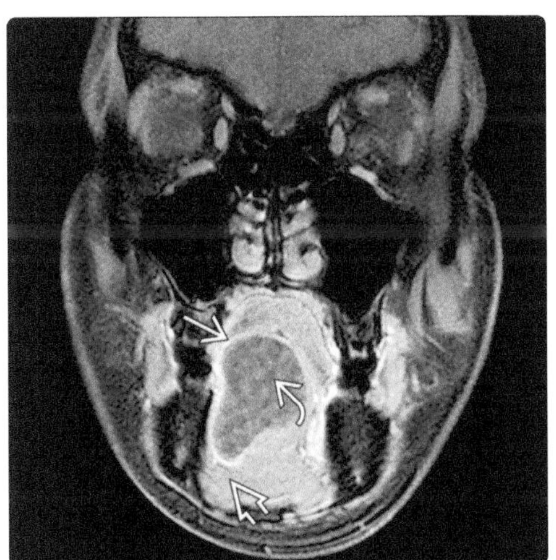

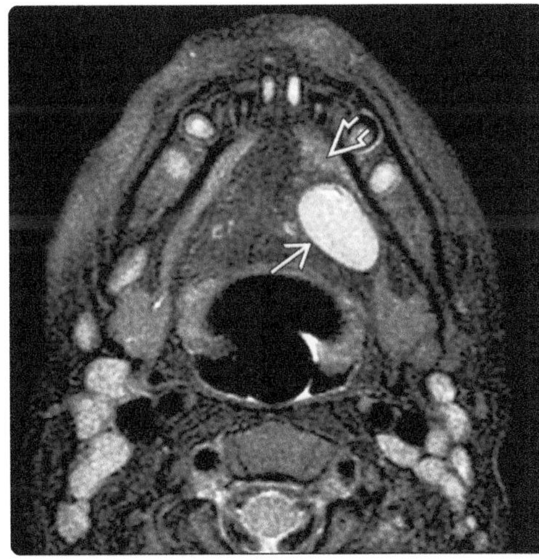

(Left) *Coronal T1 C+ FS MR shows a well-circumscribed mass with thin rim enhancement → superior to the mylohyoid muscle ⇨, confirming the sublingual location. Internal fat globules ↷ are hypointense with fat saturation, confirming dermoid cyst.* **(Right)** *Axial STIR MR shows hyperintense left SLS epidermoid →, posterior to the sublingual salivary gland ⇨. Simple fluid content of epidermoid cannot be differentiated from that of ranula or lymphatic malformation, but epidermoid may restrict diffusion.*

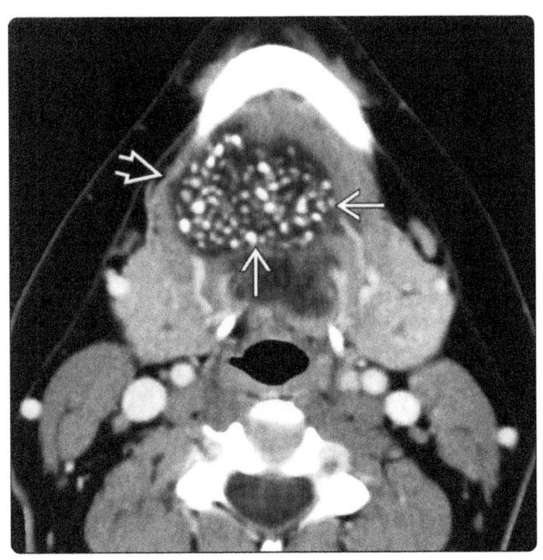

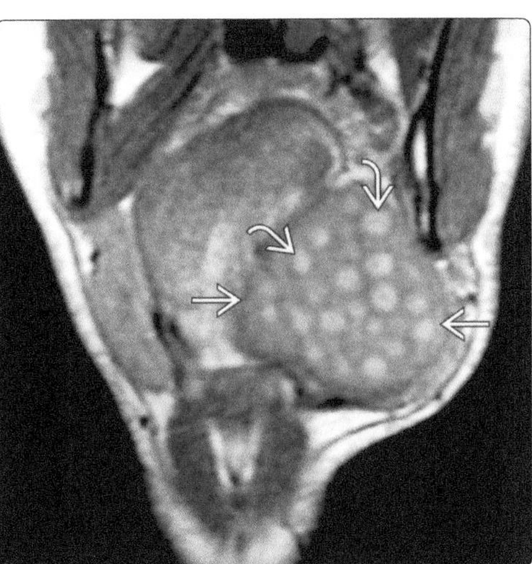

(Left) *Axial CECT reveals a well-circumscribed paramedian SLS mass → medial to attenuated mylohyoid muscle ⇨. A calcified sack of marbles appearance in otherwise heterogeneous low attenuation is consistent with a dermoid cyst.* **(Right)** *Coronal T1 MR shows a large, sublingual dermoid → stretching mylohyoid muscle laterally. Round, hyperintense foci within ↷ are fat (sack of marbles) and distinguish a dermoid from other sublingual cysts, like epidermoid, ranula, or lymphatic malformation.*

Reactive Lymph Nodes

KEY FACTS

TERMINOLOGY

- Reactive nodes: Benign, reversible enlargement of nodes in response to antigen stimulus
- Nodal involvement may be acute or subacute/chronic, unilateral or bilateral, localized or generalized

IMAGING

- Multiple well-defined, oval-shaped, or reniform nodes
- Size alone relatively poor predictor of benignity
  - In children, reactive nodes may be ≥ 2 cm
- CECT 1st-line imaging modality
  - Enhancement minimal to mild, homogeneous
  - Linear enhancement within node characteristic
- Increasing role of US elastography in differentiating benign, reactive nodes from malignancy

TOP DIFFERENTIAL DIAGNOSES

- Squamous cell carcinoma nodal metastases
- Systemic nodal metastases
- Non-Hodgkin lymphoma nodes
- Tuberculous adenitis
- Sarcoid nodes

PATHOLOGY

- Node reaction seen as specific histologic patterns of hyperplasia: Follicular, sinus, diffuse, or mixed

CLINICAL ISSUES

- Common clinical problem in pediatric age group
- Infectious mononucleosis (IMN)/kissing disease due to EBV: Associated splenic enlargement
  - Rare potential of splenic rupture, especially during sports

DIAGNOSTIC CHECKLIST

- Reactive nodes typically oval-shaped or reniform, clustered
- Adjacent cellulitis suggests bacterial infection
- Focal nonenhancement suggests suppuration or necrosis
- Supraclavicular & posterior cervical location more concerning for malignancy

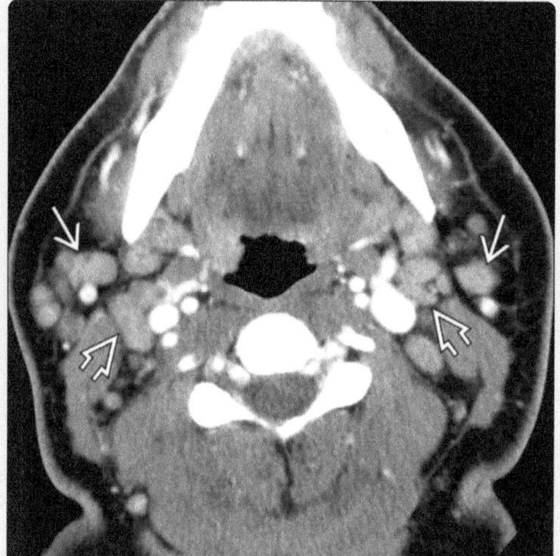

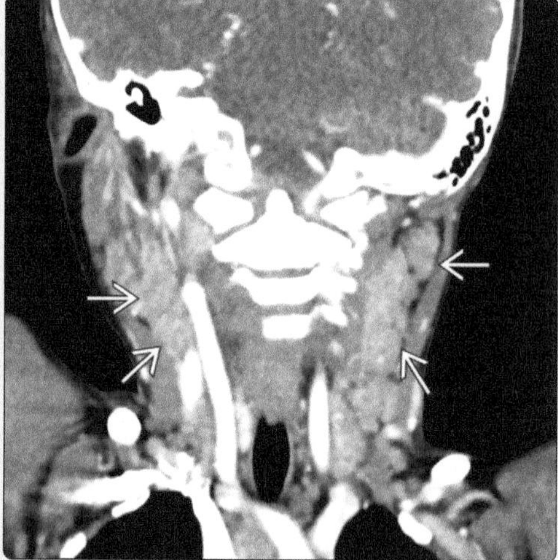

(Left) *Axial CECT reveals multiple mildly enhancing parotid tail reactive nodes ➙ & prominent high jugular oval-shaped nodes ⇨. Patient was found to have HIV adenopathy.* **(Right)** *Coronal reformatted CECT in a child with infectious mononucleosis/kissing disease (due to EBV) shows bilateral mildly hyperenhancing cervical lymphadenopathy ➙. Coronal images are very useful not to miss lymphadenopathy, as it is easier to identify enlarged lymph nodes in the background of cervical fat.*

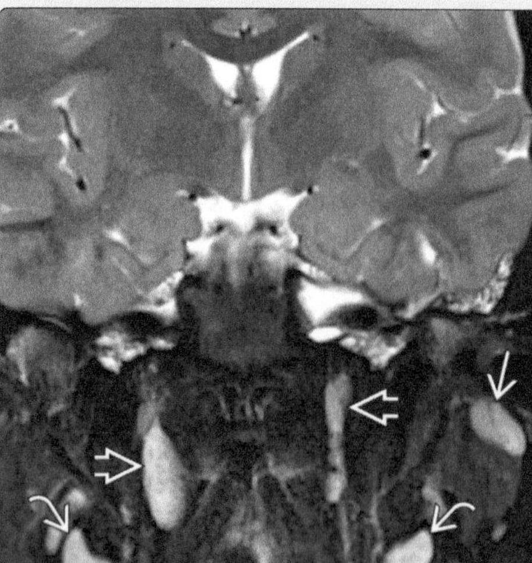

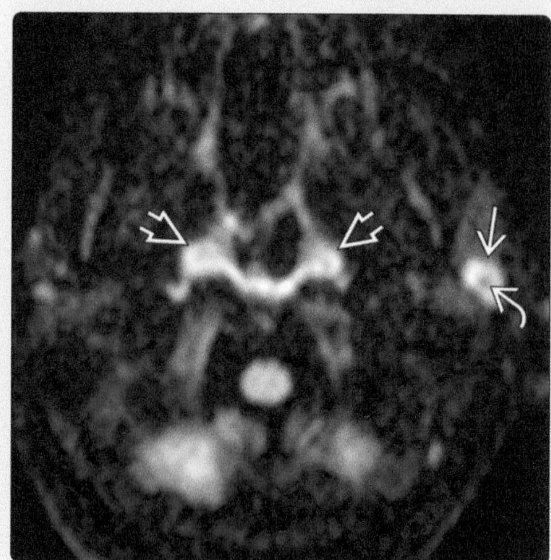

(Left) *Coronal T2 FS MR in a child with left otitis externa & media shows reactive adenopathy, including enlarged parotid ➙, retropharyngeal ⇨, & high deep cervical ↪ nodes. Reactive nodes are solid, homogeneous, & reniform in shape.* **(Right)** *Axial DWI trace MR in the same patient is sensitive for identifying lymph nodes, which are bright relative to adjacent structures. An enlarged, reactive left parotid node ➙ maintains a dark, fatty hilum ↪. Note associated adenoidal hyperplasia ⇨.*

TERMINOLOGY

Synonyms

- Reactive adenopathy, reactive lymphoid hyperplasia, nodal hyperplasia

Definitions

- **Reactive** implies **benign etiology**
- Benign, reversible enlargement of nodes in response to antigen stimulus
- **Lymphadenopathy**: Enlargement of lymph nodes
  - Due to proliferation of normal lymphatic tissue or invasion by inflammatory/neoplastic cells
- **Lymphadenitis**: Lymphadenopathy due to invasion by inflammatory cells

IMAGING

General Features

- Best diagnostic clue
  - Multiple well-defined, kidney-shaped (reniform) nodes
    - Nodes of normal size or mildly enlarged
- Location
  - Any nodal group of head & neck
- Size
  - Wide size range
    - Adult: Often up to 1.5 cm
    - Child: Reactive node may be ≥ 2 cm
  - Size alone relatively poor predictor of benignity
- Morphology
  - Reactive node: Typically oval or reniform
  - Malignant node: Rounded with cortical expansion

CT Findings

- NECT
  - Homogeneous, well-defined nodes, isodense or hypodense to muscle
  - Stranding of adjacent fat frequently associated when acute infectious cause
- CECT
  - Enhancement minimal to mild, homogeneous
  - **Linear enhancement** within node **characteristic**
  - Hyperplasia of pharyngeal lymphoid tissue (Waldeyer ring) often associated

MR Findings

- T1WI
  - Homogeneous, low to intermediate signal intensity
- T2WI
  - Homogeneous, intermediate to high signal intensity
  - Cystic change suggests suppuration or tumoral necrosis
- DWI
  - Benign nodes tend to have higher ADC values than neoplastic nodes
    - Optimal ADC thresholds remain undefined
- T1WI C+
  - Variable enhancement, usually mild & homogeneous
  - **Linear central enhancement** favors benign node
  - Tonsillar enlargement (Waldeyer ring) may be found

Ultrasonographic Findings

- Reniform nodes with echogenic vascular hilus
- Combination of B-mode US features as well as color Doppler US helps detect reactive lymph nodes
  - Individual parameters of B mode used alone not very effective to differentiate benign from malignant nodes
- Cannot be used as diagnostic method for metastatic or tubercular lymphadenopathy
  - Fine-needle aspiration cytology (FNAC)/histopathology gold standard
- High-resolution US of lymph node peripheral region to detect micrometastasis in normal-sized node
  - In subcapsular sinus, just beneath lymph node outer surface, where metastatic tumor cells deposited by afferent lymphatics grow first
- US elastography promising tool for differentiating reactive nodes from metastatic adenopathy
  - Malignant nodes demonstrate higher stiffness than benign lymph nodes

Nuclear Medicine Findings

- PET
  - Mild FDG uptake may be seen; marked uptake more likely with active granulomatous disease or tumor

Imaging Recommendations

- Best imaging tool
  - CECT 1st-line tool for evaluation of adenopathy
  - Differentiates reactive from suppurative nodes & cellulitis from abscess
  - Allows determination of node extent & evaluation for potential malignant cause

DIFFERENTIAL DIAGNOSIS

Squamous Cell Carcinoma Nodal Metastases

- Enlarged **round** node or cluster of nodes
- **Necrosis** suggestive (suppuration may mimic necrosis)
- High-resolution US to look for **micrometastasis** in **subcapsular sinus** region
- Primary pharyngeal lesion should be sought

Systemic Nodal Metastases

- Supraclavicular node suggests infraclavicular primary

Non-Hodgkin Lymphoma Nodes

- Multiple large nodes, often ≥ 1.5 cm
- Enlargement of Waldeyer ring may be seen
- Homogeneous mild contrast enhancement

Tuberculous Adenitis

- Suppurative tuberculous adenopathy in multiple neck nodes
- Rupture with adjacent phlegmon & fistula possible
- Positive chest x-ray common

Sarcoid Nodes

- Homogeneous, well-defined nodes; often > 2 cm
- Intraparotid nodes often involved
- Positive thoracic nodes common

PATHOLOGY

General Features

- Etiology
  - Response to infection, chemical, drug, or foreign antigen

    - Includes viruses, bacteria, parasites, & fungi
  - **Acute unilateral cervical lymphadenitis**: *Staphylococcus aureus* or *Streptococcus pyogenes* (group A) > 80%
    - Mostly between 1-4 years of age; submandibular & cervical lymphadenopathy; may reach up to 6 cm
    - Neonatal acute cervical lymphadenitis by *S. aureus*
    - Late-onset cellulitis-adenitis syndrome between 7 days to 3 months of age by group B *Streptococcus* (*Streptococcus agalactiae*)
  - **Acute bilateral cervical lymphadenitis**: Viral upper respiratory tract infections
    - Adeno-, entero-, influenza, & respiratory syncytial virus
    - Less commonly in group A streptococcal pharyngitis
  - **Subacute or chronic unilateral cervical lymphadenitis**: Nontuberculous mycobacteria; most commonly in immunocompetent children < 5 years age
    - *Mycobacterium avium-intracellulare* & *Mycobacterium scrofulaceum* most common
    - May drain spontaneously → sinus tract & scarring
    - *Mycobacterium tuberculosis* present with unilateral lymphadenitis & less commonly bilateral
    - Tuberculous cervical lymphadenopathy by direct spread to supraclavicular nodes from apical pleura
      - Or by tuberculous infection spread from paratracheal nodes to tonsillar & submandibular nodes
    - *Bartonella henselae* cutaneous inoculation due to lick, bite, or scratch from kittens/cats
      - Chronic unilateral tender cervical, axillary, or epitrochlear lymphadenitis (cat-scratch disease)
  - **Subacute or chronic bilateral lymphadenitis**: EBV [**infectious mononucleosis** (**IMN**)/**kissing disease**], or CMV in adolescents & school aged
    - Splenic enlargement common in IMN with relatively rare splenic rupture potential, typically within 1 month of symptom onset
      - Splenic rupture risk complicates sports participation
    - Rarely, *Toxoplasma gondii* with fatigue & cervical nodes
    - Chronic bilateral cervical adenitis uncommonly by *M. tuberculosis*, HIV, histoplasmosis, brucellosis, syphilis
- Associated abnormalities
  - Hyperplasia of pharyngeal lymphoid tissue (Waldeyer ring) often with viral infections
  - Associated findings may suggest causative agent
    - **Stranding** of adjacent fat common with bacteria, rare with atypical mycobacteria
    - **Generalized adenopathy** suggests viral infection, collagen vascular disease, or malignancy
    - Parotid lymphoepithelial lesions ± adenoidal hypertrophy suggests **HIV adenopathy**
    - Parotid adenopathy frequently seen with **sarcoid**

Gross Pathologic & Surgical Features

- Firm, rubbery, mobile, enlarged nodes

Microscopic Features

- Node reaction with different histologic patterns of **hyperplasia**: Follicular, sinus, diffuse or mixed
- Culture or staining may reveal infectious agent

CLINICAL ISSUES

Presentation

- Most common signs/symptoms
  - Firm, sometimes fluctuant, freely mobile subcutaneous nodal masses
  - Other signs/symptoms
    - Bacterial adenitis & cat-scratch disease usually painful
    - Nontuberculous mycobacteria usually nontender

Demographics

- Age
  - Any but most common in pediatric age group
    - Neonatal neck nodes not palpable
  - Children: Organisms have predilection for specific ages
    - < 1 year: *S. aureus*, group B *Streptococcus*, Kawasaki disease
    - 1-5 years: *S. aureus*, group A β-hemolytic *Streptococcus*, atypical mycobacteria
    - 5-15 years: Anaerobic bacteria, toxoplasmosis, cat-scratch disease, EBV

Natural History & Prognosis

- Bacterial infection, nontuberculous mycobacteria, & cat-scratch disease frequently progress to necrotic nodes
- Chronic inflammation may result in fatty metaplasia
  - Low-density nodal hilus mimics necrosis

Treatment

- Many reactive nodes resolve spontaneously
- Antibiotics, if bacterial cause suspected
- Nodal aspiration or biopsy if failed antibiotics, rapid increase in size, systemic adenopathy, fever, & weight loss
  - Or if malignant nodal features, such as hard, matted nodes, & supraclavicular or posterior cervical node location
- If needle aspiration shows nonspecific reactive changes, follow clinically for 3-6 months
- Persistent adenopathy requires repeat needle aspiration to rule out lymphoma, metastasis, or tuberculosis

DIAGNOSTIC CHECKLIST

Consider

- Certain locations should raise concern
  - Postauricular nodes in child > 2 years likely significant
  - Supraclavicular nodes neoplastic in ~ 60%
  - Posterior cervical nodes suggest non-Hodgkin lymphoma, skin nodal metastases, or nasopharyngeal carcinoma

Image Interpretation Pearls

- Imaging findings often nonspecific with multiple homogeneous, mildly enlarged or normal-sized nodes
- Oval-shaped nodes more likely benign & reactive
- Central linear vascular enhancement characteristic
- Focal nonenhancement within node suggests suppuration or necrosis

SELECTED REFERENCES

1. Putukian M et al: American Medical Society of Sports Medicine position statement: mononucleosis and athletic participation. Clin J Sport Med. ePub, 2023

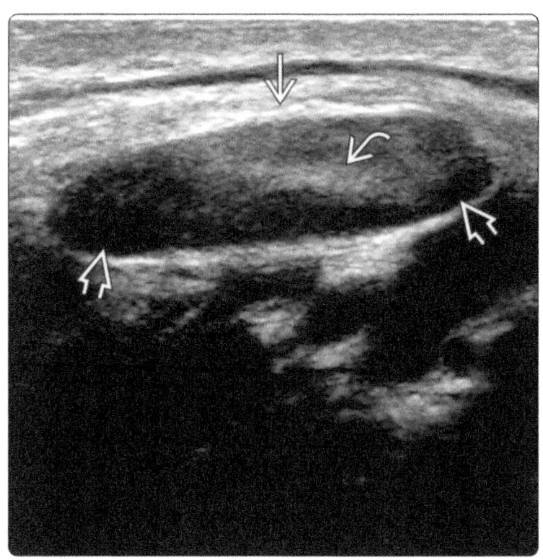

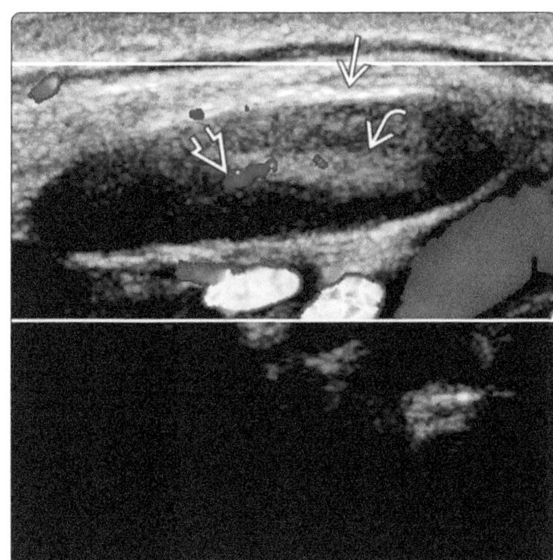

(Left) *Transverse grayscale US demonstrates the typical appearance of a reactive submandibular node ➡. Note the low internal echogenicity ➡ with echogenic fatty hilum ➡. Micrometastasis initially occurs along the periphery of a lymph node in the subcapsular sinus, where metastatic tumor cells deposited by the afferent lymphatics piercing the outer lymph node cortex first start to grow.* **(Right)** *Transverse color Doppler US in the same reactive submandibular node ➡ shows typical vascularity ➡ associated with the echogenic hilum ➡.*

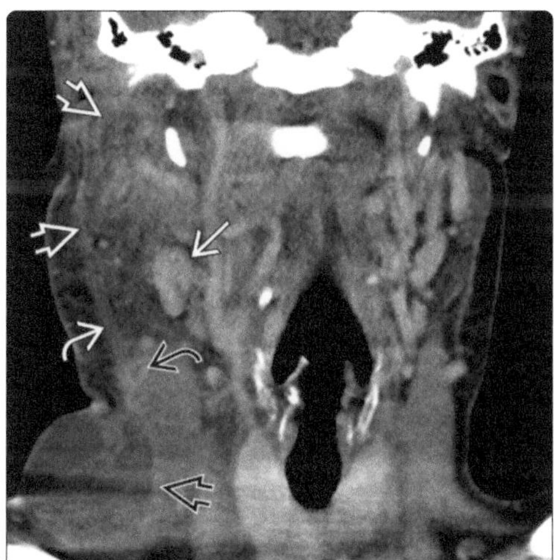

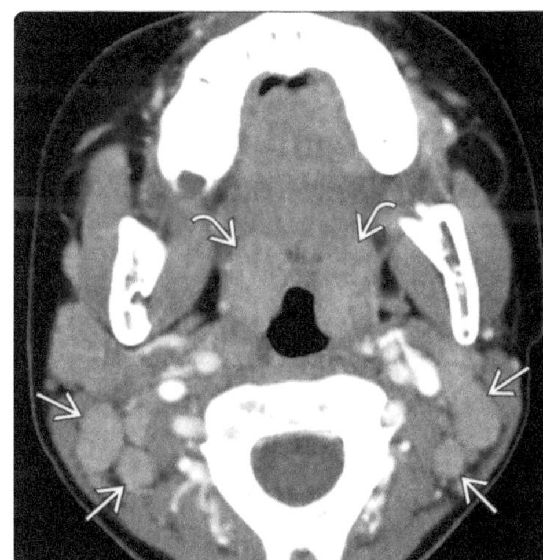

(Left) *Coronal CECT in an IV drug user shows the typical appearance of reactive level II node ➡. Reactive nodes are enlarged but maintain an ovoid or reniform morphology. Note additional diffuse edema ➡, platysma thickening ➡, rim-enhancing early abscess ➡, & septic thrombophlebitis in the external jugular vein ➡.* **(Right)** *Axial CECT in a patient with nonsuppurative tonsillopharyngitis shows bilateral, enlarged, ovoid reactive nodes ➡ without fat stranding or suppuration. Palatine tonsillar enlargement & hyperemia ➡ are evident.*

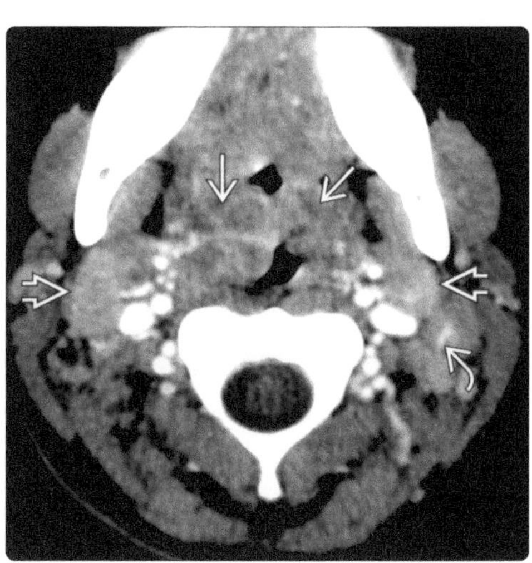

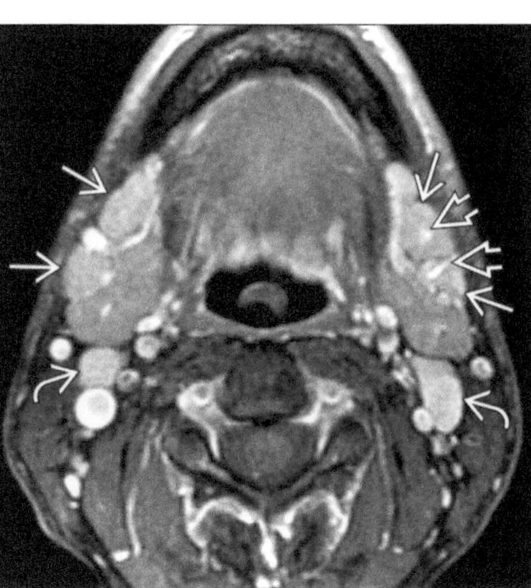

(Left) *Axial CECT in a patient with suppurative tonsillitis shows enlarged tonsils with small intratonsillar abscesses ➡ & bilateral, homogeneous, enlarged cervical nodes ➡. Nodes show mild enhancement, & some reveal central linear enhancement ➡ characteristic of reactive nodes.* **(Right)** *Axial T1 C+ FS MR shows prominent, bilateral, homogeneously enhancing reactive nodes in the upper cervical ➡ & submandibular ➡ chains. Note linear enhancement of the central vessel in some nodes ➡.*

KEY FACTS

TERMINOLOGY

- Pus formation within nodes from bacterial infection
- Synonyms: Adenitis, lymphadenitis, intranodal abscess

IMAGING

- Enlarged node(s) with internal fluid & surrounding inflammation (cellulitis)
  - Most often jugulodigastric, submandibular, or retropharyngeal
- Loss of normal nodal architecture & internal vascularity/enhancement
- Conglomeration of necrotic nodes progressing to abscess shows marked heterogeneity of irregular collection
  - Well-defined, enhancing/hyperemic wall
  - Complex hypoechoic/nonenhancing center
- US is useful to confirm true liquefaction with drainable pus
  - Swirling internal debris upon compression
- CECT best defines deep extent & complications
  - Lemierre syndrome (venous thrombophlebitis), internal carotid artery spasm or pseudoaneurysm, airway compression, mediastinal extension

TOP DIFFERENTIAL DIAGNOSES

- Nontuberculous *Mycobacterium* adenopathy
- Tuberculous adenopathy
- 2nd branchial cleft anomaly
- Rhabdomyosarcoma
- Lymphoma
- Lymphatic malformation
- Fibromatosis colli

PATHOLOGY

- *Staphylococcus* & *Streptococcus*: Most frequent organisms

DIAGNOSTIC CHECKLIST

- Look for primary infectious source on images
  - Pharyngitis, dental infection, salivary gland calculi

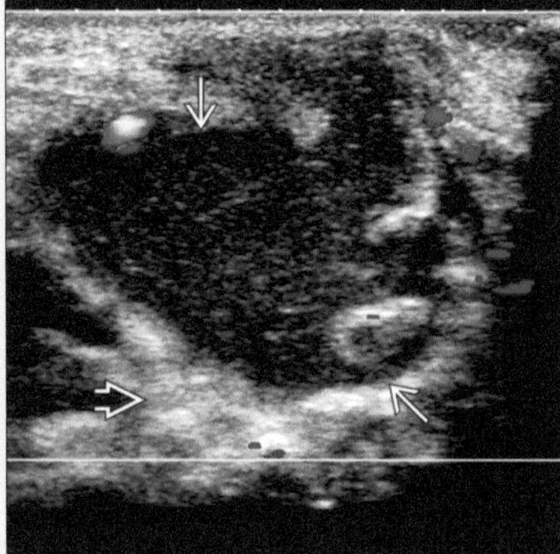

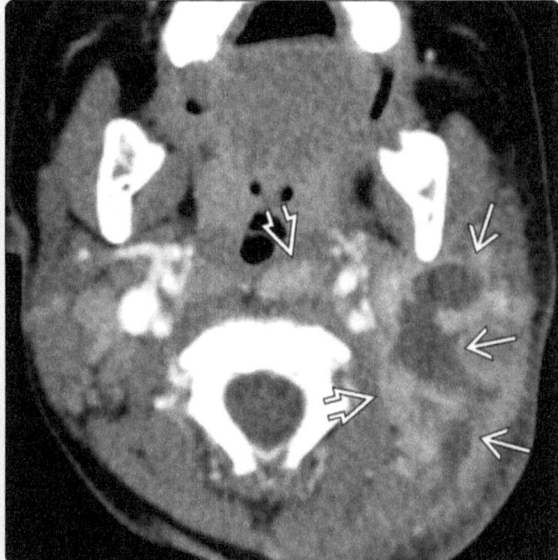

(Left) *Transverse Doppler US in a 6-year-old with fever & a tender neck mass shows an irregular hypoechoic abscess ➡ with posterior acoustic enhancement ➡ & no internal vascularity. Swirling of debris upon compression can help confirm drainability.* **(Right)** *Axial CECT in a 23-month-old with fever & neck swelling demonstrates an irregularly shaped abscess in the left neck ➡. Well-defined rim enhancement anteriorly likely represents intranodal origin of pus with posterior extranodal extension, cellulitis, & additional adenopathy ➡.*

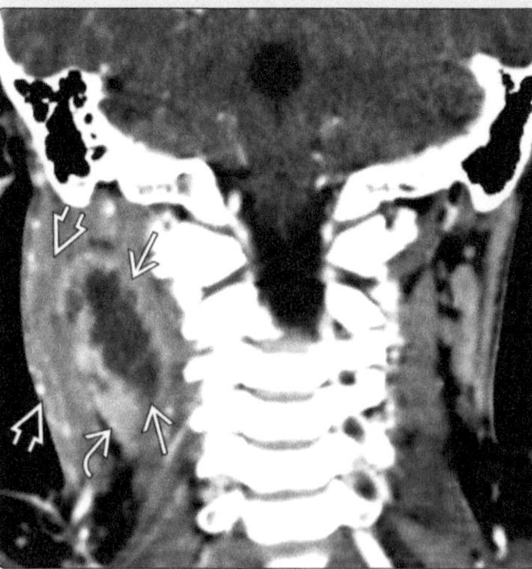

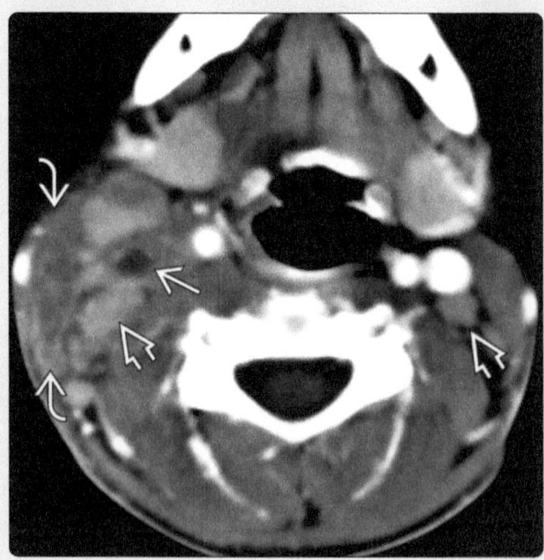

(Left) *Coronal CECT in a 6-year-old with fever & a fluctuant neck mass shows an irregular, rim-enhancing abscess ➡ with overlying myositis/cellulitis ➡ & an adjacent nonsuppurative lymph node ➡.* **(Right)** *More inferior axial CECT in the same patient shows a round focus of nonenhancement, representing a segmental clot ➡ in the right internal jugular vein, consistent with Lemierre syndrome. Note the R > L nonsuppurative nodes ➡ as well as the overlying myositis/cellulitis ➡.*

TERMINOLOGY

Synonyms

- Adenitis, acute lymphadenitis, intranodal abscess

Definitions

- Pus formation within nodes from bacterial infection

IMAGING

General Features

- Best diagnostic clue
  - Enlarged node(s) with internal fluid & surrounding inflammation (cellulitis)
- Location
  - Any nodal groups of head/neck
    - Most often: Jugulodigastric, submandibular, retropharyngeal
  - May be unilateral or bilateral
- Size
  - Enlarged single node or conglomeration of nodes
    - Often in 1- to 4-cm range
- Morphology
  - Ovoid to round, large node with central necrosis
  - Margins are often poorly defined
  - Additional adjacent solid or suppurative nodes are typically present

Ultrasonographic Findings

- Early adenitis may show enlarged ovoid foci with retained nodal architecture & hyperemia
- Loss of architecture & internal vascularity occurs with necrosis
  - Central ↓ echogenicity with ↑ through transmission
- Conglomeration of necrotic nodes progressing to abscess shows marked heterogeneity of irregular collection
  - Liquefied pus: Swirling internal debris with compression
  - ↑ peripheral vascularity
    - Very low-resistance & pulsatility indices

CT Findings

- CECT
  - Enhancing nodal wall with central hypoattenuation/lack of enhancement
  - Stranding/edema of surrounding tissues = cellulitis
  - With progression to abscess → irregular, ill-defined, peripherally enhancing, low-attenuation collection
    - Caveat: Well-defined, low-attenuation collection with rim enhancement is not necessarily pathognomonic for drainable pus → consider US
      - Represents nondrainable phlegmon in ~ 20%
  - ± myositis, Lemierre syndrome (venous thrombophlebitis), deviation of carotid sheath vessels, internal carotid artery spasm or pseudoaneurysm, retropharyngeal soft tissue edema, mass effect on airway, mediastinal extension

MR Findings

- T1WI
  - Node with central low signal intensity
  - Dampening of normal high signal intensity of surrounding fat
- STIR/T2WI FS
  - Node with diffuse or central high signal intensity
  - Edema of surrounding soft tissues
- DWI
  - Complimentary to routine pulse sequences
  - Suppurative, necrotic nodes have reduced diffusivity (bright DWI, dark ADC signal)
    - May show higher DWI & lower ADC signal relative to metastatic necrotic nodes
      - Optimal ADC thresholds remain undefined
- T1WI C+ FS
  - Marked peripheral enhancement with poorly defined margin
  - Absent central enhancement

Nuclear Medicine Findings

- PET
  - Nonspecific ↑ FDG uptake
  - Abscess shows central ↓ FDG uptake

Imaging Recommendations

- Best imaging tool
  - Ultrasound to determine phlegmon vs. abscess & guide aspiration
    - May be difficult to determine deep relationships
  - CECT is best for deep neck infections
    - Determines epicenter & total extent for aspiration or surgical planning

DIFFERENTIAL DIAGNOSIS

Nontuberculous *Mycobacterium* Adenopathy

- Asymmetric, enlarged nodes with adjacent necrotic, ring-enhancing masses
- Minimal or absent subcutaneous fat stranding
- Purified protein derivative (PPD) skin test is weakly reactive in ~ 55%
- Usually ≤ 5 years of age

Tuberculous Adenopathy

- Painless low jugular & posterior cervical low-density nodes
- Ca^{++} may be present
- Strongly reactive PPD skin test, positive interferon-γ release assay
- Systemically unwell if active pulmonary infection

2nd Branchial Cleft Anomaly

- Solitary unilocular cyst, posterior to submandibular gland
  - Anterior to sternocleidomastoid (SCM), posterolateral to carotid sheath
- Mimics suppurative node, particularly if inflamed

Rhabdomyosarcoma

- Solid, firm soft tissue neoplasm of children (typically beyond infancy) occurring in many head/neck locations
- Typically lacks surrounding edema
- ± bone destruction

Lymphoma

- Multifocal, solid, enhancing nodes, often of bilateral neck & chest
- ± enlargement of tonsillar tissue

Lymphatic Malformation

- Congenital, multicystic mass with thin rim & septations
- Variable internal echogenicity due to internal hemorrhage
- No significant internal vascularity
- Often infiltrative & transspatial, may be bilateral

Fibromatosis Colli

- Self-limited, benign reactive mass within SCM muscle of young infants, likely due to birth trauma
  - Usually appears within 2 weeks of delivery, regresses by 8 months
  - Associated torticollis in up to 30%
- Expands SCM focally or diffusely
- Ranges from homogeneous to very heterogeneous on ultrasound, CECT, & MR
  - Heterogeneous contrast enhancement is common
  - SCM muscle may be edematous surrounding mass, but further soft tissue edema is not typical
  - No adenopathy

PATHOLOGY

General Features

- Etiology
  - Primary head/neck infection: Pharyngitis, salivary gland ductal calculus, dental decay ± mandibular osteomyelitis
    - Adjacent lymph nodes enlarge secondary to pathogen: Reactive nodes
    - Intranodal exudate forms, containing protein-rich fluid with dead neutrophils (pus): Suppurative nodes
    - If untreated or incorrectly treated, suppurative nodes rupture → interstitial pus walled-off by immune system → extranodal abscess in soft tissues
  - Reactive nodes from viral pathogen may have secondary bacterial superinfection, creating suppurative nodes

Microscopic Features

- Acute inflammatory cell infiltrate in necrotic background
  - Presence of neutrophils & macrophages
  - Negative staining for acid-fast bacilli
- *Staphylococcus* & *Streptococcus* are most frequent organisms
  - ↑ incidence of MRSA
- Pediatric infections show clustering of organisms by age
  - Infants < 1 year: *Staphylococcus aureus*, group B *Streptococcus*
  - Children 1-4 years: *S. aureus*, group A β-hemolytic *Streptococcus*, atypical mycobacteria
  - 5-15 years: Anaerobic bacteria, toxoplasmosis, cat-scratch disease, tuberculosis
- Dental infections: Typically polymicrobial, predominantly anaerobic

CLINICAL ISSUES

Presentation

- Most common signs/symptoms
  - Painful neck mass
    - Overlying skin is often warm, erythematous
  - Fever, poor oral intake
  - Elevated WBC & ESR
- Other signs/symptoms
  - Symptoms referable to primary source of infection
    - Pharyngeal/laryngeal infection: Drooling, respiratory distress
    - Peritonsillar infection: Trismus
    - Retropharyngeal or paravertebral infection: Neck stiffness, torticollis
- Clinical profile
  - Young patient presents with acute/subacute onset of tender neck mass & fever
- Clinical predictors of drainable suppurative adenitis in children
  - Absence of pharyngitis, WBC > 15,000/mm³, age ≤ 3 years, anterior cervical chain, largest palpable diameter > 3 cm, prior antibiotic treatment ≥ 24 hours

Demographics

- Age
  - Most commonly seen in pediatric & young adult population
  - Odontogenic neck infections: Adults > > children

Natural History & Prognosis

- Conglomeration of suppurative nodes or rupture of node → abscess formation
  - Superficial neck abscesses: Anterior or posterior cervical space, submandibular space
  - Deep neck abscesses: Retropharyngeal or parapharyngeal space
    - Deep space abscesses can rapidly progress with airway compromise

Treatment

- Small suppurative nodes & primary infection → antibiotics
- Large suppurative nodes, abscesses, or poor response to antibiotics → incision & drainage
  - CT & US-guided aspiration for minimally invasive management
- Nodes from atypical mycobacteria → excision to prevent recurrence or fistula/sinus tract

DIAGNOSTIC CHECKLIST

Consider

- Nontuberculous mycobacterial adenitis if no significant inflammatory changes

Image Interpretation Pearls

- Look for primary infectious source on images
  - Pharyngitis, dental infection, salivary gland calculi
- Evaluate airway for compromise with any neck infection
  - More problematic in deep infections
- Evaluate vascular structures for thrombophlebitis

SELECTED REFERENCES

1. O'Brien WT Sr: Common neck and otomastoid infections in children. Neuroimaging Clin N Am. 33(4):661-71, 2023
2. Park JE et al: Cervical lymphadenopathy in children: a diagnostic tree analysis model based on ultrasonographic and clinical findings. Eur Radiol. 30(8):4475-85, 2020
3. Matos R et al: Unilateral acute cervical lymphadenitis in children: can we predict the need for surgery? Int J Pediatr Otorhinolaryngol. 127:109655, 2019
4. Kimia AA et al: Predictors of a drainable suppurative adenitis among children presenting with cervical adenopathy. Am J Emerg Med. 37(1):109-13, 2018

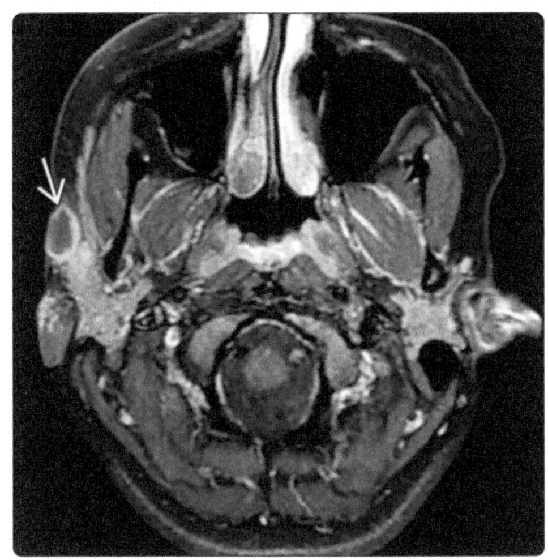

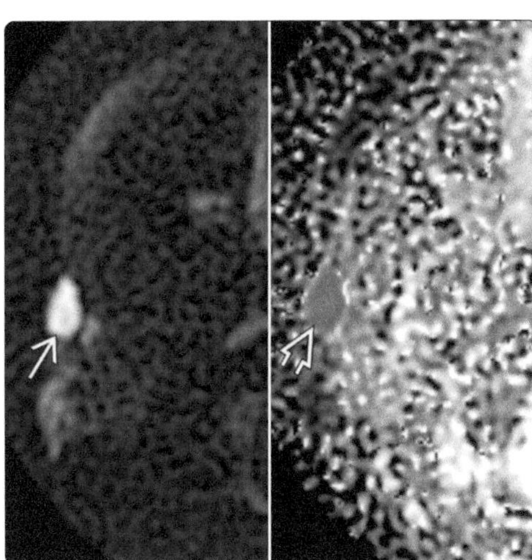

(Left) *Axial T1WI C+ FS MR in a teenager diagnosed with preauricular nonsuppurative adenopathy 1 week prior by US shows a rim-enhancing fluid collection anterior to the right parotid gland ➡.* **(Right)** *Axial DWI MR in the same patient shows diffuse hyperintense signal ➡ on DWI (left) & hypointense signal ➡ on ADC image (right), consistent with purulent fluid within periparotid suppurative lymph node.*

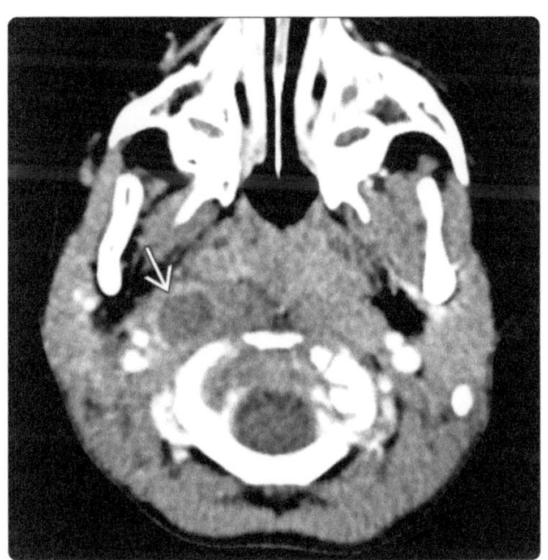

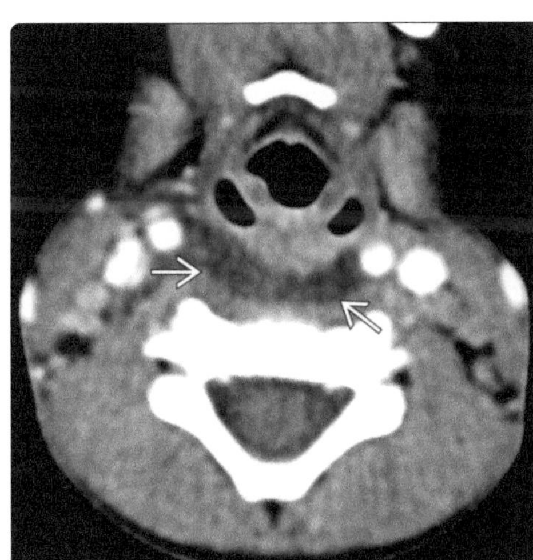

(Left) *Axial CECT in a child with fever & sore throat shows an enlarged, low-attenuation right lateral retropharyngeal lymph node with partial rim enhancement ➡, consistent with early purulence or phlegmon. Note the deviation of the right carotid sheath vessels, which are minimally ↓ in caliber compared to the left.* **(Right)** *Axial CECT in the same patient demonstrates a poorly defined prevertebral fluid collection ➡ with concave anterior margin & no rim enhancement, consistent with soft tissue edema rather than abscess.*

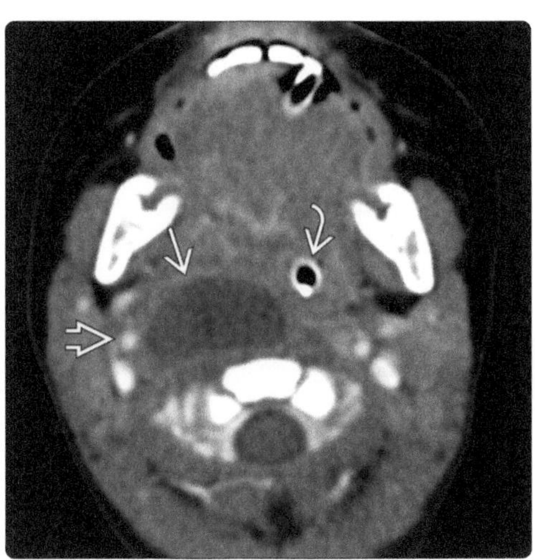

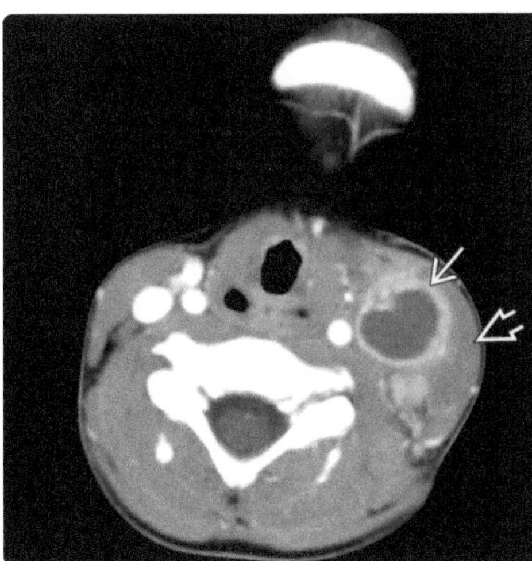

(Left) *Axial CECT in a 1-year-old shows a right lateral retropharyngeal low-attenuation abscess with peripheral enhancement ➡, secondary to suppurative adenitis. Note the mass effect on the carotid sheath ➡ & endotracheal tube ➡.* **(Right)** *Axial CECT in a child with a left neck abscess secondary to a suppurative lymph node shows a well-defined, low-attenuation mass with diffuse, thick peripheral enhancement ➡ deep to the anterior aspect of the edematous left sternocleidomastoid muscle ➡.*

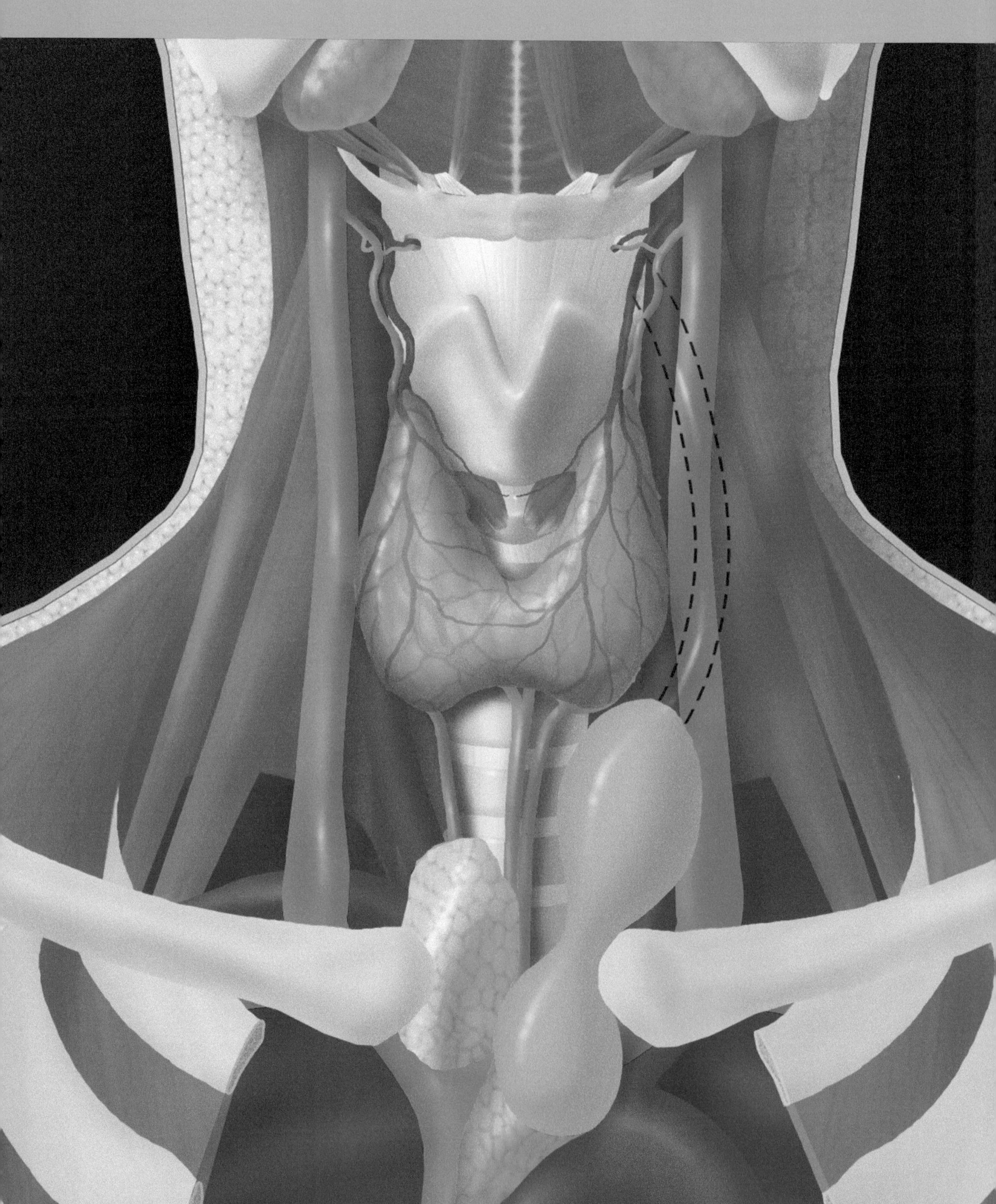

PART II
SECTION 4

Multiple Regions, Head and Neck

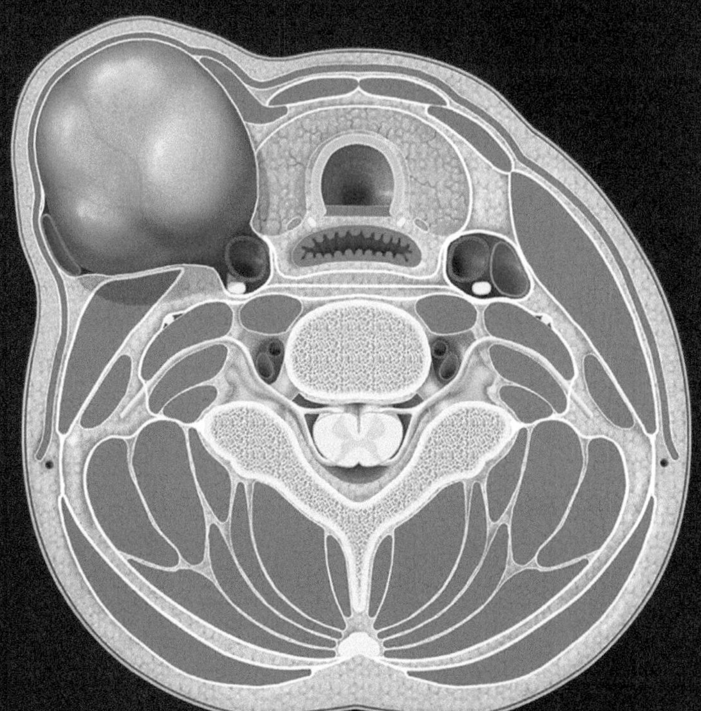

1st Branchial Cleft Cyst

KEY FACTS

TERMINOLOGY

- Most common 1st branchial cleft (BC) anomalies are cysts (BCCs) or sinus tracts

IMAGING

- Best diagnostic clue: Cystic mass near pinna & external auditory canal (EAC) or extending from EAC to angle of mandible
- CECT: Well-circumscribed, nonenhancing or rim-enhancing, low-density mass
  - If infected, may have thickened, enhancing rim

TOP DIFFERENTIAL DIAGNOSES

- Cholesteatoma, EAC
  - Submucosal mass with bone erosion
- Granulomatous infection (nontuberculous *Mycobacterium*)
  - Conglomerate parotid space necrotic nodal mass
  - Necrotic material extrudes into subcutaneous fat
- Parotitis complicated by abscess (rare)
  - Parotitis with thick-walled, ring-enhancing, cystic mass within or adjacent to parotid gland
  - Cellulitis extends to EAC & angle of mandible
- Lymphatic malformation
  - No contrast enhancement, ± fluid-fluid levels
- Venous malformation, EAC
  - Variably enhancing mass, ± phleboliths

PATHOLOGY

- **Remnant of 1st branchial apparatus**
  - Cysts > > sinus or fistula
- Most common location for 1st BCC to terminate is in EAC, between cartilaginous & bony portions

DIAGNOSTIC CHECKLIST

- Think 1st BCC in patient with chronic, unexplained otorrhea or recurrent parotid space abscess
- Look for cyst in or adjacent to EAC, pinna, parotid gland, or, rarely, parapharyngeal space

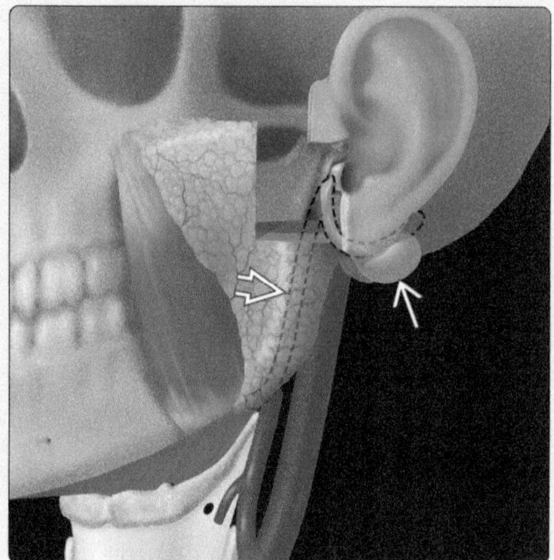

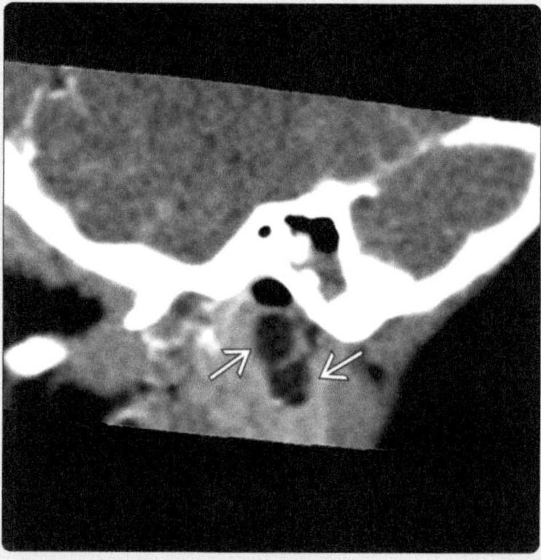

(Left) *Oblique graphic of the ear and cheek reveals a Work type I 1st branchial cleft cyst (BCC) ➡ along the tract from the bony-cartilaginous junction of the external auditory canal (EAC) situated just posteroinferior to auricle. The tract of the Work type II BCC ➡ would project inferiorly to the angle of the mandible.* **(Right)** *Sagittal CECT in a 2-year-old child shows a well-defined, hypoattenuating 1st BCC ➡ inferior to the left EAC. There is minimal rim enhancement and a single septation.*

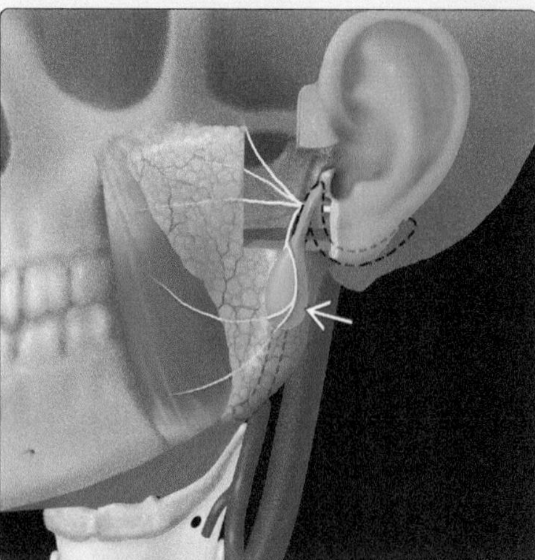

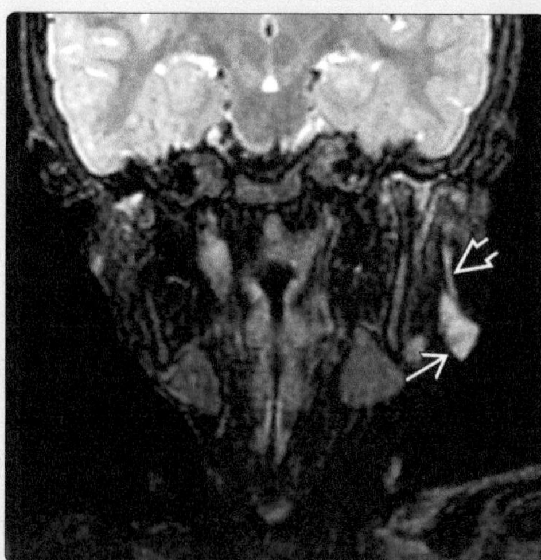

(Left) *Oblique graphic of the ear and cheek shows an example of a Work type II 1st BCC ➡ along the course of the tract from the bony-cartilaginous EAC to the angle of the mandible. Note the intimate relationship of the BCC to the facial nerve branches.* **(Right)** *Coronal T2WI FS MR demonstrates the cystic inferior component of a type II 1st branchial apparatus cyst ➡ and the sinus tract ➡ extending superiorly toward the EAC. There was a 2nd cyst just inferior to the EAC (not shown), connected to the lower cyst by the sinus tract.*

TERMINOLOGY

Abbreviations

- Branchial cleft (BC) cyst (BCC)

Synonyms

- Pharyngeal cleft anomaly = BC anomaly (BCA)
- Pharyngeal apparatus = branchial apparatus (cleft, arch, & pouch)

Definitions

- 1st BCA: Most are cysts or sinuses; fistula from skin to external auditory canal (EAC), eustachian tube, oropharynx, or middle ear rare
- 1st BCC: Benign, congenital cyst in or adjacent to parotid gland, EAC, or pinna
  - Remnant of 1st branchial apparatus: Most commonly used classification
    - Work type I: Duplication of membranous EAC; ectodermal (cleft) origin
    - Work type II: Duplication of membranous EAC & cartilaginous pinna
      - Skin (ectodermal cleft) & cartilage (mesodermal arch) origin
      - May also have contribution from 2nd arch
  - Less commonly used classification
    - Arnot type 1: Derived from buried rests of 1st BC; intraparotid cyst or sinus
    - Arnot type 2: Secondary to incomplete closure of 1st BC
      - Cyst or sinus in anterior triangle of neck ± communication with EAC
- 1st BC sinus tract opens near parotid gland, EAC, parapharyngeal space (PPS), or anterior triangle of neck

IMAGING

General Features

- Best diagnostic clue
  - Cystic mass near pinna & EAC (Work type I) or extending from EAC to angle of mandible (Work type II)
- Location
  - Type I: Periauricular cyst or sinus tract
    - Anterior, inferior, or posterior to pinna & concha
  - Type II: Periparotid cyst or sinus tract
    - More intimately associated with parotid gland, medial or lateral to CNVII
    - Superficial, parotid space, or PPS
- Size
  - Variable but usually < 3 cm
- Morphology
  - Well-circumscribed cyst

CT Findings

- CECT
  - Well-circumscribed, nonenhancing or rim-enhancing, low-density mass
  - If infected, may have thickened, enhancing rim &/or intermediate attenuation contents
    - Surrounding fat stranding suggests infection
  - 1st BCC, Work type I
    - Cyst anterior, inferior, or posterior to EAC
    - Lesion may beak toward bony-cartilaginous junction of EAC
    - Often runs parallel to EAC
  - 1st BCC, Work type II
    - May be superficial (meaning subcutaneous), in parotid space, or in PPD
    - May be as low as posterior submandibular space
    - Deep projection may beak to bony-cartilaginous junction of EAC
  - 1st BC sinus tract: Linear density courses through subcutaneous fat in vicinity of parotid, EAC, or PPS
- If previously infected, can be isodense

MR Findings

- T1WI
  - Low signal intensity, unilocular cyst
- T2WI
  - High signal intensity, unilocular cyst
  - May see sinus tract to skin, EAC, or, rarely, PPS
  - Edema in surrounding soft tissues when superinfected
- T1WI C+
  - Cyst wall normally does not enhance
  - Previous or concurrent infection may → thickened, enhancing rim

Ultrasonographic Findings

- Anechoic mass in periauricular or periparotid area

Imaging Recommendations

- Best imaging tool
  - CECT or MR for evaluation of cyst
  - MR (T2WI) for small lesions & associated sinus tract
- Protocol advice
  - Coronal reformatted images helpful to evaluate relationship to EAC

DIFFERENTIAL DIAGNOSIS

Congenital Cholesteatoma of External Auditory Canal

- Nonenhancing submucosal mass with bone erosion
- Lesion matrix may show bone fragments
- Hole in tympanic plate
- Known association with 1st BCC ± fistula to EAC & stenotic or duplicated EAC

Non-TB *Mycobacterium*, Lymph Nodes

- 4- to 6-week history of minimally tender mass with violaceous skin discoloration
- Conglomerate parotid space necrotic nodal mass
- Necrotic tissue may extrude into subcutaneous fat
- Minimal stranding of subcutaneous fat

Parotitis, Acute

- Presents with marked tenderness & fever
- Enlarged/inflamed, enhancing parotid
- Cellulitis extends to EAC & angle of mandible
- Complicating abscess is rare: Thick-walled, ring-enhancing, cystic mass within/adjacent to parotid gland

Lymphatic Malformation, Periauricular

- Congenital vascular malformation; embryonic lymphatic sacs

- Unilocular or multilocular; microcystic or macrocystic
- Single space or transspatial
- Characteristic fluid-fluid levels are common
- No contrast enhancement or phleboliths unless mixed venolymphatic malformation

Venous Malformation, Periauricular

- Congenital vascular malformation: Endothelial-lined vascular sinusoids
- Single or multiple lobulated mass ± phleboliths
- Variable enhancement pattern reflects sluggish vascular flow to & through lesion
- ± nonenhancing lymphatic component if mixed venolymphatic malformation

PATHOLOGY

General Features

- Associated abnormalities
  - May be seen in association with other 1st branchial apparatus anomalies
  - May occasionally have associated but separate EAC congenital cholesteatoma
    - Small mass in medial EAC with bony remodeling/erosion of EAC & hole in tympanic plate
    - May transgress tympanic membrane (TM) or extend from tympanic plate under TM into middle ear cavity
- Embryology/anatomy
  - Remnant of 1st branchial apparatus
    - Cleft (ectoderm) of 1st apparatus → EAC
    - Arch (mesoderm) → mandible, muscles of mastication, CNV, incus body, malleus head
    - Pouch (endoderm) → eustachian tube, middle ear cavity, & mastoid air cells
  - Branchial remnant occurs with incomplete obliteration of 1st branchial apparatus
  - Isolated BCC has no internal (pharyngeal) or external (cutaneous) communication
  - BC fistula has both internal & external connections, from EAC lumen to skin
  - BC sinus tract opens externally or (rarely) internally; closed portion ends as blind pouch
  - 2/3 of 1st BC remnants are isolated cysts

Gross Pathologic & Surgical Features

- Cystic neck mass
  - Easily dissected unless repeated infection
- Contents of cyst usually thick mucus
- Cystic remnant may split facial nerve (CNVII) trunk
- CNVII may be medial or lateral to 1st BCC
- Close proximity to CNVII makes surgery more difficult
- Most common location for 1st BCC to terminate is in EAC between cartilaginous & bony portions

Microscopic Features

- Thin outer layer: Fibrous pseudocapsule
- Inner layer: Flat squamoid epithelium
- ± germinal centers & lymphocytes in cyst wall

CLINICAL ISSUES

Presentation

- Most common signs/symptoms
  - Soft, painless, compressible mass: EAC, periauricular, intraparotid, or periparotid suprahyoid neck
- Other signs/symptoms
  - Recurrent EAC, preauricular or periparotid swelling
  - Tender mass ± fever if infected
  - EAC or skin sinus tract rare
  - Chronic purulent ear drainage if EAC sinus tract or fistula

Demographics

- Age
  - Majority present < 10 years old
  - Sinus tracts present earlier
  - When cyst only, may present later, even as adult
- Epidemiology
  - Accounts for 8% of all branchial apparatus remnants
  - Work type II > > Work type I 1st BCC

Natural History & Prognosis

- May enlarge with upper respiratory tract infection
  - Lymph follicles in wall react, wall secretes
- Often incised & drained as "abscess," only to recur
- Prognosis excellent if completely resected
- May recur if residual cyst wall remains
- If multiple BCCs are associated with craniofacial anomalies, think syndromic etiology (e.g., branchiootorenal syndrome)

Treatment

- Complete surgical resection
- Proximity to CNVII puts nerve at risk during surgery
  - Work type I: Proximal CNVII
  - Work type II: More distal CNVII branches

DIAGNOSTIC CHECKLIST

Consider

- Look for cyst in or adjacent to parotid gland, EAC, pinna, or, rarely, PPS
- Think of 1st branchial apparatus anomaly in patient with chronic, unexplained otorrhea or recurrent parotid gland abscess

SELECTED REFERENCES

1. Booth TN: Congenital cystic neck masses. Neuroimaging Clin N Am. 33(4):591-605, 2023
2. Koch BL et al: Complete first branchial fistula in a child extending from the external auditory canal to the oropharynx. Neurographics. American Society of Neuroradiology. 11(1):35-7, 2021
3. Liu H et al: Clinical manifestations, diagnosis, and management of first branchial cleft fistula/sinus: a case series and literature review. J Oral Maxillofac Surg. 78(5):749-61, 2020
4. Mehmi N et al: Importance and impact of appropriate radiology in the management of branchial cleft anomalies. Indian J Otolaryngol Head Neck Surg. 71(Suppl 1):953-9, 2019
5. Guerin JB et al: Pediatric parotid region lesions: an imaging review. Neurographics. American Society of Neuroradiology. 8(6):394-412, 2018
6. Johnson JM et al: Syndromes of the first and second branchial arches, part 1: embryology and characteristic defects. AJNR Am J Neuroradiol. 32(1):14-9, 2011
7. Johnson JM et al: Syndromes of the first and second branchial arches, part 2: syndromes. AJNR Am J Neuroradiol. 32(2):230-7, 2011
8. Koch BL: Cystic malformations of the neck in children. Pediatr Radiol. 35(5):463-77, 2005

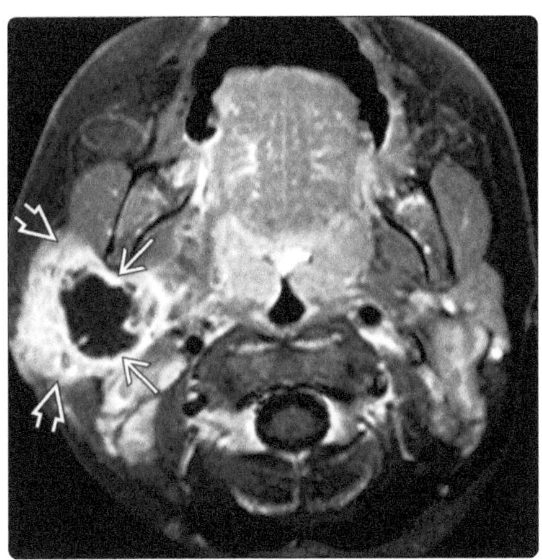

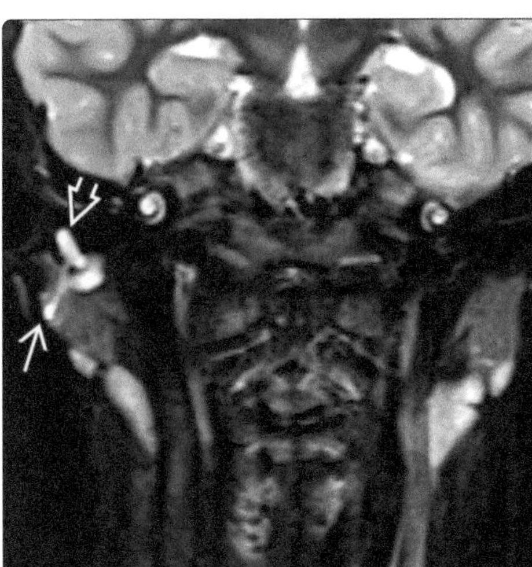

(Left) *Axial T1WI C+ FS MR demonstrates an irregularly shaped, infected 1st BCC ➔ within the right parotid gland with a thick, enhancing wall & diffuse, abnormal enhancement of the surrounding parotid gland ➔.* **(Right)** *Coronal STIR MR in a child with recurrent periauricular abscess and intermittent EAC drainage demonstrates a curvilinear tubular 1st branchial apparatus anomaly in the form of a fluid-filled fistula extending from the skin surface ➔ to the floor of the EAC ➔.*

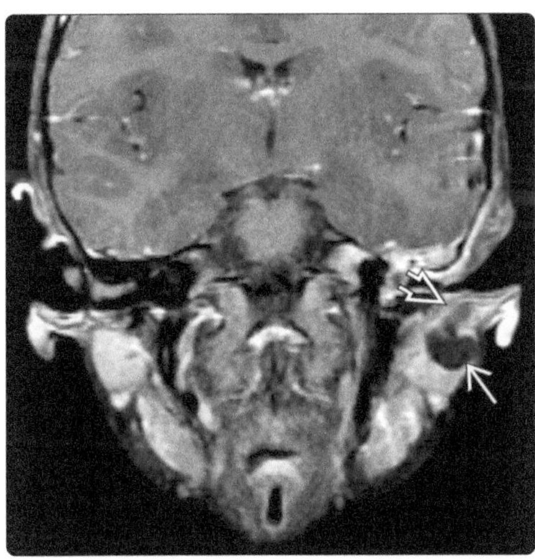

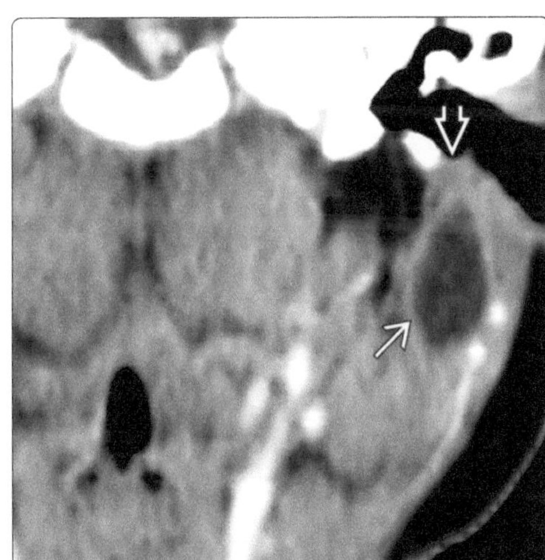

(Left) *Coronal T1WI C+ FS MR in a 3-year-old child with a palpable mass shows a lobulated, hypointense intraparotid mass ➔ with a curvilinear component ➔ extending toward the osseous-cartilaginous junction of the EAC.* **(Right)** *Coronal CECT shows a well-defined intraparotid 1st BCC ➔ with the superior aspect directed toward the bony-cartilaginous junction ➔ of the left EAC.*

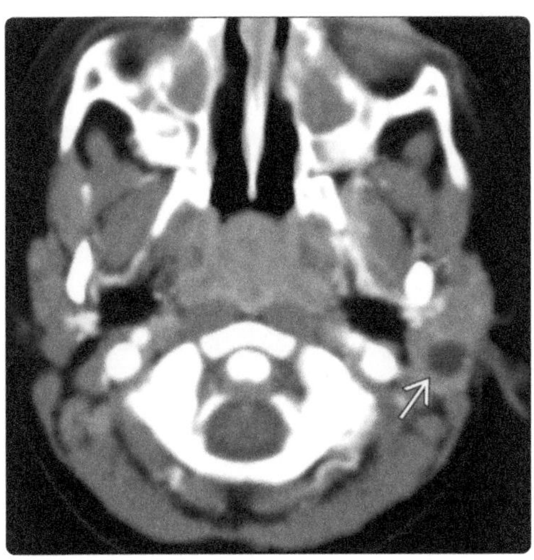

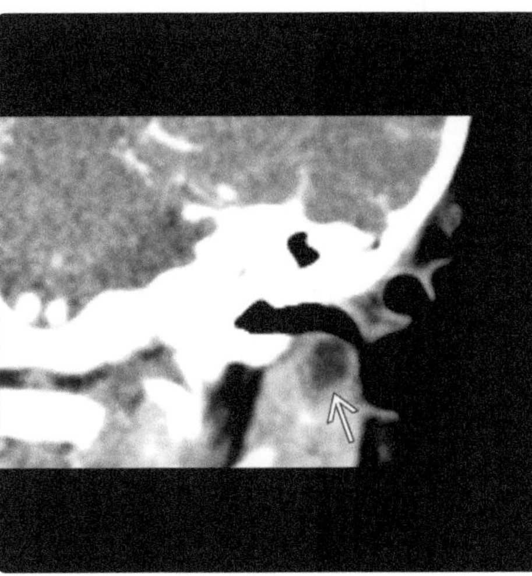

(Left) *Axial CECT in a 1-year-old with a bilobed 1st BCC shows the inferior extent of the cyst to be well defined and intraparotid in location ➔.* **(Right)** *Coronal CECT in the same patient shows the well-defined, nonenhancing upper aspect of the bilobed BCC ➔ along the inferior margin of the left cartilaginous EAC. Any cystic structure in or adjacent to the EAC or parotid gland should be imaged in its entirety and, in a child, should raise the question of a 1st branchial apparatus cyst.*

2nd Branchial Cleft Cyst

KEY FACTS

TERMINOLOGY

- Cervical sinus of His cystic remnant: 2nd, 3rd, and 4th branchial clefts and 2nd branchial arch derivative
- Synonyms
  - 2nd branchial cleft cyst (BCC) or anomaly
  - 2nd branchial apparatus cyst (BAC) or anomaly

IMAGING

- Best diagnostic clue: Cystic neck mass posterolateral to submandibular gland, lateral to carotid space, anterior (or anteromedial) to sternocleidomastoid muscle
- If infected, wall is thicker and enhances with surrounding soft tissue cellulitis

TOP DIFFERENTIAL DIAGNOSES

- Lymphatic malformation
  - Frequently transspatial
- Cervical thymic cyst
  - Remnant of 3rd pharyngeal pouch
- Lymphadenopathy/abscess
  - Presents with signs and symptoms of infection
- Cystic metastatic nodes
  - Squamous cell carcinoma (SCCa) nodal metastasis
  - Differentiated thyroid carcinoma nodal metastasis
- Carotid space schwannoma
  - Occasional large intramural cysts
  - Thick, enhancing wall
  - Rare in children

PATHOLOGY

- 2nd BAC, sinus, or fistulae
- Epidemiology: 2nd branchial apparatus anomalies (BAAs) account for up to 95% of all BAAs

DIAGNOSTIC CHECKLIST

- Beware of adult with 1st presentation of 2nd BCC
  - May be necrotic metastasis from head and neck SCCa primary tumor

(Left) *Sagittal oblique graphic shows a 2nd branchial cleft cyst (BCC) ➡ in its most common location, anterior to the sternocleidomastoid muscle (SCM) and anterolateral to the carotid space. Full tract may extend from the faucial tonsil ➡ to the low anterior neck ➡.* **(Right)** *Axial CECT in a 17-year-old boy shows a well-defined, low-attenuation mass ➡ in the typical location of a Bailey type II 2nd BCC: Anterior to the SCM ➡, lateral to the carotid sheath vessels ➡, and posterior to the submandibular gland ➡.*

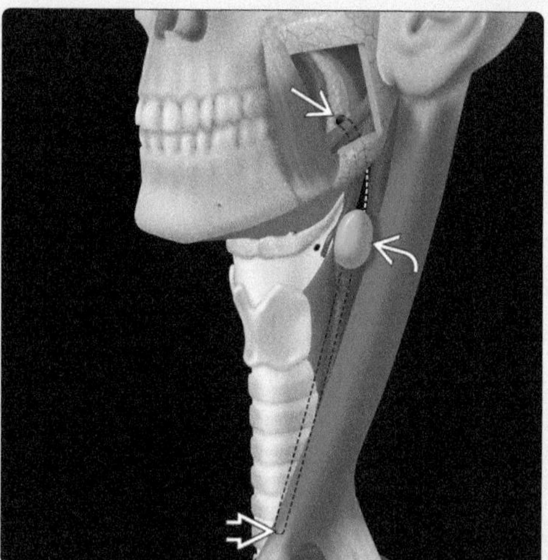

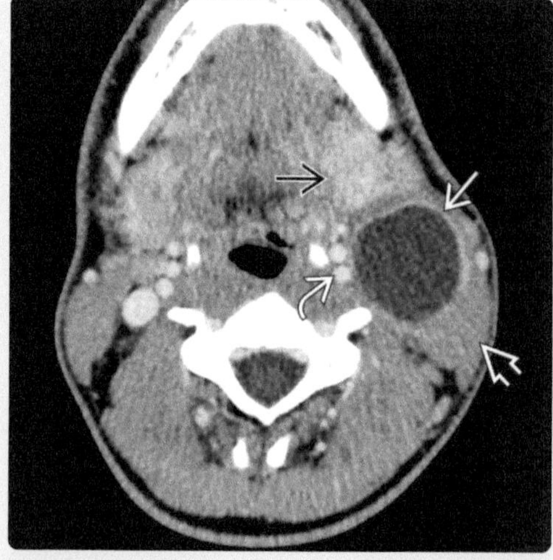

(Left) *Longitudinal US in a young adult with VACTERL association and a neck mass with signs or symptoms of infection shows a well-defined, unilocular, hypoechoic anterior right neck mass ➡ with posterior acoustic enhancement and internal echoes.* **(Right)** *Axial CECT in the same patient shows to better advantage the typical relationship of a 2nd BCC to the adjacent structures, SCM muscle ➡, submandibular gland ➡, and carotid sheath vessels ➡.*

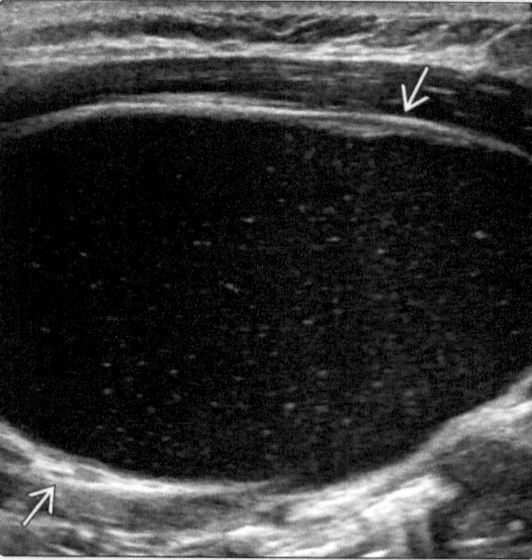

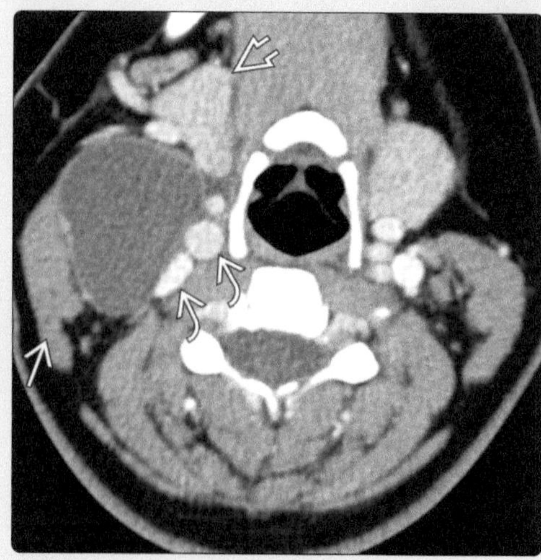

TERMINOLOGY

Abbreviations

- 2nd branchial cleft cyst (BCC)

Synonyms

- 2nd branchial apparatus cyst (BAC)
- 2nd branchial apparatus anomaly (BAA)

Definitions

- 2nd BCC
  - Most common BAC
  - Cystic remnant of cervical sinus of His: Derivative of 2nd, 3rd, and 4th branchial clefts
- Sinus
  - Usually communicates externally along anterior margin of sternocleidomastoid muscle (SCM)
  - Rarely communicates internally to tonsillar fossa
- Fistula
  - Communicates externally and internally
  - Secondary to persistence of both branchial cleft and pharyngeal pouch remnant
- Combinations
  - Cyst + sinus &/or fistula

IMAGING

General Features

- Best diagnostic clue
  - Cystic neck mass posterolateral to submandibular gland, lateral to carotid space, anterior to SCM
  - Most are at or immediately caudal to angle of mandible
- Location
  - Bailey classification of 2nd BACs
    - Type I: Deep to platysma muscle, anterior to SCM
    - Type II: Anterior to SCM, posterior to submandibular gland, lateral to carotid sheath
      - Most common
    - Type III: Protrudes between internal carotid artery (ICA) and external carotid artery (ECA), may extend to lateral pharyngeal wall or superiorly to skull base
    - Type IV: Adjacent to lateral pharyngeal wall, probably remnant of 2nd pharyngeal pouch
  - 2nd branchial apparatus fistula extends from anterior to SCM, through carotid artery bifurcation, and terminates in tonsillar fossa
- Size
  - Variable; may range from several cm to > 5 cm
- Morphology
  - Ovoid or rounded, well-circumscribed cyst
  - Focal rim of cyst may extend to carotid bifurcation

CT Findings

- CECT
  - Low-density cyst with nonenhancing wall
  - If infected, wall is thicker and enhances with surrounding soft tissue cellulitis

MR Findings

- T1WI
  - Cyst is usually isointense to CSF
  - Infection → increased signal intensity/protein content
- T2WI
  - Hyperintense cyst, no discernible wall
- FLAIR
  - Cyst is iso- or slightly hyperintense to CSF
- T1WI C+
  - No intrinsic contrast enhancement
  - Peripheral wall enhancement if infected

Ultrasonographic Findings

- Anechoic or hypoechoic, thin-walled cyst
  - May give pseudosolid US appearance
    - Real time will demonstrate mobile internal echoes to differentiate from solid lesion
- Thickened cyst wall if infected

Imaging Recommendations

- CT, US, or MR clearly demonstrate location of type I, II, and III cysts
- May be difficult to visualize type IV cysts with US
- CT or MR best demonstrates associated findings of infection and rare type IV cysts

DIFFERENTIAL DIAGNOSIS

Lymphatic Malformation

- Unilocular or multilocular
- Frequently transspatial
- Fluid-fluid levels if intralesional hemorrhage
- Isolation to same location as 2nd BAAs is uncommon

Thymic Cyst

- Remnant of thymopharyngeal duct, derivative of 3rd pharyngeal pouch
- Left side more common than right
- Up to 50% extend into superior mediastinum

Lymphadenopathy/Abscess

- Presents with signs and symptoms of infection
- Irregular, thick, enhancing wall with nonenhancing central cavity
- Surrounding soft tissue induration except with *Mycobacterium*
- Associated ipsilateral nonsuppurative adenopathy

Cystic Metastatic Nodes

- Necrotic mass with thick, enhancing wall
- Rare in children, occasional in teenagers
- Cystic squamous cell carcinoma (SCCa) nodal metastasis
- Cystic differentiated thyroid carcinoma nodal metastasis

Carotid Space Schwannoma

- Occasional large intramural cysts
- Thick, enhancing wall
- Centered in posterior carotid space

PATHOLOGY

General Features

- Embryology
  - 2nd branchial arch overgrows 2nd, 3rd, and 4th branchial clefts, forming ectodermally lined cervical sinus of His
  - Remnant of 2nd, 3rd, and 4th branchial clefts opens into cervical sinus of His via cervical vesicles

- Normally developing cervical sinus of His and vesicles involute
- Etiology
  - Remnants of 2nd branchial apparatus may form cyst, sinus, or fistula
- Associated abnormalities
  - Usually isolated lesion
  - May be part of branchiootorenal (BOR) syndrome
    - Autosomal dominant inheritance
    - Bilateral branchial fistulas or cysts and preauricular tag or pit
    - Profound mixed hearing loss
      - Tapered basal turn of cochlea with offset middle/apical turns → unwound appearance
      - Dysmorphic ossicles: Fused, malformed ossicles
      - Semicircular canal malformations, bulbous vestibular aqueduct, flared internal auditory canal
    - Renal anomalies: Cysts, dysplasia, agenesis
    - Dilated eustachian tubes
  - Branchiootic syndrome; similar to BOR syndrome without renal involvement

Gross Pathologic & Surgical Features

- Well-defined cyst in locations described by Bailey
- Filled with cheesy material or serous, mucoid, or purulent fluid

Microscopic Features

- Squamous epithelial-lined cyst
- Lymphoid infiltrate in wall, in form of germinal centers
  - Lymphoid tissue suggests epithelial rests may be entrapped within cervical lymph nodes during embryogenesis

CLINICAL ISSUES

Presentation

- Most common signs/symptoms
  - Painless, compressible lateral neck mass in child or young adult
  - May enlarge during upper respiratory tract infection
    - Probably due to response of lymphoid tissue
  - Fever, tenderness, and erythema if infected

Demographics

- Age
  - Majority < 5 years; 2nd peak in 2nd or 3rd decade
- Epidemiology
  - 2nd BAAs account for up to 95% of all BAAs

Natural History & Prognosis

- If untreated, may become repeatedly infected
- Recurrent inflammation makes surgical resection more difficult
- Excellent prognosis if lesion is completely resected

Treatment

- Complete surgical resection is treatment of choice
- Surgeon must dissect around cyst bed to exclude possibility of associated fistula or sinus
  - If fistula present, usually identified at birth
    - Mucoid secretions are emitted from skin opening
  - If tract proceeds superomedially, it passes through carotid bifurcation into palatine tonsil crypts
  - If tract courses inferiorly, it passes along anterior carotid space, reaching supraclavicular skin
- Endoscope-assisted resection via retroauricular approach feasible alternative to conventional resection

DIAGNOSTIC CHECKLIST

Consider

- If cyst wall enhances &/or associated cellulitis, consider superimposed infection
- If abscess is recognized posterior to submandibular gland, anterior to SCM, and anteromedial to carotid sheath vessels, think infected 2nd BCC
- Does cyst appear adherent to internal jugular vein or carotid sheath?

Image Interpretation Pearls

- Beware of teenager or adult with 1st presentation of 2nd BCC
  - Mass may be metastatic node from head and neck SCCa primary tumor
  - If patient > 30 years of age, 1st consider cystic nodal metastasis

SELECTED REFERENCES

1. Booth TN: Congenital cystic neck masses. Neuroimaging Clin N Am. 33(4):591-605, 2023
2. Gao S et al: Endoscopically assisted transoral resection of a Bailey type IV second branchial cleft cyst: a case report. Medicine (Baltimore). 100(3):e24375, 2021
3. Ginat DT: Imaging findings in syndromes with temporal bone abnormalities. Neuroimaging Clin N Am. 29(1):117-28, 2019
4. Hsu A et al: The unwound cochlea: a specific imaging marker of branchio-oto-renal syndrome. AJNR Am J Neuroradiol. 39(12):2345-9, 2018
5. Thottam PJ et al: Complete second branchial cleft anomaly presenting as a fistula and a tonsillar cyst: an interesting congenital anomaly. Ear Nose Throat J. 93(10-11):466-8, 2014
6. Chen LS et al: Endoscope-assisted versus conventional second branchial cleft cyst resection. Surg Endosc. 26(5):1397-402, 2012
7. Goff CJ et al: Current management of congenital branchial cleft cysts, sinuses, and fistulae. Curr Opin Otolaryngol Head Neck Surg. 20(6):533-9, 2012
8. Bajaj Y et al: Branchial anomalies in children. Int J Pediatr Otorhinolaryngol. 75(8):1020-3, 2011
9. Buchanan MA et al: Cystic schwannoma of the cervical plexus masquerading as a type II second branchial cleft cyst. Eur Arch Otorhinolaryngol. 266(3):459-62, 2009
10. Hudgins PA et al: Second branchial cleft cyst: not!! AJNR Am J Neuroradiol. 30(9):1628-9, 2009
11. Gupta AK et al: Bilateral first and second branchial cleft fistulas: a case report. Ear Nose Throat J. 87(5):291-3, 2008
12. Koch BL: Cystic malformations of the neck in children. Pediatr Radiol. 35(5):463-77, 2005
13. Lanham PD et al: Second brachial cleft cyst mimic: case report. AJNR Am J Neuroradiol. 26(7):1862-4, 2005
14. Ceruti S et al: Temporal bone anomalies in the branchio-oto-renal syndrome: detailed computed tomographic and magnetic resonance imaging findings. Otol Neurotol. 23(2):200-7, 2002
15. Shin JH et al: Parapharyngeal second branchial cyst manifesting as cranial nerve palsies: MR findings. AJNR Am J Neuroradiol. 22(3):510-2, 2001
16. Benson MT et al: Congenital anomalies of the branchial apparatus: embryology and pathologic anatomy. Radiographics. 12(5):943-60, 1992
17. Harnsberger HR et al: Branchial cleft anomalies and their mimics: computed tomographic evaluation. Radiology. 152(3):739-48, 1984

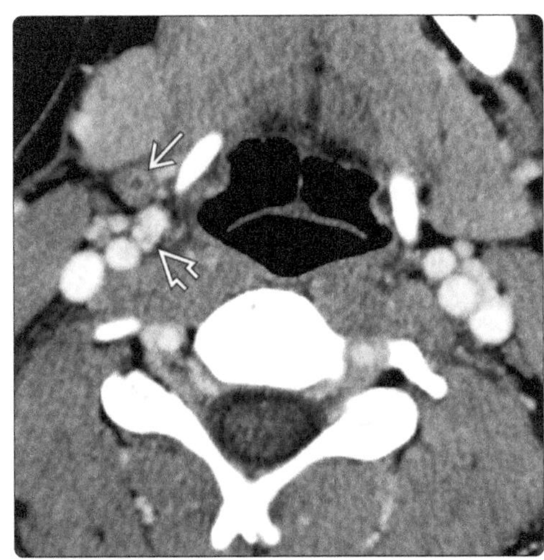

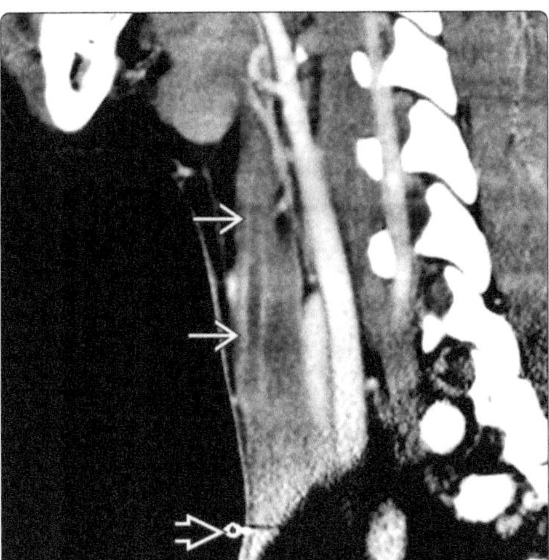

(Left) *Axial CECT in a 15-year-old boy with a pit in the lower anterior neck since birth, now draining purulent fluid, demonstrates a well-defined small lesion ➡ with a thick wall anterior to the carotid vessels ⇨ and posterior to the submandibular gland.* **(Right)** *Sagittal CT reconstruction in the same patient demonstrates the course of the infected 2nd branchial cleft sinus tract ➡, extending from the level of the pit (marked with radiodense marker ⇨) toward the faucial tonsil.*

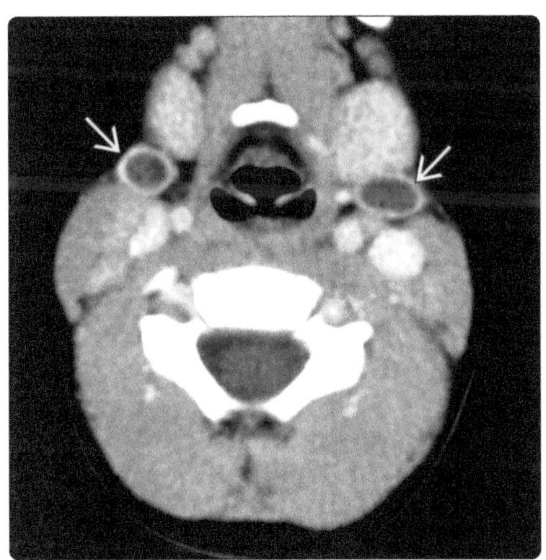

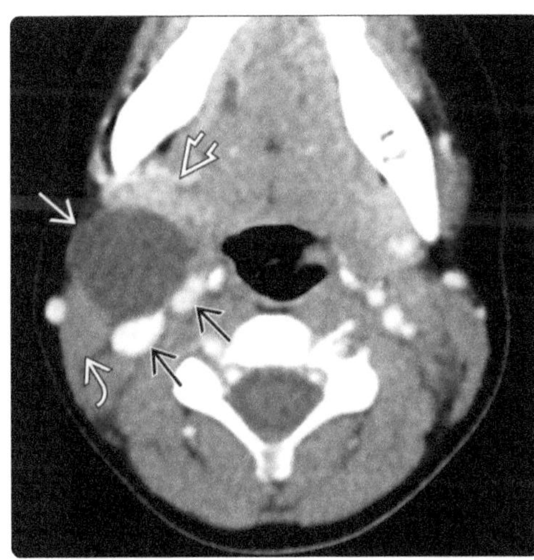

(Left) *Axial CECT in a 2-year-old boy with branchiootorenal (BOR) syndrome shows bilateral, well-defined, nonenhancing cysts ➡ in the typical location of Bailey type II 2nd BCCs.* **(Right)** *Axial CECT in a 7-year-old child shows a typical 2nd BCC ➡: Round, low attenuation with an imperceptible wall without enhancement. Location is also typical: Posterior to the submandibular gland ⇨, anterior to the SCM ↷, and anterolateral to the carotid sheath vessels ➡.*

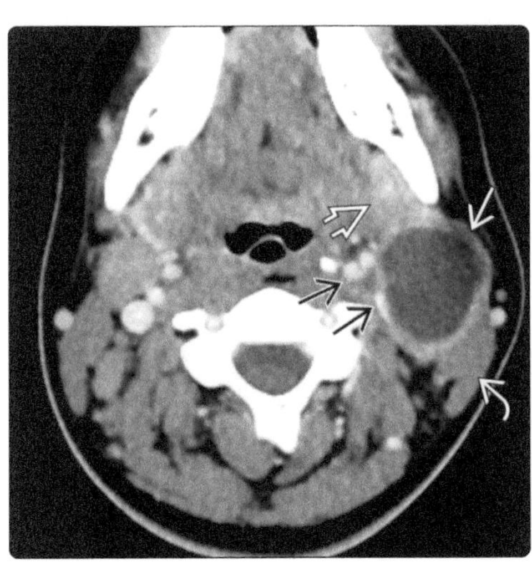

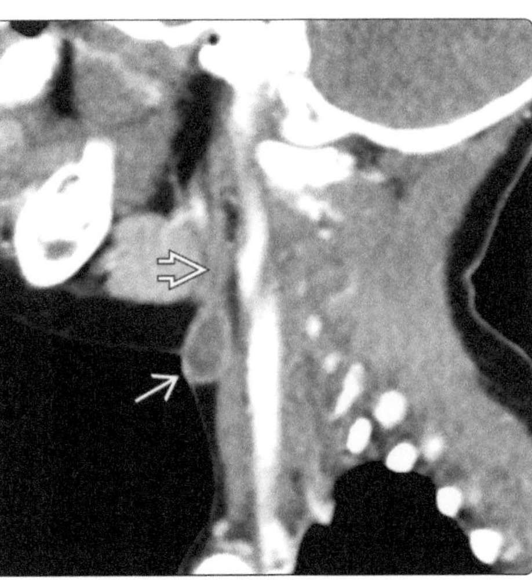

(Left) *Axial CECT shows a cyst ➡ in the typical location of a 2nd BCC: Posterior to submandibular gland ⇨, anterior to SCM ↷, and lateral to carotid sheath vessels ➡. Mildly thick wall suggests prior infection. In an adult, differential diagnosis includes a necrotic, metastatic lymph node.* **(Right)** *Sagittal CECT in a 2-year-old with BOR syndrome and bilateral anterior neck sinus tracts shows a cyst ➡ extending from the skin surface, along the left SCM, and a small sinus tract that extends superiorly toward the tonsillar fossa ⇨.*

3rd Branchial Cleft Cyst

KEY FACTS

TERMINOLOGY

- 3rd branchial cleft cyst (BCC)
  - Epithelial-lined remnant of 3rd branchial cleft

IMAGING

- CT/MR/US
  - Unilocular, thin-walled cyst in upper posterior cervical space or lower anterior neck
  - If infected, cyst wall thickens and enhances
  - ± adjacent cellulitis or myositis
- Barium or water-soluble contrast swallow may outline associated sinus or fistula

TOP DIFFERENTIAL DIAGNOSES

- 2nd BCC: Most common BCC
- Lymphatic malformation: Uni- or multilocular
- Abscess: Signs and symptoms of infection
- Cervical thymic cyst: 3rd pouch remnant
- 4th branchial apparatus anomaly: Pyriform sinus tract and left neck abscess
- Infrahyoid thyroglossal duct cyst: Embedded in strap muscles when infrahyoid
- Cystic-necrotic metastatic lymph node: Usually known primary H&N squamous cell carcinoma or systemic NHL
- External laryngocele: Communicates with laryngeal ventricle through thyrohyoid membrane

CLINICAL ISSUES

- Fluctuant mass in posterolateral upper neck
- Frequently presents in **adulthood**
- Purulent drainage from skin ostium if associated fistula

DIAGNOSTIC CHECKLIST

- Cyst in posterior cervical space of upper neck
  - Think 3rd BCC
- Abscess in posterior cervical space of upper neck
  - Think infected, preexisting, underlying 3rd BCC

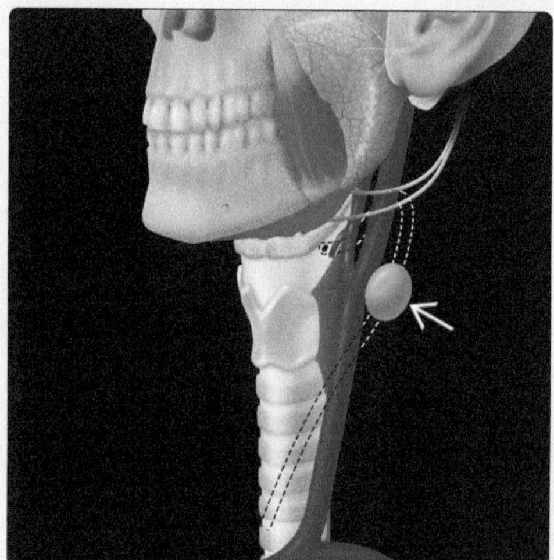

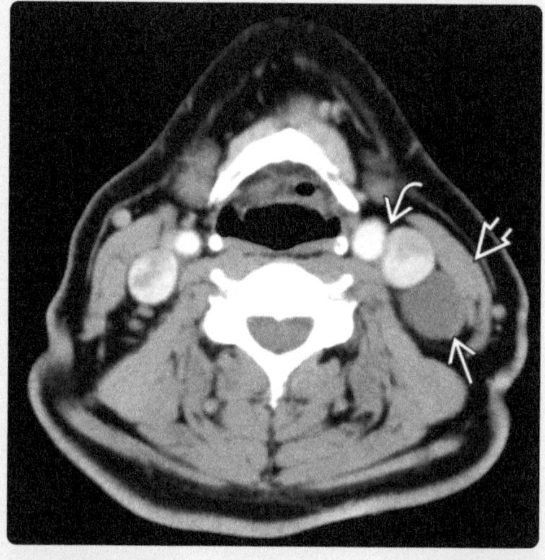

(Left) *Lateral graphic illustrates the course of a 3rd branchial anomaly (dashes), along which the 3rd branchial cleft cysts (BCCs) arise, most commonly in the upper posterior triangle ➡. **(Right)** Axial CECT in a man with a posterior left neck mass demonstrates a well-defined, thin-walled unilocular cyst ➡ in the posterior cervical space, deep to sternocleidomastoid muscle (SCM) ➡ and posterolateral to the carotid space ➡. Note that the cyst wall is imperceptible, indicating that the lesion has not been infected.*

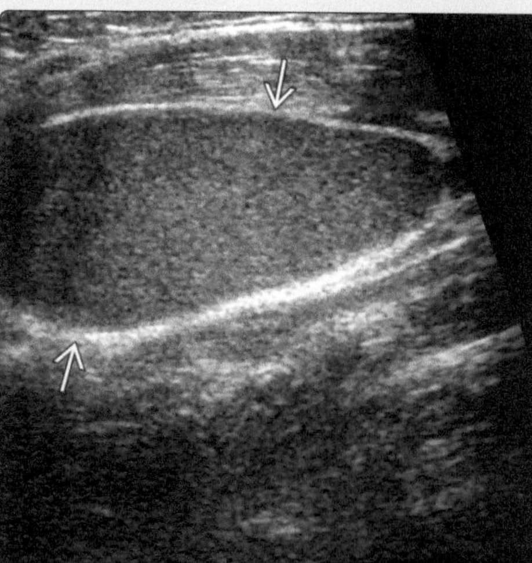

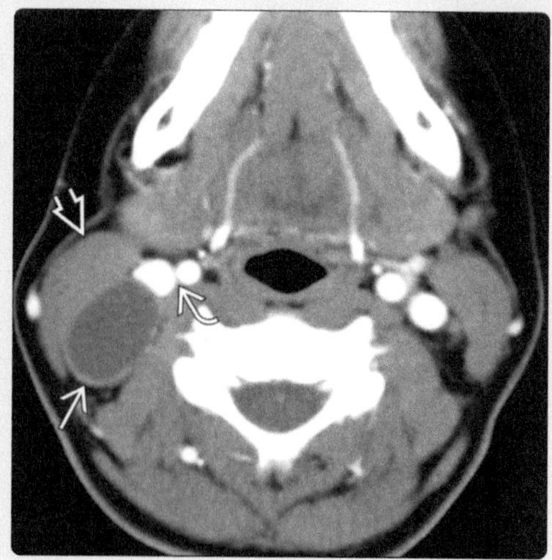

(Left) *Longitudinal US of the neck in a teenager with recent onset of a neck mass demonstrates a well-defined cyst ➡ with internal echoes in the posterior upper neck.* **(Right)** *Axial CECT in the same child demonstrates the relationship of the well-defined, nonenhancing cyst ➡ to the adjacent structures in the suprahyoid posterior neck, deep to SCM ➡ and posterolateral to carotid sheath vessels ➡. The location and appearance typical of a 3rd BCC DDx would include unilocular lymphatic malformation.*

TERMINOLOGY

Abbreviations

- 3rd branchial cleft cyst (BCC)

Synonyms

- 3rd branchial apparatus cyst (BAC)

Definitions

- Epithelial-lined cystic remnant of 3rd branchial cleft

IMAGING

General Features

- Best diagnostic clue
  - Unilocular, thin-walled cyst in upper posterior cervical space or lower anterior neck
- Location
  - Anywhere along course of 3rd branchial cleft or pouch
    - Upper neck: Posterior cervical space
    - Lower neck: Anterior border of sternocleidomastoid muscle (SCM)
    - Rarely in submandibular space, lateral to cephalad hypopharynx
  - Classically, 3rd branchial fistula would exit base of pyriform sinus and course superior to laryngeal and hypoglossal nerves, inferior to glossopharyngeal nerve
- Size
  - Variable; usually 2-3 cm at presentation
- Morphology
  - Typically ovoid or round cyst

Fluoroscopic Findings

- Barium or water-soluble contrast swallow
  - May outline associated sinus or fistula
  - Point of exit from hypopharynx
    - High lateral margin of pyriform sinus

CT Findings

- CECT
  - Round or ovoid, sharply marginated lesions with central fluid attenuation
  - Cyst wall thin; no calcifications
  - If infected, cyst wall thickens and enhances
    - ± adjacent cellulitis &/or myositis
  - SCM displaced laterally when cyst in high posterior neck
  - SCM displaced posterolaterally when cyst in low anterior neck

MR Findings

- T1WI
  - Homogeneous, hypointense fluid contents
  - Cyst wall thin or imperceptible
- T2WI
  - Homogeneous, hyperintense fluid contents
  - + edema in surrounding tissues if infected
- T1WI C+
  - Thin, uniform, minimally enhancing cyst wall
  - If infected
    - Cyst wall thickened and enhancing
    - Fluid contents hyperintense relative to CSF
    - Strand-like enhancement in soft tissues surrounding 3rd BCC

Ultrasonographic Findings

- Thin-walled, hypoechoic mass upper posterior neck or lower anterior neck
- Lacks internal vascularity

Imaging Recommendations

- Best imaging tool
  - CECT or MR best to evaluate complete extent
- Protocol advice
  - Barium (or water-soluble contrast) swallow may outline associated sinus or fistula
  - Fistula may be outlined by direct injection of cutaneous ostium

DIFFERENTIAL DIAGNOSIS

2nd Branchial Cleft Cyst

- Most common branchial apparatus anomaly
- Most common angle of mandible mass in young adult
- Usually lateral to carotid space, posterior to submandibular gland, and anteromedial to SCM
- Typically nonenhancing fluid signal/attenuation/echogenicity on MR/CT/US
  - If infected, thicker wall with enhancement and surrounding soft tissue cellulitis

Lymphatic Malformation

- Majority diagnosed < 2 years of age
- Unilocular or multilocular
- Focal or infiltrative
- Fluid-fluid levels if intralesional hemorrhage
- Alone or combined with enhancing venous malformation

Abscess

- Presents with signs and symptoms of infection
- Irregular, thick, enhancing wall; low-attenuation center
- Surrounding cellulitis
- If associated with thyroid gland, think 4th branchial pouch anomaly
- If in posterior cervical space of upper neck, think infected underlying 3rd BCC

Cervical Thymic Cyst

- 3rd branchial pouch remnant
- Along course of thymopharyngeal duct
- Left > > right
- Closely associated with carotid sheath
- ± extension to anterior mediastinum

4th Branchial Apparatus Anomaly

- Most often presents with suppurative thyroiditis in children
- Abscess closely associated with anterior left thyroid lobe, thyroiditis
- Sinus tract from pyriform sinus apex to anterior lower left neck
- Prenatal diagnosis suggested if left-sided unilocular neck cyst is identified with tapered medial margin at level of pyriform sinus
- Remnant of 4th (or 3rd) branchial pouch

Infrahyoid Thyroglossal Duct Cyst

- Midline or paramidline anterior neck cyst in child or young adult
- Infrahyoid < suprahyoid, at level of hyoid bone
  - Infrahyoid: Off-midline in strap muscles or anterior to thyroid gland

Metastases, Cystic-Necrotic Lymph Node

- Spinal accessory malignant necrotic adenopathy in posterior cervical space
- Usually known primary head and neck squamous cell carcinoma or systemic non-Hodgkin lymphoma (NHL)
- Almost always in adults; rarely in children

External Laryngocele

- Thin-walled, fluid- or air-filled cystic lesion communicating with laryngeal ventricle + extralaryngeal extension through thyrohyoid membrane
- Most commonly seen in adult glassblowers, trumpet players, or those with chronic coughs
  - Present with enlarging neck mass

PATHOLOGY

General Features

- Etiology
  - Controversial
    - Failure of obliteration of 3rd branchial cleft, portion of cervical sinus of His, or 3rd pharyngeal pouch
- Associated abnormalities
  - 3rd branchial sinus
    - Single opening
      - Endopharyngeal in high lateral hypopharynx or cutaneous opening in supraclavicular area anterior to carotid artery
  - 3rd branchial fistula
    - 2 openings
      - Endopharyngeal in high lateral hypopharynx and cutaneous opening in supraclavicular area anterior to carotid artery
      - Skin opening may be pseudofistula secondary to repeated infection or surgical incision rather than true fistula

Gross Pathologic & Surgical Features

- Smooth, thin-walled cysts
- May contain clear, watery to mucinous material
  - ± desquamated cellular debris

Microscopic Features

- Lined by squamous epithelium (occasionally by columnar epithelium)
- Lymphoid tissue in walls of cyst with reactive lymphoid follicles

CLINICAL ISSUES

Presentation

- Most common signs/symptoms
  - Fluctuant mass in posterolateral neck
  - May enlarge rapidly following upper respiratory tract infection
- Other signs/symptoms
  - Recurrent lateral neck or retropharyngeal abscesses
  - Draining fistula along anterior margin of SCM

Demographics

- Age
  - Frequently presents in adulthood
  - Presentation of cysts in neonates and infants unusual
  - When sinus or fistula present, early presentation more common
- Epidemiology
  - 3rd branchial cleft anomalies account for only **3%** of all branchial anomalies
  - 2nd BCC > 1st BCC > 3rd BCC

Natural History & Prognosis

- Good prognosis if completely resected
- May become infected and present with neck abscess

Treatment

- Surgical resection
  - If infected, treat with antibiotics prior to surgical resection
  - Surgery includes resection of cyst and any associated sinus or fistula

DIAGNOSTIC CHECKLIST

Consider

- Cyst in posterior cervical space of upper neck, think 3rd BCC
- Abscess in posterior cervical space of upper neck, think infected, preexisting, underlying 3rd BCC

SELECTED REFERENCES

1. Booth TN: Congenital cystic neck masses. Neuroimaging Clin N Am. 33(4):591-605, 2023
2. Castro PT et al: Pre and postnatal diagnosis of a third branchial cleft cyst by sonography and magnetic resonance imaging with three-dimensional virtual reconstruction. J Clin Ultrasound. 49(9):966-8, 2021
3. Li Y et al: Prenatal diagnosis of third and fourth branchial apparatus anomalies: case series and comparison with lymphatic malformation. AJNR Am J Neuroradiol. 42(11):2094-100, 2021
4. Buch K et al: MR imaging evaluation of pediatric neck masses: review and update. Magn Reson Imaging Clin N Am. 27(2):173-99, 2019
5. Mehmi N et al: Importance and impact of appropriate radiology in the management of branchial cleft anomalies. Indian J Otolaryngol Head Neck Surg. 71(Suppl 1):953-9, 2019
6. Goff CJ et al: Current management of congenital branchial cleft cysts, sinuses, and fistulae. Curr Opin Otolaryngol Head Neck Surg. 20(6):533-9, 2012
7. Thomas B et al: Revisiting imaging features and the embryologic basis of third and fourth branchial anomalies. AJNR Am J Neuroradiol. 31(4):755-60, 2010
8. Joshi MJ et al: The rare third branchial cleft cyst. AJNR Am J Neuroradiol. 30(9):1804-6, 2009
9. Koch BL: Cystic malformations of the neck in children. Pediatr Radiol. 35(5):463-77, 2005
10. Liberman M et al: Ten years of experience with third and fourth branchial remnants. J Pediatr Surg. 37(5):685-90, 2002
11. Huang RY et al: Third branchial cleft anomaly presenting as a retropharyngeal abscess. Int J Pediatr Otorhinolaryngol. 54(2-3):167-72, 2000
12. Mandell DL: Head and neck anomalies related to the branchial apparatus. Otolaryngol Clin North Am. 33(6):1309-32, 2000
13. Mukherji SK et al: Imaging of congenital anomalies of the branchial apparatus. Neuroimaging Clin N Am. 10(1):75-93, viii, 2000
14. Koeller KK et al: Congenital cystic masses of the neck: radiologic-pathologic correlation. Radiographics. 19(1):121-46; quiz 152-3, 1999
15. Benson MT et al: Congenital anomalies of the branchial apparatus: embryology and pathologic anatomy. Radiographics. 12(5):943-60, 1992

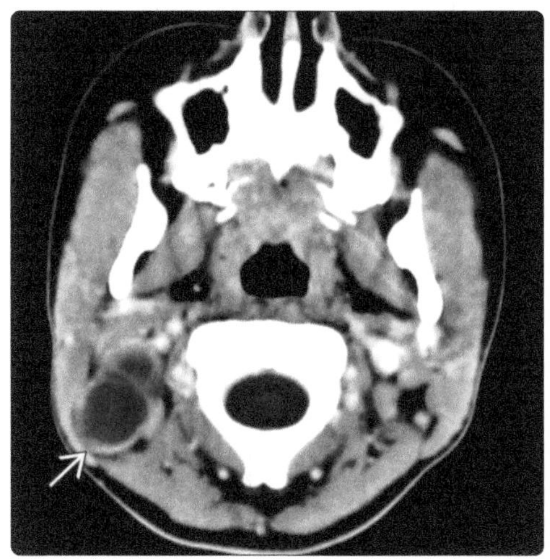

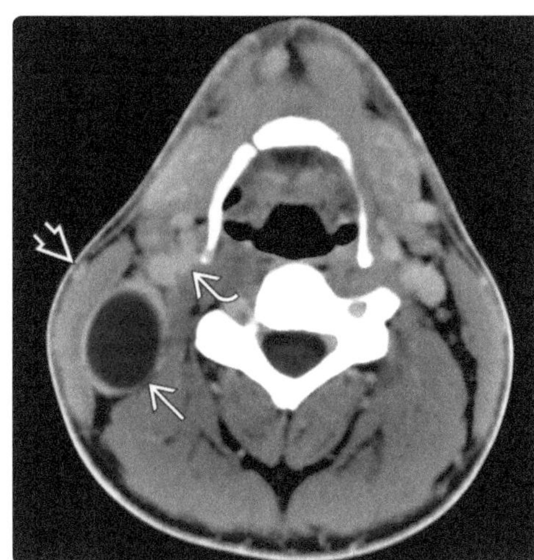

(Left) *Axial CECT demonstrates a 3rd BCC → in the posterior cervical space of the upper neck. Mild enhancement and internal septation are consistent with sequelae of superimposed infection.* **(Right)** *Axial CECT demonstrates a mildly thick-walled, infected 3rd BCC → deep to the SCM → and posterolateral to the carotid sheath →. When occurring in the upper neck, the posterior cervical space is the typical location of 3rd BCCs.*

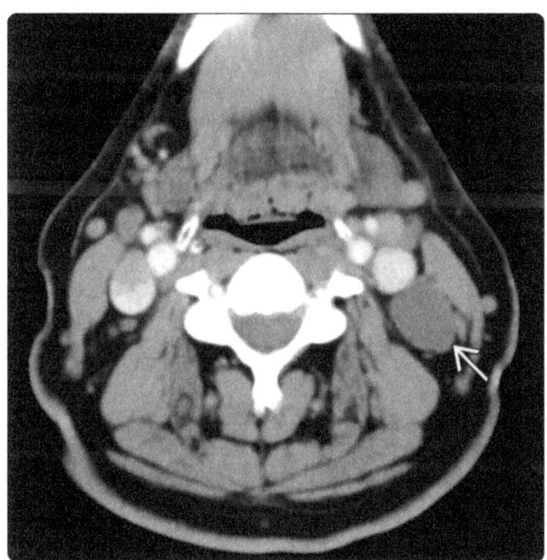

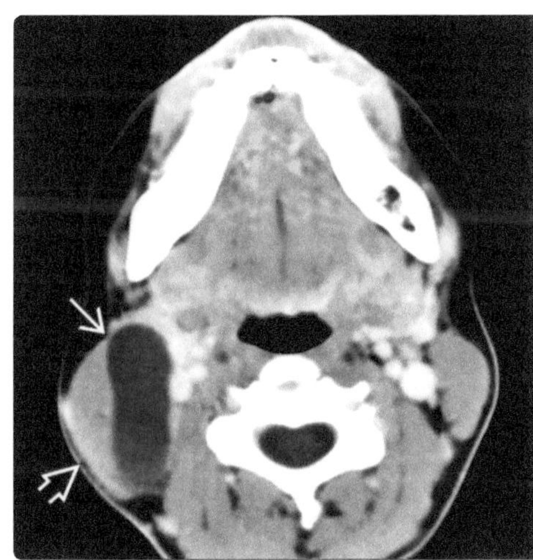

(Left) *Axial CECT shows a 3rd BCC → posterolateral to the left carotid sheath. Lack of enhancement is typical. In this location, imaging alone cannot differentiate a 3rd BCC from a macrocystic lymphatic malformation.* **(Right)** *Axial CECT shows a 3rd BCC → posterolateral to the carotid space, deviating the SCM → laterally.*

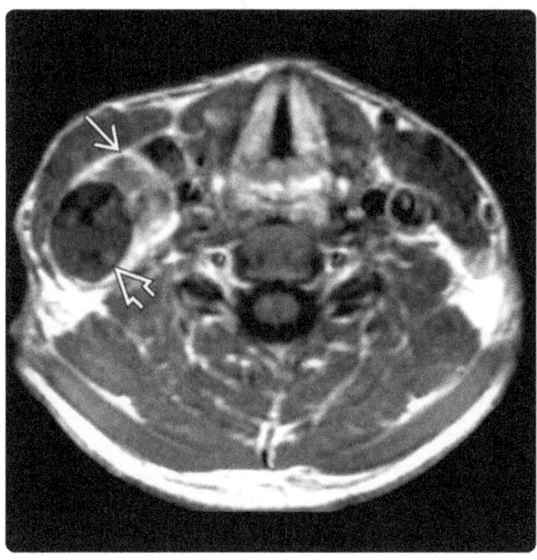

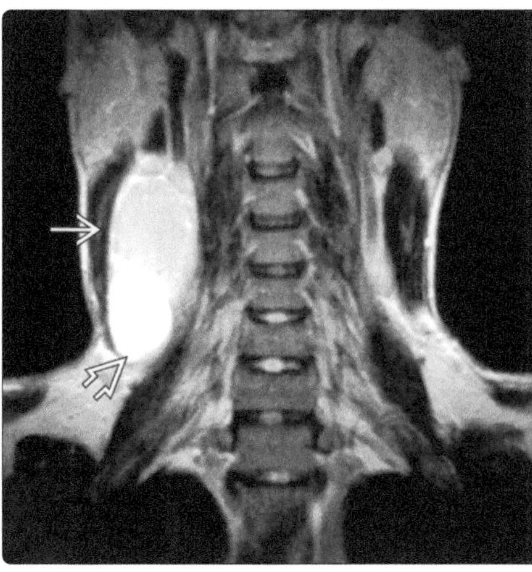

(Left) *Axial T1 C+ MR demonstrates a variant multiloculated 3rd BCC in the right posterior cervical space. The anterior portion → is hyperintense relative to the posterior portion →, indicating higher protein content secondary to prior infection or hemorrhage.* **(Right)** *Coronal T2 MR in the same patient shows the superior portion → to be hypointense relative to the inferior portion →. Lymphatic malformation should be included in the preoperative differential diagnosis.*

4th Branchial Cleft Cyst

KEY FACTS

TERMINOLOGY

- Pyriform sinus "fistula" or 4th branchial apparatus anomaly
  - Most anomalies are actually sinus tracts (not cysts) from 4th (or 3rd) pharyngeal pouch remnant
  - Course from apex of pyriform sinus to upper aspect of left thyroid lobe → abscess in anterior lower neck ± thyroid involvement

IMAGING

- Sinus tract extending from apex of pyriform sinus to lower anterior neck after barium swallow
- CECT best demonstrates phlegmon or abscess
  - Abscess in or adjacent to anterior left thyroid lobe
  - CT after barium swallow best identifies sinus tract
- Direct injection of fistula best demonstrates course of fistulous tract

TOP DIFFERENTIAL DIAGNOSES

- Cervical thymic cyst
- Lymphatic malformation
- Thyroglossal duct cyst
- Thyroid colloid cyst
- 3rd branchial cleft cyst

CLINICAL ISSUES

- Recurrent neck abscesses
- Recurrent suppurative thyroiditis
- Treatment options
  - Initial treatment is antibiotics ± incision and drainage of abscess
  - Complete resection of sinus tract or fistula
  - Thyroid lobectomy for lesions in thyroid lobe

DIAGNOSTIC CHECKLIST

- Suspect sinus tract from pyriform sinus in any child with abscess in or anterior to left thyroid lobe

(Left) *Sagittal oblique graphic shows a sinus tract ➡ from the pyriform sinus to the left thyroid lobe with associated abscess ➡ and thyroiditis secondary to a 4th pharyngeal pouch remnant.* **(Right)** *Coronal CECT shows the classic appearance of an inflammatory mass ➡ deviating the left thyroid lobe inferiorly with inflammation surrounding the sinus tract ➡, extending from the pyriform sinus apex ➡ to the phlegmonous process in the lower neck.*

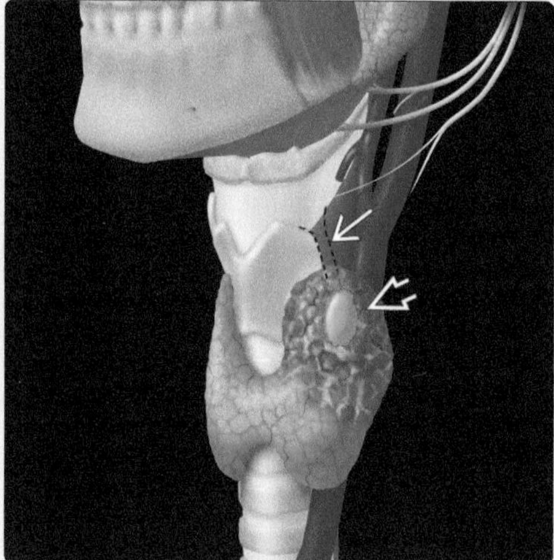

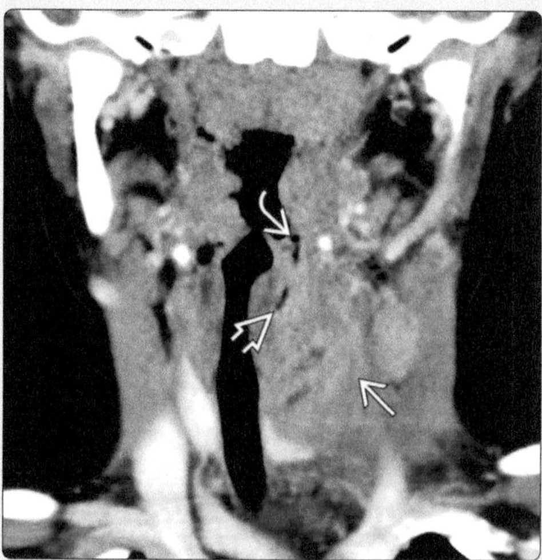

(Left) *Axial CECT in a child presenting with acute signs of infection demonstrates a phlegmonous mass ➡ in the anterior left neck, involving the left thyroid lobe ➡ and causing deviation of the airway to the right of midline.* **(Right)** *Axial CECT in the same patient shows a rim-enhancing early abscess ➡ deviating an air-filled sinus tract ➡ forward. This constellation of findings should alert the clinician to search for an opening at the apex of the pyriform sinus.*

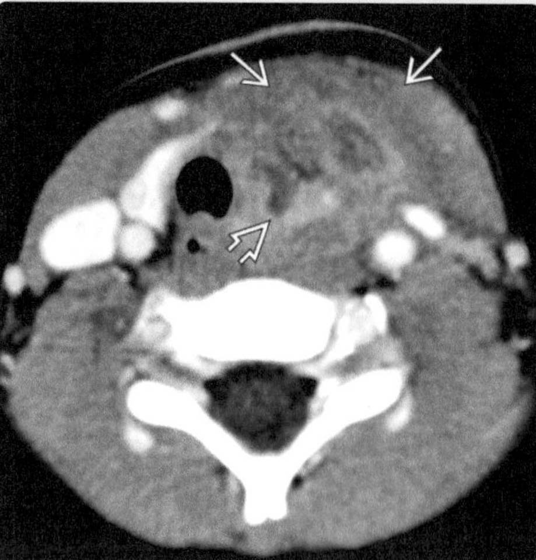

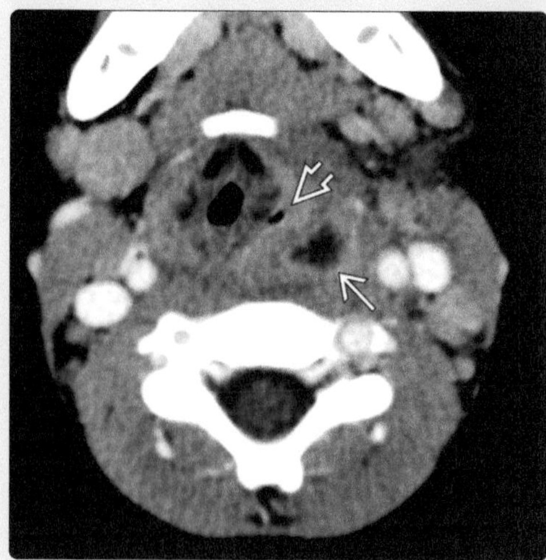

TERMINOLOGY

Synonyms

- Pyriform sinus "fistula"
  - Most 4th branchial anomalies are actually sinus tracts, not fistulas or cysts

Definitions

- 4th branchial apparatus sinus tract
  - Course from apex of pyriform sinus to upper aspect of left thyroid lobe
- Branchial sinus tract: 1 opening to skin surface, external auditory canal, pharynx or hypopharynx
- Branchial fistula: 2 openings to skin and lumen of foregut
  - Arises from epithelial-lined tract left behind when there is persistence of both branchial cleft and its corresponding pharyngeal pouch

IMAGING

General Features

- Best diagnostic clue
  - Sinus tract extending from apex of pyriform sinus to lower anterior neck after barium swallow
  - Abscess in or adjacent to anterior left thyroid lobe
- Location
  - May occur anywhere from pyriform sinus apex to thyroid lobe (> 90% left-sided)
    - Commonly against or within superior aspect of left thyroid lobe or attached to thyroid cartilage
    - Upper end may communicate with or be adherent to pyriform sinus
- Size
  - Variable
- Morphology
  - Thick-walled sinus tract ± abscess in or adjacent to left thyroid lobe

Fluoroscopic Findings

- Barium swallow
  - Barium-filled sinus tract extending from apex of pyriform sinus to anterior lower neck
  - If performed during acute infection, may not fill portions of sinus tract
  - Scarring secondary to infection may prohibit filling of sinus tract

CT Findings

- CECT
  - Phlegmonous mass or frank abscess in or adjacent to left thyroid lobe with cellulitis extending around and collapsing ipsilateral pyriform sinus
  - Air within sinus tract or thyroid lobe occasionally present
  - Rarely, fistulous tract identifiable extending to skin at anterior lower neck
- NECT after barium swallow
  - Barium-filled tract extending from apex of pyriform sinus to lower anterior neck
  - If performed during acute infection, may not fill portions of sinus tract
  - Scarring secondary to infection may prohibit filling of sinus tract

MR Findings

- Phlegmon or abscess in left anterior neck with deep neck inflammation extending to pyriform sinus
- Tubular, fluid-filled tract posterior to cricothyroid joint, extending from pyriform sinus apex to left lobe of thyroid in 40%
- Sinus tract may course through thyroid gland or posterior to thyroid gland
- Rarely see unilocular, cystic mass
- Prenatal diagnosis suggested if left-sided unilocular neck cyst is identified with tapered medial margin at level of pyriform sinus

Ultrasonographic Findings

- Heterogeneous, phlegmonous mass or thick-walled abscess with hyperemic wall anterior to or within left thyroid lobe
- Difficult to visualize extent of inflammation surrounding sinus tract communicating with pyriform sinus

Nuclear Medicine Findings

- Cold nodule on thyroid scan

Imaging Recommendations

- Best imaging tool
  - CECT best demonstrates phlegmon or abscess as well as inflammation extending craniad to level of asymmetric pyriform sinus
  - CT after barium swallow best identifies sinus tract
  - Direct injection of fistula best demonstrates course of fistula
- Protocol advice
  - Thin-section postcontrast helical CT with multiplanar reconstructions very helpful

DIFFERENTIAL DIAGNOSIS

Cervical Thymic Cyst

- Congenital cyst: Remnant of thymopharyngeal duct, derivative of 3rd pharyngeal pouch
- Left side more common than right
- Closely associated with carotid sheath
  - In lower neck: Medial to carotid sheath, posterior to thyroid
  - In upper neck or extending from upper neck to mediastinum: Splay carotid artery and jugular vein
- If confined to visceral space, may mimic 4th branchial apparatus cyst
- Up to 50% extend into superior mediastinum
- May be connected to mediastinal thymus directly or by fibrous cord

Lymphatic Malformation

- Uni- or multilocular
- Microcystic or macrocystic
- Focal or infiltrative
- Isolated or transspatial
- Fluid-fluid levels if intralesional hemorrhage
- ± enhancing venous malformation components if combined venolymphatic malformation

Thyroglossal Duct Cyst

- Anywhere along thyroglossal duct from base of tongue (foramen cecum) to lower anterior neck thyroid bed

- 20-25% in suprahyoid neck
- Almost 50% at hyoid bone
- ~ 25% in infrahyoid neck
  - Embedded in strap muscles = claw sign
  - Off-midline, anterior to thyroid lobe
  - Closely related to thyroid cartilage or strap muscles

Colloid Cyst, Thyroid

- Uncommon in young children, most occur in older children and adults
- True thyroid cysts are rare
- Most thyroid cysts = degenerating adenomas
- May appear bright on T1 MR due to hemorrhage, colloid, or high protein content

3rd Branchial Cleft Cyst

- Unilocular, thin-walled cyst
- Most arise in upper posterior cervical space
- Rarely along lower anterior margin of sternocleidomastoid muscle

PATHOLOGY

General Features

- Etiology
  - Controversial
    - Failure of obliteration of 4th branchial pouch or distal cervical sinus of His
    - Recent literature suggests course of sinus tract does not follow theoretical tract for 3rd or 4th branchial remnant
      - Sinus tract may actually be remnant of 3rd branchial pouch
- Associated abnormalities
  - 4th branchial sinus
    - When sinus connection with apex of pyriform sinus is maintained, infection is likely
    - Thyroiditis ± thyroid abscess possible in such circumstances
  - 4th branchial fistula
    - Term fistula denotes 2 openings: 1 in low anterior neck, another into pyriform sinus apex

Gross Pathologic & Surgical Features

- Anterolateral neck cellulitis, phlegmon or abscess
- Direct probing of pyriform apex frequently demonstrates fistula or sinus tract

CLINICAL ISSUES

Presentation

- Most common signs/symptoms
  - Recurrent neck abscesses
  - Recurrent suppurative thyroiditis
  - Fluctuant mass in lower 1/3 of neck anteromedial to sternocleidomastoid muscle
    - Tender if infected
  - Throat pain, dysphagia, stridor, dyspnea

Demographics

- Age
  - Most branchial sinuses and fistulae (all types) present in childhood
  - Most 4th branchial apparatus anomalies are diagnosed in infants and young children
- Sex
  - More common in female patients
- Epidemiology
  - Rarest of all forms of branchial apparatus anomalies (1-2% of all branchial anomalies)
  - Most cases arise on left

Natural History & Prognosis

- If sinus tract connection to pyriform sinus unrecognized and untreated, recurrent suppurative thyroiditis ensues
- Recurrence likely if tract contains secretory epithelium, which is not resected

Treatment

- If infected, initial treatment is antibiotics ± incision and drainage of abscess
- Complete resection of sinus tract or fistula, obliterate opening in pyriform sinus
- Thyroid lobectomy is required for lesions in thyroid lobe to prevent recurrence

DIAGNOSTIC CHECKLIST

Consider

- Suspect sinus tract from pyriform sinus in child with phlegmon or abscess in or anterior to left thyroid lobe

SELECTED REFERENCES

1. Booth TN: Congenital cystic neck masses. Neuroimaging Clin N Am. 33(4):591-605, 2023
2. Han Z et al: MRI in children with pyriform sinus fistula. J Magn Reson Imaging. 53(1):85-95, 2021
3. Li Y et al: Prenatal diagnosis of third and fourth branchial apparatus anomalies: case series and comparison with lymphatic malformation. AJNR Am J Neuroradiol. 42(11):2094-100, 2021
4. Buch K et al: MR imaging evaluation of pediatric neck masses: review and update. Magn Reson Imaging Clin N Am. 27(2):173-99, 2019
5. Prosser JD et al: Branchial cleft anomalies and thymic cysts. Otolaryngol Clin North Am. 48(1):1-14, 2015
6. Goff CJ et al: Current management of congenital branchial cleft cysts, sinuses, and fistulae. Curr Opin Otolaryngol Head Neck Surg. 20(6):533-9, 2012
7. Bajaj Y et al: Branchial anomalies in children. Int J Pediatr Otorhinolaryngol. 75(8):1020-3, 2011
8. Ibrahim M et al: Congenital cystic lesions of the head and neck. Neuroimaging Clin N Am. 21(3):621-39, viii, 2011
9. Thomas B et al: Revisiting imaging features and the embryologic basis of third and fourth branchial anomalies. AJNR Am J Neuroradiol. 31(4):755-60, 2010
10. Nicoucar K et al: Management of congenital fourth branchial arch anomalies: a review and analysis of published cases. J Pediatr Surg. 44(7):1432-9, 2009
11. Mantle BA et al: Fourth branchial cleft sinus: relationship to superior and recurrent laryngeal nerves. Am J Otolaryngol. 29(3):198-200, 2008
12. James A et al: Branchial sinus of the piriform fossa: reappraisal of third and fourth branchial anomalies. Laryngoscope. 117(11):1920-4, 2007
13. Koch BL: Cystic malformations of the neck in children. Pediatr Radiol. 35(5):463-77, 2005
14. Wang HK et al: Imaging studies of pyriform sinus fistula. Pediatr Radiol. 33(5):328-33, 2003
15. Mandell DL: Head and neck anomalies related to the branchial apparatus. Otolaryngol Clin North Am. 33(6): 1309-32, 2000
16. Park SW et al: Neck infection associated with pyriform sinus fistula: imaging findings. AJNR Am J Neuroradiol. 21(5):817-22, 2000
17. Stone ME et al: A new role for computed tomography in the diagnosis and treatment of pyriform sinus fistula. Am J Otolaryngol. 21(5):323-5, 2000
18. Benson MT et al: Congenital anomalies of the branchial apparatus: embryology and pathologic anatomy. Radiographics. 12(5):943-60, 1992

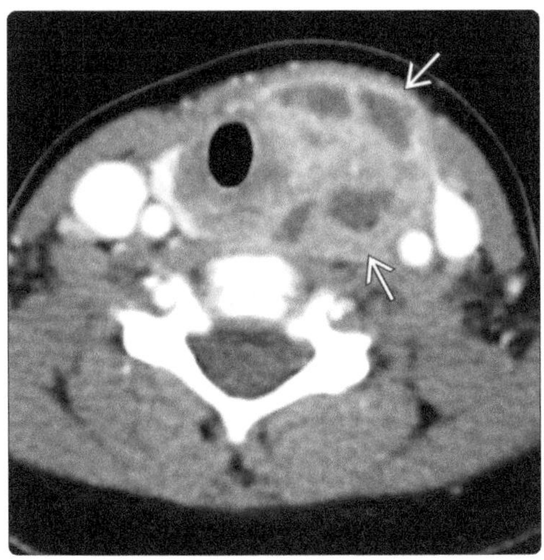

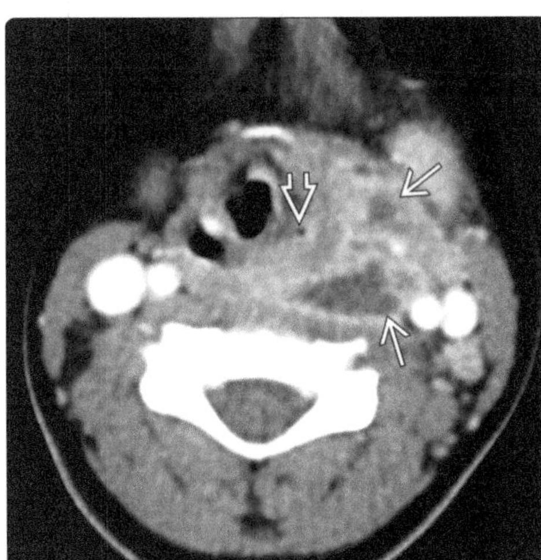

(Left) *Axial CECT in a 6-year-old child shows a multiloculated abscess in the left lower neck ➡, causing significant rightward deviation of the trachea.* **(Right)** *Axial CECT in the same patient at the level of the pyriform sinus demonstrates the uppermost aspect of the abscess ➡, posterior to the nearly effaced and anteriorly deviated pyriform sinus apex ➡. This appearance should alert the clinician to search for the opening of the sinus tract in the pyriform sinus, which, unless obliterated, may cause recurrent abscess.*

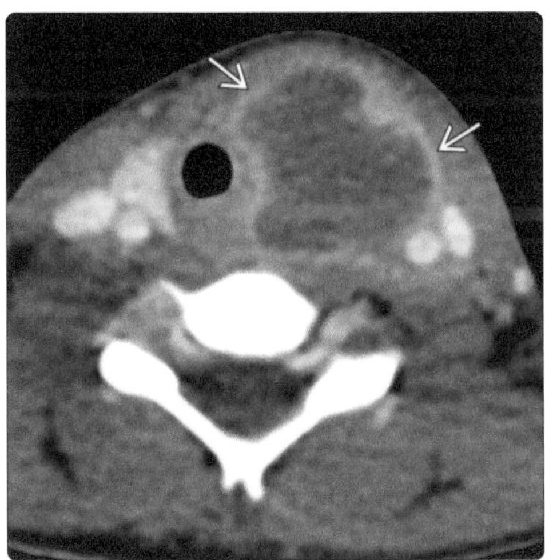

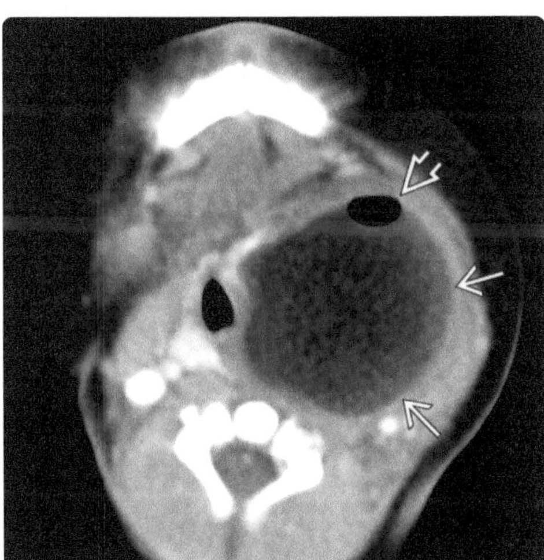

(Left) *Axial CECT in a 7-year-old child shows a well-defined, rim-enhancing collection in the left lower neck ➡ with associated myositis and cellulitis. On more inferior images, this involved the left lobe of thyroid and extended superiorly to the level of the pyriform sinus; alerting the clinician to search for the sinus tract is imperative.* **(Right)** *Axial CECT shows a large, left-sided cystic mass ➡ at the level of the left thyroid lobe with a small focus of intralesional air ➡, which should suggest connection to the aerodigestive tract.*

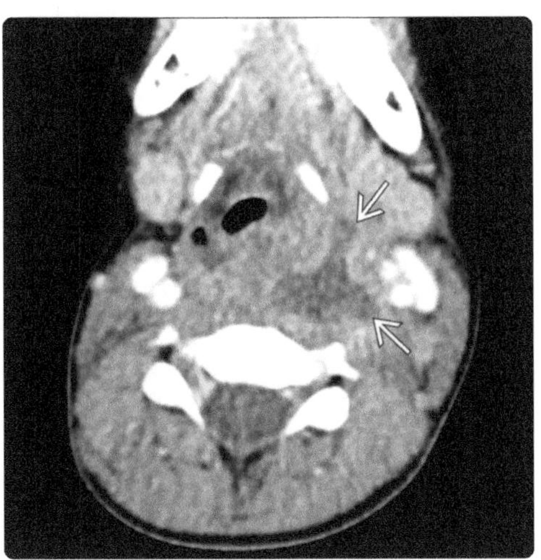

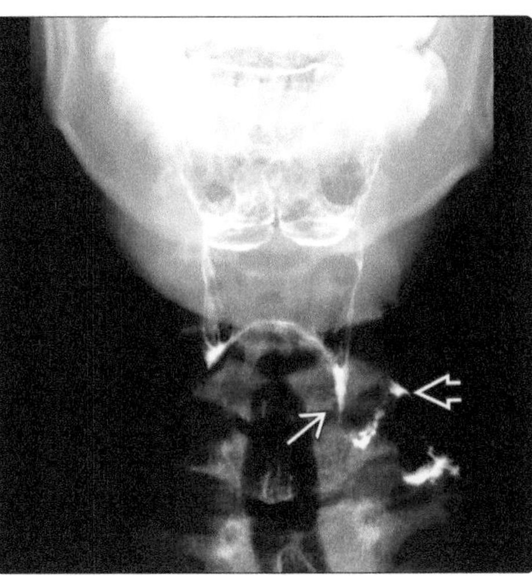

(Left) *Axial CECT in a child with fever and a left neck mass shows an irregular-shaped, heterogeneously enhancing abscess ➡ resulting in effacement of the left pyriform sinus and rightward deviation of the airway, the extent of which should raise the question of sinus tract from the pyriform sinus as a cause of the abscess.* **(Right)** *AP radiograph in a patient with a perithyroidal abscess confirms a sinus tract ➡ with barium extending from the apex of the left pyriform sinus ➡ to the soft tissues of the lower left neck.*

Thyroglossal Duct Cyst

KEY FACTS

TERMINOLOGY

- Thyroglossal duct cyst (TGDC): Cystic remnant of embryologic thyroglossal duct (TGD)

IMAGING

- Best diagnostic clue: Round or ovoid midline suprahyoid or midline/paramidline infrahyoid cystic neck mass
- Suprahyoid neck: ~ 20-25%, typically midline
- At hyoid bone: ~ 50%
- Infrahyoid neck: ~ 25%, midline or paramidline
  - Embedded in strap muscles: Claw sign
- ± wall enhancement, soft tissue stranding if infected

TOP DIFFERENTIAL DIAGNOSES

- Dermoid or epidermoid
- Lingual thyroid
- Lymphatic malformation
- 4th branchial apparatus anomaly
- Cervical thymic cyst

PATHOLOGY

- Failure of involution of TGD + persistent secretion of epithelial cells lining duct → TGDC
- Lies anywhere along TGD route of thyroid anlage descent from foramen cecum at tongue base to thyroid bed in infrahyoid neck

CLINICAL ISSUES

- Most common congenital neck lesion
- Treatment: Sistrunk procedure (excision of cyst, tract, & midline hyoid bone) → ↓ recurrences

DIAGNOSTIC CHECKLIST

- Relationship to hyoid bone important to note: Suprahyoid, hyoid, or infrahyoid in location
- Nodularity or Ca^{++} can suggest associated thyroid carcinoma
- Confirm normal thyroid by US prior to TGDC or lingual thyroid resection

(Left) *Sagittal oblique graphic shows the potential sites of a thyroglossal duct cyst (TGDC) from the foramen cecum ➡ to the thyroid bed ➡. Note the close relationship of the midportion of the hyoid bone ➡ to this pathway. A cyst can occur anywhere along this tract.* **(Right)** *Transverse US of the anterior left neck in a teenager shows a well-defined, hypoechoic left paramidline, infrahyoid TGDC ➡. The presence of internal low level echoes is not uncommon, and usually not associated with hemorrhage or infection.*

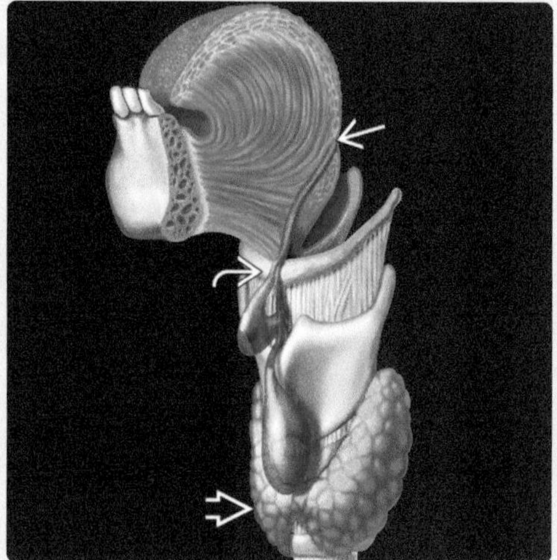

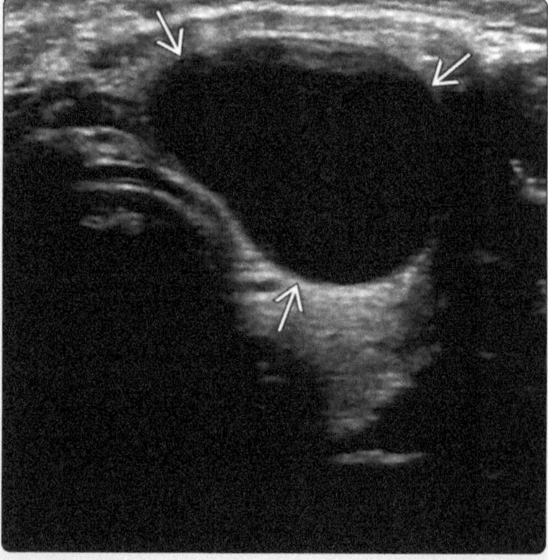

(Left) *Sagittal CECT in a child with a sore throat & difficulty swallowing shows a lobulated, rim-enhancing, fluid-attenuation mass ➡ in the midline sublingual space with a small, posterior extension at the tongue base ➡. Histologically, this proved to be an inflamed TGDC.* **(Right)** *Sagittal T2 MR incidentally shows a well-defined, hyperintense TGDC ➡ in the midline base of the tongue (at the level of the foramen cecum) in a patient imaged after posterior fossa decompression ➡ for treatment of Chiari 1.*

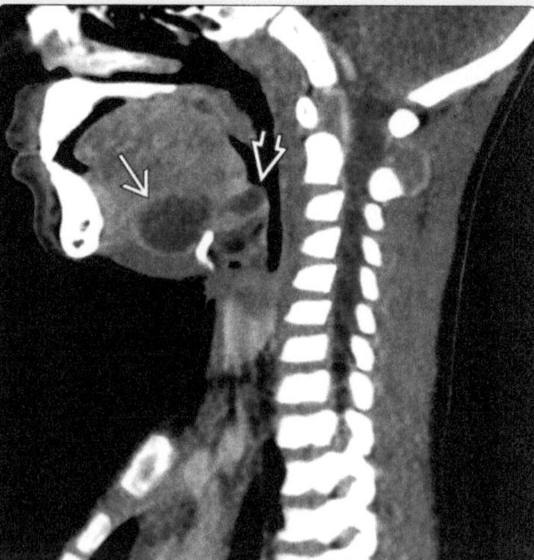

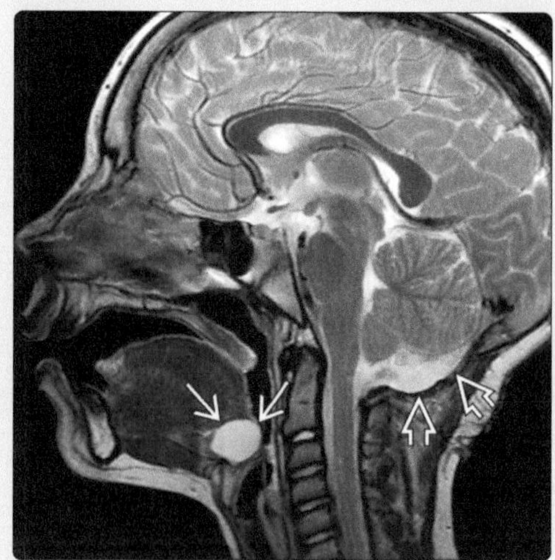

TERMINOLOGY

Abbreviations

- Thyroglossal duct cyst (TGDC)

Synonyms

- Thyroglossal duct (TGD) remnant

Definitions

- Remnant of embryologic TGD between foramen cecum at midline tongue base & thyroid bed in infrahyoid neck

IMAGING

General Features

- Best diagnostic clue
  - Anterior midline suprahyoid or midline/paramidline infrahyoid cystic neck mass
- Location
  - Suprahyoid neck: ~ 20-25%, typically midline
    - Base of tongue or within posterior floor of mouth
  - At hyoid bone: ~ 50%
    - Usually abutting anterior hyoid bone
    - May project into preepiglottic space
  - Infrahyoid neck: ~ 25%, midline or paramidline, embedded in strap muscles
    - Further inferior TGDC is more likely to be off-midline
- Size
  - Variable, usually 2-4 cm
- Morphology
  - Round or ovoid cyst
  - More likely to be irregular in shape, elongated toward tongue base, & have ill-defined margins vs. dermoid

Ultrasonographic Findings

- Anechoic or hypoechoic midline neck mass
- Internal heterogeneity, septations, & solid components are more likely in TGDC than dermoid
  - SIST score (favors TGDC over dermoid): Septations + irregular walls + solid components = TGDC
- Synchronous movement with hyoid bone
- Elongation toward tongue base
- Must image lower neck to prove presence of normal-appearing bilobed thyroid

CT Findings

- CECT
  - Low-attenuation, cystic midline neck mass with thin rim of peripheral enhancement
    - ± wall enhancement, soft tissue stranding if infected
    - Occasional septations
  - Paramidline infrahyoid TGDC embedded in strap muscles may show claw sign
  - < 1% contain associated thyroid carcinoma (usually papillary carcinoma)
    - Solid eccentric mass, often with Ca^{++}, within cyst
    - May only be microscopic & not identifiable prospectively with imaging
    - Majority occur in adults but may occur in teenagers
      - Youngest reported: 10 years old

MR Findings

- T1WI
  - Usually hypointense; hyperintense if proteinaceous fluid
- T2WI
  - Hyperintense, often homogeneous
- DWI
  - Mean ADC values of ~ 2.2×10^{-3} mm^2/s
- T1WI C+
  - Nonenhancing cyst; rim enhancement if infected

Imaging Recommendations

- US can suggest TGDC vs. other lesions & confirm normal thyroid
- Nuclear scintigraphy is helpful if ectopic thyroid is suspected

DIFFERENTIAL DIAGNOSIS

Dermoid or Epidermoid

- Dermoid: Fat, fluid, or mixed
  - ADC ~ 1.54×10^{-3} mm^2/s
- Epidermoid: Fluid
- More likely to be in subcutaneous fat
- Floor of mouth & suprasternal notch are classic locations

Lingual Thyroid

- Most common location of ectopic thyroid
- In 75% of patients, lingual thyroid is only functioning thyroid tissue
- May expand rapidly during puberty
- Solid, round, hyperattenuating mass in base of tongue on NECT; avid enhancement on CECT
- Variable T1 & T2 signal, variable enhancement on MR

Lymphatic Malformation

- Classic appearance: Multilocular & transspatial
- Microcystic or macrocystic
- Fluid-fluid levels are common secondary to hemorrhage
- Thin rim & septal enhancement unless infected, microcystic, or part of combined venolymphatic malformation

4th Branchial Apparatus Anomaly

- May present with recurrent thyroiditis
- Majority are sinus tracts from apex of left pyriform sinus to lower neck → abscess in or adjacent to left thyroid lobe
- 4th (or 3rd) pharyngeal pouch remnant

Cervical Thymic Cyst

- Congenital cyst, anywhere along thymopharyngeal duct from pyriform sinus to anterior mediastinum
  - May be bilobed with waist at thoracic inlet
- Left > right
- Close association with carotid sheath
  - May splay carotid artery & jugular vein, particularly near skull base
- May be combined solid thymic tissue & cyst

Mixed Laryngocele

- Off-midline, fluid- or air- & fluid-containing mass
- Traces back to laryngeal origin
- Not embedded within strap muscles

Delphian Chain Necrotic Node

- Can be difficult to differentiate from infected TGDC
  - Rare in children

PATHOLOGY

General Features

- Genetics
  - Thyroid developmental anomalies often occur in same family
- Associated abnormalities
  - Thyroid agenesis, ectopia, or pyramidal lobe
  - Occasionally associated with carcinoma
    - Most common: Papillary carcinoma within TGDC
- Embryology/anatomy
  - TGD originates near foramen cecum at posterior 3rd of tongue
  - Thyroid anlage arises at base of tongue → descends around or through hyoid bone → descends along strap muscles → final position in thyroid bed, anterior to thyroid cartilage or cricoid cartilage
  - At 5- to 6-gestational weeks, TGD usually involutes
    - Foramen cecum & pyramidal thyroid lobe may be left as normal remnants
  - Failure of TGD involution with persistent secretory activity of epithelial cells lining duct → TGDC
  - TGDC or ectopic thyroid tissue may occur anywhere along TGD

Gross Pathologic & Surgical Features

- Smooth, benign-appearing cyst with tract to hyoid bone ± foramen cecum

Microscopic Features

- Cyst is lined by respiratory or squamous epithelium
- Small deposits of thyroid tissue with colloid are commonly associated
- ± thyroid carcinoma (papillary carcinoma is most common)

CLINICAL ISSUES

Presentation

- Most common signs/symptoms
  - Midline or paramidline doughy, compressible, painless neck mass in child or young adult
  - Cyst elevates when tongue protrudes if TGDC is located around hyoid bone
- Other signs/symptoms
  - Recurrent midline neck mass with upper respiratory tract infections or trauma
  - ± multiple prior incision & drainage procedures for neck abscess
  - Rarely, lingual TGDC may lead to airway obstruction in infants
  - Small lesion may be recognized as incidental finding on brain MR: Majority at base of tongue

Demographics

- Age
  - < 10 years at presentation (up to 90%)
- Epidemiology
  - Most common congenital neck lesion
    - Up to 90% of nonodontogenic congenital cysts
  - At autopsy > 7% of population will have TGD remnant somewhere along course of tract

Natural History & Prognosis

- Recurrent, intermittent swelling of mass, usually following minor upper respiratory infection
- Rapidly enlarging mass suggests either infection or differentiated thyroid carcinoma (< 1%)
  - 85% papillary carcinoma

Treatment

- Complete surgical resection: Sistrunk procedure ↓ recurrence rate from 50% to < 4%
  - Tract to foramen cecum is dissected free
  - Entire cyst & midline portion of hyoid bone are resected
    - Even if imaging shows no obvious connection to hyoid bone
    - Exception: Low infrahyoid neck TGDC
  - Prognosis is excellent with complete surgical resection
- Isolated lingual TGDC may be treated endoscopically
- Recurrences (from incomplete resection) are often complicated & lateral; ↑ risk of recurrence in patients with postoperative infection
- Some reports of successful sclerotherapy in adults

DIAGNOSTIC CHECKLIST

Consider

- Relationship to hyoid bone is important to note
  - Suprahyoid, hyoid, or infrahyoid in location
- Nodularity or Ca^{++} can suggest associated thyroid carcinoma
- Image thyroid bed with US to confirm presence of normal thyroid gland prior to TGDC or lingual thyroid excision

SELECTED REFERENCES

1. Bertoni DG et al: Diagnosing midline neck masses: comparing clinical exam, the SIST score, and the 4S algorithm. Otolaryngol Head Neck Surg. 169(3):496-503, 2023
2. Booth TN: Congenital cystic neck masses. Neuroimaging Clin N Am. 33(4):591-605, 2023
3. Lee E et al: Efficacy of ethanol ablation as a treatment of benign head and neck cystic lesions. Am J Otolaryngol. 42(6):103082, 2021
4. Tokarz E et al: Proposed ultrasound algorithm to differentiate thyroglossal duct and dermoid cysts. Int J Pediatr Otorhinolaryngol. 142:110624, 2021
5. Abdel Razek AAK et al: Differentiation of sublingual thyroglossal duct cyst from midline dermoid cyst with diffusion weighted imaging. Int J Pediatr Otorhinolaryngol. 126:109623, 2019
6. Chang KV et al: Thyroglossal duct cyst: dynamic ultrasound evaluation and sonoanatomy revisited. Med Ultrason. 21(1):99-100, 2019
7. Devine CM et al: Preoperative ultrasound for the diagnosis of thyroglossal duct cysts: a validation study. Int J Pediatr Otorhinolaryngol. 122:89-92, 2019
8. Lekkerkerker I et al: Pediatric thyroglossal duct cysts: post-operative complications. Int J Pediatr Otorhinolaryngol. 124:14-17, 2019
9. Liaw J et al: Primary papillary thyroid cancer of a thyroglossal duct cyst. Ear Nose Throat J. 98(3):136-8, 2019
10. Patel S et al: Thyroglossal duct pathology and mimics. Insights Imaging. 10(1):12, 2019
11. Pitner H et al: Diagnostic accuracy of midline pediatric neck masses. Otolaryngol Head Neck Surg. 160(6):1111-7, 2019
12. Bansal AG et al: US of pediatric superficial masses of the head and neck. Radiographics. 38(4):1239-63, 2018
13. Choi HI et al: Ultrasonographic features differentiating thyroglossal duct cysts from dermoid cysts. Ultrasonography. 37(1):71-7, 2018
14. Oyewumi M et al: Ultrasound to differentiate thyroglossal duct cysts and dermoid cysts in children. Laryngoscope. 125(4):998-1003, 2015
15. Koch BL: Cystic malformations of the neck in children. Pediatr Radiol. 35(5):463-77, 2005

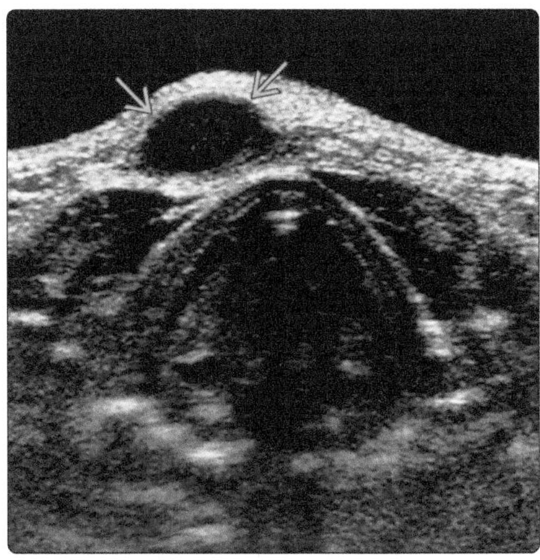

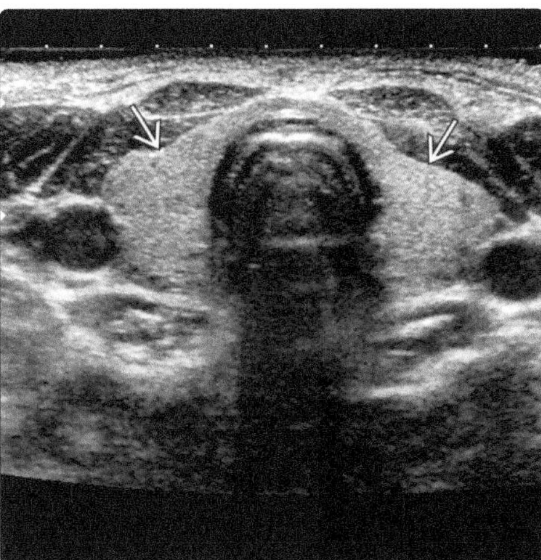

(Left) *Transverse US of the anterior neck shows a well-defined, subcutaneous, right paramidline hypoechoic mass ➙ ventral to the strap muscles. This lesion was surgically removed & confirmed to be a TGDC.* **(Right)** *Transverse US in a child with a suspected TGDC (not shown) demonstrates a normal-appearing bilobed thyroid ➙ at the expected location in the lower anterior midline neck. It is important to document the presence of normal thyroid tissue in all patients imaged for the work-up of a TGDC.*

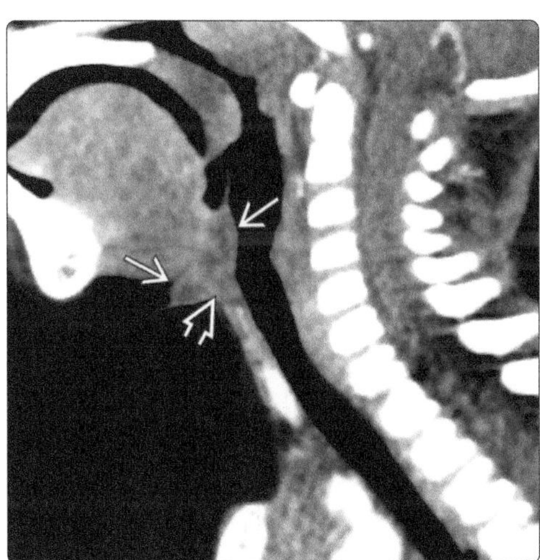

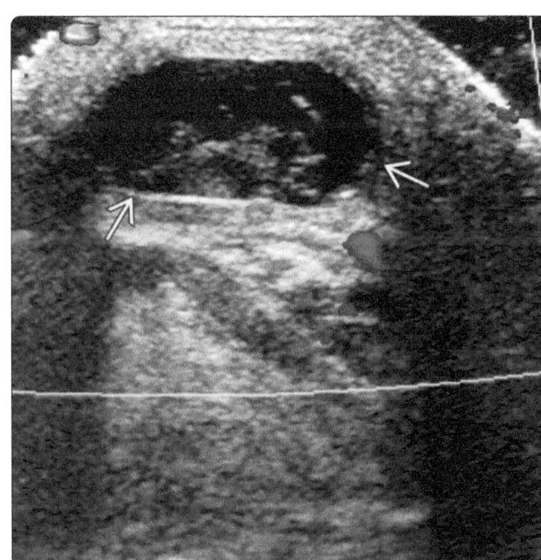

(Left) *Sagittal CECT in a child with proven recurrence of a TGDC demonstrates a lobulated, heterogeneous mass ➙ in the midline suprahyoid neck. By imaging, this is indistinguishable from a postsurgical collection. Note the absence of a midline hyoid bone ➙, consistent with a prior Sistrunk procedure.* **(Right)** *Transverse color Doppler US in a child with a new paramidline anterior left neck mass shows a hypoechoic, avascular lesion ➙ with internal echoes. Histologically, lesion proved to be uncomplicated TGDC.*

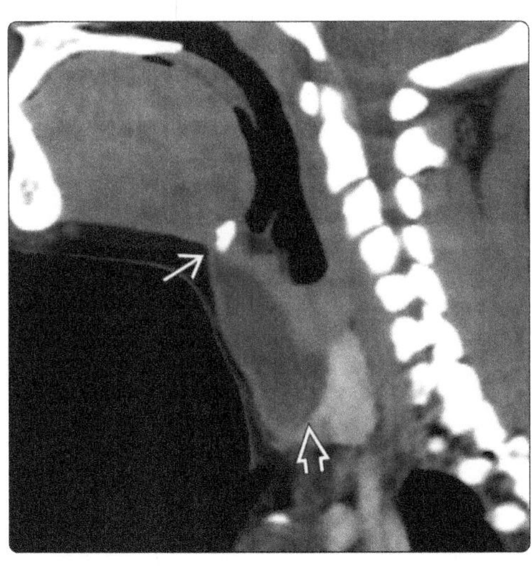

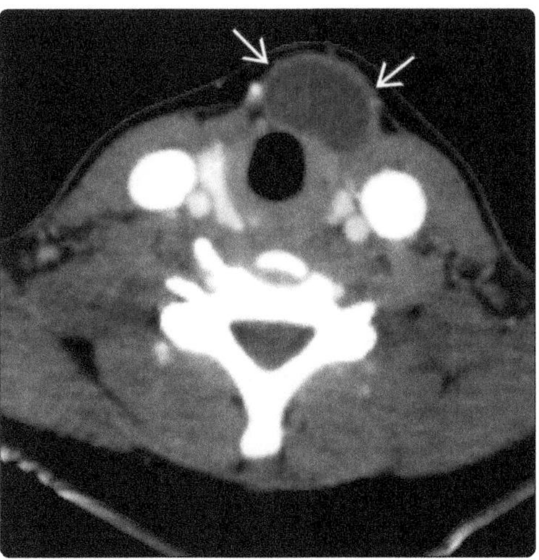

(Left) *Sagittal CECT of the neck in a teenager with the new onset of a neck mass demonstrates a low-attenuation mass extending from the undersurface of the hyoid bone ➙ to the level of the upper thyroid lobe ➙, where it causes mild mass effect on the gland.* **(Right)** *Axial CECT in the same patient demonstrates the low-attenuation, paramidline, infrahyoid anterior neck mass ➙ that is embedded within the left strap muscle, the typical location of an infrahyoid TGDC.*

KEY FACTS

TERMINOLOGY

- Cervical thymic cyst
- Cystic remnant of thymopharyngeal duct
  - Derivative of 3rd pharyngeal pouch

IMAGING

- Cystic mass closely associated with carotid sheath
- Anywhere along thymopharyngeal duct from pyriform sinus to anterior mediastinum
- Usually lateral infrahyoid neck
- Left > right side of neck
- May splay carotid artery and jugular vein
- Cyst wall may mildly enhance; solid thymic remnants may enhance similar to intrathoracic thymus

TOP DIFFERENTIAL DIAGNOSES

- 2nd branchial cleft cyst; most common: Lateral to carotid sheath, anteromedial to sternocleidomastoid muscle, posterior to submandibular gland
- 4th branchial anomaly
  - Cyst or abscess anterior to left thyroid lobe
- Lymphatic malformation
  - Unilocular or multilocular, focal or infiltrative
  - Fluid-fluid levels common
- Abscess
  - Irregular, enhancing wall with low-attenuation center
  - If associated with thyroid gland, think 4th branchial pouch anomaly

PATHOLOGY

- Hassall corpuscles in cyst wall confirm diagnosis

CLINICAL ISSUES

- Most present between 2-15 years of age
- Only 33% present after 1st decade

DIAGNOSTIC CHECKLIST

- Dumbbell-shaped cervicothoracic cystic mass highly suggestive of thymic cyst (vs. lymphatic malformation)

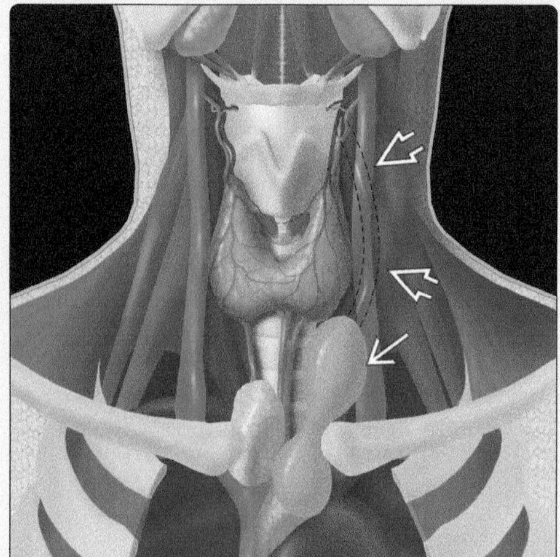

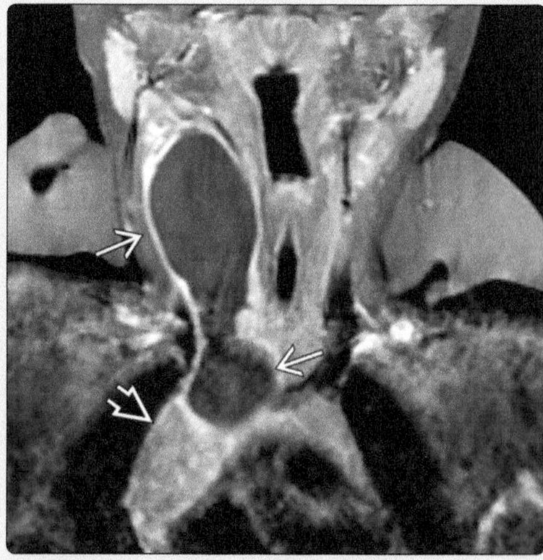

(Left) *Coronal graphic shows a typical bilobed cervical thymic cyst ➡ extending from the anterior mediastinum into the lower neck along the course of the thymopharyngeal duct ➡. Notice the close association with the carotid space.* **(Right)** *Coronal T1 C+ FS MR in a 16-month-old child shows a cystic-appearing right neck mass ➡ causing mild airway compression. The cyst extends to the otherwise normal-appearing thymus ➡. Mild, diffuse wall enhancement is consistent with chronic inflammation, identified histologically.*

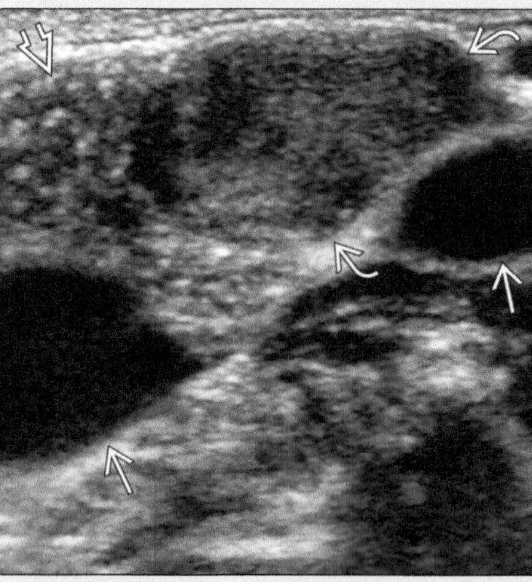

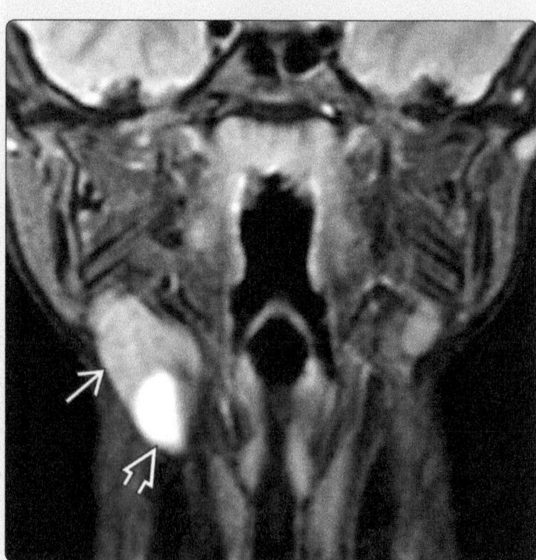

(Left) *Transverse ultrasound in a 7-year-old child demonstrates a mixed cystic and solid right thymic remnant splaying the carotid sheath vessels ➡. The lateral component demonstrates echogenicity typical of thymus ➡, and the medial component is cystic with mobile intraluminal echoes ➡ on real-time imaging.* **(Right)** *Coronal T2 MR in the same patient shows a mixed solid ➡ and cystic ➡ thymic remnant, the solid portion of which was isointense to intrathoracic thymus on all sequences.*

TERMINOLOGY

Abbreviations

- Cervical thymic cyst (CTC)

Synonyms

- Thymopharyngeal duct cyst, congenital thymic cyst

Definitions

- Cystic remnant of thymopharyngeal duct
  - Derivative of 3rd pharyngeal pouch
- Hassall corpuscles in cyst wall confirm diagnosis

IMAGING

General Features

- Best diagnostic clue
  - Cystic mass in left > right lateral infrahyoid neck, in lateral visceral space, or adjacent to carotid space
    - Closely associated with carotid sheath
      - In lower neck: Medial to carotid sheath, posterior to thyroid
      - In upper neck or extending from upper neck to mediastinum: Splay carotid artery and jugular vein
- Location
  - Anywhere along thymopharyngeal duct
    - From pyriform sinus to anterior mediastinum
  - Most common site: Lateral infrahyoid neck, at level of thyroid gland
    - Left > right
  - May parallel sternocleidomastoid muscle (SCM), close to carotid sheath
  - Cervical neck component ± extension to mediastinum
- Size
  - Variable, from several cm to very long, along course of thymopharyngeal duct
- Morphology
  - Usually large, dominant cyst
  - May be multiloculated
  - May splay carotid artery and jugular vein, especially in upper neck
  - Larger CTC may present as dumbbell-shaped cervicothoracic mass, projecting from lower lateral cervical neck into superior mediastinum

CT Findings

- CECT
  - Nonenhancing, low-attenuation, lateral neck cyst
    - Close association with carotid sheath common
    - Solid components rare = aberrant thymic tissue, lymphoid aggregates, or parathyroid tissue
    - May be connected to mediastinal thymus directly or by fibrous cord

MR Findings

- T1WI
  - Homogeneous, hypointense cyst most common
  - May be iso- to hyperintense if filled with blood products, proteinaceous fluid, or cholesterol
  - Thin wall
  - Solid nodules usually isointense to muscle and intrathoracic thymus
- T2WI
  - Homogeneously hyperintense fluid contents
- T1WI C+
  - Cystic component nonenhancing
  - Cyst wall or solid nodules may enhance
    - Solid thymic remnants enhance similar to intrathoracic thymus
  - If infected, cyst wall may be thickened and enhancing; surrounding soft tissue may be inflamed

Ultrasonographic Findings

- Thin-walled anechoic or hypoechoic lateral neck mass
- Rarely has solid nodules in wall

Imaging Recommendations

- Best imaging tool
  - CECT or MR preferable to ultrasound to demonstrate total extent of cyst
  - Ultrasound helpful if solid component has typical thymus echotexture
- Protocol advice
  - **Include upper mediastinum** to demonstrate mediastinal extension

DIFFERENTIAL DIAGNOSIS

2nd Branchial Cleft Cyst

- Most common branchial apparatus cyst
- Most common location
  - Posterolateral to submandibular gland, lateral to carotid space, anterior (or anteromedial) to SCM
- When infrahyoid, anterior to carotid space
- May mimic CTC when found in lower neck
- Rarely protrudes between internal carotid artery and external carotid artery

4th Branchial Anomaly

- Primary location: Sinus tract remnant of 4th (or 3rd) pharyngeal pouch
  - Sinus tract extends from pyriform sinus apex to anterior lower neck → left anterior neck abscess
- Often presents with suppurative thyroiditis
- Inflammation frequently extends to surround apex of pyriform sinus

Lymphatic Malformation

- May affect any space in head and neck
- When in posterior cervical space, abuts carotid space posteriorly
- Unilocular or multilocular
- Focal or infiltrative and transspatial
- Fluid-fluid levels common, secondary to intralesional hemorrhage

Abscess

- Presents with signs and symptoms of infection
- Irregular, thick, enhancing wall with low-attenuation center
- If associated with thyroid gland, think 4th branchial pouch anomaly

Colloid Cyst, Thyroid

- Primary location: Intrathyroidal, left or right
- Thin wall with smooth margins

- May be large &/or hemorrhagic colloid cyst
- Usually more medial than CTC

PATHOLOGY

General Features

- Etiology
  - Remnants of thymopharyngeal duct → CTC
  - Ectopic thymus may also occur along thymopharyngeal duct
- Embryology
  - Failure of obliteration of thymopharyngeal duct, remnant of 3rd pharyngeal pouch
  - Thymopharyngeal duct arises from pyriform sinus, descends into mediastinum
  - Persistent sequestered remnants may occur from mandible to thoracic inlet
  - Thymus and parathyroid glands arise from 3rd and 4th pharyngeal pouches, respectively
  - Embryologic migration follows caudal course along thymopharyngeal duct during 1st trimester
- No malignant association

Gross Pathologic & Surgical Features

- Smooth, thin-walled cervical cyst, often with caudal fibrous strand extending to mediastinal thymus
- Filled with brownish fluid
- Cyst wall may be nodular
- Associated with lymphoid tissue or parathyroid or thymic remnants
- Rarely may extend through thyrohyoid membrane into pyriform sinus

Microscopic Features

- Hassall corpuscles in cyst wall confirm diagnosis
  - May not always be identifiable if prior hemorrhage or infection
- Cyst wall may contain
  - Lymphoid tissue
  - Parathyroid tissue
  - Thyroid or thymic tissue
  - Cholesterol crystals and granulomas, probably from prior hemorrhage

CLINICAL ISSUES

Presentation

- Most common signs/symptoms
  - Often asymptomatic
  - Gradually enlarging, soft, compressible mid- to lower cervical neck mass
  - When large, may cause dysphagia, respiratory distress, or vocal cord paralysis
- Other presentations
  - Large, infantile, cervicothoracic thymic cyst may present with respiratory compromise
  - Rarely may be associated with disordered calcium metabolism if parathyroid component is functioning

Demographics

- Age
  - Most present between 2-15 years
  - Only 33% present after 1st decade
  - Rare reports of primary presentation in adulthood
- Sex
  - Slightly more common in male patients
- Epidemiology
  - Rare compared with other congenital neck masses
  - Left > right side of neck

Natural History & Prognosis

- Excellent prognosis if completely resected
- Recurrence common if incompletely resected

Treatment

- Complete surgical resection
- Large cervicothoracic thymic cyst may require head and neck and thoracic surgery

DIAGNOSTIC CHECKLIST

Consider

- If cystic mass is intimately associated with anterior carotid sheath, think CTC
- If cystic mass extends from anterior neck to upper mediastinum, think CTC

Image Interpretation Pearls

- Dumbbell-shaped cervicothoracic cystic mass highly suggestive of thymic cyst (vs. lymphatic malformation)
- Unilocular ovoid lesion with discrete margins; may be thymic cyst or unilocular lymphatic malformation

SELECTED REFERENCES

1. Chang A et al: Diagnosis and management of ectopic cervical thymus in children: systematic review of the literature. J Pediatr Surg. 56(11):2062-8, 2021
2. Buch K et al: MR imaging evaluation of pediatric neck masses:: review and update. Magn Reson Imaging Clin N Am. 27(2):173-99, 2019
3. Mehmi N et al: Importance and impact of appropriate radiology in the management of branchial cleft anomalies. Indian J Otolaryngol Head Neck Surg. 71(Suppl 1):953-9, 2019
4. Prosser JD et al: Branchial cleft anomalies and thymic cysts. Otolaryngol Clin North Am. 48(1):1-14, 2015
5. Goff CJ et al: Current management of congenital branchial cleft cysts, sinuses, and fistulae. Curr Opin Otolaryngol Head Neck Surg. 20(6):533-9, 2012
6. Thomas B et al: Revisiting imaging features and the embryologic basis of third and fourth branchial anomalies. AJNR Am J Neuroradiol. 31(4):755-60, 2010
7. Sturm-O'Brien AK et al: Cervical thymic anomalies--the Texas Children's Hospital experience. Laryngoscope. 119(10):1988-93, 2009
8. Statham MM et al: Cervical thymic remnants in children. Int J Pediatr Otorhinolaryngol. 72(12):1807-13, 2008
9. Mehrzad H et al: A combined third and fourth branchial arch anomaly: clinical and embryological implications. Eur Arch Otorhinolaryngol. 264(8):913-6, 2007
10. Koch BL: Cystic malformations of the neck in children. Pediatr Radiol. 35(5):463-77, 2005
11. Pereira KD et al: Management of anomalies of the third and fourth branchial pouches. Int J Pediatr Otorhinolaryngol. 68(1):43-50, 2004
12. Liberman M et al: Ten years of experience with third and fourth branchial remnants. J Pediatr Surg. 37(5):685-90, 2002
13. Ozturk H et al: Multilocular cervical thymic cyst: an unusual neck mass in children. Int J Pediatr Otorhinolaryngol. 61(3): 249-52, 2001
14. Koeller KK et al: Congenital cystic masses of the neck: radiologic-pathologic correlation. Radiographics. 19(1): 121-46; quiz 152-3, 1999
15. Benson MT et al: Congenital anomalies of the branchial apparatus: embryology and pathologic anatomy. Radiographics. 12(5):943-60, 1992

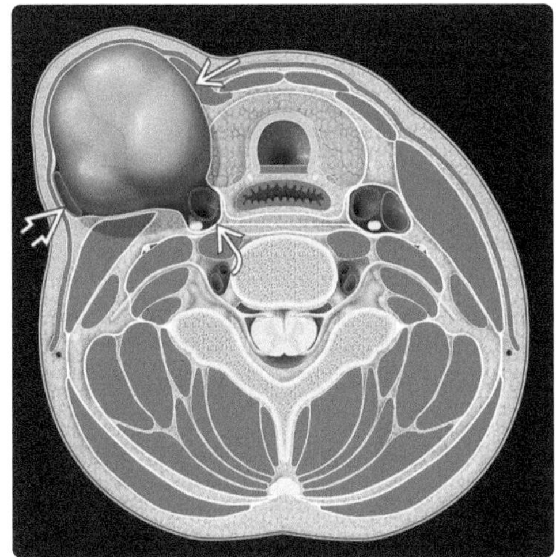

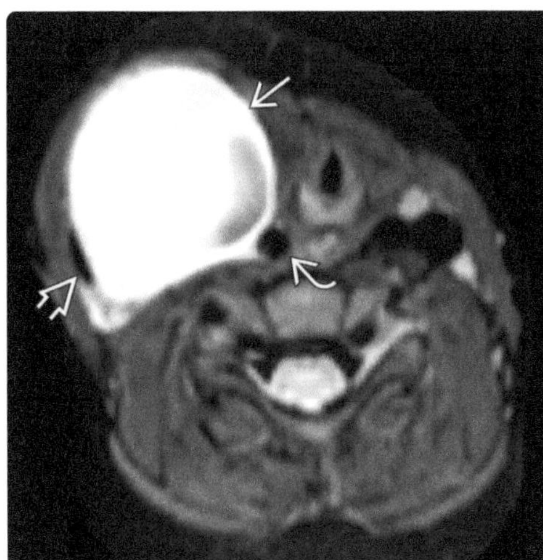

(Left) *Axial graphic of the neck depicts a large right neck cystic mass, representing a cervical thymic cyst. Note that the cyst splays the right jugular vein and carotid artery, an appearance typical of thymic cysts.* **(Right)** *Axial FSE-IR MR of the neck demonstrates hyperintense signal within a right neck cystic mass that characteristically splays the right jugular vein and carotid artery.*

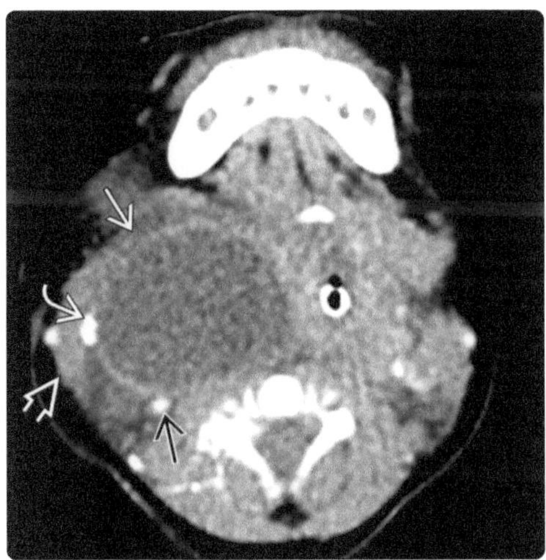

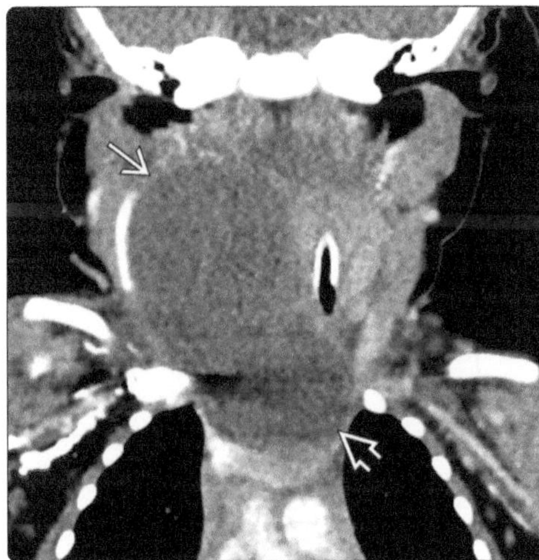

(Left) *Axial CECT in a 4-month-old infant shows a thin-walled cyst deep to the right sternocleidomastoid muscle that splays the jugular vein and carotid artery and causes significant mass effect on the airway.* **(Right)** *Coronal CECT in the same patient shows the typical bilobed appearance of a thymic cyst with a cervical component and extension of the cyst to the mediastinal.*

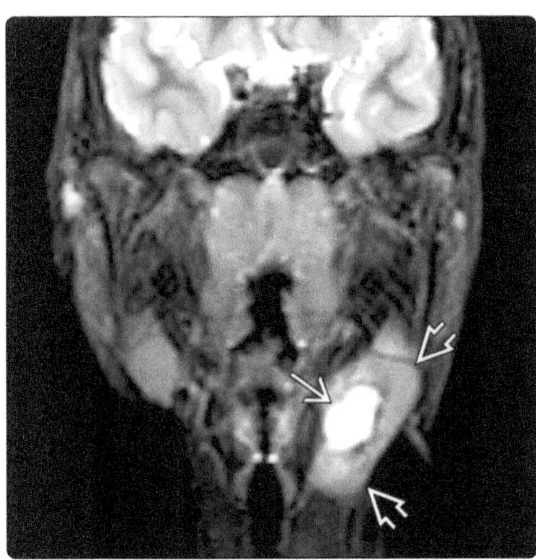

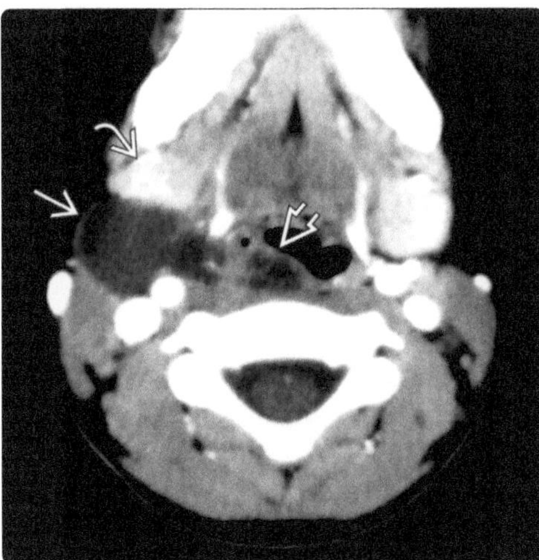

(Left) *Coronal T2 MR shows a rare association of both cystic and solid remnants of the thymus in the left neck.* **(Right)** *Axial CECT shows a rare appearance of a thymic cyst extending into the retropharyngeal space. Notice the majority of the cyst is located in the right neck posterior submandibular space, displacing the submandibular gland anteriorly.*

KEY FACTS

TERMINOLOGY

- Venous malformation (VM)

IMAGING

- Use MR & US when possible
- General imaging findings
  - Lobulated soft tissue "mass" with phleboliths
  - Solitary or multiple
  - May be circumscribed or transspatial, infiltrating adjacent soft tissue compartments
  - ± combined lymphatic malformation (LM), i.e., mixed venolymphatic malformation (VLM)
- CT findings
  - Rounded calcifications (phleboliths)
  - Osseous remodeling in adjacent bone
  - Fat hypertrophy in adjacent soft tissues
- Enhancement features
  - Variable enhancement pattern reflects sluggish vascular flow to & through lesion
  - Patchy & delayed or homogeneous & intense

TOP DIFFERENTIAL DIAGNOSES

- LM
- Infantile hemangioma
- Arteriovenous malformation
- Neurofibroma
- Dermoid & epidermoid
- Soft tissue sarcoma

PATHOLOGY

- Congenital slow- or low-flow vascular malformation
- 70% of patients with periorbital LM or VLM have intracranial vascular & parenchymal anomalies

CLINICAL ISSUES

- Presents as spongy H&N mass that grows proportionately with patient
  - May enlarge suddenly due to hemorrhage, thrombosis, or hormonal changes

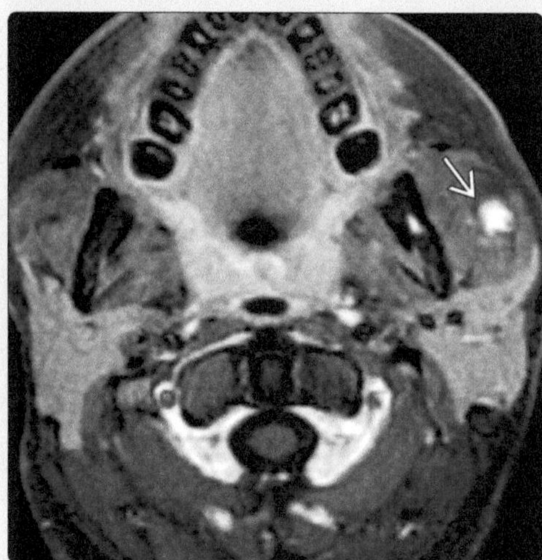

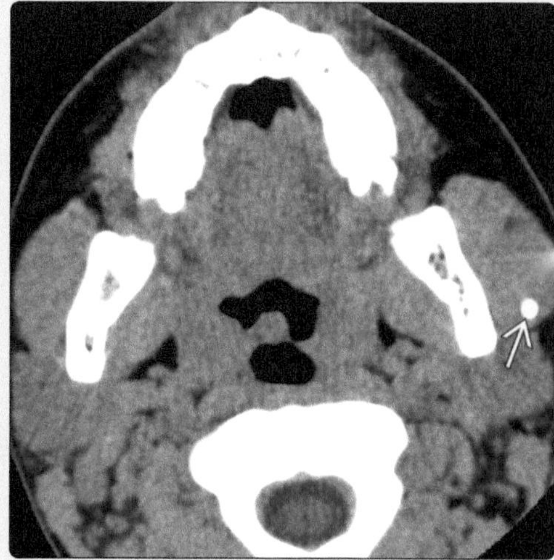

(Left) *Axial T1 C+ FS MR in a 14-year-old boy demonstrates a small focal area of enhancement ➡ in an otherwise nonspecific lesion within the left masseter muscle within the masticator space.* **(Right)** *Axial NECT in the same patient shows an ill-defined, intramuscular mass with a small phlebolith ➡ representing a calcified intraluminal thrombus, characteristic of a venous malformation (VM). This case seems to be isolated VM without mixed lymphatic malformation.*

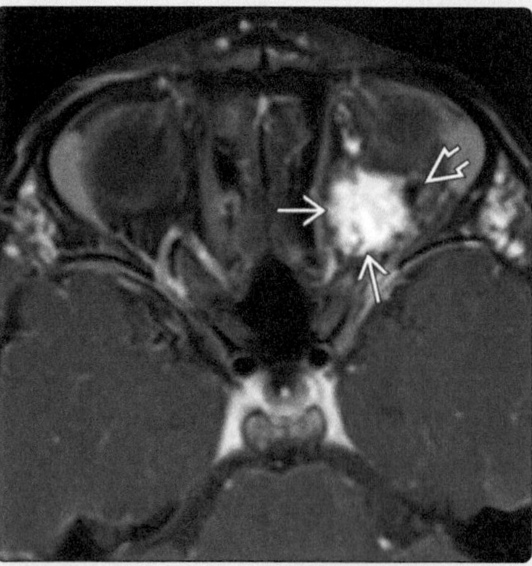

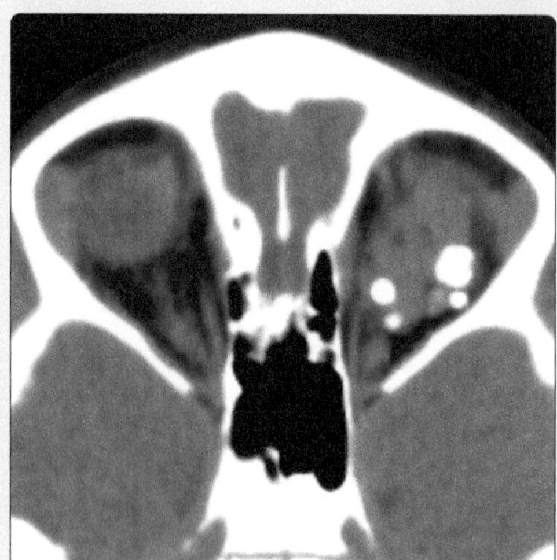

(Left) *Axial T1 C+ FS MR in a 5-year-old with proptosis shows an enhancing mass with irregular margins in the left intraconal space ➡. There is a small focus of hypointense signal in the anterolateral aspect of the mass ➡ and a few other punctate foci of nonenhancing hypointense signal that may represent a phleboliths.* **(Right)** *Axial NECT in the same child demonstrates multiple well-defined calcifications within the intraconal space of the left orbit, characteristic of phleboliths in venous vascular malformations.*

TERMINOLOGY

Abbreviations

- Venous malformation (VM) (preferred term)

Synonyms

- Cavernous malformation, cavernous hemangioma (both terms to be avoided)

Definitions

- VM: Subtype of congenital slow- or low-flow vascular malformation due to error in vein formation; not neoplastic
- Venolymphatic malformation (VLM) combined lesion with venous & lymphatic components

IMAGING

General Features

- Best diagnostic clue
  - Cluster of slow-flow serpiginous vessels + phleboliths
- Location
  - Most commonly subcutaneous &/or intramuscular
  - Focal, multifocal, or diffuse
  - H&N (40%), extremities (40%), trunk (20%)
  - May be in any space(s) in H&N
- Morphology
  - Multilobulated, solitary, or multiple
  - Well circumscribed or transspatial (multiple contiguous spaces), confluent & infiltrative
  - ± combined lymphatic malformation (LM), i.e., mixed VLM
  - ± discrete serpentine venous channels of abnormal number, size, shape, & location (phlebectasia)

Fluoroscopic Findings

- Anatomy & venous drainage best mapped via direct percutaneous injection of venous sinusoids
  - Contrast material pools within clusters of abnormal venous channels/lakes ± connections to normal or abnormal veins
  - Large channels resemble cluster of grapes; smaller channels have more cotton-wool blush appearance

CT Findings

- Lobulated soft tissue mass with fluid attenuation
- Rounded, calcified phleboliths essentially pathognomonic
- Enhancement usually evident but variable: Patchy & delayed or homogeneous & intense
- Lymphatic component of VLM does not enhance
- ± osseous remodeling in adjacent bone
- ± fat hypertrophy in adjacent soft tissues

MR Findings

- T1WI
  - Multilobulated with variable signal intensity
    - Isointense to hypointense relative to muscle typical
    - Hemorrhage, stagnant blood, &/or thrombi → ↑ signal
    - Phleboliths hypointense due to calcification
  - Regional fat hypertrophy, often with fat interspersed within & around lesion
- T2WI FS
  - Vascular channel size influences appearance
    - Large, serpentine vascular channels hyperintense, septated
      - Large varicosities may be hypointense 2° to disturbed flow; may mimic clot
    - Smaller vascular channels appear more solid & intermediate in signal intensity
  - Phleboliths appear as rounded or oval signal voids
  - ± layering fluid-fluid levels 2° to settling of blood products within stagnant cavity
- T1WI C+ FS
  - Enhancement variable: May be delayed, heterogeneous or homogeneous, & mild to intense
  - Variable enhancement pattern reflects sluggish vascular flow to & through lesion
    - No enlarged feeding arteries
    - Lesion often drained by enlarged veins
  - Thrombi &/or intermixed LM components do not enhance
- MRV
  - May show enlarged veins associated with lesion
  - Extracranial VMs may show associated intracranial venous anomalies

Ultrasonographic Findings

- Spongy, compressible mass, heterogeneous echotexture
  - Small vascular channels are more echogenic & less compressible than large, vascular lumina
- ± discrete venous channels of abnormal number, size, shape, & location in surrounding tissues
- Phleboliths = hyperechoic foci with poor acoustic shadowing & twinkle artifact
- Valsalva or compression/release of transducer will ↑ venous flow
- Lack of arterial waveforms or arterialized draining veins; 1-2 normal arteries may be encased by VM

Imaging Recommendations

- Best imaging tool
  - MR best to map full extent & identify possible combined LM/VLM
  - US to assess response to compression if lesion is superficial
  - CT & radiographs identify phleboliths
- Protocol advice
  - US &/or MR for suspected vascular malformation
  - MR with contrast, fat suppression, & gradient-echo to confirm lack of high-flow vessels

DIFFERENTIAL DIAGNOSIS

Lymphatic Malformation

- Another common slow-or low-flow lesion
- Compressible, fluid-filled, macrocystic soft tissue mass
  - Thin, enhancing internal septations, internal debris, blood-fluid levels
  - Microcystic lesions may enhance & appear solid
- No phleboliths; no enhancement unless mixed VLM or microcystic lesion
- Solitary or multiple; single space or transspatial

Infantile Hemangioma

- Characteristic life cycle: Small at birth, rapid growth during infancy, gradual involution over years
- Benign, vascular neoplasm, GLUT1(+) marker
- Prominent intralesional vessels
- Rapid, homogeneous, intense enhancement
- Typically intermediate hyperintensity on T2

Arteriovenous Malformation

- Tangle of enlarged tortuous arteries & veins
- High-flow vessels with shunting by US, MRA/MRV

Neurofibroma

- Elongated lobular masses along course of nerves
- Multiple adjacent nerves → bag of worms appearance
- Target sign: T2-hypointense center, T2-hyperintense rim
- Variable contrast enhancement

Dermoid & Epidermoid

- Rounded calcifications possible (dermoid)
  - If present, found lying within fat-containing lesion
- Lesion contents very echogenic on ultrasound (dermoid)

Soft Tissue Sarcoma

- Well-defined soft tissue mass with variable enhancement
- ± cystic foci, ± bone destruction

PATHOLOGY

General Features

- Etiology
  - Subtype of congenital slow- or low-flow vascular malformation due to error in vein formation
- Genetics
  - *TEK* mutation in many VM (50% of sporadic VM)
- Associated abnormalities
  - 70% of patients with periorbital LM or VLM have intracranial vascular & parenchymal anomalies
    - Developmental venous anomaly (DVA), cerebral cavernous malformation, dural arteriovenous malformation (AVM), pial AVM, sinus pericranii
- Staging, grading, & classification
  - 2018 revised classification of VM by International Society for Study of Vascular Anomalies
    - Common VM: Causal genes *TEK/PIK3CA*
    - Familial VM cutaneomucosal: *TEK*
      - Multifocal lesions of lips, tongue
    - Blue rubber bleb nevus syndrome: *TEK* (TIE2)
      - Multiple cutaneous, muscular, gastrointestinal VM
    - Glomuvenous malformation: Chromosome 1p
    - Cerebral cavernous malformation: *CCM1, CCM2, CCM3*
    - Familial intraosseous vascular malformation: *ELMO2*
    - Verrucous VM: *MAP3K3*

Microscopic Features

- Venous channels, variable luminal diameter, wall thickness
- Luminal thrombi, phleboliths
- Immunohistochemical markers: GLUT1(-), PROX1(-) [(+) in LM], CD31(+), CD34(+) [(-) in LM]

CLINICAL ISSUES

Presentation

- Most common signs/symptoms
  - Spongy soft tissue mass without thrill
    - Bluish skin discoloration when superficial
  - Grows proportionately with patient
  - ↑ ↑ in size with Valsalva, bending over, crying
  - May enlarge rapidly after trauma, thrombosis or under hormonal influences (puberty, pregnancy)
  - May be painful 2° to stasis, intralesional thrombus, or hemorrhage into adjacent tissues

Demographics

- Age
  - VMs are present at birth, but may not clinically manifest until adolescence, or young adulthood
- Epidemiology
  - Most common vascular malformation of H&N

Treatment

- Treatment aimed at decreasing symptoms & improving function, rather than eliminating disease
- Conservative therapy
  - Compression garments, antiinflammatory medications
  - Low-molecular-weight heparin if thrombosis risk ↑
  - Sirolimus may be helpful for lesions with mixed lymphatic components
- Percutaneous procedures
  - Direct injection with sclerosing agent under fluoroscopic/ultrasonic guidance
  - Laser ablation (Nd:YAG laser) of superficial VM
  - Endovascular ablation of varicosities
- Surgical resection of focal lesions
  - May be used in combination with percutaneous sclerotherapy

DIAGNOSTIC CHECKLIST

Consider

- Does lesion enlarge with Valsalva maneuver, crying, or when head is dependent?
  - If yes, suggests VM

Image Interpretation Pearls

- Presence of phleboliths on CT or T2-hyperintense facial mass is most specific imaging finding for VM
  - Rare spindle cell hemangioma may contain phleboliths
- Multiple fluid-fluid levels in pediatric soft tissue mass strongly suggests slow- or low-flow vascular malformation (LM > VM)

SELECTED REFERENCES

1. Tasiou A et al: Cavernous malformations of the central nervous system: an international consensus statement. Brain Spine. 3:102707, 2023
2. Cooke-Barber J et al: Venous malformations. Semin Pediatr Surg. 29(5):150976, 2020
3. Van Damme A et al: New and emerging targeted therapies for vascular malformations. Am J Clin Dermatol. 21(5):657-68, 2020
4. Mamlouk MD et al: Vascular anomaly imaging mimics and differential diagnoses. Pediatr Radiol. 49(8):1088-103, 2019
5. ISSVA: 2018 classification. Reviewed May 2018. Accessed January 10, 2024. https://www.issva.org/classification

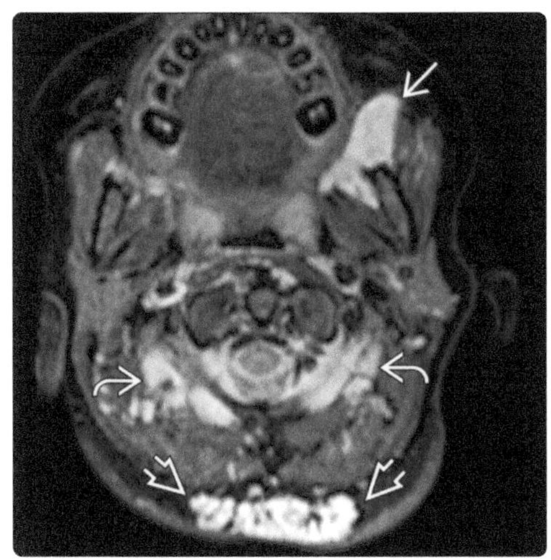

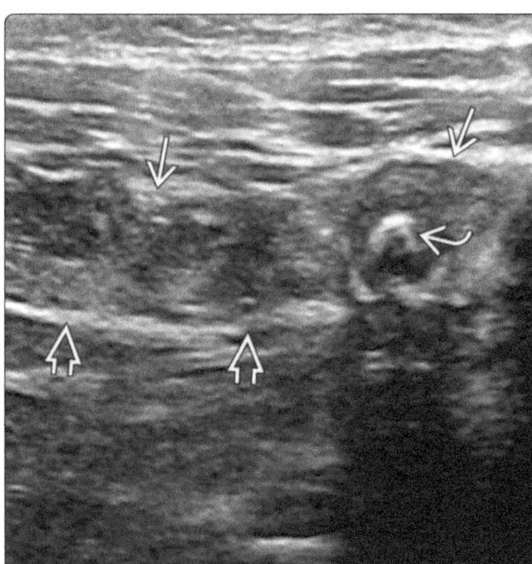

(Left) *Axial STIR MR in a 10-year-old girl with multiple VMs demonstrates hyperintense lesions in the left buccal space ➡, the midline posterior subcutaneous neck ➡, and the bilateral paraspinal soft tissues ➡.* **(Right)** *Longitudinal ultrasound in a child with known VMs demonstrates a heterogeneous mass ➡ adjacent to the mandible ➡ with a focal echogenic phlebolith ➡ that shows posterior acoustical shadowing.*

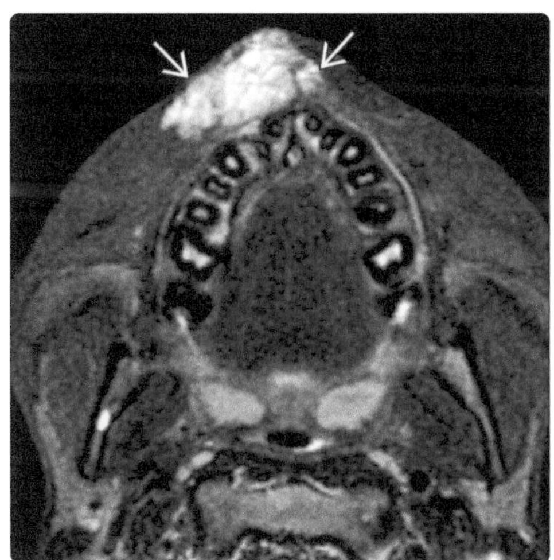

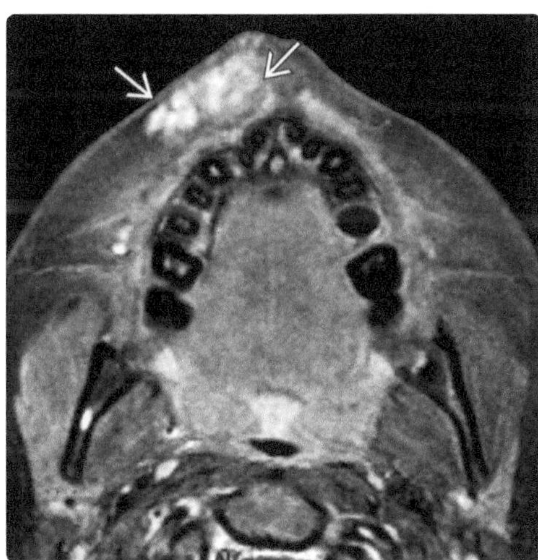

(Left) *Axial STIR MR reveals a well-defined, lobulated VM involving the subcutaneous tissues of the upper lip ➡ without an underlying osseous or dental abnormality.* **(Right)** *Axial T1 C+ FS MR in the same patient shows moderate, heterogeneous contrast within the abnormal venous lakes ➡, a typical appearance of many VMs.*

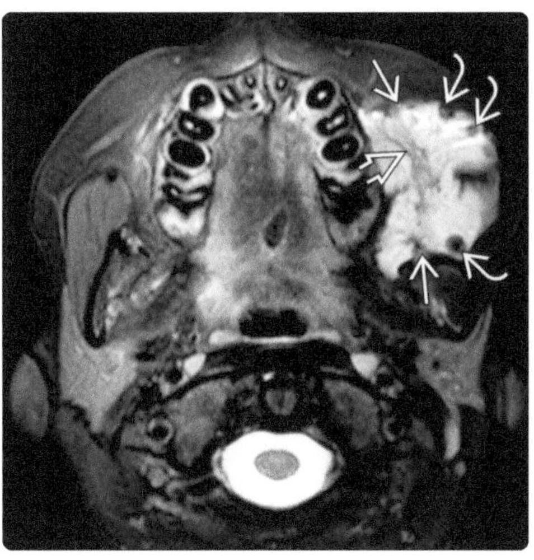

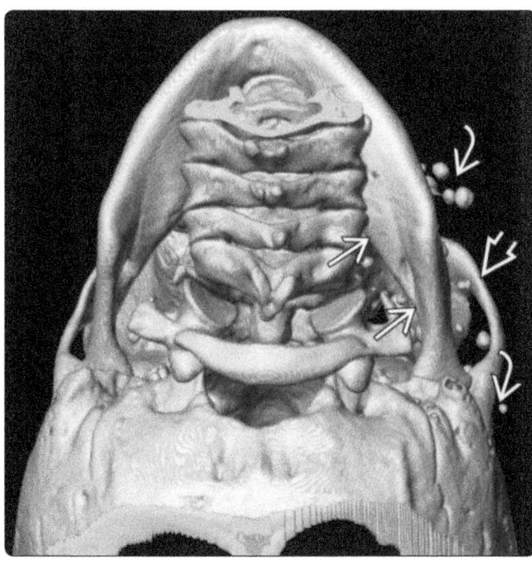

(Left) *Axial T2 TSE FS MR in a teenager demonstrates a large, hyperintense left buccal space mass ➡ that contains multiple hypointense septa ➡. Notice also multiple well-defined, round, hypointense foci ➡, typical of phleboliths and nearly pathognomonic of a VM.* **(Right)** *3D surface-rendered MR in the same patient shows mild overgrowth of the left hemimandible ➡, relative to the right, lateral bowing of the thickened left zygomatic arch ➡, and multiple soft tissue phleboliths ➡.*

KEY FACTS

TERMINOLOGY

- Lymphatic malformation (LM): Subtype of slow-/low-flow congenital vascular malformation composed of embryonic lymphatic sacs; not neoplastic
- Composed of macrocysts > 1 cm &/or microcysts < 1 cm

IMAGING

- Macrocystic LM: Multiloculated cystic neck mass with imperceptible wall, thin septations, and fluid-fluid levels
- Microcystic LM: Ill-defined, infiltrative, &/or solid-appearing
- Transspatial, often crosses midline extensively
- Insinuates between vessels and other normal structures
- T2 FS/STIR MR: Hyperintense, frequent fluid-fluid levels
  - Best defines extent, relationship to airway and vessels
- T1 FS C+ MR: No significant or minimal rim enhancement
  - Must compare with precontrast T1, as hemorrhage and protein often show hyperintensity
- US: Cysts can show varying degrees of ↑ echogenicity; Doppler shows no significant internal vascularity

TOP DIFFERENTIAL DIAGNOSES

- 2nd branchial cleft anomaly
- Thyroglossal duct cyst
- Abscess
- Thymic cyst
- Teratoma
- Neurofibroma
- Soft tissue sarcoma

CLINICAL ISSUES

- Nontender, compressible mass
  - Present since birth, grows commensurate with patient
  - May not be clinically apparent until hemorrhage, infection, or hormonal stimulation → rapid ↑ in size
- Depending on size and extent, treatment options primarily include resection, sclerotherapy (for macrocysts), and sirolimus
  - Combination therapy (often staged; may be required)

(Left) *Axial T2 FS MR in a 1-week-old infant demonstrates a multiloculated, mixed micro- and macrocystic transspatial lymphatic malformation (LM) ➡ involving the left anterior neck more than the right. A single fluid-fluid level is present in a left-sided submandibular macrocyst ➡, typical of layering blood products.* **(Right)** *Axial T1 C+ FS MR in the same child shows a typical appearance of an extensive LM. The macrocysts show only mild peripheral enhancement ➡, and the fluid-fluid level ➡ is much more difficult to discern.*

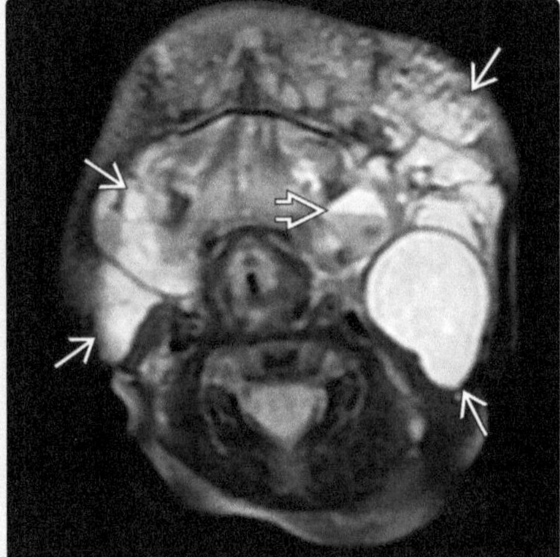

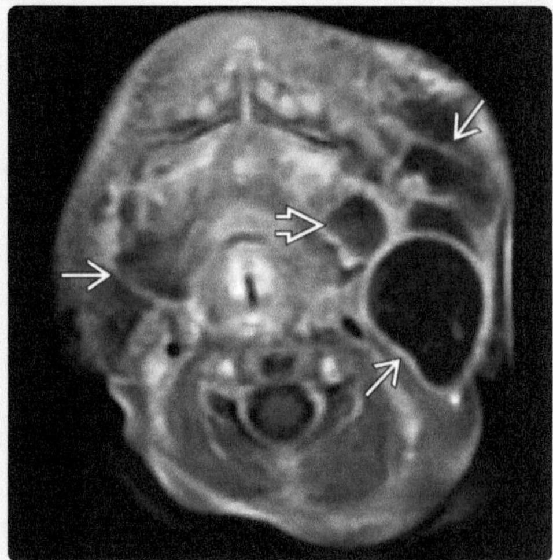

(Left) *Transverse color Doppler US in an infant with a macrocystic LM shows the typical anechoic nature of the dominant cyst ➡ with vessels ➡ identified adjacent to, but not within, the cyst. Note the thin septation ➡ peripherally.* **(Right)** *Axial T2 MR of the orbit in a 5-year-old with rapid-onset proptosis demonstrates an intraconal, multiloculated lesion with fluid-fluid levels ➡, consistent with layering blood products, resulting in moderate right-sided proptosis, secondary to the intralesional hemorrhage.*

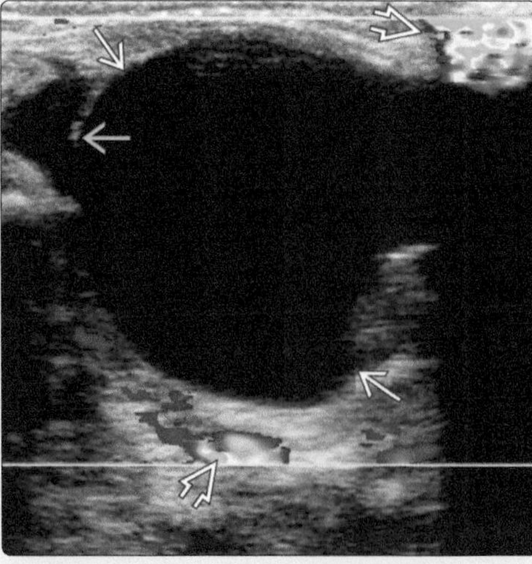

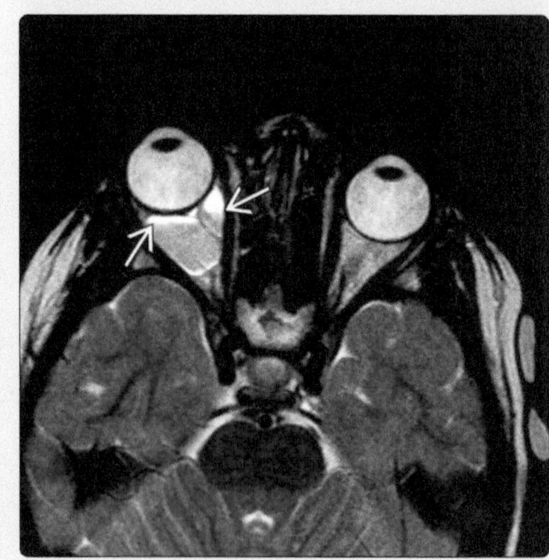

TERMINOLOGY

Synonyms

- Vascular malformation, lymphatic type; lymphatic anomaly
- Avoid incorrect terms: Cystic hygroma and lymphangioma

Definitions

- Lymphatic malformation (LM): Subtype of slow-/low-flow congenital vascular malformation composed of embryonic lymphatic sacs; not neoplastic
  - No communication with normal lymphatics
  - Composed of macrocysts > 1 cm &/or microcysts < 1 cm
- Venolymphatic malformation (VLM): Combined elements of venous malformation and LM

IMAGING

General Features

- Best diagnostic clue
  - Macrocystic LM: Multiloculated cystic neck mass with imperceptible wall, thin septations, and fluid-fluid levels
  - Microcystic LM: More ill-defined, infiltrative, &/or solid-appearing
  - Crosses tissue planes, insinuating between vessels and other normal structures
- Location
  - Any face/neck location (not intracranial)
    - Infrahyoid neck
      - Posterior cervical space most common
    - Suprahyoid neck
      - Masticator, submandibular, and parotid spaces most common
    - Orbit, tongue, floor of mouth, buccal space
  - Often in multiple contiguous spaces: Transspatial
    - Soft tissue involvement > > bone; single lesion > > multiple discontinuous lesions
  - Often crosses midline extensively
- Size
  - Individual compartments: Microcystic or macrocystic
  - Overall lesion varies from few cm to massive
  - May suddenly ↑ in size, particularly when intralesional hemorrhage occurs
- Morphology
  - Uni- or multilocular

Radiographic Findings

- LMs may cause mass effect on airway

CT Findings

- NECT
  - Low-attenuation, well-defined, or poorly circumscribed cystic neck mass
  - ± fluid-fluid levels
  - ± phleboliths in venous malformation components of VLM
- CECT
  - Unilocular or multilocular cystic mass with minimal rim &/or septal enhancement
    - In mixed VLM, venous malformation components will show patchy, gradual enhancement ± phleboliths

MR Findings

- T1WI
  - Primarily hypointense fluid; hyperintense if prior hemorrhage or high protein content (± fluid-fluid levels)
- T2WI FS or STIR
  - Best sequence to map lesion extent: Hyperintense throughout
    - Fluid-fluid levels in multiple cysts very common
  - When transspatial, often poorly marginated
- T1WI C+ FS
  - No significant enhancement (± subtle rim enhancement)
  - Patchy enhancement suggests VLM or microcystic LM

Ultrasonographic Findings

- Unilocular vs. septated and multilocular transspatial mass
- Contents predominantly hypo- or anechoic
  - Separate compartments in multicystic mass can show varying degrees of ↑ echogenicity
    - ± swirling debris &/or layering fluid-debris levels
- No true vascular flow in cysts by Doppler
  - ± flow (from encased normal vessels) in septations

Imaging Recommendations

- Best imaging tool
  - US often diagnostic of superficial components
  - MR better for defining deep extent and recognizing characteristic fluid-fluid levels
- Protocol advice
  - Fluid-sensitive sequences (T2 FS or STIR) essential
    - STIR particularly helpful for overcoming poor chemical fat suppression in neck (typical of T2)
  - T1 C+ FS helpful to detect venous malformation component of mixed lesions
    - Subtraction of precontrast T1 FS improves assessment of true enhancement (vs. pseudoenhancement from preexisting T1 shortening of protein/hemorrhage)

DIFFERENTIAL DIAGNOSIS

2nd Branchial Cleft Anomaly

- Ovoid, unilocular cyst at angle of mandible with characteristic displacement pattern

Abscess

- Fluid collection with thick, enhancing, irregular wall
- Adjacent soft tissues show cellulitis > myositis, fasciitis

Teratoma

- Solid and cystic components typical ± internal vascularity
- Frequently contain calcification
- Tend to be more unilateral and focal than LM

Thyroglossal Duct Cyst

- Anterior midline/paramidline unilocular cystic mass
- Tongue base to lower anterior neck
- Embedded in infrahyoid strap muscles

Thymic Cyst

- Unilocular lateral neck cyst
- Closely associated with carotid sheath
- May extend into anterior superior mediastinum

Neurofibroma

- ± lobular, low-attenuation foci on CT without significant enhancement
- T2 MR often confirms characteristic target sign

Soft Tissue Sarcoma

- Well-defined, typically solid; rarely predominantly cystic
  - Cystic mass with discrete solid nodules showing internal vascularity requires biopsy/excision

PATHOLOGY

General Features

- Etiology
  - Congenital error of vessel morphogenesis
  - 2 main theories
    - Failure of embryologic fusion between primordial lymph sac and venous system
    - Abnormal sequestration of embryonic lymphatic sacs
- Genetics
  - Majority sporadic
  - May be part of extensive overgrowth syndrome with capillary VLM
  - Generalized lymphatic anomaly (lymphangiomatosis), kaposiform lymphangiomatosis, and Gorham-Stout disease may have soft tissue LM in association with bone and visceral lesions
  - Confusion regarding anterior neck LM association with Turner syndrome and trisomies
    - Aneuploidy and high mortality in posterior midline cystic neck masses ("cystic hygroma") of early gestation
- Associated abnormalities
  - 70% of patients with periorbital VLM have intracranial vascular and parenchymal anomalies
    - Developmental venous anomaly, cerebral cavernous malformation, dural arteriovenous malformation (AVM), pial AVM, sinus pericranii

Staging, Grading, & Classification

- Microcystic or macrocystic
- Lymphatic alone vs. mixed venolymphatic

Microscopic Features

- Primitive embryonic lymph sacs of varying sizes separated by connective tissue stroma
- Recent recommendation: Use immunohistochemical panel of PROX1, D2-40, VEGFR3, CD31, and CD34 antibodies to differentiate LM from other vascular malformations
  - PROX1 and VEGFR3 most sensitive, specific

CLINICAL ISSUES

Presentation

- Most common signs/symptoms
  - Nontender, soft, compressible mass
  - Present since birth and grows commensurate with patient
    - May not be clinically apparent until hemorrhage, infection, or hormonal stimulation → rapid ↑ in size
  - Larger lesions detected prenatally
- Other signs/symptoms
  - LMs may infiltrate upper airway or cause extrinsic compression

Demographics

- Age
  - 90% diagnosed < 2 years of age

Natural History & Prognosis

- No clear malignant potential
- Benign disease with potential lifelong morbidity in more extensive cases
- Recurrence may be secondary to redirection of lymphatic fluid into remaining dilated spaces or to growth of truncated lymphatic channels

Treatment

- Surgical resection &/or percutaneous sclerotherapy
  - Sclerotherapy primarily for macrocystic disease
  - Extensive disease often requires combined &/or numerous staged procedures
- Some success with radiofrequency ablation of microcystic LM of oral cavity and laser therapy of tongue lesions
- Medical therapy with sirolimus
- Tracheostomy for significant airway involvement

DIAGNOSTIC CHECKLIST

Image Interpretation Pearls

- Transspatial multicystic neck mass with fluid-fluid levels highly suggestive of LM
- Multiplanar T2 FS/STIR MR: Maps extent of transspatial lesion, especially relationship to airway and vessels
- In absence of irritation by infection or hemorrhage, lesion wall should be thin and nearly imperceptible
  - True, solid nodular enhancement in cyst wall must suggest predominantly cystic soft tissue sarcoma over LM → biopsy

SELECTED REFERENCES

1. Wiegand S et al: Efficacy of sirolimus in children with lymphatic malformations of the head and neck. Eur Arch Otorhinolaryngol. 279(8):3801-10, 2022
2. Le HDT et al: Generalized lymphangiomatosis-a rare manifestation of lymphatic malformation. Radiol Case Rep. 16(1):66-71, 2021
3. Reis J 3rd et al: Ultrasound evaluation of pediatric slow-flow vascular malformations: practical diagnostic reporting to guide interventional management. AJR Am J Roentgenol. 216(2):494-506, 2021
4. Crane J et al: Kaposiform lymphangiomatosis treated with multimodal therapy improves coagulopathy and reduces blood angiopoietin-2 levels. Pediatr Blood Cancer. 67(9):e28529, 2020
5. ISSVA: 2018 classification. Published May 2018. Accessed March 14, 2021. https://www.issva.org/classification
6. Adams DM et al: Efficacy and safety of sirolimus in the treatment of complicated vascular anomalies. Pediatrics. 137(2):1-10, 2016
7. Cramer SL et al: Gorham-Stout disease successfully treated with sirolimus and zoledronic acid therapy. J Pediatr Hematol Oncol. 38(3):e129-32, 2016
8. Merrow AC et al: 2014 revised classification of vascular lesions from the International Society for the Study of Vascular Anomalies: radiologic-pathologic update. Radiographics. 36(5):1494-516, 2016
9. Elluru RG et al: Lymphatic malformations: diagnosis and management. Semin Pediatr Surg. 23(4):178-85, 2014
10. Lala S et al: Gorham-Stout disease and generalized lymphatic anomaly--clinical, radiologic, and histologic differentiation. Skeletal Radiol. 42(7):917-24, 2013
11. Shiels WE 2nd et al: Percutaneous treatment of lymphatic malformations. Otolaryngol Head Neck Surg. 141(2):219-24, 2009
12. Mulliken JB et al: Hemangiomas and vascular malformations in infants and children: a classification based on endothelial characteristics. Plast Reconstr Surg. 69(3):412-22, 1982

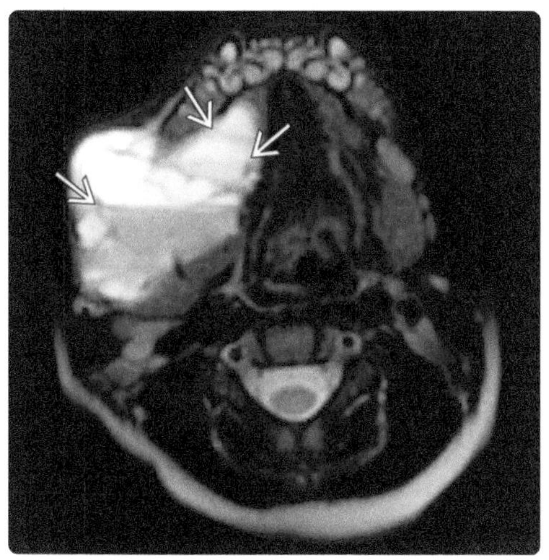

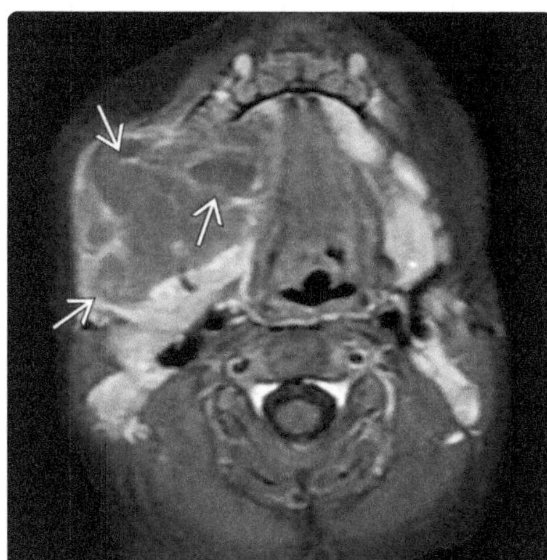

(Left) *Axial TSE FS MR in a 1-year-old child shows a multiloculated, transspatial, macrocystic LM in the right submandibular and sublingual spaces. Notice the multiple fluid-fluid levels of varying intensities, indicating intralesional blood products.* **(Right)** *Axial T1 C+ FS MR in the same child shows only minimal linear, peripheral, and septal contrast enhancement, typical of macrocystic LM. There is associated mass effect on the submandibular gland and the airway.*

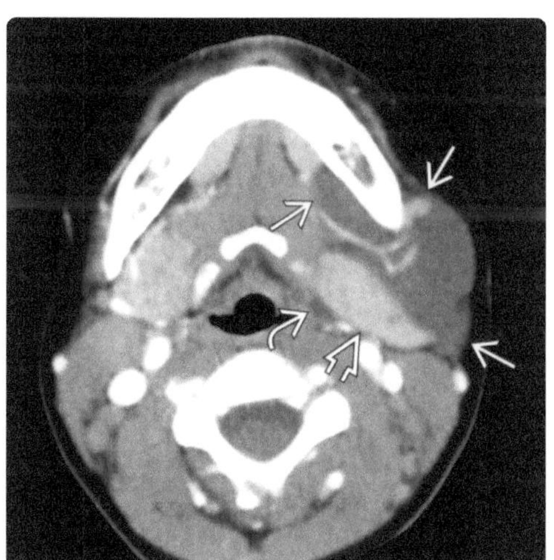

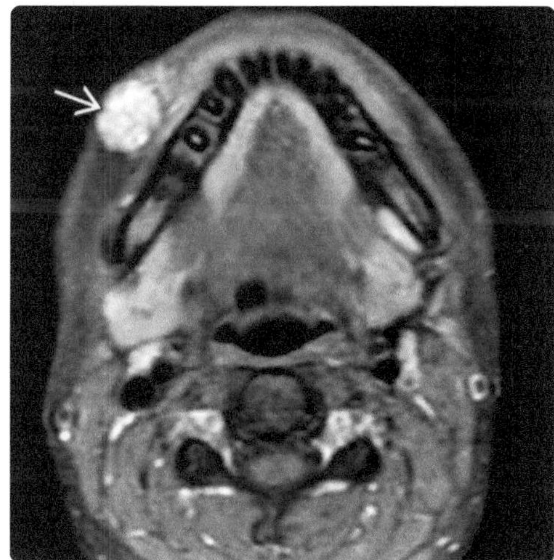

(Left) *Axial CECT in a 3-year-old shows a well-defined, hypodense, macrocystic LM in sublingual & submandibular spaces, flattening the gland, without phleboliths. There is minimal extension deep to left submandibular gland.* **(Right)** *Axial T1 C+ FS MR in a teenager with a firm, tender lump shows a lobulated, enhancing subcutaneous mass adjacent to the right mandible, proven to be a microcystic LM. The well-circumscribed morphology and enhancement could also be seen with a sarcoma, thus requiring excision.*

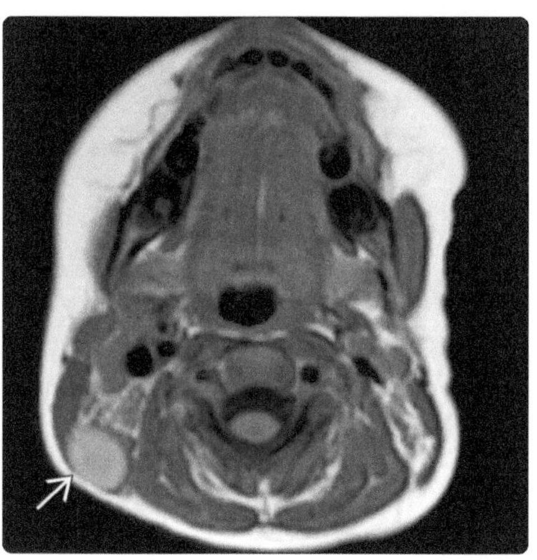

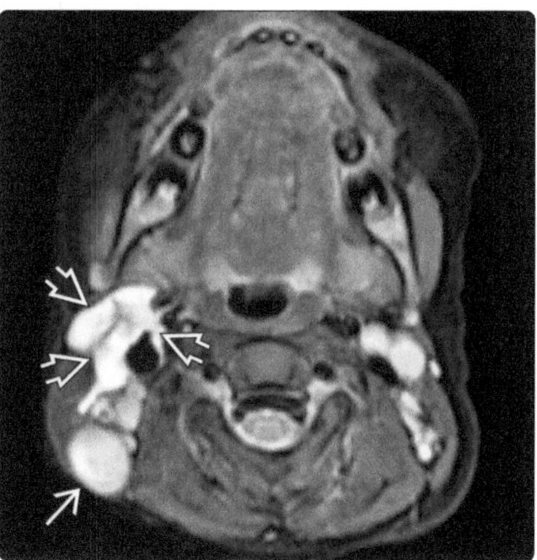

(Left) *Axial T1 MR in a 4-year-old child with an enlarging neck mass shows a multiloculated, macrocystic LM with a hyperintense locule related to recent intralesional hemorrhage.* **(Right)** *Axial FSEIR MR in the same patient shows the dominant macrocyst contains intermediate signal intensity blood products and shows to better advantage the more hyperintense, multiloculated, smaller cysts in the anterior neck with extension into the carotid space.*

Infantile Hemangioma

KEY FACTS

TERMINOLOGY

- Infantile hemangioma (IH): Benign vascular neoplasm of proliferating endothelial cells; **not** vascular malformation

IMAGING

- Doppler US (including spectral): Characteristic flow patterns
  - High vessel density (> 5/cm²) with low-resistance arterial waveforms but no arteriovenous shunting
- Contrast-enhanced CT/MR
  - Well-defined mass with diffuse and intense enhancement during proliferative phase
  - High-flow vessels in/adjacent to mass during proliferation
  - ↓ size with ↑ fatty replacement during involuting phase

TOP DIFFERENTIAL DIAGNOSES

- **Congenital hemangioma**
- **Venous malformation**
- **Soft tissue sarcoma**
- **Plexiform neurofibroma**
- **Arteriovenous malformation**

PATHOLOGY

- **GLUT1** IHC marker (+) in all phases of growth and regression
- In contrast to GLUT1(-) congenital hemangioma

CLINICAL ISSUES

- Typically inapparent at birth → appears in 1st few weeks of life → grows rapidly for months → spontaneously involutes over years
  - Typically warm, soft, raised reddish or strawberry-like cutaneous lesion
- Majority do not require treatment; propranolol 1st-line therapy in setting of ulceration or vital structure compromise (e.g., airway or orbit)
- If age, clinical/imaging appearance, or growth history are atypical for IH, biopsy recommended

(Left) *Axial T1 C+ FS MR in a 5-month-old shows a large, lobulated, intensely enhancing mass ➡ infiltrating the massively enlarged right parotid gland. Notice the prominent intralesional ⇨ and perilesional ➡ flow voids, typical of an infantile hemangioma (IH).* **(Right)** *Axial 2D SPGR flow-sensitive MR sequence in the same patient shows the typical appearance of multiple high-flow vessels within and adjacent to the primary parotid IH ➡.*

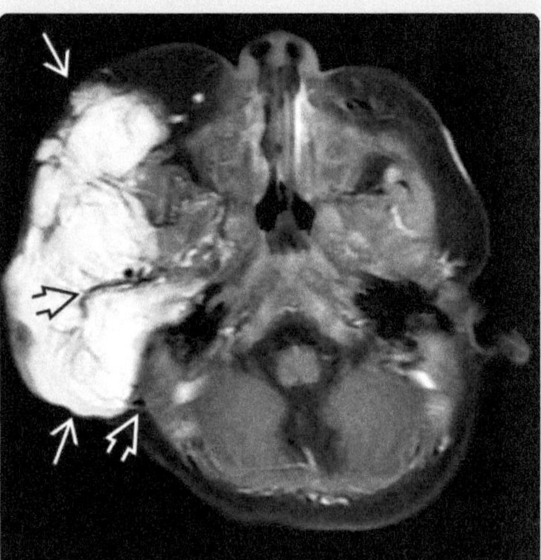

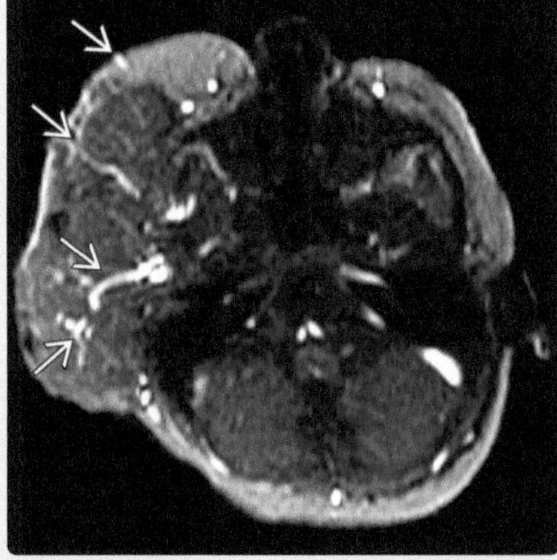

(Left) *Transverse color Doppler US in a 1-month-old child shows a lobular lesion replacing and expanding the parotid gland. Note the high vessel density ➡, typical of a proliferating IH.* **(Right)** *Transverse color Doppler US spectral tracing through the lesion in the same patient demonstrates low-resistance arterial waveforms, typical of proliferating-phase IH. The waveforms will develop a high-resistance pattern during involution, and there will be a decrease in vessel density.*

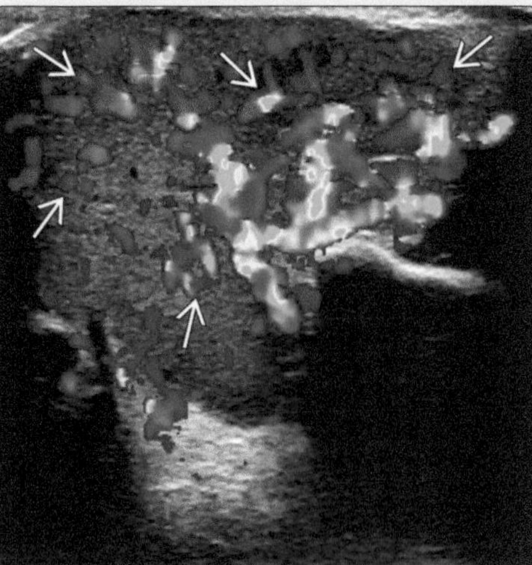

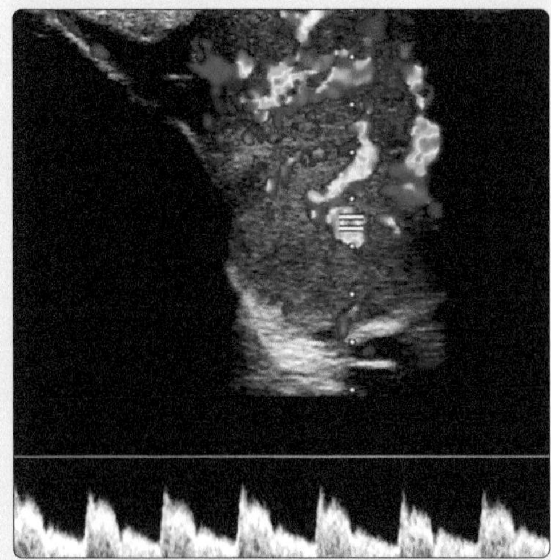

TERMINOLOGY

Synonyms

- Capillary hemangioma

Definitions

- Widespread misuse of term hemangioma in literature
- Infantile hemangioma (IH) is different entity from
  - Congenital hemangioma, spindle cell hemangioma, epithelioid hemangioma, lobular capillary hemangioma (pyogenic granuloma)
    - All benign but different vascular neoplasms
  - Hemangioendothelioma: Higher grade vascular neoplasm
  - Cavernous hemangioma, vertebral body hemangioma, and synovial hemangioma = venous malformations
- IH: Benign vascular neoplasm (not malformation) of proliferating endothelial cells
  - Most common soft tissue tumor of infancy
- **Not** vascular malformation
- 2018 revised classification by International Society for Study of Vascular Anomalies (ISSVA) retains 2 main categories
  - Vascular tumors: True neoplasms with cellular proliferation; grow out of proportion to patient
  - Vascular malformation: Congenital errors of vessel development; grow commensurate with patient

IMAGING

General Features

- Best diagnostic clue
  - During proliferative phase (PP): Lobular, well-defined mass with intense, diffuse enhancement + high-flow vessels in/adjacent to mass
  - During involuting phase (IP): ↓ size, vascularity, and enhancement with progressive fatty replacement
- Location
  - 60% occur in head and neck
    - Any space: Parotid space, orbit, nasal cavity, subglottic airway, face, neck; rarely intracranial
      - When intracranial &/or multiple, consider PHACE(S) association; typically not intramuscular
- Size
  - Depends on phase of growth and regression; predictable clinical course
    - PP: Rapid growth beginning few weeks after birth and continuing 6-24 months
    - IP: Gradual regression over next several years
    - Involuted phase: Relatively small residual lesion
- Morphology
  - Majority: Isolated, focal, well-circumscribed, lobulated lesions in subcutaneous tissues
    - Tend to displace/efface rather than encase structures
  - Occasionally multiple, transspatial, or deep
    - May be part of PHACE(S) association
      - **P**osterior fossa malformations (cerebellar hypoplasia most common)
      - **H**emangioma (infantile) of face and neck, typically segmental or midline, &/or internal auditory canal (IAC)/cerebellopontine angle (CPA)
      - **A**rterial stenosis, occlusion, aneurysm, hypoplasia, agenesis, aberrant origin
      - **C**ardiovascular defects (aortic coarctation/aneurysm/dysplasia, aberrant subclavian artery ± vascular ring, ventricular septal defect)
      - **E**ye abnormalities (persistent hyperplastic primary vitreous, coloboma, morning glory disc anomaly, optic nerve hypoplasia, peripapillary staphyloma, microphthalmia, cataract, sclerocornea)
      - **S**upraumbilical raphe and sternal clefts/defects
- CECT
  - Well-circumscribed, lobulated mass with diffuse and intense contrast enhancement in PP
    - Prominent vessels in/adjacent to mass
    - No internal calcification or surrounding edema
  - Progressive fatty infiltration of mass + ↓ size in IP
- MR
  - T1: Isointense to muscle in PP; hyperintense from fatty replacement during IP
  - T2: Mildly hyperintense relative to muscle
  - T2 FS/STIR: At least moderately hyperintense relative to muscle (but not fluid signal intensity) during PP; hypointense to muscle (follows fat) during IP
  - T1 C+ FS: Intense contrast enhancement in PP
  - GRE: High-flow vessels in/adjacent to mass in PP
    - Corresponding serpiginous flow voids in/adjacent to mass on SE/FSE sequences
  - MRA: Stenosis, occlusion, agenesis, aneurysm of craniocervical vessels [PHACE(S) association]
  - Noncontrast arterial spin-labeling (ASL) perfusion MR shows ↑ blood flow on cerebral blood flow (CBF) images
  - DWI: ADC values higher in IHs mm^2/sec vs. sarcomas $0.67\text{-}0.78 \times 10^{-3}$ mm^2/sec
- Ultrasonographic findings
  - Grayscale: Soft tissue mass with variable echogenicity and few macroscopic vessels; ↑ echogenicity during IP
  - Color/spectral Doppler
    - High vessel density (> 5 vessels/cm^2), high systolic Doppler shift (> 2 kHz), and low resistive index in arterial vessels without arterialized veins (to suggest shunting) during PP
    - Mean venous peak velocities not elevated (unlike arteriovenous malformation)
  - ↓ vessel density, ↑ resistive index in IP

Imaging Recommendations

- No imaging necessary in majority of patients; characteristic cutaneous appearance and change over time
- Best imaging tool depends on indications
  - US with spectral Doppler
    - Used to establish diagnosis of superficial lesion with atypical history, appearance, or clinical behavior
    - To identify deeper lesions without classic cutaneous manifestations
  - MR
    - To define deep extension of lesion with implications for compromise of vital structures (e.g., orbit and airway)
    - To plan/evaluate therapy pre- and post treatment (if considering medical or surgical/laser therapy)

- To evaluate for suspected PHACE(S) association (e.g., large segmental facial IH)
- Search for extracutaneous anomalies: Warranted for children with facial segmental or periorbital IH
- Protocol advice
  - Pulsed/spectral color Doppler US to document characteristic flow throughout lesion
  - MR imaging should include flow-sensitive, fluid-sensitive, and T1 C+ FS sequences

DIFFERENTIAL DIAGNOSIS

Congenital Hemangioma (Rapidly, Non-, or Partially Involuting)

- Present at birth or on prenatal imaging; do not proliferate after birth
  - Rapidly involuting congenital hemangioma (RICH): Involutes by 3-14 months
  - Noninvoluting congenital hemangioma (NICH)
  - Partially involuting congenital hemangioma (PICH)
- Solid, heterogeneous, less well-defined mass ± calcification, hemorrhage, necrosis
- GLUT1(-) on histology

Venous Malformation

- Congenital vascular malformation composed of large venous lakes
- Fluid signal intensity throughout mass; ± fluid-fluid levels, phleboliths
- Gradual, patchy fill-in with contrast

Soft Tissue Sarcoma

- Rhabdomyosarcoma, extraosseous Ewing sarcoma, undifferentiated sarcoma
- Solid or mixed cystic/solid mass, typically firm
- Mild to moderate enhancement ± osseous erosion
- Internal vascularity present but typically < < IH

Plexiform Neurofibroma

- Infiltrative, lobulated masses with target appearance in cross section
- Transspatial involvement ± poorly defined margins
- + additional stigmata of neurofibromatosis type 1

Arteriovenous Malformation

- Congenital high-flow vascular malformation
- Arteriovenous shunting through tangle of feeding arteries and large draining veins; ± other soft tissue components

PATHOLOGY

General Features

- Etiology
  - Proposed theory: Clonal expansion of angioblasts with high expression of basic fibroblast growth factors and other angiogenesis markers
- Genetics: Majority sporadic

Microscopic Features

- Prominent endothelial cells forming small vascular channels (PP), flat endothelial cells + fibrofatty replacement (IP)

Immunohistochemical Features

- GLUT1(+) during all phases of proliferation and regression

CLINICAL ISSUES

Presentation

- Most common signs/symptoms
  - Growing superficial soft tissue mass in young infant (PP); typically with warm, soft, raised reddish or strawberry-like cutaneous discoloration
  - Occasionally, deeper lesions show bluish skin discoloration secondary to prominent draining veins
- Other signs/symptoms
  - Ulceration of overlying skin
  - Airway obstruction from airway involvement
  - Proptosis from orbital lesion
  - Associated abnormalities in PHACE(S) association

Demographics

- Age
  - Median at presentation: 2 weeks; majority by 1-3 months
    - Typically inapparent at birth
    - Up to 1/3 nascent at birth (i.e., pale or erythematous macule, telangiectasia, pseudoecchymotic patch or red spot)
- Sex
  - F > M (1.5-4:1)
- Epidemiology
  - Most common head and neck tumor in infants
  - Incidence is 1-2% of neonates; 12% by 1 year of age
  - ↑ in preterm infants and low-birth-weight infants
    - Up to 30% of infants weighing < 1 kg

Natural History & Prognosis

- Majority undergo PP followed by spontaneous regression
  - 90% resolve by 9 years of age
- Large and segmental facial hemangiomas have ↑ incidence of complications if not treated

Treatment

- Majority do not require treatment
- Treatment indications: Compromise vital structures (e.g., optic nerve compression or airway obstruction); significant skin ulceration
- Treatment options: Oral propranolol (β-blocker) primary therapy (instead of oral steroids) due to low side effect profile; less common: Intralesional steroids, laser; rarely, surgical excision

SELECTED REFERENCES

1. Luu J et al: Hemangioma genetics and associated syndromes. Dermatol Clin. 40(4):393-400, 2022
2. Tanaka F et al: Pseudocontinuous arterial spin labeling: clinical applications and usefulness in head and neck entities. Cancers (Basel). 14(16), 2022
3. Maldonado FR et al: Quantitative characterization of extraocular orbital lesions in children using diffusion-weighted imaging. Pediatr Radiol. 51(1):119-27, 2021
4. Proisy M et al: PHACES syndrome and associated anomalies: risk associated with small and large facial hemangiomas. AJR Am J Roentgenol. 1-8, 2021
5. Gong X et al: Conventional ultrasonography and elastography for the diagnosis of congenital and infantile hemangiomas. J Dermatol. 47(5):527-33, 2020
6. Mamlouk MD et al: Arterial spin-labeling perfusion for PHACE syndrome. AJNR Am J Neuroradiol. 42(1):173-7, 2020
7. ISSVA: 2018 classification. Reviewed May 2018. Accessed January 10, 2024. https://www.issva.org/UserFiles/file/ISSVA-Classification-2018.pdf

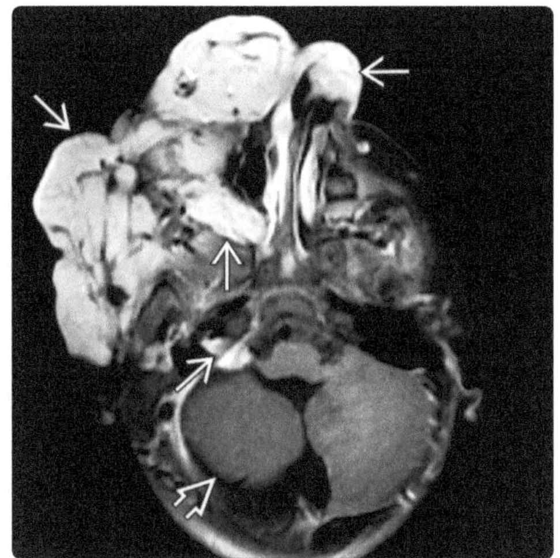

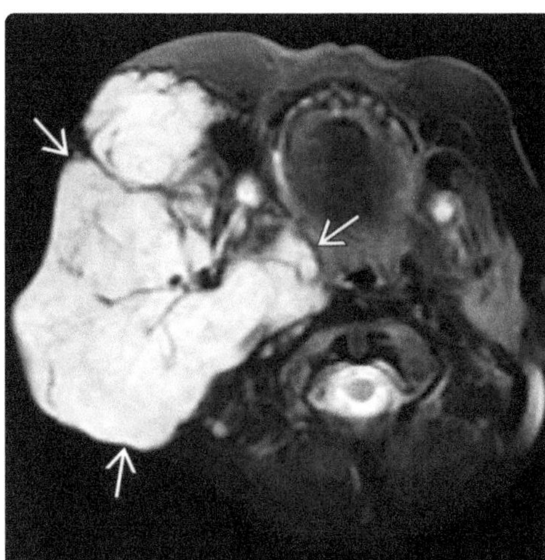

(Left) *Axial T1 C+ FS MR in a 4-month-old girl with PHACE(S) association shows multiple enhancing hemangiomas ➡ in the right parotid space, right posterior-inferior orbit, right cheek, nose, and right internal auditory canal (IAC)/cerebellopontine angle (CPA). Also note the ipsilateral right cerebellar hemisphere hypoplasia ➡.* **(Right)** *Axial T2 FS MR in a 3-month-old girl shows a holoparotid lesion ➡ with extension to the right cheek with diffuse hyperintense T2 signal and intralesional flow voids, typical of IH.*

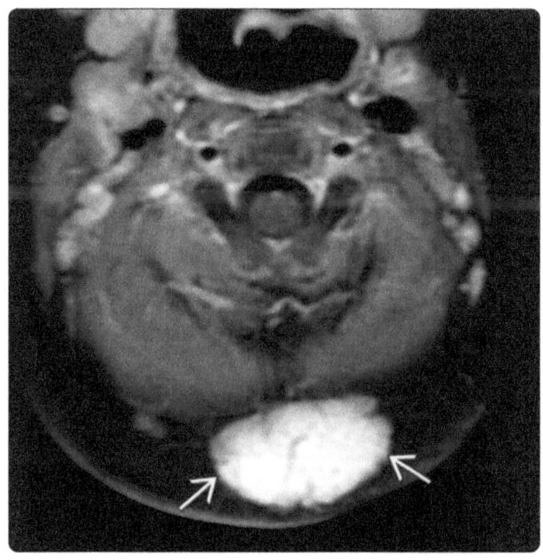

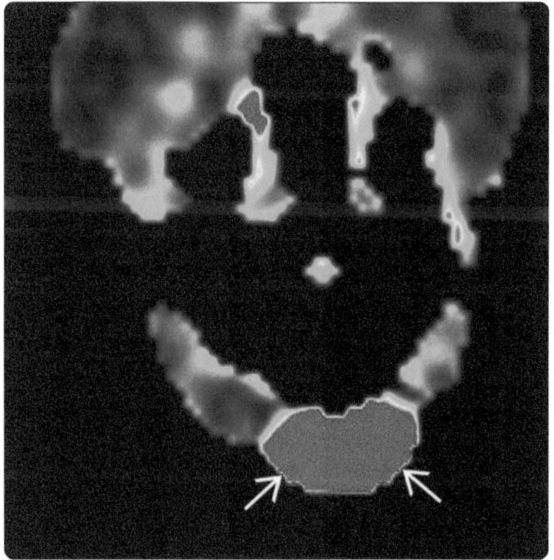

(Left) *Axial T1 C+ FS MR in a 5-month-old demonstrates the typical appearance of subcutaneous IH ➡, intensely enhancing but with only a few intralesional foci that may represent high-flow vessels.* **(Right)** *Axial noncontrast arterial spin-labeling (ASL) perfusion MR in the same patient shows increased perfusion ➡, typical of an IH.*

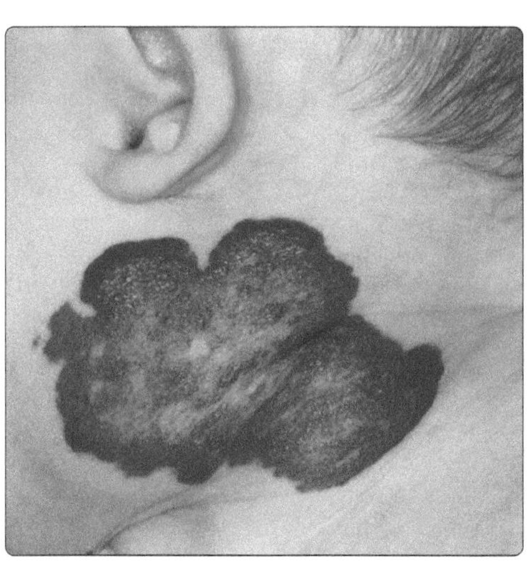

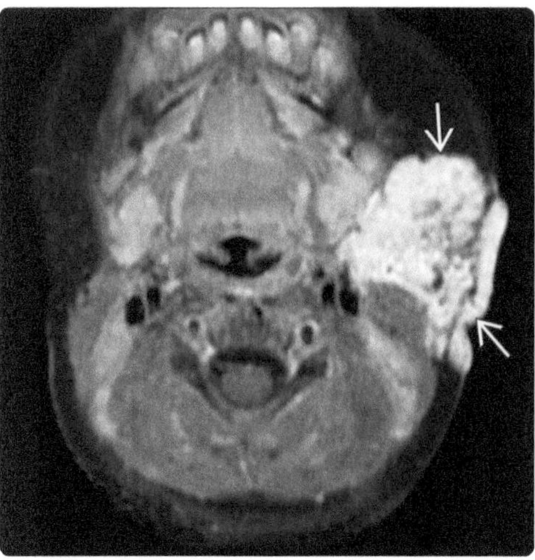

(Left) *Clinical photograph in a 6-week-old shows an intensely violaceous lesion with well-defined margins in the left neck, typical of IH.* **(Right)** *Axial T1 C+ FS MR in the same child shows the typical intense enhancement of the left face IH ➡. If there is a typical appearance and appropriate clinical scenario of a lesion not present at birth but now growing in size at a few months of age, there is no need for biopsy. If age, history, or imaging are atypical, then biopsy is imperative.*

KEY FACTS

TERMINOLOGY

- Neurofibromatosis type 1 (**NF1**)
- **Neurofibromas**: Multiple localized neurofibromas & plexiform neurofibromas (PNF) in NF1

IMAGING

- Hyperintense T2 signal
  - **Target** = ↓ signal center, ↑ signal periphery PNF
- Postcontrast CT or MR
  - Localized NF: Homogeneous or patchy enhancement, well-circumscribed fusiform mass
  - PNF: Heterogeneously enhancing, lobulated mass along course of peripheral nerve
- Most conspicuous on STIR & FS T2WI
- Other extracranial H&N manifestations of NF1
  - Orbit: **Optic pathway glioma (OPG)**, optic nerve sheath ectasia, Lisch nodules, buphthalmos, large foramina with PNFs
  - Skull & skull base: **Sphenoid dysplasia**, smooth enlargement of bony foramina with PNF infiltration, lambdoid suture defect
  - Vascular dysplasia: Internal carotid artery stenosis/occlusion & moyamoya; aneurysms & arteriovenous fistula rare

TOP DIFFERENTIAL DIAGNOSES

- Lymphatic malformation
- Venous malformation
- Rhabdomyosarcoma

DIAGNOSTIC CHECKLIST

- Patient with PNF or multiple localized neurofibromas, consider NF1
  - Look for additional findings of brain lesions, OPG, sphenoid wing dysplasia
- Transspatial neurofibroma may be hypodense on CT & mimic lymphatic malformation

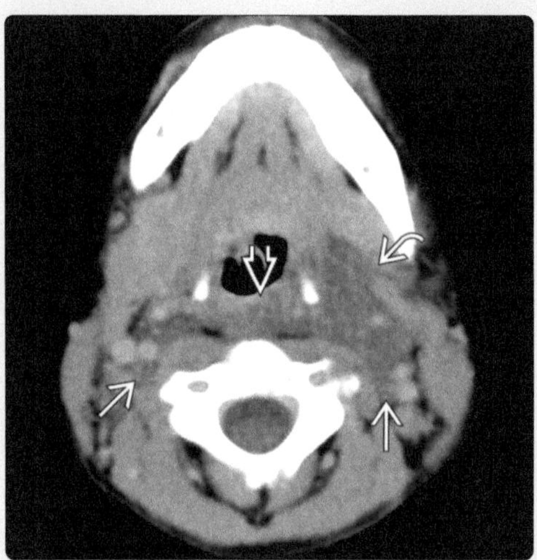

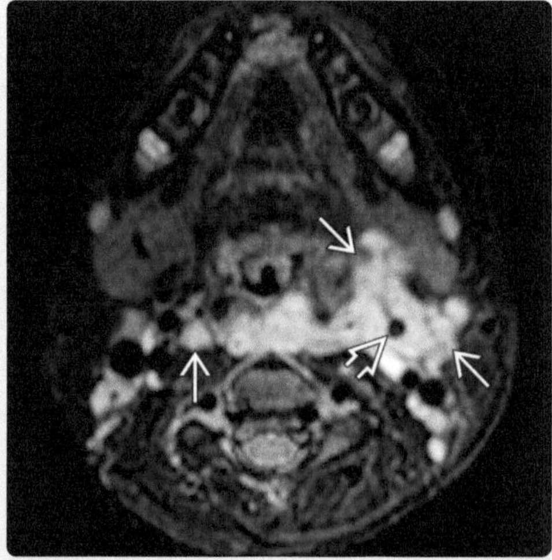

(Left) *Axial CECT in a child with neurofibromatosis type 1 (NF1) shows an ill-defined, infiltrative, transspatial plexiform neurofibroma (PNF) involving the bilateral carotid ➔, retropharyngeal ➔, and left submandibular ➔ spaces.* **(Right)** *Axial STIR MR in the same patient better defines the margins of the PNF ➔. Notice the infiltrative pattern with circumferential involvement of the left carotid artery ➔, typical of plexiform lesions.*

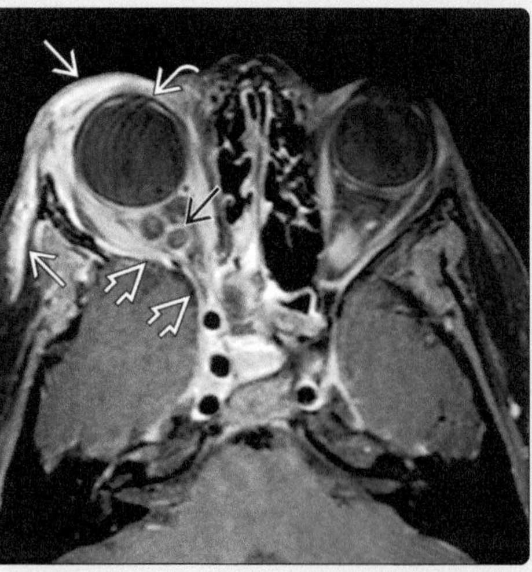

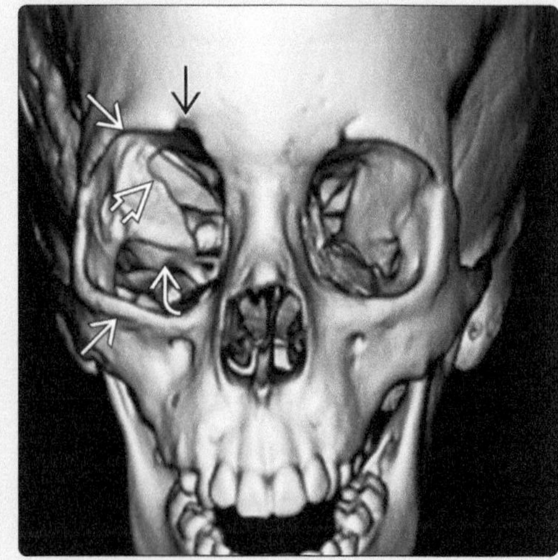

(Left) *Axial T1WI C+ FS MR shows a diffusely enhancing neurofibroma ➔ involving the right pre- and postseptal orbit and temporalis scalp. There is also sphenoid wing hypoplasia ➔, buphthalmos ➔, and a tortuous optic nerve ➔.* **(Right)** *Frontal 3D reformation in the same patient shows diffuse right orbital expansion ➔. There is also enlargement of the superior ➔ and inferior ➔ orbital fissures and supraorbital foramen ➔ related to sphenoid dysplasia and adjacent PNF.*

TERMINOLOGY

Abbreviations

- Neurofibromatosis type 1 (**NF1**)

Synonyms

- von Recklinghausen disease, autosomal dominant neurofibromatosis

Definitions

- Autosomal dominant neurocutaneous disorder (**phakomatosis**)
- Diagnostic NF1 criteria: If ≥ 2 of following present
  - > 6 café au lait spots measuring ≥ 5 mm in prepubertal & ≥ 15 mm in postpubertal patients
  - ≥ 2 neurofibromas (NFs) or 1 plexiform NF (PNF)
  - Axillary/inguinal freckling
  - Visual pathway glioma
  - ≥ Lisch nodules (optic hamartomas)
  - Distinctive bony lesion
    - Sphenoid wing dysplasia
    - Thinning of long bones
      - ± pseudoarthrosis
  - 1st-degree relative with NF1
- Peripheral nerve sheath tumor (PNST) = schwannoma, NF, & PNF
- **NFs**: Localized, plexiform, & diffuse variants

IMAGING

General Features

- Best diagnostic clue
  - **PNF**
    - Characteristic & diagnostic feature of NF1
  - **Multiple localized NFs**
- Location
  - NFs may involve **any space in H&N**
    - Most common: Carotid, retropharyngeal, & posterior cervical spaces; brachial plexus, oral cavity, cheek
  - PNST
    - Usually major nerve trunks, including brachial plexus
- Morphology
  - **Localized** NF
    - Multiple well-circumscribed, smooth, fusiform, variably enhancing masses along course of nerves
    - Paraspinal NF may be dumbbell-shaped ± smooth enlargement of bony neural foramina
    - Schwannoma may be indistinguishable from NF
  - **Diffuse** NF
    - Plaque-like or infiltrative, poorly defined, reticulated lesion in skin & subcutaneous fat
  - **PNF**
    - Transspatial, lobulated, tortuous, rope-like expansion within major nerve distribution
    - Resembles tangle of worms

CT Findings

- CECT
  - Localized NF & PNF
    - Frequently have low attenuation (5-25 HU) on pre- & postcontrast images; mimic lymphatic malformation
    - Paraspinal NF may be dumbbell-shaped
      - ± enlarged neural foramina

MR Findings

- T2WI
  - Hyperintense
  - Target sign: ↓ signal center, ↑ signal periphery PNF
    - Fascicular sign: Multiple small, irregular hypointense foci (represents fascicular bundles)
- T1WI C+
  - Localized NF: Homogeneous or patchy, heterogeneous enhancement, well-circumscribed fusiform mass
  - PNF: Heterogeneously enhancing, lobulated mass along course of peripheral nerve
  - Malignant PNST
    - Differentiation of benign from malignant PNST difficult on imaging alone
    - If large size (> 5 cm), heterogeneous with central necrosis, infiltrative margins, & rapid growth, consider malignant PNST
  - Diffuse NF: Plaque-like or infiltrative intense enhancement in skin & subcutaneous fat

Imaging Recommendations

- Best imaging tool
  - MR best to characterize & define total extent
    - Most conspicuous on STIR & FS T2WI
  - Bone CT delineates associated bone changes
    - Particularly helpful in patients with sphenoid wing dysplasia & PNF

DIFFERENTIAL DIAGNOSIS

Lymphatic Malformation

- Low attenuation
- Unilocular or multilocular, focal or infiltrative
- No enhancement unless infected or mixed venolymphatic malformation

Venous Malformation

- Phleboliths common

Rhabdomyosarcoma

- Invasive transspatial mass
- Frequently with aggressive bone destruction

PATHOLOGY

General Features

- Etiology
  - *NF1* gene (tumor suppressor gene) normally encodes production of "neurofibromin" that influences cell growth regulation
  - *NF1* gene "turned off" in NF1 → allows cellular proliferation & tumor development
- Genetics
  - **Autosomal dominant; 50% new mutations**
  - Gene locus = **chromosome 17q11.2**
    - Nonsense mutation of this gene leads to NF1
- Associated abnormalities
  - Other extracranial H&N manifestations of NF1

- Orbit: Optic pathway glioma (OPG), optic nerve sheath ectasia, Lisch nodules, **buphthalmos**, **large foramina** with PNFs
- Skull: Lambdoid suture defect
- Skull base findings
  - Sphenoid dysplasia with PNF, probably sequelae of PNF interaction with developing underlying bone
  - Smooth, corticated enlargement of skull base bony foramina with PNF infiltration
- Vascular dysplasia: Internal carotid artery stenosis/occlusion & moyamoya; aneurysms & arteriovenous fistula rare
- Neural crest tumors
  - **Pheochromocytoma** 10x ↑ in NF1 patients
  - **Parathyroid adenomas** ↑ incidence
- Other imaging manifestations of NF1
  - CNS findings
    - Cerebral gliomas, hydrocephalus, cranial nerve schwannomas
    - Nonenhancing hyperintense T2/FLAIR lesions: White matter, dentate nucleus, globus pallidus, brainstem, thalamus, hippocampus
    - Spinal cord astrocytomas

Staging, Grading, & Classification

- NFs are WHO grade 1
- Malignant PNSTs are WHO grade 3/4

Gross Pathologic & Surgical Features

- **Localized NF**: Fusiform, firm, gray/white-colored mass intermixed with nerve of origin
- **PNF**: Diffuse, tortuous, rope-like expansion of nerves resembling tangle of worms
  - Involves adjacent skin, fascia, & deeper tissues
- **Malignant PNST**: Fusiform, fleshy, tan-white mass with areas of necrosis & hemorrhage
  - Nerve proximally & distally thickened due to spread of tumor along epineurium & perineurium

Microscopic Features

- Localized NF
  - Schwann cells, fibroblasts, mast cells in matrix of collagen fibers, & mucoid substance
  - Axons usually embedded within tumor
- PNF
  - Schwann cells & perineural fibroblasts grow along nerve fascicles
- Malignant PNST
  - Fibrosarcoma-like growth of spindle cells
  - Considered high-grade sarcomas
  - PNF: 5% risk of malignant transformation

CLINICAL ISSUES

Presentation

- Most common signs/symptoms
  - Majority of NF & PNF asymptomatic
  - Cutaneous stigmata of NF1
    - > 95% have skin lesions
  - Sudden, painful ↑ size of stable NF suggests malignant transformation
- Other signs/symptoms
  - ↓ vision with OPG
  - Pulsatile buphthalmos with sphenoid wing dysplasia & PNF

Demographics

- Age
  - Any age; most common presentation in late childhood to early adulthood; new lesions may develop at any time
  - Malignant PNST: Usually in adults, rare in children
- Epidemiology
  - NF1
    - Most common autosomal dominant disorder
      - 1 in 3,000-5,000
    - **Most common neurocutaneous syndrome**
    - Most common inherited tumor syndrome
  - Localized NF
    - **90%** are solitary & not associated with NF1
    - **10%** associated with NF1 → more frequently large, multiple, & involve large deep nerves (e.g., brachial plexus)
  - Malignant PNST
    - **50% associated with NF1**
    - **5%** of patients with NF1 develop malignant PNST
  - Diffuse NF
    - Majority are in patients **without NF1**

Natural History & Prognosis

- Usually slow-growing NFs unless malignant transformation
  - Occasionally, massive enlargement in young kids

Treatment

- Resection of NFs that press on vital structures
- Solitary NF resectable; PNF generally unresectable
- mTOR &/or MEK inhibitors showing promise

DIAGNOSTIC CHECKLIST

Consider

- If patient has PNF or multiple localized NFs, consider NF1
  - Look for additional findings of brain lesions, OPG, sphenoid wing dysplasia

Image Interpretation Pearls

- Beware: Transspatial NF may be hypodense on CT & mimic lymphatic malformation

SELECTED REFERENCES

1. Nosé V et al: Update from the 5th edition of the World Health Organization classification of head and neck tumors: familial tumor syndromes. Head Neck Pathol. 16(1):143-57, 2022
2. Galvin R et al: Neurofibromatosis in the era of precision medicine: development of MEK inhibitors and recent successes with selumetinib. Curr Oncol Rep. 23(4):45, 2021
3. Abdel Razek AAK et al: Peripheral nerve sheath tumors of head and neck: imaging-based review of World Health Organization classification. J Comput Assist Tomogr. 44(6):928-40, 2020
4. Kim A et al: Targeting refractory sarcomas and malignant peripheral nerve sheath tumors in a phase i/ii study of sirolimus in combination with ganetespib (SARC023). Sarcoma. 2020:5784876, 2020
5. Ullrich NJ et al: A phase II study of continuous oral mTOR inhibitor everolimus for recurrent, radiographic-progressive neurofibromatosis type 1-associated pediatric low-grade glioma: a Neurofibromatosis Clinical Trials Consortium study. Neuro Oncol. 22(10):1527-35, 2020
6. de Blank PMK et al: Optic pathway gliomas in neurofibromatosis type 1: an update: surveillance, treatment indications, and biomarkers of vision. J Neuroophthalmol. 37 Suppl 1:S23-32, 2017

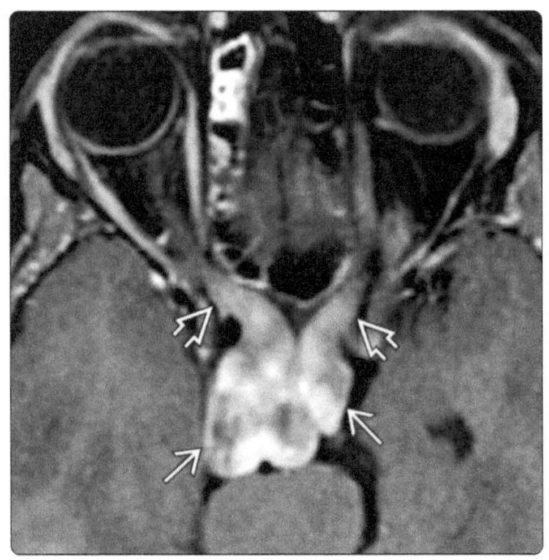

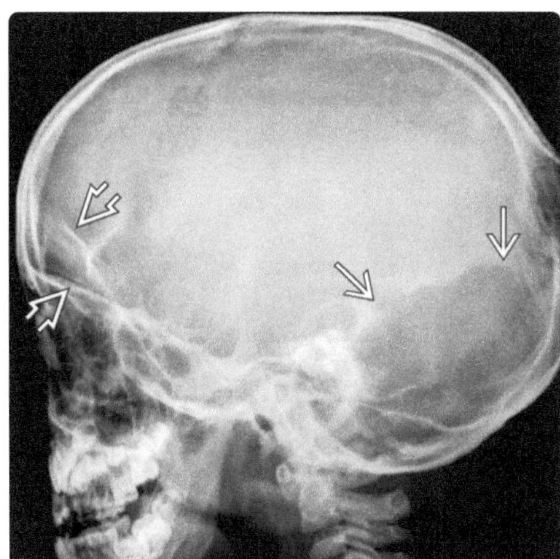

(Left) *Axial T1WI C+ MR shows a large optic pathway glioma involving the chiasm → and prechiasmatic optic nerves →* *in a child with NF1.* **(Right)** *Lateral radiograph in a child with a skull base PNF shows a large lambdoid defect →, a typical but rare lesion in children with NF1. Notice also the asymmetry in the orbital roofs →, secondary to unilateral orbital enlargement, typical of patients with sphenoid wing dysplasia and adjacent PNF.*

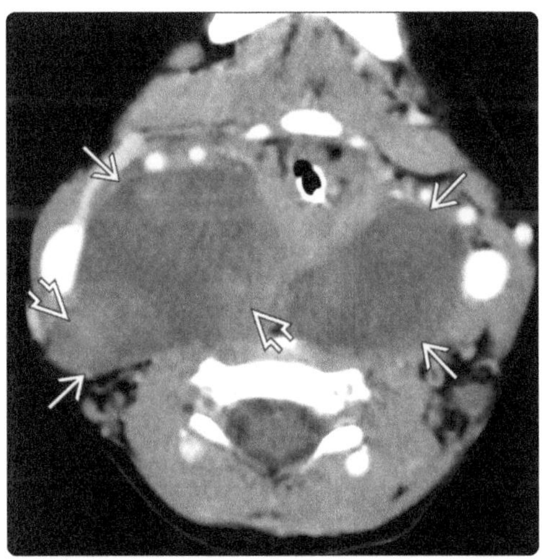

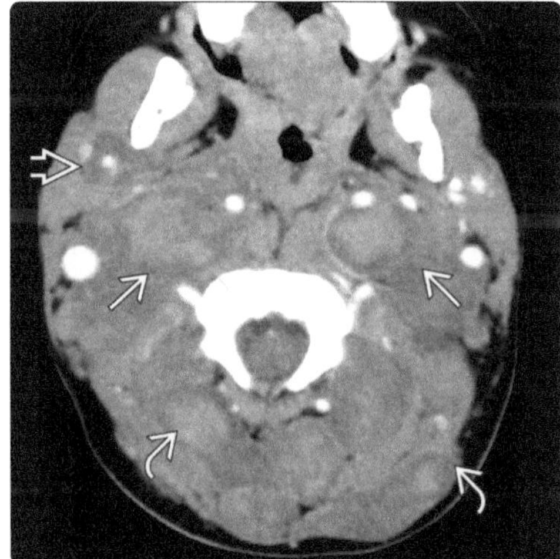

(Left) *Axial CECT in a child with NF1 shows the typical appearance of large carotid space neurofibromas →: Low in attenuation with only mild patchy contrast enhancement →.* **(Right)** *Axial CECT in a child with NF1 shows massive tumor burden with numerous neurofibromas involving the bilateral carotid spaces →, right parotid space →, and posterior cervical spaces →. Patchy central enhancement with a peripheral rim of less enhancement is not uncommon.*

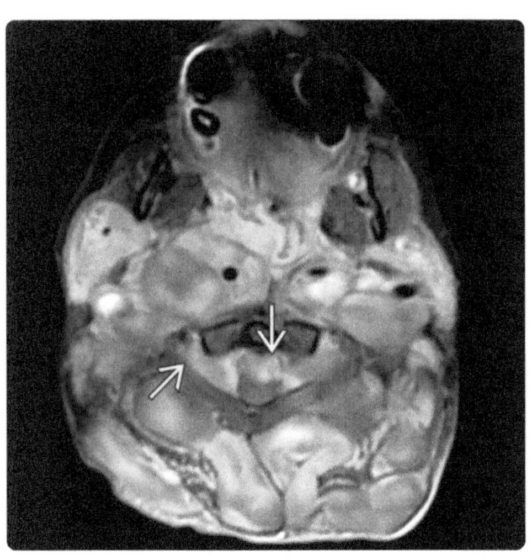

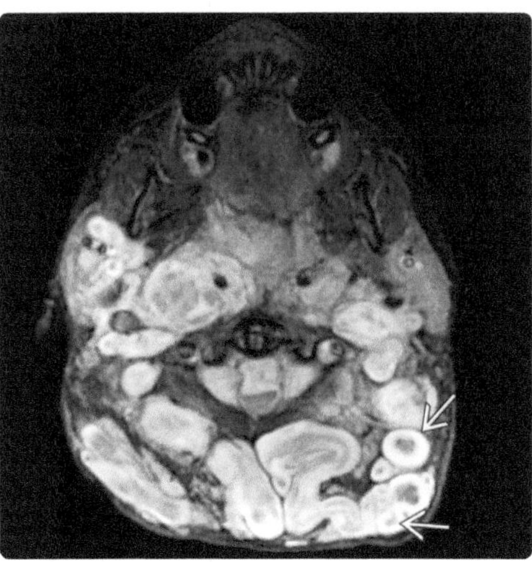

(Left) *Axial T1WI C+ FS MR in the same patient shows a similar pattern of contrast enhancement with patchy central enhancement and peripheral decreased enhancement. Notice also neural foraminal extension into the spinal canal →, compressing the upper cervical cord.* **(Right)** *All lesions are more conspicuous on axial STIR MR. Notice the typical target appearance to several lesions → and a more tram-track appearance to others, imaged along the long axis rather than a cross section through the neurofibroma.*

Brachial Plexus Schwannoma in Perivertebral Space

KEY FACTS

TERMINOLOGY

- Benign Schwann cell neoplasm that **arises from brachial plexus** (BP) in perivertebral space (PVS)

IMAGING

- Well-circumscribed, **fusiform mass** along course of BP
- Occurs along course of BP in any segment
- Intra- and extradural and neural foramen
- In PVS between anterior and middle scalene muscles
- 3D STIR with IV Gd contrast MR neurography for fat and water suppression, nerve visualization, and enhancement of lesions

TOP DIFFERENTIAL DIAGNOSES

- Systemic nodal metastases
- Neurofibroma
- Lateral meningocele
- Malignant peripheral nerve sheath tumor

PATHOLOGY

- Cystic degeneration and hemorrhage common
- Firm, encapsulated, fusiform mass
- Attaches to and displaces nerve
- Multiple schwannomas occur with multiple inherited schwannomas, meningiomas, ependymomas (MISME), and schwannomatosis

CLINICAL ISSUES

- 5% of benign soft tissue neoplasms
- Malignant degeneration rare, more common with multiple schwannoma syndromes
- Development of pain should raise suspicion for malignancy

DIAGNOSTIC CHECKLIST

- Key: Lesion localization along course of BP
- "Roots" and "trunks" of BP related to **interscalene triangle**, between anterior and middle scalene muscles

(Left) *Right parasagittal STIR MR shows an ovoid, hyperintense brachial plexus (BP) schwannoma in the perivertebral space (PVS) ➡ just lateral to the right C7 root extending outside from the right C6-C7 neural foramen.* **(Right)** *Axial non-fat-suppressed T1 C+ MR in the same patient shows that the enhancing lesion ➡ lies along the course of right BP within the interscalene triangle, splaying the anterior ⇨ and middle ⇨ scalene muscles. Note the normal left interscalene triangle fat/BP ➡ and scalene muscles.*

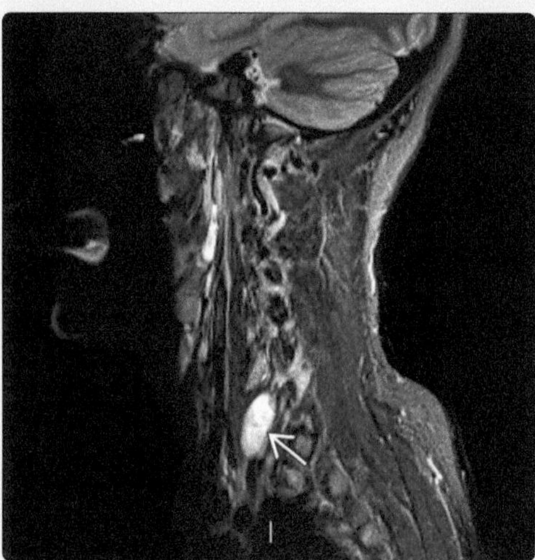

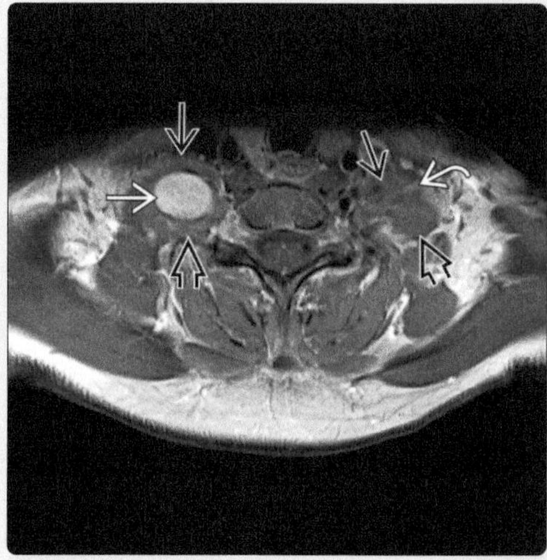

(Left) *Axial T1 C+ FS MR shows a BP schwannoma ➡ in the PVS with intense, irregular peripheral enhancement and central cystic degeneration. Note the internal jugular vein ➡ further anteriorly.* **(Right)** *Coronal STIR MR neurography in another patient demonstrates an asymmetrically enlarged right CNVIII nerve root ➡ extending from CNVII-T1 neural foramen. Note the marked hyperintensity as compared to adjacent BP elements ⇨ that the lesion parallels.*

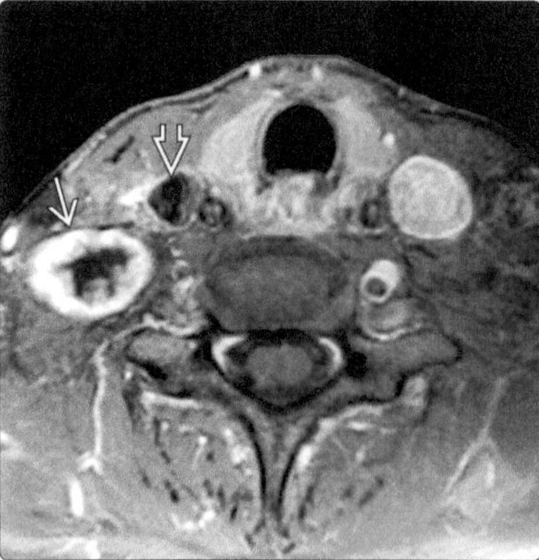

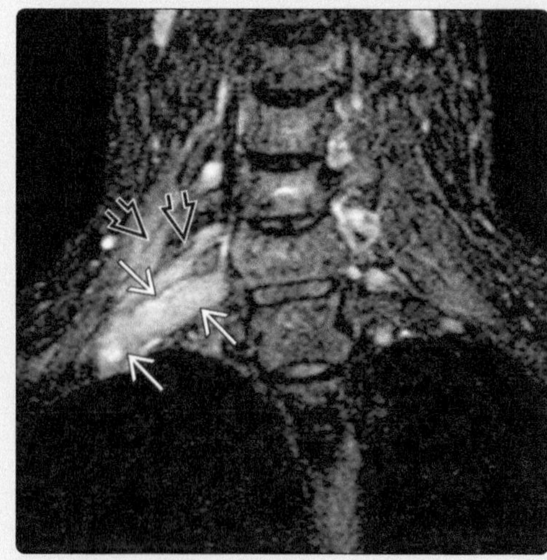

Brachial Plexus Schwannoma in Perivertebral Space

TERMINOLOGY

Abbreviations

- Brachial plexus (BP) schwannoma

Definitions

- Benign Schwann cell neoplasm that arises from BP in perivertebral space (PVS)
- PVS: Cylindrical space surrounding vertebral column bound by deep layer of deep cervical fascia (DL-DCF)
  - Subdivided at level of transverse processes into anterior prevertebral and posterior paraspinal components

IMAGING

General Features

- Best diagnostic clue
  - Well-circumscribed, fusiform mass along course of BP
- Location
  - Ventral rami of C5-T1 spinal nerves ± minor branches from C4 and T2 constitute "**roots**" **of BP**
    - Enter interscalene triangle between anterior and middle scalene muscles
    - Roots join to form "**trunks**"
  - In PVS, **C5, C6, C7 roots** of BP lie within upper aspect of **interscalene triangle** superior to subclavian artery and start forming **upper and middle trunks** as they pass through triangle
  - **C8, T1 roots** of BP first outside medial to triangle and then start forming **lower trunk** as they enter medial margin of triangle posterior to subclavian artery
- Morphology
  - Fusiform or dumbbell-shaped mass
  - Cystic degeneration and hemorrhage common

CT Findings

- NECT
  - Typically isodense to muscle; calcification uncommon
  - When paraspinal, bony neural foramen shows **smooth enlargement**
- CECT
  - Mild to moderate enhancement

MR Findings

- T1WI
  - **Fusiform mass**, isointense to muscle
- T2WI
  - Heterogeneously hyperintense
  - **Target sign**: Central hypointense, peripheral hyperintense signal
  - **Fascicular sign**: Multiple central hypointense foci
- STIR
  - 3D STIR to produce MR neurography
  - Post-Gd IV contrast STIR ↑ vascular signal suppression and ↑ nerve:muscle contrast ratio with enhanced visualization of BP and branch nerves
- T1WI C+
  - Moderate heterogeneous enhancement
    - **Intramural cysts and hemorrhage** common
  - More uniform enhancement when small

Imaging Recommendations

- Protocol advice
  - 3D STIR (fat suppression); STIR with Gd contrast (better water suppression, nerve visualization and lesion enhancement)
  - Diffusion-weighted imaging with background signal suppression (DWIBS)-based MR neurography
  - Diffusion tensor imaging (DTI) tractography

DIFFERENTIAL DIAGNOSIS

Systemic Nodal Metastases

- Supraclavicular nodes metastatic site for chest and abdominal disease
- Lower cervical nodes medial to anterior scalene muscle, adjacent to internal jugular vein

Neurofibroma

- **Most common primary tumor of BP**
  - Most common tumor of BP: Metastasis
- May be indistinguishable from schwannoma on MR
- Typically lower density on NECT, approaching water density
- **Cystic** degeneration and **hemorrhage uncommon**

Lateral Meningocele

- Fusiform cystic mass follows CSF density/intensity
- Contiguous with spinal canal

Malignant Peripheral Nerve Sheath Tumor

- Progressively enlarging, irregular, heterogeneous mass
- Typically associated with pain

PATHOLOGY

Microscopic Features

- Tumor arises from Schwann cells of nerve sheath
- Alternating regions of high cellularity (Antoni A) and loose, myxoid component (Antoni B)

CLINICAL ISSUES

Natural History & Prognosis

- Slow-growing lesion
- Malignant degeneration rare, more common with multiple schwannoma syndromes
- Development of **pain** should raise suspicion for **malignancy**

Treatment

- Surgical excision usually cures

DIAGNOSTIC CHECKLIST

Image Interpretation Pearls

- Key: Lesion localization along course of BP
- Roots and trunks of BP related to **interscalene triangle**, between anterior and middle scalene muscles

SELECTED REFERENCES

1. Szaro P et al: Magnetic resonance imaging of the brachial plexus. Part 1: anatomical considerations, magnetic resonance techniques, and non-traumatic lesions. Eur J Radiol Open. 9:100392, 2022
2. Sneag DB et al: Post-contrast 3D inversion recovery magnetic resonance neurography for evaluation of branch nerves of the brachial plexus. Eur J Radiol. 132:109304, 2020

Fibromatosis Colli

KEY FACTS

TERMINOLOGY

- **Sternocleidomastoid (SCM) tumor of infancy**
- Nonneoplastic SCM muscle enlargement in early infancy

IMAGING

- **Nontender** SCM muscle **enlargement** in infant
- No adjacent inflammation or significant adenopathy
- Location: Right > left; rarely bilateral
- US: Modality of choice when imaging required
  - Variable echogenicity
- CT: Enlarged muscle has similar attenuation to normal muscle pre- & post contrast
- MR: Variable signal, diffuse enhancement

TOP DIFFERENTIAL DIAGNOSES

- Myositis related to neck infection
  - Tenderness, cellulitis evident clinically
  - Adenopathy conspicuous
- Infantile hemangioma
  - Benign, intensely enhancing vascular neoplasm
- Systemic nodal metastases
  - Nodes deep to normal SCM muscle
- Primary cervical neuroblastoma
  - Close association with carotid sheath
- Rhabdomyosarcoma
  - More discrete mass with aggressive margins
- Teratoma
  - Often with fat, calcifications

CLINICAL ISSUES

- **Unilateral** longitudinal cervical neck mass
- Torticollis in up to 30%
- Mass appears within 2 weeks of delivery
- Usually **regresses by 8 months** of age
- ↑ in breech presentation & forceps delivery
- Occasionally, developmental dysplasia of hip
- Treatment: Physical therapy/stretching exercises to ↑ range of motion

(Left) *Longitudinal US in a 2-week-old infant shows typical fusiform enlargement of the left sternocleidomastoid (SCM) muscle with mildly increased echogenicity ➡ relative to the uninvolved portion of the muscle ⇨.* **(Right)** *Longitudinal US in a 24-day-old boy with a right-sided neck mass shows mild increase in echogenicity and fusiform enlargement of the right SCM ➡, consistent with fibromatosis colli. Compare to the normal left SCM ⇨.*

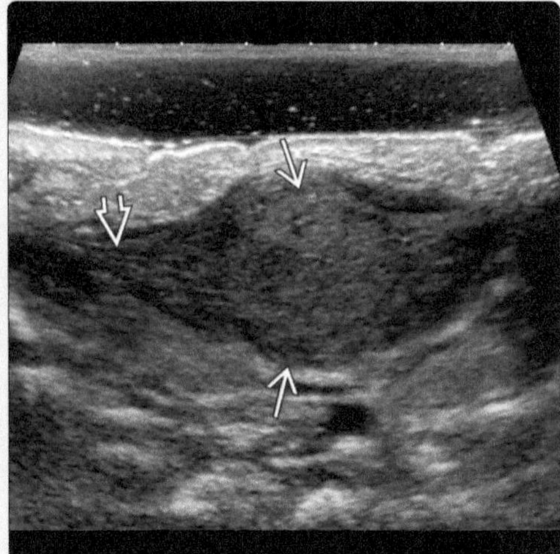

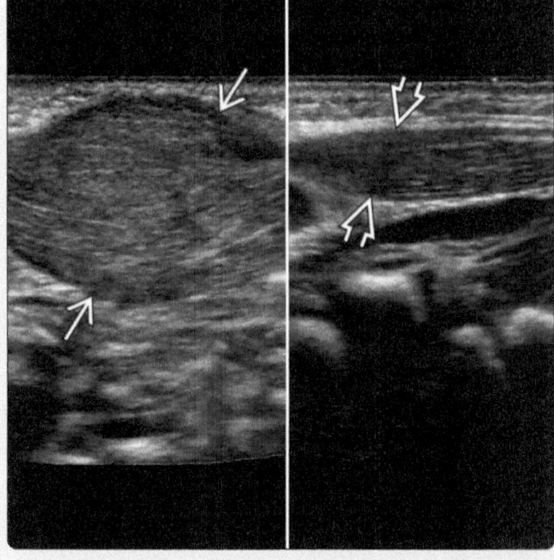

(Left) *Axial CECT in a 1-month-old girl with fibromatosis colli demonstrates diffuse enlargement of the right SCM muscle ➡ isodense to the normal contralateral SCM muscle ⇨. There is no extramuscular extension, overlying cellulitis, or associated adenopathy.* **(Right)** *Coronal T1 C+ FS MR in a 26-day-old boy shows diffuse enlargement and enhancement of the left SCM ➡ compared to the normal right SCM ⇨. Also notice mild torticollis with the head tilted to the left.*

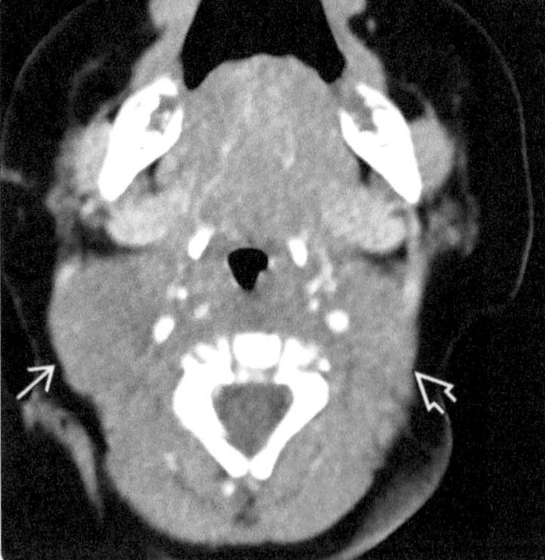

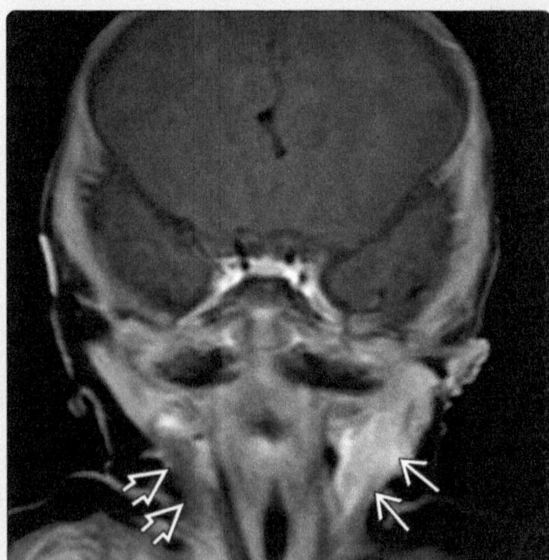

TERMINOLOGY

Synonyms

- **Sternocleidomastoid (SCM) tumor of infancy**
- **Congenital muscular torticollis**
  - Some literature includes 3 clinical subgroups
    - SCM tumor of infancy
    - Muscular torticollis: "Tightness" without mass
    - Postural torticollis: Torticollis without mass or "tightness"

Definitions

- Nonneoplastic SCM muscle enlargement in early infancy
- Postulated to be due to birth trauma, peripartum injury, in utero compartment syndrome, or maldevelopment
- Torticollis ("wry neck"): Twisting of neck such that ear on affected side is positioned lower & more midline than normal & chin turned to contralateral side

IMAGING

General Features

- Best diagnostic clue
  - **Nontender** SCM muscle enlargement in infant
  - Without extramuscular extension, inflammatory changes, or pathologic adenopathy
- Location
  - Mid to lower 1/3 of SCM muscle
    - Rarely, similar process involves trapezius muscle
  - **Right > left; rarely bilateral**
- Size
  - Variable
  - Usually spans much of cervical portion of SCM muscle
- Morphology
  - Fusiform SCM muscle enlargement, lacks surrounding inflammatory change and pathologic adenopathy

Radiographic Findings

- Radiography
  - Cervical spine radiographs may be obtained to exclude congenital or acquired bony abnormalities causing torticollis
  - Lytic changes in clavicular head at muscle attachment is rarely reported x-ray finding

Ultrasonographic Findings

- Grayscale ultrasound
  - Modality of choice when imaging is required
  - **Oval or fusiform SCM muscle enlargement**
  - Variable echogenicity
    - Hyperechoic or mixed echogenicity common
    - Hypoechoic peripheral rim may represent compressed normal muscle
  - **No** discrete extramuscular mass or adenopathy
  - Affected SCM muscle moves with respiration in same fashion as contralateral muscle
  - Affected SCM is shorter & thicker than contralateral side
    - Extended field of view imaging is useful to show entire length of SCM
    - Comparison to asymptomatic side useful
- Color Doppler
  - Variable hyperemia in acute phase, ↓ blood flow in fibrotic phase

CT Findings

- CECT
  - **Focal or fusiform enlargement of SCM muscle**
  - Similar attenuation to normal contralateral muscle
  - No inflammatory stranding in adjacent fat
  - No adenopathy or calcifications

MR Findings

- T1WI
  - **Focal or diffuse fusiform enlargement of SCM**
  - Variable signal: Iso- to hypointense vs. normal muscle
- T2WI
  - Variable signal intensity
    - Hyper- to isointense vs. other muscles
    - Zones of hypointensity at maximal enlargement, probably due to evolving fibrosis
  - Adjacent soft tissues normal
    - Be aware that incidental reactive nodal enlargement in infants is common
    - Presence of adjacent reactive nodes does not turn this pseudotumor into tumor
- T1WI C+
  - Affected muscle **enhances** heterogeneously

Imaging Recommendations

- Best imaging tool
  - Diagnosis frequently on clinical exam alone without imaging
  - US confirms clinical suspicion
  - MR recommended for atypical cases
- Protocol advice
  - Real-time US + clinical knowledge arrives at correct diagnosis

DIFFERENTIAL DIAGNOSIS

Myositis Related to Neck Infection

- Tenderness, cellulitis evident clinically
- + inflammatory changes & adenopathy

Infantile Hemangioma

- Intensely enhancing, benign vascular neoplasm with characteristic ↑ in size followed by spontaneous resolution
- Characteristic Doppler US appearance: > 5 vessels per cm^2, shows numerous low resistance arterial waveforms
- GLUT1 immunohistochemical marker **positive** in all phases of growth & regression
- If multiple, think PHACE(S) association

Systemic Nodal Metastases

- Pathologic appearance &/or number/size of cervical lymph nodes
- Non-Hodgkin lymphoma/leukemia
- Metastatic neuroblastoma

Primary Cervical Neuroblastoma

- Mild to moderately enhancing mass closely associated with carotid sheath
  - Usually posterior → anterior displacement of vessels
- ± calcification &/or adjacent metastatic lymphadenopathy

- Rarely intraspinal extension

Rhabdomyosarcoma

- Rare in newborns
- Up to 40% occur in head & neck
- Invasive soft tissue mass with variable enhancement, not confined to SCM
- ± bone erosion, metastatic adenopathy
- Transspatial mass common

Teratoma

- Complex density (CT) or signal intensity (MR) neck mass
- Solid & cystic components
- Often with fat, calcifications
- Frequently very large
  - May present with airway or feeding difficulties

Congenital Hemangioma (Rapidly, Non-, or Partially Involuting

- Present at birth or on prenatal imaging; does not proliferate after birth
- Solid, heterogeneous, less well-defined mass
- ± calcification, hemorrhage, necrosis
- GLUT1 immunohistochemical marker **negative**

Pseudomass From Contralateral Sternocleidomastoid Denervation

- CNXI injury → SCM & trapezius muscle atrophy
  - Contralateral normal SCM muscle may appear large
  - Uncommon in infants

PATHOLOGY

General Features

- Etiology
  - Unknown; several trauma theories → degeneration of fibers & fibrosis
    - Trauma → intramuscular hemorrhage &/or edema
    - Traumatic compression of neck during delivery → pressure necrosis or occlusion of venous outflow
    - Possibly precipitated by in utero head position & SCM compartment syndrome
  - ↑ in breech presentation & forceps delivery
- Associated abnormalities
  - Developmental dysplasia of hip, talipes equinovarus (clubfoot)
- When necessary, diagnosis can be confirmed by fine-needle aspiration cytology
  - Cytopathologists must be careful in interpreting cells as benign

Gross Pathologic & Surgical Features

- Seldom resected
- Fine-needle aspirates more common than excisional biopsy; both are uncommon
- Enlargement, fibrosis of affected SCM muscle

Microscopic Features

- Some skeletal muscle fibers atrophy or degenerate, & others have fibroblastic-myofibroblastic proliferation
- Cellularity variable: Early on more cellular; later develop ↑ collagen & ↓ cellularity
- Inflammatory changes rare

CLINICAL ISSUES

Presentation

- Most common signs/symptoms
  - Painless unilateral longitudinal cervical neck mass
  - Torticollis in up to 30%
- Other signs/symptoms
  - ↓ range of neck motion, facial asymmetry, plagiocephaly
- Clinical profile
  - Infant with nontender neck mass following breech or forceps delivery

Demographics

- Age
  - 70% present by 2 months of age; peak: 24 days
- Sex
  - Male patients slightly more than female patients
- Epidemiology
  - Affects 0.4% of infants

Natural History & Prognosis

- Mass appears within 2 weeks of delivery
- Mass may ↑ in size for days to weeks
  - Usually regresses by 8 months of age
- Up to 20% progress to muscular torticollis despite conservative therapy
- Patients with unsuccessfully treated torticollis may develop plagiocephaly

Treatment

- Physical therapy/stretching exercises to ↑ range of motion
- 90% full recovery with conservative treatment, physiotherapy
- Tenotomy for patients with refractory torticollis that fails conservative therapy

DIAGNOSTIC CHECKLIST

Consider

- History of traumatic birth? Mass confined to SCM muscle?
  - If answer to both is yes, DDx = fibromatosis colli
- Mass tender? Other clinical or imaging signs of inflammation?
  - If answer to both is yes, DDx likely neck infection
- Mass extending beyond margins of SCM muscle?
  - Consider rhabdomyosarcoma or other tumor

Image Interpretation Pearls

- Fusiform mass conforming to shape of SCM muscle = fibromatosis colli

SELECTED REFERENCES

1. Chauvin NA et al: Musculoskeletal imaging in neonates: use of ultrasound. Pediatr Radiol. 52(4):765-76, 2021
2. Durnford L et al: Bilateral sternocleidomastoid pseudotumors-a case report and literature review. Radiol Case Rep. 16(4):964-67, 2021
3. Rousslang LK et al: Fibromatosis colli leading to positional plagiocephaly with gross anatomical and sonographic correlation. BMJ Case Rep. 14(1), 2021
4. Navarro OM: Pearls and pitfalls in the imaging of soft-tissue masses in children. Semin Ultrasound CT MR. 41(5):498-512, 2020
5. Bansal AG et al: US of pediatric superficial masses of the head and neck. Radiographics. 38(4):1239-63, 2018

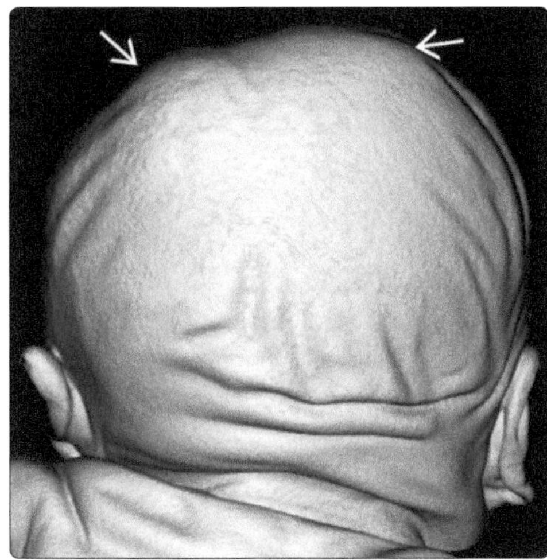

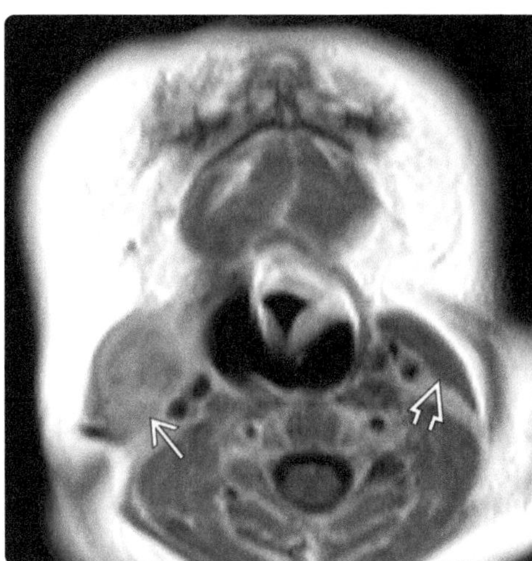

(Left) *Posterior 3D surface-rendered soft tissue CT in a child evaluated for bilateral cephalohematomas ➡ demonstrates incidental torticollis secondary to left SCM tumor of infancy (large left SCM not included).* **(Right)** *Axial T1 C+ MR shows prominent, mixed heterogenous enhancement of an enlarged right SCM muscle ➡ in a patient with fibromatosis colli who presented with a right neck mass. Note the normal left SCM muscle ➡.*

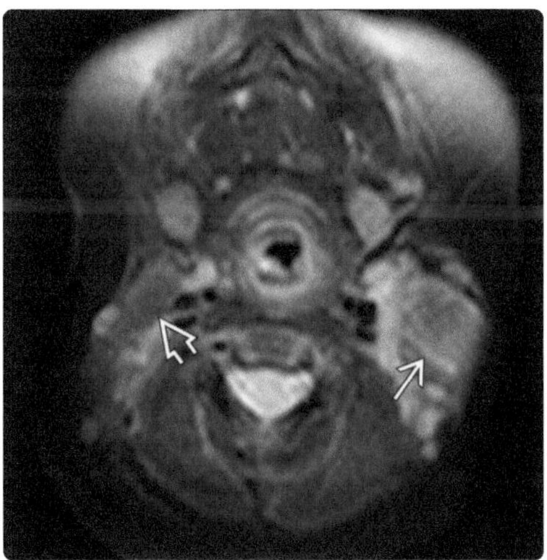

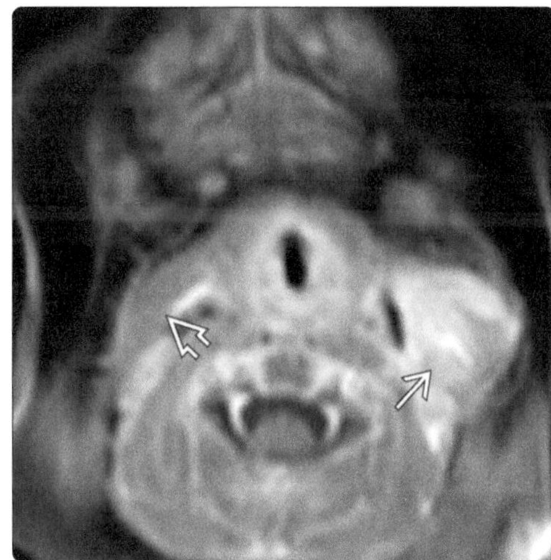

(Left) *Axial T2 TSE FS MR in a 1-month-old with a hard left neck mass without torticollis shows a heterogeneously hyperintense left SCM ➡ with a few small adjacent reactive lymph nodes. Note the normal size and signal intensity of the right SCM muscle ➡.* **(Right)** *Axial T1 C+ FS MR in the same child shows heterogeneous enhancement of the enlarged left SCM muscle ➡ compared to the normal right SCM muscle ➡.*

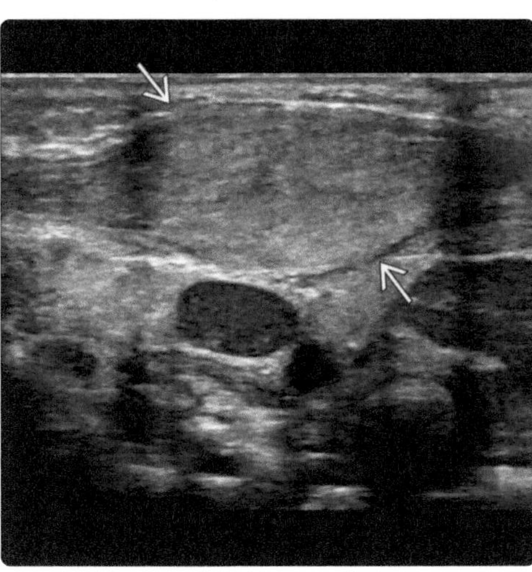

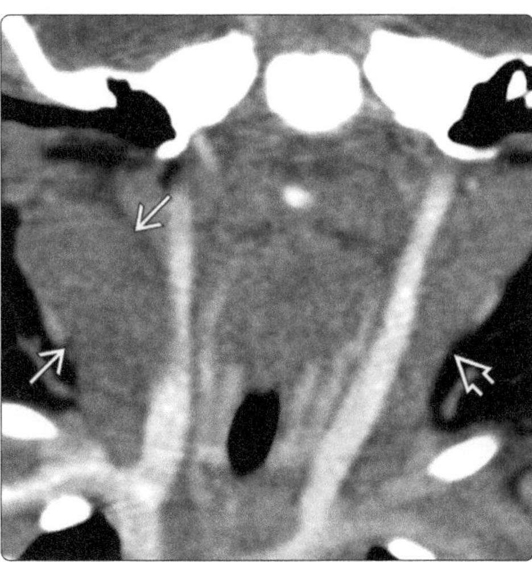

(Left) *Longitudinal US in a 21-day-old girl with a nontender neck mass shows fusiform enlargement and heterogeneous mildly hyperechoic echotexture of the SCM muscle ➡, consistent with fibromatosis colli.* **(Right)** *Coronal CECT in a 1-month-old with facial anomalies shows homogeneous thickening of the right SCM muscle ➡, isodense to the normal contralateral SCM muscle ➡. There is mild associated torticollis with asymmetry at the level of the external auditory canals.*

Rhabdomyosarcoma

KEY FACTS

TERMINOLOGY

- Rhabdomyosarcoma (RMS): Most common childhood soft tissue sarcoma

IMAGING

- Up to 40% occur in H&N
  - Orbital, parameningeal, other sites
- MR is best to
  - Characterize solid soft tissue mass
    - Often intermediate signal on T2 FS or STIR
    - Variable contrast enhancement
    - Typically restrict diffusion
  - Evaluate intracranial spread (requires contrast)
- CT is best to look for bone destruction or remodeling
- Neck imaging for cervical metastatic adenopathy
  - PET/CT may improve staging & treatment evaluation

TOP DIFFERENTIAL DIAGNOSES

- Infantile hemangioma
- Slow-flow vascular malformations
- Fibromatosis colli
- Metastatic neuroblastoma
- Langerhans cell histiocytosis
- Juvenile angiofibroma
- Nasopharyngeal carcinoma
- Non-Hodgkin & Hodgkin lymphoma
- Plexiform neurofibroma

PATHOLOGY

- 3 histologic subtypes
  - Embryonal RMS: Most common; young children
  - Alveolar RMS: 2nd most common; 15-25 years of age
  - Pleomorphic RMS: Least common; 40-60 years of age

CLINICAL ISSUES

- Presentation: 70% < 12 years of age; 40% < 5 years
- Treatment: Surgery, chemotherapy, ± radiation therapy

(Left) *Axial T2 FS MR in a 10-year-old girl shows an intermediate signal intensity mass ➔ in the superomedial right orbit, deviating the globe laterally, without bone destruction.* **(Right)** *Axial T1 C+ MR in the same patient shows heterogeneous enhancement of the mass ➔, which demonstrated moderate diffusion restriction (DWI image not shown). Biopsy confirmed embryonal rhabdomyosarcoma (RMS). The absence of bone destruction does not exclude RMS*

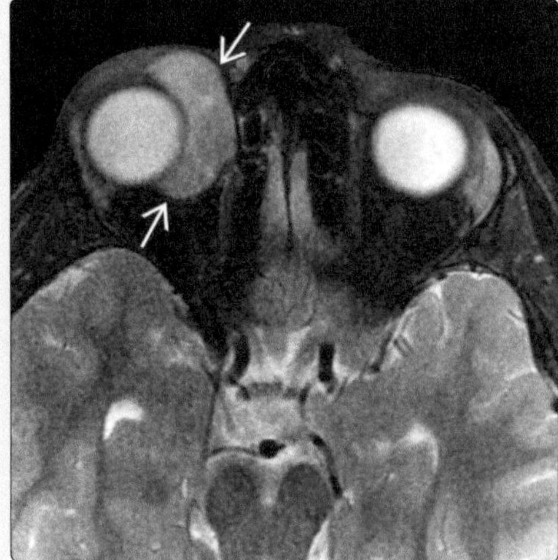

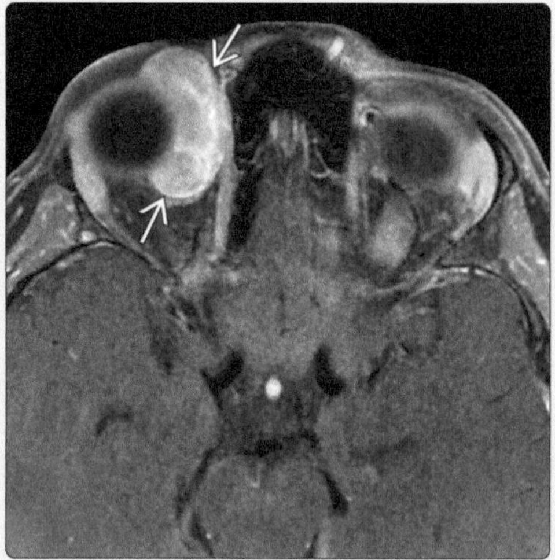

(Left) *Axial T1 C+ FS MR in a 15-month-old boy with intermittent epistaxis and swelling of the left nasal ala demonstrates a heterogeneously enhancing left intranasal/nasal alar mass ➔ obstructing the left nasal cavity.* **(Right)** *Axial STIR MR in the same patient demonstrates primarily intermediate signal intensity throughout the mass ➔ with the exception of a small cystic/necrotic region anteriorly ➔. Subsequent biopsy revealed an alveolar RMS.*

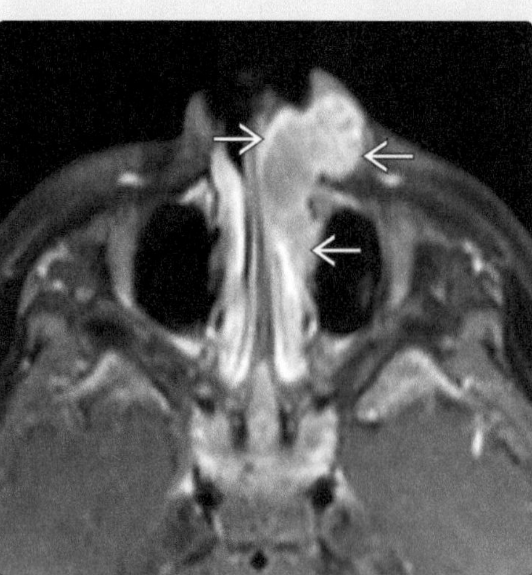

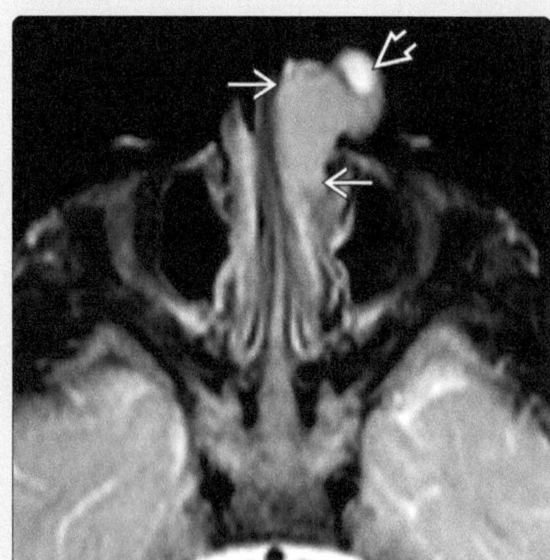

TERMINOLOGY

Definitions

- Rhabdomyosarcoma (RMS): Malignant neoplasm of mesenchymal origin
  - Most common childhood soft tissue sarcoma

IMAGING

General Features

- Best diagnostic clue
  - Solid soft tissue mass with variable enhancement
- Location
  - Up to 40% occur in H&N, including orbit, parameningeal sites, neck/face soft tissues, nasal cavity
    - Parameningeal sites: Middle ear, paranasal sinus, nasal cavity, nasopharynx, masticator space, pterygopalatine fossa, parapharyngeal space
      - Intracranial extension in up to 55%
      - Temporal bone involvement: Petrous apex & middle ear > mastoid
    - Orbit
    - All other H&N sites: Scalp, cheek, parotid, oral cavity, larynx, oropharynx, hypopharynx, thyroid/parathyroid

Ultrasonographic Findings

- Solid, firm mass with variable internal vascularity
- May show bone destruction in superficial masses

CT Findings

- Invasive soft tissue mass with variable enhancement
- Osseous erosion is common but not seen in all cases

MR Findings

- Isointense T1, hyperintense T2 signal relative to muscle
  - Not "fluid bright" unless necrotic/cystic components
- Variable contrast enhancement, often mild to moderate
  - Diffuse, intense enhancement is atypical
- Often restricts diffusion
  - ADC values range from ~ 0.5-1.3 x 10^{-3}/mm²
- ASL: Variable, but ↑ perfusion argues against benign low-flow vascular malformations

Nuclear Medicine Findings

- PET/CT
  - Hypermetabolic
    - May improve staging & posttreatment evaluation

Imaging Recommendations

- Best imaging tool
  - CT to evaluate osseous erosion
  - MR is best for soft tissue mass characterization
  - MR to evaluate perineural & intracranial spread of parameningeal RMS
    - Thickening & enhancement of nerves, leptomeninges
  - MR to distinguish between sinonasal tumor & obstructive/inflammatory disease
- Protocol advice
  - T2 FS or STIR MR: ↑ tumor conspicuity
  - Coronal T1 C+ FS MR: Detect intracranial extension
  - DWI MR: ADC values can help separate cellular tumor from benign vascular anomaly
  - Axial & coronal thin-section bone CT: Osseous erosion
  - Image neck: Rule out cervical metastatic adenopathy

DIFFERENTIAL DIAGNOSIS

Infantile Hemangioma

- Benign vascular neoplasm in infants, often with characteristic cutaneous involvement
- Intensely enhancing round or lobulated mass with high-flow vessels during proliferative phase
- ASL MR shows markedly ↑ perfusion
- ADC MR values typically range from ~ 1.3-1.6 x 10^{-3}/mm²
- No bone destruction
- Fatty infiltration during involuting phase

Slow-Flow Vascular Malformation

- May be well defined or extensive/infiltrative
- Fluid signal contents ± layering blood products, retracted clots, or phleboliths (in venous type)
- Venous type shows gradual patchy enhancement; lymphatic macrocystic type shows thin septal enhancement
- ADC values typically range from ~ 2.0-2.6 x 10^{-3}/mm²
- ASL MR will not show ↑ perfusion

Fibromatosis Colli

- Benign, self-limited, heterogeneous mass within & expanding midportion of sternocleidomastoid muscle in young infant with torticollis

Metastatic Neuroblastoma

- Most cervical disease is due to metastatic adenopathy rather than primary lesion
- Metastatic disease to skull/skull base is frequently bilateral: Enhancing masses surround aggressive osseous permeation/expansion with radiating spicules of new bone

Langerhans Cell Histiocytosis

- Enhancing soft tissue mass filling sharply marginated, punched-out lytic bone lesion
- Temporal bone: Mastoid > petrous apex & middle ear

Juvenile Angiofibroma

- Highly vascular mass causing nasal obstruction &/or epistaxis in adolescent males
- Intensely enhancing lesion with bone destruction & internal high-flow vessels
- Originates at sphenopalatine foramen on lateral nasal wall
- Often involves nasal cavity, nasopharynx, skull base, masticator space ± orbit, sinus, intracranial extension

Nasopharyngeal Carcinoma

- Nasopharyngeal mass in 2nd decade of life
- Variable contrast enhancement
- Central skull base erosion, widening of petroclival fissure, extension to pterygopalatine fossa + masticator & parapharyngeal spaces
- Unilateral or bilateral cervical & lateral retropharyngeal adenopathy

Non-Hodgkin Lymphoma

- Non-Hodgkin lymphoma (NHL) & Hodgkin lymphoma imaging findings are similar; difficult to differentiate
- Large, nonnecrotic nodes are typical

- Sinonasal, orbital, or nasopharyngeal NHL may cause osseous erosion

Plexiform Neurofibroma

- Benign peripheral nerve sheath tumor in neurofibromatosis type 1
- Lobulated masses with peripherally ↑ T2 signal & centrally ↓ T2 signal (target sign)
- Bone remodeling, typically without destruction

PATHOLOGY

General Features

- Etiology
  - Originates from primitive mesenchymal cells committed to skeletal muscle differentiation (rhabdomyoblasts)
- Genetics
  - ↑ incidence in children with *TP53* tumor suppressor gene mutation
  - PAX fusion-negative (embryonal) RMS has loss of heterozygosity at 11p15 locus
    - Up to 70% of childhood RMS
    - Better prognosis
  - PAX fusion-positive RMS is associated with balanced chromosomal translocations, most commonly t(2;13) have *FOXO1* to *PAX3* (or *PAX7*) gene fusion
- Associated abnormalities
  - ↑ incidence of RMS in Noonan syndrome
    - Hematologic malignancies & neuroblastoma are also seen
  - Rarely (~ 5%) associated with underlying cancer predisposition syndromes: Neurofibromatosis type 1, Li-Fraumeni, DICER1, Rubenstein-Taybi, Gorlin basal cell nevus, Beckwith-Wiedemann, or Costello
  - Rarely associated with hereditary retinoblastoma
  - May occur as radiation-induced 2nd primary neoplasm

Staging, Grading, & Classification

- Intergroup RMS (IRS) group classification prechemotherapy staging system
  - IRS-I: Tumor completely removed
  - IRS-II: a: Microscopic residual tumor; b: Involved regional nodes; c: Both
  - IRS-III: Gross residual tumor after incomplete resection or biopsy only
  - IRS-IV: Distant metastatic disease
- TNM: Tumor site, size, local invasion, lymph nodes, distant metastases
- Subtypes
  - PAX fusion-negative RMS (previously called embryonal RMS): Most common
    - Up to 70% of all pediatric RMS
    - Occurs in younger children
    - 70-90% occur in H&N or GU tract
  - PAX fusion-positive RMS (previously called alveolar RMS): 2nd most common
    - Usually occurs in patients 15-25 years of age
    - Most common in extremities & trunk
  - Spindle cell/sclerosing RMS
  - Pleomorphic RMS: Least common
    - Usually in adults 40-60 years of age; rarely < 15 years
    - Most arise in extremities; rarely in H&N

CLINICAL ISSUES

Presentation

- Most common signs/symptoms
  - Symptoms in H&N are variable, depend on location
    - Orbit: Mass, proptosis, ↓ vision
    - Sinonasal: Nasal obstruction, epistaxis; may present late with soft tissue facial mass
    - Temporal bone: Postauricular or external auditory canal mass, otitis media, CNVII palsy
    - Neck: Mass, pain, rarely airway compromise

Demographics

- Age
  - 70% < 12 years; 40% < 5 years

Natural History & Prognosis

- Favorable primary tumor sites: H&N, orbital, GU, biliary
- Unfavorable primary tumor sites: Parameningeal, extremities, bladder/prostate, trunk, chest wall, other sites
- Children's Oncology Group risk group assignment: Low, intermediate, & high risk
  - Based on fusion status, stage, & group
    - Fusion negative lower risk

Treatment

- Staging & risk stratification → treatment using risk-adapted approach
- Risk-group assignment based on pretreatment stage, IRS group, tumor biology, & patient age
- Chemotherapy ± surgery &/or radiotherapy
- Research ongoing in proton therapy, immunotherapy, & vaccination
- Sentinel node biopsy may improve treatment stratification

DIAGNOSTIC CHECKLIST

Consider

- Not always associated with bone destruction
  - Beware of enhancing soft tissue mass without bone destruction; may simulate infantile hemangioma (IH)
    - IH is almost always found in 1st year of life; RMS is more common > 12 months
    - IH is typically soft/compressible while RMS is more likely firm
    - IH demonstrates high density of low-resistance arterial vessels on color Doppler
    - IH enhances more intensely & homogeneously
    - IH has higher ADC values on DWI MR

SELECTED REFERENCES

1. Biswas A et al: Extraocular orbital and peri-orbital masses. Neuroimaging Clin N Am. 33(4):643-59, 2023
2. Mamlouk MD: Solid and vascular neck masses in children. Neuroimaging Clin N Am. 33(4):607-21, 2023
3. Maldonado FR et al: Quantitative characterization of extraocular orbital lesions in children using diffusion-weighted imaging. Pediatr Radiol. 51(1):119-27, 2021
4. Rogers TN et al: Management of rhabdomyosarcoma in pediatric patients. Surg Oncol Clin N Am. 30(2):339-53, 2021
5. Jawad N et al: The clinical and radiologic features of paediatric rhabdomyosarcoma. Pediatr Radiol. 49(11):1516-23, 2019

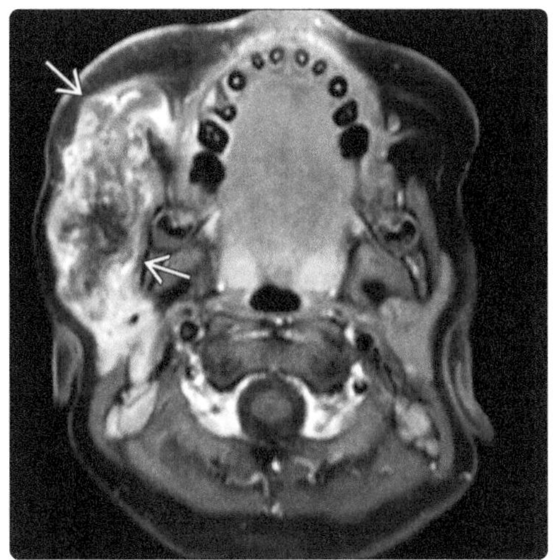

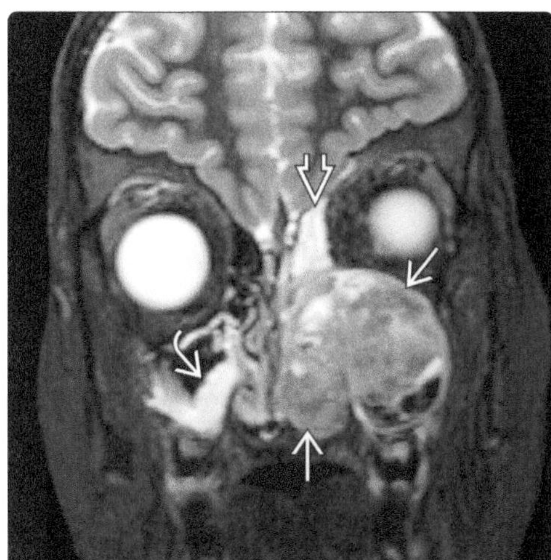

(Left) *Axial C+ FS MR in a 5-year-old with right-sided facial port-wine stain & recent facial swelling shows a necrotic mass inseparable from the right masseter muscle ➡. The lack of overlying cellulitis & reported unresponsive to antibiotics suggest that the lesion is not inflammatory & was biopsy-proven RMS.* **(Right)** *Coronal STIR MR helps differentiate tumor ➡ filling the expanded left maxillary sinus & nasal cavity from hyperintense, inflammatory mucosal disease in the left ethmoid ⇨ & right maxillary ↪ sinuses.*

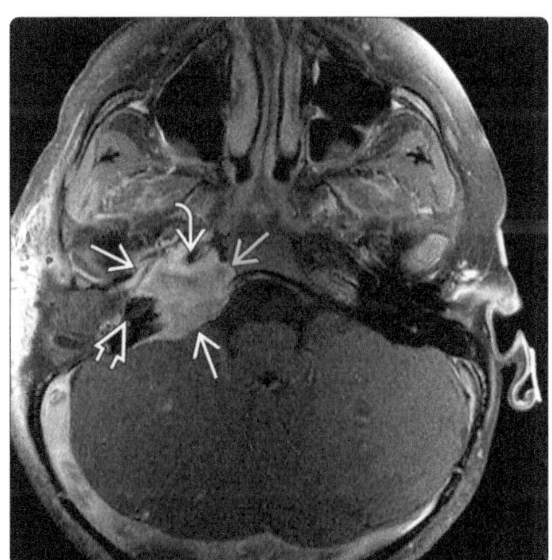

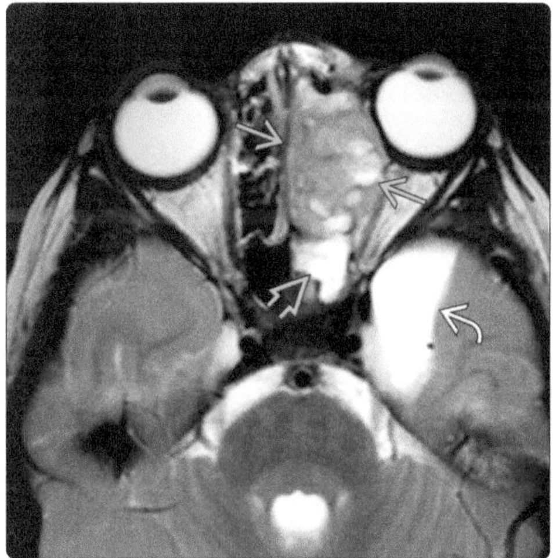

(Left) *Axial T1 C+ FS MR demonstrates a moderately enhancing RMS ➡ destroying the right petrous apex & otic capsule bone adjacent to the cochlea ⇨ & extending along margins of the internal carotid artery ↪ into the clivus ⇒.* **(Right)** *Axial T2 MR in a 5-year-old with left proptosis & palpable cervical adenopathy demonstrates a mixed intensity alveolar RMS ⇒, as compared to the hyperintense sphenoid sinus inflammatory disease ⇨ & incidental middle cranial fossa arachnoid cyst ↪.*

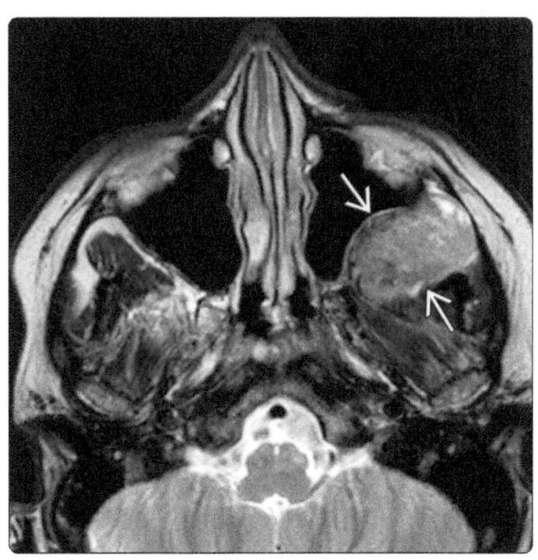

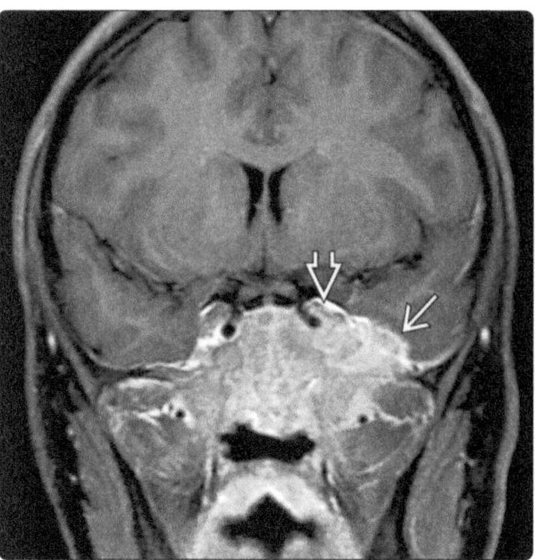

(Left) *Axial T2 MR in a 21-year-old with an embryonal RMS shows anterior bowing of the left maxillary sinus posterior wall by a heterogeneous, mildly hypointense left infratemporal fossa mass ➡, consistent with a highly cellular RMS. Although it is relatively hypointense without FS, it is hyperintense relative to skeletal muscle, typical of RMS.* **(Right)** *Coronal T1 C+ FS MR shows an extensive left skull base RMS with left middle cranial fossa extension (displacing the left temporal lobe ➡) and invasion of the left cavernous sinus ⇨.*

Melanotic Neuroectodermal Tumors

KEY FACTS

TERMINOLOGY

- Melanotic neuroectodermal tumor of infancy (MNTI): Rare, usually benign, locally aggressive pigmented tumor of infancy of neural crest cell origin
  - Rarely malignant with metastatic potential
- Synonyms: Melanotic progonoma, melanin-containing primitive neuroectodermal tumor

IMAGING

- Head, neck, CNS locations: Maxilla (most common), calvarium, mandible, orbit, CNS (vermis, pineal region)
- Plain films and CT: **Floridly ossified**, expansile occipitotemporal calvarial tumor with **hyperostosis**
- MR: **Ossification and melanosis** → pronounced tumor **hypointensity on T2WI**; may not be T1 hyperintense
- Nonossified soft tissue component in scalp and epidural space enhances

TOP DIFFERENTIAL DIAGNOSES

- **Infantile hemangioma**
  - Avidly enhancing vascular tumor; no bone destruction
- **Infantile fibrosarcoma**
  - Moderately to avidly enhancing, locally aggressive
- **Metastasis (e.g., neuroblastoma)**
  - Lytic ± permeative bony destruction

PATHOLOGY

- Brownish-black mass
- Positive neural, epithelial, and melanocytic markers

CLINICAL ISSUES

- Infant (< 1 year) with subcutaneous mass fixed to skin
- CNS tumors ± malignancy with CSF dissemination

DIAGNOSTIC CHECKLIST

- **Do not confuse** with **neurocutaneous melanosis**

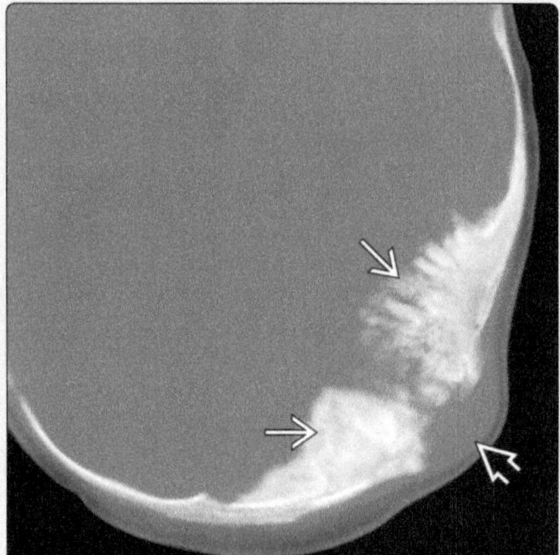

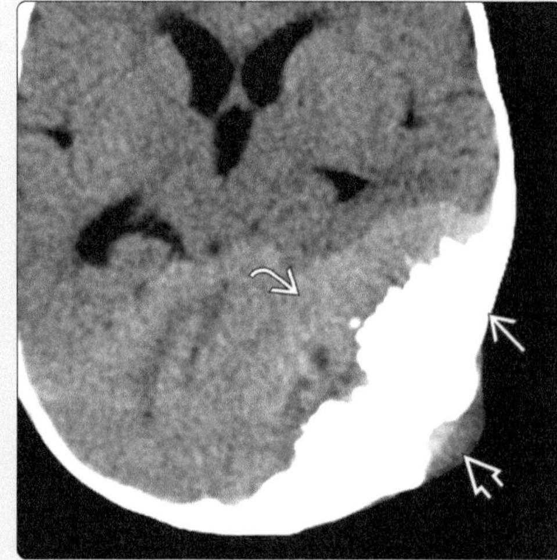

(Left) *Axial bone CT in a 6-month-old girl with melanotic neuroectodermal tumor of infancy shows an expansile tumor of the left temporal and occipital bones, which is characterized by florid, expansile new bone formation ➡. A small soft tissue component extends into the scalp ➡.* **(Right)** *Brain window NECT in the same patient shows a large, ossified tumor ➡. A soft tissue component involves the scalp ➡ with a large, isodense epidural soft tissue mass ➡ compressing the brain and causing mild hydrocephalus.*

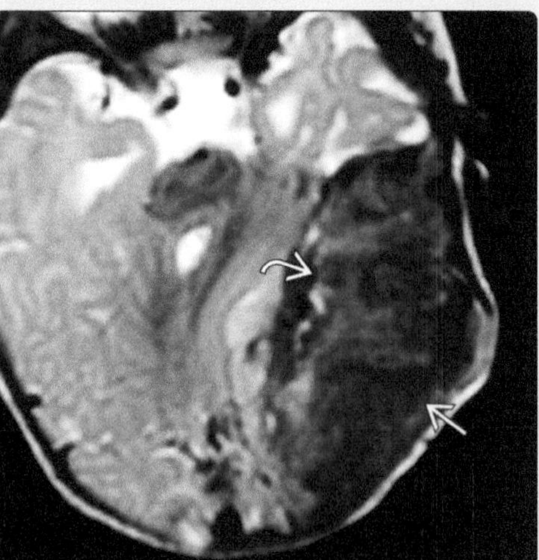

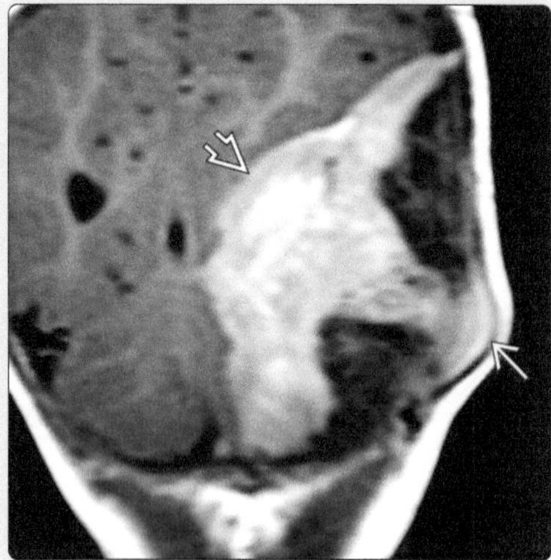

(Left) *Axial T2WI MR in the same patient interestingly shows that both the osseous ➡ and soft tissue ➡ components of the tumor display marked T2 hypointensity due to the bone and melanotic content.* **(Right)** *Coronal T1 C+ MR in the same patient distinguishes the enhancing extracranial ➡ and epidural ➡ soft tissue components from the osseous portion. These MR images also show a highly characteristic appearance for this rare and unusual tumor of infancy.*

TERMINOLOGY

Abbreviations

- Melanotic neuroectodermal tumor of infancy (MNTI)

Synonyms

- Melanotic progonoma, melanin-containing primitive neuroectodermal tumor, retinal anlage tumor

Definitions

- Rare, locally aggressive pigmented tumor of infancy
- **Do not confuse** with **neurocutaneous melanosis**

IMAGING

General Features

- Best diagnostic clue
  - Large, expansile tumor with florid ossification, hyperostosis, hypointensity on T2WI MR
- Location
  - Mainly maxilla (70%) and calvarium (11%), usually occipitotemporal and around anterior fontanelle
  - Mandible (6%), skull base, orbits, other head and neck sites, epididymis
  - Occasional CNS involvement (e.g., vermis, pineal region) ± CSF tumor dissemination

CT Findings

- Bone CT
  - Floridly ossified, expansile occipitotemporal tumor with adjacent hyperostosis
  - Soft tissue component in scalp and epidural space

MR Findings

- T1WI
  - Predominantly iso- or hypointense; rarely, only T1-hyperintense specks expected of melanin
  - Attributed to variations in amounts of melanin, connective tissue stroma, and melanosome maturity
    - Altering paramagnetic effects
- T2WI
  - Ossification and melanosis → marked tumor hypointensity; rarely, slight T2 hyperintensity
  - Look for mass effect from epidural component → hydrocephalus ± herniation
- T1WI C+ FS
  - Nonossified component enhances

Imaging Recommendations

- Best imaging tool
  - CT and plain films diagnostic
  - CT and MR provide complementary information

DIFFERENTIAL DIAGNOSIS

Infantile Hemangioma

- Avidly enhancing vascular tumor of infancy
- Bony destruction not feature apart from rare intraosseous lesion ± corticated margins

Infantile Fibrosarcoma

- Moderately to avidly enhancing, locally aggressive tumor with bony destruction

Metastasis

- Lytic ± permeative bony destruction, variable enhancement
- Neuroblastoma metastasis most common in infancy

Neurocutaneous Melanosis

- Rare congenital phakomatosis with giant or multiple cutaneous melanocytic nevi and CNS melanocytic lesions
- **CNS parenchymal** disease: **Benign melanosis** or **malignant melanoma**
  - Melanosis most common in anterior temporal lobes (amygdala), brainstem, cerebellum, and cerebral cortex
  - In hindbrain, melanosis associated with its hypoplasia
- **CNS leptomeningeal** disease: **Benign** leptomeningeal **melanosis** or **malignant** leptomeningeal **melanoma**

PATHOLOGY

Gross Pathologic & Surgical Features

- Macroscopic features: Brownish-black mass
- Microscopic features (biphasic)
  - Large, polygonal epithelioid cells with melanin deposits
  - Smaller, neuroblast-like hyperchromatic cells in dense, sclerotic fibrous stroma (neural crest origin)
- Immunohistochemical features
  - Expresses markers for tissues of neural, epithelial, and melanocytic origin
  - Cytokeratin, HMB45, S100, Ki-67, anti-CD99 and antivimentin antibodies positivity and anti-S100 antibody negativity

CLINICAL ISSUES

Presentation

- Most common signs/symptoms
  - Infant with subcutaneous mass fixed to skin
  - High urinary levels of vanillylmandelic acid (VMA) reported but not consistent finding

Natural History & Prognosis

- Usually benign but locally aggressive
- Rarely malignant with metastatic and recurrent potential

Treatment

- Complete surgical resection curative ± chemotherapy for rare malignant tumors
- No statistical correlation between locoregional tumor recurrence rate and resection margins
  - Hence, conservative surgical approach avoiding functional and aesthetic sequelae may be considered

DIAGNOSTIC CHECKLIST

Image Interpretation Pearls

- **Infant** with **floridly ossified**, expansile occipitotemporal calvarial tumor with **hyperostosis** and **enhancing**, nonossified **epidural soft tissue** component

SELECTED REFERENCES

1. Zhang C et al: Melanotic neuroectodermal tumor of infancy in the epididymis: a case report. Int J Surg Pathol. ePub, 2023
2. de Sousa ALA et al: Melanotic neuroectodermal tumor of infancy: the use of immunohistochemical analysis. Acta Stomatol Croat. 56(2):176-82, 2022

Orbital Neurofibromatosis Type 1

KEY FACTS

TERMINOLOGY

- Neurocutaneous disorder (inherited tumor syndrome) with distinct orbitocranial manifestations

IMAGING

- Constellation of features pathognomonic of NF1
  - Plexiform neurofibroma (PNF)
  - Optic nerve glioma (ONG)
  - Sphenoid dysplasia (SD)
  - Buphthalmos
  - Optic nerve sheath ectasia
- Orbitofacial NF1 typically unilateral

TOP DIFFERENTIAL DIAGNOSES

- **PNF**
  - Rhabdomyosarcoma, infantile hemangioma, Langerhans cell histiocytosis, venolymphatic malformation
- **ONG**
  - Glioma without NF1, optic nerve sheath meningioma
- **SD**
  - Congenital cephalocele, traumatic cephalocele
- **Buphthalmos**
  - Congenital glaucoma, coloboma
- **Optic nerve sheath ectasia**
  - Normal variant, intracranial hypertension

PATHOLOGY

- Autosomal dominant, 50% new mutations

CLINICAL ISSUES

- Presentation: Periorbital masses, proptosis, and ptosis
- **Lisch nodules of iris**: Pigmented melanocytic hamartomas
- Natural history: Progressive orbitofacial deformity & progressive visual & ophthalmologic dysfunction

DIAGNOSTIC CHECKLIST

- Orbital NF1 manifestations progressive, develop over time
- Rapid change in PNF concerning for malignant sarcomatous degeneration

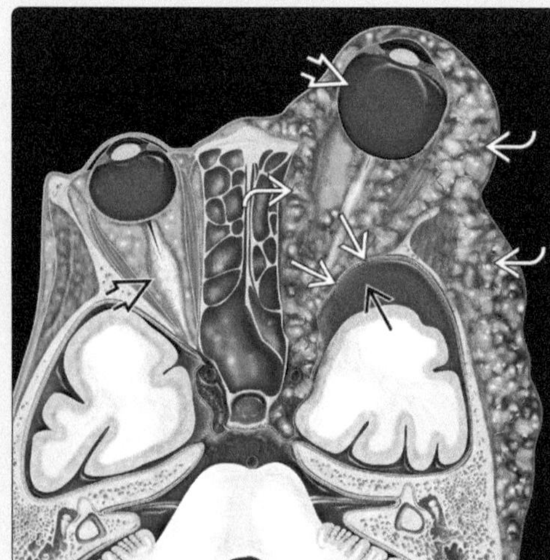

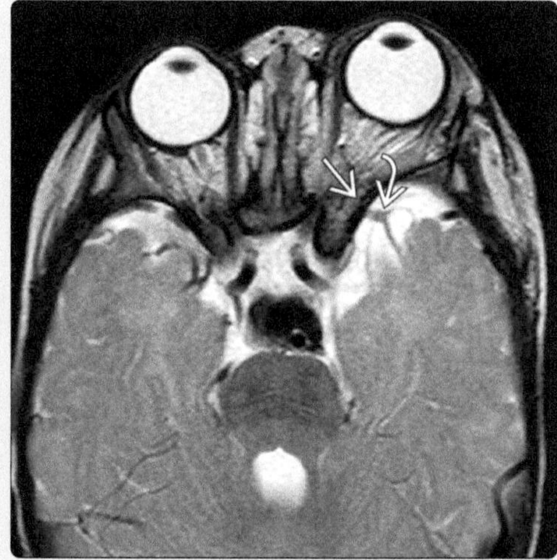

(Left) *Axial graphic depicts features of orbital neurofibromatosis type 1 (NF1), including sphenoid wing dysplasia ➡ with arachnoid cyst protruding through the bony defect ➡. Extensive plexiform neurofibromas (PNFs) are shown ➡ as well buphthalmos ➡. An optic nerve glioma ➡ is evident on the right.* **(Right)** *Axial T2WI MR in a child with NF1 shows left sphenoid wing dysplasia ➡ with proptosis and mildly enlarged eye globe. Note the prominent anterior temporal pole subarachnoid space with blood vessels ➡ traversing it.*

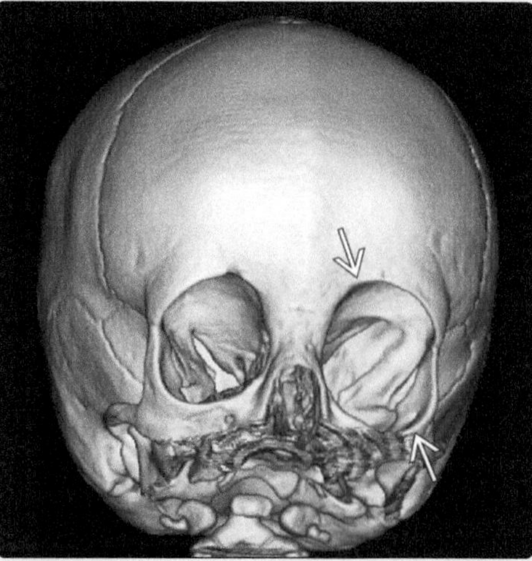

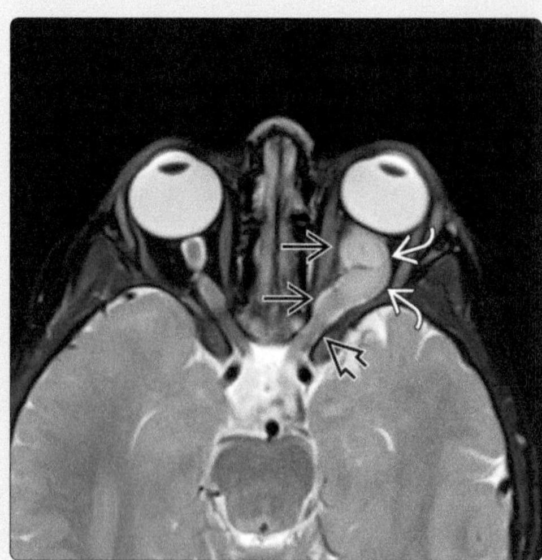

(Left) *3D bone CT in the same patient shows an enlarged left orbit with egg-shaped contour of the anterior orbital rim ➡.* **(Right)** *Axial FS T2WI MR of the orbits in a patient with NF1 shows a tortuous fusiform left optic nerve glioma involving the intraorbital ➡ and canalicular segments ➡. Notice a thin layer of slightly T2-hyperintense perineural arachnoid gliomatosis (PAG) ➡. PAG may enhance moderately (not shown) with contrast.*

TERMINOLOGY

Abbreviations

- Neurofibromatosis type 1 (NF1)

Synonyms

- von Recklinghausen disease

Definitions

- **Neurocutaneous disorder** (inherited tumor syndrome) with distinct orbitofacial & cranial manifestations

IMAGING

General Features

- Best diagnostic clue
  - Constellation of orbital, skull base, & intracranial features **pathognomonic** of NF1
- Location
  - Orbitofacial NF1 typically **unilateral**
- Morphology
  - **Plexiform neurofibroma** (PNF)
    - Serpentine, unencapsulated, infiltrative masses
    - May involve intraorbital branches of cranial nerves (III, IV, V1, VI) & sclera
    - Associated enlargement of skull base foramina
  - **Optic nerve glioma** (ONG)
    - Tubular or lobular enlargement of optic nerve (ON)
    - May involve any segment of nerve
    - May extend posterior to chiasm & brainstem
  - **Sphenoid dysplasia** (SD)
    - Bony defects, decalcification, or remodeling of greater sphenoid wing & lateral orbital wall
    - Enlargement of middle cranial fossa (MCF) with herniation of intracranial contents into orbit
    - Associated MCF arachnoid cyst common
  - **Buphthalmos (ox eye)**
    - Increased axial AP globe diameter
    - Remodeling & enlargement of anterior orbital rim
    - Thickening of uveal/scleral layer
  - **ON sheath ectasia**
    - Nontumorous enlargement of dural sheath
    - Increased CSF surrounding ON

Radiographic Findings

- Radiography
  - **Bare orbit** sign: Absence of innominate line (superior border of greater wing of sphenoid in frontal view)
  - Enlarged **egg-shaped** anterior orbital rim
  - **Harlequin eye** appearance: Innominate line appears as elevated dense ridge; rarely in NF1 SD
    - Classically, sign of coronal craniostenosis
  - Optic canal &/or superior orbital fissure enlargement

CT Findings

- NECT
  - **PNF**: Hypodense, **infiltrative** soft tissue masses
    - Overall higher CT density of orbital fat due to superimposed small PNF of cranial nerve branches
  - **ONG** or **dural ectasia**: Enlarged nerve/sheath contour
  - **SD**: Bony **defect** with **herniation** of MCF contents into orbit; proptosis may be marked

MR Findings

- T1WI
  - **PNF**: Hypointense, **ill-defined** soft tissue masses
  - **ONG**: Isointense ON mass ± **cystic** hypointensity
- T2WI
  - **PNF**: Hyperintense nodular masses with central low-signal **target sign**
  - **ONG**: Hyperintense **fusiform** ON mass
    - **Perineural arachnoid gliomatosis (PAG)**: Astrocytic proliferation in subarachnoid space (T2 hyperintense)
  - **Buphthalmos**: Enlarged globe, thickened uvea/sclera
  - **Nerve sheath ectasia**: **Increased perioptic CSF**
- T1WI C+
  - **PNF**: Irregular infiltrative **serpentine** masses; variable enhancement, may be intense
  - **ONG**: Variable enhancement; **PAG** moderately **enhances**
    - Isolated non-NF1 ONG often enhances more

Ultrasonographic Findings

- **PNF**: Irregular, compressible, **highly** reflective
- **ONG**: Smooth nerve enlargement, **minimally** reflective
- **SD**: Defect of posterior bony orbital wall
- **Buphthalmos**: Increased eye diameter

Imaging Recommendations

- Best imaging tool
  - MR ideal for assessment of orbital, extracranial, & intracranial lesions
  - CT to assess skull base defects & surgical planning

DIFFERENTIAL DIAGNOSIS

Plexiform Neurofibroma

- Rhabdomyosarcoma
- Infantile hemangioma
- Langerhans cell histiocytosis
- Leukemia
- Venolymphatic malformation

Optic Nerve Glioma

- Optic pathway glioma (isolated)
- ON sheath meningioma

Sphenoid Dysplasia

- Congenital sphenorbital cephalocele
- Posttraumatic sphenoid cephalocele

Buphthalmos

- Congenital glaucoma
- Coloboma

Optic Nerve Sheath Ectasia

- Normal variant
- Idiopathic intracranial hypertension
- ON sheath meningioma

PATHOLOGY

General Features

- Etiology
  - Disorder of histogenesis, classified as neurocutaneous inherited tumor syndrome
- Genetics

- **Autosomal dominant**; variable expression
- 50% **new mutations**; gene locus = 17q11.2
- Loss of NF1 **tumor suppressor** gene function
- Associated abnormalities
  - **CNS tumors** on brain imaging
  - Nonneoplastic foci of abnormal signal intensity **(FASI)**
  - Diffuse soft tissue neurofibromas; skeletal deformities

Gross Pathologic & Surgical Features

- **PNF**
  - Worm-like, infiltrating, tortuous masses
  - May involve eyelid, anterior periorbita, scalp, orbit, temporal fossa, & skull base
- **ONG**
  - Diffuse nerve enlargement; tan-white tumor
  - Cystic component with mucinous changes
  - 2 growth patterns: Intraneural & perineural forms; rarely, both coexist
  - **Intraneural form** shows fusiform enlargement of nerve
  - **PAG** shows astrocytic proliferation in subarachnoid space surrounding relatively preserved ON
- **SD**
  - Bony defect of posterior lateral orbit
  - MCF expansion with arachnoid cyst
- **Buphthalmos**
  - Associated with PNF in anterior orbit
  - Enlargement of anterior orbital rim

Microscopic Features

- **PNF**
  - Myxoid endoneural accumulation early
  - Schwann cell proliferation, collagen accumulation
- **ONG**
  - Spindle-shaped astrocytes with hyperplasia of fibroblasts & meningothelial cells
- **SD**
  - Bone decalcification; premature suture closure
- **Buphthalmos**
  - Periscleral infiltration by plexiform tumors

CLINICAL ISSUES

Presentation

- Most common signs/symptoms
  - Infiltrative periorbital masses, proptosis, & ptosis
  - **Lisch nodules of iris**: Clinically seen pigmented melanocytic hamartomas; incidence increases with age
    - 5% at age < 3 years; 55% at 5-6; 100% at > 21 years
- Other signs/symptoms
  - **PNF**
    - Bulky soft tissue masses; **bag-of-worms** texture
    - PNF anywhere indicative of NF1
  - **ONG**
    - Visual deficit, often relatively **mild**
    - Proptosis associated with poor vision
  - **SD**
    - **Pulsatile exophthalmos** due to orbital encroachment by middle fossa contents
  - **Buphthalmos**
    - Enlarged eye; impaired vision, glaucoma
- Clinical profile
  - Child with progressive proptosis, visual impairment, soft tissue masses, & cosmetic deformities
  - **Successive generations** of orbital NF1 have **earlier onset** & **more severe** amblyopia, expanding bony orbit & motility disorders than their parents or grandparents
    - Also associated with many **novel** NF1 gene **mutations**

Demographics

- Age
  - Findings may not be evident at birth
  - Cutaneous signs present at birth or 1st year
  - Tumors begin to appear in childhood
- Sex
  - No significant predilection
- Epidemiology
  - NF1 **most common** inherited tumor syndrome
  - Prevalence 1:2,500-5,000
  - Orbital involvement in up to 1/3 of NF1 patients

Natural History & Prognosis

- Orbital NF1 developmental lesions **progressive** over time rather than simply congenital defects
- PNF may undergo **sarcomatous degeneration** to malignant peripheral nerve sheath tumor (2-16%)

Treatment

- **PNF**
  - Generally not surgically curable due to infiltrative nature
  - Anterior orbit & eyelid procedures most common
  - Debulking may be required for vision or cosmesis
  - Radiation therapy not effective
- **ONG**
  - Observation unless vision threatened
  - Chemotherapy when progression occurs
  - Surgery challenging and performed when no useful vision or to treat corneal exposure or proptosis
  - Radiation not recommended in children
    - Risk of secondary tumors, moyamoya syndrome, & neurocognitive sequelae
- **SD**
  - Transcranial reconstruction with bone grafts for severe posterior defects
  - Management of resultant proptosis; may ultimately require enucleation
  - Debulking of associated PNF
- **Buphthalmos**
  - Medical ± surgical therapy for glaucoma

DIAGNOSTIC CHECKLIST

Consider

- Although NF1 is inherited disorder, orbital manifestations are progressive & develop over time

Image Interpretation Pearls

- Rapid change in PNF; consider sarcomatous degeneration

SELECTED REFERENCES

1. Senthilkumar VA et al: Lisch Nodules. In: StatPearls [Internet]. Treasure Island (FL): StatPearls Publishing; 2023
2. Chai P et al: Clinical characteristics and mutation Spectrum of NF1 in 12 Chinese families with orbital/periorbital plexiform Neurofibromatosis type 1. BMC Med Genet. 20(1):158, 2019

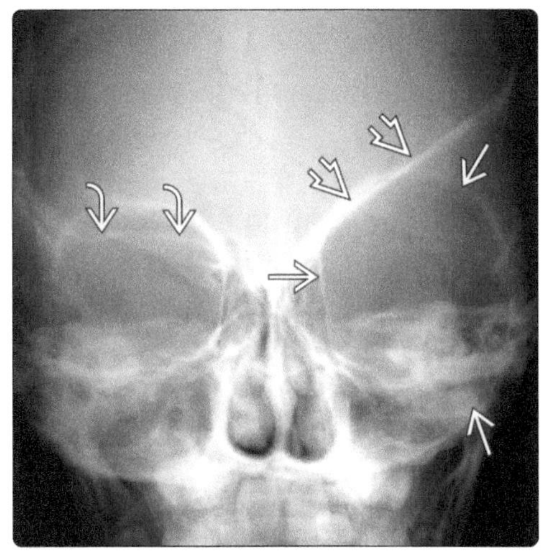

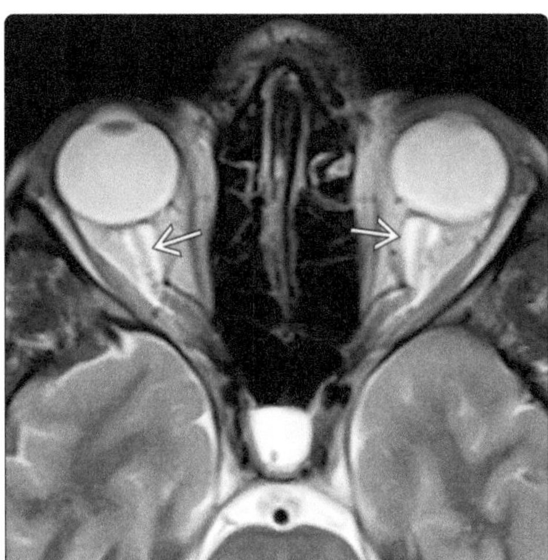

(Left) *AP radiograph in a child with NF1 and sphenoid wing dysplasia shows enlargement of the left orbital rim ➡. The normal contour of the greater wing of the sphenoid is distorted and displaced ➡ in contrast to the normal appearance on the right ➡.* **(Right)** *Axial T2WI MR in a patient with NF1 but no orbital masses shows ectasia of the optic dural sheaths, which manifest as increased CSF signal surrounding the intraorbital segments of the optic nerves bilaterally ➡.*

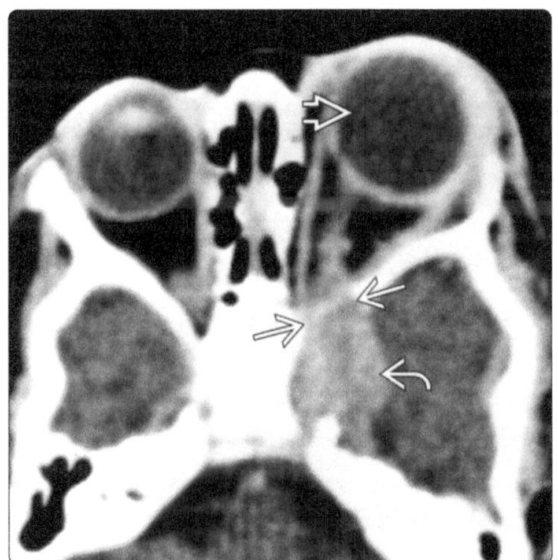

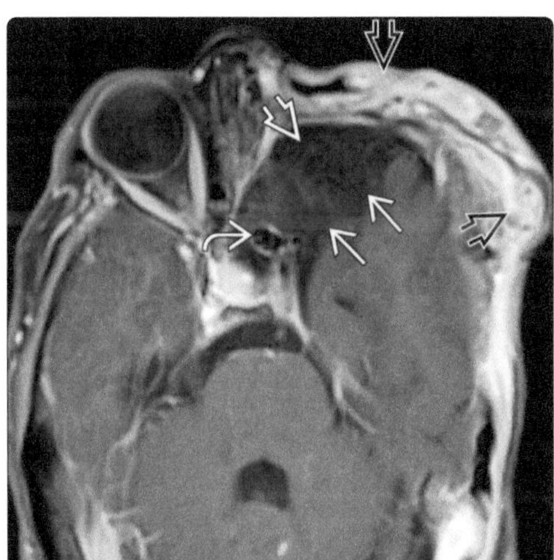

(Left) *Axial CECT in a young girl shows mild sphenoid dysplasia with widening of the superior orbital fissure ➡ and a neurofibroma extending into the central skull base ➡. The left eye globe shows buphthalmos ➡.* **(Right)** *Axial T1WI postcontrast MR in the same patient 2 decades later shows a massive sphenoid defect ➡, demonstrating the progressive nature of disease. Note herniation of a large associated arachnoid cyst ➡ (no blood vessels traversing it) into the orbit. Note soft tissue PNF ➡ & incidental internal carotid artery aneurysm ➡.*

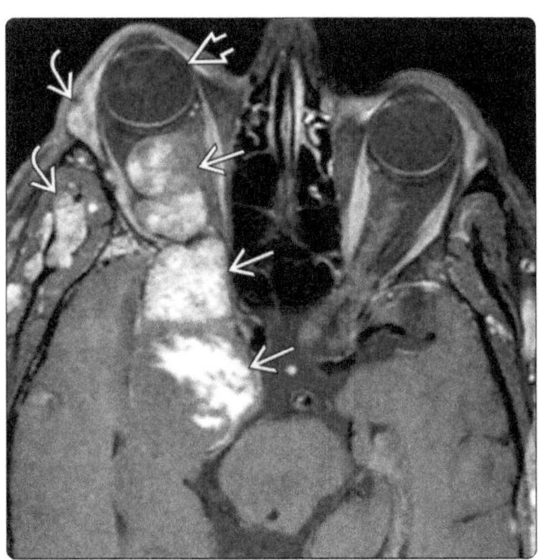

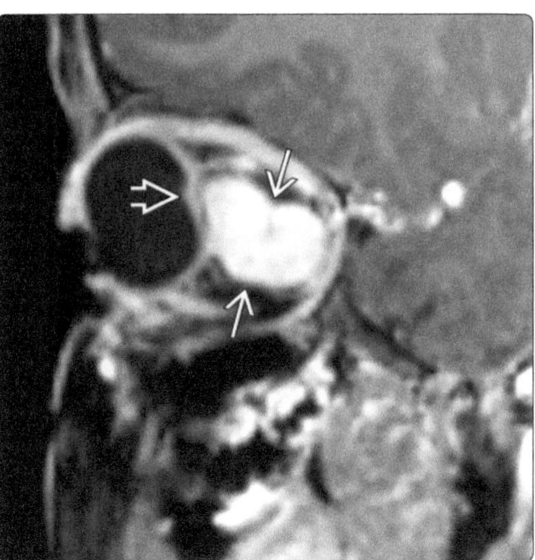

(Left) *Axial T1WI postcontrast MR in an NF1 patient shows patchy enhancement of large orbital and skull base neurofibromas ➡. Right eye globe is severely proptotic ➡. Extracranial plexiform tumors in the orbitotemporal regions ➡ are also seen.* **(Right)** *Sagittal FS T1WI MP-RAGE MR shows enhancing intraorbital optic nerve glioma ➡. Note the elevated optic papilla with a tiny enhancing focus due to papilledema ➡ (not tumor), which disappeared after chemotherapy when the lesion reduced in size (not shown).*

PART III
SECTION 1

Congenital and Genetic Disorders

Congenital

Scoliosis and Kyphosis

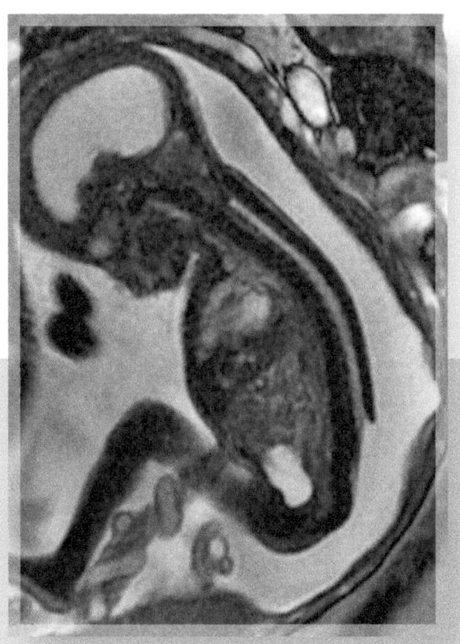

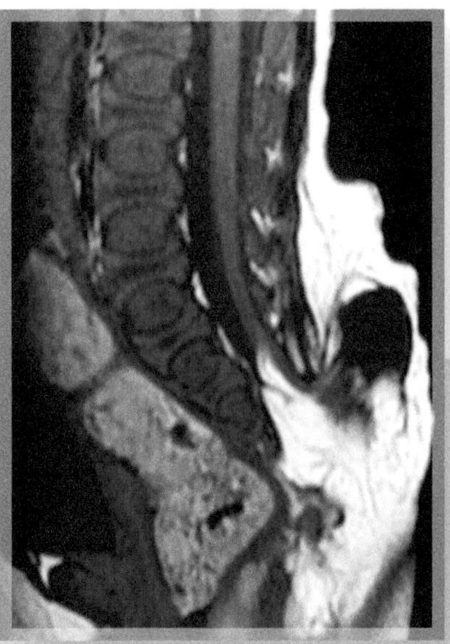

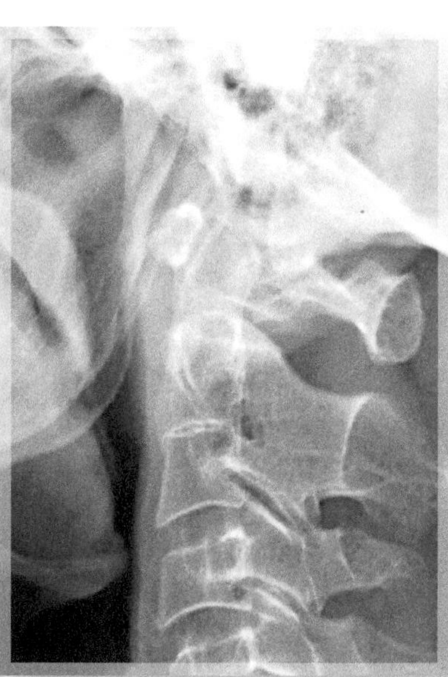

Filum Terminale Fibrolipoma

KEY FACTS

TERMINOLOGY

- Synonyms: Fibrolipoma of filum terminale, fatty filum terminale, "fat in filum"
- Asymptomatic presence of fat within otherwise normal-appearing filum terminale

IMAGING

- Linear fat signal/density within filum terminale
- Conus termination at normal position
- No additional tethered cord imaging stigmata

TOP DIFFERENTIAL DIAGNOSES

- Intraspinal lipoma
- Tethered spinal cord
- Lipomyelocele
- Epidermoid/dermoid cyst
- Subarachnoid hemorrhage
- Tumor with paramagnetic effects

PATHOLOGY

- Small focus of fat detected within otherwise normal filum terminale
  - Typical adipose tissue on gross pathology, microscopy
  - Incidentally detected in 4-6% of autopsy subjects
- No cutaneous stigmata on lower back with asymptomatic filum fibrolipoma

CLINICAL ISSUES

- Asymptomatic, incidental finding by definition
- Incidental finding in 4-6% of autopsy subjects

DIAGNOSTIC CHECKLIST

- Symptomatic patient implies diagnosis of intraspinal lipoma, not asymptomatic fibrolipoma
- Consider intraspinal lipoma if larger lesion, symptomatic, filum > 2 mm in thickness

(Left) *Sagittal graphic of the lumbosacral spine demonstrates extensive fatty infiltration* ➡ *of the filum terminale. The spinal cord conus* ⇨ *terminates at the normal L1-L2 level.* **(Right)** *Sagittal T1 MR depicts fatty infiltration of the filum terminale* ➡*. The unremarkable conus* ⇨ *terminates at normal L1-L2 level. In this case, the filum fibrolipoma was thought to be incidental, rather than causal, due to the patient presenting with gait abnormality.*

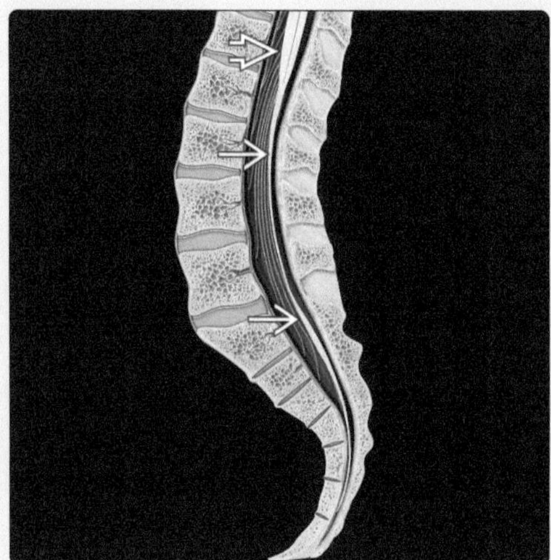

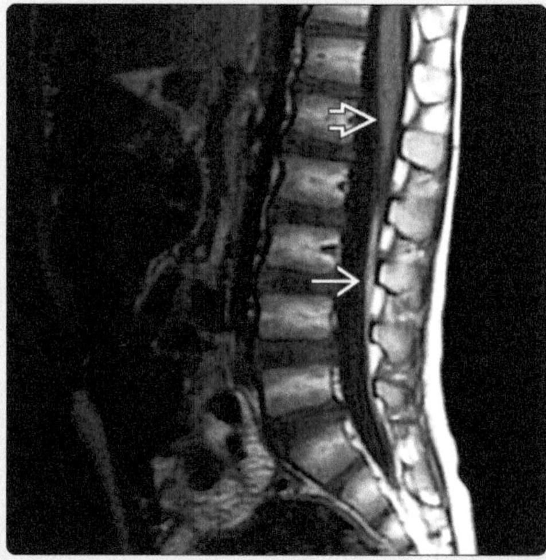

(Left) *Axial graphic of the lumbar spine shows the characteristic appearance of the fatty filum* ➡ *within the thecal sac. As depicted in this graphic, the fatty filum is dorsally located within the dural sac & produces no mass effect on the cauda equina.* **(Right)** *Axial T1 MR confirms fatty infiltration* ➡ *of the filum terminale with characteristic T1 hyperintensity & chemical shift artifact. The conus terminated at the normal L1/L2 level (not shown). In general, a fatty filum is most easily detected on axial T1 MR.*

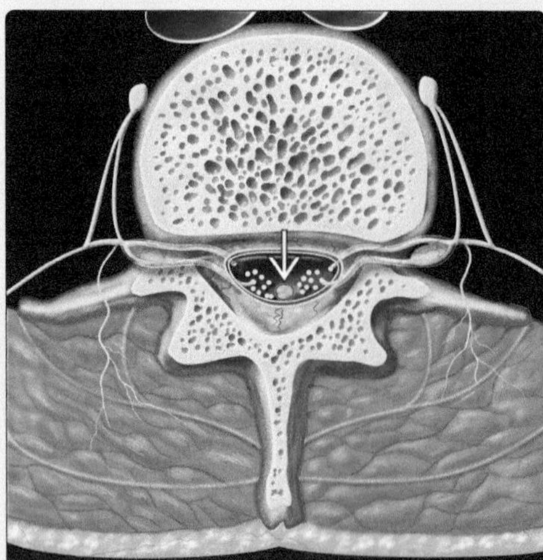

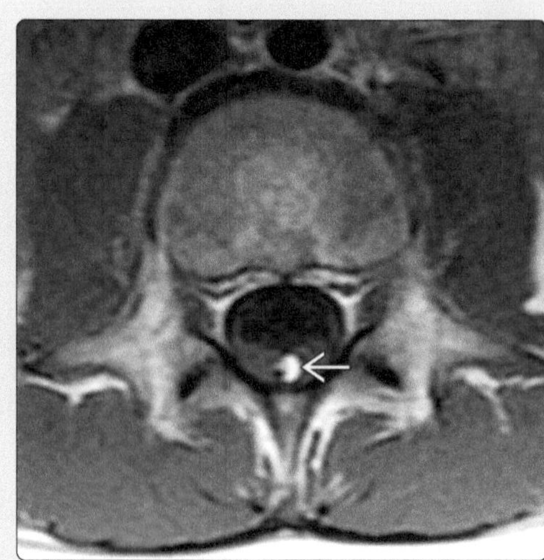

TERMINOLOGY

Synonyms

- Fibrolipoma of filum terminale, fatty filum terminale, "fat in filum"

Definitions

- Asymptomatic presence of fat within otherwise normal-appearing filum terminale
- Conus terminates at normal level without imaging stigmata of tethered spinal cord

IMAGING

General Features

- Best diagnostic clue
  - Linear fat signal/density within filum terminale
- Location
  - Filum terminale (conus level to sacrum)
- Size
  - Variable length, 1-5 mm transverse
    - Label as lipoma if > 2 mm transverse

CT Findings

- NECT
  - Punctate fat attenuation in dorsal aspect of lumbar thecal sac
  - No associated spinal dysraphism

MR Findings

- T1WI
  - Linear high signal oriented in craniocaudal direction on sagittal images
    - May occur anywhere from below conus to sacrum
  - Located in dorsal 1/2 of thecal sac in position of filum terminale
  - Signal loss on fat-suppressed sequences
- T2WI
  - Tracks fat signal

Ultrasonographic Findings

- Relatively common finding on screening ultrasound performed for simple sacral dimples
- Infrequently associated with clinical symptoms and signs

Imaging Recommendations

- Best imaging tool
  - T1 MR shows typical fat appearance, normal conus position, and morphology
- Protocol advice
  - Fat-suppressed T1 MR to define hyperintensity

DIFFERENTIAL DIAGNOSIS

Intraspinal Lipoma

- Larger lipomatous mass (> 5 mm)
- Thickening of filum terminale (> 2 mm)
- Low-lying or indistinct conus

Tethered Cord

- Thick filum, indistinct conus termination with smooth transition to filum

Lipomyelocele

- Dorsal dysraphism

Epidermoid/Dermoid Cyst

- Complex intradural mass, variable fat suppression

Subarachnoid Hemorrhage

- Fluid-fluid level in thecal sac

Tumor With Paramagnetic Effects

- Melanoma, melanotic meningioma, or schwannoma may show high signal on T1WI

PATHOLOGY

General Features

- Etiology
  - Congenital
- Associated abnormalities
  - No cutaneous stigmata on lower back with asymptomatic filum fibrolipoma
- Fatty infiltration of filum

Gross Pathologic & Surgical Features

- Small focus of fat within otherwise normal filum terminale

Microscopic Features

- Typical adipose tissue

CLINICAL ISSUES

Presentation

- Most common signs/symptoms
  - Asymptomatic by definition, incidental finding

Demographics

- Age
  - Children and adults
- Sex
  - M = F
- Epidemiology
  - Incidental finding in 4-6% of autopsy subjects

Natural History & Prognosis

- Normal variant

Treatment

- None required for asymptomatic lesion

DIAGNOSTIC CHECKLIST

Consider

- Symptomatic patient implies diagnosis of intraspinal lipoma, not asymptomatic fibrolipoma
- Intraspinal lipoma if larger lesion, symptomatic, and filum > 2 mm in thickness

SELECTED REFERENCES

1. Lalgudi Srinivasan H et al: Filum terminale lipomas-the role of intraoperative neuromonitoring. Childs Nerv Syst. 37(3):931-9, 2021
2. Oh JE et al: Filum terminale lipoma revealed by screening spinal ultrasonography in infants with simple sacral dimple. Childs Nerv Syst. 36(5):1037-42, 2019
3. Thompson EM et al: Clinical significance of imaging and histological characteristics of filum terminale in tethered cord syndrome. J Neurosurg Pediatr. 13(3):255-9, 2014

Ventriculus Terminalis

KEY FACTS

TERMINOLOGY

- Synonyms: Terminal ventricle, 5th ventricle

IMAGING

- Mild cystic dilatation of distal spinal cord canal
- No gliosis or myelomalacia
- No marginal nodularity or pathologic enhancement
- Conus terminates at normal level (T12 → L2)

TOP DIFFERENTIAL DIAGNOSES

- Transient dilatation of central spinal cord canal
- Hydrosyringomyelia
- Cystic spinal cord neoplasm
- Myelomalacia

PATHOLOGY

- Forms during embryogenesis (9th week) of caudal spinal cord by secondary neurulation
- Simple, CSF-filled cavity of conus medullaris enclosed by ependymal tissue

CLINICAL ISSUES

- No treatment indicated for classic incidental finding in asymptomatic patient
- Surgical decompression and management of associated abnormalities in rare symptomatic patients with cystic expansion

DIAGNOSTIC CHECKLIST

- Isolated, mild dilatation of distal central canal in normally located conus is nearly always incidental normal finding
- Most important imaging goal is to distinguish from cystic cord neoplasm or syrinx
    - Calcification, septations, nodules, enhancement, or eccentric location all argue against ventriculus terminalis and prompt further evaluation
- Exclude other unsuspected abnormalities predisposing to syrinx or cord tethering

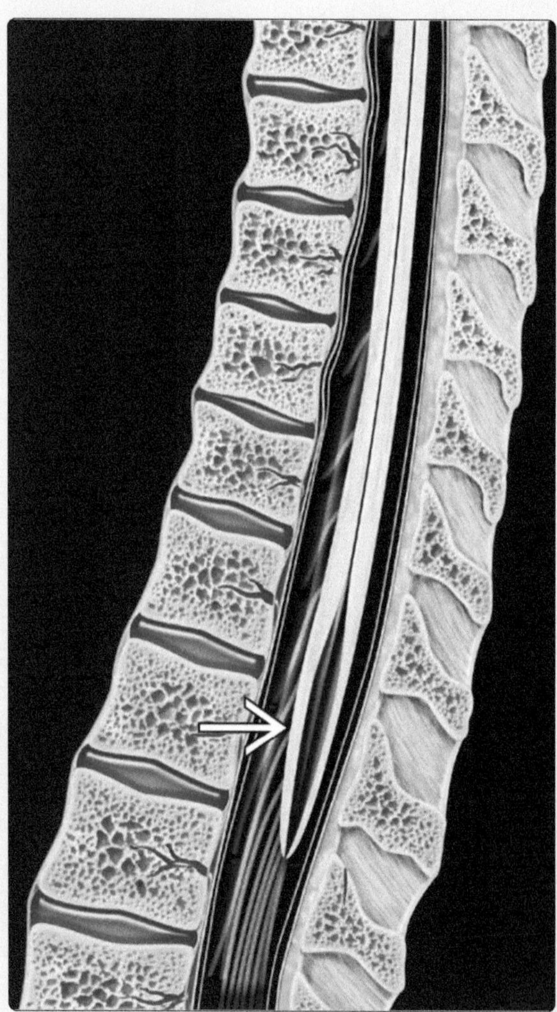

Sagittal graphic demonstrates the classic appearance of ventriculus terminalis ➡ with uncomplicated fusiform dilatation of the distal central cord canal confined to the conus.

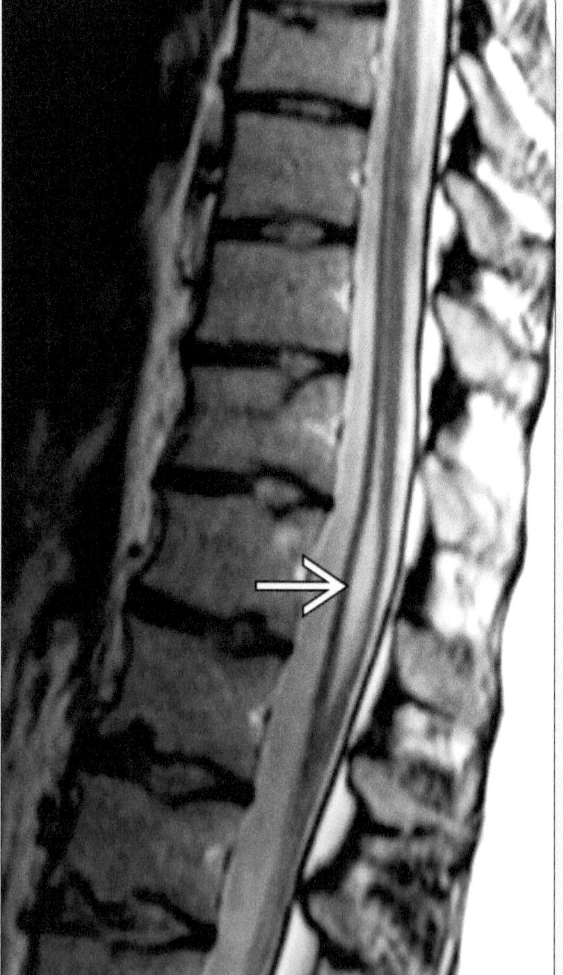

Sagittal T2WI MR shows the classic imaging appearance of ventriculus terminalis ➡ with smooth dilation of the distal spinal cord canal in the conus. Multiple vertebral endplate Schmorl nodes are an unrelated finding.

TERMINOLOGY

Synonyms

- Terminal ventricle, 5th ventricle

Definitions

- CSF signal/density within central spinal cord with central canal expansion at conus/proximal filum level

IMAGING

General Features

- Best diagnostic clue
  - Mild fusiform dilatation of distal central spinal cord canal without cord signal abnormality, nodularity, or enhancement
- Location
  - Distal spinal cord and conus medullaris
- Size
  - 2-4 mm (transverse); rarely exceeds 2 cm in length
  - < 1/3 length of spinal cord
- Morphology
  - Central intramedullary CSF signal/density dilatation with smooth regular margins and no mass
  - Conus terminates at normal level (T12 → L2)

CT Findings

- CECT
  - CSF density dilatation of distal spinal cord central canal
  - No mass lesion or enhancement

MR Findings

- T1WI
  - Hypointense CSF signal intensity dilatation of distal cord central canal
    - Beware of phase ghosting artifact imitating central canal dilatation
  - Conus terminates at normal level (T12-L2)
  - No filum terminale thickening or lipoma
- T2WI
  - Hyperintense CSF signal intensity dilatation of distal cord central canal
  - No septation of dilated central canal
- T1WI C+
  - No associated mass lesion or enhancement
    - Differentiates from cystic cord neoplasm

Ultrasonographic Findings

- Grayscale ultrasound
  - Mild, anechoic, nonseptated central canal dilatation within normally situated conus
  - Normal nerve root and conus pulsation
  - No filum terminale thickening (< 2 mm normal) or lipoma
- M-mode
  - Useful to confirm normal nerve root and conus pulsation

Imaging Recommendations

- Best imaging tool
  - Multiplanar MR imaging
- Newborns
  - Ultrasound to screen for congenital spine anomalies
    - Usually identified during characterization of sacral dimple
    - Distinguish ventriculus terminalis from syrinx or cord neoplasm
    - Abnormal or equivocal findings confirmed with MR imaging
- Children, adults, and infants (with positive ultrasound studies)
  - Thin-section sagittal T1WI and T2WI MR (3-mm slice thickness)
  - Axial T1WI and T2WI (3- to 4-mm slice thickness) distal cord to sacrum
    - Best to exclude occult dysraphism, lipoma, or thick filum
  - T1WI C+ MR in sagittal, axial planes if mass or architectural distortion identified

DIFFERENTIAL DIAGNOSIS

Transient Dilatation of Central Spinal Cord Canal

- Normal variant
- Slight dilatation of central canal in newborn
- Disappears in 1st weeks of life

Hydrosyringomyelia

- Cystic expansion of distal 1/3 (or more) of spinal cord
- Isolated finding or associated with congenital spine anomalies (up to 30% of patients)

Cystic Spinal Cord Neoplasm

- Astrocytoma
- Ependymoma
- Hemangioblastoma
- Differentiated by cord signal abnormality and expansion, contrast enhancement in solid portions

Myelomalacia

- History of trauma, vascular accident, or other cord insult
- Cord atrophy ± T2 hyperintensity (gliosis)

PATHOLOGY

General Features

- Etiology
  - Forms during embryogenesis (9th week) via secondary neurulation (formerly canalization and retrogressive differentiation) of caudal spinal cord
    - Represents point of union between central canal portion formed by primary neurulation and portion formed by secondary neurulation
    - Central canal size usually regresses during 1st weeks after birth; persistence leads to identification in children or adults
- Associated abnormalities
  - Occasionally identified in conjunction with caudal regression or tethered cord

Staging, Grading, & Classification

- Proposed classification systems for cystic ventriculus terminalis stratifies to surgical therapy based on symptoms

Gross Pathologic & Surgical Features

- Simple, CSF-filled cavity of conus medullaris enclosed by ependymal tissue
  - Normally present as either virtual cavity or ependymal residue
  - Small minority of patients demonstrate cystic expansion
- No gliosis or neoplasm
- Rare ventriculus terminalis cysts likely represent intramedullary arachnoid cysts

Microscopic Features

- Normal cord microscopic histology
  - Cystic cavity lined by ependymal cells
  - No gliosis or neoplasm

CLINICAL ISSUES

Presentation

- Most common signs/symptoms
  - Incidental finding on imaging performed for unrelated indications
    - Nearly always asymptomatic in children
    - Identification in adults usually during sciatica work-up
- Other signs/symptoms
  - Rarely becomes abnormally dilated (cystic) and symptomatic, necessitating treatment
    - Bilateral sciatica
    - Cauda equina syndrome
    - Lower extremity weakness
    - Urinary retention
- Clinical profile
  - Patient usually asymptomatic or presents with nonspecific neurologic symptoms referable to conus or cauda equina

Demographics

- Age
  - Most commonly identified < 5 years old; may occur at any age
- Sex
  - M = F in children
  - F > M more commonly reported in adults
- Epidemiology
  - 2.6% of normal children (< 5 years old) have visible ventriculus terminalis on MR
  - Less commonly identified in adults; primarily autopsy curiosity before widespread availability of MR imaging

Natural History & Prognosis

- Size variable throughout life; smallest in middle age, largest in early childhood and old age
- No effect on mortality or morbidity
  - Most commonly either stable in size or regresses; size progression rarely reported
- Rare symptomatic surgical cases usually show symptom improvement postoperatively
  - Usually when there is intrinsic cyst dilating spinal cord canal

Treatment

- No treatment indicated for classic incidental finding in asymptomatic patient
  - MR follow-up if deemed necessary based on clinical findings
- Surgical decompression and management of associated abnormalities in rare symptomatic patients with cystic expansion
  - Cyst likely represents intramedullary arachnoid cyst
  - Cyst fenestration ± cyst shunting to subarachnoid space, pleural cavity, or peritoneal cavity

DIAGNOSTIC CHECKLIST

Consider

- Most important imaging goal is to distinguish from cystic cord neoplasm or syringomyelia
- Asymptomatic patients require no further imaging evaluation
- Symptomatic patients should be monitored using clinical and MR follow-up unless degree of cyst expansion prompts surgical drainage

Image Interpretation Pearls

- Isolated mild dilatation of distal central canal in normally located conus is nearly always incidental normal finding
  - Calcification, septations, nodules, enhancement, or eccentric location all argue against ventriculus terminalis and prompt further evaluation
  - Beware of phase ghosting artifact mimicking dilated terminal ventricle or syrinx
- Exclude other unsuspected abnormalities that may predispose to syrinx or cord tethering before attributing finding to incidental dilatation of ventriculus terminalis

SELECTED REFERENCES

1. Menezes AH et al: Ventriculus terminalis cyst in an infant: a case report. J Med Case Rep. 17(1):22, 2023
2. Imamura K et al: Surgical treatment for cystic dilation of the ventriculus terminalis: a report of two cases. J Orthop Sci. 29(1):354-6, 2022
3. Kim T et al: Intradural cyst: intramedullary or extramedullary? Illustrative case. J Neurosurg Case Lessons. 2(3):CASE21327, 2021
4. Lotfinia I et al: The cystic dilation of ventriculus terminalis with neurological symptoms: three case reports and a literature review. J Spinal Cord Med. 1-7, 2018
5. Zeinali M et al: Cystic dilation of a ventriculus terminalis. Case report and review of the literature. Br J Neurosurg. 1-5, 2017
6. Zhang L et al: Cystic dilation of the ventriculus terminalis: report of 6 surgical cases treated with cyst-subarachnoid shunting using a t-catheter. World Neurosurg. 104:522-7, 2017
7. Woodley-Cook J et al: The slowly enlarging ventriculus terminalis. Pol J Radiol. 81:529-31, 2016
8. Bellocchi S et al: Multilobed cystic dilation of the ventriculus terminalis (CDVT). BMJ Case Rep. 2013, 2013
9. Ganau M et al: Cystic dilation of the ventriculus terminalis. J Neurosurg Spine. 17(1):86-92, 2012
10. de Moura Batista L et al: Cystic lesion of the ventriculus terminalis: proposal for a new clinical classification. J Neurosurg Spine. 8(2):163-8, 2008
11. Brisman JL et al: Cystic dilation of the conus ventriculus terminalis presenting as an acute cauda equina syndrome relieved by decompression and cyst drainage: case report. Neurosurgery. 58(3):E585; discussion E585, 2006
12. Sansur CA et al: Ventriculus terminalis causing back pain and urinary retention. Acta Neurochir (Wien). 148(8):919-20, 2006
13. Dullerud R et al: MR imaging of ventriculus terminalis of the conus medullaris. A report of two operated patients and a review of the literature. Acta Radiol. 44(4):444-6, 2003
14. Kriss VM et al: Sonographic appearance of the ventriculus terminalis cyst in the neonatal spinal cord. J Ultrasound Med. 19(3):207-9, 2000
15. Unsinn KM et al: US of the spinal cord in newborns: spectrum of normal findings, variants, congenital anomalies, and acquired diseases. Radiographics. 20(4):923-38, 2000

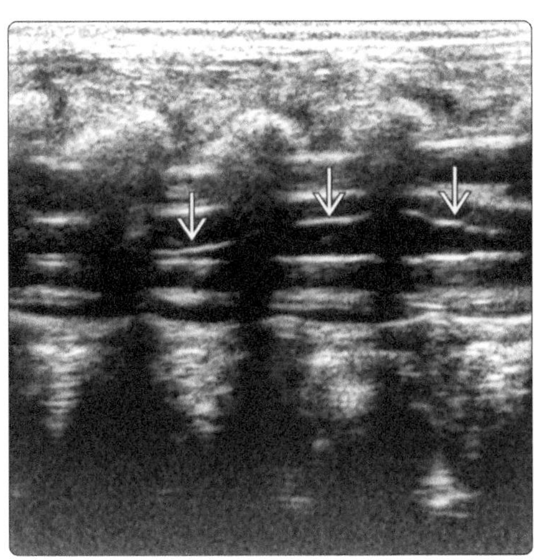

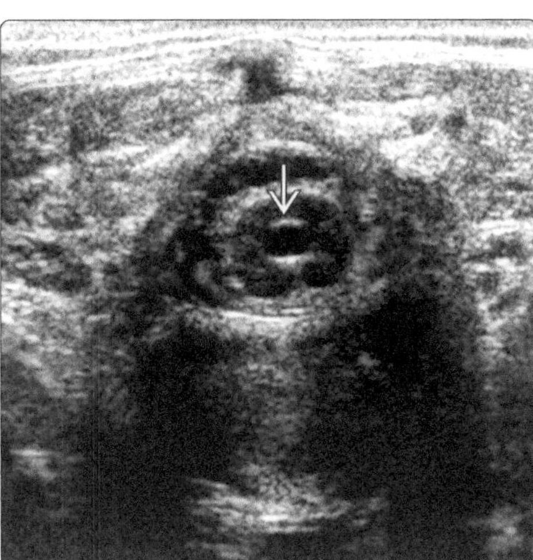

(Left) *Longitudinal ultrasound demonstrates smooth fusiform dilatation of the distal central canal ➡ localized to the conus.* **(Right)** *Transverse ultrasound reveals smooth dilation of the distal spinal cord central canal ➡ at the conus. Note the central location without eccentric cavitation or nodularity, findings that would exclude simple ventriculus terminalis.*

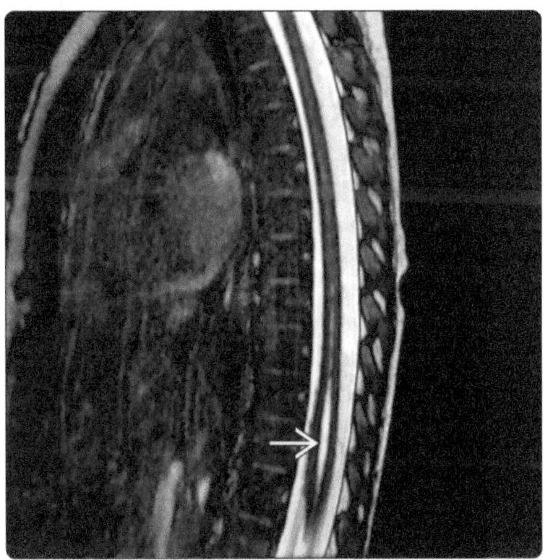

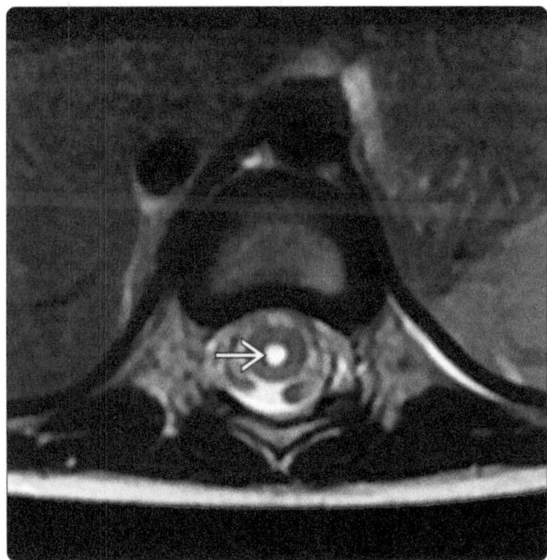

(Left) *Sagittal FIESTA MR in a 1-month-old infant imaged for simple coccygeal dimple reveals incidentally detected fluid-filled dilation ➡ of the distal spinal cord canal. A normal vestige of the closed spinal cord canal in the proximal spinal cord is present. No dermal sinus tract or tethering lesion was present (not shown).* **(Right)** *Axial T2WI MR in the same patient confirms smooth dilation of the central spinal cord canal ➡ without eccentricity or myelomalacia.*

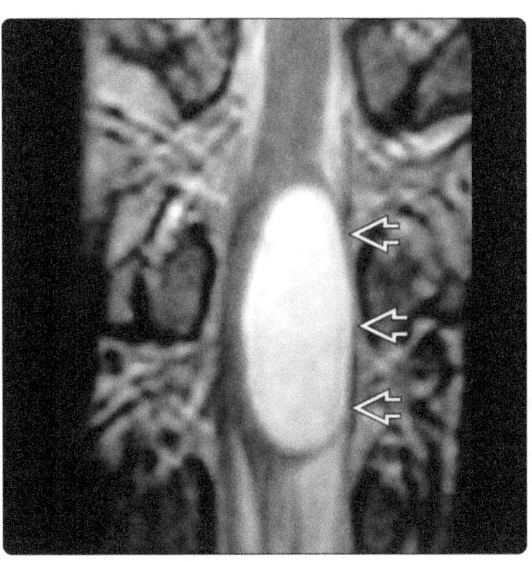

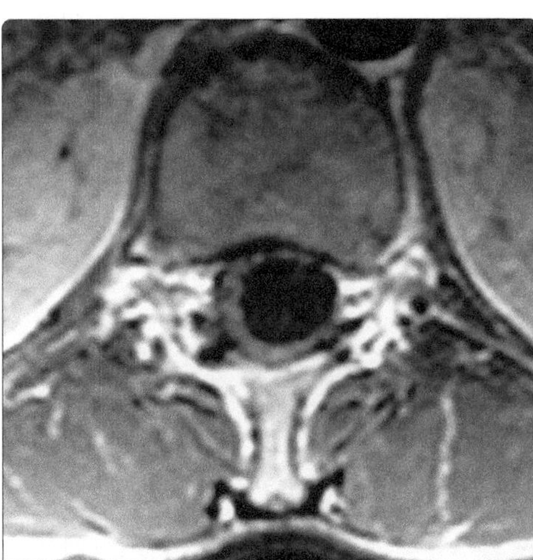

(Left) *Coronal T2WI MR reveals eccentric cystic dilatation of the central spinal cord canal confined to the conus only. Note eccentric thinning of the left lateral cord parenchyma ➡ by cyst expansion.* **(Right)** *Axial T1WI C+ MR in the same patient confirms absence of abnormal enhancement or nodularity within the eccentric terminal conus cyst. This likely represents an intramedullary arachnoid cyst.*

Chiari 1

KEY FACTS

TERMINOLOGY

- Synonyms: Chiari type 1, Chiari 1 deformity, Chiari 1 anomaly

IMAGING

- Pointed cerebellar tonsils extending ≥ 5 mm below foramen magnum (basion-opisthion/McRae line) with effacement of CSF spaces
- ± retroflexed odontoid, horizontal shortened clivus, basilar invagination, platybasia, atlantooccipital assimilation
- ± caudal descent of brainstem, brainstem compression, medullary bump
- ± syringohydromyelia, scoliosis

TOP DIFFERENTIAL DIAGNOSES

- Normal low-lying cerebellar tonsils
- Chiari 2
- Tonsillar herniation due to ↑ intracranial pressure
- Intracranial hypotension

PATHOLOGY

- Most common cause is believed to be small/underdeveloped posterior fossa; no association with open spinal dysraphism
- Can result from premature closure of sutures (craniocerebral disproportion) or chronic alterations in CSF flow dynamics (may not be considered true Chiari 1)

CLINICAL ISSUES

- Most common presenting symptom: Occipital headache
  - Up to 30% of patients are asymptomatic
- Goal of surgery in symptomatic patients: Restore normal CSF flow at foramen magnum
  - Suboccipital decompression, resection of C1 posterior arch ± duraplasty, cerebellar tonsil shrinkage/cautery

DIAGNOSTIC CHECKLIST

- Look for presence of syrinx → usually requires surgical treatment of Chiari 1 regardless of symptoms

(Left) *Sagittal graphic demonstrates pointed cerebellar tonsils extending below the foramen magnum to the inferior aspect of the C1 posterior arch. The obex ⇒ is inferiorly displaced as well.* **(Right)** *Sagittal T1 MR of a 17-year-old boy with Chiari 1 demonstrates downward displacement of the pointed cerebellar tonsils below the posterior arch of C1 and downward displacement of the obex to the same level ⇒. There is also mild retroflexion of the odontoid ➡ with mass effect on the ventral medulla.*

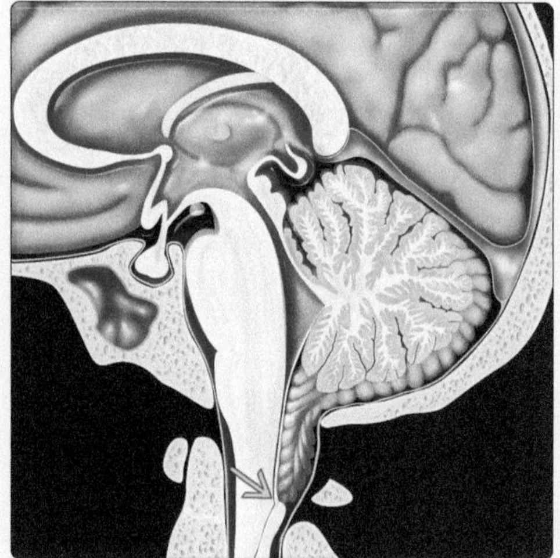

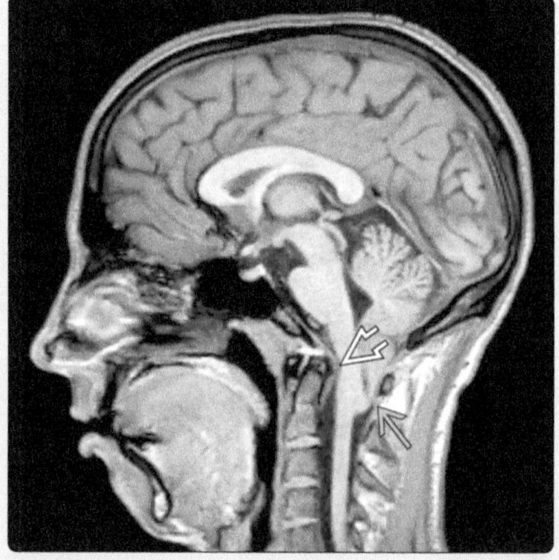

(Left) *Sagittal 3D FIESTA of the craniocervical junction in the same patient more clearly demonstrates severe foramen magnum crowding with effacement of the dorsal and ventral cisterns ⇒.* **(Right)** *Sagittal-phase contrast CSF flow study in the same patient demonstrates severe restriction of CSF flow marked by absence of black flow-related signal anterior and posterior to the herniated brainstem and cerebellar tonsils with pulsation of the cerebellar tonsils (pistoning) demonstrating intermediate signal ⇒.*

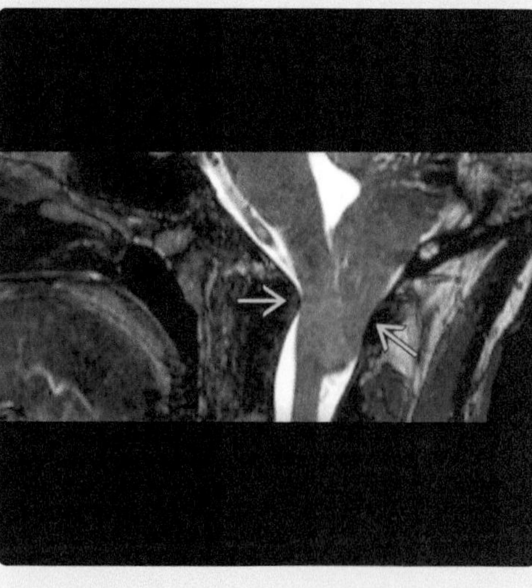

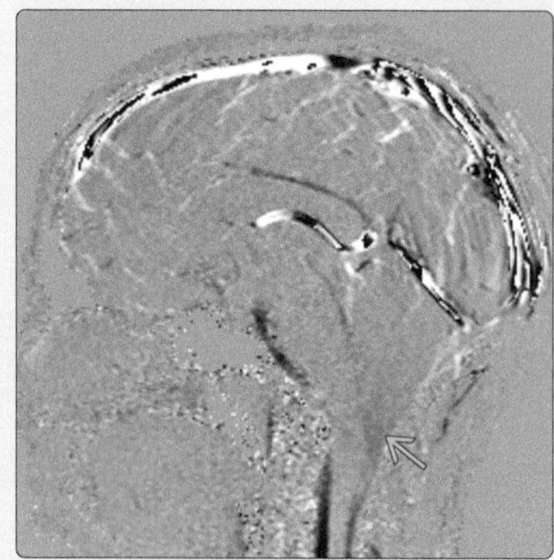

TERMINOLOGY

Definitions

- Compressed & pointed cerebellar tonsils extending below foramen magnum with effacement of CSF spaces
- Terminology somewhat controversial; some argue it is not true malformation

IMAGING

General Features

- Best diagnostic clue
  - Pointed cerebellar tonsils (unilateral or bilateral) extending ≥ 5 mm below foramen magnum (McRae line: Basion-opisthion)
    - No consensus statement on exact definition

CT Findings

- Osseous anomalies: Small posterior fossa, short horizontal clivus, retroflexed odontoid, basilar invagination, platybasia, hypoplastic occipital condyles, segmentation anomalies (such as atlantooccipital assimilation), scoliosis

MR Findings

- T1, T2, FLAIR
  - Pointed (not rounded) cerebellar tonsils extending ≥ 5 mm below foramen magnum
  - Crowded foramen magnum with small/effaced cisterns ± brainstem compression
  - ± small posterior fossa, elongated 4th ventricle
  - ± syringohydromyelia/syrinx, scoliosis
  - ± dorsal apex cervicomedullary "kinking" or "bump"
  - Ventriculomegaly/hydrocephalus uncommon complication of Chiari 1 but can happen in up to 10% of cases
- MR cine
  - Restricted CSF flow through foramen magnum ± ↑ brainstem/cerebellar tonsil motion (pistoning)

DIFFERENTIAL DIAGNOSIS

Normal Variation of Cerebellar Tonsil Position

- Tonsils may normally lie below foramen magnum

Tonsillar Herniation Due to ↑ Intracranial Pressure

- Neoplasm, hemorrhage, hydrocephalus, infarct

Intracranial Hypotension

- ± subdural hygromas

PATHOLOGY

General Features

- Etiology
  - Primary (congenital malformation) vs. secondary (acquired morphologic changes vs. chronic altered CSF flow dynamics)
  - Primary: Posterior fossa underdevelopment theory is most common
  - Secondary: Premature closure of cranial sutures &/or generalized abnormal bone formation
    - Shunted infantile hydrocephalus leading to craniocerebral disproportion
    - Calvarial thickening of bone dysplasias or thalassemia
    - Genetic syndromes (Crouzon syndrome, Pfeiffer syndrome)
  - Secondary: ↑ intracranial pressure vs. decreased spinal pressure → may not be considered true Chiari 1
    - Chiari 1 seen in up to 20% of patients with idiopathic intracranial hypertension (a.k.a. pseudotumor cerebri)

Staging, Grading, & Classification

- Described subtypes sometimes used in certain clinical practices
  - Chiari 1.5: Brainstem herniation
    - Obex located below foramen magnum
  - Complex Chiari: Retroflexed odontoid causes medullary bump, abnormally acute clival-cervical angle; ± atlantooccipital assimilation, basilar invagination, & platybasia
    - pB-C2 & clivo-axial angle (CXA) can be used to select candidates for additional surgical techniques outside standard posterior fossa decompression (PFD)
  - Chiari 0: Syrinx with posterior fossa symptoms in absence of cerebellar tonsillar ectopia
    - Surgical management of these patients is controversial

CLINICAL ISSUES

Presentation

- Most common signs/symptoms
  - Occipital headache
    - Exacerbated by cough, Valsalva, neck extension, or physical exertion
  - Less common: Cerebellar, brainstem, bulbar, otoneurologic, spinal cord symptoms

Demographics

- True prevalence is unknown given how frequently Chiari 1 is picked up incidentally

Treatment

- Conservative management for asymptomatic or minimally symptomatic children without syrinx
- PFD: Suboccipital craniectomy with C1 laminectomy ± duraplasty, arachnoid opening/dissection, cerebellar tonsillar reduction/cautery
- Complex Chiari 1 may also require odontoid resection &/or craniocervical junction (CCJ) fusion
- Scoliosis may improve from decompression alone but often requires bracing or additional surgery

DIAGNOSTIC CHECKLIST

Consider

- Degree of tonsillar descent does not always correlate with symptoms: Chiari 1 is frequently picked up incidentally

SELECTED REFERENCES

1. Pindrik J et al: Imaging in Chiari I malformation. Neurosurg Clin N Am. 34(1):67-79, 2023
2. Alford EN et al: Imaging characteristics associated with surgery in Chiari malformation type I. J Neurosurg Pediatr. 1-9, 2021
3. Barkovich AJ et al: Pediatric Neuroimaging. 6th ed. Wolters Kluwer. 550-54, 2019

KEY FACTS

TERMINOLOGY

- Constellation of intracranial findings, mainly hindbrain herniation, due to open spinal dysraphism (OSD) (either myelomeningocele or myelocele/myeloschisis)

IMAGING

- Small posterior fossa: Cerebellum herniates downward through foramen magnum & upward through incisura
- Caudal brainstem herniation with cervicomedullary kink, tectal beaking
- ± ventriculomegaly
- Falx insufficiency, thickened massa intermedia, callosal dysgenesis, ↓ white matter volume
- ± periventricular gray matter heterotopias
- Lacunar skull (lückenschädel)

TOP DIFFERENTIAL DIAGNOSES

- Chiari 1
- Chiari 3
- Intracranial hypotension
- Severe, chronic shunted hydrocephalus

PATHOLOGY

- Secondary to sequelae of chronic in utero CSF leakage through OSD (4th fetal week)

CLINICAL ISSUES

- Lower extremity paresis/spasticity, bowel/bladder dysfunction, symptoms of brainstem compression (swallowing difficulties, stridor, apnea), epilepsy
- In utero repair of OSD ↓ need for postnatal CSF diversion (shunting) & may improve neurologic outcomes in some patients

DIAGNOSTIC CHECKLIST

- Confirm history of OSD before assigning Chiari 2
- Fetal surgery results in milder Chiari 2 phenotype with less hindbrain herniation

(Left) *Sagittal BTFE/FIESTA MR from a 22-weeks-gestational age fetus referred for evaluation for fetal surgery demonstrates grade 3 Chiari 2 ➔ in the setting of a lumbosacral myelomeningocele (MMC) ➔.* **(Right)** *Axial T2 SSFSE MR of the brain in the same fetus demonstrates flattening of the bifrontal calvarium ➔ (a.k.a. lemon sign) with associated effacement of the extraaxial CSF spaces & parallel configuration of the lateral ventricles ➔.*

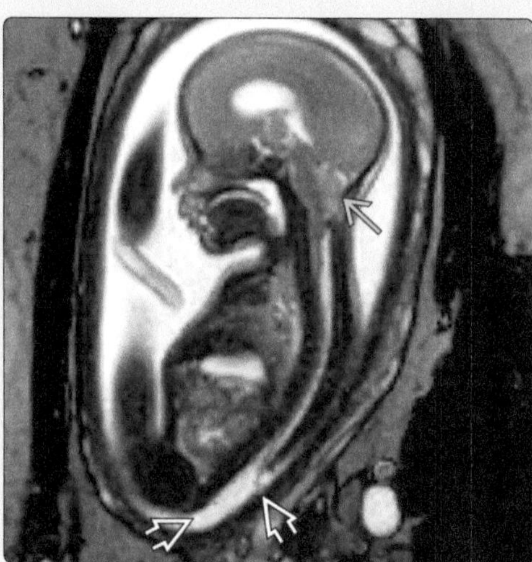

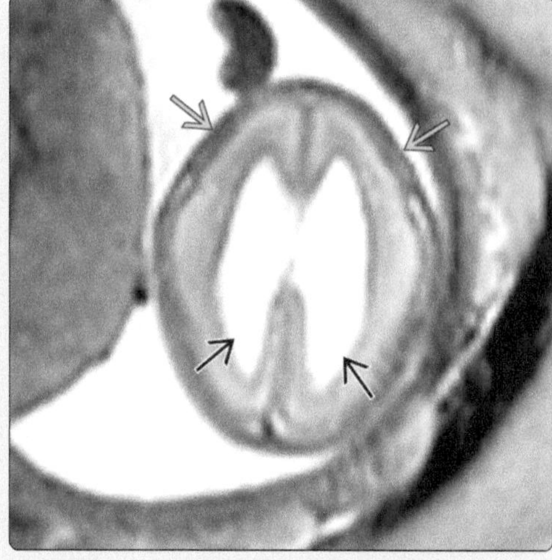

(Left) *Sagittal T2WI MR in a 1-year-old after postnatal repair of an MMC shows typical findings of Chiari 2, including cerebellar herniation ➔, elongated & effaced 4th ventricle ➔, tectal beaking ➔, enlarged massa intermedia ➔, & callosal hypogenesis ➔.* **(Right)** *Sagittal T1WI MR in a 1-month-old status post prenatal repair of an MMC shows no hindbrain herniation. Other findings of Chiari 2 are present, including callosal hypogenesis ➔, large massa intermedia ➔, & tectal beaking ➔.*

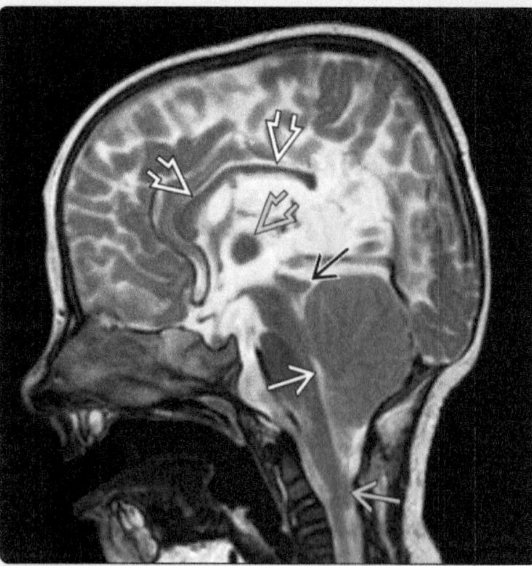

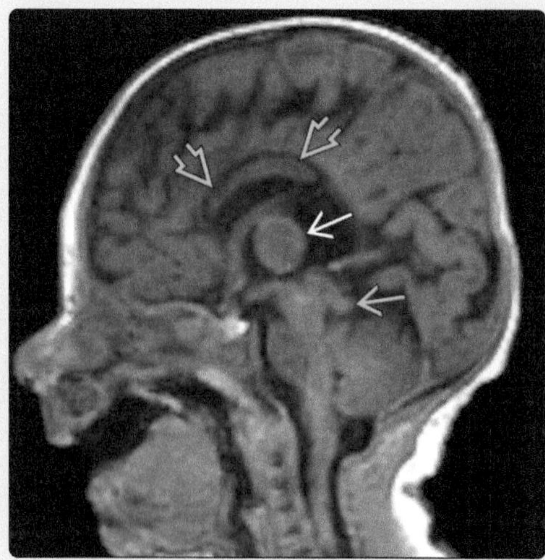

TERMINOLOGY

Definitions

- Constellation of intracranial anomalies, mainly hindbrain herniation, due to open spinal dysraphism (OSD) (either myelomeningocele or myelocele)

IMAGING

General Features

- Best diagnostic clue
  - Small posterior fossa (PF) with inferior cerebellar & brainstem herniation in presence of OSD

Radiographic Findings

- Radiography
  - Lacunar skull (lückenschädel) → numerous undulations of inner calvarium with focal thinning

MR Findings

- Infratentorial
  - Small PF with downward sloping tentorium, low torcular Herophili
  - Hindbrain herniation (postnatal repair)
    - Caudal descent of pointed cerebellar tonsils/vermis
    - Towering appearance of cerebellum with upward herniation through widened incisura
    - Elongated, effaced, inferiorly displaced 4th ventricle with flattened fastigium
    - Cerebellar hemispheres wrap around brainstem on axial images
  - Significant hindbrain herniation is unusual after prenatal repair
  - Tectal beaking, brainstem caudal displacement ± cervicomedullary kink
- Supratentorial
  - ± ventriculomegaly
  - Midline anomalies: Large massa intermedia, callosal hypogenesis/dysgenesis, absent septum pellucidum
  - ± neuronal migrational anomalies: Periventricular gray matter (GM) heterotopia (~ 25%), polymicrogyria (rare)
  - Falx insufficiency with interdigitation of hemispheric gyri
  - Stenogyria (elongated, compact gyri) after shunting (differs from polymicrogyria)

Ultrasonographic Findings

- Grayscale ultrasound
  - Prenatal US is key for early diagnosis
    - Lemon sign: Bifrontal concavity of calvarium
    - Banana sign: Cerebellum wraps around brainstem with effacement of cisterna magna

DIFFERENTIAL DIAGNOSIS

Chiari 1

- Low pointed cerebellar tonsils effacing CSF at foramen magnum
- Absence of associated OSD
- None of associated supratentorial findings seen in Chiari 2

Chiari 3

- PF contents herniate through suboccipital ± high cervical encephalocele

Intracranial Hypotension

- Dural enhancement, venous sinus engorgement, ± subdural collections
- Typically in setting of CSF leak with postural headaches

Severe Chronically Shunted Hydrocephalus

- May cause collapsed & dysmorphic brain with upward cerebellar herniation

PATHOLOGY

General Features

- Etiology
  - Folate deficiency during pregnancy is leading preventable risk factor

Staging, Grading, & Classification

- Grading system for Chari 2 on fetal MR is based on PF morphology
  - Grade 1: 4th ventricle & cisterna magna are patent
  - Grade 2: 4th ventricle is effaced, cisterna magna is patent
  - Grade 3: 4th ventricle & cisterna magna are effaced

CLINICAL ISSUES

Presentation

- Most common signs/symptoms
  - 80-90% develop hydrocephalus requiring shunting, though incidence is lower in those who undergo prenatal repair of OSD
  - Varying degrees of lower extremity paresis/spasticity, clubfoot, bowel/bladder dysfunction
  - ± epilepsy, symptoms from brainstem compression (swallowing difficulties, stridor, apnea)

Treatment

- Surgical management
  - OSD is classically repaired in first 48 hours after delivery
  - CSF diversion/shunting is classically required in 80-90%
  - PF decompression in those who do not improve with shunting
  - Fetal OSD repair in select patients
    - Must have hindbrain herniation & upper level of spinal defect T1-S1
    - Reduces need for shunting; may improve neurologic outcomes in some patients
    - Improved neurologic outcomes must be balanced with potential surgical risks (e.g., premature birth)

SELECTED REFERENCES

1. Khalaveh F et al: Myelomeningocele-Chiari II malformation-neurological predictability based on fetal and postnatal magnetic resonance imaging. Prenat Diagn. 41(8):922-32, 2021
2. Trapp B et al: A practical approach to diagnosis of spinal dysraphism. Radiographics. 41(2):559-75, 2021
3. Nagaraj UD et al: Imaging of open spinal dysraphisms in the era of prenatal surgery. Pediatr Radiol. 50(13):1988-98, 2020
4. Miller JL et al: Spinal dysraphia, Chiari 2 malformation, unified theory, and advances in fetoscopic repair. Neuroimaging Clin N Am. 29(3):357-66, 2019

KEY FACTS

TERMINOLOGY

- Chiari 3 (C3)
- Synonyms: Chiari III, rhombencephalocele

IMAGING

- Low occipital or high cervical meningoencephalocele containing cerebellum ± brainstem, meninges, vessels, CSF
- Midline bone defect within supraoccipital bone, opisthion

TOP DIFFERENTIAL DIAGNOSES

- Isolated occipital encephalocele
- Other occipital encephaloceles
  - Iniencephaly
  - Syndromic occipital encephalocele

PATHOLOGY

- Severity classified by sac contents
- Cephalocele contents: Meninges, cerebellum, brainstem ± cervical cord, occipital poles, vasculature
  - Disorganized (neuronal migration anomalies, cortical dysplasias) and gliotic brain tissue
  - Lining of sac may show gray matter heterotopias
- Associated abnormalities: Corpus callosum anomalies, gray matter heterotopia, syringohydromyelia, tethered cord

CLINICAL ISSUES

- Microcephaly, severe developmental delay, spasticity, hypotonia, seizures
- Mechanical brainstem traction, respiratory deterioration, lower cranial nerve dysfunction

DIAGNOSTIC CHECKLIST

- Occipitocervical cephalocele containing cerebellum ± brainstem in conjunction with C1-C2 spina bifida = C3
- Distinct malformation; not just Chiari 2 with encephalocele

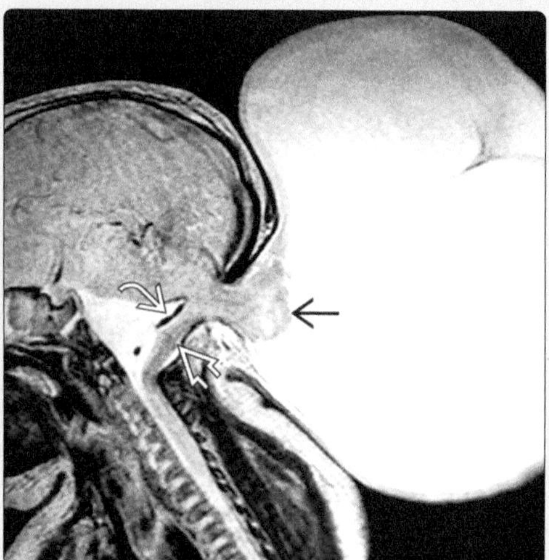

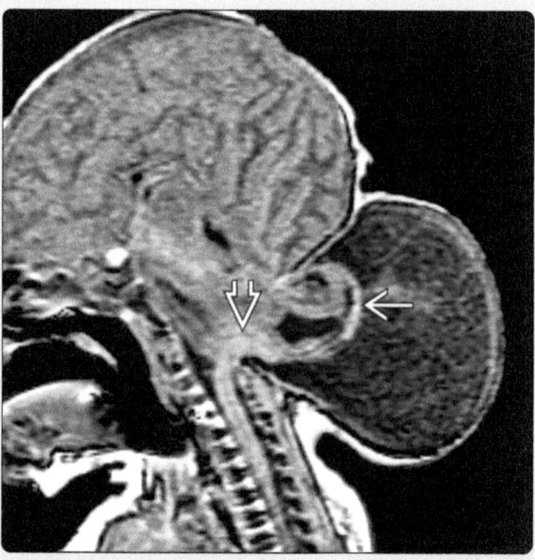

(Left) *Sagittal T2 MR reveals a large defect in the ventral chondral portion of the supraoccipital bone and opisthion of the foramen magnum. Gliotic cerebellar tissue ➡ protrudes into a large sac. Note displacement of the brainstem ➡ and basilar artery ➡.* **(Right)** *Sagittal T1 MR shows a large meningoencephalocele composed of meninges, CSF, cerebellum ➡, brainstem ➡, and upper cervical spinal cord herniated through a bone defect in the lower occiput and upper cervical spine.*

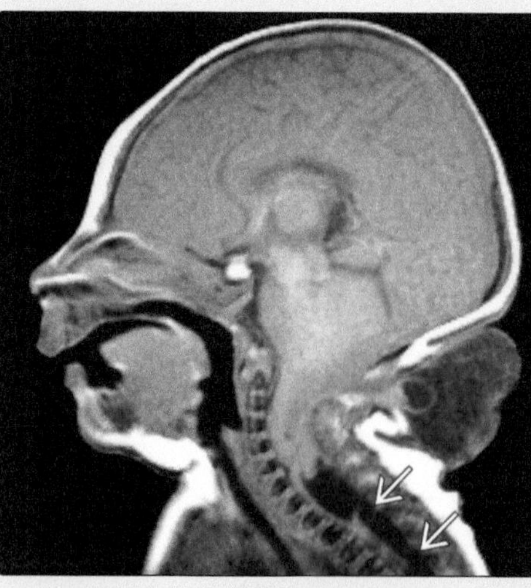

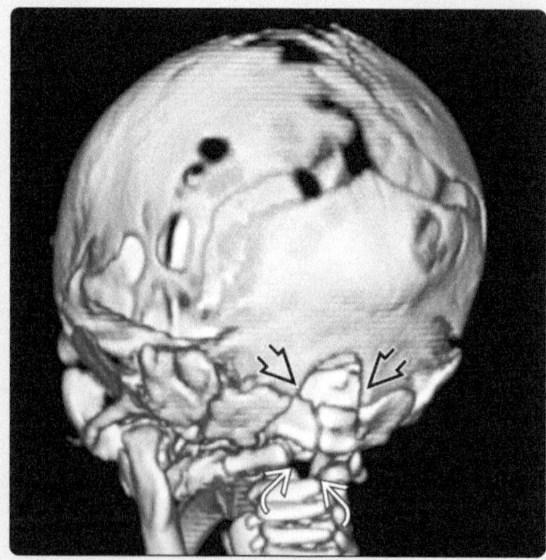

(Left) *Sagittal T1 MR demonstrates herniation of brain, CSF, and meninges through a dorsal midline bone defect at the craniocervical junction. Note also cervical spinal cord hydromyelia ➡.* **(Right)** *Bone CT 3D shaded surface rendering of the posterior calvarium/upper cervical spine in a Chiari 3 (C3) patient shows a large defect ➡ of the ventral chondral and squamous supraoccipital bones in conjunction with upper cervical spina bifida ➡.*

TERMINOLOGY

Synonyms

- Chiari III, Chiari 3 (C3) malformation rhombencephalocele

Definitions

- Originally described by Dr. Chiari as herniation of cerebellum ± brainstem through posterior C1-C2 dysraphic defect
- However, many imagers more loosely define C3 as low occipital or high cervical meningoencephalocele

IMAGING

General Features

- Best diagnostic clue
  - Skin-covered combined cephalocele + upper cervical myelocele containing cerebellum ± brainstem, meninges, vessels, CSF herniating through high cervical ± low supraoccipital bone/opisthion osseous defect

CT Findings

- NECT
  - Midline posterior cephalocele containing cerebellum
- Bone CT
  - Opisthion, upper cervical osseous dysraphic bone defect
- CTA
  - Basilar artery "pulled" into defect along with brainstem into cephalocele sac
  - ± veins/dural sinuses within cephalocele sac
  - Anomalous &/or ptotic veins, dural sinuses

MR Findings

- T1WI
  - High cervical cephalocele sac containing meninges and cerebellum ± brainstem, upper cervical cord
- T2WI
  - Tissues in cephalocele sac may be bright (gliosis), strand-like (necrotic), or hypointense (hemorrhagic)

Imaging Recommendations

- Best imaging tool
  - Multiplanar brain MR + MRV to characterize occipitocervical encephalocele, vessels
  - Multiplanar bone CT to evaluate osseous defects

DIFFERENTIAL DIAGNOSIS

Isolated Occipital Encephalocele

- Spares foramen magnum, lacks intracranial Chiari 2 findings

Other Occipital Encephaloceles

- Iniencephaly
- Syndromic occipital encephalocele
  - Meckel-Gruber, Goldenhar-Gorlin, MURCS (müllerian, renal, cervical spine), Walker-Warburg, amniotic band

PATHOLOGY

General Features

- Genetics
  - 677C → T mutation on methylenetetrahydrofolate reductase (*MTHFR*) gene (≤ 50%)
- Associated abnormalities
  - Corpus callosum anomalies, gray matter heterotopia, syringohydromyelia, tethered cord
  - Previously described in combination with intracranial Chiari 2 manifestations
    - Now thought that tectum, lower brainstem findings actually reflect distortion related to cerebellar displacement into sac

Gross Pathologic & Surgical Features

- Severity classified by cephalocele sac contents
  - 1 or more of meninges, cerebellum, brainstem ± cervical cord, occipital lobe poles, arterial and venous vessels, disorganized and gliotic brain tissue
  - Sac lining may contain gray matter heterotopia

Microscopic Features

- Disorganized (neuronal migration anomalies, cortical dysplasias, gliotic) brain tissue within sac

CLINICAL ISSUES

Presentation

- Most common signs/symptoms
  - Occipital/upper cervical cephalocele, microcephaly
  - Discovered by fetal ultrasound/MR or surprise at birth
- Other signs/symptoms
  - Mechanical brainstem traction, respiratory deterioration, lower cranial nerve dysfunction
- Clinical profile
  - Severe developmental delay, spasticity, hypotonia, seizures

Demographics

- Age
  - Newborn
- Sex
  - F > M [as in all neural tube defects (NTDs)] in most series
- Epidemiology
  - Rare; 1-4.5% of all Chiari complexes

Natural History & Prognosis

- Dependent on amount, type of herniated tissue
- Prognosis usually dismal; severe disability, early death

Treatment

- Surgical resection, encephalocele repair
  - Resect or repair sac (most structures in sac are nonfunctioning)
  - If amount of CNS tissue in sac > intracranial → not surgical candidate
- CSF diversion for hydrocephalus

DIAGNOSTIC CHECKLIST

Consider

- C3 in newborn presenting with low occipital encephalocele

SELECTED REFERENCES

1. Gabr M et al: Chiari type III: experience of outcome for 15 cases. J Korean Neurosurg Soc. 65(6):841-5, 2022
2. Ivashchuk G et al: Chiari III malformation: a comprehensive review of this enigmatic anomaly. Childs Nerv Syst. 31(11):2035-40, 2015

KEY FACTS

TERMINOLOGY

- Complex Chiari (CC), Chiari 1.5

IMAGING

- Cerebellar tonsillar herniation with low obex, dorsal medullary "bump"
  - "Bump" thought to represent aberrant clava, used as marker for cervicomedullary junction
  - Abnormal tonsillar "pistoning" motion, reduced CSF flow around foramen magnum and cerebellar tonsils
- ± syringohydromyelia, ventral cervicomedullary compression
- ± odontoid retroflexion, small posterior fossa, clival anomalies, platybasia

TOP DIFFERENTIAL DIAGNOSES

- Chiari 1
- Chiari 2

PATHOLOGY

- Medullary pyramid decussation anatomic border between spinal cord, medulla oblongata
  - Normal obex level is 10-12 mm above foramen magnum
  - Obex displaced to or below foramen magnum level in CC patients

CLINICAL ISSUES

- Headaches, myelopathy, bulbar symptoms, lethargy, failure to thrive
- Natural history is progressively severe symptoms

DIAGNOSTIC CHECKLIST

- CC considered subgroup of Chiari 1 with more severe clinical phenotype
- Consider CC in context of cerebellar tonsillar herniation, low obex, dorsal medullary "bump" + craniovertebral junction anomalies

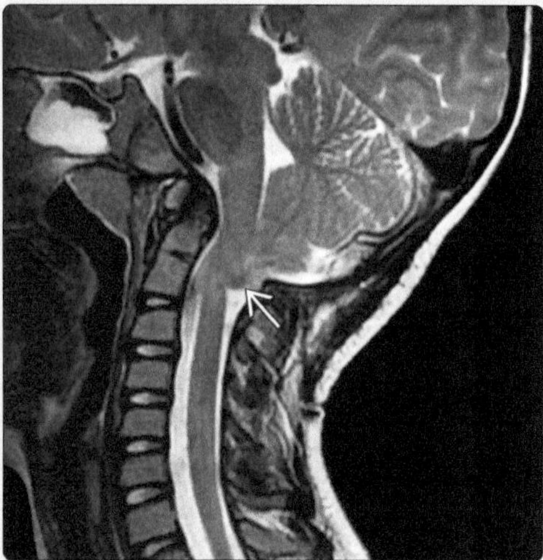

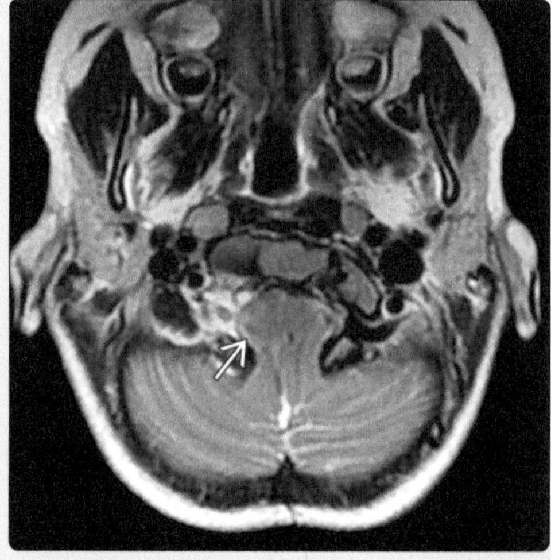

(Left) *Sagittal T2WI MR demonstrates characteristic features of complex Chiari (CC) with cervicomedullary kink with dorsal bump ➡, low obex, and craniovertebral junction (CVJ) anomalies (short clivus, reduced craniocervical angle, type II basilar invagination). Tonsillar herniation is modest. Note ventral medullary distortion.* **(Right)** *Axial T2WI MR in the same patient confirms the dorsal medullary bump ➡ and tonsillar crowding below the foramen magnum.*

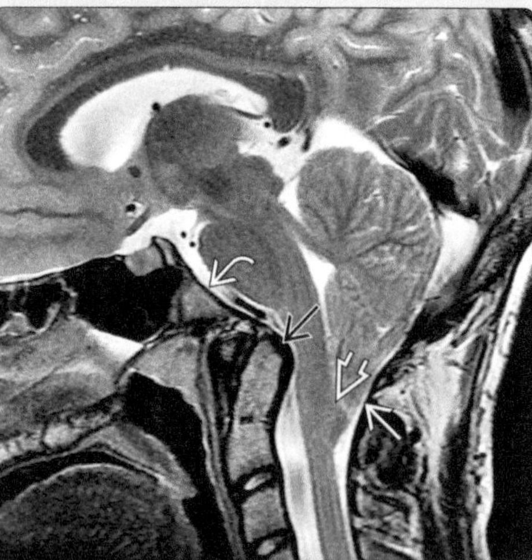

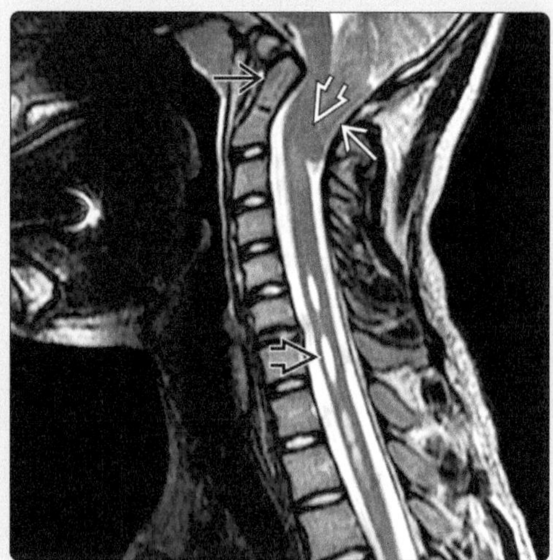

(Left) *Sagittal T2WI MR shows a prominent obex ➡ and pointed, ectopic cerebellar tonsils ➡. The odontoid process ➡ is retroflexed, and the clivus ➡ is foreshortened with a reduced craniocervical angle.* **(Right)** *Sagittal T2WI MR reveals striking odontoid ➡ retroflexion. Also note severe cerebellar tonsillar ectopia ➡ extending inferiorly to the C3 level and cervical syringohydromyelia ➡. The prominent, inferiorly displaced obex ➡ in conjunction with CVJ anomalies confirms a CC.*

TERMINOLOGY

Abbreviations

- Complex Chiari (CC)

Definitions

- Caudal cerebellar tonsil and brainstem herniation with dorsal cervicomedullary "bump" (Chiari 1.5)
- Associated craniovertebral junction (CVJ) anomalies by definition
  - Refinement of definition and terminology in evolution

IMAGING

General Features

- Best diagnostic clue
  - Cerebellar tonsillar herniation with low obex, dorsal medullary "bump"
- Location
  - Posterior fossa, CVJ
- Morphology
  - Dorsal medullary "bump" thought to represent aberrant clava, used as surrogate marker for cervicomedullary junction

CT Findings

- Bone CT
  - May show odontoid retroflexion, basilar invagination, small posterior fossa, clival anomalies, platybasia

MR Findings

- T1WI
  - Cerebellar tonsillar ectopia + low obex, dorsal medullary "bump"
    - Obex descends to or below foramen magnum
  - ± retroflexed odontoid, foreshortened clivus, basilar invagination
- T2WI
  - Same as T1WI ± syringohydromyelia, ventral cervicomedullary compression
- MR cine
  - Abnormal tonsillar "pistoning" motion, reduced CSF flow around foramen magnum and cerebellar tonsils

DIFFERENTIAL DIAGNOSIS

Chiari 1

- Cerebellar tonsillar ectopia ± low obex position
  - If obex inferiorly displaced, more modest than CC and no dorsal "bump"
  - ± syringomyelia, retroflexed odontoid process, platybasia, CVJ anomalies
- Generally less symptomatic than CC patients

Chiari 2

- Tectal beaking, cerebellar tonsil/vermis ectopia, medullary kink, other characteristic brain findings
- Associated with myelomeningocele

PATHOLOGY

General Features

- Associated abnormalities
  - Platybasia, occipital sclerotomal anomalies, Klippel-Feil spectrum

Gross Pathologic & Surgical Features

- Medullary pyramid decussation anatomic border between spinal cord, medulla oblongata
  - Pyramidal decussation difficult to image; obex position used as surrogate imaging landmark for cervicomedullary junction
  - Obex is thin band of neural tissue between area of postrema nuclei
    - Forms dorsal roof of central canal opening
    - Apex defines inferior margin of foramen of Magendie
  - Normal obex level is 10-12 mm above foramen magnum
  - Obex displaced to or below foramen magnum level in CC patients

CLINICAL ISSUES

Presentation

- Most common signs/symptoms
  - Headaches
- Other signs/symptoms
  - Myelopathy
  - Bulbar symptoms
  - Lethargy, failure to thrive

Natural History & Prognosis

- Progressively severe symptoms
- Patients frequently require more and earlier surgical intervention than typical Chiari 1
- Clinical symptoms may worsen after suboccipital decompression

Treatment

- Some patients (rarely) have minimal or no symptoms and require only observation
- Symptomatic patients generally require > 1 operation
  - Standard Chiari decompression procedure with dural patch
  - May also require dens resection, CVJ fusion to address basilar invagination, ventral cervicomedullary compression

DIAGNOSTIC CHECKLIST

Consider

- CC in context of cerebellar tonsillar herniation + low obex, dorsal medullary "bump"
- Growing repudiation of term Chiari 1.5
  - Incorrectly implies that patients reside along spectrum between Chiari 1 and Chiari 2
  - CC is best term to refer to these patients

SELECTED REFERENCES

1. Ravindra VM et al: Complex Chiari malformations: diagnosis, evaluation, and treatment. Neurosurg Clin N Am. 34(1):143-50, 2023
2. Marianayagam NJ et al: Increase in clivo-axial angle is associated with clinical improvement in children undergoing occipitocervical fusion for complex Chiari malformation: patient series. J Neurosurg Case Lessons. 2(23):CASE21433, 2021
3. Ho WSC et al: Complex Chiari malformation: using craniovertebral junction metrics to guide treatment. Childs Nerv Syst. 35(10):1847-51, 2019

Terminology

Definitions

Morphogenetic fields
- Embryologic cellular regions with potential for development into discrete anatomic structures

Gradient fields
- Describe gradually varying potential to form specific individual bones and organs within morphogenetic field

Homeobox genes
- Gene family complexes that regulate early embryologic differentiation
- Located on separate chromosomes
- Arranged linearly in same order as expression along craniocaudal axis

Imaging Protocols

Multiplanar magnetic resonance (MR) imaging best evaluates soft tissues, neural structures, and ligaments. Multidetector axial CT with sagittal and coronal reconstruction optimally defines bone anatomy.

Embryology

The spinal axis develops following a (mostly) orderly progression of steps with the vertebral axis and spinal cord developing synchronously. Embryologic spine formation begins in the occipital region, then subsequently commences at multiple other sites simultaneously. These sites progress at different rates and, thus, will be at different developmental stages at any given point in time. The cephalic spine (to approximately the conus level) forms by the process of primary neurulation, while the caudal spine forms separately by secondary neurulation (previously canalization and retrogressive differentiation). Most spinal anomalies may be explained by 1 or more events going awry during these steps.

Gastrulation

The 1st embryologic stage important for spinal development is gastrulation, when the bilaminar embryonic disk (composed of 2 distinct cell layers, epiblast and hypoblast) transforms into a trilaminar embryonic disk through interposition of a 3rd layer, the mesoderm. Subsequently, the epiblast cells migrate ventrally, forming the primitive streak. The nodular cluster at the cephalic end of the primitive streak is called the primitive node of Hensen. The notochord forms from mesodermal cells during the 2nd and 3rd gestational weeks. Spine formation proceeds concurrently with formation of other visceral structures, explaining the frequent occurrence of congenital malformations involving multiple organ systems.

Primary Neurulation

Embryonic spinal formation commences at the end of the 2nd gestational week, with formation of the Hensen node, and at the beginning of the 3rd week with the appearance of the neural plate during gastrulation (2-germ-cell-layer embryo → 3-germ-cell-layer embryo). The notochordal process forms at days 16-17 with transient communication of the amnion through the notochordal canal to the yolk sac through the neurenteric canal of Kovalevsky. Abnormalities during this stage produce the neurenteric cyst spectrum. The neural tube folds and closes at the end of the 3rd week, leaving temporary cranial and caudal openings called neuropores. The neural tube normally closes by days 25-27, signaling the end of primary neurulation. A closed neural tube is a prerequisite for normal development of the posterior neural arch.

During primary neurulation, the neural tube separates from the overlying ectoderm during the process of dysjunction. If dysjunction occurs prematurely (premature dysjunction), the perineural mesenchyme is permitted access to the neural groove and ependymal lining, differentiates into fat, and prevents complete neural tube closure, leading to the lipomatous malformation spectrum. Conversely, if dysjunction fails to occur (nondysjunction), an ectodermal-neuroectodermal tract forms that prevents mesenchymal migration, leading to focal or widespread dysraphism and the open neural tube defect spectrum, including myelomeningocele (MMC), dorsal dermal sinus, and myelocystocele. It is important to note that nondysjunction and premature dysjunction anomalies can coexist in combination simultaneously.

Spinal dysraphism (SD) refers to congenital discontinuity of the posterior elements. The etymologic origin of the term dysraphism is from the Greek words *dys* (bad) and *rhaph* (suture). Strictly speaking, this term should be applied only to primary neurulation abnormalities and not other congenital abnormalities of dorsal spinal formation. A genetic basis for SD has been described in some patients (particularly *MTHFR*).

Premature Dysjunction

Premature dysjunction of the neural tube from the overlying ectoderm allows the perineural mesenchyme to access the neural groove and differentiate into fat, physically preventing completion of neural tube closure and resulting in a spinal lipoma, ± closed posterior SD. The most commonly premature dysjunction anomalies are lipomyelomeningocele (LMMC) and intradural (juxtamedullary) lipoma. LMMC is a skin-covered, closed dysraphism anomaly in which the neural placode is complexed with a lipoma contiguous with the subcutaneous fat through a posterior dysraphic defect. In all cases, the lipoma attaches to and tethers the spinal cord. LMMC accounts for 20-56% of occult SD and 20% of skin-covered lumbosacral masses. Spinal lipoma is subdivided into intradural (juxtamedullary, subpial) and terminal lipomas. Intradural lipomas most commonly occur near the conus. Conversely, terminal lipoma is variably considered within both the premature dysjunction and abnormal caudal cell mass differentiation spectra with findings overlapping both mechanisms. Some authorities ("lumpers") combine all of the premature dysjunction disorders featuring lipomas into a lipomatous malformation spectrum for simplicity, recognizing that there is considerable overlap between the LMMC and lipoma malformations.

Nondysjunction

In contrast, anomalies resulting from nondysjunction related to teratogens or faulty notochord induction occur when the neural tube fails to dissociate from adjacent cutaneous ectoderm over either a focal or long interval. The least extensive variation is the dorsal dermal sinus, which occurs when a single connection remains, forming a fibrous cord from skin to conus or central spinal cord canal. The dermal sinus tract usually has an atypical dimple at the ostium that is remote (> 2.5 cm) from the anus, often combined with other cutaneous anomalies. They are most common in the lumbosacral spine, followed by the occipital region, and the sinus opening dermatomal level correlates with the metameric level of spinal cord attachment. All have some degree of focal dysraphism, which may be as subtle as a bifid spinous process. More extensive nondysjunction produces the open MMC lesion associated with maternal folate deficiency.

In this entity, the infant presents with an open, red, weeping skin defect. Lumbosacral and thoracolumbar MMC are most common, but cervical and thoracic MMC are observed rarely. Their association with the Chiari 2 malformation is well described.

Important mimics of the dorsal dermal sinus are the low sacral (coccygeal) dimple and pilonidal sinus. The low sacral or coccygeal dimple is common and features a low skin dimple affixed to the coccyx by a "spot weld." These dimples are found within the intergluteal cleft, never communicate with the spinal canal, and require no treatment. A pilonidal sinus has a low ostium, does not communicate with the spinal canal, and may present later with cutaneous infection.

Secondary Neurulation (Formerly Canalization and Retrogressive Differentiation)

By day 30, neural tube development below the caudal neuropore has commenced within the undifferentiated caudal cell mass of the primitive streak, which subsequently regresses. This process is inherently less precise than primary neurulation, which leads to more bizarre anomalies, and is characterized by the development of cysts in the caudal cell mass that coalesce into an ependymal-lined tubular structure that subsequently unites with the rostral neural tube. At day 48, a transient ventriculus terminalis appears in the future conus. If this persists after birth, it is noted incidentally as a persistent ventriculus terminalis or 5th ventricle, usually of no clinical significance. Failure of proper secondary neurulation leads to caudal regression spectrum, terminal myelocystocele, anterior sacral meningocele (ASM), tethered cord spectrum, or SCT. By the 3rd gestational month, the spinal cord extends the entire length of the developing spinal column. It is the more rapid elongation of the vertebral column and dura relative to the spinal cord that produces the apparent cord ascent during gestation. The conus should be at adult level soon after birth, and conus persistence below L2 after the 1st month of life in a full-term infant is probably abnormal.

Caudal cell mass anomalies are a diverse group of anomalies with a significant range of severity resulting from aberrant differentiation and retrogressive differentiation of the caudal cell mass. The etiology is postulated to be a metabolic or toxic insult to the caudal cell mass prior to the 4th gestational week. Most cases are sporadic, although a dominantly inherited defect in *HLBX9* has been recently described. 15-20% of affected caudal regression syndrome (CRS) patients are infants of diabetic mothers. Conversely, only 1% of diabetic mother offspring are afflicted with CRS. There is an association with vertebral, anal, cardiac, tracheal, esophageal, renal, and limb (VACTERL) anomalies; omphalocele; bladder extrophy; imperforate anus; and Currarino triad.

Hypogenesis or agenesis of the caudal cell mass produces CRS. Two types are described here. The more severe type I CRS shows a foreshortened terminal vertebral column with high-lying, wedge-shaped conus termination and severe associated anomalies, while the less severe type II CRS demonstrates a low-lying, tethered cord with milder associated malformations. In general, the higher the cord termination, the more severe the sacral anomalies. The most severe CRS presentations are lumbosacral agenesis, in which the spine terminates at the lower thoracic level, and severe sacral dysgenesis with fused lower extremities resulting in a so-called mermaid configuration (sirenomelia). In contrast, the mildest CRS cases manifest only a missing terminal sacral segment and are clinically asymptomatic. CRS is associated with myriad other congenital abnormalities, including renal/pulmonary hypoplasia and anorectal malformations. Other congenital spinal malformations, such as open dysraphism, segmentation and fusion anomalies (SFAs), and split cord malformations, are also commonly associated, and imaging should include a search to exclude those entities as well.

A rarer presentation of caudal cell mass dysplasia than CRS is the ASM, which is a large meningocele traversing an enlarged sacral foramen producing a presacral cystic mass. Most are sporadic, with a minority showing an inherited predisposition within the Currarino triad or in syndromes featuring dural dysplasia (neurofibromatosis type 1, Marfan syndrome). As with other caudal cell mass dysplasias, anorectal malformations, caudal dysgenesis, and dermoid/epidermoid tumors may be found as well.

Terminal myelocystocele is very rare and manifests as a hydromyelic spinal cord traversing a meningocele terminating in a skin-covered myelocystocele. Associated anorectal and other visceral anomalies are common and drive the early management as well as produce much of the morbidity and mortality.

Perhaps the most common lesion in the caudal cell mass dysplasia spectrum is tethered cord syndrome (TCS). Semantically speaking, TCS refers only to patients with a low-lying cord and thickened filum and not to patients with other spinal anomalies and cord abnormalities, even though those patients may appear tethered and clinically present similarly. It is important to consider TCS as a clinical diagnosis with imaging relegated to the role of preoperative planning rather than for establishing the primary diagnosis. On imaging, TCS manifests either as a taut spinal cord without definitive conus or low-lying conus with thickened, shortened filum and variably an associated lipomatous malformation.

Finally, if the primitive streak incompletely regresses and leaves a caudal remnant, a sacrococcygeal teratoma (SCT) may arise from the residual totipotential cell rests (Hensen node). SCTs demonstrate tissue derived from all 3 cell layers and contain varying proportions of mature and immature elements.

Vertebral Formation and Segmentation

Vertebral body formation occurs simultaneously with spinal cord development. During neurulation, the notochord induces the surrounding paraxial mesoderm derived from the primitive streak to form paired somite blocks (myotomes, sclerotomes). The myotomes form the paraspinal muscles and skin cover, while the sclerotomes divide into medial and lateral formations to produce the vertebral body, intervertebral disc, meninges, and spinal ligaments (medial) and posterior spinal elements (lateral). Failure of correct notochordal induction leads to incomplete splitting of the neural plate from the notochord and produces the split notochord syndromes [neurenteric cyst and diastematomyelia (DSM)]. At day 24, a remarkable process known as sclerotomal resegmentation commences and continues until the 5th week. During sclerotomal resegmentation, a horizontal sclerotomal cleft appears in the vertebra, and the caudal 1/2 of 1 vertebra combines with the rostral 1/2 of the vertebra below to form a "new" vertebral body. The notochord within the vertebral body subsequently degenerates, and the intervertebral notochordal remnant becomes the intervertebral disc nucleus pulposus. Between days 40-60, the vertebral body and neural arches undergo chondrification and then subsequent ossification, continuing past birth and into young adulthood. Ossification begins in the lower thoracic and upper lumbar regions and diverges cranially and caudally. In the cervical region, the vertebral primary ossification centers appear after the neural arch centers, beginning in lower cervical spine (C6, C7) and commencing rostrally. Cells of sclerotomal origin migrate dorsally to form the neural arch and condense to produce the spinous processes. The neural arches are situated intersegmentally with respect to the myotomes, so that each neural arch is associated with 2 successive myotomal segments. Absence of a ganglion at a vertebral level is postulated to allow unilateral arch fusion (congenital osseous bar).

Anomalies of vertebral formation and segmentation arise from aberrancies in vertebral column formation. These are generally divided into anomalies resulting from failure (partial or total) of vertebral formation (FVF) and failure to correctly segment after vertebral formation [vertebral segmentation failure (VSF)]. The abnormal vertebra may be supernumerary or replace a normal vertebral body. As a rule of thumb, the more severe the SFAs, the higher the incidence of concurrent visceral organ or other neuraxis anomalies. Abnormal *PAX1* expression is postulated to be etiologic in the development of the segmentation anomalies, and other visceral and neuraxis anomalies are commonly identified as well. With FVF, the degree and location of vertebral formation failure predicts morphology; unilateral chondral center deficiency and failure of ossification produce a hemivertebra, whereas central failure of ossification centers to unite produces a butterfly vertebra. Conversely, VSF presents with composite or "block" vertebra and posterior element fusions. Not surprisingly, block vertebra frequently coexist with FVF hemivertebra and butterfly vertebra, leading many to lump them together into the working term SFAs. Many clinical syndromes prominently feature SFAs, including Klippel-Feil and Jarcho-Levin (spondylothoracic dysplasia). Therefore, SFAs are not a finding that implicate a specific disorder but rather function more as an imaging marker for a possible syndromic process.

Spinal Cord

Spinal cord formation occurs in conjunction with vertebral formation. Within the spinal cord, the neuroepithelial cells (neuroblasts) around the central tube form the mantle layer, which produces the spinal cord gray matter. The outermost layer forms the marginal layer, which myelinates to produce the spinal cord white matter. The central neuroepithelial cells differentiate into ependymal cells along the central canal. Neural crest cells along each side of the neural groove form the dorsal root ganglia (DRG), autonomic ganglia, Schwann cells, leptomeninges, and adrenal medulla.

Notochordal Anomalies

Notochordal anomalies, primarily neurenteric cyst and DSM, produce some of the most bizarre congenital spinal anomalies. Neurenteric cysts, consisting of an intraspinal cyst lined by enteric mucosa, are most common in the thoracic spine, followed by the cervical spine. They arise from a putative, abnormal, persistent connection between the primitive endoderm and ectoderm during the 3rd embryonic week. Whereas, normally, the notochord separates the ventral endoderm (foregut) and dorsal ectoderm (skin, spinal cord) during embryogenesis, in a neurenteric cyst, there is failure of separation that "splits" the notochord and hinders development of mesoderm, trapping a small piece of the primitive gut within the developing spinal canal. This gut remnant may become isolated, forming a cyst, or maintain connections with the gut, skin, or both, producing the spectrum of fistulae and sinuses comprising the dorsal-enteric spinal anomalies spectrum. The most severe cases maintain communication through a primitive vertebral canal of Kovalevsky, but even mild cases usually show some kind of vertebral segmentation anomalies on close inspection.

DSM arises from a similar aberrant process to neurenteric cyst, resulting in a splitting of the spinal cord into 2 hemicords, each with 1 ventral and 1 dorsal root. The hemicords may be symmetric or asymmetric (partial DSM), and 1 or both may feature hydromyelia or tethering. Because the notochord influences vertebral development, vertebral segmentation anomalies are very commonly associated with DSM. The presence (type I) or absence (type II) of an osseous or fibrous spur and whether the cords reside in separate or a single dural tube is important for preoperative planning. Occasionally, the nerve root(s) will become adherent to the dura and tether the spinal cord, producing the so-called meningocele manqué. DSM may be isolated or found in conjunction with other spinal anomalies, particularly MMC, and it is thus critical to search for DSM prior to operative repair of a spinal anomaly or scoliosis correction.

Congenital and Developmental Anomalies of Unknown Etiology

Other uncommon but important anomalies where the etiology is not definitively known include the simple dorsal meningocele and the lateral meningocele. Dorsal meningocele by definition occurs dorsally, often in the lumbosacral spine, and, strictly defined, features a skin-covered meningocele devoid of neural elements protruding through a posterior dysraphic defect. In practice, however, it is not uncommon to find pieces of dysplastic nerve root or other neural tissue within the meningocele. Lateral meningoceles present as CSF-filled paraspinal masses contiguous with the thecal sac, extending through a neural foramen with adjacent pedicular and foraminal osseous remodeling.

Selected References

1. White C et al: Imaging of congenital spine malformations. Clin Perinatol. 49(3):623-40, 2022
2. Trapp B et al: A practical approach to diagnosis of spinal dysraphism. Radiographics. 41(2):559-75, 2021
3. Chaturvedi A et al: Malformed vertebrae: a clinical and imaging review. Insights Imaging. 9(3):343-55, 2018
4. Panagopoulos D et al: Intradural-extramedullary cervical cord lipoma: case report and literature review. World Neurosurg. 110:162-8, 2018
5. Ward L et al: The role of the notochord in amniote vertebral column segmentation. Dev Biol. 439(1):3-18, 2018
6. Scaal M: Early development of the vertebral column. Semin Cell Dev Biol. 49:83-91, 2016
7. Pang D: Sacral agenesis and caudal spinal cord malformations. Neurosurgery. 32(5):755-78; discussion 778-9, 1993
8. Pang D et al: Split cord malformation: part I: a unified theory of embryogenesis for double spinal cord malformations. Neurosurgery. 31(3):451-80, 1992

Neural Tube Embryology

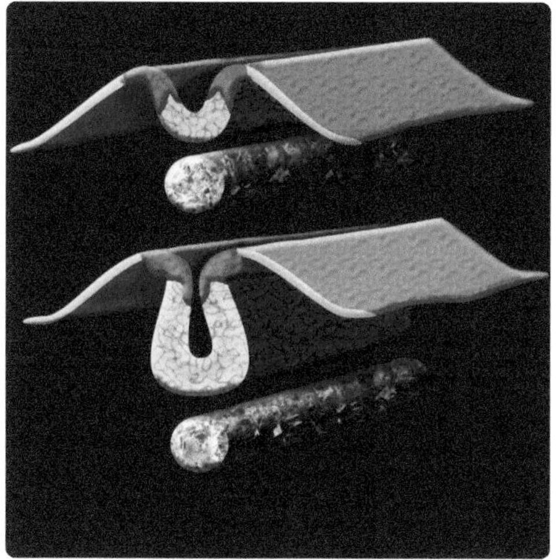

Neural Tube Embryology

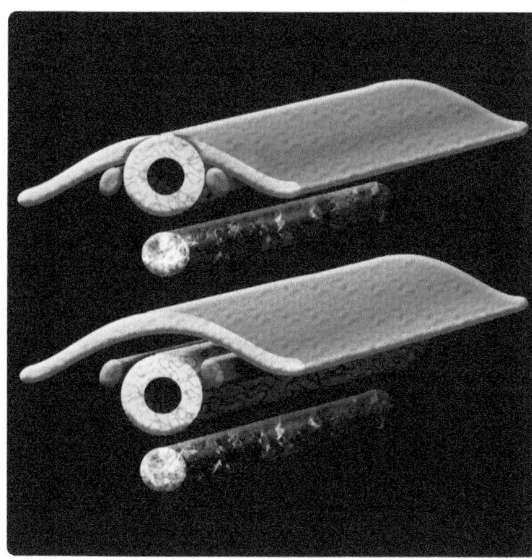

(Left) *3D graphic of neural tube embryology demonstrates normal formation of neural plate (top) and neural groove (bottom). Note the cutaneous epithelium (orange), neural crest (red), neural ectoderm (green), and notochord (gray).* **(Right)** *3D graphic of neural tube formation depicts normal neural tube closure (top) and subsequent dysjunction (bottom). Note the cutaneous epithelium (orange), neural crest (red), neural ectoderm (green), and notochord (gray).*

Lipomyelomeningocele

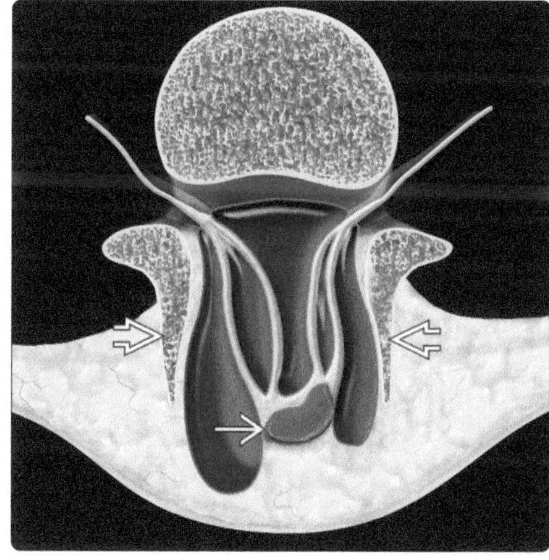

Lipomyelomeningocele

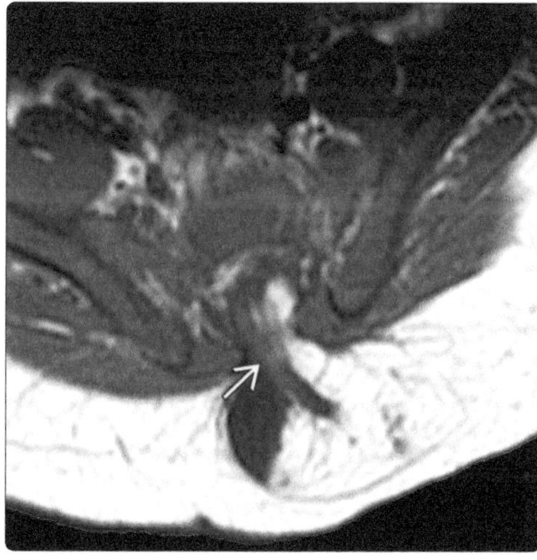

(Left) *Axial graphic illustrates premature dysjunction with a classic lipomyelomeningocele. The neural placode ➡ is displaced through the dysraphic unfused posterior elements ➡ into a meningocele sac.* **(Right)** *Axial T1WI MR demonstrates an elongated spinal cord placode ➡ inserting into a distal lipomatous malformation that "balloons" through a posterior dysraphic defect into a CSF signal cyst within the subcutaneous fat.*

Subpial Conus Lipoma

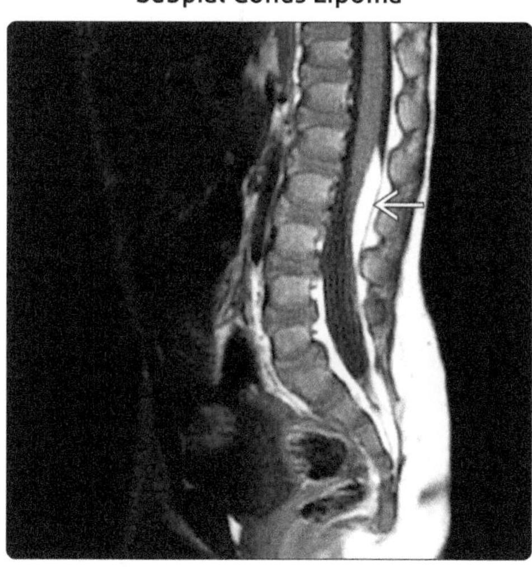

Subpial Conus Lipoma

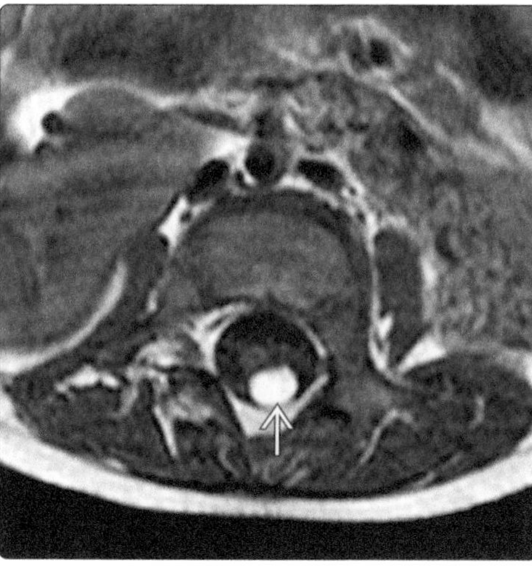

(Left) *Sagittal T1WI MR demonstrates the typical hyperintense appearance of a juxtamedullary or subpial conus lipoma ➡. The conus is low-lying at L2/L3. These lipomas classically arise from premature dysjunction.* **(Right)** *Axial T1WI MR confirms the lipoma's ➡ intradural location and close relationship with the dorsal conus surface. Additionally, the misshapen right kidney and empty left renal fossa proved to represent crossed fused renal ectopia.*

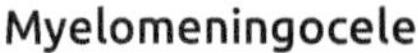

Myelomeningocele

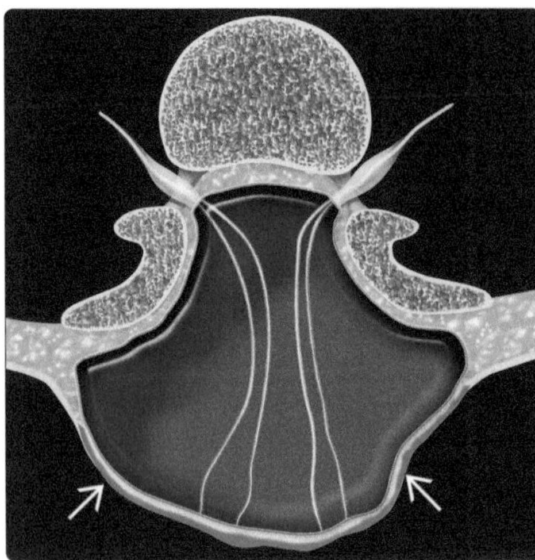

Myelomeningocele

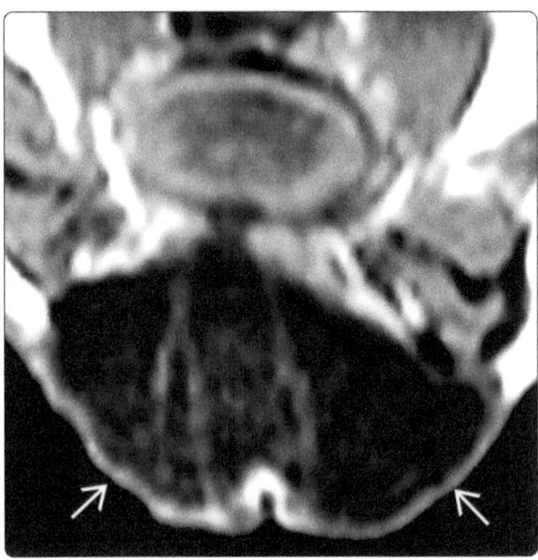

(Left) *Axial graphic shows a classic myelomeningocele, with the nerve roots traversing a large meningocele sac from the exposed neural placode* ➡, *which merges into adjacent cutaneous fat and skin. This is an example of nondysjunction.* **(Right)** *Axial T1WI MR (unrepaired lumbar myelomeningocele) demonstrates nondysjunction, characterized by open dysraphism with lack of skin covering over the neural placode* ➡. *The neural elements are in direct contact with the outside environment.*

Dorsal Dermal Sinus

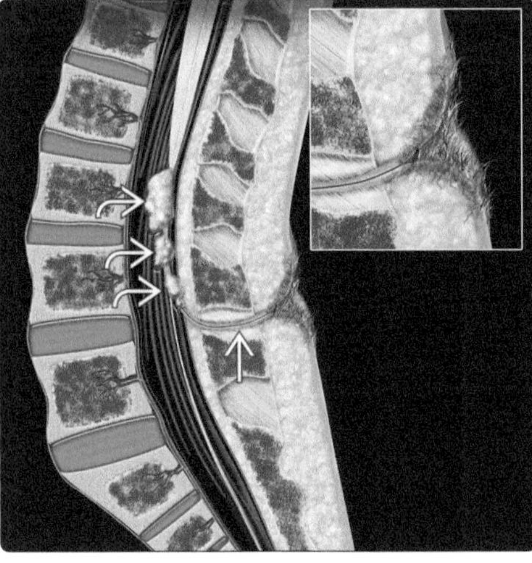

Dorsal Dermal Sinus

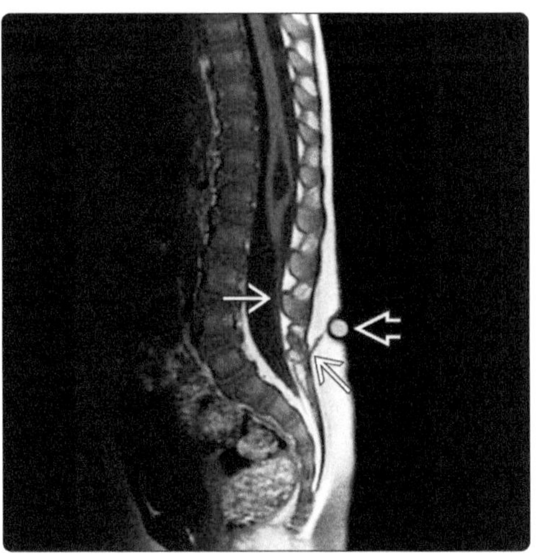

(Left) *Sagittal graphic illustrates focal nondisjunction with a dorsal dermal cutaneous sinus tract* ➡ *extending from skin surface to conus. A hairy vascular cutaneous lesion marks the sinus ostium. Note the epidermoid deposits* ➡ *along the sinus tract.* **(Right)** *Sagittal T1WI MR reveals a hypointense dermal sinus extending through the L5 posterior elements and coursing intradurally* ➡ *to tether the low-lying conus at L2/L3. A vitamin E capsule has been placed to mark the skin opening of the sinus* ➡.

Caudal Regression

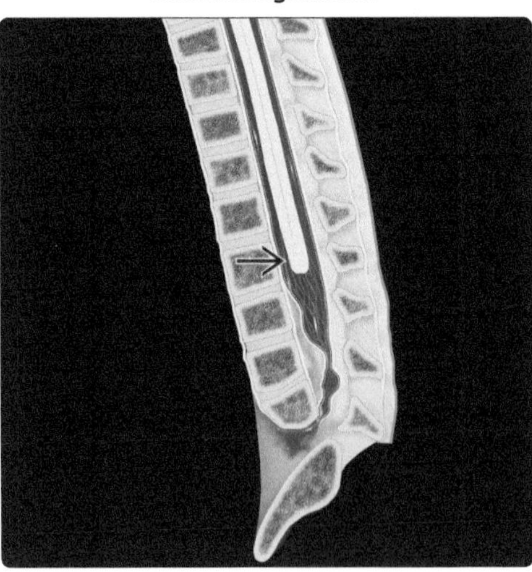

Caudal Regression

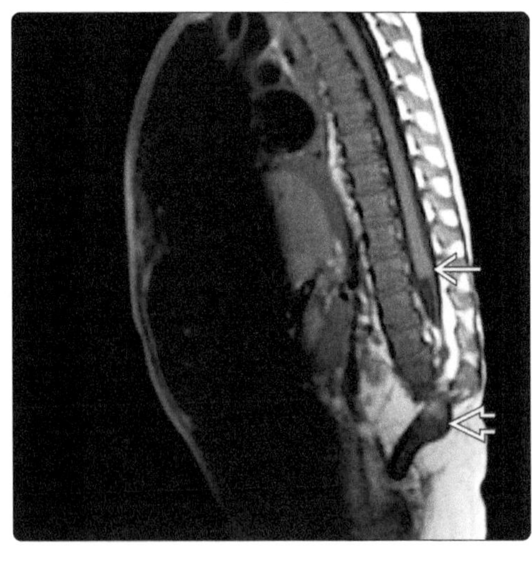

(Left) *Sagittal graphic depicts aberrant secondary neurulation resulting in severe caudal regression and vertebral column termination at the lower lumbar spine. The blunt, abnormally high conus* ➡ *is characteristic of type I caudal regression syndrome (CRS).* **(Right)** *Sagittal T1WI MR (caudal regression) reveals abnormal vertebral column termination at the low lumbar level. The abnormal conus* ➡ *shows a characteristic blunt-wedge shape. Sacral absence permits medial migration of the iliac wings* ➡.

Tethered Spinal Cord

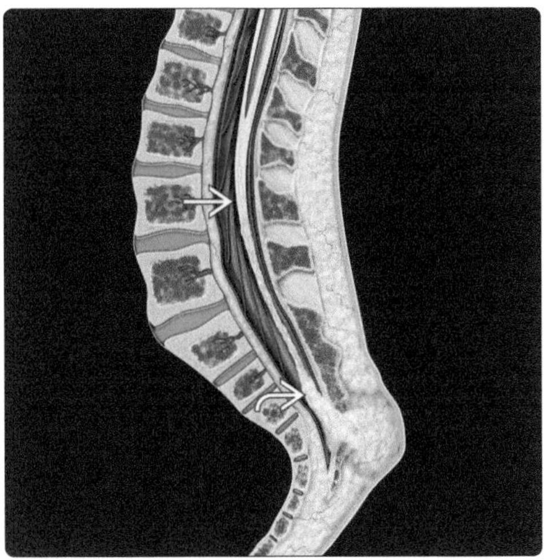

Tethered Spinal Cord

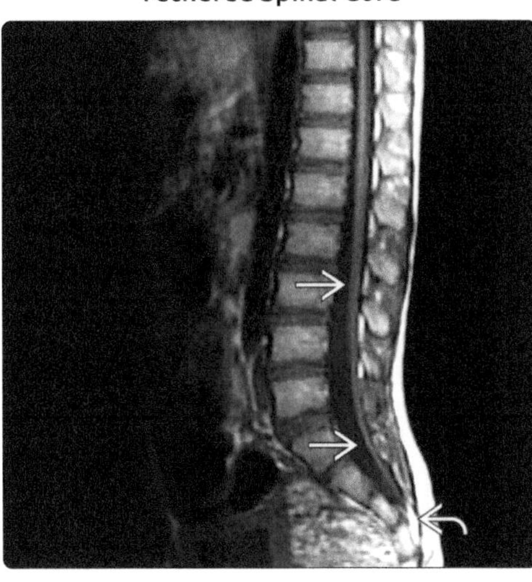

(Left) *Sagittal graphic (tethered spinal cord) demonstrates abnormal elongation of the low-lying spinal cord ➡, which inserts into a terminal lipoma ↪ at the end of a thick, shortened fatty filum.* **(Right)** *Sagittal T1WI MR (tethered spinal cord) reveals an abnormally elongated spinal cord ➡ extending to at least L5, subtly transitioning into a thickened filum terminale that terminates in a small terminal lipoma ↪. No syrinx or hydromyelia is present.*

Sacrococcygeal Teratoma

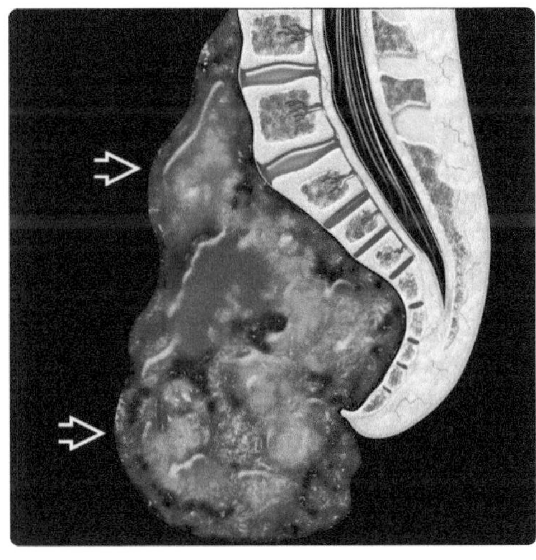

Sacrococcygeal Teratoma

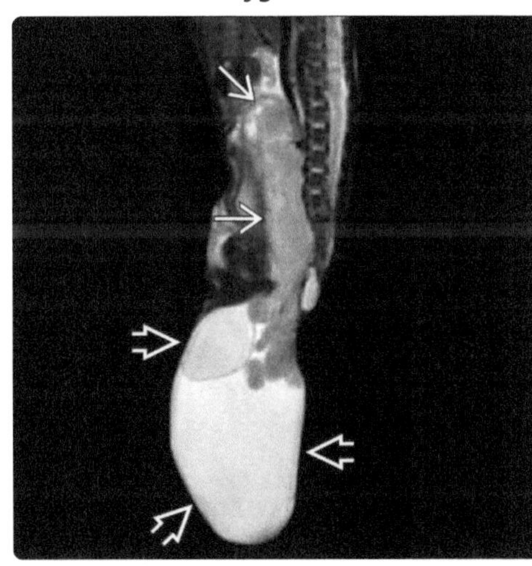

(Left) *Sagittal graphic (AAP II sacrococcygeal teratoma) shows a heterogeneous necrotic neoplasm ➡ located ventral to the sacrum. Approximately equal to external and internal components classify the tumor as AAP type II. Absence of sacral invasion is characteristic.* **(Right)** *Sagittal T2WI MR (AAP II sacrococcygeal teratoma) depicts a mixed cystic and solid pelvic mass. The internal portion ➡ is predominantly solid, whereas the external portion ➡ is more cystic.*

Anterior Sacral Meningocele

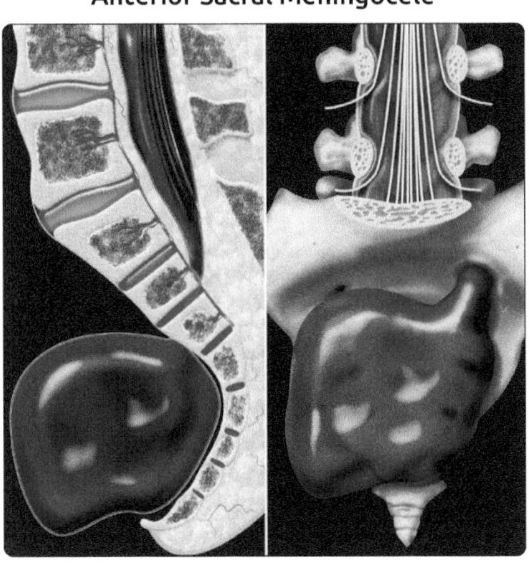

Terminal Myelocystocele

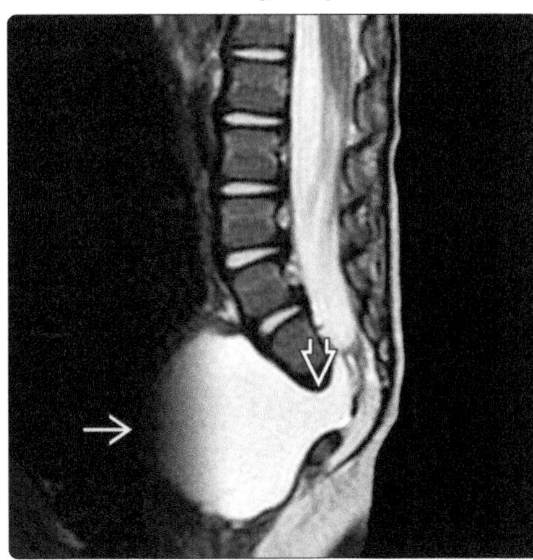

(Left) *Sagittal and coronal graphics demonstrate a classic anterior sacral meningocele. The sac enters the presacral space through an enlarged sacral neural foramina.* **(Right)** *Sagittal T2WI MR (anterior sacral meningocele) imaged parasagittal off-midline demonstrates continuity of the ventral meningocele sac ➡ with the thecal sac through an abnormally enlarged sacral foramen ➡.*

(Left) *Sagittal graphic demonstrates a typical terminal myelocystocele with posterior spinal dysraphism and classic cyst within a cyst configuration.* **(Right)** *Sagittal T2WI MR shows the classic appearance of terminal myelocystocele with a low-lying tethered spinal cord with distal hydromyelia ➔ traversing a meningocele ➔ produced by obstruction of the subarachnoid space. Also note the hypoplastic sacrum.*

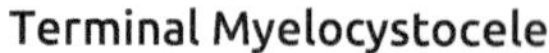

Terminal Myelocystocele

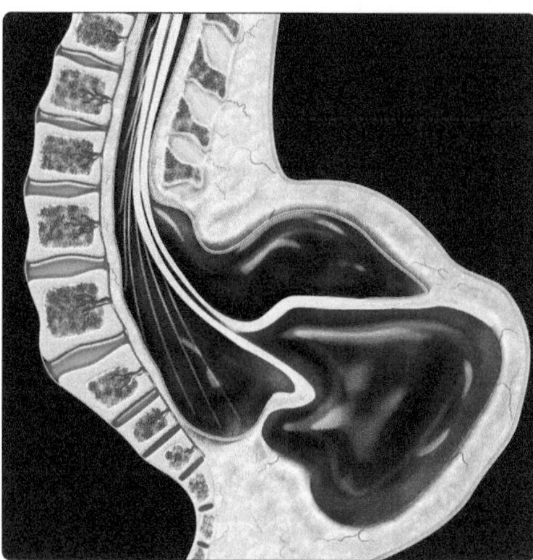

Terminal Myelocystocele

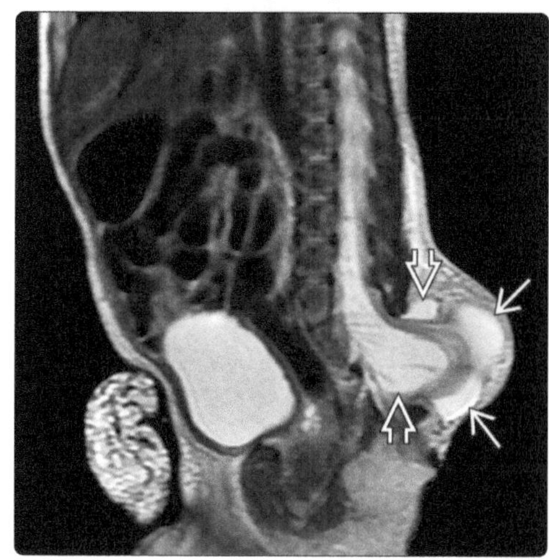

(Left) *Sagittal bone CT of the sacrum and coccyx in a 24-month-old demonstrates normal ossification of the 5 sacral vertebra and first 3 coccygeal vertebra. The underlying cartilaginous model is faintly visible as soft tissue density containing the ossified centra.* **(Right)** *Axial bone CT in a 3-day-old infant demonstrates the normal CT imaging appearance of the vertebral centrum ➔ and neural arch ➔. The primary ossification centers are separated by cartilaginous synchondroses ➔.*

Normal Ossification

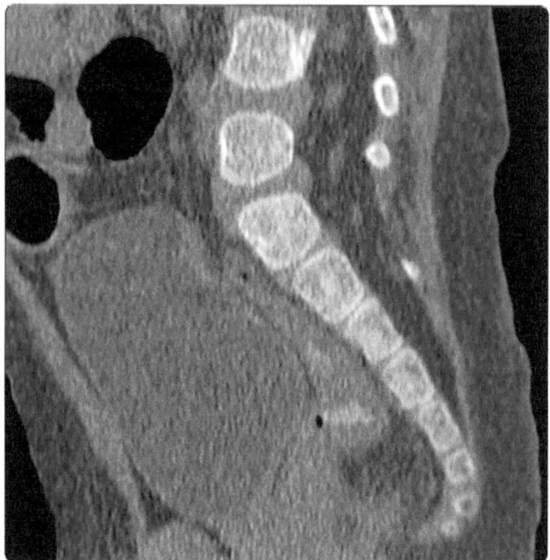

Normal Ossification

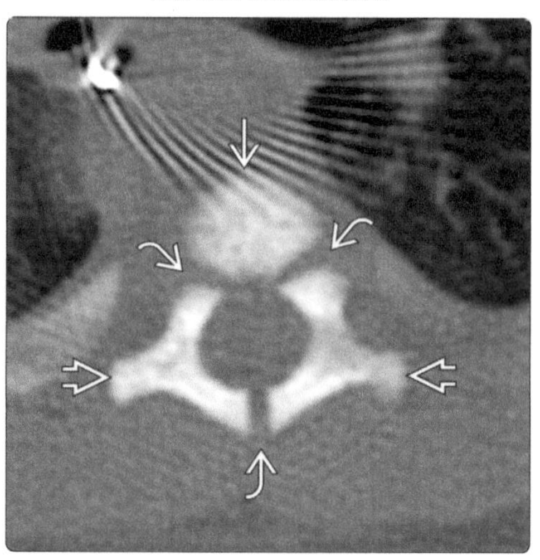

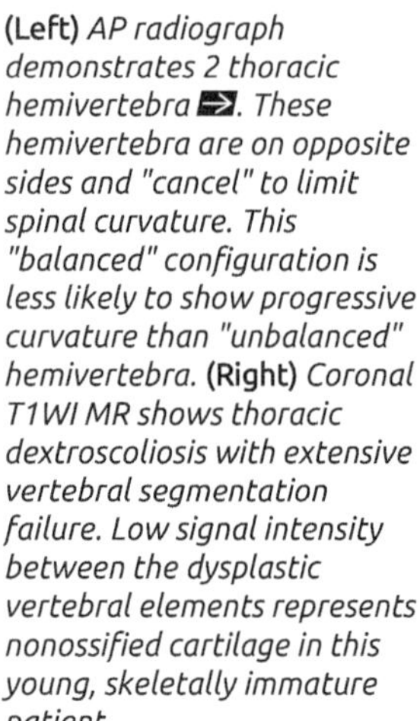

(Left) *AP radiograph demonstrates 2 thoracic hemivertebra ➔. These hemivertebra are on opposite sides and "cancel" to limit spinal curvature. This "balanced" configuration is less likely to show progressive curvature than "unbalanced" hemivertebra.* **(Right)** *Coronal T1WI MR shows thoracic dextroscoliosis with extensive vertebral segmentation failure. Low signal intensity between the dysplastic vertebral elements represents nonossified cartilage in this young, skeletally immature patient.*

Failure of Vertebral Malformation

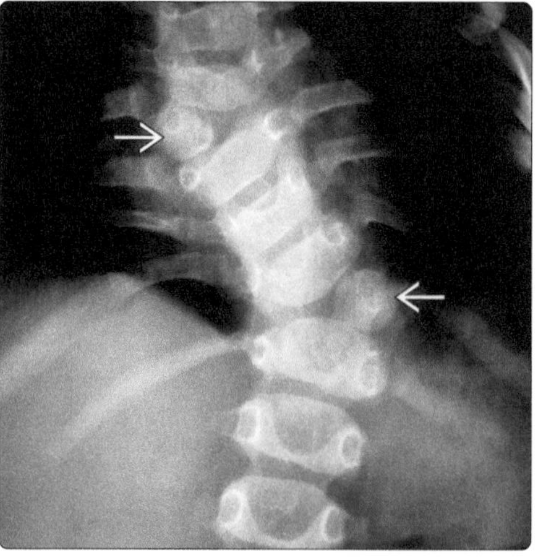

Vertebral Segmentation Failure

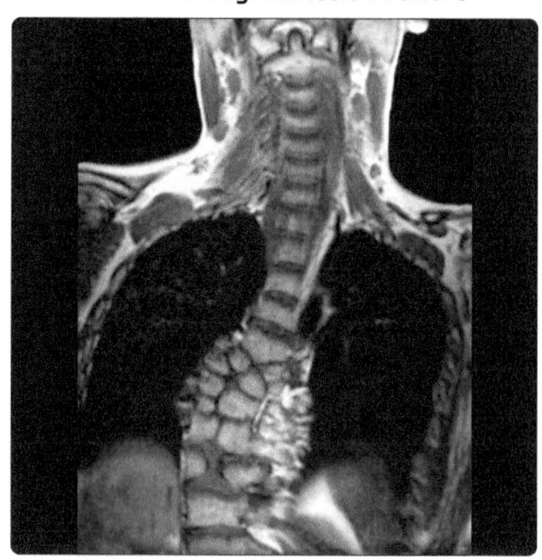

Diastematomyelia

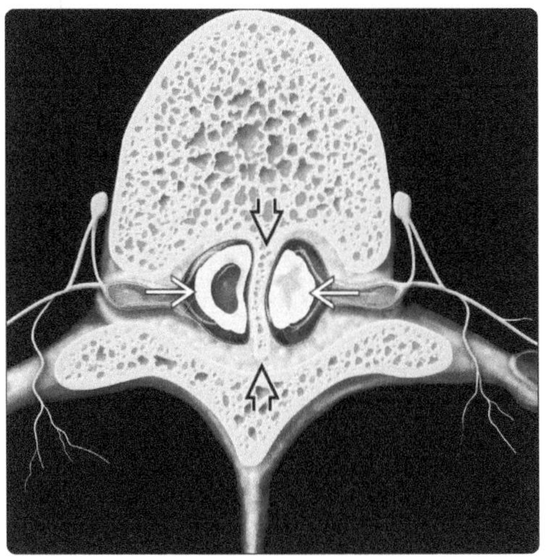

Diastematomyelia

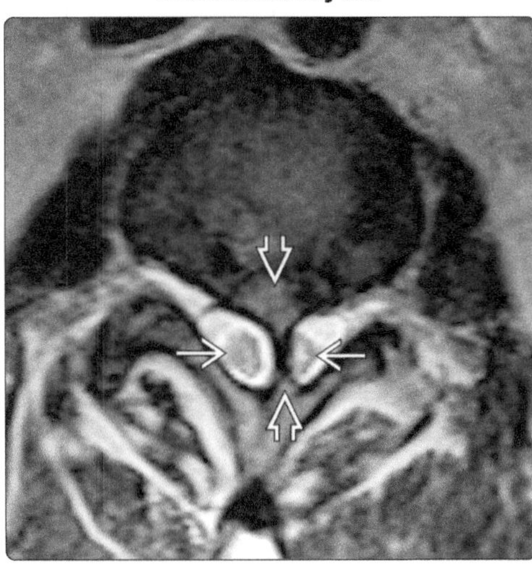

(Left) *Axial graphic demonstrates type 1 diastematomyelia with a large osseous spur ⇨ connecting the vertebral body to posterior elements and dividing the spinal cord into 2 hemicords ➡, each within a separate dural tube. The right hemicord has a syrinx.* **(Right)** *Axial T1WI MR (split notochord syndrome) depicts classic type 1 diastematomyelia with an ossified spur ⇨ dividing the dural sac and spinal cord into 2 separate hemicords ➡, each within their own dural tube.*

Split Notochord Syndrome

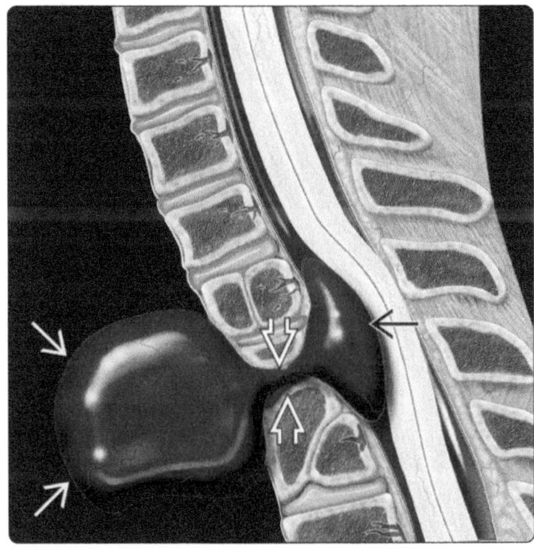

Split Notochord Syndrome

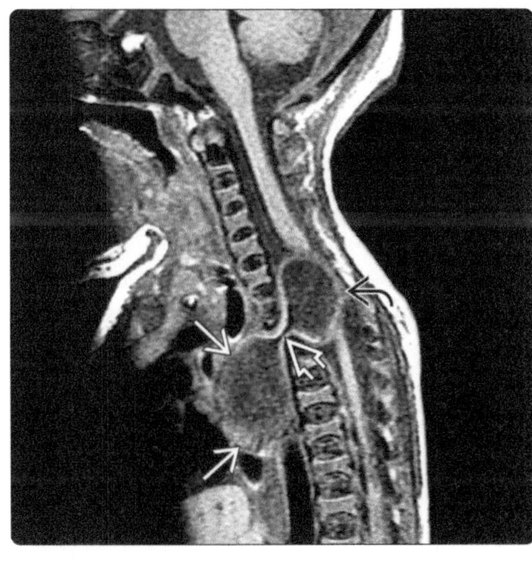

(Left) *Sagittal graphic (split notochord syndrome) shows upper thoracic vertebral segmentation anomalies with a persistent canal of Kovalevsky ⇨ permitting communication of the mediastinal enteric cyst ➡ with the extradural neurenteric cyst ➡.* **(Right)** *Sagittal T1WI MR demonstrates a large, dumbbell-shaped neurenteric cyst. The mediastinal enteric cyst ➡ extends into the ventral spinal canal through the canal of Kovalevsky ⇨ to produce an intracanalicular neurenteric cyst ➡.*

Dorsal Spinal Meningocele

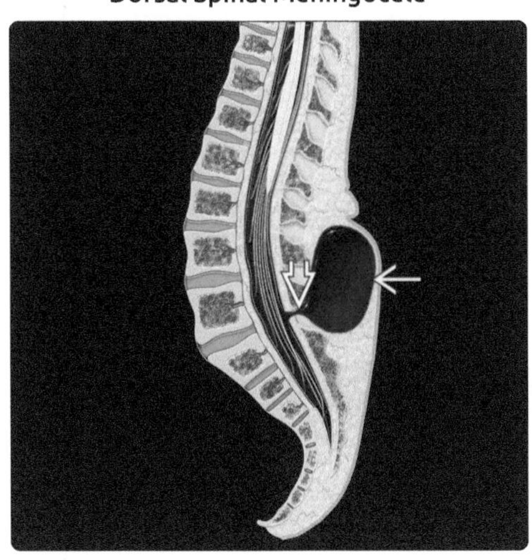

Dorsal Spinal Meningocele

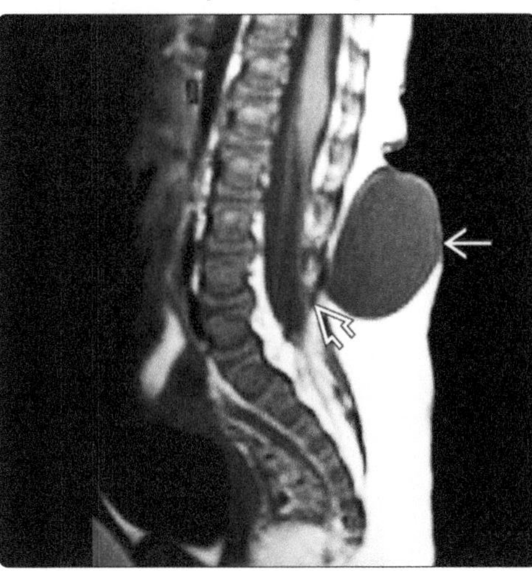

(Left) *Sagittal graphic demonstrates a dorsal spinal meningocele, a malformation of unknown etiology. The meningocele sac ➡ communicates with the dural sac by a thin isthmus ⇨. There are no neural elements within the meningocele sac.* **(Right)** *Sagittal T1WI MR shows the classic appearance of a dorsal spinal meningocele. The meningocele sac ➡ extends through the posterior elements via a thin isthmus ⇨, representing mild focal closed spinal dysraphism.*

Myelomeningocele

KEY FACTS

TERMINOLOGY

- Myelomeningocele (MMC) & myelocele (MC) comprise spectrum of open (not skin-covered) spinal dysraphisms
- MMC: Neural placode outside of spinal canal with measurable sac
- MC: Neural placode flush with skin surface or inside spinal canal

IMAGING

- Fetal US/MR: Lumbosacral dysraphism ± thin-walled MMC sac + intracranial findings of Chiari 2 (lemon sign, banana sign, ± ventriculomegaly)
- Postnatal spine imaging typically only performed after repair (need prenatal imaging or preoperative clinical confirmation of open defect)
  - Posterior osseous dysraphic defect & elongation of spinal cord persist
  - Neural placode (distal, nonneurulated segment of cord) inserts onto dorsal aspect of distal thecal sac

TOP DIFFERENTIAL DIAGNOSES

- Closed (skin-covered) spinal dysraphism
- Postoperative pseudomeningocele

CLINICAL ISSUES

- Most common neurologic deficits: Lower extremities, bowel & bladder dysfunction
- ~ 80-85% have hydrocephalus requiring CSF diversion, though lower incidence reported after fetal repair
- Mortality: 10-30% die before adulthood
  - Brainstem/cerebellar dysfunction or shunt malfunction

DIAGNOSTIC CHECKLIST

- Most common spinal cause of delayed neurologic deterioration: Cord retethering (clinical diagnosis)
  - Spine MR (± brain imaging) to look for other causes
- For postnatal spine imaging, check clinical history to confirm history of open spinal dysraphism
  - MMC vs. MC on prenatal imaging only

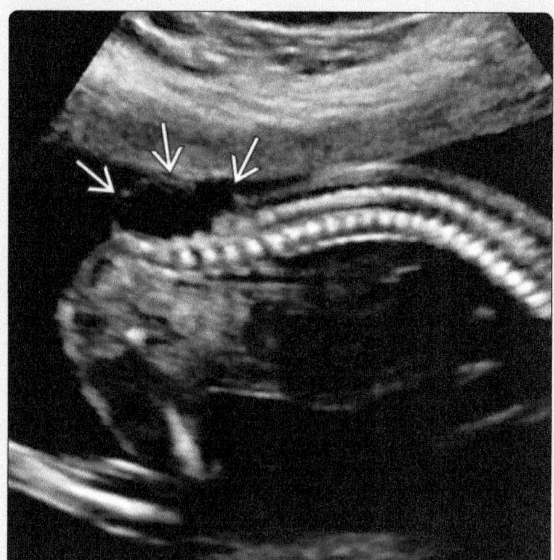

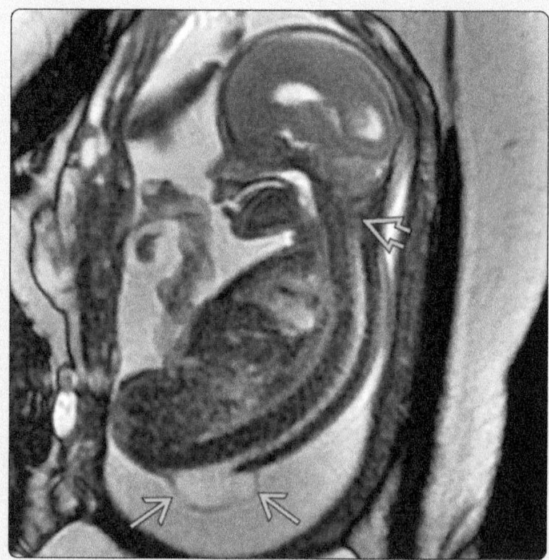

(Left) *Longitudinal US of the spine in a 20-weeks-gestation fetus shows absence of posterior lumbosacral spinal elements & a measurable sac extending beyond the expected contours of the skin, consistent with a myelomeningocele (MMC) ➡.* **(Right)** *Sagittal 2D SSFP MR in the same fetus, now at 21-weeks gestation, shows the lumbosacral MMC ⇒. There is a small posterior fossa, hindbrain herniation ⇒, & effacement of the normal 4th ventricle, consistent with Chiari 2.*

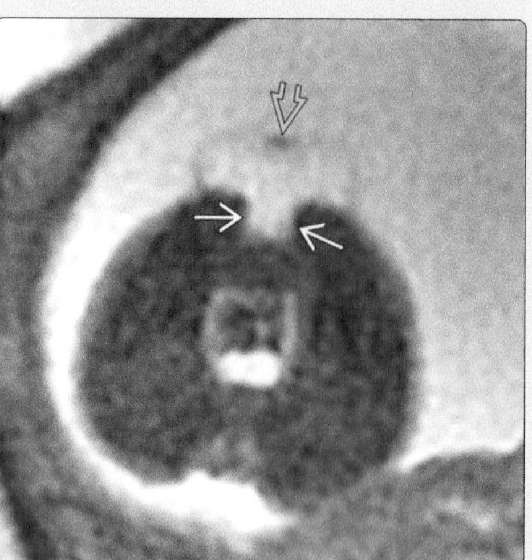

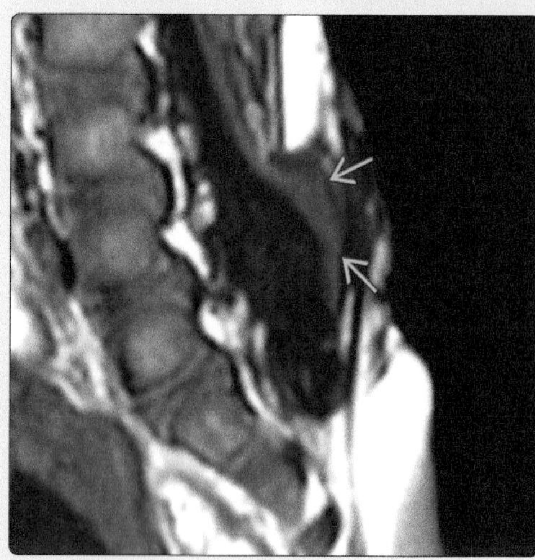

(Left) *Axial 2D SSFP MR in the lumbosacral spine from the same fetus demonstrates the neural placode ⇒ outside of the open spinal canal ➡, consistent with an MMC.* **(Right)** *Sagittal T1WI MR in the same patient at 10 months of age (status post MMC closure) shows an expected skin-covered, postoperative appearance. The neural placode is attached to the dorsal thecal sac at the repair site ⇒, which is a typical finding.*

TERMINOLOGY

Definitions

- Myelomeningocele (MMC): Open (no skin covering) spinal dysraphism in which neural placode (exposed nonneurulated end of elongated spinal cord) protrudes as sac beyond skin surface dorsal to spinal canal
- Myelocele (MC): Open spinal dysraphism with neural placode flush with skin surface or within spinal canal (no sac)
- Some refer to all open spinal dysraphisms as MMC (as MMC & MC fall along same pathologic spectrum)

IMAGING

General Features

- Best diagnostic clue
  - Absent posterior osseous elements, distorted low-lying spinal cord/roots, postoperative skin closure changes
    - Rarely imaged before repair in postnatal period due to infection risk
  - > 80% have significant hindbrain herniation in setting of Chiari 2

MR Findings

- Fetal MR
  - Abnormal elongation of spinal cord with neural placode extending into osseous dysraphism ± MMC sac
  - Intracranial findings of Chiari 2
- Postnatal MR: T1, T2
  - Postoperative soft tissue changes of MMC/MC closure
  - Elongation of spinal cord extending to flat neural placode adherent to posterior thecal sac
    - Loss of normal posterior epidural fat at level of defect
  - Postoperative complications
    - Syringohydromyelia
    - Dermoid/epidermoid or arachnoid cysts
  - Associated anomalies: Split cord malformation (31-46%), dorsal dermal sinus, segmentation anomalies, caudal agenesis

DIFFERENTIAL DIAGNOSIS

Closed (Occult) Spinal Dysraphism

- Skin-covered osseous defect

Postoperative Pseudomeningocele

- History & clinical exam allow for differentiation

PATHOLOGY

General Features

- Etiology
  - Failure of neural tube closure in 3rd-gestational week
    - Due to lack of expression of specific receptors on surface of neuroectodermal cells
    - Likely multifactorial: Folate deficiency, toxins, genetics
  - Neurologic deficits are worsened by chronic mechanical injury & amniotic fluid exposure

CLINICAL ISSUES

Presentation

- Most common signs/symptoms
  - Clinically obvious at birth: Exposed neural placode, usually leaking CSF
  - Dysfunction of bowel, bladder, & lower extremities
    - Higher level spine defect correlates with greater motor & somatosensory deficits

Natural History & Prognosis

- Stable postoperative motor deficit in majority (~ 73%)
  - Neurologic deterioration suggests complication
- ~ 2/3 have normal intelligence, ~ 23% have ≥ 1 seizure
- Bladder, bowel, & sexual dysfunction
- Lower extremity dysfunction
- Mortality: 10-30% die before adulthood

Treatment

- MMC closure < 48 hours after delivery to stabilize neurologic deficits & prevent infection
- In utero surgical repair: ↓ need for shunting, ↓ Chiari 2 findings; may improve neurologic function
  - Candidates in MOMS trial had defect T1-S1, < 30° kyphosis, & hindbrain herniation
  - MMC technically easier to repair primarily than MC because of ↑ viable skin tissue
  - MMC has worse lower extremity motor outcomes than MC → more clubfoot
- Subsequent management of postoperative complications
  - Cord untethering, CSF diversion

DIAGNOSTIC CHECKLIST

Consider

- Open spinal dysraphisms are rarely imaged before repair postnatally
- Differentiation between MMC vs. MC is on prenatal imaging & has implications for fetal surgical approach
- Hindbrain herniation is seen in majority of open spinal dysraphisms after postnatal repair but not prenatal repair
- After repair, it cannot always be determined what type of spinal dysraphism was repaired (even open vs. closed spinal dysraphism) → must be correlated with clinical history or prenatal imaging

Image Interpretation Pearls

- Cord retethering is clinical diagnosis as neural placode will always appear attached to operative site
  - Imaging is used to look for other complications causing symptoms, such as syrinx, arachnoid cyst, dermoid/epidermoid cyst

SELECTED REFERENCES

1. Patel SK et al: Effect of allograft patch closure on incidence of spinal inclusion cyst formation following open fetal myelomeningocele repair. J Neurosurg Pediatr. 32(2):141-8, 2023
2. Trapp B et al: A practical approach to diagnosis of spinal dysraphism. Radiographics. 41(2):559-75, 2021
3. Nagaraj UD et al: Imaging of open spinal dysraphisms in the era of prenatal surgery. Pediatr Radiol. 50(13):1988-98, 2020
4. Oliver ER et al: Myelomeningocele sac associated with worse lower-extremity neurological sequelae: evidence for prenatal neural stretch injury? Ultrasound Obstet Gynecol. 55(6):740-6, 2020

Lipomyelomeningocele

KEY FACTS

TERMINOLOGY

- Subtype of closed (skin-covered) spinal dysraphism characterized by lipoma with dorsal defect
  - Neural placode of elongated spinal cord attaches to lipomatous tissue in continuity with dorsal subcutaneous fat through spinal dysraphic defect, forming placode-lipoma interface
  - Placode-lipoma interface can be within spinal canal [lipomyelocele (LMC)] or protrude outside spinal canal with expansion of adjacent subarachnoid space/meninges [lipomyelomeningocele (LMMC)]

IMAGING

- Elongated spinal cord ends in neural placode attached dorsally to lipomatous tissue with dorsal osseous dysraphic defect; subarachnoid space expanded around neural placode with LMMC
- ± syrinx, split cord malformation, segmentation anomalies, caudal agenesis (group 2)

TOP DIFFERENTIAL DIAGNOSES

- Other closed spinal dysraphisms
  - With subcutaneous mass: Meningocele, terminal myelocystocele
  - Without subcutaneous mass: Intradural lipoma, dorsal dermal sinus
- Open spinal dysraphisms: Myelomeningocele, myelocele
  - Not skin covered, usually obvious at birth clinically
- Sacrococcygeal teratoma

PATHOLOGY

- Premature disjunction (separation) of neural ectoderm from cutaneous ectoderm → allows mesenchyme to enter closing neural tube, preventing neurulation to proceed

DIAGNOSTIC CHECKLIST

- Other closed spinal dysraphisms may coexist, especially caudal agenesis (look for complete formation of sacrococcygeal spine)

(Left) *Sagittal T2 MR of the spine shows closed lumbosacral spinal dysraphism with a low-lying spinal cord in association with intradural fat that is in continuity with the dorsal SQ fat through the osseous spinal defect. The placode-lipoma interface ➡ is in the spinal canal, consistent with lipomyelocele (LMC). There is also sacral hypoplasia ➡ with coccygeal aplasia, consistent with group 2 caudal agenesis.* **(Right)** *Axial T1 MR (same patient) again shows the placode lipoma interface in the spinal canal ➡, consistent with LMC.*

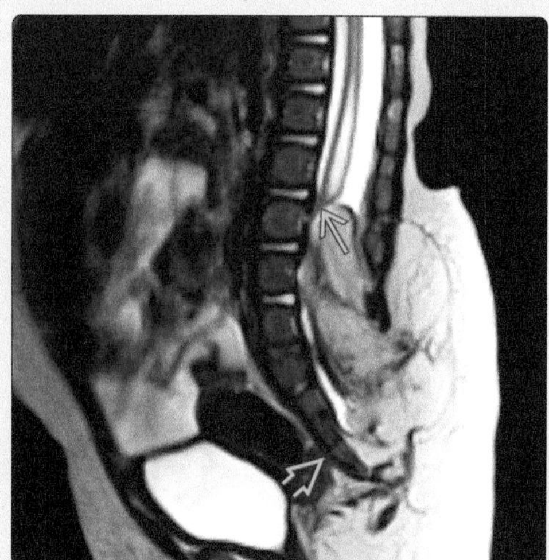

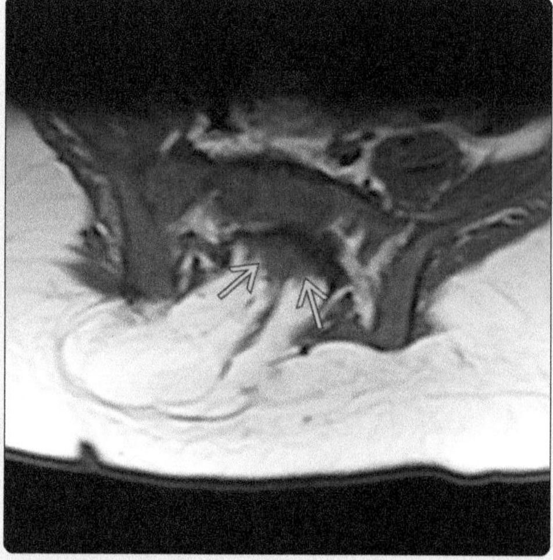

(Left) *Sagittal T1 MR of the spine shows a closed lumbosacral spinal dysraphism with elongation of the spinal cord in association with a placode-lipoma interface ➡, which extends outside the spinal canal, consistent with lipomyelomeningocele (LMMC). There is also a dorsal dermal sinus tract ➡ extending to the skin surface & marked thickening of SQ fat.* **(Right)** *Axial T2 MR of the spine (same patient) shows the placode-lipoma interface ➡ extending outside the spinal canal & mild expansion of the thecal sac ➡ dorsally.*

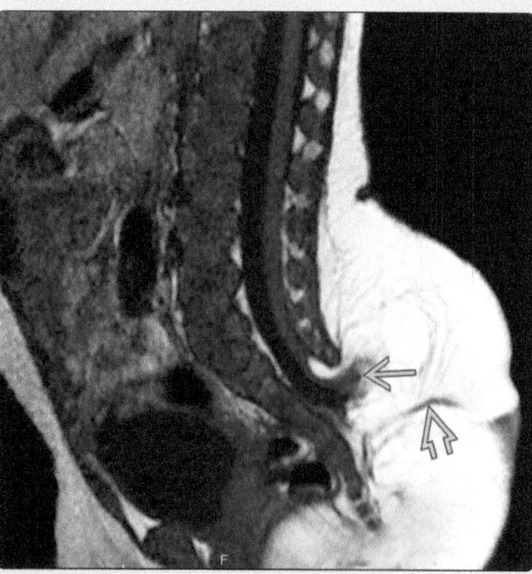

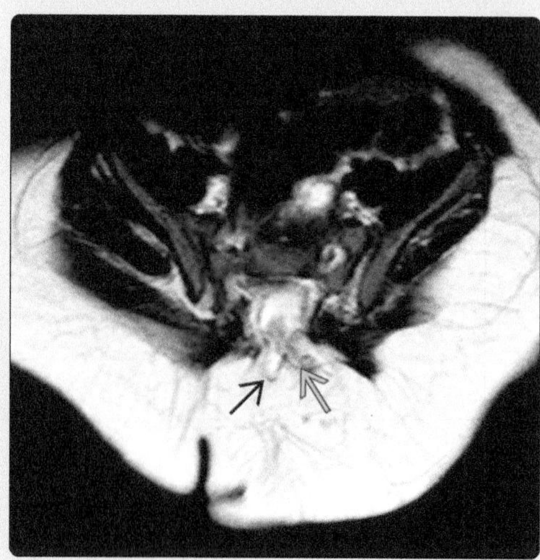

TERMINOLOGY

Abbreviations

- Lipomyelomeningocele (LMMC)

Synonyms

- Lipoma with dorsal defect [includes spectrum of lipomyeloceles (LMCs) & LMMCs]
- Lipomyeloschisis

IMAGING

General Features

- Best diagnostic clue
  - Skin-covered (closed) spinal dysraphism with elongated spinal cord terminating in lipomatous tissue (placode-lipoma interface) that is in continuity with dorsal subcutaneous fat through osseous spinal dysraphic defect
  - LMMC: Placode-lipoma interface lies outside spinal canal with expansion of surrounding subarachnoid space/thecal sac
  - LMC: Placode-lipoma interface lies within spinal canal
  - LMMC & LMC along same spectrum & may be difficult to distinguish in certain cases
- Location
  - Lumbosacral
- Size
  - Subcutaneous mass varies from nearly imperceptible (LMC) to large (LMMC)
- Morphology
  - Intradural/epidural extent of lipomatous component variable
    - Fatty tissue may be eccentric, lobulated, focal or multifocal & can surround neural placode & spinal cord

Radiographic Findings

- Radiography
  - Absence of posterior osseous spinal elements
    - Best seen on frontal view

CT Findings

- NECT
  - Hypodense dorsal lipomatous mass attached to neural placode through posterior dysraphic defect
- Bone CT
  - Multilevel posterior dysraphic defects typically involving lumbosacral spine
  - Enlarged spinal canal at placode level
  - ~ 40% with associated segmentation anomalies; sacral hypoplasia/agenesis in ~ 25%

MR Findings

- T1WI, T2WI
  - LMMC: Placode-lipoma interface outside spinal canal through dorsal dysraphic defect immediately inferior to last intact lamina
    - With herniation of meninges through defect
      - Contain variable amounts of T2-hyperintense CSF
    - Lipoma asymmetric in ~ 40% of patients, causing rotation of neural placode with unequal nerve root length
  - LMC: Placode-lipoma interface within spinal canal
    - Variable degrees of expansion of subcutaneous fat & intradural lipomatous tissue surrounding neural placode
  - Thinned conus/neural placode attached to T1-hyperintense lipomatous mass
    - Mass continuous with subcutaneous fat through osteocartilaginous defect
    - Variable extent of intramedullary, intradural, or extradural lipoma
  - Enlargement of subarachnoid space ventral to neural placode
  - Syringohydromyelia in 20-25% of cases

Imaging Recommendations

- Best imaging tool
  - Multiplanar MR
  - MR to further define anomalies preoperatively & assess complications or worsening neurologic symptoms postoperatively
- Protocol advice
  - Sagittal & axial T1 to fully delineate extent of lipoma
  - 3D BTFE/FIESTA to improve resolution of involved nerve roots & identify presence of cysts in association with neural placode
  - Consider DWI to look for coexisting dermoid/epidermoid cysts
- Ultrasound to screen neonatal distal spine if concerning cutaneous stigmata present

DIFFERENTIAL DIAGNOSIS

Other Closed Spinal Dysraphisms

- With subcutaneous mass
  - Meningocele: Herniation of CSF-filled sac lined by dura & arachnoid
  - Terminal myelocystocele: Herniation of terminal syrinx into posterior skin-covered sac
    - Can be difficult to differentiate from LMMC at times
    - Look for cyst within cyst appearance of sac or splitting of neural placode with trumpet morphology in terminal myelocystoceles
- Without subcutaneous mass
  - Intradural lipoma: Fat within intact dural sac separate from subcutaneous fat
  - Dorsal dermal sinus: Subcutaneous tract extending up to/into spinal canal, ± epidermoid/dermoid (which may contain fat)

Open Spinal Dysraphisms

- Myelomeningocele & myelocele: No skin covering neural placode
  - Clinically obvious at birth; rarely imaged in neonatal period prior to repair
  - Increasingly imaged by fetal MR for possible in utero repair
  - Postoperative appearance may resemble closed spinal dysraphism
- Usually evident Chiari 2
- No intradural lipoma

Sacrococcygeal Teratoma

- Large, heterogeneous, solid &/or cystic presacral mass
  - ± fat, Ca^{++}
- External/exophytic components often much greater than internal components
- May demonstrate intraspinal extension
- May demonstrate urinary bladder &/or bowel dilation from obstruction/dysfunction

PATHOLOGY

General Features

- Etiology
  - Neural tube normally forms by infolding & closure of neural ectoderm as it separates from cutaneous ectoderm during 3rd-4th weeks of gestation (primary neurulation & disjunction)
    - In LMMC/LMC, premature disjunction of neural ectoderm from cutaneous ectoderm → mesenchymal tissue enters incompletely closed neural tube, preventing neurulation to proceed
    - Mesenchyme becomes incorporated between neural folds
    - Neural folds remain open, forming neural placode at site of premature disjunction
    - Ependymal lining of primitive neural tube induces mesenchyme to form fat (this theory not uniformly accepted) → lipoma
- Associated abnormalities
  - Anorectal & genitourinary tract malformations in 5-10%
  - Split cord malformation in ≤ 10%
  - Less common: Dermoid/epidermoid cyst, dorsal dermal sinus, hamartoma, vascular malformation, arachnoid cyst
  - Sacral hypogenesis in ~ 25% (group 2 caudal agenesis)
  - **O**mphalocele, cloacal **e**xstrophy, **i**mperforate anus, **s**pinal defects (OEIS) complex → usually with terminal myelocystoceles
  - **P**erineal hemangioma, **e**xternal genitalia malformation, **L**MMC, **v**esicorenal abnormalities, **i**mperforate anus, & **s**kin tag (PELVIS) syndrome

Staging, Grading, & Classification

- Location of placode-lipoma interface to differentiate LMC (within spinal canal) with LMMC (outside spinal canal)
- On spectrum differentiation between 2, not always clear

Microscopic Features

- Dorsal placode surface attached to lipoma (placode-lipoma interface) has no ependymal lining
  - Covered by connective tissue mixed with islands of glial cells & smooth muscle fibers

CLINICAL ISSUES

Presentation

- Most common signs/symptoms
  - Subcutaneous fatty mass above intergluteal crease
    - May have appearance of vestigial tail
  - Some have abnormal neurologic function at birth, others present in adulthood or are symptomatic
    - Back/leg pain, lower extremity weakness, sensory loss in sacral dermatomes, bladder/bowel dysfunction
- Other signs/symptoms
  - Scoliosis, limb atrophy, orthopedic foot deformity
- Associated findings
  - OEIS complex
  - Genitourinary: Renal agenesis, bifid uterus, duplicated vagina
  - Brain: Occipital encephalocele, Chiari 1, hydrocephalus
  - Spine: Klippel-Feil, caudal agenesis, split cord malformation

Demographics

- Epidemiology
  - ~ 1/4,000 live births; true incidence unknown as some cases asymptomatic
  - Incidence not impacted by folate supplementation during pregnancy (unlike open spinal dysraphisms)

Natural History & Prognosis

- 40-60% neurologically normal at birth
- 16-88% will subsequently develop symptoms
- Some recovery has been reported after surgery (but not complete neurologic restoration)
- Late clinical deterioration reported in some patients after repair

Treatment

- Surgical repair: Remove lipoma, untether spinal cord, repair dura
- Timing of intervention controversial
  - Some advocate early prophylactic surgery (< 1 year of age)
  - Others believe in delaying 1st operation until symptoms develop

DIAGNOSTIC CHECKLIST

Consider

- Group 2 caudal agenesis spectrum is common so look for complete formation of sacrococcygeal spine & genitourinary anomalies
- Preoperative imaging is needed for accurate classification of spinal dysraphism

Image Interpretation Pearls

- LMMC & LMC are on same pathologic spectrum; description of location of placode-lipoma interface can be helpful
- LMMC & terminal myelocystoceles can be difficult to distinguish & are often both differential considerations

SELECTED REFERENCES

1. Hwang HW et al: A case of perineal hemangioma, external genitalia malformations, lipomyelomeningocele, vesicorenal abnormalities, imperforate anus, and skin tag (PELVIS) syndrome with extensive perineal infantile hemangioma. Ann Dermatol. 35(Suppl 1):S88-92, 2023
2. Trapp B et al: A practical approach to diagnosis of spinal dysraphism. Radiographics. 41(2):559-75, 2021
3. Barkovich AJ et al: Pediatric Neuroimaging. 6th ed. Wolters Kluwer. 996-8, 2019
4. Nagaraj UD et al: Differentiating closed versus open spinal dysraphisms on fetal MRI. AJR Am J Roentgenol. 207(6):1316-23, 2016

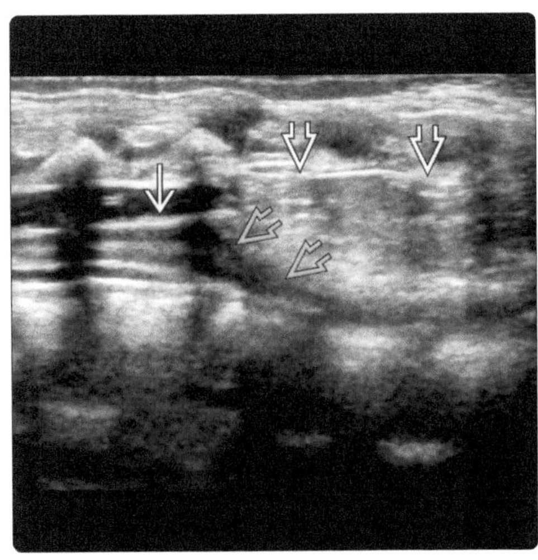

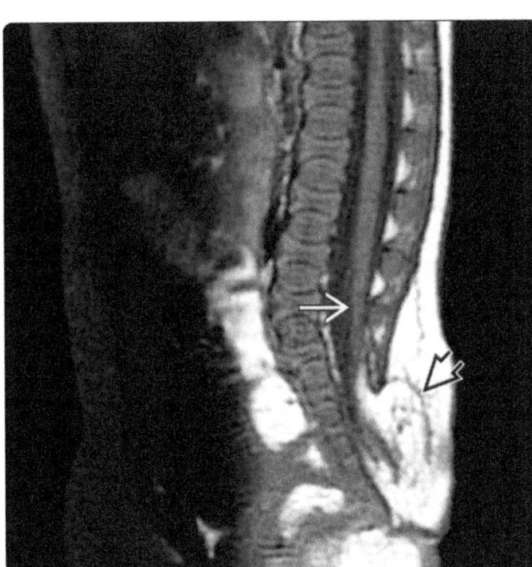

(Left) *Sagittal view from a spinal US in an infant with an LMC shows the terminal spinal cord inserting directly into an echogenic intraspinal lipomatous mass at the L2 level. The placode-lipoma interface is within the spinal canal.* **(Right)** *Sagittal T1 MR shows an LMC with a low-lying cord attached to lipoma that is contiguous with SQ fat. Of note, LMMC & LMC are on a spectrum, & it may not always be clear if the placode-lipoma interface is within the spinal canal.*

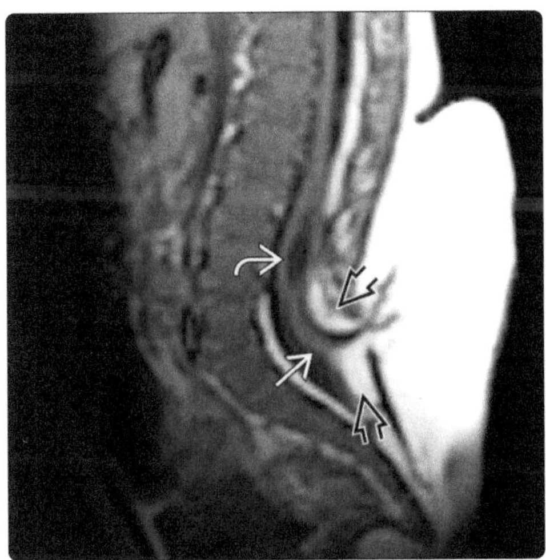

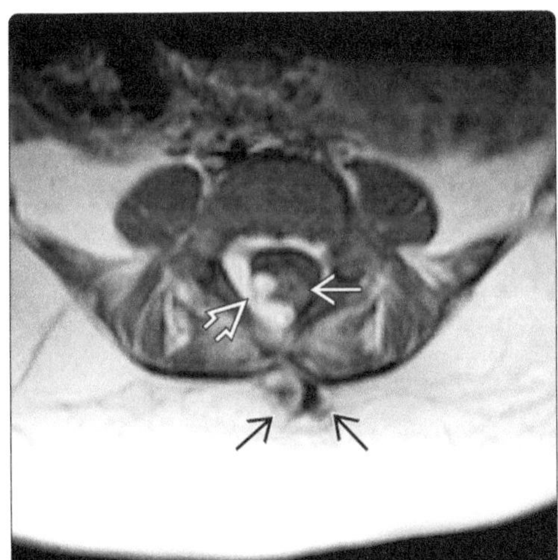

(Left) *Sagittal T1 MR shows a low-lying spinal cord inserting directly into lumbosacral lipomatous tissue that is in continuity with dorsal expanded SQ fat. The distal cord also demonstrates syringohydromyelia.* **(Right)** *Axial T1 MR (in the same patient) depicts the insertion of the distal cord into the rotated neural placode & lipoma. Portions of the placode-lipoma interface are likely within & outside the spinal canal, consistent with the LMMC/LMC spectrum.*

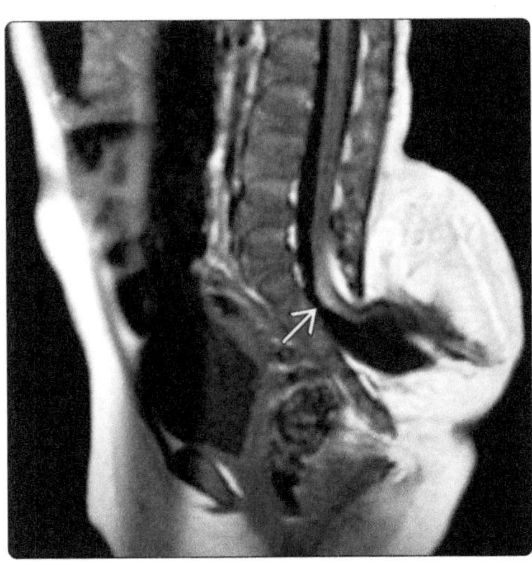

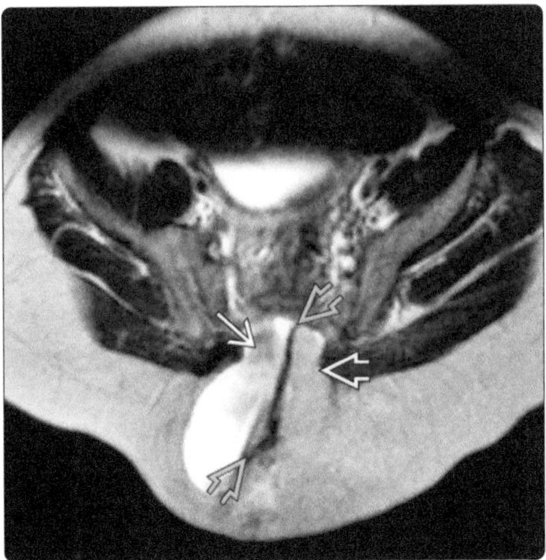

(Left) *Sagittal T1 MR shows a low-lying spinal cord inserting into lipomatous tissue that is contiguous with SQ fat through a posterior dysraphic defect. The most inferior level of complete posterior elements is at the S1 level.* **(Right)** *Axial T2 MR at the upper sacral level (same patient) demonstrates the relationship of the low-lying cord/placode with the lipoma component of the LMMC. Chemical shift artifact along the placode-lipoma interface confirms fat content.*

Terminal Myelocystocele

KEY FACTS

TERMINOLOGY

- Synonym: Terminal syringocele

IMAGING

- Complex spinal malformation → closed spinal dysraphism, large skin-covered back mass
- Hydromyelic, low-lying tethered spinal cord traverses dorsal meningocele and terminates in dilated terminal cyst (myelocystocele)
- Multiplanar MR imaging best demonstrates constellation of abnormalities

TOP DIFFERENTIAL DIAGNOSES

- Anterior sacral meningocele
- Simple dorsal meningocele
- Sacrococcygeal teratoma
- Myelomeningocele

PATHOLOGY

- Results from deranged secondary neurulation of caudal cell mass
- Associated malformations: Cloacal exstrophy, imperforate anus, omphalocele, pelvic deformities, equinovarus, ambiguous hypoplastic genitalia, and renal abnormalities

CLINICAL ISSUES

- Presents at birth with large skin-covered back mass
- Usually neurologically intact at birth; may later develop lower extremity sensorimotor deficits

DIAGNOSTIC CHECKLIST

- Early diagnosis and surgery → best chance for normal neurologic outcome
- Nonneurologic prognosis largely linked to severity of associated anomalies

(Left) *Sagittal graphic displays a low-lying, hydromyelic spinal cord ➡ piercing an expanded subarachnoid space (meningocele ➡), terminating in a myelocystocele ➡.* **(Right)** *Sagittal T1WI MR depicts a low-lying hydromyelic spinal cord ➡ traversing a meningocele ➡ and expanding into a large terminal cyst ➡. Note the hypointense dorsal fibrous band ➡ constraining the spinal cord. In this patient, the back mass is produced by both the meningocele and myelocystocele.*

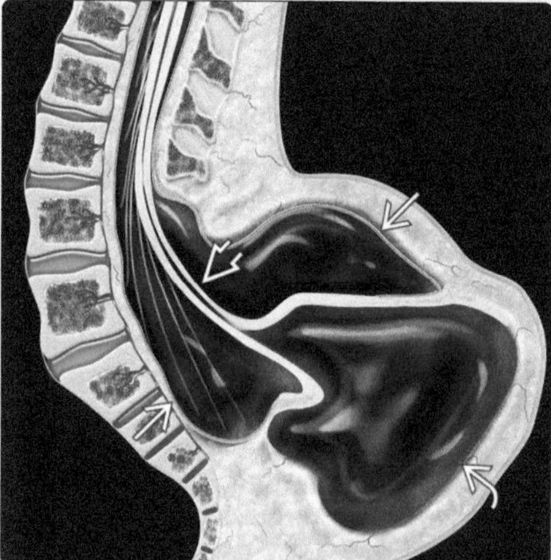

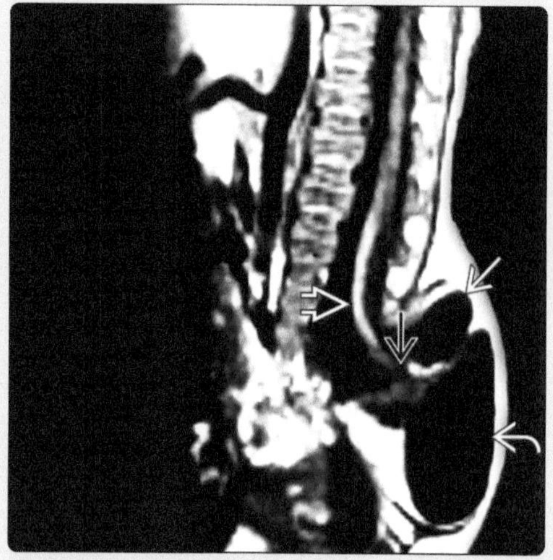

(Left) *Sagittal FIESTA cine MR demonstrates truncation of the sacrum. The spinal cord is abnormally low lying with caudal extension of the attenuated cord ➡ through a sacral cyst ➡ (meningocele). The terminal spinal cord flares into a 2nd terminal cyst ➡ within the meningocele ("cyst in a cyst") completing the terminal myelocystocele malformation.* **(Right)** *Coronal T2WI MR demonstrates flaring of terminal spinal cord ➡ and transition of central canal into the terminal myelocystocele ➡.*

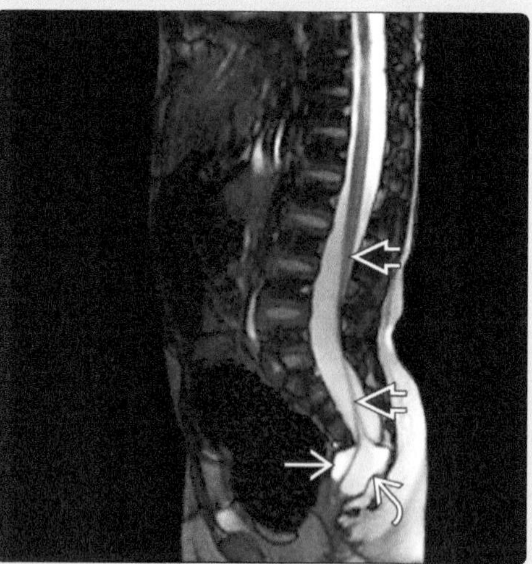

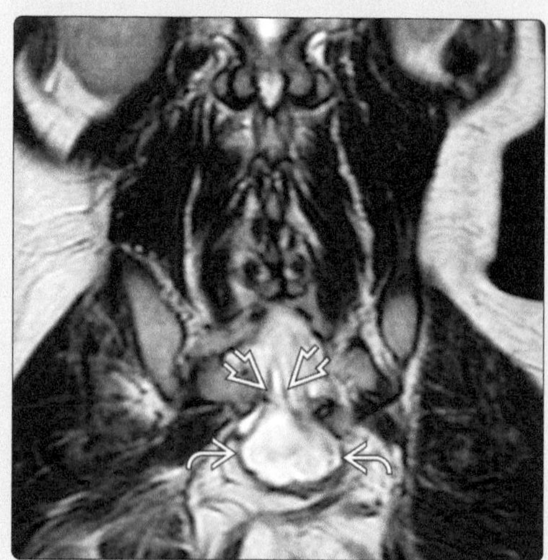

TERMINOLOGY

Synonyms

- Terminal syringocele

Definitions

- Complex spinal malformation → hydromyelic, low-lying tethered spinal cord traverses meningocele to terminate in myelocystocele

IMAGING

General Features

- Best diagnostic clue
  - Hydromyelic tethered cord traversing dorsal meningocele to terminate in dilated terminal ventricle cyst
- Location
  - Sacrum/coccyx
- Size
  - Mass varies from small to large (> 10-cm diameter)
- Morphology
  - Closed spinal dysraphism, large skin-covered mass, terminal cord cyst traversing meningocele

Radiographic Findings

- Radiography
  - Lumbosacral dysraphism ± soft tissue mass
  - ± pubic diastasis (usually + bladder exstrophy)

CT Findings

- NECT
  - Lumbosacral dysraphism
  - Hydromyelic cord penetrates meningocele sac, ends in caudal terminal cystic sac

MR Findings

- T1WI
  - Hypointense cephalic dorsal meningocele → back mass
  - Tethered distal cord shows trumpet-like flaring into hypointense caudal terminal cyst
- T2WI
  - Hypointense dorsal fibrous band at cephalic margin of meningocele constrains spinal cord
  - Fibrolipomatous tissue surrounds both sacs

Ultrasonographic Findings

- Grayscale ultrasound
  - Sagittal plane: Spinal cord passes through hypoechoic, dilated subarachnoid space (meningocele), terminates in cord cyst
  - Axial plane: Bifid hydromyelic dorsal spinal cord within meningocele

Nonvascular Interventions

- Myelography
  - Hydromyelic cord passes through meningocele, terminates in separate sac caudal to contrast-filled meningocele
  - Delayed imaging → ± contrast imbibition into hydromyelic cord/terminal cyst

Imaging Recommendations

- Best imaging tool
  - Multiplanar MR
- Protocol advice
  - Sagittal MR for diagnosis and estimating length of hydromyelia, sizing cysts, and identifying associated abnormalities
  - Axial MR to clarify extent of rachischisis, evaluate associated anomalies

DIFFERENTIAL DIAGNOSIS

Anterior Sacral Meningocele

- Anterior meningocele protrudes thorough enlarged sacral neural foramen into pelvis

Simple Dorsal Meningocele

- Dorsal meningocele protrudes through focal dysraphism
- Cord rarely tethered or hydromyelic

Sacrococcygeal Teratoma

- Similar clinical appearance of skin mass
- Distinguish by presence of solid tumor elements within cysts, calcifications

Myelomeningocele

- Open spinal dysraphism; no skin covering, clinically obvious
- Associated with Chiari 2

PATHOLOGY

General Features

- Etiology
  - Postulated to result from deranged secondary neurulation of caudal cell mass; typically associated with other caudal tail fold malformations
    - CSF unable to normally exit from early neural tube → terminal ventricle balloons into cyst → disrupts overlying dorsal mesenchyme but not superficial ectoderm
    - Posterior elements do not form normally → spina bifida with intact skin
    - Terminal ventricle dilatation → distends arachnoid cord lining → meningocele
    - Cyst bulk prevents cord ascent → tethered cord
    - Progressive distention of distal cord causes caudal bulge below end of meningocele into extraarachnoid space and results in flaring of distal spinal cord
    - Disruption of caudal motor segments → progressive symptoms that present at birth or appear later
  - Some speculate → most severe manifestation of persistent terminal ventricle (ventriculus terminalis) spectrum
  - Newer reports postulate severity spectrum between retained medullary cord (RMC) and terminal myelocystocele
    - Share same pathoembryogenic origin, failure of regression phase of secondary neurulation
- Associated abnormalities
  - Cloacal exstrophy, imperforate anus, omphalocele, pelvic deformities, equinovarus, ambiguous hypoplastic genitalia, and renal abnormalities
  - Syndromal associations

- Caudal regression syndrome
- OEIS syndrome constellation (**o**mphalocele, **e**xstrophy of bladder, **i**mperforate anus, and **s**pinal anomalies)
  - Chiari 1 and 2, hydrocephalus, and vertebral segmentation anomalies (rare)
- Classic pathologic triad
  - Skin-covered lumbosacral dysraphism
  - Arachnoid-lined meningocele directly contiguous with spinal subarachnoid space
  - Low-lying hydromyelic cord traverses meningocele, expands into large contiguous ependymal-lined terminal cyst

Gross Pathologic & Surgical Features

- Lumbosacral dysraphism with hypoplastic, widely everted laminae
- Proximal (smaller, rostral) sac resembles typical meningocele with inner surface lined by arachnoid and thick fibrous layer
- Distal spinal cord herniates under fibrous band between medial ends of most cephalic widely bifid lamina, traverses meningocele → terminal cyst (larger, caudal)
  - Cord narrowed by fibrous band where it exits spinal canal, then widens distally due to concurrent hydromyelia
  - Distal spinal nerve roots arise from ventral surface of intraarachnoid segment of spinal cord, traverse meningocele, and reenter spinal canal before exiting at their root sleeves or via bony clefts
- Terminal cyst does not communicate directly with subarachnoid space

Microscopic Features

- Meningocele lined by arachnoid, thick fibrous layer
- Terminal cyst lined by ependyma, dysplastic glia; directly contiguous with central cord canal
- Outer cord surface pia, arachnoid continuous with meningocele

CLINICAL ISSUES

Presentation

- Most common signs/symptoms
  - Presents at birth with large skin-covered back mass
    - Skin appears normal or exhibits hemangioma, nevus, or hypertrichosis
    - Rare patients without back mass present later with progressive neurologic deficits
  - Majority neurologically intact at diagnosis
- Other signs/symptoms
  - Later presentation or untreated lesion may develop progressive lower extremity paresis
- Clinical profile
  - Usually neurologically intact at birth but may present with lower extremity sensorimotor deficits
  - Large mass obliterates intergluteal cleft, extends upward from perineum for variable distance
  - ± concurrent midline cecal and paramedian bladder exstrophy, other visible anomalies

Demographics

- Age
  - Infancy
- Sex
  - F > M
- Epidemiology
  - Rare: 1-5% of skin-covered lumbosacral masses
    - Much more common in cloacal exstrophy patients
  - Sporadic; no familial incidence
  - Postulated associations with teratogens retinoic acid, hydantoin, loperamide hydrochloride
  - No known association with diabetes mellitus (unlike caudal regression syndrome)

Natural History & Prognosis

- Normal intellectual potential
- Mass size and deficits tend to progress with time; may be partially or totally reversible with prompt surgical repair
  - Main goals of neurosurgical intervention are to reduce mass size and untether cord
  - Operation soon after diagnosis indicated to prevent progression of neurologic abnormalities, cyst growth
  - Persistent neurologic deficits usually permanent
- Overall prognosis mainly related to other associated anomalies (OEIS constellation)
  - Patients without abdominal wall defects have more favorable neurologic outcome than those with ventral wall defects

Treatment

- Early diagnosis and surgical repair maximize probability of normal neurologic outcome
- Delayed recognition and operation increase odds of onset, progression of lower extremity paresis

DIAGNOSTIC CHECKLIST

Consider

- Early diagnosis and surgery → best chance for normal neurologic outcome
- Nonneurologic prognosis largely linked to severity of associated anomalies

Image Interpretation Pearls

- Tethered hydromyelic cord traversing meningocele to terminate in separate caudal cyst is unique imaging finding diagnostic of terminal myelocystocele

SELECTED REFERENCES

1. Kurogi A et al: Retained medullary cord associated with terminal myelocystocele and intramedullary arachnoid cyst. Pediatr Neurosurg. 57(3):184-90, 2022
2. Shim Y et al: Retained medullary cord and terminal myelocystocele as a spectrum: case report. Childs Nerv Syst. 38(6):1223-8, 2022
3. Kim KH et al: Cystic retained medullary cord in an intraspinal J-shaped cul-de-sac: a lesion in the spectrum of regression failure during secondary neurulation. Childs Nerv Syst. 37(6):2051-6, 2021
4. Sprenger F et al: Turbulent cerebrospinal fluid flow in enlarging terminal myelocystocele. World Neurosurg. 147:8-10, 2020
5. Takamiya S et al: Myelocystocele mimicking myelomeningocele: a case report and review of the literature. World Neurosurg. 119:172-5, 2018
6. Bansal S et al: "Giant" terminal myelocystocele: a rare variant of spinal dysraphism. Asian J Neurosurg. 10(4):350-2, 2015
7. Catala M: Terminal myelocystocele. Neurosurgery. 72(4):E697-8, 2013
8. Pang D et al: Terminal myelocystocele: surgical observations and theory of embryogenesis. Neurosurgery. 70(6):1383-404; discussion 1404-5, 2012
9. Tandon V et al: Terminal myelocystocele: a series of 30 cases and review of the literature. Pediatr Neurosurg. 48(4):229-35, 2012

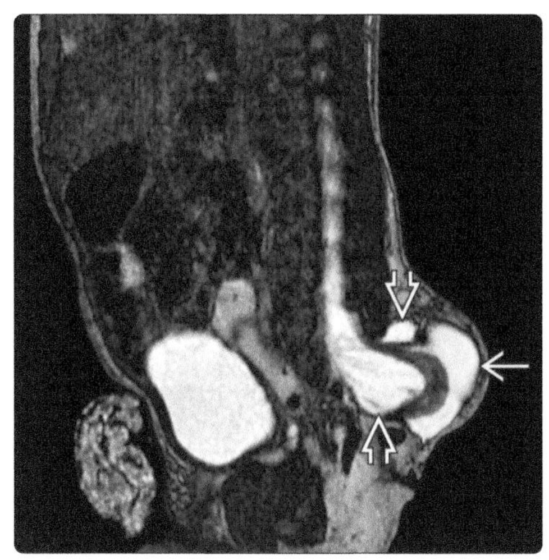

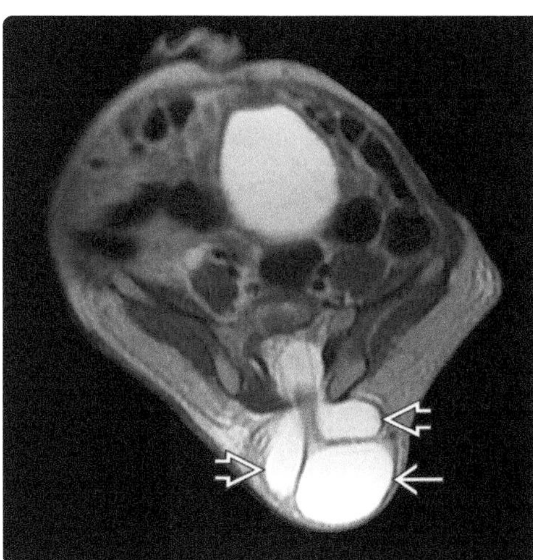

(Left) *Sagittal FIESTA MR in a 1-day-old boy with a skin-covered back mass reveals trumpeted low termination of the spinal cord into a terminal myelocystocele* ➡*. The terminal cord passes through the meningocele* ➡*.* **(Right)** *Axial T2WI MR (in the same patient) confirms the trumpeted configuration of terminal spinal cord into a myelocystocele* ➡*. Signal intensity in the meningocele* ➡ *is similar to the myelocystocele.*

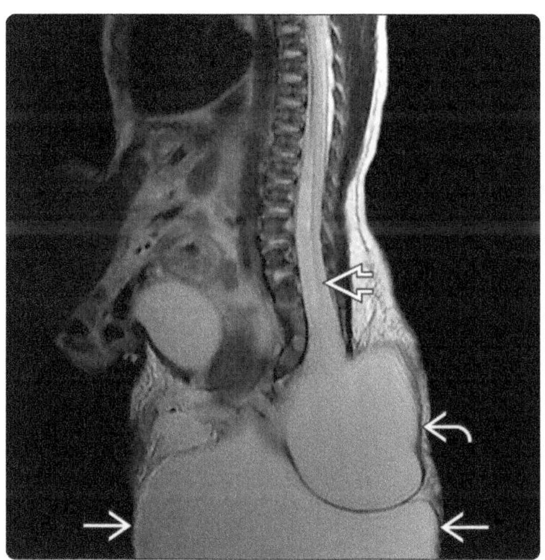

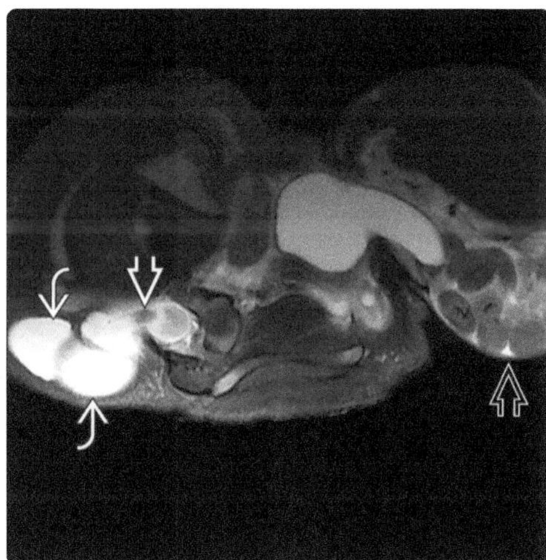

(Left) *Sagittal T2WI MR in a newborn with multiple congenital anomalies, including an omphalocele and a large skin-covered back mass, demonstrates a low-lying spinal cord* ➡ *terminating in a myelocystocele* ➡ *surrounded by a large meningocele* ➡*.* **(Right)** *Axial T2WI FS MR in the same patient shows the low-lying distal spinal cord* ➡ *passing through a posterior dysraphic defect to terminate in the myelocystocele* ➡*. A large omphalocele* ➡ *contains the urinary bladder and bowel as well as liver.*

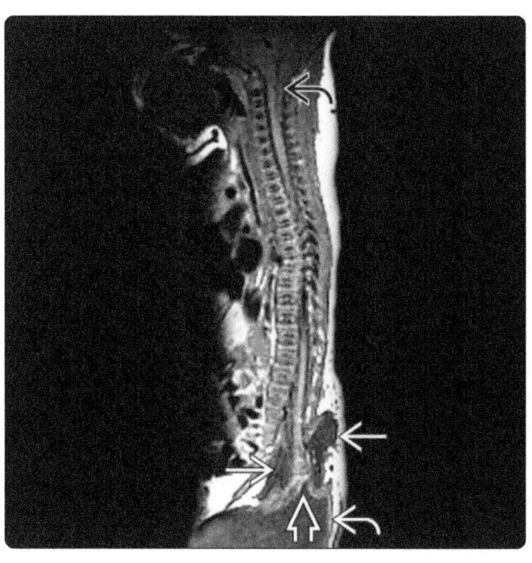

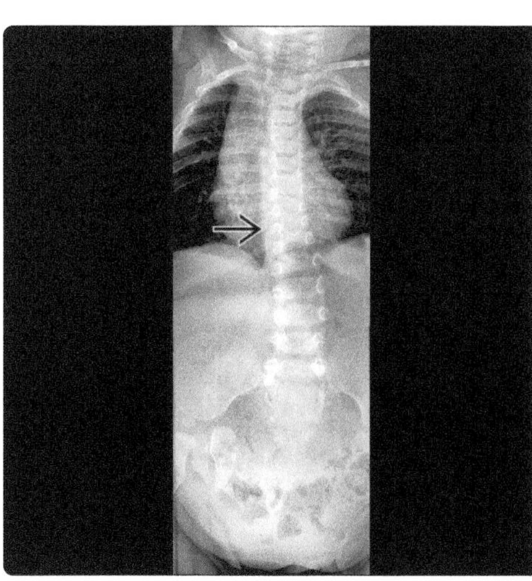

(Left) *Sagittal T1WI MR in a newborn shows the central canal of a low-lying cord traversing the meningocele* ➡ *before expanding into a large terminal cyst* ➡*. Note "trumpet splaying"* ➡ *of the terminal spinal cord. This infant also has a coexisting Chiari 1* ➡*.* **(Right)** *AP radiograph in a patient with terminal myelocystocele shows associated sacral dysgenesis, wide symphysis pubis (bladder exstrophy), unfused posterior sacral elements, and a midthoracic hemivertebra* ➡*.*

KEY FACTS

TERMINOLOGY

- Midline/paramidline subcutaneous sinus tract extending from skin surface toward spinal canal
- Located anywhere along neuraxis from cranium to intergluteal cleft; most common location (~ 70%) is lumbosacral region above intergluteal cleft

IMAGING

- Linear, midline/paramidline, sagittal T1-hypointense tract in subcutaneous tissues
- Terminates anywhere from subcutaneous tissues (blind ending) to spine (epidural, intradural/intrathecal, or even intramedullary)
- ± dermoid/epidermoid cysts along tract (~ 50%)
  - DWI or thin-section fluid-sensitive sequences are helpful for intrathecal mass visualization
- ± tethered cord with low-lying conus medullaris, intradural lipoma, or split cord malformation

TOP DIFFERENTIAL DIAGNOSES

- Coccygeal pit
- Pilonidal sinus/cyst
- Dermoid/epidermoid cyst without sinus tract
- Limited dorsal myeloschisis
- Lipomyelomeningocele (or other closed dysraphisms)

PATHOLOGY

- Closed spinal dysraphism due to incomplete disjunction of cutaneous & neural ectoderm at 3- to 8-weeks gestation

CLINICAL ISSUES

- Presentations include
  - Asymptomatic (incidentally noted skin dimple)
  - Infection (meningitis, abscess)
  - Neurologic deficits from cord tethering or compression
- Dorsal dermal sinus typically requires excision of entire tract
  - Intraspinal extension may be occult on imaging (necessitating operative exploration of dura)

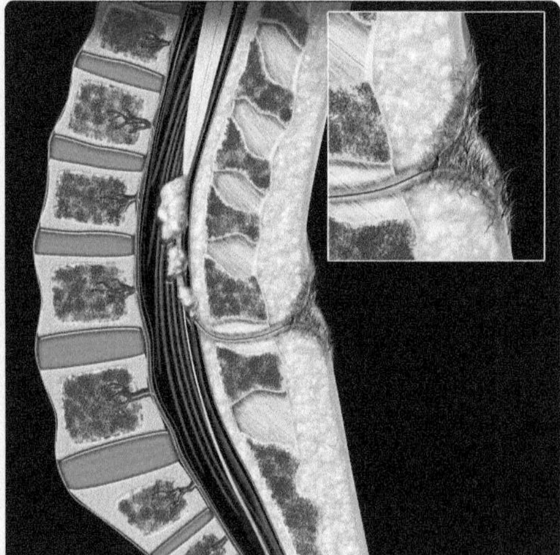

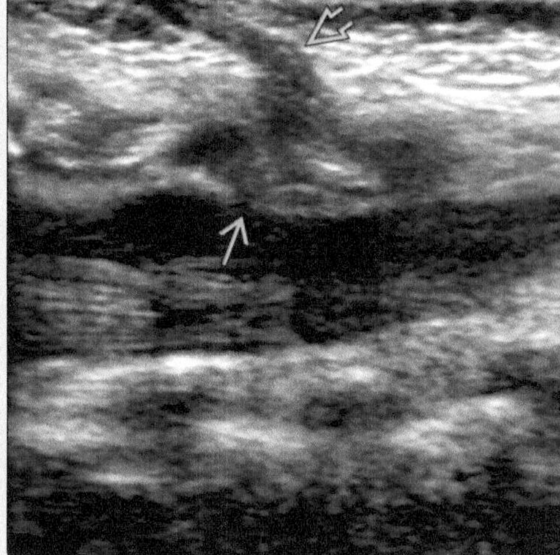

(Left) *Sagittal graphic shows a dermal sinus extending from the skin surface into the spinal canal to terminate with epidermoid cysts at the conus medullaris. In this case, the sinus opening is marked by a skin dimple with a hairy tuft & capillary malformation.* **(Right)** *Sagittal US of the spine in an infant with a cutaneous lumbar dimple demonstrates a hypoechoic dorsal dermal sinus tract ⇨ in the subcutaneous tissues. A dural defect ➔ confirms communication of the tract with the thecal sac & subarachnoid space.*

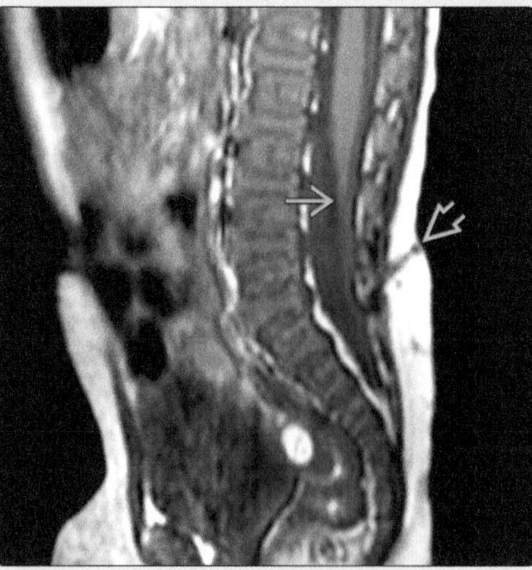

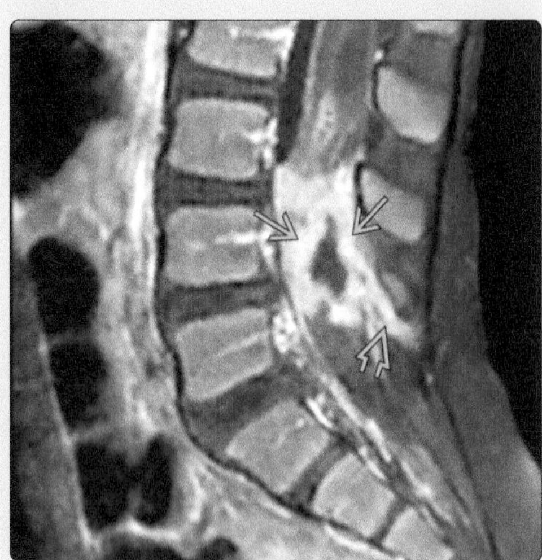

(Left) *Sagittal T1WI MR in the same patient shows a hypointense dorsal dermal sinus tract ⇨ in the subcutaneous tissues. The conus medullaris ➔ is low lying at the L4 level. No associated intraspinal mass or cyst is identified.* **(Right)** *Sagittal T1WI C+ FS MR in the same patient at 3 years of age demonstrates the interval development of a rim-enhancing intraspinal abscess ➔. Note that there is also enhancement along the dorsal dermal sinus tract ⇨ as it enters the spinal canal.*

TERMINOLOGY

Synonyms

- Dermal sinus tract (DST), congenital dermal sinus

Definitions

- Sinus tract of subcutaneous tissues lined by stratified squamous epithelium
- Tract lies above intergluteal cleft & extends deep from skin surface for variable distance
  - Tract may end in subcutaneous tissues, fascia/muscle, vertebrae, epidural space, subarachnoid space, or even intramedullary within spinal cord

IMAGING

General Features

- Best diagnostic clue
  - Sagittally oriented, linear/curvilinear, T1-hypointense tract in dorsal subcutaneous tissues deep to skin dimple
- Location
  - Can occur anywhere along craniospinal axis, usually midline (rarely paramidline)
  - Most commonly lumbosacral; up to 25% are occipital
- Morphology
  - Up to 40% can be seen with additional coexisting closed spinal dysraphism (e.g., lipomyelomeningocele, split cord malformation, tethered cord syndrome)

MR Findings

- DWI
  - ± hyperintense dermoid/epidermoid cyst
- T1WI C+
  - ± nerve root enhancement in meningitis or frank, rim-enhancing abscess (intraspinal or along tract)
  - ± enhancement of coexisting capillary malformation or hemangioma
- T1WI, T2WI
  - Sinus tract is hypointense to subcutaneous fat, may have ↑ T2 if fluid filled or inflamed
  - Dorsal dural tenting may indicate point of dural penetration
    - Intradural sinus course is often impossible to follow (i.e., indistinguishable from cauda equina, filum)
  - ± tethered cord
    - Low-lying conus medullaris, intradural lipoma
  - ± nerve root clumping (arachnoiditis)

DIFFERENTIAL DIAGNOSIS

Coccygeal Pit

- Intergluteal dorsal dermal sinus found in 2-4% of infants
- Clinically distinct entity (usually of no clinical significance)

Pilonidal Sinus/Cyst

- Result of chronic inflammatory changes involving hair follicle in intergluteal cleft near anus

Dermoid/Epidermoid Cyst Without Dermal Sinus

- Almost always acquired if spinal in location (due to surgery, repeated lumbar punctures)

Limited Dorsal Myeloschisis (a.k.a. Abortive Nonterminal Myelocystocele)

- Tract is of mesenchymal origin (not epithelium-lined) & closed

Other Closed Spinal Dysraphisms

- Can coexist with dorsal dermal sinus

PATHOLOGY

General Features

- Associated abnormalities
  - Cutaneous stigmata: Midline or paramidline dimple above gluteal cleft, hyperpigmented patch, capillary malformation or hemangioma, hairy nevus
  - Dermoid/epidermoid cyst
  - Tethered cord, intradural lipoma, split cord malformation
  - Meningitis ± epidural/subdural/subarachnoid/intramedullary abscess
- Important to differentiate true dorsal dermal sinus from intergluteal dorsal dermal sinus/coccygeal pit

CLINICAL ISSUES

Presentation

- Most common signs/symptoms
  - Asymptomatic (incidentally noted atypical skin dimple)
  - Neurologic signs/symptoms secondary to
    - Spinal cord tethering &/or compression
    - Tract infection leading to meningitis, abscess
- Clinical profile
  - Midline/paramidline dimple above intergluteal cleft ± cutaneous stigmata
    - Hyperpigmentation, capillary malformation, hypertrichosis

Treatment

- Surgical excision of sinus tract with intradural exploration, tethered cord release, treatment of complications
  - Sinus tract may not be visible on imaging & may require surgical exploration for diagnosis if there is high index of clinical suspicion

DIAGNOSTIC CHECKLIST

Consider

- Dorsal dermal sinus must be differentiated from intergluteal dorsal dermal sinus/coccygeal pit
  - Maintain high index of suspicion for all dimples above intergluteal cleft

Image Interpretation Pearls

- Sinus tract may be subtle on imaging: Consider placing vitamin E capsule over dimple for improved localization during MR imaging

SELECTED REFERENCES

1. Trapp B et al: A practical approach to diagnosis of spinal dysraphism. Radiographics. 41(2):559-75, 2021
2. Majumdar I et al: Dorsal dermal sinus presenting as quadriparesis. BMJ Case Rep. 12(6):e228503, 2019
3. Schwartz E et al: Congenital anomalies of the spine. In Barkovich A et al:. Pediatric Neuroimaging. 6th ed. Wolter Kluwer. 987-9, 2019

Dermoid Cyst, Spine

KEY FACTS

TERMINOLOGY

- Synonyms: Dermoid tumor, "dermoid"
- Benign spinal mass composed of cells embryologically composing skin and its appendages

IMAGING

- Lumbosacral or cauda equina CSF isointense/isodense mass ± interspersed fat signal intensity/density
- Focal osseous erosion, spinal canal widening, flattening of pedicles and laminae at spinal level of mass
- Less likely to show diffusion restriction than epidermoid cyst

TOP DIFFERENTIAL DIAGNOSES

- Arachnoid cyst
- Neurenteric cyst
- Epidermoid cyst

PATHOLOGY

- Congenital or acquired origin
    - Congenital cysts arise from dermal rests or focal expansion of dermal sinus
- Cyst filled with thick, cheesy, buttery, yellowish material (desquamated keratin, lipids)
- Associated anomalies include dermal sinus, vertebral segmentation anomalies, closed dysraphism

CLINICAL ISSUES

- Most commonly asymptomatic or presentation with slowly progressive compressive radiculopathy/myelopathy
- Infectious meningitis in association with dermal sinus
- Acute chemical meningitis 2° to rupture, discharge of inflammatory cholesterol crystals into CSF

DIAGNOSTIC CHECKLIST

- Often difficult to diagnose on CT and MR; presence of fat helpful to suggest diagnosis
- Requires high index of suspicion; look for mass effect on regional structures
- Diffusion-weighted imaging may be helpful

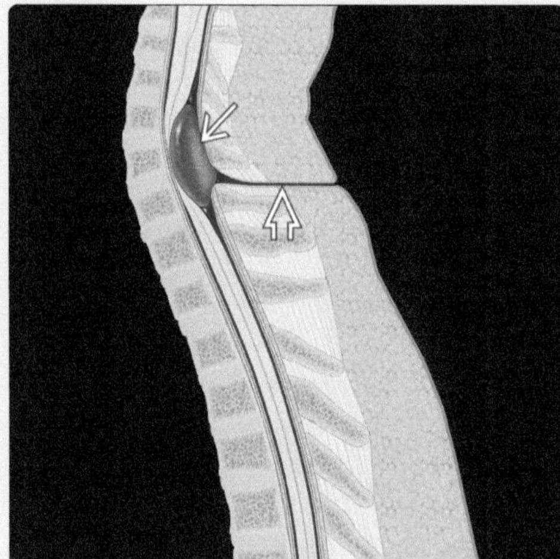

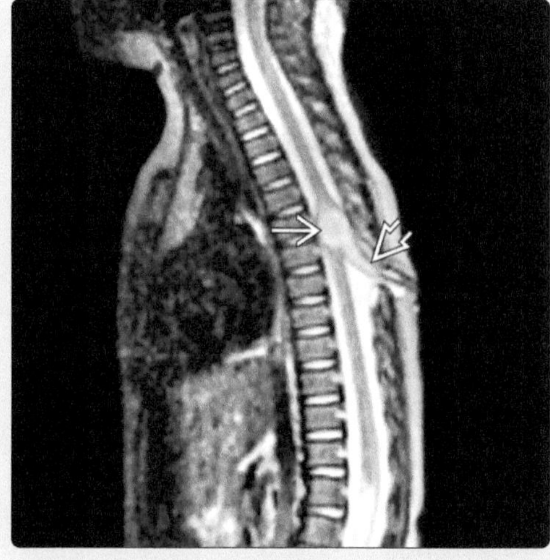

(Left) *Sagittal graphic of the cervicothoracic spine demonstrates a large dorsal dermoid cyst ➡ in association with a dermal sinus tract ➡. There is marked spinal cord compression.* **(Right)** *Sagittal T2 MR (myelopathy) demonstrates a hyperintense dermoid tumor with an intramedullary component ➡ contiguous with an extramedullary component following a dermal sinus tract ➡ to the skin surface.*

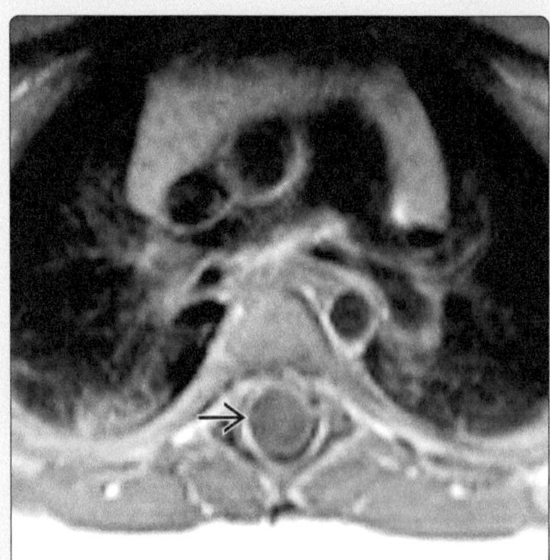

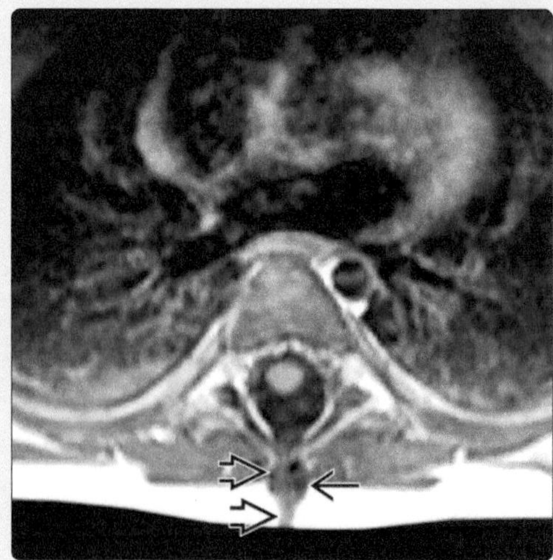

(Left) *Axial T1 MR (myelopathy) depicts a dermoid cyst ➡ with a prominent intramedullary component entirely within the spinal cord substance.* **(Right)** *Axial T1 MR (myelopathy) shows contiguous extension of a dermoid cyst along the dermal sinus tract ➡ to the skin surface. There is a small dermoid cyst ➡ within the dermal sinus tract as well.*

TERMINOLOGY

Synonyms

- Dermoid tumor, "dermoid"

Definitions

- Benign spinal mass
- Composed of cells that embryologically compose skin and its appendages (hair follicles, sweat glands, and sebaceous glands)

IMAGING

General Features

- Best diagnostic clue
  - Lumbosacral or cauda equina CSF isointense/isodense mass ± interspersed fat signal intensity/density
- Location
  - Lumbosacral (60%), cauda equina (20%)
    - 40% intramedullary, 60% extramedullary; extradural rare
  - Rare in cervical and thoracic spine
- Size
  - Range: Tiny subpial masses → huge growths
- Morphology
  - Uni- or multilobular round/ovoid mass

Radiographic Findings

- Radiography
  - Focal vertebral osseous erosion
  - Spinal canal widening
  - Flattening of pedicles and laminae
  - ± dysraphic posterior elements

CT Findings

- CECT
  - Well-demarcated isodense mass ± regions of fat hypodensity, calcification
    - ± minimal enhancement
- Bone CT
  - Focal osseous erosion, spinal canal widening, flattening of pedicles and laminae at spinal level of mass

MR Findings

- T1WI
  - Hypo- to hyperintense signal intensity mass
    - Hypointensity may reflect increased water content from sweat gland secretions
    - Fat hyperintensity is most specific for dermoid but least common appearance
      - Intrinsic T1 shortening permits differentiation of dermoid from epidermoid cyst
- T2WI
  - Hyperintense T2 signal intensity mass
- FLAIR
  - Mild hyperintensity to CSF may help detect occult dermoid tumor, differentiate from arachnoid cyst
- DWI
  - Less likely to show diffusion restriction than epidermoid cyst
- T1WI C+
  - ± mild ring enhancement; more avid surrounding contrast enhancement if infected

Ultrasonographic Findings

- Grayscale ultrasound
  - Hypoechoic mass lesion with internal echoes, focal areas of hyperechogenicity (if fat present)

Nonvascular Interventions

- Myelography
  - CSF or fat-density mass adjacent to bright CSF
  - Myelographic block common if symptomatic
  - Most useful in conjunction with CT (CT myelography)
  - Largely replaced by MR imaging
    - Primarily of utility in patients with MR contraindications (pacemaker, devices, etc.)

Imaging Recommendations

- Best imaging tool
  - MR; reserve CT myelography for patients with MR contraindications or inconclusive MR studies
- Protocol advice
  - Sagittal and axial T1WI and T2WI MR to include entire conus and cauda equina to coccyx tip

DIFFERENTIAL DIAGNOSIS

Arachnoid Cyst

- Follows CSF signal intensity/density on all sequences
- DWI MR useful to distinguish arachnoid cyst (isointense to CSF) from dermoid with restriction (hyperintense)

Neurenteric Cyst

- Intradural cyst; usually ventral to cord but may be dorsal or intramedullary
- ± vertebral anomalies, hyperdense/hyperintense proteinaceous content
- Definitive diagnosis is pathologic

Epidermoid Cyst

- Inclusion cyst, similar etiologies to dermoid cyst
- Avid diffusion restriction on DWI distinguishes from nonrestricting dermoid cyst and arachnoid cyst

PATHOLOGY

General Features

- Etiology
  - Congenital
    - Arise from dermal rests or focal expansion of dermal sinus
  - Acquired
    - Iatrogenic lesion
    - Results from implantation of viable dermal and epidermal elements following lumbar puncture (nontrocar spinal needle) or following surgery (myelomeningocele closure)
    - Cells slowly grow until large enough to cause symptoms
    - Link between lumbar puncture and subsequent epidermoid or dermoid cyst is particularly strong in neonatal period
- Associated abnormalities

- Dermal sinus (20%)
- Vertebral abnormalities (diastematomyelia, hemivertebra, scoliosis)
- Closed dysraphism (anterior sacral meningocele, spina bifida occulta): Rare
- Benign "tumor"
- Arises from cells that produce skin and its appendages (hair follicles, sweat glands, sebaceous glands)

Gross Pathologic & Surgical Features

- Well-demarcated, smooth, uni- or multilocular mass
- Cyst wall may be thickened by skin appendages or calcifications
- Cyst filled with thick, cheesy, buttery, yellowish material

Microscopic Features

- Outer connective tissue capsule lined with stratified squamous epithelium containing hair follicles, sebaceous glands, and sweat glands
- ± inflammation (if ruptured)
- Centrally contains desquamated epithelial keratin, lipid material

CLINICAL ISSUES

Presentation

- Most common signs/symptoms
  - Asymptomatic
  - Slowly progressive compressive radiculopathy/myelopathy
- Other signs/symptoms
  - Cauda equina syndrome
  - Infectious meningitis; most common in association with dermal sinus
  - Acute chemical meningitis secondary to rupture and discharge of inflammatory cholesterol crystals into CSF

Demographics

- Age
  - Usually symptomatic < 20 years
- Sex
  - M = F
- Epidemiology
  - (Epi)dermoid compose 1-2% of all spinal cord tumors, up to 10% of spinal cord tumors < 15 years of age
  - Dermoid and epidermoid occur roughly equally in spine; ~ 40% single epidermoid, 35% single dermoid, and 5% multiple dermoid or epidermoid

Natural History & Prognosis

- Symptoms slowly progress if untreated
- Complete surgical resection offers best opportunity for good neurologic outcome
  - Incomplete resection frequently recurs; malignant transformation extremely rare

Treatment

- Standard treatment is complete surgical excision

DIAGNOSTIC CHECKLIST

Consider

- Congenital lesion that usually presents during childhood/adolescence

Image Interpretation Pearls

- Often difficult to diagnose on CT and MR; presence of fat helpful to suggest diagnosis
  - Requires high index of suspicion; look for mass effect on regional structures

SELECTED REFERENCES

1. Cunha B et al: Imaging of intraspinal cystic lesions: a review. J Neuroimaging. 32(6):1044-61, 2022
2. Gupta SK et al: Infected congenital lumbosacral dermal sinus tract with conus epidermoid abscess: a rare entity. Childs Nerv Syst. 37(3):741-7, 2021
3. Prasad GL et al: Rupture of spinal dermoid cyst with intracranial dissemination: report of a case and review of the literature. Neurol India. 66(4):1195-9, 2018
4. AbouZeid AA et al: The Currarino triad: what pediatric surgeons need to know. J Pediatr Surg. 52(8):1260-8, 2017
5. Graillon T et al: Intramedullary epidermoid cysts in adults: case report and updated literature review. Neurochirurgie. 63(2):99-102, 2017
6. Garg K et al: Isolated central canal rupture of spinal dermoid. Report of 3 cases. J Neurosurg Spine. 21(3):361-6, 2014
7. Mishra SS et al: Thoracic congenital dermal sinus associated with intramedullary spinal dermoid cyst. J Pediatr Neurosci. 9(1):30-2, 2014
8. Vadivelu S et al: Infected lumbar dermoid cyst mimicking intramedullary spinal cord tumor: observations and outcomes. J Pediatr Neurosci. 9(1):21-6, 2014
9. Liu H et al: Microsurgical treatment of spinal epidermoid and dermoid cysts in the lumbosacral region. J Clin Neurosci. 19(5):712-7, 2012
10. van Aalst J et al: Intraspinal dermoid and epidermoid tumors: report of 18 cases and reappraisal of the literature. Pediatr Neurosurg. 45(4):281-90, 2009
11. Danzer E et al: Intradural inclusion cysts following in utero closure of myelomeningocele: clinical implications and follow-up findings. J Neurosurg Pediatr. 2(6):406-13, 2008
12. Ramos E et al: Congenital dermoid tumor in a child at initial myelomeningocele closure: an etiological discussion. J Neurosurg Pediatr. 2(6):414-5, 2008
13. Kasliwal MK et al: Symptomatic central canal rupture heralding the presence of an asymptomatic conus dermoid. J Neurooncol. 84(1):39-40, 2007
14. Kukreja K et al: Differentiation between pediatric spinal arachnoid and epidermoid-dermoid cysts: is diffusion-weighted MRI useful? Pediatr Radiol. 37(6):556-60, 2007
15. Muthukumar N et al: Intramedullary dermoid in a low lying conus tethered by a fatty filum - embryological implications. Acta Neurochir (Wien). 149(11):1173-5, 2007
16. Coppens JR et al: Presumed rupture of a conus medullaris dermoid cyst with cervical intramedullary fat and lipomatous infiltration of the cauda equina. Case illustration. J Neurosurg Spine. 5(2):178, 2006
17. Terai T et al: Adult onset tethered cord syndrome associated with intradural dermoid cyst. A case report. Spinal Cord. 44(4):260-2, 2006
18. Najjar MW et al: Dorsal intramedullary dermoids. Neurosurg Rev. 28(4):320-5, 2005
19. Goyal A et al: Spontaneous rupture of spinal dermoid cyst with disseminated lipid droplets in central canal and ventricles. J Neurosurg Sci. 48(2):63-5, 2004
20. Ziv ET et al: Iatrogenic intraspinal epidermoid tumor: two cases and a review of the literature. Spine. 29(1):E15-8, 2004
21. Bretz A et al: Intraspinal epidermoid cyst successfully treated with radiotherapy: case report. Neurosurgery. 53(6):1429-31; discussion 1431-2, 2003
22. Ferrara P et al: Intramedullary epidermoid cyst presenting with abnormal urological manifestations. Spinal Cord. 41(11):645-8, 2003
23. Graham D et al: Greenfield's Neuropathology. 7th ed. Arnold. 964-6, 2002
24. Kikuchi K et al: The utility of diffusion-weighted imaging with navigator-echo technique for the diagnosis of spinal epidermoid cysts. AJNR Am J Neuroradiol. 21(6):1164-6, 2000
25. Potgieter S et al: Epidermoid tumours associated with lumbar punctures performed in early neonatal life. Dev Med Child Neurol. 40(4):266-9, 1998

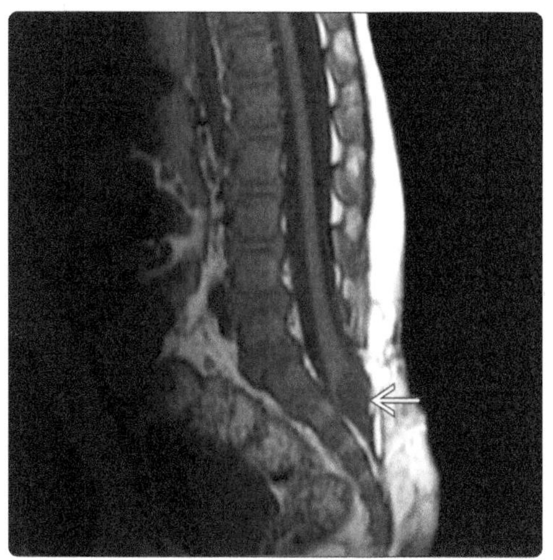

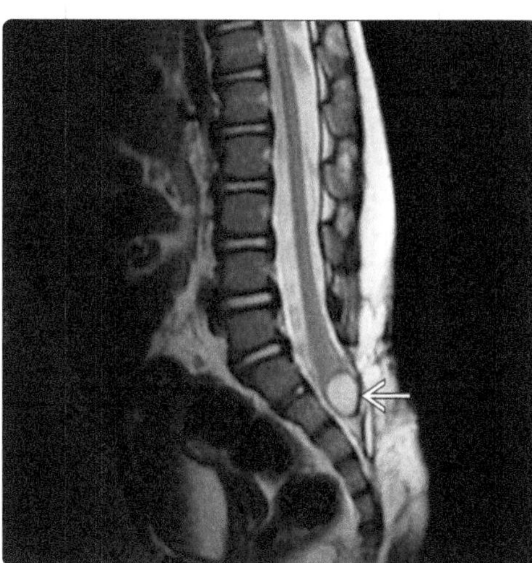

(Left) *Sagittal T1 MR in a 1-month-old girl who underwent in utero closure of a myelomeningocele reveals a low-lying spinal cord termination with intrinsic hypointense mass ➡ in the distal cord.* **(Right)** *Sagittal T2 MR in the same patient reveals hyperintense signal within the cord mass ➡. Surgical pathology revealed dermoid cyst.*

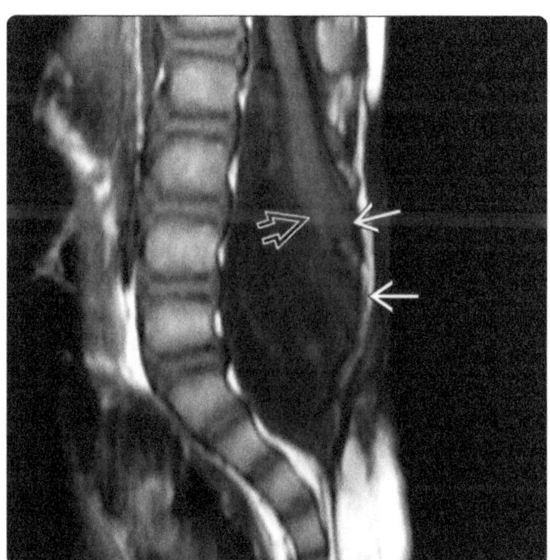

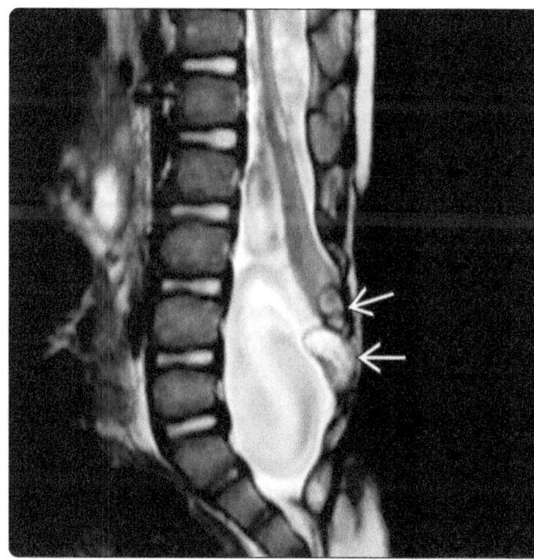

(Left) *Sagittal T1 MR in a patient with prior in utero repair of a myelomeningocele reveals 3 masses ➡ slightly hypointense to CSF at the spinal cord terminus ⇨ adjacent to the dural closure. (Courtesy B. Koch, MD.)* **(Right)** *Sagittal T2 MR in the same patient confirms heterogeneous signal within the 3 cysts ➡. Surgical pathology revealed an epidermal inclusion cyst, dermoid type. (Courtesy B. Koch, MD.)*

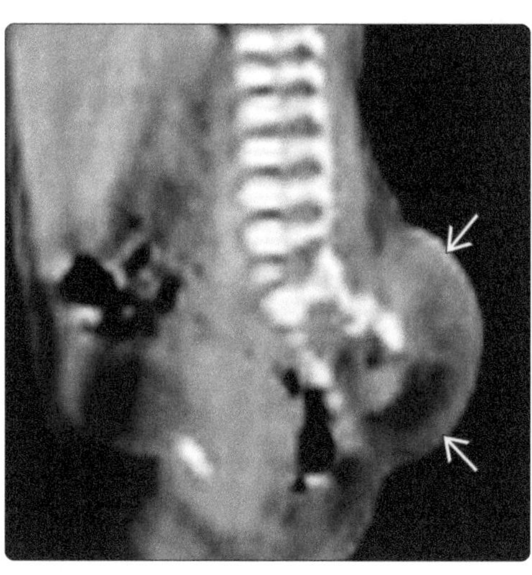

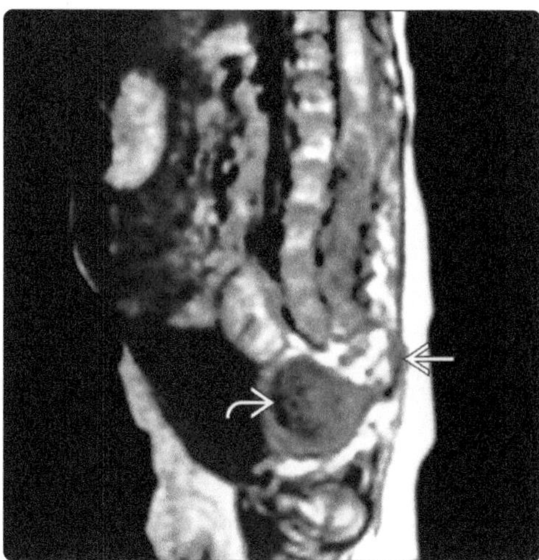

(Left) *Sagittal NECT in an infant with Currarino triad demonstrates caudal regression and a mixed density dermoid cyst ➡ contiguous with the spinal canal through a wide posterior dysraphic defect.* **(Right)** *Sagittal T1 MR in an infant with Currarino triad shows a small, mixed signal intensity dermoid "tumor" ➡ as well as a characteristic associated anterior sacral meningocele ↪.*

KEY FACTS

TERMINOLOGY

- Benign, nonneoplastic spinal mass embryologically derived from epidermal (skin) elements

IMAGING

- Lumbosacral or cauda equina CSF isointense/isodense mass
  - 40% intramedullary, 60% extramedullary
  - Acquired epidermoid cysts nearly always occur at cauda equina

TOP DIFFERENTIAL DIAGNOSES

- Arachnoid cyst
- Neurenteric cyst
- Dermoid cyst

PATHOLOGY

- Congenital (60%)
  - Arise from epidermal rests or dermal sinus
- Acquired (40%)
  - Iatrogenic, follows implantation of viable epidermal elements after lumbar puncture or surgery (myelomeningocele closure)
- Striking white, pearly sheen capsule containing creamy, waxy, pearly material

CLINICAL ISSUES

- Asymptomatic or slowly progressive compressive radiculopathy/myelopathy
- Symptoms slowly progress if untreated
- Complete surgical resection offers best opportunity for good neurologic outcome

DIAGNOSTIC CHECKLIST

- Epidermoid cysts may be congenital or acquired
  - Acquired epidermoid cysts nearly always occur in cauda equina
- Frequently difficult to identify using CT or MR
  - Diagnosis requires high index of suspicion; look for mass effect on regional structures

(Left) *Sagittal graphic of the thoracolumbar spine shows a pearly white epidermoid cyst ➡ located within the cauda equina at the conus, a typical location for a postlumbar puncture-acquired epidermoid cyst.* **(Right)** *Sagittal T1WI MR demonstrates a hypointense intradural extramedullary mass ➡ within the cauda equina in a patient who previously had a lumbar puncture as an infant. Signal intensity is slightly hyperintense to CSF, and there is no hyperintense lipid content to suggest dermoid cyst.*

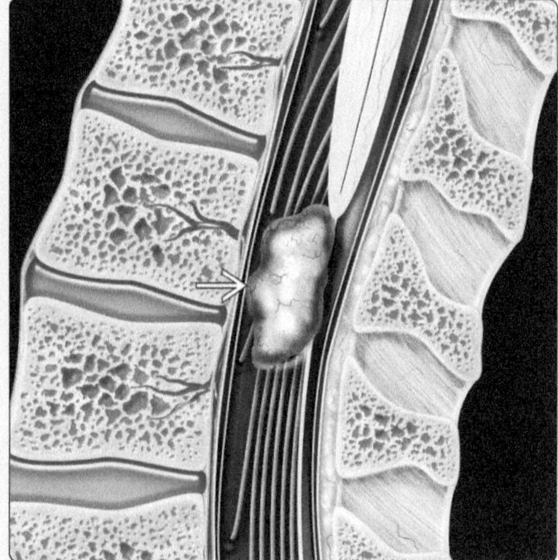

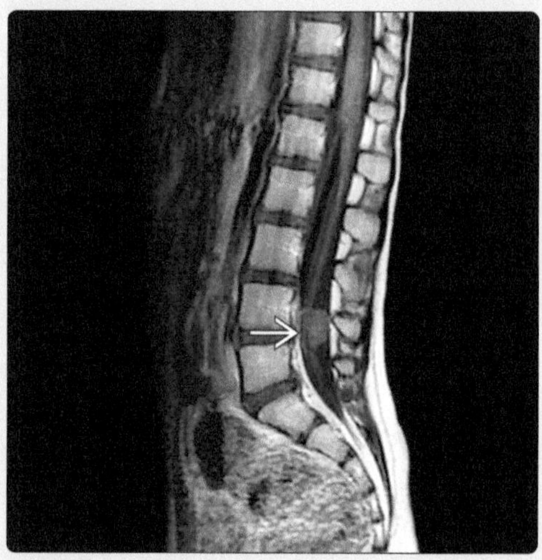

(Left) *Sagittal T2WI MR in a patient who had a lumbar puncture as an infant reveals a well-circumscribed intradural extramedullary mass ➡ within the cauda equina, which is distorted and anteriorly displaced by the cyst. Signal intensity is slightly hypointense to CSF.* **(Right)** *Axial T2WI MR shows anterior and lateral displacement of the cauda equina nerve roots ➡ by a hyperintense intradural epidermoid cyst ➡. The cyst nearly fills the spinal canal. Location is typical of a postlumbar puncture-acquired epidermoid cyst.*

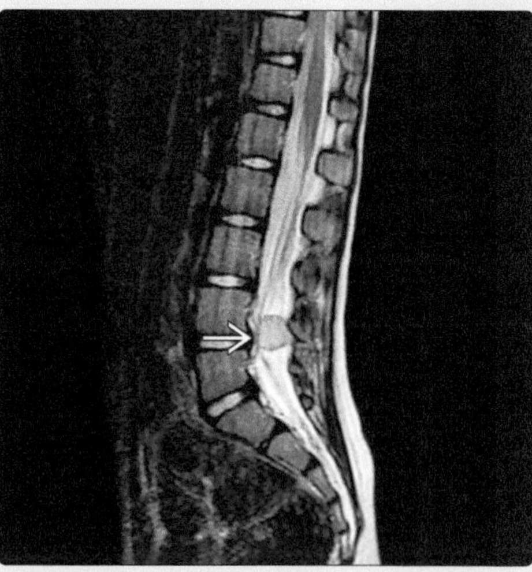

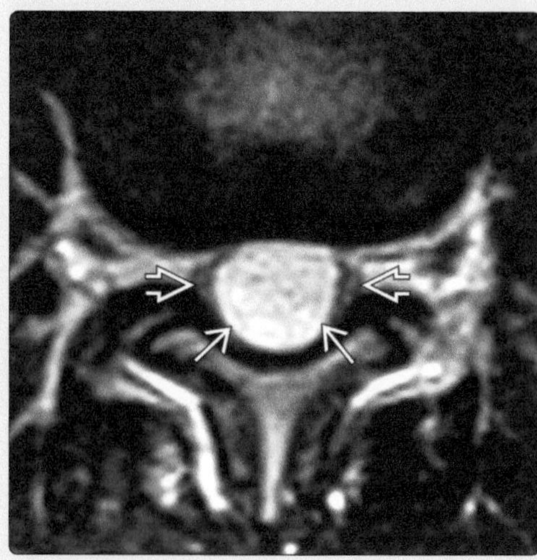

TERMINOLOGY

Synonyms

- Epidermoid tumor

Definitions

- Benign, nonneoplastic spinal mass composed of cells embryologically derived from epidermal (skin) elements

IMAGING

General Features

- Best diagnostic clue
  - Lumbosacral or cauda equina CSF isointense/isodense mass
- Location
  - 40% intramedullary, 60% extramedullary; extradural rare
    - Upper thoracic (17%), lower thoracic (26%), lumbosacral (22%), cauda equina (35%)
  - Acquired epidermoid cysts nearly always occur at cauda equina
- Size
  - Range: Tiny subpial masses → huge growths
- Morphology
  - Uni- or multilobular round/ovoid mass

Radiographic Findings

- Radiography
  - Focal vertebral osseous erosion, spinal canal widening, flattening of pedicles and laminae at spinal level of epidermoid cyst

CT Findings

- CECT
  - Well-circumscribed, hypodense mass with attenuation similar to CSF ± calcification (rare)
    - Rarely hyperdense on nonenhanced images, reflecting high protein content, hemorrhage, or cellular debris
    - Minimal to no enhancement (unless infected)
- Bone CT
  - Focal osseous erosion, spinal canal widening, flattening of pedicles and laminae at spinal level of epidermoid cyst

MR Findings

- T1WI
  - Usually isointense to CSF
  - Occasionally mildly hyperintense to CSF, reflecting protein or cellular debris (white epidermoid)
- T2WI
  - Hyperintense signal intensity to CSF
- FLAIR
  - Mildly hyperintense to CSF
    - May help detect occult epidermoid tumor, differentiate from arachnoid cyst
- DWI
  - Hyperintense diffusion restriction with concordant hypointensity on ADC map
    - Distinguishes epidermoid from arachnoid cyst (isointense to CSF)
- T1WI C+
  - ± minimal ring enhancement
  - May enhance avidly if infected

Ultrasonographic Findings

- Grayscale ultrasound
  - Hypoechoic mass lesion with subtle internal echoes

Nonvascular Interventions

- Myelography
  - CSF density mass conspicuous adjacent to bright CSF
    - Most useful in conjunction with bone CT
  - Myelographic block common in symptomatic patients
  - Has been largely replaced by noninvasive MR imaging

Imaging Recommendations

- Best imaging tool
  - Multiplanar MR
    - Reserve CT myelography for patients with MR contraindications, inconclusive MR studies
- Protocol advice
  - Sagittal and axial T1WI and T2WI MR to include entire conus and cauda equina → coccyx
  - DWI to evaluate for diffusion restriction

DIFFERENTIAL DIAGNOSIS

Arachnoid Cyst

- Follows CSF signal intensity/density on all sequences
- DWI MR useful to distinguish arachnoid cyst (isointense to CSF) from epidermoid (hyperintense)

Neurenteric Cyst

- Intradural cyst; usually ventral to cord but may be dorsal or intramedullary
- ± vertebral anomalies, hyperdense/hyperintense proteinaceous content
- Definitive diagnosis is pathologic

Dermoid Cyst

- May look exactly like epidermoid cyst or show some intrinsic fat signal intensity
- Diffusion restriction less common than with epidermoid cyst

PATHOLOGY

General Features

- Etiology
  - Congenital (60%)
    - Arise from epidermal rests or focal expansion of dermal sinus
  - Acquired (40%)
    - Iatrogenic lesion resulting from implantation of viable epidermal elements following lumbar puncture (nontrocar spinal needle) or surgery (myelomeningocele closure)
    - Cells slowly grow until large enough to produce symptoms
    - Link between lumbar puncture and subsequent epidermoid cyst development is strongest in neonatal period
- Associated abnormalities
  - Dermal sinus (20%)

- Vertebral abnormalities (diastematomyelia, vertebral segmentation anomalies, scoliosis)
- Closed spinal dysraphism (anterior sacral meningocele, spina bifida occulta): Rare

Gross Pathologic & Surgical Features

- Striking white, pearly sheen capsule; may be smooth, lobulated, or nodular
- Cyst filled with creamy, waxy, pearly material
- May be either easy to shell out or firmly affixed to regional structures (result of local inflammation)

Microscopic Features

- Outer connective tissue capsule lined with stratified squamous epithelium; calcification rare
- Centrally contains desquamated epithelial keratin, cholesterol crystals; positive staining with antibodies to EMA and cytokeratin

CLINICAL ISSUES

Presentation

- Most common signs/symptoms
  - Asymptomatic
  - Slowly progressive, compressive radiculopathy/myelopathy
- Other signs/symptoms
  - Infectious meningitis; most common in association with dermal sinus
  - Chemical meningitis secondary to rupture and discharge of inflammatory cholesterol crystals into CSF
  - Cauda equina syndrome

Demographics

- Age
  - Slower growing than dermoids; symptoms usually manifest in early adulthood (3rd-5th decades)
- Sex
  - M > F
- Epidemiology
  - Epidermoid cysts compose 1-2% of all spinal cord masses, up to 10% of spinal cord masses < 15 years of age
  - Dermoid and epidermoid cysts occur roughly equally in spine; ~ 40% single epidermoid, 35% single dermoid, and 5% multiple dermoid or epidermoid

Natural History & Prognosis

- Symptoms slowly progress if untreated
- Complete surgical resection offers best opportunity for good neurologic outcome
  - Incomplete resection frequently recurs; malignant transformation extremely rare

Treatment

- Standard treatment is complete surgical excision
- Radiotherapy not established for treatment of epidermoid cysts
  - May be alternative to palliative operation or for patients who cannot undergo surgery

DIAGNOSTIC CHECKLIST

Consider

- Epidermoid cysts may be congenital or acquired
  - Acquired epidermoid cysts nearly always occur in cauda equina
- Usually diagnosed later than dermoid (3rd-5th decades)

Image Interpretation Pearls

- Frequently difficult to identify using CT or MR
  - Diagnosis requires high index of suspicion; look for mass effect on regional structures
  - FLAIR, FIESTA, and DWI may distinguish epidermoid cyst from CSF, arachnoid cyst

SELECTED REFERENCES

1. Gupta SK et al: Infected congenital lumbosacral dermal sinus tract with conus epidermoid abscess: a rare entity. Childs Nerv Syst. 37(3):741-7, 2021
2. Rahimizadeh A et al: Spinal intramedullary epidermoid cysts: three case presentations and literature review. Surg Neurol Int. 11:17, 2020
3. Sîrbu OM et al: Spinal intramedullary epidermoid cyst: case report and updated literature review. World Neurosurg. 139:39-50, 2020
4. Prasad GL et al: Spinal intramedullary abscess secondary to dermal sinus in children. Eur J Pediatr Surg. 29(3):229-38, 2019
5. Beechar VB et al: Spinal epidermoid tumors: case report and review of the literature. Neurospine. 15(2):117-22, 2018
6. Funao H et al: A rare case of intradural and extramedullary epidermoid cyst after repetitive epidural anesthesia: case report and review of the literature. World J Surg Oncol. 15(1):131, 2017
7. Park MH et al: Iatrogenic intraspinal epidermoid cyst. Korean J Spine. 11(3):195-7, 2014
8. Yin H et al: Surgery and outcomes of six patients with intradural epidermoid cysts in the lumbar spine. World J Surg Oncol. 12(1):50, 2014
9. Velamati R et al: Meningitis secondary to ruptured epidermoid cyst: case-based review. Pediatr Ann. 42(6):248-51, 2013
10. Morita M et al: Intraspinal epidermoid tumor of the cauda equina region: seven cases and a review of the literature. J Spinal Disord Tech. 25(5):292-8, 2012
11. Gonzalvo A et al: Intramedullary spinal epidermoid cyst of the upper thoracic region. J Clin Neurosci. 16(1):142-4, 2009
12. Bernard PA: Lumbar punctures: always use a stylette. J Child Neurol. 23(8):969; author reply 969, 2008
13. Danzer E et al: Intradural inclusion cysts following in utero closure of myelomeningocele: clinical implications and follow-up findings. J Neurosurg Pediatr. 2(6):406-13, 2008
14. Piana G et al: Epidermoid-cyst of the conus medullaris: usefulness of DWI. J Neuroradiol. 35(5):304-5, 2008
15. Yen CP et al: Epidermoid cysts associated with thoracic meningocele. Acta Neurochir (Wien). 150(3):305-8; discussion 308-9, 2008
16. Gao B et al: Mollaret meningitis associated with an intraspinal epidermoid cyst. Pediatrics. 120(1):e220-4, 2007
17. Gerlach R et al: Large intramedullary abscess of the spinal cord associated with an epidermoid cyst without dermal sinus. Case report. J Neurosurg Spine. 7(3):357-61, 2007
18. Kukreja K et al: Differentiation between pediatric spinal arachnoid and epidermoid-dermoid cysts: is diffusion-weighted MRI useful? Pediatr Radiol. 37(6):556-60, 2007
19. Per H et al: Iatrogenic epidermoid tumor: late complication of lumbar puncture. J Child Neurol. 22(3):332-6, 2007
20. Refai D et al: Iatrogenic intradural epidermoid cyst after lumbar puncture. Case illustration. J Neurosurg. 106(4 Suppl):322, 2007
21. Jeong IH et al: Iatrogenic intraspinal epidermoid tumor: case report. Pediatr Neurosurg. 42(6):395-8, 2006
22. Tang L et al: Diffusion-weighted imaging distinguishes recurrent epidermoid neoplasm from postoperative arachnoid cyst in the lumbosacral spine. J Comput Assist Tomogr. 30(3):507-9, 2006
23. Lai SW et al: MRI of epidermoid cyst of the conus medullaris. Spinal Cord. 43(5):320-3, 2005
24. Bretz A et al: Intraspinal epidermoid cyst successfully treated with radiotherapy: case report. Neurosurgery. 53(6):1429-31; discussion 1431-2, 2003
25. Park JC et al: Iatrogenic spinal epidermoid tumor. A complication of spinal puncture in an adult. Clin Neurol Neurosurg. 105(4):281-5, 2003

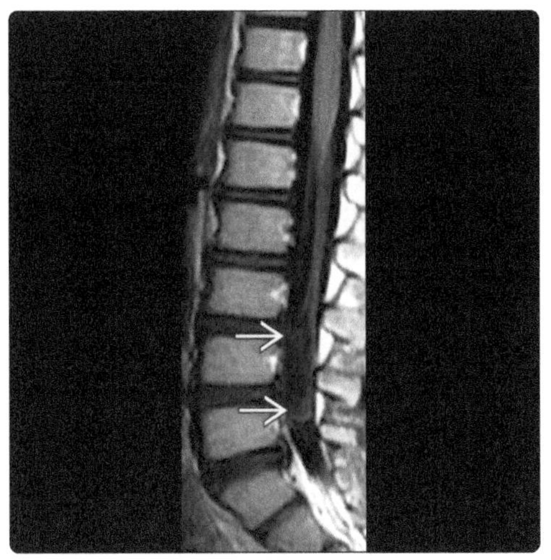

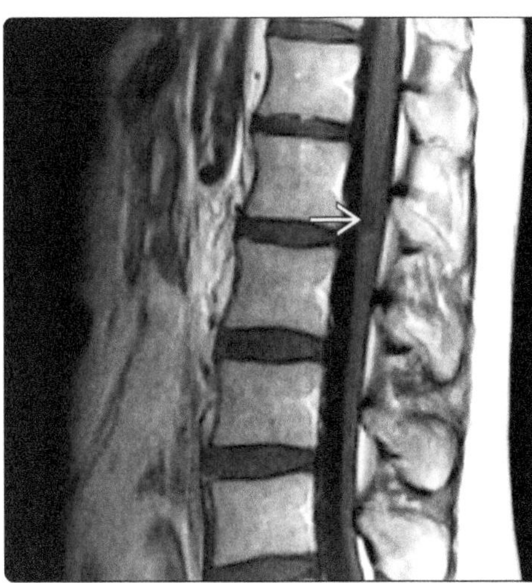

(Left) *Sagittal T1WI MR demonstrates a hypointense intradural mass ➡ nestled within the cauda equina that displaces adjacent nerve roots, compatible with a classic postlumbar puncture epidermoid cyst. Epidermoid cysts are often very subtle on standard T1 and T2 MR.* **(Right)** *Sagittal T1 C+ MR of the thoracolumbar spine demonstrates a subtle ovoid lesion ➡ nestled within the cauda equina, hypointense to the conus. The conus resides at the normal L1/L2 level.*

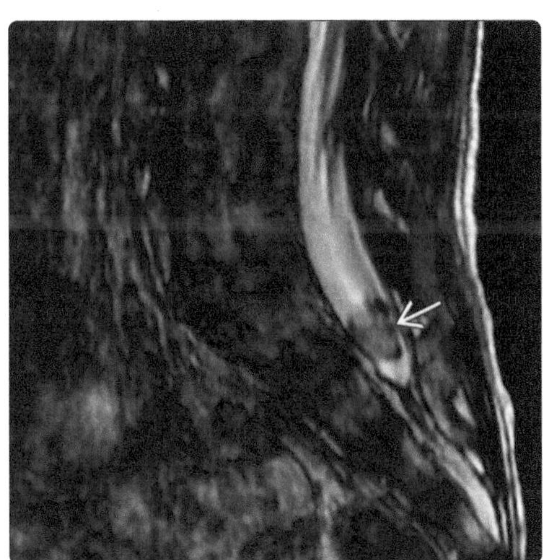

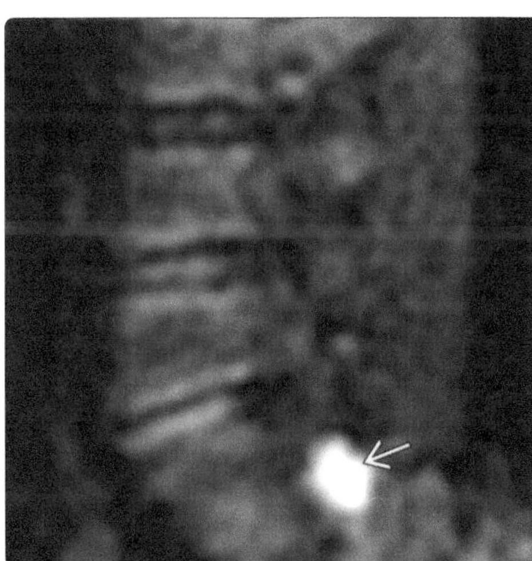

(Left) *Sagittal FIESTA MR in a pediatric patient with a myelomeningocele closed at birth reveals a hypointense mass ➡ in the caudal thecal sac. FIESTA MR is very useful for demonstrating intradural masses in the background of white CSF.* **(Right)** *Sagittal DWI MR in the same patient confirms avid mass ➡ diffusion restriction, compatible with an epidermoid cyst. ADC map (not shown) confirmed mass hypointensity.*

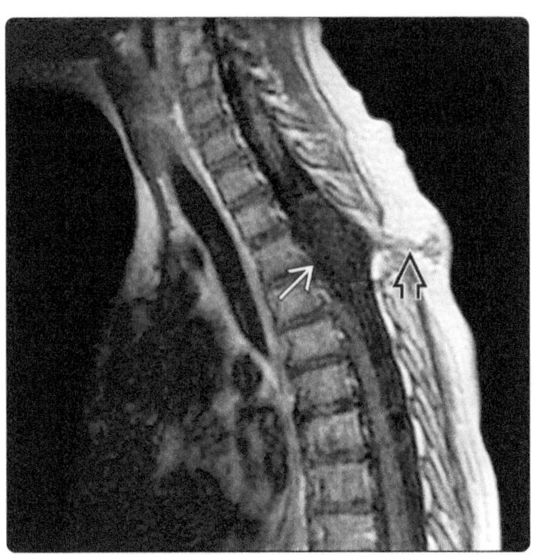

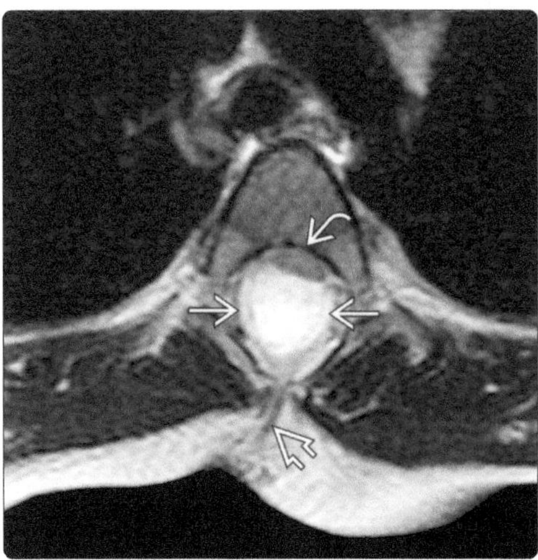

(Left) *Sagittal T1WI MR shows a thoracic dermal sinus tract ⇨ extending from the skin surface into the spinal canal, contiguous with a large intradural epidermoid cyst ➡. The epidermoid cyst displaces the spinal cord.* **(Right)** *Axial T2WI MR reveals a dermal sinus tract ➡ extending from the skin surface into the spinal canal through a bifid thoracic spinous process, connecting to an intradural epidermoid cyst ➡. Note the ventral displacement and distortion of the spinal cord ➡.*

KEY FACTS

TERMINOLOGY

- Abnormally low position & restricted mobility of conus medullaris in concert with characteristic symptoms

IMAGING

- Best clue: Low-lying conus medullaris
  - May have thickened filum terminale ± fatty infiltration or lipomatous mass
  - Accompanied by clinical signs & symptoms of tethering
- General imaging features
  - Conus below L2-L3 disc level
  - May appear taut or directly apposed to dorsal thecal sac
    - Lack of conus motion with CSF pulsations
    - Lack of dependent ventral shift of conus when prone
  - Filum > 2 mm thick (at L5-S1 on axial/transverse images)

PATHOLOGY

- Cutaneous stigmata in up to 50%
  - Hairy patch, hemangioma, skin tag, atypical dimple
- Tethering also found in clinically apparent open & closed spinal dysraphism
- Tethered filum histologically abnormal
  - ↑ connective tissue with dense collagen fibers, hyalinization, & dilated capillaries

CLINICAL ISSUES

- Lower extremity weakness, spasticity, & ↓ sensation; abnormal gait; bladder dysfunction
- Symptomatic presentation most common during rapid growth (4-8 years of age & adolescent growth spurt)
- Majority show improvement or stabilization of neurologic deficits following surgical untethering

DIAGNOSTIC CHECKLIST

- Tethered cord syndrome is clinical diagnosis
- Clinical tethering may be present despite normal conus level

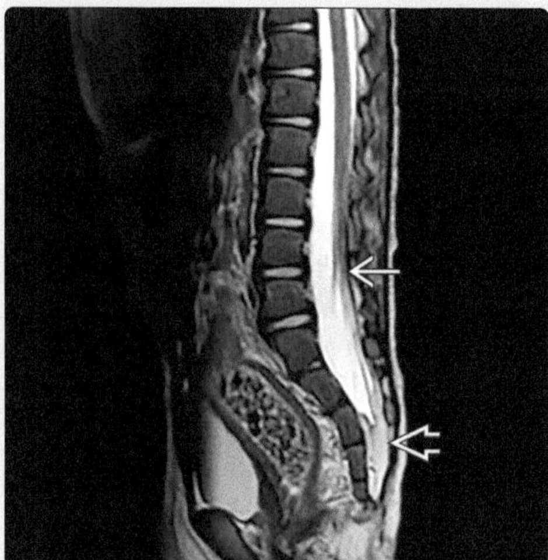

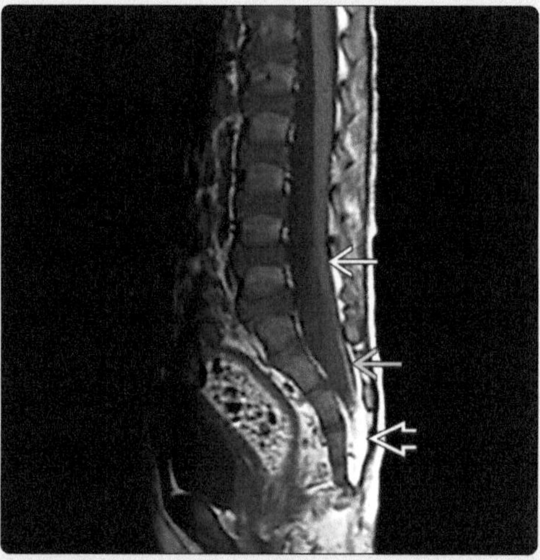

(Left) *Sagittal T2 MR in a 2-year-old with an abnormal gait demonstrates abnormal conus elongation and low termination at the L4-L5 level ➡. Note proliferation of fat in the terminal spinal canal ➡.* **(Right)** *Sagittal T1 MR in the same patient confirms abnormal low termination of the elongated conus ➡ and mild fat infiltration of the filum terminale ➡. The filum inserts into a terminal lipoma ➡.*

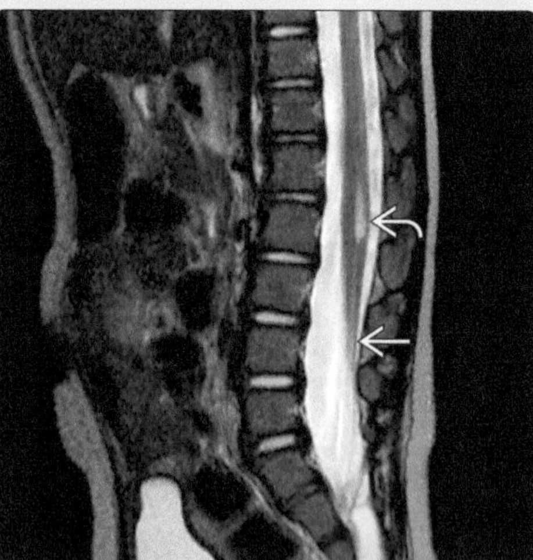

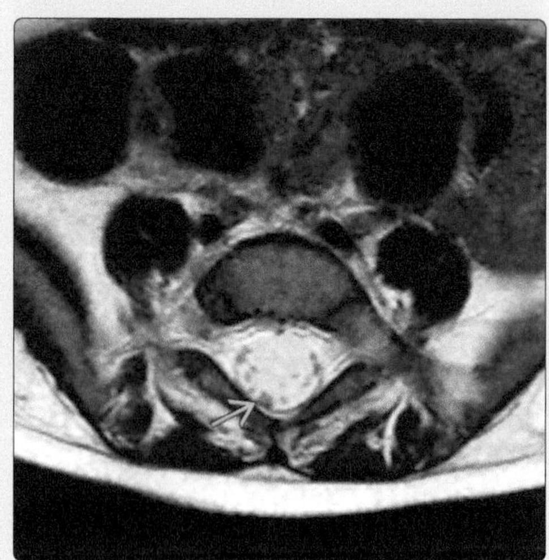

(Left) *Sagittal T2 MR in a 5-month-old with a cutaneous birthmark over the lower spine shows an abnormally low and dorsal position of the conus medullaris ➡. Also note mild syringohydromyelia of the distal spinal cord central canal ➡.* **(Right)** *Axial T2 MR at the level of L5-S1 in the same infant further demonstrates the abnormal thickening of the filum terminale ➡, which is directly apposed to the dorsal aspect of the thecal sac. These imaging findings are typical of tethering.*

TERMINOLOGY

Synonyms

- Tethered cord syndrome (TCS), tight filum terminale syndrome, retained medullary cord (RMC)

Definitions

- Abnormally low position & restricted mobility of conus medullaris in concert with characteristic symptoms

IMAGING

General Features

- Best diagnostic clue
  - Low-lying conus does not demonstrate normal anterior/ventral motion with prone positioning
    - May have thickened filum terminale ± fatty infiltration or lipomatous mass
    - Accompanied by clinical signs & symptoms of tethering
      - Lower extremity pain, weakness, spasticity; abnormal gait; abnormal deep tendon reflexes; bladder dysfunction
- Location
  - Conus terminates at or above inferior L2 vertebra in ≥ 98% of normal population
    - Conus at normal position by 0-2 months of age
    - Conus terminating below L2-L3 disc: Abnormal at any postnatal age
      - Significance questionable in absence of signs/symptoms
  - Dorsal positioning of conus medullaris & filum terminale in thecal sac
    - Persists in prone position
      - Normal spinal cord falls into anterior 2/3 of thecal sac when prone
- Size
  - Filum terminale thickened (> 2 mm at L5-S1 on axial/transverse images)

Radiographic Findings

- Radiography
  - May be normal but frequently shows localized dysraphism or incomplete posterior element fusion
  - ± scoliosis (20%), vertebral segmentation anomalies

MR Findings

- T1WI
  - Thickened filum ± hyperintense fat in or surrounding filum
    - Filum thickened at > 2 mm (L5-S1 on axial MR)
  - ± low-lying conus; may be difficult to distinguish transition from thickened filum
- T2WI
  - Fatty filum → chemical shift artifact
    - Drops signal with application of fat suppression
- MR cine
  - ± ↓ spinal cord motion
- Prone lumbar MR
  - Decreased ventral conus movement on prone compared to supine imaging reported to correlate with clinical tethering

Ultrasonographic Findings

- Grayscale ultrasound
  - ± low-lying conus, thickened filum terminale ± echogenic mass, persistent dorsal position of conus in prone position, ↓ or absent spinal cord motion with CSF pulsations

Imaging Recommendations

- Best imaging tool
  - US < 6 months of age: Excellent screening tool
    - Conus can be readily identified in children < 6 months of age
  - MR imaging > 6 months of age
    - Primary assessment of patient > 6 months of age
    - Further characterization if US abnormal in infant < 6 months of age
- Protocol advice
  - Thin-section sagittal & axial T1 & T2 MR
  - ± rapid SSFSE T2 MR in prone position or cine MR images to document motion
    - May not ↑ accuracy for tethering over conus level alone

DIFFERENTIAL DIAGNOSIS

Normal Variant: Low-Lying Conus

- Asymptomatic patient with normal filar thickness
- Clinical follow-up required

Open or Closed Spinal Dysraphism

- Varying degrees of bony & soft tissue defects ± herniation of canal contents, tethering of elongated cord into defect/mass
  - Dorsal dermal sinus tract
  - (Epi)dermoid
  - Spinal lipoma
  - Lipomyelomeningocele
  - Myelomeningocele
  - Meningocele
  - Diastematomyelia

Postsurgical Low-Lying Conus

- Persistent low position of conus after untethering procedure, irrespective of symptoms
- Cannot exclude retethering by imaging alone (requires correlation with clinical exam)

PATHOLOGY

General Features

- Etiology
  - Incomplete secondary neurulation with failure of terminal cord involution or failure of filum terminale to lengthen (RMC)
  - Tethering stretches nerve fibers, arterioles, & venules → impairs oxidative metabolism of conus & nerve roots → syringohydromyelia/myelomalacia
- Associated abnormalities
  - Cutaneous stigmata (50%)
    - Hairy patch, hemangioma, skin tag, atypical sacral dimple
  - Lumbosacral hypogenesis, VACTERL association

- Open or closed spinal dysraphism
- Scoliosis
  - Functional adaption to ↓ length of spinal cord course & ↓ intramedullary tension
- Syringohydromyelia/myelomalacia (25%)

Gross Pathologic & Surgical Features

- Thickened fibrotic filum (55%), small fibrolipoma within thickened filum (23%), filar cyst (3%)
- Conus & filum may not be distinct; elongated spinal cord may end directly in small terminal lipoma

Microscopic Features

- Tethered filum histologically abnormal, even if conus terminates at normal level
  - Normal filum: Mainly collagen fibers
  - Tethered cord filum: ↑ connective tissue with dense collagen fibers, hyalinization, & dilated capillaries

CLINICAL ISSUES

Presentation

- Most common signs/symptoms
  - Gait spasticity, weakness, muscular atrophy
  - ↓ sensation, abnormal lower extremity reflexes
  - Lower back & leg pain; worse in morning or with exertion
  - Urinary bladder dysfunction
- Other signs/symptoms
  - Orthopedic foot abnormalities (usually clubfoot)
- Clinical profile
  - Adults & children present differently
    - Children: Incontinence, scoliosis, weakness
    - Adults: Pain (secondary to degenerative changes) followed later by weakness ± incontinence

Demographics

- Age
  - Symptomatic presentation most common during rapid somatic growth (4-8 years of age & adolescent growth spurt) or secondary to kyphosis (older adults)
  - Higher prevalence in patients with anorectal malformations (ARM)
  - Prevalence in adults probably underestimated
- Sex
  - M = F
- Epidemiology
  - Prevalence unknown; probably more common than appreciated

Natural History & Prognosis

- Progressive, irreversible neurologic impairment
  - Majority of patients show improvement or stabilization of neurologic deficits following surgical untethering
    - Motor weakness (12-60%)
    - Sensory dysfunction (40-60%)
    - Pain (50-88%)
    - Bladder dysfunction (19-67%)
  - Better outcome if symptom duration shorter or conus moves to more normal level following surgery
- Postoperative symptom recurrence rare but prompts consideration for retethering

Treatment

- Symptomatic patients: Early prophylactic surgery
  - Resect tethering mass (if present), release cord, & repair dura
  - Spinal column shortening procedures in early phase of assessment to avoid physical cord detethering procedural & delayed complications
- Asymptomatic patients with radiologic tethering: Management controversial
  - Some advocate prophylactic surgery given low operative morbidity; prognosis for asymptomatic patients better than symptomatic
  - Others advocate prophylactic surgery only for asymptomatic adults who lead physically active lives
    - Some postoperative patients show eventual development of TCS symptoms

DIAGNOSTIC CHECKLIST

Consider

- TSC is clinical diagnosis
  - US for screening young infants with ↑ likelihood of spine abnormalities
    - Based on cutaneous stigmata or associated anomalies
  - MR evaluates symptomatic patients for underlying spine abnormalities affecting surgical planning
    - Distinguish cord tethering secondary to tight/thickened filum terminale vs. tethering secondary to other lesions
- Clinical tethering may be present despite normal conus level

Image Interpretation Pearls

- Determine conus level using axial images
  - Cauda equina may obscure conus tip on sagittal images, simulating elongated conus
- Measure filum thickness at L5/S1 (as stretching at more rostral levels may erroneously thin filum into normal size range)
- Recognize that scoliosis restricts normal cord mobility
  - Bowstring effect of cord draping across curvature

SELECTED REFERENCES

1. Mualem W et al: Utilizing pre- and postoperative radiological parameters to predict surgical outcomes following untethering for tethered cord syndrome in a pediatric population. J Neurosurg Pediatr. 31(2):159-68, 2023
2. Howells M et al: Detethering of MRI-demonstrated tethered cord syndrome. Pediatr Neurosurg. 57(2):85-92, 2022
3. Smith CA et al: Detection and management of tethered cord in anorectal malformation: a survey of pediatric neurosurgeons in the United States. Pediatr Neurosurg. 57(6):434-40, 2022
4. Kim KH et al: Secondary neurulation defects-1 : retained medullary cord. J Korean Neurosurg Soc. 63(3):314-20, 2020
5. Lin W et al: Spine-shortening osteotomy for patients with tethered cord syndrome: a systematic review and meta-analysis. Neurol Res. 40(5):340-63, 2018
6. Shukla M et al: Adult versus pediatric tethered cord syndrome: clinicoradiological differences and its management. Asian J Neurosurg. 13(2):264-70, 2018
7. Stamates MM et al: Magnetic resonance imaging in the prone position and the diagnosis of tethered spinal cord. J Neurosurg Pediatr. 21(1):4-10, 2018
8. Pang D et al: Retained medullary cord in humans: late arrest of secondary neurulation. Neurosurgery. 68(6):1500-19; discussion 1519, 2011

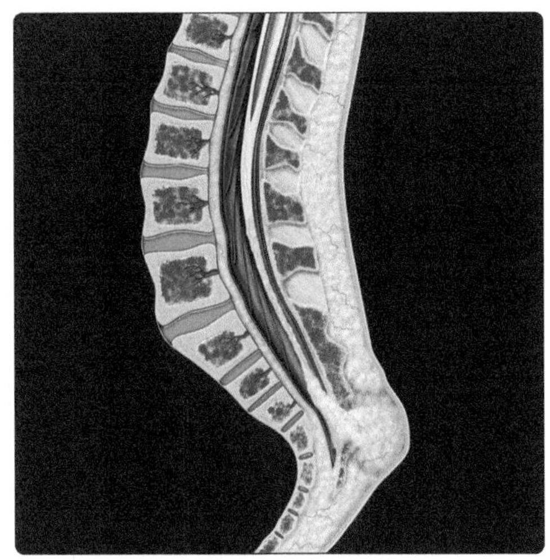

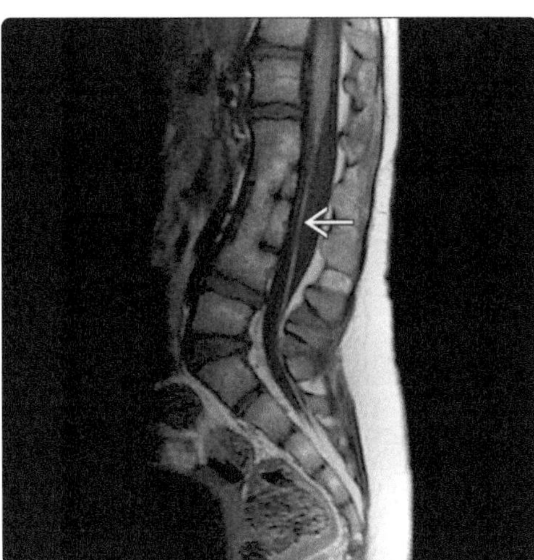

(Left) *Sagittal graphic of the lumbosacral spine shows composite TCS findings of a low-lying, hydromyelic tethered cord with thickened filum & fibrolipoma inserting into a terminal lipoma that is contiguous with subcutaneous fat through dorsal dysraphism.* **(Right)** *Sagittal T1 MR shows congenital segmentation failure at L1-L4. Spinal cord ends at the L1-L2 level but is abnormally pointed with a thickened, fatty infiltrated filum terminale ➡. The course of the filum and appearance of the conus strongly suggests tension.*

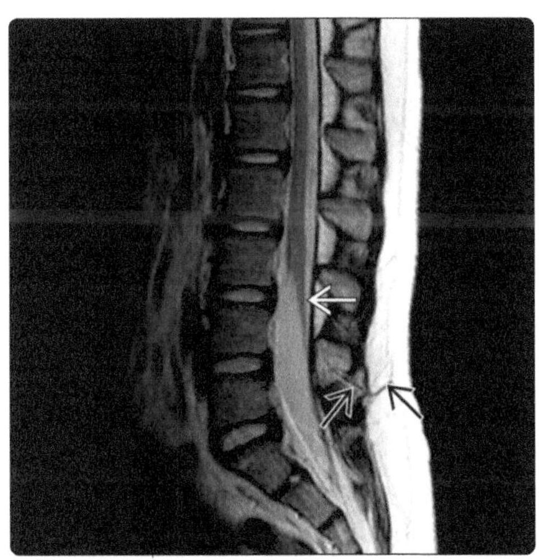

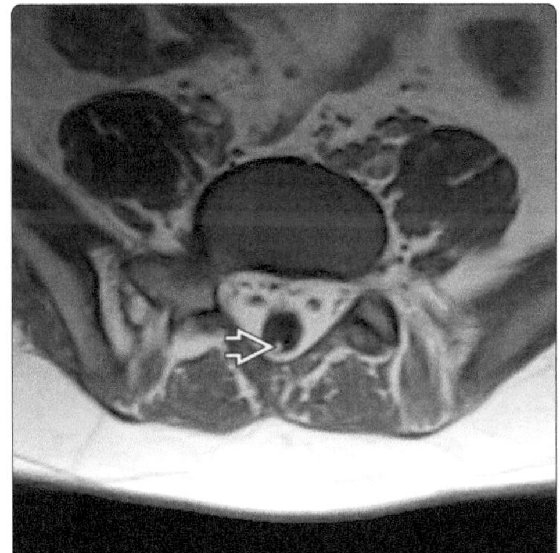

(Left) *Sagittal T2 MR reveals a taut appearance of the posteriorly positioned and low-lying conus ➡ with the tip near L4. Careful inspection of the image reveals a dermal sinus tract ⇨.* **(Right)** *Axial T1 MR in the same patient confirms the additional presence of a small filum lipoma ➡. The fibrolipoma may be an incidental observation in this patient with dorsal dermal sinus tethering the cord.*

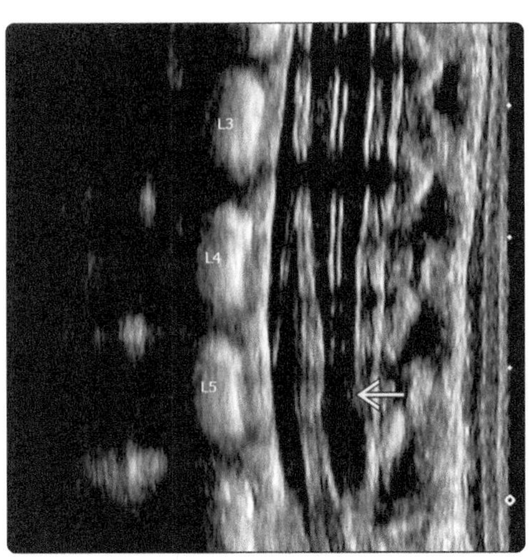

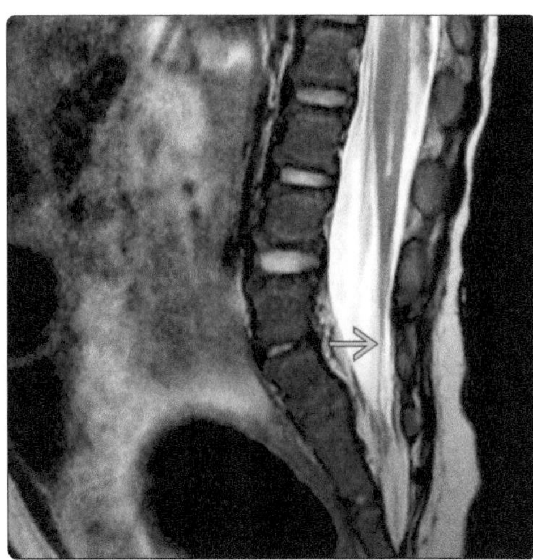

(Left) *Sagittal US of the lumbar spine in an 8-day-old infant with VACTERL association shows that the conus medullaris ➡ extends caudally to the level of L5-S1. The conus remains dorsally positioned despite the patient being prone. Configuration suggests RMC.* **(Right)** *Sagittal T2 MR in the same child again shows the inferior position of the conus with a thickened filum terminale ⇨, findings that suggest tethering. No mass is identified. Up to 40% of children with VACTERL association will be diagnosed with a tethered cord.*

KEY FACTS

TERMINOLOGY

- Segmental spinal dysgenesis (SSD), caudal regression syndrome (CRS)

IMAGING

- Localized segmental lumbar or thoracolumbar vertebral, spinal cord dysgenesis or agenesis
- Congenital acute angle kyphosis or kyphoscoliosis
- Distal spinal osseous architecture usually normal (unless concurrent CRS)

TOP DIFFERENTIAL DIAGNOSES

- Multiple vertebral segmentation disorders
- Congenital vertebral displacement
- Medial spinal aplasia
- CRS

PATHOLOGY

- Characteristic segmental vertebral, cord anomalies
    - Normal upper spinal cord
    - Hypoplastic or absent spinal cord, vertebral dysgenesis at gibbus apex
    - Bulky, thickened, low-lying cord segment within spinal canal below dysgenesis

CLINICAL ISSUES

- Thoracic or lumbar kyphosis
- Palpable bone spur at gibbus apex
- Spastic paraparesis or paraplegia
- Rarely present with normal or mildly impaired lower extremity function → subsequent deterioration

DIAGNOSTIC CHECKLIST

- SSD and CRS probably represent 2 different phenotypes along single malformation spectrum
- Morphologic severity correlates with residual spinal cord function, severity of clinical deficit

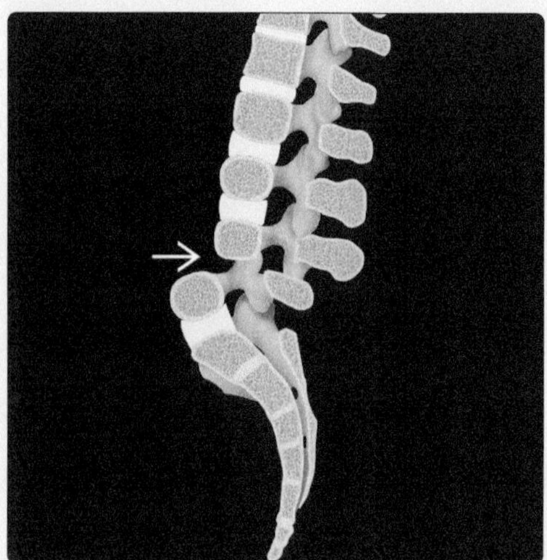

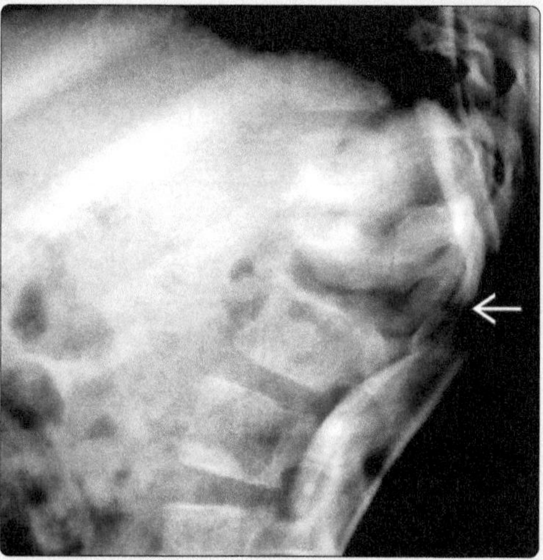

(Left) *Sagittal graphic demonstrates lower lumbar segmental spinal dysgenesis (SSD) with posterior subluxation of the upper lumbar spine relative to the segment below the dysgenetic level ➡. The spine is dysraphic at the dysgenetic level, but kyphosis has not yet developed.* **(Right)** *Lateral myelography of the thoracolumbar spine shows relatively mild SSD with focal kyphosis and severe thecal sac narrowing at the hypoplastic level ➡.*

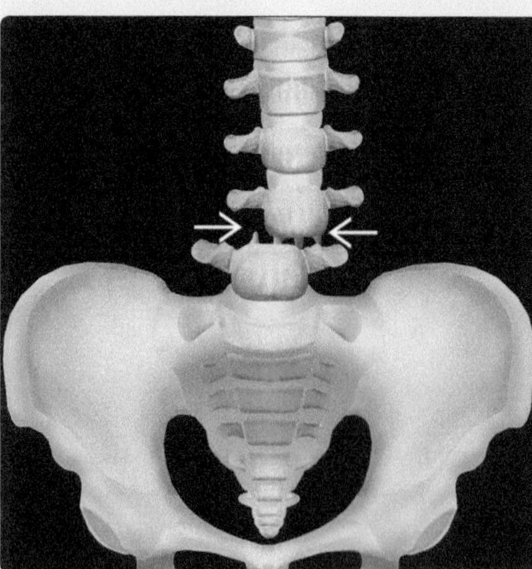

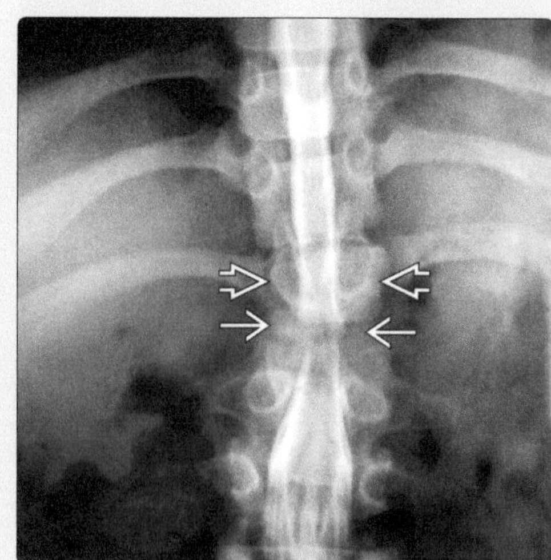

(Left) *Coronal graphic demonstrates lower lumbar SSD with lateral subluxation of the upper spine relative to the lumbosacral spine caudal to the dysgenetic level ➡.* **(Right)** *AP myelography shows hypoplasia of the lower thoracic vertebral body ➡ above the dysgenetic segment ➡ with narrowing of the myelographic column secondary to spinal canal stenosis. There is also mild focal scoliosis, probably related to segmental instability.*

TERMINOLOGY

Abbreviations

- Segmental spinal dysgenesis (SSD)

Definitions

- Complex congenital spinal malformation
  - Localized segmental agenesis or dysgenesis of lumbar or thoracolumbar spine, spinal cord
  - Distal spinal osseous architecture usually normal [unless concurrent caudal regression syndrome (CRS)]

IMAGING

General Features

- Best diagnostic clue
  - Localized segmental spinal agenesis or dysgenesis with severe congenital kyphosis or kyphoscoliosis, segmental spinal cord attenuation
- Location
  - Thoracolumbar, lumbar > lumbosacral
- Size
  - Extent variable
- Morphology
  - SSD is morphologic continuum rather than single appearance
    - Severe: Acute-angle gibbus kyphosis or kyphoscoliosis, indiscernible spinal cord at dysgenetic level, palpable spur at apex
    - Mild: Less severe kyphosis, segmental spinal cord thinning, hypoplastic spinal canal contiguous across dysgenetic segment
  - Classic spinal cord morphology
    - Upper spinal cord normal
    - Spinal cord thinned or atretic, absent nerve roots at dysgenetic level
    - Lower cord below dysgenetic level thickened, low lying
      - Nerve roots directed cephalad

Imaging Recommendations

- Best imaging tool
  - Multiplanar MR
- Protocol advice
  - Sagittal and coronal MR imaging most helpful for evaluating spinal cord
  - Multiplanar and 3D bone CT useful for characterizing vertebral anomalies, surgical planning

Radiographic Findings

- Radiography
  - Moderate to severe congenital kyphosis or kyphoscoliosis
    - Gibbus apex marks dysgenetic level of vertebral malformation
  - Segmental osseous anomalies at dysgenetic level
    - Focal canal stenosis, hypoplastic or aplastic vertebrae, spinal column subluxation (implies instability)
  - Marked stenosis or interruption of spinal canal at malformation level
    - Spinal canal superficially located at gibbus apex
  - ± costal abnormalities (bifid, fused, or absent ribs)
  - ± vertebral formation and segmentation anomalies at other levels

CT Findings

- Bone CT
  - Similar to radiography but easier to characterize vertebral anomalies

MR Findings

- T1WI
  - Significant narrowing of thecal sac, abnormal spinal cord, absent nerve roots at lesion level
  - Spinal cord always abnormal
  - Low-lying conus medullaris terminates at or below L3
  - Hypoplastic cord segment blends with filum terminale in lumbosacral SSD
- T2WI
  - Same as T1WI

Ultrasonographic Findings

- Grayscale ultrasound
  - Similar to MR findings
  - Diagnostic role limited; may be useful for neonates unable to undergo MR imaging

DIFFERENTIAL DIAGNOSIS

Multiple Vertebral Segmentation Disorders

- Short-trunk dwarfism, variably associated with costal abnormalities
  - Jarcho-Levin syndrome proper, spondylothoracic dysostosis, and spondylocostal dysostosis
- Entire spine abnormal rather than focal dysgenesis

Congenital Vertebral Displacement

- Dislocation at single vertebral level → abrupt spinal canal offset
- Vertebral pedicles present (absent in SSD)
- Spinal cord stretched/compressed but otherwise normally developed
- Closed spinal dysraphism unusual
- Neurologic deficits often mild, secondary to spinal instability ± cord compression

Medial Spinal Aplasia

- Isolated absence of spinal segments (mainly lower thoracic, lumbar)
- Congenital kyphoscoliosis + paraplegia
- Probably represents severe SSD; use of term medial spinal aplasia is discouraged

Caudal Regression Syndrome

- Malformation resulting from disturbed development of caudal cell mass
- Dysgenesis or absence of caudal spine, spinal cord
- Isolated or in conjunction with SSD

PATHOLOGY

General Features

- Etiology
  - Cause not definitively known, putative mechanisms include

- Association with maternal diabetes, medications, toxins
- Related to aberrant segmental vascular supply
- Failure of neural tube to correctly join caudal cell mass after primary and secondary neurulation (junctional neurulation)

o Embryologically, may represent inappropriately induced activation of positional apoptosis at dysgenetic level during gastrulation
- Wrongly specified cells eliminated → few or no prospective neuroectodermal cells induced to form neural plate during primary neurulation
- Abnormal primary neurulation → hypoplastic or aplastic spinal cord segment
  - Missing nerve roots at abnormal segment may be secondary to apoptotic elimination of somatic motoneurons
- Neurulation in neural plate proceeds below malformation level → lower cord segment usually present

o SSD and CRS probably represent different phenotypes along single spectrum of segmental spine/spinal cord malformations
- Segmental location(s) of derangement along embryo longitudinal axis determines malformation type
  - Intermediate segment → SSD
  - Caudal segment → CRS
  - 2 abnormal segments → double level SSD or SSD + CRS

- Associated abnormalities
  - Vertebral formation and segmentation anomalies
  - Closed spinal dysraphism (diastematomyelia, dermal sinus tract, terminal myelocystocele, lipoma, thickened filum terminale)
  - Visceral anomalies (renal, cardiac, neurogenic bladder)
  - Orthopedic anomalies (equinocavovarus feet, lower extremity deformities)
  - Cutaneous stigmata (angiomas, dermal sinus, hairy tuft)

Staging, Grading, & Classification

- Diagnostic criteria
  - Lumbar or thoracolumbar vertebral dysgenesis with kyphosis
  - Focal spinal cord hypoplasia or absence without exiting roots
  - Lower extremity deformity with paraplegia or paraparesis

Gross Pathologic & Surgical Features

- Normal upper spinal cord
- Spinal cord, vertebral malformation located at kyphotic gibbus apex
  - Vertebrae present above and below anomaly
- Bulky, thickened, low-lying cord segment within caudal spinal canal below dysgenesis

CLINICAL ISSUES

Presentation

- Most common signs/symptoms
  - Thoracic or lumbar kyphosis with palpable bone spur to gibbus apex
  - Spastic paraparesis or paraplegia
  - Neurogenic bladder
- Other signs/symptoms
  - Rarely present with normal or mildly impaired lower extremity neurologic function → subsequent deterioration
- Clinical profile
  - Infant with severely hypotrophic, deformed lower limbs, hip joint flexion-abduction, knee flexion equinocavovarus feet → "Buddha" sitting position
  - Moderate to severe motor impairment

Demographics

- Age
  - Diagnosed during infancy
- Epidemiology
  - Very rare

Natural History & Prognosis

- Progressive kyphosis
- Degree of neurologic deficit dependent on severity of hypoplasia, functionality of residual cord
  - Nearly all patients eventually progress to severe motor impairment

Treatment

- Goals include maintenance of spinal stability, arrest of progressive kyphosis
  - Early spinal fusion ± cord decompression enables patient to sit up without support
  - Bracing less effective than surgical stabilization for arresting neurologic decline
- Untethering procedures of limited utility
  - Neurologic dysfunction attributed to segmental hypoplasia or absent spinal cord, roots rather than spinal cord tethering

DIAGNOSTIC CHECKLIST

Consider

- Severity of morphologic derangement correlates with residual spinal cord function, severity of clinical deficit
- SSD and CRS probably represent 2 different phenotypes along single malformation spectrum

SELECTED REFERENCES

1. Aboughalia H et al: Multimodality imaging evaluation of fetal spine anomalies with postnatal correlation. Radiographics. 41(7):2176-92, 2021
2. Remondino RG et al: Surgical treatment of segmental spinal dysgenesis: a report of 19 cases. Spine Deform. 9(2):539-47, 2021
3. Cacciola F et al: Segmental spinal dysgenesis associated with occult dysraphism: considerations on management strategies. J Craniovertebr Junction Spine. 8(2):144-8, 2017
4. Eibach S et al: Unjoined primary and secondary neural tubes: junctional neural tube defect, a new form of spinal dysraphism caused by disturbance of junctional neurulation. Childs Nerv Syst. 33(10):1633-47, 2017
5. Morell SM et al: Segmental spinal dysgenesis: a report of early surgical intervention and outcome in a 14-month-old child. Childs Nerv Syst. 33(2):381-4, 2017
6. Pavlova OM et al: Surgical treatment of thoracolumbar segmental spinal dysgenesis: Optimal type of fusion. World Neurosurg. 106:551-6, 2017
7. Emmanouilidou M et al: Spinal segmental dysgenesis: presentation of a rare spinal congenital abnormality. Neuroradiol J. 21(3):388-92, 2008
8. Tortori-Donati P et al: Segmental spinal dysgenesis: neuroradiologic findings with clinical and embryologic correlation. AJNR Am J Neuroradiol. 20(3):445-56, 1999

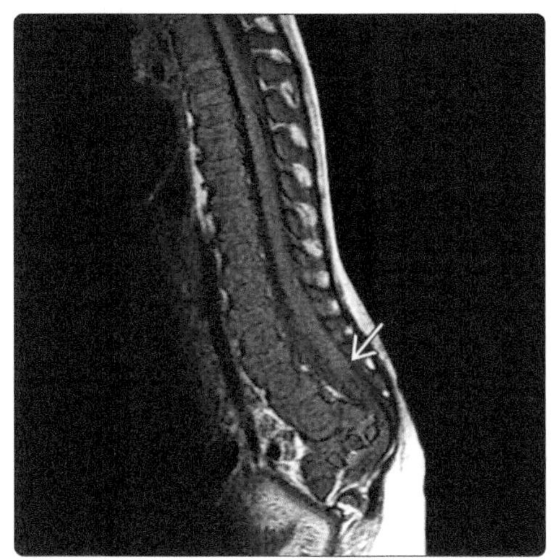

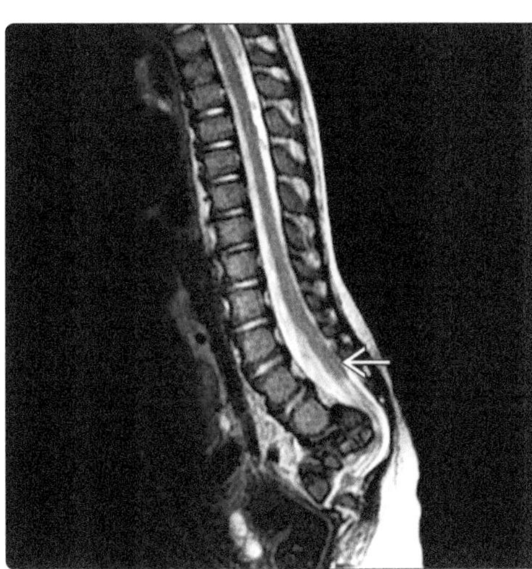

(Left) *Sagittal T1 MR (mixed SSD, caudal regression) shows relatively low (caudal) site of focal lumbosacral hypoplasia with multiple dysmorphic vertebra and focal kyphosis. Conus ➡ morphology is abnormal with a truncated, squared-off appearance.* **(Right)** *Sagittal T2 MR (mixed SSD, caudal regression) shows a relatively low dysgenetic level. The dysmorphic vertebral bodies produce acute angle focal kyphosis. Note truncated, squared-off conus ➡.*

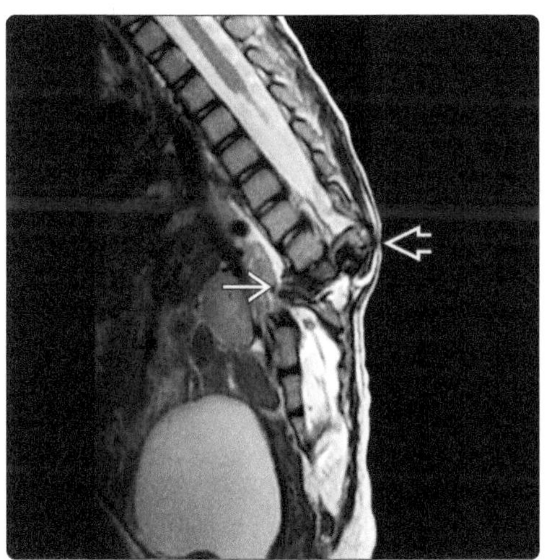

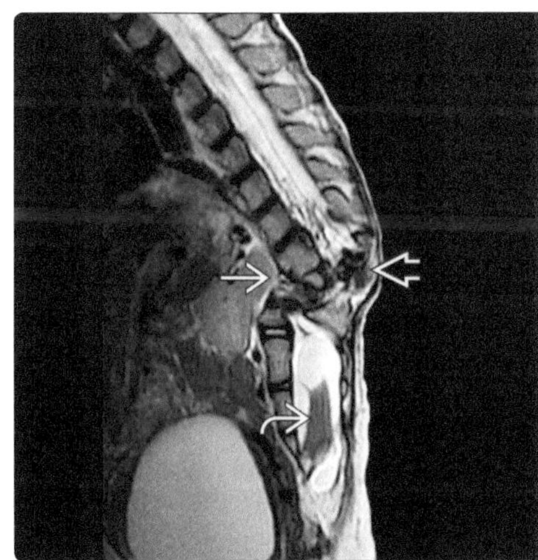

(Left) *Sagittal T2 MR shows complete disconnection of the spinal canal at the dysgenetic level ➡ with pronounced kyphosis and attenuation of the proximal spinal cord. A clinically palpable spur ➡ is conspicuous at the kyphotic apex.* **(Right)** *Sagittal T2 MR reveals complete disconnection of the spinal canal at the dysgenetic level ➡. There is pronounced kyphosis and prominent bone spur ➡ at the gibbus apex. The bulky distal cord ➡ is separate from the thoracic cord.*

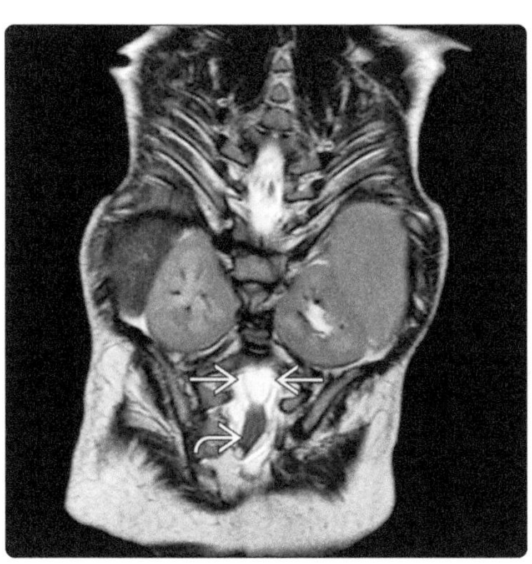

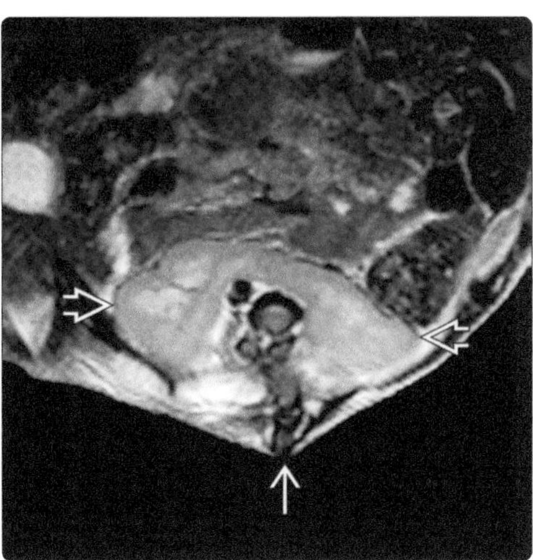

(Left) *Coronal T2 MR (severe lumbosacral SSD) shows separation of the distal spinal cord component ➡ from the thoracic spinal cord (not shown) above the dysgenetic level. The cephalad-directed nerve roots ➡ are commonly observed in lumbosacral SSD.* **(Right)** *Axial T2 MR (severe lumbosacral SSD) depicts an associated anomalous horseshoe kidney ➡. The prominent midline bone spur ➡ was clinically obvious and projects dorsally at the kyphotic gibbus apex.*

Caudal Regression Syndrome

KEY FACTS

TERMINOLOGY

- Caudal regression syndrome (CRS), sacral agenesis, lumbosacral hypogenesis

IMAGING

- Constellation of caudal developmental growth abnormalities and associated soft tissue anomalies
- Spectrum ranges in severity from absent coccyx to lumbosacral agenesis
- 2 main types
  - Group 1: Distal spinal cord hypoplasia, severe sacral osseous anomalies
  - Group 2: Tapered, low-lying, distal cord elongation with tethering, less severe sacral anomalies

TOP DIFFERENTIAL DIAGNOSES

- Tethered spinal cord
- Closed spinal dysraphism
- Occult intrasacral meningocele

PATHOLOGY

- Group 1: More severe caudal dysgenesis with high-lying, club-shaped cord terminus (↓ number of anterior horn cells)
- Group 2: Less severe dysgenesis with low-lying, tapered, distal cord tethered by tight filum, lipoma, lipomyelomeningocele, or terminal myelocystocele

CLINICAL ISSUES

- Clinical spectrum ranges from neurologically normal → severely impaired
- Symptomatic patient presentation spans mild foot disorders → complete lower extremity paralysis and distal leg atrophy

DIAGNOSTIC CHECKLIST

- Look for caudal spine anomalies in patients with genitourinary or anorectal anomalies

(Left) *Sagittal graphic of the lumbosacral spine in severe group 1 caudal regression syndrome (CRS) shows high truncation of the sacrum ➡ and medial position of the iliac wing ➡. The conus ➡ terminates abnormally high in a blunt, wedge shape.* **(Right)** *Sagittal T2WI MR (group 1 CRS) reveals severe truncation of the sacrum ➡ and abnormally high termination of the spinal cord at the T12-L1 vertebral body level with a typical blunted, wedge-shaped conus ➡.*

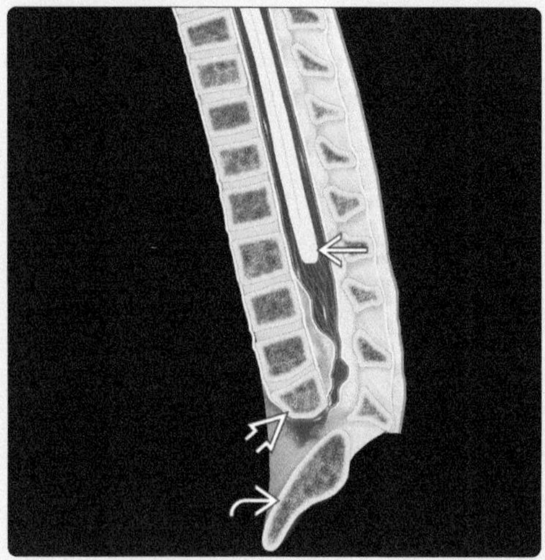

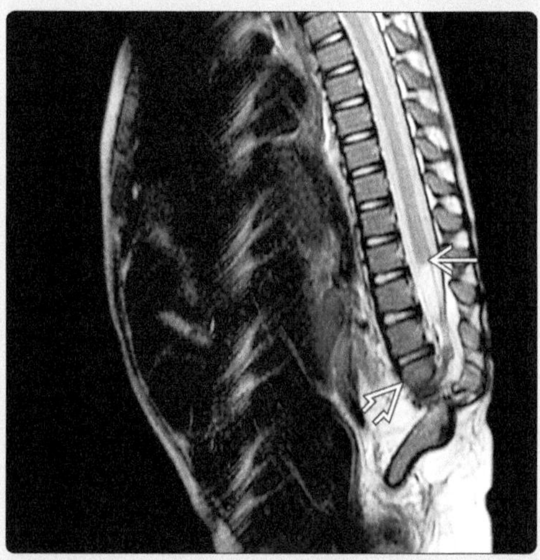

(Left) *Axial T2WI MR (group 1 CRS) obtained immediately below the conus level demonstrates abrupt conus termination with relatively normal-appearing ventral ➡ and dorsal ➡ cauda equina nerve roots.* **(Right)** *Axial T2WI MR of the pelvis (severe group 1 CRS) demonstrates bilateral abnormal hypoplastic iliac wings ➡ closely approximated in the midline secondary to complete absence of a normal sacrum at this level.*

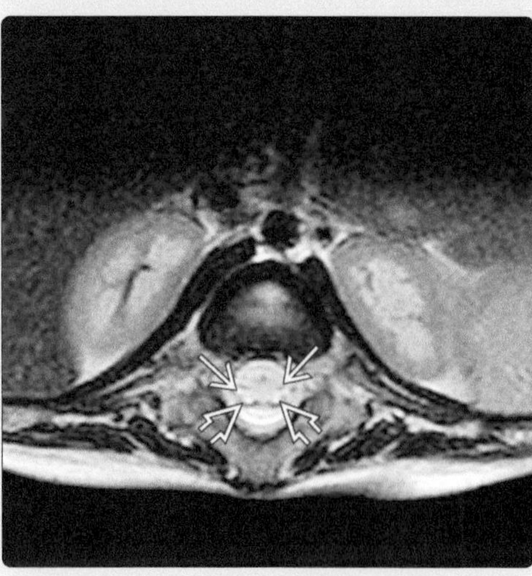

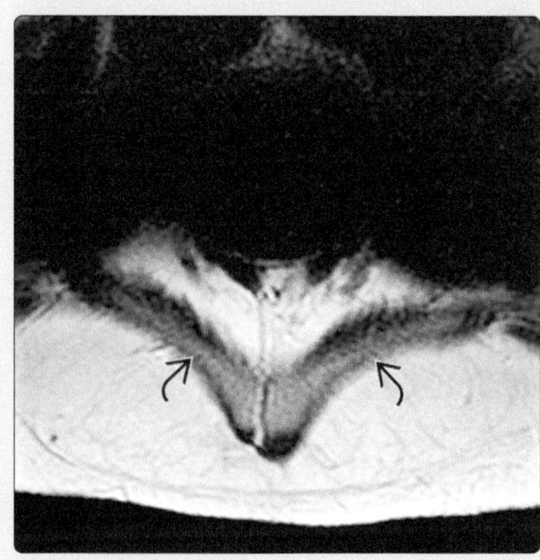

TERMINOLOGY

Abbreviations

- Caudal regression syndrome (CRS)

Synonyms

- Sacral agenesis, lumbosacral hypogenesis

Definitions

- Constellation of caudal developmental growth abnormalities and associated soft tissue anomalies

IMAGING

General Features

- Best diagnostic clue
  - Incomplete lumbosacral spine formation
  - Abnormal distal spinal cord
- Location
  - Lumbosacral spine
- Size
  - Variable diminution of caudal spine
- Morphology
  - Spectrum ranging in severity from absent coccyx to lumbosacral agenesis
    - Partial or total unilateral dysgenesis with oblique lumbosacral joint
    - Bilateral total lumbosacral hypogenesis; vertebral column terminates in thoracic spine
  - Caudal vertebral bodies often show segmentation failure
  - Severe canal narrowing rostral to last intact vertebra
    - Osseous vertebral excrescences, fibrous bands connecting bifid spinous processes, or severe distal dural tube stenosis

Radiographic Findings

- Radiography
  - Lumbosacral osseous hypogenesis

CT Findings

- CECT
  - Lumbosacral dysgenesis with distal spinal stenosis
  - ± prominent nerve/dorsal root ganglion (DRG) enhancement

MR Findings

- T1WI
  - Vertebral body dysgenesis/hypogenesis
  - Group 1: Distal spinal cord hypoplasia (wedge-shaped cord termination), severe sacral osseous anomalies
    - ± dilated central canal, conus CSF cyst
  - Group 2: Tapered, low-lying, distal cord elongation with tethering, less severe sacral anomalies
- T2WI
  - Same findings as T1WI; best for depicting dural stenosis
- T1WI C+
  - Hypertrophied DRG/nerve roots may enhance

Ultrasonographic Findings

- Grayscale ultrasound
  - Group 1: Blunt spinal cord termination above L1; central canal may be prominent
  - Group 2: Elongated conus with thick filum ± intraspinal lipoma

Nonvascular Interventions

- Myelography
  - Caudal hypogenesis ± dural stenosis; most useful in conjunction with CT

Imaging Recommendations

- Protocol advice
  - Consider US for infant screening if MR is not possible
  - MR to confirm US findings, treatment planning
    - Sagittal MR to demonstrate extent of lumbosacral deficiency, distal spinal cord morphology, and presence/absence of tethering/lipoma
    - Axial MR to detect osseous spinal narrowing, hydromyelia, and associated lesions

DIFFERENTIAL DIAGNOSIS

Tethered Spinal Cord

- Low-lying spinal cord ± thickened or fatty filum, no caudal dysgenesis
- Difficult to clinically discern from mild sacral dysgenesis
  - ± associated imaging abnormalities that may help distinguish

Closed Spinal Dysraphism

- Dorsal dysraphism without vertebral column hypogenesis (e.g., lipomyelomeningocele)

Occult Intrasacral Meningocele

- Sacrum is thinned and remodeled, sometimes imitating caudal regression
- Currently considered extradural arachnoid cyst rather than true meningocele

PATHOLOGY

General Features

- Etiology
  - Normal caudal spine development → normal secondary neurulation (formerly canalization and retrogressive differentiation)
    - Anorectal and genitourinary structures form contemporaneously to caudal spine in close anatomic proximity
  - Insult prior to 4th gestational week → caudal cell mass developmental abnormalities
    - Hyperglycemia, infectious, toxic, or ischemic insult postulated to impair spinal cord and vertebral formation
    - Signaling defects by retinoic acid and sonic hedgehog during blastogenesis and gastrulation
    - Abnormal neural tube, notochord development → impaired migration of neurons and mesodermal cells
- Genetics
  - Most cases sporadic
  - Association with variations in homeobox 2 (*CDX2*) gene in some patient
    - May also have anorectal malformations
  - Dominantly inherited form recently described; defect in *MNX1* (HLXB9) homeobox gene (chromosome 7)

 - *MNX1* also expressed in pancreas → possible association between diabetes hyperglycemia and caudal regression
- Associated abnormalities
 - Tethered cord
 - ~ 100% of CRS patients with conus terminating below L1
 - Thickened filum (65%) ± dermoid or lipoma
 - Other spinal anomalies
 - Vertebral anomalies (22%), diastematomyelia, terminal hydromyelia (10%), myelomeningocele (35-50%), lipomyelomeningocele (10-20%), terminal myelocystocele (15%), anterior sacral meningocele, terminal lipoma (< 10%)
 - Congenital cardiac defects (24%), pulmonary hypoplasia
 - Genitourinary abnormalities (24%)
 - Renal agenesis/ectopia, hydronephrosis, müllerian duct malformations, urinary bladder malformation
 - Anorectal anomalies (particularly anal atresia)
 - Higher level of anal atresia → more severe lumbosacral dysgenesis, genitourinary anomalies
 - Currarino triad: Partial sacral agenesis with intact 1st sacral vertebra, presacral mass, anorectal malformations
 - Orthopedic abnormalities; extreme cases → lower extremity fusion (sirenomelia)
- Sequela of caudal cell mass dysplasia with spectrum of severity
- Lower extremity deformities, lumbosacral agenesis, anorectal abnormalities, renal/pulmonary hypoplasia characteristic
 - Most severe cases → sirenomelia ("mermaid syndrome")
 - 20% → tethering subcutaneous lesions (group 2)

Staging, Grading, & Classification

- Group 1: More severe caudal dysgenesis with high-lying, club-shaped cord terminus (↓ number of anterior horn cells)
 - Distal cord hypoplasia with wedging is seen in all patients with partial or complete dysgenesis and termination of spinal cord above L1
 - Termination of conus above L1 is highly correlated with sacral malformations ending at S1 or above
- Group 2: Less severe dysgenesis with low-lying, tapered, distal cord tethered by tight filum, lipoma, lipomyelomeningocele, or terminal myelocystocele
 - Conus termination below L1 highly correlated with sacral malformations ending at S2 or below
 - Cord tethering more common in milder sacral dysgenesis

Gross Pathologic & Surgical Features

- Severity of vertebral dysgenesis, presence/absence of tethering, and osseous canal diameter impact surgical planning

CLINICAL ISSUES

Presentation

- Most common signs/symptoms
 - Neurogenic urinary bladder dysfunction (nearly all patients)
 - Sensorimotor paresis (group 2 > group 1)
 - Severity of motor deficit > sensory
 - Sacral sensory sparing common, even in severe cases
- Other signs/symptoms
 - Neurologically asymptomatic (group 1 > group 2)
- Clinical profile
 - Broad spectrum ranging from neurologically normal to complete lumbosacral agenesis and fusion of lower extremities (sirenomelia)
 - Always accompanied by narrow hips, hypoplastic gluteal muscles, shallow intergluteal cleft
 - Symptomatic patient presentation ranges from mild foot disorders to complete lower extremity paralysis and distal leg atrophy
 - Motor level usually higher than sensory level
 - Level of vertebral aplasia correlates with motor but not sensory level

Demographics

- Age
 - Severe cases identified in utero (obstetrical US) or at birth
 - Mild cases may not be identified until adulthood
- Sex
 - M = F
- Epidemiology
 - 1/7,500 births (milder forms > severe forms)
 - 15-20% are infants of diabetic mothers; 1% of offspring from diabetic mothers affected
 - Association with VACTERL (10%), omphalocele, exstrophy bladder, imperforate anus, spinal anomalies (10%), and Currarino triad syndromic complexes

Natural History & Prognosis

- Variable depending on severity

Treatment

- Surgical untethering if clinically symptomatic
- Surgical release/duraplasty may improve neurologic function in patients with distal spinal canal stenosis
- Orthopedic procedures to improve lower extremity functionality

DIAGNOSTIC CHECKLIST

Consider

- MR most useful imaging tool for characterizing abnormalities and surgical planning

Image Interpretation Pearls

- Caudal spine anomalies should be sought out in patients with genitourinary or anorectal anomalies and vice versa

SELECTED REFERENCES

1. Jasiewicz B et al: Caudal regression syndrome-a narrative review: an orthopedic point of view. Children (Basel). 10(3):589, 2023
2. Mwamanenge N et al: Caudal regression syndrome without maternal diabetes mellitus. BMJ Case Rep. 16(3):e253136, 2023
3. Gajagowni S et al: Diabetic embryopathies. Neoreviews. 23(10):e677-88, 2022
4. Gill KG: Congenital musculoskeletal anomalies - key radiographic findings. Pediatr Radiol. 52(4):777-85, 2022
5. Stevens SJC et al: The broader phenotypic spectrum of congenital caudal abnormalities associated with mutations in the caudal type homeobox 2 gene. Clin Genet. 101(2):183-9, 2022

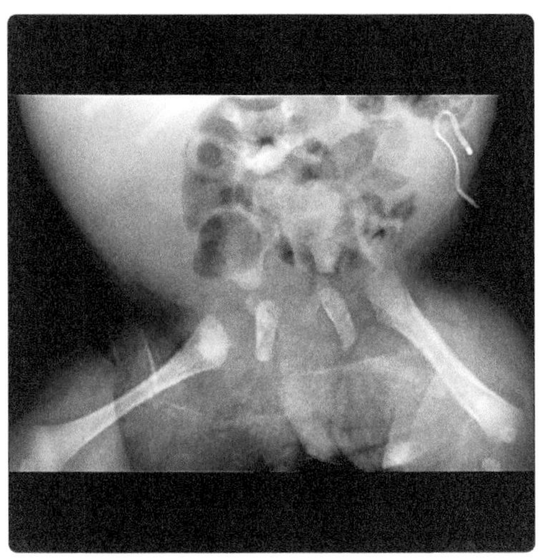

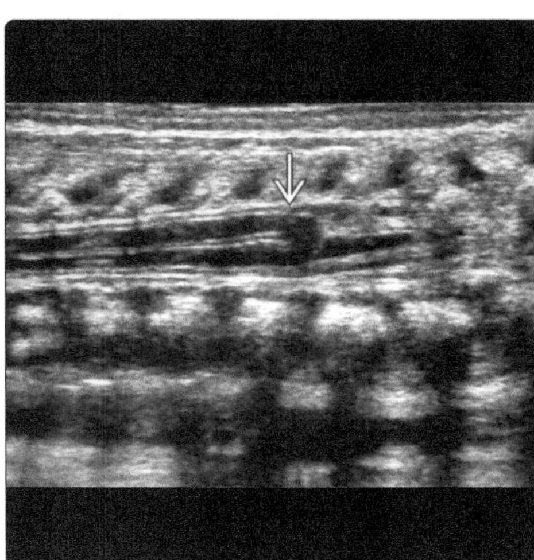

(Left) *Anteroposterior radiograph (group 1 CRS) depicts marked pelvic hypogenesis and pubic deficiency correlating with clinical bladder exstrophy and lower extremity underdevelopment.* **(Right)** *Longitudinal spinal US (group 1 CRS) shows mild distal spinal cord thinning with blunt, wedge- or club-shaped termination ➡ of the spinal cord (at T1 level, confirmed with radiography).*

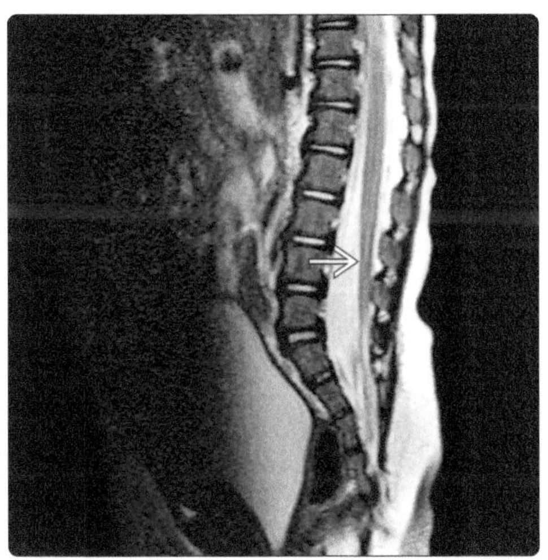

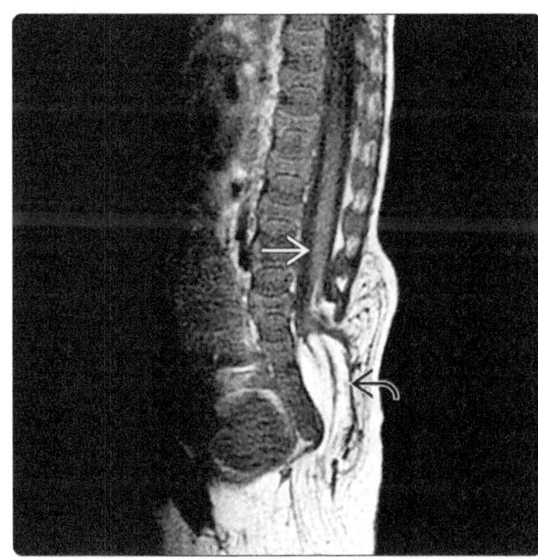

(Left) *Sagittal T2WI MR (group 2 CRS) demonstrates a milder variant of CRS. In this case, there are 4 sacral vertebra with absence of S5 and the coccyx. The spinal cord ➡ is low lying and taut, features suggesting that it is probably tethered.* **(Right)** *Sagittal T1WI MR (group 2 CRS) depicts mild sacral dysgenesis and posterior spinal dysraphism with the abnormal, low-lying, tapered spinal cord terminating ➡ into a large terminal lipoma ➡.*

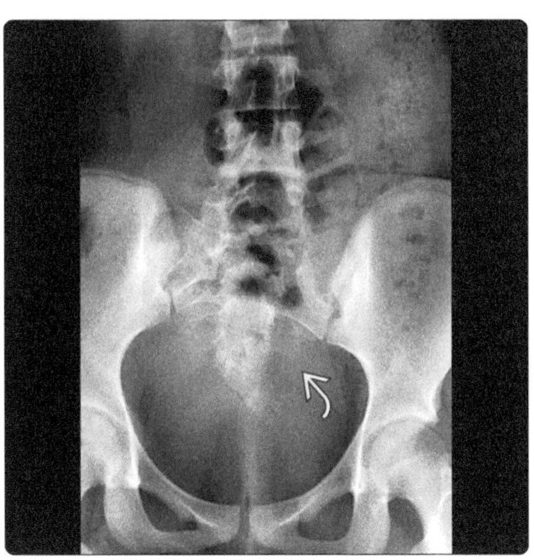

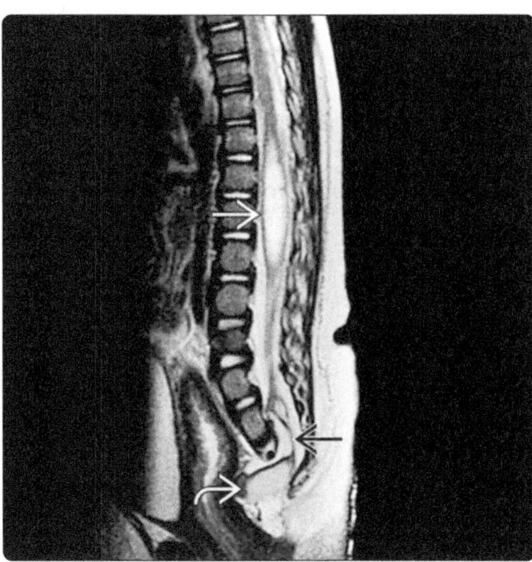

(Left) *Anteroposterior radiograph of the pelvis demonstrates partial absence of the left sacral ala ➡ in a patient with hemisacral agenesis variant of caudal regression.* **(Right)** *Sagittal T2WI MR (group 2 CRS) reveals sacral dysgenesis with barely 2 sacral vertebra. The spinal cord ➡ is low lying with prominent conus syrinx. Also confirmed was a parasagittal presacral cystic mass (anterior sacral meningocele) ➡ with a thin, fluid-filled tract ➡ communicating to the thecal sac.*

KEY FACTS

IMAGING

- Definitions
  - Closed spinal dysraphism characterized by syrinx associated with neural placode protruding outside of spinal canal through osseous dysraphic defect
  - Terminal and nonterminal subtypes
    - Terminal myelocystocele: Distal spinal cord has trumpet-shaped morphology
    - Nonterminal myelocystocele: 2 types
      - Abortive form: No visible syrinx, sac traversed by linear fibroneurovascular stalk
      - Complete form: Hydromyelic cavity within sac is continuous with ependymal canal of spinal cord
  - ± other closed spinal dysraphisms, Chiari (more common than in other closed spinal dysraphisms, though not nearly as common as in open spinal dysraphisms)

TOP DIFFERENTIAL DIAGNOSES

- Meningocele
- Lipomyelomeningocele
- Other closed spinal dysraphisms
- Sacrococcygeal teratoma
- Myelomeningocele

PATHOLOGY

- Associated malformations: Omphalocele, cloacal exstrophy, imperforate anus, spinal anomalies, caudal agenesis

CLINICAL ISSUES

- Presents at birth with lumbosacral skin-covered mass
- Can be neurologically intact at birth with progressive lower extremity sensorimotor deficits
- Early neurosurgical intervention recommended

(Left) *Sagittal graphic displays a closed (skin-covered) dysraphism with a low-lying, hydromyelic spinal cord ➡ extending into an expanded subarachnoid space ➡ and terminating in a myelocystocele ➡.* **(Right)** *Sagittal FIESTA MR of a fetus at 28-weeks gestational age demonstrates a terminal myelocystocele ➡. There are additional findings of the omphalocele, cloacal exstrophy, imperforate anus, and spinal anomalies (OEIS) complex, including a low omphalocele ➡ and an obstructed distal colon ➡.*

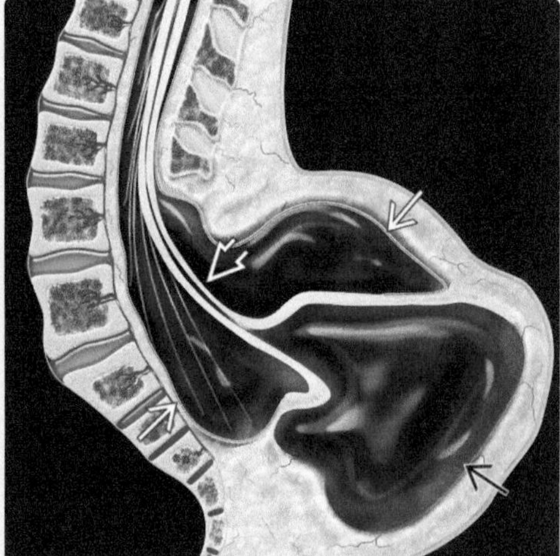

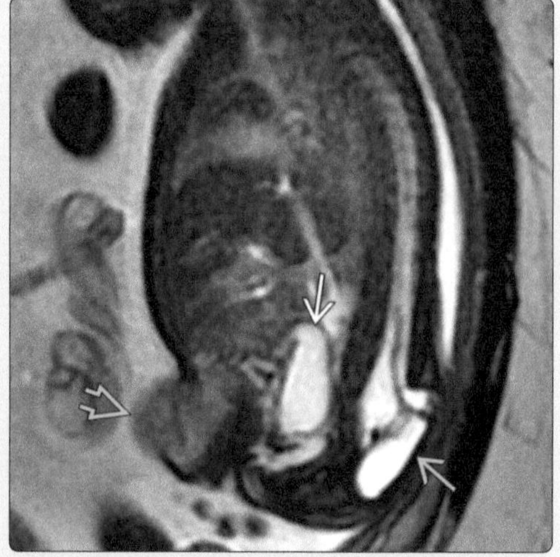

(Left) *Postnatal T1WI MR in the same patient 11 weeks after delivery confirms the presence of a skin-covered terminal myelocystocele with splaying of the neural placode ➡ around a fluid collection ➡ that does not communicate with the surrounding subarachnoid space. There is also syringohydromyelia ➡.* **(Right)** *Axial T1WI MR in the same patient shows the myelocystocele ➡, which is covered by skin and fat.*

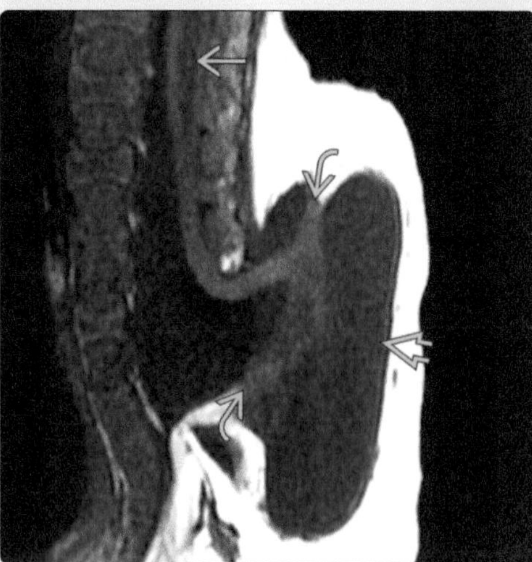

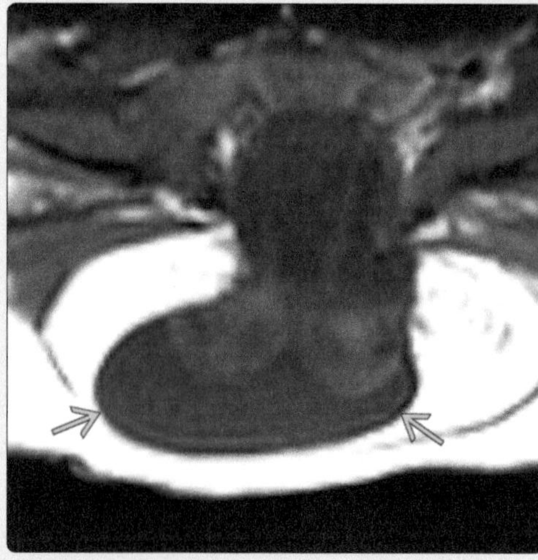

TERMINOLOGY

Synonyms

- Syringocele, lipomyelocystocele

Definitions

- Closed spinal dysraphism characterized by syrinx associated with neural placode protruding outside of spinal canal through dorsal osseous dysraphic defect
- Terminal and nonterminal subtypes
  - Terminal myelocystocele: Involves caudal-most aspect of spinal cord
  - Nonterminal myelocystocele: 2 types
    - Abortive nonterminal myelocystocele/myelocystocele manque ("limited dorsal myeloschisis")
      - Appears as meningocele crossed by fibroneurovascular stalk that extends from dorsal aspect of spinal cord to attach to dome of sac
    - Complete form
      - Hydromyelic cavity within sac is continuous with ependymal canal of spinal cord

IMAGING

General Features

- Best diagnostic clue
  - Terminal myelocystocele: Distal spinal cord has trumpet-shaped morphology
  - Nonterminal myelocystocele
    - Abortive form: No syrinx, sac contains fibroneurovascular stalk
    - Complete form: Syringohydromyelia in continuity with sac contents
  - Unlike other closed spinal dysraphisms, significant association with Chiari (as high as 40%)
- Location
  - Terminal: Lumbosacral
  - Nonterminal: Cervical, thoracic, upper lumbar
- Size
  - Subcutaneous mass varies from small to large
- Morphology
  - Closed spinal dysraphism with subcutaneous, skin-covered cystic mass

Radiographic Findings

- Posterior osseous dysraphism ± soft tissue mass
- ± scoliosis, segmentation anomalies, caudal agenesis (group 2)
- ± pubic diastasis (usually with abdominal wall defect and cloacal exstrophy)

CT Findings

- NECT
  - Posterior osseous dysraphic defects
  - ± scoliosis, segmentation anomalies, caudal agenesis (group 2)

MR Findings

- T1WI, T2WI
  - Terminal myelocystocele
    - Elongated cord with flared distal neural placode attached to subcutaneous fat within sac with dilated distal central canal
      - Creates trumpet-flaring appearance of distal cord
    - Cyst-within-cyst appearance of distal cord: Dilated central canal surrounded by expanded subarachnoid spaces
    - Fluid collection in distal spinal cord does not communicate with surrounding subarachnoid space in sac
  - Nonterminal myelocystocele
    - Sac dorsal to other portions of spinal cord other than distal cord
    - In abortive form, cord may appear near normal or slightly tethered toward sac
      - Linear fibroneurovascular stalk traverses sac
    - In complete form, fluid in sac appears continuous with cord syrinx
  - ± syringohydromyelia, can be holocord
  - ± other associated closed spinal dysraphisms
    - Intradural lipoma, dorsal dermal sinus, split cord malformation
  - ± Chiari(hindbrain herniation)

Ultrasonographic Findings

- Grayscale ultrasound
  - Terminal myelocystocele: Spinal cord passes through hypoechoic, dilated subarachnoid space and terminates in cord cyst
  - Unlikely to start with ultrasound for nonterminal myelocystoceles in postnatal period (straight to MR)

Imaging Recommendations

- Best imaging tool
  - Multiplanar MR
- Protocol advice
  - 3D SSFP images helpful in diagnosis and delineating margins of terminal myelocystocele or fibroneurovascular stalk of abortive nonterminal myelocystocele

DIFFERENTIAL DIAGNOSIS

Meningocele

- Skin-covered dorsal dural sac protruding thorough posterior osseous defect
- Sac occasionally contains herniated filum or nerve roots but not neural placode
- May be difficult to distinguish from abortive nonterminal myelocystocele

Lipomyelomeningocele

- No dilation of distal central canal

Other Closed Spinal Dysraphisms

- Lipomyelocele, intradural lipoma, tethered cord

Sacrococcygeal Teratoma

- Skin-covered solid, cystic, or mixed solid-cystic presacral mass, ± fat, Ca^{++}
- May be primarily exophytic from perineum or primarily internal (or combination)

Myelomeningocele

- In certain cases, may be difficult to differentiate in presence of hindbrain herniation/Chiari on fetal imaging

PATHOLOGY

General Features

- Etiology
  - Terminal myelocystocele
    - Believed to result from disruption in embryogenesis during later phases of secondary neurulation, during which time secondary neural tube forms
    - Arrest of normal apoptosis during retrogressive differentiation results in persistent attachment of secondary neural tube to cutaneous ectoderm, which dilates
  - Nonterminal myelocystocele
    - Partial failure of late primary neurulation → late or incomplete separation (disjunction) of cutaneous ectoderm from neural ectoderm, resulting fibroneurovascular filament or stalk
  - Postulated associations with teratogens: Retinoic acid, hydantoin, loperamide hydrochloride
- Associated abnormalities
  - Omphalocele, cloacal exstrophy, imperforate anus, and spinal anomalies (OEIS)
  - Caudal agenesis (group 2)
  - GU anomalies → cloacal exstrophy, ambiguous hypoplastic genitalia, and renal abnormalities
  - MSK anomalies → pelvic deformities (pubic symphysis diastasis), scoliosis, segmentation anomalies, clubfoot
  - Hindbrain herniation/Chiari
    - 10-40% of cases, not nearly as common as open spinal dysraphisms
    - More common than with other closed spinal dysraphisms
  - Anorectal anomalies → anal atresia

Gross Pathologic & Surgical Features

- Elongated dorsal spinal cord extends through skin-covered dorsal lumbosacral spinal dysraphism into extraspinal space and fuses with subcutaneous fat
- Fluid collection within distal spinal cord communicates with central canal
- Distal spinal cord surrounded by expanded dura
- Spinal cord fluid collection does not communicate with surrounding subarachnoid space of meningocele

CLINICAL ISSUES

Presentation

- Most common signs/symptoms
  - Presents at birth with skin-covered mass (lumbosacral in location if terminal myelocystocele)
    - Skin appears normal or exhibits hemangioma, nevus, or hypertrichosis
  - Many neurologically intact at diagnosis (nonterminal myelocystoceles)
- Other signs/symptoms
  - Later presentation or untreated lesion may develop tethered cord syndrome
  - Absent bowel and bladder control, progressive lower extremity paresis
- Clinical profile
  - ± midline cloacal and paramedian bladder exstrophy, other visible anomalies

Demographics

- Age
  - Infancy
- Sex
  - No predilection clearly established, though F > M in some small series
- Epidemiology
  - Rare: 1-5% of skin-covered lumbosacral masses
    - Much more common in cloacal exstrophy patients

Natural History & Prognosis

- Mass size and deficits tend to progress with time, may be partially or totally reversible with prompt surgical repair
- Overall prognosis mainly related to other associated anomalies (OEIS)
  - Patients without abdominal wall defects have more favorable neurologic outcome than those with ventral wall defects

Treatment

- Early diagnosis and surgical repair maximizes probability of normal neurologic outcome
- Surgery involves reduction of size of spinal cord fluid collection, terminal ventriculostomy, excision of meningocele sac, and untethering of spinal cord

DIAGNOSTIC CHECKLIST

Consider

- Can be associated with hindbrain herniation (Chiari), which can make prenatal differentiation with open spinal dysraphisms difficult in certain cases
- Nonneurologic prognosis largely linked to severity of associated anomalies

Image Interpretation Pearls

- Terminal myelocystoceles have characteristic trumpet morphology of neural placode
- Nonterminal myelocystoceles can be difficult to differentiate from simple meningoceles, particularly abortive subtype

SELECTED REFERENCES

1. Trapp B et al: A practical approach to diagnosis of spinal dysraphism. Radiographics. 41(2):559-75, 2021
2. Barkovich AJ et al: Pediatric Neuroimaging. 6th ed. Wolters Kluwer. 989-91, 1007-8, 2019
3. Nagaraj UD et al: Differentiating closed versus open spinal dysraphisms on fetal MRI. AJR Am J Roentgenol. 207(6):1316-23, 2016
4. Pang D et al: Terminal myelocystocele: surgical observations and theory of embryogenesis. Neurosurgery. 70(6):1383-404; discussion 1404-5, 2012
5. Tandon V et al: Terminal myelocystocele: a series of 30 cases and review of the literature. Pediatr Neurosurg. 48(4):229-35, 2012
6. Morioka T et al: Neurosurgical management of occult spinal dysraphism associated with OEIS complex. Childs Nerv Syst. 24(6):723-9, 2008
7. Rossi A et al: Spectrum of nonterminal myelocystoceles. Neurosurgery. 58(3):509-15; discussion 509-15, 2006
8. Tortori-Donati P et al: Spinal dysraphism: a review of neuroradiological features with embryological correlations and proposal for a new classification. Neuroradiology. 42(7):471-91, 2000

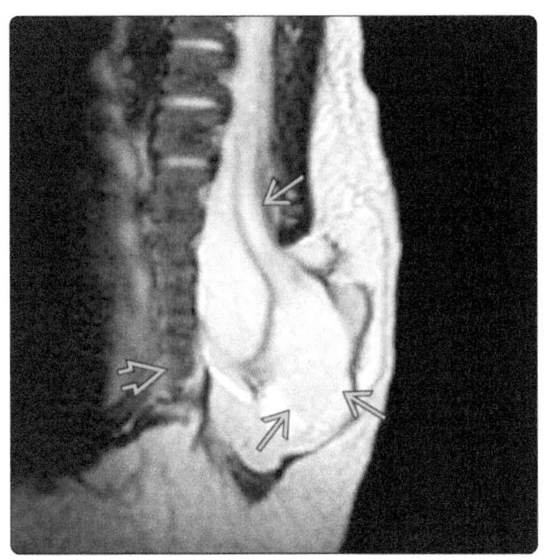

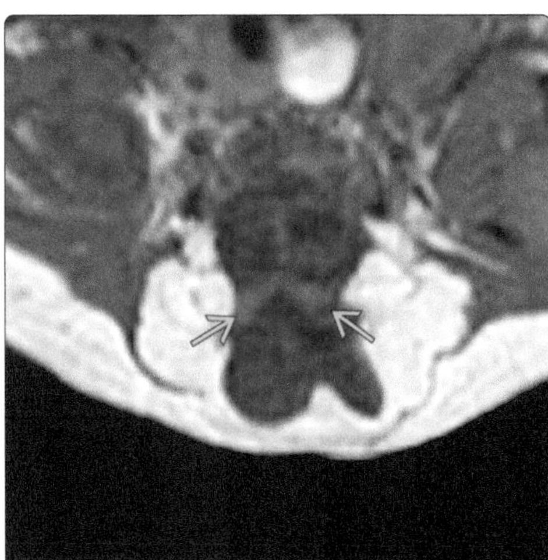

(Left) *Sagittal T2WI MR in a 2-week-old with known OEIS demonstrates classic findings of a terminal myelocystocele with a syrinx ➡ that is in continuity with the sac contents. Also note sacral hypoplasia ➡, consistent with group 2 caudal agenesis.* **(Right)** *Axial T1WI MR in the same patient demonstrates the classic flaring ➡ of the neural placode around the syrinx of this terminal myelocystocele.*

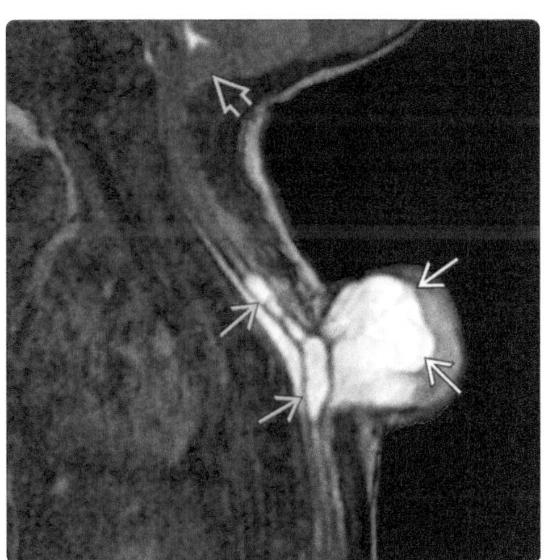

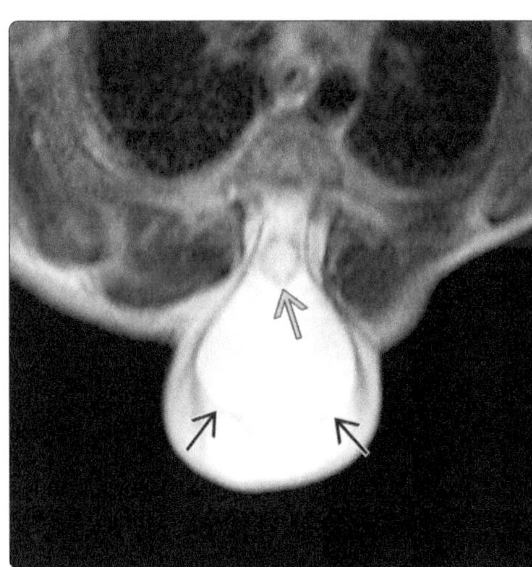

(Left) *Sagittal 3D CISS MR in a 3-day-old with a nonterminal myelocystocele, complete type, is shown. There is a syrinx ➡ in communication with the CSF space within the closed spinal dysraphism sac ➡. Also note the presence of hindbrain herniation ➡.* **(Right)** *Axial T2WI MR in the same patient demonstrates the communication of the syrinx cavity ➡ with the skin-covered sac contents ➡.*

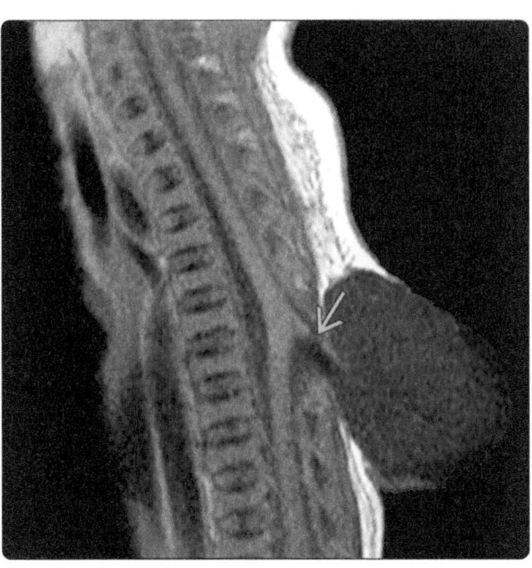

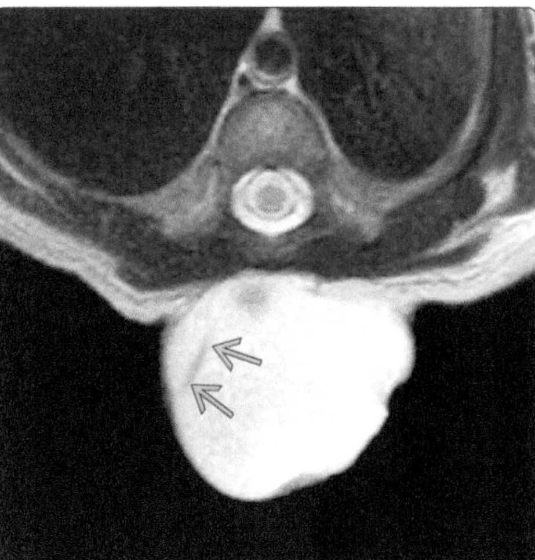

(Left) *Sagittal T1WI MR in a 2-day-old with a nonterminal myelocystocele, abortive type, is shown. Even though there is no visible syrinx, there is a neurofibrovascular stalk ➡ connecting the spinal cord to the dome of the skin-covered sac, consistent with the abortive subtype.* **(Right)** *Axial T2WI MR in the same patient demonstrates the fibroneurovascular stalk ➡ within the sac, which differentiates this from a simple meningocele.*

Anterior Sacral Meningocele

KEY FACTS

TERMINOLOGY

- Anterior sacral meningocele (ASM)
- Sacral meninges herniate anteriorly into pelvis through focal erosion or hypogenesis of sacral ± coccygeal vertebral segments

IMAGING

- Presacral cyst, contiguous with thecal sac through anterior osseous defect
- Deficient sacrum ± curved (scimitar) shape

TOP DIFFERENTIAL DIAGNOSES

- Sacrococcygeal teratoma
- Sacral chordoma
- Neurenteric cyst
- Cystic neuroblastoma
- Ovarian cyst

PATHOLOGY

- Currarino triad: Anorectal anomalies, caudal regression syndrome, epidermoid/dermoid tumor or other tethering lesion

CLINICAL ISSUES

- Constipation, urinary frequency, incontinence, dysmenorrhea, dyspareunia, low back/pelvic pain
- Most patients present with urinary or bowel complaints; ASM discovered during imaging evaluation

DIAGNOSTIC CHECKLIST

- Continuity of cyst with thecal sac necessary to ensure ASM diagnosis
- Soft tissue mass or calcification implies tumor
- Imaging recommendations
  - Ultrasound for NICU infant screening
  - MR to confirm presacral cyst location & characterize contents

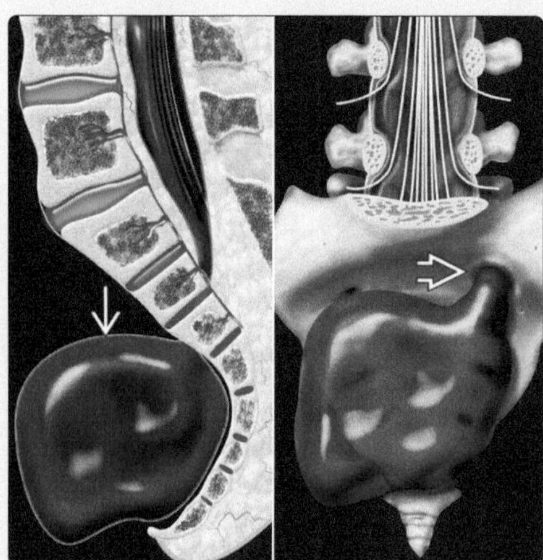

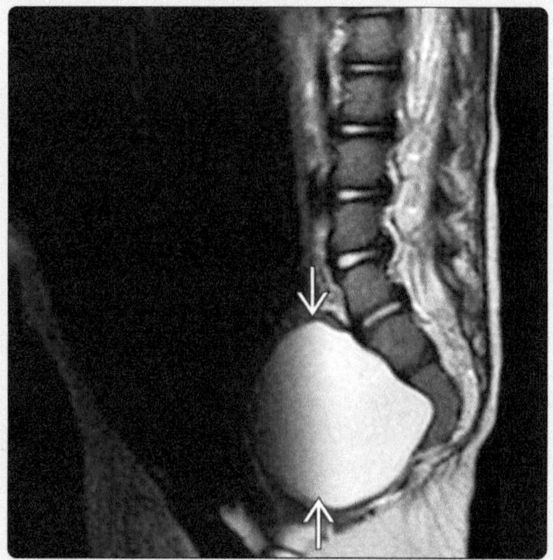

(Left) *Sagittal graphic (left) depicts characteristic anterior sacrum scimitar remodeling by a large anterior meningocele cyst* ➔. *Coronal graphic (right) shows an anterior sacral meningocele cyst origin through an enlarged neural foramen* ➔. **(Right)** *Midline sagittal T2WI MR demonstrates the classic relationship of a characteristic scimitar sacrum configuration with the adjacent presacral cyst (anterior sacral meningocele)* ➔.

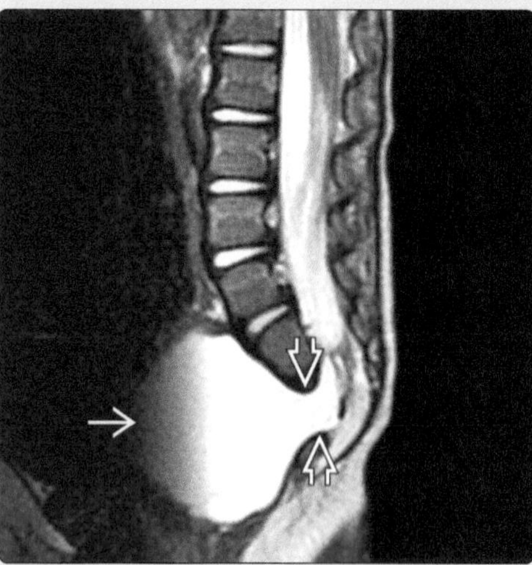

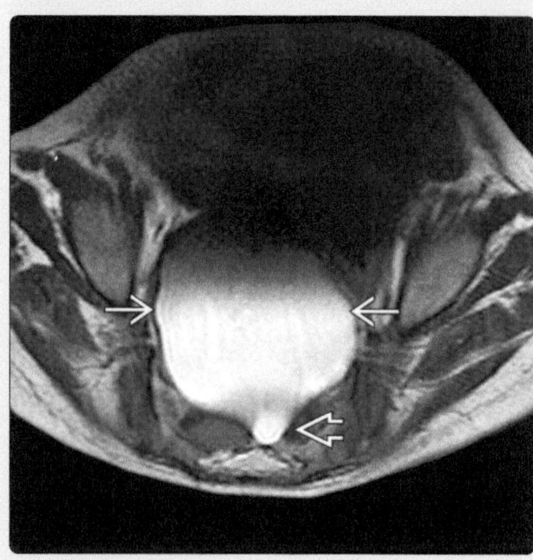

(Left) *Sagittal T2WI MR obtained off-midline parasagittal shows a large anterior presacral cyst* ➔ *contiguous with the meninges, extending from the thecal sac into the pelvis through an enlarged neural foramen* ➔. **(Right)** *Axial T2WI MR confirms unilateral left sacral neural foraminal enlargement* ➔ *permitting ventral herniation of the meninges into the pelvis to form a classic anterior sacral meningocele* ➔.

TERMINOLOGY

Abbreviations

- Anterior sacral meningocele (ASM)

Definitions

- Sacral meninges herniate anteriorly into pelvis through focal erosion or hypogenesis of sacral ± coccygeal vertebral segments

IMAGING

General Features

- Best diagnostic clue
  - Presacral cyst, contiguous with thecal sac, protruding through anterior osseous defect
- Location
  - Sacrum/coccyx
- Size
  - Variable
- Morphology
  - Uni- or multiloculated cyst; usually devoid of neural tissue but may have traversing nerve roots
  - Sacral defect 2° to neural foraminal widening
    - May be unilateral or bilateral, symmetrical or asymmetrical, single or multiple level

Radiographic Findings

- Radiography
  - Widened sacral canal & neural foramina
  - Scalloping of anterior sacrum wall
    - Curved scimitar sacrum on lateral projection
  - ± scoliosis

CT Findings

- CECT
  - Deficient sacrum with variably sized anterior cyst
    - ± nerve roots traversing sacral defect
  - ± lipoma/dermoid (hypodense)
  - Absence of enhancement

MR Findings

- T1WI
  - Deficient sacrum with variably sized presacral cyst
    - Sagittal images confirm cyst/thecal sac continuity
  - ± cord tethering, lipoma/dermoid (hyperintense)
- T2WI
  - Homogeneous, hyperintense CSF signal intensity cyst (similar to CSF in thecal sac)
  - Best sequence to identify nerve roots traversing sacral defect
- T2* GRE
  - No hypointensity (calcification) within cyst wall
    - Helps distinguish from sacrococcygeal teratoma
- DWI
  - Hypointense signal (↑ diffusivity) confirms CSF composition, excludes epidermoid cyst (hyperintense)
- T1WI C+
  - Absence of enhancement

Ultrasonographic Findings

- Grayscale ultrasound
  - Cystic hypoechoic pelvic mass anterior to sacrum
  - Complex internal echoes if prior/concurrent inflammation or infection

Nonvascular Interventions

- Myelography
  - Thecal sac communicates with cyst
    - Most useful in conjunction with CT post intrathecal contrast
  - Rarely used unless MR contraindicated or nondiagnostic

Imaging Recommendations

- Best imaging tool
  - MR confirms cyst contiguity with thecal sac
    - T1WI shows epidermoid, lipoma/dermoid if present
    - T2WI demonstrates ± entrapped neural tissue
  - CT imaging best depicts osseous defect, absence of rim calcification (that would imply sacrococcygeal teratoma)
- Protocol advice
  - Ultrasound for initial screening & characterization in NICU infants
  - Sagittal & axial MR for confirmation of positive ultrasound studies, preoperative planning, &/or postoperative surveillance

DIFFERENTIAL DIAGNOSIS

Sacrococcygeal Teratoma

- Cystic sacrococcygeal teratoma may be difficult to distinguish from ASM
- Look for soft tissue mass, enhancement, calcification
- Coccyx usually normal

Neurenteric Cyst

- Cyst usually within spinal canal ± spinal dysraphism, vertebral formation, & segmentation anomalies
- Often proteinaceous; T1 hyperintense

Cystic Neuroblastoma

- Frequently calcified
- Search for characteristic metastatic lesions

Ovarian Cyst

- Ultrasound may reveal surrounding ovarian tissue that clinches diagnosis

Sacral Chordoma

- Mixed solid/cystic destructive sacral mass
  - No communication with thecal sac
- Rare in children; peak incidence: 5th-6th decades
- Markedly hyperintense on T2WI MR
- Bone CT shows destructive margins

PATHOLOGY

General Features

- Etiology
  - Embryogenesis not definitively known; classified within caudal cell mass anomalies spectrum
    - Erosion or dysgenesis of sacral/coccygeal segments permits herniation of meningeal sac into anterior pelvis
    - 5% of retrorectal masses

- Possible associations
  - Simple form: Marfan, neurofibromatosis type 1 (NF1)
  - Complicated form: Familial, partial sacral agenesis, imperforate anus or anal stenosis, & tethered cord
- Genetics
  - Most patients sporadic
  - Minority show inherited predisposition
    - Currarino triad: Autosomal dominant with variable penetration (*MNX1* gene, chromosome 7q36)
    - Conditions where dural ectasia is prominent (NF1, Marfan, homocystinuria)
- Associated abnormalities
  - Currarino triad: Anorectal anomalies, caudal regression syndrome, epidermoid/dermoid cyst or other tethering mass lesion

Gross Pathologic & Surgical Features

- Osseous sacral remodeling in large meningoceles → classic scimitar shape
- Widened sacral dural sac communicates with pelvic cyst through narrow neck within sacral defect
- ± neural tissue within cyst sac

Microscopic Features

- Characteristic features of dural sac tissue
- May reveal signs of prior inflammation

CLINICAL ISSUES

Presentation

- Most common signs/symptoms
  - Constipation, urinary frequency, incontinence, dysmenorrhea, dyspareunia, low back/pelvic pain
    - 2° to pressure on pelvic viscera
- Other signs/symptoms
  - Sciatica, diminished rectal/detrusor tone, numbness/paresthesias in lower sacral dermatomes (nerve root pressure)
  - Intermittent positional high- or low-pressure headaches due to fluid shifts between ASM & spinal subarachnoid space
  - Superinfection ± meningitis (uncommon)
  - Rare reports of spontaneous abortions or parturition difficulties secondary to mass effect
- Clinical profile
  - Most present with urinary or bowel complaints; ASM is discovered during imaging evaluation
  - Rare finding in (low-pressure) headache patient

Demographics

- Age
  - Onset of symptoms in 2nd-3rd decades
- Sex
  - M = F in children, M < F in adults
- Epidemiology
  - Rare; less common than dorsal meningoceles

Natural History & Prognosis

- Good prognosis following successful surgical repair

Treatment

- Open posterior transsacral approach, patching of meningocele-dural sac connection
  - Easier if cyst does not contain neural elements, permitting simple ligation of cyst neck
- Endoscopic approach → lower morbidity

DIAGNOSTIC CHECKLIST

Consider

- Ultrasound for infant screening
- MR to identify & characterize cyst location & contents, confirm abnormal ultrasound findings
- Bone CT to demonstrate characteristic osseous findings that permit specific diagnosis

Image Interpretation Pearls

- Continuity of cyst with thecal sac necessary to ensure diagnosis
- Presence/absence of neural tissue within cyst important for surgical planning
- Soft tissue mass or calcification implies tumor

SELECTED REFERENCES

1. Kamal MA et al: Surgical management of anterior sacral meningoceles: an illustrated case series and review of the literature. Br J Neurosurg. 1-7, 2023
2. Pitsava G et al: Exome sequencing identifies variants in infants with sacral agenesis. Birth Defects Res. 114(7):215-27, 2022
3. Cheng C et al: Anterior sacral meningocele: a new classification and treatment using the dorsal transsacral approach. Spine (Phila Pa 1976). 45(7):444-51, 2020
4. Hollenberg AM et al: Rupture of a giant anterior sacral meningocele in a patient with Marfan syndrome: diagnosis and management. World Neurosurg. 119:137-41, 2018
5. Chakhalian D et al: Multidisciplinary surgical treatment of presacral meningocele and teratoma in an adult with Currarino triad. Surg Neurol Int. 8:77, 2017
6. Croci DM et al: Thalidomide embryopathy as possible cause of anterior sacral meningocele: a case report. Birth Defects Res. 109(17):1390-2, 2017
7. Gupta S et al: Recurrent abortion and tethered cord syndrome caused by anterior sacral meningocele: a report of a rare case with a review of the literature. World Neurosurg. 101:815.e5-7, 2017
8. Balioğlu MB et al: Sacral agenesis: evaluation of accompanying pathologies in 38 cases, with analysis of long-term outcomes. Childs Nerv Syst. 32(9):1693-702, 2016
9. Porsch RM et al: Sacral agenesis: a pilot whole exome sequencing and copy number study. BMC Med Genet. 17(1):98, 2016
10. Shastin D et al: A rare case of anterior sacral meningocoele presenting as cauda equina syndrome. Br J Neurosurg. 29(3):428-9, 2015
11. Duru S et al: Currarino syndrome: report of five consecutive patients. Childs Nerv Syst. 30(3):547-52, 2014
12. Kemp J et al: Holocord syringomyelia secondary to tethered spinal cord associated with anterior sacral meningocele and tailgut cyst: case report and review of literature. Childs Nerv Syst. 30(6):1141-6, 2014
13. Aydoseli A et al: Anterior sacral meningocele in a patient with currarino syndrome as a cause of ileus. Br J Neurosurg. 27(6):833-5, 2013
14. Beyazal M: An asymptomatic large anterior sacral meningocele in a patient with a history of gestation: a case report with radiological findings. Case Rep Radiol. 2013:842620, 2013
15. Castelli E et al: Huge anterior sacral meningocele simulating bladder retention. Urology. 81(2):e9-10, 2013
16. Polat AV et al: Anterior sacral meningocele mimicking ovarian cyst: a case report. Med Ultrason. 15(1):67-70, 2013
17. Isik N et al: The shrinking of an anterior sacral meningocele in time following transdural ligation of its neck in a case of the Currarino triad. Turk Neurosurg. 18(3):254-8, 2008
18. Miletic D et al: Giant anterior sacral meningocele presenting as bacterial meningitis in a previously healthy adult. Orthopedics. 31(2):182, 2008
19. Sánchez AA et al: Rectothecal fistula secondary to an anterior sacral meningocele. J Neurosurg Spine. 8(5):487-9, 2008
20. Trapp C et al: Laparoscopic treatment of anterior sacral meningocele. Surg Neurol. 68(4):443-8; discussion 448, 2007
21. Lee SC et al: Currarino triad: anorectal malformation, sacral bony abnormality, and presacral mass--a review of 11 cases. J Pediatr Surg. 32(1):58-61, 1997

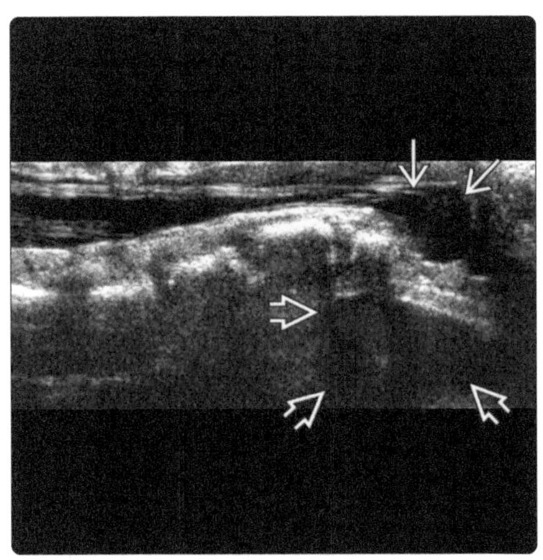
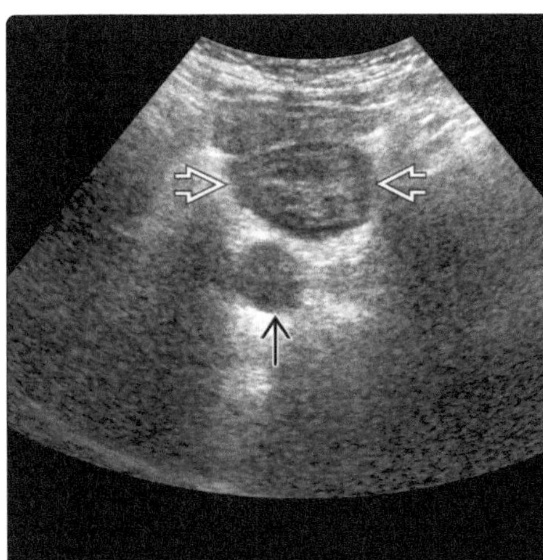

(Left) *Spinal ultrasound demonstrates cystic dilatation* ➡ *of the distal sacral thecal sac. The anterior presacral cystic mass is more difficult to appreciate* ➡ *because of its location deep in the pelvis. The connection through the foramina is not demonstrated well on this ultrasound study, but the classic scimitar configuration of the sacrum is definable.* **(Right)** *Transverse ultrasound in the same patient confirms a presacral anterior sacral meningocele* ➡ *located behind the rectum* ➡ *and below the peritoneal reflection.*

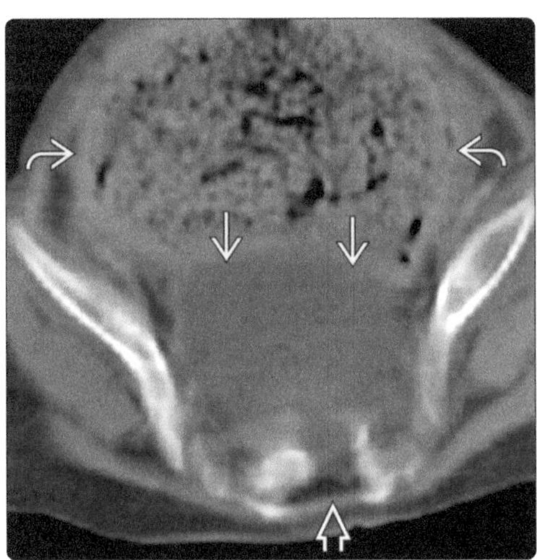
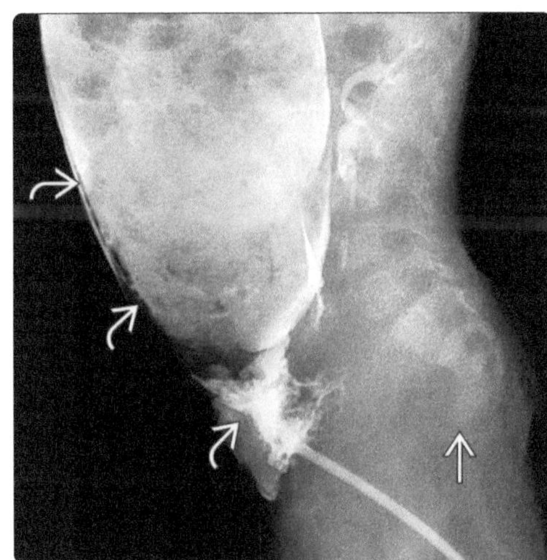

(Left) *Axial bone CT shows a large anterior sacral cyst* ➡ *contiguous with a unilateral enlarged left sacral neural foramen* ➡. *Note the anterior displacement of the markedly dilated rectum* ➡ *in this patient with severe constipation.* **(Right)** *Lateral radiograph obtained following a barium enema (performed for severe constipation) reveals the characteristic scimitar sacrum* ➡ *shape associated with anterior sacral meningocele. Note the huge obstructed large bowel* ➡ *opacified by barium.*

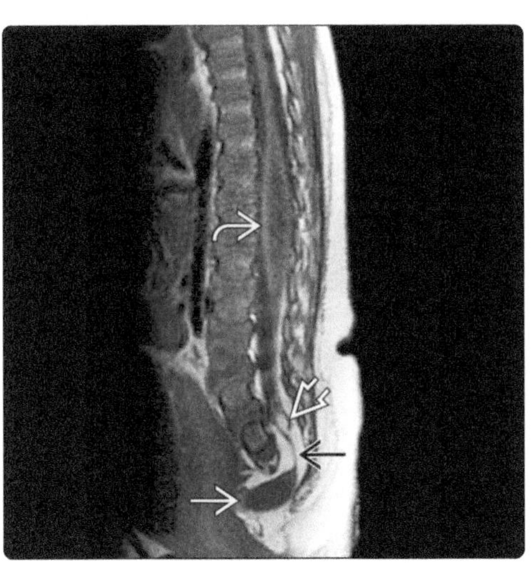
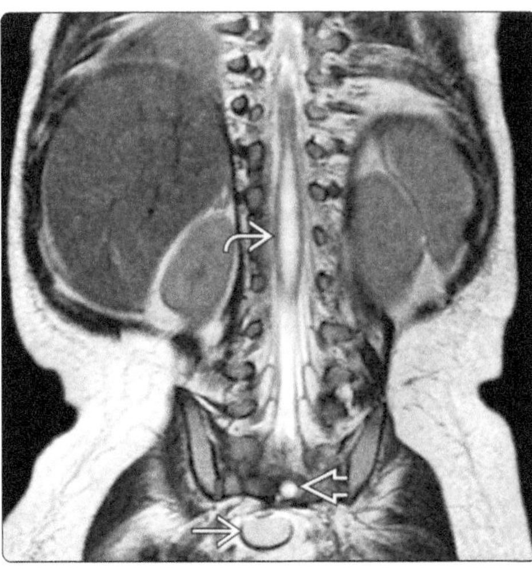

(Left) *Sagittal T1WI MR detects sacral dysgenesis with 2 sacral vertebra. The low-lying spinal cord shows a syrinx* ➡ *and terminal lipoma* ➡. *Also confirmed was a parasagittal presacral cystic mass* ➡ *with a thin fluid-filled tract* ➡ *communicating with the thecal sac through an enlarged sacral foramina.* **(Right)** *Coronal T2WI MR confirms a presacral cystic mass* ➡ *communicating with the thecal sac through an enlarged left S2 neural foramen* ➡. *Note also the terminal conus syrinx* ➡.

Sacral Extradural Arachnoid Cyst

KEY FACTS

TERMINOLOGY

- Spinal extradural arachnoid cyst (AC) located within sacrum, caudal to thecal sac termination
  - Sacral meningeal cyst, type IB meningeal cyst
- Synonym: Occult intrasacral meningocele (outdated term)

IMAGING

- Smooth enlargement of sacral spinal canal
  - Expands, but does not transgress, sacrum margins
  - No expansion or remodeling of neural foramina
- Posterior sacral vertebral scalloping characteristic
- No cyst wall enhancement

TOP DIFFERENTIAL DIAGNOSES

- Tarlov cyst
- Dorsal spinal meningocele
- Dural dysplasia

PATHOLOGY

- Diverticulum of sacral subarachnoid space expands into sacral cyst with secondary remodeling of sacral canal
- Extradural AC; no meningeal herniation (not true meningocele)
- Cyst is connected to thecal sac by thin pedicle
- No neuronal elements within cyst

CLINICAL ISSUES

- Usually asymptomatic; incidental discovery on MR
  - Asymptomatic patients need no specific treatment
  - Indications for operation include ↑ cyst size on serial exams, onset of symptoms referable to cyst

DIAGNOSTIC CHECKLIST

- AC centered in midline; cyst center over neural foramen implies Tarlov cyst
- Cyst frequently incidental finding discovered during imaging for other indications

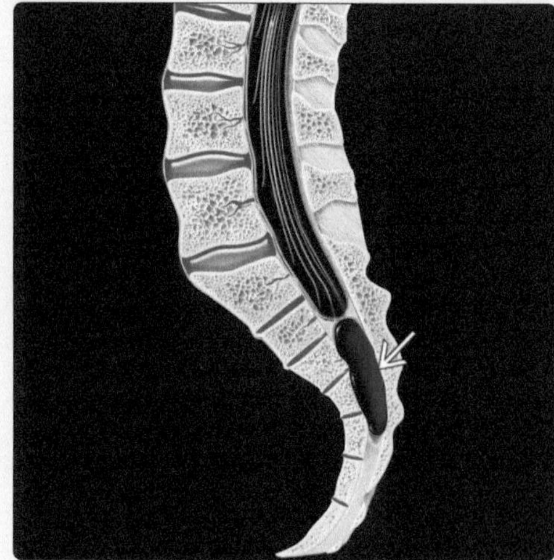

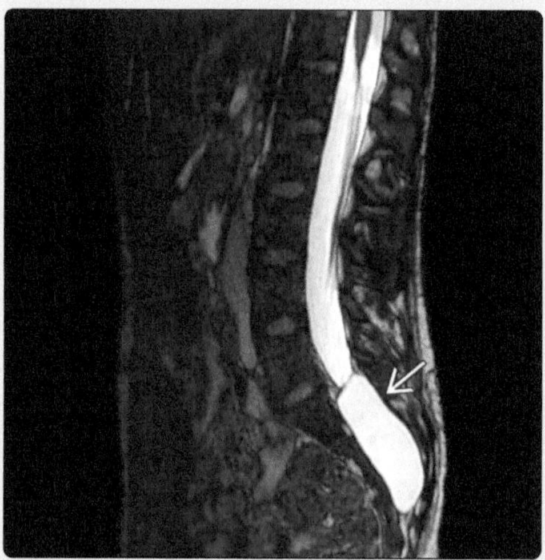

(Left) *Sagittal graphic of the lumbosacral spine demonstrates an extradural cyst ➡ within the sacral spinal canal below the thecal sac termination at S2. Note osseous remodeling of the sacral spinal canal margins.* **(Right)** *Sagittal FIESTA MR shows a large sacral extradural arachnoid cyst (type 1b meningeal cyst) ➡ that upwardly displaces the thecal sac and remodels the sacrum.*

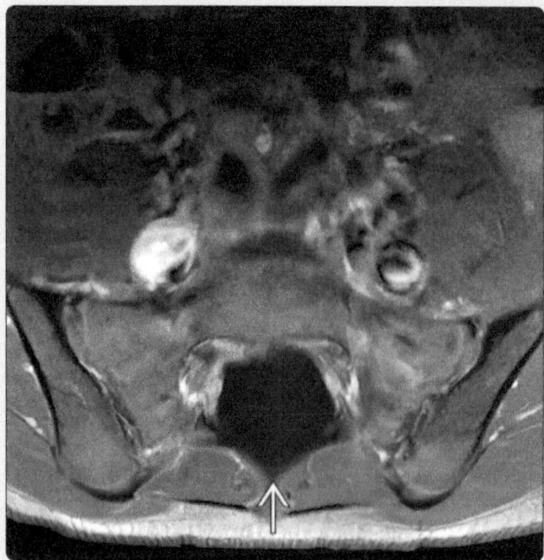

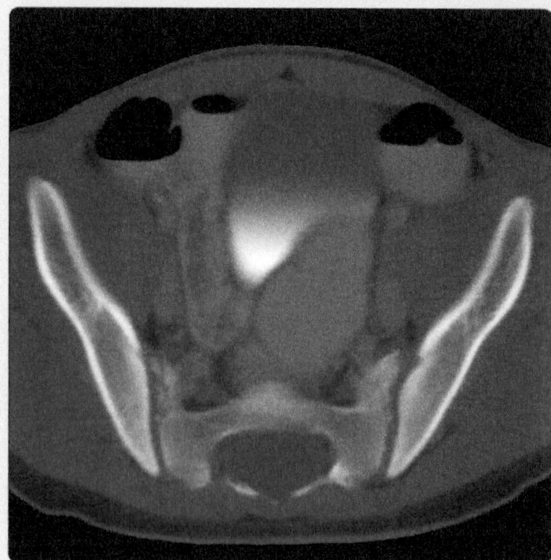

(Left) *Axial T1WI C+ MR in the same patient reveals an expansile CSF signal cyst ➡ without intrinsic neural components or enhancing tissue. This is a characteristic appearance of large type 1b meningeal cyst.* **(Right)** *Axial bone CT in the same patient confirms smooth bone remodeling of the osseous spinal canal.*

TERMINOLOGY

Synonyms

- Sacral meningeal cyst, type IB meningeal cyst (Nabors classification)

Definitions

- Spinal extradural arachnoid cyst (AC) localized to sacrum

IMAGING

General Features

- Best diagnostic clue
  - Smooth, cystic enlargement of sacral spinal canal
- Location
  - Sacrum
- Size
  - Expands, but does not transgress, margins of sacrum
- Morphology
  - Sacral extradural meningeal cyst; no internal neural elements

Radiographic Findings

- Radiography
  - Sacral canal enlargement
  - Posterior vertebral scalloping

CT Findings

- NECT
  - CSF-density cyst enlarges sacral canal
  - Nerve roots displaced by extradural cyst
- CECT
  - No cyst wall enhancement
- Bone CT
  - Smooth remodeling, enlargement of sacral canal
  - No expansion or remodeling of neural foramina

MR Findings

- T1WI
  - CSF signal intensity extradural sacral cyst adjacent to distal thecal sac
- T2WI
  - Cyst follows CSF signal intensity
  - No neural elements within cyst
- DWI
  - Hypointense signal intensity excludes epidermoid tumor
- T1WI C+
  - No cyst enhancement

Ultrasonographic Findings

- Grayscale ultrasound
  - Hypoechoic intrasacral cyst without intrinsic neural elements

Nonvascular Interventions

- Myelography
  - Enlargement of distal sacral canal, extradural compression of distal contrast-filled thecal sac
    - ± contrast opacification of cyst (if isthmus large enough)

Other Modality Findings

- CSF cine-phase contrast flow-sensitive imaging may help define cyst walls by depicting differential CSF pulsation

Imaging Recommendations

- Best imaging tool
  - MR best modality for initial diagnosis
  - CT myelography may help reveal connection between cyst and subarachnoid space
    - Delayed postmyelographic imaging may show additional cyst filling
- Protocol advice
  - Sagittal and axial T1WI and T2WI to identify cyst, clarify relationship to adjacent structures

DIFFERENTIAL DIAGNOSIS

Tarlov Cyst

- Etiologically similar to sacral extradural AC; congenital dilatation of nerve root meningeal sleeves
- Large cysts may remodel sacrum but will be eccentrically centered over neural foramen
- Frequently multiple

Dorsal Meningocele

- True meningocele; protrudes through dorsal dysraphism into subcutaneous tissues

Dural Dysplasia

- Vertebral scalloping usually present in lumbar spine as well as sacrum, ± lateral meningocele
- Search for characteristic imaging and clinical stigmata of etiologic disorder

PATHOLOGY

General Features

- Etiology
  - Diverticulum of sacral subarachnoid space that expands into sacral cyst 2° to valve-like mechanism → 2° remodeling of sacral canal
- Associated abnormalities
  - Tarlov cyst(s)
  - Posterior spinal dysraphism
  - Tethered cord syndrome
- Extradural AC
  - No herniation of meninges, hence not true meningocele
  - No neuronal elements within cyst
- Cyst is connected to thecal sac by pedicle that permits contiguous CSF flow
- CSF pulsation ± raised intraspinal pressure (across stenotic pedicle) pressure erodes and remodels sacral canal

Staging, Grading, & Classification

- Nabors classification (1988)
  - **Type I**: Extradural meningeal cyst **without** neural tissue
    - **Type Ia**: Extradural spinal AC
    - **Type Ib**: Sacral meningocele
  - **Type II**: Extradural meningeal cyst **containing** neural tissue (Tarlov cyst)
  - **Type III**: Intradural spinal AC

Gross Pathologic & Surgical Features

- Sacral laminectomy → thinned sacral vertebral laminae
  - Cyst may be attached to distal thecal sac by narrow pedicle that permits 1-way (mostly) CSF flow into cyst
  - Symptomatic cysts less likely to communicate with subarachnoid space than asymptomatic cysts

Microscopic Features

- Cyst is lined by fibrous connective tissue ± single inner layer of arachnoid membrane

CLINICAL ISSUES

Presentation

- Most common signs/symptoms
  - Asymptomatic; incidental discovery on MR
  - Symptomatic: Chronic low back pain, sciatica, perineal paresthesias, and bladder dysfunction
  - Less common signs/symptoms
    - Intermittent, severe lower back pain
    - Atypical bowel symptoms, severe constipation, and stool incontinence
    - Tethered cord syndrome
- Clinical profile
  - Specific symptoms are referable to sacral root compression
  - May be exacerbated by positional change or Valsalva maneuver

Demographics

- Age
  - Teen → older adults
  - Rarely diagnosed in children
- Sex
  - Some series report M > F; others M < F
- Epidemiology
  - Spinal meningeal cysts are uncommon
    - Comprise 1-3% of all spinal tumors
  - Prevalence of occult sacral meningocele uncertain but < prevalence of Tarlov cyst

Natural History & Prognosis

- Most patients are asymptomatic and need no specific treatment
  - Asymptomatic cysts are most commonly identified and referred to specialists following incidental discovery on MR
- Symptomatic patients or very large cysts may require surgery
  - Indications for operative intervention include ↑ cyst size on serial exams or onset of symptoms referable to cyst
  - Good prognosis for recovery following surgery

Treatment

- Conservative approach recommended for asymptomatic cysts, especially when small
- Symptomatic cysts may require treatment
  - Percutaneous cyst aspiration may relieve symptoms temporarily
    - May be used as diagnostic test prior to definitive therapy
    - Percutaneous cyst aspiration with fibrin glue therapy may produce definitive long-lasting symptom reduction
  - Operative therapy → sacral laminectomy to expose, resect cyst
    - May not be necessary to completely resect entire cyst
    - Primary goal is to close dural defect → eradicate 1-way valve communication, prevent cyst recurrence
    - If adhesions prevent full excision, may partially resect posterior wall or marsupialize cyst to subarachnoid space

DIAGNOSTIC CHECKLIST

Consider

- MR best modality for diagnosis of sacral cyst, preoperative planning
- Definitive cyst characterization based on operative inspection, histologic examination
- Cyst may be incidental finding discovered during imaging for other indications

Image Interpretation Pearls

- Classic appearance is intrasacral cyst producing smooth sacral canal expansion with outward displacement of nerve roots
- AC centered in midline; center over neural foramen implies Tarlov cyst

SELECTED REFERENCES

1. Ma Q et al: Arachnoidal diverticula of sacral extradural meningeal cyst: a novel definition and case series. World Neurosurg. 163:e106-12, 2022
2. Rahimizadeh A et al: Six cases of occult sacral meningocele. Surg Neurol Int. 13:91, 2022
3. Satyarthee GD: Pediatric symptomatic sacral extradural arachnoid cyst: surgical management review. J Pediatr Neurosci. 13(2):211-3, 2018
4. Tanaka T et al: Electrodiagnostic and advanced neuroimaging characterization for successful treatment of spinal extradural arachnoid cyst. World Neurosurg. 109:298-303, 2018
5. Habibi Z et al: Sacral extradural arachnoid cyst in association with split cord malformation. Spine J. 16(9):1109-15, 2016
6. Azad R et al: Role of screening of whole spine with sagittal MRI with MR myelography in early detection and management of occult intrasacral meningocele. Asian J Neurosurg. 8(4):174-8, 2013
7. Lohani S et al: Intrasacral meningocele in the pediatric population. J Neurosurg Pediatr. 11(6):615-22, 2013
8. Bond AE et al: Spinal arachnoid cysts in the pediatric population: report of 31 cases and a review of the literature. J Neurosurg Pediatr. 9(4):432-41, 2012
9. Vaccaro M et al: A woman with abdominal pain and headache. Neurol Sci. 30 Suppl 1:S141-3, 2009
10. Hamamcioglu MK et al: Intrasacral extradural arachnoid cysts. Neurol Med Chir (Tokyo). 48(5):223-6, 2008
11. Liu JK et al: Spinal extradural arachnoid cysts: clinical, radiological, and surgical features. Neurosurg Focus. 22(2):E6, 2007
12. Choi JY et al: Spinal extradural arachnoid cyst. Acta Neurochir (Wien). 148(5):579-85; discussion 585, 2006
13. Nishio Y et al: A case of occult intrasacral meningocele presented with atypical bowel symptoms. Childs Nerv Syst. 20(1):65-7, 2004
14. Sato K et al: Spinal extradural meningeal cyst: correct radiological and histopathological diagnosis. Neurosurg Focus. 13(4):ecp1, 2002
15. Diel J et al: The sacrum: pathologic spectrum, multimodality imaging, and subspecialty approach. Radiographics. 21(1):83-104, 2001
16. Patel MR et al: Percutaneous fibrin glue therapy of meningeal cysts of the sacral spine. AJR Am J Roentgenol. 168(2):367-70, 1997
17. Okada T et al: Occult intrasacral meningocele associated with spina bifida: a case report. Surg Neurol. 46(2):147-9, 1996
18. Nabors MW et al: Updated assessment and current classification of spinal meningeal cysts. J Neurosurg. 68(3):366-77, 1988

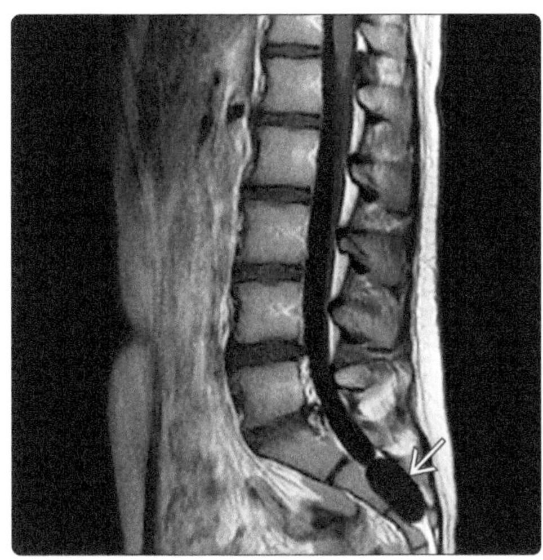

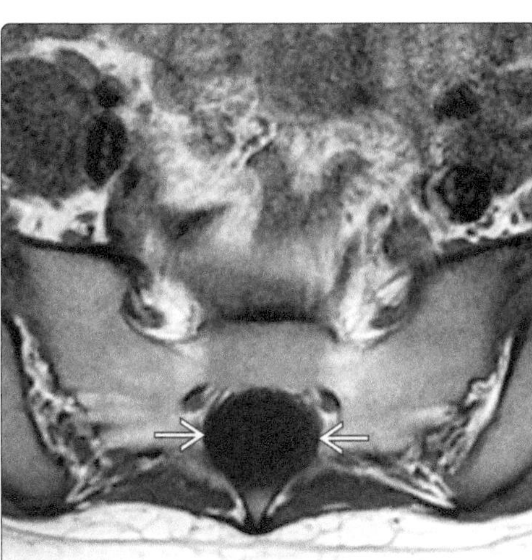

(Left) *Sagittal T1WI C+ MR demonstrates an extradural cyst ➡ located within the spinal canal at S2 and S3. It is extradural and distal to the thecal sac termination at S2. Note mild upward mass effect on the terminal thecal sac, which normally terminates at S2-S3.* **(Right)** *Axial T1WI MR confirms central arachnoid cyst ➡ location within the sacral spinal canal. There is remodeling and expansion of the adjacent vertebral body and overlying posterior elements.*

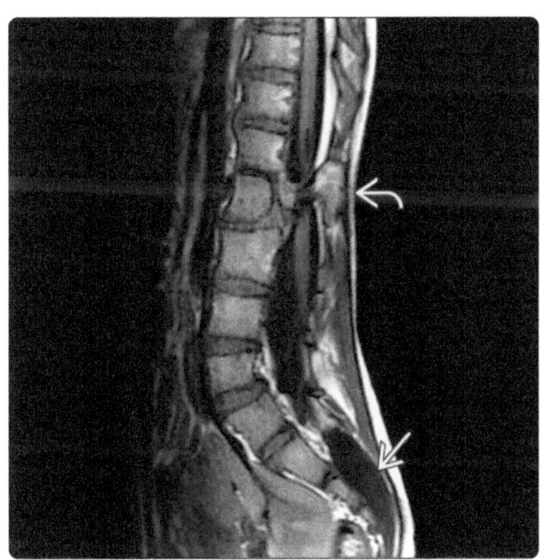

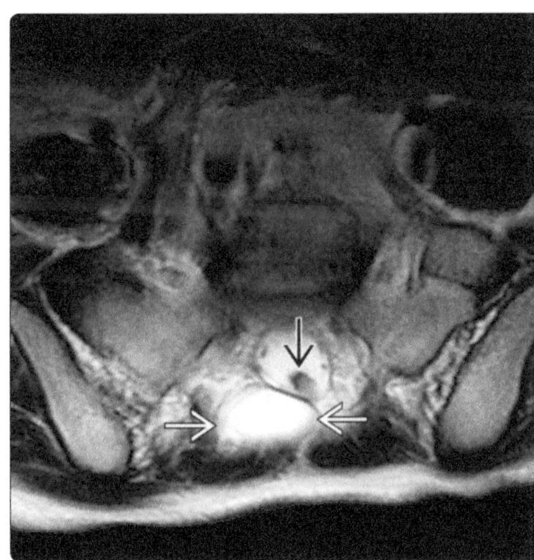

(Left) *Sagittal T1WI MR in a Klippel-Feil patient with diastematomyelia ↩ demonstrates a low-lying, hydromyelic tethered spinal cord in addition to a fluid-signal cyst ➡ in the terminal sacral canal. The cyst results in remodeling and enlargement of the sacral central canal.* **(Right)** *Axial T2WI MR reveals a low-lying, tethered spinal cord ➡ within the thecal sac, which is anterior and superior to the sacral extradural arachnoid cyst ➡ located eccentrically within the canal.*

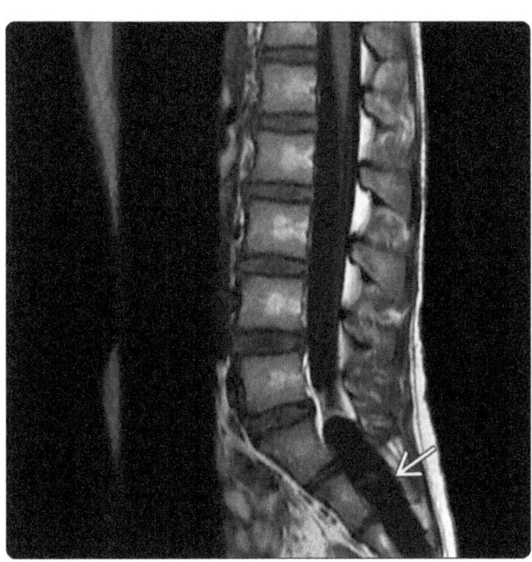

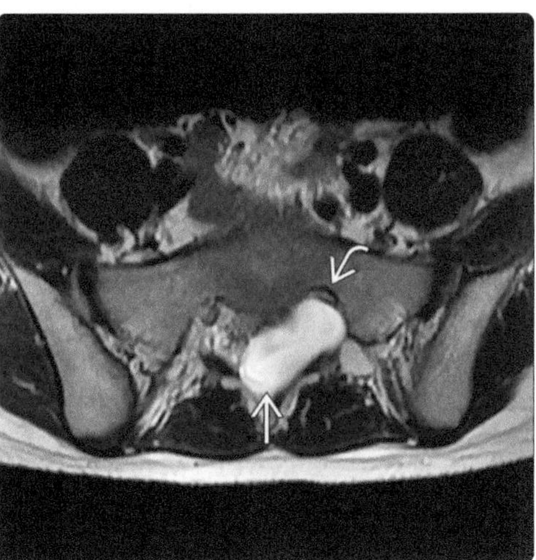

(Left) *Sagittal T1WI MR in a 12-year-old patient with back pain demonstrates a typical sacral extradural arachnoid cyst ➡ with upward displacement of the thecal sac (which normally terminates around S2).* **(Right)** *Axial T2WI MR in the same patient shows cyst ➡ remodeling of the osseous sacral spinal canal eccentric to the left. The location and absence of included neural elements (the exiting nerve root ↩ is displaced and outside the cyst) confirms type 1b meningeal cyst.*

Sacrococcygeal Teratoma

KEY FACTS

TERMINOLOGY

- Teratomas made up of various parenchymal cell types from > 1 germ layer, usually all 3
- Sacrococcygeal teratoma (SCT) arises from coccyx, potentially grows both internally & externally (with latter more common)

IMAGING

- Always with presacral components; exophytic extension more common than internal growth
- Heterogeneous mixed solid & cystic masses
  - Ca^{++}, fat, hemorrhage, cysts, various soft tissues in mass
  - Solid components may show moderate to high vascularity

TOP DIFFERENTIAL DIAGNOSES

- Pelvic rhabdomyosarcoma
- Neuroblastoma
- Myelomeningocele or myelocystocele

PATHOLOGY

- Malignant characteristics increase with age, type IV
- **American Association of Pediatric Surgery Section classification**
  - Type I (47%): Primarily external in location
  - Type II (34%): Dumbbell shape, equal pelvic & external components
  - Type III (9%): Primarily located within abdomen/pelvis
  - Type IV (10%): Entirely internal, no external component

CLINICAL ISSUES

- Prognosis excellent in patients with benign tumors after birth
- Complete surgical resection to include coccyx
- 5-15% risk of recurrence

DIAGNOSTIC CHECKLIST

- MR best for identifying intraspinal extension

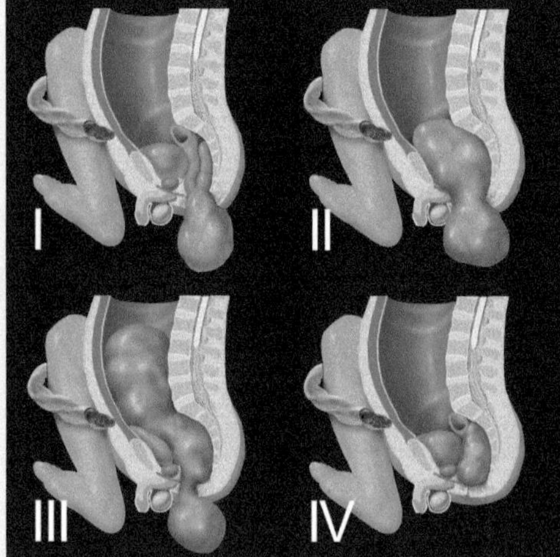

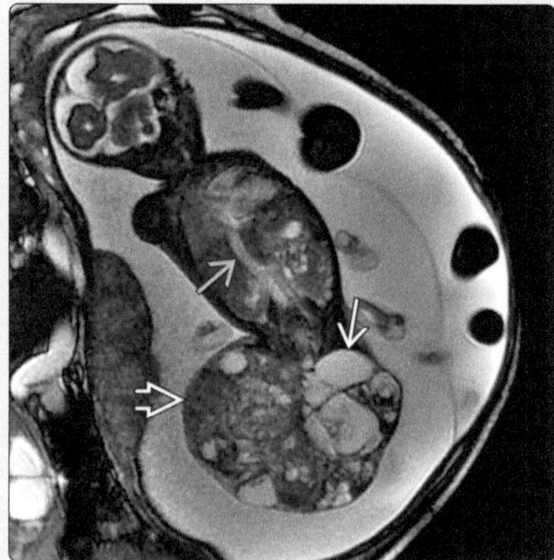

(Left) *Graphic shows tumor classification scheme: Type I is primarily exophytic, type II has equivalent-sized internal & external masses, type III has a larger intraabdominal component, & type IV is entirely internal.* **(Right)** *Coronal SSFP MR of a twin gestation shows a fetus with a large, predominantly exophytic mass extending from the perineum. Note the solid ➔ & cystic ➔ areas within the mass. The inferior vena cava → is prominent due to the amount of blood flow coursing through this tumor. However, no hydrops is seen.*

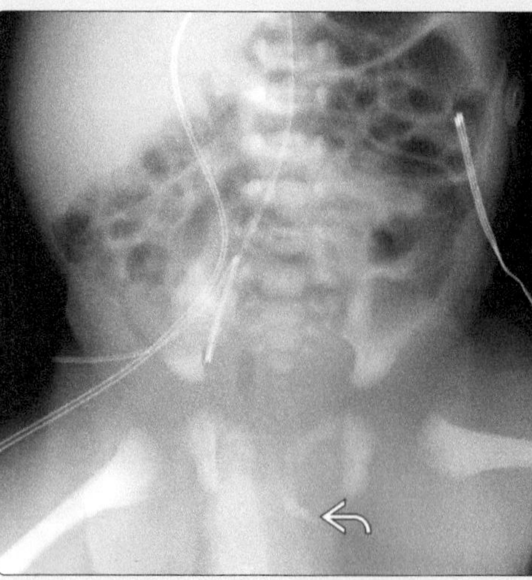

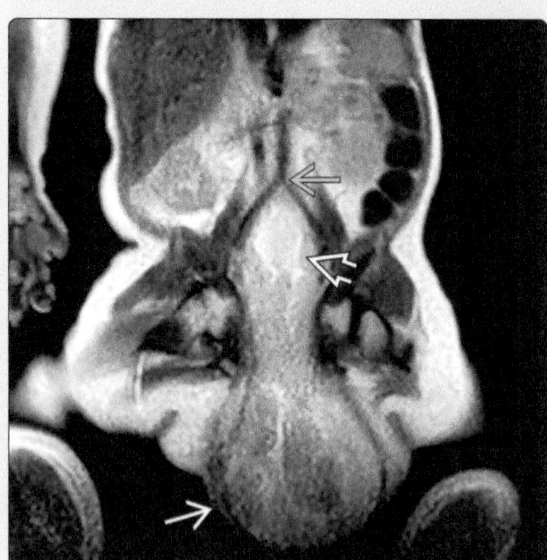

(Left) *AP radiograph in a newborn boy with a protruding buttock mass shows soft tissue fullness in the pelvis & perineum & irregular Ca^{++} ➔ below the pubic bones.* **(Right)** *Coronal T2 MR in the same infant shows a heterogeneous solid mass, which protrudes externally ➔ with dumbbell extension internally ➔, splaying the aortic bifurcation → in this case of a type II sacrococcygeal teratoma (SCT).*

TERMINOLOGY

Abbreviations

- Sacrococcygeal teratoma (SCT)

Synonyms

- Teratoma, germ cell tumor of coccyx

Definitions

- Teratomas made up of various parenchymal cell types from > 1 germ layer, usually all 3
  - Tumors may contain hair, teeth, cartilage, & fat, amongst other tissues
- SCT arises from coccyx, potentially grows both internally & externally (with latter more common)
- Both benign & malignant varieties

IMAGING

General Features

- Best diagnostic clue
  - Large solid, cystic, or mixed mass with large, exophytic perineal/buttock component & relatively small presacral component
  - May see Ca^{++}, bone, fat, fluid levels, various soft tissues in mass
- Location
  - Origin from coccyx, but growth can occur in any direction
    - Presacral components always present
  - Look for intraspinal extension
- Size
  - Ranges from only few mL to massive in volume, potentially exceeding fetal weight
- Morphology
  - Classically heterogeneous: Multiple tissue types, Ca^{++}

Radiographic Findings

- Typically show large mass extending outside infant
- Ca^{++} may be present

Fluoroscopic Findings

- Type IV SCT may be found incidentally during fluoroscopy studies for constipation or voiding problems
- Patients rarely have long-term sequela of bladder outlet obstruction

CT Findings

- NECT
  - Demonstrates fatty components, Ca^{++}, & fluid levels well
  - Heterogeneous mass wrapped around coccyx but typically without bony destruction
- CECT
  - Variable enhancement pattern in solid & cystic components

MR Findings

- Heterogeneous, similar to CT
- Fat best confirmed on T1WI with & without FS
- Variable enhancement with gadolinium that does not predict malignancy
- Best study for identifying intraspinal extension

Ultrasonographic Findings

- Grayscale ultrasound
  - Ultrasound may be limited due to large size & internal Ca^{++}
  - Heterogeneous echotexture mass
    - Ca^{++} & fat cause highly echogenic foci, while cystic areas are hypo- to anechoic
- Color Doppler
  - Solid components may show moderate to high vascularity
  - Arterial steal may be seen in nearby vessels to supply tumor

Nuclear Medicine Findings

- PET
  - Used more often in evaluation of malignant recurrence than in initial diagnosis

Imaging Recommendations

- Best imaging tool
  - Prenatal sonography most common initial diagnostic modality
  - Prenatal or postnatal MR to determine full extent of mass & aid surgical planning

DIFFERENTIAL DIAGNOSIS

Pelvic Rhabdomyosarcoma

- Solid mass without Ca^{++}, fat, or substantial cysts (usually)

Neuroblastoma

- May arise in pelvis at organ of Zuckerkandl
- Solid mass with Ca^{++}

Myelomeningocele or Myelocystocele

- Dorsal dysraphism; neural placode continuous with abnormal spinal cord

Other Intrapelvic Masses

- Consider Burkitt lymphoma, ovarian tumors, lymphatic malformation, hematometrocolpos

PATHOLOGY

General Features

- Etiology
  - Probably results from rests of pluripotential cells at caudal end of notochord/spine
- Genetics
  - Not inherited
- Associated abnormalities
  - 10% of SCTs associated with other congenital anomalies, primarily defects of hindgut & cloacal region, which exceeds baseline rate of 2.5% expected in general population
  - SCT 2nd most common lesion after anterior meningocele in familial disorder of Currarino (autosomal dominant triad of presacral mass, partial sacral agenesis, & anorectal defects)
  - Familial tendency reported, prompting some to recommend screening asymptomatic siblings
- Malignant characteristics increase with
  - Age at diagnosis

- Internal subtype (type IV is worst)
- Male sex
- Presence of necrosis or hemorrhage

Staging, Grading, & Classification

- **American Association of Pediatric Surgery Section classification**
  - Type I (47%)
    - Primarily external in location
  - Type II (34%)
    - Dumbbell shape, equal internal/external components
  - Type III (9%)
    - Primarily located within abdomen/pelvis
  - Type IV (10%)
    - Entirely internal, no external component visible

Gross Pathologic & Surgical Features

- Typical of all teratomas: Multiple tissue types in varying stages of maturation & differentiation
- Solid & cystic components common

Microscopic Features

- Tumors can be mature or immature
- Only 17% of SCTs have malignant features

CLINICAL ISSUES

Presentation

- Most common signs/symptoms
  - Frequently diagnosed in utero
    - Large fetal tumors require C-section delivery or in utero surgical intervention (open fetal surgery, radiofrequency or thermal ablation of tumor)
  - Most other tumors diagnosed within 1st few days of life
    - Exophytic masses easily diagnosed clinically
    - Entirely internal masses may have delayed diagnosis, presenting with urinary symptoms or constipation
- Other signs/symptoms
  - In utero complications: Fetal SCT can be quite vascular & grow rapidly → hydrops, intratumoral hemorrhage or rupture → fetal demise
    - Hydrops before 30-weeks gestation: > 90% mortality rate
      - Solid masses more likely to develop hydrops
      - Doppler parameters may help predict hydrops
    - Maternal mirror syndrome (preeclampsia) may develop

Demographics

- Age
  - Typically diagnosed in fetus or newborn
  - Delayed diagnoses possible in 1st year of life, rarely, even later
- Epidemiology
  - Prevalence: 1 in 14,000 (Sweden) to 40,000 births

Natural History & Prognosis

- Prognosis excellent in patients with benign tumors after birth
  - Gait abnormalities & early arthrosis reported with extensive pelvic muscle resection
- 5-15% risk of recurrence
  - Intraoperative tumor spillage & incomplete resection increase risk
- Masses diagnosed after 1st birthday & located only internally have higher malignant potential
  - Prognosis variable in malignant tumors
  - Serum α-fetoprotein is useful tumor marker postoperatively
- Malignant components may be found at presentation or at time of recurrence
  - Yolk sac tumor most common
  - Embryonal carcinoma 2nd most common
  - With intensive chemotherapy, 5-year relapse-free survival rate reported between 76-90%
- Up to 1/3 may have adverse bowel or bladder dysfunction, especially internal tumors
- Study from Netherlands showed normal fertility in adult female survivors

Treatment

- Complete surgical resection to include coccyx
- Benign tumors do not require additional therapy
- Malignant tumors treated with chemotherapy (platinum-based agents) & radiation
- Consideration of in utero intervention with development of hydrops; must weigh benefits with risks of prematurity

SELECTED REFERENCES

1. Bougie E et al: It is all about form and function: a new approach to giant neonatal sacrococcygeal teratomas. Pediatr Surg Int. 39(1):182, 2023
2. Braungart S et al: Sacrococcygeal teratoma: long-term outcomes. A UK CCLG Surgeons Group Nationwide Study. Pediatr Blood Cancer. 70(1):e29994, 2023
3. Mosleh MM et al: Sacrococcygeal teratomas: a case-based review from the perspective of individual multidisciplinary experts. Childs Nerv Syst. 39(1):57-64, 2023
4. Tosun M et al: A single-center experience of magnetic resonance imaging findings of fetal sacrococcygeal teratomas. Turk J Med Sci. 52(4):1190-6, 2022
5. Hambraeus M et al: Long-term outcome of sacrococcygeal teratoma: a controlled cohort study of urinary tract and bowel dysfunction and predictors of poor outcome. J Pediatr. 198:131-136.e2, 2018
6. Kremer MEB et al: The incidence of associated abnormalities in patients with sacrococcygeal teratoma. J Pediatr Surg. 53(10):1918-22, 2018
7. Yoon HM et al: Sacrococcygeal teratomas in newborns: a comprehensive review for the radiologists. Acta Radiol. 59(2):236-46, 2018
8. Padilla BE et al: Sacrococcygeal teratoma: late recurrence warrants long-term surveillance. Pediatr Surg Int. 33(11):1189-94, 2017
9. Hambraeus M et al: Sacrococcygeal teratoma: a population-based study of incidence and prenatal prognostic factors. J Pediatr Surg. 51(3):481-5, 2016
10. Kremer ME et al: Evaluation of chemotherapeutic sequelae and quality of life in survivors of malignant sacrococcygeal teratoma. Pediatr Surg Int. 32(3):261-8, 2016
11. Adekola H et al: The clinical relevance of fetal MRI in the diagnosis of type IV cystic sacrococcygeal teratoma--a review. Fetal Pediatr Pathol. 34(1):31-43, 2015
12. Dirix M et al: Malignant transformation in sacrococcygeal teratoma and in presacral teratoma associated with Currarino syndrome: a comparative study. J Pediatr Surg. 50(3):462-4, 2015
13. Sananes N et al: Technical aspects and effectiveness of percutaneous fetal therapies for large sacrococcygeal teratomas - a cohort study and a literature review. Ultrasound Obstet Gynecol. 47(6):712-9, 2015
14. Coleman A et al: Sacrococcygeal teratoma growth rate predicts adverse outcomes. J Pediatr Surg. 49(6):985-9, 2014
15. Garg R et al: Sacrococcygeal malignant germ cell tumor (SC-MGCT) with intraspinal extension. J Pediatr Surg. 49(7):1113-5, 2014
16. Kremer ME et al: Evaluation of pregnancy and delivery in 13 women who underwent resection of a sacrococcygeal teratoma during early childhood. BMC Pregnancy Childbirth. 14:407, 2014
17. Ladino Torres MF et al: Spine ultrasound imaging in the newborn. Semin Ultrasound CT MR. 35(6):652-61, 2014

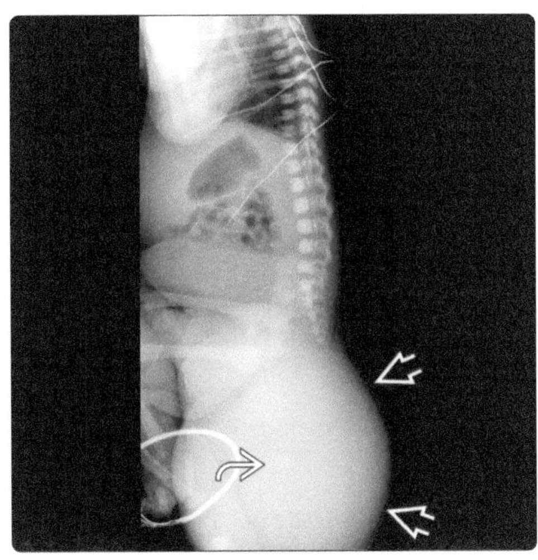

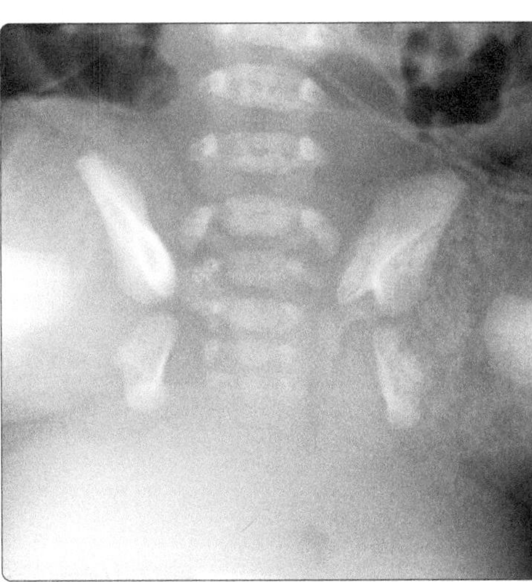

(Left) *Lateral radiograph shows a newborn infant with a large, exophytic mass ➡ extending from the sacrum & coccygeal region. A few faint Ca^{++} ➡ are visible within the mass, typical of an SCT.* **(Right)** *Frontal radiograph of the same infant shows widely spaced pubic & ischial bones, which are splayed by the large pelvic tumor.*

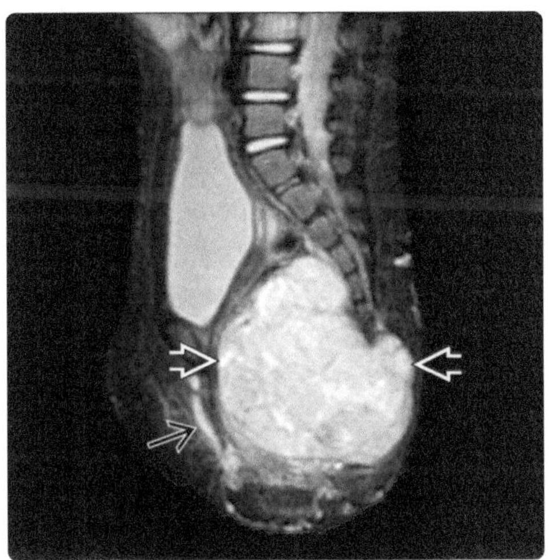

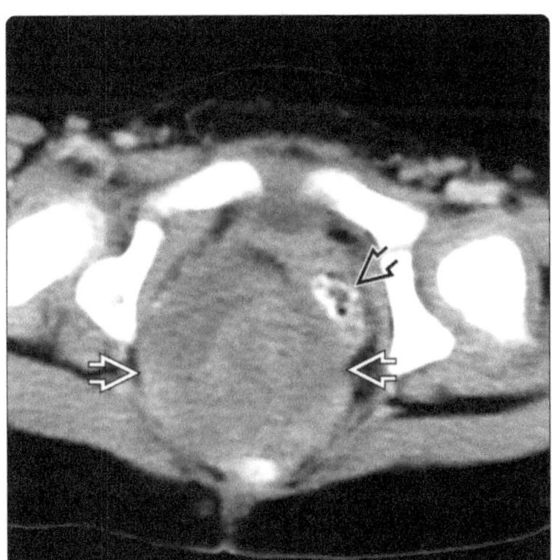

(Left) *Sagittal STIR MR (toddler girl, AAP type III) reveals a heterogeneous sacral mass ➡ that is mostly internal. The tumor anteriorly displaces the rectum & urinary bladder ➡. Note absence of abnormal sacral marrow signal or tumor extension into the spinal canal through the sacral hiatus.* **(Right)** *Axial CECT (AAP type III) reveals a heterogeneous, mildly enhancing pelvic mass ➡. Note anterior & left displacement of the rectum ➡. There is not a well-developed fat plane visible between the rectum & mass.*

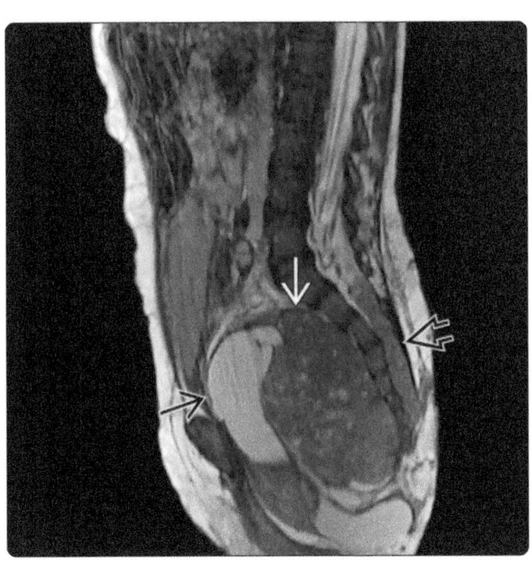

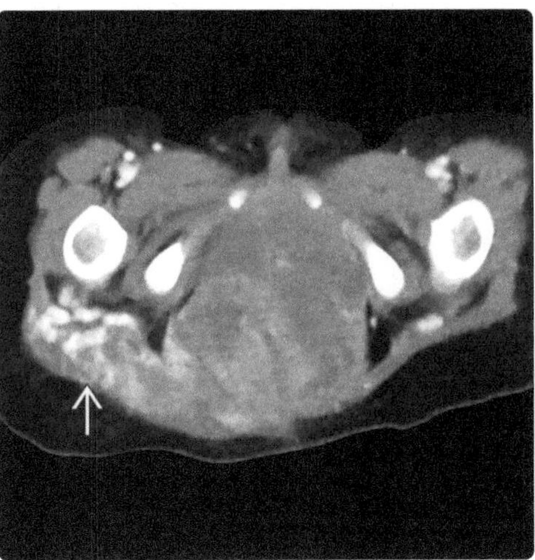

(Left) *Sagittal FIESTA in a 21-month-old with palpable buttock mass demonstrates a large internal solid mass ➡ that displaces the urinary bladder ➡ & extends into the spinal canal ➡. Surgical biopsy revealed malignant teratoma, yolk sac variant.* **(Right)** *Axial CT angiogram in the same patient shows large, enhancing vessels within the gluteal portion of the mass ➡. This represents an AAP type IV SCT that was not appreciated earlier. This patient also had lung metastases on chest CT (not shown).*

Craniovertebral Junction Variants

KEY FACTS

TERMINOLOGY

- Anomalous or variant craniovertebral junction (CVJ) anatomy

IMAGING

- Flattening or malformation of clivus/occipital condyles, anterior C1 ring, or dens
- Variable instability during dynamic flexion, extension
- ± enhancing granulation tissue mass (pannus)
    - Reducible abnormalities have largest pannus

TOP DIFFERENTIAL DIAGNOSES

- Developmental CVJ anomalies
    - Achondroplasia, Down syndrome
- Inflammatory and degenerative arthritides
- Acquired basilar impression
- Trauma

PATHOLOGY

- Congenital insult to developing CVJ neural and osseous tissue between 4th and 7th intrauterine weeks
- *PAX1* gene implicated in anomalous segmentation of proatlas
- Solid ankylosis or fibrous union in many irreducible anomalies
- Granulation tissue proliferation around motion areas in unstable or reducible anomalies

CLINICAL ISSUES

- Occipital headache or suboccipital neck pain exacerbated by flexion/extension
- Symptomatic presentation following mild trauma common

DIAGNOSTIC CHECKLIST

- Dynamic flex-extend imaging determines stability, reducibility of abnormality

(Left) *Midline sagittal bone CT (Apert syndrome) shows abnormal vertical clivus ➡ orientation with a fibrous union to the anterior C1 ring ➡. The odontoid process ➡ protrudes through the foramen magnum (basilar invagination).* **(Right)** *Sagittal bone CT demonstrates coexisting condylus tertius ➡ and os odontoideum ➡ in a patient with atlantoaxial instability. Note the osseous protrusion from the clivus tip representing the condylus tertius. The os is dystopic, and the anterior C1 ring ➡ is enlarged.*

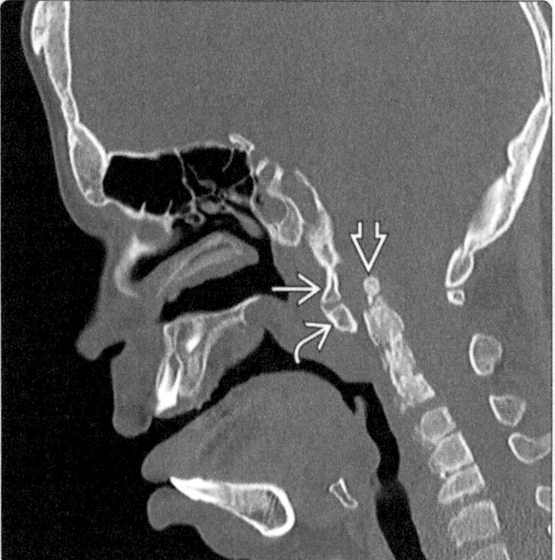

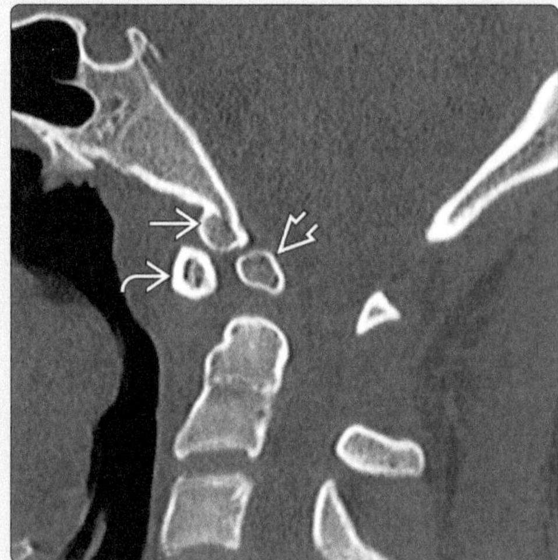

(Left) *Sagittal bone CT (os avis) reveals abnormal fusion of the os ➡ to the clivus ➡. Remodeling changes are also noted in the anterior C1 ring ➡ and os. The posterior C1 ring ➡ is hypoplastic and resides within the spinal canal just below the foramen magnum.* **(Right)** *Sagittal FLAIR MR (os avis) in the same patient reveals abnormal T2 signal within the cervical spinal cord at the C1 level, reflecting injury related to atlantoaxial instability and mild C1 ring ➡ hypoplasia.*

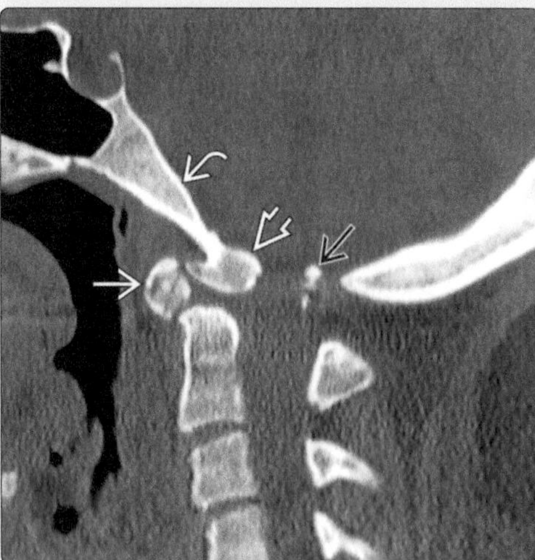

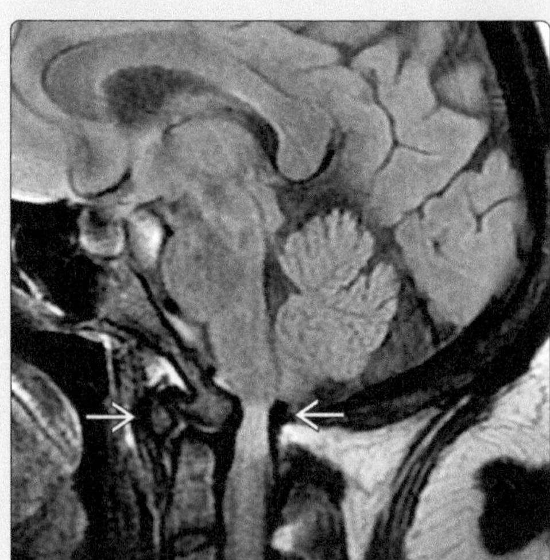

TERMINOLOGY

Abbreviations

- Craniovertebral junction (CVJ), craniocerebral junction (CCJ)

Synonyms

- CVJ anomalies, CCJ variants or anomalies

Definitions

- Anatomic variations of skull base-upper cervical spine articulation
- Many are sequelae of aberrant proatlas development

IMAGING

General Features

- Best diagnostic clue
  - Flattening or malformation of clivus/occipital condyles, anterior C1 ring, or odontoid process

Radiographic Findings

- Radiography
  - Platybasia, basilar invagination, C1 ring assimilation, asymmetrical C1/C2 articulation, backward tilt, hypoplasia/aplasia, os odontoideum of odontoid process, C2/C3 fusion (Klippel-Feil)

Fluoroscopic Findings

- Variable instability of C0/C1, C1/C2 articulations with dynamic flexion and extension

CT Findings

- Bone CT
  - Findings similar to plain radiographs; sagittal and coronal reformats minimize effect of overlapping structures

MR Findings

- T1WI
  - Osseous anomalies ± soft tissue granulation tissue, cord compression, hindbrain anomalies
- T2WI
  - Similar to T1WI; best for evaluating spinal cord
- T1WI C+
  - ± enhancing pannus
- MRA
  - Vertebral artery variants common, important for surgical planning

Imaging Recommendations

- Protocol advice
  - Dynamic flex-extend plain films to demonstrate biomechanics, uncover instability
  - Multiplanar T1WI, T2WI to evaluate cord, soft tissues; flex-extend MR optimally delineates effect of position on neural compression
  - Bone CT with multiplanar reformats to evaluate osseous structures for surgical planning

DIFFERENTIAL DIAGNOSIS

Developmental Craniovertebral Junction Anomalies

- CVJ stenosis or atlantoaxial instability 2° to
  - Achondroplasia
  - Mucopolysaccharidosis
  - Down syndrome
  - Inborn errors of metabolism

Inflammatory and Degenerative Arthritides

- ± CVJ fusion, anterior displacement of C1 ring from dens, basilar invagination → possible cord compression 2° to canal stenosis
  - Rheumatoid arthritides
  - Reactive arthritides
  - Psoriatic arthritides
  - Ankylosing spondylitis
  - Degenerative arthritis (osteoarthritis)

Acquired Basilar Impression

- Upward displacement of occipital condyles above plane of foramen magnum, radiologic protrusion of dens tip above Chamberlain line
- 2° to bone softening
  - Paget disease
  - Osteogenesis imperfecta
  - Rickets
  - Rheumatoid arthritis
  - Hyperparathyroidism

Trauma

- CVJ injuries relatively uncommon but high morbidity/mortality
- Fracture &/or ligamentous injury
- Sharp, noncorticated margins argue against congenital anomaly

PATHOLOGY

General Features

- Etiology
  - Congenital insult to developing CVJ neural and osseous tissue between 4th and 7th intrauterine weeks → hypoplasia, segmentation/fusion anomalies, CVJ ankylosis
  - *PAX1* gene implicated in anomalous segmentation of proatlas
- Associated abnormalities
  - Dwarfism, jaw anomalies, cleft palate, congenital ear deformities, short neck, Sprengel deformity, funnel chest, pes cavus, and syndactyly
- Congenital CVJ abnormalities are relatively uncommon
  - Severity ranges from benign, asymptomatic to potentially fatal instability → cord/brainstem compression
- Type and severity of anomaly determined by anatomy relative to 1 or more standard "lines of reference"
  - Chamberlain line: Line drawn from opisthion to dorsal margin of hard palate
  - McGregor line: Line drawn from upper posterior hard palate to most caudal point of occiput
  - Foramen magnum plane: Line drawn from basion to opisthion
  - Craniovertebral angle (CVA): Angle between lines drawn from posterior C2 body to posterior dens and posterior dens to sphenoclival synchondrosis

Staging, Grading, & Classification

- Occipital sclerotome malformations
  - Most occiput anomalies associated with ↓ skull base height ± basilar invagination (odontoid tip > 5 mm above McGregor line)
    - Condylus tertius, condylar hypoplasia, basiocciput hypoplasia, atlantooccipital assimilation, bifid clivus
    - Platybasia = congenital flattening of craniocervical angle > 135°
    - Associated with hindbrain herniation, syringomyelia (≤ 30%)
- C1 ring anomalies
  - C1 assimilation (occipitalized C1): Segmentation failure → fibrous or osseous union between 1st spinal sclerotome and 4th occipital sclerotome
    - ± occipitocervical synostosis; most C1 ring assimilations asymptomatic, more likely to be symptomatic if retroodontoid AP canal diameter < 19 mm
  - C1 malformation: Aplasia, hypoplasia, cleft C1 arch, "split atlas" (anterior and posterior arch rachischisis)
  - Association with Klippel-Feil, basilar invagination, Chiari 1
- C2 anomalies: C1/C2 segmentation failure, dens dysplasia
  - Majority confined to odontoid process; partial (hypoplasia) → complete absence (aplasia), ossiculum terminal persistens, os odontoideum
    - Ossiculum terminale persistens: Ossification failure of terminal ossicle → incidental "notch" in dens tip
    - Os odontoideum: Well-defined ossicle at dens tip + anterior C1 arch enlargement
  - Odontoid anomalies in association with ligamentous laxity → atlantoaxial instability
    - Incompetence of cruciate ligament → C1/C2 instability, possible neurologic deficit, or death
    - Most common in Down syndrome, Morquio syndrome, Klippel-Feil syndrome, and skeletal dysplasias

Gross Pathologic & Surgical Features

- Solid ankylosis or fibrous union in many irreducible anomalies
- Granulation tissue proliferation around motion areas in unstable or reducible anomalies

Microscopic Features

- Variable components of histologically normal bone, fibrous tissue, and granulation tissue

CLINICAL ISSUES

Presentation

- Most common signs/symptoms
  - Suboccipital neck pain (85%); may clinically mimic basilar migraine
  - Posterior occipital headache exacerbated by flexion/extension
- Other signs/symptoms
  - Myelopathy, brainstem/cranial nerve deficits, weakness, lower extremity ataxia
  - Vascular symptoms (15-20%); TIA, vertigo, visual symptoms with rotation or head manipulation
    - May reflect positional vascular occlusion or vertebral artery dissection
- Clinical profile
  - Usually normal clinical appearance; obvious clinical dysmorphism implies syndromal association
  - Symptomatic presentation following mild trauma common

Demographics

- Age
  - Infancy → late adulthood, depending on severity
- Sex
  - M = F
- Epidemiology
  - Relatively uncommon: 0.14-0.25% of pediatric population

Natural History & Prognosis

- Usually gradual onset of neurologic symptoms with localizing signs; some patients asymptomatic throughout life
- Occasionally, neurologic presentation is fulminant → quadriplegia, sudden death
- Undetected anomalies at risk for injury during minor trauma, anesthesia
- Early diagnosis permits treatment before symptoms or permanent neurologic sequelae

Treatment

- Conservative approach initially unless unstable or neural deficits present
  - Traction, cervical orthosis, activity restriction
- Symptomatic, refractory to conservative management
  - Skeletal traction to distinguish reducible from irreducible abnormalities, relieve symptoms preoperatively
  - Correction of underlying biomechanical abnormality with decompression ± fusion

DIAGNOSTIC CHECKLIST

Consider

- Look for combinations of anomalies based on known association patterns
- Do not forget to look for associated brain anomalies (e.g., Chiari 1)
- Vertebral artery variants common, important for surgical planning

Image Interpretation Pearls

- Dynamic flex-extend imaging determines stability, reducibility of abnormality
- CT with reformats valuable for evaluating osseous abnormalities

SELECTED REFERENCES

1. Dlouhy BJ et al: Management of ventral brainstem compression in Chiari malformation type I. Neurosurg Clin N Am. 34(1):119-29, 2023
2. Garg K et al: Craniovertebral junction anomalies: an overlooked cause of 'posterior circulation stroke'. Neurol India. 70(Supplement):S149-59, 2022
3. Prajapati HP et al: Surgical, clinical, and radiological outcomes analysis of craniovertebral junction anomalies cases: an institutional experience. Asian J Neurosurg. 17(4):568-76, 2022
4. Menezes AH et al: Atlas assimilation: spectrum of associated radiographic abnormalities, clinical presentation, and management in children below 10 years. Childs Nerv Syst. 36(5):975-85, 2020

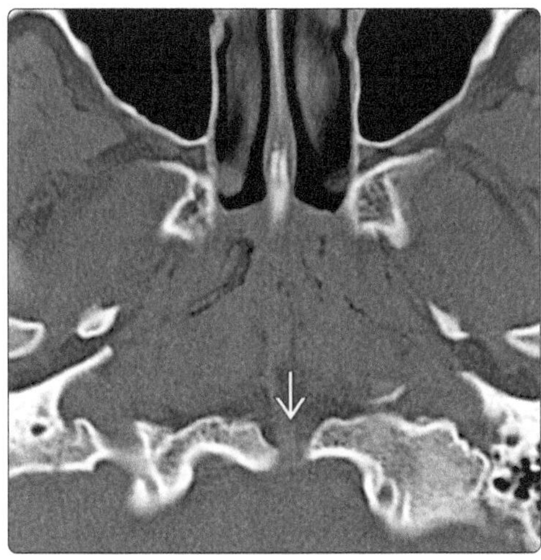

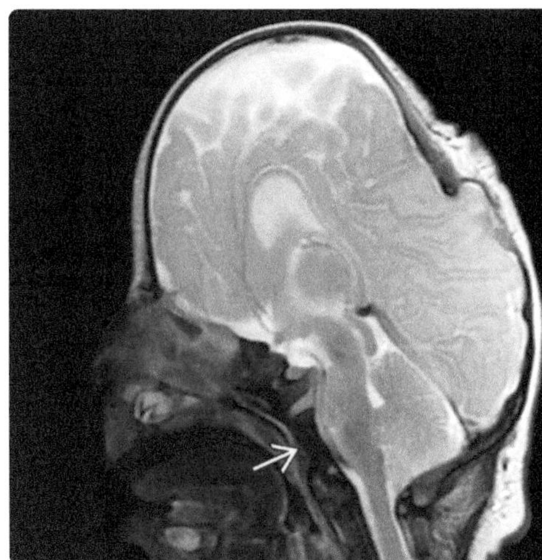

(Left) *Axial bone CT (platybasia) reveals an aberrant, flattened clivus with unusual coronal orientation. Also demonstrated is a prominent midline osseous cleft defect* ➡. **(Right)** *Sagittal T2 MR in a newborn with Apert syndrome demonstrates marked reduction of the craniovertebral angle with nearly vertical clivus* ➡ *orientation and turricephalic head shape, typical of multiple sutural craniosynostosis.*

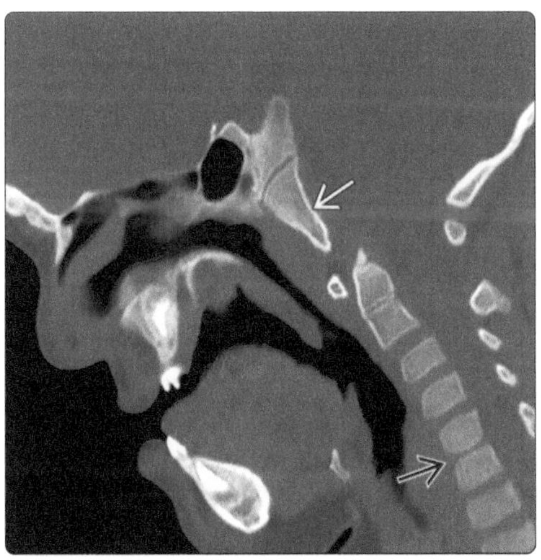

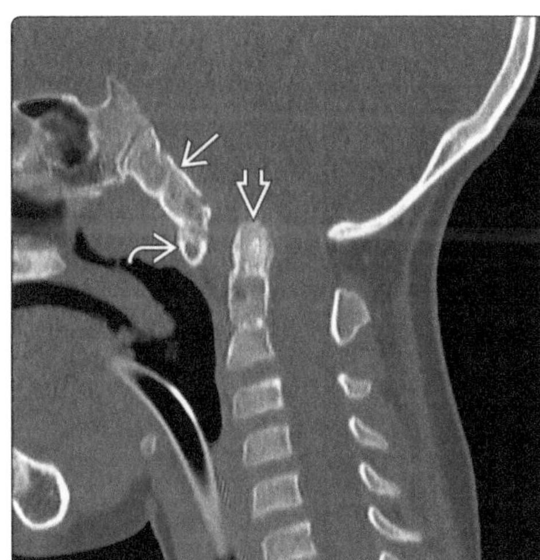

(Left) *Sagittal bone CT in a patient with multiple sutural craniosynostosis (Apert syndrome) shows characteristic vertical orientation of the clivus* ➡. *C5-C6 segmentation failure* ➡ *is relatively subtle in this young patient.* **(Right)** *Sagittal bone CT in a patient with myelopathy demonstrates aberrant thickened clivus* ➡ *with C1 anterior ring* ➡ *incorporation (atlantooccipital assimilation) and an abnormal bulbous elongated odontoid process* ➡.

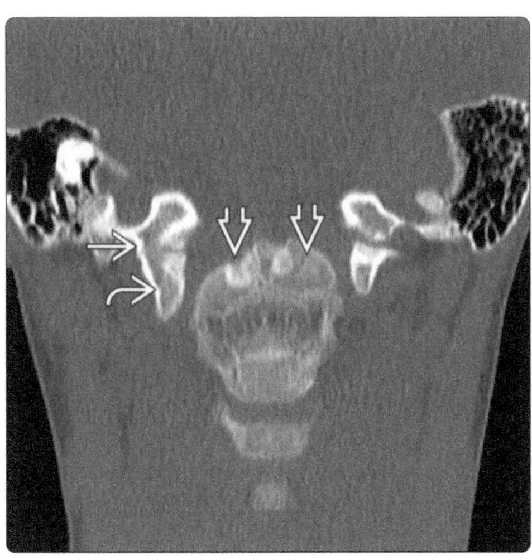

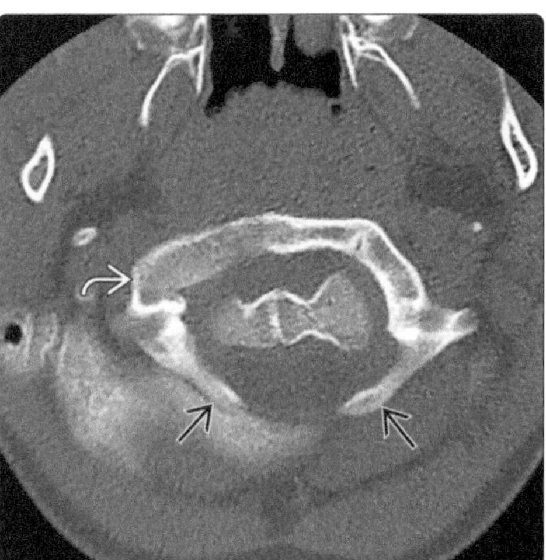

(Left) *Coronal bone CT in the same patient demonstrates unilateral incorporation of the right C1 lateral mass* ➡ *with the occipital condyle* ➡ *as well as a bizarre short and wide odontoid process* ➡. **(Right)** *Axial bone CT performed in the same patient shows the unusually wide C1 vertebra with thickened anterior ring* ➡ *and deficient posterior ring* ➡.

(Left) *Sagittal bone CT obtained in flexion shows assimilation of the anterior C1 ➡ with the basion and partial assimilation of the posterior C1 arch ➡ with the opisthion. There is a widened atlantodental interval and mild basilar invagination.* **(Right)** *Sagittal bone CT in a different patient reveals congenital assimilation of the anterior C1 ring ➡ with the clivus as well as fusion of the posterior C1 ring to the C2 spinous process ➡. This CVJ anatomic variation would be expected to produce reduced CVJ dynamic motion.*

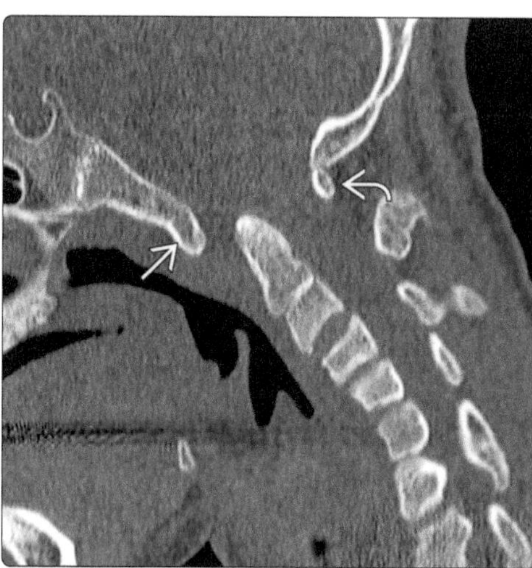

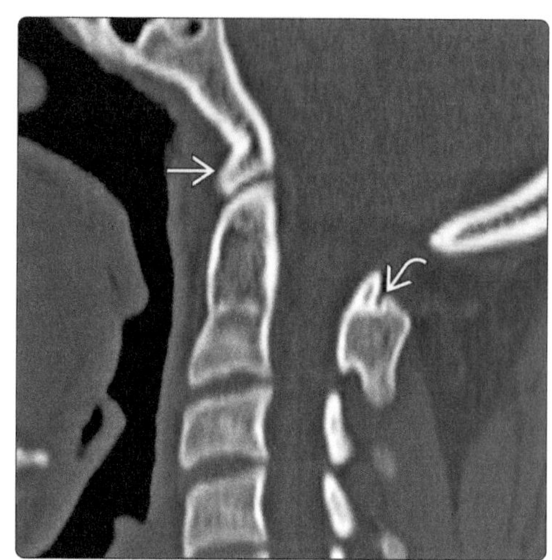

(Left) *Sagittal bone CT of the cervical spine shows fusion of the anterior C1 ring ➡ and an os odontoideum ➡. There is irregular margination of the inferior os and the odontoid base, suggesting that this finding may represent sequelae of unrecognized remote trauma.* **(Right)** *Axial bone CT in the same patient demonstrates the solid fusion of the os ➡ and the C1 ring ➡.*

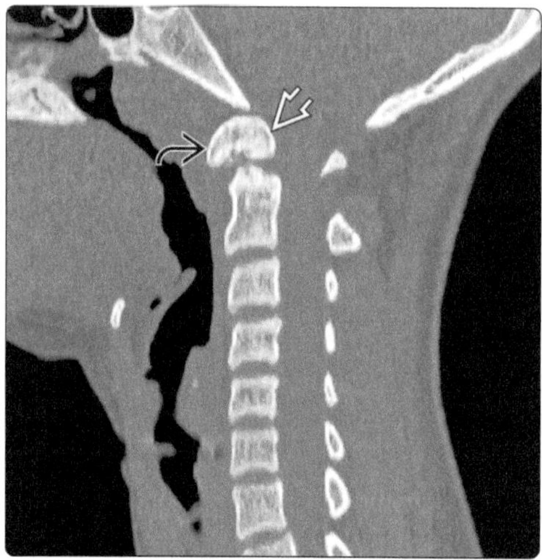

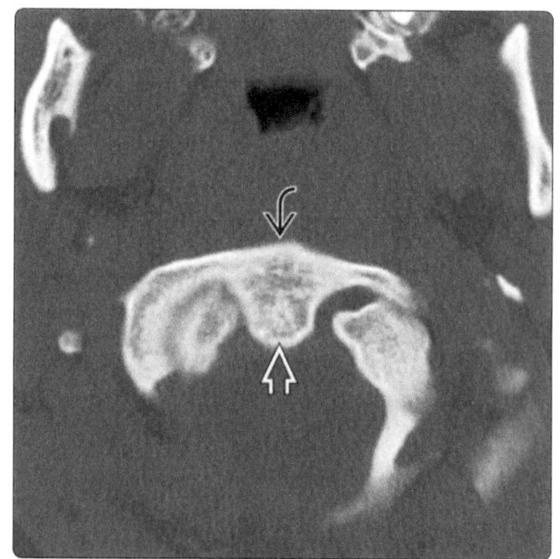

(Left) *Axial T1 MR (VACTERL) demonstrates moderately severe central canal stenosis at the C1 secondary to complete C1 ring hypoplasia. Note that the AP canal diameter is particularly reduced compared to transverse diameter.* **(Right)** *Axial bone CT depicts congenital fusion failure of the C1 ring with both anterior and posterior ring clefts ➡. Despite its bizarre appearance, this constellation of findings does not necessarily predispose to cervical instability.*

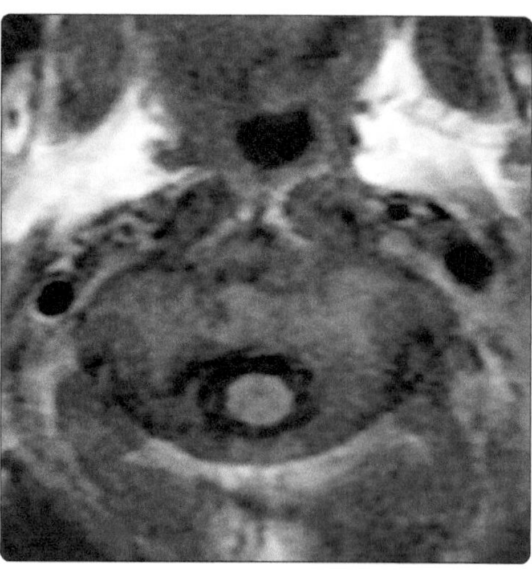

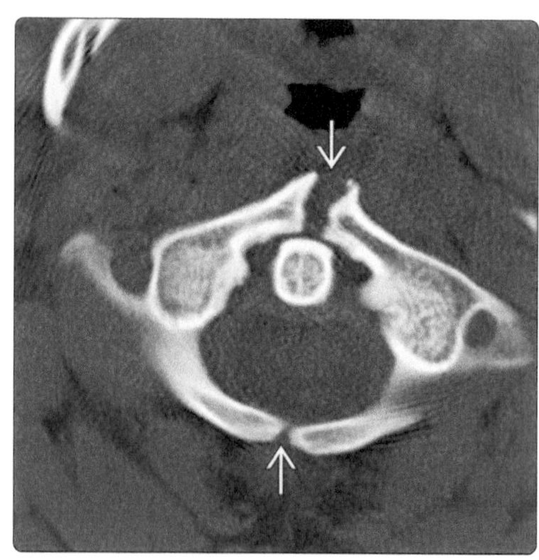

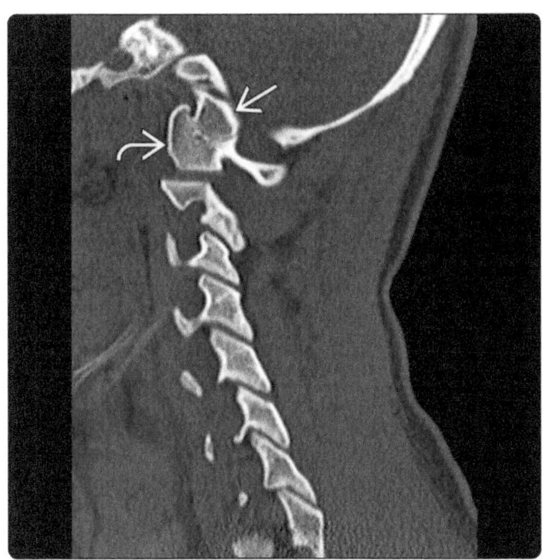

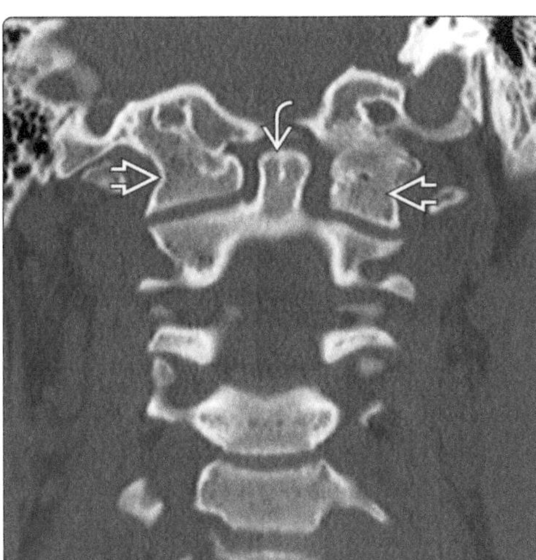

(Left) *Sagittal bone CT (Chiari 1, syringomyelia) depicts congenital craniocervical segmentation failure with "fusion" of the occipital condyles ➡ with the C1 lateral masses ➡. This is also known as atlantooccipital assimilation.* **(Right)** *Coronal bone CT in the same patient confirms congenital craniocervical segmentation failure with bilateral "fusion" of the occipital condyles and C1 lateral masses ➡. The odontoid process ➡ is mildly tilted to the left.*

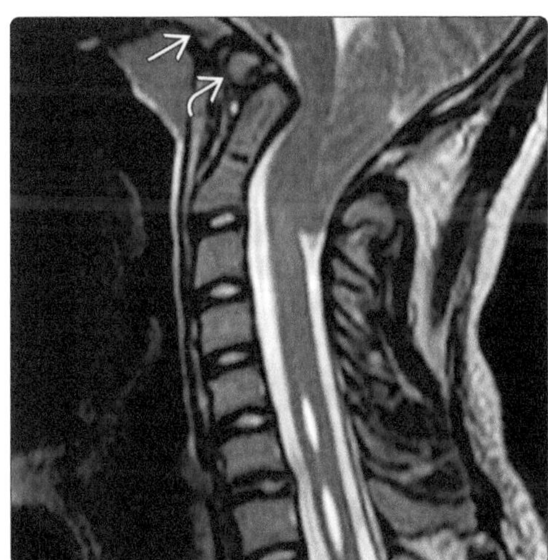

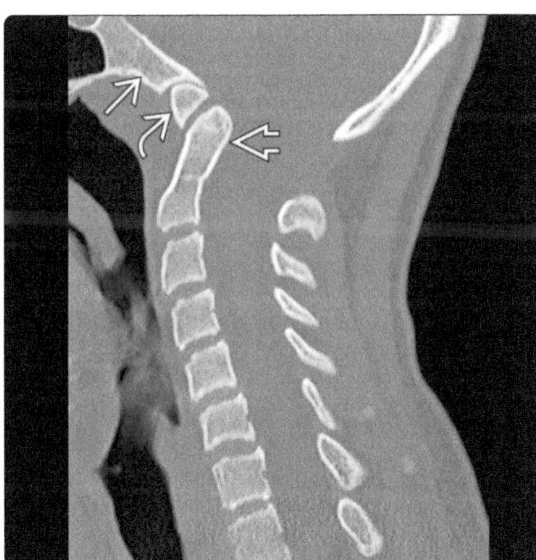

(Left) *Sagittal T2 MR (complex Chiari) demonstrates severe tonsillar ectopia, low-lying obex and prominent dorsal cervicomedullary "bump" (Chiari 1.5), and odontoid retroflexion with C1 anterior ring ➡ remodeling the clivus ➡.* **(Right)** *Sagittal midline bone CT in the same patient demonstrates aberrant odontoid retroflexion ➡ in conjunction with an abnormally large anterior C1 ring ➡ that articulates with and erodes the remodeled clivus ➡.*

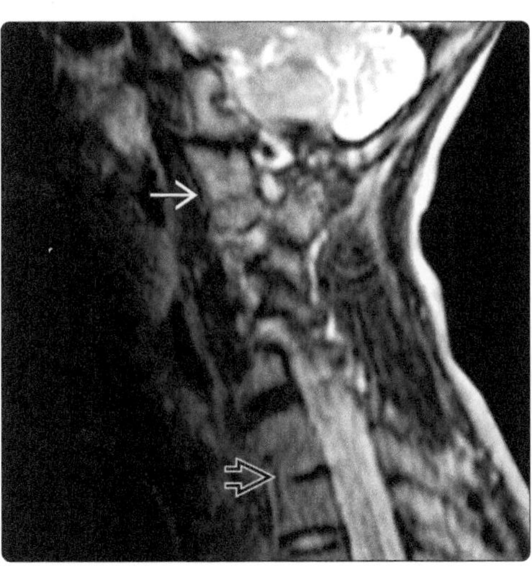

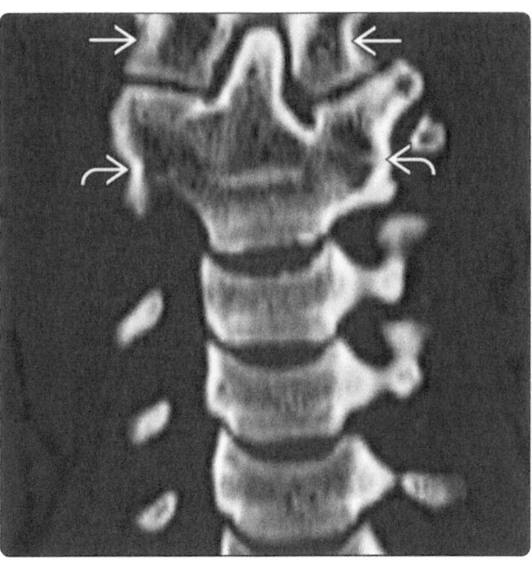

(Left) *Sagittal T2 MR (Klippel-Feil syndrome, atlantoaxial assimilation) obtained off-midline demonstrates multiple levels of upper cervical posterior element segmentation failure ➡ as well as lower cervical segmentation failure ➡.* **(Right)** *Coronal bone CT depicts congenital fusion of the C1 and C2 lateral masses ➡ (atlantoaxial assimilation). The occipital condyles ➡ show an abnormally flattened articular surface, and the odontoid process is tilted to the left.*

Klippel-Feil Spectrum

KEY FACTS

TERMINOLOGY

- Synonyms: Klippel-Feil syndrome
- Congenital spinal malformation characterized by segmentation failure of ≥ 2 cervical vertebrae ± thoracic, lumbar segmentation failure

IMAGING

- Single- or multiple-level congenital cervical segmentation and fusion anomalies
- C2-C3 (50%) > C5-C6 (33%) > craniovertebral junction (CVJ), upper thoracic spine
- Vertebral bodies usually smaller than normal
- Vertebral body narrowing ("wasp waist") at fused rudimentary disc space ± fusion of posterior elements

TOP DIFFERENTIAL DIAGNOSES

- Juvenile idiopathic arthritis
- Surgical fusion
- Chronic sequelae of discitis
- Ankylosing spondylitis

PATHOLOGY

- No universally accepted etiology; embryonic insult postulated between 4th and 8th weeks
- Sporadic; familial genetic component with variable expression identified in many patients

CLINICAL ISSUES

- Classic triad (33-50%): Short neck, low posterior hairline, and limited cervical motion
- In practice; however, wide variation in clinical, anatomic expression

DIAGNOSTIC CHECKLIST

- Much Klippel-Feil spectrum morbidity and nearly all mortality related to visceral system dysfunction
- Look for instability, progressive degenerative changes, cord/brainstem compression

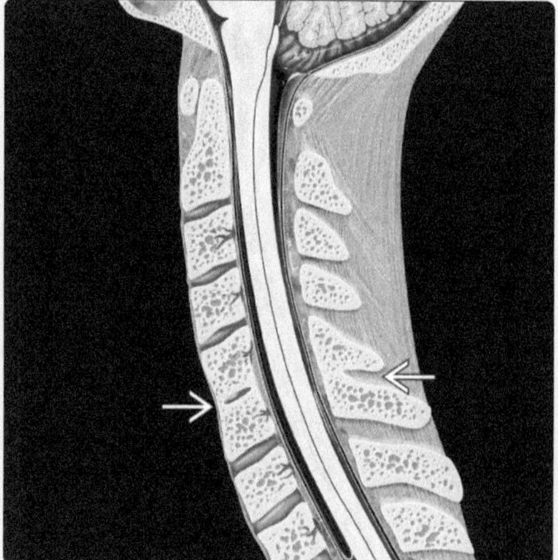

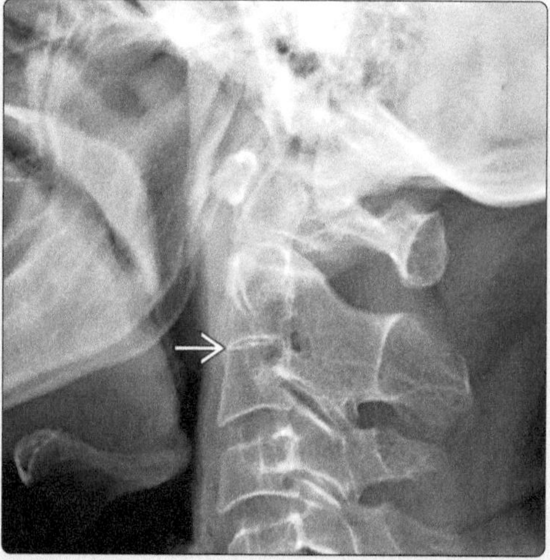

(Left) *Sagittal graphic of Klippel-Feil spectrum (KFS) type 2 shows congenital segmentation failure (fusion) ➡ of the C5-C6 vertebrae and spinous processes with characteristic rudimentary disc space and a distinctive "waist."* **(Right)** *Lateral radiograph (KFS type 2) demonstrates typical C2/C3 congenital segmentation failure (fusion) with characteristic rudimentary disc space ➡ and fusion of the facets and spinous processes. The disc space appearance helps distinguish from operative fusion.*

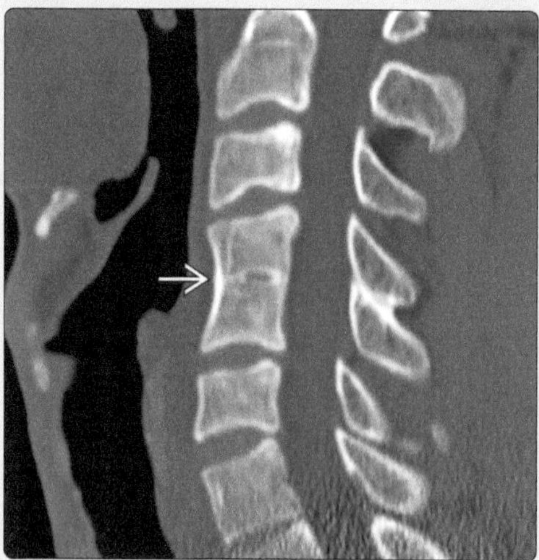

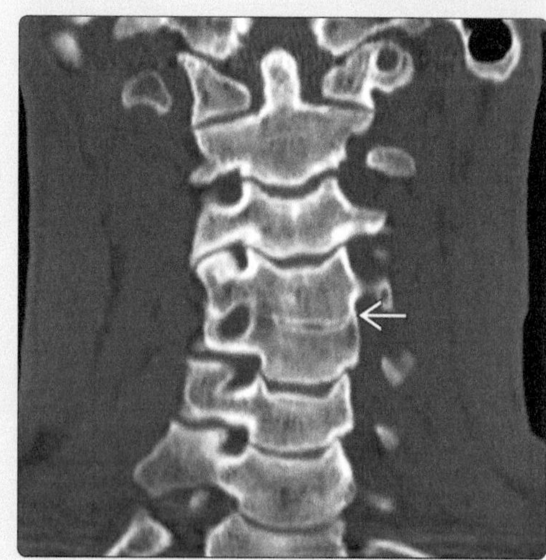

(Left) *Sagittal bone CT (KFS type 2) demonstrates single-level segmentation failure at C4-C5 ➡ with fusion of the spinous processes.* **(Right)** *Coronal bone CT in the same patient shows that C4-C5 disc space development ➡ is slightly less rudimentary on the left, resulting in convex left cervical curvature.*

TERMINOLOGY

Abbreviations

- Klippel-Feil spectrum (KFS)

Definitions

- Congenital spinal malformation characterized by segmentation failure of ≥ 2 cervical vertebrae ± thoracic, lumbar segmentation failure

IMAGING

General Features

- Best diagnostic clue
  - Single- or multiple-level congenital cervical segmentation and fusion anomalies
- Location
  - C2-C3 (50%) > C5-C6 (33%) > craniocervical junction (CVJ), upper thoracic spine
- Size
  - Vertebral bodies < normal size with tapered contour at fused disc space
  - Rudimentary disc space reduced in height, diameter
- Morphology
  - Vertebral body narrowing ("wasp waist") at fused rudimentary disc space ± fusion of posterior elements

Radiographic Findings

- Radiography
  - 1 or more fused vertebral levels with rudimentary, narrow disc space(s)
    - Disc space always abnormal; frequently fused facets and spinous processes
    - Adjacent disc spaces at mobile levels ± degenerative changes
  - ± omovertebral bone
  - Flexion/extension films → lack of motion between fused segments, ↑ mobility at nonfused levels

CT Findings

- Bone CT
  - Typical osseous findings ± degenerative changes
  - Sagittal, transverse spinal canal diameter usually normal
    - Narrowing reflects secondary degenerative changes adjacent to fused segments
    - Canal enlargement → consider syringomyelia

MR Findings

- T1WI
  - Cervical fusion(s); vertebral bodies ± facets, posterior elements
  - ± degenerative changes; spondylosis, disc herniations common (especially lower cervical spine)
  - ± CVJ osseous anomalies, Chiari 1
- T2WI
  - Osseous findings same as T1WI; normal marrow signal
  - ± cord or nerve root compression, syringomyelia, brainstem abnormalities, myeloschisis

Imaging Recommendations

- Best imaging tool
  - Radiography to evaluate and follow instability, degenerative changes
  - MR to exclude cord compression, detect degenerative changes
- Protocol advice
  - Serial neutral and flex/extend plain radiographs to detect progressive instability, degenerative disease
  - Multiplanar MR to evaluate canal compromise, cord compression, soft tissue degenerative changes
  - Ultrasound or CECT to detect and characterize associated visceral organ abnormalities

DIFFERENTIAL DIAGNOSIS

Juvenile Idiopathic Arthritis

- Difficult to distinguish from cervical block vertebra
- Search for other affected joints, appropriate history

Surgical Intervertebral Fusion

- No disc space "waist," facets infrequently ankylosed
- Surgical history key to making diagnosis

Chronic Sequelae of Discitis

- Irregular endplate margins, no "waist," ± kyphosis
- Confirm history of prior spinal infection

Ankylosing Spondylitis

- Delicate contiguous syndesmophytes ("bamboo spine") + symmetric sacroiliac joint disease
- HLA-B27 positive (95%)

PATHOLOGY

General Features

- Etiology
  - No universally accepted etiology; embryonic insult postulated between 4th and 8th weeks
    - Underlying molecular etiology remains largely unknown because of genetic, phenotypic heterogeneity
    - Association with other syndromes (fetal alcohol, Goldenhar, Wildervanck: Cervicoocculoacoustic)
    - Putative environmental causative factors include teratogens, maternal alcoholism
- Genetics
  - Sporadic; familial genetic component with variable expression identified in many patients
    - C2/C3 fusion (type 2) → autosomal dominant with variable penetrance
    - C5/C6 fusion (type 2) → autosomal recessive
  - *SGMI* (chromosome 8) → 1st Klippel-Feil gene identified; gene expression overlaps all 3 KFS types
  - Other associated genes include *GDF6, MEOX1, GDF3, MYO18B*, and *RIPPLY2*
- Associated abnormalities
  - Hemivertebrae, butterfly vertebrae, spina bifida
  - Scoliosis (usually congenital) ± kyphosis (60%)
  - Odontoid dysplasia, basilar impression, C1 assimilation, occipitocervical instability
  - Syringomyelia, diastematomyelia (20%), Chiari 1 (8%), neurenteric cyst or dermoid (rare)
  - Cervicomedullary neuroschisis ± synkinesis (20%)
  - Sprengel deformity ± omovertebral bone (15-30%); unilateral or bilateral

- Sensorineural hearing loss (30%), external ear anomalies, genitourinary tract abnormalities (35%), congenital heart disease (14%), upper extremity deformity, facial anomalies
- KFS often colloquially used for all patients with cervical congenital fusion anomalies regardless of extent
- Congenital cervical fusion 2° to failure of normal segmentation of cervical somites (3rd-8th weeks)

Staging, Grading, & Classification

- Type 1 (9%): Massive fusion of cervical, upper thoracic spine → severe neurologic impairment, frequent associated abnormalities
- Type 2 (84%): Fusion of ≥ 1 cervical vertebral interspaces
- Type 3 (7%): Fusions involve cervical and lower thoracic/lumbar vertebra

Gross Pathologic & Surgical Features

- Surgical observations correlate to imaging findings

Microscopic Features

- Histologically normal bone, disc

CLINICAL ISSUES

Presentation

- Most common signs/symptoms
  - Cosmesis complaints, neck or radicular pain, slowly progressive or acute myelopathy
    - Massive fusions often noted in infancy/early childhood 2° to cosmetic deformity
  - Neurologic problems in infancy, childhood usually 2° to CVJ abnormalities
  - Lower cervical fusions (unless massive) usually present ≥ 3rd decade when degenerative changes or instability of adjacent segments manifests
- Other signs/symptoms
  - Vocal impairment (usually > 1-level fusion)
  - Synkinesia (mirror movements): 20%, upper > lower extremity, diminish with time
- Clinical profile
  - Classic triad (33-50%): Short neck, low posterior hairline, and limited cervical motion
  - Wide variation in clinical and anatomic expression
    - Many patients have normal clinical appearance despite severity of involvement
    - Cervical motion limitation is most consistent clinical finding

Demographics

- Age
  - 2nd-3rd decades; spans entire range of life expectancy
- Sex
  - M ≤ F
- Epidemiology
  - 1/42,000 births

Natural History & Prognosis

- Progressive accelerated degenerative changes adjacent to fused segments
- 3 patterns at greatest risk for future instability
  - C0 → C3 fusion with occipitocervical synostosis
  - Long cervical fusion + abnormal C0/C1 junction
  - Single open interspace between 2 fused segments
- ↑ risk of neurologic injury following minor trauma 2° to hypermobility of cervical segments
  - High-risk patients: 2 sets of block vertebrae, occipitalization of atlas + basilar invagination, and cervical fusion + spinal stenosis
- 4 distinct phenotypes are significantly associated with surgical intervention necessity
  - Predominantly subaxial cervical spine fusions + thoracic spine abnormalities → thoracolumbar/sacral spine surgery
  - Axial cervical spine anomalies + cervical subluxation → cervical spine surgery
  - Chiari 1 → cranial surgery (suboccipital decompression)
  - Thoracic vertebral anomalies and associations with sacral agenesis and scoliosis → thoracolumbar/sacral spine surgery

Treatment

- Avoidance of contact sports, occupations, and recreational activities at risk for head or neck trauma
- Activity modification, bracing, and traction may reduce symptoms
- Neurologic lesion, significant pain despite conservative therapy, or progressive instability → decompression ± spinal fusion

DIAGNOSTIC CHECKLIST

Consider

- Much KFS morbidity and nearly all mortality related to visceral system dysfunction

Image Interpretation Pearls

- Look for instability, progressive degenerative changes, cord/brainstem compression

SELECTED REFERENCES

1. Courvoisier A: Congenital cervical spinal deformities. Orthop Traumatol Surg Res. 109(1S):103459, 2023
2. Motwani G et al: Cervical myelopathy in a child with Sprengel shoulder and Klippel-Feil syndrome. Spine Deform. 9(1):303-d9, 2021
3. Li Z et al: The mutational burden and oligogenic inheritance in Klippel-Feil syndrome. BMC Musculoskelet Disord. 21(1):220, 2020
4. Öner A et al: Sprengel deformity: comprehensive evaluation of concomitant spinal and extraspinal anomalies in 90 patients. Spine (Phila Pa 1976). 45(18):E1150-7, 2020
5. Nouri A et al: Demographics, presentation and symptoms of patients with Klippel-Feil syndrome: analysis of a global patient-reported registry. Eur Spine J. 28(10):2257-65, 2019
6. Gruber J et al: The prevalence of Klippel-Feil syndrome: a computed tomography-based analysis of 2,917 patients. Spine Deform. 6(4):448-53, 2018
7. Stelzer JW et al: Klippel-Feil syndrome with Sprengel deformity and extensive upper extremity deformity: a case report and literature review. Case Rep Orthop. 2018:5796730, 2018
8. Saker E et al: The intriguing history of vertebral fusion anomalies: the Klippel-Feil syndrome. Childs Nerv Syst. 32(9):1599-602, 2016
9. Jasper A et al: The multiple associations of Klippel-Feil syndrome. Acta Neurol Belg. 115(2):157-9, 2014
10. McLaughlin N et al: Klippel-Feil syndrome associated with a craniocervico-thoracic dermoid cyst. Surg Neurol Int. 4(Suppl 2):S61-6, 2013
11. Ogihara N et al: Surgical treatment of Klippel-Feil syndrome with basilar invagination. Eur Spine J. 22 Suppl 3:S380-7, 2013
12. Kumar D et al: Klippel-Feil syndrome with unilateral renal agenesis and renal failure. J Assoc Physicians India. 60:68-9, 2012
13. Apaydin M et al: Partial posterior split cervical spinal cord with Klippel-Feil syndrome. JBR-BTR. 93(1):30, 2010

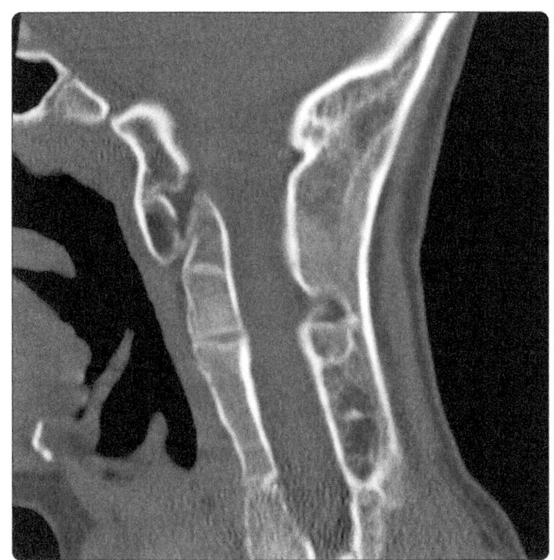

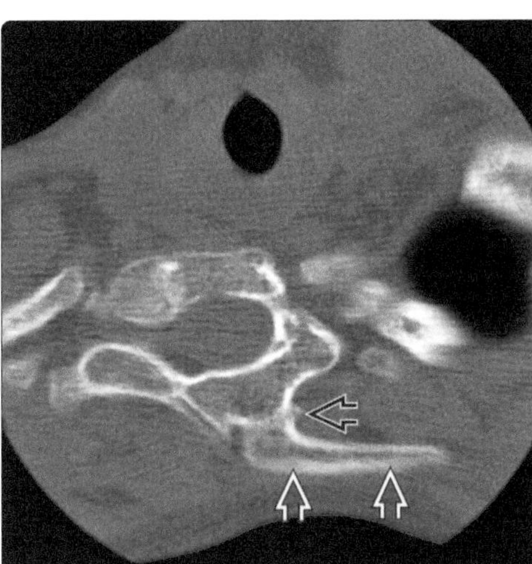

(Left) *Sagittal bone CT (KFS type 1) reveals extensive fusion of all cervical vertebrae and posterior elements with the characteristic hypoplastic appearance of the vertebrae and intervertebral disc spaces. Additionally in this patient, there is incorporation of C1 into the skull base ("occipitalization of the atlas").* **(Right)** *Axial bone CT of KFS type 1, severe segmentation anomalies demonstrates the vertebral articulation of a unilateral left omovertebral bone.*

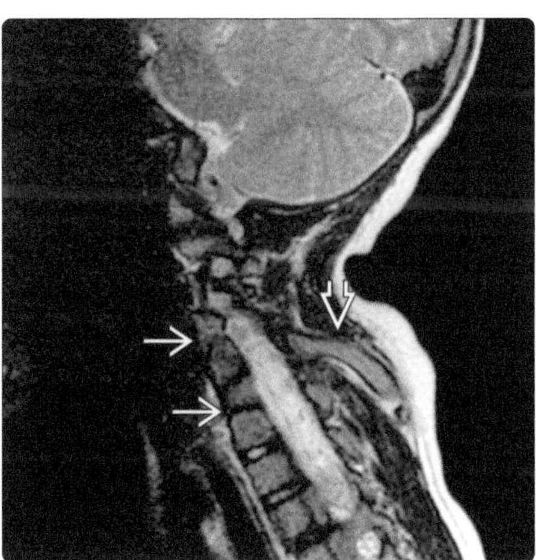

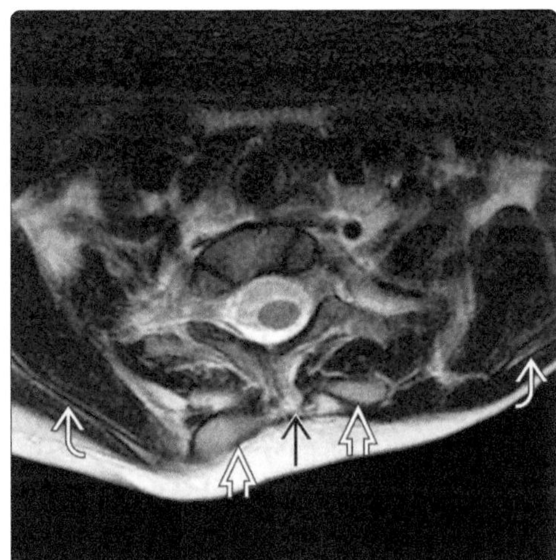

(Left) *Sagittal T2 MR of KFS type 1, bilateral omovertebral bones shows abnormal straightening of cervical lordosis and multiple vertebral segmentation anomalies. The omovertebral bone resides within the dorsal subcutaneous soft tissues and articulates with the posterior elements.* **(Right)** *Axial T2 MR of KFS type 1 depicts the MR appearance of bilateral omovertebral bones extending from the posterior spinal elements to the scapulae.*

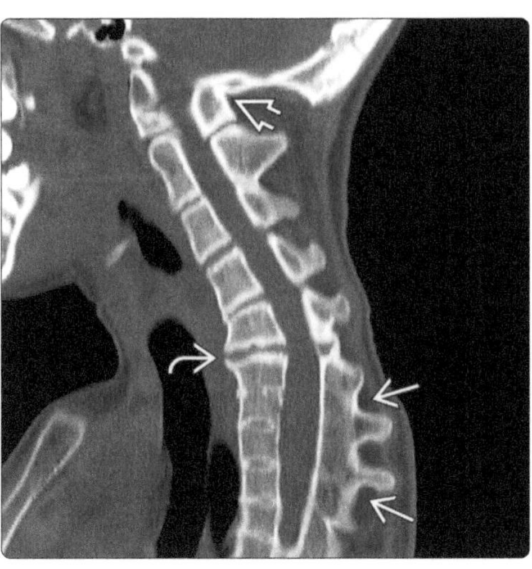

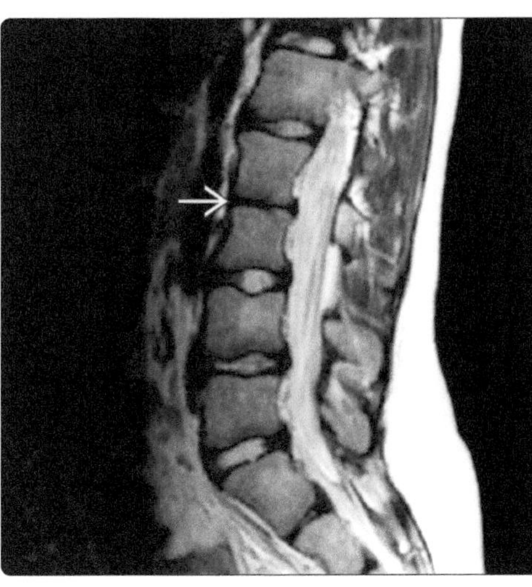

(Left) *Sagittal reformatted bone CT of the cervicothoracic spine shows extensive lack of segmentation in both the cervical and thoracic spinal column. Note the C1 spinous process fused to the occiput and fusion of bodies and posterior elements of C6-T4. There is accelerated disc degeneration at C5-C6, which is not fused.* **(Right)** *Sagittal T2 MR of KFS type 3 of the lumbar spine confirms that anomalous segmentation failure involves the lumbar spine as well as the cervical and thoracic spine (not shown).*

Failure of Vertebral Formation

KEY FACTS

TERMINOLOGY

- Vertebral dysplasia, segmentation and fusion anomaly (SFA), "disorganized spine"
- Partial or complete failure of vertebral formation

IMAGING

- Sharply angulated, single curve, or focal (kypho)scoliosis
- Hemivertebra, butterfly vertebra generally smaller than normal vertebra

TOP DIFFERENTIAL DIAGNOSES

- Vertebral fracture, history critical
- Inherited spinal dysplasias

PATHOLOGY

- Many genetic syndromes manifest vertebral dysplasia
  - However, no single gene explanation for vertebral formation anomalies
  - Nonisolated hemivertebra associated with diverse spectrum of cytogenetic abnormalities and single gene disorders
- Associated anomalies include dysraphism, split notochord syndromes, visceral anomalies (61% of congenital scoliosis patients)

CLINICAL ISSUES

- Many asymptomatic or detected during scoliosis evaluation
- Syndromal patients usually detected in infancy
  - Abnormal spine curvature ± neural deficits, limb or visceral abnormalities
  - Respiratory failure (impeded chest movement 2° to fused ribs, kyphoscoliosis)

DIAGNOSTIC CHECKLIST

- Important to look for and characterize associated visceral anomalies
- Type of deformity determines propensity for scoliosis progression

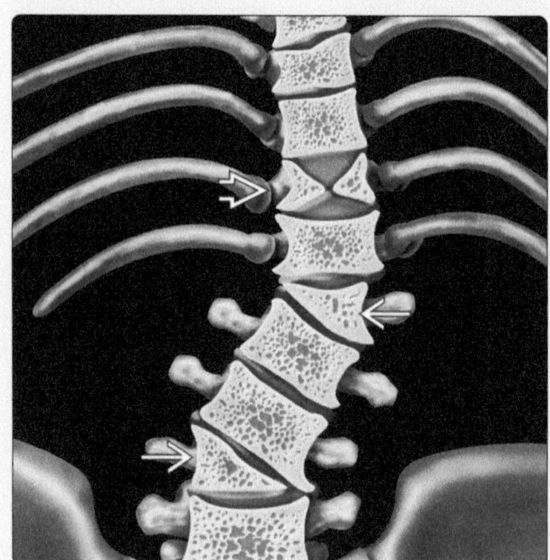

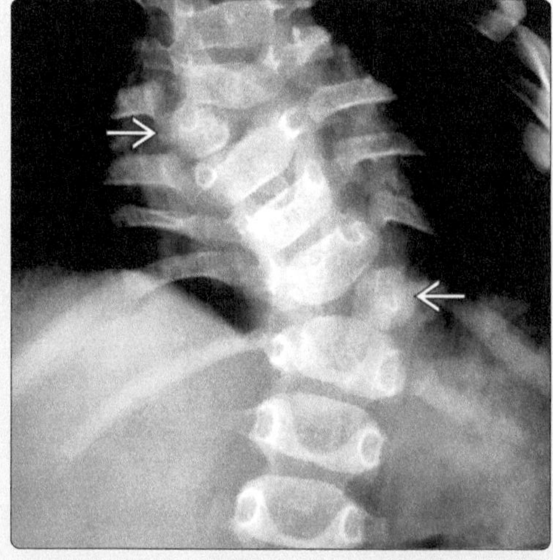

(Left) *Coronal graphic of the thoracolumbar spine demonstrates several different types of vertebral formation failure with segmented "balanced" L1 and L4 hemivertebrae ➡ and a T11 butterfly vertebra ➡.* **(Right)** *Anteroposterior radiograph shows segmented right T7 and left T11 hemivertebrae ➡ producing focal scoliotic curves. Because they mostly cancel each other's curve, this configuration is considered "balanced" for prognostic and treatment planning.*

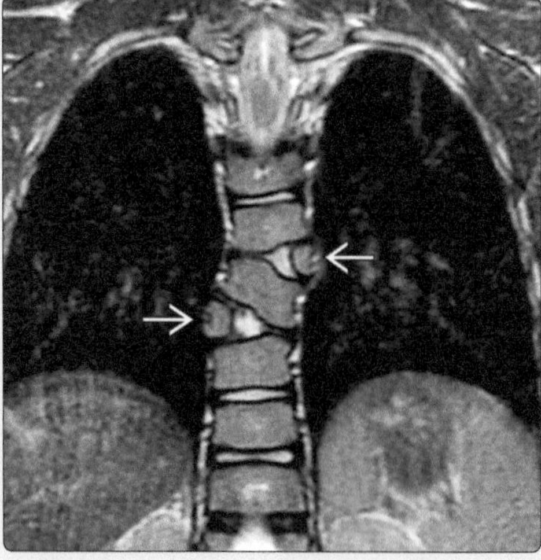

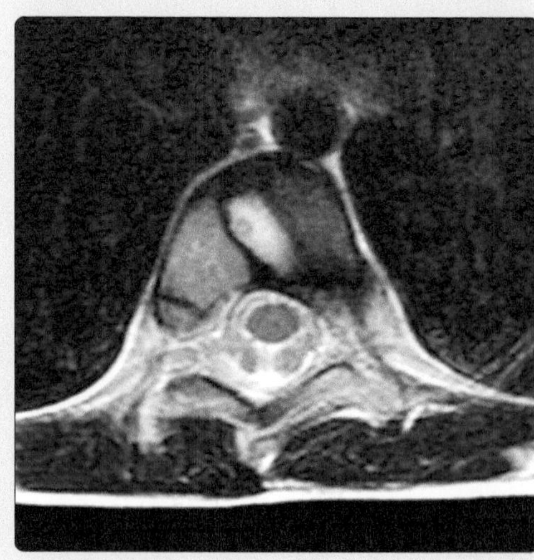

(Left) *Coronal T2WI MR demonstrates left T6 and right T8 hemivertebrae ➡. There is only minimal resultant leftward curvature because the hemivertebrae "balance" each other, and this curvature would not be expected to be rapidly progressive.* **(Right)** *Axial T2WI MR depicts the abnormal intervertebral disc-space appearance in the presence of a hemivertebra. Diagnosing a hemivertebra is most straightforward in the coronal plane and often difficult in the sagittal and axial planes.*

TERMINOLOGY

Synonyms

- Vertebral dysplasia, segmentation and fusion anomaly (SFA), "disorganized spine"

Definitions

- Partial or complete failure of vertebral formation (FVF)
  - Partial formation failure → wedge vertebra
  - Complete formation failure → vertebral aplasia, hemivertebra, butterfly vertebra

IMAGING

General Features

- Best diagnostic clue
  - Sharply angulated, single-curve, or focal scoliosis with deformed vertebral bodies
- Location
  - Thoracolumbar most common
- Size
  - Hemivertebra, butterfly vertebra generally smaller than normal vertebra
- Morphology
  - Incompletely formed vertebra; may be missing front, back, side, or middle of vertebral body

Radiographic Findings

- Radiography
  - Vertebral formation failure anomalies
  - ± scoliosis
    - Paired right and left hemivertebra → "balanced," scoliotic curves cancel out
    - 1 or more unilateral hemivertebra → "unbalanced," uncompensated scoliotic curve
  - Best modality for "counting" vertebral levels, determining presence and severity of scoliosis

CT Findings

- Bone CT
  - Sagittal or coronal vertebral clefts, hemivertebra, butterfly vertebra
    - Abnormal vertebra difficult to evaluate in axial plane; sagittal, coronal reformats helpful
  - ± posterior element dysraphism, fusion anomalies
    - Most readily evaluated in axial plane
  - 3D CT reformatted images best demonstrate vertebral anomalies for surgical planning

MR Findings

- T1WI
  - Vertebral formation failure anomalies
  - Normal marrow, disc signal intensity
- T2WI
  - Similar findings to T1WI
  - ± lipoma, tethered cord, diastematomyelia, spinal cord compression

Imaging Recommendations

- Best imaging tool
  - MR
- Protocol advice
  - Long-cassette weightbearing radiographs → quantitate scoliosis, "counting" to definitively localize abnormal vertebral level
  - Multiplanar T1WI, T2WI MR → identify vertebral anomalies, evaluate spinal cord and soft tissues
    - Most vertebral and spinal cord anomalies seen best in coronal, sagittal planes
  - 3D bone CT useful to characterize scoliosis and vertebral anomalies for preoperative planning

DIFFERENTIAL DIAGNOSIS

Vertebral Fracture, History Critical

- Pathologic
- Traumatic
- 2 pedicles per level
- Noncorticated irregular fracture margins ± soft tissue edema, cord injury

Inherited Spinal Dysplasias

- Mucopolysaccharidosis
- Achondroplasia
- Distinguish by characteristic imaging, clinical, and laboratory findings

PATHOLOGY

General Features

- Etiology
  - Total aplasia: Both chondral centers fail to develop early in development
  - Lateral hemivertebra: 1 chondral center does not develop; ossification center subsequently fails to develop on that side
  - Sagittal cleft (butterfly) vertebra: Separate ossification centers form (but fail to unite) in each paired paramedian chondrification center
  - Coronal cleft vertebra: Formation and persistence of separate ventral and dorsal ossification centers
  - Posterior hemivertebra: Later failure at ossification stage
- Genetics
  - Many genetic syndromes manifest vertebral dysplasia
  - Some result from deranged *PAX1* gene expression in developing vertebral column
  - WNT, fibroblast growth factor (FGF), and Notch signaling pathways also important for spine embryologic development
  - However, no single gene explanation for vertebral formation anomalies
    - Nonisolated hemivertebra associated with diverse spectrum of cytogenetic abnormalities and single gene disorders
- Associated abnormalities
  - Dysraphism, split notochord syndromes
    - Diastematomyelia, syrinx, tethered cord/fatty filum, congenital tumor, visceral organ anomalies
  - Other developmental vertebral abnormalities
    - Partial duplication (supernumerary hemivertebra)
    - Segmentation failure (block vertebra, posterior element dysraphism, pediculate bar, neural arch fusion)

- Visceral abnormalities; 61% of congenital scoliosis patients
  - Tracheoesophageal fistula common association (part of VACTERL)
  - Butterfly vertebra associated with Alagille syndrome
- Concurrent intraspinal anomalies reported more common in vertebral segmentation failure (VSF) and mixed anomalies than FVF
- Normal vertebral formation occurs over 3 sequential periods
  - Membrane development: Segmental formation of medial sclerotome (vertebral bodies) and lateral myotome (paraspinal muscles)
  - Chondrification: Sclerotomes separate transversely and join with adjacent sclerotomal halves → paired chondrification sites develop in vertebral bodies and neural arches
  - Ossification: Chondral skeleton ossifies from single ossification center
- Segmentation and fusion anomalies result from aberrant vertebral column formation
  - Abnormal vertebrae may be supranumerary or replace normal vertebral body
  - More severe SFA → higher likelihood of associated visceral anomalies
- Imaging appearance of vertebral formation failure determined by deficient vertebral body portion
  - Anterior formation failure (common) → sharply angulated kyphosis
  - Posterior formation failure (rare) → hyperlordotic curve
  - Lateral formation failure (common) → classic hemivertebrae of congenital scoliosis
- Hemivertebra variants subclassified as incarcerated, nonincarcerated, segmented, nonsegmented, or semisegmented
  - Incarcerated: Vertebral bodies above and below shaped to accommodate hemivertebrae → do not generally produce scoliosis
  - Nonincarcerated: Found at scoliosis apex, curve magnitude depends on size of wedged segment
  - Segmented ("free"): Normal discs above and below hemivertebra → progressive scoliosis due to unbalanced growth
  - Nonsegmented: Lack disc spaces between wedged, normal adjacent vertebral bodies
  - Semisegmented: Normal disc space on 1 side, nonsegmented on other side
- Segmental spinal dysgenesis (SSD) = rare congenital abnormality in which 1 segment of vertebral column/spinal cord fails to develop properly
  - Spinal cord thinned or indiscernible at abnormality level; bulky, low-lying cord segment caudad to focal abnormality in most cases
  - Severity of morphologic derangement correlates with residual spinal cord function, severity of clinical deficit

Gross Pathologic & Surgical Features

- Normal bone density unless concurrent metabolic abnormality
- Surgical observations of vertebral configuration matches imaging findings

Microscopic Features

- Normal bone histology unless concurrent metabolic abnormality

CLINICAL ISSUES

Presentation

- Most common signs/symptoms
  - Asymptomatic
  - Abnormal spine curvature ± neural deficits, limb or visceral abnormalities
- Other signs/symptoms
  - Respiratory failure (impeded chest movement 2° to fused ribs, kyphoscoliosis) → rare
- Clinical profile
  - Most are asymptomatic or detected during scoliosis evaluation
  - Syndromal patients usually detected in infancy

Demographics

- Age
  - Usually diagnosed in infancy to early childhood
  - Mild cases may present in adulthood
- Sex
  - M ≈ F
- Epidemiology
  - Isolated or syndromal, singular or multiple
  - Incidence increased with parental consanguinity, concurrent multisystem anomalies

Natural History & Prognosis

- Scoliosis is frequently progressive
  - Expectant watching, early intervention if warranted to prevent development of severe deformities

Treatment

- Conservative in mild cases (orthotics, observation)
- Surgical resection &/or fusion to arrest/reverse kyphoscoliosis in moderate to severe cases

DIAGNOSTIC CHECKLIST

Consider

- Syndromal origin or association → important to look for and characterize visceral anomalies

Image Interpretation Pearls

- Look for concurrent segmentation failure, other neural and visceral anomalies
- Type of deformity determines propensity for scoliosis progression

SELECTED REFERENCES

1. Gao R et al: Medium-term and long-term follow-up surgical outcomes of the 1-stage posterior-only lumbosacral hemivertebra resection with short-segment fusion in children. J Pediatr Orthop. 43(2):e120-6, 2023
2. Gill KG: Congenital musculoskeletal anomalies - key radiographic findings. Pediatr Radiol. 52(4):777-85, 2022
3. Powel JE et al: Genetics of non-isolated hemivertebra: a systematic review of fetal, neonatal, and infant cases. Clin Genet. 102(4):262-87, 2022
4. Aboughalia H et al: Multimodality imaging evaluation of fetal spine anomalies with postnatal correlation. Radiographics. 41(7):2176-92, 2021
5. Johal J et al: Hemivertebrae: a comprehensive review of embryology, imaging, classification, and management. Childs Nerv Syst. 32(11):2105-9, 2016

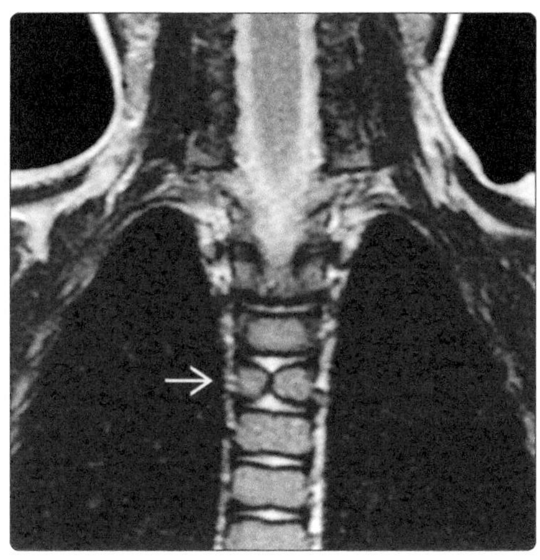

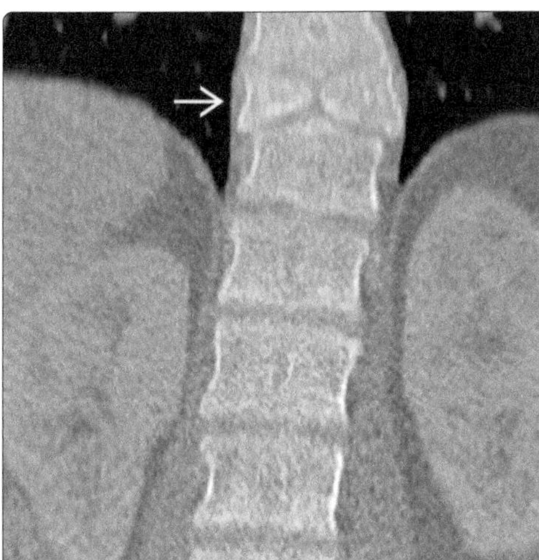

(Left) *Coronal T2WI MR from a thoracic spine MR depicts a typical thoracic butterfly vertebra ➡. This was an incidental finding. A butterfly vertebra typically results in no scoliotic curvature and may be asymptomatic. In a patient with cholestasis, consider Alagille syndrome.* **(Right)** *Coronal bone CT obtained during a trauma evaluation demonstrates an incidentally detected thoracic butterfly vertebra ➡. The characteristic shape and corticated margins distinguish a butterfly vertebra from an acute fracture.*

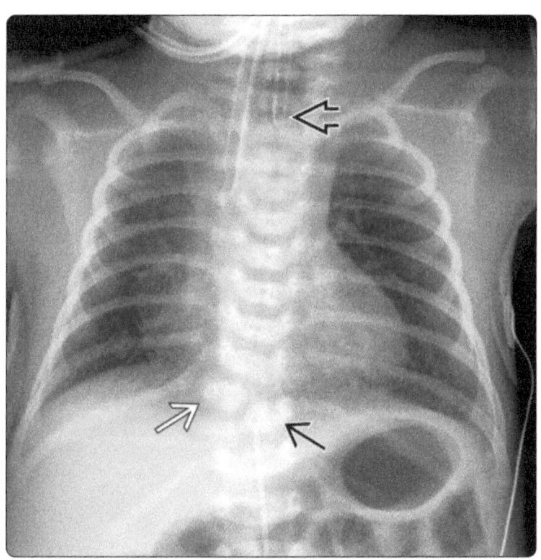

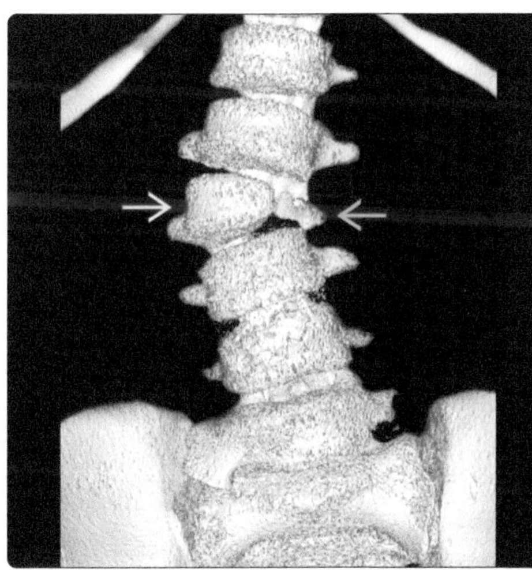

(Left) *AP radiograph of the chest in a newborn with tracheoesophageal fistula (Replogle tube in proximal esophageal pouch ⇨) shows right T10 ➡ and left T11 ⇨ hemivertebra with associated rib dysplasia. These findings led to a diagnosis of VACTERL association.* **(Right)** *Coronal 3D bone CT demonstrates an unbalanced right L3 hemivertebra ➡, resulting in focal convex right congenital scoliotic curvature. In this instance, there are rudimentary left L3 pedicle and posterior elements ⇨.*

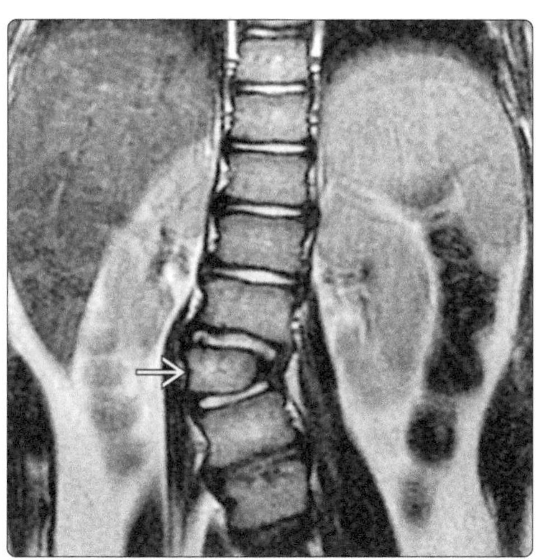

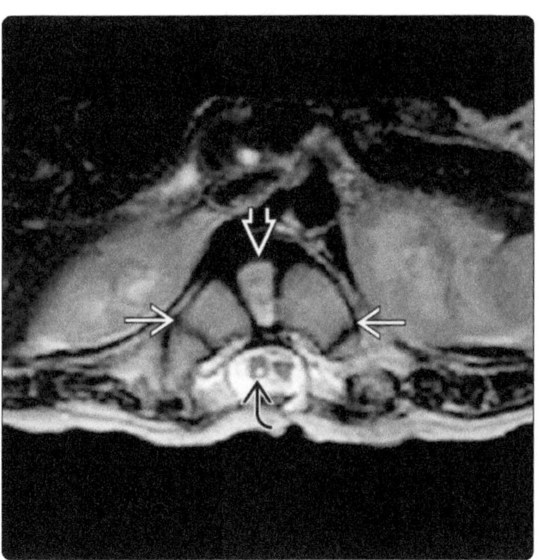

(Left) *Coronal T2WI MR of the thoracolumbar spine obtained for a scoliosis evaluation reveals a segmented, unbalanced right L3 hemivertebra ➡. The unilateral unbalanced configuration produces convex right focal congenital scoliosis.* **(Right)** *Axial T2WI MR (myelomeningocele, diastematomyelia) at the T10 level shows a bizarre, abnormally widened vertebra representing a butterfly vertebra ➡ with an abnormal intervertebral disc ➡. Note that the right hemicord ⇨ shows syringomyelia.*

Vertebral Segmentation Failure

KEY FACTS

TERMINOLOGY

- Synonyms: Segmentation anomaly, segmentation & fusion anomaly (SFA), block vertebra

IMAGING

- Sharply angulated, focal scoliotic curvature with abnormal fused vertebra
  - Ranges single level → extensive multilevel involvement
  - Lumbar > cervical > thoracic
- May have scoliosis, kyphosis, cord compression
- Search for related fused pedicles, ribs, posterior elements

TOP DIFFERENTIAL DIAGNOSES

- Juvenile chronic arthritis
- Surgical vertebral fusion
- Chronic sequelae of discitis
- Ankylosing spondylitis

PATHOLOGY

- Deranged *PAX1* gene expression → abnormal notochord signaling in developing vertebral column
- Many syndromes associated with SFA
- Associations include other neuraxis anomalies, renal, gastrointestinal, congenital cardiac defects

CLINICAL ISSUES

- Usually asymptomatic or present with kyphoscoliosis
- Less commonly, neural deficit, limb or visceral anomalies, respiratory failure
- Scoliosis frequently progressive

DIAGNOSTIC CHECKLIST

- Clinical manifestations variable, determined by type of SFA & syndromal association
- Block vertebra usually larger than single normal vertebral body

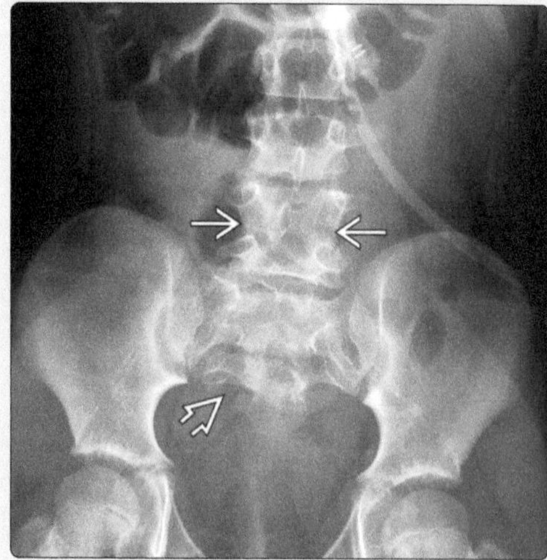

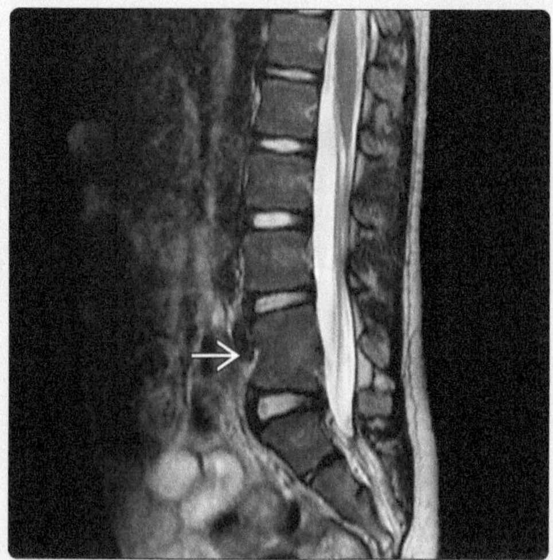

(Left) *AP radiograph demonstrates segmentation failure of L4 and L5 ➡, producing a block vertebra. Additionally, the right hemisacrum is hypoplastic ⇨.* **(Right)** *Sagittal T2WI MR of the lumbar spine depicts congenital segmentation failure at L4-L5 ➡. There is relative underdevelopment of the anterior vertebral body relative to the posterior vertebral body, resulting in mild kyphotic angulation and straightening of lumbar lordosis. Sacral hypoplasia is also noted.*

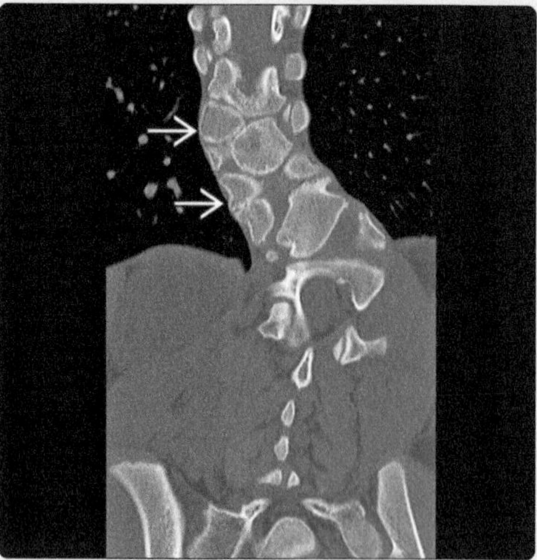

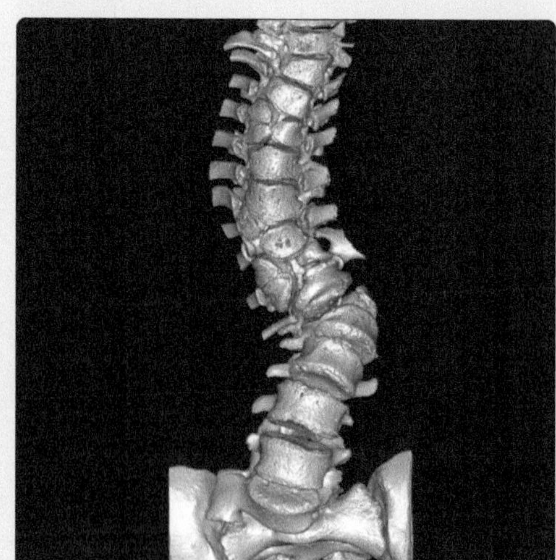

(Left) *Coronal bone CT shows multiple examples of vertebral segmentation failure with several right-sided hemivertebra ➡ that have failed to successfully segment, producing a jumble of malformed vertebra.* **(Right)** *Coronal 3D bone CT reformat shows convex right thoracic and convex left thoracolumbar kyphoscoliosis, resulting from multiple levels of vertebral segmentation failure. 3D CT is best for fully characterizing contribution of the various anomalous vertebra to scoliosis and kyphosis for treatment planning.*

TERMINOLOGY

Synonyms

- Segmentation anomaly, segmentation & fusion anomaly (SFA), block vertebra, disorganized spine

Definitions

- Vertebral column malformations (block vertebra, neural arch fusion, pediculate bar) resulting from deranged embryologic development → failure of normal segmentation

IMAGING

General Features

- Best diagnostic clue
  - Sharply angulated, focal scoliotic curvature with abnormal fused vertebra
- Location
  - Lumbar > cervical > thoracic
- Size
  - Ranges from single level → extensive multilevel involvement
  - Block vertebra usually larger than single normal vertebral body
- Morphology
  - Incomplete vertebral body segmentation, fused posterior elements, & large, misshapen vertebral bodies incorporating 1 or more levels

Radiographic Findings

- Radiography
  - Deformed, fused vertebra ± scoliosis, kyphosis
  - Upright images with lateral & AP bending assess weightbearing effect on scoliosis

CT Findings

- Bone CT
  - Incomplete vertebral body segmentation
    - Large, misshapen vertebral bodies incorporating 1 or more levels
    - ± fused pedicles, ribs, posterior elements

MR Findings

- T1WI
  - Deformed, fused vertebral bodies & posterior elements
  - ± scoliosis
  - Normal marrow signal intensity
- T2WI
  - Findings similar to T1WI
  - ± scoliosis, cord compression

Imaging Recommendations

- Best imaging tool
  - Weightbearing plain radiographs to evaluate scoliosis, "count" abnormal vertebral levels
  - MR
    - Multiplanar T1WI to evaluate vertebral anatomy
      - ▫ Vertebral anomalies seen best in coronal, sagittal planes
    - T2WI to evaluate spinal cord pathology, compression
  - 3D CT reformats to characterize osseous structures, preoperative planning

DIFFERENTIAL DIAGNOSIS

Juvenile Chronic Arthritis

- Difficult to distinguish from cervical block vertebra
- Search for other affected joints, appropriate clinical history

Surgical Fusion

- No "waist" at disc space level; facets infrequently ankylosed
- Surgical history key to making diagnosis

Chronic Sequelae of Discitis

- Cortical endplate margins irregular, "waist" absent
- Search for history of prior spinal infection

Ankylosing Spondylitis

- Delicate contiguous syndesmophytes ("bamboo spine") + symmetric sacroiliac (SI) joint disease
- HLA-B27 positive (95%)

PATHOLOGY

General Features

- Etiology
  - Segmentation & fusion anomalies result from aberrant vertebral column formation
  - Mildest (& most common) form is indeterminate (transitional) vertebrae at thoracolumbar, lumbosacral transition
- Genetics
  - Deranged *PAX1* gene expression → abnormal notochord signaling in developing vertebral column
  - Vertebral formation regulated by WNT, FGF, & Notch signaling pathways
    - Each somite is later subdivided into ventromedial sclerotome (forms vertebral body) & dorsolateral dermomyotome (forms body skeletal muscles & dorsal dermis)
    - Any defect of paraxial mesoderm or somite formation may contribute to congenital vertebral malformations
  - Many syndromes associated with SFA
    - Klippel-Feil (cervical SFA): Common, gene locus 8q22.2
    - Spondylothoracic dysplasia (Jarcho-Levin): Thoracic spine segmentation failure in crab-like array with multiple rib fusions
    - VACTERL (V = vertebral malformations, A = anal abnormalities, C = cardiac malformations, TE = tracheoesophageal fistula, & L = limb malformations)
- Associated abnormalities
  - Other neuraxis anomalies (40%)
    - Dysraphism, split notochord syndrome
    - Partial or complete failure of formation (vertebral aplasia, hemivertebra, butterfly vertebra)
    - Partial duplication (supernumerary hemivertebra)
  - Scoliosis
  - Renal, gastrointestinal, congenital cardiac defects
- Normal embryology: Vertebral formation occurs over 3 sequential periods
  - Membrane development: Segmental formation of medial sclerotome (vertebral bodies) & lateral myotome (paraspinal muscles)

- Chondrification: Sclerotomes separate transversely & join with adjacent sclerotomal halves → paired chondrification sites develop in vertebral bodies, neural arches
- Ossification: Chondral skeleton ossifies from single ossification center

Staging, Grading, & Classification

- Block vertebra: Failure of ≥ 2 vertebral somites to segment
  - Combined vertebrae may be normal height, short, or tall
  - Disc space frequently rudimentary or absent
  - Frequent association with hemivertebra/absent vertebra above or below block level, posterior element fusion
- Posterior neural arch anomalies
  - Failure to unite in midline → dysraphism (± unilateral pedicle aplasia/hypoplasia)
  - Unfused spinous processes; L5, S1 > C1 > C7 > T1 > lower thoracic spine
  - Multiple level posterior fusion → congenital vertebral bar

Gross Pathologic & Surgical Features

- Normal bone density unless concurrent metabolic abnormality
- Surgical observations of vertebral configuration matches imaging findings

Microscopic Features

- Normal bone histology unless concurrent metabolic abnormality

CLINICAL ISSUES

Presentation

- Most common signs/symptoms
  - Asymptomatic
  - Kyphoscoliosis
- Other signs/symptoms
  - Neural deficits (usually myelopathic), limb or visceral anomalies
  - Respiratory failure (rare, 2° impeded chest movement due to severe scoliosis, rib cage fusion)
- Clinical profile
  - Asymptomatic incidental detection or presents for evaluation of abnormal spine curvature

Demographics

- Age
  - Severe cases detected during infancy/childhood; mild cases may present as adults
- Sex
  - M ~ F; dependent on syndromal association
- Epidemiology
  - Isolated or syndromal, singular or multiple
  - SFAs account for 18% of scoliosis; incidence higher with multisystem abnormalities, parental consanguinity

Natural History & Prognosis

- Scoliosis frequently progressive
  - Unilateral unsegmented bar with contralateral hemivertebrae → rapidly progressive, severely deforming congenital scoliosis
  - Isolated block vertebra rarely produce scoliosis
- Abnormal segments may continue to fuse

Treatment

- Conservative in mild cases (orthotics, observation)
- Surgical fusion to arrest/reverse kyphoscoliosis in moderate to severe cases

DIAGNOSTIC CHECKLIST

Consider

- Clinical manifestations variable, determined by type of SFA & syndromal association

Image Interpretation Pearls

- Coronal MR, AP radiography best for detecting & characterizing SFAs, "counting" abnormal vertebral levels

SELECTED REFERENCES

1. Wu N et al: Retrospective analysis of associated anomalies in 636 patients with operatively treated congenital scoliosis. J Bone Joint Surg Am. 105(7):537-48, 2023
2. Krenn VA et al: The morphological consequences of segmentation anomalies in the human sacrum. Am J Biol Anthropol. 177(4):690-707, 2022
3. Aboughalia H et al: Multimodality imaging evaluation of fetal spine anomalies with postnatal correlation. Radiographics. 41(7):2176-92, 2021
4. Chaturvedi A et al: Malformed vertebrae: a clinical and imaging review. Insights Imaging. 9(3):343-55, 2018
5. Pahys JM et al: What's new in congenital scoliosis? J Pediatr Orthop. 38(3):e172-9, 2018
6. Tian Y et al: "Sandwich deformity" in Klippel-Feil syndrome: a "full-spectrum" presentation of associated craniovertebral junction abnormalities. J Clin Neurosci. 53:247-9, 2018
7. Chen W et al: Progress and perspective of TBX6 gene in congenital vertebral malformations. Oncotarget. 7(35):57430-41, 2016
8. Gupta N et al: Vertebral and intraspinal anomalies in Indian population with congenital scoliosis: a study of 119 consecutive patients. Asian Spine J. 10(2):276-81, 2016
9. Johal J et al: Hemivertebrae: a comprehensive review of embryology, imaging, classification, and management. Childs Nerv Syst. 32(11):2105-9, 2016
10. Trenga AP et al: Patterns of congenital bony spinal deformity and associated neural anomalies on X-ray and magnetic resonance imaging. J Child Orthop. 10(4):343-52, 2016
11. Ghandhari H et al: Vertebral, rib, and intraspinal anomalies in congenital scoliosis: a study on 202 Caucasians. Eur Spine J. 24(7):1510-21, 2015
12. Ramadorai U et al: Incidental findings on magnetic resonance imaging of the spine in the asymptomatic pediatric population: a systematic review. Evid Based Spine Care J. 5(2):95-100, 2014
13. Solomon BD et al: An approach to the identification of anomalies and etiologies in neonates with identified or suspected VACTERL (vertebral defects, anal atresia, tracheo-esophageal fistula with esophageal atresia, cardiac anomalies, renal anomalies, and limb anomalies) association. J Pediatr. 164(3):451-7.e1, 2014
14. Xue X et al: Klippel-Feil syndrome in congenital scoliosis. Spine (Phila Pa 1976). 39(23):E1353-8, 2014
15. Eckalbar WL et al: Scoliosis and segmentation defects of the vertebrae. Wiley Interdiscip Rev Dev Biol. 1(3):401-23, 2012
16. Thawait GK et al: Spine segmentation and enumeration and normal variants. Radiol Clin North Am. 50(4):587-98, 2012
17. Kawakami N et al: Classification of congenital scoliosis and kyphosis: a new approach to the three-dimensional classification for progressive vertebral anomalies requiring operative treatment. Spine (Phila Pa 1976). 34(17):1756-65, 2009
18. Menezes AH: Craniocervical developmental anatomy and its implications. Childs Nerv Syst. 24(10):1109-22, 2008
19. Tsirikos AI et al: Congenital anomalies of the ribs and chest wall associated with congenital deformities of the spine. J Bone Joint Surg Am. 87(11):2523-36, 2005
20. Arlet V et al: Congenital scoliosis. Eur Spine J. 12(5):456-63, 2003
21. Cornier AS et al: Controversies surrounding Jarcho-Levin syndrome. Curr Opin Pediatr. 15(6):614-20, 2003
22. Isono M et al: Limited dorsal myeloschisis associated with multiple vertebral segmentation disorder. Pediatr Neurosurg. 36(1):44-7, 2002
23. Kim YJ et al: Surgical treatment of congenital kyphosis. Spine. 26(20):2251-7, 2001

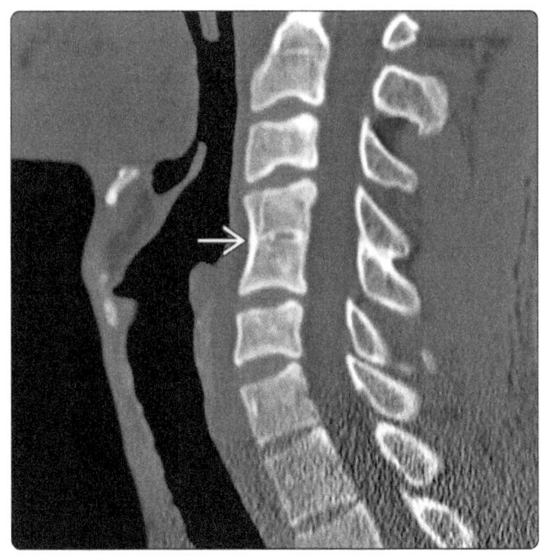

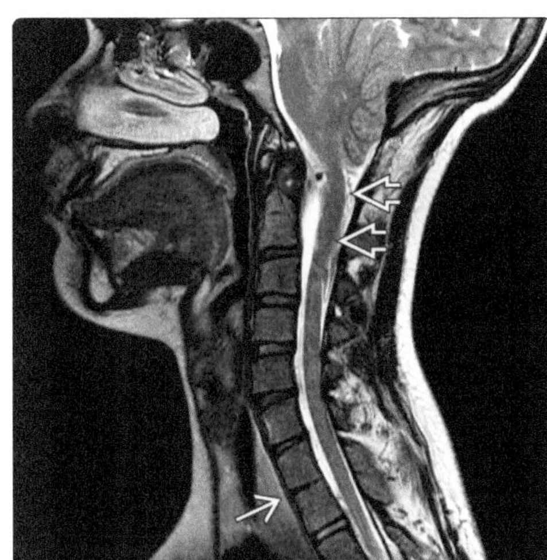

(Left) *Sagittal bone CT in a patient with Klippel-Feil syndrome shows mild single-level congenital segmentation failure at C4-C5 ➡. A narrow "waist" at the rudimentary disc space and fused spinous processes is typical.* **(Right)** *Sagittal T2WI MR in a patient with Chiari 2 shows characteristic posterior fossa malformation findings with vermian extension ➡ into the upper cervical spinal canal and vertebral segmentation failure of C7 and T1 ➡ with fusion of the spinous processes and facets.*

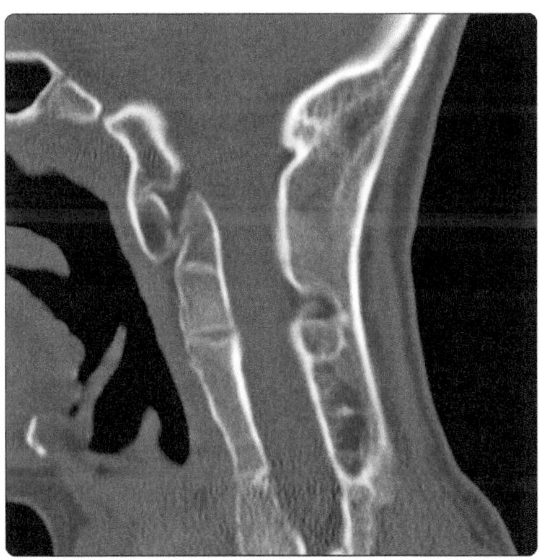

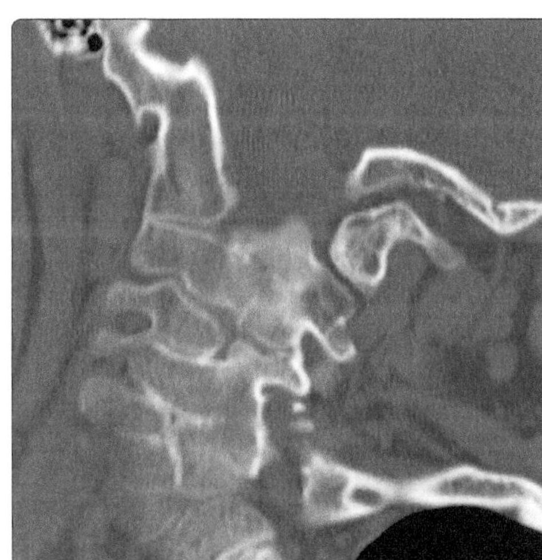

(Left) *Sagittal bone CT in a patient with severe Klippel-Feil syndrome reveals fusion at all cervical levels as well as incorporation of C1 into the skull base. The narrow vertebrae are typical of congenital segmentation failure.* **(Right)** *Coronal bone CT in a patient with severe Klippel-Feil spectrum show dens hypoplasia and fusion of the right occipital condyle, C1 lateral mass, and C2 lateral mass. The left C1 lateral mass is not incorporated into either the occipital condyle or C2 lateral mass.*

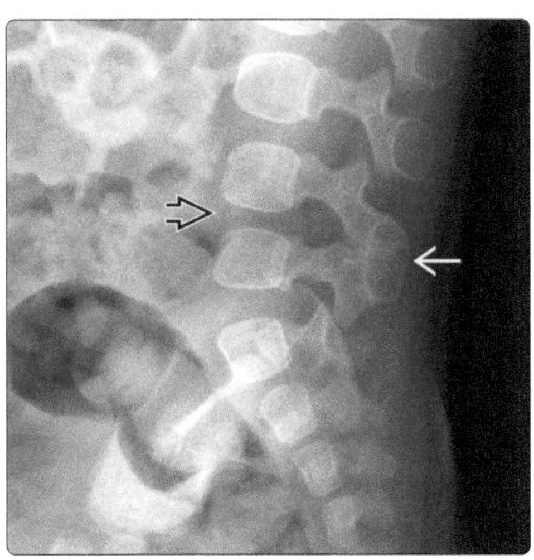

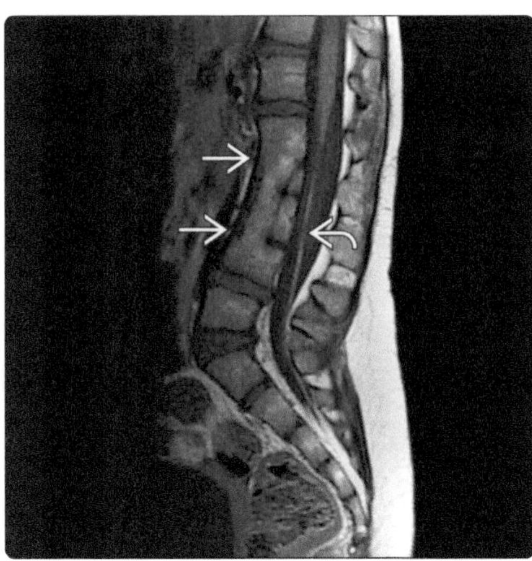

(Left) *Lateral radiograph demonstrates single-level segmentation failure of the L4 and L5 spinous processes and lamina ➡. The L4/L5 intervertebral disc space ⇨ is also abnormally narrowed and hypoplastic relative to adjacent disc spaces.* **(Right)** *Sagittal T1WI MR shows congenital segmentation failure at L1-L4 ➡. There are rudimentary residual disc spaces and abnormal lumbar kyphosis. The spinal cord ends at L1-L2 but is tethered by a thickened, fatty, infiltrated filum terminale ↪.*

Partial Vertebral Duplication

KEY FACTS

TERMINOLOGY

- Partial duplication of vertebral column → 1 or more supranumerary ("extra") vertebra

IMAGING

- Atypical scoliosis (sharply angulated, single curve, or focal) with 1 or more "extra" hemivertebra
- "Extra" hemivertebra frequently associated with focal scoliotic curvature

TOP DIFFERENTIAL DIAGNOSES

- Butterfly vertebra
- Vertebral fracture

PATHOLOGY

- Derangement of normal vertebral ossification → hemivertebra
- Cervicothoracic or thoracolumbar junction segmentation variation → "extra" counted hemivertebra
- Supernumerary hemivertebra may be incorporated into adjacent vertebra, producing unbalanced block vertebra, focal scoliosis

CLINICAL ISSUES

- May be asymptomatic or present with neuromuscular scoliosis
- Respiratory failure 2° to impeded chest movement from severe scoliosis (rare)
- Natural history variable: Scoliosis may progress with somatic growth, require treatment

DIAGNOSTIC CHECKLIST

- Patient may either appear normal or present with scoliosis ± stigmata of congenital disorder
- Supranumerary hemivertebra demonstrates "missing" pedicle on hypoplastic side; distinguishes from fracture

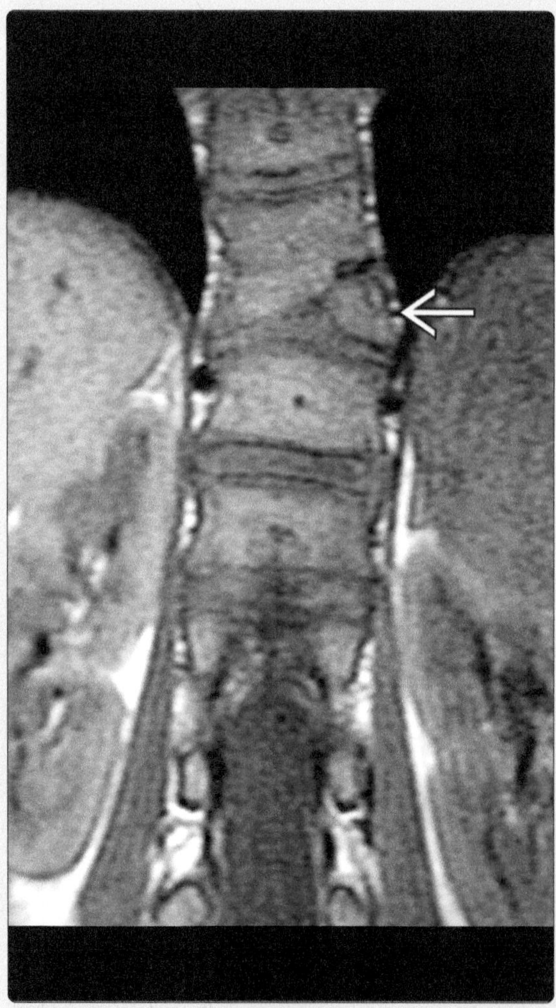

Coronal T1WI MR depicts a small left thoracic supernumerary hemivertebra ➡ producing minimal convex left lower thoracic scoliosis.

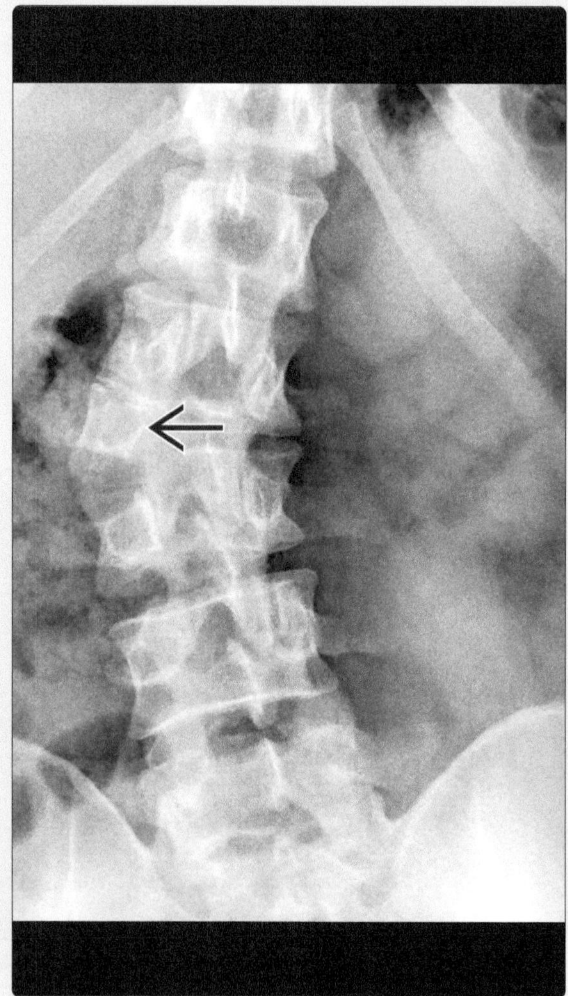

AP radiography depicts a typical supernumerary hemivertebra ➡ positioned between the right L2 and L3 vertebral levels, resulting in convex right scoliotic curvature. Note that there is only 1 pedicle at this level.

Partial Vertebral Duplication

TERMINOLOGY

Synonyms

- Supranumerary vertebra

Definitions

- Partial duplication of vertebral column → 1 or more supranumerary ("extra") vertebra

IMAGING

General Features

- Best diagnostic clue
  - Atypical scoliosis (sharply angulated, single curve, or focal) with 1 or more "extra" hemivertebra
- Location
  - Thoracolumbar > cervical

Radiographic Findings

- Radiography
  - Lateral hemivertebra with focal scoliosis
  - "Extra" vertebra on counting of thoracic and lumbar vertebra

CT Findings

- Bone CT
  - Supranumerary lateral hemivertebra

MR Findings

- T1WI
  - Supranumerary lateral hemivertebra ± dysraphism, spinal cord anomalies
- T2WI
  - Same as T1WI

Imaging Recommendations

- Protocol advice
  - AP plain film for "counting" to localize abnormal vertebral level
  - Long-cassette standing weight-bearing radiograph to quantitate scoliosis
  - Multiplanar MR imaging to evaluate vertebral anatomy, assess for associated neurologic abnormalities

DIFFERENTIAL DIAGNOSIS

Butterfly Vertebra

- 2 pedicles; appears as bilateral hemivertebra with central cleft
- Separate bilateral ossification centers fail to unite

Vertebral Fracture

- Pathologic or traumatic (history critical)
- Noncorticated irregular margins ± soft tissue edema, spinal cord injury
- 2 pedicles at abnormal level

PATHOLOGY

General Features

- Etiology
  - Derangement of normal vertebral ossification → hemivertebra
  - Cervicothoracic or thoracolumbar junction segmentation variation → "extra" counted hemivertebra
- Associated abnormalities
  - Dysraphism, split notochord syndromes, caudal regression, other vertebral segmentation anomalies, visceral organ anomalies

Gross Pathologic & Surgical Features

- Hemivertebra may be incorporated into adjacent vertebra → unbalanced block vertebra

CLINICAL ISSUES

Presentation

- Most common signs/symptoms
  - Asymptomatic
  - Neuromuscular scoliosis; usually progressive
- Other signs/symptoms
  - Respiratory failure 2° to impeded chest movement from severe scoliosis (rare)
  - Neural deficits, limb/visceral defects

Demographics

- Age
  - More severe cases detected in infancy or childhood
  - Milder cases detected in adolescence during school scoliosis checks, by pediatrician, or incidentally during imaging
- Epidemiology
  - Isolated or syndromal, singular or multiple
    - Many syndromes associated with segmentation and fusion anomalies
    - Increased incidence when multisystem congenital anomalies, parental consanguinity present

Natural History & Prognosis

- Variable: Scoliosis may progress with somatic growth, require treatment

Treatment

- Conservative management in mild cases
- Surgical management to arrest/reverse scoliosis in more severe cases

DIAGNOSTIC CHECKLIST

Consider

- Exclude associated abnormalities

Image Interpretation Pearls

- Supranumerary hemivertebra "missing" pedicle on hypoplastic side; distinguishes from fracture
- Probably represents "counting error" related to transitional thoracolumbar or lumbosacral anatomy rather than true "extra" hemivertebra

SELECTED REFERENCES

1. Vinha A et al: Lumbosacral transitional vertebrae: prevalence in a southern European population and its association with low back pain. Eur Spine J. 31(12):3647-53, 2022
2. Johal J et al: Hemivertebrae: a comprehensive review of embryology, imaging, classification, and management. Childs Nerv Syst. 32(11):2105-9, 2016

Diastematomyelia

KEY FACTS

TERMINOLOGY

- Synonyms: Split cord malformation (SCM), "diastem"

IMAGING

- Sagittal division of spinal cord into 2 hemicords, each with 1 central canal, dorsal horn, and ventral horn
  - Hemicords usually reunite above and below cleft
  - ± fibrous or osseous spur
- Frequently associated vertebral segmentation anomalies
- Imaging evaluation
  - Consider ultrasound to screen infants with skin dimple or cutaneous marker
  - MR imaging most definitive for characterization
  - Supplement with bone CT ± myelography to optimally define spur anatomy for surgical planning

TOP DIFFERENTIAL DIAGNOSES

- Duplicated spinal cord (diplomyelia)

PATHOLOGY

- Split notochord syndrome is spectrum of diastematomyelia (DSM), dorsal enteric fistula/sinus, and dorsal enteric cysts/diverticula
- Spinal cord split into symmetric or asymmetric hemicords
- Either 1 (type II) or 2 (type I) dural tubes

CLINICAL ISSUES

- May be clinically indistinguishable from other causes of tethered spinal cord in absence of cutaneous stigmata
  - Cutaneous stigmata indicate DSM level (> 50%); "fawn's tail" hair patch most common

DIAGNOSTIC CHECKLIST

- Search for DSM in patients with cutaneous stigmata, intersegmental fusion of posterior elements, clinical tethered cord
- Presence of spur = type I SCM; more severe symptoms and anomalies, worse prognosis

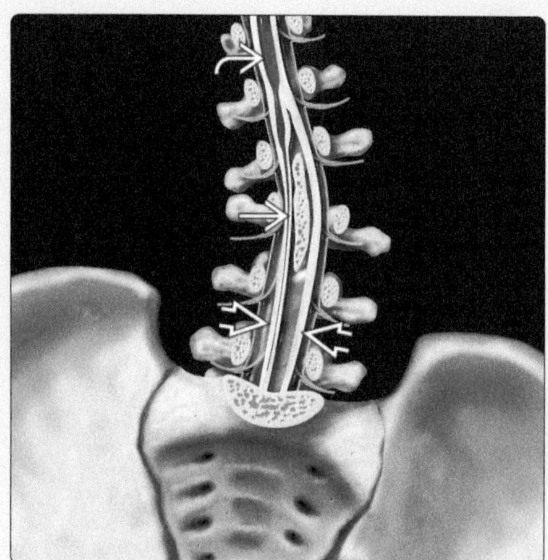

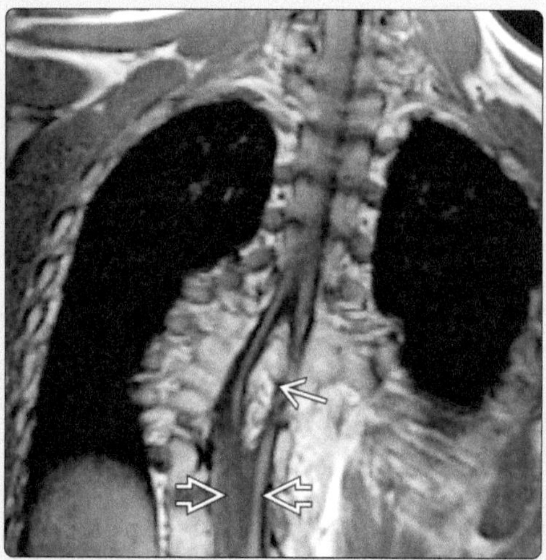

(Left) *Coronal graphic of the lumbar spine demonstrates a type I split cord malformation (SCM) with an osseous spur ➡ splitting the low-lying syringomyelic ➡ spinal cord. Both hemicords ➡ continue into the sacrum.* **(Right)** *Coronal T1 MR (type I SCM) reveals multiple vertebral segmentation anomalies with large midline marrow containing an osseous spur ➡ that splits the thoracic spinal cord into 2 hemicords ➡. Note the associated multiple posterior element and rib fusions.*

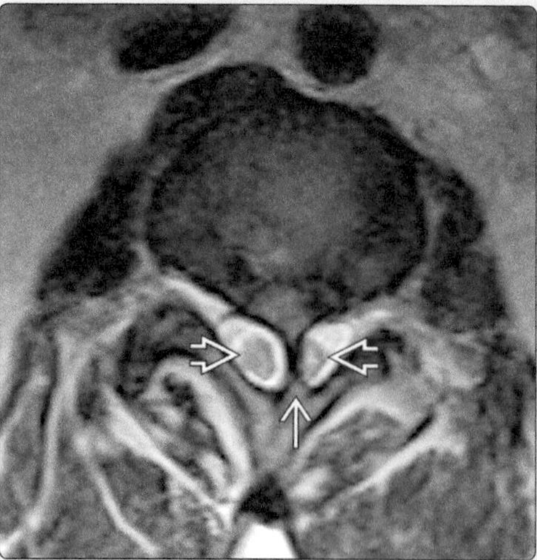

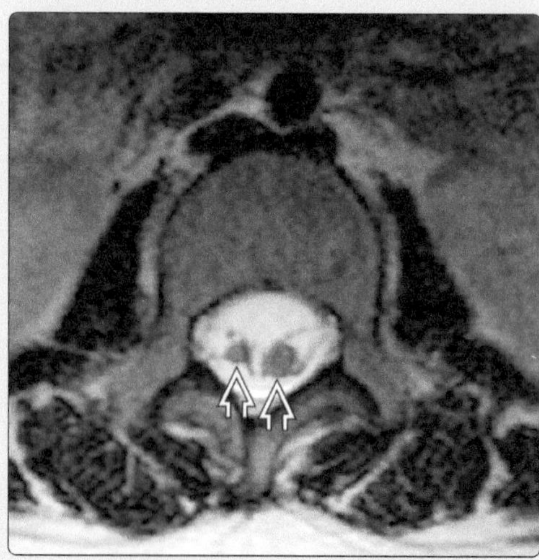

(Left) *Axial T2 MR depicts 2 hemicords ➡ within individual dural tubes separated by an osseous spur ➡ (type I SCM). The left hemicord demonstrates syringomyelia.* **(Right)** *Axial T2 MR (type II SCM) depicts 2 separate hemicords ➡ residing within a single dural tube. No osseous or fibrous septum is identified. The left hemicord is asymmetrically larger, but each hemicord has 1 ventral and 1 dorsal root.*

TERMINOLOGY

Synonyms

- Split cord malformation (SCM), "diastem"

Definitions

- Sagittal division of spinal cord into 2 hemicords, each with 1 central canal, dorsal horn, and ventral horn

IMAGING

General Features

- Best diagnostic clue
  - Fibrous or osseous spur splits spinal cord into 2 hemicords
    - Split cord and spur often occur in conjunction with intersegmental vertebral fusion
- Location
  - Thoracolumbar cleft (85% between T9 and S1) > > upper thoracic, cervical clefts
- Size
  - Range focal → extensive
- Morphology
  - Hemicords usually reunite above and below cleft
  - ± spur (fibrous, osteocartilaginous, or osseous), thickened filum, cord tethering

Radiographic Findings

- Radiography
  - Quantify kyphoscoliosis, "count" level of vertebral segmentation anomalies
  - Detects spur in < 50% of cases

CT Findings

- NECT
  - Osseous spur often visible; fibrous spurs frequently occult
  - Vertebral segmentation anomalies

MR Findings

- T1WI
  - 2 hemicords ± syringohydromyelia (50%)
  - ± isointense (fibrous) or hyperintense (osseous) spur
- T2WI
  - 2 hemicords ± syringohydromyelia (50%) in 1 or both cords, surrounded by bright CSF
  - Hypointense (fibrous or osseous) spur; fibrous spur best seen in axial or coronal plane
- T2* GRE
  - Myelographic effect produces bright CSF adjacent to dark bones, highlights hypointense spur

Ultrasonographic Findings

- Grayscale ultrasound
  - Obstetrical ultrasound → "extra" posterior echogenic focus, splaying of fetal posterior spinal elements
  - Postnatal imaging → spur, tethered cord

Nonvascular Interventions

- Myelography
  - Split cord; 1 or 2 dural tubes
  - Excellent delineation of spur location and meningocele manqué (if present); most useful in conjunction with CT

Imaging Recommendations

- Best imaging tool
  - Multiplanar spine MR imaging
- Protocol advice
  - Consider ultrasound to screen infants with skin dimple or cutaneous marker
  - MR imaging most definitive
    - Coronal, axial images best demonstrate hemicords, spur
    - T1WI to evaluate for filum lesions (e.g., fibrolipoma), vertebral anomalies
    - T2WI to determine number of dural sacs, ± syringohydromyelia
    - T2* GRE to detect spur
- Supplement with bone CT ± myelography to optimally define spur anatomy for surgical planning
  - Sagittal, coronal reformats excellent for depicting osseous anatomy, extent of spur

DIFFERENTIAL DIAGNOSIS

Duplicated Spinal Cord (Diplomyelia)

- 2 complete spinal cords, each with 2 anterior and 2 posterior horns and roots
  - Exceedingly rare, seen only in presence of spinal canal duplication; many authors dispute its true existence, believe it represents severe form of diastematomyelia (DSM)

PATHOLOGY

General Features

- Etiology
  - Split notochord syndrome spectrum
    - Congenital splitting of notochord → split notochord syndrome spectrum; DSM, dorsal enteric fistula/sinus, and dorsal enteric cysts/diverticula
  - Notochord directly influences vertebral body formation → segmentation anomalies
    - Lateral notch produces hemivertebra
    - Cleft produces butterfly vertebra
- Genetics
  - Sporadic; rare familial cases described
- Associated abnormalities
  - Other split notochord syndromes (20%)
  - Congenital spinal deformities (85%)
    - Segmentation and fusion anomalies (SFA)
    - Intersegmental laminar fusion (60%); virtually pathognomonic for DSM
    - Spinal dysraphism (myelocele/myelomeningocele 15-25%, hemimyelocele 15-20%)
    - Tethered spinal cord (75%); thickened filum terminale (40-90%)
    - Syringohydromyelia (50%) in 1 or both hemicords, usually above DSM
    - Congenital scoliosis (79%)
    - 15-20% of Chiari 2 malformations
    - Spinal lipoma (26%)
    - Dermoid cyst (13%)
- Septum inhibits normal spinal cord movement during activity → symptom progression

- Spinal cord damage occurs via direct pressure and by traction → cord ischemia
- Cleft splits cord with single cord above and below split
  - Most (91%) hemicords reunite caudally to terminate in single filum terminale
- Roots may adhere to dura → meningocele manqué

Staging, Grading, & Classification

- Pang type I SCM
  - Separate dural sac, arachnoid space surrounds each hemicord
  - Osseous/fibrous spur
  - More commonly symptomatic than type II
- Pang type II SCM
  - Single dural sac, arachnoid space
  - No osseous spur; ± adherent fibrous bands tether cord
  - Rarely present with symptoms unless hydromyelia, tethering

Gross Pathologic & Surgical Features

- Sagittal spinal cord split into symmetric or asymmetric hemicords, residing in either 1 or 2 dural tubes
  - Symmetric: Each hemicord contains 1 central canal, dorsal horn/root, and 1 ventral horn/root surrounded by pial layer
  - Asymmetric: Division of anterior or posterior hemicord ("partial DSM")
- 2 dural tubes, each with own pial, arachnoid, and dural sheaths for several spinal segments (50%)
  - Bony or cartilaginous spur at inferior cleft, originating from lamina or vertebral body
  - Vertebral anomalies more severe (block or butterfly vertebrae, hemivertebrae, and posterior spina bifida)
  - Hydromyelia common
- Single dural tube, subarachnoid space (50%)
  - No bony spur; nearly always have fibrous band coursing through inferior cleft inserting into dura → tethers cord
  - Vertebral anomalies less severe (usually butterfly vertebrae)
  - Nerve roots may become adherent to dura and tether cord → meningocele manqué

Microscopic Features

- Single ependymal-lined central canal, ventral horn/root, and dorsal horn/root per hemicord
- Septal spur may be composed of mainly cortical bone (most common), mainly cancellous bone, or bone + soft tissues

CLINICAL ISSUES

Presentation

- Most common signs/symptoms
  - Clinically indistinguishable from other causes of tethered cord
  - Cutaneous stigmata high on back indicates DSM level (> 50%); "fawn's tail" hair patch most common
  - Other signs/symptoms
    - Progressive kyphoscoliosis in older children, adults
    - Orthopedic foot problems (50%); especially clubfoot
    - Urologic dysfunction
- Clinical profile
  - Mild cases normal ± cutaneous stigmata
  - Severe cases → kyphoscoliosis, neurologic and musculoskeletal abnormalities

Demographics

- Age
  - Diagnosis in childhood; adult presentation uncommon
- Sex
  - Pediatric: F > > M
  - Adult: M < F (1:3.4)
- Epidemiology
  - 5% of congenital scoliosis

Natural History & Prognosis

- Stable or progressive disability if untreated
  - Late onset or previously stable patients may become symptomatic following relatively minor back injury or surgery requiring spinal manipulation
- ≥ 90% of patients stabilize or improve following surgery
  - Caveat: Scoliosis rarely affected by surgical untethering

Treatment

- Surgical tethered cord release, spur resection, and dural repair for progressive symptoms, prophylactic precursor to scoliosis surgery (particularly type I SCM)

DIAGNOSTIC CHECKLIST

Consider

- Scrutinize images for presence of spur; type I DSM generally has more severe symptoms and anomalies, worse prognosis
- Search for DSM in patients with cutaneous stigmata, intersegmental fusion of posterior elements, clinical tethered cord

Image Interpretation Pearls

- Segmentation anomalies with intersegmental laminar fusion virtually pathognomonic for DSM

SELECTED REFERENCES

1. Xu L et al: A heterozygous mutation in the ALPL gene in an adolescent with Chiari malformation type I accompanied by scoliosis, tethered cord and diastematomyelia. Acta Neurol Belg. 123(6):2387-9, 2023
2. Jasiewicz B et al: Spine duplication or split notochord syndrome - case report and literature review. J Spinal Cord Med. 43(4):544-7, 2020
3. Laurent D et al: Pediatric pathology all grown up - an interesting case of adult tethered spinal cord. Surg Neurol Int. 11:362, 2020
4. Morioka T et al: Neurosurgical pathology of limited dorsal myeloschisis. Childs Nerv Syst. 34(2):293-303, 2018
5. Lee SM et al: Limited dorsal myeloschisis and congenital dermal sinus: comparison of clinical and MR imaging features. AJNR Am J Neuroradiol. 38(1):176-82, 2017
6. Schmidt C et al: Meningocele manqué: a comprehensive review of this enigmatic finding in occult spinal dysraphism. Childs Nerv Syst. 33(7):1065-71, 2017
7. McComb JG: A practical clinical classification of spinal neural tube defects. Childs Nerv Syst. 31(10):1641-57, 2015
8. Alzhrani GA et al: Multi-level split cord malformation: do we need a new classification? J Clin Imaging Sci. 4:32, 2014
9. Burnei G et al: L3-L5 Teratological spondylolysis with diastematomyelia and L4 radicular syndrome followed by spondyloschisis without myelomeningocele due to somato-arcuate shifting. Spine J. 5(1):202-4, 2014
10. Muroi A et al: Split medulla in association with multiple closed neural tube defects. Childs Nerv Syst. 26(7):967-71, 2010
11. Liu W et al: Characteristics of osseous septum of split cord malformation in patients presenting with scoliosis: a retrospective study of 48 cases. Pediatr Neurosurg. 2009;45(5):350-3. Epub 2009 Nov 11. Erratum in: Pediatr Neurosurg. 45(5):406, 2009

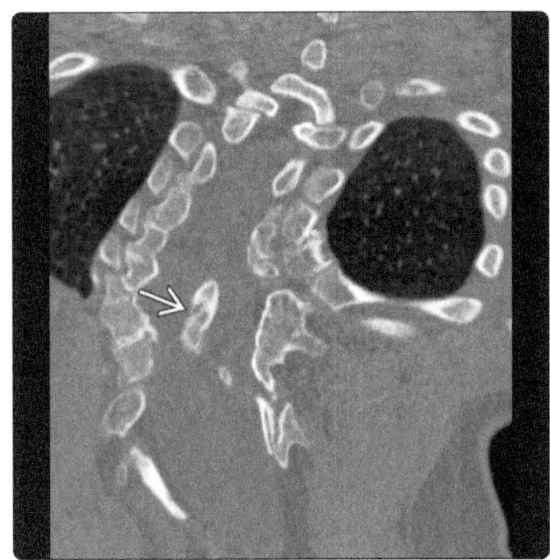

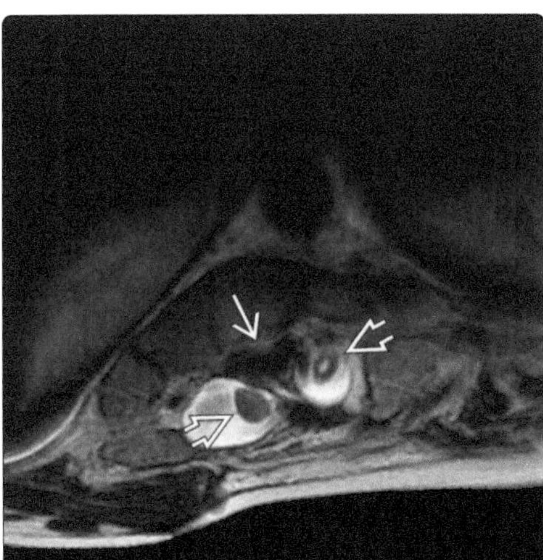

(Left) *Coronal bone CT in a patient with extensive thoracic vertebral formation and segmentation anomalies demonstrates typical marrow containing an diastematomyelia osseous spur ➔ (type I SCM).* **(Right)** *Axial T2 MR of the thoracic spine shows an aberrant wide vertebral body with a prominent ossific spur ➔ dividing the spinal canal (type I SCM). Two hemicords ➔ are noted within separate dural tubes. Note mild syringohydromyelia of the left hemicord.*

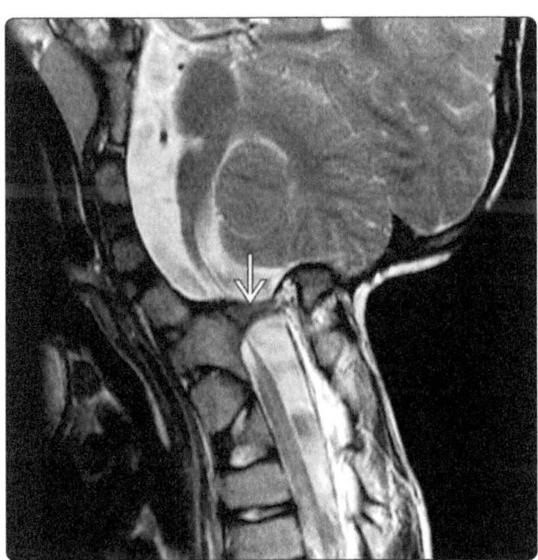

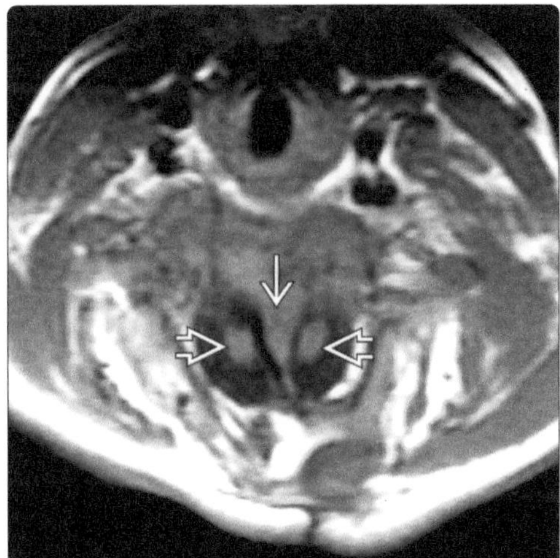

(Left) *Sagittal T2 MR (type I SCM) demonstrates severe craniocervical vertebral segmentation failure and a prominent osseous spur ➔ that pierces the high cervical dural tube. The 2 hemicords are laterally displaced out of this slice.* **(Right)** *Axial T1 MR (type I SCM) reveals a prominent cervical osseous spur ➔ piercing the dural sac and splitting the 2 cervical hemicords ➔.*

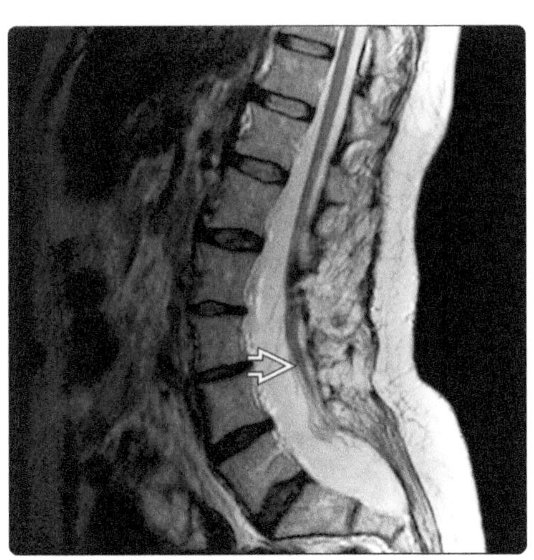

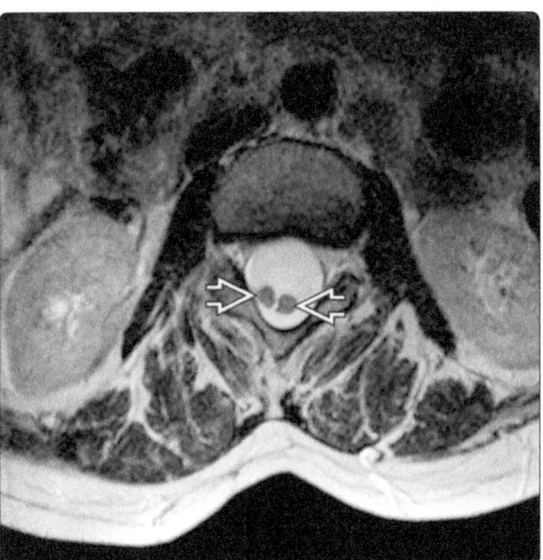

(Left) *Sagittal T1 MR (type II SCM, myelomeningocele closed at birth) demonstrates the expected postoperative findings of the dorsal lumbar spine following myelomeningocele closure with a patulous distal thecal sac and adherence of the elongated spinal cord placode ➔ to the dorsal thecal sac closure at L4-L5.* **(Right)** *Axial T2 MR (type II SCM, repaired myelomeningocele) shows splitting of the spinal cord into 2 hemicords ➔ without intervening osseous or a fibrous spur.*

KEY FACTS

TERMINOLOGY

- Spina bifida occulta is outdated term that should be abandoned
- Spinous process/lamina unfused in midline without underlying neural or dural abnormality

IMAGING

- Spinous process/lamina fail to fuse in midline
  - No abnormal neural, dural, or lipomatous tissue within posterior osseous defect
  - Normal dural sac, conus position, and filum thickness
- Lumbosacral junction (L5 > S1) > > cervical (C1 > C7 > T1), thoracic

TOP DIFFERENTIAL DIAGNOSES

- Closed spinal dysraphism
- Surgical laminectomy defect
- Normal progression of incomplete ossification

PATHOLOGY

- Etiology unknown
  - Probably not linked to abnormal neurulation process

CLINICAL ISSUES

- Most commonly, patient presents with low back or leg pain; finding is incidentally noted during imaging
- Occasionally, skin dimple observed on back
- Usually asymptomatic if no cutaneous stigmata

DIAGNOSTIC CHECKLIST

- Incomplete posterior fusion is incidental finding that is very rarely of neurologic significance
  - Plain films economic screening tool, but positive finding rarely significant
  - MR best for exclusion of significant underlying abnormality, but yield is exceedingly low in absence of cutaneous stigmata or neurologic deficits

(Left) *Anteroposterior radiograph of the lumbosacral spine (imaging performed for low back pain) demonstrates incidental incomplete fusion of the S1 lamina ➡.* **(Right)** *Axial T1WI MR reveals typical incomplete fusion of the posterior elements ➡ in the midline. This finding was incidentally observed during MR imaging for low back pain.*

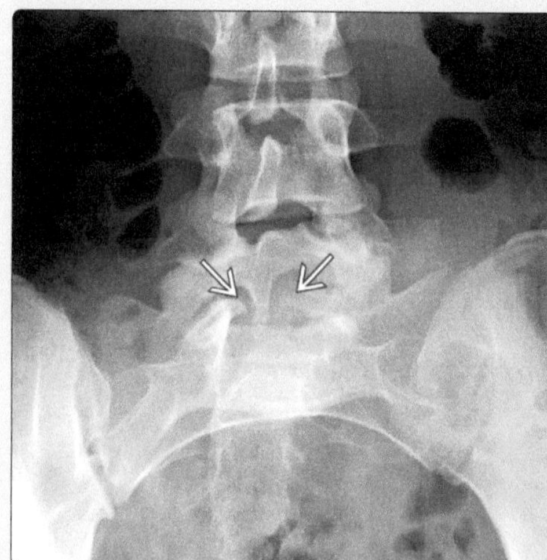

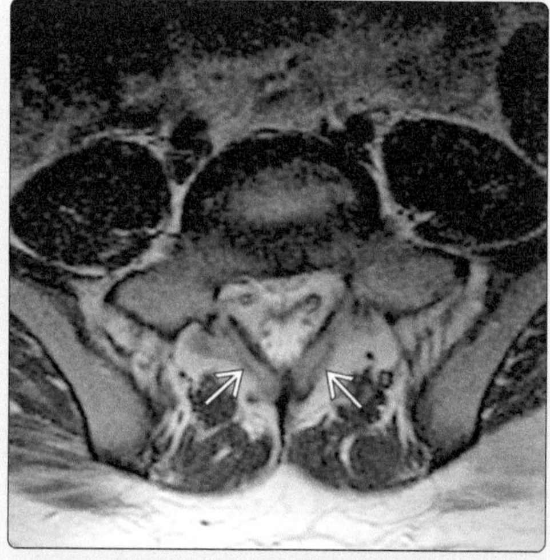

(Left) *Coronal bone CT demonstrates oblique asymmetric rotation of the L5 lamina ➡ with overlap, a configuration thought to produce rotational stresses that may lead to premature facet degenerative changes as an adult.* **(Right)** *Axial bone CT at the lumbosacral junction in a patient with oblique asymmetric rotation and incomplete fusion of the posterior elements additionally demonstrates nondisplaced L5 pars defects ➡, possibly related to rotational stress on the pars interarticularis.*

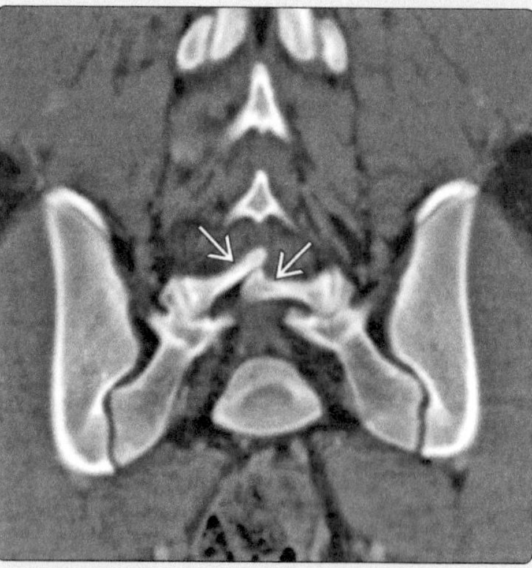

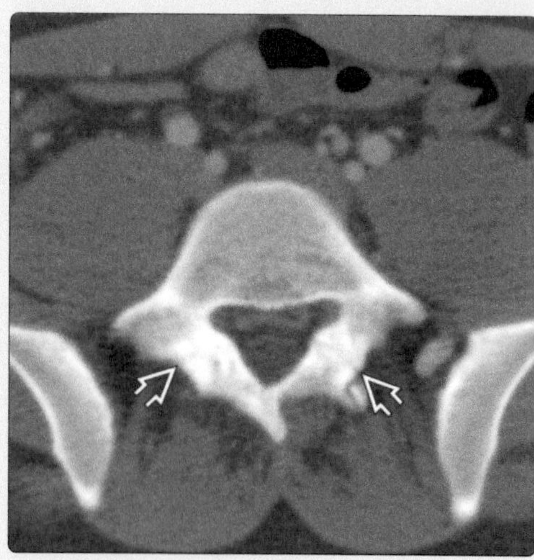

Incomplete Fusion, Posterior Element

TERMINOLOGY

Synonyms

- Spina bifida occulta is outdated term but still commonly used

Definitions

- Spinous process/lamina unfused in midline without underlying neural or dural abnormality

IMAGING

General Features

- Best diagnostic clue
  - Incomplete lumbosacral posterior element fusion
- Location
  - Lumbosacral junction (L5 > S1) > > cervical (C1 > C7 > T1), thoracic
- Size
  - Defect usually small
- Morphology
  - Posterior elements do not fuse in midline; margins are rounded, well corticated, and may overlap

Radiographic Findings

- Radiography
  - Unfused spinous process/lamina approximate at midline

CT Findings

- Bone CT
  - Unfused spinous process/lamina

MR Findings

- T1WI
  - Normal dural sac, conus position, and filum thickness
  - No abnormal neural, dural, or lipomatous tissue within posterior osseous defect
- T2WI
  - Same as T1WI

Imaging Recommendations

- Best imaging tool
  - Plain films most economic screening tool
  - MR best for definitive exclusion of significant underlying abnormality

DIFFERENTIAL DIAGNOSIS

Closed Spinal Dysraphism

- Lipoma, tethered cord, lipomyelomeningocele, dorsal meningocele, dorsal dermal sinus

Surgical Laminectomy Defect

- Surgical history present; look for incision scar, denervation of paraspinal muscles, laminectomy defect

Normal Progression of Ossification

- Normal L5 laminae may remain unfused until 5-6 years of age

PATHOLOGY

General Features

- Etiology
  - Unknown; probably not linked to neurulation process aberrations

Gross Pathologic & Surgical Features

- Nonfused spinous processes and lamina overlie normal dural sac

Microscopic Features

- Histologically normal corticated bone in lamina

CLINICAL ISSUES

Presentation

- Most common signs/symptoms
  - Usually asymptomatic if no cutaneous stigmata
  - Lumbar back pain in adolescent
  - Occasionally, skin dimple on back
    - Dimples within gluteal cleft need no further evaluation
    - Dimples above gluteal cleft have ↑ incidence of associated abnormalities; merit further evaluation with MR
- Other signs/symptoms
  - Association with lower urinary tract dysfunction and nocturnal enuresis described but not universally accepted
- Clinical profile
  - Patient presents with low back or leg pain; finding is incidentally noted during imaging

Demographics

- Age
  - All
- Sex
  - F > M
- Epidemiology
  - Up to 30% of USA population
  - 16.2% asymptomatic Turkish military recruits

Natural History & Prognosis

- Usually incidental finding of no clinical significance
- Does not appear to represent risk factor for early lumbar spine degeneration or disc herniation in children and adolescents with lumbar back pain

Treatment

- Conservative

DIAGNOSTIC CHECKLIST

Consider

- Incomplete posterior fusion is incidental finding that is very rarely of neurologic significance
- Relationship to low back pain and lumbar degenerative disease still actively debated, particularly in adult patients with asymmetric lamina and spinous processes

SELECTED REFERENCES

1. Fidan F et al: The incidence of congenital lumbosacral malformations in young male Turkish military school candidates population. J Orthop Sci. 27(6):1167-71, 2022
2. Illeez OG et al: The effect of transitional vertebrae and spina bifida occulta on disc herniation, disc degeneration, and end-plate changes in pediatric patients with low back pain. Acta Orthop Belg. 88(2):275-83, 2022

KEY FACTS

TERMINOLOGY

- Cyst along neuraxis lined with mucin-secreting cuboidal or columnar epithelium resembling alimentary tract
  - Derived from displaced endodermal tissue
- Synonyms: Enteric, enterogenous, or endodermal cyst

IMAGING

- Cyst along neuraxis (usually intraspinal) ± vertebral anomalies
- Most are intradural, extramedullary simple unilocular cysts ventral to spinal cord
- Can be associated with other closed spinal dysraphisms
- ± associated fistulae & mediastinal/abdominal cysts

TOP DIFFERENTIAL DIAGNOSES

- Arachnoid cyst
- (Epi)dermoid cyst
- Anterior spinal meningocele

PATHOLOGY

- Enteric & spinal structures connected through persistent neurenteric canal (a.k.a. canal of Kovalevsky)
- Subgroup of split notochord syndrome spectrum
  - Sporadic or syndromic (Klippel-Feil, VACTERL, OEIS)
  - Associated with vertebral anomalies, split cord malformation, lipoma, dermal sinus tract, & tethered spinal cord

CLINICAL ISSUES

- Usually present in adolescents; not typically symptomatic in infants unless large
- Best treatment (not always possible): Complete excision

DIAGNOSTIC CHECKLIST

- Location, size of cyst, degree of cord compression, & severity of associated anomalies determine prognosis
- Look for associated mediastinal or abdominal cysts, connecting fistulae, or vertebral anomalies

(Left) *Sagittal graphic shows a large, mediastinal enteric cyst ➔ extending into the ventral spinal canal through a persistent neurenteric canal (a.k.a. canal of Kovalevsky) ➲. There is dorsal displacement and compression of the thoracic spinal cord.* **(Right)** *Sagittal T2 MR in a 4-year-old with a history of repaired cervical myelocystocele ➔ shows cyst ventral to lower cervical spine ➔, communicating though an osseous defect ➲. This was subsequently resected with pathology consistent with neurenteric cyst.*

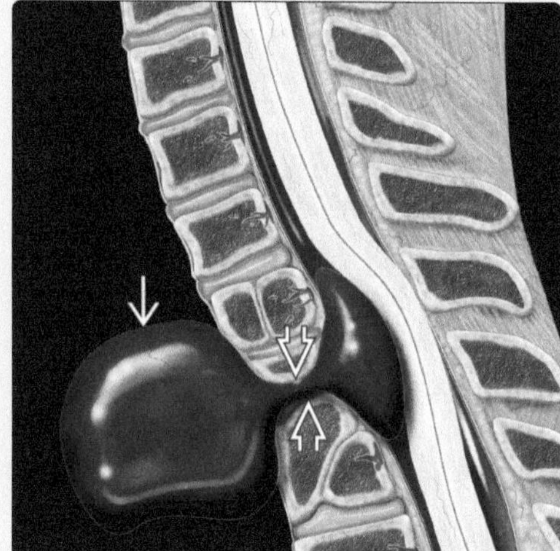

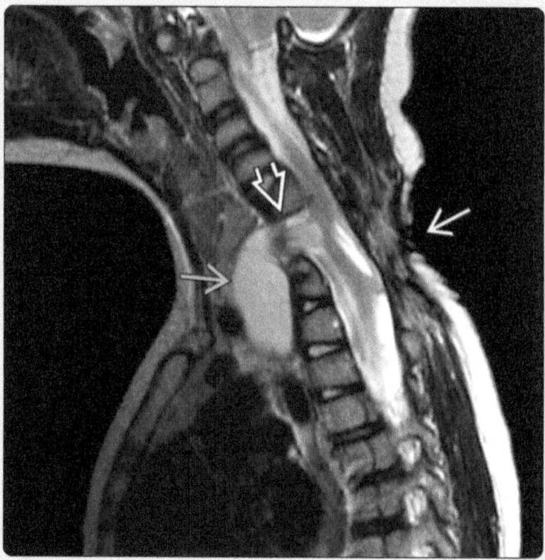

(Left) *Coronal T2 MR in the same patient demonstrates the neurenteric cyst ➔ in association with the ventral osseous defect ➲ and multiple segmentation anomalies ➔ in the cervical and thoracic spine.* **(Right)** *Axial T2 MR in the same patient shows the neurenteric cyst ➔ anterior to the osseous defect ➲ and anterior tethering of the spinal cord with a syrinx ➔.*

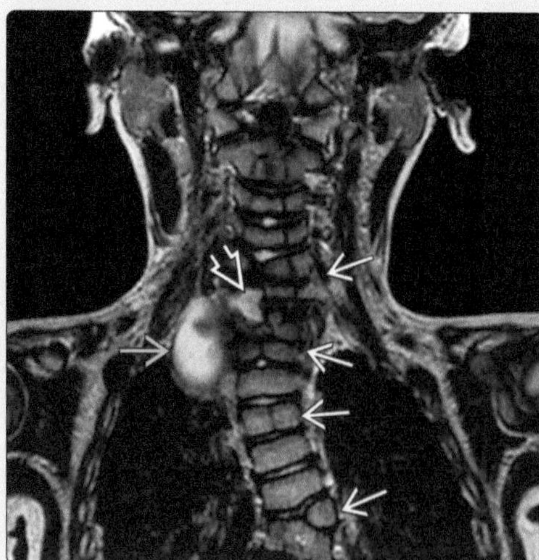

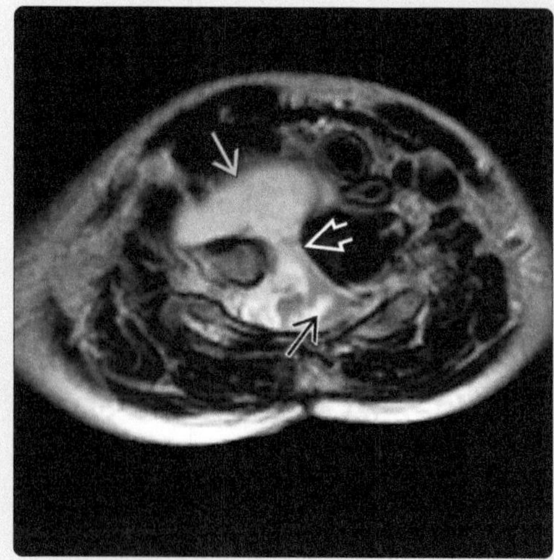

TERMINOLOGY

Synonyms

- Enteric cyst, enterogenous cyst, endodermal cyst

Definitions

- Cyst along neuraxis lined with mucin-secreting cuboidal or columnar epithelium resembling alimentary tract
  - Derived from displaced endodermal tissue
  - In spine, this is classified as complex closed spinal dysraphism without subcutaneous mass

IMAGING

General Features

- Best diagnostic clue
  - Intraspinal cyst ± vertebral abnormalities
  - Pathologic diagnosis, though can be suggested in presence of vertebral anomalies
- Location
  - Usually intraspinal: Majority in lower cervical or upper thoracic spine
    - Can be posterior mediastinal/intraabdominal or both with communication through vertebral body defect
  - Most intradural, extramedullary
    - 10-15% have intramedullary component
  - Ventral > > dorsal to spinal cord
  - Can be intracranial (~ 10-25%)
    - Most intracranial neurenteric cysts in posterior fossa (70-90%)
- Size
  - Range from small to large
- Morphology
  - Single smooth-walled, unilocular cyst

Radiographic Findings

- Radiography
  - Enlarged spinal canal with widening of interpedicular distance
  - Segmentation anomalies
  - Scoliosis

CT Findings

- Bone CT
  - Enlarged spinal canal
  - Segmentation anomalies (~ 50%)
  - Posterior spinal dysraphic defects

MR Findings

- T1WI, T2WI
  - Well-circumscribed, fluid-intensity, unilocular cystic lesion ± vertebral anomalies
  - Variable fluid signal within cyst; can parallel CSF or have proteinaceous/hemorrhagic components (↑ T1, ↓ T2)
  - Mass effect on spinal cord, associated myelomalacia
  - ± associated fistulae & mediastinal/abdominal cysts
  - ± other associated closed spinal dysraphisms: Split cord malformation, lipomyelomeningocele, intradural lipoma, dorsal dermal sinus tract, tethered cord
- T1WI C+
  - Mild to no rim enhancement
- DWI
  - Cyst contents may show mild diffusion restriction

Ultrasonographic Findings

- Grayscale ultrasound
  - Hypoechoic intraspinal cyst

Nuclear Medicine Findings

- Tc-99m cyst uptake (gastric mucosa) confirms diagnosis

Imaging Recommendations

- Best imaging tool
  - Multiplanar T1WI, T2WI to assess for vertebral anomalies, cord compression, & cyst relationship to adjacent structures
  - Bone CT/3D CT to characterize osseous anomalies, surgical planning

DIFFERENTIAL DIAGNOSIS

Arachnoid Cyst

- CSF density/intensity on all pulse sequences
- Dorsal > ventral spinal canal
- Vertebral anomalies uncommon

(Epi)dermoid Cysts

- Most common at conus/cauda equina level
- ↑ T1 fat signal (dermoid), + diffusion restriction (epidermoid)
- ± sinus tract, cord tethering, skin dimple

Anterior Spinal Meningocele

- Anterior dumbbell shape, contiguous with dural sac
- Associated with ventral osseous defect

Cystic Neoplasm

- Look for more than thin rim enhancement on postcontrast images; nodular enhancement should raise concern

Schwannoma

- Intense enhancement, rarely midline, usually associated with nerve roots or cranial nerves

PATHOLOGY

General Features

- Etiology
  - Etiology not entirely understood, though few theories exist
  - Failure of primitive endodermal cells to separate from ectodermal counterparts, multiple proposed mechanisms
    - Splitting of notochord by endodermal tissue or diverticulum
    - Adhesion between notochord & endodermal tissue
    - Failure of complete obliteration of neurenteric canal (a.k.a. canal of Kovalevsky) resulting in persistent connection between notochord & foregut
      - □ Neurenteric canal: Transient connection between amniotic cavity & yolk sac during 3rd & 4th weeks of embryogenesis
      - □ Degree of tract persistence predicts severity of abnormality
    - Incomplete "escalation" of notochord
    - Ectopic endoderm trapped in developing spinal canal

- Supratentorial neurenteric cysts (rare)
  - Believed to be remnants of Seessel pouch: Transient diverticulum of oropharyngeal membrane of cranial end of foregut
  - Common origin with Rathke cleft cysts & colloid cysts
- Associated abnormalities
  - Other coexisting closed spinal dysraphisms ± cutaneous stigmata
    - Split cord malformation, lipoma, dorsal dermal sinus tract, tethered spinal cord
  - Klippel-Feil syndrome
  - Malformations of gastrointestinal tract
    - Duplication, fistula, anal atresia
  - VACTERL association, omphalocele, exstrophy (of bladder), imperforate (anus), & spinal abnormalities (OEIS), cardiac anomalies, renal malformations

Staging, Grading, & Classification

- WHO classification: Other malformative tumors & tumor-like lesions
- 3 types based on histology (Wilkins & Odum)
  - Type A: Single layer of pseudostratified cuboidal or columnar epithelium resembling respiratory &/or gastrointestinal epithelium
  - Type B: Type A + mucous or serous glands, smooth muscle connective tissue, lymphoid tissue or nervous tissue
  - Type C: Type A + ependymal or other glial elements
- Types have no association with other associated clinical parameters (site, size, outcome after resection)
- Benign cystic lesions, malignant transformation extremely rare

Gross Pathologic & Surgical Features

- Single smooth, unilocular (rarely multilocular) cyst containing clear or proteinaceous fluid (milky, cream-colored, yellowish, xanthochromic)
  - ± cyst connection with spinal cord &/or vertebrae
  - Dorsal spinal-enteric tract traverses cartilage-lined canal of Kovalevsky through small, dysplastic vertebra

CLINICAL ISSUES

Presentation

- Most common signs/symptoms
  - Depends on location, size, degree of cord CNS compression
    - Headaches
    - Neck/radicular pain worse with elevated intraspinal pressure
    - Gait disturbance, progressive quadriparesis/paresthesias (cord compression)
    - Cranial neuropathies, sensorimotor deficits
- Other signs/symptoms
  - Acute presentation rare, usually from infection → meningitis
  - Can also be found incidentally

Demographics

- Age
  - Most present in adolescents
    - Usually not symptomatic in infants (unless large)
    - Cysts with associated malformations present earlier than isolated cysts
- Sex
  - M:F = 2:1
- Epidemiology
  - Rare: 0.7-1.3% of spinal "tumors"

Natural History & Prognosis

- Some asymptomatic → diagnosis at autopsy
- Most show progressive neurologic deterioration
- Significant symptomatic improvement following resection in many patients
- Rare cases of malignant transformation reported in adulthood

Treatment

- Treatment of choice: Complete microsurgical excision
  - Complete excision not always achieved either because of ventral location of cyst or adherence to surrounding structures (intramedullary lesions)
  - Symptomatic recurrence reported in up to 1/3 of partially resected cases

DIAGNOSTIC CHECKLIST

Consider

- Location, size of cyst, degree of cord compression, & severity of associated anomalies determine disease course & prognosis
- Important to define cyst in relation to cord

Image Interpretation Pearls

- Look for associated mediastinal or abdominal cysts, connecting fistulae, or vertebral anomalies

SELECTED REFERENCES

1. Behbahani M et al: Cutaneous Stigmata of the Spine: A Review of Indications for Imaging and Referral. Pediatr Clin North Am. 68(4):895-913, 2021
2. Anderson T et al: Intracranial neurenteric cyst: a case report and differential diagnosis of intracranial cystic lesions. Radiol Case Rep. 15(12):2649-54, 2020
3. Barkovich AJ et al: Pediatric Neuroimaging. 6th ed. Wolters Kluwer. 1012-3, 2019
4. Kozak J et al: Neurenteric cysts, incidence and surgical treatment. Bratisl Lek Listy. 120(9):680-5, 2019
5. Baek WK et al: Comprehensive review of spinal neurenteric cysts with a focus on histopathological findings. Cureus. 10(9):e3379, 2018
6. Kitamura Y et al: Supratentorial neurenteric cyst with spontaneous repetitive intracystic hemorrhage mimicking brain abscess: a case report. Neurosurg Rev. 37(1):153-9, 2014
7. Al-Ahmed IH et al: Neurosurgical management of neurenteric cysts in children. J Neurosurg Pediatr. 11(5):511-7, 2013
8. Gauden AJ et al: Intracranial neuroenteric cysts: a concise review including an illustrative patient. J Clin Neurosci. 19(3):352-9, 2012
9. Jhawar SS et al: Intramedullary spinal neurenteric cyst with fluid-fluid level. J Neurosurg Pediatr. 9(5):542-5, 2012
10. Savage JJ et al: Neurenteric cysts of the spine. J Craniovertebr Junction Spine. 1(1):58-63, 2010
11. Theret E et al: Huge intramedullar neurenteric cyst with intrathoracic development in a 1 month-old boy: excision though the anterior approach. A case report and review of the literature. Acta Neurochir (Wien). 152(3):481-3, 2010
12. Aydin AL et al: Prenatal diagnosis of a large, cervical, intraspinal, neurenteric cyst and postnatal outcome. J Pediatr Surg. 44(9):1835-8, 2009

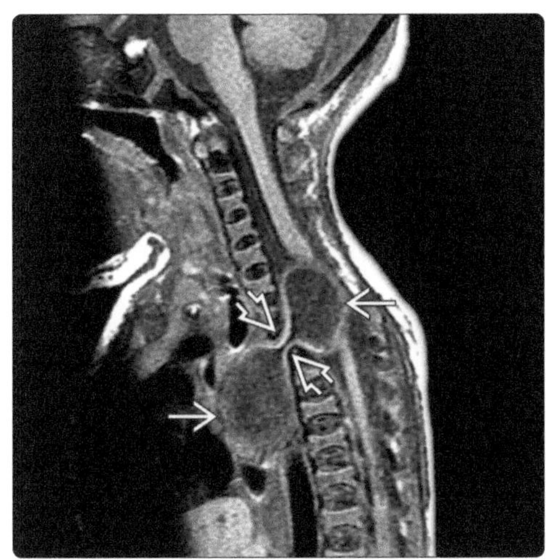

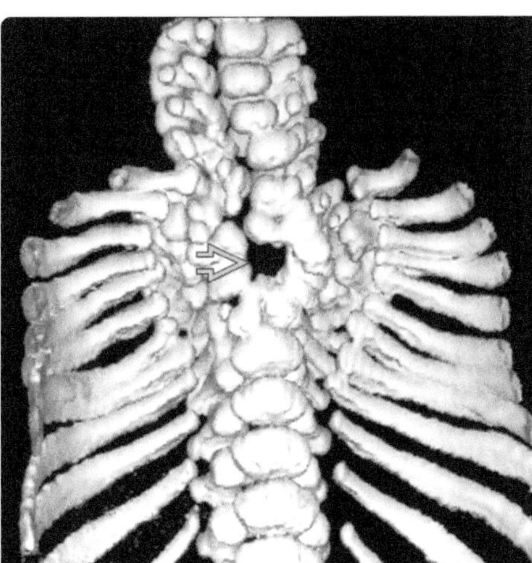

(Left) *Sagittal T1 MR demonstrates a large, dumbbell-shaped neurenteric cyst* ➡ *extending from the mediastinum into the spinal canal through a persistent neurenteric canal* ➡*. There is marked spinal cord compression.* **(Right)** *3D coronal bone CT in the same patient with a complex thoracic enteric cyst and spinal canal extension shows extensive vertebral segmentation anomalies, multiple abnormal fused ribs, and a large, persistent neurenteric canal* ⇨*. (Courtesy S. Blaser, MD.)*

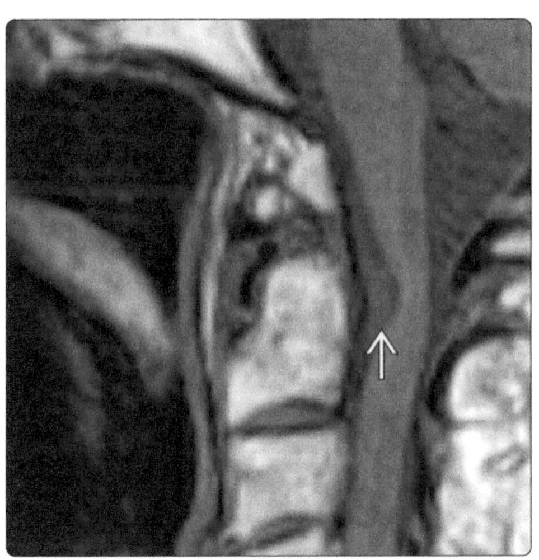

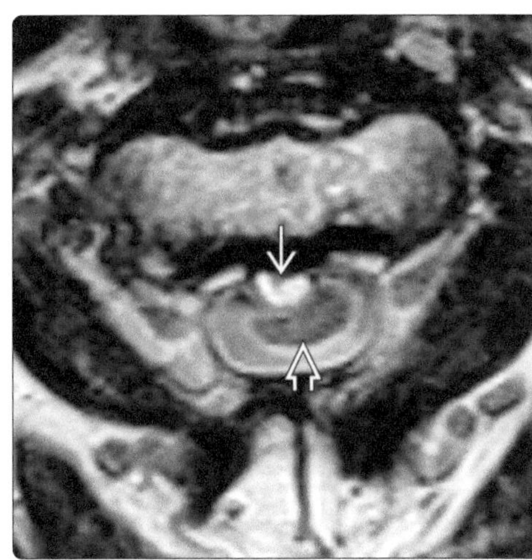

(Left) *Sagittal T1 MR in a patient with Klippel-Feil syndrome demonstrates a small, extramedullary neurenteric cyst* ➡ *associated with a vertebral defect and craniovertebral variation of os odontoideum producing mild compression of the ventral spinal cord.* **(Right)** *Axial T2 MR in a patient with Klippel-Feil syndrome reveals a small, hyperintense, intradural extramedullary neurenteric cyst* ➡ *that produces distortion and posterior displacement of the cervical spinal cord* ➡*.*

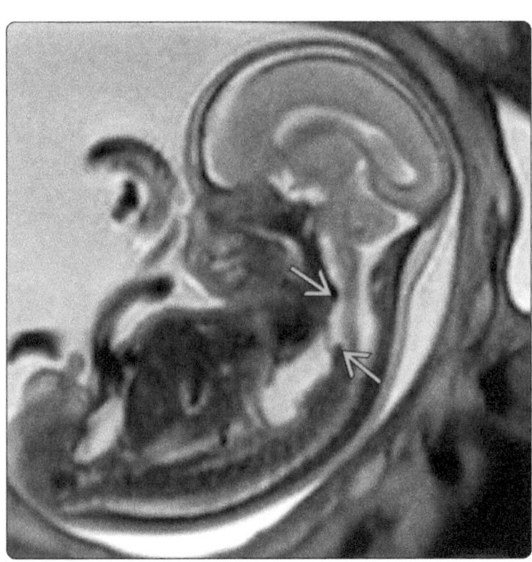

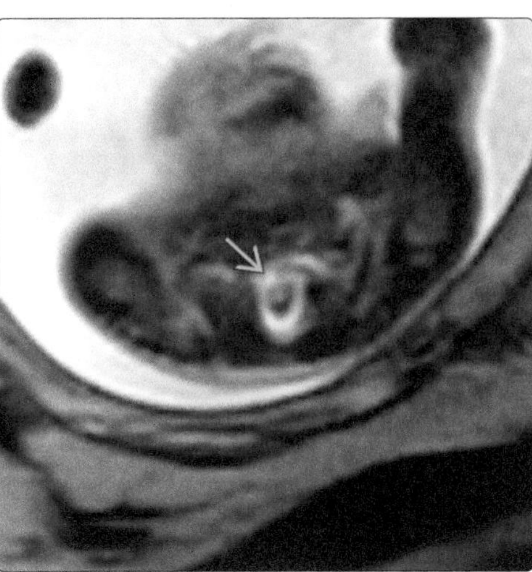

(Left) *Sagittal T2 SSFSE from a fetal MR in a 23-weeks-gestation fetus demonstrates a large, ventral cervicothoracic spinal dysraphic defect* → *with a thin wall partially separating the spinal canal from the intrathoracic stomach, which is associated with a congenital diaphragmatic hernia.* **(Right)** *Axial FIESTA MR in the same fetus shows the defect in the cyst wall allowing direct communication* → *with the spinal canal and intrathoracic stomach in this presumed neurenteric cyst.*

Lateral Meningocele

KEY FACTS

TERMINOLOGY

- Lateral meningocele (LM), lateral thoracic meningocele (LTM), lateral lumbar meningocele (LLM)

IMAGING

- CSF-filled dural/arachnoidal sac protrudes laterally through neural foramen
- Pedicular erosion, foraminal enlargement, dural dysplasia
- Bilateral meningoceles: Consider neurofibromatosis type 1 (NF1), Marfan syndrome
- Scalloping of pedicles, laminae, and vertebral bodies adjacent to meningocele
- Enlarged central spinal canal, neural foramina

TOP DIFFERENTIAL DIAGNOSES

- Nerve sheath tumor
- Radicular (meningeal) cyst
- Chronic inflammatory demyelinating polyneuropathy
- Foregut duplication cyst

PATHOLOGY

- Etiology secondary to primary meningeal dysplasia

CLINICAL ISSUES

- Asymptomatic (most common) or nonspecific motor or sensory symptoms referable to cord/nerve root compression
- Most remain asymptomatic unless very large or scoliosis causes symptoms
- Very large meningoceles may → respiratory embarrassment (meningocele fills hemithorax)

DIAGNOSTIC CHECKLIST

- CSF density/signal intensity mass extending laterally through enlarged neural foramen
- LM prompts search for history/stigmata of NF1 or connective tissue disorder

(Left) *Axial graphic depicts a large left lateral thoracic meningocele ➔ producing pedicular erosion ➔, transverse process remodeling, and widening of the neural foramen.* **(Right)** *Axial CECT of the chest in a patient with neurofibromatosis type 1 (NF1) demonstrates a large lateral meningocele ➔. Note complete erosion of the ipsilateral pedicle with widening of the neural foramen.*

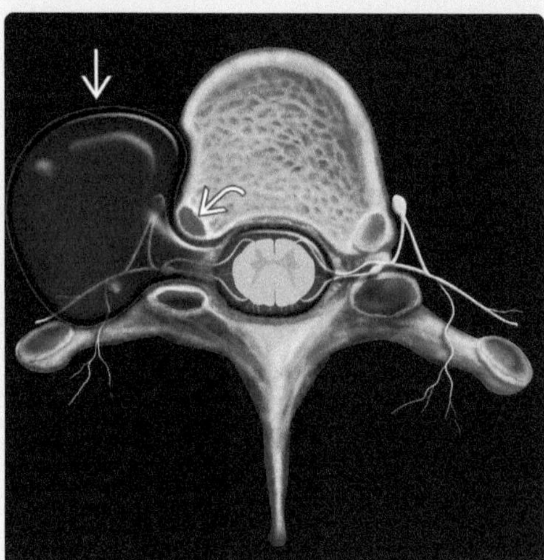

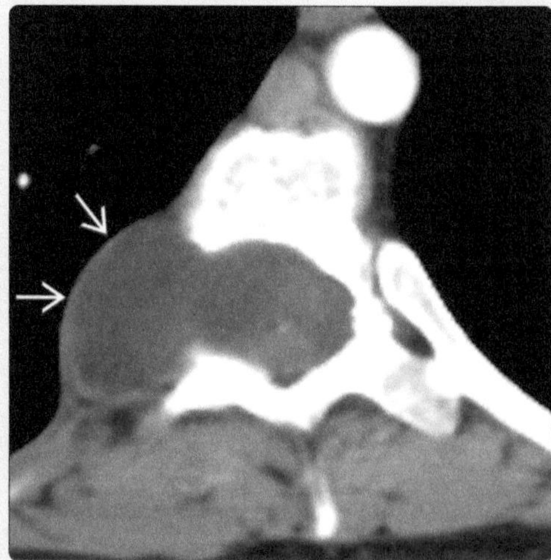

(Left) *Axial NECT following myelography in a patient with NF1 reveals a large, left lateral lumbar meningocele ➔ and extensive vertebral scalloping from dural dysplasia ➔, resulting in marked left pedicular erosion and enlargement of the ipsilateral neural foramen.* **(Right)** *Axial T2WI MR in a patient with NF1 shows a large, left lateral lumbar meningocele ➔ in conjunction with extensive dural dysplasia, vertebral remodeling ➔, and marked left pedicular erosion.*

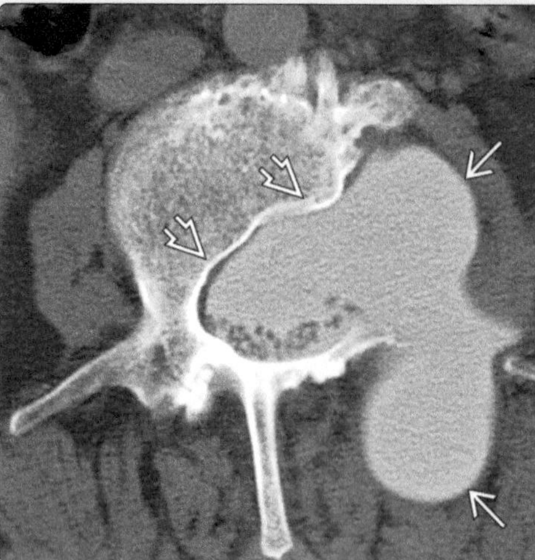

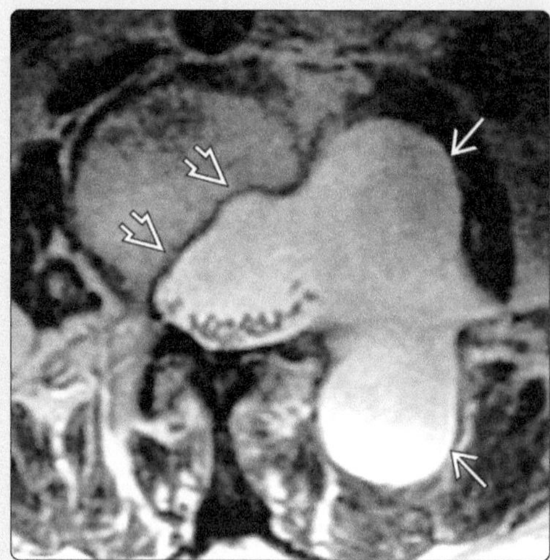

TERMINOLOGY

Abbreviations

- Lateral meningocele (LM)

Synonyms

- Lateral thoracic meningocele (LTM), lateral lumbar meningocele (LLM)

Definitions

- Meningeal dysplasia → CSF-filled dural/arachnoidal sac protrudes laterally through neural foramen

IMAGING

General Features

- Best diagnostic clue
  - CSF signal/density meningeal protrusion through neural foramen into adjacent intercostal/extrapleural space
- Location
  - Thoracic > lumbar spine
  - R > L; 10% bilateral
    - Bilateral meningoceles usually associated with neurofibromatosis type 1 (NF1) but may be seen in Marfan syndrome
- Size
  - Typically 2-3 cm; range from tiny to huge
- Morphology
  - CSF signal/density "cyst" adjacent to spine
    - Contiguous with neural foramen
    - ± sharply angled scoliosis at meningocele level

Radiographic Findings

- Radiography
  - Pedicular erosion ± neural foraminal enlargement
    - Often accompanied by scalloping of posterior vertebral bodies (dural ectasia)
    - ± sharply angled kyphosis/scoliosis (meningocele is near apex of deformity on convex side)

CT Findings

- CECT
  - CSF density mass extends through enlarged neural foramen
  - No enhancement; useful to distinguish from nerve sheath tumor, nerve inflammation [chronic inflammatory demyelinating polyneuropathy (CIDP)]
- CTA
  - ± aortic aneurysm, dissection in context of systemic connective tissue disorder
- Bone CT
  - Wide neural foramen; ± pedicular thinning, posterior vertebral scalloping (usually)
  - Reformatted images may show focal scoliosis (coronal plane) and dural ectasia (sagittal plane)

MR Findings

- T1WI
  - CSF signal intensity (hypointense) mass in contiguity with thecal sac
  - Pedicular thinning, neural foraminal widening ± posterior vertebral scalloping
- T2WI
  - CSF signal intensity (hyperintense) mass in contiguity with thecal sac; rarely see neural elements within meningocele
- T1WI C+
  - No enhancement; distinguishes from nerve sheath tumor or inflammation (CIDP)

Ultrasonographic Findings

- Grayscale ultrasound
  - Posterior mediastinal or lumbar hypoechoic paraspinal cystic mass contiguous with expanded spinal canal
    - Displaces and compresses adjacent spinal cord
  - Ultrasound is primary diagnostic tool in utero, screening newborn infants
- Pulsed Doppler
  - No vascular flow pattern
- Color Doppler
  - Avascular hypoechoic mass

Nonvascular Interventions

- Myelography
  - Intrathecal contrast fills cyst from dural sac through enlarged neural foramen
    - Confirms contiguity with thecal sac
    - Delayed imaging may be required
    - Consider placing patient with meningocele(s) dependently to improve contrast filling

Imaging Recommendations

- Best imaging tool
  - MR
- Protocol advice
  - Consider sonography for newborn screening; follow-up with MR to clarify positive ultrasound study
  - MR imaging for diagnosis, preoperative planning
  - Bone CT to evaluate pedicles, vertebral bodies (particularly if surgery is contemplated)

DIFFERENTIAL DIAGNOSIS

Nerve Sheath Tumor

- Less hyperintense than CSF on T2WI, higher signal intensity than CSF on T1WI
- Contrast enhancement implies tumor
  - Caveats: Some schwannomas may appear cystic, and some neurofibromas minimally enhance

Radicular (Meningeal) Cyst

- CSF signal intensity/density cyst within neural foramen
  - Cyst separate from dural sac, unlike meningocele
- Nerve root definable as discrete structure within or adjacent to cyst

Chronic Inflammatory Demyelinating Polyneuropathy

- Solid fusiform nerve root enlargement, enhancement
- Clinical and laboratory findings characteristic

Foregut Duplication Cyst

- Bronchogenic most common; may contain GI mucosa
  - Seldom contiguous with neural foramen
- Proximity to spinal canal ± vertebral anomalies = neurenteric cyst

PATHOLOGY

General Features

- Etiology
  - Meningocele 2° to primary meningeal dysplasia
    - Meningeal weakness permits dural sac to focally stretch in response to repetitive CSF pulsation → enlarged neural foramina
    - Secondary osseous remodeling permits further herniation
  - Posterior vertebral scalloping with dural dysplasia → same etiology
- Genetics
  - Strong association with NF1 (85%)
    - Most common posterior mediastinal mass
  - Less common with Ehlers-Danlos, Marfan syndromes
  - LM syndrome (Lehman Syndrome)
    - Connective tissue disorder associated with truncating mutations within exon 33 of *NOTCH3*
    - LM(s), distinctive craniofacial features, joint hypermobility
- Associated abnormalities
  - Occasionally isolated finding
  - ± coexistent lumbar and thoracic LMs
  - ± findings specific to hereditary disorder
    - NF1: Dural ectasia, nerve sheath tumors, CNS neoplasms, pheochromocytomas, interstitial pulmonary fibrosis, skin, and subcutaneous neurofibromas
    - Marfan syndrome: Dural ectasia, vascular dissection/aneurysm, lens dislocation, joint laxity
- Dural sac diverticulum, pedicular erosion, neural foraminal widening, and posterior vertebral scalloping

Gross Pathologic & Surgical Features

- Scalloping of pedicles, laminae, and vertebral bodies adjacent to meningocele
- Enlarged central spinal canal, neural foramina
- Cord position variable; usually displaced away from meningocele
- Scoliosis convex toward meningocele

Microscopic Features

- Dura/arachnoid lined outpouching of thecal sac

CLINICAL ISSUES

Presentation

- Most common signs/symptoms
  - Asymptomatic (most common)
  - Nonspecific motor or sensory symptoms referable to cord/nerve root compression
- Other signs/symptoms
  - Respiratory embarrassment (neonates); very large meningocele fills thoracic cavity
- Clinical profile
  - Asymptomatic patient (incidental discovery)
  - ± scoliosis evaluation
  - NF1: Cutaneous café au lait spots, cutaneous and subcutaneous neurofibromas, ± kyphoscoliosis
  - Connective tissue disorder: Frequently tall, joint hypermobility, lens dislocation, ± normal intelligence, ± scoliosis

Demographics

- Age
  - Most commonly present during 4th-5th decades of life
- Sex
  - M = F
- Epidemiology
  - Uncommon in NF1 and inherited connective tissue disorders but substantially more common than occurrence as isolated lesion

Natural History & Prognosis

- Most remain asymptomatic unless very large or scoliosis causes symptoms
- Most static in size; occasionally grow slowly
- May disappear after hydrocephalus shunting
- Excellent prognosis after surgical resection

Treatment

- Options, risks, complications
  - Surgical ligation of dural sac neck, resection of meningocele
  - Correction/stabilization of scoliosis

DIAGNOSTIC CHECKLIST

Consider

- LM prompts search for history/stigmata of NF1 or connective tissue disorder

Image Interpretation Pearls

- MR shows nonenhancing CSF signal intensity/density mass extending through enlarged neural foramen

SELECTED REFERENCES

1. Han Y et al: Management of lateral meningocele syndrome in a child without neurological symptoms and literature review. Childs Nerv Syst. 38(5):903-7, 2022
2. Yamada M et al: Early diagnosis of lateral meningocele syndrome in an infant without neurological symptoms based on genomic analysis. Childs Nerv Syst. 38(3):659-63, 2022
3. Amuthabarathi M et al: Infantile presentation of lehman syndrome with multiple lateral meningoceles, dural ectasias, and herniation of conus: a rare case report. J Pediatr Neurosci. 15(2):111-5, 2020
4. Cappuccio G et al: Expansion of the phenotype of lateral meningocele syndrome. Am J Med Genet A. 182(5):1259-62, 2020
5. Cuoco JA et al: Neurosurgical management of lateral meningocele syndrome: a clinical update for the pediatric neurosurgeon. Pediatr Neurosurg. 55(1):2-11, 2020
6. Brown EC et al: Neurosurgical management in lateral meningocele syndrome: case report. J Neurosurg Pediatr. 19(2):232-8, 2017
7. Prasad GR et al: Lateral meningomyelocele in a neonate: a case report. J Neonatal Surg. 5(1):4, 2016
8. Gripp KW et al: Truncating mutations in the last exon of NOTCH3 cause lateral meningocele syndrome. Am J Med Genet A. 167A(2):271-81, 2015
9. Alves D et al: Lateral meningocele syndrome: additional report and further evidence supporting a connective tissue basis. Am J Med Genet A. 161A(7):1768-72, 2013
10. Kumar BE et al: Bilateral multiple level lateral meningocoele. J Clin Imaging Sci. 3:1, 2013
11. Kumar V et al: Spontaneous subarachnoid pleural fistula: a rare complication of lateral thoracic meningocele. Neurol India. 58(3):466-7, 2010
12. Haddad R: Multiple asymptomatic lateral thoracic meningocele. Eur J Cardiothorac Surg. 33(1):113, 2008
13. Yen CP et al: Epidermoid cysts associated with thoracic meningocele. Acta Neurochir (Wien). 150(3):305-8; discussion 308-9, 2008

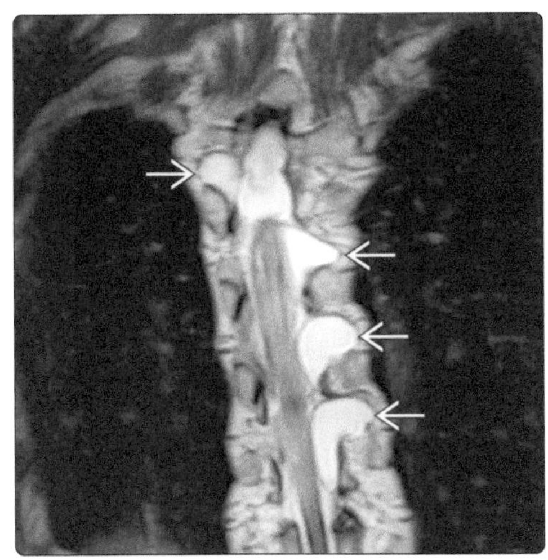

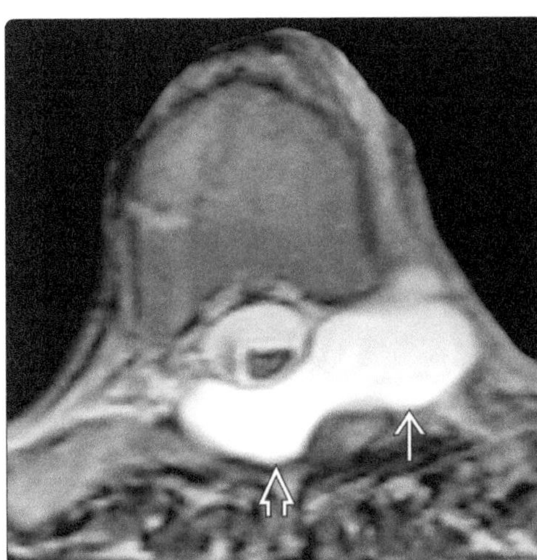

(Left) *Coronal T2WI MR in a patient with Marfan syndrome and scoliosis demonstrates multiple CSF signal lateral thoracic meningoceles ➡ extending into the adjacent enlarged neural foramina.* **(Right)** *Axial T2WI MR in a patient with Marfan syndrome reveals a large, left lateral thoracic meningocele ➡ extending through an enlarged, remodeled neural foramen. The contiguous intraspinal extradural component of the meningocele ➡ displaces the thecal sac anteriorly.*

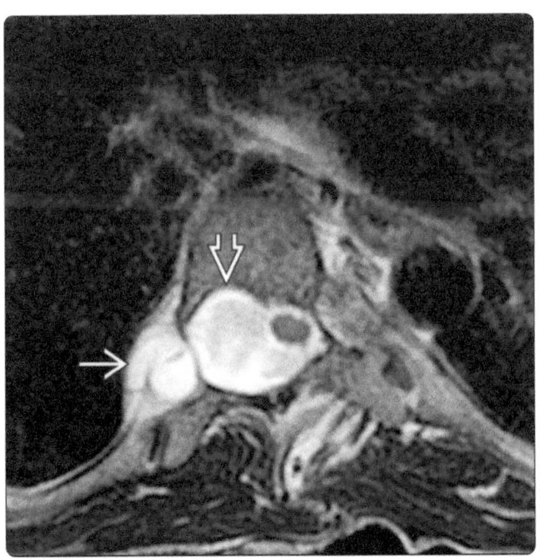

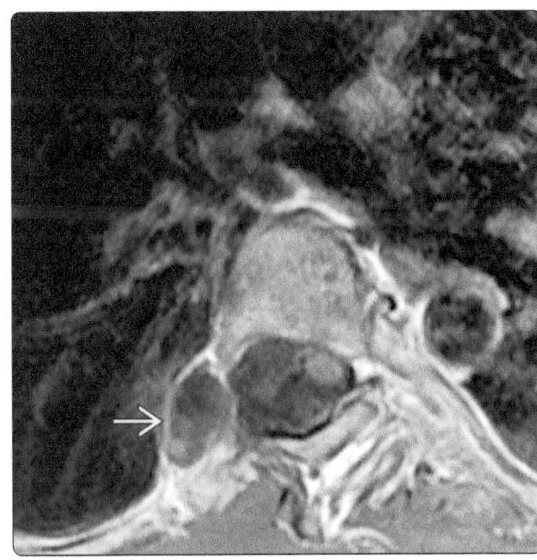

(Left) *Axial T2WI MR in a patient with NF1 demonstrates characteristic osseous remodeling of dural ectasia involving the midthoracic thecal sac ➡ with a right lateral meningocele ➡ projecting into right paraspinal soft tissue through an enlarged neural foramen.* **(Right)** *Axial T1 C+ MR in a patient with NF1 reveals extension of a lateral thoracic meningocele ➡ through an enlarged neural foramen. No abnormal tissue enhancement to indicate neurofibroma is demonstrated.*

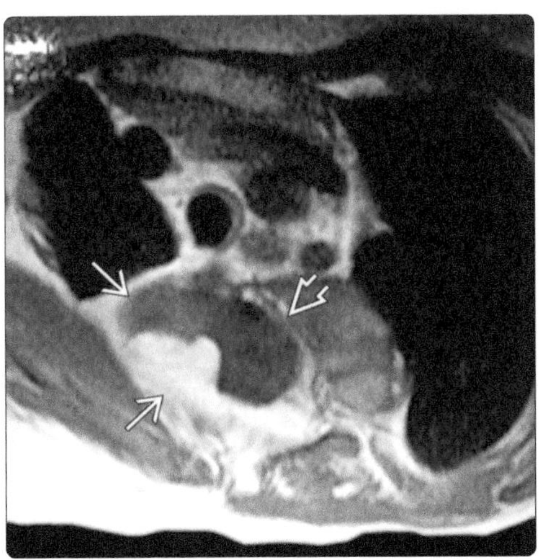

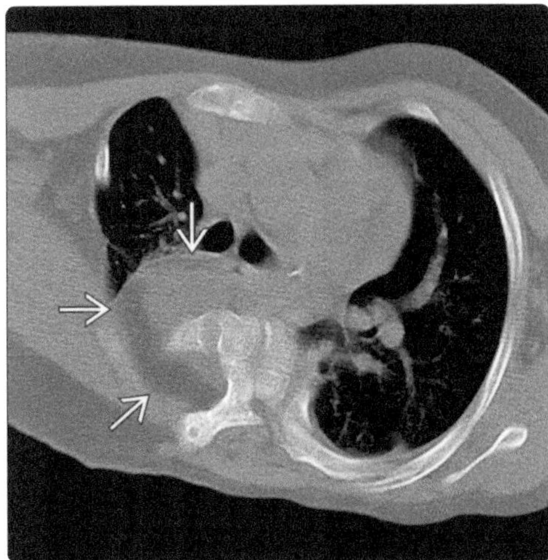

(Left) *Axial T1WI MR demonstrates lateral extension of a complex, fat-containing lateral thoracic meningocele ➡ into the right paraspinal tissues. Note scalloping of the posterior vertebral body ➡ and absence of the right pedicle.* **(Right)** *Axial bone CT shows lateral extension of a complex, fat-containing lateral thoracic meningocele ➡ around the vertebral body with enlargement of the neural foramen and absence of the right thoracic pedicle at the meningocele level.*

Dorsal Spinal Meningocele

KEY FACTS

TERMINOLOGY

- Synonyms: Simple meningocele, simple spinal meningocele, posterior meningocele

IMAGING

- Skin-covered dorsal dural sac protruding through posterior osseous defect
  - Dorsal herniation of dura, arachnoid, and CSF into spinal subcutaneous tissue
  - Occasional herniation of filum or nerve roots into defect
- Conus medullaris low or normal in position

TOP DIFFERENTIAL DIAGNOSES

- Lipomyelomeningocele
- Terminal myelocystocele
- Myelomeningocele
- Limited dorsal myeloschisis

PATHOLOGY

- ± hydromyelia, tethered cord, diastematomyelia
- Meningocele always skin covered; skin may be dysplastic, ulcerated

CLINICAL ISSUES

- Palpable, skin-covered mass or incidental discovery during imaging for other indications
  - Patients usually neurologically normal
- Cervical, thoracic meningoceles more likely to be symptomatic than lumbar meningocele

DIAGNOSTIC CHECKLIST

- Imaging goals are lesion detection, determination of simple or complex morphology, and exclusion of other spinal anomalies
  - Important to determine whether neural elements reside within sac prior to surgery

(Left) *Sagittal graphic of the lumbosacral spine shows a typical dorsal spinal meningocele sac ➡ protruding through the dysraphic posterior elements with a thin isthmus ➡ connecting to the thecal sac.* **(Right)** *Sagittal T1 MR reveals a borderline low-lying conus at L2 and a large, skin-covered, CSF signal mass ➡ in the subcutaneous tissues. The mass (dorsal meningocele) communicates with the thecal sac via a very thin fluid signal pedicle traversing the posterior elements ➡.*

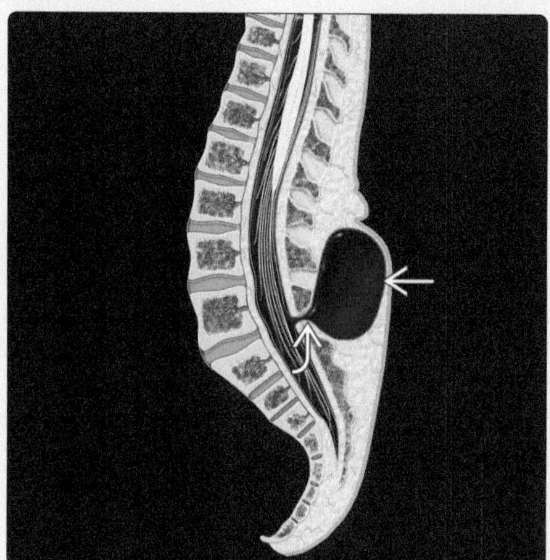

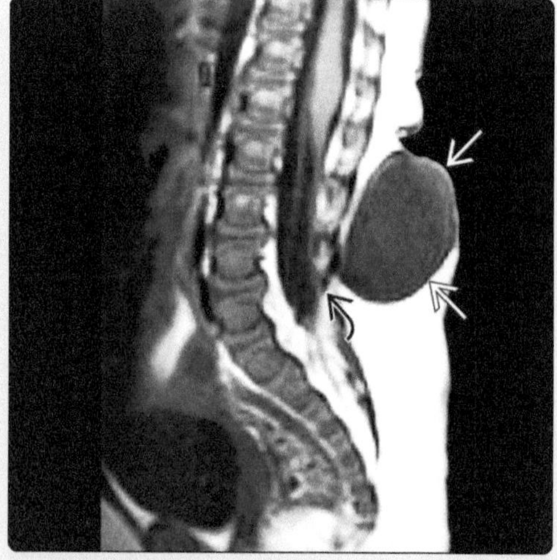

(Left) *Sagittal T2 MR of an infant with a skin-covered back mass demonstrates a large dorsal meningocele ➡ contiguous with the dural sac through a thin CSF-filled isthmus ➡. Note focal posterior spinal dysraphism ➡.* **(Right)** *Axial T2 MR demonstrates a large CSF signal dorsal spinal meningocele ➡ traversing a focal posterior spinal dysraphism ➡. Note the flow jet within the thin isthmus ➡.*

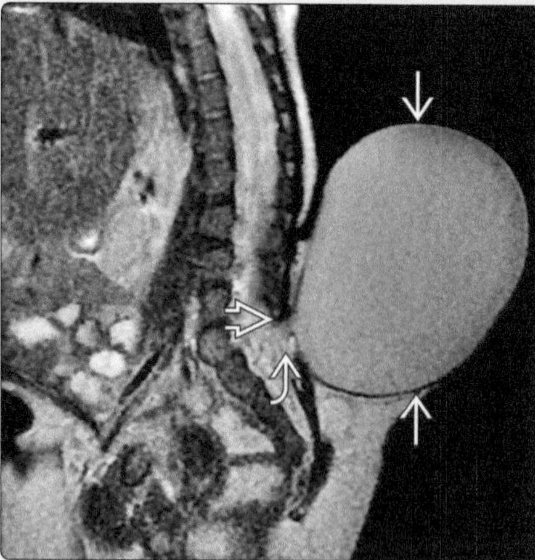

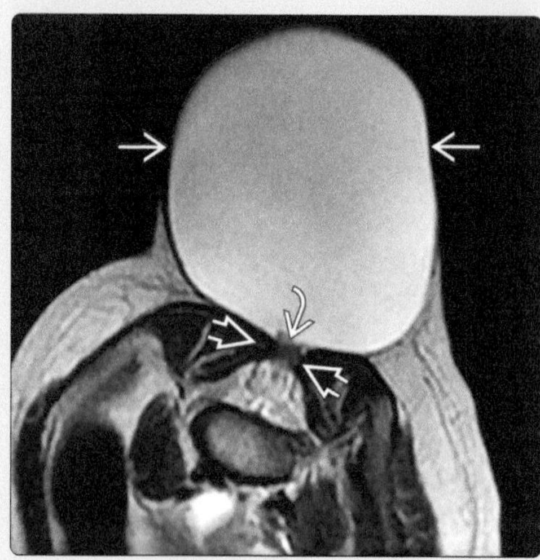

TERMINOLOGY

Synonyms

- Simple meningocele, simple spinal meningocele, posterior meningocele

Definitions

- Dorsal herniation of dura, arachnoid, and CSF into spinal subcutaneous tissue

IMAGING

General Features

- Best diagnostic clue
  - Skin-covered dorsal dural sac protruding thorough posterior osseous defect
- Location
  - Anywhere along dorsal spinal canal; lumbosacral junction, sacrum > > cervical, thoracic
- Size
  - Small and localized to large, encompassing multiple spinal levels
- Morphology
  - Sessile or pedunculated CSF intensity/density sac with spinal dysraphism
  - May (complex) or may not (simple) contain neural tissue

Radiographic Findings

- Radiography
  - Dorsal dysraphism; defect usually confined to 1-2 vertebrae
  - Widening of spinal canal, increased interpedicular distance

CT Findings

- NECT
  - Hypodense CSF dural sac
  - Overlying skin intact; may be ulcerated
- Bone CT
  - Dysraphism ± spinal canal widening, increased interpedicular distance
    - Mild cases may show only absent spinous process or localized spina bifida
    - More severe cases show multisegmental spina bifida, spinal canal enlargement

MR Findings

- T1WI
  - Skin-covered hypointense dural sac
  - Conus medullaris low or normal in position
  - Occasional herniation of filum or nerve roots into defect
- T2WI
  - Hyperintense dural sac
  - Low or normal conus medullaris position
  - ± filum terminale or nerve roots within defect

Ultrasonographic Findings

- Grayscale ultrasound
  - Hypoechoic CSF-filled sac protrudes through posterior defect ± entrapped nervous tissue
  - Demonstrates conus termination level and periodic motion
  - Primary utility for in utero or neonatal screening
    - Obstetric ultrasound may detect large meningocele in utero → altered delivery planning
    - Less useful in older children/adults due to spinal column ossification → posterior acoustic shadowing

Nonvascular Interventions

- Myelography
  - Dorsal dysraphism, widening of spinal canal, increased interpedicular distance
  - Dural sac herniates through dysraphic posterior elements
    - Dural sac communicates with subarachnoid space
      - May change size with position, Valsalva maneuver
    - ± neural elements, filum terminale within defect
  - Myelography mostly replaced by MR
    - Primary utility is for patients with MR contraindications and to answer discrepancies between MR and clinical findings

Imaging Recommendations

- Best imaging tool
  - MR best shows dural sac characteristics, associated vertebral or spinal cord anomalies
- Protocol advice
  - Sagittal and axial T1 and T2 MR
    - Sagittal useful to evaluate cord
    - Axial T1 most useful to evaluate size of dysraphic defect and to exclude lipoma
    - Axial T2 best for detecting nervous tissue within sac

DIFFERENTIAL DIAGNOSIS

Limited Dorsal Myeloschisis

- Characterized by 2 invariable features: Focal-closed neural tube defect and fibroneural stalk that links saccular or flat spinal skin lesion to underlying spinal cord
- Neuroglial tissue within fibrocollagenous band is central limited dorsal myeloschisis (LDM) stalk histopathologic feature
- Patients generally have favorable outcome following stalk untethering from spinal cord

Lipomyelomeningocele

- Skin-covered back malformation
- Distinguish by presence of neural tissue and fat within defect in addition to cyst

Terminal Myelocystocele

- Skin-covered back malformation
- Hydromyelic, low-lying cord protrudes through meningocele

Myelomeningocele

- Open spinal dysraphism; clinical appearance is diagnostic

PATHOLOGY

General Features

- Etiology
  - Unknown
    - No universally accepted unifying theory explains pathogenesis

- Associated abnormalities
  - ± hydromyelia, tethered cord, diastematomyelia
  - Chiari 2 malformation; much less common than with myelomeningocele
- Classically, simple meningoceles are considered isolated abnormality with normal conus termination level
  - However; some authors report low conus termination and other spinal anomalies with meningocele and question whether meningocele is ever truly isolated lesion
- Meningocele is always skin covered
  - Skin may be dysplastic or ulcerated
- Cervical lesions considered within cervical myelocystocele spectrum

Gross Pathologic & Surgical Features

- Nearly always contain aberrant nerve roots, ganglion cells, &/or glial nodules at surgery, gross pathology
- Herniated meningocele sac contains both dura and arachnoid
- Overlying tissue intact unless secondary skin ulceration

Microscopic Features

- Meningocele lined by arachnoid and thin-walled blood vessels
  - Arachnoidal adhesions may obstruct sac neck
- Overlying skin shows atrophic epidermis; lacks rete pegs and normal skin appendages

CLINICAL ISSUES

Presentation

- Most common signs/symptoms
  - Palpable, skin-covered mass
    - May be incidental discovery during imaging for other indications
- Other signs/symptoms
  - Back pain
  - Meningitis (ruptured or leaking meningocele)
  - Headache, other signs/symptoms of alternating high and low intracranial pressure
- Clinical profile
  - Patients are usually neurologically normal and present for imaging of palpable back mass
  - Cervical, thoracic meningoceles more likely to be symptomatic than lumbar meningocele

Demographics

- Age
  - In utero to adult life
- Sex
  - M = F
- Epidemiology
  - 1 per 10,000 live births

Natural History & Prognosis

- Variable; depends on cyst size and contents, status of overlying skin, presence or absence of meningitis
- Skin covering permits more "elective" surgical correction
  - Most newborns require operation before release from nursery to home

Treatment

- Asymptomatic patients may warrant conservative observation
- Symptomatic patients require surgical resection, repair of dural defect

DIAGNOSTIC CHECKLIST

Consider

- Ultrasound in infants to determine cord level, presence or absence of neural elements in meningocele
- MR is best modality to definitively characterize meningocele, evaluate for other spinal abnormalities
  - Use steady-state technique (CISS/FIESTA) to best visualize nerve roots/adhesions/masses

Image Interpretation Pearls

- Imaging goals are lesion detection, determination of simple or complex morphology, and exclusion of other spinal anomalies
  - Important to determine whether neural elements reside within sac prior to surgery
  - Meningocele may be most obvious abnormality that masks other less obvious, but clinically more important lesions

SELECTED REFERENCES

1. Morioka T et al: Retained medullary cord with sacral subcutaneous meningocele and congenital dermal sinus. Childs Nerv Syst. 36(2):423-7, 2020
2. Lafitte AS et al: A case of prenatally diagnosed limited dorsal myeloschisis with good prognosis. J Clin Ultrasound. 46(4):282-5, 2018
3. Morioka T et al: Neurosurgical pathology of limited dorsal myeloschisis. Childs Nerv Syst. 34(2):293-303, 2018
4. Murakami N et al: Retained medullary cord extending to a sacral subcutaneous meningocele. Childs Nerv Syst. 34(3):527-33, 2018
5. Lee SM et al: Limited dorsal myeloschisis and congenital dermal sinus: comparison of clinical and MR imaging features. AJNR Am J Neuroradiol. 38(1):176-82, 2017
6. Schmidt C et al: Meningocele manqué: a comprehensive review of this enigmatic finding in occult spinal dysraphism. Childs Nerv Syst. 33(7):1065-71, 2017
7. McComb JG: A practical clinical classification of spinal neural tube defects. Childs Nerv Syst. 31(10):1641-57, 2015
8. Kole MJ et al: Currarino syndrome and spinal dysraphism. J Neurosurg Pediatr. 13(6):685-9, 2014
9. Moriyama T et al: Postoperative spinal cord herniation with pseudomeningocele in the cervical spine: a case report. Spine J. 13(10):e43-5, 2013
10. Le TC et al: Dorsal thoracic spinal cord herniation: report of an unusual case and review of the literature. Spine J. 12(10):e9-12, 2012
11. Singh N et al: Multiple neural tube defects in a child: a rare developmental anomaly. Surg Neurol Int. 3:147, 2012
12. Rao ZX et al: Congenital spinal intradural arachnoid cyst associated with intrathoracic meningocele in a child. J Zhejiang Univ Sci B. 11(6):429-32, 2010
13. Duz B et al: Cervical congenital midline meningoceles in adults. Neurosurgery. 63(5):938-44; discussion 944-5, 2008
14. Sanli AM et al: Giant true dorsal thoracic meningocele in a school-age child. Case report. J Neurosurg Pediatr. 1(5):399-401, 2008
15. Rossi A et al: Spinal dysraphism: MR imaging rationale. J Neuroradiol. 31(1):3-24, 2004
16. Graham D et al: Greenfield's Neuropathology. 7th ed. Arnold. 380, 2002
17. Ersahin Y et al: Is meningocele really an isolated lesion? Childs Nerv Syst. 17(8):487-90, 2001
18. Unsinn KM et al: US of the spinal cord in newborns: spectrum of normal findings, variants, congenital anomalies, and acquired diseases. Radiographics. 20(4):923-38, 2000
19. Steinbok P et al: Cervical meningoceles and myelocystoceles: a unifying hypothesis. Pediatr Neurosurg. 23(6):317-22, 1995

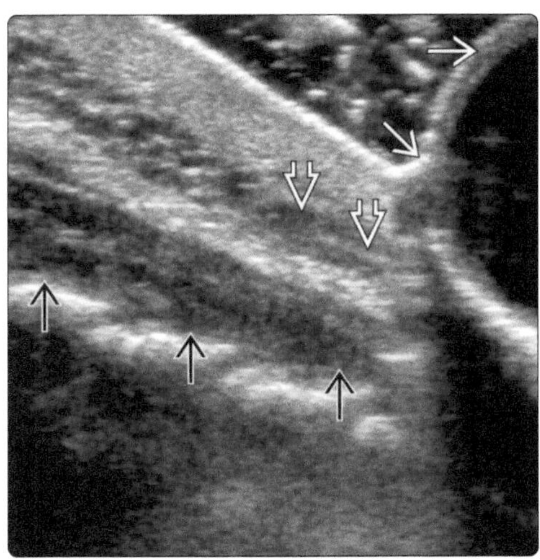

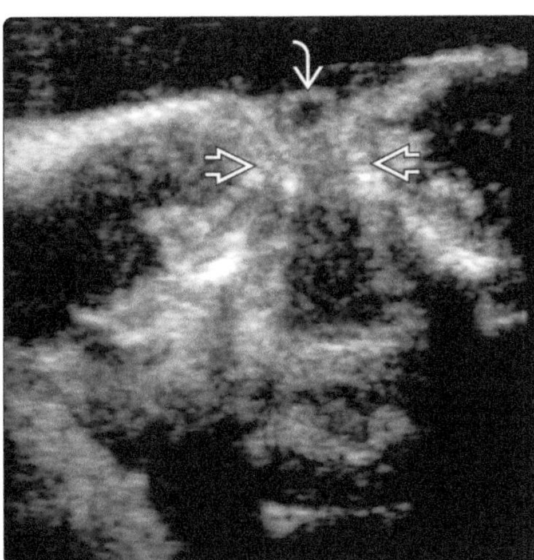

(Left) *Longitudinal ultrasound shows a skin-covered cystic mass ➡ with internal hypoechogenicity protruding from the midline back. The last intact posterior elements ➡ are demonstrated well. The distal spinal cord ➡ is low lying and tethered by the meningocele.* **(Right)** *Transverse ultrasound confirms posterior spinal dysraphism ➡ with fluid-filled extension ➡ of the dural sac through the osseous defect into the dorsal soft tissues.*

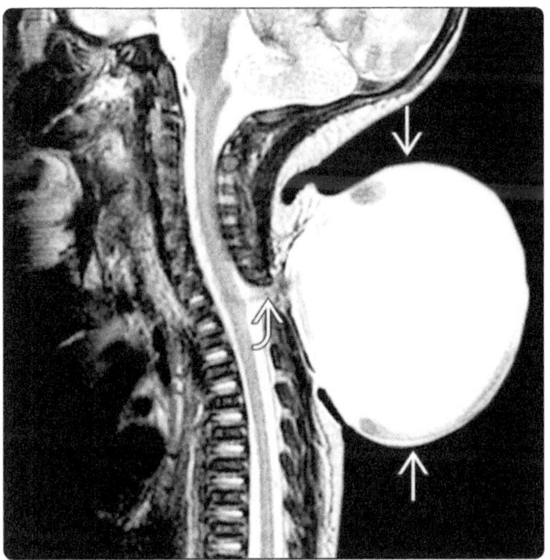

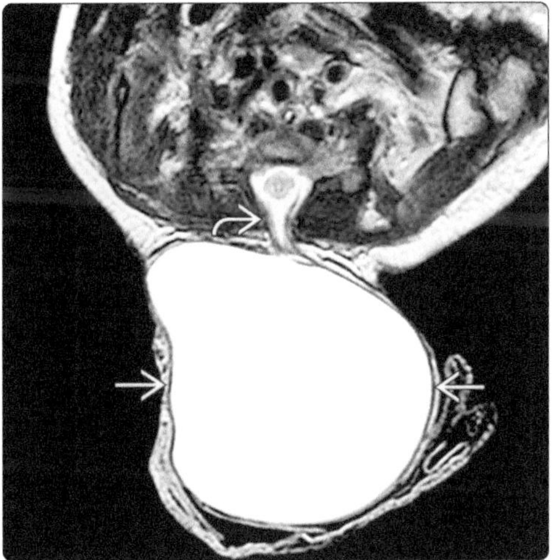

(Left) *Sagittal T2 MR demonstrates a large, cervicothoracic dorsal meningocele ➡ extending into the subcutaneous tissues through a thin dysraphic isthmus. There is a hypointense CSF flow jet ➡ through the isthmus into the sac.* **(Right)** *Axial T2 MR shows a large, cervicothoracic dorsal meningocele extending into the subcutaneous tissues through a thin dysraphic isthmus ➡. Conforming to strict definition, the sac ➡ contains no neural elements, and the cervical spinal cord is normal.*

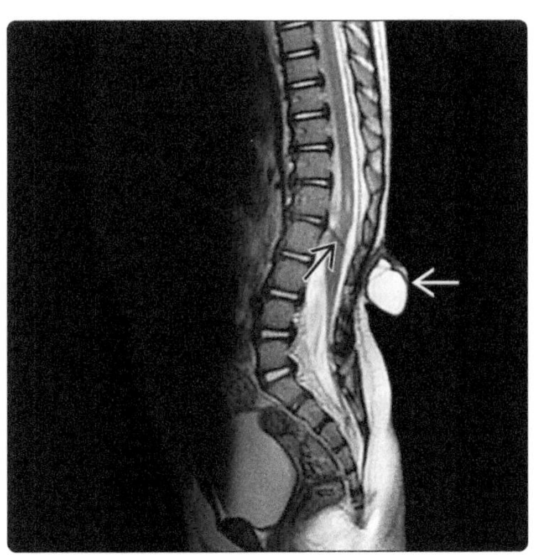

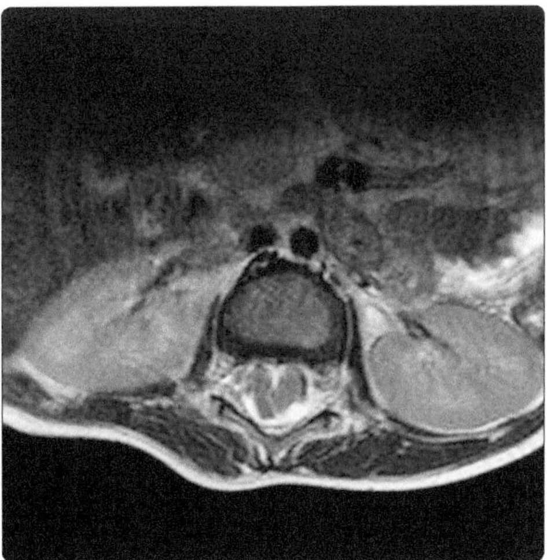

(Left) *Sagittal T2 MR shows a skin-covered cystic back mass ➡ at the lower lumbar level. The spinal cord is low lying with the conus terminating at the L5 level. An obliquely oriented, hypointense, fibrous band ➡ traverses the spinal cord and enters the cystic back mass.* **(Right)** *Axial T2 MR reveals spinal cord distortion as the fibrous band traverses the cord parenchyma above the meningocele level, representing a short segmental diastematomyelia (surgically proven).*

KEY FACTS

TERMINOLOGY

- Synonym: Dural ectasia

IMAGING

- Smooth remodeling of posterior vertebral body, expansion of osseous spinal canal, ± kyphoscoliosis
  - Pedicular attenuation, widened interpediculate distance, erosion of anterior and posterior elements
- Patulous, expansile dural sac enlargement
- Easiest to appreciate on sagittal images

TOP DIFFERENTIAL DIAGNOSES

- Congenital vertebral dysplasia
- Spinal tumor or syrinx
- Cauda equina syndrome of ankylosing spondylitis

PATHOLOGY

- Etiologies include NF1, connective tissue disorders (Marfan syndrome, Ehlers-Danlos syndrome, Loeys-Dietz syndrome, homocystinuria), idiopathic
- Association with lateral thoracic or lumbar meningocele, anterior sacral meningocele, kyphoscoliosis, joint hypermobility, lens abnormalities, aneurysm, arterial dissection, and peripheral or central neoplasms
- Dura in ectatic areas is extremely thin, fragile

CLINICAL ISSUES

- Most commonly presents with back pain ± radiculopathy
- Other complaints include headache, incontinence, pelvic symptoms
- May present at any age depending on severity, underlying etiology

DIAGNOSTIC CHECKLIST

- Recognition of specific imaging clues and integration of available clinical data permits more specific diagnosis
- Important to determine underlying disorder for treatment planning, genetic counseling, and determining prognosis

(Left) *Sagittal graphic of the lumbosacral spine demonstrates scalloping of the posterior vertebral bodies and central spinal canal enlargement. Note that the dural sac generally fills the concavity produced in the posterior vertebral body. Also conspicuous (inset) are bilateral lumbar lateral meningoceles.* **(Right)** *Sagittal T2 MR (Marfan syndrome) reveals marked posterior thoracolumbar vertebral scalloping at multiple levels, resulting in increased canal diameter.*

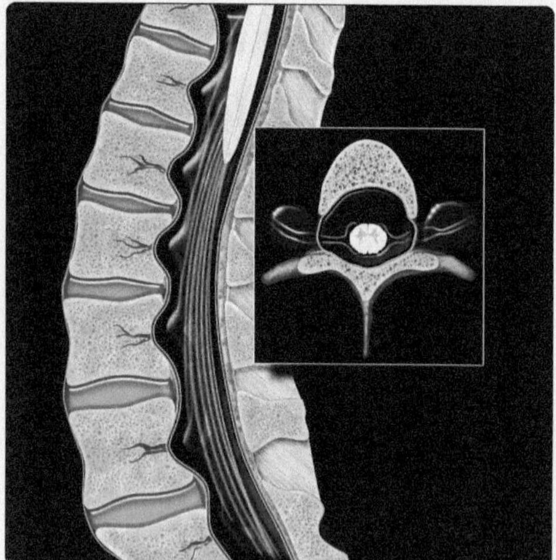

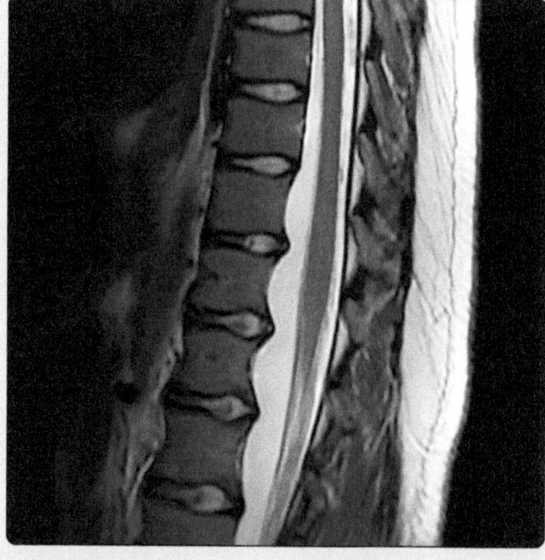

(Left) *Axial T2 MR in the same patient reveals eccentric canal expansion associated with posterior vertebral scalloping. There is also widening of the left neural foramen, suggesting the beginning of lateral meningocele formation.* **(Right)** *Axial T2 MR in the same patient obtained more caudally shows more symmetric enlargement of the spinal canal with pedicular thinning.*

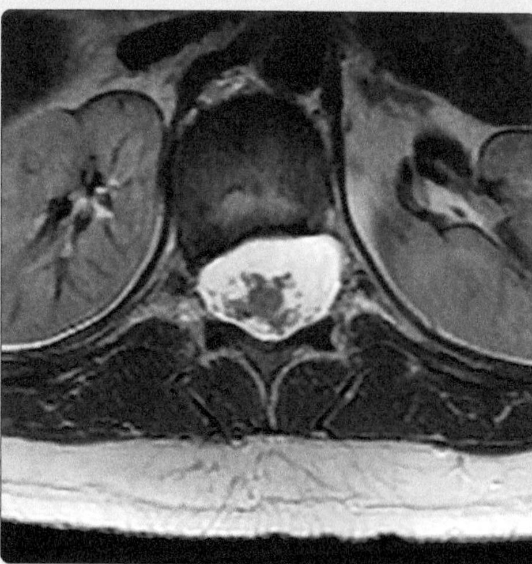

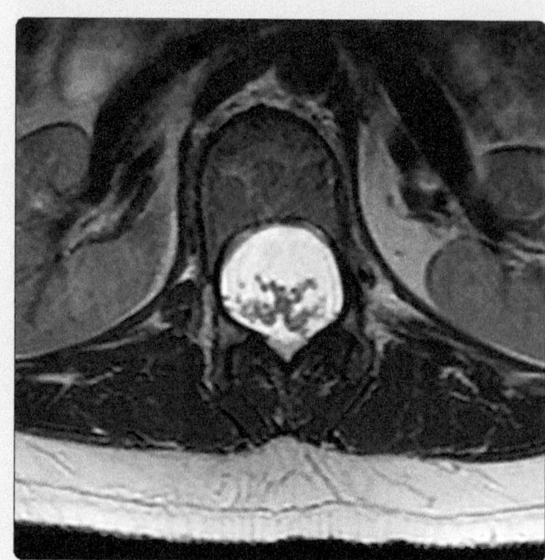

TERMINOLOGY

Synonyms

- Dural ectasia

Definitions

- Patulous dural sac with posterior vertebral scalloping

IMAGING

General Features

- Best diagnostic clue
  - Smooth, C-shaped scalloping of posterior vertebral bodies with patulous dural sac
- Location
  - Lumbar > cervical, thoracic
- Size
  - Mild → extensive deformity
- Morphology
  - Expansile dural sac, spinal canal remodeling with posterior vertebral scalloping

Radiographic Findings

- Radiography
  - Smooth remodeling of posterior vertebral body, expansion of osseous spinal canal, ± kyphoscoliosis
  - Osteopenia (homocystinuria)

CT Findings

- CECT
  - Posterior vertebral scalloping → spinal canal enlargement; easiest to appreciate on sagittal images
  - Pedicular attenuation, widened interpediculate distance, erosion of anterior and posterior elements, patulous CSF density dural sac
- CTA
  - ± arterial dissection or aneurysm; implicates Marfan or Ehlers-Danlos syndrome as underlying etiology

MR Findings

- T1WI
  - Posterior vertebral scalloping, expansion of osseous spinal canal, patulous dural sac, ± kyphoscoliosis
  - ± pedicular thinning, lateral meningocele(s)
- T2WI
  - Similar findings to T1WI
  - Best evaluates position of neural elements relative to dural ectasia
- MRA
  - ± arterial dissection or aneurysm (Marfan, Ehlers-Danlos syndrome)

Ultrasonographic Findings

- Grayscale ultrasound
  - Hypoechoic patulous dural sac, widening of spinal canal

Angiographic Findings

- Conventional: Not useful for imaging spine deformity; primary utility is detecting associated vascular anomalies
  - Ascending aortic aneurysm (tulip bulb configuration) suggests Marfan syndrome

Nonvascular Interventions

- Myelography
  - Posterior vertebral scalloping, contrast fills enlarged dural sac, ± lateral meningocele(s)

Imaging Recommendations

- MR shows osseous abnormalities well
- Additionally, MR most useful modality to exclude syrinx or tumor as cause of canal enlargement before attributing to dural ectasia

DIFFERENTIAL DIAGNOSIS

Congenital Vertebral Dysplasia

- Achondroplasia
- Mucopolysaccharidosis
- Osteogenesis imperfecta (tarda)
- Search for appropriate family history, clinical stigmata

Spinal Tumor or Syrinx

- Astrocytoma
- Ependymoma
- Nerve sheath tumor
- Syrinx
- Characteristic imaging findings lead to correct diagnosis

Cauda Equina Syndrome of Ankylosing Spondylitis

- Irregular lumbar canal expansion
- Proposed etiology for dural ectasia; proliferative inflammatory synovium → cauda equina symptoms
- Imaging and clinical stigmata of ankylosing spondylitis typically present

PATHOLOGY

General Features

- Etiology
  - Genetic disorder
    - Neurofibromatosis type 1 (NF1): Primary mesenchymal disorder
    - Marfan syndrome: Primary connective tissue resulting from mutation in fibrillin-1 (*FBN1*) gene
    - Ehlers-Danlos: > 10 different types of collagen synthesis defects
    - Homocystinuria: Cystathionine β-synthetase deficiency
  - Idiopathic
- Genetics
  - NF1: Autosomal dominant (chromosome 17q12)
  - Marfan: Autosomal dominant
  - Homocystinuria: Autosomal recessive
  - Ehlers-Danlos: Autosomal dominant
- Associated abnormalities
  - Lateral thoracic or lumbar meningocele, anterior sacral meningocele; Kyphoscoliosis
  - Joint hypermobility, lens abnormalities, aneurysm, arterial dissection (connective tissue disorders)
  - Peripheral and central neoplasms (NF1)
- Genetic predisposition → primary meningeal dysplasia → weakness in meninges → expansion, secondary remodeling of posterior vertebral body and pedicular thinning → further dural sac expansion

Gross Pathologic & Surgical Features

- Enlarged CSF thecal sac, remodeled posterior vertebral bodies; dura in ectatic areas is extremely thin, fragile

Microscopic Features

- Dural thinning in ectatic areas
  - Increased risk of CSF leak → intracranial hypotension

CLINICAL ISSUES

Presentation

- Most common signs/symptoms
  - Back pain → radiculopathy
    - Moderate to severe back pain in > 50% of Marfan patients; presence, degree of dural ectasia associated with back pain
    - High prevalence of dural ectasia (41%) in Marfan patients without back pain; however, mere presence of dural ectasia does not necessarily mean patient is symptomatic
  - Other signs/symptoms
    - Headache related to intracranial hypotension
    - Incontinence, pelvic symptoms
- Clinical profile
  - NF1: Plexiform neurofibromas, kyphoscoliosis, optic nerve gliomas and other astrocytomas, café au lait spots, axillary freckling, extremity pseudoarthrosis
  - Marfan: Tall, joint hypermobility, arachnodactyly, kyphoscoliosis, joint and lens dislocations
  - Homocystinuria: Tall, arachnodactyly, scoliosis, intellectual disability, seizures, lens dislocations
  - Ehlers-Danlos: ± tall, thin hyperelastic skin, hypermobile joints, fragile connective tissue

Demographics

- Age
  - May present at any age, depending on severity
- Sex
  - M = F
- Ethnicity
  - NF1: All ethnicities; higher in Arab-Israeli subpopulations
  - Marfan: All races, ethnicities
  - Homocystinuria: Northern European descent
  - Ehlers-Danlos: White patients, European descent
- Epidemiology
  - NF1: 1/4,000; 50% new mutations; dural ectasia common
  - Marfan: 1/5,000 (USA); dural ectasia present in > 60%
  - Homocystinuria: 1/344,000 worldwide; dural dysplasia less common than Marfan
  - Ehlers-Danlos: 1/400,000 (worldwide); dural dysplasia less common than Marfan

Natural History & Prognosis

- Variable; dependent on underlying etiology
- Morbidity and mortality primarily related to vascular pathology
  - Vascular fragility → predisposition to arterial dissection or aneurysm → premature death

Treatment

- Treatment directed toward addressing underlying etiology
- Meningocele repair, scoliosis surgery for more severe cases

DIAGNOSTIC CHECKLIST

Consider

- 3 disease categories produce posterior vertebral scalloping
  - Dural ectasia
  - Increased intraspinal pressure
  - Congenital vertebral dysplasia
- Important to determine underlying disorder for treatment planning, genetic counseling, and determining prognosis

Image Interpretation Pearls

- Recognition of specific imaging clues and integration of available clinical data permits more specific diagnosis
- Look for imaging stigmata of etiologic diseases
  - "Tulip bulb" aortic aneurysm → Marfan syndrome
  - Osteoporosis → homocystinuria
  - Pseudoarthrosis, CNS/PNS tumors → NF1

SELECTED REFERENCES

1. Han Y et al: Management of lateral meningocele syndrome in a child without neurological symptoms and literature review. Childs Nerv Syst. 38(5):903-7, 2022
2. Kang E et al: Whole-body MRI evaluation in neurofibromatosis type 1 patients younger than 3 years old and the genetic contribution to disease progression. Orphanet J Rare Dis. 17(1):24, 2022
3. Ito K et al: Increase in dural ectasia size in scoliosis patients with Marfan syndrome. J Pediatr Orthop B. 30(3):235-8, 2021
4. Well L et al: Phenotyping spinal abnormalities in patients with neurofibromatosis type 1 using whole-body MRI. Sci Rep. 11(1):16889, 2021
5. Pichott A et al: Dural ectasia and intracranial hypotension in Marfan syndrome. Rev Chil Pediatr. 91(4):591-6, 2020
6. Shah S et al: The association of spinal deformity with dural ectasia in neurofibromatosis type 1. Br J Neurosurg. 33(6):620-3, 2019
7. Kohns DJ: Interventional spine considerations for dural ectasia in a patient with Marfan syndrome. Am J Phys Med Rehabil. 97(1):e6-8, 2018
8. Razek AAKA: MR imaging of neoplastic and non-neoplastic lesions of the brain and spine in neurofibromatosis type I. Neurol Sci. 39(5):821-7, 2018
9. Sheridan GA et al: Dural ectasia associated with Mounier-Kuhn syndrome: a novel association in the context of spinal stenosis. BMJ Case Rep. 2017, 2017
10. Elgafy H et al: Sacral erosion and insufficiency fracture secondary to dural ectasia in patient with Marfan syndrome. Spine J. 16(5):e301-2, 2016
11. Kow CY et al: Incidental dural ectasia associated with scoliosis. Spine J. 16(1):e25-6, 2016
12. Jain VV et al: Dural ectasia in a child with Larsen syndrome. J Pediatr Orthop. 34(7):e44-9, 2014
13. Kono AK et al: Prevalence of dural ectasia in Loeys-Dietz syndrome: comparison with Marfan syndrome and normal controls. PLoS One. 8(9):e75264, 2013
14. Mesfin A et al: Ten-year clinical and imaging follow-up of dural ectasia in adults with Marfan syndrome. Spine J. 13(1):62-7, 2013
15. Sznajder M et al: Spinal imaging contributes to the diagnosis of Marfan syndrome. Joint Bone Spine. 77(5):445-50, 2010
16. García-Estevez DA et al: [Dural ectasia in the cervical spine and neurofibromatosis type 1.] Rev Neurol. 48(1):51, 2009
17. Sanz-Ayan MP et al: [Dural ectasia and lumbar pain associated with Marfan syndrome.] Rev Neurol. 47(10):559-60, 2008
18. Kotil K et al: Lumbar radiculopathy in ankylosing spondylitis with dural ectasia. J Clin Neurosci. 14(10):981-3, 2007
19. Knirsch W et al: Dural ectasia in children with Marfan syndrome: a prospective, multicenter, patient-control study. Am J Med Genet A. 140(7):775-81, 2006
20. Reitman CA et al: Neurologic and morphologic features of dural ectasia in ankylosing spondylitis and rheumatoid arthritis: a case report. Am J Orthop (Belle Mead NJ). 35(11):530-1, 2006
21. Habermann CR et al: MR evaluation of dural ectasia in Marfan syndrome: reassessment of the established criteria in children, adolescents, and young adults. Radiology. 234(2):535-41, 2005
22. Knirsch W et al: Normal values of the sagittal diameter of the lumbar spine (vertebral body and dural sac) in children measured by MRI. Pediatr Radiol. 35(4):419-24, 2005

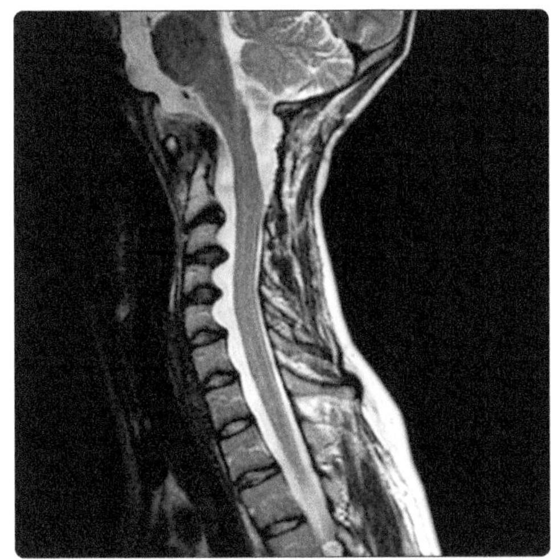

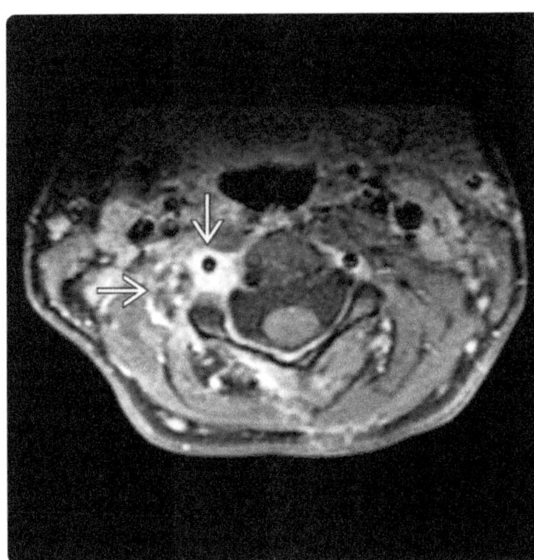

(Left) *Sagittal T2 MR (neurofibromatosis type 1) demonstrates striking posterior vertebral scalloping (C2-C6) related to dural dysplasia, producing widening of the AP canal diameter. No intradural or foraminal neurofibromas are identified at the affected levels.* **(Right)** *Axial T1 C+ FS MR confirms AP canal enlargement as well as an infiltrating, enhancing plexiform neurofibroma ➔, diagnostic of neurofibromatosis type 1.*

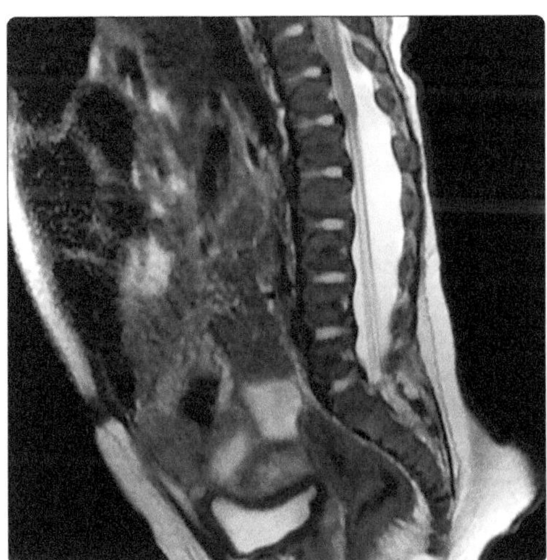

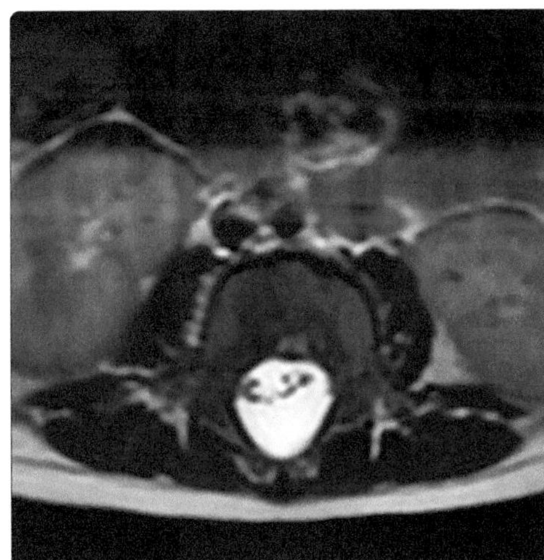

(Left) *Sagittal T2 MR in a 3-month-old with chondrodysplasia punctata demonstrates posterior dural body and posterior element remodeling, resulting in a patulous dural sac appearance.* **(Right)** *Axial T2 MR in the same patient confirms patulous widening of the lumbar spinal canal and scalloping of the posterior vertebral body. The nerve roots are anteriorly positioned because of reduced lumbar lordotic curvature.*

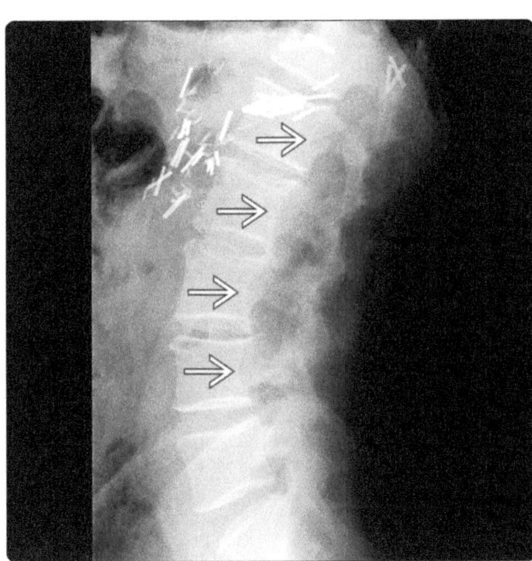

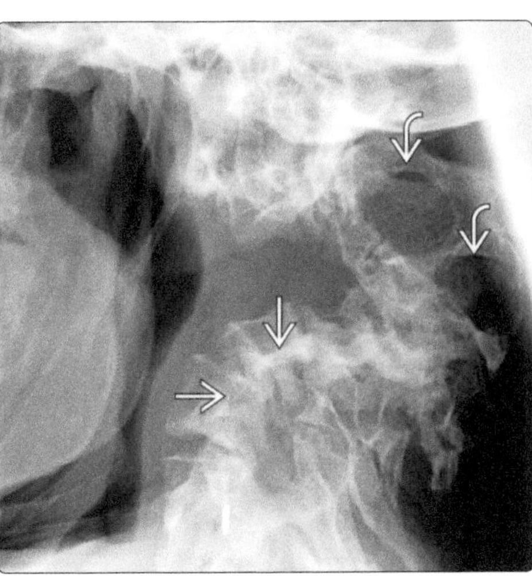

(Left) *Lateral plain radiograph (neurofibromatosis type 1) demonstrates curved posterior vertebral body remodeling ➔ at multiple lumbar vertebral levels, characteristic of dural dysplasia. Vascular clips indicate site of prior pheochromocytoma resection.* **(Right)** *Lateral radiograph (neurofibromatosis type 1) shows striking posterior vertebral scalloping ➔, extreme focal kyphosis, and marked neural foraminal enlargement ➔.*

KEY FACTS

TERMINOLOGY

- Synonyms: von Recklinghausen disease, peripheral neurofibromatosis
- Mesodermal dysplasia with neurofibromas, spinal deformity, neoplastic and nonneoplastic brain lesions, and cutaneous stigmata

IMAGING

- Kyphoscoliosis ± multiple nerve root tumors, plexiform NF (PNF), dural ectasia/lateral meningocele
- Tumors range from tiny to very large

TOP DIFFERENTIAL DIAGNOSES

- Neurofibromatosis type 2 (NF2) (central neurofibromatosis)
- Chronic inflammatory demyelinating polyneuropathy
- Congenital hypertrophic polyradiculoneuropathies

PATHOLOGY

- Autosomal dominant
- Characteristic lesion is PNF, although 3 types of spinal NF seen in NF1
  - Localized NF (90% of all NFs)
  - Diffuse NF
  - PNF (pathognomonic for NF1)

CLINICAL ISSUES

- Pigmentation anomalies (café au lait, axillary freckling, Lisch nodules)
- Focal or acute angle kyphoscoliosis ± myelopathy
- Palpable spinal or cutaneous masses
- Severity of clinical phenotype highly variable

DIAGNOSTIC CHECKLIST

- Multiple nerve sheath tumors, ≥ 1 NF, bizarre kyphoscoliosis with deformed vertebra → consider NF1
- Absence of visible stigmata does not exclude NF1
- Characteristic PNF appearance best displayed using fat-saturated T2 or STIR MR

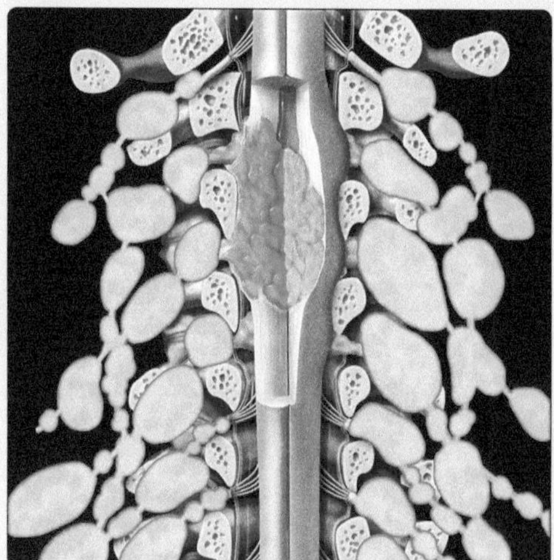

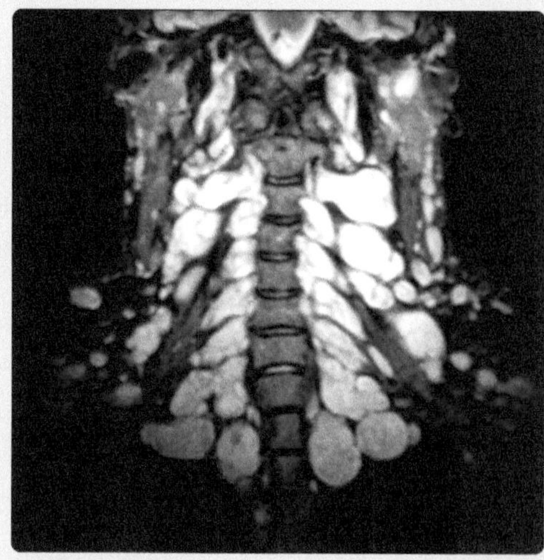

(Left) *Coronal graphic demonstrates several features of neurofibromatosis type 1 (NF1). There is an expansile intramedullary mass as well as bilateral plexiform neurofibromatas (PNFs) involving the entire brachial plexus.* **(Right)** *Coronal STIR MR reveals extensive PNF involving the bilateral brachial plexus. Some of these tumors show a characteristic central low-signal target, a pathognomonic finding for PNF.*

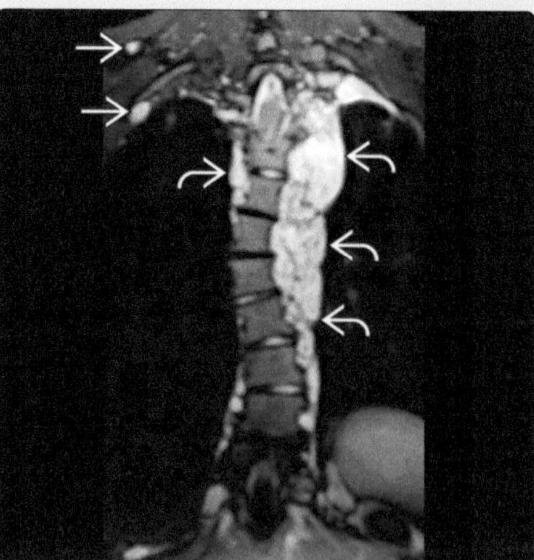

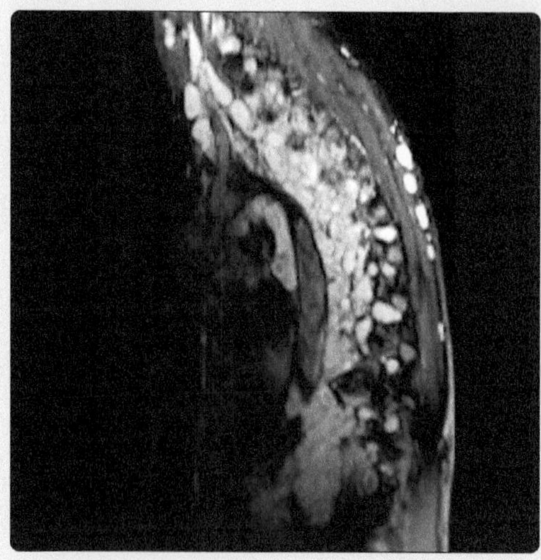

(Left) *Coronal STIR MR reveals extensive PNF ➢ involving the bilateral paraspinal sympathetic chains as well as involvement of multiple intercostal nerves ➡.* **(Right)** *Sagittal STIR MR obtained off-midline demonstrates innumerable T2-hyperintense PNFs involving the spinal nerves, sympathetic chains, and bilateral brachial plexus as well as multiple cutaneous nerves.*

TERMINOLOGY

Abbreviations

- Neurofibromatosis type 1 (NF1)

Synonyms

- von Recklinghausen disease, peripheral NF, nerve root neurofibroma

Definitions

- Autosomal dominant mesodermal dysplasia characterized by plexiform and NFs, spinal deformity, neoplastic and nonneoplastic brain lesions, and cutaneous stigmata

IMAGING

General Features

- Best diagnostic clue
  - Kyphoscoliosis ± multiple nerve root tumors, plexiform NF (PNF), dural ectasia/lateral meningocele
- Location
  - Entire craniospinal axis
- Size
  - Tumors range from tiny to very large
- Morphology
  - Kyphosis/kyphoscoliosis often severe and bizarre
  - Neurogenic tumors localized to nerve roots as well as within plexiform nerve masses, cutaneous lesions

Radiographic Findings

- Radiography
  - Kyphosis/scoliosis, scalloped vertebra, hypoplastic pedicles and posterior elements, "ribbon" ribs

CT Findings

- NECT
  - Hypodense fusiform or focal nerve root enlargement ± heterogeneous spinal cord expansion (glial tumor)
  - Dural ectasia ± CSF density lateral meningocele(s)
- CECT
  - Variable mild/moderate tumor enhancement
- Bone CT
  - Vertebral findings similar to radiography; canal, foraminal widening 2° to dural ectasia ± spinal cord tumor

MR Findings

- T1WI
  - NF: Intramedullary glial cord tumors hypo- to isointense to normal spinal cord, nerve roots, muscle
- T2WI
  - NF: Cord tumors hyperintense to normal spinal cord, nerve roots
    - NF: Target sign (hyperintense rim, low/intermediate signal intensity center) suggests neurogenic tumor; PNF > NF > malignant peripheral nerve sheath tumor (MPNST)
  - Occasional foci of T2 hyperintensity; not well studied but postulated to be spine equivalent of similar brain lesions
- STIR
  - NF: Cord tumors hyperintense to normal nerve root, cord, muscle
- T1WI C+
  - Variable mild to moderate NF, cord tumor enhancement

Nuclear Medicine Findings

- PET
  - FDG standard uptake value (SUV) MPNST > benign tumors

Imaging Recommendations

- Best imaging tool
  - MR
- Protocol advice
  - Radiography to quantitate and follow kyphosis, scoliosis
  - Multiplanar enhanced MR (especially STIR, fat-saturated T2, and T1 C+ MR) to evaluate cord, nerve pathology
  - Bone CT to optimally define osseous anatomy for surgical planning
  - May be future role for whole-body MR to characterize NF1 disease burden

DIFFERENTIAL DIAGNOSIS

Neurofibromatosis Type 2 (Central Neurofibromatosis)

- Multiple intracranial schwannomas and meningiomas and spinal schwannomas and meningiomas
- Spinal deformity uncommon
- Clinical, laboratory, and genetic testing findings distinguish from NF1

Chronic Inflammatory Demyelinating Polyneuropathy

- Repeated episodes of demyelination, remyelination → "onion skin" spinal, peripheral nerve enlargement
- Mimics PNF on imaging studies
- No cutaneous stigmata of NF1

Congenital Hypertrophic Polyradiculoneuropathies

- Charcot-Marie-Tooth, Dejerine-Sottas disease
- Nerve root enlargement mimics PNF on imaging studies
- No cutaneous stigmata of NF1

PATHOLOGY

General Features

- Etiology
  - Postulated that *NF1* tumor suppression gene "switched off" → tissue proliferation, tumor development
- Genetics
  - Autosomal dominant; chromosome 17q12, penetrance → 100%
    - *NF1* gene product (neurofibromin) is tumor suppressor
  - ~ 50% new mutations (paternal germline; paternal age 35 years → 2x ↑ in new mutations)
- Associated abnormalities
  - Brain abnormalities: Macrocephaly, focal areas of signal abnormality (FASI), sphenoid wing dysplasia, glial tumors, intellectual disability, epilepsy, hydrocephalus, aqueductal stenosis
  - ↑ risk of other neuroendocrine tumors (pheochromocytoma, carcinoid tumor), chronic myelogenous leukemia (CML)

- Congenital bowing, pseudoarthrosis of tibia and forearm, massive extremity overgrowth
- ↑ fibromuscular dysplasia, intracranial aneurysms, multiple sclerosis
- PNF is hallmark of NF1
- Kyphoscoliosis is most common NF1 osseous abnormality; variable severity mild, nonprogressive → severe curvature
  - Dystrophic scoliosis: Short segment, sharply angulated, < 6 spinal segments, tendency → severe deformity
  - Nondystrophic scoliosis: Similar to adolescent idiopathic curvature, usually 8-10 spinal segments, right convex
  - Severe cervical kyphosis highly suggestive of NF1
- Dural ectasia: 1° bone dysplasia; some cases 2° to pressure erosion from intraspinal tumors
- "Ribbon" ribs 2° to bone dysplasia ± intercostal NF

Staging, Grading, & Classification

- Consensus Development Conference on Neurofibromatosis (NIH, 1987)
  - 2 or more of following criteria
    - > 6 café au lait spots measuring ≥ 15 mm in adults or 5 mm in children
    - ≥ 2 NFs of any type or ≥ 1 PNF
    - Axillary or inguinal freckling, optic glioma
    - ≥ 2 Lisch nodules (iris hamartomas)
    - Distinctive osseous lesion (sphenoid wing dysplasia, thinning of long bone ± pseudoarthrosis)
    - 1st-degree relative with NF1

Gross Pathologic & Surgical Features

- 3 types of spinal NF recognized in NF1
  - Localized NF (90% of all NFs)
    - Most common NF in both NF1, non-NF1 patients
    - Cutaneous and deep nerves, spinal nerve roots
    - NF1: Larger, multiple, more frequently involve large deep nerves (sciatic nerve, brachial plexus)
    - Malignant transformation rare
  - Diffuse NF
    - Infiltrating subcutaneous tumor; rarely affects spinal nerves, majority (90%) unassociated with NF1
  - PNF (pathognomonic for NF1)
    - Diffuse enlargement of major nerve trunks/branches → bulky, rope-like ("bag of worms") nerve expansion with adjacent tissue distortion
    - Commonly large, bilateral, multilevel with predilection for sciatic nerve, brachial plexus
    - ~ 5% risk malignant degeneration → sarcoma

Microscopic Features

- Neoplastic Schwann cells + perineural fibroblasts grow along nerve fascicles
  - Collagen fibers, mucoid/myxoid matrix, tumor, nerve fascicles intermixed
  - S100 (+) mitotic figures rare unless malignant degeneration

CLINICAL ISSUES

Presentation

- Most common signs/symptoms
  - Skeletal deformity common (25-40%)
    - Focal or acute angle kyphoscoliosis ± myelopathy
    - Extremity bowing or overgrowth
  - Palpable spinal or cutaneous mass
  - Pigmentation anomalies (café au lait, axillary freckling, Lisch nodules) in ≥ 90% of NF1 patients
- Clinical profile
  - Severity of clinical appearance highly variable
  - Classic NF1 triad: Cutaneous lesions, skeletal deformity, and mental deficiency

Demographics

- Age
  - Childhood diagnosis; minimally affected patients may be diagnosed as adults
- Sex
  - M = F
- Ethnicity
  - ↑ frequency in Arab-Israeli populations
- Epidemiology
  - Common (1:4,000)

Natural History & Prognosis

- Kyphosis, scoliosis frequently progressive
- NF growth usually slow; rapid growth associated with pregnancy, puberty, or malignant transformation

Treatment

- Conservative observation; intervention dictated by clinical symptomatology, appearance of neoplasm
- Surgical resection of symptomatic localized NF, spinal cord tumors
- PNF invasive, rarely resectable; observation ± biologic or chemotherapeutic (thalidomide, antihistamines, maturation agents, antiangiogenic drugs) intervention
- Spinal fusion reserved for symptomatic or severe kyphoscoliosis

DIAGNOSTIC CHECKLIST

Consider

- Multiple nerve sheath tumors, ≥ 1 NF, bizarre kyphoscoliosis with deformed vertebra → consider NF1
- Absence of visible stigmata does not exclude NF1

Image Interpretation Pearls

- Characteristic PNF appearance best displayed using fat-saturated T2 or STIR MR

SELECTED REFERENCES

1. Sial M et al: A review of spinal lesions in neurofibromatosis type 1 in a large neurofibromatosis type 1 center. World Neurosurg. 169:e157-63, 2023
2. Xu AL et al: Consensus-based best practice guidelines for the management of spinal deformity and associated tumors in pediatric neurofibromatosis type 1: screening and surveillance, surgical intervention, and medical therapy. J Pediatr Orthop. 43(7):e531-7, 2023
3. Jiménez-Zapata HD et al: Cervical spine ganglioneuroma and its relationship with neurofibromatosis type 1. Cir Cir. 90(4):534-9, 2022
4. Well L et al: Phenotyping spinal abnormalities in patients with neurofibromatosis type 1 using whole-body MRI. Sci Rep. 11(1):16889, 2021
5. Crawford AH et al: Management of cervical instability as a complication of neurofibromatosis type 1 in children: a historical perspective with a 40-year experience. Spine Deform. 6(6):719-29, 2018
6. D'Amico A et al: Medullary unidentified bright objects in neurofibromatosis type 1: a case series. BMC Pediatr. 18(1):91, 2018
7. Rüegger AD et al: Spinal cord hyperintensities in neurofibromatosis type 1: are they the cord equivalent of unidentified bright objects in the brain? Pediatr Neurol. 86:63-5, 2018

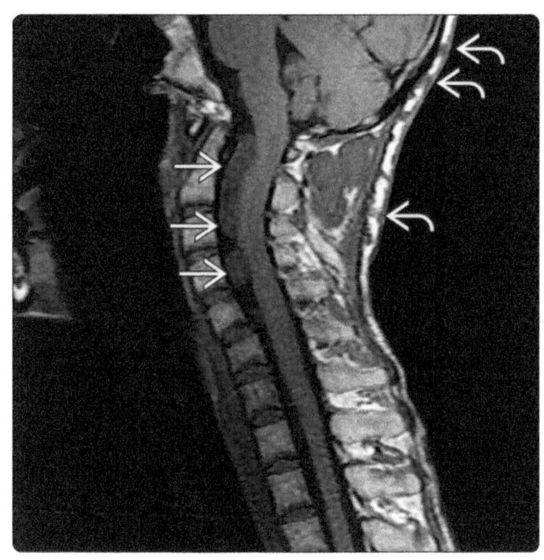

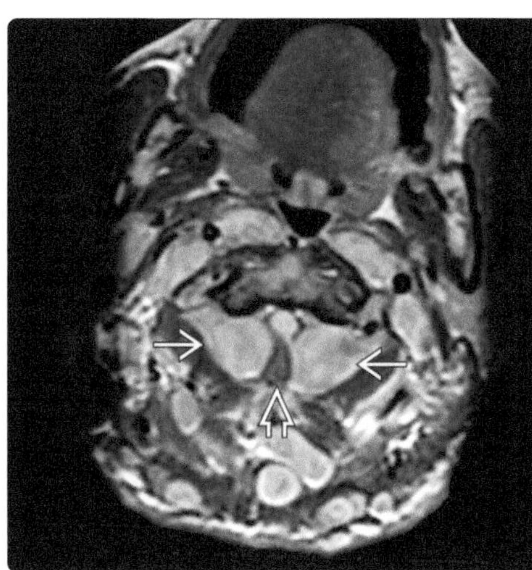

(Left) *Sagittal T1 MR shows extensive intradural extramedullary neurofibromas ➡ located ventral to the spinal cord, displacing the cord posteriorly. Numerous subcutaneous soft tissue neurofibromas ➡ are also present posteriorly.* **(Right)** *Axial T1 C+ MR of the upper cervical spine demonstrates marked extent of involvement by innumerable soft tissue and spinal neurofibromas. Note severe spinal cord ➡ compression produced by bilateral C2 neurofibromas ➡.*

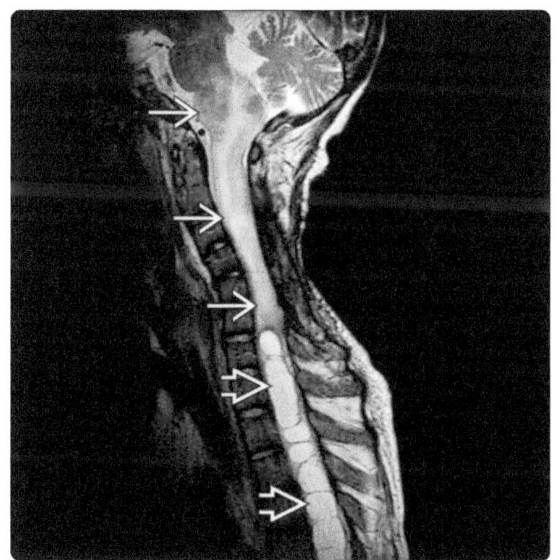

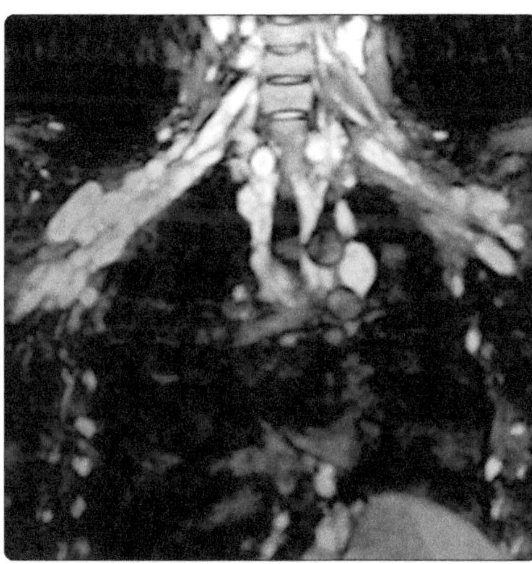

(Left) *Sagittal T2 MR demonstrates a large, expansile intramedullary primary spinal cord neoplasm (astrocytoma) ➡ expanding into the brainstem. A large neoplastic syrinx ➡ is present. Note also cervical lordosis reversal, probably secondary to laminectomy for cord biopsy.* **(Right)** *Coronal STIR MR reveals the typical appearance of innumerable PNF involving the bilateral spinal nerves, sympathetic chains, and bilateral brachial plexus as well as extensive involvement of multiple intercostal nerves.*

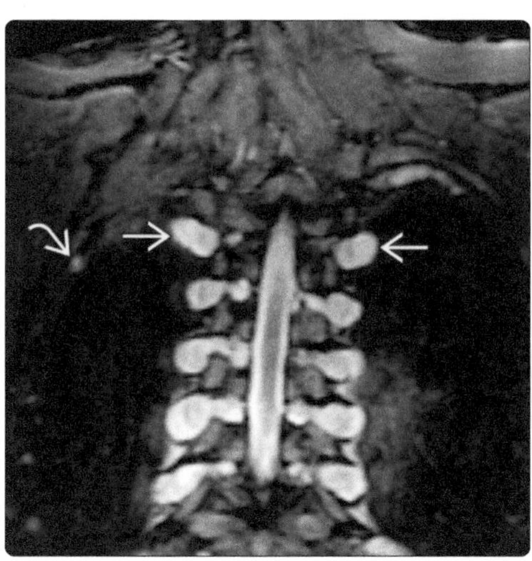

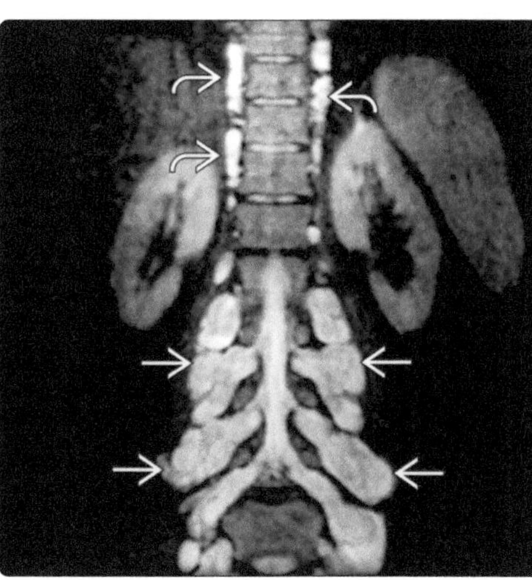

(Left) *Coronal STIR MR depicts bilateral thoracic nerve root neurofibromas ➡ extending through the neural foramina into the paraspinal tissues. Small intercostal neurofibromatas ➡ are also common. Neurofibromas are moderately hyperintense on STIR MR.* **(Right)** *Coronal STIR MR demonstrates multiple bilateral lumbar nerve root neurofibromatas ➡ extending through the neural foramina into the adjacent paraspinal soft tissues. Note the small plexiform neurofibromas ➡ of the sympathetic chain.*

Neurofibromatosis Type 2, Spine

KEY FACTS

TERMINOLOGY

- Rare autosomal dominant disease from chromosomal 22 defect in which all patients develop CNS tumors

IMAGING

- Schwannoma: Intradural, extramedullary; occurs anywhere
- Meningioma: Intradural, extramedullary; typically involving thoracic spine but occurs anywhere
- Ependymoma: Intramedullary; typically upper cervical cord or conus but occurs anywhere

TOP DIFFERENTIAL DIAGNOSES

- Hemangioblastomas
- Nonsyndromic schwannoma
- Nonsyndromic meningioma
- Nonsyndromic ependymoma

PATHOLOGY

- 22q12 deletion correlates with loss of *NF2* gene product merlin (a.k.a. schwannomin)
- Definite diagnosis of neurofibromatosis type 2 (NF2)
    - Bilateral CNVIII (vestibular) schwannomas
    - 1st-degree relative with NF2 + either unilateral early-onset vestibular schwannoma or any 2 of meningioma, glioma, schwannoma, or juvenile posterior subcapsular lenticular opacity
- Presumptive diagnosis of NF2
    - Early-onset unilateral CNVIII schwannomas (age < 30 years) + 1 of following
        - Meningioma, glioma, schwannoma, juvenile posterior subcapsular lenticular opacity
    - Multiple meningiomas (> 2) + unilateral vestibular schwannoma or 1 of following
        - Glioma, schwannoma, juvenile posterior subcapsular lenticular opacity

DIAGNOSTIC CHECKLIST

- Screen using C+ MR of brain and entire spine

(Left) *Sagittal graphic illustrates multiple rounded schwannomas (brown) ➡ distributed along the cauda equina as well as flat dural-based meningiomas (red) ➡ impinging on the conus.* **(Right)** *Sagittal T1 C+ MR in a patient with neurofibromatosis type 2 (NF2) with extensive tumor burden demonstrates multiple small, enhancing schwannomas ➡ within the cauda equina, typical of NF2.*

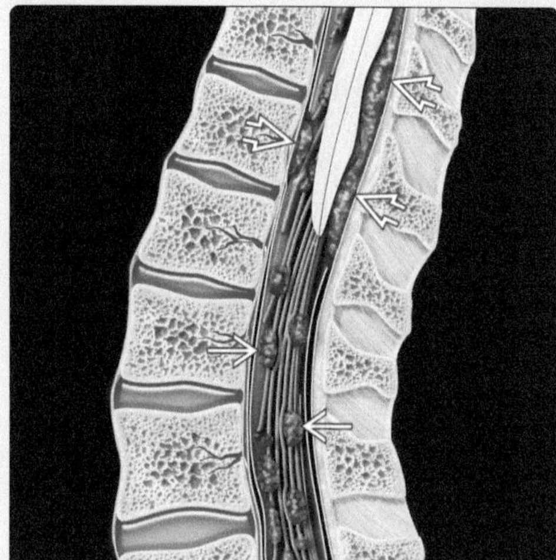

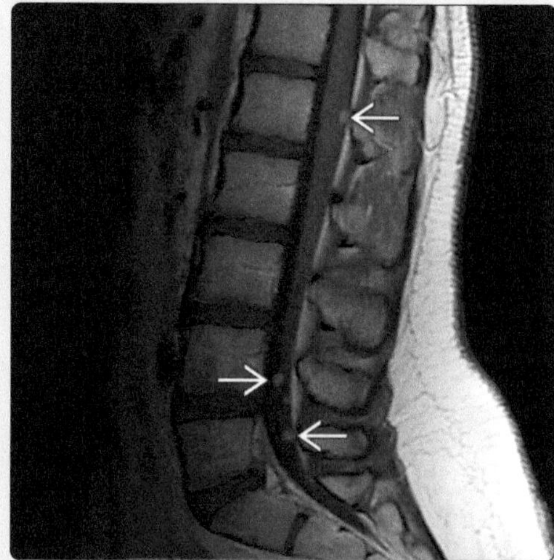

(Left) *Axial T2 MR in the same patient reveals a mildly hyperintense signal within 1 of the schwannomas ➡ originating from a cauda equina nerve.* **(Right)** *Axial T1 C+ MR in the same patient confirms avid enhancement of the cauda equina nerve schwannoma ➡. The mass is more conspicuous on T1 C+ MR than on T2 MR.*

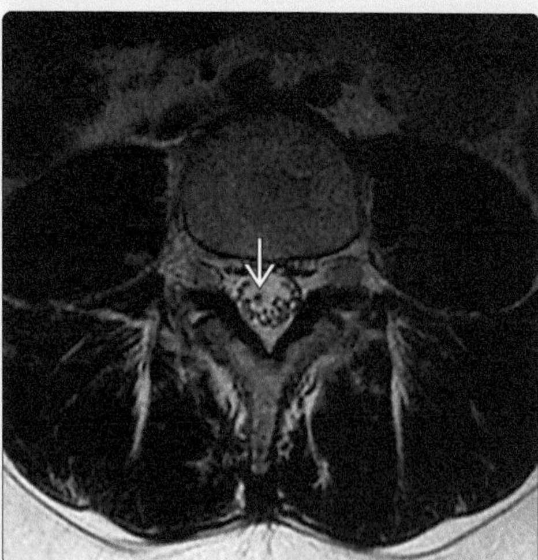

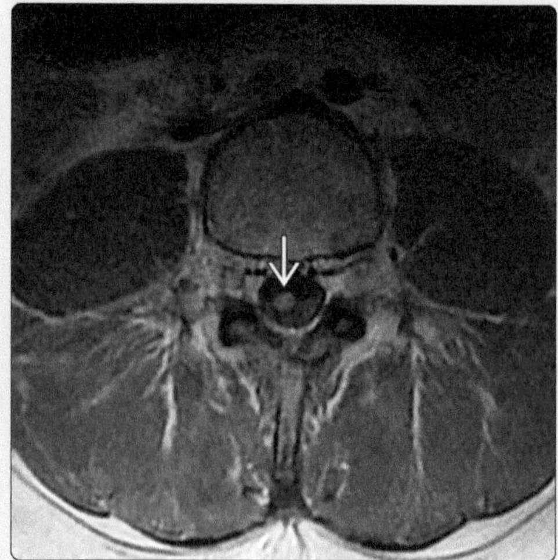

TERMINOLOGY

Abbreviations

- Neurofibromatosis type 2 (NF2)
  - Older term, less preferred because of confusion with neurofibromatosis type 1 (NF1) (unrelated disease)

Synonyms

- NF2-related schwannomatosis (SWN): Currently preferred term
- Bilateral acoustic neurofibromatosis, central neurofibromatosis (both obsolete)

Definitions

- Autosomal dominant disease from chromosomal 22 defect in which all patients develop CNS tumors
- Mnemonic for NF2 tumors: **M**ultiple **i**nherited **s**chwannomas, **m**eningiomas, and **e**pendymomas (MISME)

IMAGING

General Features

- Best diagnostic clue
  - Multiple spinal tumors of various histologic types
- Location
  - Schwannomas
    - Intradural, extramedullary; occur anywhere
    - Rarely intramedullary; arise primarily or secondarily extend from nerve root tumor
    - May extend extradurally
  - Meningiomas: Intradural, extramedullary; typically involving thoracic spine but occur anywhere
  - Ependymomas: Intramedullary; typically upper cervical cord or conus but occur anywhere

MR Findings

- T1WI
  - Schwannomas
    - Well-delineated, rounded, intermediate-signal mass
  - Meningiomas: Mid- to low intensity
  - Ependymomas
    - Iso- to slightly hyperintense
    - Centrally located with cord expansion
- T2WI
  - Schwannomas
    - Well-delineated, rounded, hyperintense mass
    - May undergo hemorrhage or cystic degeneration
  - Meningiomas
    - May be heterogeneous
    - Best defines high occurrence of cord compression
  - Ependymomas: Hyperintense; centrally located with cord expansion
    - Ill-defined, hyperintense lesion may be low-grade astrocytoma
    - Any intramedullary lesion may have syrinx
- T1WI C+
  - Schwannomas: Enhance intensely; homogeneously when small, heterogeneously when large and cystic
  - Meningiomas: Enhance intensely (often to lesser degree than schwannomas) and homogeneously
  - Ependymomas: Enhancing, centrally located mass

Imaging Recommendations

- Best imaging tool
  - Multiplanar MR + gadolinium

DIFFERENTIAL DIAGNOSIS

Hemangioblastoma

- Often associated with von Hippel-Lindau
- Originate from leptomeninges, associated cyst

Nonsyndromic Schwannoma

- Focal, usually solitary lesion

Nonsyndromic Meningioma

- Isolated dura-based mass

Nonsyndromic Ependymoma

- Usually solitary with imaging identical to syndromic tumors

Schwannomatosis

- Very rare disorder (1:40,000 to 1:1.7 million) with similarities to NF1, NF2
- NF2 and SWN are genetically distinct tumor predisposition syndromes with overlapping phenotypes
- Characterized by multiple peripheral nerve schwannomas
- Vestibular schwannoma, meningioma, ependymoma very uncommon (unlike NF2)

Lymphoma

- May coat spinal cord surface

Metastases

- Eccentrically placed, rarely within center of cord
- Cord lesions tend to have extensive edema

PATHOLOGY

General Features

- Etiology
  - Chromosomal 22 deletion with eventual inactivation of merlin functionality
    - 1st event is 22 chromosomal loss
    - 2nd-hit theory: Remaining single *NF2* copy is mutated; vast majority are null mutations
    - Results in truncated, poorly functioning, or nonfunctional merlin protein
- Genetics
  - Inherited autosomal dominant syndrome
  - 22q12 deletion correlates with loss of *NF2* gene product merlin (a.k.a. schwannomin)
- NF2 is now classified along with other forms of schwannoma predisposition, such as *SMARCB1* and *LZTR1*-related SWN
  - Genetically different disorders with phenotypic overlap

Staging, Grading, & Classification

- Definite diagnosis of NF2
  - Bilateral CNVIII (vestibular) schwannomas
  - 1st-degree relative with NF2 and either unilateral early-onset vestibular schwannoma (age < 30 years) or any 2 of following
    - Meningioma, glioma, schwannoma, juvenile posterior subcapsular lenticular opacity
- Presumptive diagnosis of NF2

- Early-onset unilateral CNVIII schwannomas (age < 30 years) and 1 of following
  - Meningioma, glioma, schwannoma, juvenile posterior subcapsular lenticular opacity
- Multiple meningiomas (> 2) and unilateral vestibular schwannoma or 1 of following
  - Glioma, schwannoma, juvenile posterior subcapsular lenticular opacity

- Germline study findings support genotype-phenotype correlation of tumor grading
  - Nonsense and frameshift mutations
    - Usually associated with severe disease phenotype
    - Higher percentage of these patients have intramedullary tumors
    - Have higher numbers of all spinal tumors; intramedullary and extramedullary
    - Younger at onset of symptoms, diagnosis of NF2, and presentation for imaging
  - Missense mutations and large gene deletions are found with mild phenotype
  - Splice site mutations; severe or mild phenotype
    - Dependent on intron involved and its affect on protein functionality

Gross Pathologic & Surgical Features

- Multiple tumors of different histiologic types

Microscopic Features

- Merlin associates at cell cytoskeleton near plasma membrane and inhibits cell proliferation, adhesion, and migration
- Merlin monoclonal antibody immunohistochemistry exhibits consistent immunostaining of Schwann cells
- NF2 histopathology no different than that of nonsyndromic tumors; exception is multiplicity

CLINICAL ISSUES

Presentation

- Most common signs/symptoms
  - Generally presents around puberty or early adulthood
  - Nearly 1/2 initially present with hearing loss
  - Up to 45% with extramedullary tumors exhibit signs/symptoms of cord compression
    - Varies depending on location
    - Weakness and sensory loss at or below level
    - Spasticity, pain, loss of bowel/bladder control
- Clinical profile
  - Detection rates for genetic testing ~ 65%
  - Juvenile subcapsular lens opacities common
  - Retinal and choroidal hamartomas in 10-20%
  - Café au lait spots < 50%
  - Minimal to no cutaneous neurofibromas
  - Cutaneous schwannomas in 67%

Demographics

- Age
  - Genetic disease present at conception
  - Become symptomatic in 2nd-3rd decades
- Sex
  - M = F
- Ethnicity
  - No predilection
- Epidemiology
  - 1 in 50,000 live births worldwide
  - Intradural spinal tumors are present in up to 65% of patients at initial presentation for imaging
    - 84% have intramedullary tumors
    - 87% have intradural extramedullary tumors

Natural History & Prognosis

- Many have relatively normal life spans
- Few patients require therapeutic intervention for intramedullary tumors, which often remain quiescent
- Intradural extramedullary tumors frequently lead to surgical intervention
  - Percentage of patients with extramedullary tumors who undergo surgery is ~ 5x higher than percentage of patients with intramedullary tumors
  - Higher surgical rate is result of high number of tumors and frequent occurrence of cord compression
  - Schwannomas are present more often and in higher numbers than meningiomas and have more surgical procedures overall
  - Meningiomas account for disproportionate number of symptomatic lesions
    - Meningiomas compose ~ 12% of extramedullary tumors, yet account for 37% of extramedullary tumors requiring excision
    - Suggests NF2 meningiomas are more aggressive

Treatment

- Tumor resection is mainstay of NF2 treatment
- Intramedullary tumors: Monitor with regular imaging and appropriate clinical correlation
  - Relatively indolent course of most intramedullary tumors and anticipated burden from other spinal/intracranial tumors must be considered
  - Standard aggressive management may not be warranted, even in symptomatic patient
- Intradural extramedullary tumors: Early removal of rapidly growing or symptomatic tumors
- 1st-degree relatives need to be evaluated

DIAGNOSTIC CHECKLIST

Consider

- Presence of multiple and different pathologic types of spinal tumors is highly suggestive of NF2

Image Interpretation Pearls

- Screen using C+ MR of brain and entire spine
- Imaging follow-up of patients with spinal tumors should be based on knowledge of tumor location, number, and suspected histologic type

SELECTED REFERENCES

1. Halliday D et al: Updated protocol for genetic testing, screening and clinical management of individuals at risk of NF2-related schwannomatosis. Clin Genet. 103(5):540-52, 2023
2. Burns R et al: Genetic testing to gain diagnostic clarity in neurofibromatosis type 2 and schwannomatosis. Am J Med Genet A. 188(8):2413-20, 2022
3. Moualed D et al: Prevalence and natural history of schwannomas in neurofibromatosis type 2 (NF2): the influence of pathogenic variants. Eur J Hum Genet. 30(4):458-64, 2022

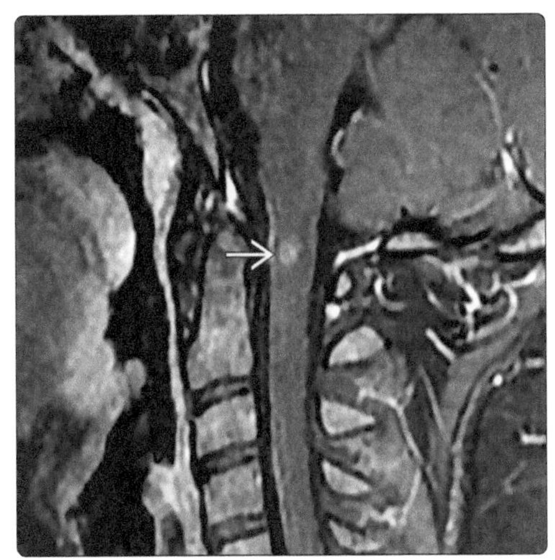

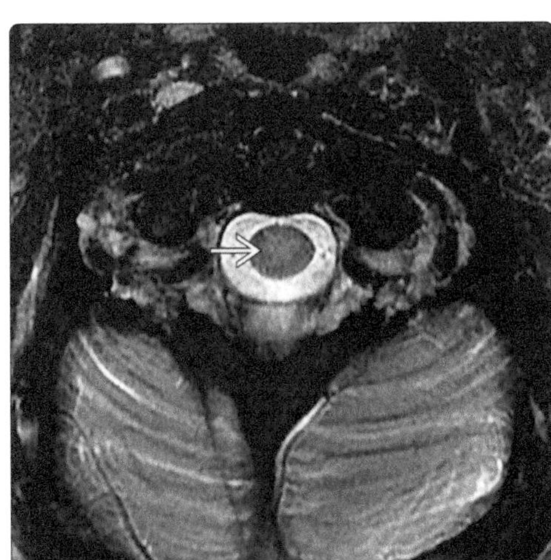

(Left) *Sagittal T1 C+ FS MR reveals a small, enhancing intramedullary lesion ➡ within the cervical spinal cord. These small cellular ependymomas are often incidental asymptomatic discoveries and amenable to imaging surveillance.* **(Right)** *Axial T2 FS MR in the same patient demonstrates a mild tumor lesion ➡ hyperintensity with minimal mass effect. No cystic cap is seen in this small ependymoma.*

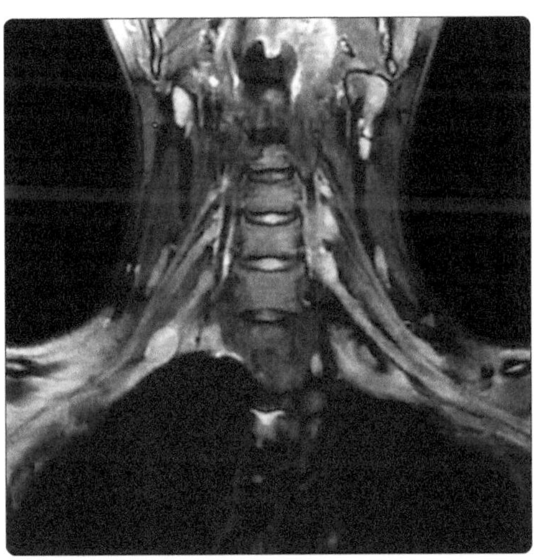

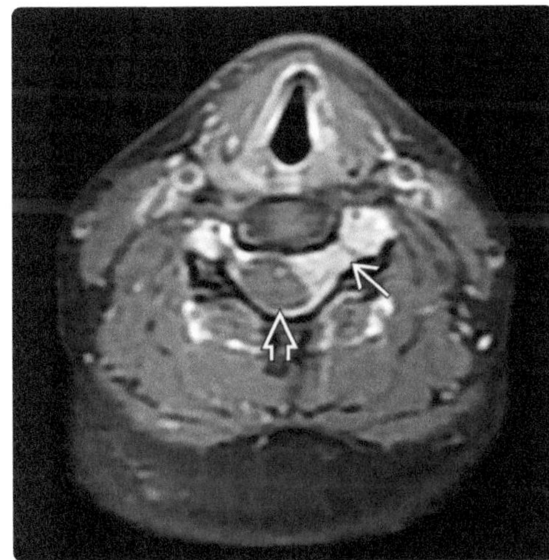

(Left) *Coronal 3D T2 FS MR in a patient with extensive stigmata of NF2 demonstrates bilateral enlargement and hyperintensity of the brachial plexus elements, compatible with multiple brachial plexus schwannomas.* **(Right)** *Axial T1 C+ FS MR in a patient with extensive NF2-related neoplasms reveals a large, dumbbell-shaped cervical schwannoma ➡ extending through the adjacent neural foramen. The tumor produces mass effect on, and displacement of, the adjacent spinal cord ⇨.*

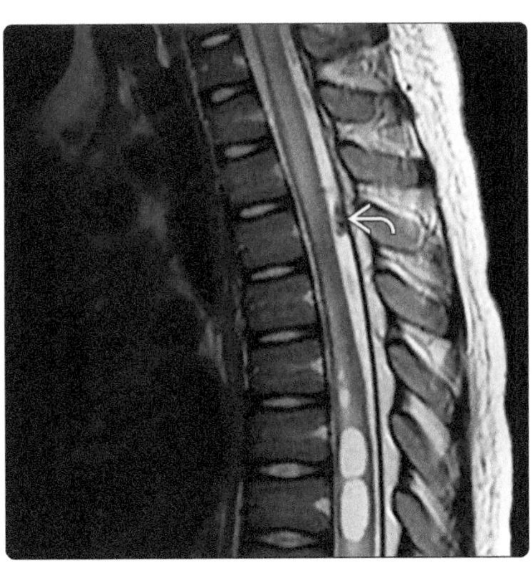

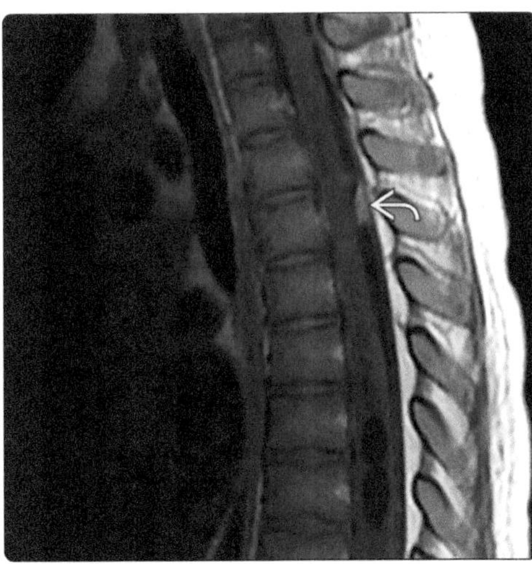

(Left) *Sagittal T2 MR in a patient with NF2 reveals spinal cord edema and syringohydromyelia attributed to Chiari 1 deformity (not shown). Incidentally noted is a hypointense, dural-based lesion ↪, compatible with meningioma, that produces mild regional mass effect on the spinal cord.* **(Right)** *Sagittal T2 MR in the same patient confirms avid enhancement within the dural-based thoracic meningioma ↪.*

Achondroplasia

KEY FACTS

TERMINOLOGY

- Autosomal dominant dwarfism affecting spine and extremities

IMAGING

- Shortened vertebral pedicles
  - Decreasing interpediculate distance toward lower levels of lumbar spine
- Mildly flattened &/or anteriorly wedged vertebral bodies
- Thoracolumbar kyphosis and lumbar hyperlordosis
- Small foramen magnum
- Other
  - Short proximal limbs (rhizomelic dwarfism)
  - "Champagne glass" pelvis and squared iliac wings

TOP DIFFERENTIAL DIAGNOSES

- Pseudoachondroplasia
- Hypochondroplasia
- Diastrophic dysplasia
- Spondyloepiphyseal dysplasia
- Thanatophoric dysplasia
- Osteogenesis imperfecta

PATHOLOGY

- Defect in *FGFR3*, responsible gene mapped to 4p16.3
- Usually spontaneous mutation (80%)
- Results in defective enchondral bone formation
- Autosomal dominant transmission

CLINICAL ISSUES

- Most common nonlethal skeletal dysplasia
- High morbidity from spinal stenosis
  - Surgical correction of progressive/unresolving kyphosis
  - Surgical decompression of foramen magnum in severe cases; usually symptoms resolve

DIAGNOSTIC CHECKLIST

- Most likely cause of short-limbed dwarfism with normal ossification detected in 3rd trimester

(Left) *Coronal graphic shows progressive narrowing of interpediculate distance in the caudad direction. Axial insert on the left shows spinal stenosis related to short pedicles and decreased interpediculate distance.* **(Right)** *AP radiograph of the lumbar spine shows narrowing of the interpediculate distance and progressive interpedicular narrowing between L1 ➙ and L4 ➙, causing narrowing of the lumbar canal in the transverse dimension. Shunt tubing reflects hydrocephalus management related to foramen magnum stenosis.*

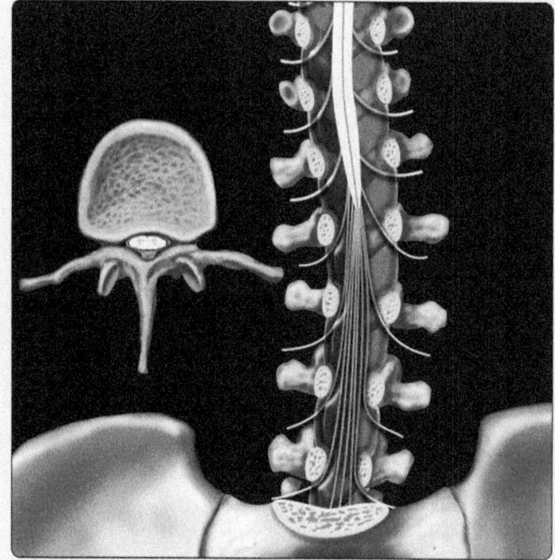

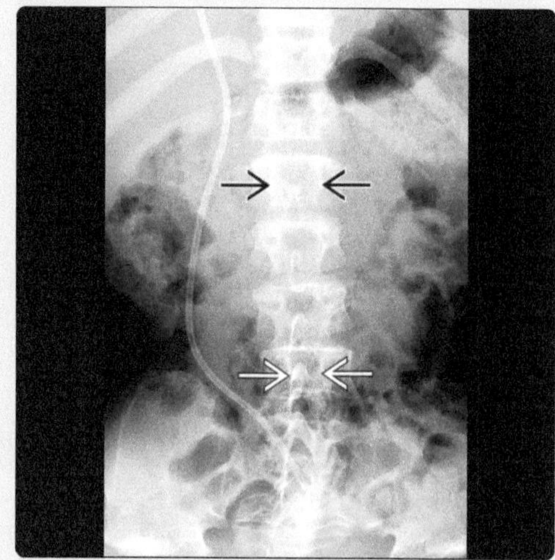

(Left) *Sagittal T2 MR in a 21-month-old patient with achondroplasia reveals spinal canal narrowing ➙ at the craniovertebral junction due to foramen magnum stenosis and C1 ring hypoplasia ➙. There is associated ventriculomegaly due to relative CSF flow obstruction at the foramen magnum.* **(Right)** *Axial T2 MR at the level of C1 in the same patient shows minimal CSF signal surrounding the spinal cord, reflecting effaced subarachnoid space.*

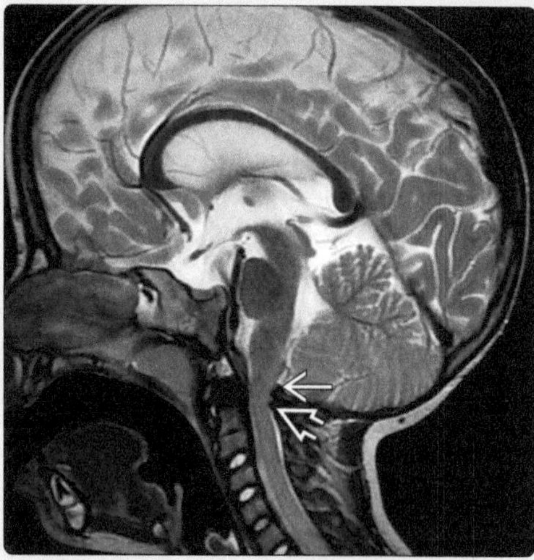

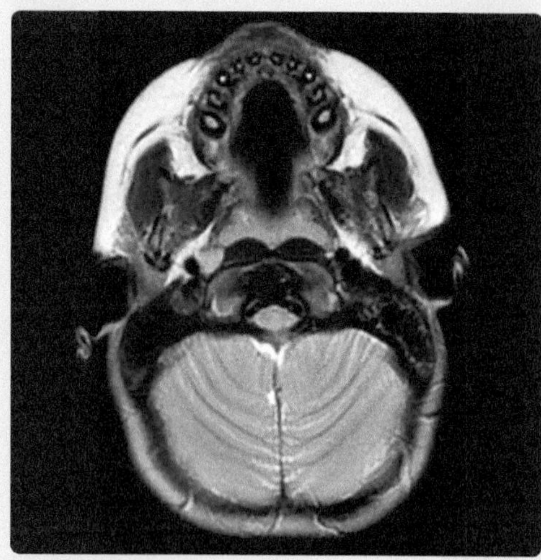

TERMINOLOGY

Synonyms

- Achondroplastic dwarfism

Definitions

- Autosomal dominant dwarfism affecting spine and extremities
- OMIM #100800

IMAGING

General Features

- Best diagnostic clue
  - Flattened vertebral bodies with short pedicles
  - Interpediculate distance of lumbar spine decreases in caudal direction (reversal of normal relationship)
- Location
  - Characteristic skeletal changes in spine, skull, pelvis, extremities
- Morphology
  - Severe dwarfism involves trunk and extremities
    - Growth disturbance more obvious in proximal limbs (rhizomelic dwarfism)
  - Vertebral bodies mildly flattened
  - Shortened pedicles
  - Lumbar hyperlordosis
  - Thoracolumbar kyphosis

Radiographic Findings

- Radiography
  - Thickened, short lumbar pedicles
    - Decreasing interpediculate distance toward lower levels of lumbar spine
  - Dysmorphic vertebral bodies
    - Bullet-shaped (anteriorly blunted) in childhood
    - Mildly flattened &/or mildly anteriorly wedged
  - Thoracolumbar kyphosis
    - Initially flexible deformity, located T10 through L4
    - Resolves as child begins to walk independently
  - Lumbar hyperlordosis
  - Mild scoliosis may be present
  - C1-C2 instability rare
  - Extraspinal findings
    - "Champagne glass" pelvis: Pelvic inlet is flat and broad
    - Squared iliac wings
    - Shortened long bones, most prominent in proximal limbs ("rhizomelic")
    - "Trident hand": 2nd, 3rd, and 4th digits equal in length
    - Enlarged skull with constricted skull base
  - Bone mineral density normal

CT Findings

- NECT
  - Small foramen magnum
  - Mildly flattened (adult) or bullet-shaped (child) vertebral bodies
  - Shortened vertebral pedicles with narrowing of interpediculate distances
    - Predisposition to significant canal and neural foraminal stenosis with otherwise mild degenerative change
  - Posterior vertebral body scalloping
  - Deformity may lead to stress fractures

MR Findings

- Morphologic changes as described for CT
- Disc herniations common
- T2WI/STIR
  - Compression of cervicomedullary junction, spinal cord, nerve roots → myelopathic signal changes (hyperintensity) in spinal cord
- Dynamic MR best evaluates craniovertebral junction (CVJ) stability and positional cord compression

Nonvascular Interventions

- Myelography
  - Spinal stenosis; spinal cord and nerve root compression
  - Disc herniations common

Imaging Recommendations

- Best imaging tool
  - Single AP "babygram" at birth shows characteristic skull, spine, pelvic abnormalities
- Protocol advice
  - Axial, sagittal MR through foramen magnum in all infants and children to assess for stenosis

Ultrasonographic Findings

- Homozygous form can be diagnosed by 2nd trimester
- Growth disturbance evident in 3rd-trimester ultrasound

DIFFERENTIAL DIAGNOSIS

Pseudoachondroplasia

- Facial features and skull normal
- Usually detected in early childhood rather than at birth
- Vertebral body flattening variably seen

Hypochondroplasia

- Midface hypoplasia
- Similar to but milder than achondroplasia: Narrowed foramen magnum, decreased interpediculate distances

Diastrophic Dysplasia

- Facial features marked by micrognathia
- Flattened vertebral bodies; narrowed interpediculate distances
- Scoliosis and kyphosis
- C1-C2 instability
- Subluxations in extremities ("hitchhiker's thumb")
- Clubfoot

Spondyloepiphyseal Dysplasia

- Facial features and skull normal
- Severe vertebral body flattening
- C1-C2 instability and odontoid hypoplasia
- Delayed ossification and flattening of epiphyses
- Shortened long bones
- Absent pubic ossification in infants

Thanatophoric Dysplasia

- Lethal dwarfism
- Severe platyspondyly
- Long, narrow trunk
- Bell-shaped thorax

Osteogenesis Imperfecta

- Infantile form has short, thick bones, multiple fractures
- Milder forms present in childhood or adulthood with short stature, platyspondyly, osteopenia, fractures, bone deformities

PATHOLOGY

General Features

- Etiology
  - Fibroblast growth factor receptor 3 (FGFR-3) abnormality
  - Defect in enchondral bone formation
  - Early fusion of pedicles to vertebral bodies
  - Short, thickened pedicles; reduction of spinal canal diameter in transverse and anteroposterior dimensions
    - Symptomatic spinal stenosis, common by 3rd or 4th decade of life
  - Neural foramina often narrowed
- Genetics
  - Gene mapped to chromosome 4p16.3
    - Same chromosome as hypochondroplasia, thanatophoric dwarfism
  - Usually spontaneous mutation (80%)
  - Autosomal dominant transmission
  - Homozygous form rare, much more severe than heterozygous
- Associated abnormalities
  - Sleep apnea, sudden infant death
    - Secondary to compression of brainstem by CVJ stenosis
  - Chest wall deformity may lead to respiratory difficulties
  - Limb-lengthening procedures can lead to neurologic symptoms

Gross Pathologic & Surgical Features

- Spinal stenosis
  - Short pedicles, thickened laminae
  - Disc bulges and herniations contribute to stenosis
  - Can occur at all spinal levels
  - Significant cause of morbidity in adults
- Foramen magnum stenosis
  - Found in almost all children with achondroplasia
  - Often resolves functionally as child grows
- Thoracolumbar kyphosis
  - Related to hypotonia in infants
  - Often resolves as child begins independent ambulation and trunk muscles strengthen
  - Up to 94% prevalence in childhood, decreases to 11% by 10 years of age, then increases to 35% at 4th or 5th decade

CLINICAL ISSUES

Presentation

- Most common signs/symptoms
  - Dwarfism, characteristic facies evident at birth
  - Other signs/symptoms
    - Infantile hypotonia
    - Sleep apnea in infants and children due to compression of cord at foramen magnum
    - Thoracolumbar kyphosis
    - Spinal stenosis
- Clinical profile
  - Rhizomelic dwarfism apparent at birth
  - Frontal bossing and depressed nasal bridge characteristic
  - Intelligence normal
  - Obesity common clinical problem
  - Clinically overdiagnosed in infants as cause of skeletal dysplasia

Demographics

- Age
  - Congenital; diagnosis usually made in infancy
- Sex
  - M = F
- Epidemiology
  - Most common nonlethal skeletal dysplasia (1:26,000 live births)

Natural History & Prognosis

- High morbidity from spinal stenosis

Treatment

- Options, risks, complications
  - Infantile kyphosis may be treatable with sitting modification ± thoracolumbar bracing
  - Surgical correction of progressive/unresolving kyphosis
  - Surgical decompression of foramen magnum in severe cases; symptoms usually resolve
  - Surgical decompression for spinal stenosis
  - Growth hormone to lengthen long bones
  - Ilizarov limb-lengthening procedure controversial

DIAGNOSTIC CHECKLIST

Consider

- Most likely cause of short-limbed dwarfism with normal ossification detected in 3rd trimester

Image Interpretation Pearls

- Spine imaging must include foramen magnum to evaluate for stenosis

SELECTED REFERENCES

1. Cabet S et al: New insights in craniovertebral junction MR changes leading to stenosis in children with achondroplasia. Childs Nerv Syst. 38(6):1137-45, 2022
2. Stender M et al: Comprehensive literature review on the prevalence of comorbid conditions in patients with achondroplasia. Bone. 162:116472, 2022
3. Smid CJ et al: Craniocervical junction issues after infancy in achondroplasia. Am J Med Genet A. 185(1):182-9, 2021
4. Calandrelli R et al: Quantitative approach to the posterior cranial fossa and craniocervical junction in asymptomatic children with achondroplasia. Neuroradiology. 59(10):1031-41, 2017
5. Khan BI et al: Prevalence of scoliosis and thoracolumbar kyphosis in patients with achondroplasia. Spine Deform. 4(2):145-8, 2016

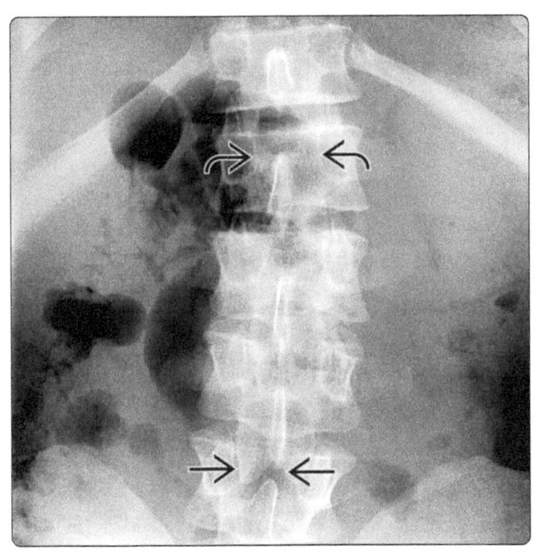

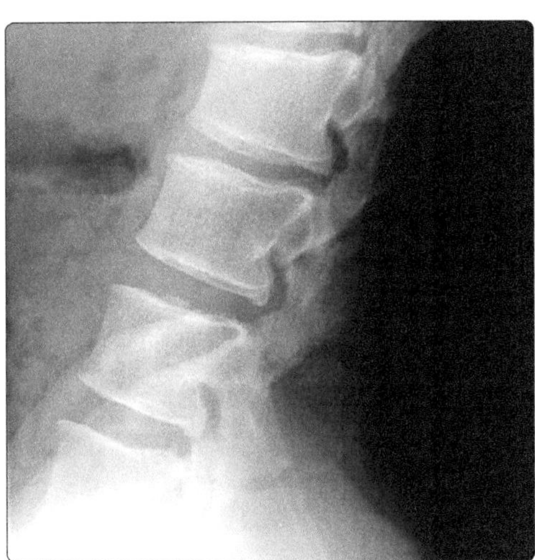

(Left) *AP radiograph shows characteristic diminishing interpediculate distance between L1* ➔ *and L4* ➔*, narrowing the spinal canal in the transverse dimension.* **(Right)** *Lateral radiograph demonstrates mild vertebral body flattening and posterior scalloping with shortened pedicles, resulting in spinal stenosis.*

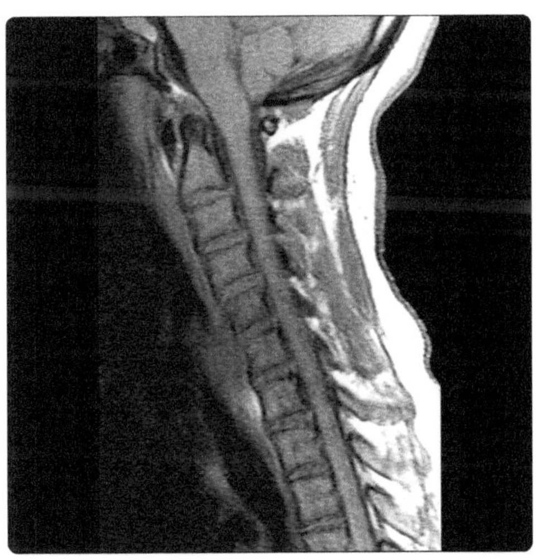

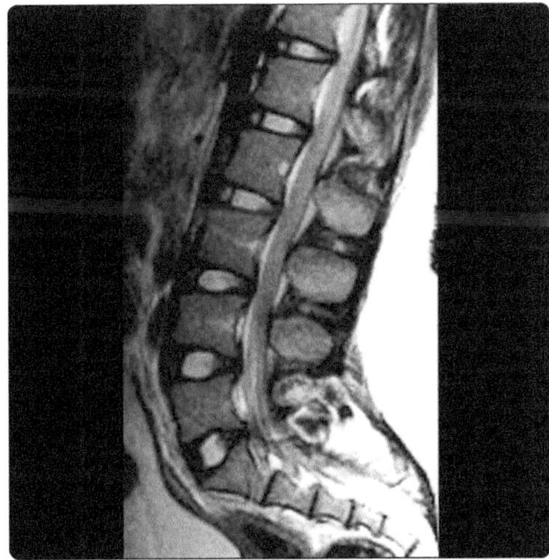

(Left) *Sagittal T1WI MR of the cervical spine depicts diffuse congenital spinal stenosis with very minimal subarachnoid space CSF surrounding the spinal cord. There is not substantial craniovertebral junction narrowing in this patient, however.* **(Right)** *Sagittal T2WI MR in the same patient confirms that diffuse congenital spinal stenosis extends into the lumbar spine with characteristic short pedicles and posterior vertebral scalloping. Minimal subarachnoid space fluid is detected at the conus and cauda equina.*

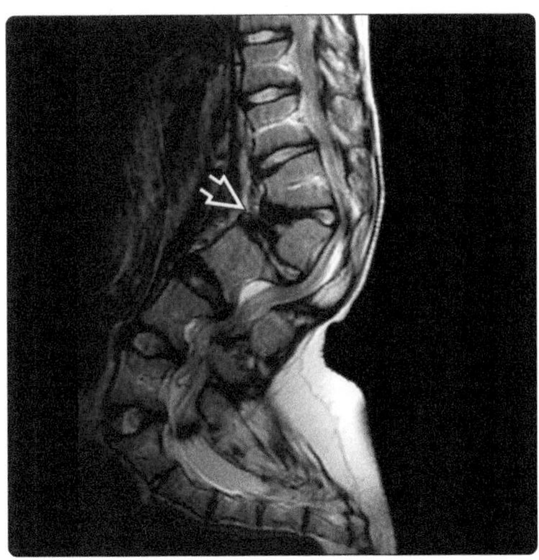

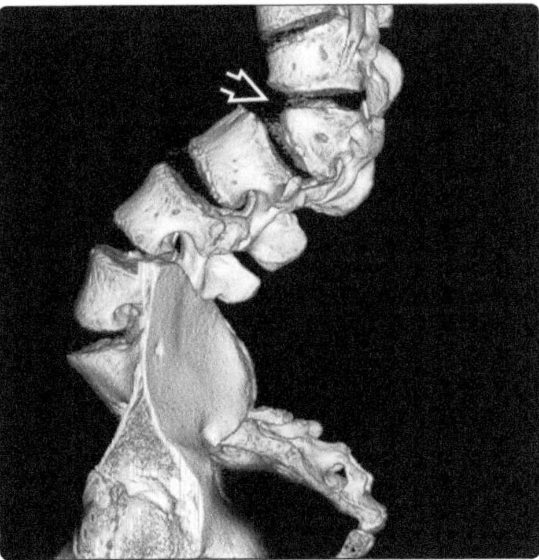

(Left) *Sagittal T2WI MR of the lumbar spine depicts congenital L2 anterior vertebral hypoplasia* ➔*, producing focal congenital kyphosis that accentuates congenital spinal stenosis from short pedicles. The remaining lumbar vertebral bodies show characteristic posterior vertebral scalloping.* **(Right)** *Sagittal 3D reformatted bone CT in the same patient confirms marked anterior L2 vertebral hypoplasia* ➔*. 3D bone CT demonstrates osseous relationships for surgical planning.*

KEY FACTS

TERMINOLOGY

- Mucopolysaccharidoses (MPS) are inherited lysosomal storage disorders

IMAGING

- Craniocervical spine
  - Craniovertebral junction (CVJ) stenosis, dens hypoplasia, ligamentous laxity, atlantoaxial instability, thickened dural ring at foramen magnum
- Thoracolumbar spine
  - Kyphoscoliosis, platyspondyly, anterior vertebral beaking, ± thoracolumbar gibbus deformity

TOP DIFFERENTIAL DIAGNOSES

- GM1 gangliosidosis
- Mucolipidosis III (pseudo-Hurler polydystrophy)
- Achondroplasia
- Trisomy 21 (Down syndrome)
- Spondyloepiphyseal dysplasia

PATHOLOGY

- Inherited lysosomal enzyme deficiency → storage disorder
  - Autosomal recessive (except MPS II Hunter; X-linked recessive)
- Glycosaminoglycan (GAG) accumulates in organs and ligaments

CLINICAL ISSUES

- Gradual progressive myelopathy
- Clinical neurologic symptoms attributable to brain GAG deposition, myelination abnormalities, spinal deformities, peripheral nerve entrapment

DIAGNOSTIC CHECKLIST

- Successful diagnosis requires combination of clinical, imaging, and genetic/biochemical information
- Dens hypoplasia with mass and dural thickening suggests MPS syndrome
- Vertebral beaking pattern may permit specific diagnosis

(Left) *Sagittal T2WI MR in a 5-year-old patient with mucopolysaccharidoses (MPS) type I, Hurler syndrome (MPS I-H) shows severe stenosis at the foramen magnum secondary to bone and ligament overgrowth related to abnormal deposition. The tectorial membrane ➡ and ligamentum flavum ➡ are markedly thickened. Note also cord myelomalacia.* **(Right)** *Sagittal bone CT in the same patient reveals markedly delayed vertebral ossification. There is also inferior beaking of some of the vertebra.*

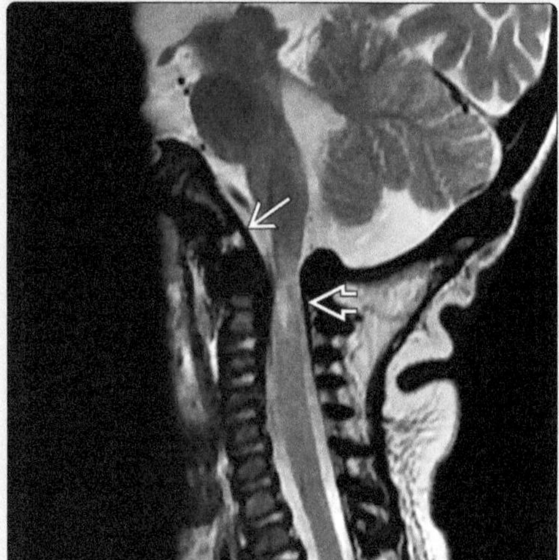

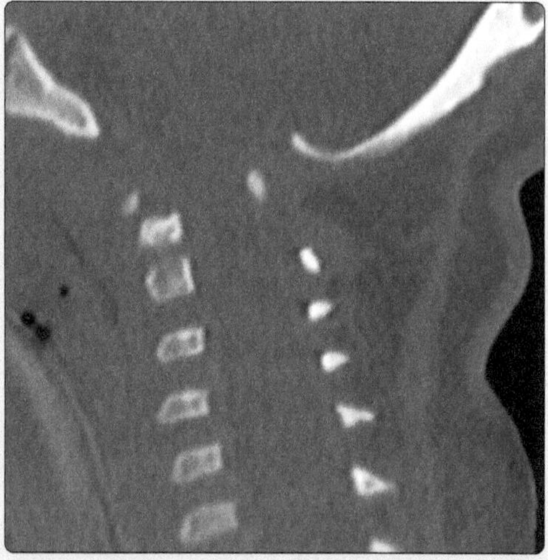

(Left) *Sagittal T2WI MR in a patient with MPS IV, Morquio syndrome demonstrates hypoplasia and flattening of all thoracic vertebral bodies as well as focal kyphosis and mild spinal canal narrowing at the thoracolumbar junction. The kyphosis results from focal anterior vertebral hypoplasia ➡ at the thoracolumbar junction.* **(Right)** *Sagittal bone CT in a patient with MPS VI, Maroteaux-Lamy syndrome reveals mild vertebral hypoplasia and inferior beaking ➡ at the thoracolumbar junction, producing focal kyphosis.*

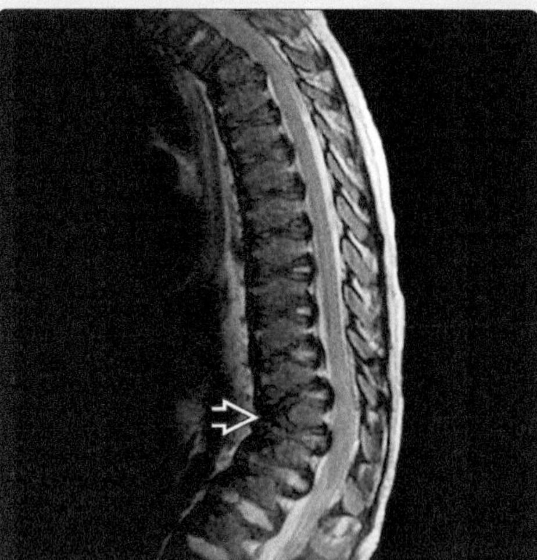

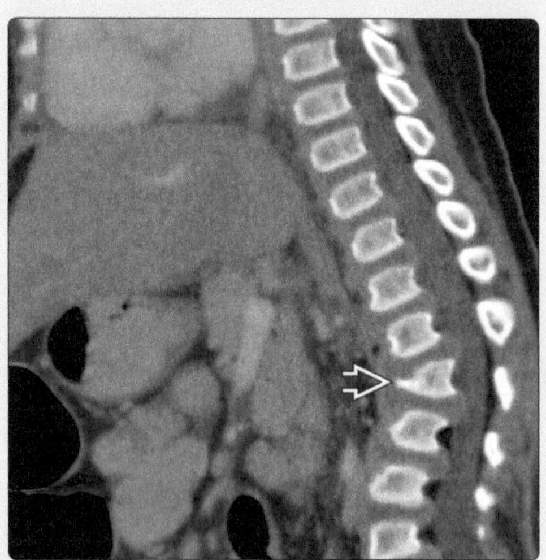

TERMINOLOGY

Abbreviations

- Mucopolysaccharidosis (MPS)

Synonyms

- Gargoylism (not politically correct terminology)

Definitions

- Multiple inherited lysosomal storage disorders
  - Specific enzyme deficiency → inability to break down specific glycosaminoglycans (GAG)
  - Failure to break down GAG → intracellular accumulation and toxicity

IMAGING

General Features

- Best diagnostic clue
  - Dens hypoplasia, craniovertebral junction (CVJ) stenosis, and thickened dural ring at foramen magnum
- Location
  - Spine: CVJ, thoracolumbar spine, pelvis
  - Extraspinal: Brain, visceral organ deposition
- Size
  - Odontoid soft tissue mass varies from small to large; larger masses usually found in older patients
- Morphology
  - Craniocervical spine
    - Skull base thickening, occipital hypoplasia, short posterior C1 arch, odontoid hypoplasia ± os odontoideum, ligamentous laxity, dural sac stenosis, and atlantoaxial instability
  - Thoracolumbar spine
    - Kyphosis, kyphoscoliosis
      - May be related to vertebral beaking/hypoplasia at those levels
    - Platyspondyly, anterior beaking + thoracolumbar gibbus deformity [MPS type I, Hurler syndrome (MPS I-H) and MPS IV]

Radiographic Findings

- Radiography
  - Odontoid dysplasia ± atlantoaxial subluxation
  - Dysplastic blunted spinous processes, wedged vertebral bodies, and spinal canal stenosis
  - Thoracolumbar inferior (MPS I-H) or central (MPS IV) vertebral beaking, gibbus deformity

Fluoroscopic Findings

- ± dynamic CVJ instability on flexion/extension

CT Findings

- CECT
  - CVJ central and foraminal narrowing, marked dural thickening without abnormal enhancement
- Bone CT
  - Abnormal dens ossification, marked laminar thickening, enlargement of medullary cavity

MR Findings

- T1WI
  - Hypo- to isointense periodontoid soft tissue mass, hypointense thickened dura
- T2WI
  - Hypoplastic dens and periodontoid soft tissue mass
  - Hypointense, thickened dura ± cyst formation due to meningeal thickening (MPS I-H, II)
  - ± cord compression with hyperintense signal abnormality
- T1WI C+
  - No abnormal enhancement, even if mass present
- MRS
  - Brain proton MRS may show diminished NAA:choline ratio, elevated glutamine/glutamate, and inositol peak areas

Imaging Recommendations

- Best imaging tool
  - Multiplanar MR
- Protocol advice
  - Spine MR to elucidate cause/site of cord compression
  - Plain radiographs to characterize osseous spine and limb abnormalities
  - Flexion/extension radiographs or fluoroscopy to detect craniovertebral instability

DIFFERENTIAL DIAGNOSIS

GM1 Gangliosidosis

- Shares features of vertebral beaking, upper lumbar gibbus, and dens hypoplasia
- Distinguish on clinical, genetic criteria

Mucolipidosis III (Pseudo-Hurler Polydystrophy)

- Shares features of vertebral beaking, upper lumbar gibbus, and dens hypoplasia
- Distinguish on clinical, genetic criteria

Achondroplasia

- Autosomal dominant disorder of enchondral bone formation
- Short, broad pedicles and thickened laminae → spinal stenosis
- Distinguish on genetic, clinical criteria

Down Syndrome

- ± dens hypoplasia without soft tissue dens mass or marrow deposition features
- Distinguish using genetic and clinical information

Spondyloepiphyseal Dysplasia

- Flattening of vertebral bodies, dens hypoplasia, scoliosis present at birth
- Minimal hand and foot involvement

PATHOLOGY

General Features

- Etiology
  - Inherited lysosomal enzyme deficiency
- Genetics
  - Autosomal recessive (except MPS II Hunter; X-linked recessive)
- GAG accumulates in most organs and ligaments
  - Coarse facies (hence name gargoylism)

- Hepatosplenomegaly, umbilical hernia
- Skeletal dysostosis multiplex, joint contractures
- Arterial wall (midaortic stenosis), cardiac valve thickening
- Upper airway obstruction (38%); very difficult intubations
- Odontoid hypoplasia, GAG deposition, ± ligamentous laxity with reactive change produce soft tissue mass around dens
- Biconvex ovoid, bullet-shaped or rectangular vertebral bodies, vertebral beaking, posterior vertebral slip (MPS IV), large disc protrusions (MPS VI)

Staging, Grading, & Classification

- Hurler (MPS I-H) (OMIM #607014), Hurler-Scheie (MPS IH/S): α-L-iduronidase (4p16.3)
- Hunter (MPS II) (OMIM #309900): Iduronate 2-sulfatase (Xq28)
- Sanfilippo (MPS IIIA) (OMIM #252900): Heparin N-sulfatase (17q25.3)
- Morquio (MPS type IVA) (OMIM #253000): Galactose 6-sulfatase (16q24.3)
- Scheie (MPS IS) (MPS V, formerly) (OMIM #607016): α-L-iduronidase (4p16.3)
- Maroteaux-Lamy (MPS VI) (OMIM #253200): Arylsulfatase B (5q11-q13)
- Sly (MPS VII) (OMIM #253220): β-glucuronidase (7q11.21)

Gross Pathologic & Surgical Features

- CVJ stenosis → neurovascular compression, altered CSF dynamics → hydrocephalus, hydrosyringomyelia
- Dilated enlarged laminae medullary cavities
- Thickened dura may appear normal at surgery

Microscopic Features

- Epidural/dural mucopolysaccharide deposition with elastic and collagenous proliferation

CLINICAL ISSUES

Presentation

- Most common signs/symptoms
  - Gradual subtle progressive myelopathy (often falsely attributed to lower extremity deformities)
    - Common with MPS I-H, II, III, and VII; uncommon with MPS IV, I H/S, VI unless associated with musculoskeletal deformities
    - Reduced exercise tolerance; may be earliest symptom
  - Clinical neurologic symptoms attributable to brain GAG deposition, myelination abnormalities, spinal deformities, and peripheral nerve entrapment
- Clinical profile
  - Coarse facies with macroglossia, bushy eyebrows, flat nasal bridge (mild in MPS VI, VII)
  - Corneal clouding (except MPS II)
  - Significant intellectual disabilities (except in MPS I H/S, IIb, IV)
  - Joint contractures, dysostosis multiplex (dominates in MPS IV, VI)
- Laboratory diagnosis: Measurement of specific urinary GAG
- Clinical diagnostic algorithm
  - Age, IQ, ± corneal clouding, urinary GAG excretion, and specific clinical findings

Demographics

- Age
  - Usually diagnosed in childhood; occasional mild cases diagnosed as adults
- Sex
  - M = F, except MPS II (boys only → X linked)
- Epidemiology
  - MPS I-H (1:10,000 births), MPS IV (1:40,000 births) most common

Natural History & Prognosis

- Premature death is rule; rate of deterioration depends on specific enzymatic deficiency
- Slowly progressive cord compression → quadriparesis, sensory loss without treatment; surgical results poor when performed late in disease course
- High spinal cord compression is major spinal cause of MPS complications and death; apnea and sudden death may follow relatively minor trauma

Treatment

- Conservative (mild symptoms): External spinal bracing
- Surgical (more severe symptoms)
  - Posterior occipitocervical decompression/stabilization
  - Transoral odontoid resection/posterior stabilization for symptomatic odontoid mass effect
- Bone marrow transplant (BMT) or intravenous recombinant human enzyme
  - Decreases GAG accumulation in organs; ameliorates some, but not all, manifestations

DIAGNOSTIC CHECKLIST

Consider

- Successful diagnosis requires combination of clinical, imaging, and genetic/biochemical information

Image Interpretation Pearls

- Dens hypoplasia with mass and dural thickening suggests MPS syndrome
- Vertebral beaking pattern may permit specific diagnosis

SELECTED REFERENCES

1. Jan YT et al: Adjunct diagnostic value of radiological findings in mucopolysaccharidosis type IVa-related thoracic spinal abnormalities: a pilot study. Orphanet J Rare Dis. 17(1):296, 2022
2. Pontesilli S et al: Evidence of treatment benefits in patients with mucopolysaccharidosis type I-Hurler in long-term follow-up using a new magnetic resonance imaging scoring system. J Pediatr. 240:297-301.e5, 2022
3. Guffon N et al: Long term disease burden post-transplantation: three decades of observations in 25 Hurler patients successfully treated with hematopoietic stem cell transplantation (HSCT). Orphanet J Rare Dis. 16(1):60, 2021
4. Lins CF et al: MRI findings of the cervical spine in patients with mucopolysaccharidosis type VI: relationship with neurological physical examination. Clin Radiol. 75(6):441-7, 2020
5. Bulut E et al: Evaluation of spinal involvement in children with mucopolysaccharidosis VI: the role of MRI. Br J Radiol. 91(1085):20170744, 2018
6. Nicolas-Jilwan M et al: Mucopolysaccharidoses: overview of neuroimaging manifestations. Pediatr Radiol. 48(10):1503-20, 2018
7. Reichert R et al: Neuroimaging findings in patients with mucopolysaccharidosis: what you really need to know. Radiographics. 36(5):1448-62, 2016
8. Żuber Z et al: Cervical spine MRI findings in patients with mucopolysaccharidosis type II. Pediatr Neurosurg. 50(1):26-30, 2015

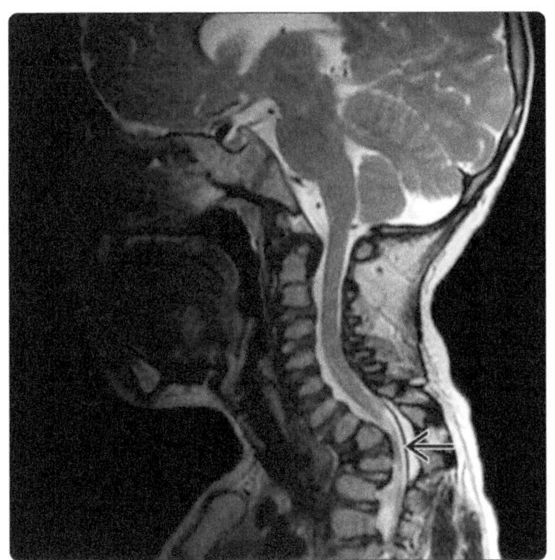

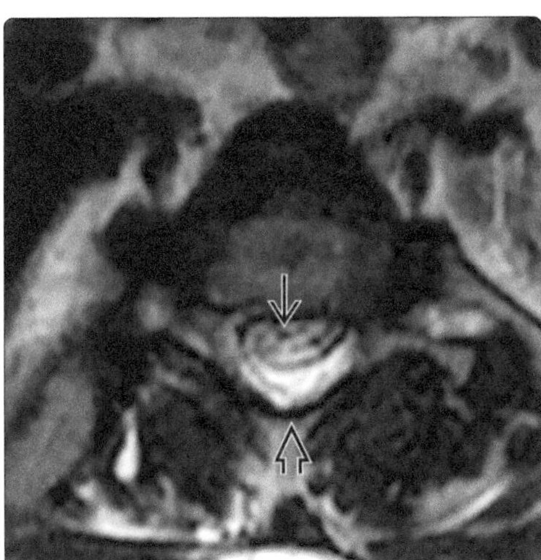

(Left) *Sagittal T2WI MR in a patient with MPS I-H reveals marked cervicothoracic kyphosis in conjunction with inferior vertebral beaking and vertebral hypoplasia. The spinal cord is markedly atrophic ➔ at the upper thoracic level.* **(Right)** *Axial T2WI MR in the same patient confirms severe spinal cord myelomalacia ➔. There is generalized coarsening of the osseous elements and thickening of the ligamentum flavum ➔.*

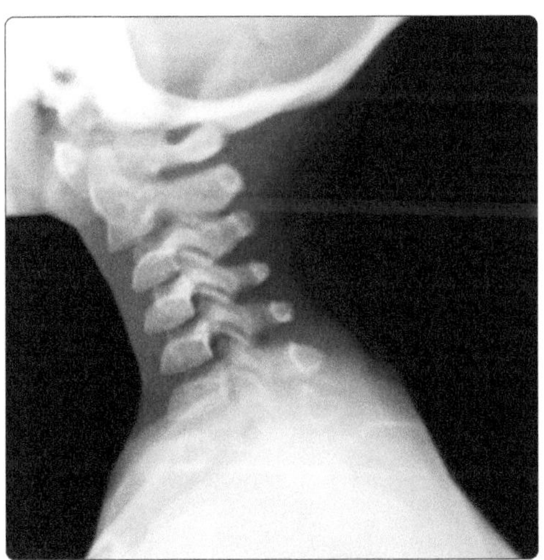

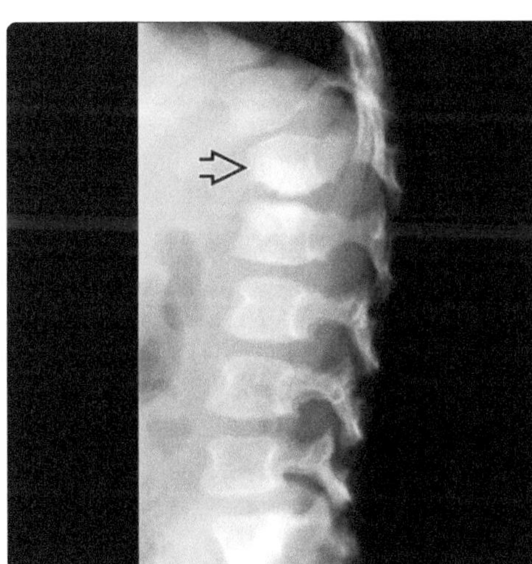

(Left) *Lateral plain radiograph of the cervical spine in a patient with Hunter syndrome, MPS II shows mild anterior inferior vertebral beaking. As a general rule, the imaging (and clinical) findings of Hunter syndrome are similar to MPS I-H but usually less severe and slower to progress.* **(Right)** *Lateral radiograph of the thoracolumbar spine in a patient with Hunter syndrome, MPS II reveals inferior vertebral beaking as well as a hypoplastic L1 vertebra ➔ producing focal kyphosis.*

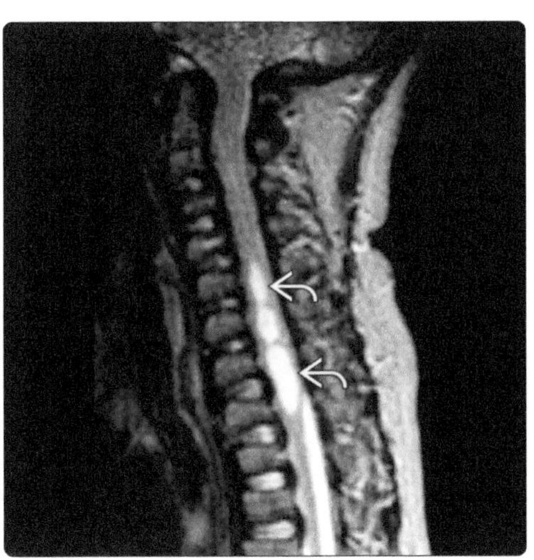

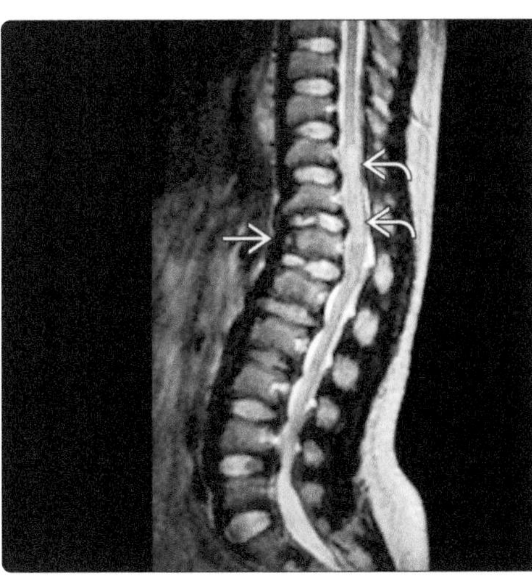

(Left) *Sagittal T2WI MR in a patient with MPS VI demonstrates mildly abnormal vertebral body morphology. In addition, there is segmental syringohydromyelia ➔ extending from C5 to T1.* **(Right)** *Sagittal T2WI MR in a patient with MPS VI reveals mild lumbar kyphosis centered at the hypoplastic T12 vertebra ➔ with multiple other abnormal anteriorly beaked vertebral bodies. Note also moderate narrowing of the thoracolumbar spinal canal at the apex of the kyphosis and abnormal spinal cord T2 signal intensity ➔.*

Sickle Cell Disease, Spine

KEY FACTS

TERMINOLOGY

- Hereditary hemoglobinopathy resulting in anemia and RBCs that deform (sickle) and occlude blood vessels

IMAGING

- Spine involvement in 43-70% of patients
- Bone infarction
  - Patchy or diffusely sclerotic bones
  - Central endplate compression deformities in spine, resulting in H-shaped vertebral bodies
- Osteopenia, osteoporotic compression fractures
- Tower vertebra: Compensatory vertical growth of vertebral body adjacent to infarcted/collapsed vertebra
- Osteomyelitis: Rare in spine

TOP DIFFERENTIAL DIAGNOSES

- Thalassemia
- Renal osteodystrophy
- Osteopetrosis
- Spondyloepiphyseal dysplasia (SED)
- Diffuse osseous metastases

PATHOLOGY

- Autosomal recessive inheritance
  - African, Middle Eastern, and Eastern Mediterranean
- Associated abnormalities
  - Moyamoya disease, multiple infarcts
  - Femoral head and humeral head infarcts
  - Growth disturbance
  - Cholelithiasis (bilirubin stones)
  - Hemosiderosis due to multiple transfusions

CLINICAL ISSUES

- Sickle cell crisis: Oxygen, hydration, pain management, blood transfusion
- High incidence of infections

DIAGNOSTIC CHECKLIST

- H-shaped vertebra strongly suggests diagnosis

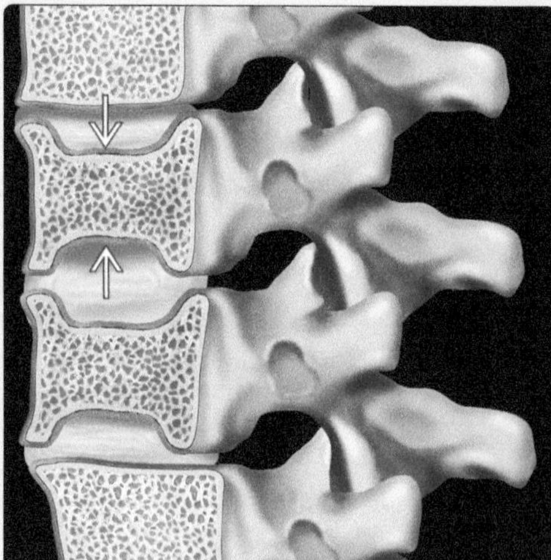

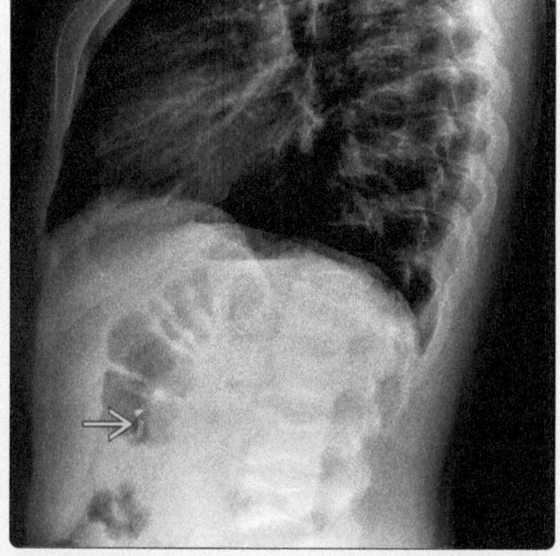

(Left) *Sagittal graphic shows central collapse of the vertebral endplates ➡ due to bone infarcts, which tends to affect the central portion of the vertebral body. Peripherally, height is preserved, yielding an H-shaped vertebra.* **(Right)** *Lateral radiography in an adolescent with sickle cell disease (SCD) and back pain reveals many H-shaped vertebra throughout the thoracic and lumbar spine. Note also abdominal clips ⇨ following cholecystectomy for cholelithiasis.*

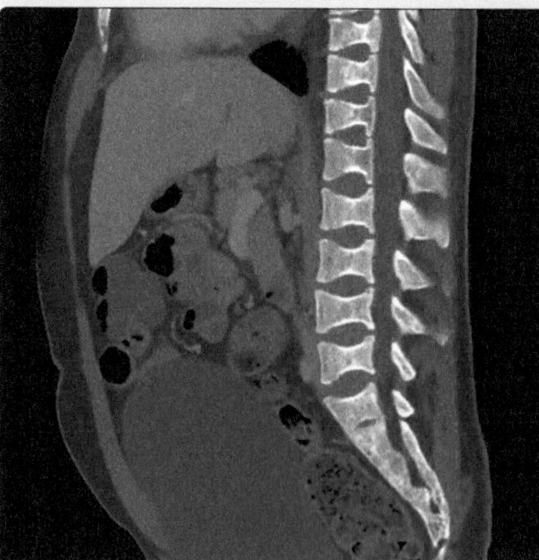

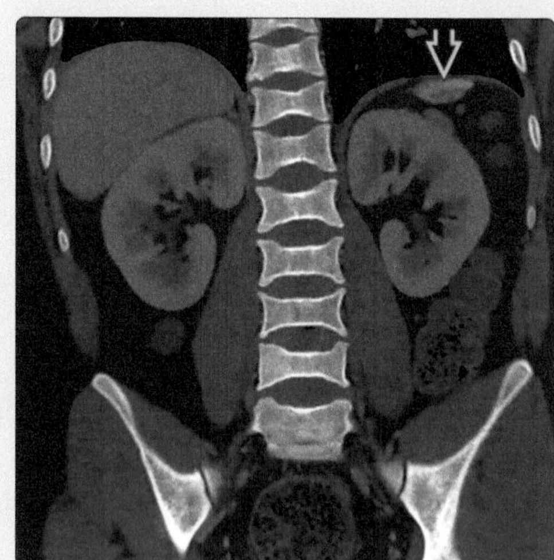

(Left) *Sagittal bone CT in the same patient with SCD confirms an H-shaped configuration of all vertebra in the lower thoracic and lumbar spine. Patchy areas of sclerosis in some of the vertebra suggest a prior bone infarction.* **(Right)** *Coronal bone CT in the same patient demonstrates conspicuous central vertebral height loss in the coronal plane as well. Note also that the spleen ⇨ is very small secondary to prior splenic infarctions (autosplenectomy).*

TERMINOLOGY

Synonyms

- Sickle cell anemia, HbSS disease

Definitions

- Hereditary hemoglobinopathy resulting in anemia and RBCs that deform (sickle) and occlude blood vessels
- Homozygous: HbSS (sickle cell anemia)
- Heterozygous: HbSA (sickle cell trait, asymptomatic), HbSC (less severe form)
- Sickle cell crisis: Acute episode of severe bone, abdomen, chest pain

IMAGING

General Features

- Best diagnostic clue
  - H-shaped vertebral bodies (on sagittal imaging) due to central endplate compression deformities
- Location
  - Spine involvement in 43-70% of patients
  - Bone infarcts much more commonly involve long bones of appendicular skeleton

Radiographic Findings

- Radiography
  - Bone infarction
    - Patchy or diffusely sclerotic bones due to chronic, repeated bone infarcts
    - Central endplate compression deformities in spine, resulting in H-shaped vertebral bodies
  - Osteopenia
    - Osteoporotic vertebral compression fractures with biconcave or wedged morphology
  - Tower vertebra
    - Compensatory vertical growth of vertebral body adjacent to infarcted/collapsed vertebra
  - Osteomyelitis
    - Rare in spine

CT Findings

- NECT
  - Mottled sclerosis in medullary spaces of axial skeleton
  - Central endplate compression deformities (on sagittal or coronal reconstructed images), resulting in H-shaped vertebral bodies
  - Osteoporotic compression fractures

MR Findings

- T1WI
  - Low T1 signal intensity marrow due to: Hyperplastic marrow, sclerosis due to chronic bone infarcts, infection, iron deposition with transfusion-dependent HbSS disease
  - Round, paravertebral soft tissue masses reflect extraosseous hematopoiesis; may be seen with severe, chronic anemia
- T2WI, STIR
  - Hyperplastic (hematopoietic) marrow: Intermediate to low T2 signal intensity
  - Iron deposition with transfusion-dependent HbSS disease: Very low T2 signal intensity
  - Acute bone infarct: Diffuse area of hyperintense marrow signal
  - Osteomyelitis: Diffuse area of hyperintense marrow signal
  - Round, paravertebral soft tissue masses reflect extraosseous hematopoiesis; may be seen with severe, chronic anemia
- T1WI C+
  - Bone infarct: Thin, serpentine rim of enhancement
  - Osteomyelitis: Diffuse enhancement or coarse peripheral rind of enhancement
    - Adjacent soft tissue enhancement with focal cortical defect/enhancement

Imaging Recommendations

- Best imaging tool
  - Radiography

Nuclear Medicine Findings

- Bone scan
  - Bone infarct: Acutely photopenic with increased activity during healing and revascularization
  - Osteomyelitis: Increased activity
- Tc-99m sulfur colloid
  - Acute bone infarct: Diminished or absent marrow uptake
  - Osteomyelitis: Normal or decreased marrow uptake
    - Marrow uptake may be normal in very early phase (< 1 week) of infection
- Ga-67 scintigraphy
  - Acute bone infarct: Congruent uptake relative to Tc-99m sulfur colloid marrow scan
  - Osteomyelitis: Increased uptake or incongruently increased relative to Tc-99m sulfur colloid marrow scan
- Labeled leukocyte scintigraphy
  - Osteomyelitis: Increased activity without corresponding activity on Tc-99m sulfur colloid marrow scan

DIFFERENTIAL DIAGNOSIS

Thalassemia

- Avascular necrosis less common than in sickle cell anemia

Radiographic Mimics

- Renal osteodystrophy
  - Thickened, dense vertebral endplates
- Osteopetrosis
  - Diffuse bone sclerosis
  - Bone-in-bone sign
- Spondyloepiphyseal dysplasia (SED)
  - Vertebrae with cup-shaped endplates
- Diffuse osseous metastases
  - Diffuse low-signal marrow on T1WI MR, intermediate to hyperintense T2WI MR
  - Leukemia, lymphoma
  - Neuroblastoma

PATHOLOGY

General Features

- Etiology

- Abnormal B-chain of hemoglobin tetramer
- Tendency for RBCs to deform (sickle) on deoxygenation
  - Decreased RBC pliability → capillary obstruction → ischemia and infarction
- Splenomegaly (RBC sequestration, destruction) → atrophy (autoinfarction)
  - Autoinfarction leads to decreased host resistance to encapsulated bacteria
    - *Salmonella typhi, Streptococcus pneumoniae, Haemophilus influenzae, Neisseria meningitidis, Klebsiella pneumoniae*
  - Pneumonia
  - Osteomyelitis
  - Meningitis
  - Sepsis
- H-shaped vertebral bodies
  - Central endplate bone vascular supply from long branches of vertebral nutrient artery
    - More susceptible to vasoocclusive effects of sickled RBCs
  - Peripheral portion of endplate supplied by short perforating branches of periosteal vessels
  - Central osteonecrosis → central collapse → H-shaped vertebral body in sagittal plane
- High prevalence of abnormal bone mineral density (BMD), especially in lumbar spine
  - Increased BMD due to healed bone infarcts
  - Decreased BMD due to chronic, severe anemia
    - Hyperplasia of marrow elements causes decreased trabecular bone and osteopenia
    - Osteonecrosis
  - One series reported 79.6% incidence of low BMD in sickle cell disease, irrespective of age or sex
  - Osteoporotic vertebral compression fractures
  - Other insufficiency fractures

- Genetics
  - Autosomal recessive inheritance
  - Structural defect in hemoglobin HbS: Glutamic acid in position 6 substituted with valine
- Associated abnormalities
  - Moyamoya disease, multiple infarcts
  - Femoral head and humeral head infarcts
  - Growth disturbance
    - Limb length discrepancy
  - Cholelithiasis (bilirubin stones)
  - Hemosiderosis due to multiple transfusions

CLINICAL ISSUES

Presentation

- Most common signs/symptoms
  - Sickle cell crisis
    - Painful episode due to vasoocclusive crisis, most commonly involving bone
  - Hemolytic anemia
- Clinical profile
  - Recurrent pain crises, jaundice, growth restriction, stroke
  - High incidence of infections
    - Pneumococcal septicemia, meningitis
    - Osteomyelitis usually seen in children

Demographics

- Age
  - Children protected during first 6 months by elevated levels of fetal Hb (HbF)
- Ethnicity
  - African, Middle Eastern, and Eastern Mediterranean ethnic heritage
- Epidemiology
  - 1% of Black populations are homozygous HbSS; 8-13% are heterozygous HbSA (asymptomatic)
  - 3% of Black populations are HbS carriers
  - In one series, 26% of all sickle cell bony crises resulted in hospital admission involving spine
    - 2nd most common site of bony involvement (after lower extremity)

Natural History & Prognosis

- Death < 50 years in homozygous form

Treatment

- Sickle cell crisis: Oxygen, hydration, pain management, blood transfusion
- Prophylactic vaccinations to prevent infection

DIAGNOSTIC CHECKLIST

Consider

- H-shaped vertebra strongly suggests diagnosis

SELECTED REFERENCES

1. Abreu VS et al: Neuroimaging findings in paediatric patients with sickle cell disease. Clin Radiol. 78(7):509-17, 2023
2. Lins CF et al: Quantitative MRI evaluation of bone marrow in sickle cell disease: relationship with haemolysis and clinical severity. Clin Radiol. 78(3):e268-78, 2023
3. De Luna G et al: High bone mineral density in sickle cell disease: prevalence and characteristics. Bone. 110:199-203, 2018
4. Eid R et al: Spinal cord infarction in hemoglobin SC disease as an amusement park accident. Pediatrics. 138(3), 2016
5. Nix JS et al: Spinal bone marrow necrosis with vertebral compression fracture: differentiation of BMN from AVN. Skeletal Radiol. 43(9):1337-40, 2014
6. Das D et al: MRI appearances of extramedullary haematopoiesis presenting with cauda equina syndrome in sickle cell disease. Clin Radiol. 66(12):1219-22, 2011
7. Gupta R et al: Pattern of bone mineral density in sickle cell disease patients with the high-Hb F phenotype. Acta Haematol. 123(1):64-70, 2010
8. Porter JB: Pathophysiology of transfusional iron overload: contrasting patterns in thalassemia major and sickle cell disease. Hemoglobin. 33 Suppl 1:S37-45, 2009
9. Sarrai M et al: Bone mass density in adults with sickle cell disease. Br J Haematol. 136(4):666-72, 2007
10. Kim SK et al: Natural history and distribution of bone and bone marrow infarction in sickle hemoglobinopathies. J Nucl Med. 43(7):896-900, 2002
11. Lonergan GJ et al: Sickle cell anemia. Radiographics. 21(4):971-94, 2001
12. Skaggs DL et al: Differentiation between bone infarction and acute osteomyelitis in children with sickle-cell disease with use of sequential radionuclide bone-marrow and bone scans. J Bone Joint Surg Am. 83-A(12):1810-3, 2001
13. States LJ: Imaging of metabolic bone disease and marrow disorders in children. Radiol Clin North Am. 39(4):749-72, 2001
14. Umans H et al: The diagnostic role of gadolinium enhanced MRI in distinguishing between acute medullary bone infarct and osteomyelitis. Magn Reson Imaging. 18(3):255-62, 2000
15. Roger E et al: Sickle cell disease of the spine in children. Can J Surg. 42(4):289-92, 1999
16. Marlow TJ et al: "Tower vertebra": a new observation in sickle cell disease. Skeletal Radiol. 27(4):195-8, 1998
17. Kahn CE Jr et al: Combined bone marrow and gallium imaging. Differentiation of osteomyelitis and infarction in sickle hemoglobinopathy. Clin Nucl Med. 13(6):443-9, 1988

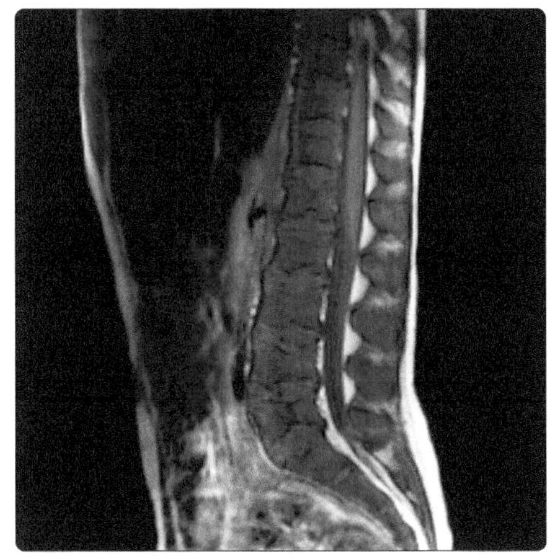

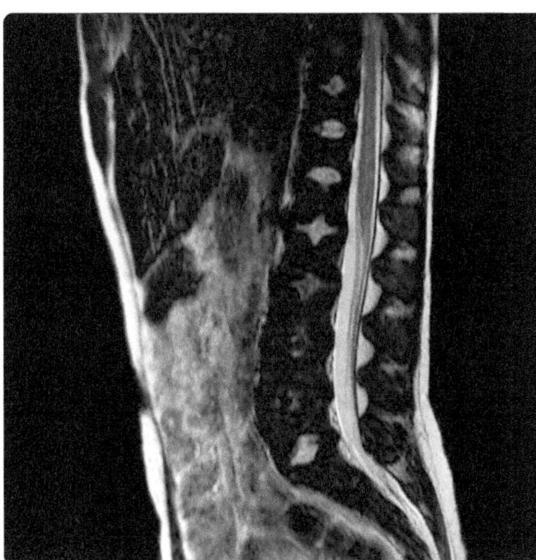

(Left) *Sagittal T1 MR in a child with severe anemia secondary to SCD reveals hypointense cellular marrow and multiple levels of central vertebral collapse resulting in H-shaped vertebra. Marrow involvement in all vertebral levels is typical of systemic disease.* **(Right)** *Sagittal T2 MR in same patient shows marked diffuse marrow hypointensity at all levels. This is frequently a reflection of both marrow cellularity secondary to anemia and iron deposition from multiple blood transfusions. H-shaped vertebra are noted at every level.*

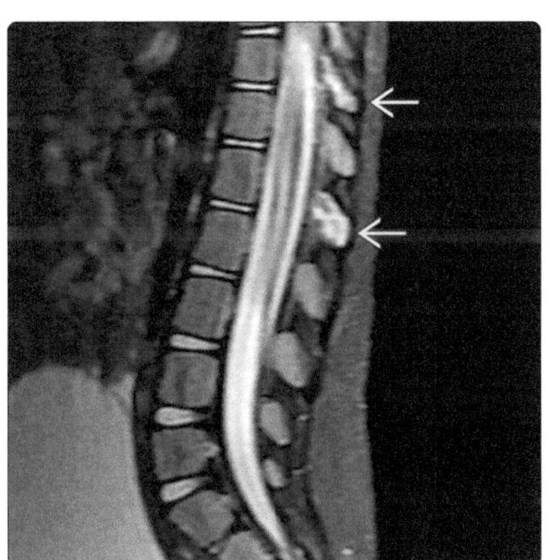

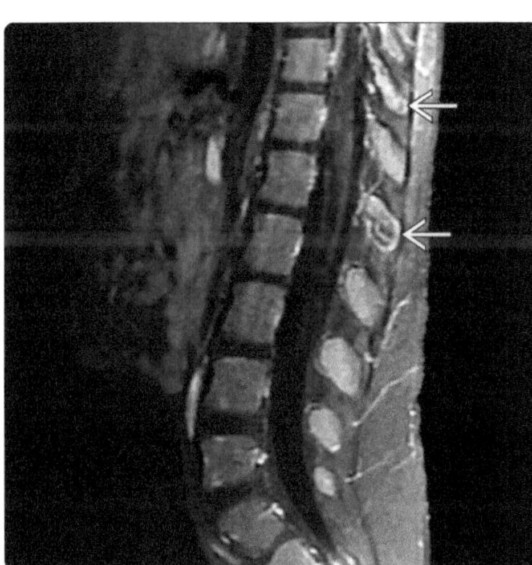

(Left) *Sagittal STIR MR in a child with SCD and acute back pain reveals abnormal hyperintensity ➔ in multiple spinous processes reflecting bone infarctions. Note that the vertebral bodies show normal height.* **(Right)** *Sagittal T1 C+ FS MR in the same patient confirms abnormal marrow enhancement within the abnormal spinous processes ➔ suggesting subacute ischemia. The other vertebral levels show a normal appearance. This young child has not yet accumulated iron within the vertebral marrow.*

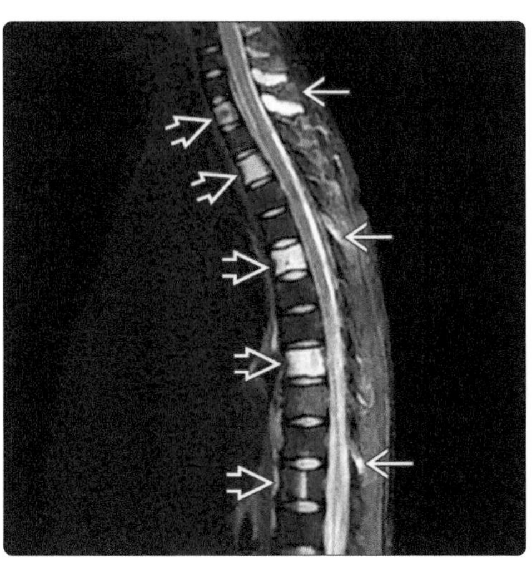

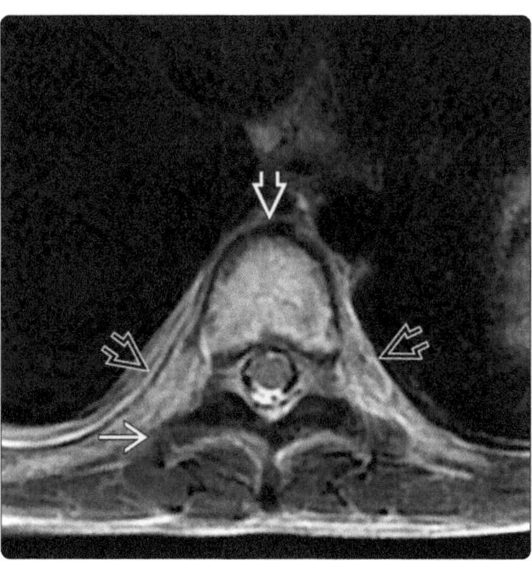

(Left) *Sagittal STIR MR in a child with SCD and severe recurrent back pain demonstrates multiple vertebra ➔ with abnormal hyperintensity reflective of bone infarcts. Several spinous processes ➔ also demonstrate bone infarcts.* **(Right)** *Axial T2 MR in the same patient shows abnormal marrow signal in both the vertebral body ➔ and medial ribs ➔. The spinous and transverse processes ➔ reveal hypointense cellular marrow signal.*

Osteogenesis Imperfecta

KEY FACTS

TERMINOLOGY

- Genetic disorder of type I collagen resulting in bone fragility
- Classified into 4 types based on clinical, genetic, and radiographic criteria

IMAGING

- Severe osteopenia
- Vertebral fractures, kyphoscoliosis
- Multiple long bone, rib fractures
- Enlarged epiphyses, popcorn metaphyseal calcifications
- Medullary cavity nearly entirely filled with fat
  - Primary trabeculae sparse but normally oriented
  - Secondary trabeculae nearly absent

TOP DIFFERENTIAL DIAGNOSES

- Nonaccidental trauma (NAT)
- Congenital dwarfism
- Osteoporosis

PATHOLOGY

- Numerous type I collagen mutations → "brittle" bone
  - Most autosomal dominant
  - Inherited or spontaneous mutation
- Associated anomalies include blue sclerae, early hearing loss, brittle teeth, thin fragile skin, joint laxity

CLINICAL ISSUES

- Short stature secondary to multiple spinal and extremity fractures, kyphoscoliosis, growth plate abnormalities
- Diagnosis suggested by radiographs, confirmed with ancillary testing

DIAGNOSTIC CHECKLIST

- Important to differentiate from NAT
- Basilar impression and other spinal complications may be difficult to detect on radiographs
  - Consider MR or CT

(Left) *Sagittal bone CT demonstrates platybasia ➡ and severe basilar impression with upward displacement of the remodeled odontoid process ➡ and anterior C1 ring ➡ through the foramen magnum. Metallic posterior spinal hardware ➡ has been placed to arrest basilar impression.* **(Right)** *Sagittal T2WI MR reveals severe cranial settling and platybasia with basilar impression of the odontoid process ➡ into the foramen magnum, producing ventral cervicomedullary compression.*

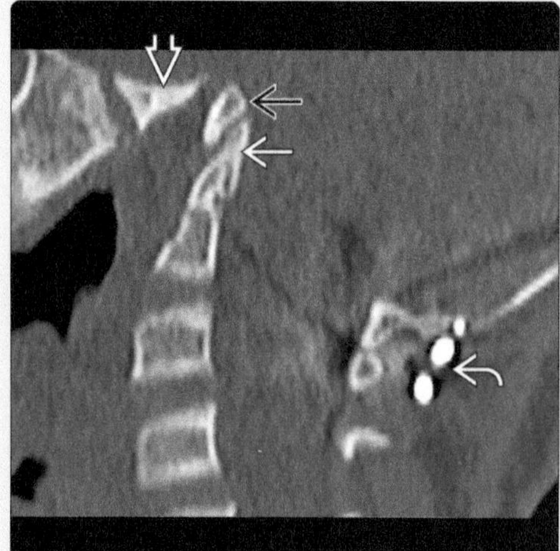

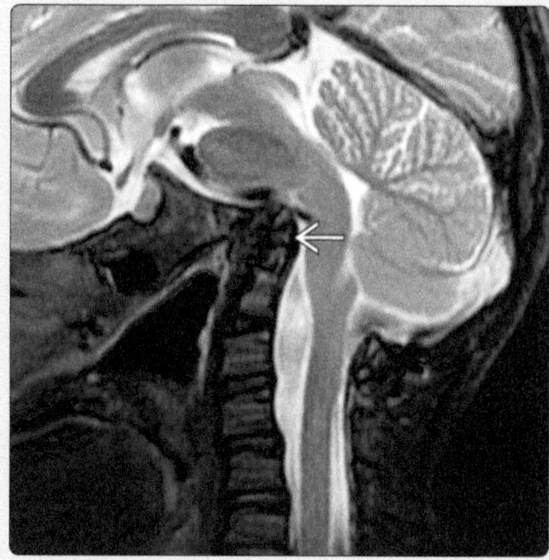

(Left) *Coronal T2WI MR confirms upward sloping of the medial skull base ➡ related to bone softening and severe basilar impression. This results in compression of the brainstem and cerebellar hemispheres.* **(Right)** *Axial T2WI MR confirms medullary distortion ➡ by the clivus ➡ related to cranial settling. Metallic susceptibility artifact ➡ reflects spinal surgical fusion hardware intended to arrest cranial settling.*

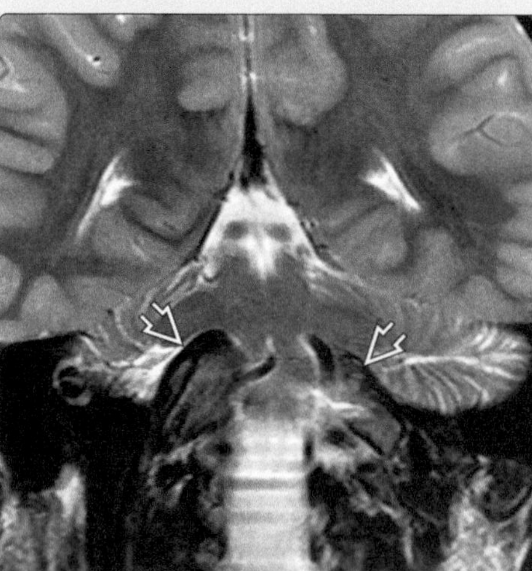

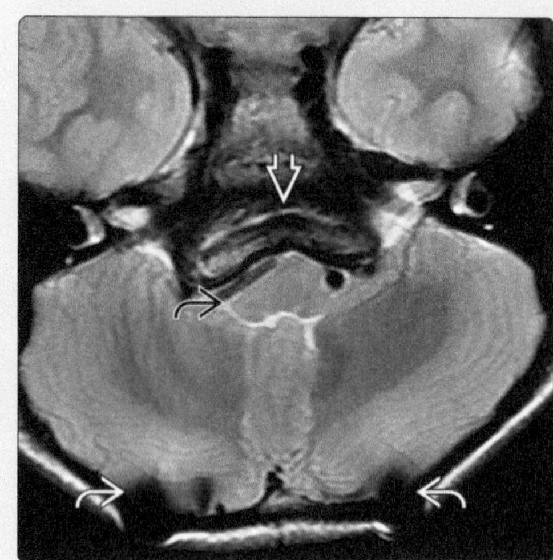

TERMINOLOGY

Synonyms

- Brittle bone disease

Definitions

- Genetic disorder of type I collagen resulting in bone fragility
- Classified into 4 types based on clinical, genetic, and radiographic criteria
  - Severe forms: Bones short, thickened due to multiple fractures in utero and early childhood
  - Milder forms: Bones thin and gracile

IMAGING

General Features

- Best diagnostic clue
  - Severe osteopenia with multiple fractures, kyphoscoliosis
- Location
  - Entire axial and appendicular skeleton
- Morphology
  - Multiple skeletal fractures common

Radiographic Findings

- Radiography
  - Osteoporosis
    - Cortical thinning, resorption of secondary trabeculae with prominent primary trabeculae
  - Kyphoscoliosis
  - Vertebral fractures, vertebra plana, codfish vertebrae
    - Codfish vertebra: Cupping of superior and inferior vertebral body endplates
  - Multiple fractures of long bones and ribs with increased anteroposterior chest diameter
    - Bowing deformity due to microfracture as well as radiographically evident fractures
  - Enlarged epiphyses
  - Popcorn metaphyseal calcifications
    - Calcified cartilage nodules due to fragmentation of growth plate from trauma
  - Pelvis: Protrusio acetabulae, coxa vara

CT Findings

- Bone CT
  - Thin bony cortices
  - Medullary cavity nearly entirely filled with fat
    - Primary trabeculae sparse but normally oriented
    - Secondary trabeculae nearly absent
  - Kyphoscoliosis
  - Basilar impression
  - Otospongiosis (temporal bone)

MR Findings

- T1WI
  - Kyphoscoliosis
  - Abnormal marrow signal intensity related to fractures, fatty infiltration
- T2WI
  - Same as T1WI
  - ± spinal cord compression, syringohydromyelia

Ultrasonographic Findings

- Grayscale ultrasound
  - Poorly ossified skull, short ribs, short deformed limbs
  - Antenatal diagnosis possible during 2nd trimester

Nuclear Medicine Findings

- Bone scan
  - Increased radiotracer uptake at fracture sites

Other Modality Findings

- Decreased bone density on dual-energy x-ray absorptiometry (DEXA) or CT
  - Used to aid diagnosis (mild forms), follow response to medical treatment

Imaging Recommendations

- Best imaging tool
  - Radiography for diagnosis, kyphoscoliosis characterization
  - MR best to evaluate for spinal cord compression, basilar impression

DIFFERENTIAL DIAGNOSIS

Nonaccidental Trauma

- Normal bone mineral density
- Fractures may otherwise appear identical to osteogenesis imperfecta (OI)
- Careful history, family evaluation required
- Genetic testing may be necessary

Congenital Dwarfism

- Loss of vertebral body height
- Short stature
- Scoliosis
- Bone density variable
- Common etiologies
  - Achondroplasia
  - Thanatophoric dwarfism
  - Spondyloepiphyseal dysplasia

Osteoporosis

- Thinned bone cortices, accentuation of primary trabeculae, resorption of secondary trabeculae
- Radiography insensitive for diagnosis; better evaluated by bone densitometry
- Codfish vertebrae, compression fractures common
- Myriad etiologies

PATHOLOGY

General Features

- Etiology
  - Numerous type I collagen mutations → abnormal type I collagen, brittle bone
    - Type I collagen found in bone, skin, sclerae
- Genetics
  - Most autosomal dominant
  - Inherited or spontaneous mutation
- Associated abnormalities
  - Blue sclerae
  - Early hearing loss

- Brittle teeth
- Thin, fragile skin
- Joint laxity
- Respiratory, cardiac problems

Staging, Grading, & Classification

- Type I: Most common
  - Thin, gracile long bones
  - High fracture risk in childhood, decreases after puberty
  - Kyphoscoliosis, wormian bones
  - Blue sclerae
- Type II: Often lethal early in life
  - Short, broad, deformed bones at birth due to multiple fractures
- Type III: Autosomal recessive; rare
  - Fractures at birth, kyphoscoliosis
- Type IV: Similar to type I
  - Kyphoscoliosis, wormian bones
  - Sclerae usually normal in adulthood, may be blue in childhood
- Recently types V-XII have been proposed; not distinguishable radiographically
  - These types do not localize to genes for type I collagen; etiology unknown
- Terms congenita and tarda no longer used

Gross Pathologic & Surgical Features

- Thin, eggshell-like bone cortices
- Decreased medullary trabeculae
- Recent or healed fractures

Microscopic Features

- Lack of organized trabeculae
- Prominent osteoid seams
- Increased numbers of morphologically normal osteoblasts
- Growth plate fragmentation

CLINICAL ISSUES

Presentation

- Most common signs/symptoms
  - Multiple spinal and extremity fractures
  - Kyphoscoliosis
- Other signs/symptoms
  - ± deafness, blue sclerae
- Clinical profile
  - Short stature secondary to fractures, kyphoscoliosis, growth plate abnormalities
  - Diagnosis suggested by radiographs, confirmed with ancillary testing
    - Skin biopsy
    - Genetic testing
    - Caveat: Both tests may be false-negative

Demographics

- Age
  - Findings often evident at birth
  - Mild cases may present in adulthood
- Sex
  - M = F
- Epidemiology
  - 4/100,000 births

Natural History & Prognosis

- Severe forms, previously lethal, now may survive to adulthood
- Growth restriction varies with severity of disease
- Fractures less common after puberty

Treatment

- Conservative management
  - Bisphosphonates variably successful for medical therapy
    - Some studies show that diphosphonates decrease scoliosis rate of progression
  - Prolonged immobilization avoided because of resultant worsened osteoporosis
- Surgical management
  - Spinal fusion for kyphoscoliosis
    - Aggressive surgical decompression stabilization procedures may halt basilar impression progression and facilitate good long-term functional outcome
    - Increasing use of magnetic "growing rods" for scoliosis
      - High risk of hardware mechanical failure
    - May be future role for kyphoplasty as alternative management
  - Intramedullary rod placement for long bone fractures
    - Least invasive internal fixation for rapid mobilization
    - Helps prevent progression of deformity, further fractures

DIAGNOSTIC CHECKLIST

Consider

- Important to differentiate from nonaccidental trauma
- Basilar impression and other spinal complications may be difficult to detect on radiographs
  - Consider MR or CT

SELECTED REFERENCES

1. Hirata K et al: Successful helmet therapy in an infant with positional brachycephaly associated with perinatal severe osteogenesis imperfecta. Pediatr Int. 65(1):e15512, 2023
2. Rabau O et al: Scoliosis in osteogenesis imperfecta: results of posterior spinal fusion in 39 patients. Eur Spine J. 32(4):1146-52, 2023
3. Rapoport M et al: The patient clinical journey and socioeconomic impact of osteogenesis imperfecta: a systematic scoping review. Orphanet J Rare Dis. 18(1):34, 2023
4. Sienko S et al: Surgical outcomes for spinal deformity in osteogenesis imperfecta. Spine Deform. 11(2):391-8, 2023
5. Shur NE et al: Genetic causes of fractures and subdural hematomas: fact versus fiction. Pediatr Radiol. 51(6):1029-43, 2021
6. Kashii M et al: Development of scoliosis in young children with osteogenesis imperfecta undergoing intravenous bisphosphonate therapy. J Bone Miner Metab. 37(3):545-53, 2019
7. Gardner A et al: The use of magnetically controlled growing rods in paediatric osteogenesis imperfecta with early onset, progressive scoliosis. J Surg Case Rep. 2018(3):rjy043, 2018
8. Liu G et al: The genetic implication of scoliosis in osteogenesis imperfecta: a review. J Spine Surg. 3(4):666-78, 2017
9. Persiani P et al: Association between spondylolisthesis and L5 fracture in patients with osteogenesis imperfecta. Eur Spine J. 26(12):3106-11, 2017
10. Wallace MJ et al: The spine in patients with osteogenesis imperfecta. J Am Acad Orthop Surg. 25(2):100-9, 2017
11. Costa FW et al: Clinical aspects, imaging features, and considerations on bisphosphonate-related osteonecrosis risk in a pediatric patient with osteogenesis imperfecta. Case Rep Dent. 2014:384292, 2014
12. Khandanpour N et al: Craniospinal abnormalities and neurologic complications of osteogenesis imperfecta: imaging overview. Radiographics. 32(7):2101-12, 2012

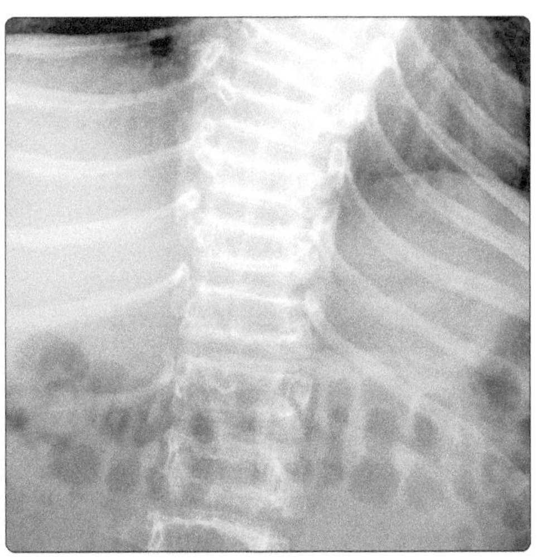

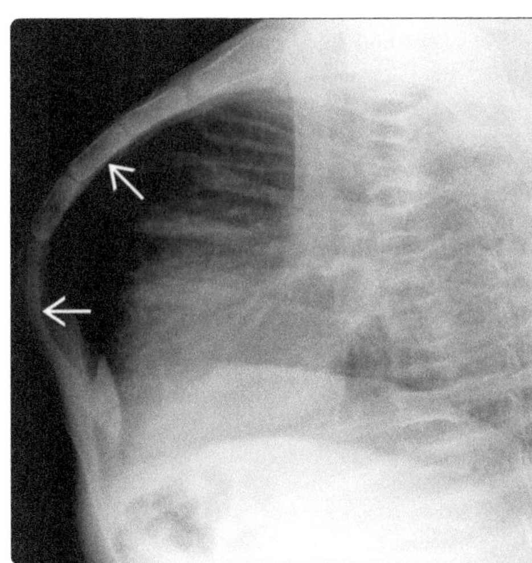

(Left) *Anteroposterior radiograph shows severe osteopenia, platyspondyly, scoliosis, gracile ribs, small, irregular pedicles, and sclerotic bands (due to bisphosphonate therapy), all characteristic of severe treated osteogenesis imperfecta (OI).* **(Right)** *Lateral radiograph in the same patient further demonstrates pectus carinatum ➡ and confirms platyspondyly with abnormal straightening of thoracic kyphosis.*

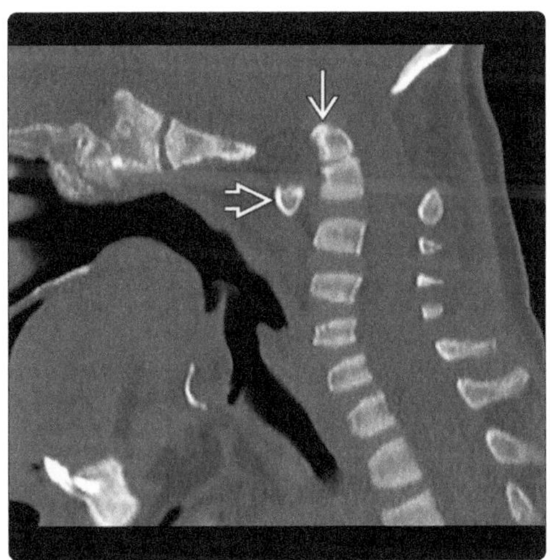

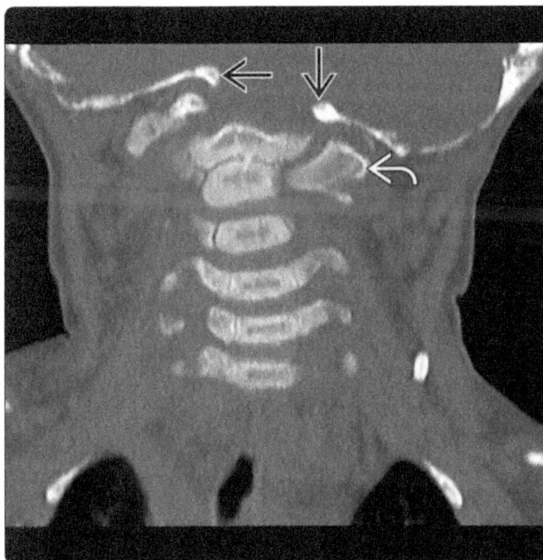

(Left) *Sagittal bone CT in a 5-year-old patient with OI reveals severe cranial settling with the odontoid process ➡ extending through the foramen magnum plane. The craniovertebral angle is flattened, and the anterior C1 ring ➡ resides at the C2/C3 level.* **(Right)** *Coronal bone CT in the same patient confirms that the left C1 lateral mass ➡ has slipped off of the C2 lateral mass, producing head tilt. Additionally, there is upward curvature of the softened skull base ➡ contributing to cranial settling.*

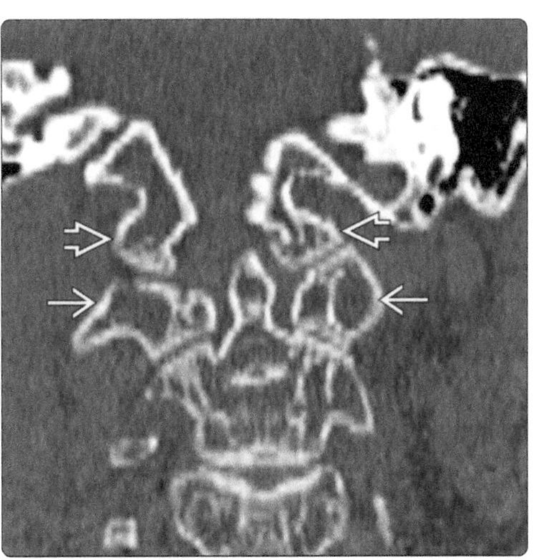

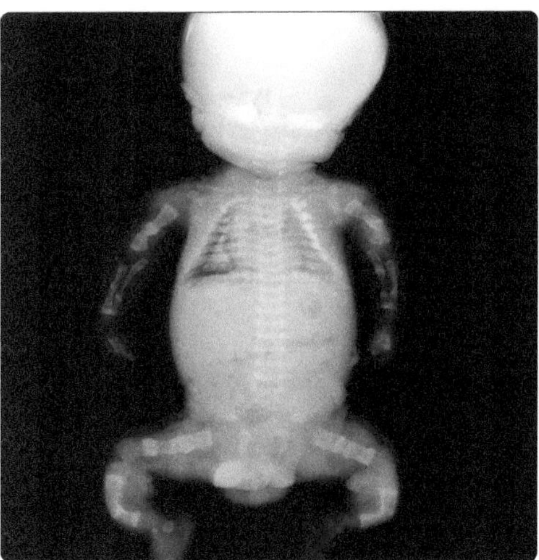

(Left) *Coronal bone CT of the cervical spine performed to evaluate severe headaches (type I OI) confirms diffuse severe osteopenia. No collapse of the occipital condyles ➡ or C1 lateral masses ➡ is confirmed.* **(Right)** *Frontal radiograph of a fetus obtained during fetal imaging autopsy demonstrates numerous fractures of all extremities and the ribs in varying states of repair as well as characteristic platyspondyly and underossification of the calvarium.*

Developmental Spinal Stenosis

KEY FACTS

TERMINOLOGY

- Reduced AP canal diameter secondary to short, squat pedicles and laterally directed laminae

IMAGING

- Central canal diameter is smaller than normal
- Short, thick pedicles
- Trefoil-shaped lateral recesses
- Laterally directed laminae

TOP DIFFERENTIAL DIAGNOSES

- Acquired spinal stenosis
- Inherited spinal stenosis
  - Achondroplasia
  - Mucopolysaccharidoses

PATHOLOGY

- Cervical spine
  - Torg ratio (AP canal diameter:AP vertebral body diameter): < 0.8
  - Absolute diameter: < 14 mm
- Lumbar spine
  - AP canal diameter at L1 < 20 mm, L2 < 19 mm, L3 < 19 mm, L4 < 17 mm, L5 < 16 mm, S1 < 16 mm

CLINICAL ISSUES

- Symptomatic cervical or lumbar stenosis symptoms at younger age than typical of degenerative stenosis
- Athletes present with temporary neurologic deficit following physical contact that subsequently resolves ("stinger")

DIAGNOSTIC CHECKLIST

- Recognition of short, thick pedicles, AP canal diameter reduction key to diagnosis
- Patients present at younger age than typical for degenerative spine disease

(Left) *Sagittal graphic of the cervical spine demonstrates marked developmental AP narrowing of the central spinal canal, resulting in cord deformation.* **(Right)** *Axial graphic depicts developmental cervical AP spinal stenosis with generalized narrowing of the subarachnoid space. The pedicles ➡ are thick and laterally directed.*

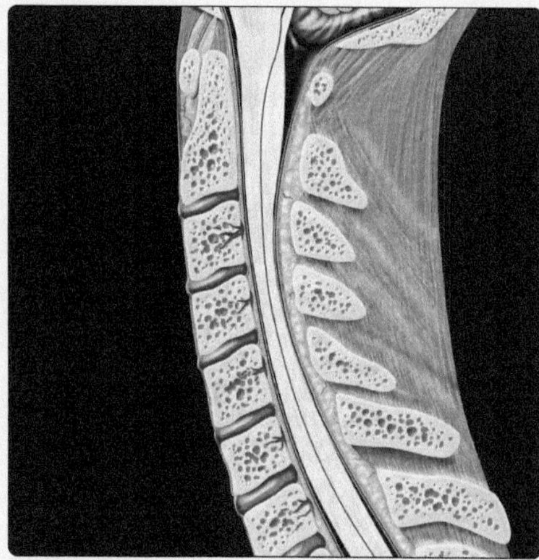

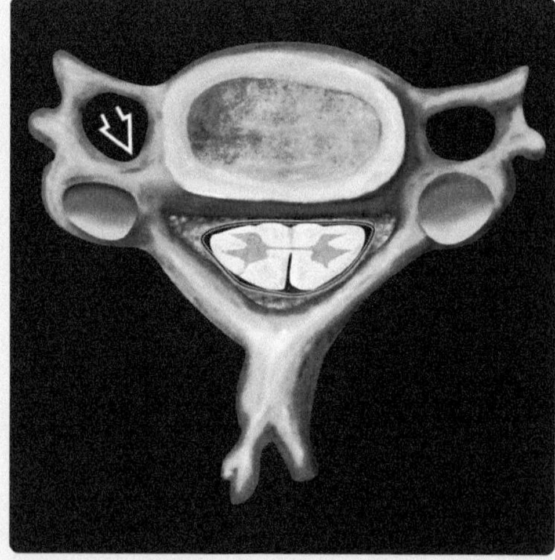

(Left) *Sagittal T2WI MR shows marked developmental stenosis at C3 due to abnormally short pedicles and dysmorphic C3 vertebra. Cord T2 hyperintensity ➡ corresponds to myelomalacia with clinical myelopathy. This football player had a "stinger" after a tackle.* **(Right)** *Axial bone CT in the same patient demonstrates marked AP canal reduction attributable to developmentally short pedicles ➡ and flattened, laterally oriented laminae ➡.*

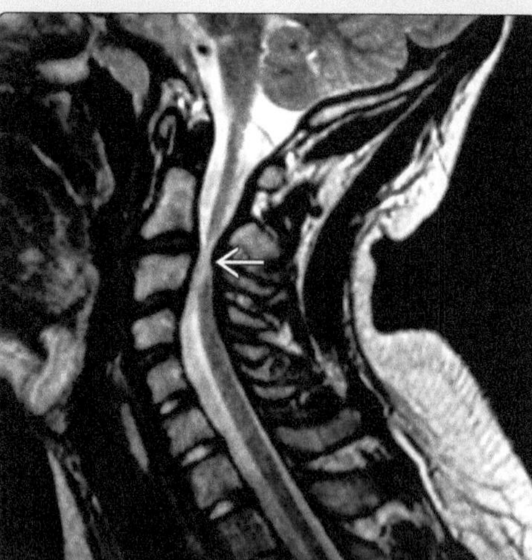

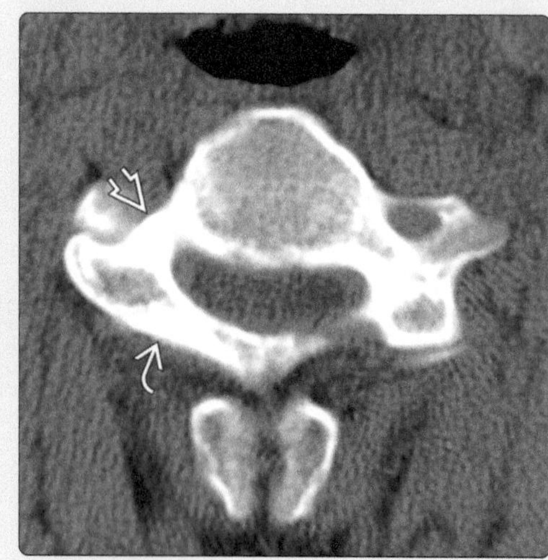

TERMINOLOGY

Abbreviations

- Developmental spinal stenosis (DSS)

Synonyms

- Short pedicle syndrome, congenital short pedicles, congenital spinal stenosis

Definitions

- Reduced AP canal diameter secondary to short, squat pedicles and laterally directed laminae

IMAGING

General Features

- Best diagnostic clue
  - Short, thick pedicles producing narrowed AP spinal canal diameter
- Location
  - Lumbar > cervical > thoracic spine
- Size
  - Central bony canal diameter is smaller than normal
    - Cervical spine: Absolute AP diameter < 14 mm
    - Lumbar spine: Critical stenosis at L4 < 14 mm, L5 < 14 mm, S1 < 12 mm
- Morphology
  - Short, thick pedicles
  - Trefoil-shaped lateral recesses
  - Laterally directed laminae

Radiographic Findings

- Radiography
  - Shortened AP distance between posterior vertebral body and spinolaminar line
    - ± superimposed degenerative disc, facet disease
  - Lateral radiograph normally shows articular pillar ending before spinolaminar line
    - Imaging pearl: If articular pillar takes up entire AP canal dimension on lateral radiograph, central canal stenosis is present

CT Findings

- Bone CT
  - Short, thick pedicles, trefoil-shaped lateral recesses, and laterally directed laminae
    - ± acquired disc, facet degenerative changes
  - Sagittal plane useful to survey extent of congenital narrowing
  - Axial plane best demonstrates reduced AP canal diameter, short, thick pedicles

MR Findings

- T1WI
  - Short AP diameter ± superimposed acquired facet, disc degenerative changes
  - ± hypointense facet, vertebral body marrow changes indicative of superimposed degenerative changes
- T2WI
  - Similar osseous findings to T1WI MR
  - ± cord compression
- T2* GRE
  - Best depicts osseous structures
  - Caveat: Overestimates true degree of canal narrowing secondary to susceptibility blooming artifact

Nonvascular Interventions

- Myelography
  - Confirms shortened AP dimension, clarifies severity of neural compression

Imaging Recommendations

- CT with sagittal and coronal reformats to evaluate osseous structures
  - Axial plane best for degree of narrowing and neural compromise
- MR to assess degree/presence of spinal cord, dural sac compression
  - Also demonstrates osseous anatomy well; permits complete imaging assessment with single imaging study
  - Sagittal MR best demonstrates AP canal narrowing; assesses for cord/cauda equina compression
  - Axial MR confirms pedicle configuration, assesses severity of canal narrowing

DIFFERENTIAL DIAGNOSIS

Acquired Spinal Stenosis

- Normal pedicle length
- ± subluxation
- ± spondylolysis
- ± disc degenerative changes
- ± facet degenerative changes

Inherited Spinal Stenosis

- Genetic predisposition; most common
  - Achondroplasia
  - Mucopolysaccharidoses (MPS)
    - Frequently associated with characteristic brain, visceral, &/or extremity abnormalities enabling specific diagnosis
    - MPS IV (Morquio) is prototype

PATHOLOGY

General Features

- Etiology
  - Idiopathic
- Associated abnormalities
  - Superimposed acquired (degenerative) stenosis
  - Ligamentum flavum redundancy
- Short, thickened pedicles

Staging, Grading, & Classification

- Cervical spine
  - Torg ratio (AP canal diameter:AP vertebral body diameter): < 0.8
  - Absolute diameter: < 14 mm
- Lumbar spine
  - Spinal stenosis present if AP canal diameter at L1 < 20 mm, L2 < 19 mm, L3 < 19 mm, L4 < 17 mm, L5 < 16 mm, S1 < 16 mm
  - Lumbar spine: Critical stenosis where surgery required at L4 < 14 mm, L5 < 14 mm, S1 < 12 mm

Gross Pathologic & Surgical Features

- Sagittal canal narrowed secondary to short pedicles, thick laminae, and protrusion of inferior facet articular processes
- Lateral recess often narrowed secondary to coexistent hypertrophic superior facet articular processes

Microscopic Features

- Histologically normal bone

CLINICAL ISSUES

Presentation

- Most common signs/symptoms
  - Lumbar
    - Low back pain, radiating leg pain (unilateral or bilateral), ± bladder and bowel dysfunction
    - Neurogenic claudication: Radiating leg pain with walking, relieved by rest, bending forward
    - Cauda equina syndrome (rare): Bilateral leg weakness, urinary retention due to atonic bladder
  - Cervical
    - Radiating arm pain or numbness
    - Progressive myelopathy (spinal cord dysfunction) or reversible acute neurologic deficits ("stingers")
- Clinical profile
  - Symptomatic cervical or lumbar stenosis symptoms at younger age than typical of degenerative stenosis
    - These patients typically lack complicating medical problems (diabetes or vascular insufficiency)
  - Athletes present with temporary neurologic deficit following physical contact that subsequently resolves

Demographics

- Age
  - Symptoms may arise in teens; more common in 4th-5th decades
- Sex
  - M ≥ F
- Ethnicity
  - No predilection
- Epidemiology
  - Prevalence in general population difficult to establish; up to 30% of surgically proven lumbar stenosis in one study
    - Not uncommonly seen in clinical practice during routine cervical or lumbar spine evaluation
    - Congenital cervical stenosis reported in 7.6% of 262 high school and college football players
  - Symptomatic at earlier age than expected

Natural History & Prognosis

- May be incidental finding in younger patients
  - Borderline cases are usually asymptomatic until superimposed acquired spinal degenerative disease occurs
- Many patients eventually develop symptomatic spinal stenosis
  - Minor superimposed acquired abnormalities (bulge, herniation, osteophyte) cause severe neurologic symptoms
- Early surgical treatment important for best outcome
  - Surgical decompression usually relieves symptoms effectively
  - Long-term pain relief following surgery common

Treatment

- Lumbar: Decompressive laminectomy, posterior foraminotomy at involved levels
  - Risk of complications increases with more levels of decompression, diabetes, and long-term steroid use
- Cervical: Posterior cervical laminectomy or laminoplasty
  - Same risk factors for complication as lumbar decompression

DIAGNOSTIC CHECKLIST

Consider

- Patients present at younger age than typical for degenerative spine disease
- Congenital spinal stenosis may not produce symptoms until superimposed acquired degenerative changes accumulate

Image Interpretation Pearls

- Recognition of short, thick pedicles, AP canal diameter reduction key to diagnosis
- Look for superimposed degenerative changes

SELECTED REFERENCES

1. Wang Y et al: The correlation between lumbar interlaminar space size on plain radiograph and spinal stenosis. Eur Spine J. 32(5):1721-8, 2023
2. Bai Q et al: Current understanding of tandem spinal stenosis: epidemiology, diagnosis, and surgical strategy. EFORT Open Rev. 7(8):587-98, 2022
3. Lai MKL et al: The profile of the spinal column in subjects with lumbar developmental spinal stenosis. Bone Joint J. 103-B(4):725-33, 2021
4. Kitab S et al: Redefining lumbar spinal stenosis as a developmental syndrome: does age matter? J Neurosurg Spine. 31(3):357-65, 2019
5. Cheung JPY et al: Etiology of developmental spinal stenosis: a genome-wide association study. J Orthop Res. 36(4):1262-8, 2018
6. Kitab S et al: Redefining lumbar spinal stenosis as a developmental syndrome: an MRI-based multivariate analysis of findings in 709 patients throughout the 16- to 82-year age spectrum. J Neurosurg Spine. 1-7, 2018
7. Cheung JPY et al: Radiographic indices for lumbar developmental spinal stenosis. Scoliosis Spinal Disord. 12:3, 2017
8. Iclal ET et al: A practical radiographic visual estimation technique for the prediction of developmental narrowing of cervical spinal canal. Br J Radiol. 90(1078):20170286, 2017
9. Nagata K et al: the prevalence of tandem spinal stenosis and its characteristics in a population-based MRI study: the Wakayama Spine Study. Eur Spine J. 26(10):2529-35, 2017
10. Nouri A et al: Cervical cord-canal mismatch: a new method for identifying predisposition to spinal cord injury. World Neurosurg. 108:112-7, 2017
11. Cheung JP et al: Defining clinically relevant values for developmental spinal stenosis: a large-scale magnetic resonance imaging study. Spine (Phila Pa 1976). 39(13):1067-76, 2014
12. Kanno H et al: Dynamic change of dural sac cross-sectional area in axial loaded magnetic resonance imaging correlates with the severity of clinical symptoms in patients with lumbar spinal canal stenosis. Spine (Phila Pa 1976). 37(3):207-13, 2012
13. Schizas C et al: Qualitative grading of severity of lumbar spinal stenosis based on the morphology of the dural sac on magnetic resonance images. Spine (Phila Pa 1976). 35(21):1919-24, 2010
14. Singh K et al: Congenital lumbar spinal stenosis: a prospective, control-matched, cohort radiographic analysis. Spine J. 5(6):615-22, 2005
15. Brigham CD et al: Permanent partial cervical spinal cord injury in a professional football player who had only congenital stenosis. A case report. J Bone Joint Surg Am. 85-A(8):1553-6, 2003
16. Allen CR et al: Transient quadriparesis in the athlete. Clin Sports Med. 21(1):15-27, 2002
17. Oguz H et al: Measurement of spinal canal diameters in young subjects with lumbosacral transitional vertebra. Eur Spine J. 11(2):115-8, 2002
18. Boockvar JA et al: Cervical spinal stenosis and sports-related cervical cord neurapraxia in children. Spine. 26(24):2709-12; discussion 2713, 2001
19. Bey T et al: Spinal cord injury with a narrow spinal canal: utilizing Torg's ratio method of analyzing cervical spine radiographs. J Emerg Med. 16(1):79-82, 1998

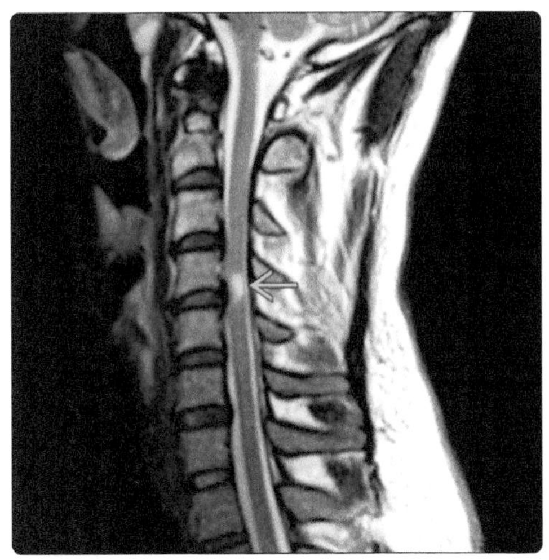

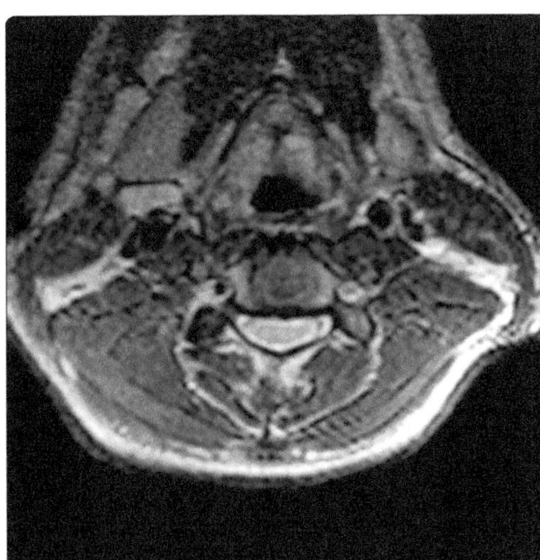

(Left) *Sagittal T2WI MR reveals moderate developmental AP canal narrowing exacerbated by C4-C5 disc herniation. The disc protrusion produces spinal cord T2 hyperintensity ⇒, corresponding to clinical myelopathy.* **(Right)** *Axial T2WI MR demonstrates moderate narrowing of the cervical AP canal diameter. No disc herniation or osseous degenerative changes are noted. Typical cervical findings include reduced AP canal diameter and short, laterally oriented pedicles.*

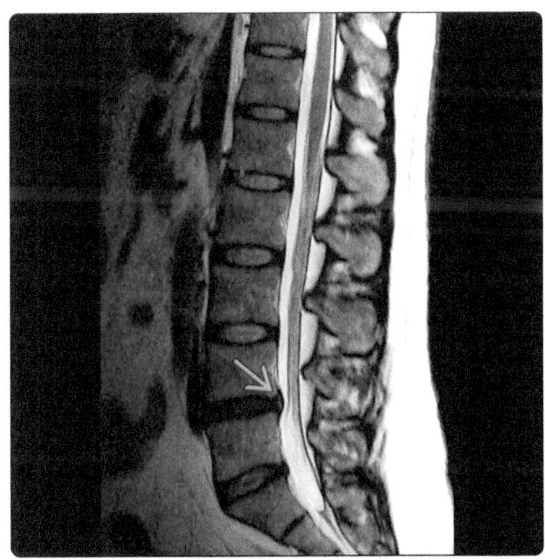

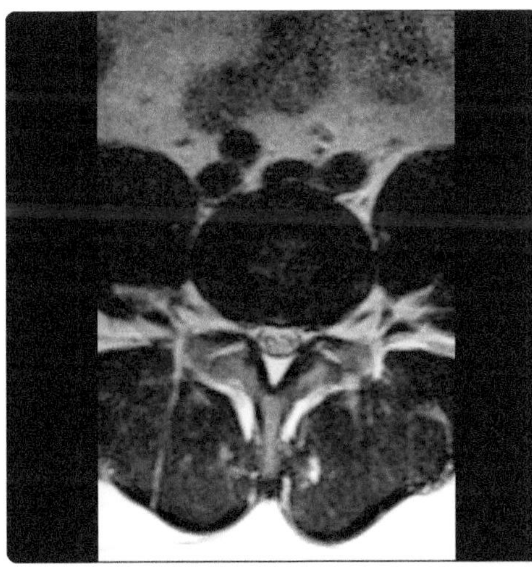

(Left) *Sagittal T2WI MR depicts diffuse narrowing of the AP diameter of the subarachnoid space in this patient with diffuse developmental spinal canal stenosis. Note the mild superimposed acquired stenosis at L4-L5 ⇒ with bulging of the anulus and disc degeneration with signal loss.* **(Right)** *Axial T2 TSE in the same patient reveals the typical appearance of developmental spinal stenosis with facets closely opposed to the intervertebral disc due to short pedicles.*

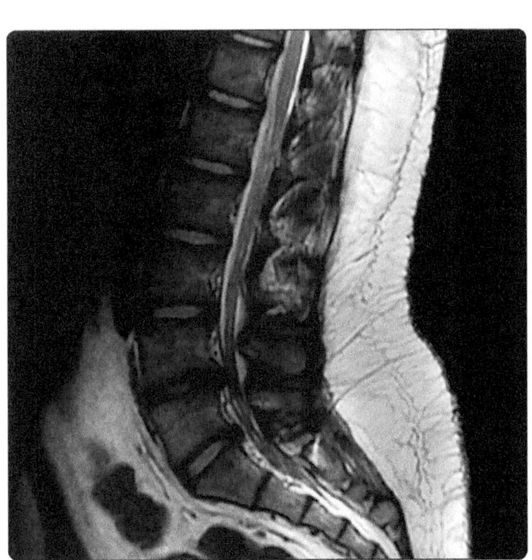

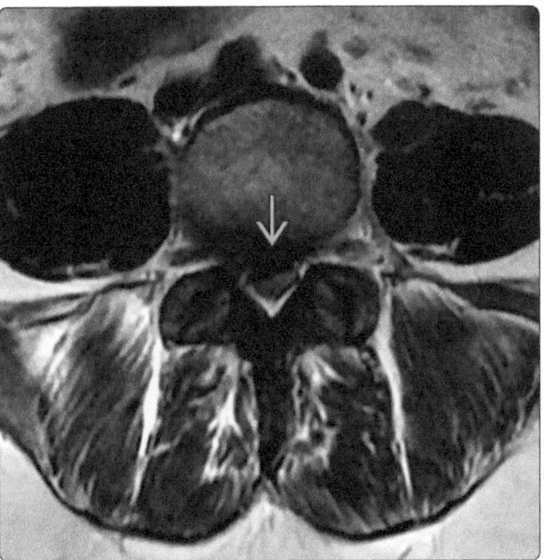

(Left) *Sagittal T2WI MR in an adolescent boy with low back pain demonstrates developmental spinal stenosis with marked AP canal reduction. A superimposed disc herniation at L4-L5 and disc bulge at L5-S1 compound canal stenosis.* **(Right)** *Axial T2WI MR in the same patient confirms right parasagittal disc herniation ⇒ with accentuated central canal and right lateral recess stenosis and facet degenerative changes compounding developmental spinal stenosis.*

KEY FACTS

TERMINOLOGY

- Scoliosis due to neurologic or myopathic diseases

IMAGING

- Most common pattern: Long, single curve thoracolumbar scoliosis
- Thoracolumbar kyphosis common
- Normal vertebral morphology, ± wedging at curve apex
- Osteopenia often present

TOP DIFFERENTIAL DIAGNOSES

- Idiopathic scoliosis
- Congenital scoliosis
- Scheuermann disease
- Scoliosis related to congenital syndromes
- Limb length inequality

PATHOLOGY

- Associated with syringomyelia, spinal dysraphism, tethered cord

CLINICAL ISSUES

- Rapidly progressive curvature
- Onset in infancy or childhood; may progress in adulthood
- 20% of cerebral palsy patients
- Progresses rapidly → respiratory compromise
- Most difficult scoliosis to treat
- Surgical fusion has higher complication rate than other scoliosis types

DIAGNOSTIC CHECKLIST

- MR of entire spine to exclude spinal cord or osseous abnormalities prior to scoliosis correction

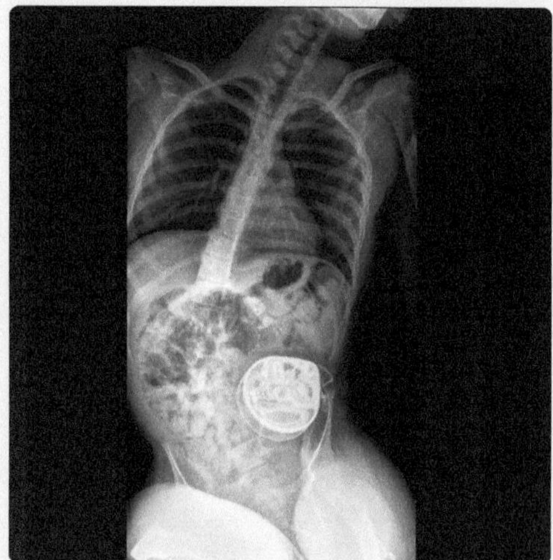

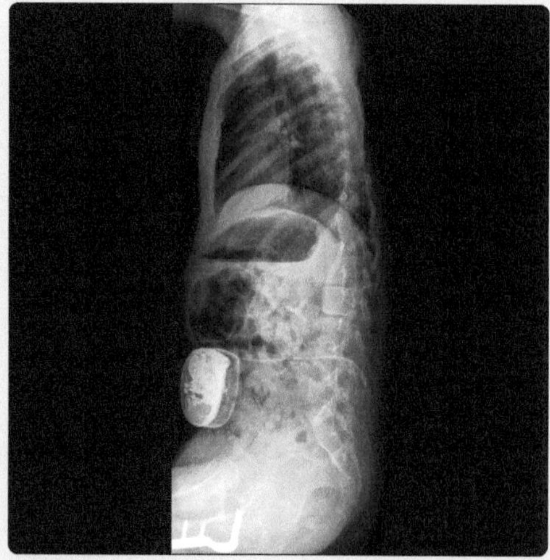

(Left) *Anteroposterior radiograph in a non-weight-bearing patient with cerebral palsy demonstrates typical C-shaped convex right neuromuscular scoliosis. An intrathecal Baclofen infusion catheter system is in place for treatment of spasticity.* **(Right)** *Lateral radiograph of the thoracolumbar spine in a cerebral palsy patient with neuromuscular scoliosis reveals flattening of lumbar lordosis. A Baclofen infusion system and prior femoral osteotomies are clues to a cerebral palsy diagnosis.*

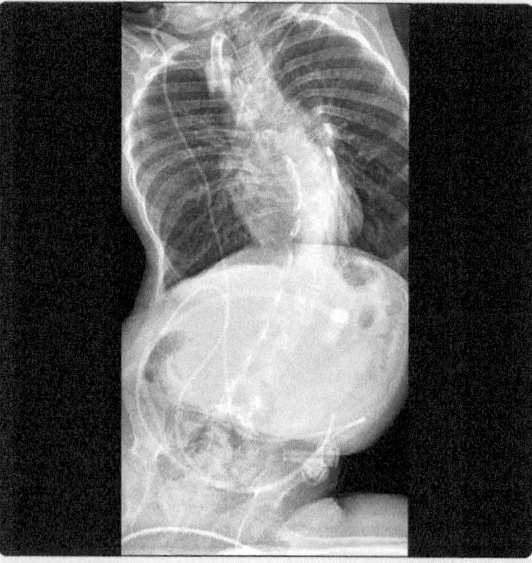

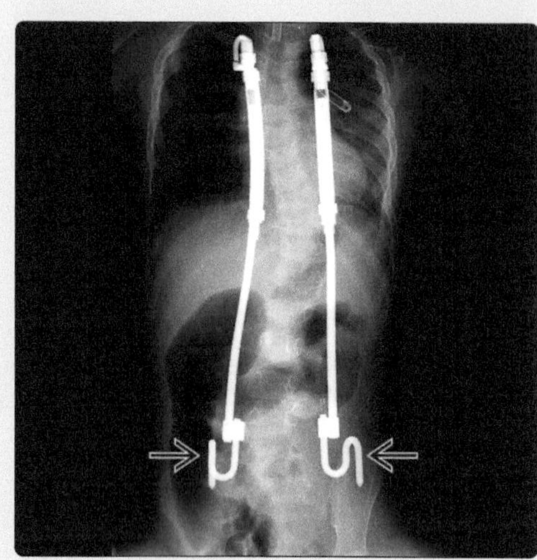

(Left) *Anteroposterior radiograph in a patient with extensive thoracolumbar myelomeningocele with posterior spinal dysraphism shows typical smooth thoracolumbar scoliotic curve. Patient is imaged sitting (non-weight-bearing).* **(Right)** *Anteroposterior thoracolumbar radiograph in a myelomeningocele patient shows levoscoliosis treated with paired titanium expandable rods. The pelvic attachment points ⇨ are a relatively common location for hardware construct failure.*

TERMINOLOGY

Synonyms

- Neurogenic scoliosis

Definitions

- Scoliosis due to neurologic or myopathic diseases

IMAGING

General Features

- Best diagnostic clue
  - Most common pattern: Long, single curve scoliosis

Radiographic Findings

- Single, long C-shaped curve
- Usually centered at thoracolumbar junction
- ± persistent infantile pattern of thoracolumbar kyphosis
- Normal vertebral morphology, ± wedging at apex
- Osteopenia often present
- Curve often unbalanced in sagittal, coronal planes
  - Normally, T1 should be centered above L5

MR Findings

- Same as plain radiography
- ± syrinx, tethered spinal cord

Ultrasonographic Findings

- Useful for assessing expansion settings for magnetic expandable rods

Imaging Recommendations

- Protocol advice
  - Sagittal T1WI and STIR, coronal T1WI through entire spine, including craniocervical junction
  - Axial T2WI through conus, syringomyelia (if present)

DIFFERENTIAL DIAGNOSIS

Idiopathic Scoliosis

- S-shaped or C-shaped curve

Congenital Scoliosis

- Vertebral anomalies present

Scheuermann Disease

- Mild scoliosis, abnormal vertebral endplates

Scoliosis Related to Congenital Syndromes

- Neurofibromatosis
- Marfan syndrome
- Osteogenesis imperfecta
- Diastrophic dwarfism
- Ehlers-Danlos syndrome

Limb-Length Inequality

- Compensatory scoliosis; look for uneven iliac crest levels to diagnose

PATHOLOGY

General Features

- Etiology
  - Neurogenic causes
    - Cerebral palsy
    - Spinal cord tumor
    - Syringomyelia
    - Traumatic paralysis
    - Poliomyelitis
    - Myelomeningocele
    - Hereditary sensorimotor neuropathies
  - Myopathic causes
    - Duchenne muscular dystrophy
    - Spinal muscular atrophy
    - Friedreich ataxia
    - Arthrogryposis multiplex congenita
- Associated abnormalities
  - Syringomyelia, spinal dysraphism, tethered cord
  - Kyphosis or lordosis

Staging, Grading, & Classification

- Cobb angle
  - Minor curve: < 20°
  - Significant curve: > 20°

CLINICAL ISSUES

Presentation

- Most common signs/symptoms
  - Rapidly progressive thoracolumbar curvature
- Other signs/symptoms
  - Respiratory compromise

Demographics

- Age
  - Onset usually in infancy or childhood
  - May progress in adulthood
- Sex
  - M = F
- Epidemiology
  - 20% of cerebral palsy patients

Natural History & Prognosis

- Progresses rapidly → respiratory compromise
- Most difficult scoliosis to treat

Treatment

- Bracing for minor curves; usually does not halt progression
- Surgical fusion for more severe curvature or respiratory embarrassment
  - Higher operative complication rate than for other types of scoliosis
  - Magnetic expandable rods can allow for patient growth

DIAGNOSTIC CHECKLIST

Consider

- MR of entire spine to exclude spinal cord or osseous abnormalities prior to scoliosis correction

SELECTED REFERENCES

1. Zheng JL et al: Current trends in surgical magnitude of neuromuscular scoliosis curves: a study of 489 operative patients with non-ambulatory cerebral palsy. Spine Deform. 11(2):399-405, 2023
2. von der Höh NH et al: [Etiology, epidemiology, prognosis and biomechanical principles of neuromuscular scoliosis.] Orthopade. 50(8):608-13, 2021

Idiopathic Scoliosis

KEY FACTS

TERMINOLOGY

- Scoliosis of undetermined etiology without underlying bony or neuromuscular abnormalities
- Flexible curvature: Curvature that resolves when patient bends to contralateral side
- Structural curvature: Curvature that does not change when patient bends to contralateral side

IMAGING

- Coronal + sagittal plane curve + rotation
- Can progress to > 90°
- Most common pattern: Thoracic dextroscoliosis
- 2nd most common: Thoracic dextroscoliosis with lumbar levoscoliosis

TOP DIFFERENTIAL DIAGNOSES

- Neuromuscular scoliosis
- Scoliosis due to tumor
- Congenital scoliosis
- Scoliosis due to congenital syndromes
- Scheuermann disease
- Degenerative scoliosis

PATHOLOGY

- Infantile type: Onset before age of 4
- Juvenile type: Onset from ages 4 to 9
- Adolescent type: Onset from 10 years to skeletal maturity

CLINICAL ISSUES

- Curve often progresses during growth spurts
- Curve usually will not progress after skeletal maturity unless > 40-50°

DIAGNOSTIC CHECKLIST

- Thoracic levoscoliosis: Higher incidence of syringomyelia, spinal cord tumors
- Preoperative multiplanar MR imaging to identify anatomic abnormalities that would alter surgical treatment

(Left) *Frontal radiograph of a patient with adolescent idiopathic scoliosis depicts convex right thoracic scoliosis away from normal left aortic arch and lumbar levoscoliosis. Terminal vertebrae ➡ are at each end of the scoliosis. Transition vertebra ➡ marks the transition from the thoracic to the lumbar curve.* **(Right)** *PA radiograph in the same patient shows dextroscoliosis improves from the neutral position (left) when the patient bends to the right (right). Residual curve indicates structural component of scoliosis.*

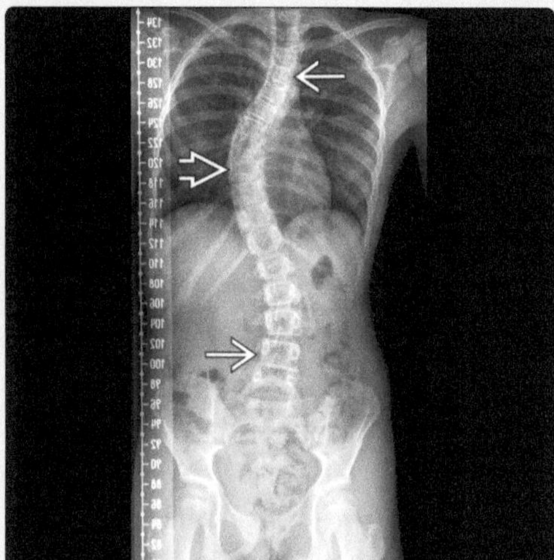

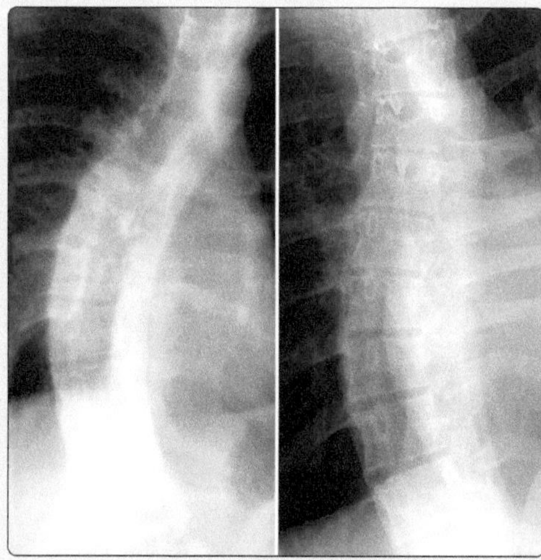

(Left) *Coronal T2 MR of a patient with infantile idiopathic scoliosis shows atypical convex left thoracic curvature. No vertebral segmentation or formation anomalies were seen.* **(Right)** *Sagittal T1 MR of a patient with infantile idiopathic scoliosis shows normal conus termination at the L1-L2 level. No syringohydromyelia or tethering lesion was identified.*

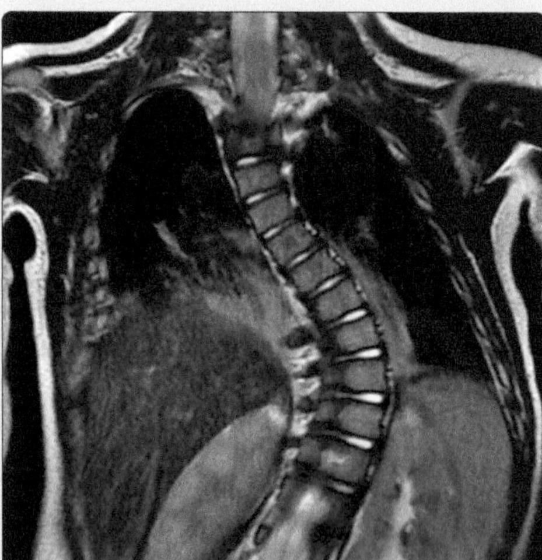

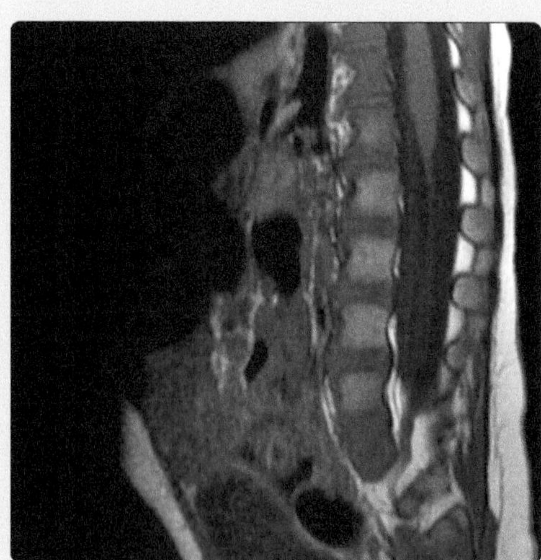

TERMINOLOGY

Definitions

- Scoliosis of undetermined etiology without underlying bony or neuromuscular abnormalities
- Flexible curvature: Curvature that resolves when patient bends to contralateral side
- Structural curvature: Curvature that does not change when patient bends to contralateral side

IMAGING

General Features

- Location
  - Most common pattern: Thoracic dextroscoliosis
  - 2nd most common: Thoracic dextroscoliosis with lumbar levoscoliosis
    - Balanced, S-shaped curve
  - Less common: Lumbar curvature without thoracic curvature
  - Thoracic levoscoliosis uncommon → increased association with underlying abnormalities
  - Occasionally involves cervical spine
- Morphology
  - Coronal + sagittal plane curve + rotation
    - Tend to have lordosis at apex of curve

Radiographic Findings

- Mild lateral wedging of vertebrae on concave aspect of curve common
- Lateral radiograph shows sagittal plane deformity
  - Usually see lordosis at apex of thoracic curvature

CT Findings

- Exclude vertebral anomalies, tumors

MR Findings

- Exclude vertebral anomalies, tumor
- Evaluate for syrinx
- Evaluate for tethered cord, lipoma of filum terminale

DIFFERENTIAL DIAGNOSIS

Neuromuscular Scoliosis

- Usually single, long thoracolumbar curve
- Contributing neurologic diagnosis

Scoliosis Due To Tumor

- Short curve, painful
- ± vertebral destruction

Congenital Scoliosis

- Congenital anomalies of vertebral formation and segmentation

Scoliosis Due To Infection

- Short curve, painful
- Endplate destruction, disc space narrowing

Scheuermann Disease

- Scoliosis seen in 15%
- Kyphosis, multiple Schmorl nodes, vertebral wedging

Scoliosis Due To Congenital Syndromes

- Look for other stigmata of syndrome

Scoliosis Due To Trauma

- Short curve scoliosis, characteristic vertebral body deformity

Scoliosis Due To Radiation

- Short curve scoliosis, vertebral hypoplasia, history of radiation

Limb Length Inequality

- Check heights of iliac wings on standing films

Degenerative Scoliosis

- Arises later in adulthood, usually lumbar

PATHOLOGY

Staging, Grading, & Classification

- Infantile type: Onset before age of 4
  - Rare, ± tethered cord, Chiari
- Juvenile type: Onset from ages 4 to 9 (uncommon)
- Adolescent type: Onset from 10 years of age to skeletal maturity (most common)
- Skeletal maturity (Risser staging) assessed to predict risk of progression

CLINICAL ISSUES

Demographics

- Sex
  - F:M = 7:1

Natural History & Prognosis

- Often progresses during growth spurts
- Also will progress to variable degree following cessation of bracing
- Usually will not progress after skeletal maturity unless > 40-50°
- Severe scoliosis → respiratory compromise

Treatment

- Options, risks, complications
  - Observation used for curves < 20-25°
  - Bracing 1st treatment option
  - Fusion if severe (> 40°) or rapidly progressive

DIAGNOSTIC CHECKLIST

Consider

- Thoracic levoscoliosis: Higher incidence of syringomyelia, spinal cord tumors
- Preoperative multiplanar MR imaging to identify anatomic abnormalities that would alter surgical treatment

SELECTED REFERENCES

1. Luhmann S et al: The natural history of curve behavior after brace removal in adolescent idiopathic scoliosis: a literature review. Spine Deform. 11(3):567-78, 2023
2. Parent EC et al: Prediction of future curve angle using prior radiographs in previously untreated idiopathic scoliosis: natural history from age 6 to after the end of growth (SOSORT 2022 award winner). Eur Spine J. 32(6):2171-84, 2023

Idiopathic Kyphosis

KEY FACTS

TERMINOLOGY

- Synonyms: Postural kyphosis, round back deformity
- Thoracic kyphosis without underlying structural abnormality

IMAGING

- Thoracic kyphosis > ~ 40°
  - Measured from superior endplate of T3 to inferior endplate of T12
- Primarily involves upper to midthoracic spine
- Smooth, nonangular curvature
- Rarely severe
- Vertebral morphology usually normal
  - May have mild anterior wedging with normal endplates
- Lateral radiograph in hyperextension to evaluate flexibility of curve

TOP DIFFERENTIAL DIAGNOSES

- Scheuermann kyphosis
- Congenital kyphosis
- Posttraumatic kyphosis
- Insufficiency fractures
- Ankylosing spondylitis
- Neuromuscular disease
- Infection

PATHOLOGY

- Etiology: Secondary to poor posture

CLINICAL ISSUES

- Premature development of thoracic degenerative disc disease

DIAGNOSTIC CHECKLIST

- Diagnosis of exclusion
- Congenital bars causing kyphosis may be occult on radiography; evaluate with MR

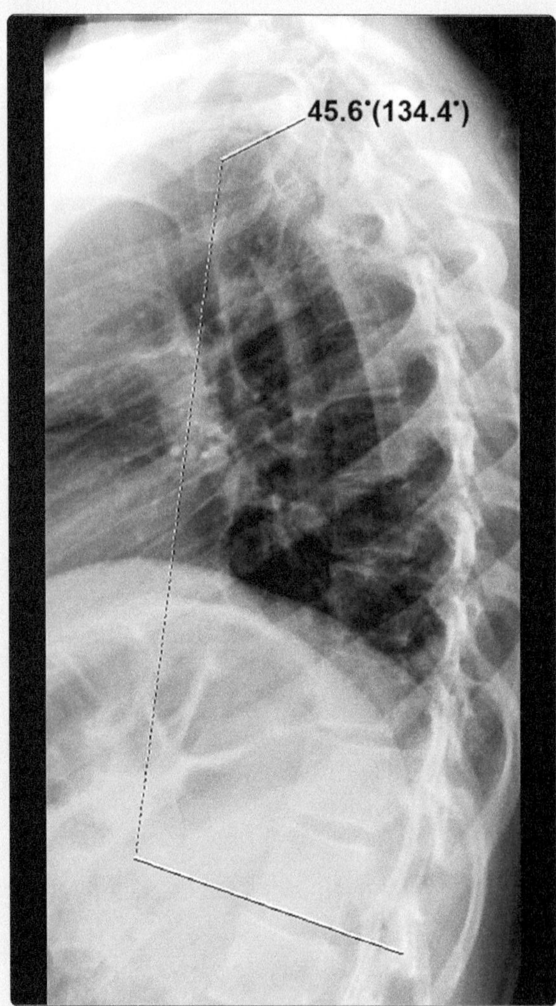

Upright lateral thoracic radiograph in a patient with postural kyphosis demonstrates the technique for measurement of overall thoracic kyphosis from superior margin of T3 to inferior margin of T12. The angle measures 45° (normal < 40°).

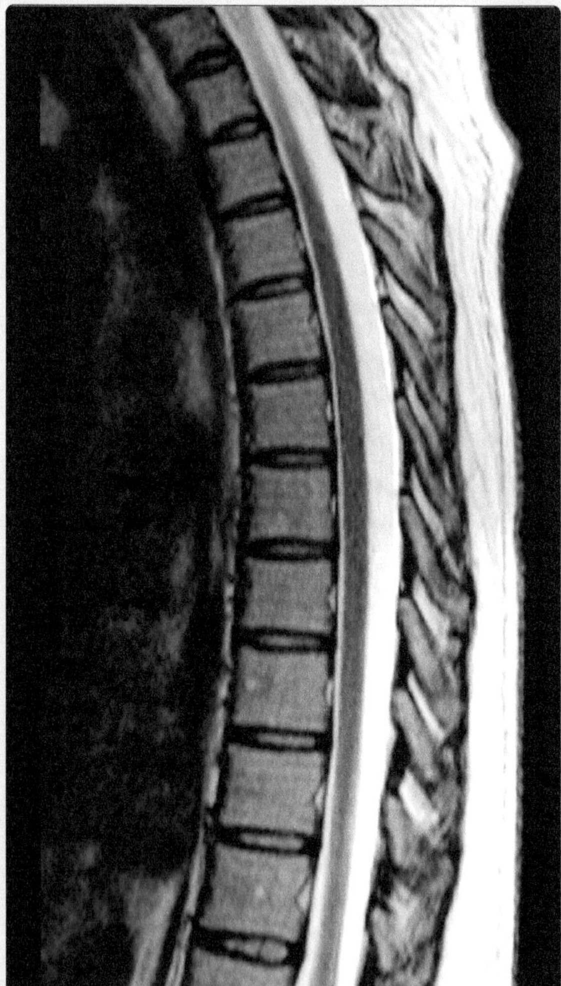

Sagittal T2 MR in the same patient performed in supine position shows reduction of kyphosis, reflecting predominant postural component of kyphotic curvature. No anatomic abnormality was present.

TERMINOLOGY

Synonyms

- Postural kyphosis, round back deformity

Definitions

- Thoracic kyphosis without underlying structural abnormality

IMAGING

General Features

- Best diagnostic clue
  - Thoracic kyphosis > ~ 40°
- Location
  - Upper to midthoracic spine
- Morphology
  - Smooth, nonangular curvature
  - Rarely severe

Radiographic Findings

- Radiography
  - Posteroanterior (PA) and lateral full spine or thoracic spine
    - Patient upright
    - PA to exclude scoliosis
  - Vertebral morphology usually normal
    - May have mild anterior wedging with normal endplates
  - Kyphosis measured from superior endplate of T3 to inferior endplate of T12
    - Wide variability in normal thoracic kyphosis
    - Kyphosis is normally less pronounced in children, increases in adolescence
    - < 40° normal in adulthood
  - Lateral radiograph in hyperextension to evaluate flexibility of curve
  - Premature degenerative disc disease often present

CT Findings

- Endplates are normal, and vertebral anomalies are absent

MR Findings

- May see premature degenerative disc disease

Imaging Recommendations

- Best imaging tool
  - Radiography for curve measurement
- Protocol advice
  - Multiplanar MR or CT to exclude underlying bone or neural abnormality

DIFFERENTIAL DIAGNOSIS

Scheuermann Kyphosis

- Presents in adolescence
- Wedging of 3 adjacent vertebral bodies > 5°, endplate irregularities, Schmorl nodes

Congenital Kyphosis

- Associated with congenital anomalies of vertebral formation and segmentation
- Note: Anterior bony intervertebral bars may not present until adolescence

Posttraumatic Kyphosis

- Vertebral body traumatic deformity

Insufficiency Fractures

- Deformity of anterior vertebral cortex

Ankylosing Spondylitis

- Thin syndesmophytes between vertebrae, facet ankylosis

Neuromuscular Disease

- Persistence of infantile kyphosis

Infection

- Short curve, vertebral endplate destruction
- ± paraspinous mass

PATHOLOGY

General Features

- Etiology
  - Secondary to poor posture ± muscle imbalance

CLINICAL ISSUES

Presentation

- Most common signs/symptoms
  - Asymptomatic
  - Stooped shoulders

Natural History & Prognosis

- Premature development of thoracic degenerative disc disease

Treatment

- Exercise
- Brace decreases kyphosis, but kyphosis tends to recur

DIAGNOSTIC CHECKLIST

Consider

- Diagnosis of exclusion

Image Interpretation Pearls

- Congenital bars causing kyphosis may be occult on radiography; evaluate with MR

SELECTED REFERENCES

1. Cici H et al: Balance control and plantar pressure distribution in hyperkyphotic adolescent and young adults. Turk Neurosurg. 33(3):451-7, 2023
2. Moustafa IM et al: Is thoracic kyphosis relevant to pain, autonomic nervous system function, disability, and cervical sensorimotor control in patients with chronic nonspecific neck pain? J Clin Med. 12(11):3707, 2023
3. Bayartai ME et al: Differences in spinal posture and mobility between children/adolescents with obesity and age-matched normal-weight individuals. Sci Rep. 12(1):15570, 2022
4. Huang Y et al: Influence of long-term participation in amateur sports on physical posture of teenagers. PeerJ. 10:e14520, 2022
5. Kiebzak WP et al: Alignment of the sternum and sacrum as a marker of sitting body posture in children. Int J Environ Res Public Health. 19(23):16287, 2022
6. Miladi L: Round and angular kyphosis in paediatric patients. Orthop Traumatol Surg Res. 99(1 Suppl):S140-9, 2013
7. Nowotny-Czupryna O et al: Postural habits of young adults and possibilities of modification. Ortop Traumatol Rehabil. 15(1):9-21, 2013

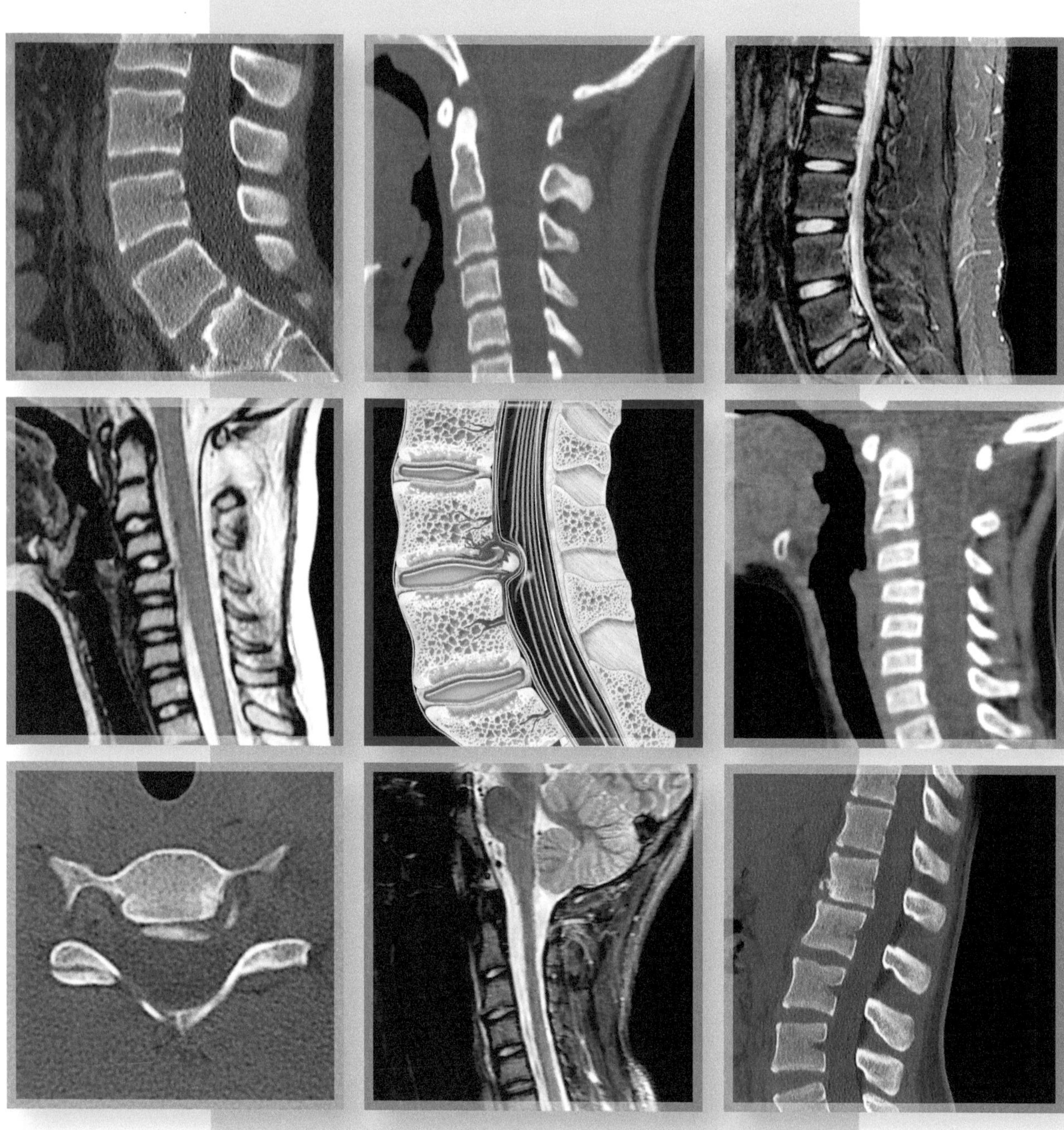

PART III
SECTION 2

Trauma

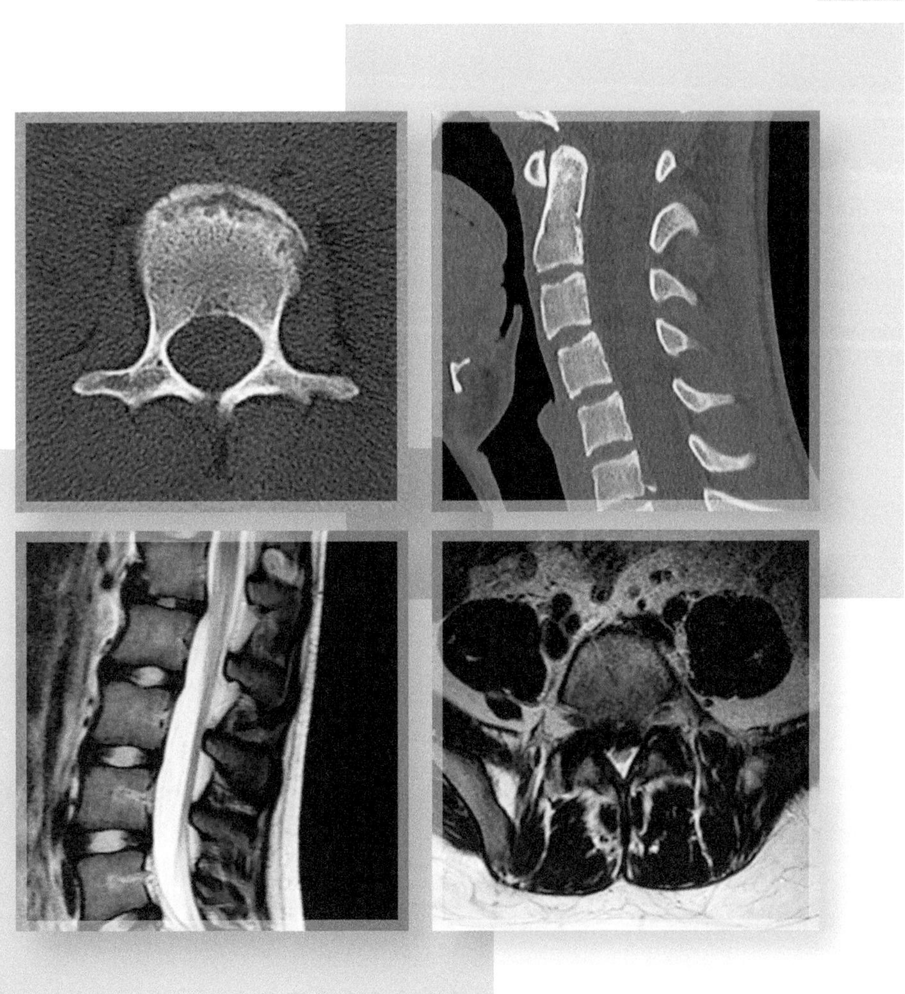

Apophyseal Ring Fracture

KEY FACTS

TERMINOLOGY

- Fracture (Fx) or avulsion of vertebral ring apophysis (RA) following injury in immature skeleton

IMAGING

- Concentric bone fragment displaced from vertebral endplate margin in skeletally immature patient
- Inferior or superior endplate may be involved; limbus vertebra (LV) usually superior
- Fractured apophyseal fragment usually midline

TOP DIFFERENTIAL DIAGNOSES

- Flexion teardrop Fx of anterior endplate corner
- Schmorl node
- Disc calcification or ossification
- Calcified disc fragment; posterior osteophyte
- Disc herniation

PATHOLOGY

- LV: Herniation of nucleus pulposus (NP) between RA and vertebral body
- Posterior apophyseal ring Fx (PAR-Fx): 2 possible mechanisms described
    - Same as LV
    - Herniating NP spares Sharpey fibers, avulses RA

CLINICAL ISSUES

- Back pain in acute (adolescent) cases
- Adolescent athlete with acute low back pain
- Majority of patients with PAR-Fx/LV report engagement in sporting activities

DIAGNOSTIC CHECKLIST

- MR more sensitive than radiographs or CT in young children (because RA not ossified)
- T2WI FS/STIR MR essential to assess for associated ligamentous injury

(Left) *Sagittal graphic demonstrates an acute lumbar apophyseal ring fracture ➡ involving the posterior inferior vertebral body corner with displacement and associated hemorrhage. There is compression of the adjacent thecal sac.* **(Right)** *Sagittal T1 MR in an adolescent athlete with acute onset of lumbar back pain demonstrates what initially appeared as an L4-L5 disc herniation with subligamentous disc fragment ➡.*

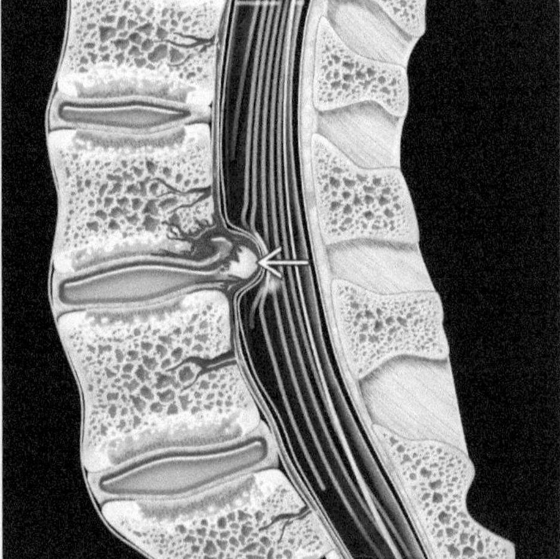

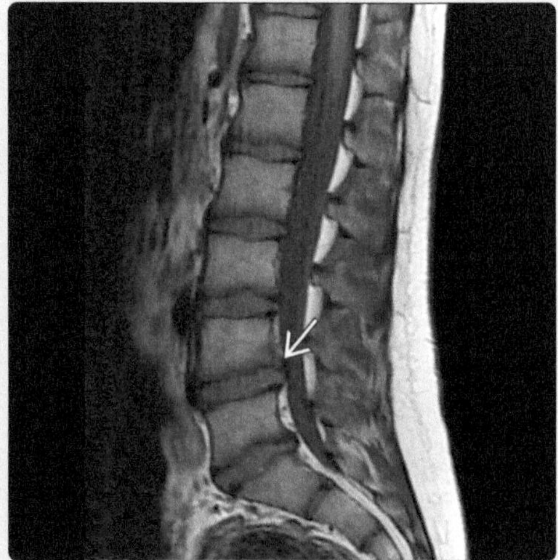

(Left) *Sagittal STIR MR in the same patient clarifies that the fragment ➡ represents a posterior inferior ring apophysis fracture with marrow edema at the donor site ➡.* **(Right)** *Axial T2 MR in the same patient reveals ventral mass effect on the thecal sac from the displaced apophyseal ring fragment ➡. Marrow edema at the donor site ➡ is also clearly defined.*

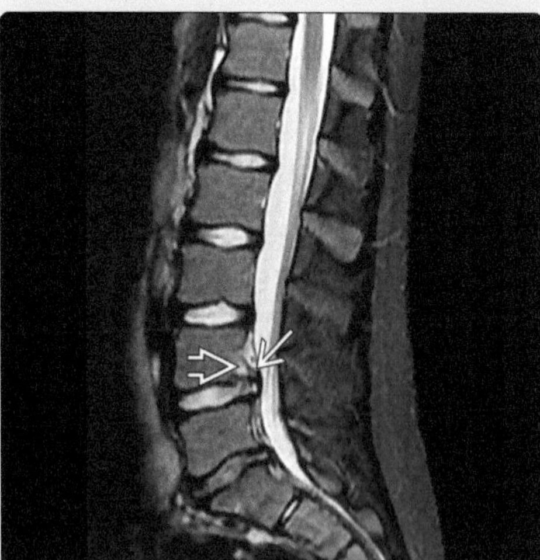

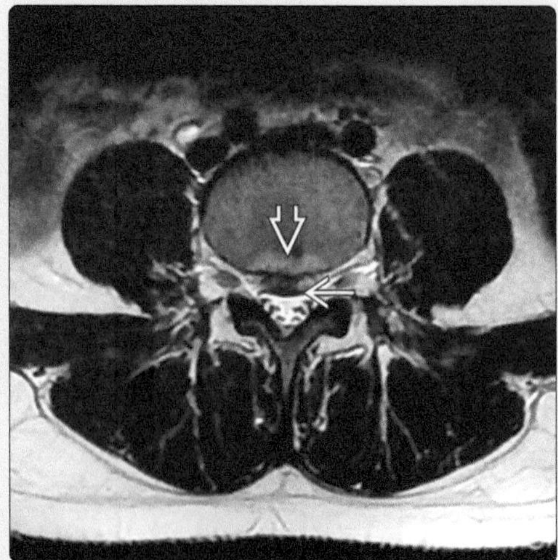

Apophyseal Ring Fracture

TERMINOLOGY

Synonyms

- Vertebral apophyseal fracture (Fx), limbus vertebra (LV), endplate avulsion Fx, corner Fx, slipped vertebral apophysis, lumbar posterior marginal node

Definitions

- Fx or avulsion of vertebral ring apophysis (RA) following injury in immature skeleton
  - Fx of anterior ring termed LV
  - Fx of posterior ring termed posterior apophyseal ring Fx (PAR-Fx)

IMAGING

General Features

- Best diagnostic clue
  - Concentric bone fragment displaced from vertebral endplate margin in skeletally immature patient
- Location
  - Lumbosacral spine most common; rare in thoracic, cervical
    - L3-S1
    - PAR-Fx commonly L4, S1
  - Inferior or superior endplate may be involved; LV usually superior
  - Fractured apophyseal fragment usually midline
- Size
  - Fragment size variable
- Morphology
  - Rim-like morphology typical, but fragment(s) may be amorphous

Radiographic Findings

- Radiography
  - Bone fragment displaced from corner defect of endplate
  - Bone fragment not identified > 50% (cartilaginous or resorbed)

CT Findings

- Bone CT
  - Acute
    - PAR-Fx: Arc-shaped or rectangular bone fragment posterior to dorsal endplate margin
    - Vertebral donor site usually identified
    - LV: Same as PAR-Fx, except located anteriorly, ± mild kyphosis
  - Subacute or chronic
    - Sclerosis of fragment and donor site margins
    - Donor defect often enlarges (particularly LV)

MR Findings

- T1WI
  - Corner defect in marrow of parent vertebral body (VB) with disc extending into defect
  - Hypointense bone fragment merges with adjacent ligaments
  - PAR-Fx fragment + Sharpey fibers = Y or 7 shape on sagittal MR
- T2WI
  - Defect in endplate; hyperintense disc between fragment and VB
  - Disc height loss common ± disc desiccation
    - Both ↑ over time
  - High signal in subjacent marrow in acute cases
- STIR
  - Same as T2WI, edema accentuated
- T2* GRE
  - Accentuation of sclerotic bone margins in chronic lesions
- T1WI C+
  - Enhancement of donor site marrow if acute Fx

Nonvascular Interventions

- Myelography
  - Epidural defect on contrast column in PAR-Fx

Nuclear Medicine Findings

- Bone scan
  - ↑ radionuclide uptake in acute lesions

Other Modality Findings

- Discography (LV): Contrast diffuses into space between fragment and VB

Imaging Recommendations

- Best imaging tool
  - Multiplanar CT in bone and soft tissue algorithm
- Protocol advice
  - Sagittal and axial reformatted images key for making diagnosis

DIFFERENTIAL DIAGNOSIS

Flexion Fracture of Anterior Endplate Corner

- Seen in older children, adults after apophysis fused
- Spinal cord injury more common than in apophyseal ring Fx

Schmorl Node

- Endplate defect is within interspace, not at endplate corner
- Associated edema and contrast enhancement when acute

Disc Calcification or Ossification

- Painful childhood nucleus pulposus (NP) calcification of unknown etiology
  - Multilevel common, cervical > thoracic, occasionally asymptomatic
  - Spontaneous resolution of calcifications and symptoms

Calcified Disc Fragment; Posterior Osteophyte

- Sequelae of longstanding degenerative disc disease, uncommon in children
- Fragment at level of disc, not above or below
- May see marrow if ossified

Disc Herniation

- Uncommon in adolescents; rare (traumatic) in 1st decade

PATHOLOGY

General Features

- Etiology
  - LV: Herniation of NP between RA and VB
  - PAR-Fx: 2 possible mechanisms described
    - Same as LV

- Herniating NP spares Sharpey fibers, avulses RA
- Genetics
  - Often seen with Scheuermann disease
- Associated abnormalities
  - Disc herniation
  - Kyphosis
- Embryology/anatomy
  - Superior and inferior surface of developing VB covered by thin, peripherally thickened cartilage plate → cartilaginous marginal ridge
  - Endochondral ossification of marginal ridge begins at 7-9 years → RA
  - RA seen as small bony triangles at corners of VB (XR, sagittal/coronal CT reconstruction)
  - RA separated from VB by thin cartilage layer until apophysis fuses to VB at 18-20 years → relative weak point in disc/VB complex until fusion occurs
  - Outermost fibers of anulus fibrosus (Sharpey fibers) embedded in RA, attaching disc to spine

Staging, Grading, & Classification

- Modified Takata classification
  - Type I: Avulsion posterior cortical vertebral rim (most common)
  - Type II: Central cortical and cancellous bone Fx
  - Type III: Lateralized chip Fx
  - Type IV: Spans entire posterior vertebral margin

Gross Pathologic & Surgical Features

- Displaced bony/cartilaginous rim fragment ± disc material
- Sharpey fibers and posterior longitudinal ligament usually intact

Microscopic Features

- Cancellous bone, hyaline cartilage, and acellular hyaline tissue (disc)
- Basophilic degeneration and foci hemorrhage in hyaline cartilage common

CLINICAL ISSUES

Presentation

- Most common signs/symptoms
  - Back pain in acute (adolescent) cases
- Clinical profile
  - Adolescent athlete with acute low back pain
  - Majority of patients with PAR-Fx/LV report engagement in sporting activities
- PAR-Fx: Principal presentation
  - Acute > > prolonged history of central low back pain ± sciatica
    - 66% had minor trauma or lifting event (weightlifting, gymnastics)
  - Physical exam (PE) findings: Similar to herniated NP
- LV: No inciting event; chronic history back pain; occasionally incidental finding
  - PE: ↓ range of motion ± kyphosis and pain with palpation of spinous processes

Demographics

- Age
  - Late childhood through adolescence
- Sex
  - M > F (up to 85% of males in PAR-Fx group)
- Epidemiology
  - 20% prevalence of PAR-Fx teen lumbar disc surgeries (33% in 14-17 years)

Natural History & Prognosis

- LV: Symptoms resolve in months (usual) to years (rare)
  - Reports document evolution of LV into anteriorly located Schmorl node
- PAR-Fx: Good to excellent with surgery; occasional mild, short-term deficits

Treatment

- LV: Conservative; analgesics and limitation of physical activity in acute symptomatic setting
- PAR-Fx: Surgical therapy is mainstay; conservative rarely successful
  - Uni- or bilateral laminotomy with removal of bone fragment, ± disc

DIAGNOSTIC CHECKLIST

Image Interpretation Pearls

- MR more sensitive than radiography, CT in young children (RA not ossified)
- T2WI FS/STIR MR essential to assess for associated ligamentous injury

SELECTED REFERENCES

1. Wu H et al: Percutaneous endoscopic interlaminar discectomy for posterior ring apophyseal fracture accompanied with lumbar disc herniation in a 12-year pediatric diver: a case report. Childs Nerv Syst. 39(1):275-8, 2023
2. Yuan S et al: Posterior apophyseal ring fracture in adult lumbar disc herniation: an 8-year experience in minimally invasive surgical management of 48 cases. Neurospine. 19(3):586-93, 2022
3. Manabe H et al: Role of growth plate (apophyseal ring fracture) in causing modic type changes in pediatric low back pain patients. Eur Spine J. 30(9):2565-9, 2021
4. Seo YN et al: The characteristics and incidence of posterior apophyseal ring fracture in patients in their early twenties with herniated lumbar disc. Neurospine. 15(2):138-43, 2018
5. Kadam G et al: Traumatic lumbar vertebral ring apophysis fracture with disk herniation in an adolescent. Radiol Case Rep. 12(2):427-30, 2017
6. Singhal A et al: Ring apophysis fracture in pediatric lumbar disc herniation: a common entity. Pediatr Neurosurg. 49(1):16-20, 2013
7. Wu X et al: A review of current treatment of lumbar posterior ring apophysis fracture with lumbar disc herniation. Eur Spine J. 22(3):475-88, 2013
8. Wu XY et al: Posterior lumbar ring apophysis fracture. Orthop Surg. 3(1):72-7, 2011
9. Chang CH et al: Clinical significance of ring apophysis fracture in adolescent lumbar disc herniation. Spine (Phila Pa 1976). 33(16):1750-4, 2008
10. Sairyo K et al: Three-dimensional finite element analysis of the pediatric lumbar spine. Part I: pathomechanism of apophyseal bony ring fracture. Eur Spine J. 15(6):923-9, 2006
11. Asazuma T et al: Lumbar disc herniation associated with separation of the posterior ring apophysis: analysis of five surgical cases and review of the literature. Acta Neurochir (Wien). 145(6):461-6; discussion 466, 2003
12. Mendez JS et al: Limbus lumbar and sacral vertebral fractures. Neurol Res. 24(2):139-44, 2002
13. Bonic EE et al: Posterior limbus fractures: five case reports and a review of selected published cases. J Manipulative Physiol Ther. 21(4):281-7, 1998
14. Martinez-Lage JF et al: Avulsed lumbar vertebral rim plate in an adolescent: trauma or malformation? Childs Nerv Syst. 14(3):131-4, 1998

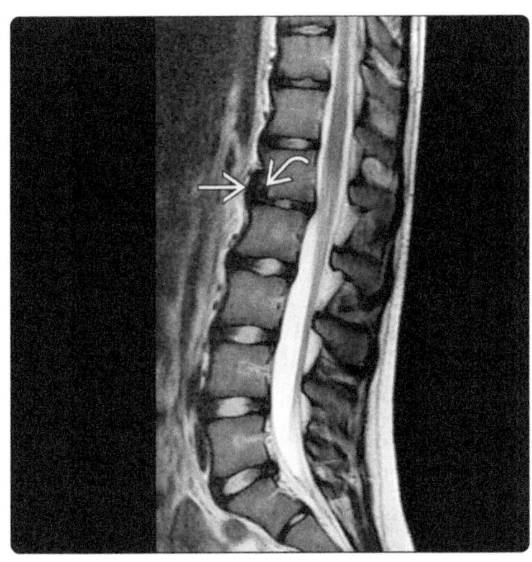

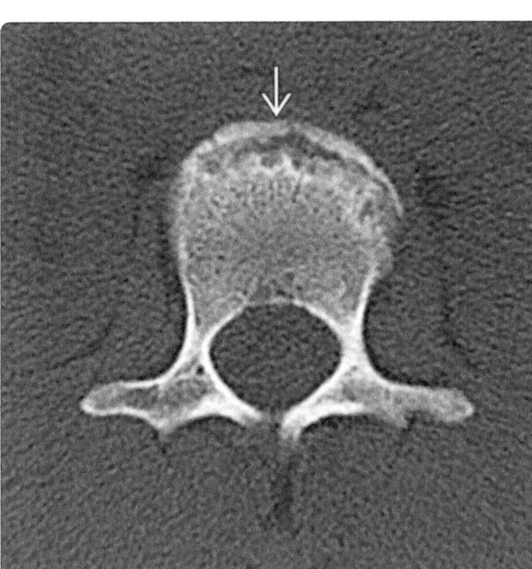

(Left) *Sagittal T2 MR (chronic lumbar ring apophysis fracture) shows displacement and remodeling of the anteroinferior L1 ring apophysis ➡, compared to normal ring apophyses at adjacent levels. Note interposition of disc material ➡ between the displaced apophysis and L1 vertebra.* **(Right)** *Axial bone CT in the same patient characterizes displaced ring apophysis ➡ more specifically as a ring apophysis fracture rather than an isolated anterior disc herniation.*

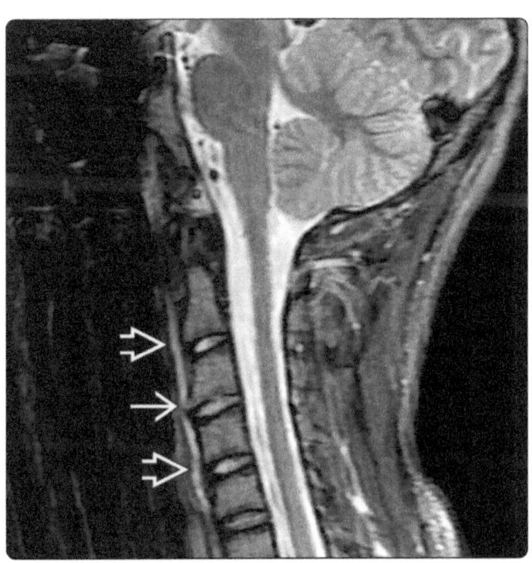

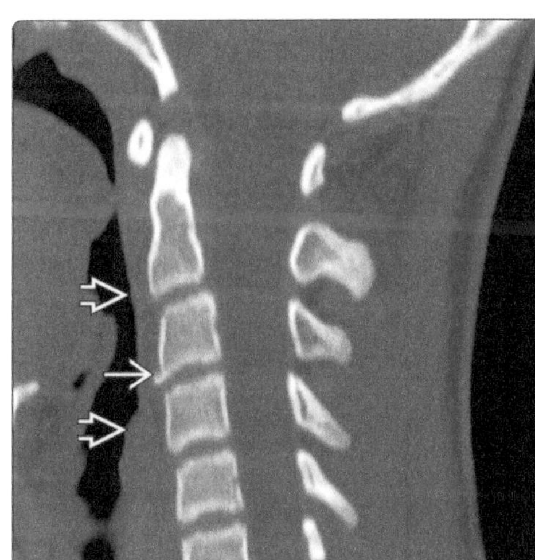

(Left) *Sagittal STIR MR (acute cervical ring apophysis fracture) shows marrow edema and avulsion of the anteroinferior corner of the C3 vertebra ➡. Note also prevertebral edema ➡ related to acute injury. The anterior longitudinal ligament (ALL) is intact.* **(Right)** *Sagittal bone CT in the same patient clearly demonstrates avulsion of the anteroinferior C3 ring apophysis ➡. The prevertebral soft tissues are widened ➡ with anterior displacement of the airway, confirming acute injury.*

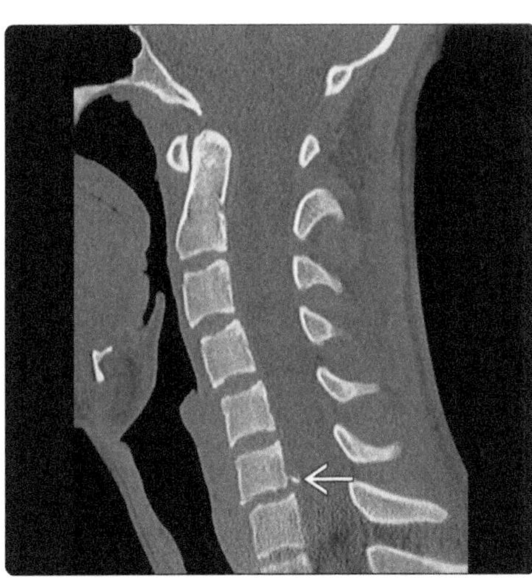

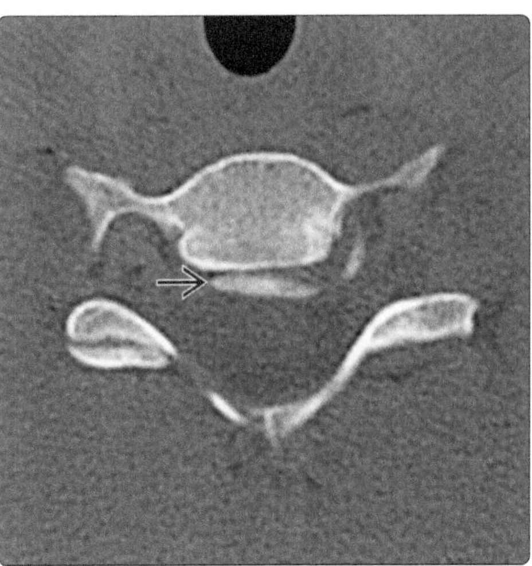

(Left) *Sagittal bone CT (cervical posterior apophyseal ring fracture) demonstrates a small posteroinferior C6 vertebral fracture fragment ➡ with associated mild C6/C7 anterolisthesis. The small osseous fragment is noted to represent the displaced posteroinferior C6 ring apophysis (empty donor site visible on comparison to other levels).* **(Right)** *Axial bone CT in the same patient confirms that the C6 osseous fragment ➡ represents the displaced C6 ring apophysis.*

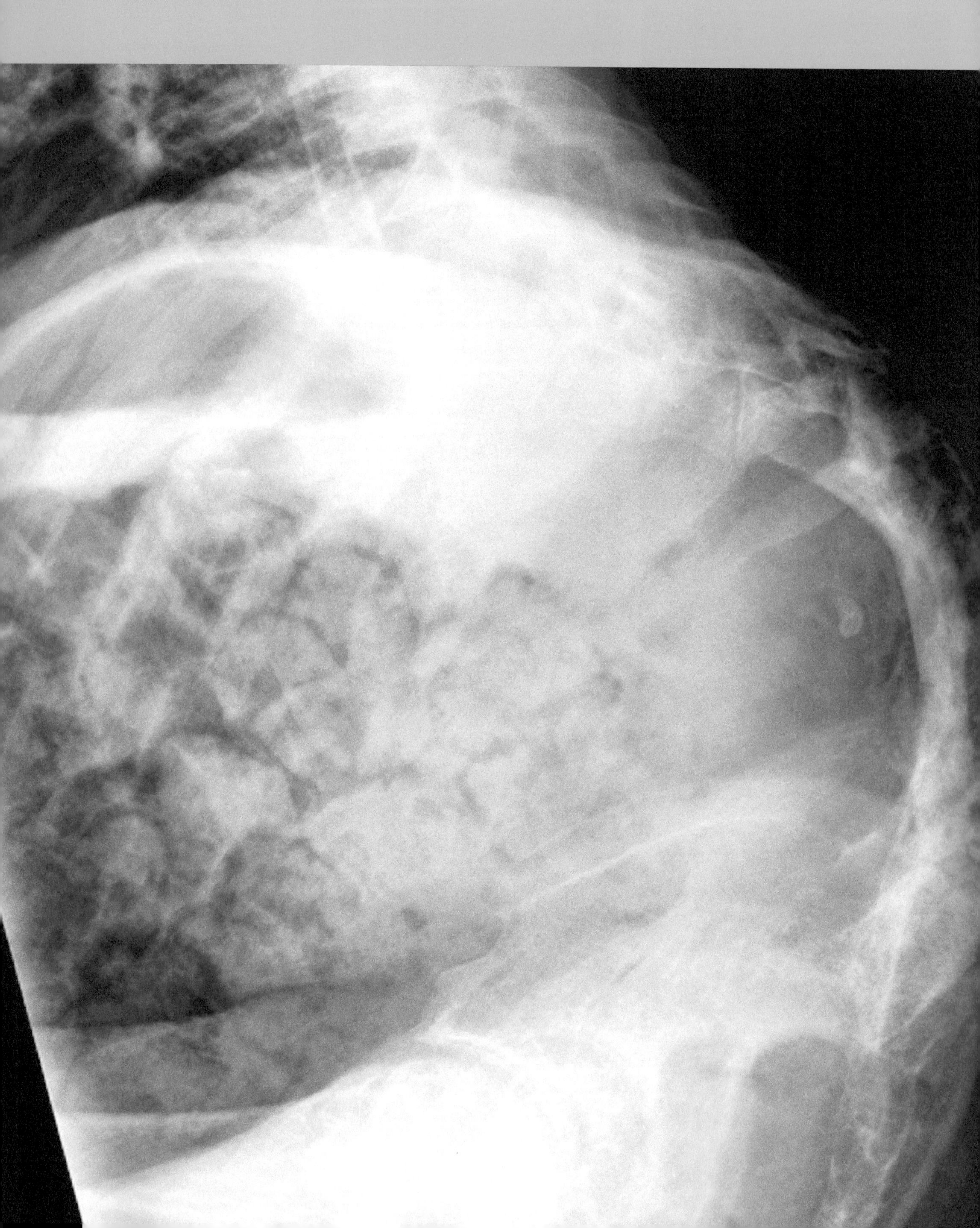

PART III
SECTION 3

Developmental and Degenerative Diseases

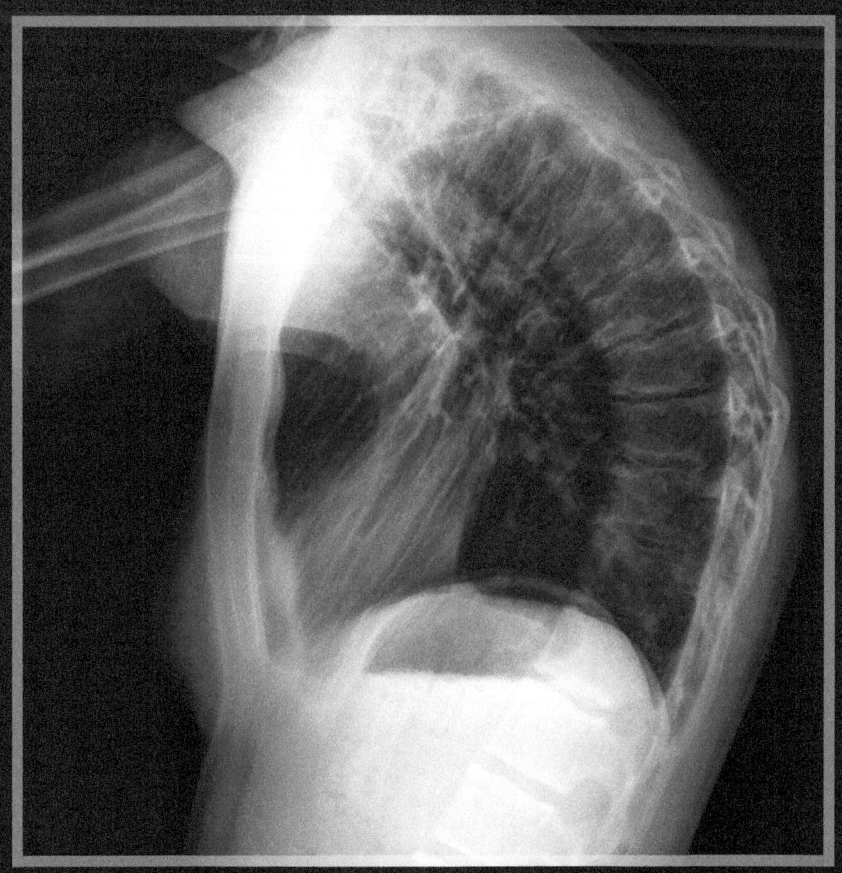

Schmorl Node

KEY FACTS

TERMINOLOGY

- Definition: Node within vertebral body due to vertical disc extension (intravertebral disc herniation) through vertebral endplate

IMAGING

- Focal invagination of endplate by disc material surrounded by sclerotic (old) or edematous (acute) bone
- Plain films
  - Contour defect within endplate, extending from disc space into vertebral body spongiosa with well-corticated margins
- CT
  - Island of low density surrounded by condensed bone on axial slice through vertebral body
- MR
  - Focal defect in endplate filled by disc ± adjacent marrow edema, fatty marrow conversion

TOP DIFFERENTIAL DIAGNOSES

- Acute compression fracture
- Degenerative endplate change
- Discitis
  - Both endplates show defect
- Limbus vertebrae
  - Seen at vertebral body corners
- Bone island
  - Sclerotic nodule
- Focal metastasis
  - No contiguity with parent disc

CLINICAL ISSUES

- Seen in up to 75% of all normal spines
- Conservative management

DIAGNOSTIC CHECKLIST

- Schmorl node (SN) is always contiguous with parent disc

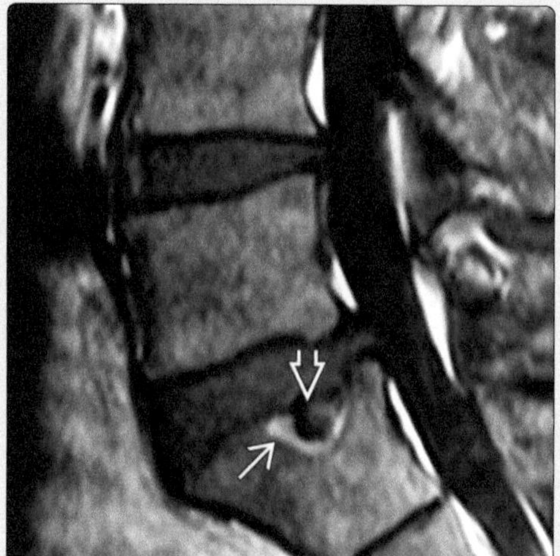

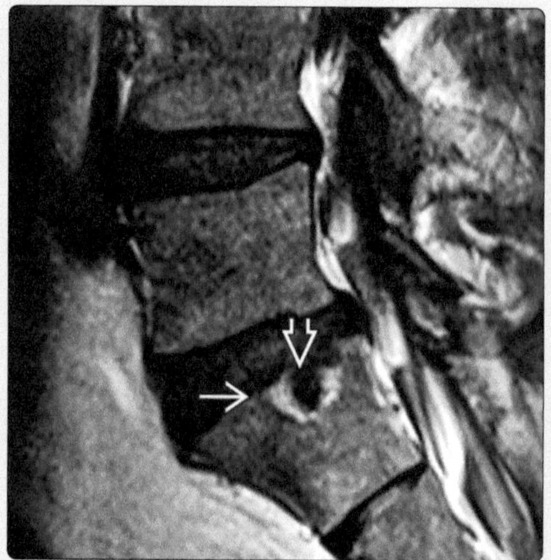

(Left) *Sagittal T1 MR shows a well-defined focus of low signal ⇨ involving the superior endplate of S1 due to endplate herniation. There is a thin rind of fatty marrow conversion adjacent to the Schmorl node (SN) ⇨.* **(Right)** *Sagittal T2 MR in the same patient demonstrates the typical pattern of fatty marrow ⇨ outlining chronic endplate herniation ⇨.*

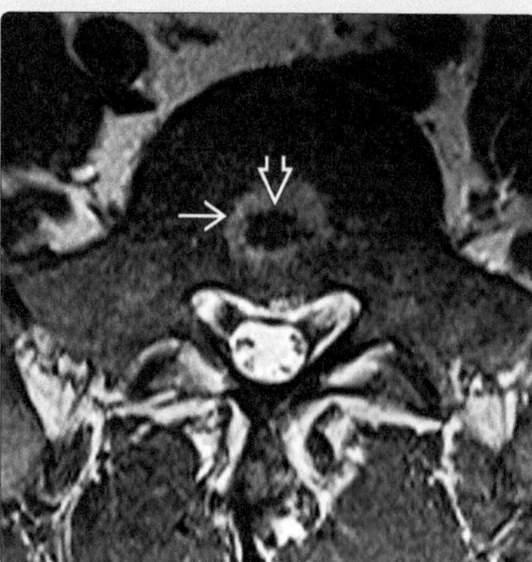

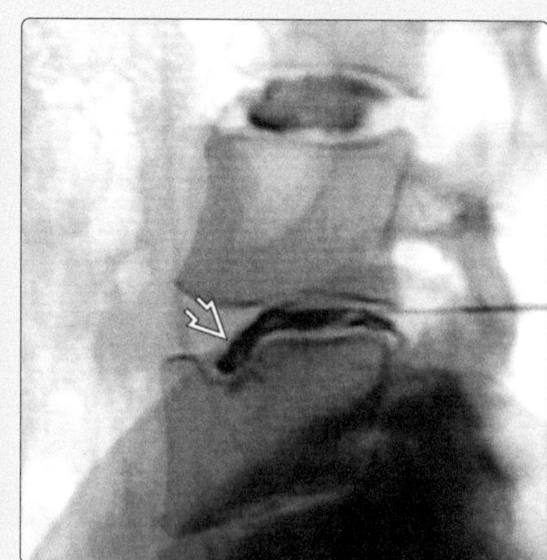

(Left) *Axial T2 MR in the same patient shows a well-defined focus of low signal ⇨ in the superior S1 endplate, representing an SN. There is a thin, concentric rind of fatty marrow conversion ⇨ surrounding the SN.* **(Right)** *Lateral fluoroscopy during discography reveals a superior endplate SN ⇨. Contrast injected into the contiguous intervertebral disc fills the herniated disc within the vertebral SN defect.*

TERMINOLOGY

Abbreviations

- Schmorl node (SN)

Synonyms

- Intravertebral disc herniation

Definitions

- Node within vertebral body due to vertical disc extension through weakened vertebral body endplate

IMAGING

General Features

- Best diagnostic clue
  - Focal invagination of endplate by disc material surrounded by either sclerotic (old) or edematous (acute) bone
- Location
  - T8-L1 region most common
- Size
  - Varies from several mm to giant
- Morphology
  - Typically upwardly round or cone-shaped defect contiguous with disc space

Radiographic Findings

- Radiography
  - Contour defect within endplate, extending from disc space into vertebral body spongiosa with well-corticated margins

CT Findings

- NECT
  - Island of low density surrounded by condensed bone on axial slice through vertebral body
  - Sagittal reformation shows endplate defect contiguous with disc space, capped by sclerotic bone
- Bone CT
  - Same as NECT
  - SN may calcify

MR Findings

- T1WI
  - Focal defect in endplate filled by disc
  - Low signal in adjacent marrow if acute
- T2WI
  - Defect in endplate filled by disc
  - Normal marrow signal if chronic
  - High signal in adjacent marrow if acute
- STIR
  - Edema in adjacent vertebral body if acute
- T1WI C+
  - Localized marginal contrast enhancement in subacute stage
  - Diffuse marrow enhancement in acute stage
  - May show central enhancement of cartilaginous component associated with disc degeneration

Nuclear Medicine Findings

- Bone scan
  - Increased uptake in acute cases

Imaging Recommendations

- Best imaging tool
  - MR with contrast will show endplate lesion and exclude concurrent pathology
- Analyze contiguity with parent disc on all sequences

DIFFERENTIAL DIAGNOSIS

Acute Compression Fracture

- Simulates diffuse edema of acute SN; may, in fact, predispose to its ultimate formation
- Lacks imploded disc nodule within abnormal marrow

Degenerative Endplate Change

- Seen as reactive change to disc degeneration; typically both adjacent vertebral bodies affected
- Represent granulation tissue and edema incited by degenerating disc
- Edema replaced by fat on follow-up studies
- No focal endplate defect

Discitis

- Both endplates show defect
- Disc signal diffusely abnormal and enhances after contrast

Limbus Vertebrae

- Seen only at vertebral body corners
- Truncated anterior margin of vertebral body
- Bone fragments anterior to defect

Bone Island

- Sclerotic nodule
- No endplate defect

Focal Fatty Marrow

- Hyperintense on T1WI

Focal Metastasis

- Does not show contiguity with parent disc or its signal intensity

PATHOLOGY

General Features

- Etiology
  - Developmental, degenerative, traumatic, and disease influences
  - Typically repetitive stress of gravity on immature endplate
  - Acute axial traumatic load can lead to SN formation with focal back pain
  - Osteoporosis, neoplasm, and infection can weaken endplate
- Genetics
  - Twin studies show SN common in middle-aged women (30%) and strongly genetically determined
    - Associated with lumbar degenerative change
    - Not independent risk factor for back pain
    - Heritability is > 70%
- Cartilaginous disc tissue with degenerative or inflammatory changes
  - Pathologic staging mirrors that of focal endplate fracture

- Typical SN is healed focal endplate fracture
- Embryology/anatomy
  - Anulus actually biomechanically more resistant to mechanical failure than endplate in young individuals
  - Focal weakness of endplate predisposes to SN formation
  - Associated with endplate weakening of Scheuermann disease

Staging, Grading, & Classification

- Edema of vertebral body next to endplate with acute trauma, pain, no endplate defect on initial MR
- Subsequent formation of chronic and asymptomatic SN on follow-up MR

Gross Pathologic & Surgical Features

- Identical to endplate fracture

Microscopic Features

- Fibrocartilaginous tissue surrounded by marrow with sclerotic cancellous bone or inflammatory changes
- Osteonecrosis may also be present beneath cartilaginous endplate
  - Increased reactive woven bone with thickened trabeculae and prominent osteoclasts and osteoblasts

CLINICAL ISSUES

Presentation

- Most common signs/symptoms
  - Sudden-onset, localized, nonradiating pain and tenderness in acute cases
  - Most cases found incidentally as chronic, burned-out lesions
- Other signs/symptoms
  - Rare cause of spinal cord infarction from nucleus pulposis vascular access
- Clinical profile
  - Teenager involved in axial-loading sports
  - Acute onset of localizing pain

Demographics

- Age
  - Adolescents and young adults
- Sex
  - M > F; up to 9:1 ratio
- Epidemiology
  - Seen in up to 75% of all normal spines
  - Most acute cases occur in individuals 11-30 years of age
  - Can occur with single traumatic episodes

Natural History & Prognosis

- Self-limited
- Good prognosis, unless systemic osteoporosis leads to recurrent compression fractures

Treatment

- Observational with pain management in symptomatic cases

DIAGNOSTIC CHECKLIST

Consider

- Follow-up MR in cases of unexplained vertebral body edema and localized pain

Image Interpretation Pearls

- Always contiguous with parent disc

SELECTED REFERENCES

1. Mallow GM et al: ISSLS PRIZE in Clinical Science 2022: epidemiology, risk factors and clinical impact of juvenile Modic changes in paediatric patients with low back pain. Eur Spine J. 31(5):1069-79, 2022
2. Quinn JN et al: Spinal cord infarction due to fibrocartilaginous embolism: a report of 3 cases. J Stroke Cerebrovasc Dis. 28(6):e66-7, 2019
3. Karstens S et al: A palaeopathological analysis of skeletal remains from Bronze Age Mongolia. Homo. 69(6):324-34, 2018
4. Sandelich SM et al: An unusual cause of back pain in a 10-year-old girl. Pediatr Emerg Care. 33(5):352-55, 2017
5. Tomasian A et al: Benign spine lesions: advances in techniques for minimally invasive percutaneous treatment. AJNR Am J Neuroradiol. 38(5):852-61, 2017
6. Mattei TA et al: Schmorl's nodes: current pathophysiological, diagnostic, and therapeutic paradigms. Neurosurg Rev. 37(1):39-46, 2014
7. Abu-Ghanem S et al: Acute schmorl node in dorsal spine: an unusual cause of a sudden onset of severe back pain in a young female. Asian Spine J. 7(2):131-5, 2013
8. Nagashima M et al: Risk factors for lumbar disc degeneration in high school American football players: a prospective 2-year follow-up study. Am J Sports Med. 41(9):2059-64, 2013
9. Mok FP et al: ISSLS prize winner: prevalence, determinants, and association of Schmorl nodes of the lumbar spine with disc degeneration: a population-based study of 2449 individuals. Spine (Phila Pa 1976). 35(21):1944-52, 2010
10. Dar G et al: Demographical aspects of Schmorl nodes: a skeletal study. Spine (Phila Pa 1976). 34(9):E312-5, 2009
11. Wu HT et al: Edematous Schmorl's nodes on thoracolumbar MR imaging: characteristic patterns and changes over time. Skeletal Radiol. 35(4):212-9, 2006
12. Coulier B: Giant fatty Schmorl's nodes: CT findings in four patients. Skeletal Radiol. 34(1):29-34, 2005
13. Peng B et al: The pathogenesis of Schmorl's nodes. J Bone Joint Surg Br. 85(6):879-82, 2003
14. Yamaguchi T et al: Schmorl's node developing in the lumbar vertebra affected with metastatic carcinoma: correlation magnetic resonance imaging with histological findings. Spine. 28(24):E503-5, 2003
15. Hauger O et al: Giant cystic Schmorl's nodes: imaging findings in six patients. AJR Am J Roentgenol. 176(4):969-72, 2001
16. Wagner AL et al: Relationship of Schmorl's nodes to vertebral body endplate fractures and acute endplate disk extrusions. AJNR Am J Neuroradiol. 21(2):276-81, 2000
17. Grive E et al: Radiologic findings in two cases of acute Schmorl's nodes. AJNR Am J Neuroradiol. 20(9):1717-21, 1999
18. Silberstein M et al: Spinal Schmorl's nodes: sagittal sectional imaging and pathological examination. Australas Radiol. 43(1):27-30, 1999
19. Fahey V et al: The pathogenesis of Schmorl's nodes in relation to acute trauma. An autopsy study. Spine. 23(21):2272-5, 1998
20. Seymour R et al: Magnetic resonance imaging of acute intraosseous disc herniation. Clin Radiol. 53(5):363-8, 1998
21. Swischuk LE et al: Disk degenerative disease in childhood: Scheuermann's disease, Schmorl's nodes, and the limbus vertebra: MRI findings in 12 patients. Pediatr Radiol. 28(5):334-8, 1998
22. Tribus CB: Scheuermann's kyphosis in adolescents and adults: diagnosis and management. J Am Acad Orthop Surg. 6(1):36-43, 1998
23. Stabler A et al: MR imaging of enhancing intraosseous disk herniation (Schmorl's nodes). AJR Am J Roentgenol. 168(4):933-8, 1997
24. Takahashi K et al: Schmorl's nodes and low-back pain. Analysis of magnetic resonance imaging findings in symptomatic and asymptomatic individuals. Eur Spine J. 4(1):56-9, 1995
25. Hamanishi C et al: Schmorl's nodes on magnetic resonance imaging. Their incidence and clinical relevance. Spine. 19(4):450-3, 1994
26. Jensen MC et al: Magnetic resonance imaging of the lumbar spine in people without back pain. N Engl J Med. 331(2):69-73, 1994
27. Takahashi K et al: A large painful Schmorl's node: a case report. J Spinal Disord. 7(1):77-81, 1994
28. Sward L: The thoracolumbar spine in young elite athletes. Current concepts on the effects of physical training. Sports Med. 13(5):357-64, 1992
29. Walters G et al: Magnetic resonance imaging of acute symptomatic Schmorl's node formation. Pediatr Emerg Care. 7(5):294-6, 1991
30. McFadden KD et al: End-plate lesions of the lumbar spine. Spine. 14(8):867-9, 1989
31. Kagen S et al: Focal uptake on bone imaging in an asymptomatic Schmorl's node. Clin Nucl Med. 13(8):615-6, 1988

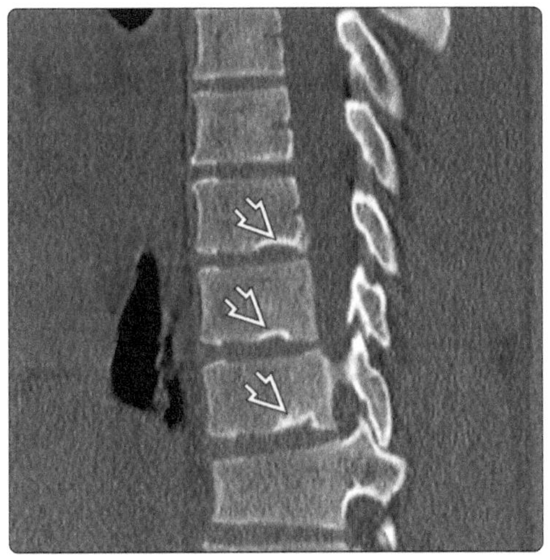

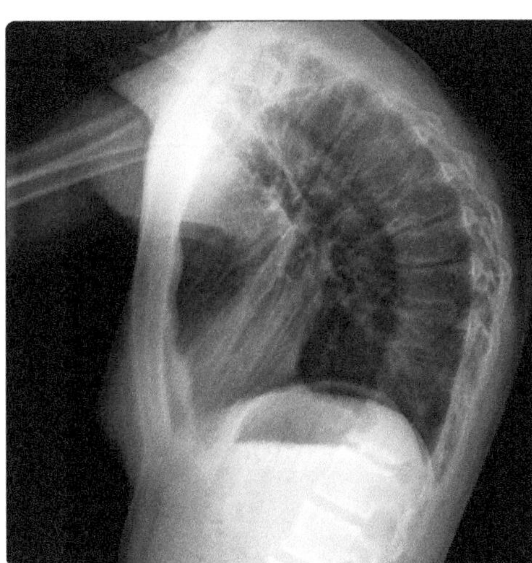

(Left) *Sagittal bone CT shows multiple SNs of varying sizes* ➡. *There is marginal sclerosis adjacent to each node, representing reparative bone changes. Straightening of thoracic kyphosis excludes Scheuermann disease because there are not 3 adjacent levels with at least 5° of anterior wedging.* **(Right)** *Lateral radiograph of the thoracic spine in a young woman with back pain and kyphosis shows the typical findings of Scheuermann kyphosis with multiple levels of vertebral wedging and numerous SNs.*

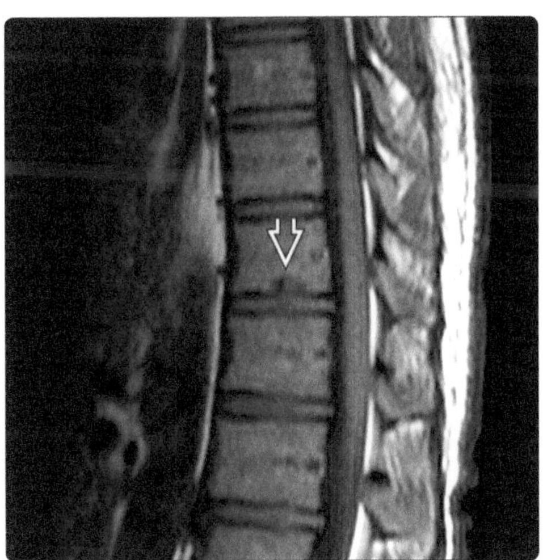

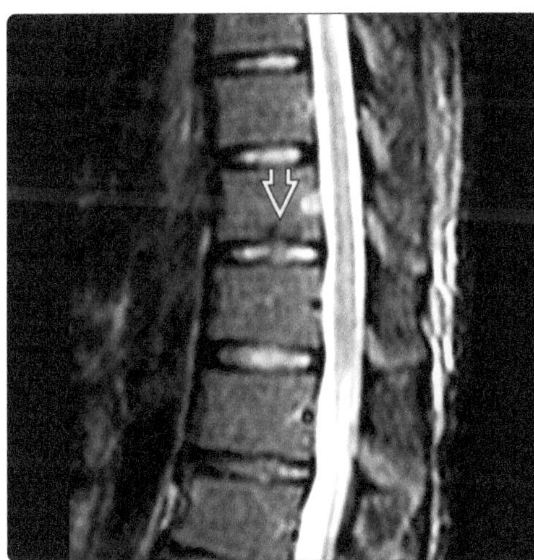

(Left) *Sagittal T1 MR shows a small, inferior endplate SN* ➡. *There is no marrow edema or fatty conversion surrounding this nonacute SN.* **(Right)** *Sagittal STIR MR confirms absence of marrow edema surrounding an asymptomatic SN* ➡ *incidentally discovered on MR performed for other reasons. The remaining intervertebral disc spaces are normal.*

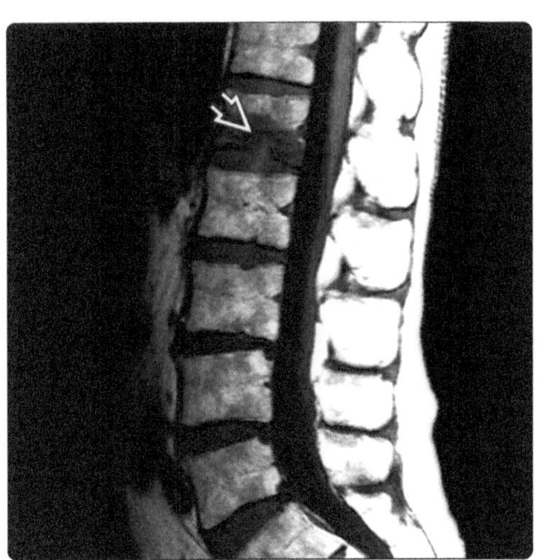

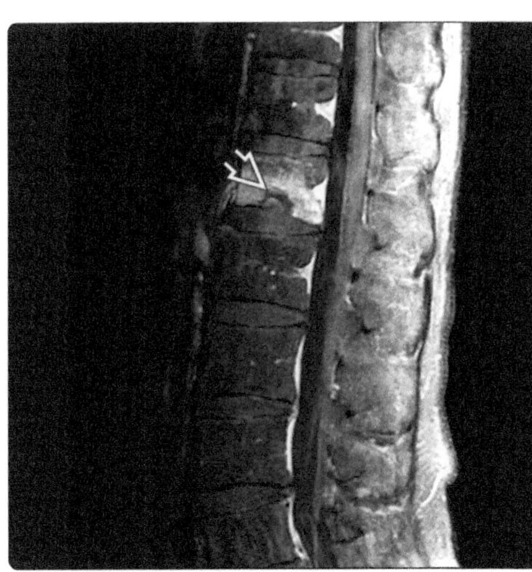

(Left) *Sagittal T1 MR demonstrates a focal undersurface endplate defect* ➡ *filled by disc material, representing an SN. There is prominent low signal intensity within adjacent marrow, representing a recent injury in this patient with focal back pain.* **(Right)** *Sagittal T1 C+ MR with fat saturation in the same patient depicts diffuse marrow enhancement surrounding the inferior endplate SN* ➡, *suggesting a subacute time point.*

Scheuermann Kyphosis

KEY FACTS

TERMINOLOGY

- Juvenile kyphosis, Scheuermann kyphosis
- Kyphosis secondary to multiple Schmorl nodes → vertebral body wedging

IMAGING

- Wedged-shaped thoracic vertebrae with irregular endplates
  - ≥ 3 contiguous vertebrae, each showing ≥ 5° of kyphosis
  - Undulation of endplates secondary to extensive disc invaginations
  - Disc spaces narrowed with greatest narrowing anteriorly
  - Well-defined Schmorl nodes

TOP DIFFERENTIAL DIAGNOSES

- Postural kyphosis
- Wedge compression fractures
- Congenital kyphosis
- Tuberculosis
- Osteogenesis imperfecta
- Neuromuscular disease

PATHOLOGY

- Disc extrusions through weakened regions of vertebral endplates
- Weightlifting, gymnastics, and other spine-loading sports may contribute

CLINICAL ISSUES

- Thoracic spine pain worsened by activity
- Kyphosis develops in adolescence; may present later in life
- Peak incidence: 13-17 years
- Initial treatment includes observation, bracing
- Surgical treatment for > 75° kyphosis in skeletally immature person

DIAGNOSTIC CHECKLIST

- Schmorl nodes without anterior wedging are not indicative of Scheuermann disease

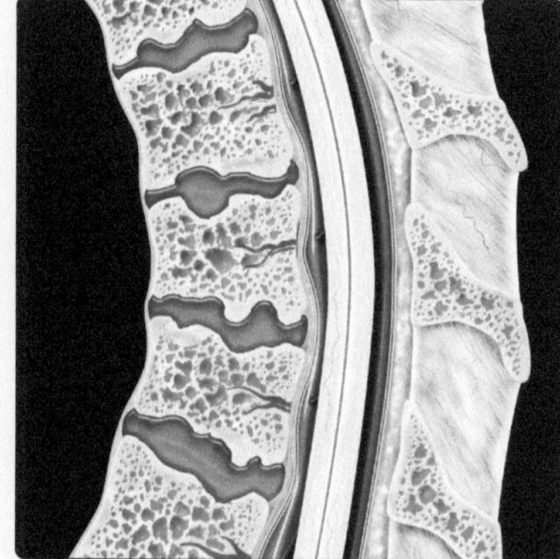
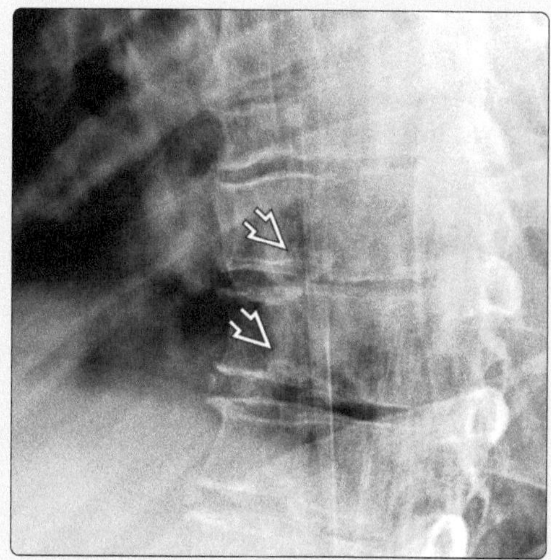

(Left) *Sagittal graphic demonstrates anterior vertebral wedging and herniation of disc material through the vertebral endplates, creating focal subcortical bone defects in conjunction with thoracic kyphotic deformity. Undulation of endplates reflects sequelae of the osseous reparative process.* **(Right)** *Lateral radiography reveals anterior wedging deformity and undulation of vertebral endplates with multiple Schmorl nodes at each level* ➡*.*

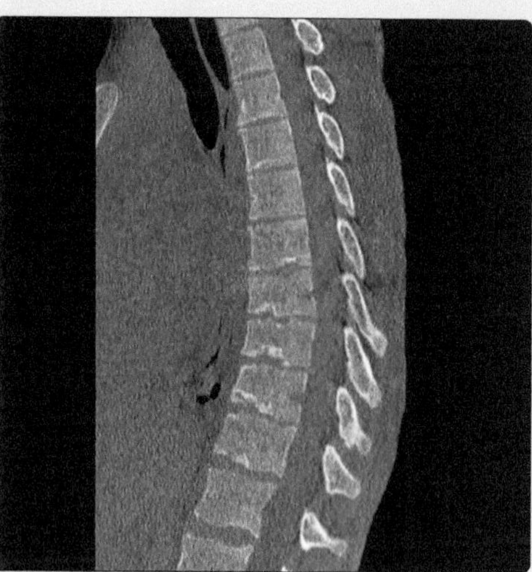
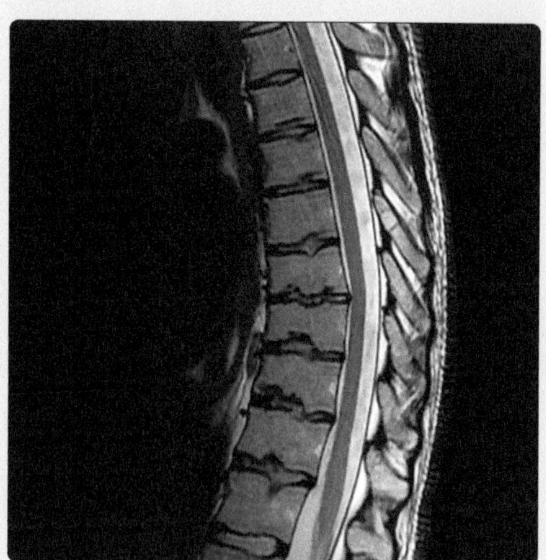

(Left) *Sagittal bone CT shows loss of anterior vertebral height and endplate irregularity involving multiple thoracic discs. There are multiple (> 3) contiguous levels of endplate irregularities (Schmorl node) and increased thoracic kyphosis.* **(Right)** *Sagittal T2WI MR in the same patient confirms loss of disc height and signal intensity at multiple thoracic levels. The thoracic spinal cord is normal, and there are no associated thoracic disc herniations into the spinal canal.*

TERMINOLOGY

Abbreviations

- Scheuermann kyphosis (SK)

Synonyms

- Juvenile kyphosis, Scheuermann disease

Definitions

- Kyphosis secondary to vertebral body wedging with multiple Schmorl nodes
- Schmorl node: Invagination of disc material through vertebral body endplate

IMAGING

General Features

- Best diagnostic clue
  - ≥ 3 wedged thoracic vertebrae with irregular endplates
- Location
  - 75% thoracic
  - 20-25% thoracolumbar
  - < 5% lumbar only
  - Rarely, cervical
- Size
  - Normal kyphosis of thoracic spine increases with age
  - Kyphosis > 40° considered abnormal

Radiographic Findings

- Radiography
  - ≥ 3 contiguous vertebrae, each showing ≥ 5° of kyphosis
  - Undulation of endplates secondary to extensive disc invaginations
  - Disc spaces narrowed with greatest narrowing anteriorly
  - Well-defined Schmorl nodes
  - Thoracic spine: Measure kyphosis from T3-T12
  - Thoracolumbar or lumbar involvement
    - Measure sagittal plane deformity from 1 vertebra above affected vertebrae to 1 vertebra below
    - This method of measuring gives better estimate of functional kyphosis
    - Loss of normal lumbar lordosis functionally significant
  - ± limbus vertebrae
  - 15% have scoliosis as well as kyphosis
    - Hyperextension lateral radiograph to assess flexibility of kyphosis

CT Findings

- Bone CT
  - Endplate abnormalities more apparent than on radiography

MR Findings

- T1WI
  - Schmorl nodes, disc herniation with low signal intensity
  - ± discogenic sclerosis
- T2WI
  - Disc degeneration seen in 50% of involved discs
  - Disc herniations
  - Schmorl nodes may be low or high signal intensity
    - ± bone marrow edema adjacent to Schmorl nodes

Nuclear Medicine Findings

- Bone scan
  - May be normal or show increased activity

Other Modality Findings

- Bone mineral density normal (DEXA, CT bone densitometry)

Imaging Recommendations

- Plain film for diagnosis
- MR to exclude disc herniations

DIFFERENTIAL DIAGNOSIS

Postural Kyphosis

- Vertebral endplates normal
- Deformity usually corrects in hyperextension (unless longstanding)

Wedge Compression Fractures

- May involve contiguous levels
- Anterior vertebral cortex often shows angular deformity
- MR shows fracture lines, bone marrow edema

Congenital Kyphosis

- Vertebral anomalies present

Tuberculosis

- Kyphosis often severe
- Endplate destruction ± vertebral fusion

Osteogenesis Imperfecta

- Platyspondyly
- Severe osteopenia

Neuromuscular Disease

- Persistence of infantile thoracolumbar kyphosis in nonambulatory patients
- Kyphoscoliosis

Ankylosing Spondylitis

- Fusion of vertebral bodies
- Abnormalities of sacroiliac joints

Spondyloepiphyseal Dysplasia Tarda

- Platyspondyly throughout spine
- Epiphyses abnormal

PATHOLOGY

General Features

- Etiology
  - Unknown
    - Weightlifting, gymnastics, and other spine-loading sports may contribute
  - Disc extrusions through weak regions of vertebral endplates
    - Disc space loss
    - Limbus vertebrae
    - Schmorl node
  - Delayed growth in anterior portion of vertebrae causes wedging
- Genetics
  - Familial tendency

- Danish twin registry showed major genetic contribution
- Associated abnormalities
  - Lordosis of cervical and lumbar segments

Gross Pathologic & Surgical Features

- Schmorl nodes invaginate into vertebral bodies through fissures in weakened growth plates
- Limbus vertebrae occur when disc material protrudes through growth plate of ring apophysis

Microscopic Features

- Vertebral body growth plates
  - Abnormal chondrocytes
  - Loose cartilage matrix
  - Diminished number or thickness of collagen fibers
  - Increased proteoglycan content
- Osteonecrosis, osteochondrosis not seen

CLINICAL ISSUES

Presentation

- Most common signs/symptoms
  - Kyphosis
  - Other signs/symptoms
    - Thoracic spine pain and tenderness worsened by activity
    - Neurologic symptoms from kyphosis or disc herniations
    - Fatigue

Demographics

- Age
  - Develops in adolescence; may present later in life
- Sex
  - Slight male predominance
- Epidemiology
  - Prevalence: 0.4-8.0%
  - Peak incidence: 13-17 years

Natural History & Prognosis

- Increases in magnitude during adolescent growth spurt
- Mild progression after growth is complete
- Severe deformity uncommon
- Kyphosis > 70° has poor functional result
- Premature disc degeneration
- Disc herniations related to degeneration, mechanical stress from spine deformity

Treatment

- Observation
  - Indications
    - Growth still remains; kyphotic deformity < 50°
  - Elimination of specific strenuous activity
  - Analgesics
  - Spine exercises
  - Follow-up until growth plate fuses (~ 25 years of age)
- Brace treatment
  - Indications
    - At least 1 year of growth remains
    - < 70° kyphosis
    - At least partial correction of kyphosis on hyperextension
    - Efficacious in skeletally immature patients
- Surgical treatment
  - Uncommonly felt to be necessary
  - Indications
    - > 75° kyphosis in skeletally immature person
    - > 60° kyphosis in mature person
    - Excessive pain
    - Neurologic deficit
  - Posterior instrumentation and fusion
  - Anterior and posterior fusion for more severe kyphosis

DIAGNOSTIC CHECKLIST

Image Interpretation Pearls

- Schmorl nodes without anterior wedging are not indicative of Scheuermann disease
- Radiography may show undulating endplates rather than discrete Schmorl nodes

SELECTED REFERENCES

1. Debnath UK et al: Long-term outcome after surgical treatment of Scheuermann's kyphosis (SK). Spine Deform. 10(2):387-97, 2022
2. Sarwahi V et al: Scheuermann kyphosis patients have a similar revision and infection rate to adolescent idiopathic scoliosis patients. Spine (Phila Pa 1976). 47(7):E290-5, 2022
3. Zloof Y et al: The hereditary nature of adolescent spinal deformities: a study of over 600,000 adolescents. Spine (Phila Pa 1976). 47(12):841-6, 2022
4. Demiroz S et al: Intraspinal anomalies in individuals with Scheuermann's kyphosis: is the routine use of magnetic resonance imaging necessary for preoperative evaluation? Asian Spine J. 12(4):697-702, 2018
5. Gaudé M et al: Long term prognosis of Scheuermann's disease: the association with fragility fracture - the MINOS cohort. Bone. 117:116-22, 2018
6. Lorente A et al: Severe hyperkyphosis reduces the aerobic capacity and maximal exercise tolerance in patients with Scheuermann disease. Spine J. 19(2):330-8, 2018
7. Ristolainen L et al: Progression of untreated mild thoracic Scheuermann's kyphosis - radiographic and functional assessment after mean follow-up of 46 years. J Orthop Sci. 22(4):652-7, 2017
8. Gokce E et al: Radiological imaging findings of scheuermann disease. World J Radiol. 8(11):895-901, 2016
9. Palazzo C et al: Scheuermann's disease: an update. Joint Bone Spine. 81(3):209-14, 2014
10. Makurthou AA et al: Scheuermann disease: evaluation of radiological criteria and population prevalence. Spine (Phila Pa 1976). 38(19):1690-4, 2013
11. Sugrue PA et al: Rapidly progressive Scheuermann's disease in an adolescent after pectus bar placement treated with posterior vertebral-column resection: case report and review of the literature. Spine (Phila Pa 1976). 38(4):E259-62, 2013
12. d'Hemecourt PA et al: Spinal deformity in young athletes. Clin Sports Med. 31(3):441-51, 2012
13. Jagtap SA et al: Scheuermann disease presenting as compressive myelopathy. Neurology. 78(16):1279, 2012
14. Damborg F et al: Genetic epidemiology of Scheuermann's disease. Acta Orthop. 82(5):602-5, 2011
15. Tsirikos AI et al: Scheuermann's kyphosis; current controversies. J Bone Joint Surg Br. 93(7):857-64, 2011
16. Lowe TG: Scheuermann's kyphosis. Neurosurg Clin N Am. 18(2):305-15, 2007
17. Lowe TG et al: Evidence based medicine: analysis of Scheuermann kyphosis. Spine (Phila Pa 1976). 32(19 Suppl):S115-9, 2007
18. Soo CL et al: Scheuermann kyphosis: long-term follow-up. Spine J. 2(1):49-56, 2002
19. Stotts AK et al: Measurement of spinal kyphosis: implications for the management of Scheuermann's kyphosis. Spine. 27(19):2143-6, 2002
20. Wenger DR et al: Scheuermann kyphosis. Spine. 24(24):2630-9, 1999
21. Swischuk LE et al: Disk degenerative disease in childhood: Scheuermann's disease, Schmorl's nodes, and the limbus vertebra: MRI findings in 12 patients. Pediatr Radiol. 28(5):334-8, 1998
22. Tribus CB: Scheuermann's kyphosis in adolescents and adults: diagnosis and management. J Am Acad Orthop Surg. 6(1):36-43, 1998
23. Platero D et al: Juvenile kyphosis: effects of different variables on conservative treatment outcome. Acta Orthop Belg. 63(3):194-201, 1997

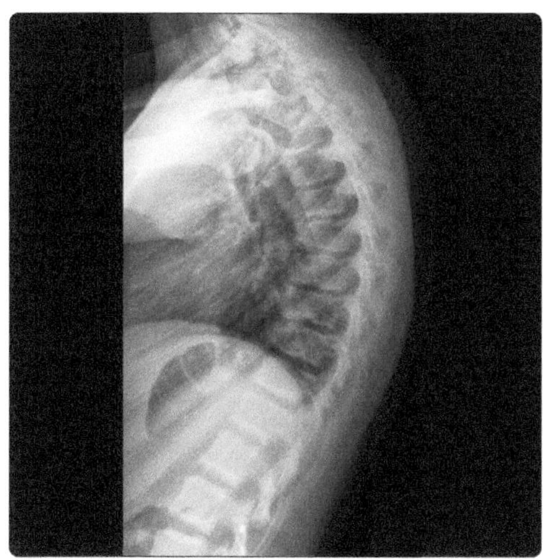

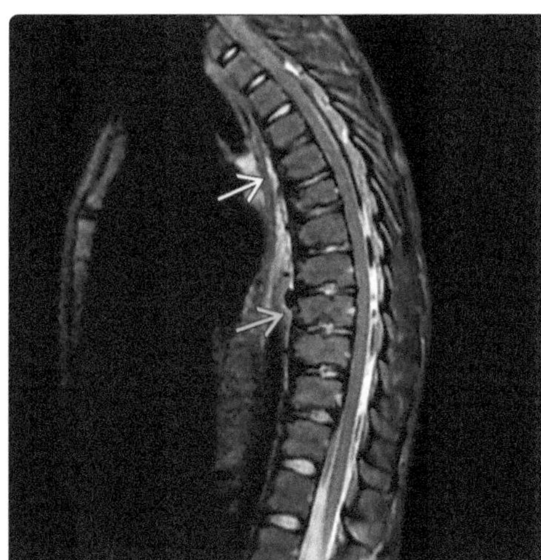

(Left) *Lateral radiograph in a 15-year-old girl with kyphosis and back pain demonstrates a smooth, rounded kyphotic thoracic curvature. Closer inspection reveals anterior wedging and endplate irregularity of multiple thoracic vertebra.* **(Right)** *Sagittal STIR MR in the same patient confirms multilevel anterior thoracic vertebral wedging and Schmorl nodes, compatible with Scheuermann kyphosis. Note the rostral ➡ and caudal ⇨ extent of abnormal vertebra.*

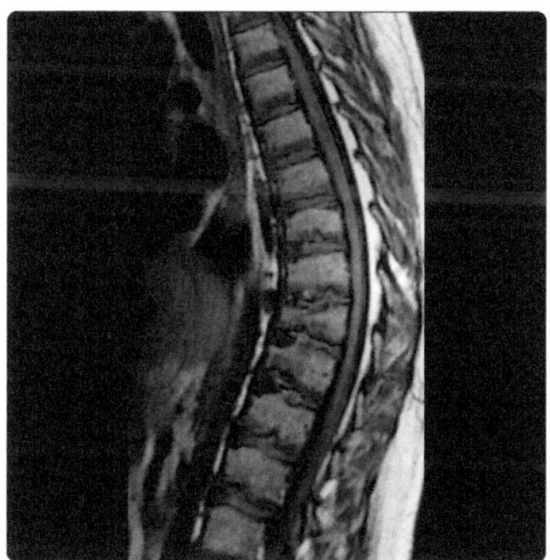

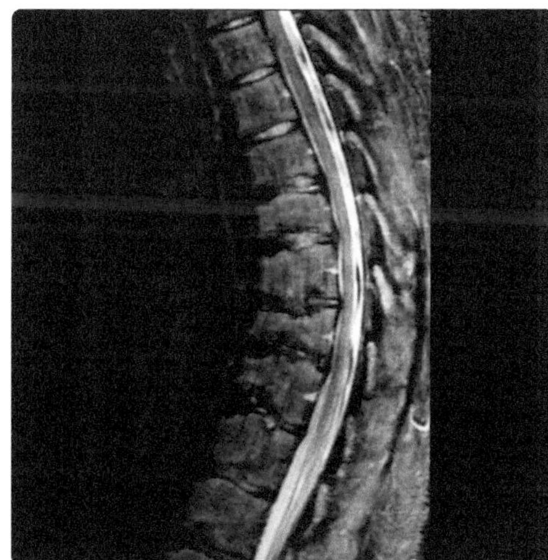

(Left) *Sagittal T1WI MR in a teen rodeo rider with back pain demonstrates multilevel thoracic vertebral anterior wedging with endplate undulations, Schmorl nodes, and kyphosis, characteristic of fairly severe Scheuermann disease.* **(Right)** *Sagittal STIR MR in the same patient confirms multilevel thoracic vertebral anterior wedging, endplate undulations, Schmorl nodes, and fairly severe kyphosis.*

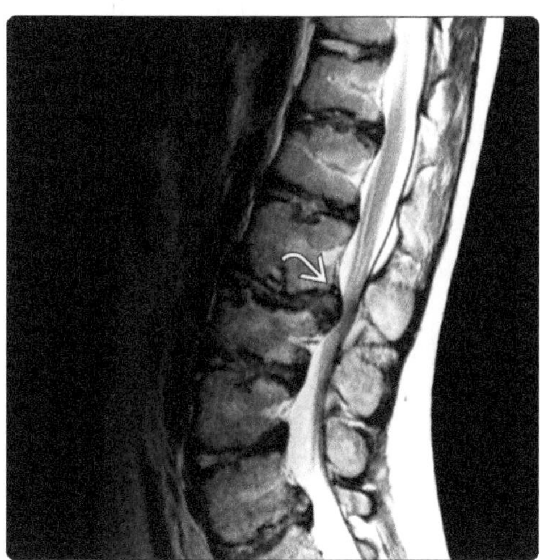

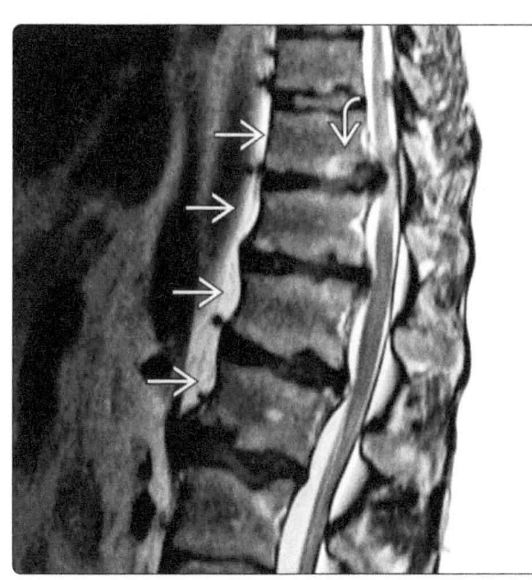

(Left) *Sagittal T2WI MR illustrates lumbar variant of Scheuermann disease with diffuse loss of intervertebral disc signal, wedging of vertebral bodies, undulation of endplates, and discrete Schmorl nodes. Note the large disc extrusion ⮫.* **(Right)** *Sagittal T2WI MR depicts multiple level endplate irregularity with Schmorl nodes and disc degeneration throughout visualized spine. Multiple contiguous levels ➡ are identified. Type I degenerative endplate changes ⮫ are present as well.*

Congenital Scoliosis and Kyphosis

KEY FACTS

TERMINOLOGY

- Spinal curvature secondary to vertebral anomalies
- Hemivertebra: Unilateral or anterior vertebral hypoplasia
- Butterfly vertebra: Central vertebral cleft due to failure of central vertebral body development
- "Fused" vertebrae: Embryologic failure of segmentation rather than fusion
- Klippel-Feil syndrome: Multiple vertebral segmentation anomalies

IMAGING

- Usually short-curve scoliosis &/or kyphosis
- May have multiple curves if multiple anomalies present

TOP DIFFERENTIAL DIAGNOSES

- Traumatic scoliosis
- Idiopathic scoliosis
- Neuromuscular scoliosis
- Scoliosis due to infection
- Scoliosis due to syndromes

PATHOLOGY

- Fetal insult in 1st trimester causing abnormal development &/or segmentation of vertebrae
- Abnormalities due to failure of development &/or failure of segmentation

CLINICAL ISSUES

- May be isolated anomaly or associated with multisystem anomalies (VACTERL)
- Present at birth but may not be evident clinically until later in childhood or adolescence

DIAGNOSTIC CHECKLIST

- Image entire spine to exclude additional bone, spinal cord abnormalities
- Vertebral bars may be cartilaginous in young children

(Left) *Coronal graphic illustrates butterfly vertebra ➔ and balanced hemivertebrae ➔. Hemivertebrae that are not fused to the adjacent vertebrae are not restricted in growth and are most likely to cause progressive scoliosis.* **(Right)** *AP radiograph shows a right-sided hemivertebra ➔ causing an angular, short-curve scoliosis, typical of congenital scoliosis. Note fusion of the pars interarticularis ➔ between the hemivertebra and the vertebra above.*

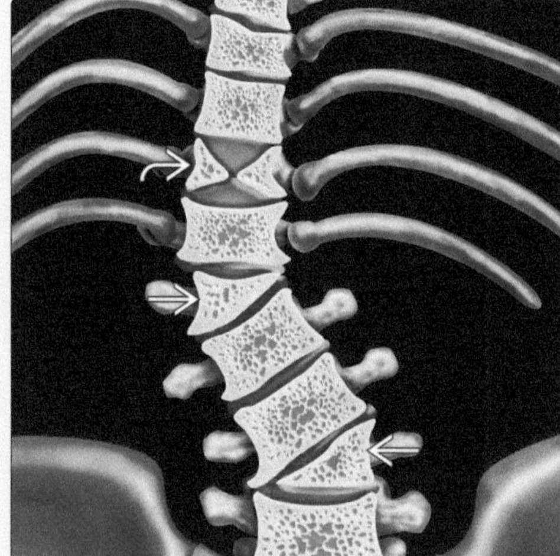

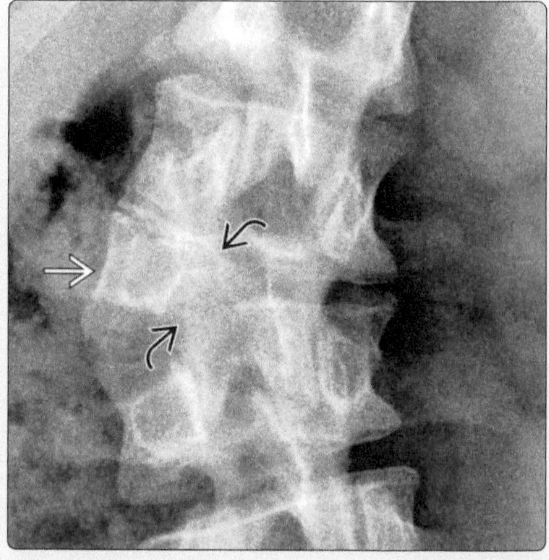

(Left) *AP 3D reformation from a bone CT confirms a right hemivertebra ➔, resulting in an angular short-curve congenital dextroscoliosis.* **(Right)** *Lateral 3D reformation from a bone CT shows a posterior hemivertebra ➔ fused to the vertebra below ➔, resulting in severe short-curve kyphoscoliosis. Complicated congenital kyphoscoliosis like this may be most easily appreciated on 3D reformations.*

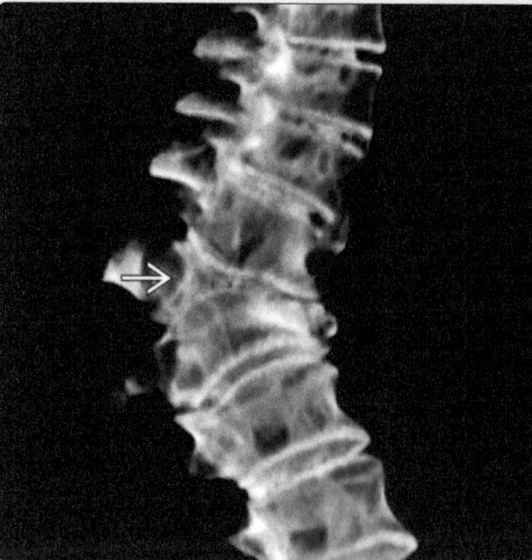

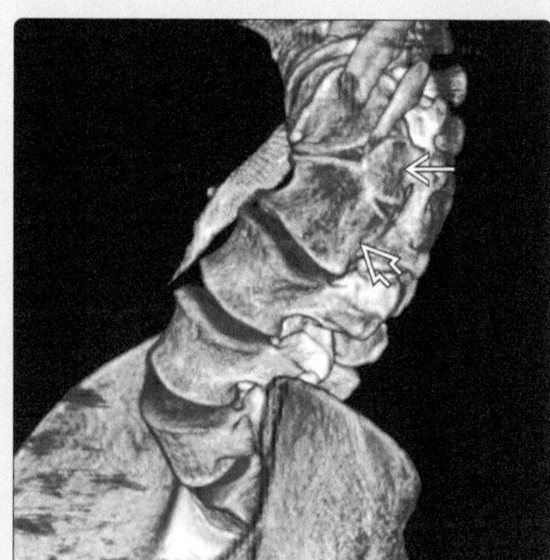

TERMINOLOGY

Definitions

- Spinal curvature secondary to vertebral anomalies
- Klippel-Feil syndrome: Multiple cervical segmentation anomalies

IMAGING

General Features

- Best diagnostic clue
  - Vertebral anomaly in patient with scoliosis or kyphosis
- Location
  - Most common in thoracic spine but can occur at any level
- Morphology
  - Butterfly vertebra: Central vertebral cleft due to failure of central vertebral body development
  - Hemivertebra: Unilateral or anterior vertebral hypoplasia
  - "Fused" vertebrae: Embryologic failure of segmentation rather than fusion
    - a.k.a. block vertebrae; may affect vertebral body, posterior elements, or both
    - Affected vertebrae narrow in mediolateral and AP dimensions
    - Rudimentary disc may be present
  - Vertebral bar
    - Bony or cartilaginous connection between adjacent vertebrae
    - Often associated with rib fusions

Radiographic Findings

- Large, small, or asymmetric vertebral bodies, hemivertebrae, fused ribs
- Fused vertebrae often have decreased AP dimension
  - Helps to distinguish from fusion occurring in adulthood
- Short-curve scoliosis
- Single or multiple curves
- Vertebral anomalies often difficult to see; use coned-down radiographs, MR, or CT to clarify

CT Findings

- Improved visualization of anomalous vertebrae compared to radiographs
- Coronal and sagittal reformatted images essential
  - 3D imaging helpful for surgical planning

MR Findings

- T1WI
  - Can be useful to determine any distortion of spinal cord
  - Only if question of neurologic impairment
- T2WI
  - Useful to look for myelomalacia if neurologic impairment
- Steady-state sequences (FIESTA, CISS) most useful for assessing central canal, nerve roots

Imaging Recommendations

- Best imaging tool
  - CT preferable for surgical planning in adults because of superior spatial resolution
  - Multiplanar MR best modality to evaluate full spine in children
    - Avoids CT radiation dose, excludes associated neural axis abnormalities
- Protocol advice
  - Coronal and sagittal images of entire spine necessary
  - Use T1WI or PD MR to evaluate bone morphology, exclude tumor or Chiari 1
  - T2WI, STIR to evaluate for tethered cord, syrinx, tumor

DIFFERENTIAL DIAGNOSIS

Traumatic Scoliosis

- Short-curve scoliosis, vertebral body deformity

Idiopathic Scoliosis

- Single or S-shaped curve, no anomalies

Neuromuscular Scoliosis

- Usually single, long thoracolumbar curve

Scoliosis Due to Infection

- Short curve, painful
- May result in vertebral body fusion

Scoliosis Due to Syndromes

- e.g., neurofibromatosis
- Marfan syndrome
- Osteogenesis imperfecta
- Diastrophic dwarfism
- Ehlers-Danlos syndrome

Scoliosis Due to Radiation in Childhood

- Short-curve scoliosis, vertebral hypoplasia, history of radiation
- Rarely occurs today

Limb Length Inequality

- Check heights of iliac wings on standing films
- Use lifts under foot to equalize lengths, evaluate true scoliosis

Idiopathic Kyphosis

- Vertebral anomalies absent

Scheuermann Kyphosis

- Wedging of ≥ 3 vertebral bodies, undulation of endplates
- 15% have scoliosis as well as kyphosis

Osteomyelitis, Granulomatous

- Kyphosis may be severe (gibbus) deformity
- Spinal fusion may develop
- Paraspinous cold abscess, endplate destruction

Juvenile Idiopathic Arthritis

- Affects cervical but not thoracic or lumbar spine
- Vertebral fusion ± scoliosis or kyphosis
- Onset in childhood

PATHOLOGY

General Features

- Etiology
  - Fetal insult in 1st trimester causing abnormal development &/or segmentation of vertebrae

- Abnormalities due either to failure of development &/or failure of segmentation at sclerotome stage of development
- Failure of vertebral body development
  - Hypoplastic vertebrae anteriorly or on 1 side (wedge vertebra)
  - Aplastic vertebrae anteriorly or on 1 side (hemivertebra)
  - Butterfly vertebra: Central cleft
- Failure of vertebral segmentation
  - Vertebral body forms from 1/2 of 2 adjacent sclerotomes
  - Therefore, apparent congenital fusion of vertebrae is really failure of segmentation
  - May involve vertebral body, posterior elements, or both
- Failure of development and of segmentation may both be present
  - Hemivertebra may be fused to adjacent vertebra
  - Underlying cause of hemivertebrae development unknown

- Genetics
  - Sometimes associated with chromosomal abnormalities
  - Usually not inherited
- Associated abnormalities
  - Klippel-Feil may be associated with craniocervical and brainstem anomalies
  - Cord abnormalities: Syringohydromyelia, diastematomyelia, tethered cord
  - Caudal regression
  - Component of **v**ertebral, **a**nal, **c**ardiac, **t**racheal, **e**sophageal, **r**enal, **l**imb (VACTERL) anomalies/abnormalities association
    - Incidence of VACTERL: 1.6/10,000 live births
    - Defective mesodermal development in early embryogenesis
    - Some cases inherited, some due to fetal insult
    - Patients have at least 3 of following
      - Vertebral anomalies (37%)
      - Anal atresia (63%)
      - Cardiac anomalies (77%)
      - Tracheoesophageal fistula (40%)
      - Renal and genitourinary anomalies (72%)
      - Radial ray hypoplasia (58%)
    - Hydrocephalus may occur
- Supernumerary hemivertebrae

CLINICAL ISSUES

Presentation

- Most common signs/symptoms
  - Visible spinal axis deformity
- Clinical profile
  - May be isolated anomaly or associated with multisystem anomalies (VACTERL)

Demographics

- Age
  - Present at birth but may not be evident clinically until later in childhood or adolescence
- Sex
  - M = F
- Epidemiology
  - Sporadic, uncommon

Natural History & Prognosis

- Kyphosis
  - Tends to progress without treatment; fusion during childhood indicated
  - May lead to
    - Cord compression
    - Paralysis
- Scoliosis
  - Difficult to predict which curves will progress
  - Balanced anomalies may grow fairly normally
    - e.g., contralateral hemivertebrae at adjacent levels
  - Scoliotic curve tends to progress rapidly when
    - Hemivertebrae not fused to vertebrae at adjacent levels
    - Hemivertebrae are associated with contralateral failure of segmentation

Treatment

- Close clinical observation of scoliosis for progression
- Brace is of limited utility
- Fusion of congenital kyphosis to prevent paralysis
- Surgery for scoliotic curves progressing > 10° per year
  - Anterior or posterior fusion with instrumentation
  - Resection of vertebral bars, hemivertebrae
  - Hemiepiphysiodesis: Fuse growth plate on 1 side to prevent progression of curve

DIAGNOSTIC CHECKLIST

Consider

- Both CT (with 3D reformations) and MR are often necessary to completely characterize spine and spinal cord

Image Interpretation Pearls

- Neural arch not fused in midline until ~ 2 years old; cleft on AP radiograph must not be confused with spinal anomaly
- Image entire spine to exclude additional bone or cord abnormalities, Chiari 1
- Vertebral bars may be cartilaginous in young children

SELECTED REFERENCES

1. Wu N et al: Retrospective analysis of associated anomalies in 636 patients with operatively treated congenital scoliosis. J Bone Joint Surg Am. 105(7):537-48, 2023
2. Canaz H et al: Surgical treatment of patients with myelomeningocele-related spine deformities: study of 26 cases. Childs Nerv Syst. 34(7):1367-74, 2018
3. Lonstein JE: Long-term outcome of early fusions for congenital scoliosis. Spine Deform. 6(5):552-9, 2018
4. Mackel CE et al: A comprehensive review of the diagnosis and management of congenital scoliosis. Childs Nerv Syst. 34(11):2155-71, 2018
5. Pijpker PAJ et al: Three-dimensional planning and use of individualized osteotomy guiding templates for surgical correction of kyphoscoliosis: a technical case report. World Neurosurg. 119:113-7, 2018
6. Soliman HAG: Health-related quality of life of adolescents with severe untreated congenital kyphosis and kyphoscoliosis in a developing country. Spine (Phila Pa 1976). 43(16):E942-8, 2018
7. Giampietro PF et al: Clinical, genetic and environmental factors associated with congenital vertebral malformations. Mol Syndromol. 4(1-2):94-105, 2013
8. McMaster MJ et al: Prognosis for congenital scoliosis due to a unilateral failure of vertebral segmentation. J Bone Joint Surg Am. 95(11):972-9, 2013

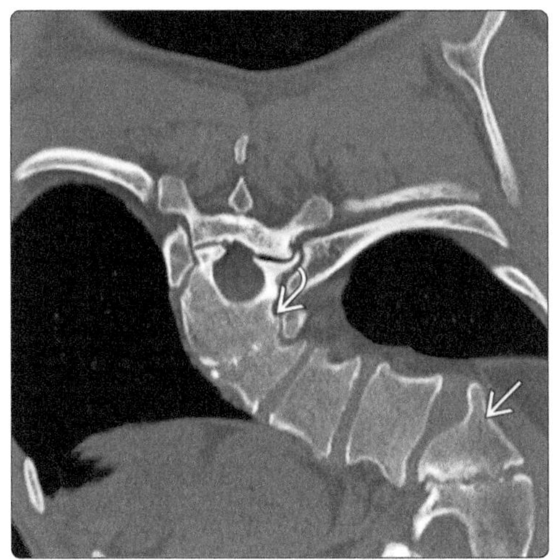

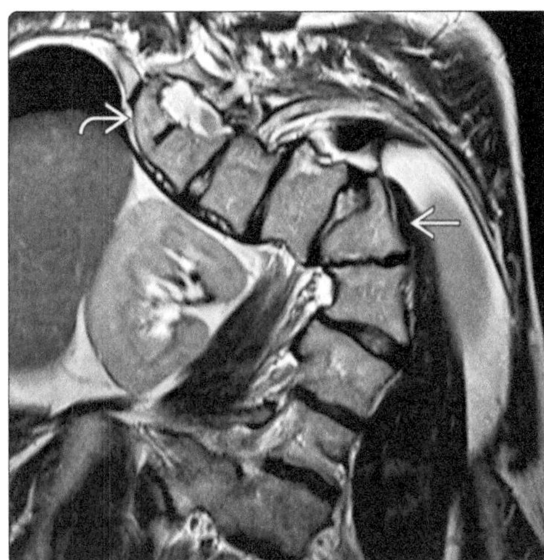

(Left) *Coronal bone CT shows 2 levels of a fusion anomaly, causing a complex kyphoscoliosis. A midthoracic vertebra ➡ is markedly rotated with its anterior cortex fused to the superior endplate of the vertebral body below. The left lumbar hemivertebra ➡ is fused to vertebra below.* **(Right)** *Coronal T2WI MR in the same patient also demonstrates the thoracic ➡ and lumbar ➡ vertebral anomalies well. There is marked acute angle congenital levoscoliosis.*

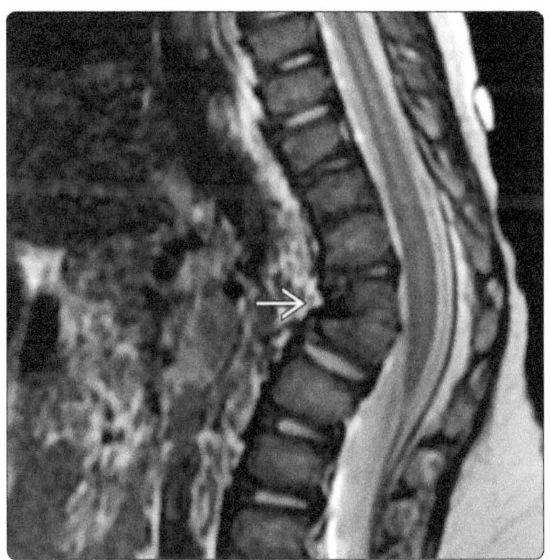

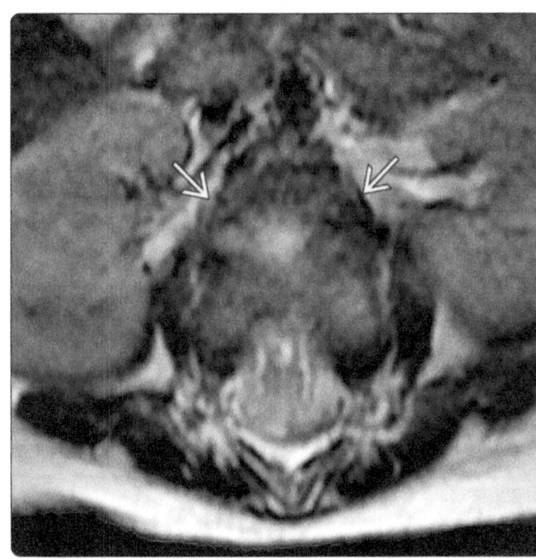

(Left) *Sagittal T2WI MR demonstrates focal short-curve thoracolumbar kyphosis secondary to a combination of anterior vertebral hypoplasia and segmentation failure of T12 and L1 ➡.* **(Right)** *Axial T2WI MR shows abnormal appearance of the vertebra ➡ in this patient with vertebral hypoplasia and segmentation failure at T12 and L1, resulting in congenital kyphosis. Axial images are relatively unhelpful for characterizing kyphosis but can help evaluate spinal canal and cord.*

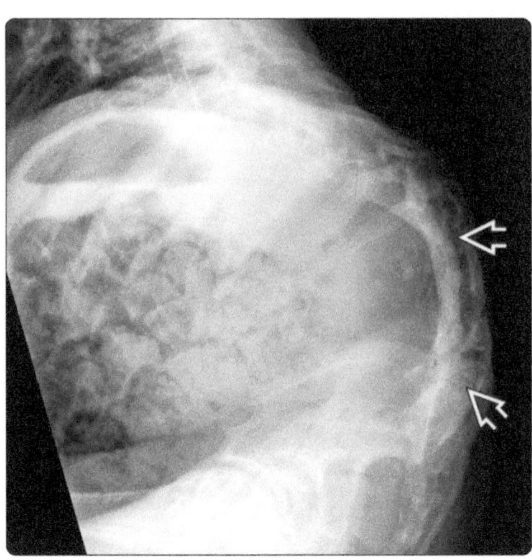

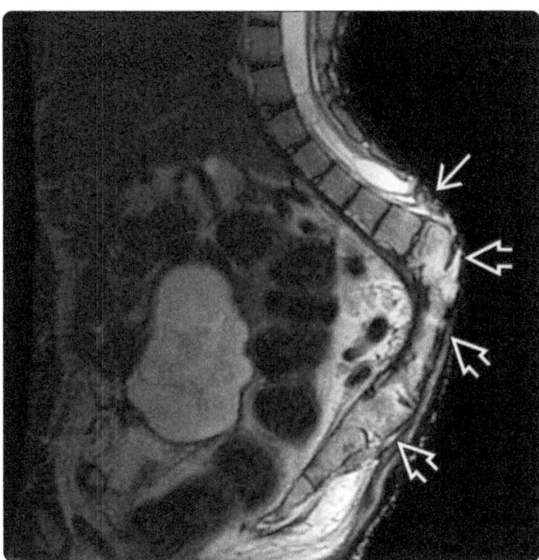

(Left) *Lateral radiograph (high myelomeningocele) reveals severe congenital kyphosis at the thoracolumbar junction with segmentation failure of multiple lumbar vertebra ➡.* **(Right)** *Sagittal T1WI MR in the same patient shows termination of the attenuated distal spinal cord at the thoracolumbar junction myelomeningocele repair site ➡. There are extensive areas of congenital vertebral segmentation failure ➡ contributing to the congenital kyphosis.*

KEY FACTS

TERMINOLOGY

- Spondylolysis: Defect/break in pars interarticularis
  - Repetitive microtrauma likely etiology
- Spondylolisthesis: Spondylolysis + anterior slippage of vertebra in relation to vertebra below

IMAGING

- Bone CT
  - Linear lucency or defect in pars interarticularis
    - Sagittal or oblique sagittal reformatted imaging vital in assessment
  - Incomplete ring sign on axial imaging ± distraction
    - May simulate "extra" or double facet joints
    - May be confused with facet joint
      - Lysis located anterior to facet joint
      - Lysis more transverse in orientation on axial images compared to facet joint, which is more oblique
      - Facet joint is smooth, while lysis typically is irregular/fragmented
  - Spondylolisthesis & foraminal narrowing on sagittal reformatted images
  - Secondary finding of sclerosis &/or hypertrophy of contralateral pedicle & lamina
- SPECT bone scan imaging helpful for diagnosis
  - Intense focal uptake in posterior elements, unilateral or bilateral
  - Remote or healed may be occult (normal)
- MR for lysis: Adjust spine protocol towards musculoskeletal system by adding STIR/T2 FS (↑ conspicuity of marrow & soft tissue edema)

CLINICAL ISSUES

- 40% incidence in children with lower back pain (LBP)
  - L5: 85%; L4: 5-15%

DIAGNOSTIC CHECKLIST

- Sagittal or oblique sagittal bone CT reformats & sagittal STIR/T2 FS MR images most important for diagnosis

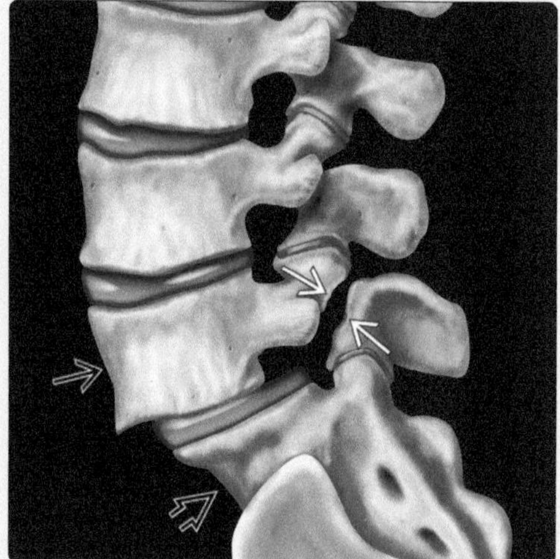

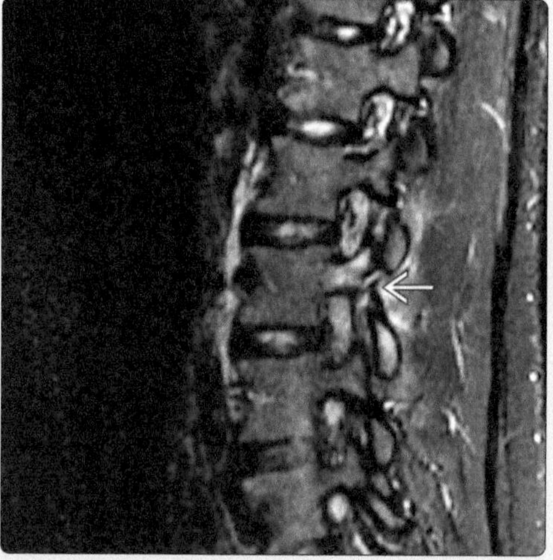

(Left) *Lateral graphic shows a separated defect within the L5 pars interarticularis (spondylolysis) ➡. Notice the resultant anterior slippage (spondylolisthesis) of L5 ➡ on S1 ➡.* **(Right)** *Sagittal STIR MR in a 14-year-old with back pain shows a pars defect ➡ with edema in the marrow of the posterior elements & adjacent soft tissues. STIR images can be helpful in detecting marrow edema associated with spondylolysis.*

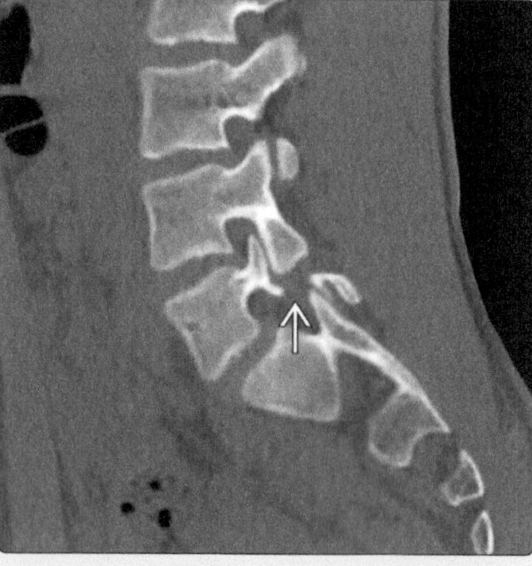

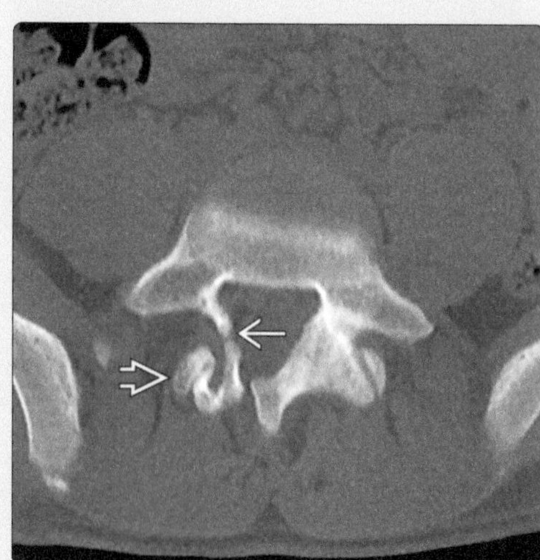

(Left) *Sagittal bone CT in a young athlete with lumbar back pain reveals a unilateral L5 spondylolysis ➡ (the opposite was normal, not shown). The margins of the pars defect are gracile and rounded, suggesting a dysplastic rather than traumatic origin.* **(Right)** *Axial bone CT in the same patient reveals a dysplastic-appearing right facet joint ➡ as well as an abnormal gracile, elongated pars interarticularis ➡, confirming dysplastic spondylolysis. This patient also had spondylolisthesis (not shown).*

TERMINOLOGY

Synonyms

- Lysis, isthmic spondylolysis

IMAGING

General Features

- Location
  - Lumbar
    - L5: 85%; L4: 5-15%
    - 10-15% unilateral
  - Cervical spine usually congenital

Radiographic Findings

- Classic: Break in neck of Scotty dog (pars interarticularis defect on oblique views of standing lumbar spine)
  - ± anterolisthesis
  - Positive predictive value of 57%

MR Findings

- T1WI: Discontinuity (sagittal images best), ↓ signal in pars interarticularis
- T2WI: ↓ signal in pars interarticularis (reactive sclerosis), ↑ signal in pars interarticularis (marrow edema)
- STIR/T2 FS: ↑ conspicuity of surrounding marrow & soft tissue edema, suggesting spondylolysis at classic location even if fracture not seen
- MR for lysis: Sensitivity: 57-86%; specificity: 81-82%

Nuclear Medicine Findings

- ↑ uptake best seen on SPECT bone scan

Imaging Recommendations

- Best imaging tool
  - If suspicious for this diagnosis
    - Targeted helical/volumetric bone CT with multiplanar reformats
    - Bone scan SPECT/CT better than SPECT alone
      - Anatomic & physiologic confirmation
  - If source of back pain not clear, MR may be more beneficial
    - Include STIR or T2 FS MR for marrow & soft tissue edema

DIFFERENTIAL DIAGNOSIS

Spectrum of Radiologic Findings in Back Pain

- Musculoskeletal
  - Normal (muscular)
  - Scoliosis, vertebral or sacral fracture, spinous process avulsion, Baastrup disease, facet degeneration, Bertolotti syndrome, degenerative disc disease, ring apophyseal injury, Scheuermann disease
- Infection
  - Discitis, osteomyelitis, sacroiliitis, paraspinal inflammation/abscess, pyelonephritis, pelvic inflammatory disease
- Tumor
  - Osteoid osteoma, osteoblastoma, Langerhans cell histiocytosis, leukemia, lymphoma, metastatic disease, neurofibroma
- Inflammatory
  - Ankylosing spondylitis, psoriatic arthritis, Reiter disease, inflammatory bowel disease

PATHOLOGY

General Features

- Etiology
  - Believed to be caused by repetitive microtrauma, resulting in stress fracture
  - Participation in gymnastics, weightlifting, wrestling, cricket, & football at young age
- Associated abnormalities
  - Spondylolisthesis (50%), scoliosis, Scheuermann disease, spina bifida occulta

CLINICAL ISSUES

Presentation

- Most common signs/symptoms
  - Asymptomatic (80%)
  - 40% incidence in children with lower back pain (LBP)
- Other signs/symptoms
  - Tight hamstring muscles
    - Waddling gait secondary to tight hamstring muscles
  - Back spasms or radiating pain
  - Back pain exacerbated by rigorous activities
  - Radiculopathy & cauda equina syndrome in lysis with high-grade spondylolisthesis

Demographics

- Sex
  - M:F = 2-4:1
- Epidemiology
  - Incidence: 3-6% of White population
  - Higher incidence in competitive athletes, especially male patients

Treatment

- Mainly conservative initially; surgical if conservative treatment fails or subluxation progresses

DIAGNOSTIC CHECKLIST

Image Interpretation Pearls

- Sagittal or oblique sagittal bone CT reformats & sagittal STIR/T2 FS MR most important for diagnosis
- Identify complete ring at each lumbar level on axial bone CT or MR
- Typical bone scan findings with normal radiographs or bone CT suggests stress reaction or early spondylolysis

SELECTED REFERENCES

1. Koucheki R et al: Surgical management of high-grade paediatric spondylolisthesis: meta-analysis and systematic review. Eur Spine J. 32(2):436-46, 2023
2. Choi JH et al: Management of lumbar spondylolysis in the adolescent athlete: a review of over 200 cases. Spine J. 22(10):1628-33, 2022
3. Tatsumura M et al: Posterior lumbar interbody fusion for dysplastic lumbar spondylolisthesis with high-grade slippage in two adolescent siblings: two case reports. J Med Case Rep. 16(1):331, 2022
4. Dhouib A et al: Diagnostic accuracy of MR imaging for direct visualization of lumbar pars defect in children and young adults: a systematic review and meta-analysis. Eur Spine J. 27(5):1058-66, 2018
5. Lemoine T et al: The prevalence of lumbar spondylolysis in young children: a retrospective analysis using CT. Eur Spine J. 27(5):1067-72, 2018

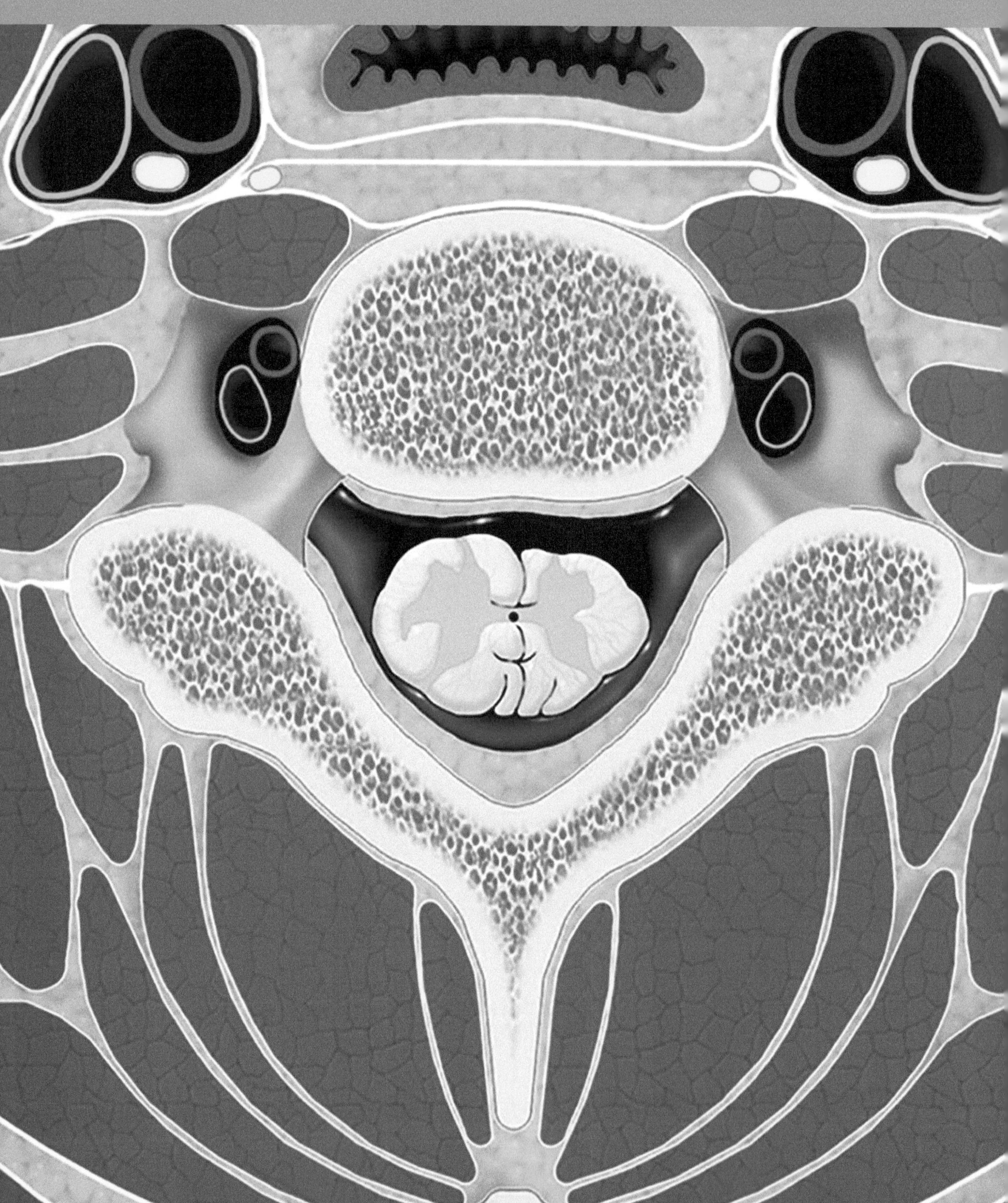

Part III
SECTION 4

Infection and Inflammatory Disorders

Infections

Inflammatory and Autoimmune Disorders

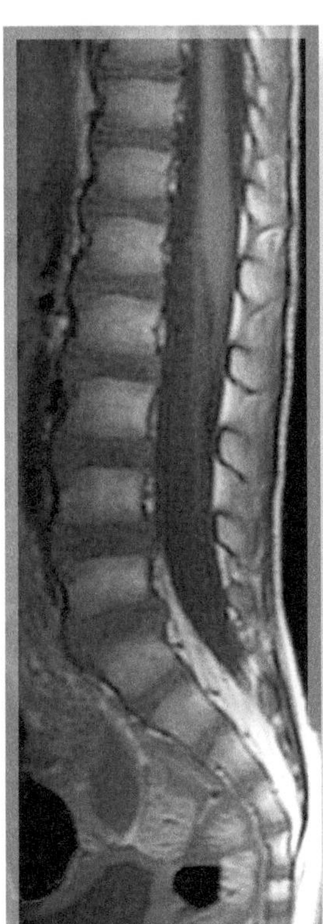
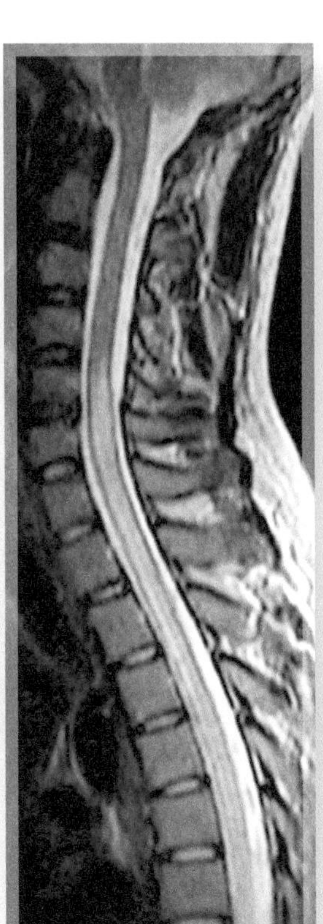
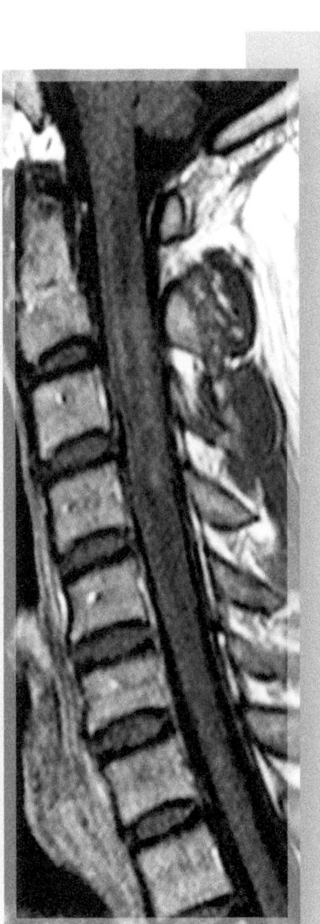
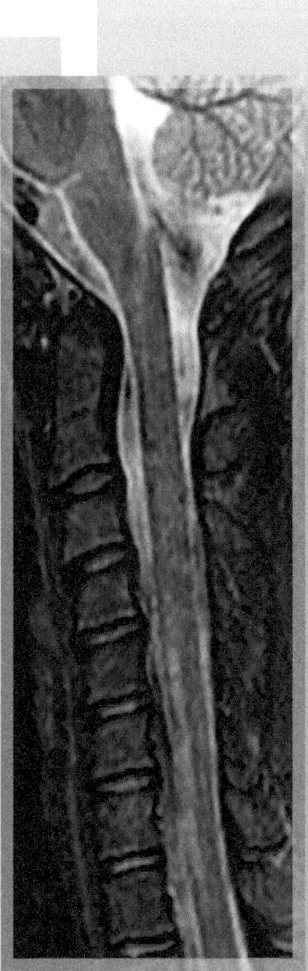

Pyogenic Osteomyelitis

KEY FACTS

TERMINOLOGY

- Bacterial suppurative infection of vertebrae & intervertebral disc

IMAGING

- Ill-defined, hypointense T1 vertebral marrow with loss of endplate definition on both sides of disc
- Loss of disc height & abnormal disc signal
- Destruction of vertebral endplate cortex
- Vertebral collapse
- Paraspinal ± epidural infiltrative soft tissue ± loculated fluid collection

TOP DIFFERENTIAL DIAGNOSES

- Degenerative endplate changes
- Tuberculous vertebral osteomyelitis
- Spinal neuropathic arthropathy

PATHOLOGY

- Predisposing factors
  - Intravenous drug use
  - Immunocompromised state
  - Chronic medical illnesses (renal failure, cirrhosis, cancer, diabetes)
- *Staphylococcus aureus* is most common pathogen

CLINICAL ISSUES

- Acute or chronic back pain
- Focal spinal tenderness
- Fever
- ↑ ESR, ↑ CRP, ↑ WBC

DIAGNOSTIC CHECKLIST

- Diffusely enhancing disc, adjacent vertebral marrow, soft tissue with endplate erosion highly suggestive
- Imaging remains abnormal long after patient clinically improves

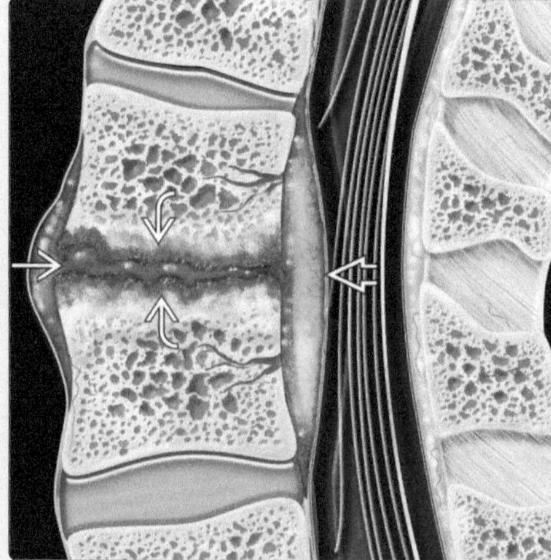

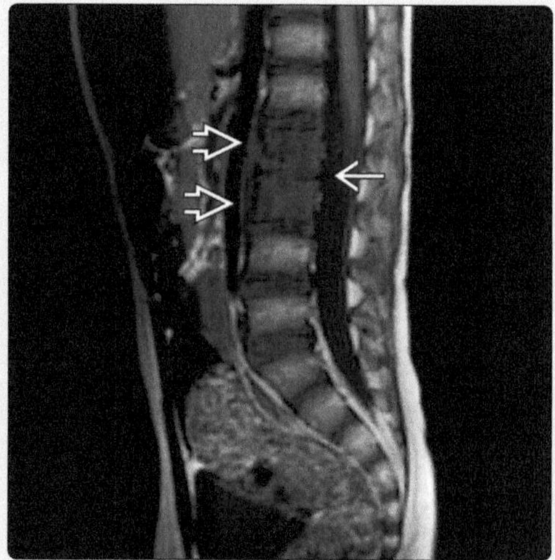

(Left) *Sagittal graphic of the lumbar spine demonstrates pyogenic infection within the intervertebral disc space ➡ with epidural extension ➡ and endplate destruction ➡.* **(Right)** *Sagittal T1 MR in a pediatric patient with fever and back pain demonstrates narrowing of the L2/L3 disc space ➡ with marrow edema in the L2 and L3 vertebra. Prevertebral soft tissue inflammation ➡ confirms extradural extension.*

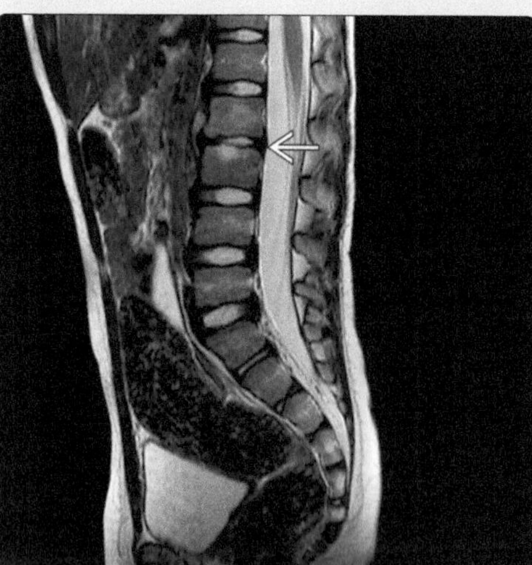

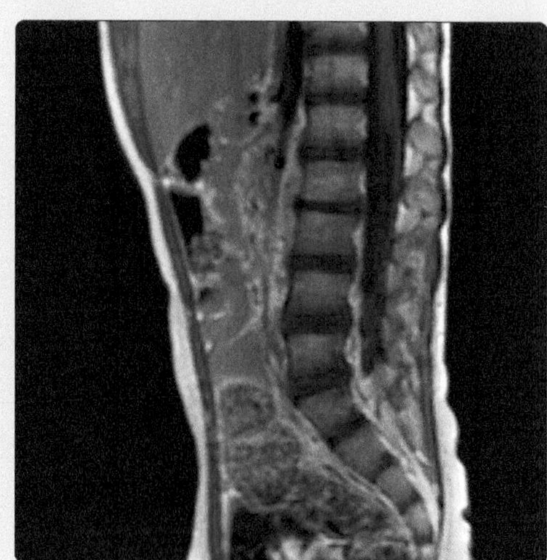

(Left) *Sagittal T2 MR in the same patient depicts narrowing of the L2/L3 disc space ➡ with relatively subtle marrow edema in the L2 and L3 vertebra, compared to T1 MR.* **(Right)** *Sagittal T1 C+ MR in the same patient confirms marrow and prevertebral soft tissue enhancement. Marrow edema is frequently most obvious on unenhanced T1 MR and may be difficult to recognize on T2 MR and T1 C+ MR if fat suppression techniques are not used.*

TERMINOLOGY

Synonyms

- Pyogenic spondylodiscitis, disc space infection

Definitions

- Bacterial suppurative infection of vertebrae & intervertebral disc

IMAGING

General Features

- Best diagnostic clue
  - Ill-defined, hypointense vertebral marrow on T1WI with loss of endplate definition on both sides of disc
- Location
  - All spinal segments involved
    - Lumbar (48%) > thoracic (35%) > cervical spine (6.5%)
- Morphology
  - Loss of disc height
  - Abnormal disc signal
  - Destruction of vertebral endplate cortex
  - Ill-defined marrow signal alteration
  - Vertebral collapse
  - Paraspinal ± epidural infiltrative soft tissue ± loculated fluid collection
    - Present in 75% of pyogenic vertebral osteomyelitis

Radiographic Findings

- Radiography
  - Negative up to 2-8 weeks after onset of symptoms
  - Initial endplate & vertebral osteolysis followed by increased bone density
  - Paraspinal soft tissue density & loss of fat planes
  - Fusion across disc space late in disease course

CT Findings

- NECT
  - Endplate osteolytic/osteosclerotic changes
  - Spinal deformity best seen on coronal & sagittal reformation
  - Increase in paraspinal soft tissue
- CECT
  - Enhancing disc, marrow, & paravertebral soft tissue

MR Findings

- Disc space
  - Hypointense on T1WI
  - Variable, typically hyperintense on T2WI
  - Diffuse or rim enhancement with gadolinium
  - Loss of height
- Vertebral marrow signal abnormality abutting disc
  - Hypointense on T1WI
  - Hyperintense on fat-saturated T2WI or STIR
  - Avid enhancement with gadolinium
- Paraspinal & epidural phlegmon or abscess
  - Isointense to muscle on T1WI
  - Hyperintense on T2WI
  - Diffuse or rim enhancement
- Cord compression
- DWI
  - Acute: Vertebral bodies, endplates, & discs hyperintense
  - Chronic: Hypointense
- Follow-up MR
  - No single MR finding was associated with clinical status
  - Less paraspinal inflammation & less epidural enhancement compared with baseline
  - Vertebral body, disc space enhancement, & bone marrow edema equivocal or worse compared with baseline

Nuclear Medicine Findings

- Bone scan
  - 3-phase Tc-99m diphosphonate scan shows increased activity in all phases
- Gallium scan
  - Increased uptake of gallium citrate (Ga-67)
    - Increased sensitivity with SPECT
- WBC scan
  - Often false-negative in patients with chronic vertebral osteomyelitis

Imaging Recommendations

- Best imaging tool
  - Sagittal & axial T2WI & T1WI MR
    - Sensitivity (96%), specificity (92%), accuracy (94%)
  - SPECT Ga-67 scan good alternative
    - Sensitivity & specificity in low 90%
- Protocol advice
  - STIR or FSE T2 with fat suppression most sensitive for marrow edema, epidural involvement
  - Postgadolinium T1WI with fat suppression also improves MR sensitivity
    - Improves evaluation of epidural & soft tissues

DIFFERENTIAL DIAGNOSIS

Degenerative Endplate Changes

- Most common mimic
- Disc desiccation
  - Hypointense on T1WI & T2WI
  - Minimal or absent enhancement with gadolinium
- Vertebral endplates preserved

Tuberculous Vertebral Osteomyelitis

- Midthoracic or thoracolumbar > lumbar or cervical
- Vertebral collapse, gibbus deformity
- ± endplate destructive changes
- Large dissecting paraspinal abscesses out of proportion to vertebral involvement

Spinal Neuropathic Arthropathy

- Sequela of spinal cord injury
- Disc space loss/T2 hyperintensity, endplate erosion/sclerosis, osteophytosis, soft tissue mass
  - Present in both spondylodiscitis & neuropathic spine
- Vacuum disc/rim enhancement, facet involvement, spondylolisthesis, debris, disorganization

Chronic Hemodialysis Spondyloarthropathy

- Cervical spine most common
- Disc space loss, endplate erosion, vertebral destruction
- Vertebral marrow hypointense on both T1WI & T2WI

- Low to intermediate disc signal intensity on T2WI

Spinal Metastases

- Discrete or ill-defined vertebral lesions
  - Hypointense on T1WI
  - Hyperintense on T2WI
  - Postgadolinium enhancement
- Posterior elements commonly affected
- Disc space preserved

PATHOLOGY

General Features

- Etiology
  - Predisposing factors
    - Intravenous drug use
    - Immunocompromised state
    - Chronic medical illnesses (renal failure, cirrhosis, cancer, diabetes)
  - *Staphylococcus aureus* is most common pathogen in children & adults
    - *Escherichia coli* most common within gram-negative bacilli
    - *Salmonella* more common in patients with sickle cell disease
    - *Klebsiella kingae* in children 6 months to 4 years of age
  - Bacteremia from extraspinal primary source
    - Most common route of infection
    - GU or GI tract, pulmonary, cardiac, mucous/cutaneous sources
    - Vascularized subchondral bone adjacent to endplate seeded primarily
    - Secondary infection of intervertebral disc, adjacent vertebra
    - Intervertebral disc 1st site of infection in children due to presence of vascularity
  - Direct inoculation from penetrating trauma, surgical intervention, or diagnostic procedures
  - Extension from adjacent infection
    - Diverticulitis, appendicitis, inflammatory bowl disease
    - Pyelonephritis
- Associated abnormalities
  - Spinal meningitis
  - Vascular compromise of cord & myelitis

CLINICAL ISSUES

Presentation

- Most common signs/symptoms
  - Acute or chronic back pain
  - Focal spinal tenderness
  - Fever
- Other signs/symptoms
  - Myelopathy if cord compromised
  - Elevated ESR, CRP, WBC
- Clinical profile
  - Average duration of symptoms for 7 weeks before diagnosis

Demographics

- Age
  - Bimodal distribution
    - Pediatric patients
    - 6th-7th decades
- Epidemiology
  - 2-7% of all osteomyelitis occurs in spine

Natural History & Prognosis

- Mortality rate: 2-12%
- Favorable outcome; resolution of symptoms if prompt diagnosis & treatment
  - Residual functional deficits may be present in 15% of patients
- Recurrence due to incomplete treatment (2-8%)
- Irreversible neurologic deficits
  - Delay in diagnosis & neurologic impairment at diagnosis significant predictors of neurologic deficit at follow-up
  - Previous spinal surgery associated with adverse outcome: Readmission within 1 year of discharge following 1st spinal infection
  - Independent predictors of long-term disability
    - Neurologic impairment at time of diagnosis, time to diagnosis ≥ 8 weeks, & debilitating disease
- Improvement in imaging findings may lag behind clinical improvement

Treatment

- CT-guided or open biopsy yields causative organism more often than blood cultures (77% vs. 58%)
  - Previous antibiotic treatment significantly lowers yield (23% vs. 60%)
- Early empiric antibiotics, broad spectrum coverage until causative pathogen isolated
- Organism-specific parenteral antibiotics for 6-8 weeks
- Spinal immobilization with bracing for 6-12 weeks
- Surgical treatment
  - Laminectomy, debridement, ± stabilization
  - Especially if epidural abscess, instability present

DIAGNOSTIC CHECKLIST

Image Interpretation Pearls

- Diffusely enhancing disc, adjacent vertebral marrow, soft tissue with endplate erosion highly suggestive of vertebral osteomyelitis

SELECTED REFERENCES

1. Kim J et al: The epidemiology of concurrent infection in patients with pyogenic spine infection and its association with early mortality: a nationwide cohort study based on 10,695 patients. J Infect Public Health. 16(6):981-8, 2023
2. Holzmann J et al: Difficulties in diagnosing vertebral osteomyelitis in a child. BMJ Case Rep. 14:e236037, 2021
3. Kim UJ et al: Comparison of pyogenic postoperative and native vertebral osteomyelitis. Spine J. 19(5):880-7, 2019
4. Boody BS et al: Evaluation and management of pyogenic and tubercular spine infections. Curr Rev Musculoskelet Med. 11(4):643-52, 2018
5. Dayer R et al: Spinal infections in children: a multicentre retrospective study. Bone Joint J. 100-B(4):542-8, 2018
6. Lemaignen A et al: Characteristics of and risk factors for severe neurological deficit in patients with pyogenic vertebral osteomyelitis: a case-control study. Medicine (Baltimore). 96(21):e6387, 2017
7. Fantoni M et al: Epidemiological and clinical features of pyogenic spondylodiscitis. Eur Rev Med Pharmacol Sci. 16 Suppl 2:2-7, 2012

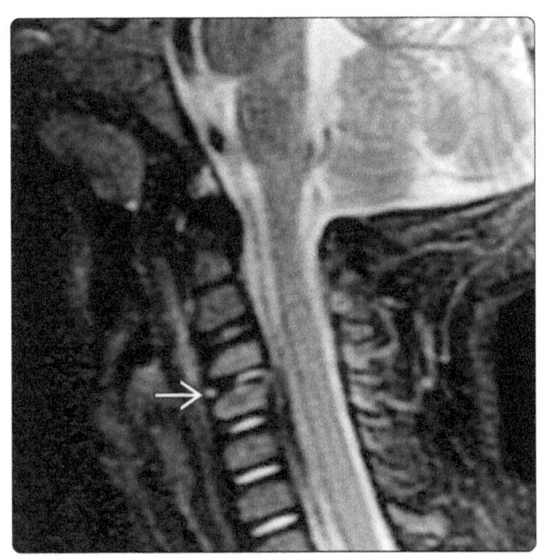

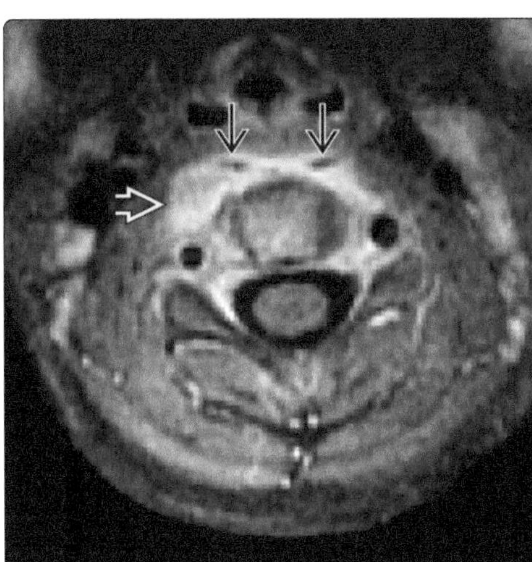

(Left) *Sagittal STIR MR in a preschool child with neck pain shows fluid signal and height loss of the C3/C4 interspace ➡ with mild focal kyphosis. There is mild vertebral marrow edema. No cord compression is evident.* **(Right)** *Axial T1 C+ FS MR confirms robust prevertebral and epidural enhancement ➡. Small, nonenhancing foci ➡ within the prevertebral inflammation represent anteriorly displaced longus coli muscles.*

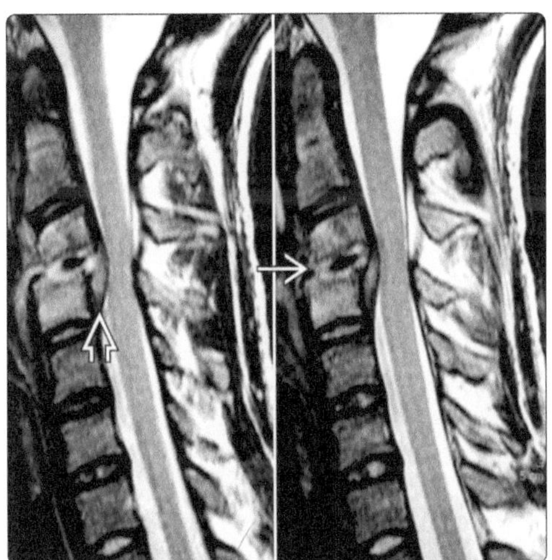

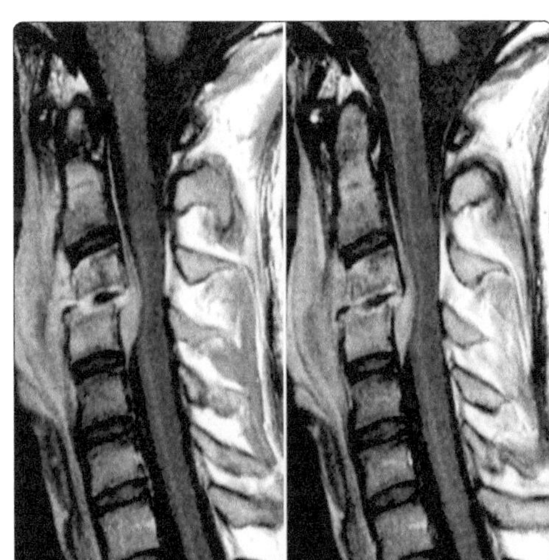

(Left) *Sagittal T2 MR in a school-aged child with severe neck pain reveals fluid signal within the C3/C4 interspace ➡ and retrolisthesis of C3 on C4. Epidural inflammation ➡ in conjunction with listhesis results in mild cord compression.* **(Right)** *Sagittal T1 C+ MR in the same patient confirms robust marrow, disc space, and epidural enhancement.*

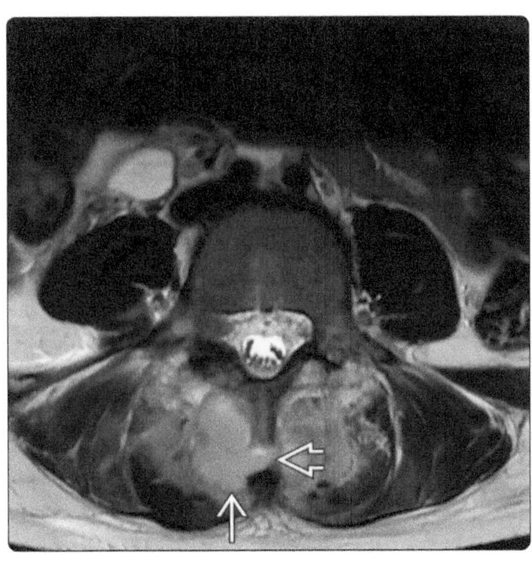

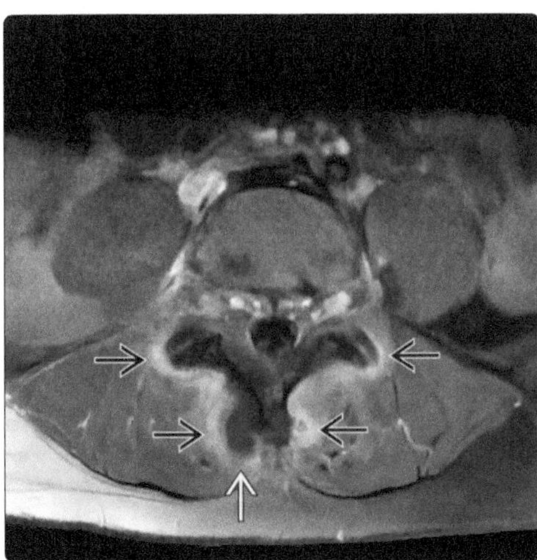

(Left) *Axial T2 MR in a 9-year-old with worsening back pain and fever after a spinous process avulsion fracture reveals bilateral paraspinal muscle edema and fluid collection ➡ communicating with the fracture site ➡.* **(Right)** *Axial T1 C+ FS MR in the same patient confirms robust enhancement of inflamed paraspinal soft tissue ➡ as well as rim enhancement surrounding the paraspinal abscess collection ➡. Abscess aspiration grew methicillin-resistant Staphylococcus aureus (MRSA) bacteria.*

KEY FACTS

TERMINOLOGY

- Tuberculous spondylitis (TS)
- Granulomatous infection of spine and adjacent soft tissue secondary to tuberculosis

IMAGING

- Gibbus vertebrae with relatively intact intervertebral discs, large paraspinal abscesses
- Midthoracic or thoracolumbar > lumbar, cervical
- Isolated posterior element involvement possible
- Sagittal STIR or FSE T2 with fat saturation most sensitive for bone marrow edema, epidural involvement
  - MR best modality to evaluate extent of disease, assess response to treatment

TOP DIFFERENTIAL DIAGNOSES

- Pyogenic spondylitis
  - Initial infection in subchondral bone
  - Intervertebral discs typically affected
- Fungal spondylitis
- Spinal metastases
  - Extraosseous epidural or paraspinal extension
  - Disc space preserved
- Brucellar spondylitis

PATHOLOGY

- Hematogenous or lymphatic spread
- Initial inoculum in anterior vertebral body
- Spread to noncontiguous vertebral bodies beneath longitudinal ligaments

CLINICAL ISSUES

- Chronic back pain, focal tenderness, fever
- Neurologic deficits more common with TS than other granulomatous infections

DIAGNOSTIC CHECKLIST

- Thoracic spondylitis with posterior element involvement, large paraspinal abscesses suggests TS

(Left) *Sagittal graphic through the lumbar spine depicts multifocal granulomatous osteomyelitis. Frank abscesses are present at the L3-L4 disc space ➡ and between spinous process of L2 and L3 ➡.* **(Right)** *Sagittal T2 MR in a 7-year-old patient with tuberculous spondylitis and gibbus deformity shows destructive changes of 2 consecutive thoracic vertebra ➡. There is anterior subligamentous spread ➡. Note that the adjacent discs are spared. The spinal cord shows mild compression.*

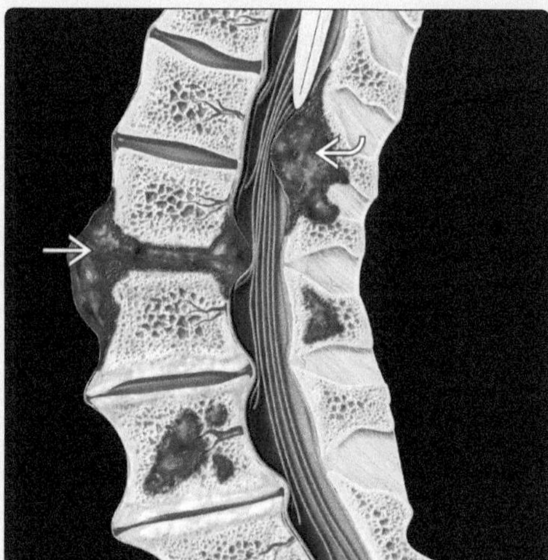

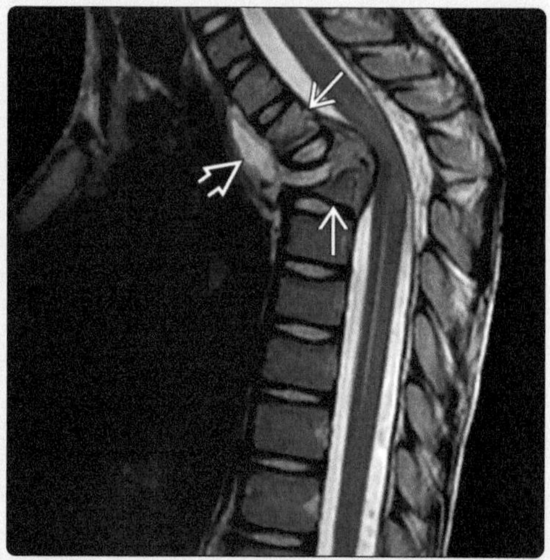

(Left) *Sagittal T1 C+ MR in the same patient confirms avid enhancement within areas of inflammation. There is both epidural ➡ and anterior subligamentous ➡ spread as well as tracking along the spinous processes ➡. The epidural component contributes to cord compression along with kyphosis.* **(Right)** *Sagittal bone CT performed for surgical planning confirms bone destruction leading to the focal kyphotic curvature. The spinous processes show more chronic bone changes ➡.*

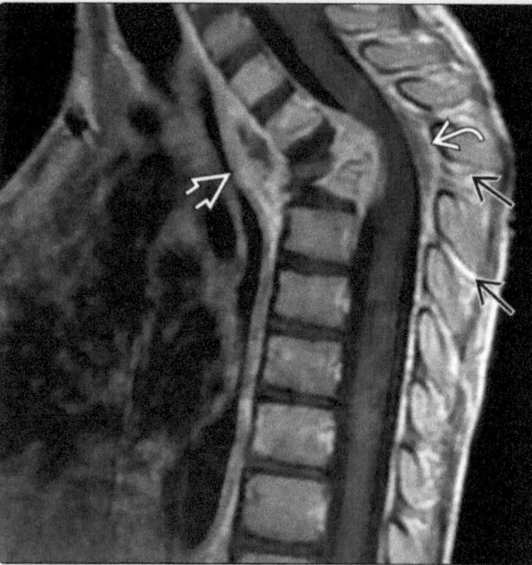

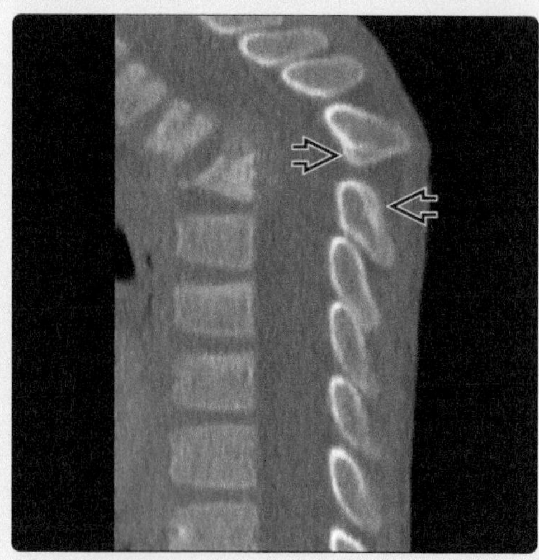

TERMINOLOGY

Definitions

- Granulomatous infection of spine and adjacent soft tissue secondary to tuberculosis (TB)

IMAGING

General Features

- Best diagnostic clue
  - Gibbus vertebrae with relatively intact intervertebral discs, large paraspinal abscesses
- Location
  - Midthoracic or thoracolumbar > lumbar, cervical
  - Anterior vertebral body
  - Isolated posterior element involvement possible
  - Laminae > pedicles > spinous process > transverse process
- Size
  - Multiple (non)contiguous vertebrae
- Morphology
  - Vertebral collapse, gibbus deformity
  - ± destruction of intervertebral discs
  - Epidural soft tissue mass
  - Large dissecting paraspinal abscesses over considerable distance
  - Tuberculous spondylitis (TS) has higher rate of psoas abscess and involvement of posterior elements compared to brucellar spondylitis (BS)

Radiographic Findings

- Radiography
  - Endplate irregularity, osteolysis
  - Diffuse vertebral sclerosis
  - Fusion across disc space in late TS
  - Findings may not be present until weeks after onset of infection

CT Findings

- NECT
  - Endplate destruction with vertebral body fragmentation
  - Calcified chronic paravertebral abscesses: TS > BS
- CECT
  - Diffuse or peripherally enhancing epidural and paraspinal soft tissue

MR Findings

- T1WI
  - Hypointense marrow in contiguous vertebrae
  - Hypointense intraosseous, extradural, paraspinal abscesses
- T2WI
  - Hyperintense marrow, disc, phlegmon/abscess
- STIR
  - Hyperintense marrow, disc, phlegmon/abscess
- DWI
  - Vertebral bodies, endplates, and discs: Acute → hyperintense; chronic → hypointense
- T1WI C+
  - Marrow, subligamentous, discal, dural enhancement
  - Diffusely enhancing soft tissue (phlegmon)
  - Peripherally enhancing soft tissue (abscess)
- Epidural abscess → cord displacement or compression
- May have extradural infection without bone destruction
- Atypical findings in TS
  - Isolated vertebral body or posterior element involvement
    - Posterior element TB: 3-5% of TS
      - Potential for coronal decompensation
  - Sacral involvement

Nuclear Medicine Findings

- Bone scan
  - Increased spinal radionuclide uptake
  - Sensitive but not specific
- Gallium scan: Increased radionuclide uptake in spine and paraspinal soft tissue
  - Highly sensitive and specific for vertebral osteomyelitis

Imaging Recommendations

- Best imaging tool
  - Sagittal and axial T1WI, T2WI, and T1 C+ MR
    - Evaluate extent of disease, assess response to treatment
- Protocol advice
  - Sagittal STIR or FSE T2 with fat saturation most sensitive for bone marrow edema, epidural involvement

DIFFERENTIAL DIAGNOSIS

Pyogenic Osteomyelitis

- Peak incidence in older patients
- Predilection for lower lumbar spine
- Initial infection in subchondral bone adjacent to endplate
  - Intervertebral discs typically affected
- Posterior element involvement less common
- Soft tissue calcifications and spinal deformity infrequent

Fungal Osteomyelitis

- May be indistinguishable from TS

Brucellar Spondylitis

- Anterosuperior epiphysitis at L4 with associated sacroiliitis
- In general, lower severity of vertebral destruction, vertebral posterior convex deformity, dead bone, and abscess scope compared to TS
  - May be indistinguishable from TS

Lytic and Blastic Osseous Metastases

- T1-hypointense, T2-hyperintense signal
  - Postgadolinium enhancement
  - Posterior elements typically involved
- Extraosseous epidural or paraspinal extension
- Pathologic compression fractures
- Disc space preserved
- May be difficult to distinguish from isolated tuberculous, fungal, or BS

Degenerative Disc Disease

- Modic type 1 changes may mimic infection
  - T1-hypointense, T2-hyperintense signal
  - Inflammatory marrow change

PATHOLOGY

General Features

- Etiology
  - Hematogenous spread or through lymphatics from pulmonary origin
  - Initial inoculum in anterior vertebral body
  - Spread to noncontiguous vertebral bodies beneath longitudinal ligaments
  - Sparing of intervertebral disc secondary to lack of proteolytic enzymes
  - Paraspinal, subarachnoid dissemination of disease
  - Other pathogens causing granulomatous osteomyelitis (*Streptomyces*, *Madurella*) uncommon
- Associated abnormalities
  - Intramedullary abscess
  - Arachnoiditis
- Granulomatous destruction of spinal column with adjacent soft tissue infection

Microscopic Features

- Caseating granulomas, nonspecific inflammatory reaction
- Acid-fast bacilli isolated < 50% of time

CLINICAL ISSUES

Presentation

- Most common signs/symptoms
  - Chronic back pain (~ 95%), focal tenderness, fever
  - Radicular pain
- Other signs/symptoms
  - Paraparesis, kyphosis, sensory disturbance
  - Bladder and bowel dysfunction
  - Osseoligamentous destruction at craniovertebral junction → atlantoaxial instability and compression of cervicomedullary junction
    - → quadriparesis, bulbar dysfunction, and respiratory insufficiency
  - Systemic toxemia
- Clinical profile
  - Gradual, insidious onset of symptoms results in diagnostic delay
  - Fever relatively infrequent in TS
  - Neurologic deficits more common with TS than other granulomatous infections, such as BS
  - TS has significant high rate of accompanying chronic renal failure, constitutional symptoms, history of TB, increased ESR, ± surgical treatment
  - QuantiFERON assay: Interferon-γ release assay
    - Sensitivity (84%), specificity (95%)
    - Combination of radiologic criteria, bone scan, ELISA, QuantiFERON assay is 90% predictive of TS

Demographics

- Age
  - Most prevalent in 5th decade
- Sex
  - M = F in TS
- Epidemiology
  - Spinal TB accounts for 2% of all TB cases
    - Rising incidence of TB in past 2 decades
    - Trend toward increased incidence in parallel with growing number of immunocompromised patients
  - Concomitant pulmonary TB in ~ 10% of patients
  - Reactivation of latent TB with anti-TNF therapies
  - TB-associated immune reconstitution inflammatory syndrome (TB-IRIS) → complication in HIV-1-infected TB patients on antiretroviral treatment
    - Neurologic manifestations occur in > 10% of TB-IRIS cases
  - Evidence for increased risk of serious local infections after kyphoplasty in patients with history of systemic infection
  - TS more aggressive in children
    - Kyphosis, cord compression more common

Natural History & Prognosis

- Prognosis depends on early diagnosis and institution of appropriate therapy
- Proper treatment leads to
  - Favorable outcome with resolution of symptoms
    - Particularly favorable if early presentation and lack of neurologic deficits or spinal deformity
- No treatment leads to
  - Progressive vertebral collapse
  - Irreversible neurologic deficits
  - Death

Treatment

- Long-term antituberculous medication for at least 1 year
- Surgical decompression in setting of neurologic deficits ± spinal deformity
  - Indicated in 10-25% of TS
  - Laminectomy and debridement in absence of vertebral destruction
  - Debridement and fusion if spinal deformity present

DIAGNOSTIC CHECKLIST

Image Interpretation Pearls

- Thoracic spondylitis with posterior element involvement, large paraspinal abscesses suggests TS

SELECTED REFERENCES

1. Abdallah A et al: Surgical outcome of spinal subdural abscesses: a report of four consecutive patients and brief review of the literature. J Neurol Surg A Cent Eur Neurosurg. 84(1):77-90, 2023
2. Igbokwe V et al: Post-tuberculosis sequelae in children and adolescents: a systematic review. Lancet Infect Dis. 23(4):e138-50, 2023
3. Kafle G et al: Diagnostic yield of image-guided biopsy in patients with suspected infectious spondylodiscitis : a prospective study from a tuberculosis-endemic country. Bone Joint J. 104-B(1):120-6, 2022
4. Guo H et al: Differentiating brucella spondylitis from tuberculous spondylitis by the conventional MRI and MR T2 mapping: a prospective study. Eur J Med Res. 26(1):125, 2021
5. Zeng H et al: Analysis of clinical characteristics of 556 spinal tuberculosis patients in two tertiary teaching hospitals in Guangxi province. Biomed Res Int. 2021:1344496, 2021
6. Liang W et al: Comparison of the clinical efficacy of 3 surgical methods for treating spinal tuberculosis in children. Med Sci Monit. 26:e926142, 2020
7. Patel AR et al: Spinal epidural abscesses: risk factors, medical versus surgical management, a retrospective review of 128 cases. Spine J. 14(2):326-30, 2014

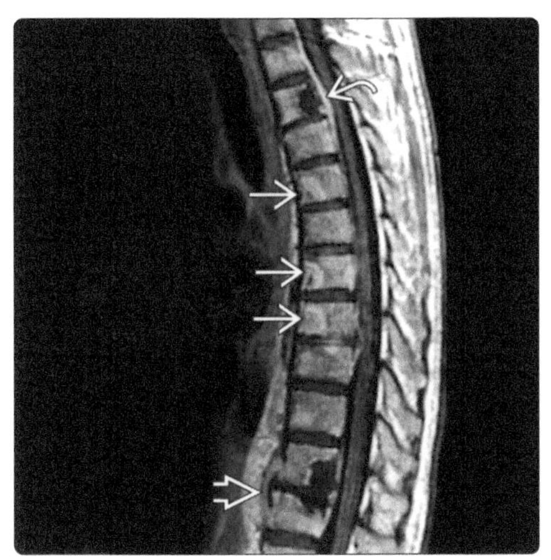

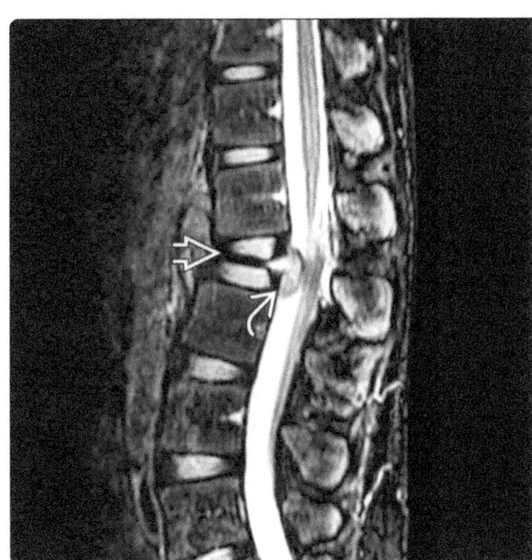

(Left) *Sagittal T1 C+ MR in tuberculosis (TB) shows contiguous vertebral body extension with subligamentous abscess spread and partial disc involvement ➡. Note multiple other focal bone lesions ➡ with mild epidural extension ➡, which can mimic metastases.* **(Right)** *Sagittal T2 FS MR demonstrates collapse of the L2 vertebral body ➡. Adjacent intervertebral discs are now contiguous with each other. There is a focal abscess collection ➡ protruding posteriorly with compression of thecal sac contents.*

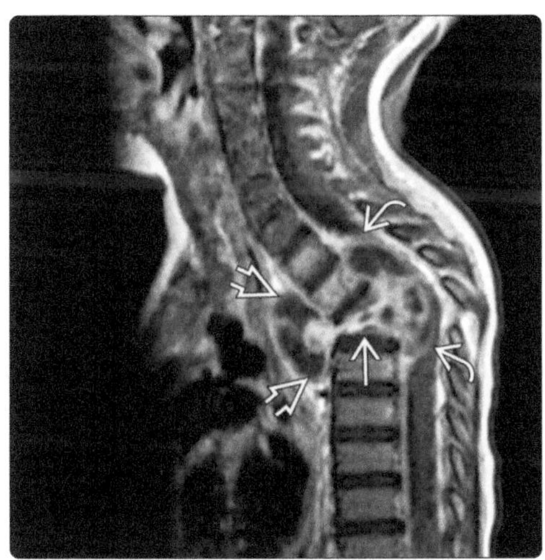

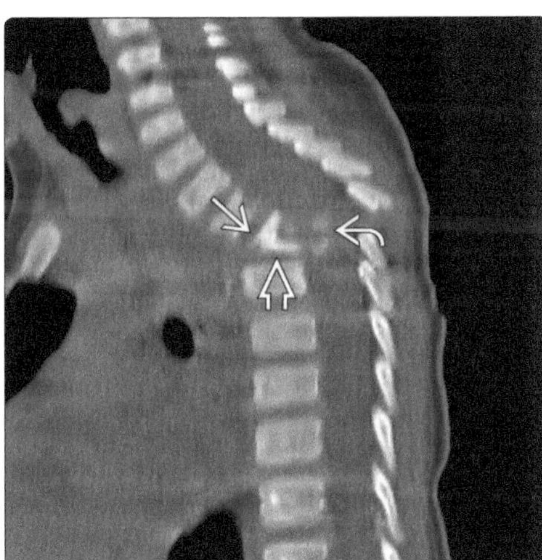

(Left) *Sagittal T1 C+ MR illustrates thoracic spinal TB with abnormally enhancing vertebral bodies and kyphotic deformity ➡. Large epidural abscess causes severe cord compression ➡. The paraspinal abscess shows typical peripheral enhancement ➡.* **(Right)** *Sagittal CT exhibits destruction of the T4-T6 bodies with kyphotic deformity and extension of calcific abscess/bone into the paravertebral region and spinal canal ➡. Only residual T4 ➡ and T6 ➡ endplates remain after T5 destruction.*

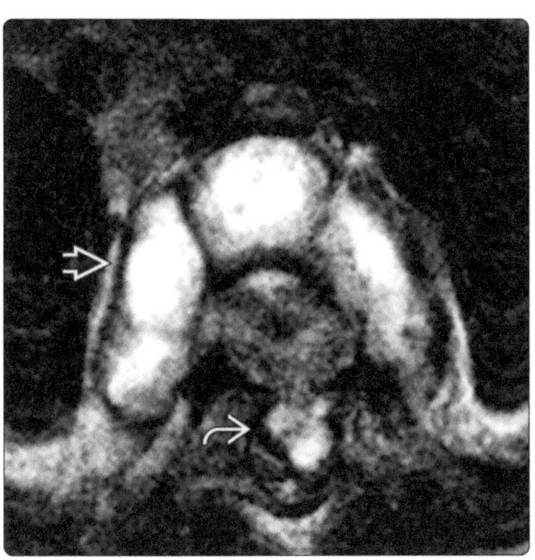

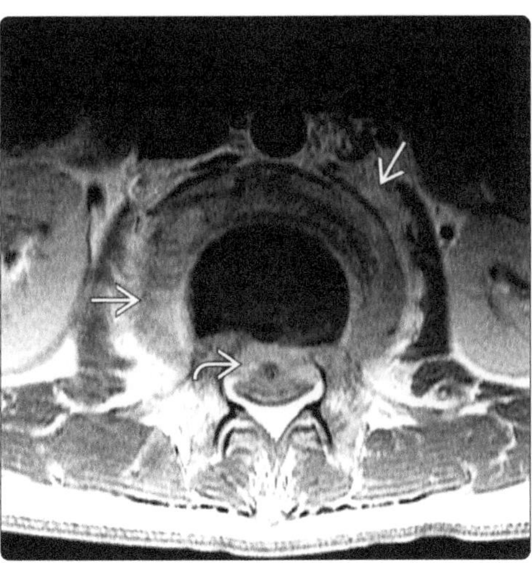

(Left) *Axial T2 MR of a patient with thoracic TB demonstrates a large prevertebral abscess ➡ with extension into the spinal canal ➡, which causes mild mass effect on the thecal sac.* **(Right)** *Axial T1 C+ MR illustrates a focal abscess collection ➡ protruding posteriorly with compression of thecal sac contents. Inflammatory soft tissue surrounds the disc ➡ and extends into the adjacent psoas muscles. Pott disease, named after Percivall Pott, is extrapulmonary TB affecting the spine.*

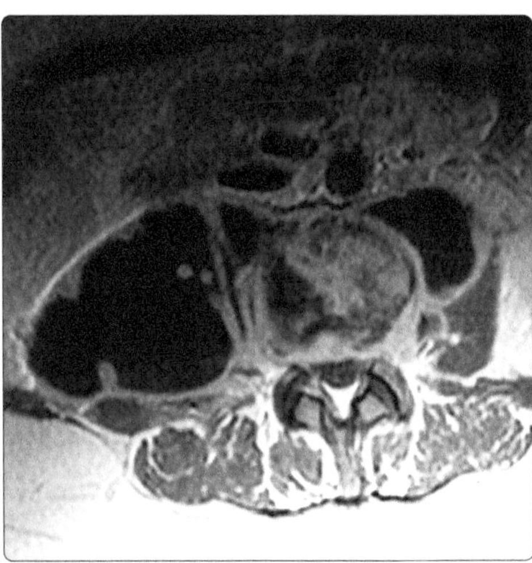

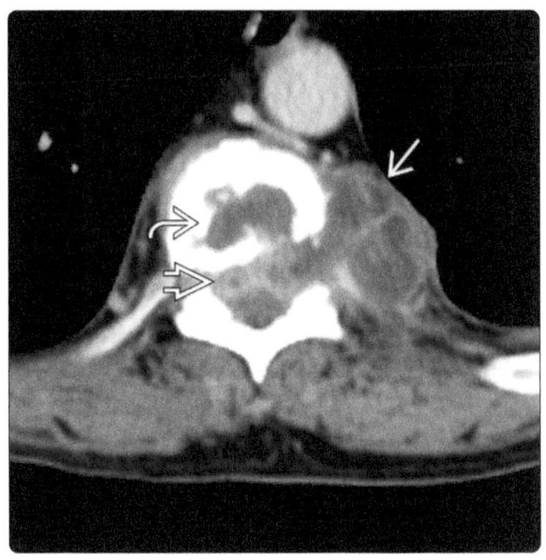

(Left) *Axial T1 C+ MR shows bilateral large psoas abscesses, right much larger than left, in this patient with tuberculous spondylitis.* **(Right)** *Axial CECT shows a rim-enhancing abscess ➡ with central low attenuation. Enhancing material is present in the epidural space with cord compression ➡. Large erosions are present in the vertebral body ➡.*

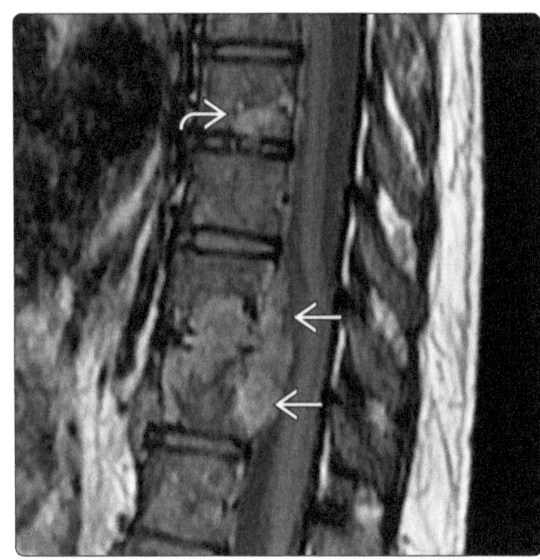

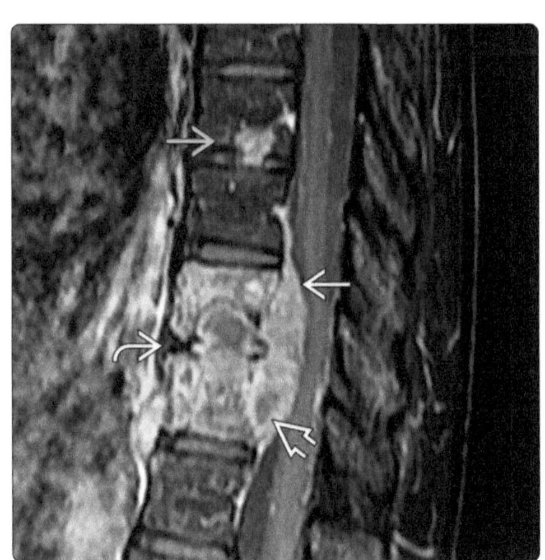

(Left) *Sagittal T1 MR without contrast shows the typical pattern of disc space infection with large ventral epidural phlegmon ➡ in this patient with tuberculous spondylitis. Note the 2nd area of vertebral body involvement ➡.* **(Right)** *Sagittal T1 C+ FS MR shows diffuse enhancement of the large ventral epidural phlegmon ➡ with a small focus of nonenhancing abscess ➡. There is disc space and adjacent vertebral body involvement ➡. Note the 2nd vertebral body focus ➡.*

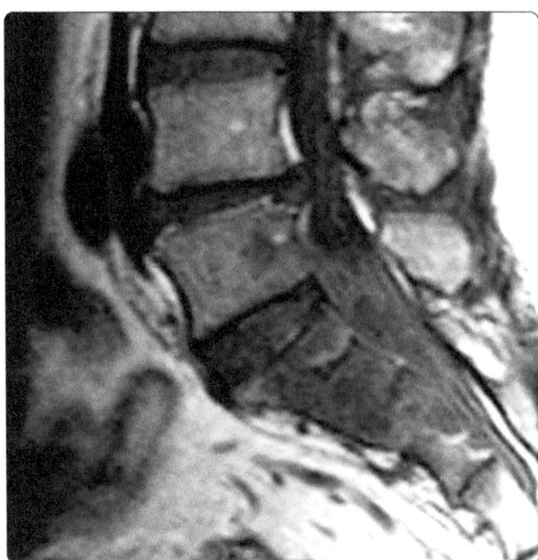

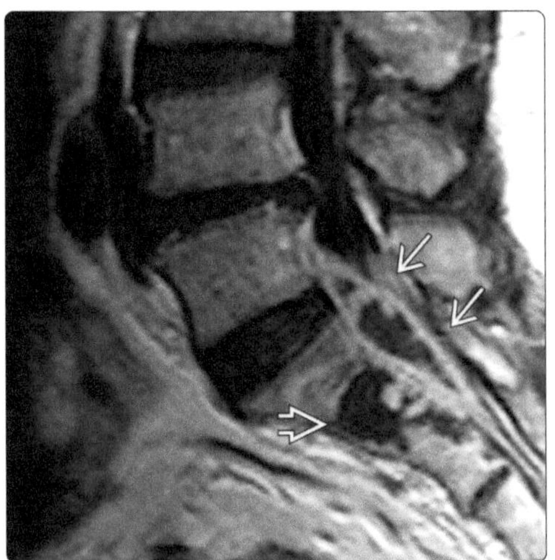

(Left) *Sagittal T1 MR shows abnormal low signal from posterior L5, S1, and S2 bodies and obscuration of the thecal sac below the L5 disc level. There is sparing of the L5 disc. This patient was diagnosed with tuberculous spondylitis.* **(Right)** *Sagittal T1 C+ MR shows a large nonenhancing area of bone abscess/necrosis ➡ with extension of large abscess into ventral epidural space compressing distal sac ➡.*

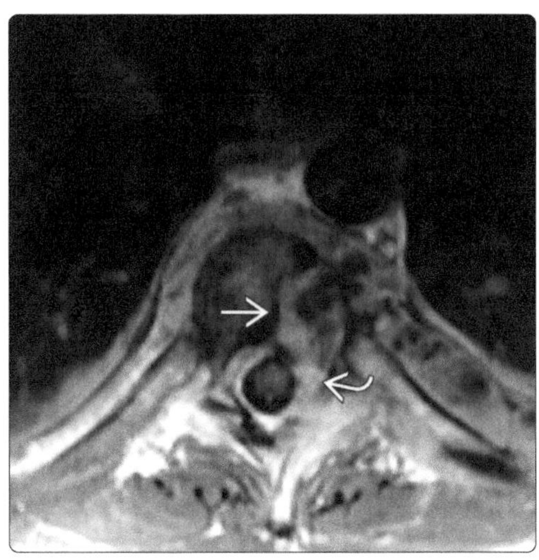

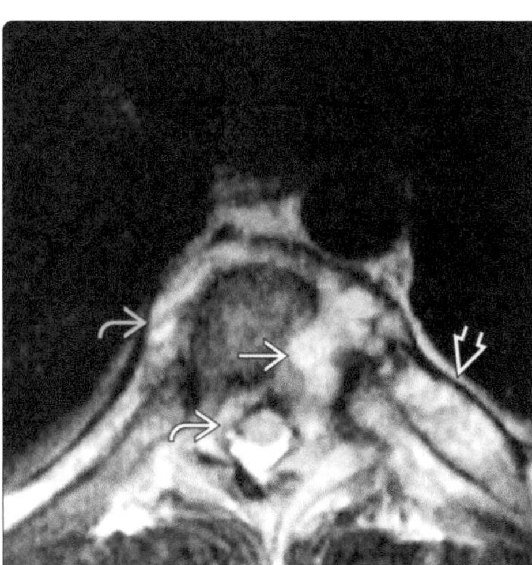

(Left) *Axial T1 C+ MR in this patient with brucellar osteomyelitis shows bone destruction ➔ with diffuse enhancing phlegmon within the epidural space ➔ and paravertebral region.* **(Right)** *Axial T2 MR in this patient with brucellar osteomyelitis shows abnormal increased signal with bone destruction ➔ and expansion ➔. There is involvement of epidural space ➔ and paravertebral region ➔.*

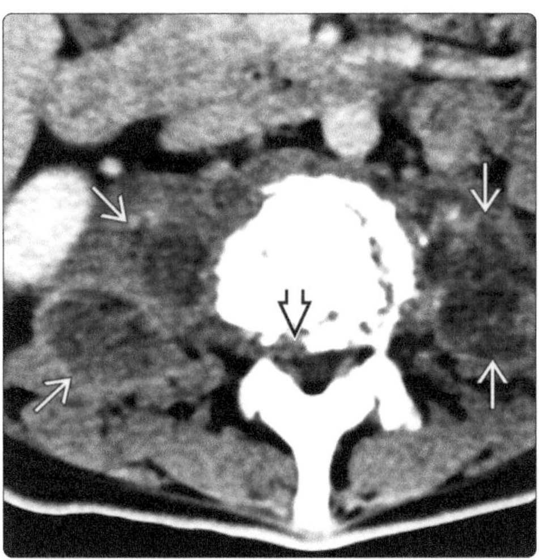

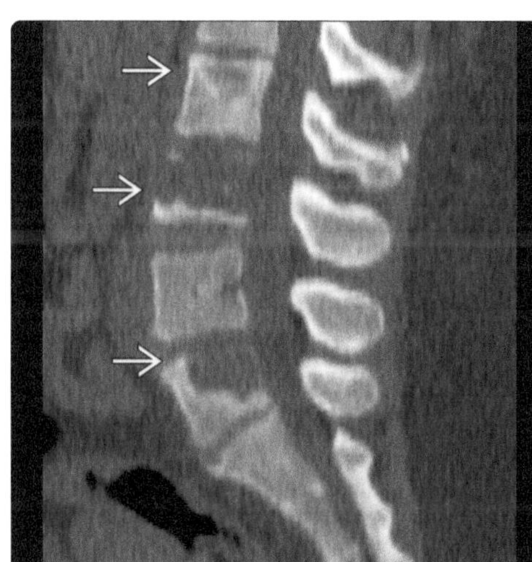

(Left) *Axial CECT reveals a case of brucellosis granulomatous discitis-osteomyelitis. There is vertebral destruction and bilateral psoas abscesses present ➔. There is also epidural extension narrowing the central spinal canal ➔.* **(Right)** *Sagittal NECT shows multiple focal areas of bone destruction involving L2, L3, and L5 ➔ with preservation of the disc spaces and minimal prevertebral soft tissue in this patient with coccidioidomycosis.*

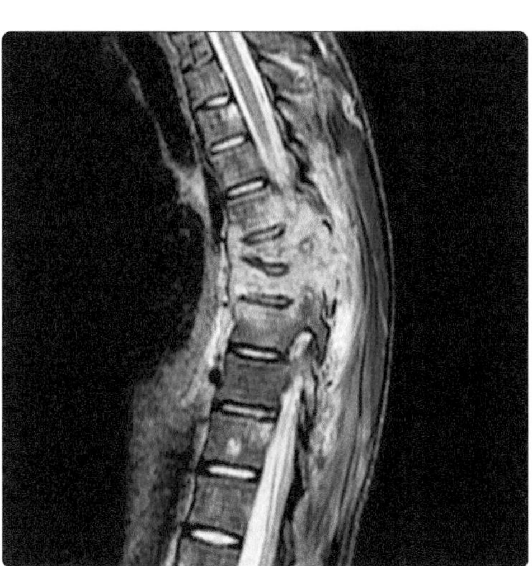

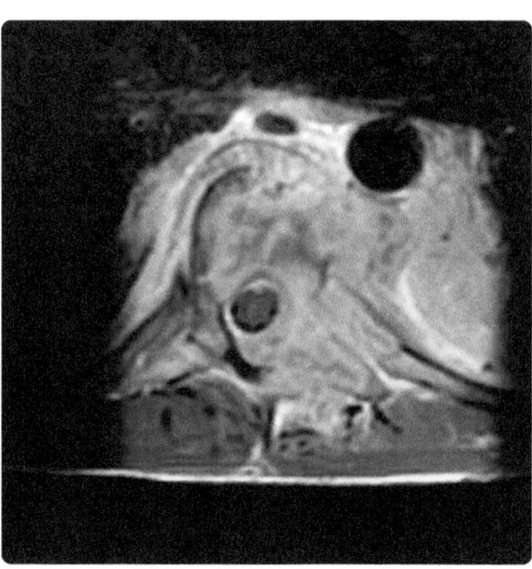

(Left) *Sagittal STIR MR shows diffuse abnormal T2 signal from bone destruction and soft tissue phlegmon involving multiple thoracic bodies and posterior elements, conspicuously sparing the intervertebral discs. Pathology was coccidioidomycosis.* **(Right)** *Axial T1 C+ MR shows soft tissue enhancement and involvement of both vertebral body and posterior elements with epidural extension. Note the paraspinal and adjacent lung extension. This patient had disseminated coccidioidomycosis.*

Idiopathic Acute Transverse Myelitis

KEY FACTS

TERMINOLOGY

- Inflammatory disorder involving both halves of spinal cord, resulting in bilateral motor, sensory, and autonomic dysfunction

IMAGING

- Central cord expansile lesion > 2 vertebral segments in length ± variable eccentric enhancement

TOP DIFFERENTIAL DIAGNOSES

- Multiple sclerosis
- Neuromyelitis optica spectrum disorders
- Myelin oligodendrocyte glycoprotein antibody disease
- Spinal cord neoplasm
- Spinal cord infarction

PATHOLOGY

- Autoimmune phenomenon with formation of antigen-antibody complexes

CLINICAL ISSUES

- Inclusion criteria
  - Sensory, motor, or autonomic dysfunction attributable to spinal cord
  - Bilateral signs/symptoms with well-defined sensory level
  - Compressive etiology excluded by neuroimaging
  - Cord inflammation confirmed by CSF pleocytosis, elevated IgG index, or gadolinium enhancement
- Exclusion criteria
  - History of spinal radiation within past 10 years
  - Cord ischemia/infarction, arteriovenous malformation
  - Connective tissue diseases
  - CNS infections, sarcoidosis, systemic lupus erythematosus (SLE), or Sjögren syndrome

DIAGNOSTIC CHECKLIST

- Central cord lesion > 2 vertebra in length, eccentric enhancement → consider acute transverse myelitis

(Left) *Sagittal T2WI MR in a patient with acute transverse myelitis demonstrates mild, multilevel cervical cord expansion with confluent intramedullary T2 hyperintensity* ➡ *extending over 5 vertebral levels.* **(Right)** *Sagittal T1WI MR in the same patient reveals mild cervical cord expansion with subtle central intramedullary hypointensity* ➡*. Lesion extent on T1 MR is usually less conspicuous than on T2 MR.*

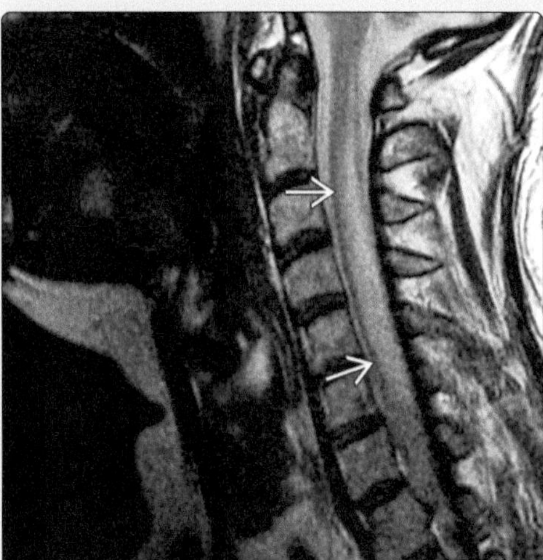

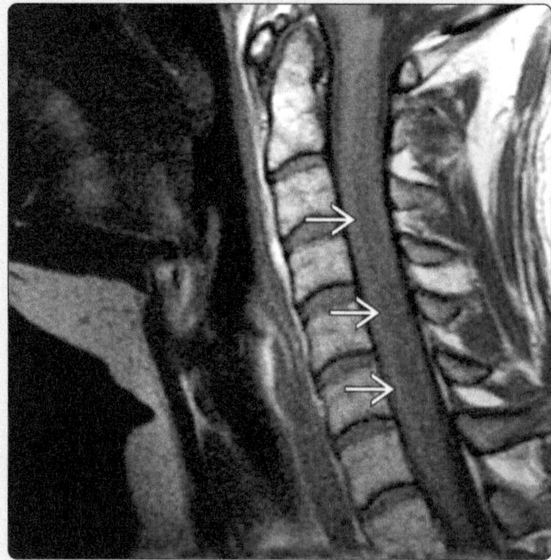

(Left) *Axial T1WI C+ MR in the same patient illustrates patchy, bilateral, central heterogeneous cervical spinal cord enhancement* ➡ *involving both gray and white matter in both hemicords.* **(Right)** *Sagittal T1WI C+ MR in the same patient confirms extensive parenchymal enhancement within the abnormal dorsal cervical spinal cord* ➡*.*

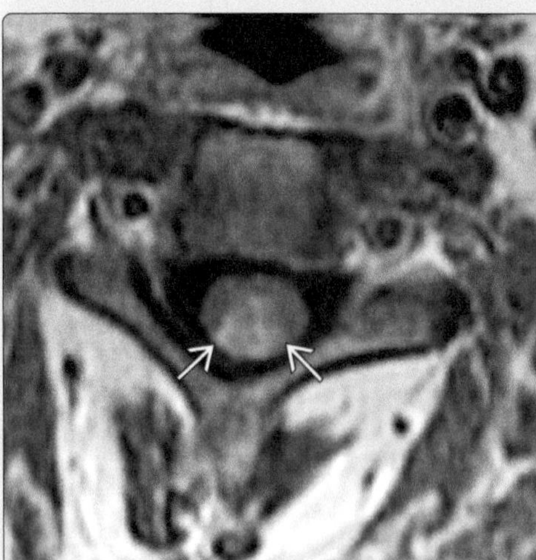

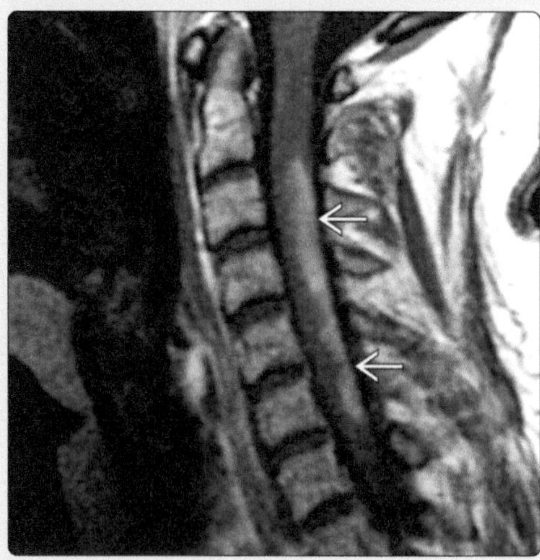

TERMINOLOGY

Abbreviations

- Idiopathic acute transverse myelitis (IATM)

Synonyms

- Idiopathic transverse myelopathy

Definitions

- Inflammatory disorder involving both halves of spinal cord, resulting in bilateral motor, sensory, and autonomic dysfunction
- Diagnosis of exclusion

IMAGING

General Features

- Best diagnostic clue
  - Central cord lesion > 2 vertebral segments in length with eccentric enhancement
- Location
  - Thoracic most common
  - 10% in cervical cord
  - Central cord location on axial imaging
- Size
  - > 2 vertebral segments in length
    - Commonly 3-4 segments
  - > 2/3 of cross-sectional area of cord on axial imaging
- Morphology
  - Well circumscribed

MR Findings

- T1WI
  - Smooth cord expansion in acute phase
    - Less extensive than T2 signal abnormality
  - Iso- to hypointense
  - Cord atrophy in late stage
- T2WI
  - Hyperintense cord expansion
  - Central dot sign
    - Central gray matter surrounded by edema
- STIR
  - Hyperintense cord expansion
- DWI
  - Significantly ↓ fractional anisotropy (FA) in lesions and distal (normal-appearing) spinal cord
  - FA ↓ in distal normal-appearing spinal cord might be related to clinical outcome
- T1WI C+
  - Variable appearance postgadolinium enhancement
    - No enhancement in up to 40-50% cases
    - Enhancement more common when cord enlargement present
      - More frequent in subacute than acute or chronic stages
        - Resolves over time
      - Enhancing area less extensive than T2 hyperintensity
    - Solitary or multifocal lesions
      - Focal, nodular, subtle, or patchy enhancement
      - Peripheral lesion enhancement
    - ± meningeal enhancement
  - Enhancement not predictive of clinical course

Imaging Recommendations

- Best imaging tool
  - Multiplanar spinal MR with sagittal and axial T2WI, T1WI C+ MR

DIFFERENTIAL DIAGNOSIS

Multiple Sclerosis

- < 2 vertebral segments in length, peripheral location
- < 1/2 of cord cross-sectional area
- 90% have associated intracranial lesions
- Relapsing and remitting clinical course

Neuromyelitis Optica Spectrum Disorders

- Autoimmune inflammatory disorder involving neuronal myelin of optic nerves and spinal cord
- Extensive (> 3 vertebral segments) cord T2 hyperintensity + optic nerve enhancement
- Limited brain involvement

Spinal Cord Neoplasm

- Cord expansion and extensive peritumoral edema invariably present
- Cystic ± hemorrhage components
- Diffuse or nodular contrast enhancement
- Slower clinical progression

Myelin Oligodendrocyte Glycoprotein Antibody Disease

- MOG-IgG positive
- Optic neuritis, longitudinally extensive transverse myelitis (LETM), &/or acute disseminated encephalomyelitis (ADEM)-like encephalopathy presentation
- Mimics IATM, neuromyelitis optica (NMO) spectrum disorder

Spinal Cord Infarction

- Ventral or central cord location, less mass effect initially
- Patients present more often with motor signs than sensory signs
- Immediate onset (minutes, rather than hours, days)

Acute Flaccid Myelitis

- Abnormal T2 signal in central gray matter favoring anterior horn cells
- Motor weakness, **flaccid** paralysis/paresis
- May be asymmetric

PATHOLOGY

General Features

- Etiology
  - Autoimmune phenomenon with formation of antigen-antibody complexes
  - Small vessel vasculopathy results in cord ischemia
  - Associated demyelinating process
  - Neoplastic, paraneoplastic, collagen vascular, and iatrogenic etiologies
    - Not considered idiopathic in those cases

- Association with previous viral infection or vaccination postulated in some cases
- Associated abnormalities
  - Depression
    - Lifetime risk (> 50%), correlates with severity of sensory symptoms
- Perivascular inflammation
- Demyelination

Microscopic Features

- Gray and white matter necrosis
- Destruction of neurons, axons, and myelin
- Astrocytic gliosis
- Perivascular lymphocytic infiltrate

CLINICAL ISSUES

Presentation

- Most common signs/symptoms
  - Sensory deficit
    - Loss of pain and temperature sensation
    - Clearly defined upper level
    - Band-like dysesthesia at lesion level
    - Ascending paresthesia in bilateral lower extremities
  - Other signs/symptoms
    - Paraplegia or quadriplegia
    - Back ± radicular pain
    - Bladder and bowel dysfunction
    - Hypotonia and hyporeflexia initially
    - Spasticity and hyperreflexia over time
- Clinical profile
  - Prodrome of generalized body aches
  - Preceding viral-like illness
  - Rapid progression to maximal neurologic deficits within days
- Transverse Myelitis Consortium Working Group
  - Inclusion criteria
    - Sensory, motor, or autonomic dysfunction attributable to spinal cord
    - Bilateral signs and symptoms
    - Well-defined sensory level
    - Cord inflammation confirmed by CSF pleocytosis, elevated IgG index, or gadolinium enhancement
    - Progression to nadir between 4 hours and 21 days from onset
    - Symptoms must progress if present upon awakening
    - Compressive etiology excluded by neuroimaging
    - May repeat MR ± lumbar puncture between 2-7 days if signs of inflammation absent initially
  - Exclusion criteria
    - History of spinal radiation within past 10 years
    - Cord ischemia and infarction due to anterior spinal artery thrombosis
    - Cord arteriovenous malformation
    - Connective tissue disorder [sarcoidosis, systemic lupus erythematosus (SLE), or Sjögren syndrome]
    - CNS infections (syphilis, Lyme disease, mycoplasma, HIV, HTLV-1, or other viral infections)
    - Brain MR suggestive of multiple sclerosis (MS) or other demyelinating process
    - Clinical optic neuritis
  - 2005 modifications
    - Acute partial transverse myelitis
      - Small cord lesions, associated with MS
    - Acute complete transverse myelitis
      - Associated with LETM
      - Within spectrum of NMO, as antiaquaporin 4 antibody is present in 1/2 of recurrent cases of IATM

Demographics

- Age
  - Any, but peaks at 10-19 and 30-39 years
- Epidemiology
  - Incidence 2 per 500,000 population

Natural History & Prognosis

- Typically monophasic
  - Recurrence rate reported between 24-40%
  - If recurrent, must consider
    - MS: Progression to MS in 2-8% of cases of transverse myelitis
    - SLE, antiphospholipid syndrome
    - Vascular malformation
- 1/3 of patients experience good to complete recovery
  - Symptomatic improvement 2-12 weeks after onset
  - Children have slightly better prognosis than adults
- 1/3 of patients experience fair recovery
  - Residual spasticity and urinary dysfunction
- 1/3 of patients experience poor recovery
  - Persistent complete deficits
  - Assistance required in activities of daily living
- Factors portending poor prognosis
  - Back pain
  - Rapid clinical deterioration
  - Spinal shock: Loss of motor, sensation, sphincter control, and areflexia
  - MR signal alteration > 10 spinal segments
  - Significant denervation on electromyogram or abnormal somatosensory evoked potential
  - Presence of antiaquaporin 4 antibody

Treatment

- High-dose intravenous steroid pulse therapy
- Physical therapy

DIAGNOSTIC CHECKLIST

Image Interpretation Pearls

- IATM is diagnosis of exclusion with multiple differential diagnostic possibilities
- Central enhancement in peripherally located T2 hyperintensity more characteristic of MS

SELECTED REFERENCES

1. Choudhary A et al: Etiological spectrum, clinico-radiological profile and treatment outcomes of longitudinally extensive transverse myelitis - a prospective study from Northwest India. J Neuroimmunol. 351:577456, 2021
2. Ganelin-Cohen E et al: Prognostic parameters of acute transverse myelitis in children. J Child Neurol. 35(14):999-1003, 2020
3. Maillart E et al: Outcome and risk of recurrence in a large cohort of idiopathic longitudinally extensive transverse myelitis without AQP4/MOG antibodies. J Neuroinflammation. 17(1):128, 2020

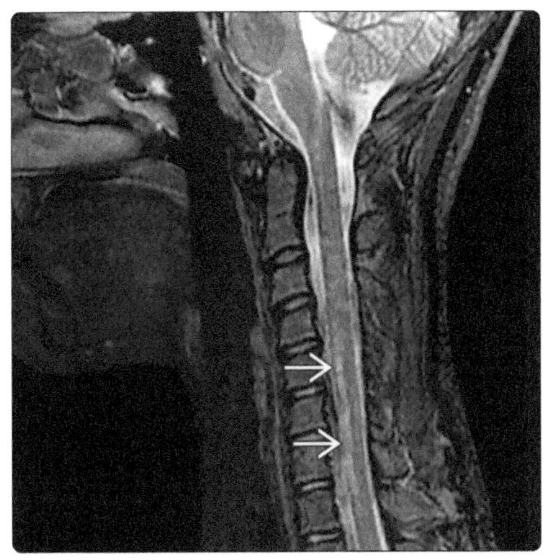

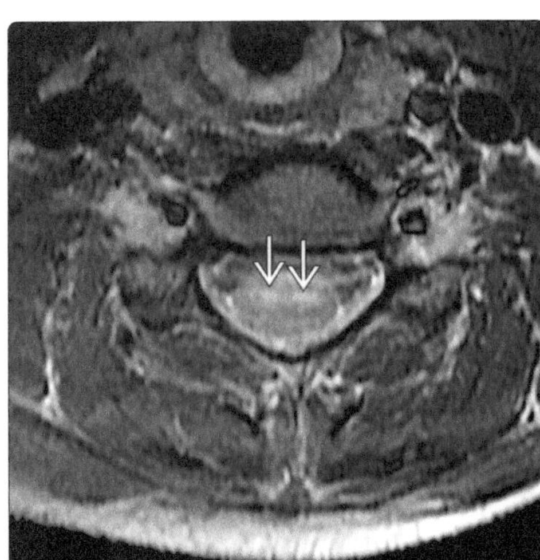

(Left) *Sagittal STIR MR (acute upper extremity weakness) demonstrates patchy, predominantly ventral T2 hyperintensity in the cervical spinal cord over > 3 vertebral segments.* **(Right)** *Axial T2WI MR in the same patient confirms ill-defined abnormal T2 hyperintensity within the cervical spinal cord. Blurred involvement of both gray and white matter helps distinguish from acute flaccid myelitis.*

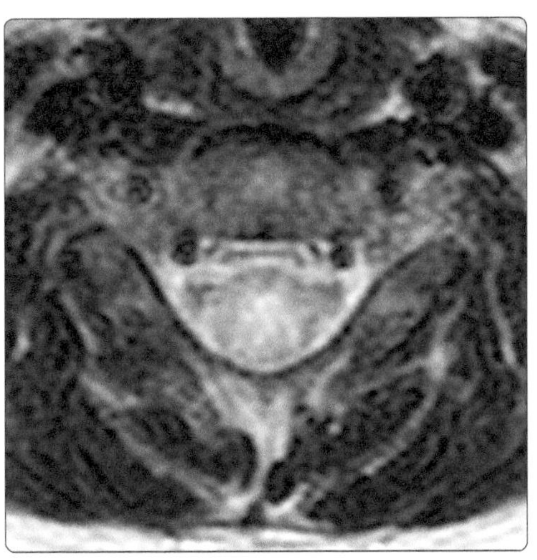

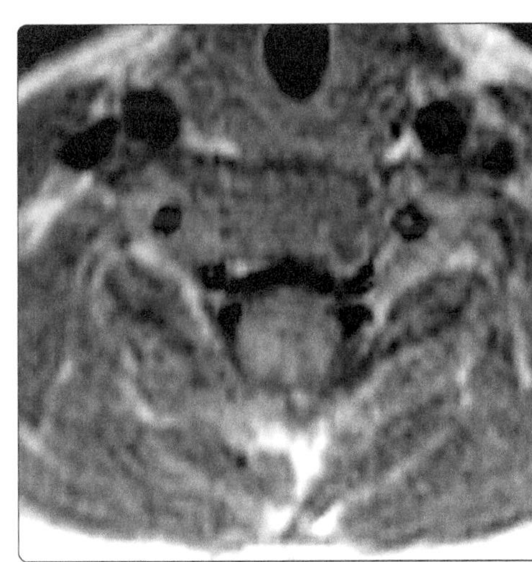

(Left) *Axial T2WI MR reveals abnormal intramedullary T2 hyperintensity involving both gray and white matter. Thoracic MR (not shown) confirmed extension to the conus. The areas of abnormality are patchy rather than contiguous.* **(Right)** *Axial T1WI C+ MR in the same patient confirms heterogeneous enhancement within the areas of abnormal spinal cord T2 hyperintensity.*

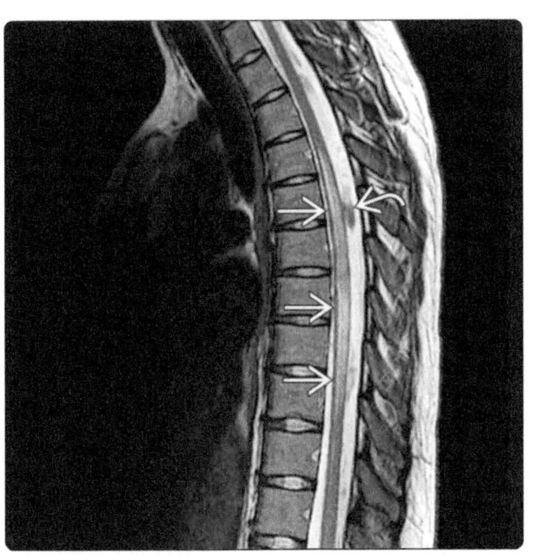

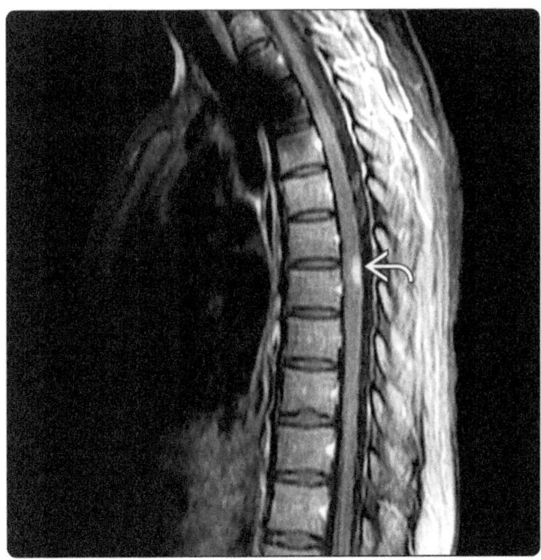

(Left) *Sagittal T2WI MR demonstrates long-segment T2 hyperintensity within the thoracic cord spanning 6 levels. This is a typical central edema pattern for acute transverse myelitis with relative sparing of the cord periphery. CSF dephasing, a common artifact, mimics an intradural extramedullary lesion.* **(Right)** *Sagittal T1WI C+ FS MR in the same patient reveals a single focus of enhancement within the abnormal thoracic spinal cord segment that is much smaller than the extent of T2 signal abnormality.*

Neuromyelitis Optica

KEY FACTS

TERMINOLOGY

- Synonyms: Devic disease, optic-spinal multiple sclerosis
- Autoimmune inflammatory disorder involving myelin of neurons of optic nerves and spinal cord with limited brain parenchymal involvement

IMAGING

- Longitudinally extensive (> 3 vertebral segments) T2 hyperintensity within cord + enhancement of optic nerves (85% of cases)
- T2 abnormality tends to involve entire cross section of cord unlike more focal involvement of MS

TOP DIFFERENTIAL DIAGNOSES

- Inflammatory etiologies
  - Multiple sclerosis
  - Acute disseminated encephalomyelitis (ADEM)
  - Parainfectious myelitis (viral, bacterial)
- Systemic autoimmune disease
- Noninflammatory mimics
  - Dural fistula, tumor
- Idiopathic acute transverse myelitis

PATHOLOGY

- Autoimmune disease targeting water channel proteins (AQP4)
- Originally considered subtype of multiple sclerosis but now known to be separate entity

CLINICAL ISSUES

- Recurrent optic neuritis (ON), recurrent transverse myelitis, simultaneous attacks of ON + myelitis
- **Revised International Consensus Criteria (2011)**
  - Recognition of AQP4-Ab (-) neuromyelitis optica (NMO) disorders, particularly in children

DIAGNOSTIC CHECKLIST

- Simultaneous ON and myelitis → NMO cannot be distinguished from ADEM at 1st attack

(Left) *Sagittal T2WI MR shows a long segment of cervical spinal cord enlargement with T2 hyperintensity ➡.* **(Right)** *Sagittal T1WI C+ MR shows cord enlargement and ill-defined enhancement ➡. Neuromyelitis optica (NMO) is an autoimmune disease possibly targeting the aquaporin-4 transmembrane water channel. The vasculocentric distribution of antigen of NMO-IgG correlates with the sites of immunoglobulin and complement deposition seen in spinal cord lesions of patients with NMO.*

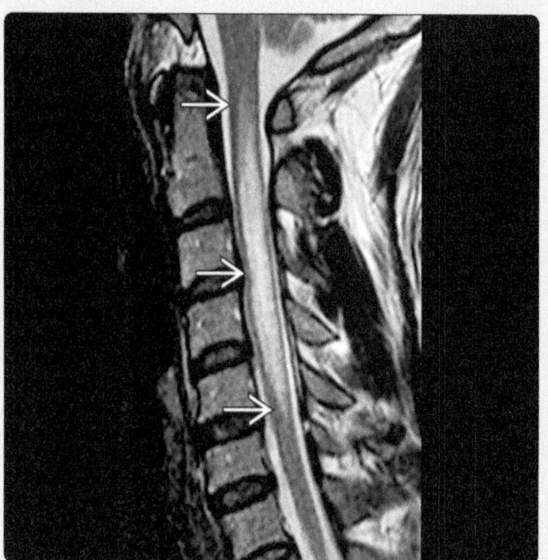

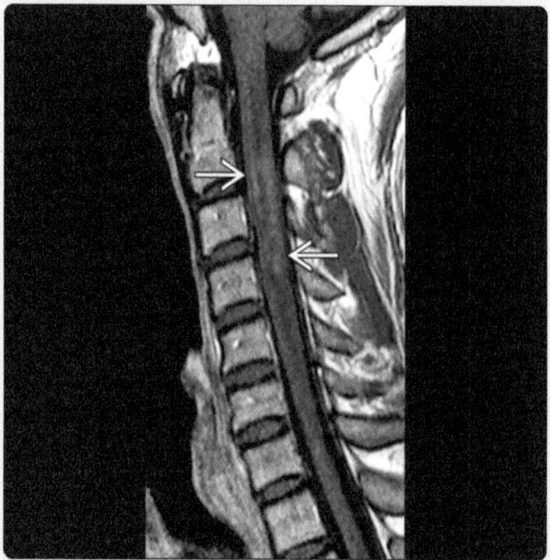

(Left) *Axial T1WI C+ FS MR in the same patient reveals intense enhancement and mild enlargement of the intracanalicular and prechiasmatic segments of the right optic nerve ➡.* **(Right)** *Coronal T1WI C+ FS MR in the same patient confirms intense enhancement and mild enlargement of the intracanalicular and prechiasmatic segments of the right optic nerve ➡. This is the classic appearance of NMO involving the optic nerves and spinal cord with no brain parenchymal abnormalities.*

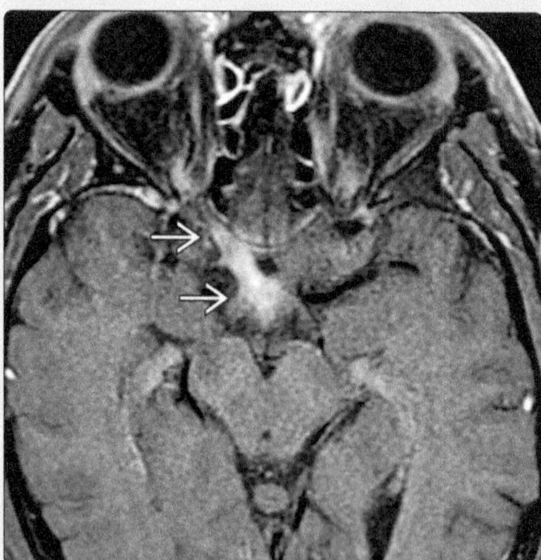

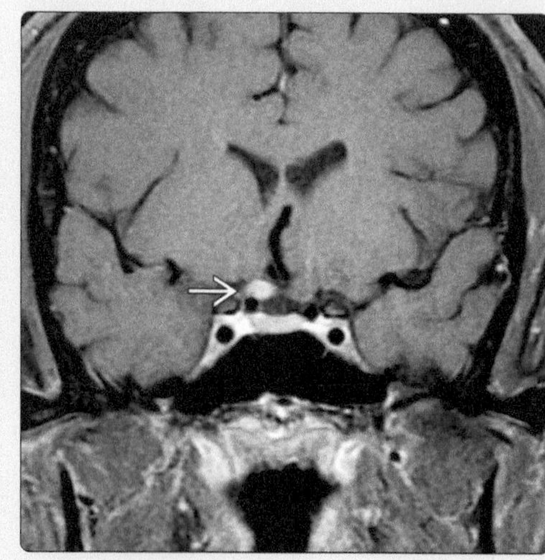

TERMINOLOGY

Abbreviations

- Neuromyelitis optica (NMO)

Synonyms

- Devic disease, Devic syndrome, Devic NMO

Definitions

- Autoimmune inflammatory disorder involving myelin of optic nerve and spinal cord neurons with limited brain parenchymal involvement

IMAGING

General Features

- Best diagnostic clue
  - Longitudinally extensive (LTE) (> 3 vertebral segments) T2 hyperintensity within cord + enhancement of optic nerves (85% of cases)
- Location
  - Spinal cord + optic nerves/chiasm
  - Studies have reported multiple sclerosis (MS)-like lesions in 10-30% of NMO patients; brain MR is usually normal
- Size
  - > 3 segments of T2 abnormality more likely in NMO or acute transverse myelitis than in classic MS
    - Most specific nonserologic feature to differentiate NMO from MS
- Morphology
  - T2 abnormality tends to involve entire cross section of cord, unlike more focal involvement of MS

Imaging Recommendations

- Best imaging tool
  - STIR, T2WI MR, C+ MR of cord/brain
- Protocol advice
  - Proton density or STIR imaging of cord; sole use of heavily T2WI will lower sensitivity to cord lesions

MR Findings

- T1WI
  - Hypointense cord lesions
- T2WI
  - Lesions more linear than in MS patients
- DWI
  - Mean diffusivity (MD) and fractional anisotropy (FA) in patients with relapsing NMO are significantly different from those in patients with relapsing MS

DIFFERENTIAL DIAGNOSIS

Inflammatory Etiologies

- **Multiple sclerosis**
  - < 1 vertebral segment length of cord T2 signal abnormality
  - Tends to involve cord periphery; multiple cord lesions
  - Associated typical periventricular white matter (WM) lesions
- **Acute disseminated encephalomyelitis**
  - Encephalopathy
  - May be indistinguishable from MS on imaging
  - Thalamic involvement
  - Monophasic
- **Myelin Oligodendroglial Glycoprotein Antibody Disease**
  - Immune-mediated inflammation directed towards myelin oligodendrocyte glycoprotein (MOG)
  - Characteristic presentation with optic neuritis (ON), acute disseminated encephalomyelitis (ADEM)-like encephalopathy, &/or longitudinally extensive transverse myelitis (LETM)
  - MOG-IgG AB (+)
- **Parainfectious Myelitis (Viral, Bacterial)**
  - Long segment of T2 signal abnormality
  - Usually prominent irregular enhancement (not ring-shaped)
- **Systemic Autoimmune Disease**
  - Sjögren, SLE, antiphospholipid syndrome

Noninflammatory Mimics

- Tumor
  - Irregular enhancement
  - Cord expansion; may be asymmetric

Idiopathic Acute Transverse Myelitis

- Diagnosis of exclusion
- Cord lesion may be indistinguishable from NMO
- Monophasic

PATHOLOGY

General Features

- Etiology
  - Originally considered subtype of MS but now known to be separate entity
  - Autoimmune disease → possibly targeting of AQP4
    - Aquaporins = family of transmembrane channel proteins highly selective for water transport
    - AQP4-predominant water channel expressed in brain
    - Localized to astrocytic foot processes surrounding cerebral capillary endothelium
    - NMO-IgG binds to abluminal face of microvessels, pia, and Virchow-Robin sheath
  - LETM may confer high risk of conversion into NMO
- Associated abnormalities
  - Brain WM lesions
    - Recurrent ON, myelitis with normal brain MR, or when several brain WM lesions fail MS criteria, NMO very likely
    - WM lesions relatively common in patients with otherwise typical NMO (60%)
      - Asymptomatic brain lesions common in NMO, but symptomatic brain lesions do not exclude diagnosis of NMO
    - Children with NMO are more susceptible to atypical brain lesions than adults
      - Lesions are usually large (> 2 cm), localize to areas of high AQP4 expression [periventricular regions of III (diencephalic) and IV ventricles (brainstem)], supratentorial and infratentorial WM, midbrain, and cerebellum
  - Other concomitant or associated immunologic diseases
    - Prior viral infection
    - ANA (+) (10%)
    - Autoimmune thyroiditis (9%)

- Myasthenia gravis (2%)
- Sjögren syndrome

- Anti-MOG (MOG-Abs) found in some patients with AQP4-Ab (-) NMO-like disorders as well as other demyelinating disorders
  - Relationship appears to be reciprocal; no patients reported to have both MOG and AQP4 antibodies

Gross Pathologic & Surgical Features

- Optic nerves show nonspecific segments of demyelination + atrophy
- Spinal cord shows perivascular inflammatory demyelination with necrosis
- May show ↑ neutrophils + eosinophils (not seen in MS)

Microscopic Features

- Prominent vasculocentric IgG and C9 neoantigen deposits
- Eosinophilic and neutrophilic inflammatory infiltrates, necrosis, vascular hyalinization, and extensive vasculocentric immunoglobulin and complement deposition

CLINICAL ISSUES

Presentation

- Most common signs/symptoms
  - Recurrent ON, recurrent transverse myelitis, simultaneous attacks of ON + myelitis
  - Bilateral simultaneous ON or sequential ON more suggestive of NMO than MS
  - Respiratory failure due to extensive cervical myelitis in up to 1/3 of cases (very uncommon in MS)
  - Radicular pain in 35% (uncommon in MS)
  - L'hermitte symptom common in MS (40%) and NMO (35%)
  - CSF in NMO may show prominent pleocytosis (especially with myelitis) compared to MS
    - Oligoclonal bands in 20-30% (vs. 85% with MS)
- Other signs/symptoms
  - **Diagnostic neurology criteria**, Wingerchuk **(2006)**
    - ON, myelitis, and at least 2 of 3 supportive criteria: MR evidence of contiguous spinal cord lesion 3 or more segments in length, brain MR findings nondiagnostic for MS, or NMO-IgG seropositivity
      - CNS involvement beyond optic nerves and spinal cord is compatible with NMO
    - NMO-IgG seropositivity 76% sensitive and 94% specific for NMO
  - **Revised International Consensus Diagnostic Criteria** (International Panel for NMO Diagnosis, **2011**)
    - Recognition of AQP4-Ab (-) NMO disorders, particularly in children
    - Propose NMO spectrum disorder (NMOSD) as term to define entire spectrum of typical NMO [AQP4-Ab (+)], ON, acute myelitis, brain syndrome, and combinations
    - Diagnostic criteria currently same for adults and children but under investigation

Demographics

- Age
  - Mean range: 30-40 years, but seen in nearly all age groups
  - Presentation uncommon in pediatric age group, accounting for 3-5% of cases
- Sex
  - F > M (4:1)
- Ethnicity
  - NMO greater proportion of CNS demyelinating disease in people of non-White background

Natural History & Prognosis

- Outcome worse than in MS
  - > 50% children with AQP4-IgG seropositive NMOSD develop permanent disability, particularly in visual, motor domains
- Frequent and early relapses (annual relapse rate of 1.3%)
  - ↑ risk of relapse during pregnancy in NMO
- Compared with MS, NMO patients have older age at onset (depending on ethnicity), female patients more frequently affected, course more severe
  - Vision/ambulation impaired within 5 years of onset in 50%
  - 20% succumb to respiratory failure
- Some reports state predictor of poor evolution is high number of MR brain lesions at diagnosis → predictive of residual visual acuity

Treatment

- Intravenous steroids used as 1st-line treatment of ON/myelitis
- Immunosuppressive medications
  - 1st-line treatment options in pediatrics include rituximab, azathioprine, and mycophenolate mofetil
- Plasmapheresis as rescue therapy

DIAGNOSTIC CHECKLIST

Consider

- Simultaneous ON and myelitis → NMO cannot be distinguished from ADEM at 1st attack
- Brain MR should be normal or near normal (≤ 2 lesions)
- Longitudinally extensive cord T2 hyperintensity in 85%
- Best diagnostic combination (99% sensitive and 90% specific)
  - At least 2 of 3 elements: LTE cord lesion, onset brain MR nondiagnostic for MS, or NMO-IgG seropositivity

SELECTED REFERENCES

1. Poisson K et al: Pediatric neuromyelitis optica spectrum disorder. Semin Pediatr Neurol. 46:101051, 2023
2. Pandit L et al: Incidence and prevalence of neuromyelitis optica spectrum disorders in the background of International Consensus Diagnostic Criteria - a systematic review. Neurol India. 70(5):1771-9, 2022
3. Tarhan B et al: A comparison of pediatric- and adult-onset aquaporin-4 immunoglobulin G-positive neuromyelitis optica spectrum disorder: a review of clinical and radiographic characteristics. J Child Neurol. 37(8-9):727-37, 2022
4. Baghbanian SM et al: A comparison of pediatric and adult neuromyelitis optica spectrum disorders: a review of clinical manifestation, diagnosis, and treatment. J Neurol Sci. 388:222-31, 2018
5. Akaishi T et al: Neuromyelitis optica spectrum disorders. Neuroimaging Clin N Am. 27(2):251-65, 2017
6. Chitnis T et al: Clinical features of neuromyelitis optica in children: US Network of Pediatric MS Centers report. Neurology. 86(3):245-52, 2016
7. Tenembaum S et al: Neuromyelitis optica spectrum disorders in children and adolescents. Neurology. 87(9 Suppl 2):S59-66, 2016

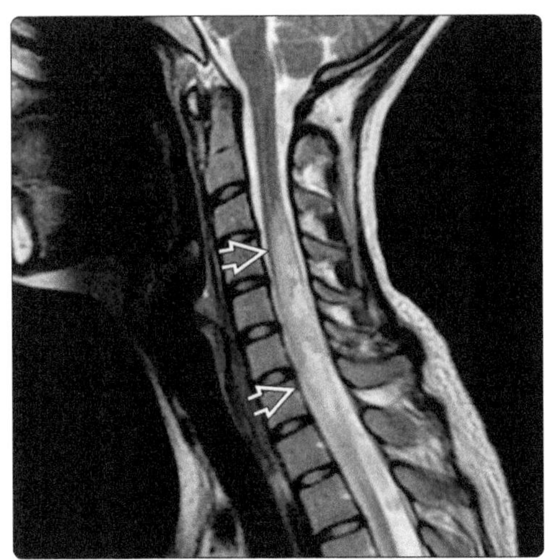

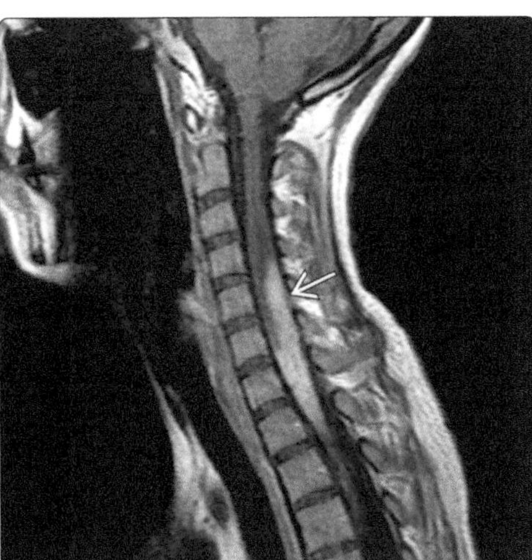

(Left) *Sagittal T2WI MR shows fusiform expansion of the cervical spinal cord* ➡ *with longitudinally extensive T2 signal abnormality > 3 vertebral segments in this patient with NMO spectrum disorder (NMOSD).* **(Right)** *Sagittal T1WI C+ MR in the same patient depicts extensive diffuse enhancement* ➡ *of the cervical spinal cord in addition to fusiform spinal cord expansion characteristic of the long-segment cord involvement of NMOSD.*

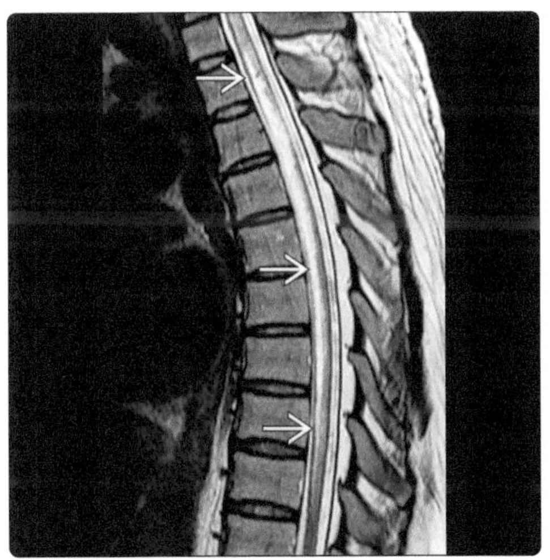

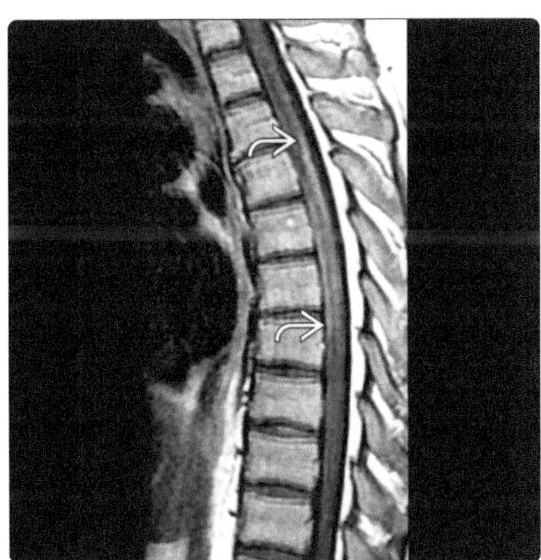

(Left) *Sagittal T2WI MR depicts a longitudinally extensive focus of hyperintensity within the thoracic spinal cord* ➡ *with slight fusiform expansion.* **(Right)** *Sagittal T1WI C+ MR in the same patient exhibits long-segment diffuse enhancement* ➡. *This initial pattern is nonspecific, and DDx would include other acute transverse myelopathies, such as the noninflammatory group (dural fistula, cord infarct, and radiation change) and the inflammatory group (MS, NMO, ADEM, SLE, and other connective tissue disorders).*

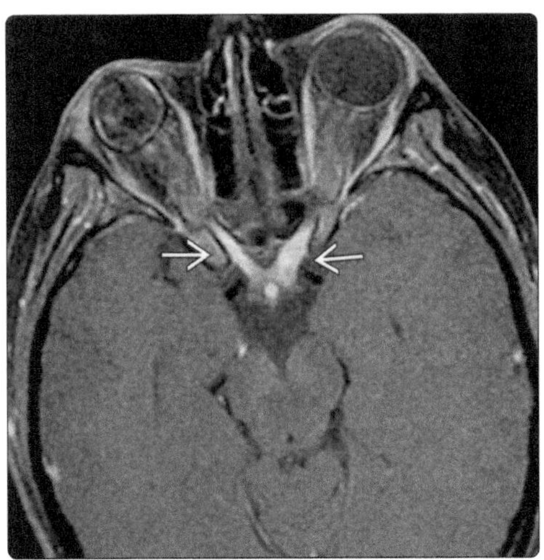

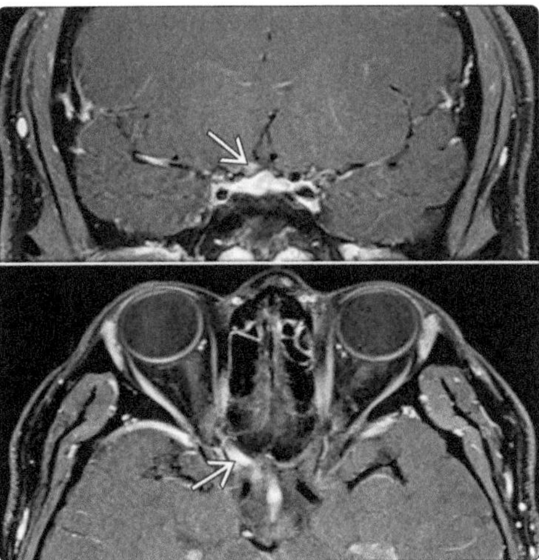

(Left) *Axial T1WI C+ FS MR of the optic nerves in a patient with NMOSD shows marked enhancement of both optic nerves* ➡ *and optic chiasm. There is also phthisis bulbi on the right.* **(Right)** *T1WI C+ FS MR images demonstrate mild enlargement and enhancement of the intracanalicular right optic nerve* ➡. *Systemic autoimmune disorders and autoantibodies may coexist in NMO (e.g., thyroid disease, myasthenia gravis, celiac disease, systemic lupus erythematosus, and Sjögren syndrome).*

KEY FACTS

TERMINOLOGY

- Primary demyelinating disease of CNS with multiple lesions disseminated over time & space
  - Concomitant intracranial lesions in periventricular, subcallosal, brainstem, or cerebellar white matter

IMAGING

- Isolated spinal cord disease (10-20%)
- Cervical segment is most commonly affected
  - Dorsolateral aspect of cord
  - < 1/2 of cross-sectional area of spinal cord
  - < 2 vertebral segments in length
- Sagittal & axial T1WI/T2WI sequences with gadolinium
  - Lesions typically oval, peripheral, & asymmetric
  - Discrete vs. vague hyperintense lesions

TOP DIFFERENTIAL DIAGNOSES

- Acute disseminated encephalomyelitis
- Neuromyelitis optica spectrum disorders
- Myelin oligodendrocyte glycoprotein antibody disorder
- Idiopathic transverse myelitis
- Intramedullary neoplasm
- Spinal cord infarct

PATHOLOGY

- Autoimmune, cell-mediated inflammatory process focused on CNS myelin

CLINICAL ISSUES

- Peak onset: 20-40 years
- Multiple clinical presentations
  - Relapsing remitting (RR)
  - Secondary progressive (SP)
  - Primary progressive (PP)
  - Progressive relapsing (PR)

DIAGNOSTIC CHECKLIST

- Imaging findings must be correlated with clinical & laboratory features to confirm diagnosis

(Left) *Sagittal graphic depicts multiple sclerosis (MS) demyelinating plaques within the cervical spinal cord. Lesions are focal and < 2 vertebral bodies in length, typical of MS.* **(Right)** *Sagittal T2WI MR (left) demonstrates a solitary active MS plaque ➔ at the C6-C7 level with focal T2 hyperintensity but without significant cord enlargement. Sagittal T1WI C+ FS MR (right) confirms ring enhancement of the focal lesion, consistent with an active MS plaque.*

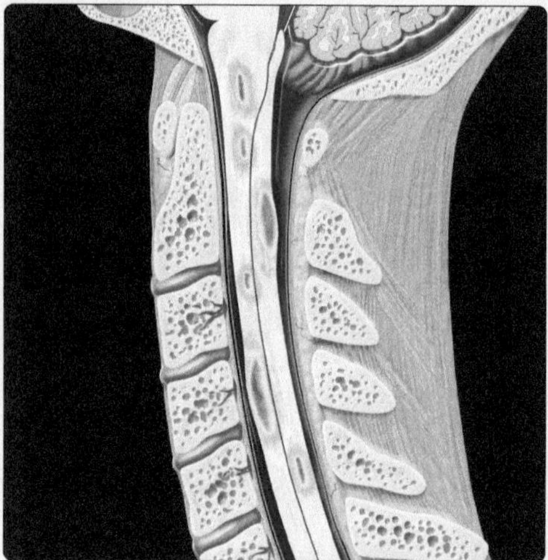

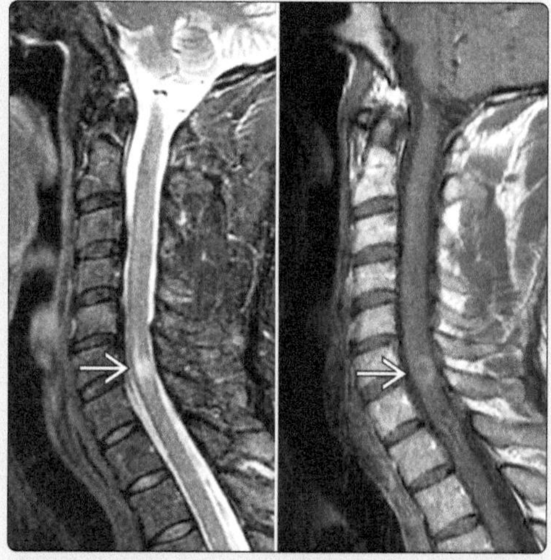

(Left) *Sagittal T2WI (left), PD (middle), and STIR (right) MR images show multiple short-segment MS plaques within the thoracic spinal cord ⇨. Note the relatively improved conspicuity of the plaques on PD and STIR relative to the routine T2 sequence.* **(Right)** *Sagittal STIR (left), T2WI (middle), and T1WI C+ FS (right) MR images of the thoracic spine show multiple short-segment foci of T2 hyperintensity ➔ in a different patient with MS. Multiple lesions ⇨ show solid enhancement.*

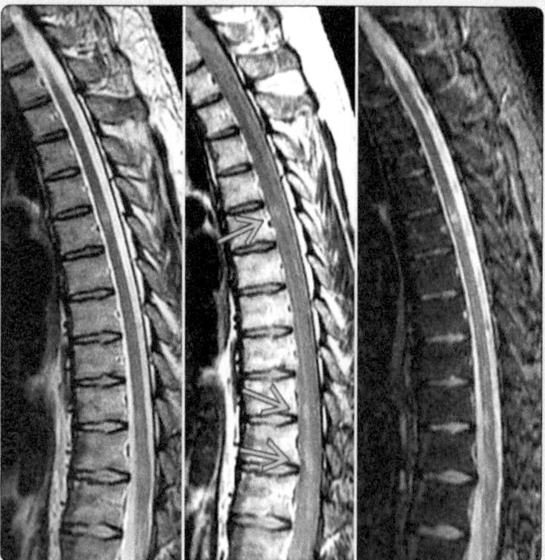

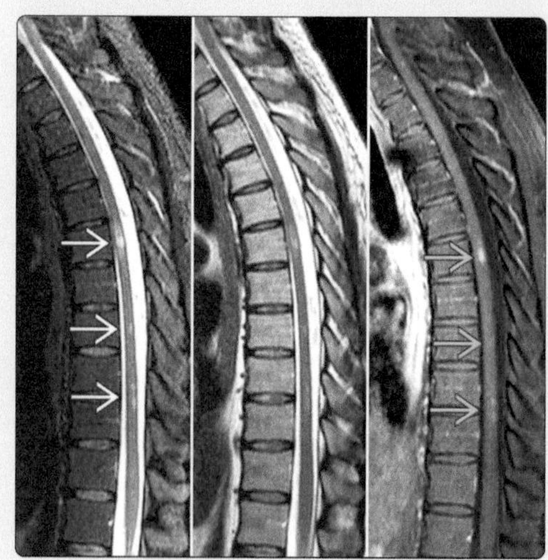

TERMINOLOGY

Definitions

- Primary demyelinating disease of CNS with multiple lesions disseminated over time & space

IMAGING

General Features

- Location
  - Lesions solitary or multifocal
    - Isolated spinal cord disease in 10-20%
  - Cervical segment is most commonly affected (2/3 of cord lesions)
  - Lesions frequently in dorsolateral cord
- Size
  - < 1/2 of cross-sectional area of spinal cord
  - < 2 vertebral segments in length

MR Findings

- T1WI
  - Iso- to hypointense lesions
- T2WI
  - Discrete or ill-defined hyperintense lesions
  - Lesions typically oval, peripheral, & asymmetric
- STIR
  - Improved lesion detection, more artifact
- DWI
  - ↑ mean diffusivity, ↓ fractional anisotropy in plaques & areas without T2 abnormality
- T1WI C+
  - Variable

DIFFERENTIAL DIAGNOSIS

Acute Disseminated Encephalomyelitis

- Para-/postinfectious immune-mediated inflammatory disorder of spinal cord white matter
- Frequently preceding infection 4-12 days before onset

Neuromyelitis Optica Spectrum Disorders

- Longitudinally extensive cord T2 hyperintensity + optic nerve enhancement
- T2 abnormality involves entire cross section of cord

Myelin Oligodendrocyte Glycoprotein Antibody Disease

- Autoimmune inflammatory disorder involving neuronal myelin of brain, optic nerves, &/or spinal cord
- Often longitudinally extensive

Idiopathic Transverse Myelitis

- Longitudinally extensive, > 2/3 of cord cross-sectional area
- No associated intracranial lesions
- Diagnosis of exclusion

Intramedullary Neoplasm

- Cord expansion, peritumoral edema, cystic ± hemorrhagic components
- Entire cross section of spinal cord
- Diffuse or partial enhancement

Spinal Cord Infarction

- Sudden onset of symptoms
- Positive diffusion restriction

PATHOLOGY

General Features

- Etiology
  - Autoimmune, cell-mediated inflammatory process focused on CNS myelin
    - Infectious agents may play primary or secondary role
- Associated abnormalities
  - 90% incidence of associated intracranial lesions

Staging, Grading, & Classification

- McDonald criteria (2001, revised in 2005 & 2017) widely used for adult MS diagnosis
  - Has also been shown to be useful for pediatric MS diagnosis
- Relies on lesion dissemination in both time & space

CLINICAL ISSUES

Presentation

- Most common signs/symptoms
  - Cord lesions asymptomatic
  - Paresthesia
- Other signs/symptoms
  - Muscle weakness, hyperreflexia, gait disturbance
  - Bladder/bowel dysfunction

Demographics

- Age
  - Peak onset: 20-40 years
  - Onset < 18 years in 3-5% of MS cases
- Sex
  - Women more susceptible than men (1.7:1)
- Ethnicity
  - Western Europeans have higher risk

Treatment

- Multiple approved medications include interferon, chemotherapy agents, monoclonal antibodies
- Supportive therapy
- Physical therapy

DIAGNOSTIC CHECKLIST

Consider

- Multiplanar spine contrast MR ± contrast, including STIR MR

Image Interpretation Pearls

- Imaging findings must be correlated with clinical & laboratory features to confirm diagnosis
- Acute MS can mimic cord neoplasm

SELECTED REFERENCES

1. Bower A et al: Radiologically isolated syndrome and the multiple sclerosis prodrome in pediatrics: early features of the spectrum of demyelination. Semin Pediatr Neurol. 46:101053, 2023
2. Ciccarelli O et al: Spinal cord involvement in multiple sclerosis and neuromyelitis optica spectrum disorders. Lancet Neurol. 18(2):185-97, 2019

KEY FACTS

TERMINOLOGY

- Para-/postinfectious immune-mediated inflammatory disorder of white matter
  - Antibodies to pathogens exhibit cross immunoreactivity with myelin basic protein

IMAGING

- Multifocal white matter lesions with relatively little mass effect or vasogenic edema
  - Flame-shaped lesions with slight cord swelling
  - May see gray matter involvement
  - Variable enhancement, depending on stage of disease

TOP DIFFERENTIAL DIAGNOSES

- Inflammatory etiologies
  - Acquired demyelinating diseases
    - Multiple sclerosis
    - Neuromyelitis optica
  - Parainfectious myelitis
  - Systemic autoimmune (vasculitis)
- Noninflammatory mimics
  - Vascular malformation
  - Infarction, spinal cord
  - Tumor and cysts
- Idiopathic acute transverse myelitis

PATHOLOGY

- Autoimmune process producing inflammatory reaction

CLINICAL ISSUES

- Usually monophasic illness lasting from 2-4 weeks
  - Encephalopathy, paresis
- Typically childhood or young adult onset

DIAGNOSTIC CHECKLIST

- Repeat MR if initially negative and strong clinical suspicion
- Typically, delay between clinical onset and appearance of imaging findings

(Left) *Sagittal T2WI MR in a 5-year-old patient with encephalopathy and myelopathy following a viral respiratory illness demonstrates T2-hyperintense lesions at C3 ➡ and T2 ⇨ that produce focal cord swelling. Brain imaging (not shown) revealed typical findings of acute disseminated encephalomyelitis (ADEM).* **(Right)** *Axial T1WI C+ MR in the same patient shows eccentric enhancement ➡ in the right lateral hemicord.*

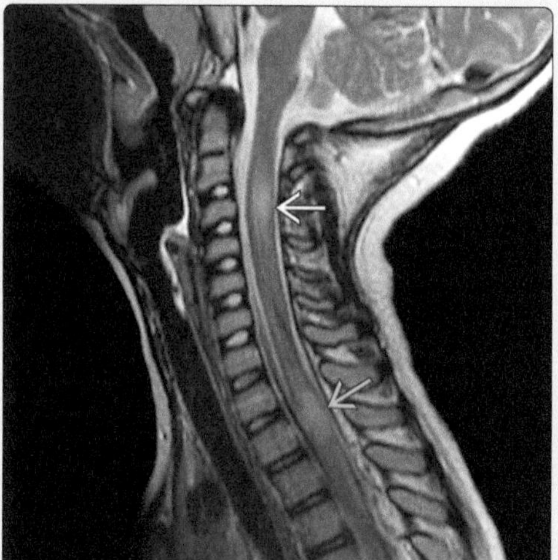

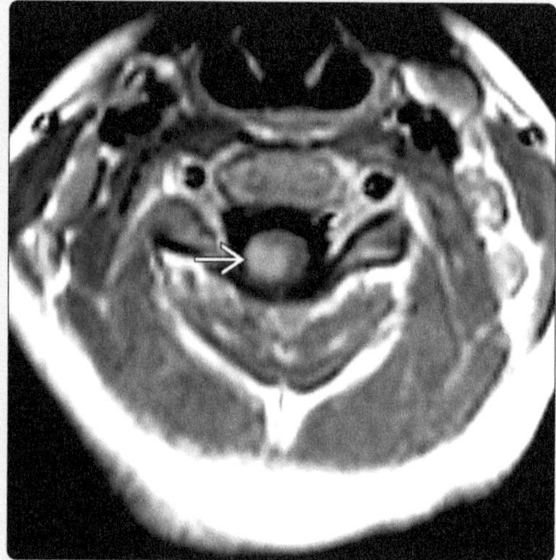

(Left) *Sagittal T2WI MR in an ADEM patient with encephalopathy and myelopathy demonstrates a vague intramedullary focus of T2 hyperintensity ➡. There is mild cord expansion at the affected level.* **(Right)** *Sagittal T1WI C+ MR in the same patient illustrates an ovoid intramedullary focus of enhancement in the upper thoracic cord ➡ at the site of T2 hyperintensity.*

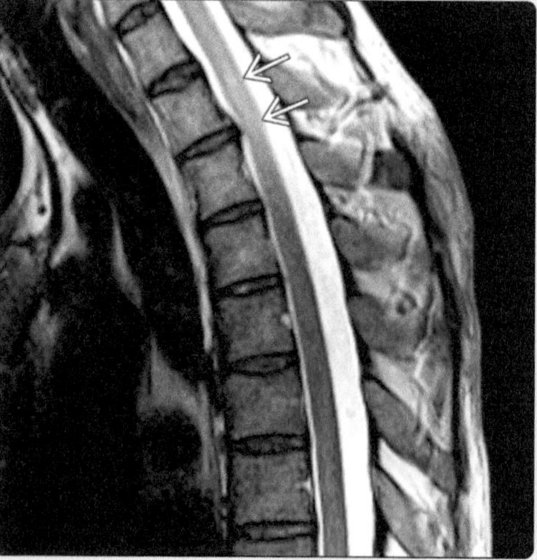

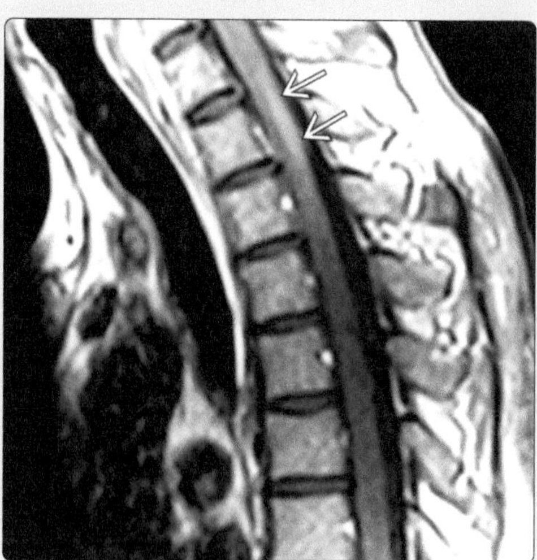

TERMINOLOGY

Abbreviations

- Acute disseminated encephalomyelitis (ADEM)

Definitions

- Para-/postinfectious immune-mediated inflammatory disorder of spinal cord white matter

IMAGING

General Features

- Best diagnostic clue
  - Multifocal white matter lesions with relatively little mass effect or vasogenic edema
- Size
  - May be short and focal or extensive [longitudinally extensive transverse myelitis (LETM)]

MR Findings

- T1WI
  - Focal (often subtle) low signal, slight cord swelling
- T2WI
  - Multifocal flame-shaped white matter lesions with slight cord swelling
- T1WI C+
  - Enhancement varies from absent to punctate, ring-shaped, or fluffy
  - May see nerve enhancement

Imaging Recommendations

- Multiplanar MR with T2WI and T1WI pre- and postcontrast

DIFFERENTIAL DIAGNOSIS

Inflammatory Etiologies

- Other acquired demyelinating diseases
  - **Multiple sclerosis**
    - Indistinguishable on single study
    - Brain MR findings may help differentiate
  - **Neuromyelitis optica spectrum disorders**
    - Little clinical involvement beyond optic nerves and spinal cord
- **Parainfectious myelitis**
- **Systemic autoimmune (vasculitis)**

Noninflammatory Mimics

- **Vascular malformation**
  - High-flow arteriovenous malformation (AVM) demonstrates obvious serpentine structures with flow void at periphery of abnormal cord
- **Infarction, spinal cord**
  - Stroke-like, acute presentation
  - Focal, segmental gray matter lesion
- **Spinal cord neoplasm**
  - Diffuse or nodular contrast enhancement
  - Cystic and hemorrhagic components
  - Peritumoral edema

Idiopathic Acute Transverse Myelitis

- Diagnosis of exclusion
- Usually single lesion

PATHOLOGY

General Features

- Etiology
  - Autoimmune process producing inflammatory reaction
    - Antibodies to pathogens exhibit cross immunoreactivity with white matter myelin basic protein
  - Frequently preceding predisposing infection 4-12 days before ADEM onset

Gross Pathologic & Surgical Features

- Slight swelling to tumefactive necrosis

Microscopic Features

- Acute myelin loss
  - Perivenous demyelination → pathologic hallmark of ADEM; confluent demyelination → hallmark of acute multiple sclerosis

CLINICAL ISSUES

Presentation

- Most common signs/symptoms
  - Encephalopathy
  - Other signs/symptoms
    - Paresis
    - Voiding dysfunction, urinary retention
- Clinical profile
  - Usual prodromal phase
    - Fever, malaise, myalgia
  - Abnormal CSF evaluation
    - Increased protein, leukocytosis, no oligoclonal bands (usually)

Demographics

- Age
  - Typically childhood or young adult

Natural History & Prognosis

- Typically monophasic illness lasting from 2-4 weeks
- 50-60% recover completely
- Neurologic sequelae in 30-40%

Treatment

- Immunomodulation, supportive
  - Steroid treatment with intravenous methylprednisolone is treatment of choice, immunoglobulin therapy

DIAGNOSTIC CHECKLIST

Consider

- Repeat MR if initially negative and strong clinical suspicion

Image Interpretation Pearls

- ADEM can mimic cord neoplasm!

SELECTED REFERENCES

1. Cautilli F et al: Case report: a case of acute disseminated encephalomyelitis after SARS-CoV-2 infection in pediatric patients. Front Neurol. 14:1099458, 2023
2. Marin SE et al: The magnetic resonance imaging appearance of monophasic acute disseminated encephalomyelitis: an update post application of the 2007 consensus criteria. Neuroimaging Clin N Am. 23(2):245-66, 2013

Myelin Oligodendrocyte Glycoprotein Antibody-Associated Disease, Spine

KEY FACTS

TERMINOLOGY

- CNS immune-mediated demyelination with positive myelin oligodendrocyte glycoprotein (MOG)-IgG antibody test

IMAGING

- Patterns of cord involvement
  - Primarily central gray matter involvement
    - Sagittal plane: Pseudodilatation of central canal
    - Axial plane: H sign
  - Diffuse central T2 hyperintensity affecting gray and white matter
    - Appearance indistinguishable from AQP4-IgG myelitis

TOP DIFFERENTIAL DIAGNOSES

- Multiple sclerosis
- Neuromyelitis optica spectrum disorders
- Idiopathic transverse myelitis (TM)
- Spinal cord neoplasm
- Viral myelitis
- Spinal cord infarct

PATHOLOGY

- New diagnostic criteria for MOG antibody-associated disease (MOGAD) (March 2023)
  - 1 of 6 core clinical demyelinating events (optic neuritis, TM, acute disseminated encephalomyelitis, cerebral monofocal or polyfocal deficits, brainstem/cerebellar deficits, or cerebral cortical encephalitis)
  - Positive MOG-IgG antibody test
  - Exclusion of better diagnosis

CLINICAL ISSUES

- Limb weakness, sensory loss
- Neurogenic bowel, bladder, &/or sexual dysfunction (especially if conus involved)

DIAGNOSTIC CHECKLIST

- Consider MOGAD when bilateral optic neuritis and longitudinally extensive TM, particularly if conus involved

(Left) *Sagittal STIR MR in a 7-year-old with longitudinally extensive transverse myelitis (LETM) demonstrates abnormal long-segment cervicothoracic cord swelling and abnormal hyperintensity. This patient demonstrates the pseudodilatation of the central canal sign. Faint enhancement was also noted on contrast imaging (not shown).* **(Right)** *Axial T2WI MR in the same patient demonstrates the H sign with abnormal signal intensity in the central gray matter with hazy, fainter surrounding signal intensity.*

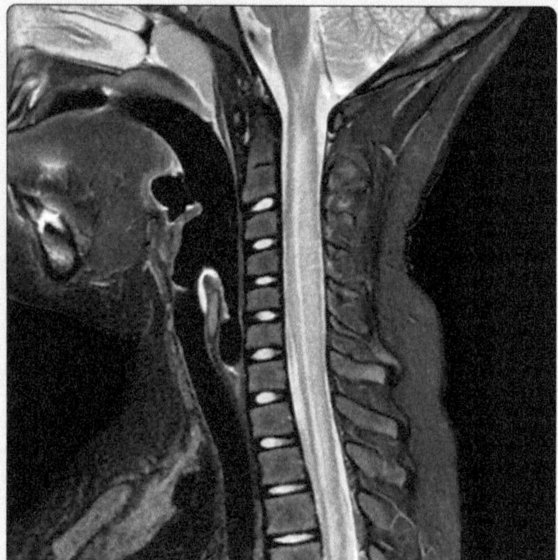

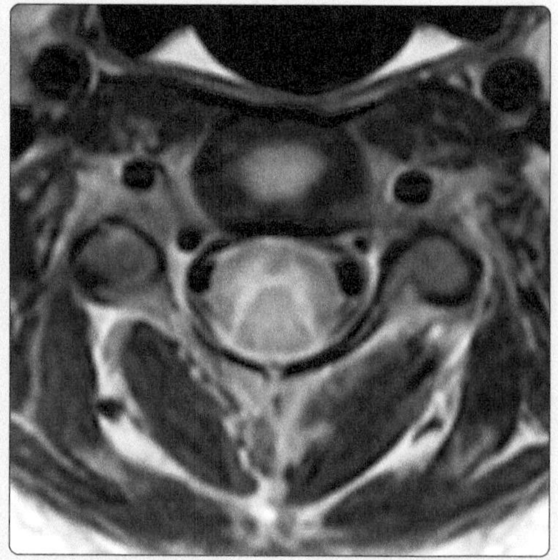

(Left) *Sagittal STIR MR in a 10-year-old girl presenting with lower extremity weakness and urinary retention demonstrates a focal hyperintense lesion ➡ in the conus. The patient also presented with bilateral optic neuritis but no encephalopathy. Subsequent brain imaging revealed metachronous development of characteristic demyelinating lesions (not shown). Serum MOG-Ab testing was positive.* **(Right)** *Sagittal T1WI C+ FS MR in the same patient shows no lesion enhancement.*

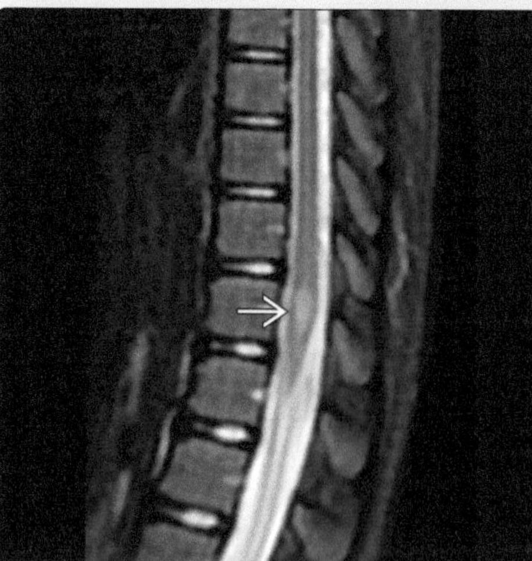

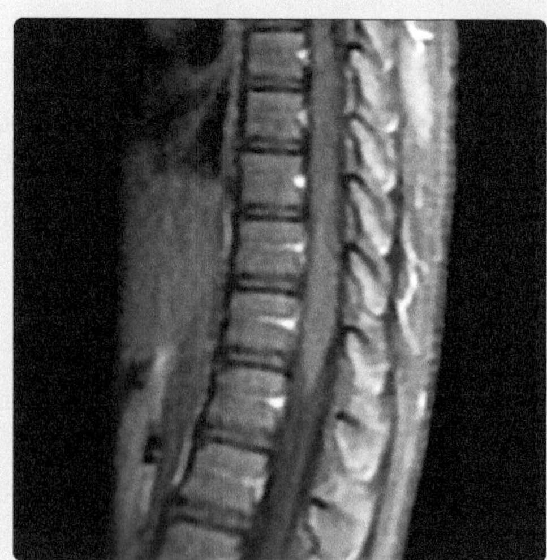

TERMINOLOGY

Abbreviations

- Myelin oligodendrocyte glycoprotein (MOG)
- MOG antibody-associated disease (MOGAD)

Definitions

- Inflammatory disease of CNS characterized by attacks of immune-mediated demyelination
- Serum MOG-IgG antibody positive

IMAGING

General Features

- Best diagnostic clue
  - Bilateral anterior optic pathway neuritis + longitudinally extensive transverse myelitis (LETM)
- Location
  - Spinal cord
    - LETM > 70% of MOGAD patients
    - Primarily cervical ± thoracic cord
    - Predilection for conus involvement
- Size
  - Longitudinally extensive lesion, ≥ 3 vertebral bodies in length common
  - May also see short lesions (< 2 vertebral bodies in length)

MR Findings

- T1WI
  - Lesions often isointense to cord parenchyma
- T2WI
  - Primarily central gray matter (GM) involvement
    - Sagittal plane: Pseudodilatation of central canal sign
      - Hyperintense line surrounded by hazy T2-hyperintense signal in anterior, posterior GM horns
      - ≈ 28% of MOGAD cases, highly suggestive of diagnosis
    - Axial plane: H sign
      - Central GM hyperintensity with fainter surrounding signal
  - Diffuse central T2 hyperintensity affecting GM and white matter (WM)
    - Appearance indistinguishable from AQP4-IgG myelitis
- T1WI C+
  - ± lesion enhancement

Imaging Recommendations

- Best imaging tool
  - MR with contrast, of orbits, brain, spinal cord

DIFFERENTIAL DIAGNOSIS

Multiple Sclerosis

- Short-segment cord involvement
- Peripheral location, often in dorsolateral tracts
- CSF oligoclonal bands

Neuromyelitis Optica Spectrum Disorders

- Central spinal cord location, longitudinally extensive
- Most patients positive for AQP4-IgG antibodies [seropositive neuromyelitis optica spectrum disorders (NMOSD)]

Idiopathic Transverse Myelitis

- Similar appearance to MOGAD, NMOSD
- Diagnosis of exclusion

Spinal Cord Neoplasm

- Look for heterogeneity, hemorrhage, cystic changes
- Occupies entire diameter of cord

Viral Myelitis

- Signal abnormalities often confined to GM (especially ventral GM)
- Consider West Nile, poliomyelitis, other neurotropic viruses

Spinal Cord Infarct

- Onset of flaccid paralysis usually rapid
- Diffusion-weighted imaging reveals acute restriction

PATHOLOGY

General Features

- MOG is myelin protein expressed on outer surface of oligodendrocytes and myelin sheath

Laboratory Evaluation

- Serum testing for MOG-IgG antibody
- Serum AQP4-IgG testing to evaluate for NMOSD
- CSF analysis with testing for oligoclonal bands to evaluate for MS

CLINICAL ISSUES

Presentation

- Most common signs/symptoms
  - Limb weakness, sensory loss
- Other signs/symptoms
  - Neurogenic bowel, bladder, &/or sexual dysfunction (especially if conus involved)

Demographics

- Age
  - Any age; median age of onset: 20-30 years
  - Children account for ~ 50% of MOGAD cases

Treatment

- Glucocorticoid or immunomodulatory therapy

DIAGNOSTIC CHECKLIST

Consider

- Consider MOGAD when bilateral optic neuritis and LETM, particularly if conus involved

SELECTED REFERENCES

1. Banwell B et al: Diagnosis of myelin oligodendrocyte glycoprotein antibody-associated disease: International MOGAD Panel proposed criteria. Lancet Neurol. 22(3):268-82, 2023
2. Gadde JA et al: Rate of leptomeningeal enhancement in pediatric myelin oligodendrocyte glycoprotein antibody-associated encephalomyelitis. J Child Neurol. 36(11):1042-6, 2021
3. Shahriari M et al: MOGAD: how it differs from and resembles other neuroinflammatory disorders. AJR Am J Roentgenol. 216(4):1031-9, 2021
4. Armangue T et al: Associations of paediatric demyelinating and encephalitic syndromes with myelin oligodendrocyte glycoprotein antibodies: a multicentre observational study. Lancet Neurol. 19(3):234-46, 2020
5. Dubey D et al: Clinical, radiologic, and prognostic features of myelitis associated with myelin oligodendrocyte glycoprotein autoantibody. JAMA Neurol. 76(3):301-9, 2019

Guillain-Barré Syndrome

KEY FACTS

TERMINOLOGY

- Group of disorders characterized by acute onset of weakness & diminished reflexes secondary to inflammatory polyradiculopathy

IMAGING

- Smooth pial enhancement of cauda equina & conus medullaris
  - Ventral roots > dorsal roots
  - May be slightly thickened but not nodular
- May see cranial nerve enhancement (Miller-Fisher variant)

TOP DIFFERENTIAL DIAGNOSES

- Physiologic nerve root enhancement
- CSF-disseminated metastases
- Hereditary polyneuropathies
- Subacute & chronic demyelinating polyneuropathies

PATHOLOGY

- Inflammatory immune-mediated demyelination
  - Cross reactivity of antibodies to pathogen with specific gangliosides & glycolipids
- Antecedent event or trigger in 70% of cases
- Subtypes include
  - Acute inflammatory demyelinating polyradiculoneuropathy: Most common form in USA
  - Acute motor axonal neuropathy: Pure motor form
  - Miller-Fisher variant: Ophthalmoplegia, ataxia, areflexia, normal extremity strength, & CSF protein

CLINICAL ISSUES

- Acute flaccid paralysis or distal paraesthesias rapidly followed by ascending paralysis

DIAGNOSTIC CHECKLIST

- Anterior cauda nerve root & pial conus enhancement without significant enlargement or nodularity suggestive

(Left) *Sagittal T1 MR in a patient with lower extremity flaccid weakness reveals a normal appearance of the conus and cauda equina.* **(Right)** *Sagittal T2 MR in the same patient confirms the normal appearance of the conus and cauda equina. No subjective root thickening or nodularity is seen.*

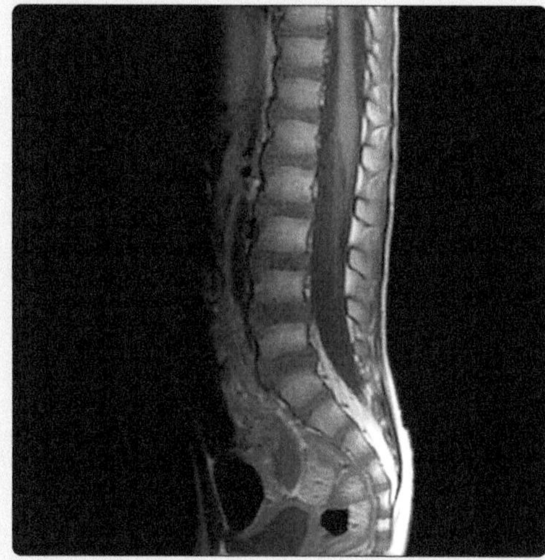

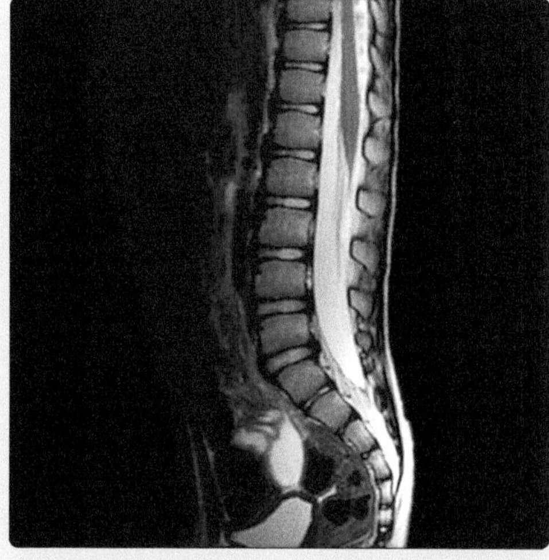

(Left) *Sagittal T1 C+ MR in the same patient reveals abnormal nerve root enhancement of both the ventral and dorsal cauda equina, providing a more specific imaging diagnosis.* **(Right)** *Axial T1 C+ MR in the same patient confirms that there is more enhancement of the ventral ➡ than the dorsal roots of the cauda equina, a characteristic but not absolute finding in Guillain-Barré syndrome (GBS).*

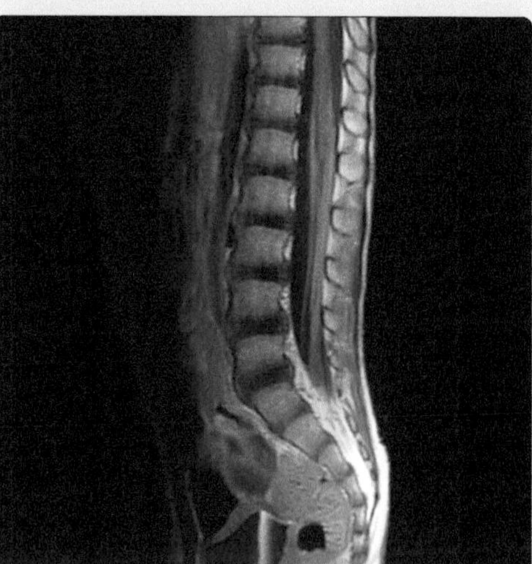

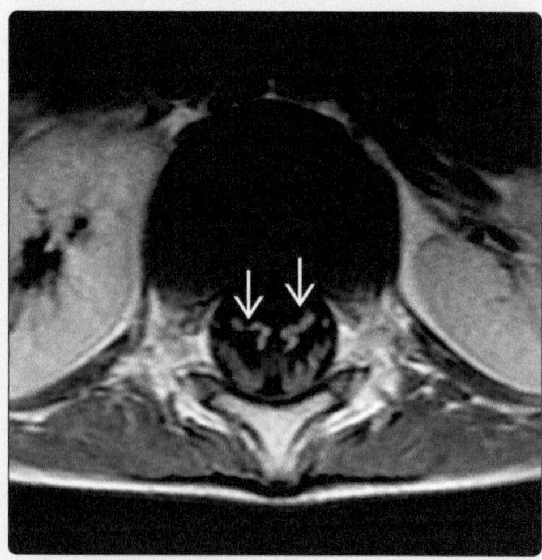

TERMINOLOGY

Abbreviations

- Guillain-Barré syndrome (GBS)

Synonyms

- Acute inflammatory demyelinating polyradiculoneuropathy (AIDP)

Definitions

- Group of disorders characterized by acute development of weakness & diminished reflexes secondary to inflammatory polyradiculopathy
  - Several subtypes exist
    - AIDP
    - Acute motor axonal neuropathy
    - Acute motor sensory axonal neuropathy
    - Miller-Fisher syndrome
- Primarily clinical diagnosis with supporting imaging findings

IMAGING

General Features

- Best diagnostic clue
  - Smooth prominent enhancement of cauda equina nerve roots
- Location
  - Ventral roots > dorsal roots
  - Lesions are scattered throughout peripheral nerves, nerve roots, & cranial nerves
- Size
  - Nerve roots may be slightly enlarged
- Morphology
  - Symmetric, smooth appearance of roots

CT Findings

- CECT
  - May rarely see symmetric enhancement of lumbar roots

MR Findings

- T2WI
  - Normal conus
  - May see slight prominence of root size
- T1WI C+
  - Avid enhancement of cauda equina: Ventral roots > dorsal roots; may be slightly thickened (but not nodular)
  - Pial surface of distal cord & conus enhances variably; conus not enlarged
  - Cranial nerve enhancement in Miller-Fisher variant

Nonvascular Interventions

- Myelography
  - May see symmetric enlargement of cauda equina roots
  - Lumbar puncture typically done in early stages to assess spinal fluid chemistry, protein levels, bacteriology

Imaging Recommendations

- Best imaging tool: Sagittal & axial T1WI with contrast

DIFFERENTIAL DIAGNOSIS

Physiologic Nerve Root Enhancement

- Much more subtle enhancement of normal roots
- Absent clinical syndrome

CSF-Disseminated Metastases

- Typically more nodular
- Conus deposits frequently cause T2 signal abnormality

Hereditary Polyneuropathies

- Charcot-Marie-Tooth, Dejerine-Sottas

Subacute or Chronic Demyelinating Polyneuropathies

- Clinical syndromes of inflammatory demyelinating polyradiculoneuropathy that have slower onset & longer duration than GBS
  - Chronic inflammatory demyelinating polyradiculoneuropathy (CIDP)
    - Chronic equivalent of AIDP
    - Slower onset, more protracted course
    - Minimum duration of symptoms until patients reach nadir: 2 months
  - Subacute inflammatory demyelinating polyradiculoneuropathy (SIDP)
    - Patients who fall between 4 weeks & 2 months

Acute Transverse Myelitis

- Cranial nerves always spared

Chemical or Postsurgical Arachnoiditis

- Hemorrhage-induced arachnoidal inflammation
- Systemic chemotherapy → vincristine neuropathy

Vasculitic Neuropathy

- Polyarteritis nodosa or Churg-Strauss most commonly
- Cranial nerves & respiratory nerves frequently spared

Bacterial or Granulomatous Meningitis

- Acute onset
- Fever, headache, + lumbar puncture

Anterior Lumbar Radiculopathy

- Transient or permanent paraplegia uncommon complication following intrathecal chemotherapy
- Smooth linear enhancement of ventral cauda equina & conus pia

Postradiation Radiculopathy

- Smooth enhancement of both ventral & dorsal cauda equina nerve roots
- History of prior radiation therapy

PATHOLOGY

General Features

- Etiology
  - Inflammatory immune-mediated demyelination; cross reactivity of antibodies to pathogen with specific gangliosides & glycolipids
    - Both cell-mediated & humoral mechanisms involved in pathogenesis
  - Antecedent event or trigger in 70% of GBS cases
    - *Campylobacter jejuni* infection: 1/3 to 2/3 of cases
    - CMV infection: Up to 15% of cases

- Multiple other infectious agents have been associated: EBV, HIV, *Mycoplasma*, varicella-zoster virus, Zika
- Etiologic correlation between SARS-CoV-2 & GBS established during COVID pandemic
- Temporal link has been suggested with vaccines but no correlation has been shown
- Genetics
  - May be 1st presentation of genetic or hereditary disorders
    - 17p12 mutation
    - Reported association with HLA typing & GBS subtypes (possible HLA DR2)

Staging, Grading, & Classification

- AIDP: Most common form in USA
  - Monophasic, nonfebrile with ascending weakness & hyporeflexia
- Acute motor axonal neuropathy
  - Pure motor form; 1/3 may be hyperreflexic
- Acute motor sensory axonal neuropathy
  - Sensory root involvement; muscle wasting common
- Miller-Fisher variant
  - Cranial nerve involvement; ophthalmoplegia, ataxia, areflexia, normal extremity strength, & CSF protein
  - 5% of all cases of GBS
- Acute panautonomic neuropathy
  - Affects sympathetic & parasympathetic nervous systems
- Pure sensory GBS
  - Sensory loss, ataxia, & areflexia
- Chronic polyneuropathies
  - SIDP
    - Disease course between 4 weeks & 2 months
    - Bridge from AIDP to CIDP
  - CIDP: Insidious onset over weeks or months; relapsing & remitting course
    - Associated with HIV, lymphoma, diabetes

Gross Pathologic & Surgical Features

- Thickened nerve roots

Microscopic Features

- Focal segmental demyelination
- Perivascular & endoneural lymphocytic/monocytic (macrophages) infiltrates
- Axonal degeneration in conjunction with segmental demyelination in severe cases
- Antiganglioside antibodies play pathogenic role
  - Nerve injury 2° to complement activation or dysfunction of molecules, such as voltage-gated sodium & calcium channels

CLINICAL ISSUES

Presentation

- Acute flaccid paralysis or distal paraesthesias rapidly followed by ascending paralysis
  - Ascent up to brainstem may involve cranial nerves
  - Frequently bilateral & symmetric
- Sensory loss common but less severe
- Autonomic disturbances

Demographics

- Epidemiology
  - Most common cause of paralysis in Western countries
  - Incidence: 1.2-3.0 cases per 100,000 people per year
  - Affects all ages, races, socioeconomic statuses
    - Typically children, young adults
- Clinical factors associated with poor outcome
  - ↑ age, presence of preceding diarrhea, severity of disability in early course of disease

Natural History & Prognosis

- Clinical nadir at 4 weeks
- Most patients somewhat better by 2-3 months
  - 30-50% have persistent symptoms at 1 year
  - Permanent deficits in 5-10%
- Relapse in 2-10%
  - Early relapse occurring < 9 weeks after onset more common in patients with GBS
  - 6% develop chronic course resembling CIDP
  - Earliest stages of SIDP & CIDP may be indistinguishable clinically from GBS
- Mortality in up to 8%

Treatment

- Medical management with plasma exchange or intravenous immunoglobulin (IVIg)
  - Severe GBS may benefit from plasma exchange after IVIg
  - Plasma exchange should be considered early in cases with axonal involvement & in recurrent or familial GBS forms
- Corticosteroids given alone do not significantly hasten recovery from GBS or affect long-term outcome
- May require prolonged respiratory support in severe cases

DIAGNOSTIC CHECKLIST

Consider

- Clinical setting critical in forming differential diagnosis

Image Interpretation Pearls

- Anterior cauda nerve root & pial conus enhancement without significant enlargement or nodularity strongly suggestive

SELECTED REFERENCES

1. Akçay N et al: Recurrent GBS with COVID-19 in a child: a case report. Pediatr Infect Dis J. 42(4):e129-30, 2023
2. Devi AK et al: Long-term neurological, behavioral, functional, quality of life, and school performance outcomes in children with Guillain-Barré syndrome admitted to PICU. Pediatr Neurol. 140:18-24, 2023
3. Orak SA et al: Two case reports and a literature review of typical GBS and rare GBS variants associated with COVID-19. Arch Pediatr. 30(4):236-9, 2023
4. Jaffry M et al: No significant increase in Guillain-Barré syndrome after COVID-19 vaccination in adults: a vaccine adverse event reporting system study. Vaccine. 40(40):5791-7, 2022
5. Michev A et al: Bickerstaff brainstem encephalitis and overlapping Guillain-Barré syndrome in children: report of two cases and review of the literature. Eur J Paediatr Neurol. 23(1):43-52, 2019
6. Chung A et al: Guillain-Barré syndrome. Pediatr Rev. 39(1):53-4, 2018
7. Fontes CA et al: Magnetic resonance imaging findings in Guillain-Barré syndrome caused by Zika virus infection. Neuroradiology. 58(8):837-8, 2016
8. Heikema AP et al: Campylobacter jejuni capsular genotypes are related to Guillain-Barré syndrome. Clin Microbiol Infect. 21(9):852.e1-9, 2015

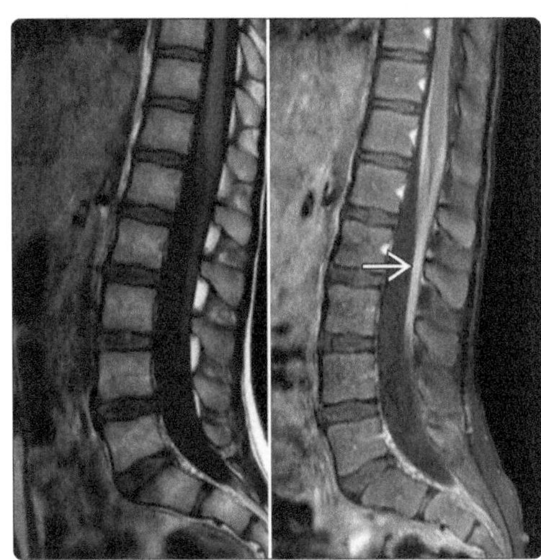

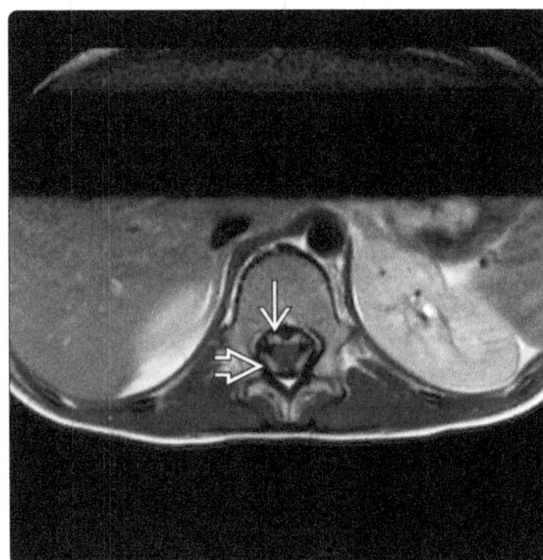

(Left) *Sagittal T1 (left) and T1 C+ FS (right) MR images show marked enhancement of the cauda equina nerve roots ➡ in this 10-year-old patient with GBS.* **(Right)** *Axial T1 C+ MR in the same patient shows a striking degree of enhancement of both ventral ➡ and dorsal ➡ cauda equina nerves relative to the conus medullaris. Some nerve root enhancement can be normal, but this degree of enhancement is not physiologic.*

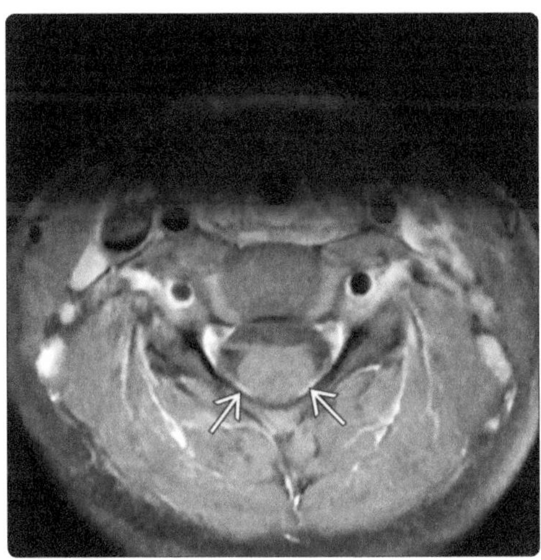

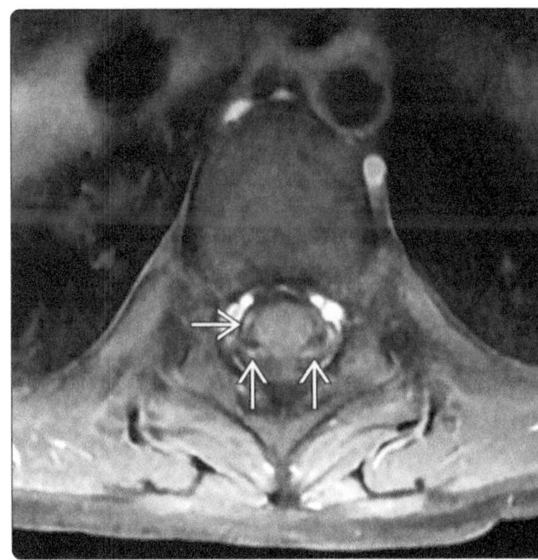

(Left) *Axial T1 C+ FS MR in a GBS patient with cranial nerve and upper extremity neuropathy reveals abnormal enhancement of multiple cervical nerve roots ➡. This patient also had cranial nerve and cauda equina enhancement (not shown).* **(Right)** *Axial T1 C+ FS MR in the same patient also reveals multiple enhancing thoracic nerves ➡.*

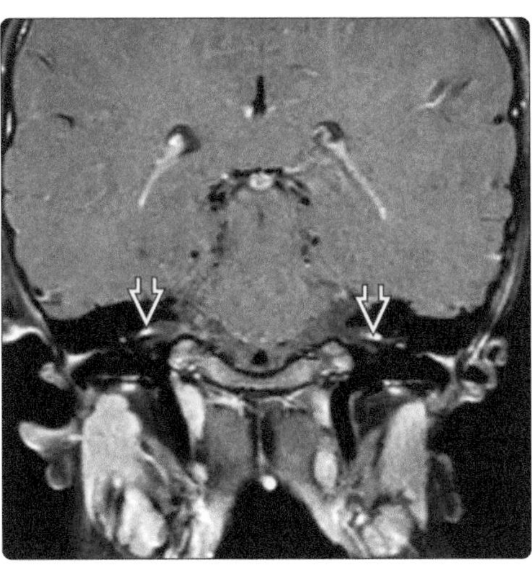

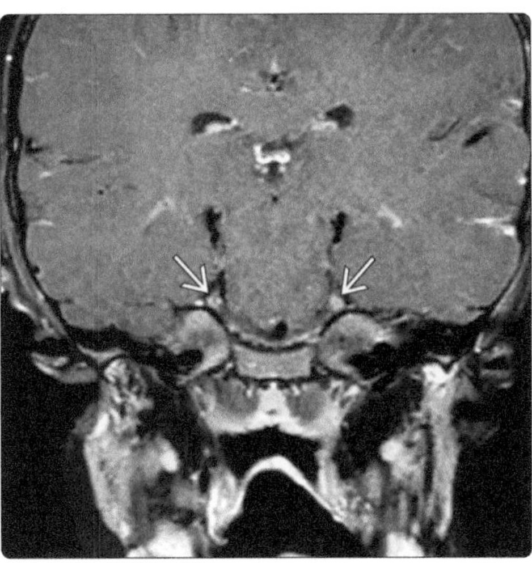

(Left) *Coronal T1 C+ FS MR through the internal auditory canals in a 3-year-old patient with the Miller-Fisher variant of GBS shows abnormal enhancement of the facial nerve on each side ➡.* **(Right)** *Coronal T1 C+ FS MR more anteriorly in the same patient shows bilateral and symmetric abnormal enhancement of the trigeminal nerves ➡ as well.*

Acute Flaccid Myelitis

KEY FACTS

TERMINOLOGY

- Synonyms: Acute flaccid paralysis, poliomyelitis-like paralytic syndrome

IMAGING

- Longitudinal T2 and FLAIR hyperintensity in spinal cord gray matter (cervical + variable inferior extension)
- Preference for ventral gray matter but may involve entirety of spinal cord gray matter in affected sections
  - Acute imaging shows involvement of either ventral or entire cord gray matter
  - Subacute imaging favors ventral gray matter
  - Cord lesions rarely enhance
- ± T2 hyperintensity in brainstem, medial cerebellum
- ± spinal nerve root, cranial nerve enhancement

TOP DIFFERENTIAL DIAGNOSES

- Guillain-Barré syndrome
- Acute transverse myelitis
- Paralytic poliomyelitis
- Poliomyelitis-like conditions

PATHOLOGY

- CSF: Lymphocytic or mixed pleocytosis

CLINICAL ISSUES

- Presentation with acute flaccid limb weakness but minimal or no sensory symptoms
  - May involve any combination of limbs but preference for upper extremities
  - Weakness frequently asymmetric
- > 80% cases have prodromal illness (median 5 days before onset)

DIAGNOSTIC CHECKLIST

- Localization to spinal cord ventral gray matter highly suggestive of acute flaccid myelitis
- Imaging findings frequently regress or resolve on long-term imaging follow-up

(Left) *Axial graphic of the cervical spinal cord demonstrates abnormal enlargement and edema in the central cord gray matter with greater involvement of the ventral horns compared to dorsal horns.* **(Right)** *Axial T2 MR of the cervical cord in an acute flaccid myelitis (AFM) patient with asymmetric arm weakness reveals abnormal enlargement and T2 hyperintensity within the central cord gray matter. Note the greater involvement of the ventral horns compared to dorsal horns.*

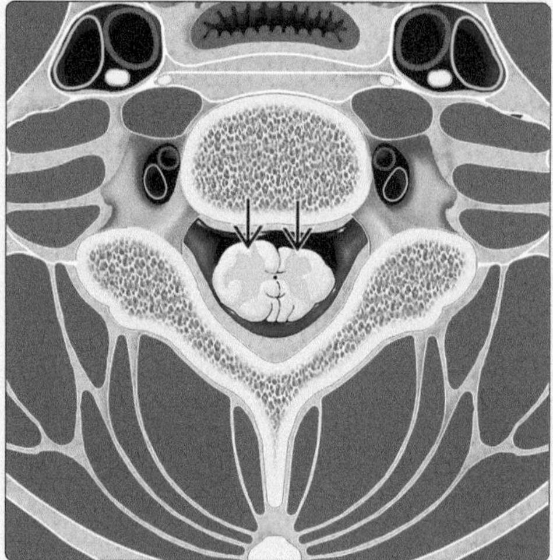

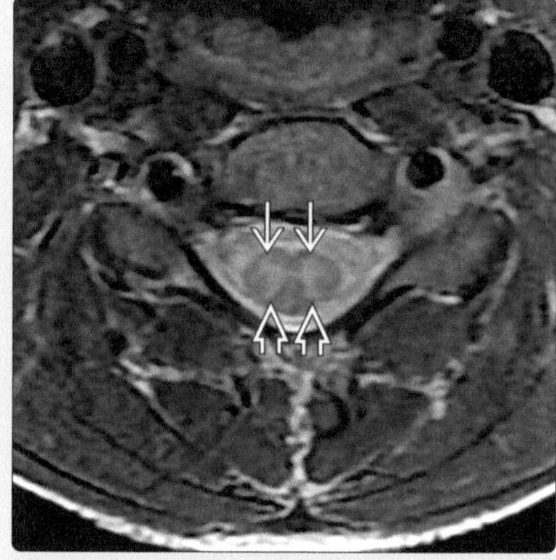

(Left) *Sagittal T2 MR in the same patient shows long-segment ventral intramedullary signal abnormality within the cervical spinal cord that extended into upper thoracic cord (not shown), conforming to findings on axial imaging.* **(Right)** *Axial T1 C+ MR in the same patient reveals mild contrast enhancement within the anterior gray matter, corresponding to more severe areas of T2 hyperintensity. Contrast enhancement is rare but has been reported in some subacute cases.*

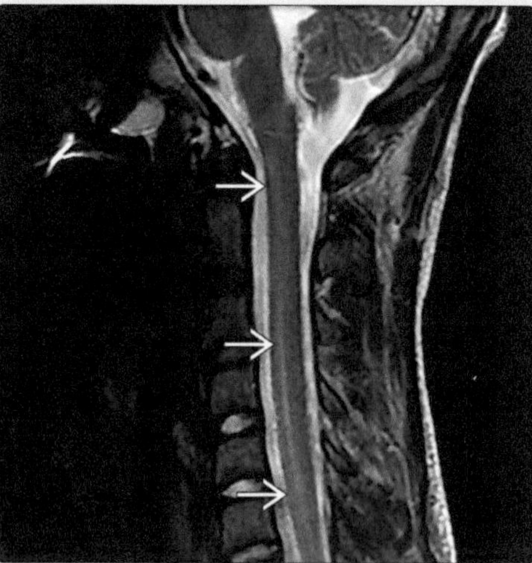

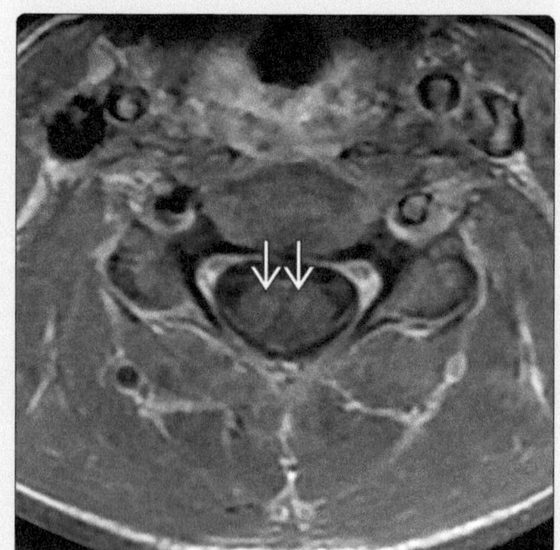

TERMINOLOGY

Abbreviations

- Acute flaccid myelitis (AFM)

Synonyms

- Acute flaccid paralysis
- Poliomyelitis-like paralytic syndrome

IMAGING

General Features

- Best diagnostic clue
  - Enlargement and abnormal T2 hyperintensity of spinal cord gray matter (ventral vs. entire) in affected segments
- Location
  - Spinal cord gray matter (cervical + variable inferior extension)
    - Preference for ventral gray matter
    - May involve entirety of spinal cord gray matter in affected sections
  - ± brainstem, medial cerebellum (dentate nuclei)
  - Spares supratentorial brain
- Morphology
  - Restricted to central cord gray matter
    - ± edema or enlargement

Radiographic Findings

- No routine role

CT Findings

- No routine role

MR Findings

- T1WI
  - Normal to mildly hypointense central cord signal in affected segments
- T2WI
  - Longitudinal T2 and FLAIR hyperintensity within spinal cord gray matter
    - Acute imaging shows involvement of either ventral or entire cord gray matter
    - Subacute imaging favors ventral gray matter
  - Some patients show abnormal T2 hyperintensity within brainstem, medial cerebellum
    - Pontine tegmentum > midbrain, medulla (rare)
    - Cerebellar dentate nuclei
  - Imaging findings frequently regress or resolve on long-term imaging follow-up
- T1WI C+
  - ± spinal nerve root, cranial nerve enhancement (subacute phase)
  - Cord lesions enhance rarely

Ultrasonographic Findings

- No routine role

Imaging Recommendations

- Best imaging tool
  - Multiplanar MR imaging of entire spinal cord
- Protocol advice
  - Sagittal and axial T2, axial T1 C+ MR most helpful

DIFFERENTIAL DIAGNOSIS

Guillain-Barré Syndrome

- Typically presents with ascending paralysis
  - May be associated with facial paralysis and sensory symptoms
- Enhancement of **dorsal** nerve rootlets, conus pia, cauda equina
- CSF cytoalbuminologic dissociation (high CSF protein, usually < 6 WBCs)

Acute Transverse Myelitis

- Presents with weakness and prominent sensory loss, often with demonstrable spinal sensory level
  - In contrast, majority of children with AFM show minimal or no sensory symptoms
- Involvement of both gray matter and white matter
- Supratentorial lesions common
- Lymphocytic or mixed CSF pleocytosis

Paralytic Poliomyelitis

- Human enterovirus (EV) C group (types 1, 2, and 3): All types produce motor neuron disease
- Most paralytic disease caused by poliovirus type 1 in prevaccination era
- Disease due to wildtype poliovirus infection (as of 2018) limited to Afghanistan and Pakistan
- Rare cases of vaccine-associated paralytic polio continue to occur in countries that use live attenuated oral polio vaccine for routine infant immunization and control of wildtype polio
- Imaging features overlap with AFM, West Nile virus

Poliomyelitis-Like Conditions

- West Nile virus, nonpolio EVs, herpes zoster, rabies
- Imaging findings overlap with AFM

PATHOLOGY

General Features

- Etiology
  - USA outbreak of acute flaccid paralysis reported in spring/summer of 2014
  - Association with EV-D68 (North America) and EV-A71 (Southeast Asia) nonpolioviruses postulated, but causal link not definitively proved
    - Outbreak coincided with spike in EV-D68 respiratory infections
    - EV-A71 and EV-D70 produce similar clinical illness
    - EV-A71 also associated with severe form of brainstem encephalitis affecting young children
  - Suspected to reflect immune response to prior infectious illness rather than direct infectious myelitis
    - CDC has created task force to investigate relationship to EV-D68 or autoimmune reaction to prior viral stimulus
  - Human EV comprises 4 species (A, B, C, and D) and 64 human serotypes
    - Single-stranded RNA genome
    - Viruses target motor neurons in brainstem, spinal cord
    - Polioviruses part of human EV C group
- Associated abnormalities

- CSF: Lymphocytic or mixed pleocytosis
  - ~ 70-80% of children with AFM have moderate CSF pleocytosis, median cell count ~ 100 WBCs
  - EV-D68 detection in CSF rare (< 10%)

Gross Pathologic & Surgical Features

- Rarely fatal; gross pathology and histopathology not described

CLINICAL ISSUES

Presentation

- Most common signs/symptoms
  - Lower motor neuron paralysis with hyporeflexia/areflexia, hypotonia
    - Patients present with acute flaccid limb weakness
      - May involve any combination of limbs with preference for upper extremities
    - Paralysis onset is rapid (hours to days) and frequently asymmetric
    - Maximum paralysis occurs within 4 days of onset
  - Minimal or no sensory symptoms
  - > 80% cases have prodromal illness
    - Median 5 days before paralysis onset
    - Illness usually includes fever and respiratory or gastrointestinal symptoms
- Other signs/symptoms
  - Motor cranial nerve deficits (~ 30%)
  - Variable bowel/bladder dysfunction
  - Sensory impairment unusual; generally mild and transient

Demographics

- Sex
  - M ≥ F
- Epidemiology
  - Outbreaks since identification seem to be biennial (2014, 2016, 2018)
    - 2020 and 2022 seemed to have much lower incidence of outbreak
      - Speculated due to changes in masking and socializing due to SARS CoV-2
  - Seasonal predilection for summer and fall
  - Estimated 22-35 cases EV-D68-associated AFM cases per year from 2015-2017
    - Relationship to EV-D68 varies with geographical area
  - Primarily affects children; median age 6 years

Natural History & Prognosis

- Motor deficits common at follow-up despite therapy with intravenous immunoglobulin, corticosteroids, or plasma exchange
- Intensive rehabilitation may improve functional outcome
  - Recovery is frequently incomplete; motor deficits and muscle atrophy persist in most children at 1 year
- EMG findings correlate better with outcome than imaging findings

Treatment

- Currently no specific acute treatment with demonstrated efficacy
- Intravenous immunoglobulin, corticosteroids, and plasma exchange all investigated
  - Ineffective; 9/10 (90%) children in one study had motor deficits at follow-up

DIAGNOSTIC CHECKLIST

Consider

- AFM is unique subset of acute flaccid paralysis distinct from GBS and transverse myelitis
  - Prominent motor involvement, limited sensory symptoms, and high probability of residual motor deficits compared to other forms of acute flaccid paralysis

Image Interpretation Pearls

- Lesion localization to spinal cord ventral gray matter in correct clinical context highly suggestive of AFM

SELECTED REFERENCES

1. Kozlowski J et al: Acute flaccid myelitis: review of clinical features, diagnosis, and management with nerve transfers. Plast Reconstr Surg. 151(1):85e-98e, 2023
2. Helfferich J et al: Epidemiology of acute flaccid myelitis in children in the Netherlands, 2014 to 2019. Euro Surveill. 27(42), 2022
3. Ma KC et al: Increase in acute respiratory illnesses among children and adolescents associated with rhinoviruses and enteroviruses, including enterovirus D68 - United States, July-September 2022. MMWR Morb Mortal Wkly Rep. 71(40):1265-70, 2022
4. Kramer R et al: Acute flaccid myelitis caused by enterovirus D68: case definitions for use in clinical practice. Eur J Paediatr Neurol. 23(2):235-9, 2019
5. Messacar K et al: Enterovirus D68-associated acute flaccid myelitis: rising to the clinical and research challenges. JAMA. 321(9):831-2, 2019
6. Bitnun A et al: Acute flaccid paralysis and enteroviral infections. Curr Infect Dis Rep. 20(9):34, 2018
7. Chong PF et al: Clinical features of acute flaccid myelitis temporally associated with an enterovirus D68 outbreak: results of a nationwide survey of acute flaccid paralysis in Japan, August-December 2015. Clin Infect Dis. 66(5):653-64, 2018
8. Dyda A et al: The association between acute flaccid myelitis (AFM) and enterovirus D68 (EV-D68) - what is the evidence for causation? Euro Surveill. 23(3), 2018
9. Messacar K et al: Enterovirus D68 and acute flaccid myelitis-evaluating the evidence for causality. Lancet Infect Dis. 18(8):e239-47, 2018
10. Andersen EW et al: Acute flaccid myelitis in childhood: a retrospective cohort study. Eur J Neurol. 24(8):1077-83, 2017
11. Ben Achour N et al: Comment on 'acute flaccid myelitis in childhood: a retrospective cohort study'. Eur J Neurol. 24(11):e81-2, 2017
12. Bonwitt J et al: Acute flaccid myelitis among children - Washington, September-November 2016. MMWR Morb Mortal Wkly Rep. 66(31):826-9, 2017
13. Esposito S et al: Acute flaccid myelitis associated with enterovirus-D68 infection in an otherwise healthy child. Virol J. 14(1):4, 2017
14. Hopkins SE: Acute flaccid myelitis: Etiologic challenges, diagnostic and management considerations. Curr Treat Options Neurol. 19(12):48, 2017
15. Martin JA et al: Outcomes of Colorado children with acute flaccid myelitis at 1 year. Neurology. 89(2):129-37, 2017
16. McCoy DB et al: MRI atlas-based measurement of spinal cord injury predicts outcome in acute flaccid myelitis. AJNR Am J Neuroradiol. 38(2):410-7, 2017
17. Yoder JA et al: Pediatric acute flaccid paralysis: enterovirus D68-associated anterior myelitis. J Emerg Med. 53(1):e19-23, 2017
18. Aliabadi N et al: Enterovirus D68 infection in children with acute flaccid myelitis, Colorado, USA, 2014. Emerg Infect Dis. 22(8):1387-94, 2016
19. Messacar K et al: Acute flaccid myelitis: a clinical review of US cases 2012-2015. Ann Neurol. 80(3):326-38, 2016
20. Nelson GR et al: Recognition and management of acute flaccid myelitis in children. Pediatr Neurol. 55:17-21, 2016
21. Sejvar JJ et al: Acute flaccid myelitis in the United States, August-December 2014: results of Nationwide Surveillance. Clin Infect Dis. 63(6):737-45, 2016
22. Maloney JA et al: MRI findings in children with acute flaccid paralysis and cranial nerve dysfunction occurring during the 2014 enterovirus D68 outbreak. AJNR Am J Neuroradiol. 36(2):245-50, 2014

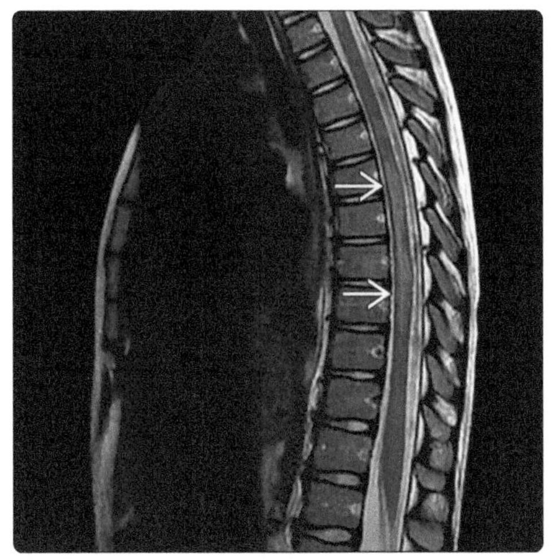

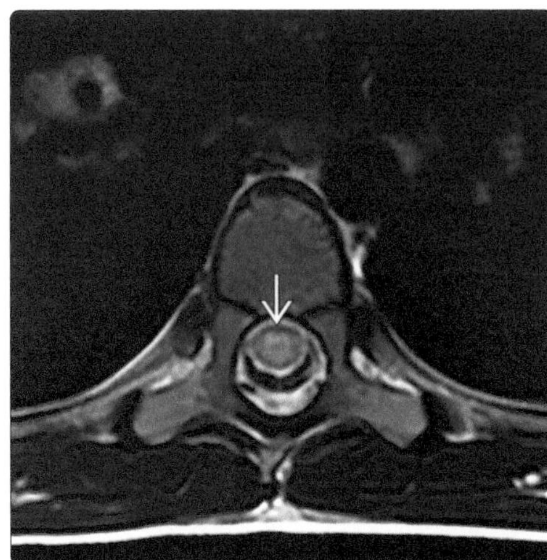

(Left) *Sagittal T2 MR in a patient with relatively rapid onset of lower extremity paralysis and urinary bladder retention reveals segmental thoracic cord enlargement and abnormal T2 hyperintensity ➡.* **(Right)** *Axial T2 MR in the same patient reveals abnormal T2 hyperintensity within the thoracic spinal cord gray matter favoring the anterior horns ➡. T1 C+ MR (not shown) revealed no abnormal contrast enhancement.*

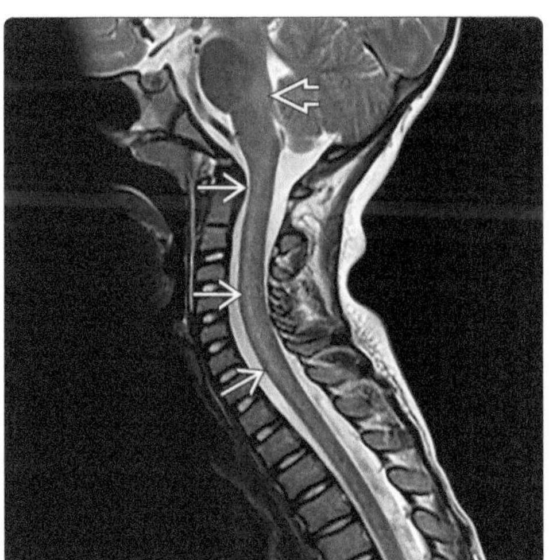

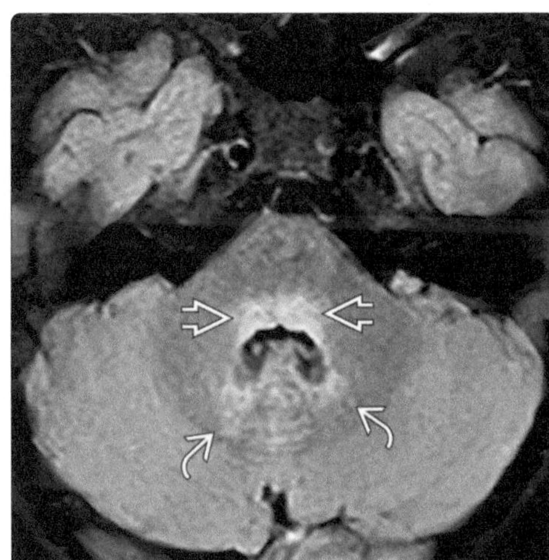

(Left) *Sagittal T2 MR in a patient with bilateral (asymmetric) weakness reveals abnormal central cervical cord T2 hyperintensity ➡. Note also abnormal T2-hyperintense signal within the medulla and pontine tegmentum ⇨.* **(Right)** *Axial FLAIR MR in the same patient confirms abnormal T2 hyperintensity within the pontine tegmentum ⇨ as well as within the deep cerebellar white matter ↪, reflecting characteristic brain manifestations seen in some AFM patients.*

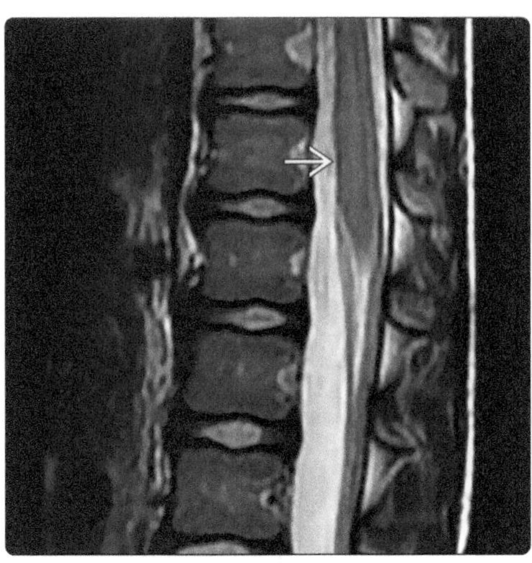

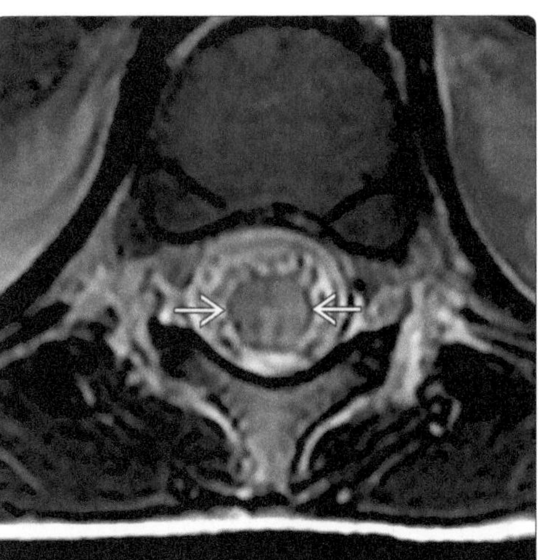

(Left) *Sagittal T2 MR in a patient with acute-onset asymmetric (left worse than right) lower extremity paralysis reveals abnormal enlargement and T2 hyperintensity ➡ within the conus.* **(Right)** *Axial T2 MR in the same patient confirms abnormal conus gray matter enlargement and T2 hyperintensity ➡, anterior worse than posterior, and left greater than right involvement.*

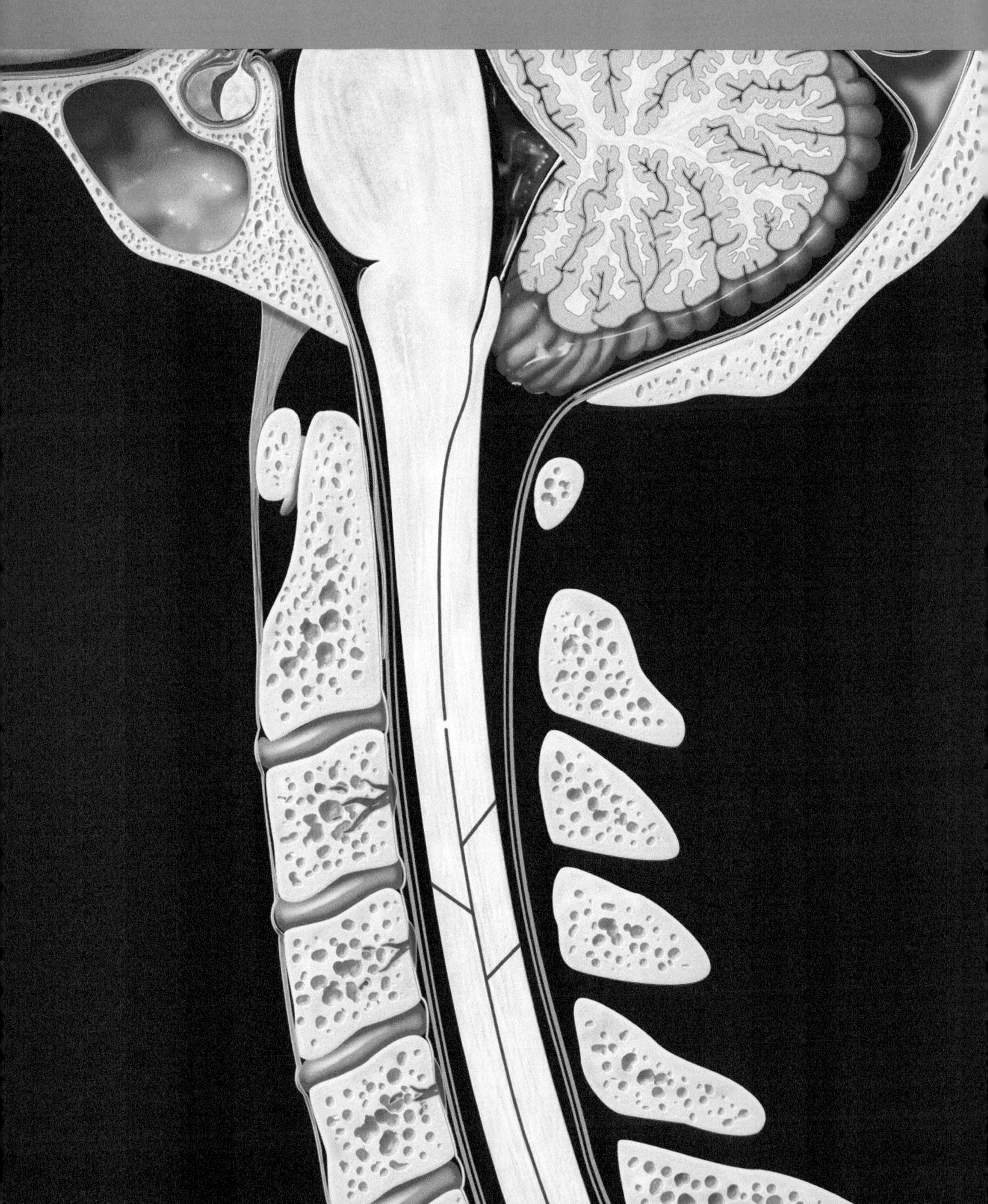

PART III
SECTION 5

Neoplasms, Cysts, and Other Masses

Neoplasms

Nonneoplastic Cysts and Tumor Mimics

KEY FACTS

TERMINOLOGY

- Benign osteoid-producing tumor < 1.5 cm in size
- Tumor often called "nidus" to distinguish it from surrounding reactive zone due to host response

IMAGING

- 10% of osteoid osteomas (OOs) occur in spine, in neural arch
- Focal scoliosis, concave on side of tumor
- Central nidus
  - Variable amount of ossification
- Reactive zone
  - Dense sclerosis, edema around nidus
  - Involves much larger area than tumor
  - Periosteal reaction variably present
  - Soft tissue mass or pleural thickening/effusion
  - Low signal on T1WI, high signal on T2WI, STIR
  - Enhances with gadolinium, iodinated contrast

TOP DIFFERENTIAL DIAGNOSES

- Osteoblastoma
- Stress fracture of pedicle or lamina
- Unilateral spondylolysis
- Unilateral absent pedicle or pars interarticularis
- Sclerotic metastasis
- Lymphoma
- Osteomyelitis
- Ewing sarcoma

CLINICAL ISSUES

- Night pain relieved by aspirin, NSAIDs
- 70% have scoliosis related to muscle spasm, concave on side of tumor

DIAGNOSTIC CHECKLIST

- Thin-section CT most accurate in visualizing nidus
- Edema on MR mimics infection, malignancy

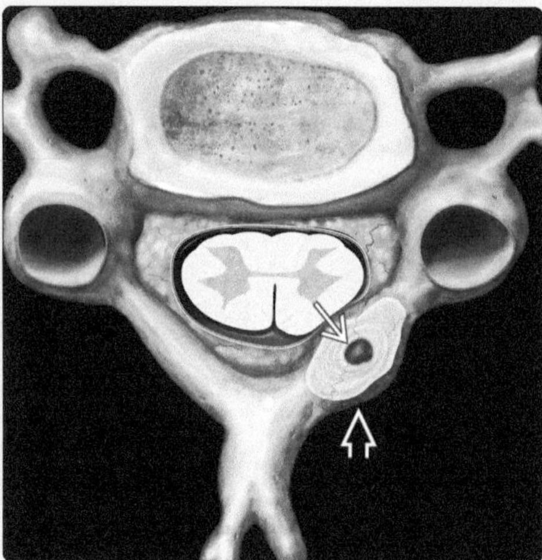

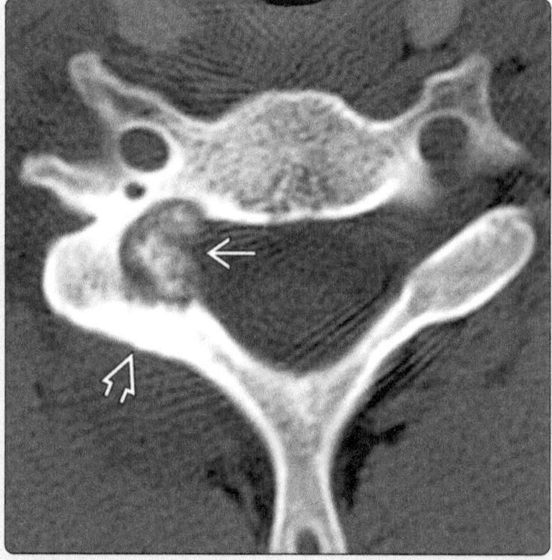

(Left) *Axial graphic shows a small, highly vascular tumor nidus ➡ of an osteoid osteoma (OO) in the left lamina surrounded by dense reactive bone ⇨.* **(Right)** *Axial bone CT in the same patient shows a sclerotic C6 OO nidus ➡. The nidus may range from purely radiolucent to completely sclerotic. The lesion is sharply demarcated and surrounded by reactive sclerosis ⇨. The lesion was missed on a prior routine cervical spine MR.*

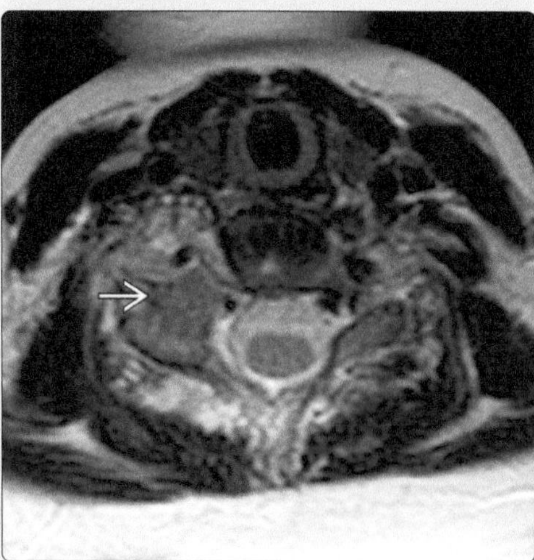

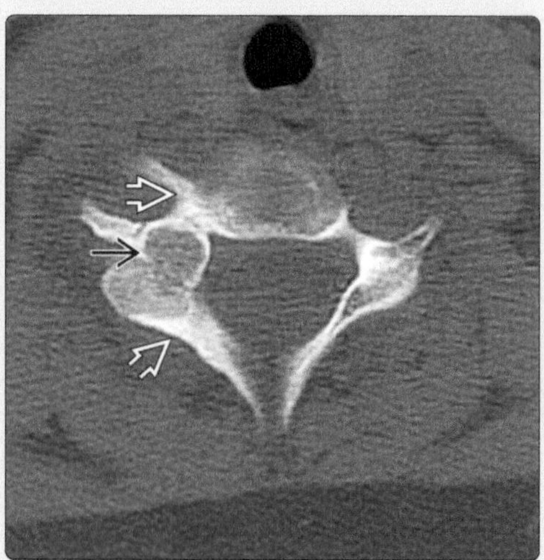

(Left) *Axial T2WI MR shows an ill-defined intermediate signal intensity mass in the right C6 neural foramen ➡. The mass appears poorly marginated, mimicking malignancy. Because of the patient's age, OO was considered, and a CT scan was performed.* **(Right)** *Axial bone CT in the same patient confirms a lytic OO nidus ➡ with surrounding host sclerosis ⇨ accounting for reactive edema noted on MR.*

TERMINOLOGY

Abbreviations

- Osteoid osteoma (OO)

Definitions

- Benign osteoid-producing tumor < 1.5 cm in size
- Tumor often called "nidus" to distinguish it from surrounding reactive zone due to host response

IMAGING

General Features

- Best diagnostic clue
  - Small, radiolucent tumor nidus with surrounding sclerosis
- Location
  - 10% of OOs occur in spine
  - Almost all involve neural arch
  - 59% lumbar, 27% cervical, 12% thoracic, 2% sacrum
- Size
  - < 1.5 cm nidus; larger lesions called osteoblastoma
- Morphology
  - Nidus round or oval

Radiographic Findings

- Radiography
  - Central lucent tumor nidus often obscured by reactive sclerosis
  - Focal scoliosis concave on side of tumor

CT Findings

- CECT
  - Variable enhancement of nidus and reactive zone
    - Contrast administration may obscure bony matrix
- Bone CT
  - Central nidus
    - Variable amount of ossification in nidus
    - Nidus usually predominantly lucent
    - Occasionally, nidus is sclerotic
  - Reactive zone
    - Dense sclerosis around tumor
    - Periosteal reaction variably present, usually unilaminar
    - Soft tissue mass or pleural thickening/effusion often seen
    - Bones adjacent to OO may show sclerosis, periosteal reaction
      - Ribs, adjacent vertebrae affected
    - Ossification of ligamentum flavum has been reported

MR Findings

- Central nidus
  - Low signal intensity on T1WI
  - Variable low to high signal intensity on T2WI, STIR
  - Avid, rapid enhancement with gadolinium
- Reactive zone
  - Edema surrounding nidus due to prostaglandin release
    - Low signal on T1WI, high signal on T2WI, STIR
    - Enhances with gadolinium
      - Dynamic scan may show delayed enhancement relative to nidus
  - Involves much larger area than tumor
  - May lead to misdiagnosis of malignancy or infection
  - Periosteal reaction and cortical thickening common
  - May extend to adjacent vertebrae, ribs, and paraspinous soft tissues
    - Pleural thickening, enhancement, and effusion common with thoracic OO
- Literature reports high rate of missed MR diagnosis of OO
  - Lesion may not be seen due to small size of nidus
    - Thin shape, oblique orientation of posterior elements
    - Partial volume averaging with adjacent structures
    - Improve visualization with thin slices, 3.0-3.5 mm
    - Axial, coronal, and sagittal planes
  - Lesion misidentified based on appearance of reactive zone rather than nidus
    - Misdiagnosis of infection or malignancy common

Nuclear Medicine Findings

- Bone scan
  - Positive on all 3 phases of Tc-99m MDP bone scan

Imaging Recommendations

- Best imaging tool
  - CT

DIFFERENTIAL DIAGNOSIS

Osteoblastoma

- Larger (> 1.5 cm)
- Expansile lesion of neural arch/pedicle

Stress Fracture of Pedicle or Lamina

- Sclerosis around fracture mimics reactive sclerosis around OO
- CT with reformatted images or high-resolution MR will show fracture line
- May occur in patients with preexisting scoliosis due to altered stresses
- Pain related to activity, improves at night

Unilateral Spondylolysis

- Linear defect pars interarticularis
- Contralateral side is sclerotic
- Painful
- Presents in young patients
- Scoliosis may develop
- May be diagnosed on oblique radiographs, CT

Unilateral Absent Pedicle or Pars Interarticularis

- Contralateral side is sclerotic
- Congenital absence of pedicle or pars interarticularis confirmed on CT

Sclerotic Metastasis

- Older patients

Lymphoma

- Older patients
- Often involves pedicle, destroys posterior body cortex
- Poorly defined, wide zone of transition
- Associated soft tissue mass common
- Often presents with night pain relieved by aspirin, NSAIDs

Osteomyelitis

- Sequestrum or focal abscess can mimic nidus of OO
  - Tends to have irregular shape, unlike round OO nidus
- Usually involves vertebral bodies rather than neural arch
- CT usually shows endplate destruction or destructive arthritis of facet joints
- Often presents with night pain relieved by aspirin, NSAIDs

Ewing Sarcoma

- Marrow replacement looks similar on MR
  - Centered in vertebral body
  - Diffuse edema may involve adjacent vertebrae and ribs

PATHOLOGY

General Features

- Etiology
  - Benign tumor of osteoblastic origin

Gross Pathologic & Surgical Features

- Sharply demarcated, round, pink-red mass (nidus)
- Nidus can be shelled out from surrounding sclerotic reactive bone that does not contain tumor

Microscopic Features

- Web of osteoid trabeculae showing variable amounts of mineralization
- Vascular fibrous connective tissue
- Histologically similar to osteoblastoma
- No malignant potential
- Reactive zone may contain lymphocytes and plasmocytes

CLINICAL ISSUES

Presentation

- Most common signs/symptoms
  - Night pain relieved by aspirin, NSAIDs
- Clinical profile
  - 70% have scoliosis related to muscle spasm, concave on side of tumor
  - Gait disturbance, muscle atrophy, torticollis sometimes seen

Demographics

- Age
  - Majority occur in 2nd decade of life
  - Reported as late as 7th decade, but very rare
- Sex
  - M:F = 2-3:1
- Epidemiology
  - 12% of all benign skeletal neoplasms

Natural History & Prognosis

- Resection is curative in most cases
  - Entire nidus must be removed or recurrence is probable
  - Radionuclide labeling can be used to localize intraoperatively
- Spontaneous healing has been reported

Treatment

- Open excision
  - Proximity to vertebral artery should be noted in cervical OOs
- CT-guided percutaneous excision
- Thermo-/photocoagulation (radiofrequency ablation)
- Conservative observation (patients with well-controlled symptoms)

DIAGNOSTIC CHECKLIST

Consider

- Important cause of painful scoliosis in child or young adult

Image Interpretation Pearls

- Thin-section CT most accurate in visualizing nidus
- Edema on MR mimics infection, malignancy

SELECTED REFERENCES

1. Zairi M et al: Structural scoliosis secondary to thoracic osteoid osteoma: a case report of delayed diagnosis. Spine Deform. 11(1):247-51, 2023
2. Sagoo NS et al: Radiofrequency ablation for spinal osteoid osteoma: a systematic review of safety and treatment outcomes. Surg Oncol. 41:101747, 2022
3. Filippiadis D et al: Percutaneous computed tomography-guided radiofrequency ablation of a spinal osteoid osteoma abutting the dura: a case report and review of the literature. Eur J Orthop Surg Traumatol. 31(8):1625-30, 2021
4. Pipola V et al: Surgery Versus radiofrequency ablation in the management of spinal osteoid osteomas: a spine oncology referral center comparison analysis of 138 cases. World Neurosurg. 145:e298-304, 2021
5. Ono T et al: Osteoid osteoma can occur at the pars interarticularis of the lumbar spine, leading to misdiagnosis of lumbar spondylolysis. Am J Case Rep. 19:207-13, 2018
6. Tomasian A et al: Spinal osteoid osteoma: percutaneous radiofrequency ablation using a navigational bipolar electrode system. AJR Am J Roentgenol. 211(4):856-60, 2018
7. Tomasian A et al: Benign spine lesions: advances in techniques for minimally invasive percutaneous treatment. AJNR Am J Neuroradiol. 38(5):852-61, 2017
8. Earhart J et al: Radiofrequency ablation in the treatment of osteoid osteoma: results and complications. Pediatr Radiol. 43(7):814-9, 2013
9. Liu PT et al: The vascular groove sign: a new CT finding associated with osteoid osteomas. AJR Am J Roentgenol. 196(1):168-73, 2011
10. Chai JW et al: Radiologic diagnosis of osteoid osteoma: from simple to challenging findings. Radiographics. 2010 May;30(3):737-49. Erratum in: Radiographics. 30(4):1156, 2010
11. Hoffmann RT et al: Radiofrequency ablation in the treatment of osteoid osteoma-5-year experience. Eur J Radiol. 73(2):374-9, 2010
12. Kan P et al: Osteoid osteoma and osteoblastoma of the spine. Neurosurg Clin N Am. 19(1):65-70, 2008
13. Liu PT et al: Imaging of osteoid osteoma with dynamic gadolinium-enhanced MR imaging. Radiology. 227(3):691-700, 2003
14. Davies M et al: The diagnostic accuracy of MR imaging in osteoid osteoma. Skeletal Radiol. 31(10):559-69, 2002
15. Scuotto A et al: Unusual manifestation of vertebral osteoid osteoma: case report. Eur Radiol. 12(1):109-12, 2002
16. Lefton DR et al: Vertebral osteoid osteoma masquerading as a malignant bone or soft-tissue tumor on MRI. Pediatr Radiol. 31(2):72-5, 2001
17. Cove JA et al: Osteoid osteoma of the spine treated with percutaneous computed tomography-guided thermocoagulation. Spine. 25(10):1283-6, 2000
18. Gangi A et al: Percutaneous laser photocoagulation of spinal osteoid osteomas under CT guidance. AJNR Am J Neuroradiol. 19(10):1955-8, 1998
19. Radcliffe SN et al: Osteoid osteoma: the difficult diagnosis. Eur J Radiol. 28(1):67-79, 1998
20. Assoun J et al: Osteoid osteoma: MR imaging versus CT. Radiology. 191(1):217-23, 1994
21. Zambelli PY et al: Osteoid osteoma or osteoblastoma of the cervical spine in relation to the vertebral artery. J Pediatr Orthop. 14(6):788-92, 1994
22. Greenspan A: Benign bone-forming lesions: osteoma, osteoid osteoma, and osteoblastoma. Clinical, imaging, pathologic, and differential considerations. Skeletal Radiol. 22(7):485-500, 1993
23. Woods ER et al: Reactive soft-tissue mass associated with osteoid osteoma: correlation of MR imaging features with pathologic findings. Radiology. 186(1):221-5, 1993
24. Klein MH et al: Osteoid osteoma: radiologic and pathologic correlation. Skeletal Radiol. 21(1):23-31, 1992

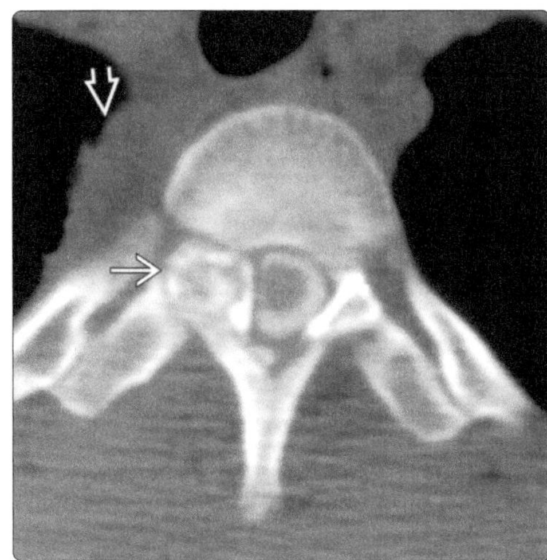

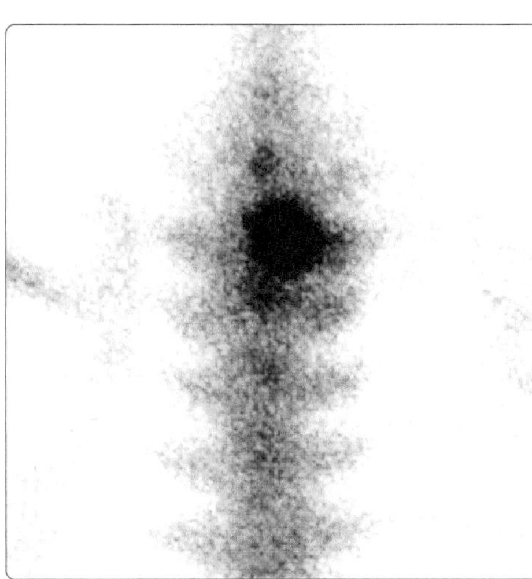

(Left) *Axial CT myelogram shows the characteristic, sharply demarcated tumor nidus ➡ of OO. Local pleural reaction ➡ is commonly seen in thoracic OOs.* **(Right)** *Posterior bone scan shows not only marked uptake by the tumor itself but a "corona" of increased uptake involving the adjacent bones. This reflects the local response to prostaglandin secreted by the tumor.*

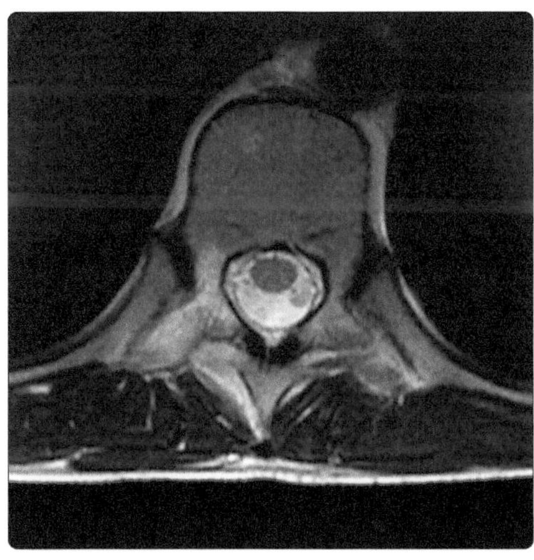

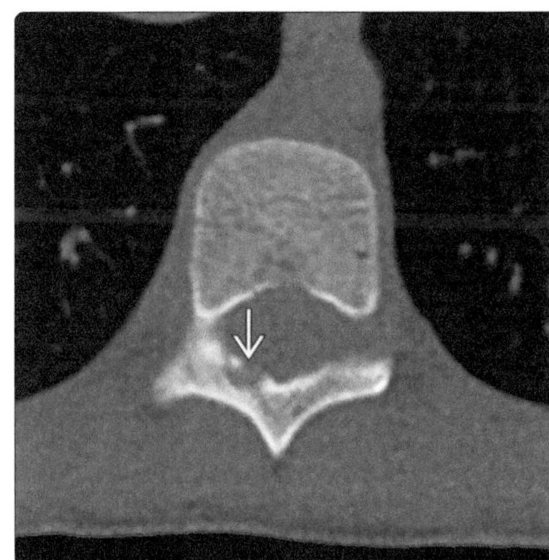

(Left) *Axial T2WI MR in an adolescent patient with thoracic back pain shows marrow edema in the right pedicle and transverse pedicle at the symptomatic level. It is very difficult to appreciate an underlying lesional cause.* **(Right)** *Axial bone CT in the same patient shows a characteristic lucent nidus ➡ in the right lamina, indicative of OO. In the presence of significant edema and sclerosis, an OO can be occult on MR imaging. Consider CT if there is high suspicion.*

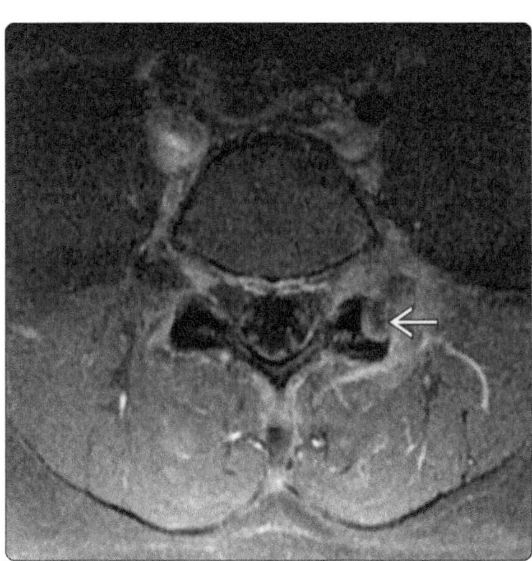

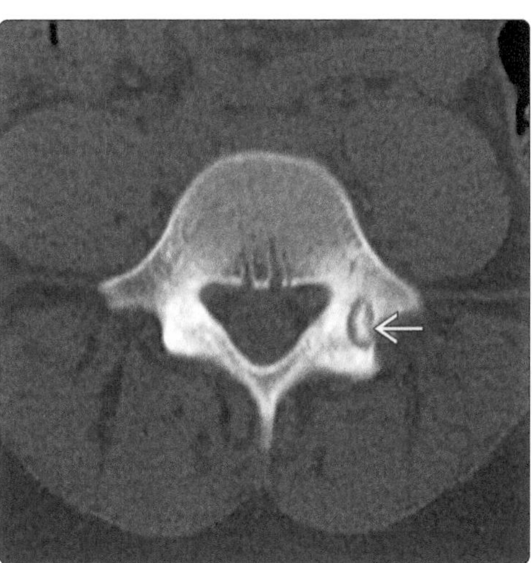

(Left) *Axial T1WI C+ FS MR in a teenager with lumbar back pain shows a rounded enhancing focus ➡ with central low signal in the left L5 pedicle. The left-sided facets also appear overgrown.* **(Right)** *Axial bone CT in the same patient performed to better evaluate the lesion shows a characteristic lucent lesion ➡ with central calcification compatible with an OO. Note how the pedicle and facet are overgrown and sclerotic.*

Osteoblastoma

KEY FACTS

TERMINOLOGY

- Osteoblastoma (OB): Benign tumor that forms osteoid
  - Differentiated grossly from osteoid osteoma by larger size (> 1.5 cm)

IMAGING

- 40% of OBs occur in spine
- Well-circumscribed, expansile lesion of neural arch
  - Frequent extension into vertebral body
  - Narrow zone of transition, sclerotic rim
- Periosteal inflammatory response of adjacent ribs, pleural thickening, effusion
- Peritumoral edema (flare phenomenon)
  - Edema enhances, obscures tumor margins, mimics malignancy (MR)

TOP DIFFERENTIAL DIAGNOSES

- Osteoid osteoma
- Aneurysmal bone cyst
- Metastasis
- Osteogenic sarcoma
- Chordoma
- Infection

PATHOLOGY

- Tumor prostaglandins release causes extensive peritumoral edema

CLINICAL ISSUES

- 90% in 2nd-3rd decades of life
- Dull, localized pain
- Painful scoliosis
- Neurologic symptoms due to compression of cord, nerve roots

DIAGNOSTIC CHECKLIST

- May be occult on radiographs; consider MR in young patients with painful scoliosis

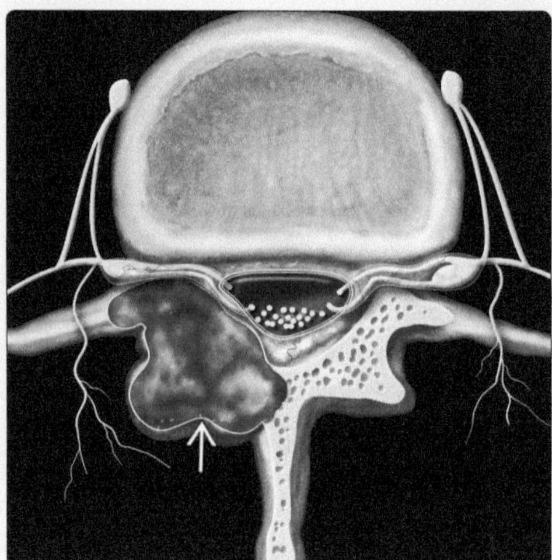

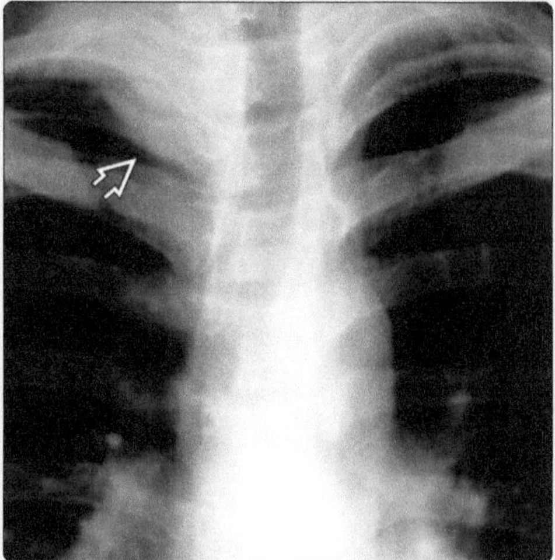

(Left) *Axial graphic shows an expansile, highly vascular osteoblastoma (OB) ➡ arising in the right lamina and impinging on the exiting nerve root.* **(Right)** *AP radiograph shows focal levoscoliosis secondary to upper thoracic OB. The tumor is not visible. Note focal pleural thickening ➡, a secondary sign of OB. The patient also had upper thoracic pain. This combination of symptoms and radiographic findings should prompt CT evaluation.*

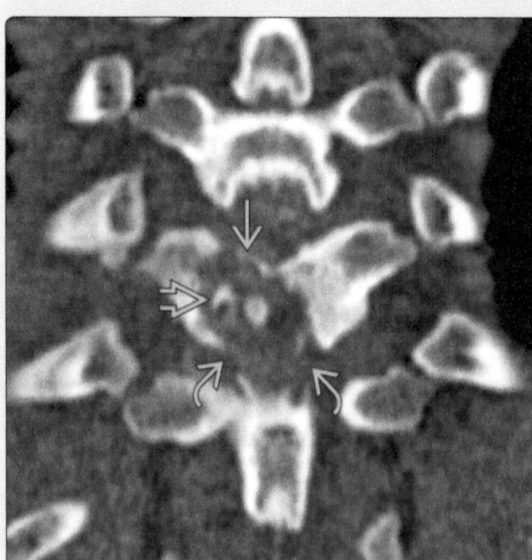

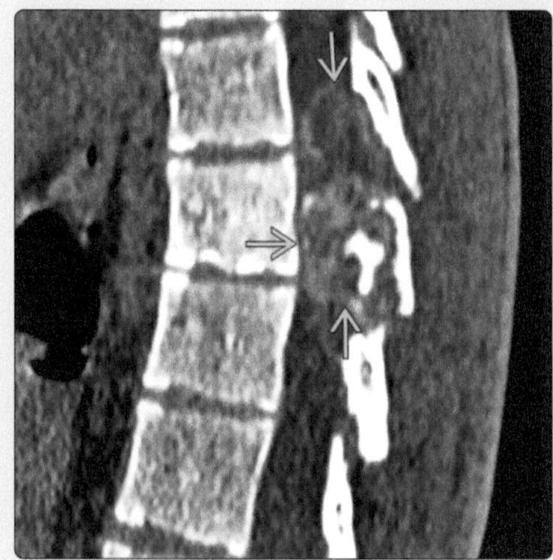

(Left) *Coronal bone CT shows expansile OB ➡ of the right lamina. The matrix ➡ mimics "rings and arcs" of chondroid matrix. Cortical breakthrough ➡ is evident at the inferior tumor margin.* **(Right)** *Sagittal bone CT shows an expansile lower thoracic OB ➡ extending from the lamina into the spinal canal. The lesion is sharply circumscribed and bilobed, involving 2 adjacent levels.*

TERMINOLOGY

Definitions

- Osteoblastoma (OB): Benign tumor that forms osteoid
  - Differentiated grossly from osteoid osteoma by larger size (> 1.5 cm)

IMAGING

General Features

- Best diagnostic clue
  - Expansile mass occurring in posterior elements
- Location
  - 40% of OBs occur in spine
    - 40% cervical, 25% lumbar, 20% thoracic, 15-20% sacrum
  - Originates in neural arch
    - May be centered in pedicle, lamina, transverse or spinous process, articular pillar, or pars interarticularis
  - Often extends into vertebral body
- Size
  - > 1.5 cm (by definition)

Radiographic Findings

- Radiography
  - Geographic, expansile lesion
  - Matrix often not visible on spine radiographs, better seen on CT
  - Usually radiolucent, occasionally sclerotic
  - Subtle imaging findings
    - Compare posterior elements to contralateral side and to levels above and below area of concern
  - AP radiograph
    - Lucent or sclerotic pedicle
    - Expansion of transverse process
    - Scoliosis in 50-60% of cases
    - Scoliosis concave on side of tumor
  - Lateral radiograph
    - Expanded pedicle, lamina, or spinous process
    - Sharply demarcated lucency in posterior portion of vertebral body

CT Findings

- CECT
  - Heterogeneous enhancement obscures bone matrix
- Bone CT
  - Most common appearance
    - Well-circumscribed, expansile lesion of neural arch
    - Often extends into vertebral body
    - Narrow zone of transition, sclerotic rim
  - Aggressive OB
    - Cortical breakthrough, wide zone of transition
    - Difficult differential diagnosis with osteosarcoma
  - Matrix mineralization
    - Variable amount of mineralization
    - May see small, irregular trabeculae
    - Can be difficult to distinguish from calcified cartilage of chondrosarcoma, enchondroma
  - Inflammatory response may spread far beyond lesion
    - Widespread, ill-defined sclerotic bone around lesion
    - Periosteal reaction of adjacent ribs
    - Pleural thickening &/or effusion
    - Ossification of ligamentum flavum

MR Findings

- T1WI
  - Low/intermediate signal intensity
- T2WI
  - Low to high signal intensity
    - Depending on extent of ossification in tumor
  - Periosteal reaction common in involved or adjacent bone
    - Due to prostaglandin excretion
  - Bone matrix is often not visible
    - May see small, irregularly shaped areas of low signal intensity on all sequences
  - Pleural effusion is common
- STIR
  - Low to high signal intensity
  - Peritumoral edema is prominent (flare phenomenon)
    - Due to prostaglandin secretion
    - May mimic malignancy
    - May involve adjacent bones and soft tissues
    - Tumor margins often obscured by surrounding bone marrow edema
      - ▫ Better seen on CT
- T1WI C+
  - Variable enhancement
  - Peritumoral edema can enhance, obscure tumor margins

Angiographic Findings

- Intense tumor blush
- Mostly used for preoperative embolization

Nuclear Medicine Findings

- Bone scan
  - Positive 3-phase bone scan

Imaging Recommendations

- Bone CT with multiplanar reformations

DIFFERENTIAL DIAGNOSIS

Osteoid Osteoma

- Same age group
- Smaller (< 1.5 cm) by definition
- Round nidus with surrounding sclerotic bone
- Pain is usually more intense than OB
- Scoliosis is common

Aneurysmal Bone Cyst

- Expansile lesion of posterior elements
- Aneurysmal bone cyst (ABC) component present in 10-15% of OBs
- ABC may also be isolated or associated with other tumors
- Multiple blood-filled cavities with fluid-fluid levels
- Matrix absent in ABC without OB

Metastasis

- Older patients
- Usually destroys cortex rather than expanding
- May be expansile, especially in renal cell carcinoma
- Involves posterior elements &/or vertebral body

Osteogenic Sarcoma

- Rare in spine
- Sarcoma containing bone matrix
- More aggressive appearance on radiographs, CT than OB
  - Wider zone of transition
  - Cortical breakthrough rather than cortical expansion
- Involves neural arch &/or vertebral body

Chordoma

- Involves vertebral body rather than posterior elements
- Common in sacrum, rare in vertebrae
- No matrix; purely lytic tumor
- Hyperintense on T2WI

Infection

- MR appearance of OB may mimic infection because of inflammatory change in adjacent bones
- Distinction between OB and infection best made on bone CT

Fibrous Dysplasia

- Rare in spine
- Expansile lesion of posterior elements
- May be lytic or contain ground-glass matrix or tiny trabeculae of bone

Chondrosarcoma

- Rare in spine
- Involves vertebral body &/or posterior elements
- May have fairly nonaggressive features on imaging studies
- Cartilage Ca^{++} in arcs and rings

PATHOLOGY

General Features

- Prostaglandins released by tumor cause extensive peritumoral edema
- Pain usually less intense than with osteoid osteoma
- Rarely coexist with ABC

Staging, Grading, & Classification

- Classic OB
- Aggressive OB
  - Borderline lesion with osteosarcoma
  - Locally aggressive but does not metastasize

Gross Pathologic & Surgical Features

- Friable, highly vascular tumor
- Red color due to vascularity
- Well demarcated from surrounding host bone

Microscopic Features

- Prominent osteoblasts
- Rims of osteoblasts along trabeculae
- Vascular fibrous stroma
- Woven bone matrix of variable quantity
- ABC component found in 10-15%
- "Aggressive" OB
  - Same features as above, plus
    - More nuclear pleomorphism
    - Epithelioid osteoblasts

CLINICAL ISSUES

Presentation

- Most common signs/symptoms
  - Dull, localized pain
  - Neurologic symptoms due to compression of cord, nerve roots
- Painful scoliosis

Demographics

- Age
  - 90% in 2nd-3rd decades of life
  - Diagnosed in patients up to 7th decade of life
- Sex
  - M:F = 2-2.5:1

Natural History & Prognosis

- Grow slowly
- 10-15% recurrence for typical OB
- 50% recurrence for aggressive OB

Treatment

- Curettage with bone graft or methylmethacrylate placement
- Preoperative embolization may be helpful

DIAGNOSTIC CHECKLIST

Consider

- May be occult on radiographs; consider MR in young patients with painful scoliosis
- Occasionally associated with ABC
  - Look for fluid-fluid levels

Image Interpretation Pearls

- Aggressive OB is difficult on imaging and histology to distinguish from osteogenic sarcoma
  - Wide zone of transition suspicious for osteogenic sarcoma
  - Cortical breakthrough is common in OB
    - Without wide transition zone, should not be considered indication of malignancy

SELECTED REFERENCES

1. Laverde Mächler A et al: Osteoblastoma of the lumbar spine: findings in SPECT/CT. Clin Nucl Med. 47(1):e87-8, 2022
2. Chen K et al: Typical and atypical radiographic features of symptomatic osteoblastoma in the spine. World Neurosurg. 145:e209-15, 2021
3. Lazaro FA et al: Aneurysmal bone cyst and osteoblastoma: an extremely rare combination in the pediatric spine. Spine Deform. 9(2):615-20, 2021
4. Jia Q et al: Factors affecting prognosis of patients with osteoblastoma of the mobile spine: a long-term follow-up study of 70 patients in a single center. Neurosurgery. 86(1):71-9, 2020
5. López-Puerta JM et al: Spinal osteoid osteoma recurring as an aggressive osteoblastoma. Neurocirugia (Astur : Engl Ed). 31(3):146-50, 2020
6. Mishra A et al: Cervical spine osteoblastoma with an aneurysmal bone cyst in a 2-year-old child: a case report. Pediatr Neurosurg. 54(1):46-50, 2019
7. Galgano MA et al: Osteoblastomas of the spine: a comprehensive review. Neurosurg Focus. 41(2):E4, 2016
8. Orguc S et al: Primary tumors of the spine. Semin Musculoskelet Radiol. 18(3):280-99, 2014
9. Ruggieri P et al: Osteoblastoma of the sacrum: report of 18 cases and analysis of the literature. Spine (Phila Pa 1976). 39(2):E97-103, 2014
10. Li Z et al: Clinical features and surgical management of spinal osteoblastoma: a retrospective study in 18 cases. PLoS One. 8(9):e74635, 2013

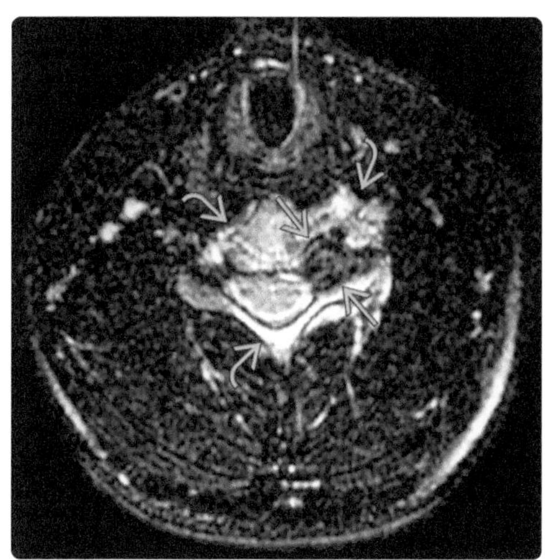

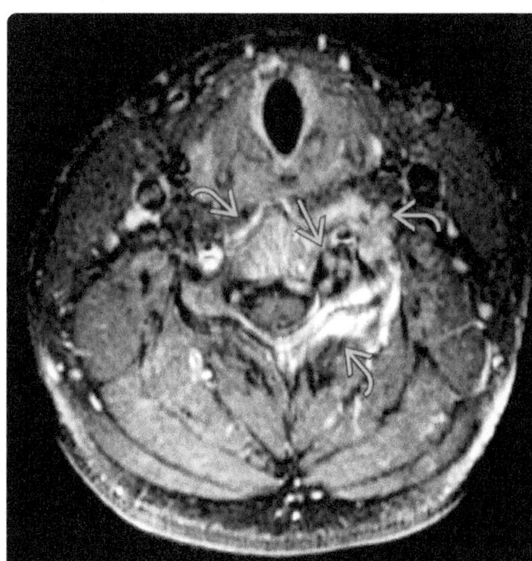

(Left) *Axial T2WI FS MR shows a low signal intensity, densely ossified mass expanding the left pedicle. The central, densely ossified tumor* ➡ *remains low signal intensity, while the surrounding edema* ➡ *is high signal intensity. Extensive reactive edema in the adjacent posterior elements, vertebral body, and soft tissues mimics a more aggressive tumor.* **(Right)** *Axial T1WI C+ FS MR in the same patient shows enhancement of nonossified portions of tumor* ➡ *as well as the peritumoral edema* ➡*.*

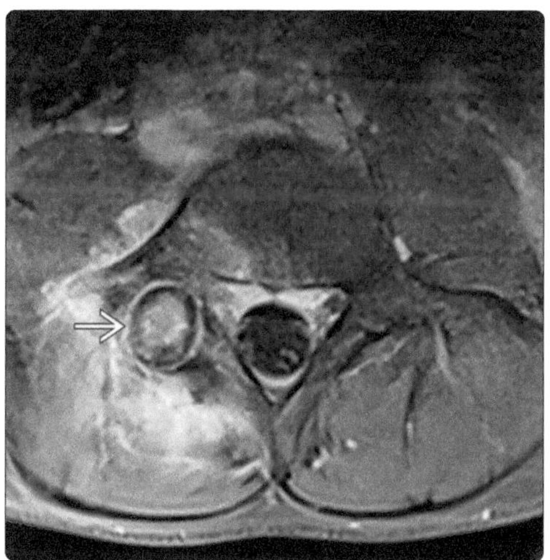

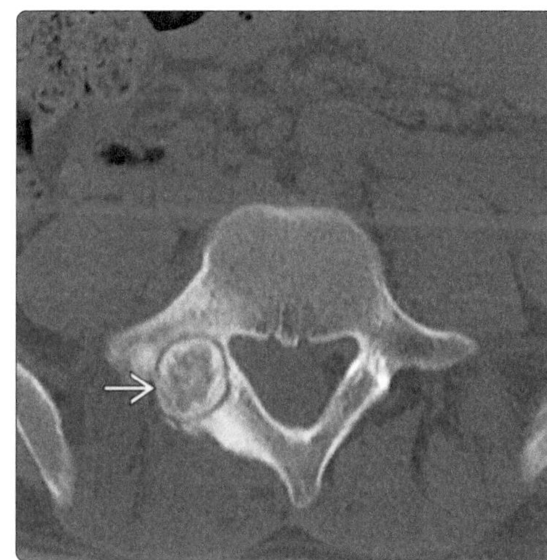

(Left) *Axial T1WI C+ FS MR in a teen with lumbar back pain demonstrates a rounded lesion* ➡ *centered within the right L5 lamina. The tumor has an enhancing center with hypointense (sclerotic) rim and marked surrounding enhancing edema.* **(Right)** *Axial bone CT in the same patient reveals a well-circumscribed mass* ➡ *that measured 2 cm in diameter, distinguishing it from osteoid osteoma. Note thickening and sclerotic changes of the right neural arch bone.*

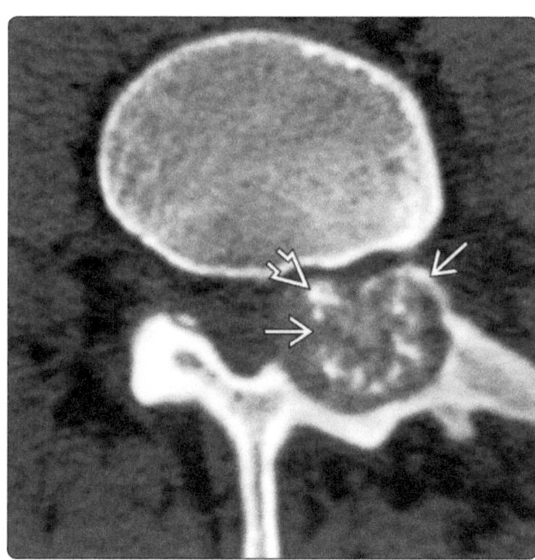

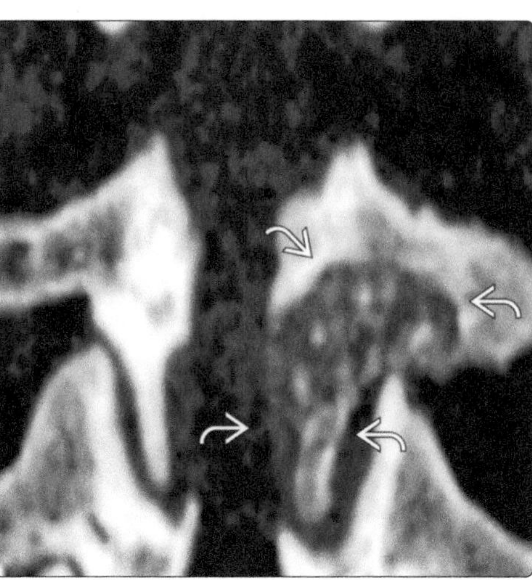

(Left) *Axial bone CT in the same patient shows an expansile mass* ➡ *containing thin, irregular bone trabeculae* ➡*, characteristic of OB. Although cortical breakthrough is present, the zone of transition to adjacent bone is narrow and sclerotic.* **(Right)** *Coronal bone CT in the same patient is useful to confirm the tumor extent* ➡ *from the transverse process to the inferior articular facet. Compare this image to the AP radiograph to better understand the radiographic findings.*

Aneurysmal Bone Cyst

KEY FACTS

IMAGING

- Balloon-like expansile bone remodeling
  - Thinned, eggshell cortex
  - Narrow, nonsclerotic zone of transition with adjacent bone
  - Focal cortical destruction common
- Centered in neural arch, extends into vertebral body
- Absent pedicle sign: Expansion of pedicle results in loss of pedicle contour on AP radiographs
- Contains multiple round cysts with fluid-fluid levels
  - Caused by hemorrhage, blood product sedimentation
  - Blood-filled cysts separated by septa of varying thickness

TOP DIFFERENTIAL DIAGNOSES

- Osteoblastoma
- Telangiectatic osteogenic sarcoma
- Metastases
- Giant cell tumor
- Tarlov cyst

PATHOLOGY

- Spongy, red mass with multiple blood-filled spaces
- Divided into primary and secondary types
  - Primary aneurysmal bone cyst (ABC) is isolated neoplasm of bone
  - Secondary ABC is associated with another tumor
- Now considered true neoplasm since cytogenetic abnormalities found in > 50%
  - Translocation between chromosomes 16 and 17

CLINICAL ISSUES

- Young patient with back pain of insidious onset

DIAGNOSTIC CHECKLIST

- Absent pedicle sign caused by ABC, osteoblastoma, lytic osteogenic sarcoma, metastasis, trauma, congenital absence of pedicle
- Evaluation of pedicles on AP radiograph should be part of routine on every patient

(Left) *Axial graphic demonstrates aneurysmal bone cyst with an expansile, multicystic mass in the posterior vertebral body and pedicle extending into epidural space. Fluid-fluid levels are characteristic.* **(Right)** *Axial T2WI MR shows aneurysmal bone cyst of T12 with multiple fluid-fluid levels due to layering blood products. The zone of transition ⤻ to normal bone is narrow and sclerotic. There is cortical breakthrough as well as extension into the spinal canal ⇨, compressing the spinal cord.*

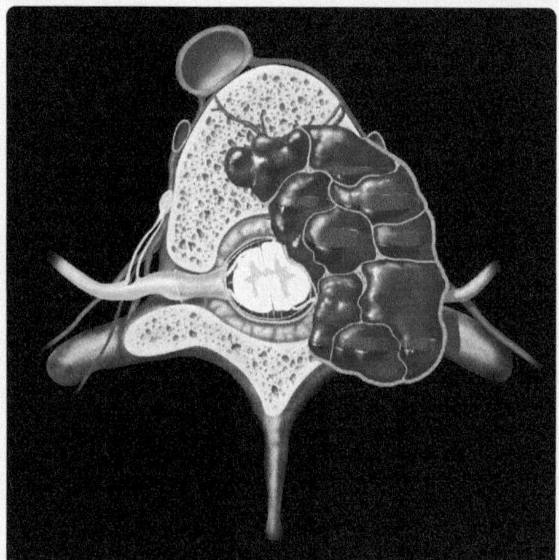

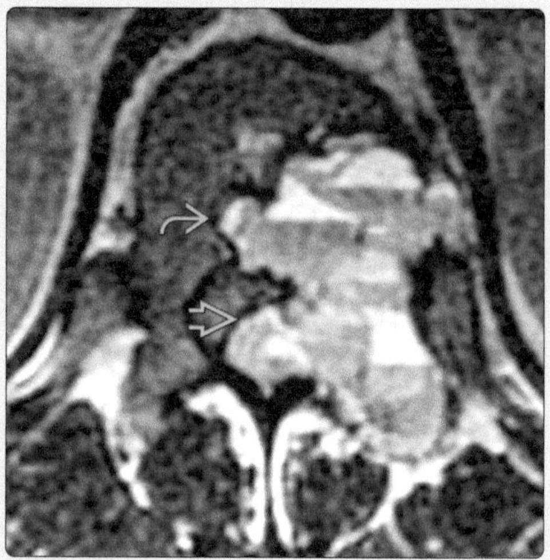

(Left) *Sagittal T2WI MR in the same patient shows extension into the vertebral body → and spinal canal ⇨. Determining the center of origin of a bone tumor is critical in differential diagnosis.* **(Right)** *AP radiography in the same patient reveals more subtle depiction of an aneurysmal bone cyst of T12 on plain radiography. Note the absent pedicle sign ⇨. The superior and inferior extent of tumor is shown by bone destruction →, which involved the vertebral body as well as the neural arch.*

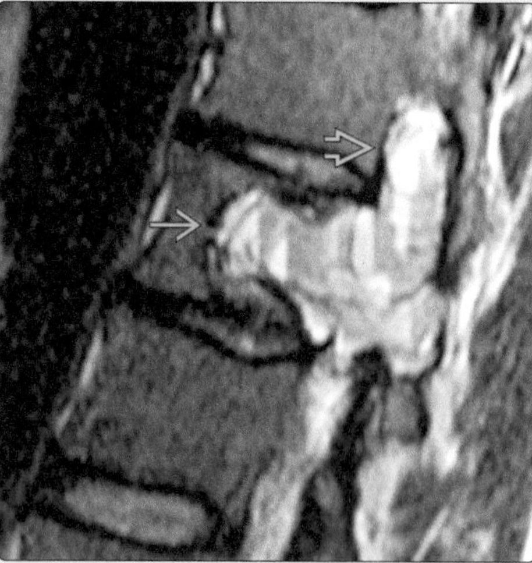

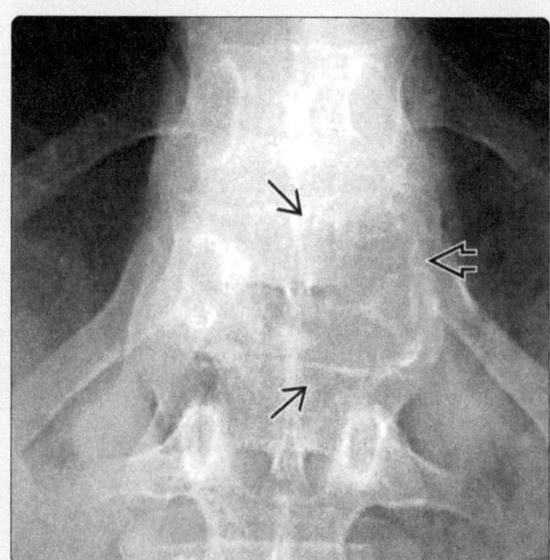

TERMINOLOGY

Abbreviations

- Aneurysmal bone cyst (ABC)

Definitions

- Expansile benign neoplasm containing thin-walled, blood-filled cavities

IMAGING

General Features

- Best diagnostic clue
  - Multiple fluid-fluid levels in expansile mass
- Location
  - 10-30% of ABCs occur in spine/sacrum
    - Arise in neural arch
    - 75-90% extend into vertebral body
- Morphology
  - Bone cannot truly expand
  - Expansile appearance reflects containment of tumor by appositional periosteal new bone

Radiographic Findings

- Radiography
  - Balloon-like expansile remodeling of bone
    - Centered in neural arch, extends into vertebral body
  - Cortical thinning
  - Focal cortical destruction common
  - Absent pedicle sign: Expansion of pedicle results in loss of pedicle contour on AP radiographs
  - Rare: Vertebral body collapse (vertebra plana)
  - Rare: Extends to > 1 vertebral level
  - Rare: Involves adjacent ribs

CT Findings

- Balloon-like expansile mass centered on posterior elements
  - Commonly extends into epidural space, may severely narrow spinal canal
- Contains rounded cysts that show fluid-fluid levels
  - Caused by hemorrhage, blood product sedimentation
- Calcified tumor matrix absent
  - Thin, bony septa may be present
- Narrow, nonsclerotic zone of transition with adjacent bone
- Thinned, eggshell cortex
- Focal cortical destruction common
- Periphery of tumor, septa between cysts enhance
- Solid ABC variant enhances diffusely

MR Findings

- Lobulated neural arch mass ± extension into vertebral body
- Well-defined rim of low signal intensity around mass
  - Reflects periosteum &/or pseudocapsule
- Peritumoral edema
  - High signal intensity on T2WI; STIR extends beyond tumor margins
  - Enhances with gadolinium (Gd)
- Cystic spaces of varying sizes within mass
  - Contain fluid-fluid levels due to blood products
  - Signal intensity variable
  - Cysts separated by septa of varying thickness
  - Gd enhancement at periphery, septa between cysts
- Part or all of mass may be solid (solid ABC)
  - Diffuse contrast enhancement of solid portions

Angiographic Findings

- Conventional
  - Hypervascular
  - Vessels more prominent at periphery, drape around lesion

Nuclear Medicine Findings

- Bone scan
  - Positive 3-phase bone scan
    - May have rim of activity around photopenic region (donut sign)

Imaging Recommendations

- CT best for diagnosis based on specific imaging features
- CT best to differentiate from telangiectatic osteogenic sarcoma
  - Narrow zone of transition in ABC
  - Absence of infiltration into surrounding soft tissues
- MR shows epidural extent, cord compromise

DIFFERENTIAL DIAGNOSIS

Osteoblastoma

- Same age range
- Expansile lesion of neural arch
- Bone matrix visible on plain films or CT
- May be associated with ABC

Telangiectatic Osteogenic Sarcoma

- Same age range or older
- Involves vertebral body &/or neural arch
- Also shows fluid-fluid levels
- Has more permeative bone destruction
- Wider zone of transition
- Infiltrates into surrounding soft tissues

Metastases

- Older patients
- Involves vertebral body ± neural arch
- Destructive lesion with associated soft tissue mass
- Rare: Vascular metastasis can have fluid-fluid levels
- Usually destroys bone cortex rather than expanding it
- Renal cell carcinoma can have soap bubble expansile appearance

Giant Cell Tumor

- Slightly older patients
- Originates in vertebral body rather than neural arch
- Expansile lytic lesion ± soft tissue mass
- May be associated with ABC

Plasmacytoma

- Older patients, usually > 40 years old
- Involves vertebral body, usually spares neural arch
- May expand vertebral body

Tarlov Cyst

- Perineural cyst occurring in sacrum
- Arises in neural foramina or spinal canal

- Causes bone remodeling
- No enhancement
- Simple fluid on all pulse sequences

Simple Bone Cyst

- In peripheral bones, simple bone cyst is another cystic lesion
- May have fluid-fluid levels
- Not seen in spine

PATHOLOGY

General Features

- Etiology
  - Now considered true neoplasm since cytogenetic abnormalities found in > 50%
    - Previously thought to result from trauma or local circulatory disturbance
  - Divided into primary and secondary types
    - Primary ABC is isolated neoplasm of bone
    - Secondary ABC is associated with another tumor
      - Most commonly giant cell tumor or osteoblastoma

Gross Pathologic & Surgical Features

- Spongy, red mass
- Multiple blood-filled spaces

Microscopic Features

- Typical
  - Cystic component predominates
    - Cavernous blood-filled cysts of variable sizes
    - Lined by fibroblasts, giant cells, histiocytes, hemosiderin
  - Solid components
    - Septations interposed between blood-filled spaces
    - Contain bland stroma with fibrous tissue, reactive bone, giant cells
- Solid ABC is rare variant
  - 5-8% of all ABCs
  - Solid component predominates
  - Propensity for spine

Genetics

- Translocation t(16;17)(q22;p13)
- Results in fusion of promoter region of osteoblast cadherin 11 gene (*CDH11*) on chromosome 16q22 to ubiquitin protease gene (*USP6*) on chromosome 17p13
  - Promoter swapping mechanism
  - Upregulates transcription of *USP6*
  - Immature cells of osteoblast lineage likely involved in overexpression

CLINICAL ISSUES

Presentation

- Most common signs/symptoms
  - Back pain, most severe at night
  - Other signs/symptoms
    - Scoliosis
    - Neurologic signs and symptoms from root &/or cord compression
    - Pathologic fracture
- Clinical profile
  - Young patient with back pain of insidious onset

Demographics

- Age
  - 80% < 20 years old
- Sex
  - Slightly more common in female patients
- Epidemiology
  - 1-2% of primary bone tumors are ABC
    - Familial incidence has been reported
  - 0.15 per million individuals in general population

Natural History & Prognosis

- Long-term history of untreated ABC variable
  - Grows initially, then usually stabilizes
  - No malignant degeneration
- Recurrence rate 20-30% (increased if incomplete excision)

Treatment

- Embolization
  - Curative as sole therapy in some cases
  - Can also be used preoperatively
- Surgical excision or curettage
- Role for preoperative sclerotherapy (doxycycline, Sotradecol) in some lesions
- Early data suggest role for denosumab, primarily as adjunct treatment for cases not curable by surgery/embolization
- May require instrumentation for stabilization of spine
- Radiation therapy may predispose to radiation-induced sarcoma

DIAGNOSTIC CHECKLIST

Consider

- Absent pedicle sign caused by ABC, osteoblastoma, lytic osteogenic sarcoma, metastasis, trauma, congenital absence of pedicle

Image Interpretation Pearls

- Evaluation of pedicles on AP radiograph should be part of routine on every patient

SELECTED REFERENCES

1. Aljamaan YM et al: Unusual presentation of aneurysmal bone cyst with scoliosis: a case report. J Med Case Rep. 16(1):446, 2022
2. Giantini-Larsen AM et al: The role of neoadjuvant denosumab in the treatment of aneurysmal bone cysts: a case series and review of the literature. J Neurosurg Pediatr. 30(6):547-54, 2022
3. Maximen J et al: Denosumab in the management of aneurysmal bone cyst. Joint Bone Spine. 89(1):105260, 2022
4. Wong MN et al: Doxycycline sclerotherapy of cervical spine aneurysmal bone cysts: single-institution 13-year experience. Pediatr Radiol. 52(8):1528-38, 2022
5. Bazzocchi A et al: Fluid-fluid levels in aneurysmal bone cysts. J Pediatr. 204:317, 2018
6. Girolami M et al: Do multiple fluid-fluid levels on MRI always reveal primary benign aneurysmal bone cyst? J Neurosurg Sci. 62(2):234-36, 2018
7. Palmerini E et al: Denosumab in patients with aneurysmal bone cysts: a case series with preliminary results. Tumori. 104(5):344-51, 2018
8. Protas M et al: Cervical spine aneurysmal bone cysts in the pediatric population: a systematic review of the literature. Pediatr Neurosurg. 52(4):219-24, 2017
9. Dubory A et al: Interest of denosumab for the treatment of giant-cells tumors and aneurysmal bone cysts of the spine. About nine cases. Spine (Phila Pa 1976). 41(11):E654-60, 2016

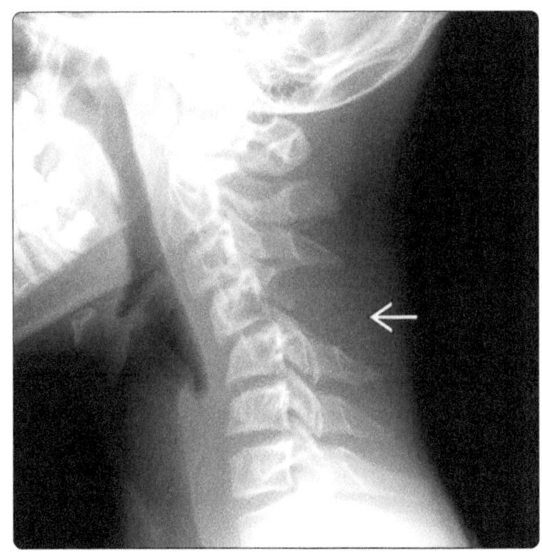

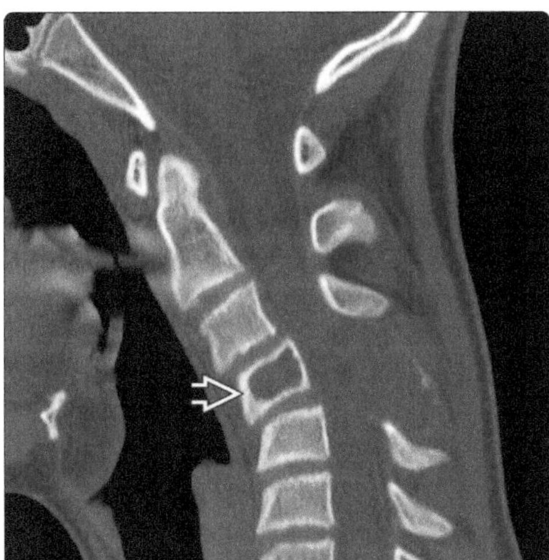

(Left) *Lateral cervical radiograph demonstrates a lytic expansile mass of the C4 spinous process ➡. Extension into the lateral masses and posterior vertebral body is more subtle. There is focal kyphosis secondary to mass effect from the spinous process mass.* **(Right)** *Sagittal bone CT in the same patient through the midline cervical spine confirms that there is lytic bone loss of the C4 vertebral body ➡ as well as expansile changes within the posterior elements.*

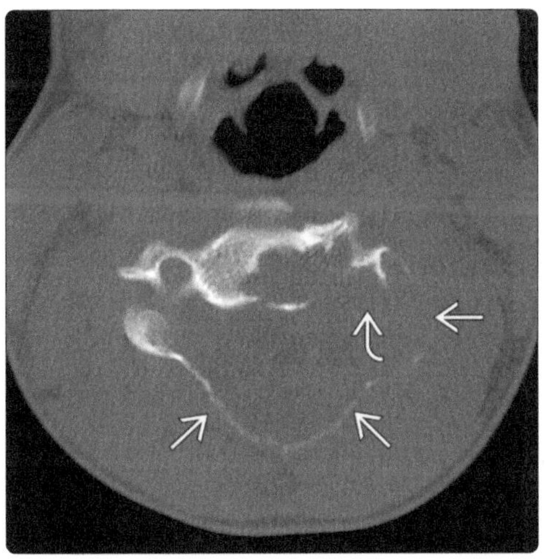

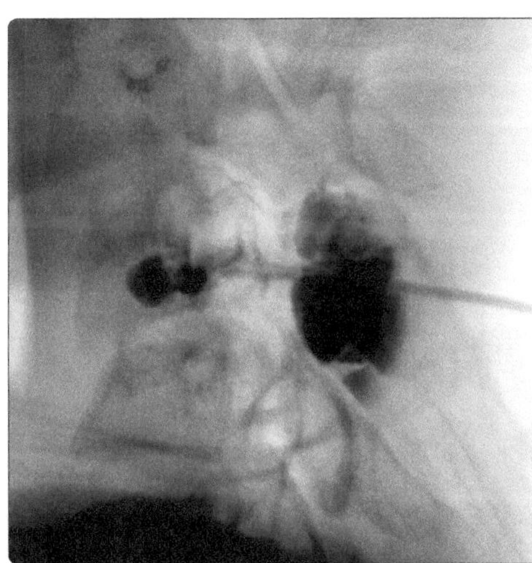

(Left) *Axial bone CT in an ABC patient depicts the pronounced posterior element expansile bone changes ➡ well. Left osseous vertebral artery canal ➡ is nearly effaced, indicating that the tumor encircles the artery.* **(Right)** *Lateral DSA image obtained during preoperative sclerotherapy shows injection of radiopaque sclerosis agent (Sotradecol) directly into the spinous process and C4 vertebral lesion portions.*

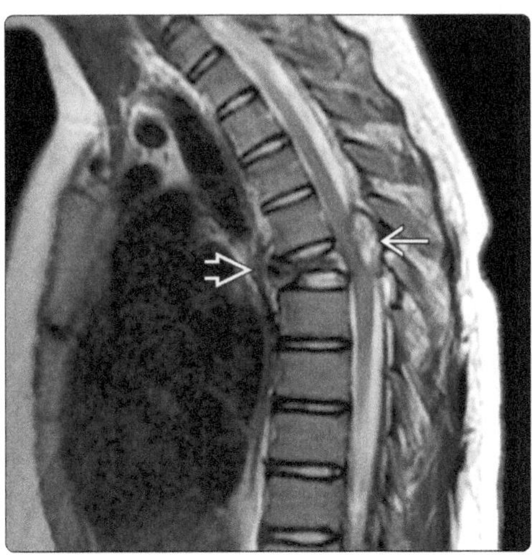

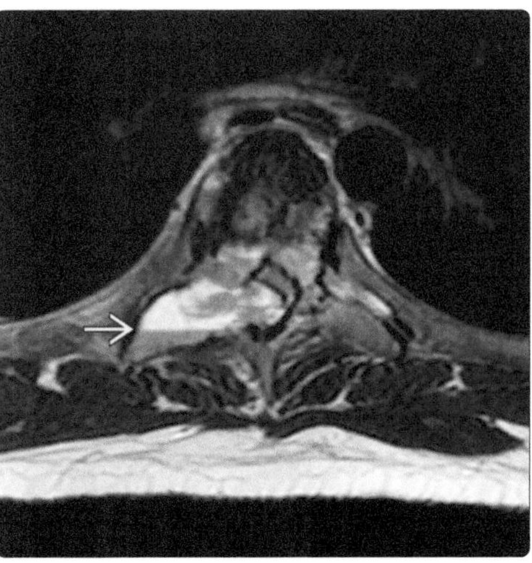

(Left) *Midline sagittal T2WI MR in a 14-year-old boy with back pain demonstrates a dorsal epidural mass ➡ and an associated pathologic thoracic vertebral fracture (vertebra plana) ➡.* **(Right)** *Axial T2WI MR in the same patient confirms an expansile mass ➡ centered in the neural arch extending into the right transverse process. Multiple fluid-fluid levels are demonstrated with a narrow zone of transition and hypointense ossified borders compatible with ABC.*

Osteochondroma

KEY FACTS

TERMINOLOGY

- Osteochondroma (OC)
- Osteocartilaginous exostosis, exostosis
- Cartilage-capped osseous growth contiguous with parent bone

IMAGING

- Sessile or pedunculated osseous "cauliflower" lesion
- Continuity of bony cortex and medullary space between lesion and underlying bone
- May see chondroid calcifications in cartilage cap
- Center follows normal marrow signal on MR
- Cartilage cap of similar intensity to cord on T1WI, hyperintense on T2WI

TOP DIFFERENTIAL DIAGNOSES

- Chondrosarcoma
- Osteoblastoma
- Aneurysmal bone cyst
- Tumoral calcinosis
- Enthesopathy

PATHOLOGY

- Idiopathic, trauma, perichondrial ring deficiency
- Radiation-induced OC
- Syndromic: Hereditary multiple exostoses (HME)
- Vertebral OC rare; 1-5% of sporadic OC, 1-9% OC in HME

CLINICAL ISSUES

- Often asymptomatic; incidental diagnosis on radiography
- Palpable mass
- Mechanical impingement of joint, muscle
- Cord compression, radiculopathy unusual
- Peak age: 10-30 years

DIAGNOSTIC CHECKLIST

- Multiplicity → consider HME
- Cartilage cap > 1.5 cm in adults raises concern for malignant transformation (chondrosarcoma)

(Left) *Axial graphic of the cervical spine depicts a typical osteochondroma (exostosis) ➡ with thin cartilage cap protruding into the spinal canal, resulting in canal stenosis and cord compression.* **(Right)** *Axial bone CT in a patient with myelopathy demonstrates a typical exostosis ➡ protruding into the central spinal canal resulting in severe stenosis. Marrow contiguity with vertebral body is characteristic.*

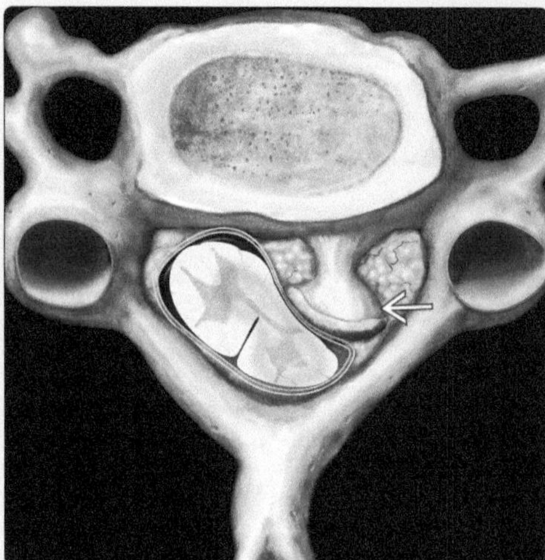

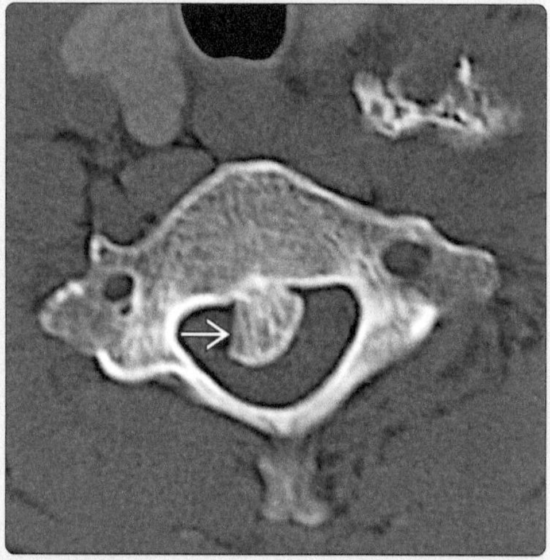

(Left) *Axial bone CT shows a pedunculated osseous lesion ➡ extending into the canal from the right pedicle with cortical and medullary continuity. There is resulting canal stenosis. The right pedicle and superior facet are irregularly enlarged ➡ due to the sessile component of the osteochondroma.* **(Right)** *Axial T2 FS MR in the same patient confirms medullary continuity of the osseous mass with the right pedicle ➡ and a hyperintense cartilaginous cap ➡. The spinal cord ➡ is displaced and compressed.*

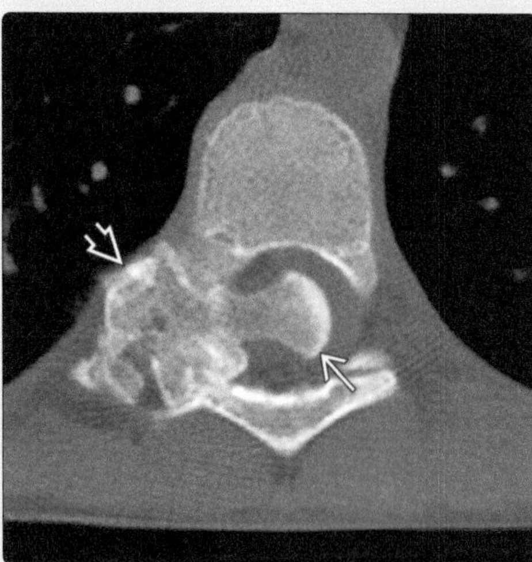

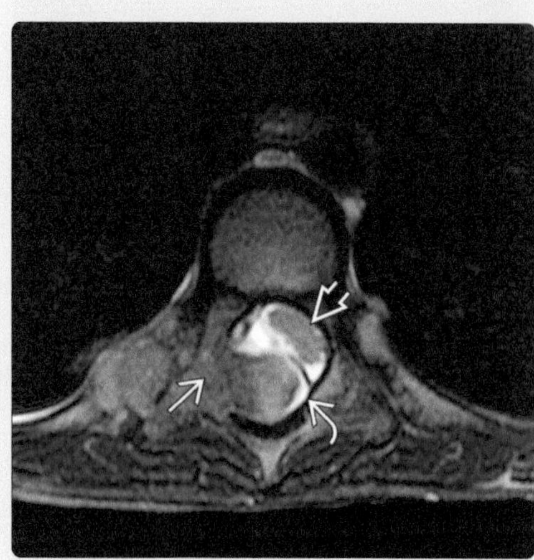

TERMINOLOGY

Abbreviations

- Osteochondroma (OC)

Synonyms

- Osteocartilaginous exostosis, exostosis
- Hereditary multiple exostoses (HME), a.k.a. diaphyseal aclasis, multiple cartilaginous exostoses
- Multiple hereditary exostoses (MHE)

Definitions

- Cartilage-capped osseous excrescence contiguous with parent bone

IMAGING

General Features

- Best diagnostic clue
  - Sessile or pedunculated osseous "cauliflower" lesion with parent bone corticomedullary continuity
- Location
  - Bones forming through endochondral ossification
    - Metaphysis of long tubular bones (85%) common, particularly knee
    - Iliac wing
  - < 5% occur in spine
    - Cervical (50%, C2 predilection) > thoracic (T8 > T4 > other levels) > lumbar > > sacrum
    - Spinous/transverse processes, lamina > vertebral body
- Size
  - Varies dramatically at time of presentation; 1-10 cm

Radiographic Findings

- Radiography
  - Sessile/pedunculated osseous protuberance with flaring of parent bone cortex at OC attachment
  - Cartilage cap visible only if extensively mineralized

CT Findings

- NECT
  - Sessile or pedunculated osseous lesion
  - Cortex and medullary cavity continuous with attached bone
  - May see chondroid calcifications in cartilage cap
- CECT
  - May see peripheral, septal enhancement in cartilage cap

MR Findings

- T1WI
  - Central hyperintensity (marrow) surrounded by hypointense cortex
  - Hypo-/isointense hyaline cartilage cap
- T2WI
  - Central iso- to hyperintense signal (marrow) surrounded by hypointense cortex
  - Hyperintense hyaline cartilage cap
- T1WI C+
  - May see peripheral, septal enhancement in cartilage cap

Ultrasonographic Findings

- Grayscale ultrasound
  - Hypoechoic nonmineralized cartilage cap easily distinguished from adjacent fat, muscle
  - Cartilage cap mineralization and osseous stalk → posterior acoustic shadowing

Nuclear Medicine Findings

- Bone scan
  - Variable; direct correlation with enchondral bone formation
    - ↑ radionuclide uptake = metabolically active OC
    - No ↑ radionuclide uptake = quiescent OC

Imaging Recommendations

- Best imaging tool
  - MR
- Protocol advice
  - MR to measure cartilage cap, determine status of regional neural and musculoskeletal tissue
  - Bone CT to assess mineralization, confirm continuity with vertebral marrow space

DIFFERENTIAL DIAGNOSIS

Chondrosarcoma

- Isolated or secondary to malignant OC degeneration
- Lytic destructive lesion with sclerotic margins, soft tissue mass
- Chondroid matrix ("rings and arcs," 50%)

Osteoblastoma

- Expansile lesion, typically involving posterior elements
- Lytic lesion with osseous matrix, narrow zone of transition

Aneurysmal Bone Cyst

- Expansile, lytic lesion
- Multicystic, fluid-fluid levels

Tumoral Calcinosis

- Calcific periarticular mass
- Spinal involvement uncommon

Enthesopathy

- DISH, ankylosing spondylitis, psoriatic arthropathy, disorders of calcium metabolism

PATHOLOGY

General Features

- Etiology
  - Idiopathic, trauma, perichondrial ring deficiency
    - Peripheral portion of epiphyseal cartilage herniates out of growth plate
    - Metaplastic cartilage is stimulated; enchondral bone formation → bony stalk
  - Radiation-induced OC
    - Most common benign radiation-induced tumor
      - Prevalence 6-24%
    - Radiation dose 1,500-5,500 cGy; occur at treatment field periphery
      - Patients generally < 2 years old at time of XRT
      - Latent period 3-17 years
    - Pathologically and radiographically identical to other exostoses

- Genetics
  - HME
    - Autosomal dominant transmission
    - Exostoses (multiple) 1 gene (a.k.a. *EXT1*) on long arm of chromosome 8; produces exostosin 1
    - Exostoses (multiple) 2 gene (a.k.a. *EXT2*) on short arm of chromosome 11; produces exostosin 2
    - Exostoses (multiple) 3 gene (a.k.a. *EXT3*) on short arm of chromosome 19
    - Inactivation of 1 EXT gene → exostosis; subsequent inactivation of 2nd EXT gene → malignant transformation
- Benign cartilaginous bone tumor
  - 9% of all bone tumors, most common benign bone tumor (30-45%)
  - Rapid growth, new pain, and continued growth of cartilage cap > 1.5-cm thickness after skeletal maturity imply malignant transformation to chondrosarcoma
  - OC complications include deformity, fracture, vascular compromise, neurologic sequelae, overlying bursa formation, and malignant transformation
- Vertebral OC rare; 1-5% of sporadic OC, 1-9% OC in HME
  - Narrow stalk (pedunculated) or broad attachment base (sessile) contiguous with vertebral cortex, medullary space
  - Hyaline cartilage cap thickness proportional to patient age
- Many spinal OC are asymptomatic
  - May cause mechanical impingement
  - May compress spinal cord or nerve root

Gross Pathologic & Surgical Features

- Osseous excrescence with corticomedullary contiguity with parent bone
- Cartilage cap ranges from thick, bosselated, glistening blue-gray surface (young patients) to several millimeters thick or entirely absent (adults)

Microscopic Features

- Mature cartilaginous, cancellous, and cortical bone
- Cartilage cap histology reflects classic growth plate zones

CLINICAL ISSUES

Presentation

- Most common signs/symptoms
  - Often asymptomatic; incidental diagnosis on radiography
  - Palpable mass
  - Mechanical impingement of joint, muscle
- Other signs/symptoms
  - Myelopathy or radiculopathy, more common with HME
  - Canal stenosis may predispose to cord injury with mild trauma
  - Cranial nerve deficits
  - Pharyngeal mass
  - Scoliosis

Demographics

- Age
  - Peak: 10-30 years
    - Solitary spinal OC most commonly diagnosed in adolescents and adults
  - Most HME patients diagnosed by 5 years of age; virtually all by 12 years of age
- Sex
  - M:F = 3:1
- Epidemiology
  - Prevalence of solitary OC unknown since many asymptomatic
  - Prevalence of HME 1:50,000-100,000 in Western populations; up to 1:1,000 in ethnic Chamorro population

Natural History & Prognosis

- Postsurgical local recurrence rate < 2%
- Benign lesions; no propensity for metastasis
- Malignant transformation < 1% solitary lesions; 3-5% HME
  - Growth or new pain after skeletal maturity, ↑ cartilage cap thickness (> 1.5 cm in adults)

Treatment

- Conservative management in asymptomatic patients
- Surgical excision, deformity correction in symptomatic patients

DIAGNOSTIC CHECKLIST

Consider

- Multiplicity → consider HME
- Interpret cartilage thickness in context of patient age

Image Interpretation Pearls

- Cartilage cap > 1.5 cm in adults raises concern for malignant transformation (chondrosarcoma)
- Radiologic features pathognomonic, reflect pathologic appearance

SELECTED REFERENCES

1. Assan BR et al: Surgical outcomes of spinal osteochondroma in children: a multicentre observational study. Orthop Traumatol Surg Res. 108(6):103239, 2022
2. Carlos-Escalante JA et al: Primary benign tumors of the spinal canal. World Neurosurg. 164:178-98, 2022
3. Kumar P et al: Rib osteochondroma presenting as acute paraparesis. J Cancer Res Ther. 18(6):1807-8, 2022
4. Mamdouhi T et al: Solitary pediatric osteochondroma of the spine with cord compression. Cureus. 14(3):e23342, 2022
5. Akhaddar A et al: Multiple hereditary exostoses with tetraparesis due to cervical spine osteochondroma. World Neurosurg. 116:247-8, 2018
6. Ganesh S et al: Solitary facet joint osteochondroma of the upper thoracic spine: an unusual cause of cord compression in the pediatric age group. Neurol India. 66(2):555-6, 2018
7. Garg B et al: Solitary anterior osteochondroma of cervical spine: an unusual cause of dysphagia and review of literature. J Clin Orthop Trauma. 9(Suppl 2):S5-7, 2018
8. Yakkanti R et al: Solitary osteochondroma of the spine-a case series: review of solitary osteochondroma with myelopathic symptoms. Global Spine J. 8(4):323-39, 2018
9. Raswan US et al: A solitary osteochondroma of the cervical spine: a case report and review of literature. Childs Nerv Syst. 33(6):1019-22, 2017
10. Ruivo C et al: Spinal chondrosarcoma arising from a solitary lumbar osteochondroma. JBR-BTR. 97(1):21-4, 2014
11. Rustagi T et al: C2 compressive osteochondroma with transient neurologic symptoms in a pediatric patient. Spine J. 14(10):2516-7, 2014
12. Aldea S et al: Acute spinal cord compression in hereditary multiple exostoses. Acta Neurochir (Wien). 148(2):195-8; discussion 198, 2006
13. Moon KS et al: Osteochondroma of the cervical spine extending multiple segments with cord compression. Pediatr Neurosurg. 42(5):304-7, 2006

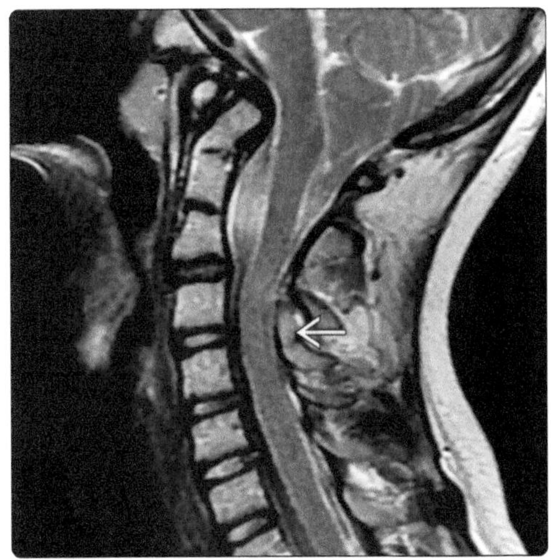

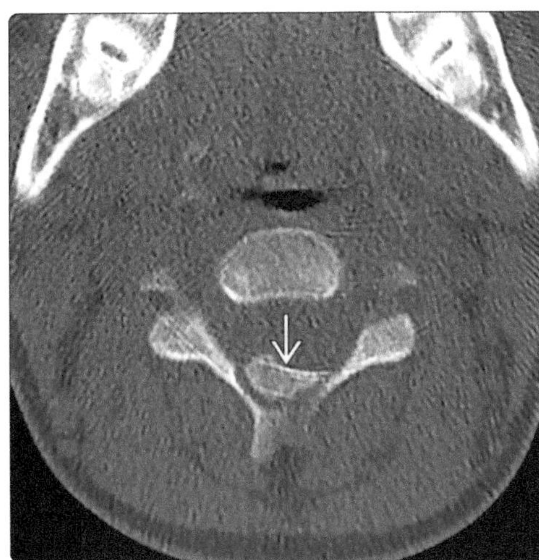

(Left) *Sagittal T2 MR in an 11-year-old patient with hereditary multiple exostoses (HME) reveals a laminar osteochondroma* ➡ *arising from C5 that dorsally compresses the cervical spinal cord. This patient also incidentally demonstrates C2/C3 segmentation failure and a retroflexed odontoid process.* **(Right)** *Axial bone CT in the same patient shows that the osteochondroma* ➡ *arises from the left C5 lamina, narrowing the osseous spinal canal.*

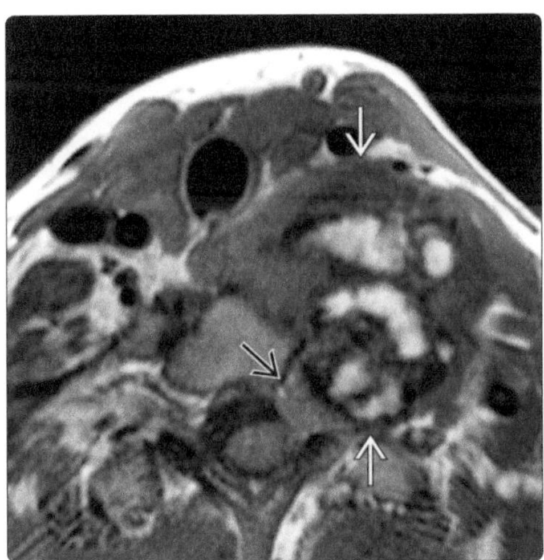

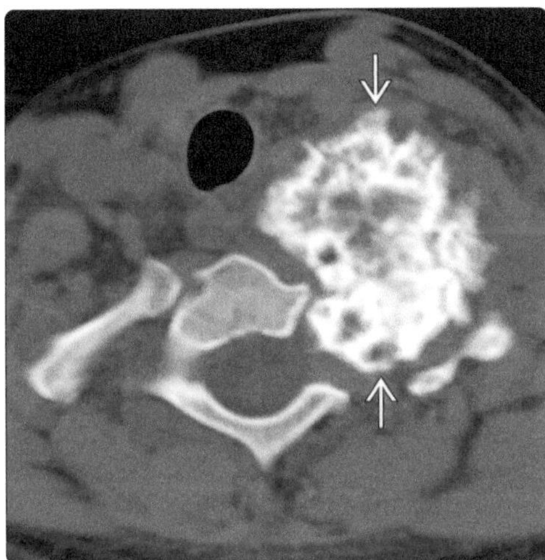

(Left) *Axial T1 MR shows a large left T1 osteochondroma* ➡ *presenting with brachial plexopathy in a patient with HME. The tumor fills the left C7/T1 foramen* ⇨*. Cartilage cap thickness was < 1.5 cm* **(Right)** *Axial bone CT in the same patient shows large left T1 exostosis with typical cauliflower ossification* ➡*. This patient presented with brachial plexopathy secondary to regional neural compression. Note how CT and MR are complimentary for depicting the different tissue elements.*

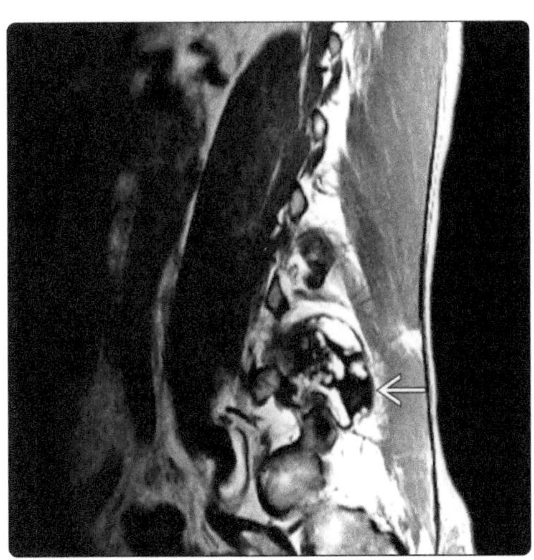

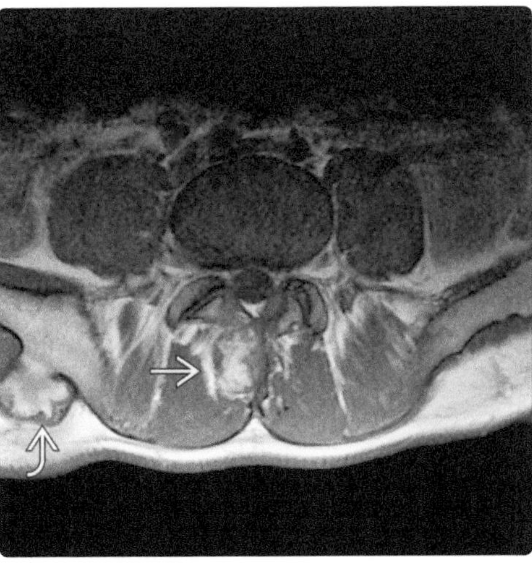

(Left) *Sagittal T1 MR in a patient with back pain and a palpable mass shows a cauliflower-like, heterogeneous signal osteochondroma* ➡ *arising from the left L5-S1 facet joint. T1 hyperintensity reflects marrow elements.* **(Right)** *Axial T1 MR shows a large osteochondroma originating from the L4 spinous process* ➡ *with hyperintense marrow centrally and a peripheral isointense cartilage cap. Another osteochondroma with more classic cauliflower morphology is noted at the right iliac crest* ⮫*.*

Osteogenic Sarcoma

KEY FACTS

TERMINOLOGY

- Sarcoma containing osteoid matrix produced directly by malignant cells

IMAGING

- Permeative or moth-eaten appearance
- Cortical breakthrough
- Bone sclerosis due to production of immature bone
- Wide zone of transition
- Discontinuous periosteal reaction, usually multilaminar
- Soft tissue mass; fluid-fluid levels seen in telangiectatic osteogenic sarcoma (OGS)

TOP DIFFERENTIAL DIAGNOSES

- Sclerotic metastasis
- Osteoblastoma
- Aneurysmal bone cyst
- Chordoma
- Osteomyelitis
- Ewing sarcoma
- Chondrosarcoma
- Lymphoma
- Malignant giant cell tumor

PATHOLOGY

- 4% of all primary OGSs occur in spine and sacrum
- Majority of OGSs of unknown etiology = primary OGS
- Association with retinoblastoma (*RB1* gene mutation)

CLINICAL ISSUES

- Insidious onset of back pain, greatest at night
- Neurologic symptoms, including radicular pain, weakness
- 3% of 10-year survivors of all OGSs develop 2nd malignancy

DIAGNOSTIC CHECKLIST

- CT scan best method for evaluation of tumor matrix, zone of transition
- All telangiectatic OGSs are lytic on radiographs and CT, but not all lytic OGSs are telangiectatic

(Left) *Axial graphic shows an osteosarcoma arising in a lumbar vertebral body, destroying cortex, and invading adjacent soft tissues. The soft tissue mass in osteosarcoma usually contains ossification.* **(Right)** *Sagittal T2 MR shows an aggressive mass (telangiectatic osteosarcoma) arising within the S1 vertebral body ⇨ with extension into the posterior elements and spinal canal ➡. Note tumor fluid-fluid levels ➡.*

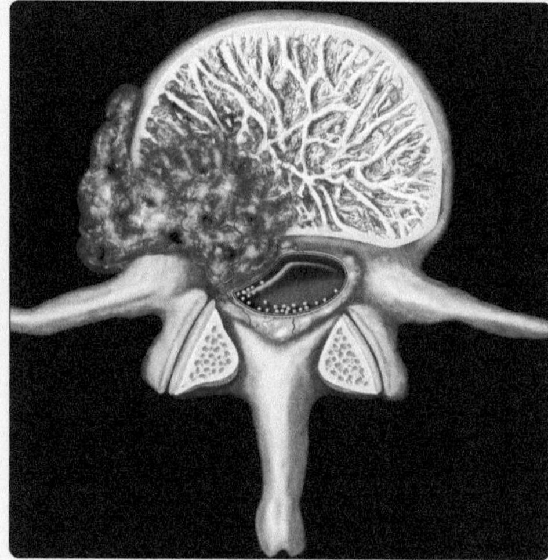

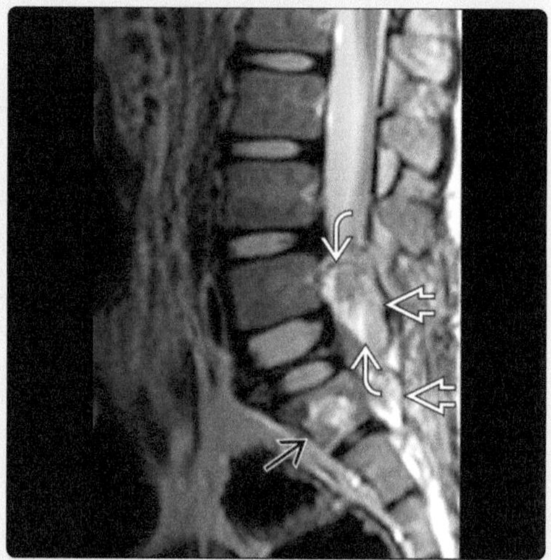

(Left) *Axial T2 FS MR (telangiectatic osteosarcoma) reveals an aggressive-appearing sacral mass demonstrating multiple fluid-fluid levels ➡ within the tumor.* **(Right)** *Axial T1 C+ FS MR further characterizes the aggressive destructive sacral mass ➡ (telangiectatic osteosarcoma). Note the wide zone of tumor transition with adjacent bone. There is enhancement of solid components surrounding nonenhancing, low-signal cystic areas.*

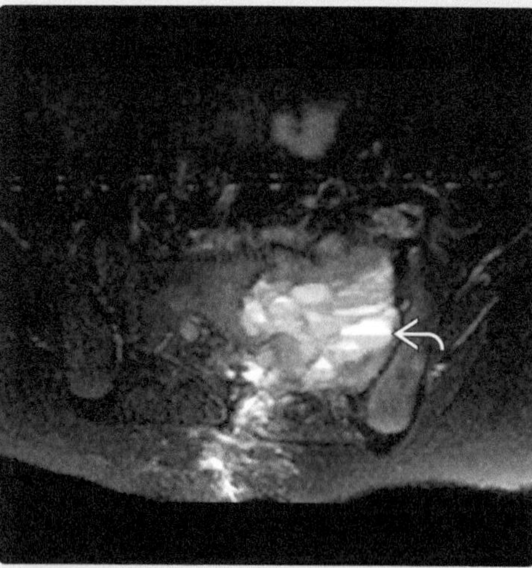

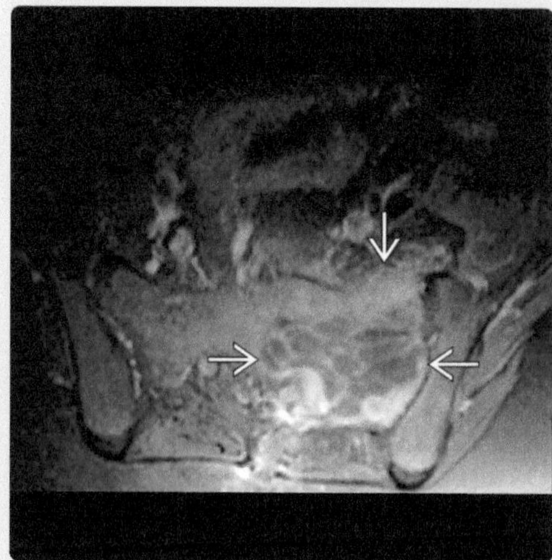

TERMINOLOGY

Abbreviations

- Osteogenic sarcoma (OGS)

Definitions

- Sarcoma containing osteoid produced directly by malignant cells

IMAGING

General Features

- Best diagnostic clue
  - Aggressive-appearing lesion forming immature bone
- Location
  - 4% of all primary OGSs occur in spine and sacrum
  - 79% arise in posterior elements
  - 17% involve 2 adjacent spinal levels
  - 84% invade spinal canal

Radiographic Findings

- Permeative or moth-eaten appearance
  - Multiple small areas of bone destruction
  - Best visualized at tumor periphery
- Wide zone of transition
  - Difficult to demarcate where tumor ends and normal bone begins
- Bone sclerosis due to production of immature bone
  - 80%: Bone matrix seen on radiographs or CT scan
  - 20%: Lytic appearance without visible bone matrix
- Cortical breakthrough
  - Usually extensive
- Discontinuous periosteal reaction, usually multilaminar
- Soft tissue mass
  - Often contains immature bone
- May cross sacroiliac joint or disc space

CT Findings

- Same as on radiographs but better detail
- Best method to evaluate tumor matrix
  - OGS matrix is cloud-like, amorphous
- Contrast administration tends to obscure bone matrix and is not recommended

MR Findings

- Aggressive, heterogeneous mass similar to other malignancies
- Matrix difficult to see, CT more specific
- Densely ossified portions of tumor ↓ signal intensity on all sequences
- Nonossified tumor ↓ signal on T1WI, ↑ on T2WI, STIR
- Fluid-fluid levels seen in telangiectatic OGS

Nuclear Medicine Findings

- Bone scan
  - ↑ uptake on all 3 phases
  - Used for staging, detection of skip lesions, metastases

Imaging Recommendations

- Best imaging tool
  - CT scan
- Protocol advice
  - Avoid IV contrast on bone CT to allow visualization of tumor matrix
  - MR useful to evaluate for cord, nerve root impingement
  - Staging should also include bone scan and chest CT scan

DIFFERENTIAL DIAGNOSIS

Sclerotic Metastasis

- Most commonly prostate, breast, gastrointestinal
  - Medulloblastoma in pediatric patients
- Sclerosis rarely extends beyond borders of bone
- Often multiple

Osteoblastoma

- Expansile, bone-forming lesion in posterior elements
- Can extend into vertebral body
- Cortical breakthrough often seen
- Narrow zone of transition
- Aggressive osteoblastoma mimics OGS on imaging studies

Aneurysmal Bone Cyst

- Fluid-fluid levels similar to telangiectatic OGS
- Expansile lesion centered in posterior elements
- Cortical breakthrough often seen
- Narrow zone of transition

Chordoma

- Most common in sacrum
- Arises in midline
- Lytic, aggressive mass; no sclerosis; T2 hyperintense

Osteomyelitis

- Occasionally sclerotic
- Usually involves 2 contiguous vertebrae and intervening disc space

Ewing Sarcoma

- Sometimes sclerotic
- Tends to permeate through cortex rather than cause large visible area of destruction

Chondrosarcoma

- Ring and arc calcification

Lymphoma

- Moth-eaten, lytic bone destruction
- Can rarely be sclerotic

Malignant Giant Cell Tumor

- Rare entity, most common in sacrum
- Lytic, aggressive mass without bone matrix formation
- Histologically similar to giant cell-rich OGS

Giant Bone Island

- Sclerotic focus in medullary bone
- Mature cortical bone
- Shows "brush border": Trabeculae merge with adjacent bone

PATHOLOGY

General Features

- Etiology
  - Majority of OGSs of unknown etiology = primary OGS

- Associated with retinoblastoma (*RB1* gene mutation)
- Secondary osteosarcoma associated with
  - Paget disease
  - Bone infarct
  - Radiation

Staging, Grading, & Classification

- Classified by predominant cell type histologically
  - Osteoblastic (conventional), chondroblastic, fibroblastic, telangiectatic, small cell, giant cell, epithelioid
- AJCC staging based on size, grade, and metastases

Gross Pathologic & Surgical Features

- Heterogeneous mass with ossified and nonossified components
- Ossified areas: Yellow-white, firm, may be as hard as cortical bone
- Less ossified areas: Soft, tan with foci of hemorrhage and necrosis
- Necrosis common
- Cortical breakthrough
- Often large, extraosseous tumor mass

Microscopic Features

- Pluripotential neoplasm
- Malignant cells produce some osteoid in all subtypes, but it may be difficult to find
  - Osteoid is immature
- Classic: High-degree anaplasia, high mitotic rate
  - Tumor cells may be spindled or round
  - Size of cells ranges from small to giant
- Telangiectatic OGS
  - Dilated vascular channels lined by multinucleated giant cells
  - Stroma forms osteoid, which may not be prominent feature
- Other malignant tumors (e.g., chondrosarcoma) may contain reactive bone, but osteoid is not produced by malignant cells

CLINICAL ISSUES

Presentation

- Most common signs/symptoms
  - Insidious onset of back pain, greatest at night
  - Neurologic symptoms, including radicular pain, weakness
- Clinical profile
  - Pathologic fracture
  - Most common sites of metastases are liver, lung, bone, and lymph nodes
    - Metastases often show calcification
  - Pulmonary metastases may result in pneumothorax
  - Increased serum alkaline phosphatase

Demographics

- Age
  - Spine OGS has peak incidence in 4th decade
    - Later than for appendicular OGS
  - Range: 8-80 years in one large series
- Sex
  - M = F
- Epidemiology
  - 2nd most common primary bone malignancy (after multiple myeloma)

Natural History & Prognosis

- Median survival: 23 months in recent series
- Survival rate lower than for peripheral OGS due to difficulty of surgical resection
- 3% of 10-year survivors of all OGS develop 2nd malignancy
- Patients should have close CT (or PET/CT) surveillance

Treatment

- Neoadjuvant chemotherapy ± radiation therapy
- Surgical resection with wide margins provides survival benefit in selected patients
- Biopsies must be planned with future tumor excision in mind

DIAGNOSTIC CHECKLIST

Consider

- CT scan best method for evaluation of tumor matrix, zone of transition
- Patients may present with multiple synchronous tumors (osteosarcomatosis)

Image Interpretation Pearls

- All telangiectatic OGS are lytic on radiographs and CT, but not all lytic OGS are telangiectatic

SELECTED REFERENCES

1. Egea-Gámez RM et al: Case report: giant cell-rich osteosarcoma of the cervical spine in the pediatric age. A rare entity to consider. Front Surg. 9:1001149, 2022
2. Huang Z et al: Clinical features, risk factors, and prediction nomogram for primary spinal osteosarcoma: a large-cohort retrospective study. Global Spine J. ePub, 2022
3. Rae M et al: Atypical presentation of primary osteosarcoma of the lumbar spine with caval tumor thrombus in a 17-year-old male: a case report. Curr Sports Med Rep. 21(11):391-4, 2022
4. Tang C et al: Surgery has positive effects on spinal osteosarcoma prognosis: a population-based database study. World Neurosurg. 164:e367-86, 2022
5. Pillai SS: Long-term survival following resection of extracompartmental osteosarcoma of the spine - a case report and literature review. Surg Neurol Int. 12:545, 2021
6. Chen DJ et al: Lumbar spinal canal osteosarcoma: a case report. Medicine (Baltimore). 97(25):e11210, 2018
7. Shankar GM et al: The role of revision surgery and adjuvant therapy following subtotal resection of osteosarcoma of the spine: a systematic review with meta-analysis. J Neurosurg Spine. 27(1):97-104, 2017
8. Dekutoski MB et al: Osteosarcoma of the spine: prognostic variables for local recurrence and overall survival, a multicenter ambispective study. J Neurosurg Spine. 25(1):59-68, 2016
9. Groves ML et al: Epidemiologic, functional, and oncologic outcome analysis of spinal sarcomas treated surgically at a single institution over 10 years. Spine J. 15(1):110-4, 2014
10. Bhatia R et al: Osteosarcoma of the spine: dismal past, any hope for the future? Br J Neurosurg. 28(4):495-502, 2013
11. Katonis P et al: Spinal osteosarcoma. Clin Med Insights Oncol. 7:199-208, 2013
12. Lim JB et al: Primary osteosarcoma of the spine: a review of 10 cases. Acta Orthop Belg. 79(4):457-62, 2013
13. Schiller MD et al: A case of intradural osteosarcoma of the spine. Spine J. 13(8):e55-8, 2013
14. Zils K et al: Osteosarcoma of the mobile spine. Ann Oncol. 24(8):2190-5, 2013
15. Ilaslan H et al: Primary vertebral osteosarcoma: imaging findings. Radiology. 230(3):697-702, 2004

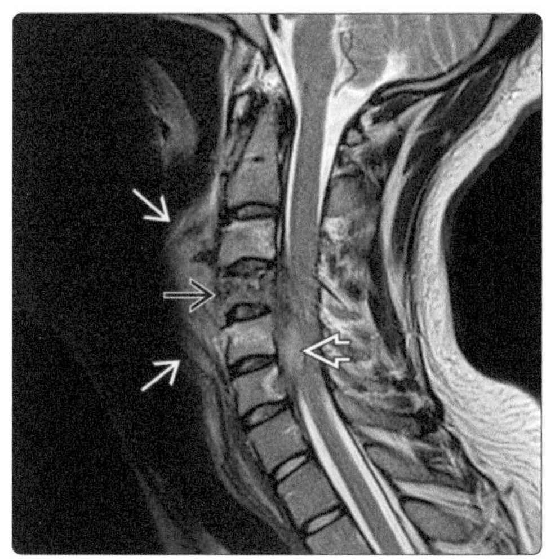

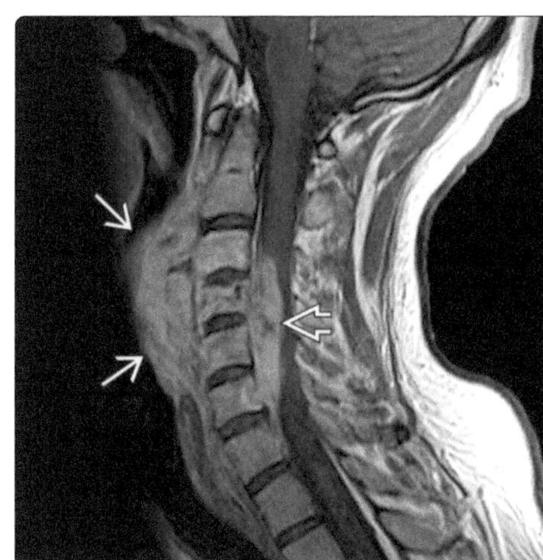

(Left) *Sagittal T2 MR (epithelioid osteosarcoma) shows a very large soft tissue mass, which shows relatively low T2 signal, consistent with a highly cellular tumor. The mass involves multiple vertebral bodies but probably arises from C4. Note epidural extension with cord displacement.* **(Right)** *Sagittal T1 C+ MR (epithelioid osteosarcoma) confirms diffuse soft mass enhancement with bulky prevertebral/paravertebral and epidural tumor extension.*

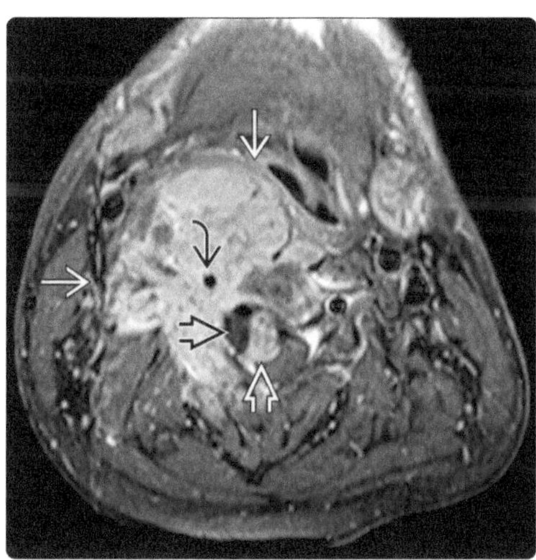

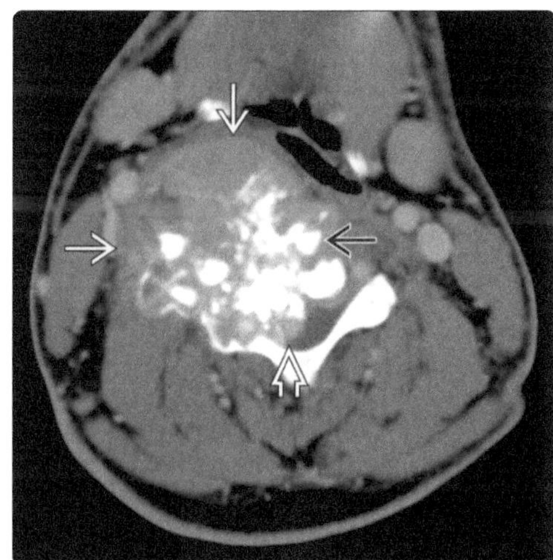

(Left) *Axial T1 C+ FS MR (epithelioid osteosarcoma) confirms a large, diffusely enhancing soft tissue mass. Note prevertebral and paravertebral extension, epidural extension, and right vertebral artery encasement with spinal cord compression.* **(Right)** *Axial CECT (epithelioid osteosarcoma) shows a very aggressive-appearing, large soft tissue mass. There is immature-appearing osteoid matrix within areas of frank bone destruction.*

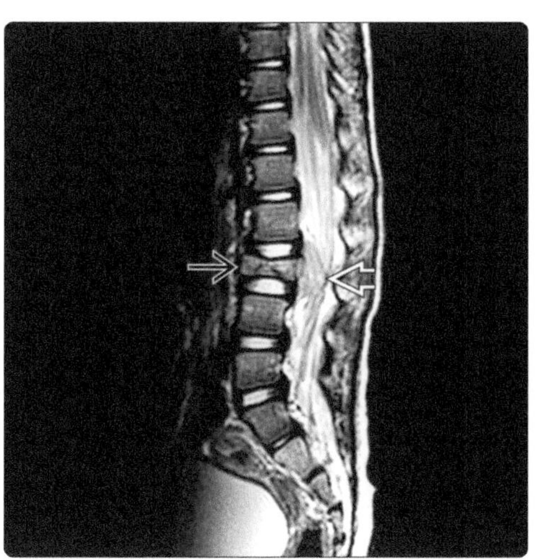

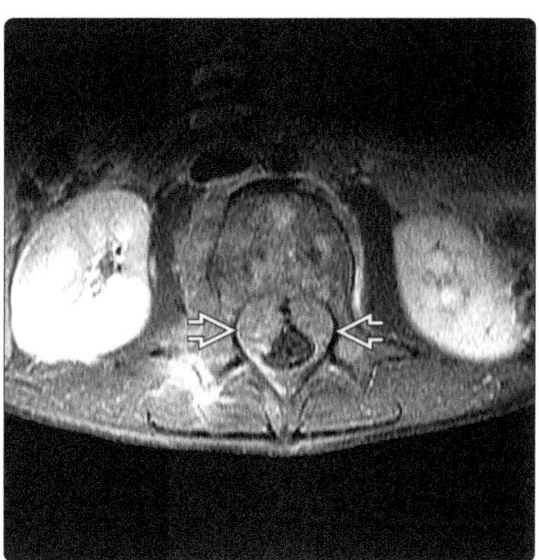

(Left) *Sagittal STIR MR demonstrates a pathologic L3 vertebral body fracture with height loss. Note posterior epidural mass extension producing cauda equina compression. Bone matrix is poorly seen on MR.* **(Right)** *Axial T1 C+ FS MR in the same patient confirms a large, diffusely enhancing tumor, which permeates through cortex into the spinal canal and paraspinous soft tissues. Note extensive epidural extension with the curtain sign.*

KEY FACTS

TERMINOLOGY

- Malignant tumor arising from notochord remnants

IMAGING

- Clival > sacrococcygeal in children
- Osseous destruction with disproportionately large soft tissue mass
- Circumscribed, scalloped, or sclerotic bony margins
- Amorphous intratumoral calcifications
- Hyperintense to disc on T2WI with multiple septa
- May extend into disc space, involve 2 or more adjacent vertebrae

TOP DIFFERENTIAL DIAGNOSES

- Chondrosarcoma
- Giant cell tumor
- Metastases
- Plasmacytoma

PATHOLOGY

- Lobulated, soft, grayish gelatinous (myxoid) mass
- Areas of calcification and hemorrhage

CLINICAL ISSUES

- Skull base
  - Diplopia
  - Headaches
  - Facial pain
- Mobile spine: Cord compression, radiculopathy (50%)
- Sacral: Altered sacrogluteal sensation
- Symptoms tend to be longstanding (4-24 months)
- Recurrence common

DIAGNOSTIC CHECKLIST

- High signal intensity mass on T2WI with septations, little enhancement is chordoma or chondrosarcoma
- Recurrence (seeding) along operative tract not uncommon; modify field of view to include operative approach

(Left) *Sagittal graphic of the cervical spine shows extradural soft tissue mass (chordoma) with the epicenter within the posterior aspect of the C2 body, causing bone destruction and epidural extension with cord compression.* **(Right)** *Sagittal T2 MR in an adolescent patient with neck pain and myelopathy reveals a very hyperintense mass ➡ centered at C2/C3 producing extrinsic cord compression. There is mild heterogeneous increased marrow signal in the C2 and C3 vertebra.*

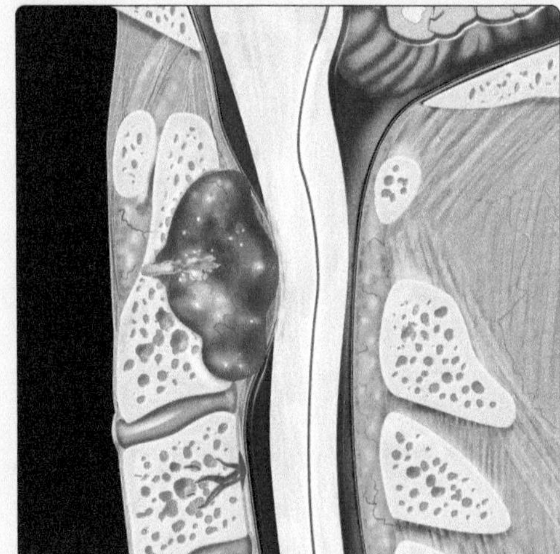

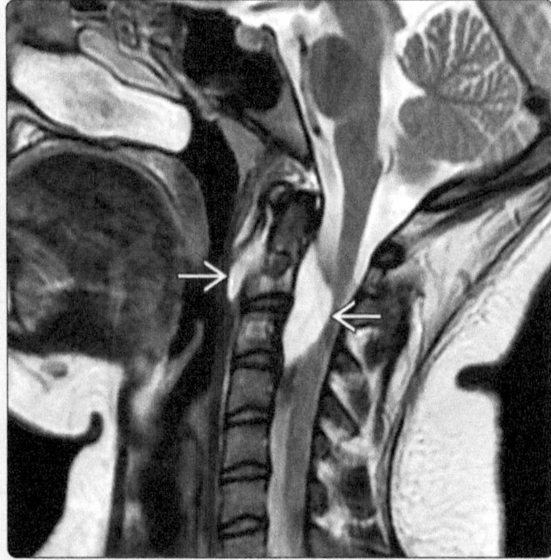

(Left) *Axial T2 MR in the same patient demonstrates well-circumscribed tumor ➡ expansion into the left paraspinal soft tissues with bone destruction and lateral displacement of the left vertebral artery ➡. Marrow abnormality in the vertebra is typically posterior because of anatomic location of notochord remnant.* **(Right)** *Axial T1 C+ FS MR in the same patient reveals characteristic low mass T1 signal intensity without significant mass contrast enhancement.*

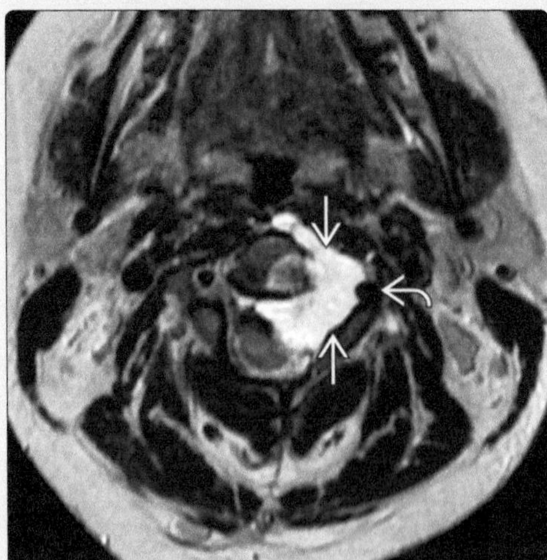

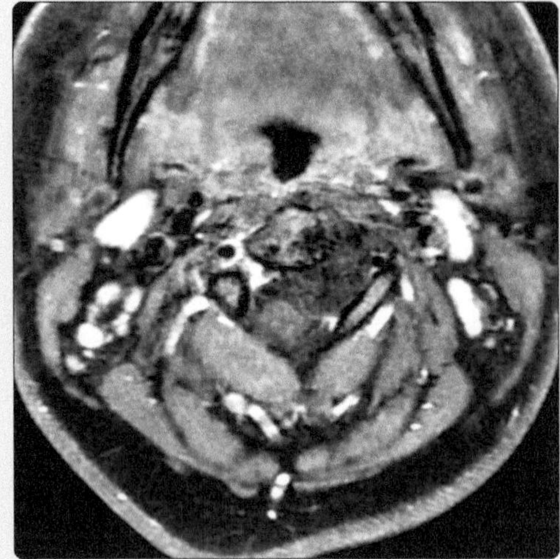

TERMINOLOGY

Definitions

- Malignant tumor arising from notochord remnants

IMAGING

General Features

- Best diagnostic clue
  - Destructive process with disproportionately large soft tissue mass
  - Located in clivus or sacrum
  - Mass is hyperintense to disc on T2WI with multiple septa
- Location
  - Craniovertebral junction > sacrococcygeal in children
  - Sacrococcygeal > craniovertebral junction > mobile spine in adults
- Size
  - Variable
  - Sacrococcygeal chordomas can be huge at presentation
- Morphology
  - Midline lobular soft tissue mass with osseous destruction

Radiographic Findings

- Radiography
  - Heterogeneous destructive mass of sacrum or vertebral body
  - May extend into disc space, involve 2 or more adjacent vertebrae
  - May enlarge neural foramen
  - Osseous sclerosis in up to 60% of cases
    - Solitary sclerotic "ivory" vertebra (rare)

CT Findings

- NECT
  - Destructive, lytic lesion
  - Soft tissue mass usually present
    - Often disproportionately large relative to bony destruction
  - Amorphous intratumoral calcifications
    - Sacrum: > 70%
    - Vertebra: 30%
- CECT
  - Mild to moderate enhancement
  - ± inhomogeneous areas (cystic necrosis, hemorrhage)

MR Findings

- T1WI
  - Heterogeneous, hypo- to isointense (compared to marrow)
- T2WI
  - Hyperintense to CSF, intervertebral discs ("light bulb")
  - May have low-signal septations (fibrous)
- T1WI C+
  - Variable enhancement: Blush → intense enhancement

Nuclear Medicine Findings

- Bone scan
  - Normal or decreased uptake within tumor
- PET/CT
  - Moderate, heterogeneous tumor F-18 FDG uptake
    - F-18 FDG PET/CT may be useful for staging, evaluating treatment response, and assessing for recurrent or metastatic disease

Imaging Recommendations

- Best imaging tool
  - MR for soft tissue (STIR/fat-saturated T2WI, contrast-enhanced T1WI)
  - Bone CT for bone detail

DIFFERENTIAL DIAGNOSIS

Chondrosarcoma

- Neural arch > vertebral body
- Chondroid matrix (rings and arcs)
- Mild peripheral and internal septal enhancement
- Similar MR characteristics

Giant Cell Tumor

- Heterogeneous, intermediate to hyperintense T2 signal
- May infiltrate disc space with spread to adjacent vertebral body

Metastases

- Hypointense T1, variably hyperintense T2WI lesion(s)
- Often multiple, involving vertebral bodies and posterior elements

Plasmacytoma

- Destructive vertebral body lesion, similar appearance to lytic metastases

Lymphoma

- Multifocal disease; heterogeneous T2 signal

Sacrococcygeal Teratoma

- Heterogeneous MR signal
- Areas of macroscopic fat hyperintense on T1WI
- Pediatric patients

Ecchordosis Physaliphora (Rare)

- Benign, nonneoplastic ectopic notochordal remnant(s)
- Usually at skull base/C2 but can occur anywhere (including intradural)

PATHOLOGY

General Features

- Etiology
  - Arises from notochord remnants
- Genetics
  - Losses on chromosomal arms 3p (50%) and 1p (44%)
  - Gains on 7q (69%), 20 (50%), 5q (38%), and 12q (38%)
  - *SMARCB1* (INI1) deletion in pediatric undifferentiated chordoma
- Location
  - 2-4% of primary malignant bone tumors
  - Sacrococcygeal (50%), sphenooccipital (35%), mobile spine (15%)
  - Mobile spine: Cervical (20-50%) > lumbar > thoracic
- Embryology/anatomy
  - Tumor arises from notochordal remnants
    - Notochord (column of cells ventral to neural tube) arises 3rd gestational week, disappears by 7th week

      - Rest of notochord cells occur in axial skeleton from coccyx to dorsum sellae

Staging, Grading, & Classification

- Enneking system for staging musculoskeletal sarcomas
  - Grade of biologic aggressiveness
  - Anatomic setting
  - Presence of metastasis

Gross Pathologic & Surgical Features

- Lobulated, soft, grayish gelatinous (myxoid) mass
- Areas of calcification and hemorrhage

Microscopic Features

- 3 types described
  - Typical: Lobules, sheets, and cords of clear cells with intracytoplasmic vacuoles (physaliphorous cells); abundant mucin
  - Chondroid: Hyaline cartilage (usually sphenooccipital region)
  - Dedifferentiated: Sarcomatous elements (rare, highly malignant)
- Immunohistochemistry: Positive for S100, keratin (AE1/AE3; CK8, CK19, and often CK5), HBME-1, epithelial membrane antigen; usually negative for CK7, CK20

CLINICAL ISSUES

Presentation

- Most common signs/symptoms
  - Location dependent
    - Clival
      - Diplopia
      - Headaches
      - Facial pain
    - Sacral
      - Weakness
      - Sacral mass
      - Altered sacrogluteal sensation
      - Bowel/bladder/sexual dysfunction
    - Spinal
      - Cord compression, radiculopathy (50%)
      - Cervical spine chordomas may present with airway obstruction, dysphagia
  - Symptoms tend to be longstanding (4-24 months)
- Clinical profile
  - Middle-aged man presenting with pain, neurologic dysfunction

Demographics

- Age
  - Peak incidence: 5th-6th decades (rare in children)
- Sex
  - M:F = 2:1 in adults, female predominance in children
    - More equal sex distribution for clival chordoma
- Ethnicity
  - Rare in Black populations
- Epidemiology
  - 2-4% of primary malignant bone neoplasms
  - Most common primary nonlymphoproliferative malignancy of spine
  - Incidence rate of 0.08 per 100,000
  - Rare among patients < 40 years old

Natural History & Prognosis

- Slow growing
- Overall survival
  - 5-year survival up to 67-84%
  - 10-year survival: 40%
- Distant metastases 5-40% (lung, liver, lymph nodes, bone)
- Poor prognostic factors
  - Large size
  - Subtotal resection, local recurrence
  - Microscopic necrosis
  - Ki-67 index > 5%
  - Young or old age
- Dedifferentiation into high-grade sarcoma portends worse prognosis

Treatment

- Surgical resection with adjuvant XRT
  - En bloc resection yields best outcome
- Recurrence common
  - Local (90%)
  - Regional lymph nodes (5%)
  - Distant metastases (5%); lung, bone
  - 5-year survival: 50-68%; 10-year survival: 28-40%

DIAGNOSTIC CHECKLIST

Consider

- High signal intensity mass on T2WI with septations, little enhancement is chordoma or chondrosarcoma

Image Interpretation Pearls

- Recurrence (seeding) along operative tract is not uncommon; modify field of view to include operative approach

SELECTED REFERENCES

1. Olson JT et al: Chordoma: 18F-FDG PET/CT and MRI imaging features. Skeletal Radiol. 50(8):1657-66, 2021
2. Reardon T et al: Clinical management of pediatric chordomas: a comprehensive review. Acta Neurol Belg. 121(6):1407-14, 2021
3. Rekhi B et al: Poorly differentiated chordoma showing loss of SMARCB1/INI1: clinicopathological and radiological spectrum of nine cases, including uncommon features of a relatively under-recognized entity. Ann Diagn Pathol. 55:151809, 2021
4. Hung YP et al: Dedifferentiated chordoma: clinicopathologic and molecular characteristics with integrative analysis. Am J Surg Pathol. 44(9):1213-23, 2020
5. Antonelli M et al: SMARCB1/INI1 involvement in pediatric chordoma: a mutational and immunohistochemical analysis. Am J Surg Pathol. 41(1):56-61, 2017
6. Ramesh S et al: Multicentric chordoma in a child. J Pediatr Neurosci. 12(2):156-9, 2017
7. Zhou J et al: Prognostic factors in patients with spinal chordoma: an integrative analysis of 682 patients. Neurosurgery. 81(5):812-23, 2017
8. Sebro R et al: Differences in sex distribution, anatomic location and MR imaging appearance of pediatric compared to adult chordomas. BMC Med Imaging. 16(1):53, 2016
9. Tsitouras V et al: Management and outcome of chordomas in the pediatric population: the Hospital for Sick Children experience and review of the literature. J Clin Neurosci. 34:169-76, 2016
10. Sciubba DM et al: Chordoma of the spinal column. Neurosurg Clin N Am. 19(1):5-15, 2008
11. Boriani S et al: Chordoma of the mobile spine: fifty years of experience. Spine (Phila Pa 1976). 31(4):493-503, 2006
12. Takeyama J et al: Notochordal remnant-derived mass: ecchordosis physaliphora or chordoma? Pathology. 38(6):599-600, 2006

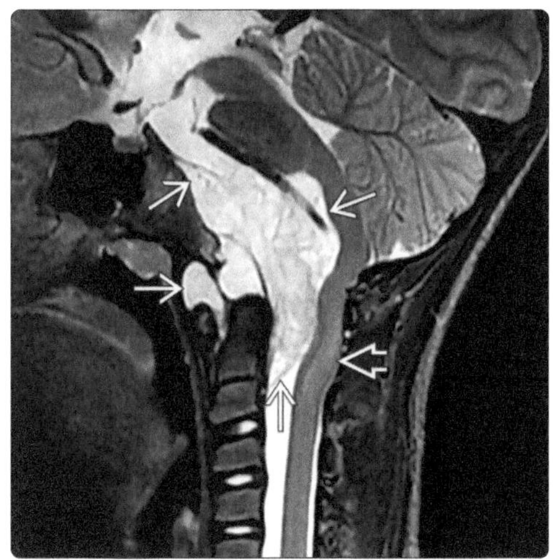

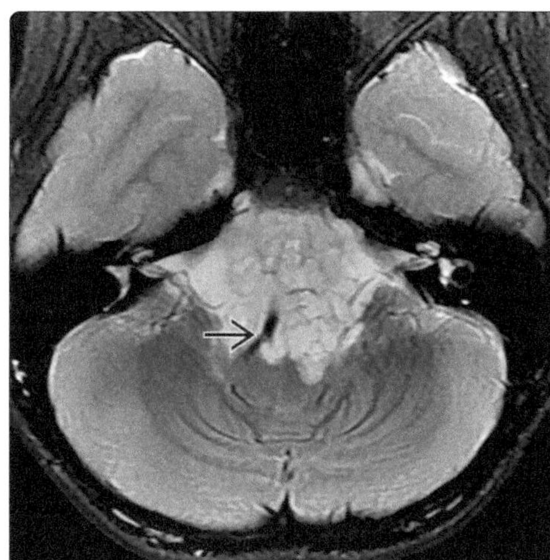

(Left) *Sagittal T2 FS MR reveals a large craniovertebral junction chordoma* ➔ *arising from the distal clivus. Note displacement and distortion of the cervicomedullary junction with intramedullary signal abnormality in the cervical cord* ➔. **(Right)** *Axial T2 FS MR in the same patient presenting with quadriparesis shows a light bulb-bright signal within the tumor mass. The mass engulfs the vertebrobasilar arterial junction* ⇨.

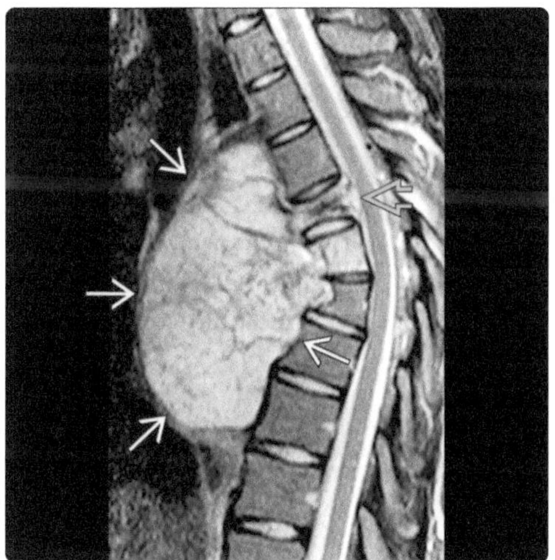

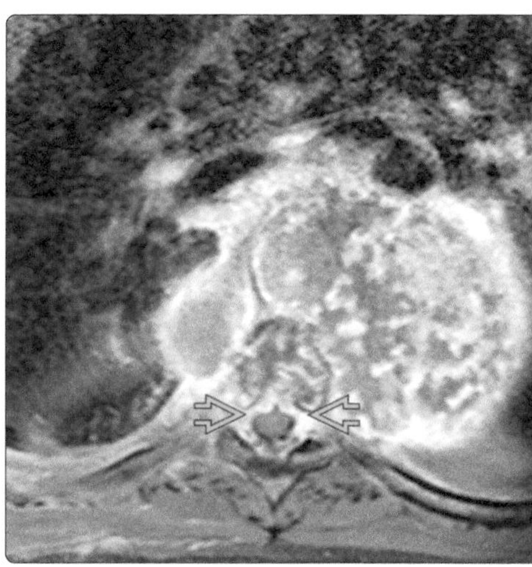

(Left) *Sagittal T2 FS MR shows a large posterior mediastinal mass* ➔ *with involvement of 4 adjacent thoracic vertebral bodies. The mass is hyperintense with fine septations. Note the pathologic compression fracture of the top vertebra with ventral epidural tumor* ⇨. **(Right)** *Axial T1 C+ FS MR in the same patient confirms heterogeneous enhancement within the large posterior mediastinal mass. Note epidural spread with the characteristic curtain sign* ⇨.

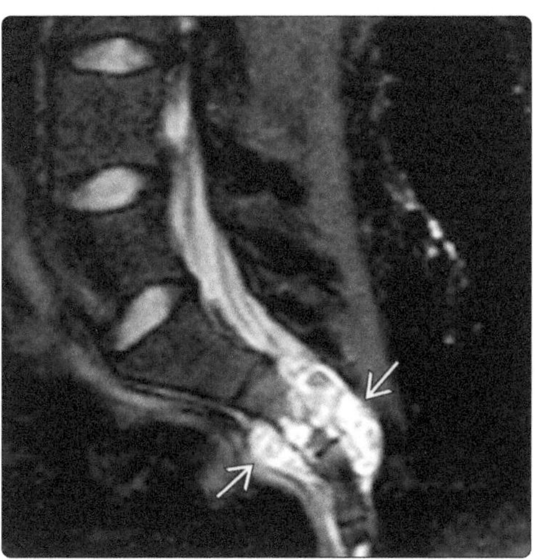

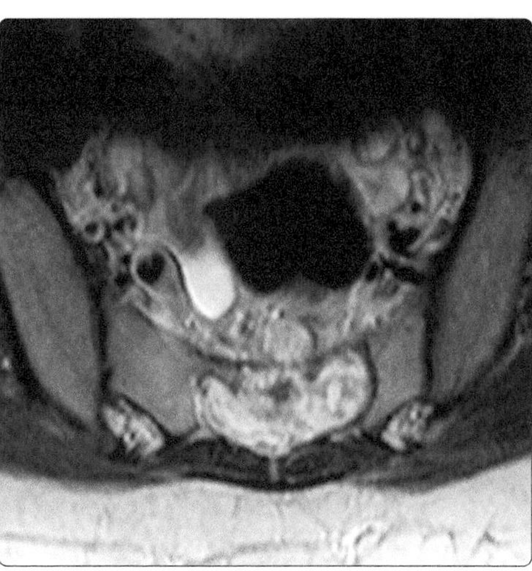

(Left) *Sagittal STIR MR of the lumbosacral spine reveals a destructive, T2-hyperintense mass* ➔ *originating in the S2 vertebra with epidural extension into the central spinal canal.* **(Right)** *Axial T2 MR in the same patient confirms expansion of the osseous sacral canal by the T2-hyperintense tumor mass.*

KEY FACTS

TERMINOLOGY

- Ewing sarcoma family of tumors (ESFT)
- Aggressive childhood cancer family that includes Ewing sarcoma, Askin tumor, and peripheral primitive neuroectodermal tumor (PNET)

IMAGING

- Spine: 5% of all Ewing tumors
  - Sacrum most common spinal site
- May originate in epidural or paraspinous soft tissues
- Permeative/moth-eaten bone destruction
- MR best shows involvement of adjacent bones and soft tissues, which can be underestimated on CT scan
- CT useful to confirm absence of tumor matrix, distinguish from osteogenic sarcoma (OGS)

TOP DIFFERENTIAL DIAGNOSES

- PNET
- Langerhans cell histiocytosis
- Osteosarcoma
- Metastatic neuroblastoma
- Osteomyelitis

PATHOLOGY

- Exact progenitor cell debated, not definitively known
- Reciprocal translocation between *EWSR1* gene on chromosome 22 and ETS-like genes on chromosome 11 t(11;22)

CLINICAL ISSUES

- 90% of all Ewing sarcoma patients present before 20 years
- Fever, leukocytosis, elevated ESR (simulating osteomyelitis)
- Spine and sacral lesions often in older patients than in peripheral Ewing sarcoma

DIAGNOSTIC CHECKLIST

- Always consider osteomyelitis and other small round cell tumors in imaging differential diagnosis

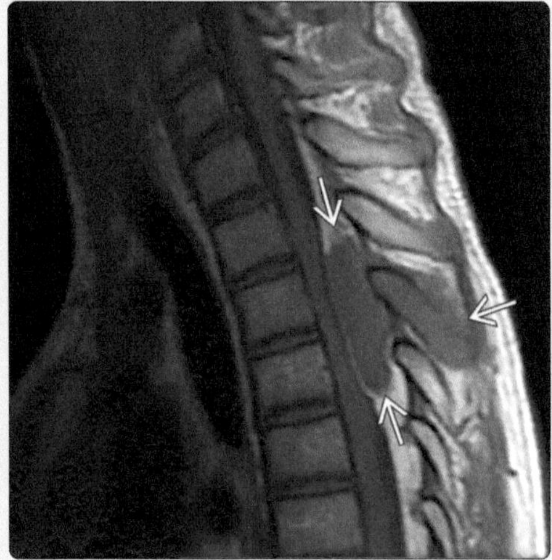

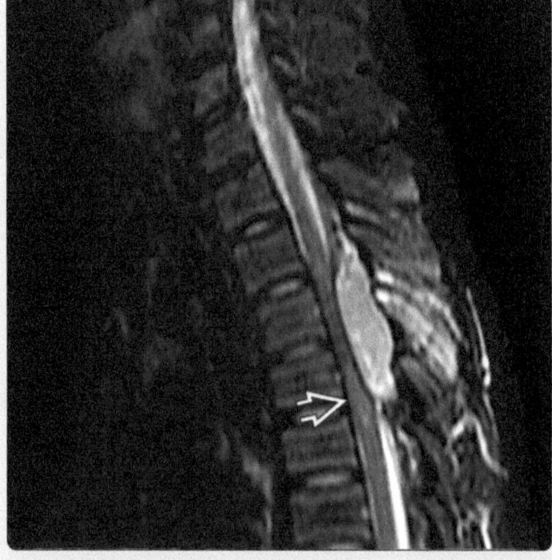

(Left) *Sagittal T1WI MR of the cervicothoracic spine demonstrates an extradural mass ➡ originating within the T4 spinous process. Epidural extension is illustrated by a cap of epidural fat above and below the mass.* **(Right)** *Sagittal STIR MR in the same patient confirms mass cellular signal intensity. There is cord compression with abnormal intramedullary signal ➡ noted.*

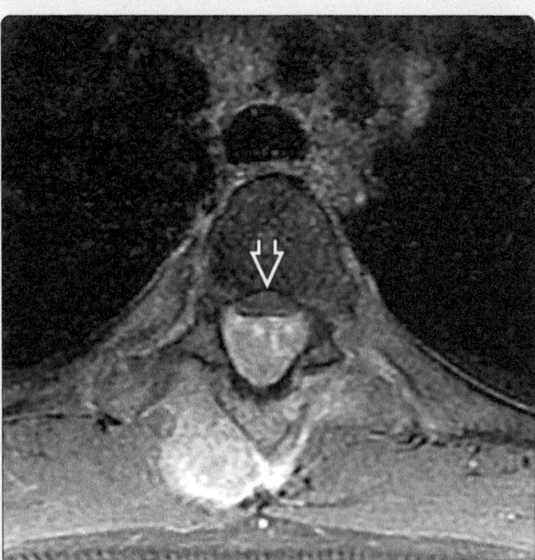

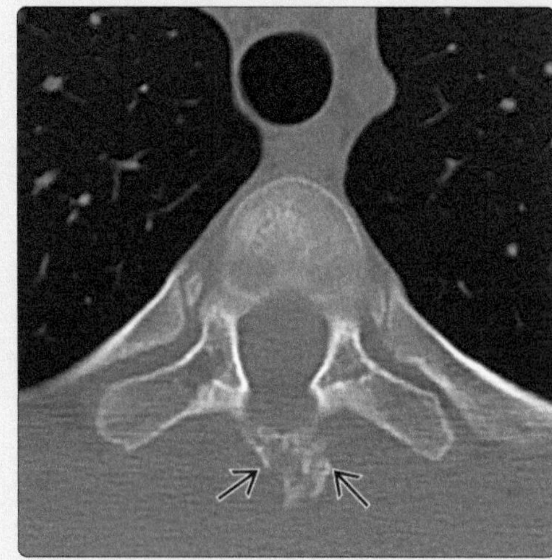

(Left) *Axial T1WI C+ FS MR in the same patient confirms moderate mass enhancement. The spinal cord ➡ is compressed and anteriorly displaced by the epidural tumor extension into the spinal canal.* **(Right)** *Axial bone CT in the same patient shows mottled bone destruction ➡ within the T4 spinous process at the site of tumor origination.*

TERMINOLOGY

Synonyms

- Ewing sarcoma family of tumors (ESFT)
- Round cell sarcoma of bone

Definitions

- Aggressive childhood cancer that includes Ewing sarcoma, Askin tumor, and peripheral primitive neuroectodermal tumor (PNET)

IMAGING

General Features

- Best diagnostic clue
  - Permeative lytic lesion of vertebral body or sacrum
- Location
  - Spine: 5% of all Ewing tumors
  - Involves vertebral body before neural arch
  - Sacrum most common spinal site
  - May involve adjacent bones: Vertebrae, ribs, or ilium
  - Spreads along peripheral nerves
  - May originate in epidural or paraspinous soft tissues

Radiographic Findings

- Radiography
  - Centered in vertebral body or sacrum
  - Permeative/moth-eaten bone destruction
  - Wide zone of transition
    - Difficult to identify tumor margin
  - Cortical destruction difficult to see
    - Tiny perforations of cortex better seen on CT
  - 50% have extraosseous, noncalcified soft tissue mass
  - 5% sclerotic (represents host reaction, not tumor matrix)
  - May cause vertebra plana
  - May involve 2 or more adjacent bones
  - If adjacent vertebrae involved, do not see disc height loss and endplate erosions as in osteomyelitis

CT Findings

- Permeative intramedullary mass ± soft tissue mass
- Areas of central necrosis common
- "Percolates" through tiny perforations in cortex
  - Usually do not see large areas of cortical breakthrough
- Heterogeneous contrast enhancement
- Rarely sclerotic, due to reactive new bone formation
  - Mimics osteogenic sarcoma (OGS)
  - Ossification is not present in soft tissue component
- Soft tissue Ewing sarcoma is nonspecific mass

MR Findings

- Poorly defined lesion originating in bone or soft tissue
  - Lower signal intensity than disc or muscle on T1WI
  - May be isointense to red marrow on T2WI
  - Intermediate to high signal intensity on STIR
- Central necrosis often present
  - Heterogeneous enhancement with gadolinium (Gd)
    - Cannot reliably distinguish between tumor and peritumoral edema
      - Peritumoral edema enhances with Gd
- Bone cortex often visible despite soft tissue extension of bone mass
  - Has smudged appearance due to perforation of tumor through cortex

Nuclear Medicine Findings

- Bone scan
  - Positive 3-phase bone scan
- PET
  - Increased FDG uptake of tumor, metastases

Imaging Recommendations

- Best imaging tool
  - MR best shows involvement of adjacent bones and soft tissues, which can be underestimated on CT scan
    - May overestimate tumor size due to peritumoral edema
- Protocol advice
  - MR to determine extent of tumor
    - Sagittal T1WI
    - Axial and sagittal STIR, postcontrast T1WI
  - CT useful to confirm absence of tumor matrix, distinguish from OGS

DIFFERENTIAL DIAGNOSIS

Peripheral Primitive Neuroectodermal Tumor

- Clinically/radiologically identical to Ewing sarcoma
- May occur in bone or soft tissue
- Greater neuroectodermal differentiation of tumor cells

Langerhans Cell Histiocytosis

- May have identical radiographic appearance to Ewing sarcoma
- More classically discrete geographic lytic lesion
- Vertebra plana common

Lymphoma and Leukemia

- Same radiographic appearance as Ewing sarcoma
- Ill-defined lytic lesion showing permeative pattern
- Involves vertebral body more than neural arch
- Often involves multiple vertebrae

Metastatic Neuroblastoma

- Adrenal or extraadrenal primary
- Occurs in children
- Identical appearance in bone

Osteosarcoma

- Ill-defined lytic lesion showing permeative pattern
- 80% show bone matrix on radiographs or CT
- Involves vertebral body or neural arch
- May involve adjacent vertebral body
- Tends to have cortical destruction rather than permeation through cortex

Osteomyelitis

- Ill-defined lytic lesion showing permeative pattern
- May be more geographic (intraosseous abscess with peripheral enhancement)
- Involves vertebral body more than neural arch
- Discocentric: Extends from 1 vertebral body to adjacent vertebra across disc

- Disc height loss, enhancement of disc on MR, endplate erosions
- Soft tissue mass common

Multiple Myeloma

- Occurs in older patients
- Usually multiple vertebrae

Chordoma

- Most common in sacrum
- Originates in midline
- Bone expansion and destruction

Giant Cell Tumor

- Originates in vertebral body
- Narrow zone of transition
- Focal cortical destruction

Chondrosarcoma

- Usually show areas of chondroid matrix
  - Rings and arcs of Ca^{++}

PATHOLOGY

General Features

- Etiology
  - Mesenchymal cells with slight differentiation toward neuroectodermal cells
  - Exact progenitor cell debated, not definitively known
- Genetics
  - Reciprocal translocation between *EWSR1* gene on chromosome 22 and erythroblast transformation-specific (ETS)-like genes on chromosome 11 t(11;22)

Staging, Grading, & Classification

- No internationally recognized risk classification scheme for Ewing sarcoma patients

Gross Pathologic & Surgical Features

- Grayish-white tumor
- Poorly demarcated
- Areas of hemorrhage, cyst formation, necrosis

Microscopic Features

- Small, round cells (2-3x larger than lymphocytes), meager cytoplasm
- Cell outlines indistinct
- Round nuclei, frequent indentations, high mitotic rate
- Solid sheets of cells divided into irregular masses by fibrous strands

CLINICAL ISSUES

Presentation

- Most common signs/symptoms
  - Localized pain
  - Fever, leukocytosis, elevated ESR (simulating osteomyelitis)
  - Neurologic symptoms ranging from radiculopathy to paralysis
  - Vertebra plana

Demographics

- Age
  - 90% of all Ewing sarcoma patients present before 20 years
  - 2nd (smaller) peak at 50 years
  - Spine and sacral lesions often in older patients than in peripheral Ewing sarcoma
- Sex
  - M:F = 2:1
- Epidemiology
  - Annual incidence of Ewing sarcoma (all locations): 3/1 million White children < 15 years old
  - 6th most common malignant bone tumor

Natural History & Prognosis

- Metastases to lung, regional lymph nodes, and other bones in 30% at presentation
- Prognosis worse in spinal than peripheral Ewing sarcoma due to difficulty of surgical resection
- Significant risk of 2nd malignancy
- Current treatments yield long-term survival in > 50% of patients with localized disease at presentation
- Complications common > 5 years after treatment
  - Local recurrence
  - Metastases
  - 2nd malignancies

Treatment

- Surgery or radiotherapy; without chemotherapy, universally fatal
- Neoadjuvant chemotherapy given prior to surgery
- Surgical resection with wide margins
- Radiation therapy for surgically inaccessible lesions, stage III disease, poor response to chemotherapy

DIAGNOSTIC CHECKLIST

Consider

- Often metastatic at time of presentation

Image Interpretation Pearls

- Always consider osteomyelitis and other small round cell tumors in imaging differential diagnosis

SELECTED REFERENCES

1. Indelicato DJ et al: Modern therapy for spinal and paraspinal ewing sarcoma: an update of the University of Florida experience. Int J Radiat Oncol Biol Phys. 113(1):161-5, 2022
2. Shapira Rootman M et al: Tumours involving the neural foramina in children: beyond neuroblastoma. Clin Radiol. 77(1):e33-9, 2022
3. Soni A et al: Primary extra-skeletal Ewing's sarcoma presenting as an epidural soft tissue lesion causing cauda equina syndrome in an adolescent girl: a case report. Spinal Cord Ser Cases. 8(1):13, 2022
4. Amelot A et al: Primary extraosseous spinal Ewing sarcomas: should we be more aware about diagnosis? Spine (Phila Pa 1976). 46(5):313-21, 2021
5. Berger GK et al: Outcomes in different age groups with primary Ewing sarcoma of the spine: a systematic review of the literature. J Neurosurg Spine. 1-10, 2019
6. Hesla AC et al: Ewing sarcoma of the mobile spine; predictive factors for survival, neurological function and local control. A Scandinavian sarcoma group study with a mean follow-up of 12 years. J Bone Oncol. 14:100216, 2019
7. Charest-Morin R et al: Ewing sarcoma of the spine: prognostic variables for survival and local control in surgically treated patients. Spine (Phila Pa 1976). 43(9):622-9, 2018
8. Murphey MD et al: From the radiologic pathology archives: Ewing sarcoma family of tumors: radiologic-pathologic correlation. Radiographics. 33(3):803-31, 2013

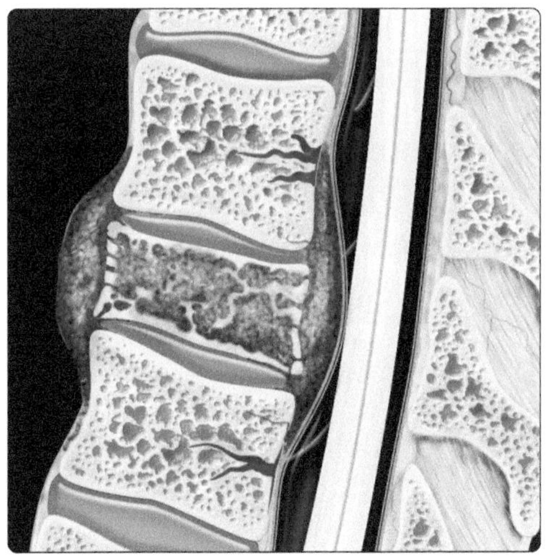

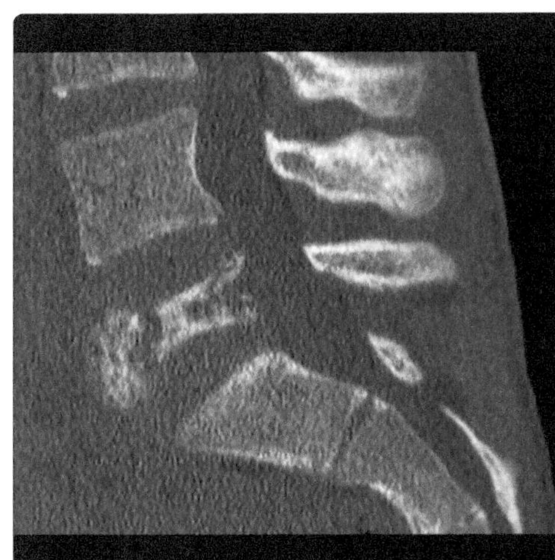

(Left) *Sagittal graphic shows vertebral body replacement by Ewing sarcoma, resulting in mild vertebral collapse. The tumor extends into adjacent soft tissues through small perforations in bone cortex.* **(Right)** *Sagittal bone CT in an adolescent patient with acute low back pain shows a pathologic fracture through an abnormal L5 vertebra secondary to permeative Ewing sarcoma.*

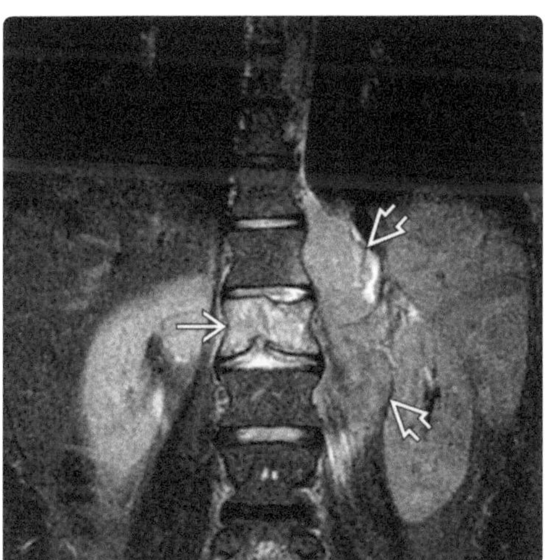

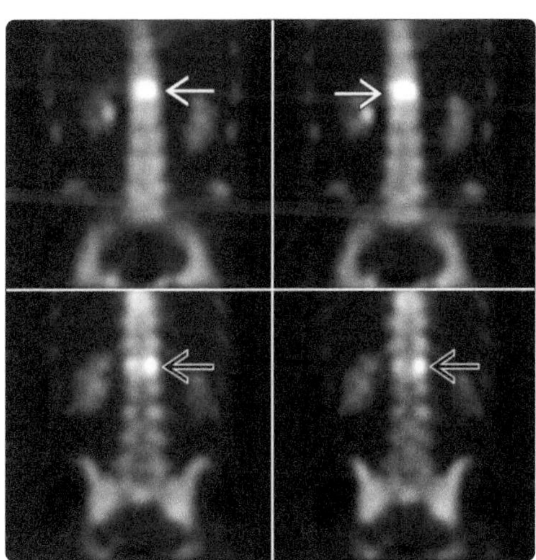

(Left) *Coronal T2WI FS MR demonstrates a destructive L1 vertebral body mass ➡ with a large left paraspinal epidural tumor mass ⮕. Note mild loss of vertebral body height related to a pathologic compression fracture.* **(Right)** *Coronal SPECT bone scans reveal focal increased uptake at the abnormal L1 vertebra ➡ extending into the left L1 pedicle ⇨. No metastatic lesions were detected.*

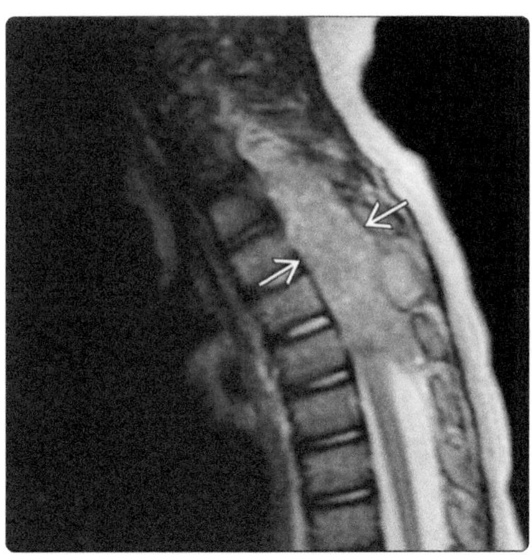

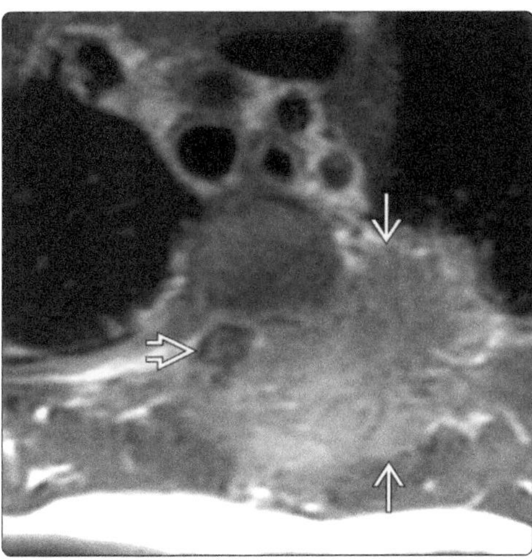

(Left) *Sagittal T2WI MR in a 6-month-old with progressive paraparesis demonstrates a large extradural mass ➡ filling the spinal canal, resulting in severe cord compression. Prebiopsy prediction was neuroblastoma given the age and appearance.* **(Right)** *Axial T1WI C+ MR in the same patient confirms a large enhancing extradural mass ➡ displacing and compressing the thoracic spinal cord ⮕. Pathology was typical for Ewing sarcoma with characteristic genetic translocation.*

KEY FACTS

TERMINOLOGY

- Acute or chronic myeloid or lymphoid WBC neoplasia with spinal involvement as component of systemic disease

IMAGING

- Radiographs/CT
  - Diffuse osteopenia with multiple vertebral fractures ± lytic spine lesions
  - Variable enhancing isodense soft tissue mass with adjacent bone destruction
- MR
  - T1WI: Hypointense marrow and focal tumor masses
  - T2WI: Hyperintense marrow ± focal vertebral mass, cord signal abnormality
  - T1WI C+: Abnormal enhancement of marrow, focal lesion, or leptomeninges

TOP DIFFERENTIAL DIAGNOSES

- Metastases
- Lymphoma
- Ewing sarcoma
- Langerhans cell histiocytosis

CLINICAL ISSUES

- Localized or diffuse bone pain
- Symptomatic patients present with fever, ↑ ESR, hepatosplenomegaly, lymphadenopathy, joint effusions, petechial and retinal hemorrhage, anemia, frequent infections

DIAGNOSTIC CHECKLIST

- Marrow infiltration in child with osteoporosis raises suspicion for leukemia
- Consider leukemia in patient with unexplained compression fractures

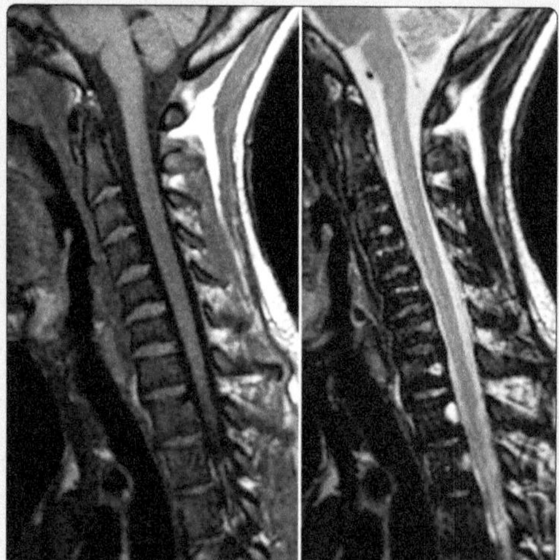

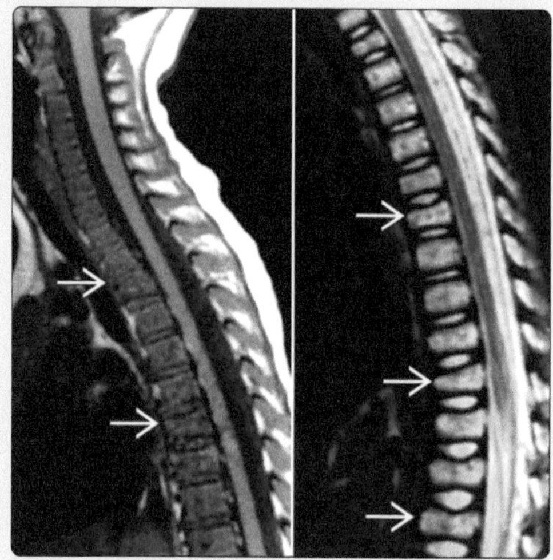

(Left) *Sagittal T1WI (left) and T2WI (right) MR images of the cervical spine demonstrate diffuse abnormal hypointense signal intensity within the vertebra. Signal intensity is lower than the adjacent disc spaces.* **(Right)** *Sagittal T1WI (left) and STIR (right) MR images illustrate abnormal hypointense and hyperintense marrow signal, respectively. Numerous compression fractures ➡ are present. This represents a case of leukemic marrow infiltration precipitating initial leukemia presentation with compression fractures.*

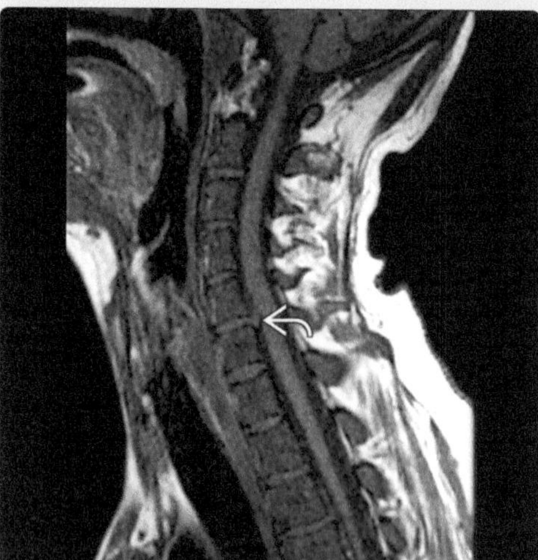

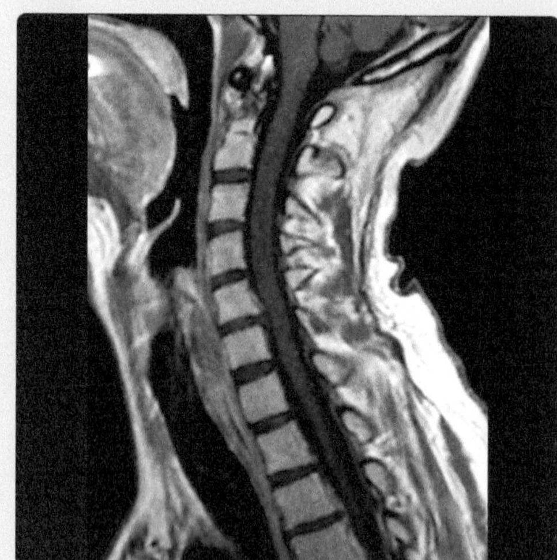

(Left) *Sagittal T1WI MR in a chronic myelogenous leukemia (CML) patient demonstrates marked diffuse marrow hypointensity relative to adjacent discs. Incidental disc herniation ➡ was the etiology of neck pain, prompting imaging.* **(Right)** *Sagittal T1WI C+ MR depicts avid diffuse marrow enhancement, reflecting CML marrow infiltration. Normal marrow would be expected to minimally enhance.*

TERMINOLOGY

Synonyms

- Acute lymphocytic leukemia (ALL), chronic lymphocytic leukemia (CLL), acute myelogenous leukemia (AML), chronic myelogenous leukemia (CML), granulocytic sarcoma (GS), chloroma, myeloid sarcoma (MS)

Definitions

- Acute or chronic myeloid or lymphoid WBC neoplasia with spinal involvement as component of systemic disease

IMAGING

General Features

- Best diagnostic clue
  - Diffuse osteopenia with multiple vertebral fractures ± lytic spine lesions
- Location
  - Children: Multiple long bones and spine (14%)
  - Adults: Predominately axial skeleton
- Morphology
  - Osteopenia ± moth-eaten bone destruction of multiple vertebral bodies, leptomeningeal enhancement, focal mass (chloroma)

Radiographic Findings

- Radiography
  - Diffuse vertebral long bone osteopenia
    - Coarse cancellous trabeculation ± pathologic vertebral compression fractures
    - Radiographs may look normal, even if extensive disease
  - ± leukemic lines (horizontal vertebral bands)
  - GS: Focal lytic mass

CT Findings

- NECT
  - Isodense soft tissue mass with adjacent bone destruction
  - Leptomeningeal disease: ↑ density of subarachnoid with lumbar nerve root enlargement
  - GS: Isodense to muscle
- Bone CT
  - Permeative bone destruction ± focal lytic lesions, pathologic vertebral fractures

MR Findings

- T1WI
  - Leukemic marrow, focal tumor masses relatively hypointense
  - GS: Isointense
- T2WI
  - ↑ leukemic marrow signal intensity ± focal vertebral mass, cord signal abnormality
  - GS: Hyperintense (mild to moderate)
- STIR
  - Hyperintense leukemic marrow
- T1WI C+
  - Abnormal enhancement of marrow, focal lesion, or leptomeninges
  - GS: Variable enhancement; peripheral rim enhancement may mimic abscess
  - Dynamic, contrast-enhanced MR (DCE-MR) based on time-intensity curves can be used to distinguish between highly cellular hematopoietic marrow and highly cellular neoplastic infiltration

Nuclear Medicine Findings

- Bone scan
  - ± ↑ radiotracer uptake; often underestimates disease extent, especially in absence of significant cortical destruction

Imaging Recommendations

- Protocol advice
  - Multiplanar T1WI, T2WI (+ fat saturation) or STIR, T1 C+ MR
  - Whole-body STIR MR proposed for staging, assessing lesion burden
  - Bone CT with multiplanar reformats to delineate osseous lesions, quantitate compression fractures

DIFFERENTIAL DIAGNOSIS

Metastases

- Metastatic neuroblastoma or rhabdomyosarcoma in children, carcinomas in adults
- Multifocal bone involvement similar to leukemia

Langerhans Cell Histiocytosis

- Lytic lesion with periosteal reaction, endosteal scalloping, soft tissue mass
- May have systemic symptoms similar to leukemia

Osteomyelitis, Pyogenic

- Bacterial suppurative infection of vertebrae and intervertebral disc
- Soft tissue extension
- May have systemic symptoms similar to leukemia

Osteomyelitis, Granulomatous

- Gibbus vertebrae with relatively intact intervertebral discs, large paraspinal abscesses

Lymphoma

- Older patient with large soft tissue mass; predilection for paraspinal, epidural locations
- Systemic lymphomatous metastasis or primary vertebral lesion

Ewing Sarcoma

- Marked periosteal reaction + soft tissue mass
- No metaphyseal lucent lines
- May have systemic symptoms similar to leukemia

PATHOLOGY

General Features

- Etiology
  - External factors: Alkylating drugs, ionizing radiation, chemicals (benzene)
  - Internal factors: Chromosomal abnormalities
  - Predisposing hematologic disorders: Aplastic anemia, chronic myeloproliferative disorders

- GS: Bone involvement may be via migration of leukemia cells through the Haversian canal, from bone marrow to periosteum and dura
  - CNS involvement may occur via perivascular or perineural routes from direct dural extension or through capillary migration
- Genetics
  - Strong association with chromosomal abnormalities
    - ALL: Trisomy 21, chromosomal translocations
    - CLL: Trisomy 12
    - CML: 90% have Philadelphia chromosome t(9;22)
- Associated abnormalities
  - Diagnosis of acute leukemia established by bone marrow aspirate showing at least 30% blast cells
  - Long bone periostitis (12-25%), leukemic metaphyseal lines
  - Focal destruction of flat/tubular bones, pathologic fractures
- Neuropathologic features include
  - Spinal manifestations of primary disease: Fractures, marrow or meningeal infiltration
  - Treatment effects [radiation therapy, chemotherapy, bone marrow transplant (BMT)]: Secondary neoplasms (usually aggressive CNS tumors), hemorrhage, anterior lumbosacral radiculopathy (intrathecal methotrexate toxicity)
  - Immunosuppression complications: Fungal or other opportunistic infection
- GS/MS (chloroma): Extramedullary neoplasm of immature granulocytic cells → focal lytic mass
  - Most common in AML (concurrent presentation ≤ 9.1% AML cases)
  - Multiple soft tissue masses in CNS, subcutaneous tissues, and genitourinary system

Microscopic Features

- Diffuse bone marrow infiltration by poorly differentiated hematologic cells
  - ALL: Infiltrates of small blue cells
  - AML: Auer rods (condensed lysosomal, cytoplasmic, rod-shaped structures) are diagnostic
  - CML: Leukocytosis with ↑ in basophils, eosinophils, neutrophils; Philadelphia chromosome t(9;22)
  - CLL: Mature lymphocytes, < 55% atypical cells

CLINICAL ISSUES

Presentation

- Most common signs/symptoms
  - Localized or diffuse bone pain
  - Recurrent paraarticular arthralgias (75%)
- Other signs/symptoms
  - CSF of patients with neoplastic meningitis shows ↑ molecules involved in CNS penetration, tumor cell tropism, and angiogenesis
  - GS: Mass effect from soft tissue lesions may produce symptoms similar to cauda equina syndrome
- Clinical profile
  - Chronic leukemia may be asymptomatic
  - Symptomatic patients present with fever, ↑ ESR, hepatosplenomegaly, lymphadenopathy, joint effusions, petechial and retinal hemorrhage, anemia, frequent infections

Demographics

- Age
  - ALL: Peak 2-10 years
  - AML: Peak > 65 years
  - CML: Rare in childhood (< 5%), peak > 40 years
  - CLL: Peak 50-70 years
- Sex
  - M:F = 2:1
- Epidemiology
  - Most common malignancy of childhood (ALL: 75%, AML: 15-20%, CML: 5%)
  - 20th most common cause of cancer death (all age groups)

Natural History & Prognosis

- 5-year survival (all leukemias): 25-30%
  - Children with ALL: 90% complete remission, 80% 5-year disease-free survival
  - Adults with ALL: Remission in 60-80%, 20-30% 5-year disease-free survival
  - AML: 45% 5-year survival
  - CLL: 6-year median survival
  - CML: 5-year median survival

Treatment

- Chemotherapy: Induction phase, consolidation phase, maintenance therapy phase
  - Systemic chemotherapy with cytarabine and methotrexate
  - Intrathecal chemotherapy for CNS involvement
  - ↓ bone marrow density with chemotherapy, ↑ fracture risk
- Radiation therapy
- BMT

DIAGNOSTIC CHECKLIST

Consider

- Marrow infiltration in child with osteoporosis raises suspicion for leukemia
- Laboratory CSF evaluation > > MR sensitivity for leptomeningeal metastases

Image Interpretation Pearls

- Consider leukemia in patient with unexplained compression fractures
- Leukemic marrow changes are diffuse, lymphoma often more focal

SELECTED REFERENCES

1. Al-Chalabi M et al: Acute lymphoblastic leukemia masquerading as Guillain-Barré syndrome. Neurologist. 27(5):263-5, 2022
2. Sanchez-Mostiero DO et al: Low back pain as an unusual presentation in a child with acute lymphoblastic leukaemia. BMJ Case Rep. 15(3), 2022
3. Nguyen JC et al: Pre-treatment MRI of leukaemia and lymphoma in children: are there differences in marrow replacement patterns on T1-weighted images? Eur Radiol. 31(10):7992-8000, 2021

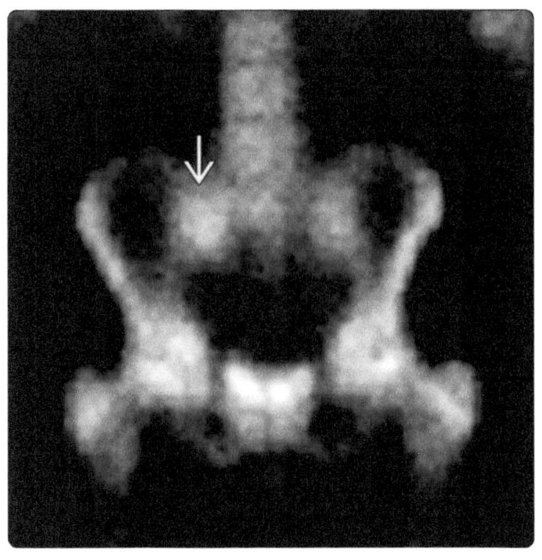

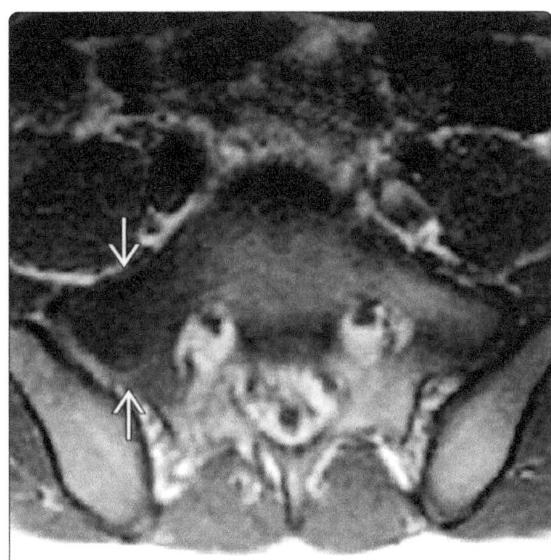

(Left) *Coronal planar bone scan of the pelvis reveals abnormal increased uptake within the right sacral ala ➡ in this case of focal leukemic metastasis to the axial skeleton. Note that a bone scan may underestimate the extent of disease, especially in the absence of significant cortical destruction.* **(Right)** *Axial T1WI MR of the sacrum in the same patient clarifies the right sacral alar metastatic lesion ➡. There is abnormal marrow signal but no definitive cortical breakthrough.*

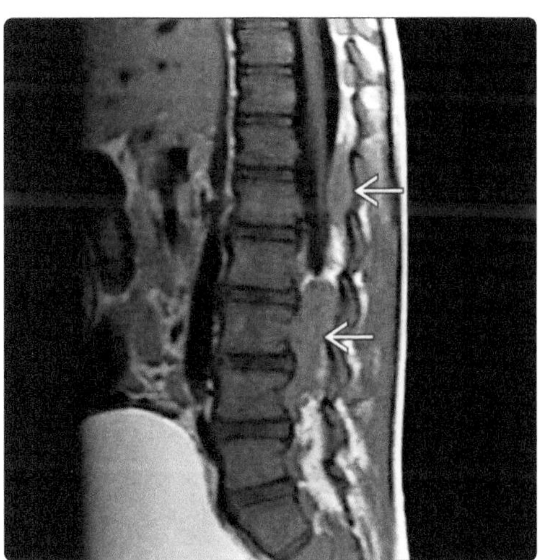

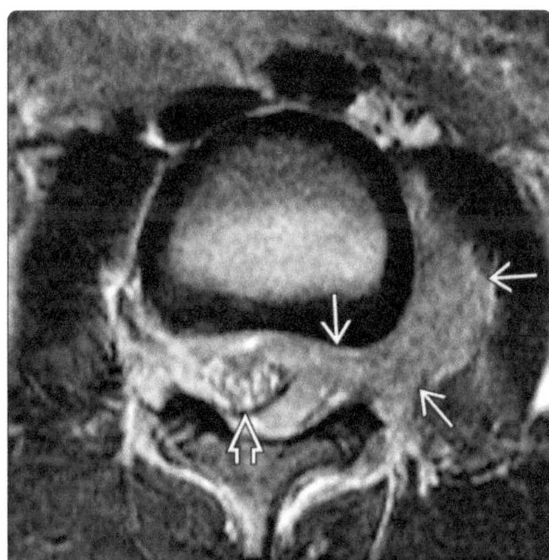

(Left) *Sagittal T1WI MR reveals diffuse abnormal vertebral marrow hypointensity. There are additional multifocal epidural masses ➡, representing leukemic involvement of the extradural space.* **(Right)** *Axial T2WI MR in the same patient demonstrates a left paraspinal soft tissue mass ➡, slightly hyperintense to muscle, infiltrating into the epidural space from the left paraspinal region. The mass causes mild mass effect on the thecal sac ➡, which is displaced medially.*

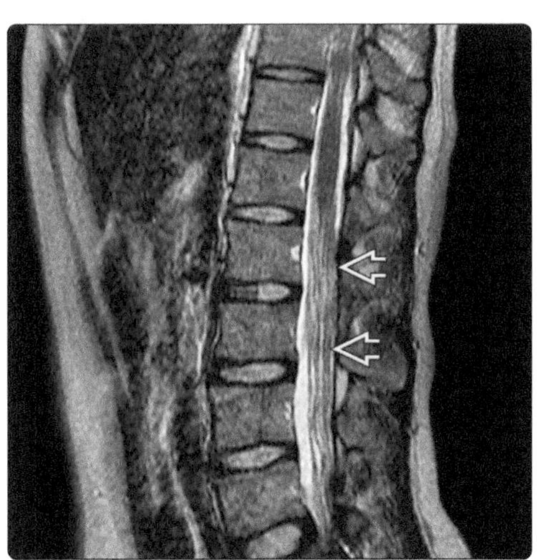

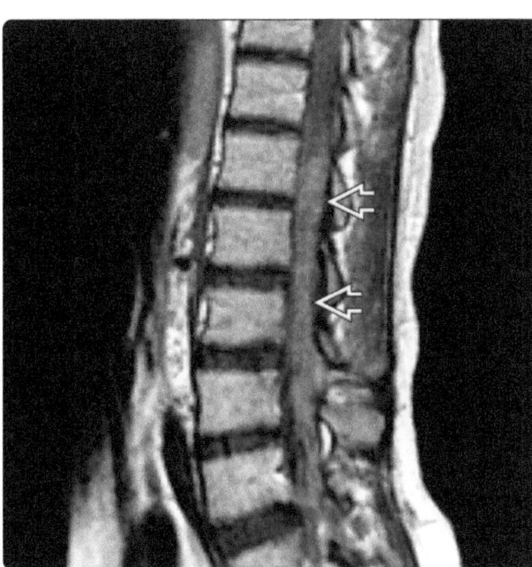

(Left) *Sagittal T2WI MR demonstrates nodular cauda equina infiltration ➡, representing CSF leukemia cell dissemination, producing abnormal cauda equina nerve root thickening.* **(Right)** *Sagittal T1WI C+ MR confirms diffuse leptomeningeal enhancement from disseminated intrathecal leukemic metastasis ➡ encircling the caudal spinal cord and infiltrating the cauda equina.*

KEY FACTS

TERMINOLOGY

- Embryonal tumors derived from primordial neural crest cells that form sympathetic nervous system
- Neuroblastic tumors = ganglioneuroma (GN), ganglioneuroblastoma (GNB), and neuroblastoma (NB)

IMAGING

- Abdominal (adrenal, paraspinal ganglia) > thoracic > pelvic > cervical
- Radiographs
  - Widened paraspinal soft tissues, stippled calcifications
- CT
  - Widened neural foramina and intercostal spaces, pedicle erosion, adjacent rib splaying (GN, GNB) or destruction (NB)
- MR for diagnosis, presurgical planning
  - T1WI: Hypo-/isointense paraspinal mass
  - T2WI: Hypo-/hyperintense paraspinal mass
  - Variable enhancement ± internal hemorrhage, necrosis
- MIBG for NB staging, posttreatment surveillance

TOP DIFFERENTIAL DIAGNOSES

- Ewing sarcoma
- Vertebral metastasis
- Lymphoma

PATHOLOGY

- International Neuroblastoma Staging System (INSS)
  - Considers surgical resectability, radiologic findings, and lymph node and bone marrow involvement

CLINICAL ISSUES

- Abdominal mass/pain, bone pain, fatigue, weight loss, blanching subcutaneous nodules
- Paraparesis/paraplegia (cord compression)

DIAGNOSTIC CHECKLIST

- Critical to determine whether tumor extends into spinal canal or neural foramina

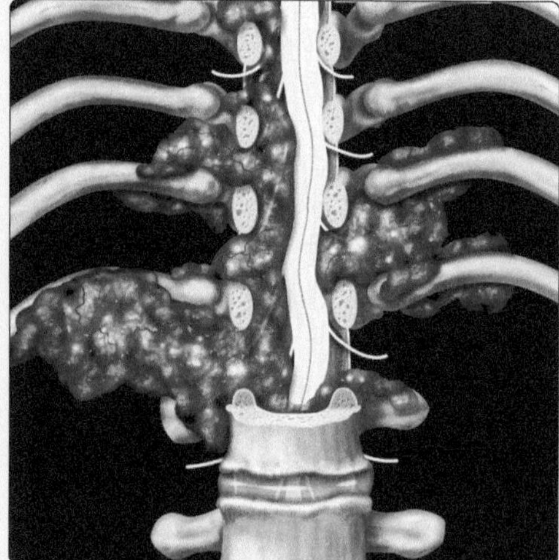

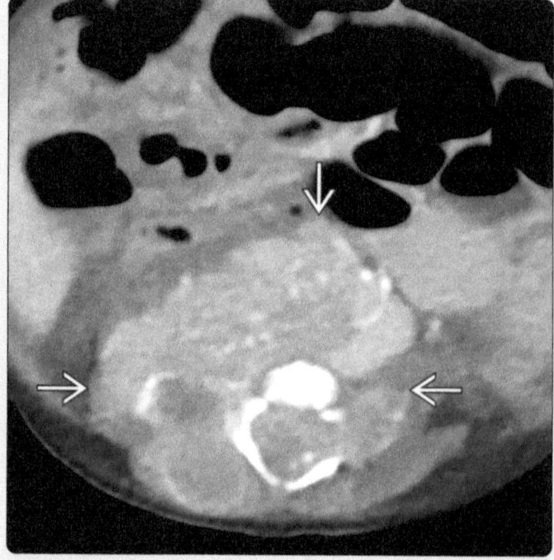

(Left) *Coronal graphic depicts a vascular paraspinal neuroblastoma (NB) originating on the right with spread across the midline to the left (Evans stage 3). Note also neural foraminal invasion into the spinal canal.* **(Right)** *Axial CECT obtained in an infant with a palpable abdominal mass and leg weakness demonstrates a large paraspinal mass with intrinsic calcifications ➡ that invades through the neural foramina to nearly completely fill the spinal canal.*

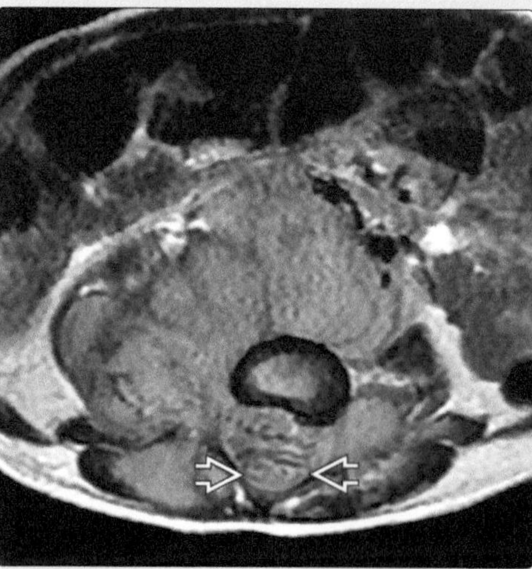

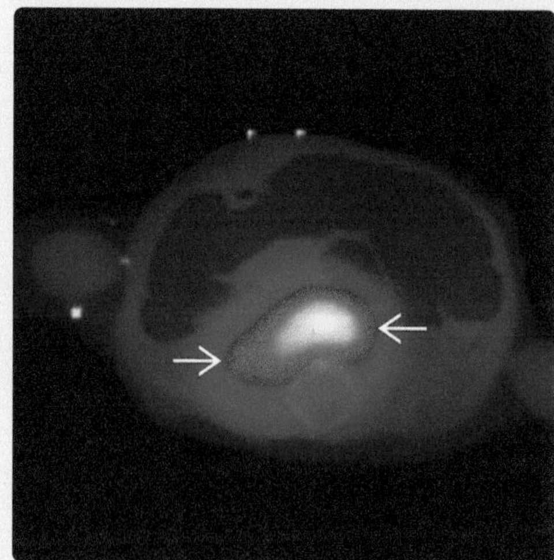

(Left) *Axial T2 MR in the same patient reveals a cellular-appearing, hypointense mass. The tumor extends through the neural foramina to fill much of the spinal canal. The thecal sac ➡ is compressed, but the individual nerve roots of the cauda equina are visible and surrounded by CSF.* **(Right)** *Axial MIBG SPECT confirms avid radiotracer uptake within the tumor ➡. Surgical resection of the abdominal component was performed with pathology confirming NB.*

TERMINOLOGY

Abbreviations

- Opsoclonus myoclonus ataxia syndrome (OMAS)

Definitions

- Neuroblastic tumors = ganglioneuroma (GN), ganglioneuroblastoma (GNB), and neuroblastoma (NB)
  - Embryonal tumors derived from neural crest cells

IMAGING

General Features

- Best diagnostic clue
  - Abdominal or thoracic paraspinal mass ± intraspinal extension, calcification
- Location
  - Adrenal (40%) > paraspinal ganglia (25%) > thoracic (15%) > pelvic (5%) > cervical (3%); miscellaneous (12%)
- Size
  - Variable: 1-10 cm diameter
- Morphology
  - Marrow replacement, dumbbell-shaped paraspinal-intraspinal tumor

Radiographic Findings

- Radiography
  - Widened paraspinal soft tissues ± scoliosis
    - Rigid, progressive curve & atypical left curve in skeletally immature adolescent should undergo further investigation
  - ± stippled abdominal or mediastinal calcifications

CT Findings

- CECT
  - Enhancing paraspinal mass ± epidural extension, finely stippled calcifications
- Bone CT
  - Widened neural foramina & intercostal spaces, pedicle erosion, adjacent rib splaying (GN, GNB) or destruction (NB)

MR Findings

- T1WI
  - Hypo-/isointense paraspinal mass ± epidural extension through neural foramina
  - ± hypointense marrow replacement
- T2WI
  - Hypo-/hyperintense paraspinal mass ± epidural extension, spinal cord compression
- DWI
  - Diffusion restriction in NB helpful to distinguish from GN/GNB
- T1WI C+
  - Variable enhancement ± internal hemorrhage, necrosis

Nuclear Medicine Findings

- Bone scan
  - Tc-99m MDP uptake in osseous metastatic lesions
- PET
  - Avid FDG uptake
- Metaiodobenzylguanidine (MIBG)
  - Uptake by sympathetic catecholaminergic cells
    - I-123 MIBG for NB staging, posttherapy surveillance
    - I-131 MIBG shows early therapeutic promise for NB treatment

Imaging Recommendations

- Best imaging tool
  - MR for diagnosis, presurgical planning
  - MIBG for staging, posttreatment surveillance
- Protocol advice
  - Multiplanar enhanced MR for tumor evaluation
  - Bone CT with multiplanar reformats to evaluate bone disease, detect calcifications

DIFFERENTIAL DIAGNOSIS

Ewing Sarcoma

- Small round blue cell tumor; relatively T2 hypointense
- Arises from adjacent flat bones (rib, chest wall, pelvis) → 2° to vertebral invasion

Vertebral Metastasis

- Variable signal intensity; imaging characteristics follow primary tumor
- Multifocal disease common

Nerve Sheath Tumor

- Contiguous with neural foramen ± dumbbell configuration

Lymphoma

- Systemic metastasis or primary vertebral lesion; predilection for paraspinal, epidural locations

Wilms Tumor

- Majority arise from renal parenchyma; distinctive histopathology; slightly older patient age facilitates distinction from NB

PATHOLOGY

General Features

- Etiology
  - No specific environmental exposure or risk factors definitively identified
- Genetics
  - 1p chromosomal deletion in 70-80% of NB patients
  - *MYCN* (protooncogene chromosome 2p) amplification → rapid tumor progression, poor outcome
  - Gain on chromosome arm 17q linked with advanced-stage tumors
  - *HER2/neu* oncogene overexpression is unfavorable prognostic indicator
  - ↑ CD44 (glycoprotein on surface of NB cells) and expression of TrkA (nerve growth factor) correlate with better prognosis
- Associated abnormalities
  - Orbit/skull/mandible osseous/dural metastases, "hair on end" periostitis, primary brain NB (primitive neuroectodermal tumors)
- Arise from primordial neural crest cell derivatives along sympathetic chain
  - GN = most benign, differentiated stromal and cellular components, mature ganglion cells (100%)

- GNB = intermediate malignant potential, varying proportions of NB and mature ganglion cells (> 50%)
- NB = malignant small round blue cell tumor, < 50% differentiated elements

Staging, Grading, & Classification

- International Neuroblastoma Risk Group Staging System (INRGSS)
  - Developed to establish consensus approach for pretreatment risk stratification
    - L1: Localized tumor not involving vital structures as defined by list of image-defined risk factors and confined to 1 body compartment
    - L2: Locoregional tumor with presence of 1 or more image-defined risk factors
    - M: Distant metastatic disease (except stage MS)
    - MS: Metastatic disease in children < 18 months old with metastases confined to skin, liver, &/or bone marrow

Gross Pathologic & Surgical Features

- GN, GNB: Firm, gray-white nodules
- NB: Soft, gray-tan nodules ± hemorrhage, necrosis, calcification

Microscopic Features

- GN: Mature ganglion cells, Schwann cells, neuritic processes
- GNB: Internal spectrum ranging from GN → NB
- NB: Undifferentiated neuroblasts, ganglion cells

CLINICAL ISSUES

Presentation

- Most common signs/symptoms
  - Abdominal mass/pain, bone pain, fatigue, weight loss, blanching subcutaneous nodules
  - Paraparesis/paraplegia (cord compression)
- Other signs/symptoms
  - Diarrhea due to vasoactive intestinal peptide (VIP)
  - Proptosis, periorbital/conjunctival ecchymoses ("raccoon eyes")
  - Opsoclonus-myoclonus-ataxia (OMAS) paraneoplastic syndrome (2-3%)
  - Horner syndrome (cervical NB)
  - Cauda equina syndrome
  - Children with malignancies have higher proportion of abnormal ribs (18%)
    - Homeobox genes, involved in vertebral and rib sequencing, are abnormally expressed in many different malignancies
  - Laboratory findings
    - > 90% ↑ urine homovanillic acid (HVA) ± vanillylmandelic acid (VMA)
      - HVA: Metabolite of dopamine, elevated in more mature NBs and GNBs
      - VMA: Less mature metabolite of epinephrine and norepinephrine
      - VMA:HVA ratio: Indicator of maturity; ratio < 1 favorable; ratio > 1 poor prognosis
- Clinical profile
  - Kerner-Morrison syndrome: Intractable secretory diarrhea 2° to VIP secretion (GN, GNB > NB)
  - Pepper syndrome: Infant with overwhelming liver metastatic NB → respiratory compromise
  - Blueberry muffin baby: Infant with subcutaneous metastatic NB
  - Hutchinson syndrome: Widespread bone metastasis → bone pain, limping, pathologic fractures
  - Nonaccidental trauma mimic: Metastatic retrobulbar NB → rapidly progressive painless proptosis, periorbital ecchymosis

Demographics

- Age
  - 40% < 1 year, 35% 1-2 years, and 25% > 2 years at diagnosis; rare > 10 years
- Sex
  - M > F (1.3:1)
- Epidemiology
  - 7-10 new NB cases/1 million children (USA); true incidence of GNB, GN unknown because many asymptomatic

Natural History & Prognosis

- GN prognosis excellent after surgical resection
- GNB prognosis dependent on proportion of GN, NB
- NB 5-year survival ~ 83% for infants, 55% for children 1-5 years, and 40% for children > 5 years
  - Favorable: Locoregional, stage 4S, ↓ *MYCN* amplification, hyperdiploid DNA
  - Unfavorable: Stage 4 disease, ocular and CNS involvement, ↑ serum levels of neuron-specific enolase (NSE) and ferritin, ↑ urine VMA/HVA

Treatment

- Chemotherapy, surgery, radiation, steroids
- No differences in neurologic improvement in patients with spinal cord compression treated with radiotherapy, laminectomy, or chemotherapy alone

DIAGNOSTIC CHECKLIST

Consider

- NB presentation depends on patient age, primary site, metastatic burden, metabolically active products
- Infants more often present with thoracic, cervical tumors; older children present with abdominal tumors

Reporting Tips

- Critical to determine preoperatively whether tumor extends into spinal canal or neural foramina, as epidural extension complicates surgical management

SELECTED REFERENCES

1. Bacchus MK et al: Neuroblastic tumor recurrence associated with opsoclonus myoclonus ataxia syndrome relapse a decade after initial resection and treatments. J Pediatr Hematol Oncol. 45(3):152-4, 2023
2. Qian LD et al: (18)F-FDG PET/CT imaging of pediatric peripheral neuroblastic tumor: a combined model to predict the International Neuroblastoma Pathology Classification. Quant Imaging Med Surg. 13(1):94-107, 2023
3. Maughan NM et al: Failure modes and effects analysis of pediatric I-131 MIBG therapy: program design and potential pitfalls. Pediatr Blood Cancer. 69(12):e29996, 2022
4. Chen AM et al: A review of neuroblastoma image-defined risk factors on magnetic resonance imaging. Pediatr Radiol. 48(9):1337-47, 2018
5. Del Campo Braojos F et al: Practical application of the International Neuroblastoma Risk Group Staging System: a pictorial review. Curr Probl Diagn Radiol. 48(5):509-18, 2018

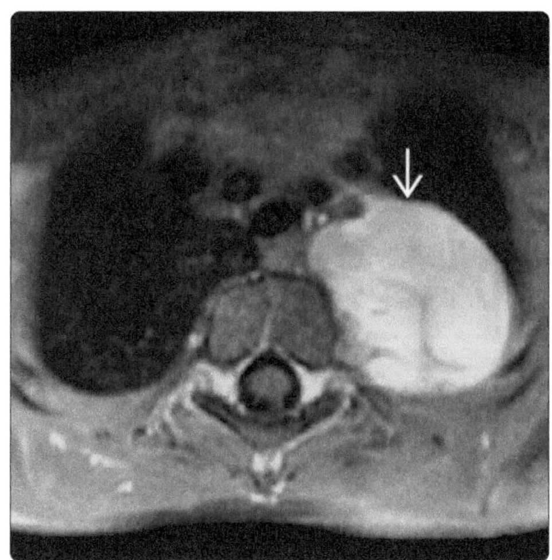

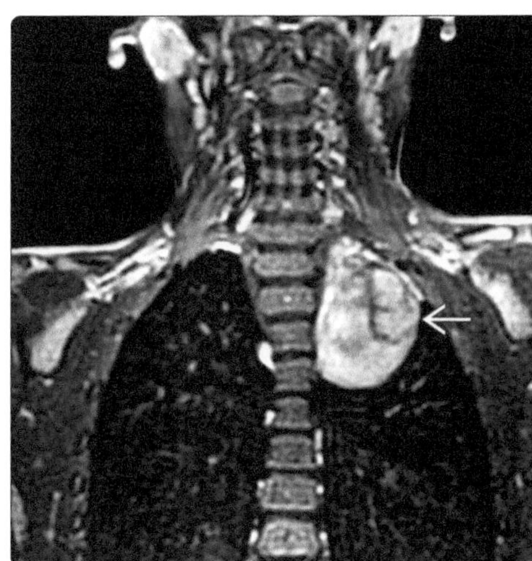

(Left) *Axial T1 C+ MR reveals a large, left, surgically proven paraspinal ganglioneuroma ➔. No vertebral or neural foraminal invasion was detected. This lesion demonstrates fairly avid enhancement. Ganglioneuroma tumoral enhancement ranges from minimal to avid.* **(Right)** *Coronal T1 C+ FS MR in a patient with a surgically proven ganglioneuroblastoma reveals an avidly enhancing, posterosuperior mediastinal mass ➔.*

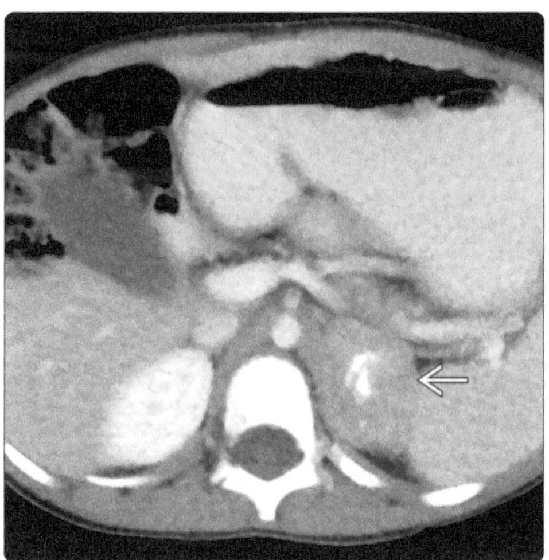

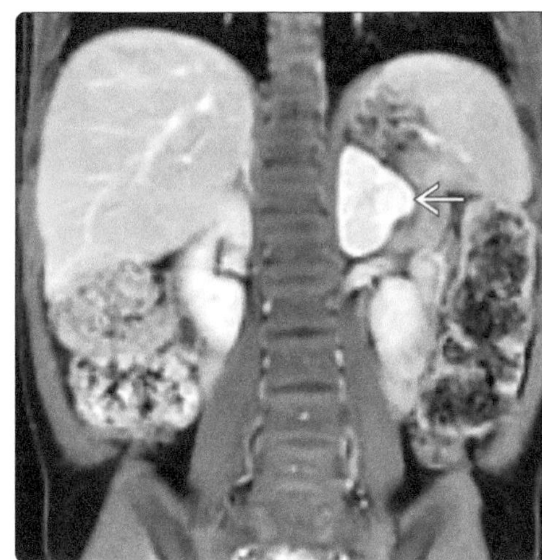

(Left) *Axial CECT in a pediatric patient reveals a well-circumscribed left adrenal mass ➔ with intrinsic calcification. Location within the adrenal gland and the presence of calcium are strongly suggestive of a neuroblastic tumor.* **(Right)** *Coronal T1 FS MR in the same patient reveals moderate enhancement that is similar to the kidneys in the well-circumscribed adrenal mass ➔. Surgical resection was performed with pathology confirming ganglioneuroblastoma.*

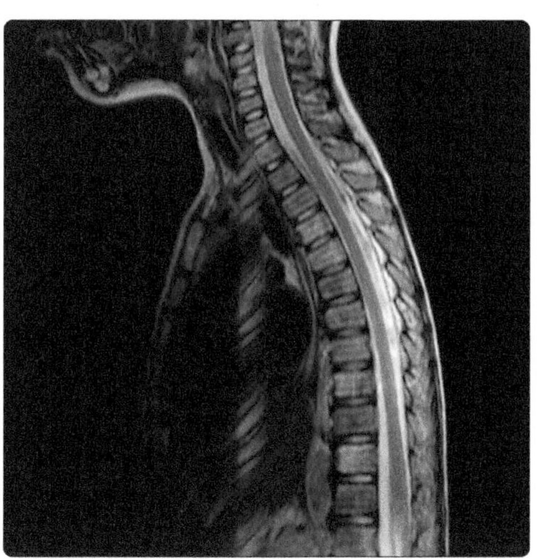

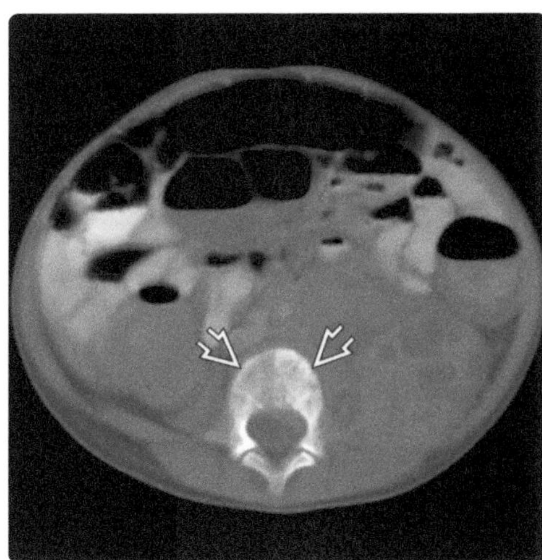

(Left) *Sagittal T2 MR in a patient with stage IV NB demonstrates extensive hematogenous vertebral metastases at nearly every level.* **(Right)** *Axial NECT bone window of a stage IV large, metastatic NB, retroperitoneal primary tumor reveals osseous vertebral metastases ➔ featuring mixed blastic and lytic changes, a common imaging appearance of metastatic NB.*

KEY FACTS

TERMINOLOGY

- Abnormal histiocyte proliferation producing granulomatous skeletal lesions

IMAGING

- Calvarium > mandible > long bones > vertebrae
- Spinal involvement greater in children
  - Thoracic > lumbar > cervical
- Destructive lytic lesion ± pathologic fracture, paraspinal/epidural mass, spinal canal extension
- ± vertebra plana (adjacent discs, posterior elements rarely involved)

TOP DIFFERENTIAL DIAGNOSES

- Ewing sarcoma
- Metastases
- Neuroblastoma
- Hemopoietic malignancies

PATHOLOGY

- Restricted Langerhans cell histiocytosis (LCH)
  - Only skin lesions
  - Osseous lesions ± diabetes insipidus (DI), adjacent lymph node involvement, or rash
- Extensive LCH
  - Visceral organ involvement ± bone lesions, DI, adjacent lymph node involvement, ± rash, ± hemopoietic organ system dysfunction

CLINICAL ISSUES

- Asymptomatic or localized pain due to medullary expansion or pathologic fracture
- ± fever, leukocytosis

DIAGNOSTIC CHECKLIST

- Vertebra plana with relative absence of epidural mass, disc abnormalities classic for LCH

(Left) *Sagittal graphic demonstrates diffuse vertebral marrow infiltration with a pathologic fracture producing vertebra plana sparing the disc spaces. Epidural extension results in ventral cord compression.* **(Right)** *Sagittal T1 C+ FS MR of the lumbar spine demonstrates intense homogeneous enhancement of a pathologic L3 fracture ➡ resulting in vertebra plana and an epidural mass. Note that the intervertebral disc spaces are preserved.*

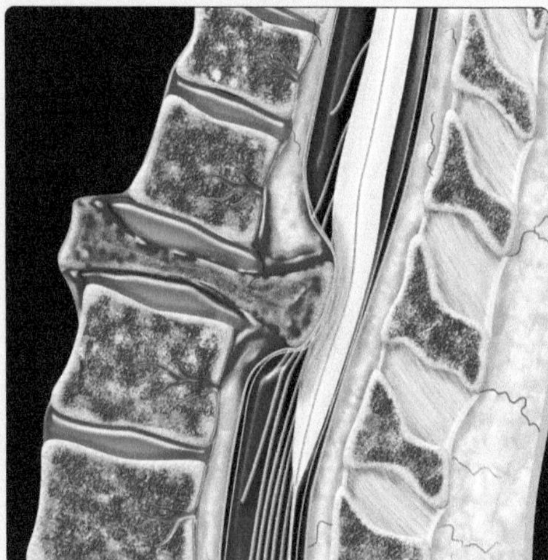

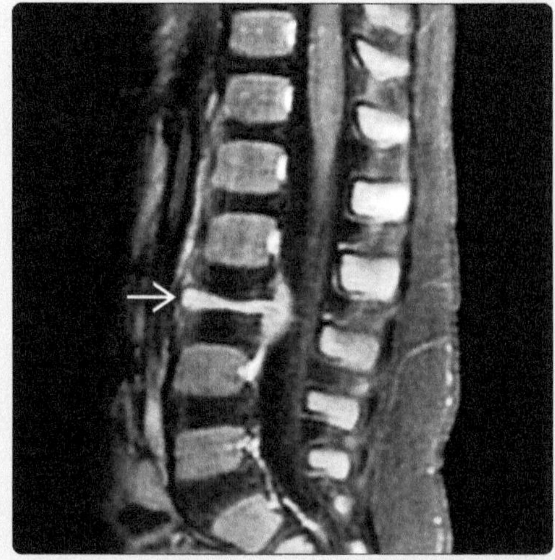

(Left) *Coronal T1 C+ FS MR illustrates vertebral plana of L3 ➡. The vertebral body shows avid homogeneous enhancement.* **(Right)** *Axial T1 C+ FS MR reveals relatively mild abnormal enhancement of the flattened L3 vertebra (volume averaging with disc space) with posterior extension into the epidural space.*

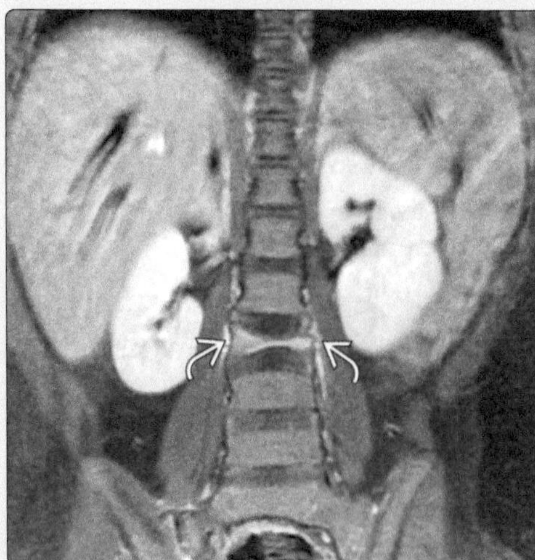

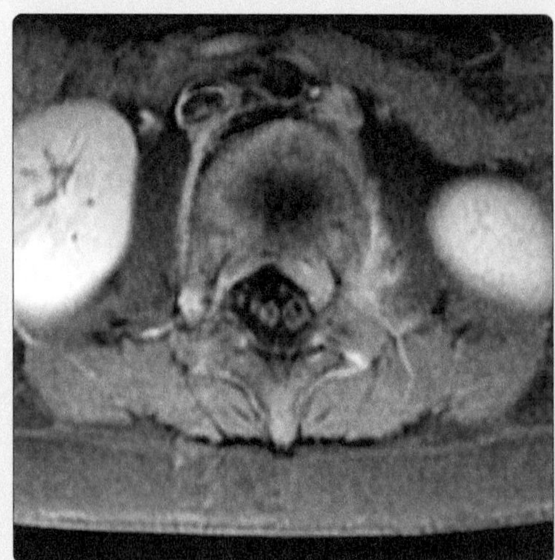

TERMINOLOGY

Synonyms

- Langerhans cell histiocytosis (LCH), Langerhans cell granulomatosis, eosinophilic granuloma (EG), histiocytosis X

Definitions

- Group of idiopathic histiocytic disorders featuring granulomatous skeletal lesions that contain abnormal cells similar to bone marrow-derived Langerhans cells

IMAGING

General Features

- Best diagnostic clue
  - ± vertebra plana sparing disc space
- Location
  - Calvarium > mandible > long bones > ribs > pelvis > vertebrae
  - Spinal involvement
    - Thoracic (54%) > lumbar (35%) > cervical (11%)
    - Children > adults
- Morphology
  - Destructive lytic lesion ± pathologic fracture, soft tissue mass, spinal canal extension

Radiographic Findings

- Radiography
  - Lytic, nonsclerotic, destructive vertebral lesion
    - ± vertebra plana (adjacent discs, posterior elements rarely involved)
    - ± scoliosis; kyphosis uncommon

CT Findings

- CECT
  - Lytic, nonsclerotic, destructive vertebral lesion with enhancing soft tissue mass ± paraspinal, epidural extension
- Bone CT
  - Lytic vertebral lesion ± collapsed vertebral body (vertebra plana)

MR Findings

- T1WI
  - Hypointense vertebral soft tissue mass ± pathologic fracture
- T2WI
  - Heterogeneously hyperintense soft tissue mass ± pathologic fracture
  - Disc spaces generally spared
- T1WI C+
  - Homogeneous enhancement

Nuclear Medicine Findings

- Bone scan
  - Variable uptake; bone lesions may be hot, cold, or mixed ("ring") activity
  - False-negatives common (35%)

Imaging Recommendations

- Protocol advice
  - Multiplanar enhanced MR to evaluate soft tissues, determine epidural extension
  - Bone algorithm CT with multiplanar reformats to define osseous destruction &/or vertebral height loss

DIFFERENTIAL DIAGNOSIS

Ewing Sarcoma

- Permeative bone destruction ± pathologic fracture
- More likely than LCH to have large soft tissue mass, adjacent bone destruction

Metastases

- Extension of primary tumor to spine
  - Bone production > destruction (blastic)
  - Bone destruction > production (lytic)

Neuroblastic Tumors

- Abdominal or thoracic paraspinal mass ± intraspinal extension

Hemopoietic Malignancies

- Multifocal disease; may be indistinguishable from LCH
- Widespread abnormal marrow signal, enhancement with extensive disease

Pyogenic Osteomyelitis

- Abnormal marrow signal ± vertebral collapse
- Hyperintense narrowed disc ± fluid signal

Giant Cell Tumor

- Expansile, lytic vertebral lesion + soft tissue mass
- Usually older patient (> 30 years of age)

PATHOLOGY

General Features

- Etiology
  - Dysregulated growth, activity, and trafficking of Langerhans cells
  - Unknown cause; infectious agents (especially viruses), immune system dysfunction, neoplastic mechanisms, genetic factors, cellular adhesion molecules proposed
  - Ongoing debate whether LCH is reactive or neoplastic process; neoplastic currently favored
- Genetics
  - *BRAF* V600E mutations are associated with disease relapse and worse prognosis
    - *BRAF* V600E (+) mutations more likely present in systemic LCH than isolated lesions
    - Potential treatment target with BRAF inhibitors
- Associated abnormalities
  - Pituitary-hypothalamic axis → diabetes insipidus (DI)
  - Purulent otitis media → deafness
  - Orbital involvement → proptosis
  - Cutaneous LCH (≤ 50%)
  - Pulmonary involvement (20-40%); male predominance, older age (20-40 years), smoking association
  - Gastrointestinal bleeding, liver/spleen abnormalities
  - Lymph node enlargement ± suppuration, chronic drainage (30%)
- < 1% of biopsy-proven primary bone lesions; vertebral involvement (6%)
  - Most common cause of vertebra plana in children

- Variable vertebral body restoration occurs over months to years
- Pedicles often involved; posterior elements, adjacent disc spaces usually spared
- PCR-based assay demonstrates all LCH forms are clonal → LCH probably clonal neoplastic rather than reactive disorder, as previously believed

Staging, Grading, & Classification

- Classic categorization of LCH based on age, severity, and extent of involvement
  - EG
  - Hand-Schüller-Christian disease
  - Letterer-Siwe disease
- Revised LCH classification according to disease extent
  - Restricted LCH
    - Skin lesions without other site of involvement
    - Monostotic lesion ± DI, adjacent lymph node involvement, or rash
    - Polyostotic lesions involving several bones or ≥ 2 lesions in 1 bone ± DI, adjacent lymph node involvement, or rash
  - Extensive LCH
    - Visceral organ involvement ± bone lesions, DI, adjacent lymph node involvement, &/or rash
      - ± lung, liver, or hemopoietic organ system dysfunction

Microscopic Features

- Light microscopy → abnormal granulomatous histiocytes (Langerhans cells) with folded nuclei, cytoplasmic S100 reactivity, areas of bone necrosis
- EM: Birbeck granule cytoplasmic inclusions

CLINICAL ISSUES

Presentation

- Most common signs/symptoms
  - Asymptomatic
  - Localized pain due to medullary expansion or pathologic fracture, reduced mobility, swelling, fever, or leukocytosis
  - Myelopathy or radiculopathy
- Clinical profile
  - EG (70%)
    - Localized form (bone lesions only), older children (5-15 years), good prognosis
    - Back pain, stiffness, scoliosis, neurologic complications, fever, leukocytosis
  - Hand-Schüller-Christian disease (20%)
    - Chronic disseminated osseous and visceral lesions, younger children (1-5 years), intermediate prognosis (fatal 10-30%)
    - Triad of DI, exophthalmos, osteolytic lesions
  - Letterer-Siwe disease (10%)
    - Acute form, rapid visceral organ dissemination, infants (< 3 years), poor prognosis
    - Fever, cachexia, anemia, hepatosplenomegaly, lymphadenopathy, rash, gum hyperplasia
    - Most patients die ≤ 1-2 years
  - Multisystem disease represents > 2/3 (68.6%) of total cases among adult patients with LCH
    - Skin and pulmonary involvement representing 51% and 62% of cases, respectively

Demographics

- Age
  - Predominantly affects children, adolescents, or young adults but may occur at any age
    - Most severe manifestations peak at younger ages
- Sex
  - M:F = 2:1

Natural History & Prognosis

- Variable depending on presentation age, extent of systemic disease
  - Single-system disease 5-year event-free survival: 100%
  - Isolated pulmonary manifestation: 87.8% survival
  - Multisystem disease: 91.7% survival
- Spontaneous remission of lesions common, but relapse or reactivation possible
  - Lesions usually begin to regress after ~ 3 months but may take up to 2 years to resolve
  - Lower rate of recurrence in skeletally immature
- Vertebra plana prognosis favorable for symptomatic improvement, vertebral height restoration with conservative orthopedic treatment
  - Vertebral height restoration varies 18.2% → 63.8% before, 72.2% → 97% after skeletal maturity

Treatment

- Conservative management initially with observation ± bracing
  - Limited disease has excellent prognosis, usually without need for systemic therapy
- Multifocal skeletal involvement, refractory cutaneous lesions, and disseminated or recurrent organ disease benefit from systemic treatment
  - Combined chemotherapy options for multisystem disease
- Advanced-stage disease: Local treatment, radiation therapy, chemotherapy, immunomodulation, and liver, lung, and stem cell transplantation
- ± surgical intervention (partial intralesional curettage, fusion), external beam radiotherapy, chemotherapy, steroids in patients with neurologic deficits, conservative treatment failure

DIAGNOSTIC CHECKLIST

Consider

- Vertebra plana much more common in children than adults
- Unexplained vertebral compression fractures in children or adolescents merit evaluation to exclude LCH or leukemia

Image Interpretation Pearls

- Vertebra plana with relative absence of epidural mass, disc abnormalities classic for LCH

SELECTED REFERENCES

1. Baratto L et al: Comparison of whole-body DW-MRI with 2-[(18)F]FDG PET for staging and treatment monitoring of children with Langerhans cell histiocytosis. Eur J Nucl Med Mol Imaging. 50(6):1689-98, 2023
2. Morimoto A et al: Bone lesions of Langerhans cell histiocytosis triggered by trauma in children. Pediatr Int. 64(1):e15199, 2022

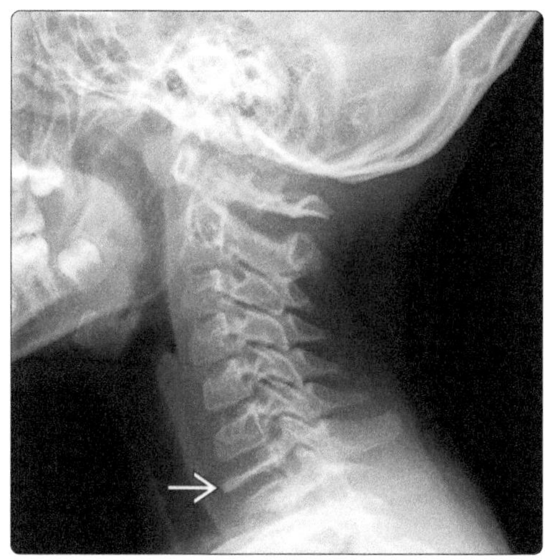

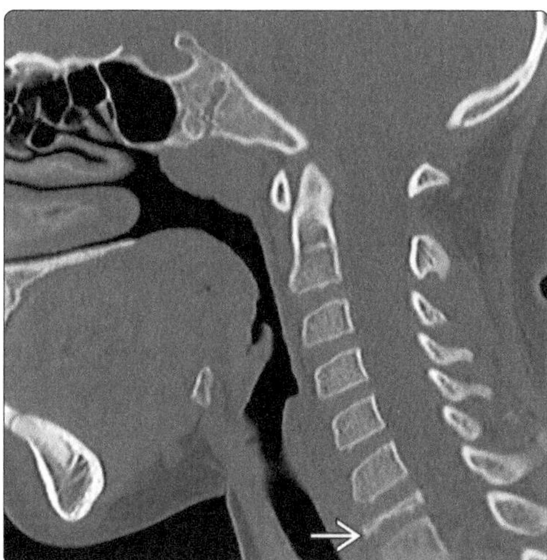

(Left) *Lateral cervical radiograph reveals marked vertebra plana of the C7 vertebra ➡ in this 7-year-old patient with neck pain. Note how flattened the abnormal vertebra is compared to adjacent normal vertebra.* **(Right)** *Sagittal bone CT in the same patient confirms flattening of the C7 vertebra ➡ with normal appearance of the other cervical vertebra.*

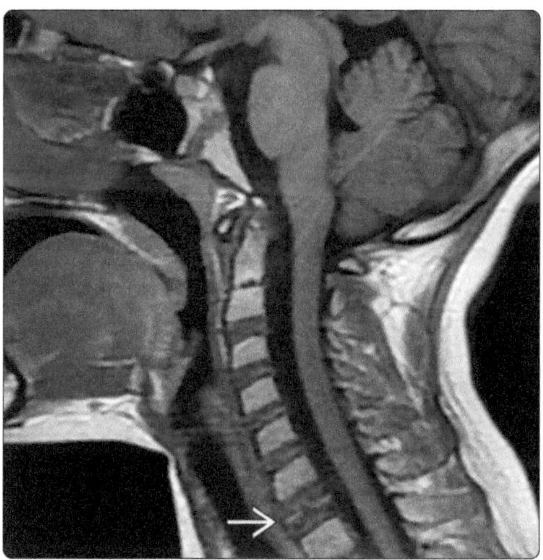

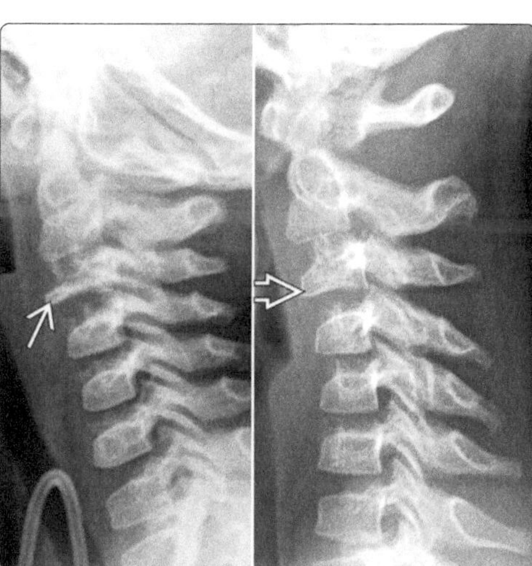

(Left) *Sagittal T1 MR in the same patient shows preservation of marrow signal in the flattened C7 vertebra ➡ and absence of associated soft tissue mass. The adjacent intervertebral discs are normal.* **(Right)** *Lateral radiographs show acute C3 vertebra plana ➡ (left) with marked loss of vertebral height. Follow-up (right), 3 years later, exhibits substantial height reconstitution ➡. Reconstitution of vertebral height results from endochondral ossification at the apophyseal plate.*

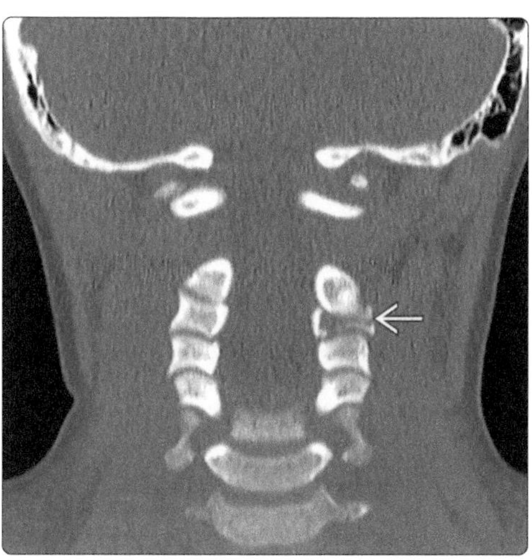

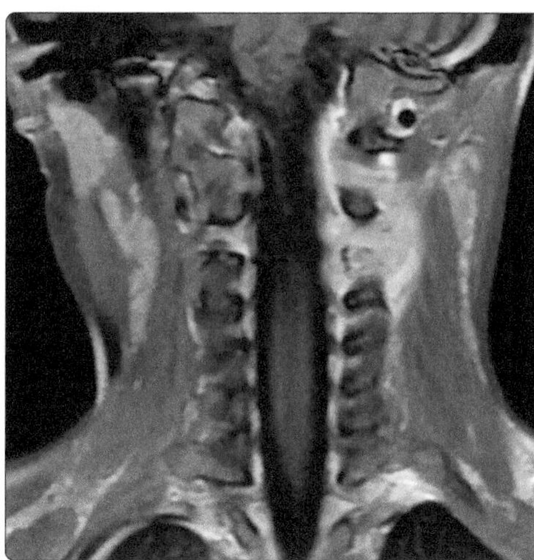

(Left) *Coronal bone CT in a 6-year-old patient with neck pain reveals lytic changes and height loss within the left C3 lateral mass ➡, compatible with pathologic fracture.* **(Right)** *Coronal T1 C+ FS MR reveals avid marrow and soft tissue enhancement. The amount of soft tissue mass prompted consideration of Ewing sarcoma and other malignancies, but biopsy proved Langerhans cell histiocytosis.*

Angiolipoma

KEY FACTS

TERMINOLOGY

- Benign tumor of adipose and vascular elements

IMAGING

- Extradural mass with fat attenuation (-20 to -60 HU) with scattered soft tissue reticulation on CT
- Thoracic predominance; usually extends over 1-4 vertebral body segments
- Hyperintense on unenhanced T1WI, + enhancement on fat-suppressed T1WI MR
  - Inhomogeneous signal (attributed to vascular channels)
- Spine involvement uncommon: Extradural
  - Degree of central hypointensity on T1WI MR is predictive of degree of vascularity
- Mildly increased signal relative to CSF on T2WI/STIR

TOP DIFFERENTIAL DIAGNOSES

- Lipoma
- Liposarcoma
- Hematoma
- Abscess, epidural, paravertebral
- Epidural lipomatosis

PATHOLOGY

- Infiltrating form more common in anterior epidural space; may destroy adjacent bone
- Focal form more common in posterior thoracic epidural space; no bone destruction

CLINICAL ISSUES

- Slowly progressive paraparesis with back pain

DIAGNOSTIC CHECKLIST

- Fat-suppressed T1WI MR most useful for lesion definition as it shows heterogeneous enhancement
- Not to be confused with angiomyolipoma, which is found in kidney of tuberous sclerosis patients

(Left) *Sagittal T1WI MR shows a large, predominantly T1-hyperintense mass involving a long segment of the thoracic dorsal epidural space with moderate spinal cord ➡ compression. Intermixed with the fatty component are islands of intermediate T1 signal (angiomatous tissue).* **(Right)** *Axial T1WI C+ MR of a large thoracic dorsal epidural angiolipoma demonstrates cord ➡ compression. Within the fatty component is the angiomatous component ➡ of the lesion, which exhibits hypointense signal.*

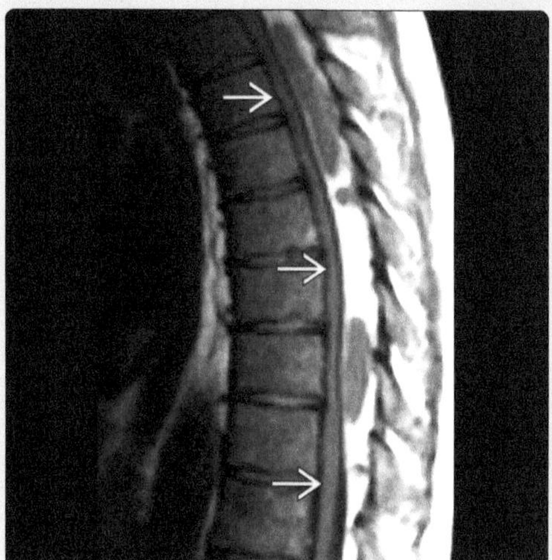

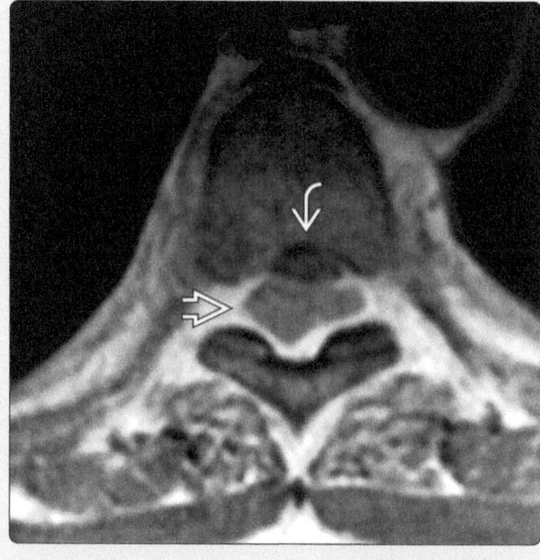

(Left) *Sagittal STIR MR depicts a lobulated, heterogeneous dorsal epidural mass ➡. The fatty component suppresses on STIR; the vascular component remains hyperintense ➡.* **(Right)** *Sagittal T1WI MR (left) reveals a heterogeneous lesion ➡ within the dorsal epidural space at the L3-L4 level. Sagittal T1 C+ MR (right) confirms mild heterogeneous enhancement ➡ of the angiomatous portions.*

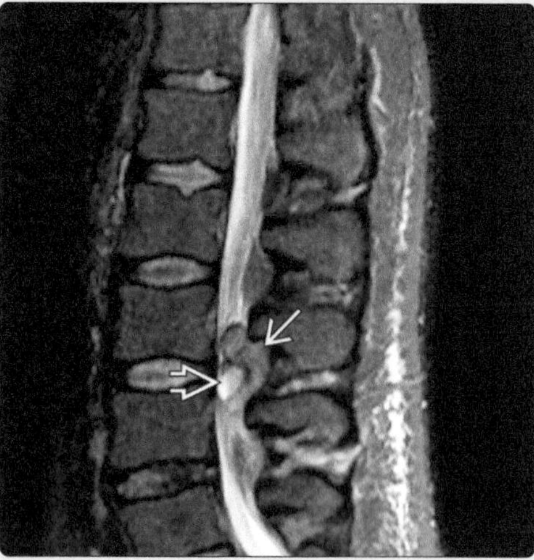

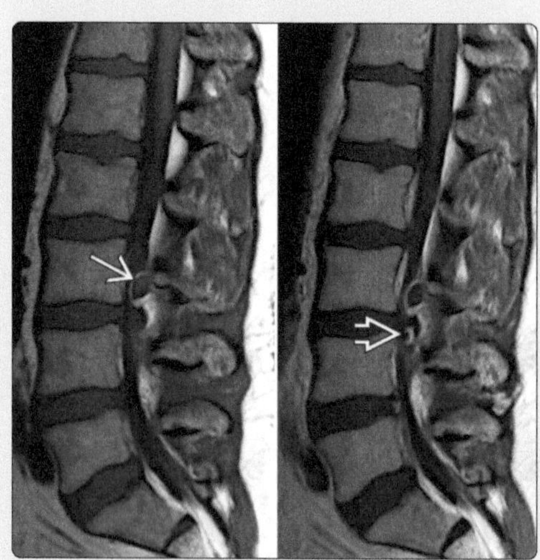

TERMINOLOGY

Abbreviations

- Spinal angiolipoma (SAL)

Synonyms

- Vascular lipoma, hemangiolipoma, fibromyolipoma

Definitions

- Benign tumor of adipose and vascular elements

IMAGING

General Features

- Best diagnostic clue
  - Hyperintense mass on unenhanced T1WI MR showing enhancement on fat-suppressed T1WI MR
- Location
  - Uncommon tumors of extremities, trunk, neck
  - Spine involvement uncommon: Extradural
    - Thoracic predominance may be result of regional variation in blood supply
      - Midthoracic spine is least perfused
    - Intramedullary SAL is **extremely rare**
  - SAL can infiltrate from paravertebral areas into spinal canal
  - Rare reports of mediastinal angiolipoma with spinal canal extension
- Size
  - Extends over 1-4 vertebral body segments
  - Average extent > 2 vertebral bodies in length
- Morphology
  - Focal or infiltrating mass showing heterogeneous fat signal

Radiographic Findings

- Often negative
- Some cases show erosions of pedicle and widening of spinal canal
- Infiltrating tumors cause trabeculation of affected vertebral body

CT Findings

- NECT
  - Extradural mass of fat attenuation (-20 to -60 HU) with scattered soft tissue reticulation
  - Slight enhancement
  - Rare calcification
  - Rare bony remodeling

MR Findings

- T1WI
  - Hyperintense with inhomogeneous signal
  - Heterogeneity thought to be related to vascular channels
  - Prominence of vascular component may give more isointense T1 signal
- T2WI
  - Mild increased signal relative to CSF
- PD/intermediate
  - Increased signal relative to CSF, but decreased signal relative to fat
- T1WI C+
  - Fat-suppressed T1WI most useful for lesion definition as it shows heterogeneous enhancement

Nonvascular Interventions

- Myelography
  - Nonspecific extradural mass
  - May show block with aggressive lesion

Imaging Recommendations

- Best imaging tool
  - Fat-suppressed contrast-enhanced T1WI MR
- Protocol advice
  - Axial, sagittal T1, STIR, T2WI MR precontrast
  - Axial, sagittal postcontrast fat-suppressed T1WI MR

Nuclear Medicine Findings

- PET
  - SAL can be detected by using F18 FDG PET

DIFFERENTIAL DIAGNOSIS

Lipoma

- Little or no enhancement, minimal septations
- May be intradural, extradural, or subcutaneous
- Distinguishable microscopically with angiolipoma showing vessels branching pattern and fibrous scarring

Liposarcoma

- May have irregular thickened septa with areas of T2 hyperintensity
- Liposarcoma shows cellular pleomorphism and mitotic activity
- May show considerable T1-isointense tissue

Hematoma

- No suppression with fat saturation
- No enhancement unless more chronic
- May show low signal on T2* images

Abscess, Epidural, Paravertebral

- May show heterogeneous T1 signal within epidural fat with focal areas of low signal
- Prominent peripheral enhancement
- May show heterogeneous signal and enhancement like angiolipoma

Epidural Lipomatosis

- Homogeneous fat signal without enhancement
- ± history of steroid use or obesity
- Typical dorsal thoracic epidural location

PATHOLOGY

General Features

- Etiology
  - Unknown with several theories
    - May originate from primitive pluripotential mesenchymal cells
    - Congenital malformation
    - Hamartomatous lesion, enlarging in response to injury/inflammation
- Genetics

- Subcutaneous angiolipomas show predominantly normal karyotype
  - vs. characteristic chromosomal aberrations in other lipomatous lesions, such as lipoma, lipoblastoma, hibernomas
- Rare familial occurrence of angiolipomas
- Benign tumor usually found in extremities, trunk, or neck
- Spine angiolipomas rare
- May occur as focal or infiltrating forms
  - Infiltrating form more common in anterior epidural space; may destroy adjacent bone
  - Focal form more common in posterior thoracic epidural space; no bone destruction
    - May occur at multiple sites in subcutaneous tissues

Gross Pathologic & Surgical Features

- Gross features of fatty tissue, although may show port-wine or dark brown coloration

Microscopic Features

- Presence of fat and vascular tissues
  - Vascular proliferation with microthrombi
  - Consistent marker of angiolipomas is presence of fibrin microthrombi in vascular channels associated with disrupted endothelial cells
- SAL is distinct from cutaneous angiolipoma in that caliber of its predominant vascular component is far larger than that of fat cells
- Vessels variously described as sinusoids, thin walled, thick walled with smooth muscle proliferation
- Mitoses and pleomorphism not present
- Features vary
  - Predominantly lipomatous with few small angiomatous regions
  - Predominantly vascular with small lipomatous component

CLINICAL ISSUES

Presentation

- Most common signs/symptoms
  - Nonspecific back pain
  - Other signs/symptoms: Cord compression
    - Progressive paraparesis
    - Symptoms may progress with pregnancy
      - May be associated with weight gain
      - Increase in tumor volume resulting in impaired spinal venous drainage
      - Hormonal changes resulting in increased extravascular fluid volume
    - Obesity may lead to symptoms induced by greater fatty component
    - Prolonged neurologic course can suddenly deteriorate
      - Vascular engorgement
      - Enlarging or degenerated blood vessels
      - Vascular steal phenomenon
      - Venous stasis with thrombosis
      - Hemorrhage into lesion
- Clinical profile
  - Slowly progressive paraparesis with back pain

Demographics

- Age
  - 4th-5th decades, although may occur in children
  - Mean: 42 years
- Sex
  - F > M
- Epidemiology
  - Rare (~ 0.14-1.2% of all spinal tumors)
  - 2-3% of extradural tumors
  - Focal form more common in spine
  - Typically midthoracic level but can occur anywhere in spine
  - CNS involvement rare, but 90% occur in spine

Natural History & Prognosis

- Slowly progressive
- Bone infiltration associated with more aggressive behavior and worse prognosis

Treatment

- Surgical excision for painful, symptomatic lesions
  - Focal form: Encapsulated; low rate of recurrence following excision
  - Infiltrative form: 50% recurrence rate
    - Wider resection followed by radiotherapy should be considered
- Partial resection may give good symptomatic relief in infiltrative form
- Degree of hypointensity on T1WI MR predictive of degree of vascularity encountered at surgery

DIAGNOSTIC CHECKLIST

Consider

- Not to be confused with angiomyolipoma, which is seen in tuberous sclerosis and occurs in kidney

Image Interpretation Pearls

- Angiolipomas do not show vascular flow voids

SELECTED REFERENCES

1. Wang K et al: Clinical features and surgical outcomes of spinal epidural angiolipomas. Acta Neurol Belg. 123(1):115-20, 2023
2. Somrani K et al: A rare case report of sacral epidural angiolipoma: diagnosis and treatment. Surg Neurol Int. 13:38, 2022
3. Umana GE et al: Thoracic spinal angiolipomas: a systematic review. J Neurol Surg A Cent Eur Neurosurg. 83(2):161-72, 2022
4. Zhang X et al: Spinal angiolipomas: clinical characteristics, surgical strategies and prognosis. J Korean Neurosurg Soc. 65(1):49-56, 2022
5. Shen G et al: PET/CT and MR features of infiltrating spinal angiolipoma. Clin Nucl Med. 44(3):e148-50, 2019
6. Lacour M et al: Sudden paraplegia due to spontaneous bleeding in a thoracic epidural angiolipoma and literature review. Neurochirurgie. 64(1):73-5, 2018
7. Yang X et al: Spinal extradural angiolipoma: a report of two cases and review of literature. J Spine Surg. 4(2):490-5, 2018
8. Kang HI et al: Angiolipoma on the lumbar spine. Korean J Spine. 14(3):112-4, 2017
9. Sandvik U et al: Spinal cavernous extradural angiolipoma manifesting as a spontaneous spinal epidural hematoma in a child. Childs Nerv Syst. 31(8):1223-6, 2015
10. Si Y et al: Spinal angiolipoma: etiology, imaging findings, classification, treatment, and prognosis. Eur Spine J. 23(2):417-25, 2014
11. Hu S et al: MRI features of spinal epidural angiolipomas. Korean J Radiol. 14(5):810-7, 2013
12. Reyes D et al: Thoracolumbar spinal angiolipoma demonstrating high signal on STIR imaging: a case report and review of the literature. Spine J. 13(11):e1-5, 2013

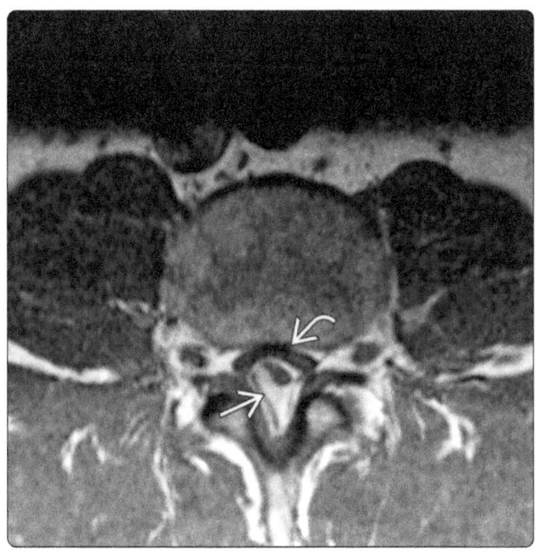

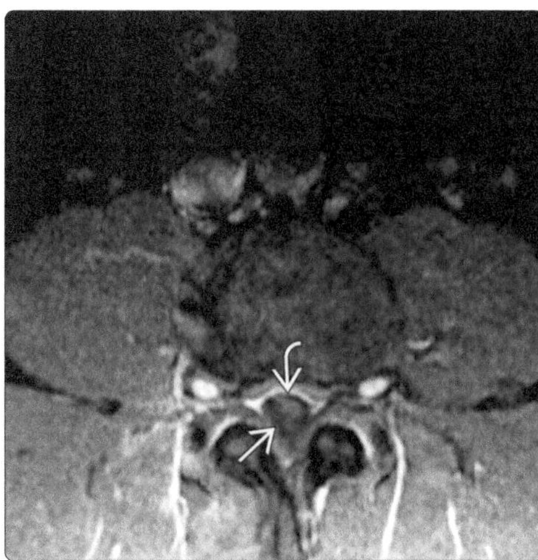

(Left) *Axial T1WI MR illustrates thecal sac compression ➔ by a heterogeneous extradural spinal angiolipoma (SAL) ➔. The degree of central hypointensity on T1WI MR is predictive of the degree of vascularity likely to be encountered at surgery.* **(Right)** *Axial T1WI C+ FS MR reveals minimal peripheral enhancement ➔ of the posterior angiolipoma. The fatty lesion elements ➔ appear dark due to fat suppression.*

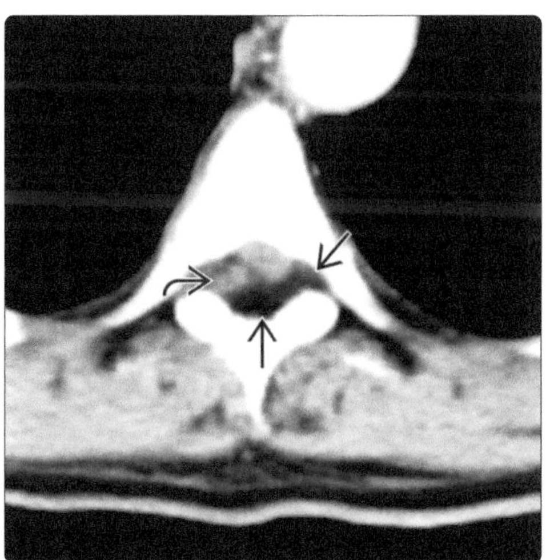

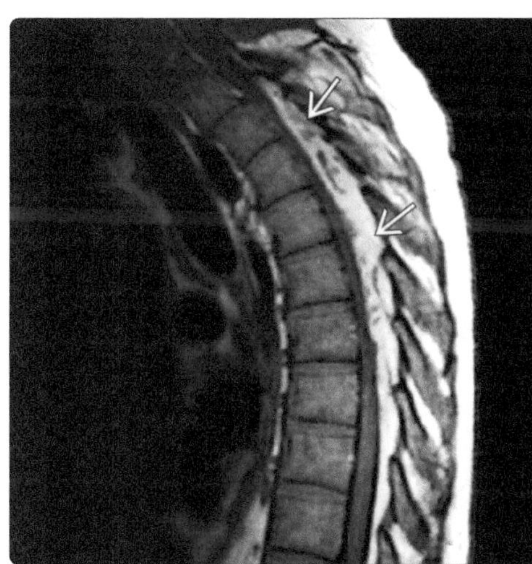

(Left) *Axial CECT through the thoracic spine demonstrates a fat-attenuation dorsal epidural mass ➔ with a soft tissue component ➔ filling much of the spinal canal.* **(Right)** *Sagittal T1WI MR demonstrates a large, heterogeneous, predominantly T1-hyperintense dorsal epidural mass ➔ producing regional spinal cord compression.*

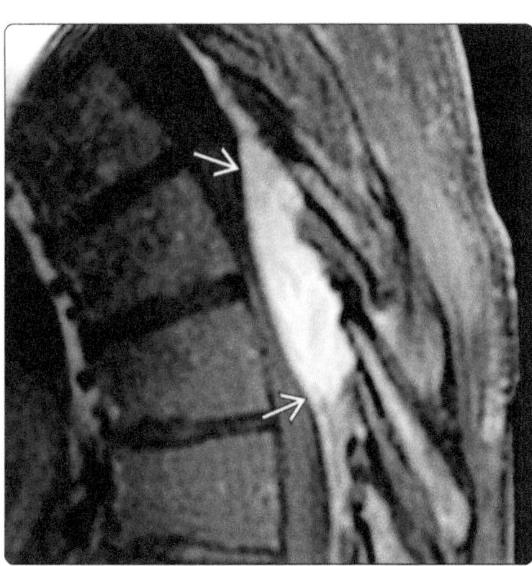

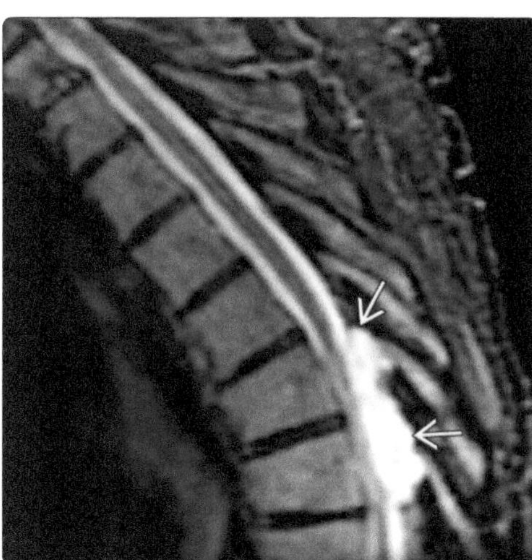

(Left) *Sagittal T1WI C+ FS MR reveals a slightly heterogeneous, intensely enhancing epidural mass ➔ involving the dorsal upper thoracic spine with cord compression. This is a nonspecific MR appearance of a dorsal epidural mass, and preoperative diagnosis of SAL can be difficult.* **(Right)** *Sagittal STIR MR depicts a lobulated, hyperintense dorsal epidural mass ➔ involving the upper thoracic spine with cord compression.*

CSF Disseminated Metastases

KEY FACTS

TERMINOLOGY

- Spread of malignant tumor through subarachnoid spaces of brain and spinal cord

IMAGING

- Smooth or nodular enhancement along cord, cauda equina
- 4 basic patterns
  - Solitary focal mass at bottom of thecal sac
  - Diffuse, thin, sheet-like coating of cord/roots (carcinomatous meningitis)
  - Rope-like thickening of cauda equina
  - Unifocal or multifocal discrete nodule(s)

TOP DIFFERENTIAL DIAGNOSES

- Multifocal primary tumor
- Pyogenic meningitis
- Granulomatous meningitis
- Chemical meningitis
- Blood products from recent lumbar puncture
- Congenital hypertrophic polyradiculoneuropathies
- Thick nerve roots/cauda equina

PATHOLOGY

- Hematogenous dissemination from solid tumors
- Drop metastases from patients with primary CNS tumor
- Leukemia, lymphoma
- False-negative CSF cytology in up to 40%

CLINICAL ISSUES

- Adults: Typically seen in advanced cancer cases
- Children: Minority of patients with certain intracranial tumor types
- Portends worse prognosis

DIAGNOSTIC CHECKLIST

- MR more sensitive than CSF cytology
- Remember to check distal thecal sac
- Postoperative or postchemotherapy meningeal enhancement can mimic leptomeningeal tumor spread

(Left) *Sagittal FIESTA (CISS) MR in a patient with metastatic posterior fossa ependymoma reveals numerous nodular CSF drop metastases, the largest ➡ compressing the conus. CISS/FIESTA imaging is very sensitive for detecting drop metastases and is recommended for all patients.* **(Right)** *Sagittal T1 C+ FS MR confirms avid enhancement of the drop metastases. These enhancing lesions are easy to detect, but nonenhancing metastatic deposits may be very difficult to identify on T2 and contrast T1 MR.*

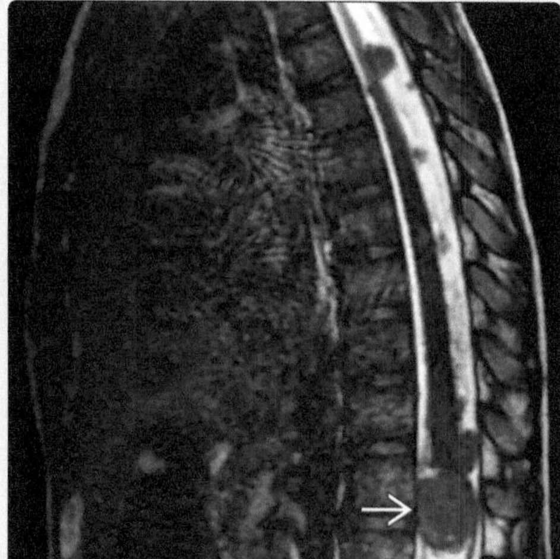

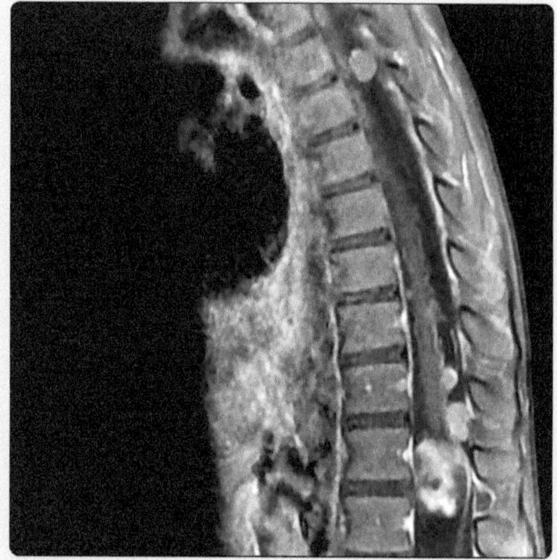

(Left) *Axial T2 MR confirms that the conus ➡ is displaced to the right by the large CSF metastasis ➡ but shows normal signal intensity. Axial images are essential to evaluate for regional cord compression, which can be overestimated on sagittal imaging.* **(Right)** *Axial T1 C+ FS MR at a different level shows a smaller metastatic lesion ➡ that invaginates into the ventrally displaced spinal cord ➡.*

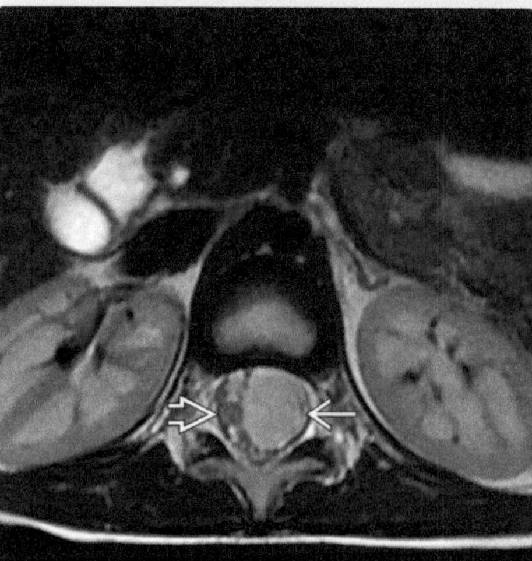

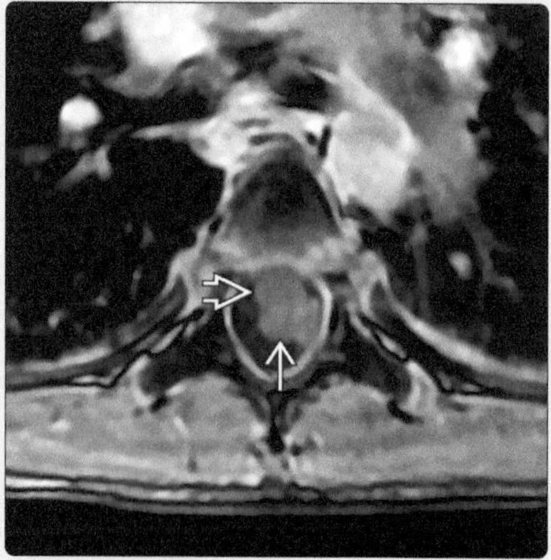

TERMINOLOGY

Synonyms

- Leptomeningeal carcinomatosis
- Carcinomatous meningitis
- Neoplastic meningitis
- Drop metastases

Definitions

- Spread of malignant tumor through subarachnoid spaces of brain and spine

IMAGING

General Features

- Best diagnostic clue
  - Smooth or nodular enhancement in basilar cisterns, along cord (especially dorsally), and cauda equina
- Location
  - Any point along CSF pathways
- Size
  - Variable
- Morphology
  - 4 basic patterns
    - Multifocal discrete nodules along cord/roots
    - Solitary focal mass at bottom of thecal sac or along cord surface
    - Diffuse, thin, sheet-like coating of cord/roots (carcinomatous meningitis)
    - Rope-like thickening of cauda equina
  - Intramedullary nodule(s)
    - Rare with CSF spread, impossible to distinguish from hematogenous metastatic disease

CT Findings

- NECT
  - Often appears normal because metastases similar density to cord
- CECT
  - Frequently appears normal
  - May be able to appreciate enhancement of cauda equina in some cases

MR Findings

- T1WI
  - Metastases usually isointense with cord, roots
  - Tumor may fill thecal sac, increasing normally low CSF signal
    - Nerve roots, dura appear blurred or smudged
    - CSF has ground-glass, hazy appearance
- T2WI
  - Thickened nerve roots
  - Tumor isointense or hyperintense to cord, nerve roots
  - May see vasogenic edema within cord
- DWI
  - Cellular tumors show diffusion restriction
    - Can detect very small metastases if tumor restricts
    - Spine DWI tends to follow diffusion appearance of primary brain tumor
- T1WI C+
  - Variable enhancement
    - Single or multiple enhancing, nodular masses
    - "Sugar coating" of cord, roots
    - Rounded intramedullary mass (very rare)
- CISS/FIESTA
  - Very sensitive for identifying metastases on cord surface
  - More sensitive than T1 C+ MR, especially if lesion < 3 mm or nonenhancing

Nonvascular Interventions

- Myelography
  - Expanded cord, thickened nerve roots
  - Nodular or mass-like filling defects in contrast column
  - Myelographic block: Contrast fails to pass beyond metastasis

Imaging Recommendations

- Protocol advice
  - With high-risk CNS tumors, image entire neuraxis for metastatic disease prior to craniotomy
    - High-resolution T2WI and STIR
    - Contrast-enhanced T1WI without fat suppression (2D or 3D technique)
      - Usually not necessary to obtain T1WI before contrast for intradural metastasis evaluation
    - 3D CISS/FIESTA ± DWI

Nuclear Medicine Findings

- Radionuclide cisternography
  - Communicating hydrocephalus
  - CSF flow obstruction in spinal canal, skull base from subarachnoid tumor

DIFFERENTIAL DIAGNOSIS

Multifocal Primary Tumor

- Hemangioblastoma
- Astrocytoma (rare)
- Myxopapillary ependymoma

Pyogenic Meningitis

- Typically chronic bacterial or fungal meningitis
- Subdural empyema
- Clinical/laboratory findings helpful

Granulomatous Meningitis

- Tubercular meningitis
- Fungal meningitis
- Sarcoidosis

Chemical Meningitis

- Postoperative change
- Subarachnoid blood, adhesions can mimic leptomeningeal metastasis

Recent Lumbar Puncture

- Leptomeningeal, dural enhancement

Congenital Hypertrophic Polyradiculoneuropathies

- Charcot-Marie-Tooth
- Dejerine-Sottas

Thick Nerve Roots/Cauda Equina

- Guillain-Barré syndrome
  - Postviral or vaccinial ascending paralysis

- Predominantly motor signs
- Immunosuppression-associated polyneuropathy (e.g., CMV)
- Chemotherapy-associated polyneuropathy
- Chronic interstitial demyelinating polyneuropathy (CIDP)

PATHOLOGY

General Features

- Etiology
  - Hematogenous spread (Batson plexus, arterial) from solid tumors (1-5%)
    - Most common: Adenocarcinomas (lung, breast), melanoma, small cell lung carcinoma
    - Unknown primary in 1-7%
  - Drop metastases from patients with primary CNS tumor (1-2%)
    - Adults: Anaplastic astrocytoma, glioblastoma multiforme (GBM) (0.5-1% of cases), ependymoma
    - Children: Medulloblastoma most common
      - Others: Germinoma, atypical teratoid/rhabdoid tumor (AT/RT), ependymoma, choroid plexus papilloma/carcinoma
  - Leukemia, lymphoma (5-15%)
- Associated abnormalities
  - Elevated CSF protein, leukocytes; decreased glucose

Microscopic Features

- Varies with histology of primary neoplasm
- CSF cytology negative in up to 40% of patients with autopsy-proven leptomeningeal carcinomatosis
  - Yield increases with
    - 2 samples
    - Adequate CSF volumes (> 10.5 cc)
    - Sampling from point on neuraxis near to clinical/radiographic disease

CLINICAL ISSUES

Presentation

- Most common signs/symptoms
  - Headache
  - Confusion, cognitive impairment, seizures
  - Cranial nerve dysfunction
    - Diplopia, especially CNVI
    - Trigeminal neuralgia, anesthesia
    - Optic neuropathy
    - Deafness
  - Weakness, legs more frequently than arms
  - Dermatomal or segmental sensory loss
  - Radicular pain
  - Nuchal rigidity (15%)
  - Disturbance of bowel, bladder function
- Other signs/symptoms
  - Abnormal CSF flow dynamics in 30-70% with obstruction at level of
    - Spine
    - Skull base
    - Arachnoid granulations (communicating hydrocephalus)
- Clinical profile
  - Adults: Typically seen in advanced cancer cases
  - Children: Minority of patients with certain intracranial tumor types

Demographics

- Epidemiology
  - 5% of all spinal metastases
  - Prevalence in adult patients is increasing, as cancer patients are living longer

Natural History & Prognosis

- Portends worse prognosis
- Relentless progression typical, although remission and cure possible

Treatment

- Radiation therapy for focal tumor
- Intravenous ± intrathecal chemotherapy
- Surgical decompression for cord compression if radiation therapy fails or acute paraplegia

DIAGNOSTIC CHECKLIST

Consider

- MR more sensitive than CSF cytology; especially CISS/FIESTA and T1 C+ MR

Image Interpretation Pearls

- Postoperative or postchemotherapy meningeal enhancement can mimic leptomeningeal tumor spread
- Do not forget to inspect distal thecal sac for drop metastases

SELECTED REFERENCES

1. Afshari FT et al: Molecular subgroup of medulloblastoma: evaluation of contribution to CSF diversion following tumour resection. Childs Nerv Syst. 39(3):563-8, 2023
2. Freret ME et al: Early detection of leptomeningeal metastases among patients undergoing spinal stereotactic radiosurgery. Adv Radiat Oncol. 8(2):101154, 2023
3. Chen R et al: Fast-developing fatal diffuse leptomeningeal dissemination of a pineal germinoma in a young child: a case report and literature review. Br J Neurosurg. 36(2):262-9, 2022
4. Schmid D et al: Diagnostic biomarkers from proteomic characterization of cerebrospinal fluid in patients with brain malignancies. J Neurochem. 158(2):522-38, 2021
5. Li Z et al: Practical applications of CISS MRI in spine imaging. Eur J Radiol Open. 6:231-42, 2019
6. Buch K et al: Balanced steady-state free precession sequence (CISS/FIESTA/3D driven equilibrium radiofrequency reset pulse) increases the diagnostic yield for spinal drop metastases in children with brain tumors. AJNR Am J Neuroradiol. 39(7):1355-61, 2018
7. Diaz-Aguilar D et al: Simultaneous cerebrospinal fluid and hematologic metastases in a high-grade ependymoma. Surg Neurol Int. 9:93, 2018
8. Tanaka H et al: Embryonal brain tumor with unknown primary lesion and massive cerebrospinal fluid dissemination: a case report. J Clin Neurosci. 54:125-8, 2018
9. Yao H et al: Leukaemia hijacks a neural mechanism to invade the central nervous system. Nature. 560(7716):55-60, 2018
10. Kralik SF et al: Radiological diagnosis of drop metastases from paediatric brain tumours using combination of 2D and 3D MRI sequences. Clin Radiol. 72(10):902.e13-19, 2017
11. Groves MD: Leptomeningeal disease. Neurosurg Clin N Am. 22(1):67-78, vii, 2011
12. Singh SK et al: MR imaging of leptomeningeal metastases: comparison of three sequences. AJNR Am J Neuroradiol. 23(5):817-21, 2002

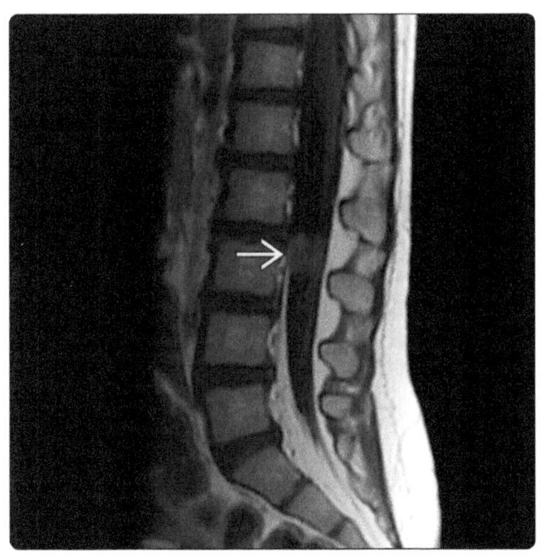

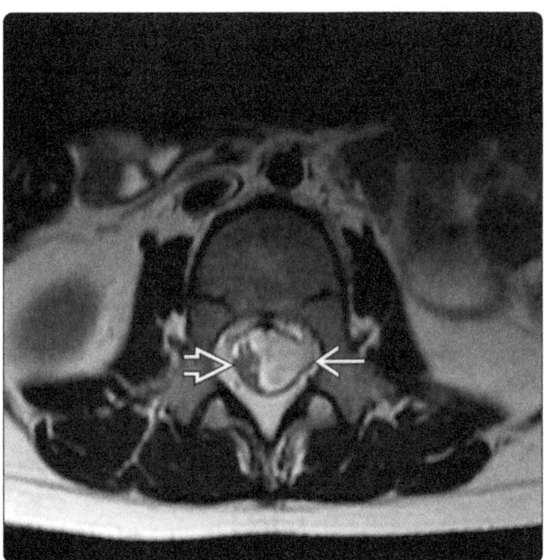

(Left) *Sagittal T1 C+ MR in a patient with intracranial diffuse midline glioma demonstrates a large drop metastasis ➡ in the caudal thecal sac. Enhancement is minimal, and lesion is subtle for its size.* **(Right)** *Axial T2 MR in the same patient shows mass effect on the cauda equina ➡ by the large metastasis ➡.*

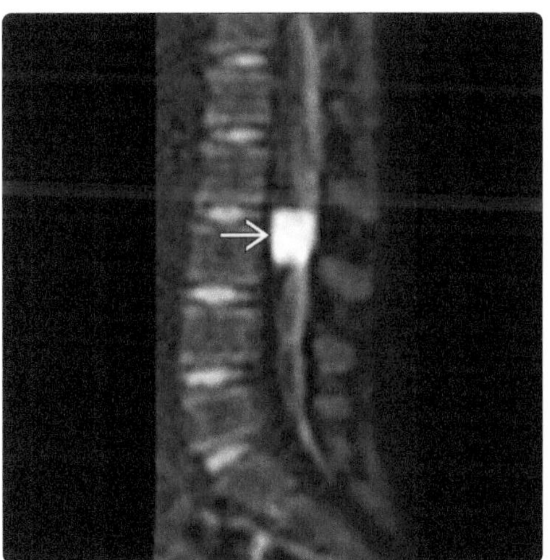

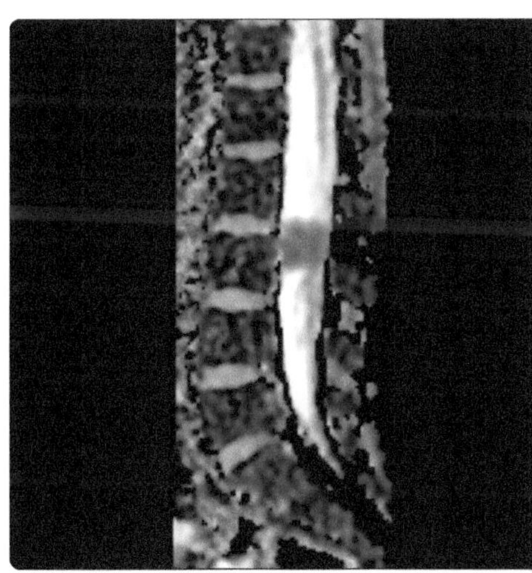

(Left) *Sagittal DWI MR demonstrates avid mass ➡ diffusion restriction (similar to the primary tumor, not shown). The lesion is much more conspicuous than on contrast T1 MR.* **(Right)** *Sagittal ADC map in the same patient confirms hypointensity of true diffusion restriction. DWI MR is a very useful addition to spinal metastasis surveillance protocols if primary tumor restricts. It adds little if primary tumor does not restrict.*

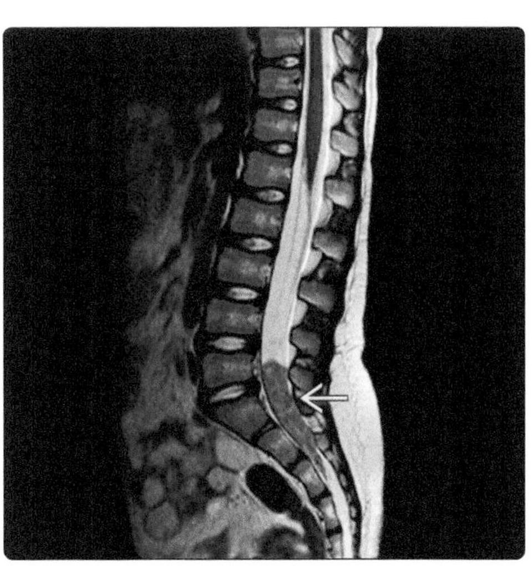

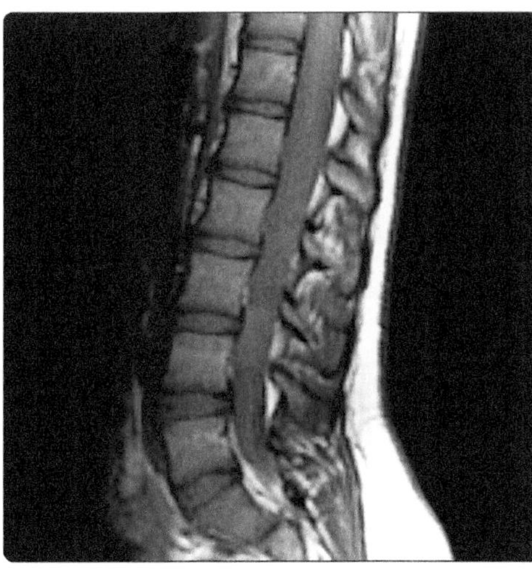

(Left) *Sagittal T2 MR in a patient with 4th ventricle ependymoma depicts a different imaging appearance for nodular drop metastasis ➡. This mass resides in the caudal thecal sac, a common location for CSF metastases to settle dependently. It is important to always carefully evaluate this location.* **(Right)** *Sagittal T1WI MR in a patient with intracranial glioma shows diffusely increased CSF T1 signal. Other imaging (not shown) confirmed leptomeningeal carcinomatosis completely filling the thecal sac.*

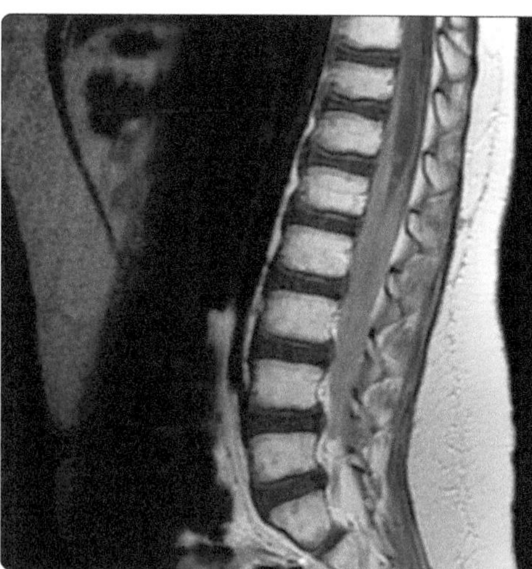

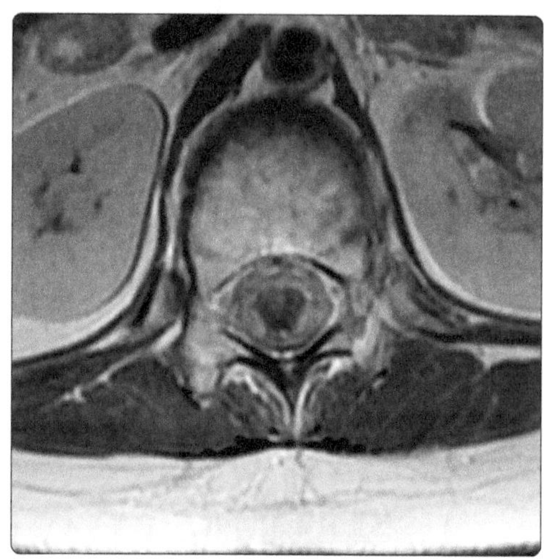

(Left) *Sagittal T1 C+ MR in a 7-year-old with a posterior fossa atypical teratoid/rhabdoid tumor (AT/RT) reveals diffuse smooth enhancement filling the thecal sac, reflecting diffuse CSF spread of the tumor.* **(Right)** *Axial T1 C+ MR in the same AT/RT patient confirms filling of the thecal sac with enhancing tumor.*

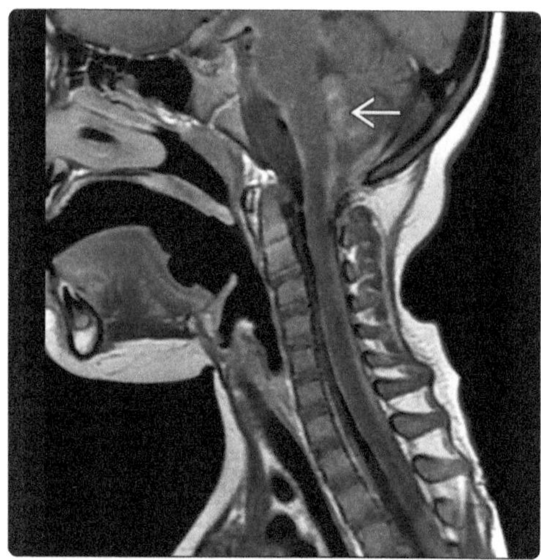

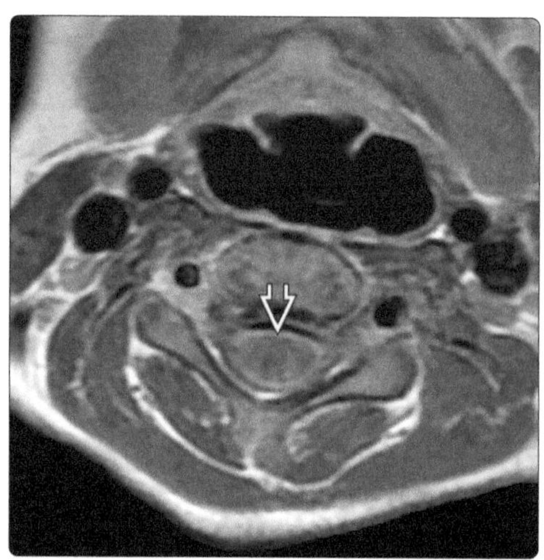

(Left) *Sagittal T1 C+ MR in a 4-year-old with a glioneuronal spinal cord tumor demonstrates a smooth, abnormal enhancing tumor coating the brain surfaces with an additional nodular tumor mass within the 4th ventricle* ➡. **(Right)** *Axial T1 C+ MR in the same patient confirms a smooth enhancing tumor surrounding the spinal cord* ➡ *and filling the dural sac.*

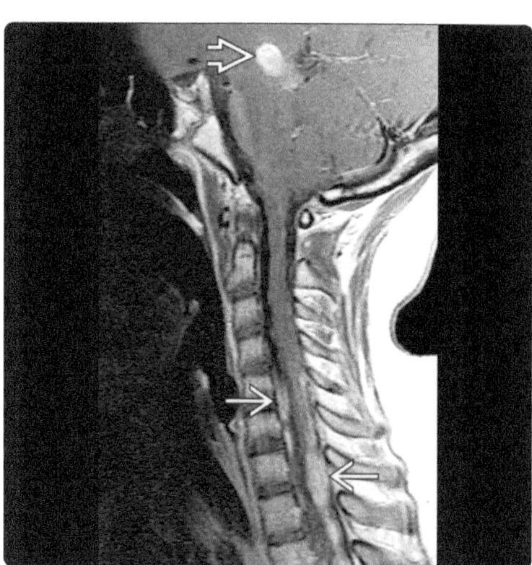

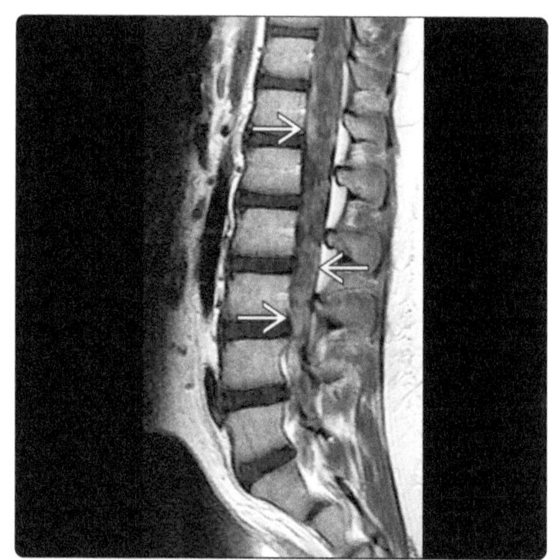

(Left) *Sagittal T1 C+ MR of the cervical spine shows an enhancing high-grade oligodendroglioma in the midbrain* ➡. *Enhancing, nodular, and confluent drop metastases* ➡ *can be seen compressing the cord in the cervical spine.* **(Right)** *Sagittal T1 C+ MR of the lumbar spine in the same patient confirms bulky nodular as well as confluent drop metastases* ➡ *in the lumbar canal, intermingling throughout the fibers of the cauda equina.*

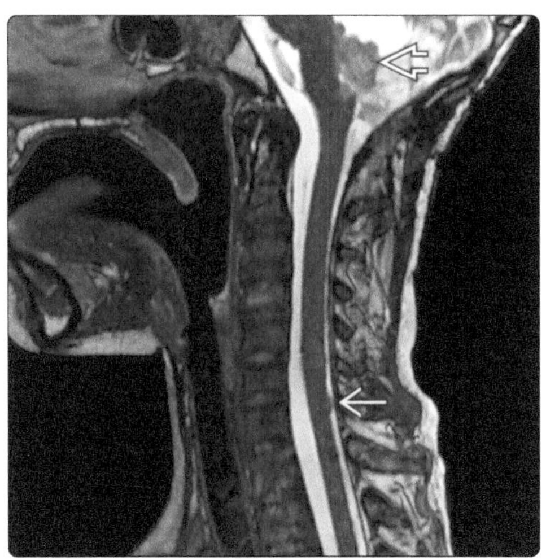

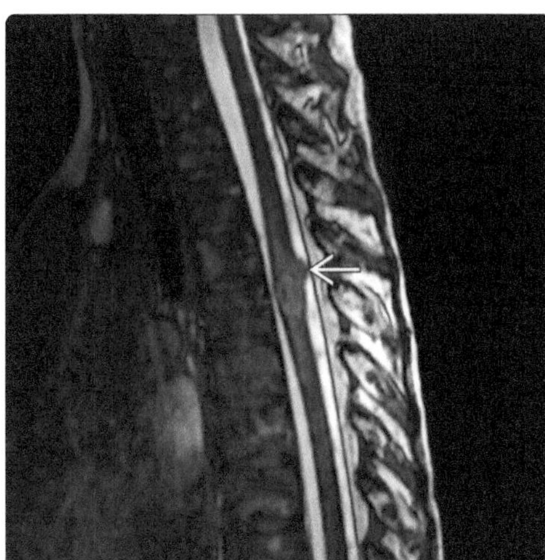

(Left) *Sagittal FIESTA MR in a patient with recurrent ependymoma ➡ reveals a subtle dorsal CSF drop metastasis ➡ that was occult on contrast T1 imaging (not shown). CISS/FIESTA is the most sensitive sequence for detecting small metastases.* **(Right)** *Sagittal FIESTA MR in the same patient shows a different large metastasis ➡ invaginating into and expanding the thoracic spinal cord.*

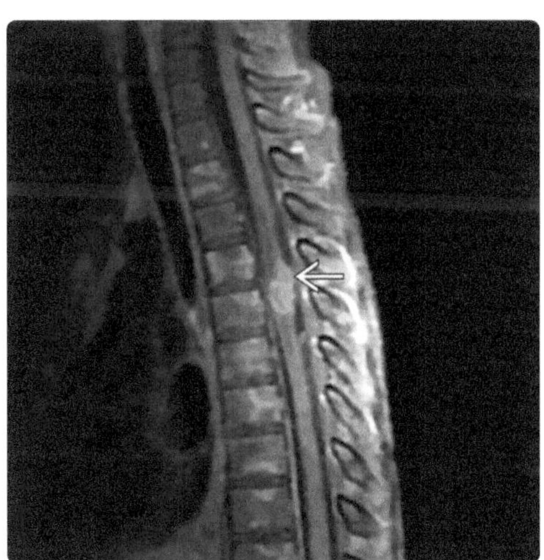

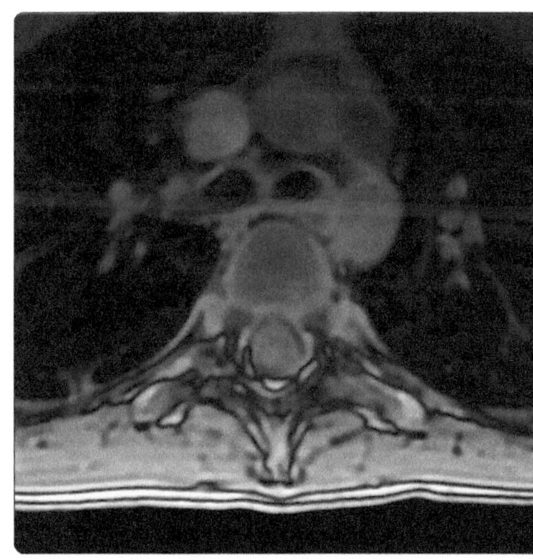

(Left) *Sagittal T1 C+ FS MR shows avid enhancement of the metastasis ➡. The spinal cord is focally enlarged at the lesion site. Note also the heterogeneous vertebral body bone marrow enhancement, reflecting prior radiation therapy.* **(Right)** *Axial T1 C+ MR (LAVA technique) shows that the cord mass fills the central osseous spinal canal.*

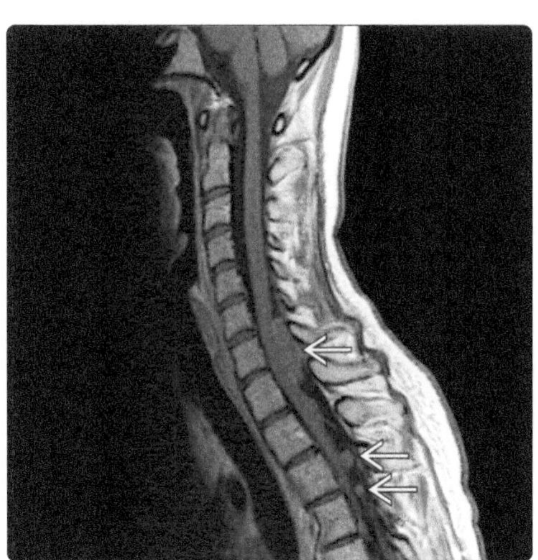

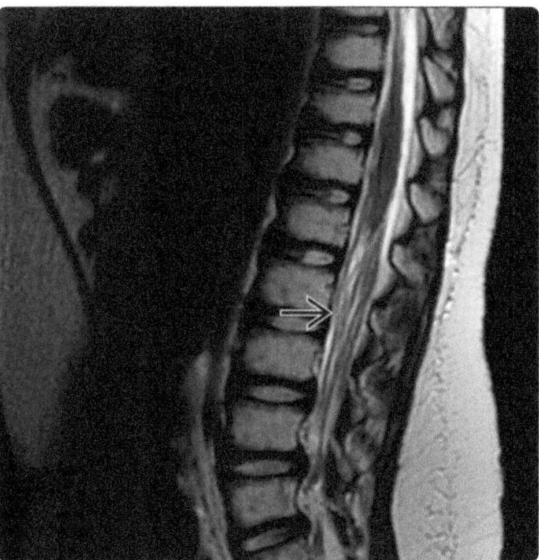

(Left) *Sagittal T1 C+ MR of the spine, performed during posttreatment follow-up after resection of a nonenhancing glioblastoma multiforme (GBM) of the right insula, shows multiple nonenhancing drop metastases along the cord surface ➡. Diffusion imaging (not commercially available at time of this imaging study) likely would have shown restriction.* **(Right)** *Sagittal T2 MR (intracranial AT/RT) shows a different imaging appearance of drop metastases with thickened, ropy appearance of the cauda equina ➡.*

KEY FACTS

TERMINOLOGY

- Slow-growing glioma arising from ependymal cells of conus, filum terminale, cauda equina

IMAGING

- Usually spans 2-4 vertebral segments
  - May fill entire lumbosacral thecal sac
- Ovoid, lobular, sausage-shaped
- CT/radiographs
  - ± osseous canal expansion, thinned pedicles, vertebral scalloping
  - May enlarge, extend through neural foramina
- T1WI: Isointense → hyperintense to cord
- T2WI: Almost always hyperintense to cord
  - Hypointensity at tumor margin = hemosiderin
- T1WI C+: Intense enhancement

TOP DIFFERENTIAL DIAGNOSES

- Nerve sheath tumor (NST)
- Intradural metastases
- Meningioma
- Paraganglioma

PATHOLOGY

- Majority are WHO grade 1
- May have local seeding or subarachnoid dissemination
- Subarachnoid hemorrhage

CLINICAL ISSUES

- Symptoms mimic disc herniation
- Back pain most common
- Other issues include paraparesis, radiculopathy, or bladder and bowel dysfunction

DIAGNOSTIC CHECKLIST

- Slow tumor growth may delay diagnosis
- Always image conus in patients presenting with back pain

(Left) *Sagittal graphic shows a multilevel cauda equina myxopapillary ependymoma. The mass is vascular with old intratumoral hemorrhage and acute subarachnoid hemorrhage along the dorsal conus. Indolent tumor growth has an enlarged spinal canal and remodeled posterior vertebral cortex.* **(Right)** *Sagittal T1 C+ MR illustrates a mildly enhancing, well-delineated, intradural extramedullary mass in the lumbar spine ➡. The mass likely arose within the filum terminale.*

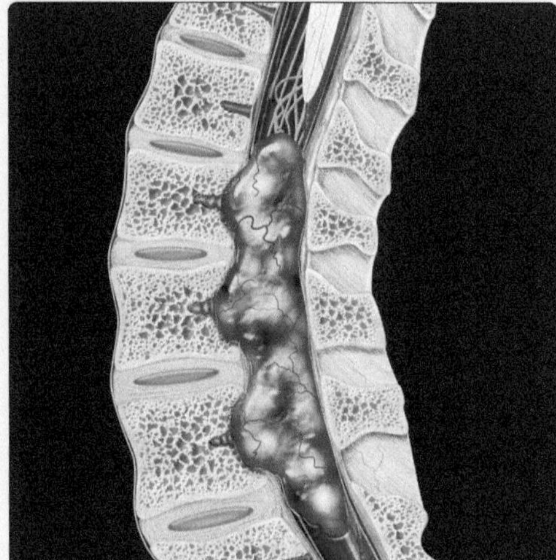

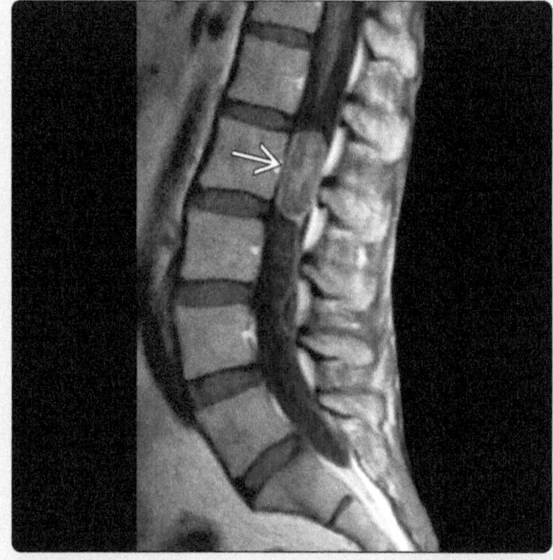

(Left) *Coronal T1 MR in the same patient confirms a well-delineated, intradural extramedullary mass ➡ in the lumbar spine. The lesion is predominantly isointense with cord and nerves. Almost 70% of filum terminale masses are ependymomas, mostly myxopapillary type.* **(Right)** *Intraoperative photograph in the same patient following dural retraction with exposure of an intradural myxopapillary ependymoma ➡ is shown. Note the mildly ↑ vasculature on the mass surface.*

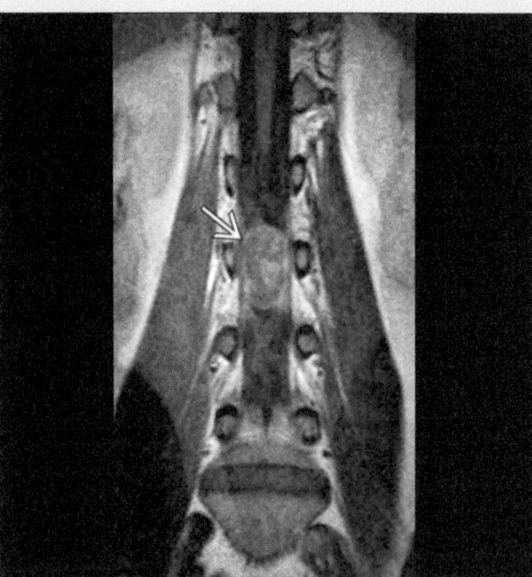

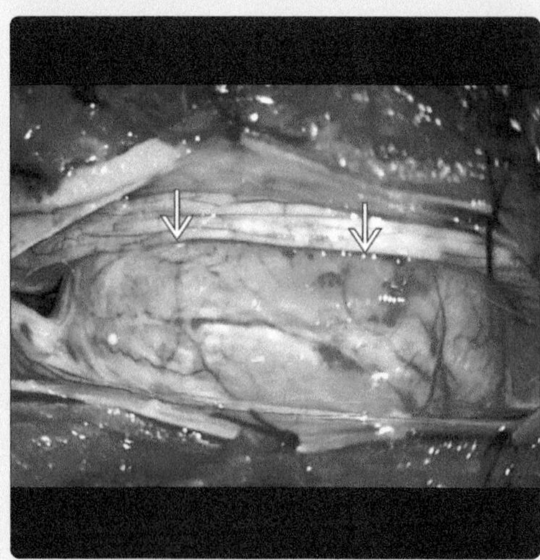

TERMINOLOGY

Abbreviations

- Myxopapillary ependymoma (ME)

Definitions

- Slow-growing glioma arising from ependymal cells of filum terminale

IMAGING

General Features

- Best diagnostic clue
  - Enhancing cauda equina mass with hemorrhage
- Location
  - Almost exclusively in conus, filum terminale, or cauda equina
  - Ependymomas outside of CNS are rare
    - Metastases or direct extension of primary CNS lesion after surgery
    - Direct extension to sacrococcygeal area from cord ependymoma or ME
    - Primary presacral, pelvic, or abdominal lesion
    - Primary ME of skin or subcutaneous tissue in sacrococcygeal region
      - Originates from ectopic ependymal remnants
- Size
  - Usually spans 2-4 vertebral segments
    - May fill entire lumbosacral thecal sac
- Morphology
  - Well circumscribed
  - Ovoid, lobular, sausage-shaped

Radiographic Findings

- Radiography
  - Vertebral remodeling changes
    - Widened interpediculate distance
    - Eroded pedicles
    - Posterior vertebral scalloping
    - Intervertebral foraminal widening

CT Findings

- NECT
  - Isodense intradural mass
- CECT
  - Homogeneous, avid enhancement
- Bone CT
  - ± osseous canal expansion
    - Thinned pedicles
    - Widened interpediculate distance
    - Scalloped vertebral bodies
    - May enlarge and extend through neural foramina

MR Findings

- T1WI
  - Usually isointense with cord
  - Hyperintensity attributed to mucin accumulation
- T2WI
  - Nearly always hyperintense to cord
  - Hypointensity at tumor margin = hemosiderin
    - 70% of intradural spine tumors with hemorrhage are ependymomas
  - May see flow voids
- STIR
  - Hyperintense
- T1WI C+
  - Intense enhancement
    - Reports of heterogeneous enhancement reflect unencapsulated tumors
      - Unencapsulated tumors may have extensive tumor necrosis, intratumoral hemorrhage, and progressive perivascular hyalinization → variable signal characteristics

Imaging Recommendations

- Best imaging tool
  - Multiplanar MR with contrast
- Protocol advice
  - Always image conus in patients presenting with back pain

DIFFERENTIAL DIAGNOSIS

Nerve Sheath Tumor

- Small tumor associated with nerve root rather than filum terminale
- Large, multilevel nerve sheath tumor (NST) may be indistinguishable
- Often extends through neural foramina
- Hemorrhage less common

Intradural Metastases

- Smooth or nodular enhancement along conus, nerve roots
- Enhancing mass(es), frequently multiple

Acquired Epidermoid Cyst

- Hypointense on T1WI
- Hyperintense on T2WI: Similar to CSF
- No enhancement
- Typically small

Meningioma

- Usually isointense with cord on T1WI and T2WI
- More common in thoracic, cervical spine
  - Conus/filum location unusual
- Hemorrhage uncommon
- Osseous remodeling rare

Paraganglioma

- Rare tumor of cauda equina
- May be highly vascular
  - Indistinguishable from ME, although usually smaller

PATHOLOGY

General Features

- Etiology
  - Originates from ependymal cells of filum terminale
  - Subcutaneous sacrococcygeal ME arises from coccygeal medullary vestige
    - Ependyma-lined cavity of caudal neural tube at postanal pit
- Genetics
  - Spinal ependymomas genetically different from intracranial ependymomas

- Associated abnormalities
  - Acute nonaneurysmal subarachnoid hemorrhage
  - Superficial siderosis
- 4 ependymoma subtypes: Cellular, myxopapillary, clear cell, tanycytic
  - Cellular most common intramedullary tumor subtype
  - ME most common subtype to hemorrhage
  - 10-40% of MEs are multiple

Staging, Grading, & Classification

- Majority are WHO grade 1
  - Rare anaplastic subtypes have been reported
- May have local seeding, subarachnoid dissemination
- No malignant degeneration

Gross Pathologic & Surgical Features

- Soft, lobulated, ovoid
- Grayish white surface
- Noninfiltrating, often encapsulated
- May be highly vascular

Microscopic Features

- Spindle, columnar, cuboidal tumor cells radially arranged in papillary manner around vascularized stromal cores
- Fibrous, mucoid matrix
- Cysts, hemorrhage, Ca^{++} common
- Absent, low mitotic activity
  - MIB (marker of cell proliferation): 0.4-1.6%
- Rare anaplastic types distinguished by presence of elevated mitotic activity and necrosis
- Immunohistochemistry: Glial fibrillary acidic protein, S100, vimentin positive
  - Cytokeratin negative

CLINICAL ISSUES

Presentation

- Most common signs/symptoms
  - Back pain
- Other signs/symptoms
  - Paraparesis
  - Radiculopathy
  - Bladder and bowel dysfunction: 20-25%
- Clinical profile
  - Symptoms mimic disc herniation
  - Slow tumor growth may delay diagnosis
    - ~ 2-year duration of symptoms prior to diagnosis

Demographics

- Age
  - Broad range: Reported at all ages
    - Peak: 30-40 years
- Sex
  - M:F = 2:1
- Epidemiology
  - Ependymoma: 4% of all primary CNS neoplasms in adults
    - 30% of ependymomas are spinal
  - Cord ependymoma: Most common primary spinal cord tumor in adults
    - 60% of primary spinal cord neoplasms
  - ME: 27-30% of all ependymomas
    - Most common tumor of conus, filum terminale, cauda equina
    - 90% of filum terminale tumors

Natural History & Prognosis

- Excellent prognosis with complete resection
  - Late recurrence, distant metastases uncommon after complete resection
- Risk of local recurrence if incomplete resection
  - CSF dissemination if tumor capsule is violated
- Gross characteristics appear to be of greater prognostic significance than histologic features
  - Encapsulated tumors amenable to total surgical removal have lower recurrence rate (~ 10%) than those removed either piecemeal or subtotally (~ 19%)
  - Overall survival is related to residual disease
    - Total removal of tumor results in longer survival than subtotal resection
- Pediatric patients more likely to develop metastases and display more aggressive disease
  - Higher rate of local recurrence and tumor dissemination within neural axis
  - Rare anaplastic variants associated with more aggressive clinical course

Treatment

- Resection
  - Gross total resection in > 85% of cases
- Radiotherapy for recurrence or subtotal resection
  - MEs are radiosensitive
- Closer surveillance, adjuvant therapy for multifocal lesions and anaplastic variants

DIAGNOSTIC CHECKLIST

Consider

- Scanning up to at least midthoracic spine if conus lesion is found
- Slow tumor growth may delay clinical presentation, diagnosis

Image Interpretation Pearls

- T1-/T2-hyperintense, enhancing, hemorrhagic mass associated with filum terminale is highly suggestive of ME

SELECTED REFERENCES

1. Khristov V et al: Myxopapillary ependymoma with anaplastic features: a case series and review of the literature. World Neurosurg. 158:e735-45, 2022
2. Eschbacher KL et al: Pediatric myxopapillary ependymomas: a clinicopathologic evaluation. J Pediatr Hematol Oncol. 43(8):e1194-200, 2021
3. Liu Y et al: Pediatric extraspinal subcutaneous sacrococcygeal myxopapillary ependymoma: case report and minireview. Am J Dermatopathol. 43(12):e273-6, 2021
4. Khalid SI et al: Pediatric spinal ependymomas: an epidemiologic study. World Neurosurg. 115:e119-28, 2018
5. Kraetzig T et al: Metastases of spinal myxopapillary ependymoma: unique characteristics and clinical management. J Neurosurg Spine. 28(2):201-8, 2018
6. Rogers S et al: Unusual paediatric spinal myxopapillary ependymomas: unique molecular entities or pathological variations on a theme? J Clin Neurosci. 50:144-8, 2018
7. Lucchesi KM et al: Primary spinal myxopapillary ependymoma in the pediatric population: a study from the surveillance, epidemiology, and end results (SEER) database. J Neurooncol. 130(1):133-40, 2016

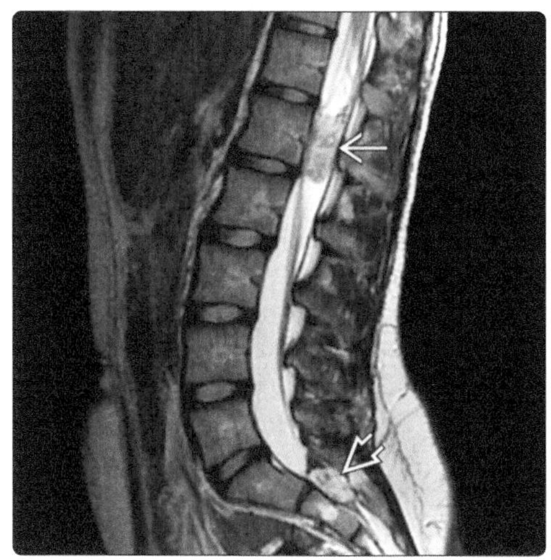

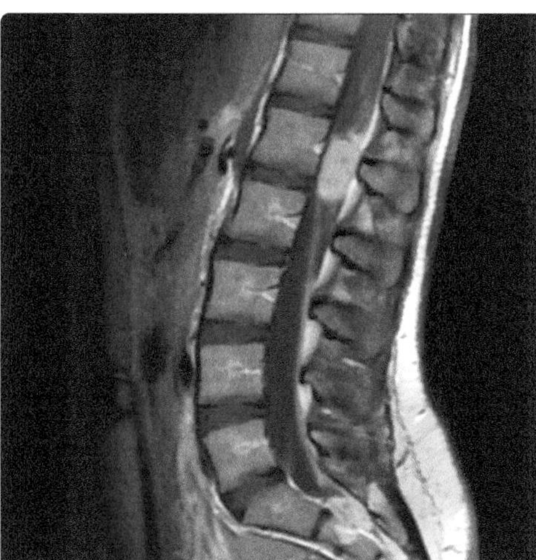

(Left) *Sagittal T2 MR in a pediatric patient with severe back pain reveals a T2-hyperintense mass ➡ arising just below the conus. It is always prudent to inspect the distal thecal sac for intradural metastasis with intradural tumors, revealing a 2nd lesion ⇨.* **(Right)** *Sagittal T1 C+ MR confirms avid enhancement of both lesions. Surgical resection of the conus lesion confirmed WHO grade 1 myxopapillary ependymoma.*

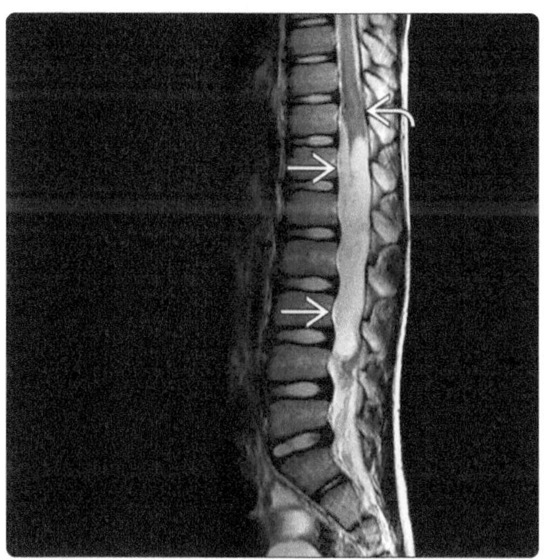

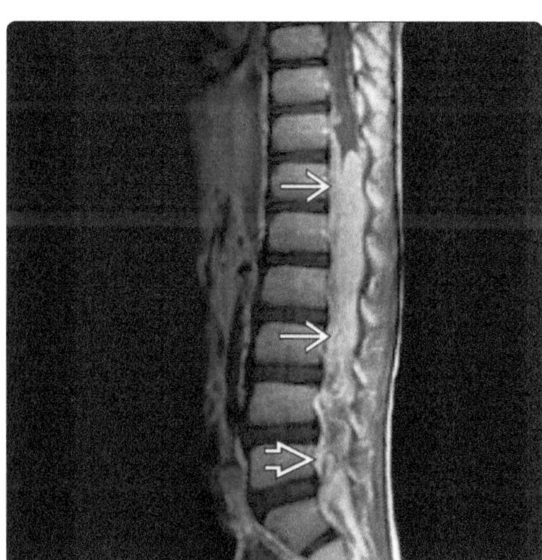

(Left) *Sagittal T2 MR reveals an extensive hyperintense tumor ➡ in the thecal sac that distorts the normal conus and cauda equina. A disseminated appearance, rather than a single mass, indicates diffuse intradural tumor seeding. The conus ↪ shows T2-hyperintense edema.* **(Right)** *Sagittal T1 C+ MR shows avid homogeneous tumor ➡ enhancement. Note diffuse intradural tumor seeding ⇨. Smaller tumors tend to displace the cauda equina nerve roots, whereas large tumors often compress or encase them.*

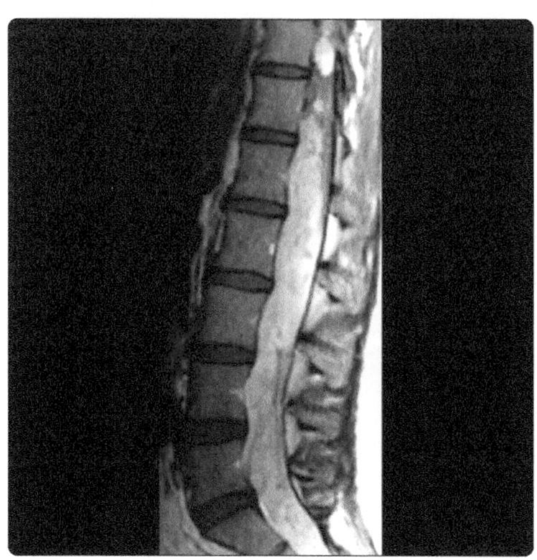

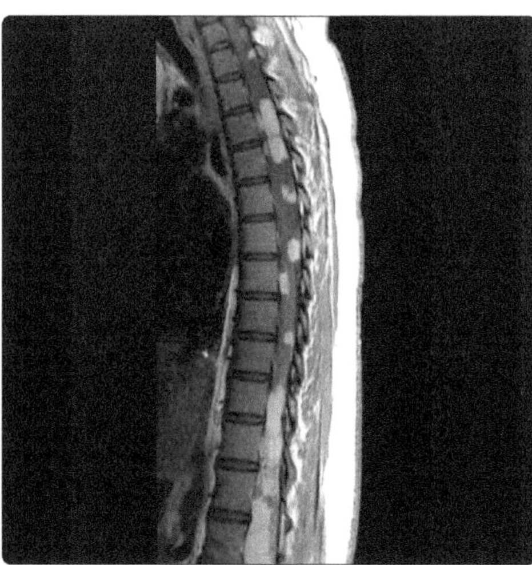

(Left) *Sagittal T1 C+ MR shows multiple extensive enhancing intradural masses distributed throughout the lumbar and thoracic spinal canal, reflecting CSF disseminated metastatic myxopapillary ependymoma.* **(Right)** *Sagittal T1 C+ MR of the thoracic spine shows multiple enhancing intradural masses throughout the lumbar and thoracic spine from CSF dissemination of metastatic ependymoma.*

KEY FACTS

TERMINOLOGY

- Primary spinal cord neoplasm of astrocytic origin

IMAGING

- Fusiform expansion of cord with enhancing component of variable morphology
  - Almost always enhances
- Cervical > thoracic
- Usually ≤ 4 segments
  - Occasionally multisegmental, even holocord (more common with pilocytic astrocytoma)
- ± cyst/syrinx (fluid slightly T1 hyperintense to CSF)
- Hyperintense on proton density and T2WI MR
- Myelopathy should be evaluated with contrast-enhanced MR

TOP DIFFERENTIAL DIAGNOSES

- Ependymoma
- Hemangioblastoma
- Syringohydromyelia
- Autoimmune or inflammatory myelitis

PATHOLOGY

- Low grade: 80-90%
- High grade: 10-15%

CLINICAL ISSUES

- Slow onset of myelopathy
- May cause painful scoliosis
- Most are slow growing
  - Malignant tumors may cause rapid neurologic deterioration
- Most common intramedullary tumor in children and young adults
- Overall, ependymomas > astrocytomas (2:1)

DIAGNOSTIC CHECKLIST

- Myelopathy should be evaluated with MR

(Left) *Sagittal T1 MR in a 2-year-old with decreasing arm function and gait abnormality reveals a mildly hypointense, expansile intramedullary mass ➡ within the cervicothoracic spinal cord.* **(Right)** *Sagittal T1 C+ MR in the same patient confirms patchy, heterogeneous mass enhancement. Diffuse astrocytomas generally show a patchy, rather than homogeneous, enhancement pattern.*

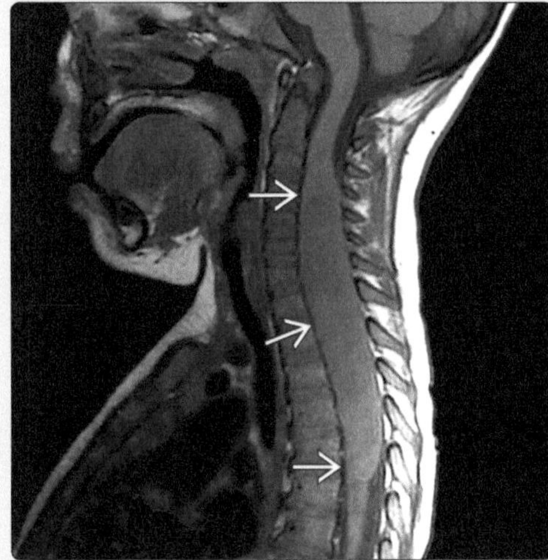

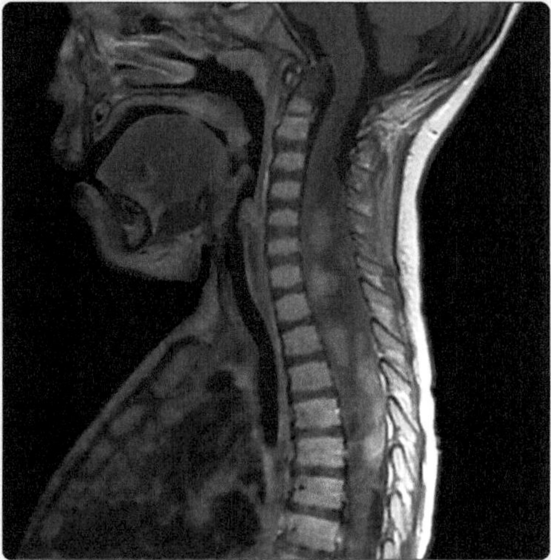

(Left) *Sagittal T2 MR in the same patient confirms heterogeneous mass increased T2 signal intensity as well as cord expansion filling the spinal canal. Note mild enlargement of the spinal canal suggesting chronicity.* **(Right)** *Axial T2 MR in the same patient confirms diffuse spinal cord enlargement as well as expansile remodeling of the osseous spinal canal. Surgical biopsy revealed diffuse WHO grade 2 astrocytoma.*

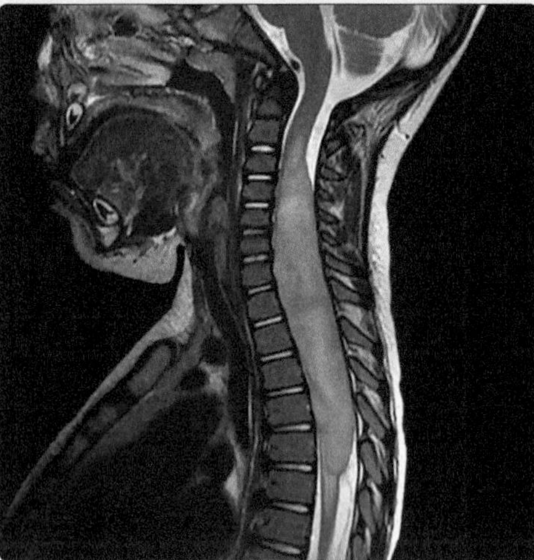

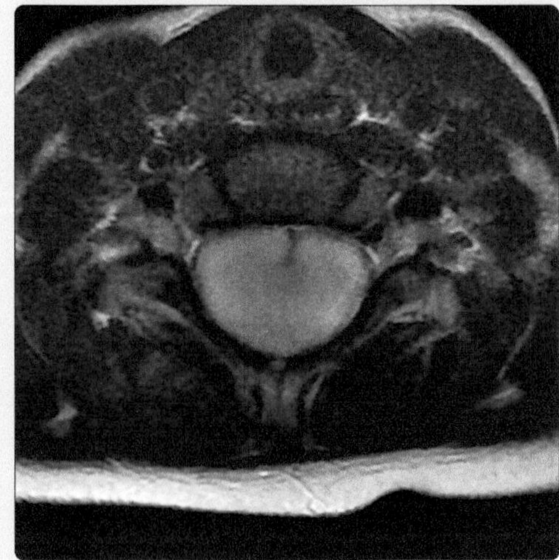

TERMINOLOGY

Definitions

- Primary neoplasm of astrocytic origin within spinal cord (SC)

IMAGING

General Features

- Best diagnostic clue
  - Enhancing infiltrating mass expanding SC
- Location
  - Cervical > thoracic
- Size
  - Usually ≤ 4 segments
  - May be extensive, especially with pilocytic histology
- Morphology
  - Fusiform spinal expansion with enhancing component of variable morphology
  - Occasionally asymmetric, even exophytic
    - Eccentric > central growth pattern

Radiographic Findings

- Radiography
  - ± scoliosis
  - ± expansion of osseous canal

CT Findings

- NECT
  - Enlarged SC
  - ± expansion, remodeling of osseous canal
- CECT
  - Mild/moderate enhancement

MR Findings

- T1WI
  - Cord expansion
    - Usually < 4 segments
    - Occasionally multisegmental, even holocord [more common with pilocytic astrocytoma (PA)]
  - ± cyst/syrinx fluid slightly hyperintense to CSF
  - Solid portion hypo-/isointense
    - Minority of cases may have areas of hyperintensity (methemoglobin)
- T2WI
  - Hyperintense
- T2* GRE
  - Hyperintense
  - Minority of cases may have hypointense areas if hemorrhagic products
- DWI
  - ↓ fractional anisotropy, ↑ ADC
  - Diffusion tensor imaging with fiber tracking (DTT) shows promise for evaluating tumor malignancy and extent
- T1WI C+
  - Usually enhance (partial > total)
  - Mild/moderate > intense enhancement
  - Heterogeneous/infiltrating > homogeneous/sharply delineated

Nuclear Medicine Findings

- Anaplastic astrocytomas demonstrate high uptake of F-18 FDG and C-11 methionine

Imaging Recommendations

- Best imaging tool
  - Contrast-enhanced multiplanar MR
- Protocol advice
  - Sagittal and axial T2WI and T1WI C+ MR

DIFFERENTIAL DIAGNOSIS

Ependymoma

- Intense, sharply delineated enhancement
- Central > eccentric growth pattern
- More often seen in low thoracic cord
- Cystic or necrotic component, hemorrhage common
- Typically older patients than those with astrocytoma

Other Neoplasms

- **Ganglioglioma**
  - Mixed T1 signal intensity due to solid, cystic components
  - Homogeneous > heterogeneous T2 hyperintensity
- **Lymphoma**
  - Intramedullary form presents as poorly defined, enhancing lesion
- **Metastasis**
  - Intramedullary nidus of enhancement much more focal with extensive edema
  - Pial metastasis can simulate hemangioblastoma
  - Usually older patients
- **Hemangioblastoma**
  - Focal, enhancing pial/subpial nodule
  - Associated syrinx simulates astrocytoma

Syringohydromyelia

- Cyst fluid similar to CSF; no enhancement

Autoimmune or Inflammatory Myelitis

- Demyelinating disease (± patchy, ill-defined enhancement if acute)
  - Multiple sclerosis
    - Cord may show mild focal swelling, flame-shaped
    - Typically multifocal
  - Transverse myelitis
    - Long cord segment ± patchy enhancement
  - Infectious myelitis
    - Viral myelitis, granulomatous osteomyelitis, bacterial meningitis
    - Rapid onset, constitutional signs
- SC infarction
  - Abrupt onset
  - Risk factors: Atherosclerosis, hypertension, diabetes
  - Clinical setting: Aortic dissection, abdominal aortic aneurysm, or surgery
- Dural vascular malformation
  - Typically, cord shows mild edema and enlargement
  - Prominent pial vessels
  - Slow onset of upper leg weakness

PATHOLOGY

Staging, Grading, & Classification

- Low grade: 80-90%
  - PA = WHO grade 1

    - Focal or diffuse cord-enlarging, irregularly shaped masses with cystic elements and hydromyelia
    - Propensity for thoracic and cervical regions
    - Different degrees of enhancement, high water diffusivity
  - Fibrillary astrocytoma = WHO grade 2
  - Pilomyxoid astrocytoma (similar to PA but with distinct histopathologic characteristics)
    - Rare in SC
    - More aggressive behavior than PA
    - ± CSF dissemination at presentation
  - Pleomorphic xanthoastrocytoma
    - Rare in SC
    - Favorable prognosis; however, 15-20% undergo progressive anaplastic transformation
    - Superficially located and partly infiltrates leptomeninges
  - Ganglioglioma, mixed gliomas
- High grade: 10-15%
  - Most are anaplastic astrocytomas (WHO grade 3)
  - Glioblastoma (GBM) (WHO grade 4), diffuse midline glioma (H3K27M mutant) uncommon
    - Distinguished by molecular testing
  - Higher grades (WHO grades 3-4) exhibit high rate of local and distant recurrence throughout neuraxis

Microscopic Features

- Fibrillary astrocytoma
  - Hypercellularity, variable atypia/mitoses
  - Parenchymal infiltration
- PA
  - Rosenthal fibers, glomeruloid/hyalinized vessels
  - Low prevalence of nuclear atypia/mitoses
- Anaplastic astrocytoma
  - Hypercellularity
  - Nuclear atypia and mitotic activity
  - Absent microvascular proliferation and necrosis
- GBM
  - Vascular proliferation, cellular pleomorphism, necrosis, and high mitotic activity (similar to intracranial GBM)

CLINICAL ISSUES

Presentation

- Most common signs/symptoms
  - Slow onset of myelopathy
- Other signs/symptoms
  - Painful scoliosis
  - Radiculopathy
  - Sensory or motor deficits
  - Incontinence
- Clinical profile
  - Insidious onset of myelopathy in adolescents or young adults

Demographics

- Age
  - Most common intramedullary tumor in children/young adults
  - 60% of intramedullary SC tumors (IMSCTs) in children are astrocytomas; 30% are ependymomas
- Sex
  - M:F = 1.3:1
- Epidemiology
  - 2nd most common SC neoplasm overall
  - IMSCTs = 5-10% of all CNS tumors
    - 20% of intraspinal neoplasms in adults
    - 30-35% of intraspinal neoplasms in children
  - 90-95% of IMSCTs are gliomas
    - Overall, ependymomas > astrocytomas (2:1)
    - Compared to PAs in other sites, cord PAs occur in older patients and comprise large proportion (58%) of spinal astrocytic tumors
  - M:F = 1.3:1
  - Association with NF2

Natural History & Prognosis

- Most slow growing
- Malignant tumors may cause rapid neurologic deterioration
- Survival varies with tumor histology/grade and gross total resection (GTR)
  - 5-year survival: 80% for low grade; 30% for high grade
  - Modern surgical techniques resulting in more GTR, longer progression-free survival (PFS)
- Postoperative neurologic function determined largely by degree of preoperative deficit

Treatment

- Serial monitoring for asymptomatic individuals
- Molecular subtype evaluation may reveal actionable targets
- Resection reserved for progressive neurologic decline
- Microsurgical resection (low-grade tumors)
- Adjuvant therapy
  - Option for WHO grades 3-4 astrocytomas
  - No evidence that radiation therapy and chemotherapy improve long-term outcome

DIAGNOSTIC CHECKLIST

Consider

- Myelopathy should be evaluated with MR

Image Interpretation Pearls

- Axial and sagittal T1WI C+ FS MR to exclude dural or pial lesion inciting syringomyelia

SELECTED REFERENCES

1. Bansal S et al: Holocord metastasis from supratentorial glioblastoma multiforme: an uncommon manifestation of a common tumor. Childs Nerv Syst. 39(1):13-5, 2023
2. Chai RC et al: Genomic profiling and prognostic factors of H3 K27M-mutant spinal cord diffuse glioma. Brain Pathol. e13153, 2023
3. Chalif EJ et al: Impact of extent of resection and adjuvant therapy in diffuse gliomas of the spine. Spine J. 23(7):1015-27, 2023
4. Hersh AM et al: Surgical approaches to intramedullary spinal cord astrocytomas in the age of genomics. Front Oncol. 12:982089, 2022
5. Park SH et al: Pathological classification of the intramedullary spinal cord tumors according to 2021 World Health Organization classification of central nervous system tumors, a single-institute experience. Neurospine. 19(3):780-91, 2022
6. Snyder MH et al: Primary spinal cord astrocytomas: two-center clinical experience of low- and high-grade lesions. World Neurosurg. 167:e1006-16, 2022
7. Kim DH et al: Differentiation between intramedullary spinal ependymoma and astrocytoma: comparative MRI analysis. Clin Radiol. 69(1):29-35, 2014

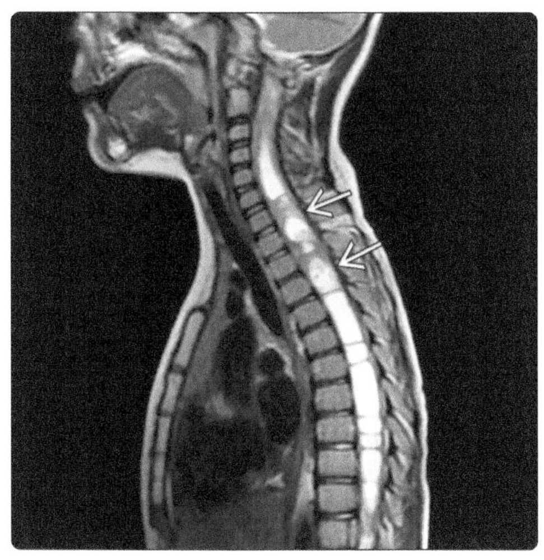

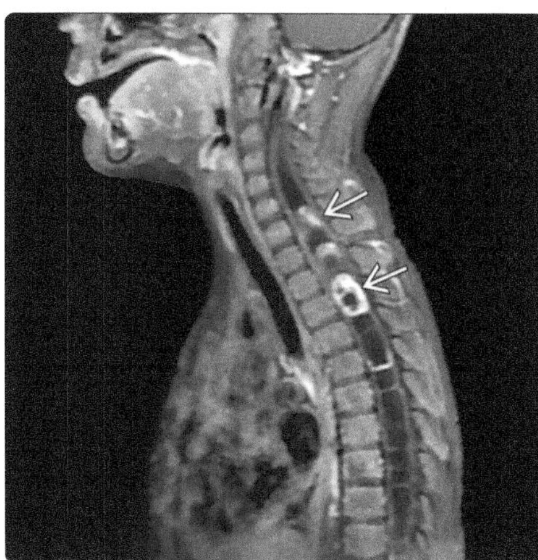

(Left) *Sagittal T2 MR in a 6-year-old patient with myelopathy reveals a heterogeneous intramedullary mass* ➡ *with extensive syrinx formation above and below the mass.* **(Right)** *Sagittal T1 C+ FS MR in the same patient reveals heterogeneous enhancement within the solid portions* ➡*. Surgical pathology was WHO grade 1 pilocytic astrocytoma, and the surgeon successfully performed a gross total resection of the enhancing tumor.*

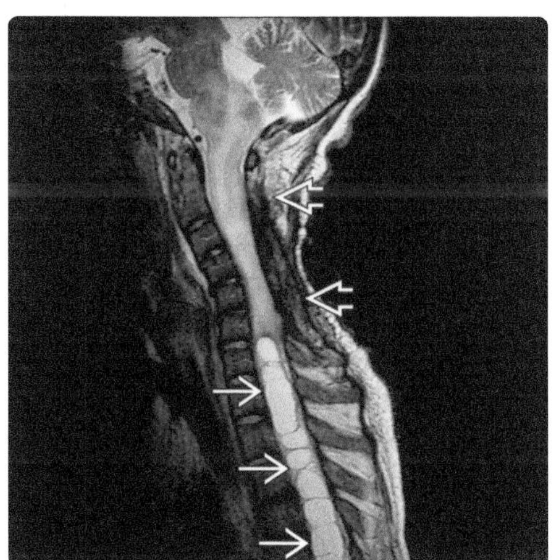

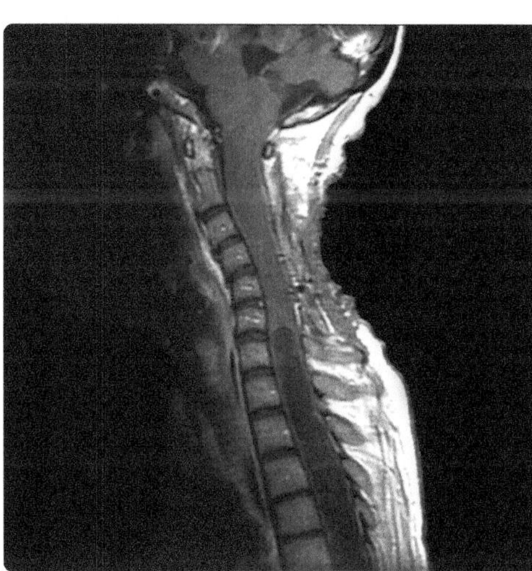

(Left) *Sagittal T2 MR (spinal cord diffuse WHO grade 2 astrocytoma, NF1) reveals an extensive, hyperintense intramedullary lesion with septated neoplastic syrinx* ➡*. Note postoperative laminectomy changes* ➡ *from biopsy.* **(Right)** *Sagittal T1 C+ MR in the same patient reveals minimal intrinsic tumor enhancement. Diffuse tumor infiltration, absence of hemorrhage, and intrinsic neoplastic syrinx cavity favor astrocytoma over ependymoma in this NF1 patient.*

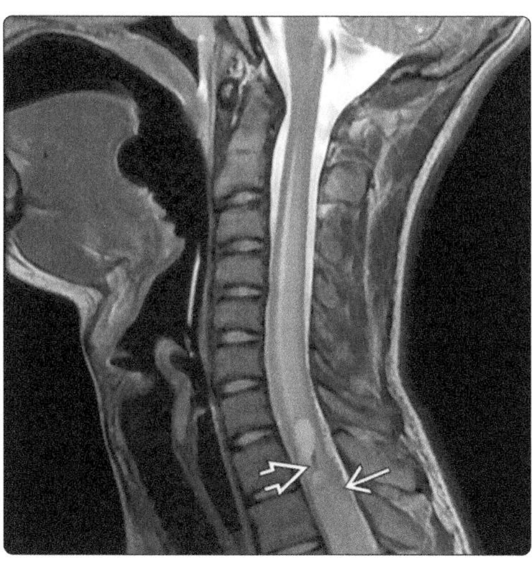

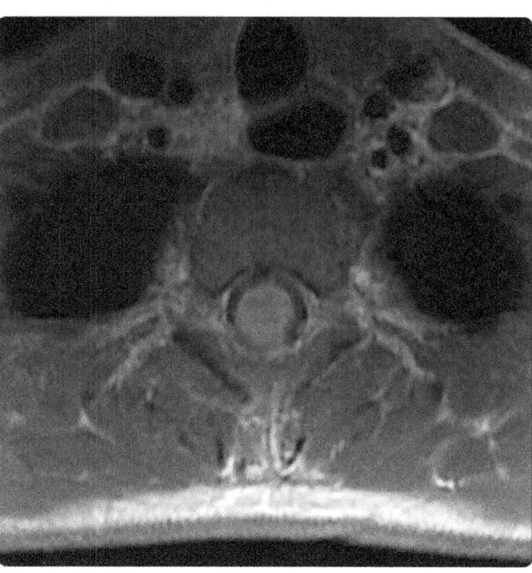

(Left) *Sagittal T2 MR in a 12-year-old patient presenting with back pain and myelopathy reveals an intrinsic intramedullary tumor* ➡ *with solid and cystic portions as well as a small focus of hemorrhage* ➡*. Extensive cord edema above and below (not shown) the lesion was present.* **(Right)** *Axial T1 C+ MR through a solid portion of the tumor reveals contrast enhancement. Biopsy was performed revealing WHO grade 4 diffuse midline glioma, H3K27M mutant. Surgical resection was not indicated.*

KEY FACTS

TERMINOLOGY

- Neoplasm arising from ependyma lining spinal cord central canal

IMAGING

- Circumscribed, enhancing hemorrhagic cord mass with surrounding edema
- Cervical > thoracic > conus
- Associated cysts common
- Cap sign: Hemosiderin at cranial or caudal margin
- Most tumors enhance

TOP DIFFERENTIAL DIAGNOSES

- Astrocytoma
- Hemangioblastoma
- Demyelinating disease
- Idiopathic transverse myelitis

PATHOLOGY

- Arises from ependymal cells of central cord canal
  - Most intramedullary
  - Rarely, can be intradural extramedullary
- Most spinal ependymomas (SP-EPNs) are WHO grade 2
- SP-EPN with *MYCN* amplification (SP-MYCN) defined by spinal localization, presence of *MYCN* amplification
  - Clinically more aggressive course than SP-EPN
- Association with neurofibromatosis type 2

CLINICAL ISSUES

- Most common presentation
  - Neck or back pain
- Other presentations
  - Progressive paraparesis, paresthesias

DIAGNOSTIC CHECKLIST

- Spinal cord neoplasm with associated peripheral hemorrhage suggestive of cellular ependymoma

(Left) *Coronal graphic depicts an intramedullary spinal ependymoma mildly expanding the cervical cord. Associated cranial and rostral cysts as well as hemorrhagic products are classic findings for this mass.* **(Right)** *Sagittal T2WI MR shows a large cervical intramedullary mass lesion ➡ with diffuse, relatively low signal intensity and very well-defined margins. Note the well-defined, tumor-associated cysts ↪ superior and inferior to the intramedullary mass.*

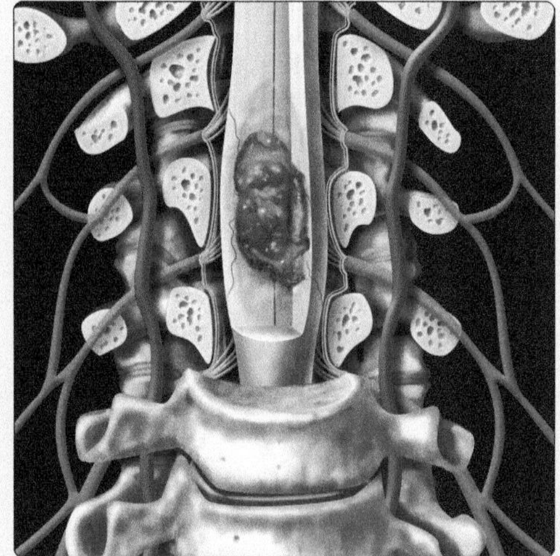

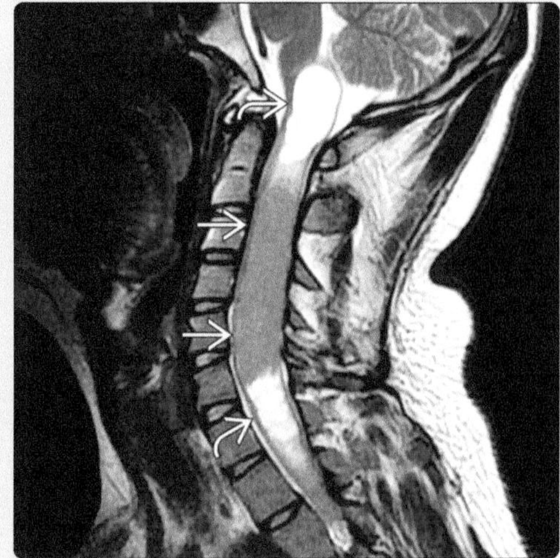

(Left) *Sagittal T1WI MR in the same patient reveals homogeneous signal intensity within the mass ➡, similar to normal brainstem. Polar cysts ↪ are hypointense but higher signal than CSF, indicating protein content.* **(Right)** *Sagittal T1WI C+ MR confirms avid homogeneous enhancement within the well-circumscribed intramedullary mass ➡.*

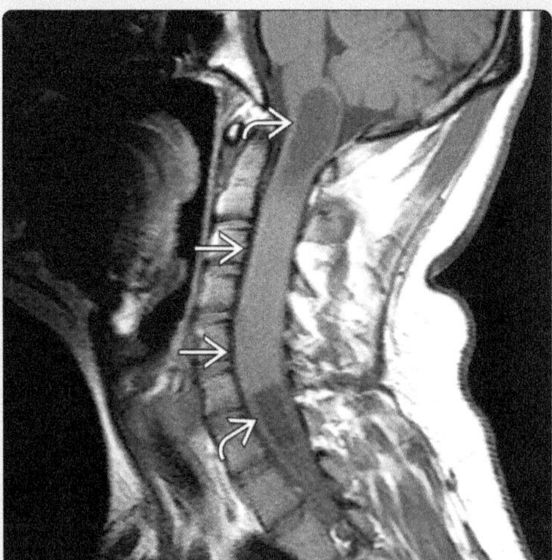

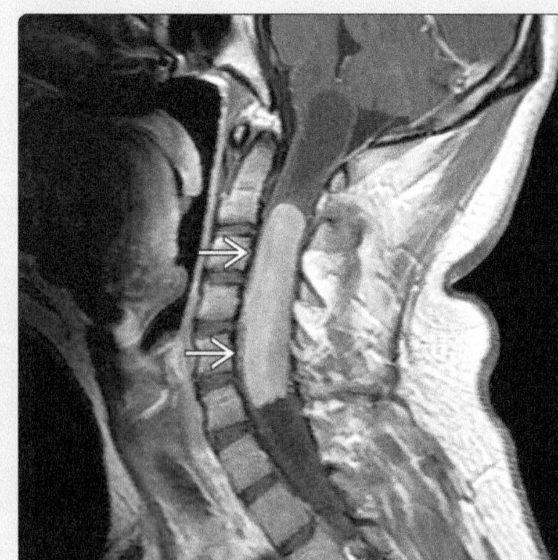

TERMINOLOGY

Definitions

- Neoplasm arising from ependyma lining spinal cord central canal
- Spinal cord ependymal tumors comprise 4 distinct tumor types
  - Spinal ependymoma (SP-EPN)
  - SP-EPN with *MYCN* amplification (SP-MYCN)
  - Myxopapillary ependymoma (MPE)
  - Subependymoma (SE)
- SP-EPN defined by spinal localization and absence of morphologic features of either MPE or SE

IMAGING

General Features

- Best diagnostic clue
  - Circumscribed, enhancing hemorrhagic cord mass
- Location
  - Cervical > thoracic > conus
- Size
  - Multisegmental: Typically 3-4 segments
- Morphology
  - Symmetric cord expansion
  - Well circumscribed
  - ± exophytic component

Radiographic Findings

- Radiography
  - Osseous spinal canal widening: 20%
  - Erosion of medial pedicles, posterior vertebral scalloping
  - ± scoliosis

CT Findings

- Bone CT
  - Osseous spinal canal widening (particularly lower spinal canal)
    - Thinned pedicles
    - Widened interpediculate distance
    - Posterior vertebral scalloping

MR Findings

- T1WI
  - Mass isointense or slightly hypointense to spinal cord
  - Hemorrhage hyperintense
  - Cord atrophy may be present
    - Correlates with surgical morbidity
- T2WI
  - Mass hyperintense relative to spinal cord
  - Focal hypointensity: Hemosiderin
    - Cap sign: Hemosiderin at cranial or caudal margin
    - 20-64% of cord ependymomas
  - Surrounding cord edema
  - 3 types of cyst (50-90%): Tumoral cyst; rostral or caudal cyst; central canal reactive dilatation (syrinx)
    - Tumoral cyst: Arises from degeneration, necrosis, and liquefaction within neoplasm
      - Contains mixture of protein, old hemorrhage, and necrotic tumoral tissue
      - Inhomogeneous composition → variable signal
      - Lined by abnormal glial cells
    - Rostral/caudal cyst
      - Location at pole(s) of neoplastic mass
    - Syrinx: Likely related to partial obstruction of central canal by tumor mass
      - Central location within spinal cord
      - CSF-equivalent signal
      - Location beyond tumor margins (above &/or below)
    - Extensive regions of cord enlargement may be caused by polar cysts or by reactive dilatation of central canal
- T2* GRE
  - Hypointensity (hemorrhage)
    - May be 2° to highly vascular connective tissue stroma
    - May be 2° to lack of intervening neural tissue; therefore, vulnerable interface between tumor and normal cord substance
- T1WI C+
  - Tumor enhancement patterns
    - Intense, well-delineated homogeneous enhancement (50%)
    - Nodular, peripheral, or heterogeneous enhancement
    - Minimal or no enhancement (rare)
  - Peripheral enhancement of tumoral cysts
  - Polar cysts and syrinx do not demonstrate contrast enhancement around borders

Imaging Recommendations

- Best imaging tool
  - Multiplanar MR ± contrast

DIFFERENTIAL DIAGNOSIS

Astrocytoma

- May be indistinguishable from ependymoma
  - Often longer, may be holocord
  - More often eccentric, infiltrative with indistinct margins
- Hemorrhage uncommon
- Tumor cysts, syrinx less common
- Most common primary cord neoplasm in children

Hemangioblastoma

- Cyst with enhancing highly vascular nodule
  - Flow voids often prominent
- Extensive surrounding edema relative to tumor size
- Thoracic > cervical
- 1/3 with von Hippel-Lindau disease

Demyelinating Disease

- Multiple sclerosis, acute disseminated encephalomyelitis (ADEM), myelin oligodendrocyte glycoprotein antibody-associated disease (MOGAD)
- Lesions more often peripheral, posterolateral, multifocal
  - 90% have concurrent brain lesions
- Typically < 2 vertebral segments in length
- Faint nodular or patchy enhancement

Infarction, Spinal Cord

- Sudden onset of symptoms
- Posterior columns typically spared in anterior spinal infarct

Idiopathic Transverse Myelitis

- Cord expansion less pronounced than ependymoma
- Centrally located, 3-4 vertebral segments in length
- Variable enhancement
- Thoracic > cervical

PATHOLOGY

General Features

- Etiology
  - Arises from ependymal cells of central cord canal
- Genetics
  - Cord ependymomas are genetically different from intracranial lesions
    - Chromosome copy number aberrations using comparative genomic hybridization: Gain on chromosomes 2, 7, 12, etc.
    - Structural abnormalities on chromosomes 1, 6, 17, etc.
  - Ependymoma associated with neurofibromatosis type 2 (NF2); deletions, translocations of chromosome 22
- Associated abnormalities
  - Subarachnoid hemorrhage (especially papillary type)
  - Superficial siderosis
  - NF2: Schwannomas, meningiomas

Staging, Grading, & Classification

- Currently, clinical utility of histologic grading is controversial and debated
  - WHO classification 2021 continues to recommend including information on histologic features (especially anaplasia extent) into integrated diagnosis
  - Most SP-EPNs are WHO grade 2 and, rarely, WHO grade 3 (anaplastic ependymoma)
- However, risk stratification based on distinct molecular ependymoma subtypes shown superior to histopathologic grading
- SP-MYCN defined by spinal localization and presence of *MYCN* amplification
  - Clinically aggressive ependymoma type, typically showing early metastases, rapid progression after relapse, leptomeningeal dissemination, and poor response to multimodal treatment strategies compared to SP-EPN

Gross Pathologic & Surgical Features

- Soft red or grayish purple mass
  - Small blood vessels on tumor surface
- Well circumscribed
  - May be encapsulated
- Cystic change common
- Hemorrhage at tumor periphery

Microscopic Features

- Immunohistochemistry: Positive for GFAP, S100, vimentin
- 4 histologic subtypes: Cellular, papillary, clear cell, tanycytic
  - Cellular most common intramedullary tumor subtype
  - Tanycytes: Precursors of astrocytes and ependymal cells
- Papillary, clear cell, and tanycytic morphologic variants are no longer listed as ependymoma subtypes
  - Instead listed as patterns in histopathologic description of ependymoma

CLINICAL ISSUES

Presentation

- Most common signs/symptoms
  - Neck or back pain
- Other signs/symptoms
  - Progressive paraparesis
  - Paresthesia
- Clinical profile
  - Delay in diagnosis due to slow tumor growth
    - Average duration of symptoms before diagnosis: 2.5 years

Demographics

- Age
  - Median of diagnosis: 41 years; range: 11-59 years
- Epidemiology
  - Ependymomas: 4% of all primary CNS neoplasms in adults
    - 30% of ependymomas are spinal
  - Most common primary spinal cord tumor in adults
    - 60% of primary spinal cord neoplasms
  - 2nd most common primary spinal cord tumor in children

Natural History & Prognosis

- Less preoperative neurologic deficit at presentation, better postoperative outcome
- Thoracic tumors have worse surgical outcome
- Metastasis rare
  - Lung, skin, kidney, lymph nodes
- 5-year survival: 85%

Treatment

- Surgical resection
  - Gross total resection in > 85% of cases
  - Very low risk of local and intracranial recurrence
- Radiotherapy for subtotal resection or recurrent disease
  - Typical doses of radiation therapy range from 4,000-5,400 cGy
  - No dose-response relationship

DIAGNOSTIC CHECKLIST

Image Interpretation Pearls

- Associated peripheral hemorrhage suggestive of cord ependymoma

SELECTED REFERENCES

1. Farooqi S et al: Clinical characteristics, management, and outcomes of intramedullary spinal cord ependymomas in adults: a systematic review. World Neurosurg. 173:237-50.e8, 2023
2. Zhang D et al: Clinical characteristics and treatment outcomes of long-level intramedullary spinal cord tumors: a consecutive series of 43 cases. Neurospine. 20(1):231-9, 2023
3. Kresbach C et al: Updates in the classification of ependymal neoplasms: the 2021 WHO classification and beyond. Wiley Online Library. Published March 21, 2022. Accessed January 17, 2024. https://onlinelibrary.wiley.com/doi/10.1111/bpa.13068
4. Pennington Z et al: Impact of tumor-associated syrinx on outcomes following resection of primary ependymomas of the spinal cord. J Neurooncol. 160(3):725-33, 2022
5. Louis DN et al: TheReferences 2021 WHO Classification of Tumors of the Central Nervous System: a summary. Neuro Oncol. 23(8):1231-51, 2021
6. Khalid SI et al: Pediatric spinal ependymomas: an epidemiologic study. World Neurosurg. 115:e119-28, 2018

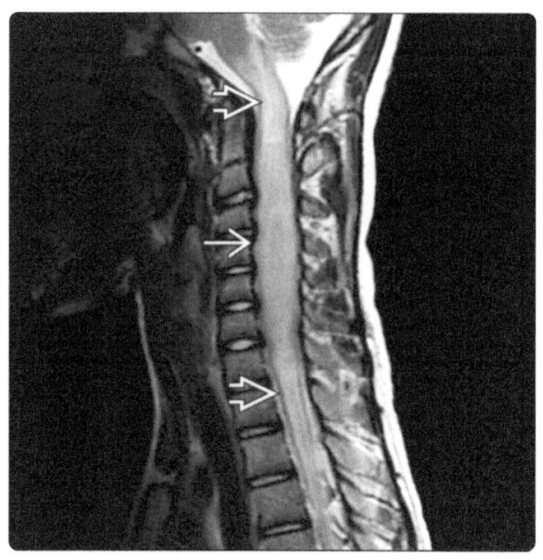

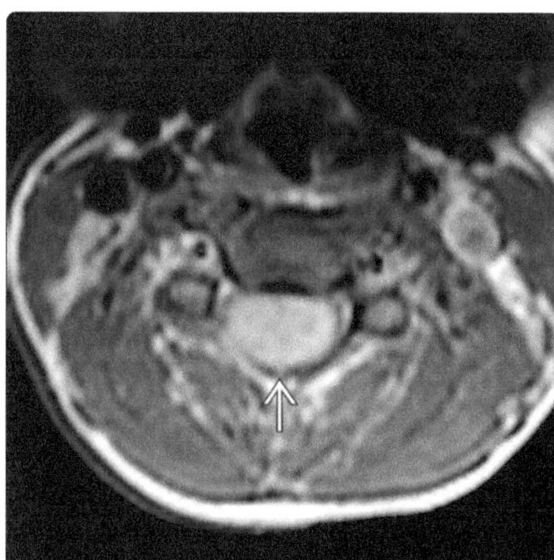

(Left) *Sagittal T2WI MR reveals marked fusiform enlargement of the cervical cord ➔ from the foramen magnum to the upper thoracic spine. Cord edema ➔ extends superiorly and inferiorly within the cord and brainstem. Note mild posterior vertebral scalloping.* **(Right)** *Axial T1WI C+ MR confirms avid intramedullary mass ➔ enhancement that nearly entirely fills the osseous spinal canal.*

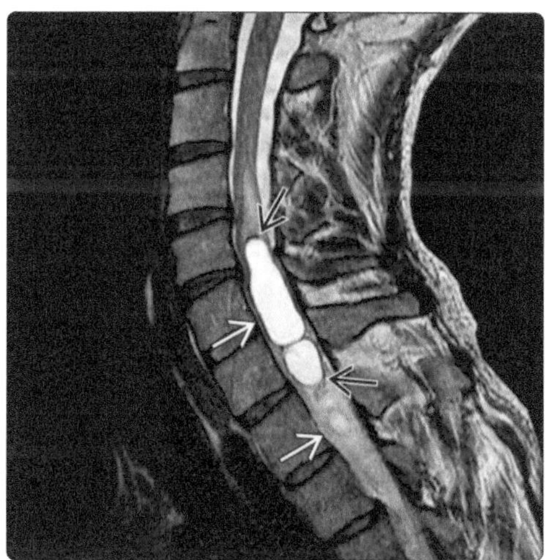

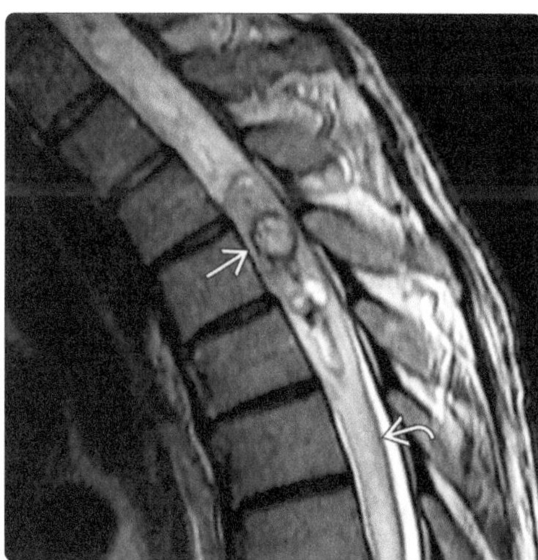

(Left) *Sagittal T2WI MR shows a large, heterogeneous, expansile mass ➔ involving the cervicothoracic spinal cord with cyst formation and low-signal hemosiderin ➔, reflecting prior hemorrhage capping the margins of the lesion.* **(Right)** *Sagittal T2WI MR depicts a large cord ependymoma ➔ with cyst formation and prior hemorrhage. Areas of low signal reflect hemosiderin deposition from prior hemorrhage. Note extensive caudal spinal cord edema ➔.*

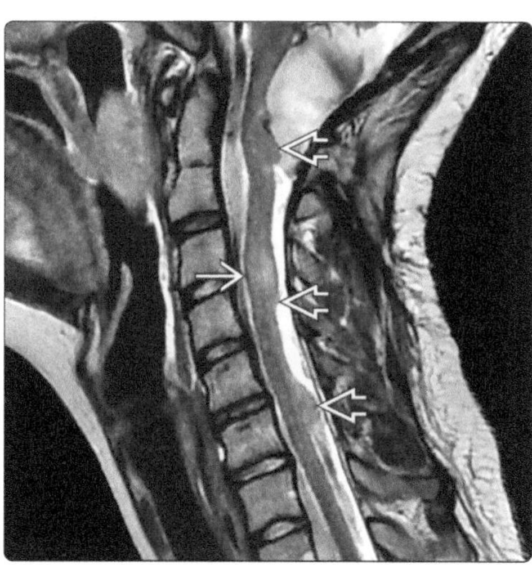

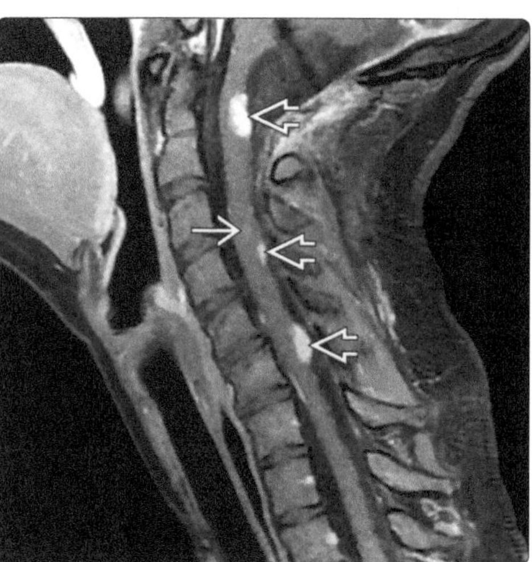

(Left) *Sagittal T2WI MR in a neurofibromatosis type 2 (NF2) patient with multiple inherited schwannomas, meningiomas, ependymomas (MISME), and prior surgeries for schwannoma resection shows a growing cervical hyperintense intramedullary mass ➔. Other surface masses represent schwannomata ➔.* **(Right)** *Sagittal T1WI C+ FS MR in the same NF2 patient shows minimal enhancement within the ependymoma ➔ but avid schwannoma enhancement ➔.*

KEY FACTS

TERMINOLOGY

- Hydromyelia, syringohydromyelia, syrinx

IMAGING

- Overlap between incidental (nonprogressive) & pathologic central canal dilation
  - Diameter of normal central canal can be up to 4 mm
  - Do not label central canal of 1-2 mm as syrinx
- Extent & morphology best demonstrated on T2 MR
  - Hyperintense intramedullary cavity ± adjacent gliosis, myelomalacia
  - Axial images more reliable for measurement
  - Carefully examine for features suggesting neoplastic or inflammatory etiology
    - Nodularity/mass, signal abnormality in adjacent cord
    - Give contrast if atypical features present

PATHOLOGY

- Lesions obstructing both central canal & subarachnoid space (SAS) can cause syrinx
  - Tumor, inflammation, Chiari 1 or 2
    - Up to 45% of primary spinal cord tumors have syrinx at presentation
- Posttraumatic or postinflammatory myelomalacia can lead to cavitation
- Majority of pediatric causes congenital
  - 10-15% of children with Chiari 1 present with syrinx

CLINICAL ISSUES

- Distal upper extremity weakness, gait instability
- Cloak-like pain & temperature sensory loss

DIAGNOSTIC CHECKLIST

- Image entire CNS for associated abnormalities

(Left) *The normal central canal has multiple small obstructions ⇒, but it also has small channels → that lead from the central canal to the subarachnoid space, allowing for the transmission of CSF between the 2 compartments. Because of this, flow must be impeded in both compartments for a syrinx to develop.* **(Right)** *Sagittal T2WI MR (Chiari 1) reveals a large holocord syringomyelia that effaces subarachnoid CSF and expands the cord filling the spinal canal.*

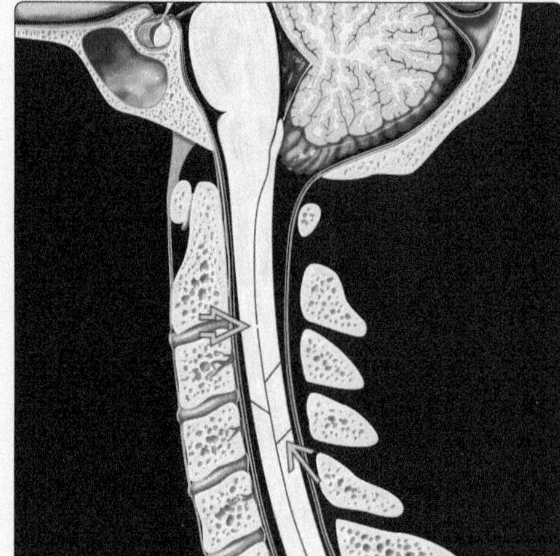

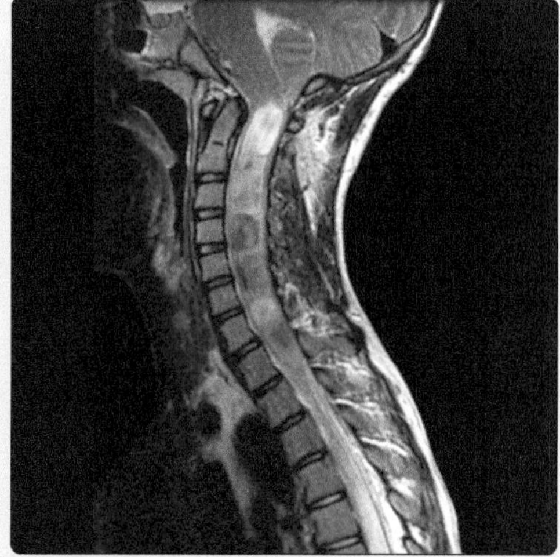

(Left) *Sagittal FIESTA MR in a patient with Dandy-Walker malformation and syringomyelia demonstrates a multiseptated syrinx in the cervical and upper thoracic spinal cord. A large posterior fossa cyst is postulated to produce aberrant CSF flow at the craniovertebral junction.* **(Right)** *Axial T2WI MR in the same patient reveals multiseptated dilation of the central spinal cord with parenchymal thinning, compatible with syringomyelia.*

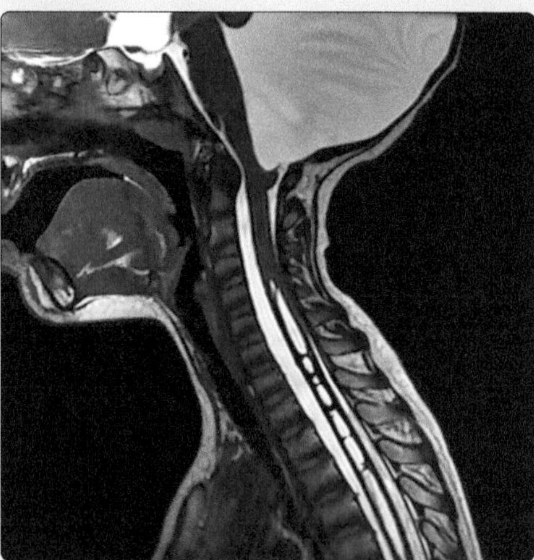

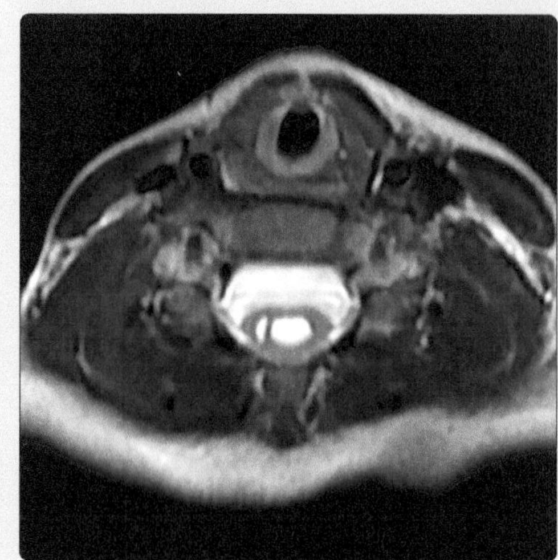

TERMINOLOGY

Definitions

- Hydromyelia: Cystic dilation of spinal cord central canal
- Syringomyelia: Cystic spinal cord cavity not contiguous with central canal
- Syringohydromyelia: Features of both syringomyelia & hydromyelia
- Syringobulbia: Extension of syrinx/cavity into brainstem
- Presyrinx state: Reversible spinal cord edema produced by alterations in CSF flow dynamics

IMAGING

General Features

- Location
  - Intramedullary spinal cord
  - Thoracic > cervicothoracic > cervical
- Size
  - Cavity diameter: Small → markedly dilated
  - Cavity length: Short segment (1 or 2 levels) to holocord

MR Findings

- T2WI
  - Hyperintense cystic intramedullary cavity ± adjacent gliosis, myelomalacia
  - ± flow artifact with poorly defined, heterogeneously hypointense signal throughout larger cavities
- T1WI C+
  - Simple syrinx does not enhance; enhancement suggests inflammatory or neoplastic lesion

Imaging Recommendations

- Best imaging tool
  - MR: Although syrinx may be seen on CT, extent & associated abnormalities best assessed by MR
- Protocol advice
  - Extent & morphology best demonstrated on T2WI
    - Axial plane most reliable for diameter measurement

DIFFERENTIAL DIAGNOSIS

Ventriculus Terminalis

- Asymptomatic (normal) dilation of terminal cord central canal only

Cystic Spinal Cord Tumor

- Cord expansion; cystic cavity surrounded by abnormal T2 signal, nodular enhancement

Myelomalacia

- Cord volume loss, gliosis
- No CSF signal cavitation on T1WI MR

PATHOLOGY

General Features

- Syringomyelia: Paracentral spinal cord cavitation lined by gliotic parenchyma independent of central canal
- Hydromyelia: Dilated ependymal-lined central canal
  - Spinal cord hydrocephalus
  - Central canal patency determines syrinx location, extent
- Presyrinx state
  - Reversible cervical spinal cord edema may precede syrinx development
  - Analogous to transependymal edema in brain
- Associated abnormalities
  - Congenital anomalies (frequent in children)
    - Chiari 1 (not always congenital)
      - 10-15% of children with Chiari 1 present with syrinx
    - Chiari 2
    - Dandy-Walker continuum
  - Scoliosis
  - Tumors
    - Up to 45% of primary spinal cord tumors have syrinx at presentation
      - Most common in hemangioblastoma, ependymoma

CLINICAL ISSUES

Presentation

- Distal upper extremity weakness, gait instability
- Cloak-like pain & temperature sensory loss
- May be asymptomatic

Natural History & Prognosis

- Variable; dependent on underlying etiology
  - Those associated with underlying malformations (Chiari 1 or 2, tethering lesions) more likely to progress
  - Spontaneous resolution rare

Treatment

- Suboccipital decompression can reverse/resolve syrinx associated with Chiari
- Consider syrinx drainage with indwelling catheter only if other efforts to restore normal cord CSF dynamics unsuccessful

DIAGNOSTIC CHECKLIST

Consider

- Image entire CNS for associated abnormalities
- Syrinx etiology influences treatment approach
- Distinction between syringomyelia & hydromyelia often not clinically relevant

Image Interpretation Pearls

- Do not label central canal of 1- to 2-mm diameter as syrinx
- Simple syringomyelia does not require contrast
  - Give contrast if associated cord signal abnormalities, complex morphology, focal mass, or off-midline location

SELECTED REFERENCES

1. Heiss JD: Cerebrospinal fluid hydrodynamics in Chiari I malformation and syringomyelia: modeling pathophysiology. Neurosurg Clin N Am. 34(1):81-90, 2023
2. Holste KG et al: Epidemiology of Chiari I malformation and syringomyelia. Neurosurg Clin N Am. 34(1):9-15, 2023
3. Spennato P et al: Fourth ventricle to spinal subarachnoid space stenting in pediatric patients with refractory syringomyelia: case series and systematic review. Neurosurg Rev. 46(1):67, 2023
4. Vinje V et al: Fluid dynamics in syringomyelia cavities: effects of heart rate, CSF velocity, CSF velocity waveform and craniovertebral decompression. Neuroradiol J. 31(5):482-9, 2018
5. Timpone VM et al: MRI of a syrinx: is contrast material always necessary? AJR Am J Roentgenol. 204(5):1082-5, 2015

KEY FACTS

TERMINOLOGY

- Intradural (juxtamedullary, subpial) or terminal lipoma

IMAGING

- Lipoma intimately associated with spinal cord (intradural) or distal cord/filum insertion (terminal)
- Lipoma follows fat signal intensity, density, and echogenicity

TOP DIFFERENTIAL DIAGNOSES

- Lipomyelocele/lipomyelomeningocele
- Filum fibrolipoma
- Dermoid cyst

PATHOLOGY

- Follows premature separation (premature disjunction) of cutaneous ectoderm from neuroectoderm during primary neurulation
  - Surrounding mesenchyme enters ependyma-lined central spinal canal, impedes neural tube closure → open placode
  - Mesenchyme differentiates into fat
- Skin closed over malformation (closed neural tube defect)

CLINICAL ISSUES

- Symptoms referable to lipoma level, presence of spinal cord compression
- Small lipomas may grow dramatically during infancy

DIAGNOSTIC CHECKLIST

- Profound hypodensity on CT myelography and T1 hyperintensity distinctively characteristic of lipoma
- Use chemical fat-saturation or inversion recovery MR technique to confirm fat content

(Left) *Axial graphic of the thoracic spine demonstrates incomplete closure of the dorsal spinal cord ➡ around a dorsal juxtamedullary conus lipoma ➡, encompassing the dorsal spinal nerve roots.* **(Right)** *Axial T1 MR performed in an infant with a dermal sinus tract (DST) (not shown here) reveals a dorsal conus lipoma ➡. This would be classified as type 1 using embryologic criteria given the presence of dural discontinuity and limited dysraphism associated with the DST. Note that the patient also has a solitary right kidney ➡.*

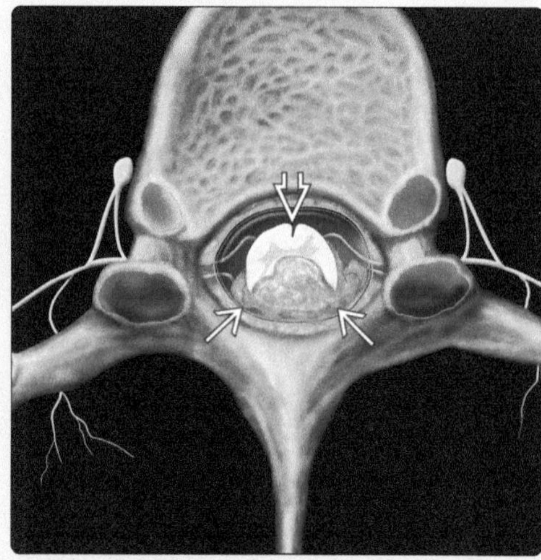

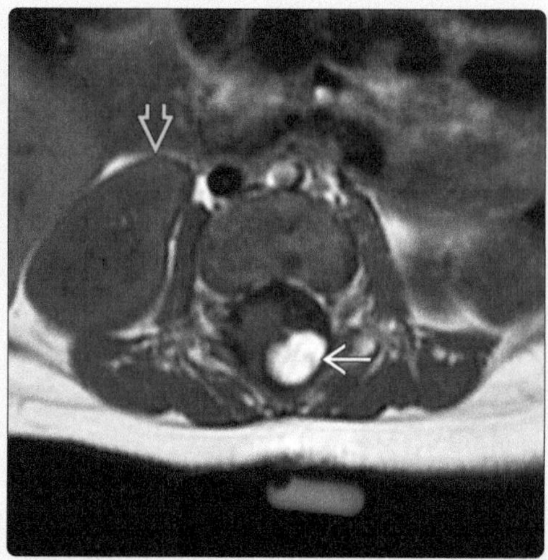

(Left) *Axial T2 MR in the same patient reveals signal intensity similar to subcutaneous fat with a prominent hypointense border on the right ➡ representing chemical shift artifact in the frequency encoding direction, strongly suggesting fat. There is no dysraphic defect.* **(Right)** *Axial T1 C+ FS MR in the same patient confirms complete signal loss with fat saturation ➡, confirming lipoma. The solitary right kidney enhances normally without hydronephrosis.*

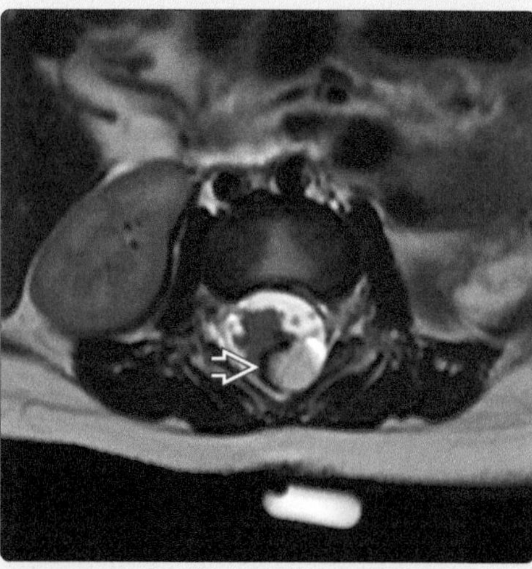

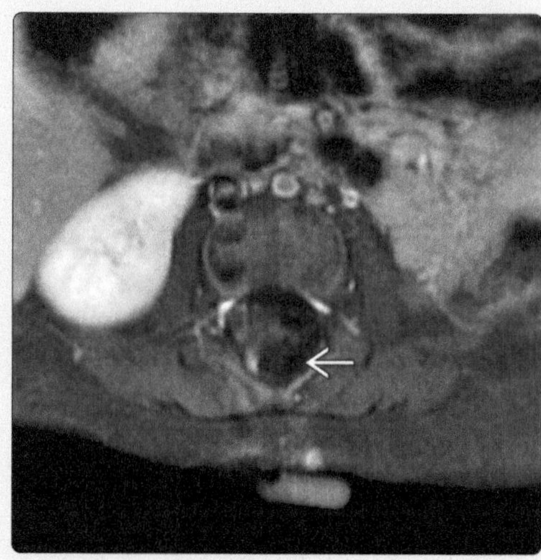

TERMINOLOGY

Synonyms

- Intradural (juxtamedullary, subpial) or terminal lipoma

Definitions

- Spinal lipoma intimately associated with spinal cord (intradural) or distal cord/filum insertion (terminal)

IMAGING

General Features

- Best diagnostic clue
  - T1-hyperintense intradural mass
- Location
  - Intradural
    - Thoracic (30%) > cervicothoracic (24%) > cervical (12%) > lumbosacral spine
    - Dorsal (73%) > lateral/anterolateral (25%) > anterior (2%)
  - Terminal
    - Lumbosacral
- Size
  - Range: Tiny → huge
- Morphology
  - Wide spectrum of lesions ranging from simple filum lipomas → complex malformations

Radiographic Findings

- Radiography
  - Intradural lipoma
    - Hypodense mass ± dysraphism; posterior elements generally intact but show focal canal widening 2° to bony erosion
  - Terminal lipoma
    - Hypodense mass ± posterior dysraphism

CT Findings

- NECT
  - Intradural lipoma: Focal, lobulated, hypodense intradural mass ± central canal, neural foraminal widening at lipoma level
  - Terminal lipoma: Elongated, hypodense mass at filum termination; may extend into subcutaneous fat through dysraphic defect

MR Findings

- T1WI
  - Intradural lipoma
    - Lobulated, ovoid/rounded, hyperintense intradural mass intimately associated with cord
    - ± canal widening, local dysraphism
    - ↓ signal intensity on fat-saturation sequences
  - Terminal lipoma
    - Hyperintense mass attached to distal cord/filum; extends through lumbosacral dysraphism → subcutaneous fat
    - Thin, "stretched" cord usually tethered ± syrinx
- T2WI
  - Similar signal intensity, imaging appearance to T1WI
  - ± spinal cord compression (intradural) → hyperintense cord signal
- STIR
  - ↓ signal intensity confirms fat
- T1WI C+
  - No lipoma enhancement

Ultrasonographic Findings

- Grayscale ultrasound
  - Echogenic intraspinal mass ± reduced conus motion

Imaging Recommendations

- Best imaging tool
  - Multiplanar MR
- Protocol advice
  - Ultrasound in infants for screening; confirm with MR if positive
  - Sagittal, axial T1WI MR to define extent of lipoma(s) and relationship to neural placode, adjacent tissues

DIFFERENTIAL DIAGNOSIS

Lipomyelocele/Lipomyelomeningocele

- Skin-covered (closed) neural placode-lipoma complex contiguous with subcutaneous fat through dysraphic defect
- Mass often palpable ± cutaneous stigmata

Filum Fibrolipoma

- Common (4-6% of population); mostly asymptomatic but symptomatic patients present with "tethered cord"
- Hyperintense/hypodense mass in filum ± tethering, low-lying conus
- Prophylactic detethering low risk but necessity remains debated

Dermoid Cyst

- Mixed-density/signal-intensity mass; lack of homogeneous hyperintensity ± dermal sinus help to distinguish

PATHOLOGY

General Features

- Etiology
  - Arise from premature separation (disjunction) of cutaneous ectoderm from neuroectoderm during primary neurulation
    - Surrounding mesenchyme enters ependyma-lined central spinal canal, impeding closure of neural folds → open placode
    - Mesenchyme differentiates into fat
    - Similar mechanism (nondisjunction) → dermal sinus tract; explains their frequent association
- Associated abnormalities
  - Intradural lipoma: ± localized dysraphism at lipoma level; segmentation anomalies rare
  - Terminal lipoma: Sacral hypogenesis, anorectal malformations, GU malformations (5-10%), terminal diastematomyelia, epidermoid, dermal sinus, angioma, arachnoid cyst
    - Sacral anomalies much more likely if GU, anorectal malformations present (≥ 90%)

Staging, Grading, & Classification

- Traditional classification divides into intradural and terminal lipomatous malformations
  - Ambiguous and confusing; many lipomatous malformations fall along spectrum between lipoma and lipomyelomeningocele
  - Intradural lipoma
    - Partially encapsulated sessile (55%) or exophytic (45%) juxtamedullary fatty mass entirely enclosed within dural sac
    - Midline spinal cord "open"; subpial lipoma nestled between open lips
  - Terminal lipoma
    - Delicately encapsulated fatty mass attached to cord/filum; frequently contiguous with subcutaneous fat through dorsal lumbosacral dysraphism
    - Cord almost always tethered; stretched and thinned ± hydrosyringomyelia (20%)
- Classification scheme dividing lipomas into 2 groups of lipomatous malformations based on presence or absence of dural defect (2009)
  - Better accounts for differences in embryology, clinical presentation, operative findings, complications, and prognosis than traditional classification
  - Lipomas without dural defect
    - Filum lipoma, caudal lipoma without dural defect, intramedullary lipoma
  - Lipomas with dural defect
    - Dorsal lipoma, caudal lipoma with dural defect, transitional lipoma, lipomyelocele, lipomyelomeningocele
- Classification of spinal lipoma types based on embryologic stage (2017)
  - Type 1: Pure primary neurulation failure with dorsal posterior elements/dural defect
  - Type 2: Ranges primary to secondary neurulation failure with posterior elements/dural defect
  - Type 3: Secondary neurulation failure, early phase with intact posterior elements/dura
  - Type 4: Secondary neurulation failure, late phase with lipoma confined to filum

Gross Pathologic & Surgical Features

- Composed of normal fat
  - Fat cells ↑ in size considerably during infancy; tiny lipomas in neonates may grow substantially during infancy
  - Conversely, lipomas ↓ in size if patient loses weight

Microscopic Features

- Homogeneous mass of mature fat separated into globules by strands of fibrous tissue
  - ± calcification, ossification, muscle fibers, nerves, glial tissue, arachnoid, ependyma

CLINICAL ISSUES

Presentation

- Most common signs/symptoms
  - Cervical, thoracic intradural lipoma: Slow ascending mono- or paraparesis, spasticity, cutaneous sensory loss, deep sensory loss
  - Lumbosacral intradural lipoma: Flaccid lower extremity paralysis, sphincter dysfunction
  - Terminal lipoma: Bowel/bladder dysfunction, lower extremity weakness/sensory abnormality, foot deformity, scoliosis
- Other signs/symptoms
  - Symptoms may be exacerbated by pregnancy
- Clinical profile
  - Intradural lipoma: Patient complains of weakness and sensory anomalies referable to lesion level
    - Overlying skin usually looks normal; no cutaneous stigmata
  - Terminal lipoma: Patient presents with clinical appearance of "tethered cord" syndrome and (frequently) cutaneous stigmata

Demographics

- Age
  - 3 age peaks for presentation
    - < 5 years (24%)
    - 2nd → 3rd decades (55%)
    - 5th decade (16%)
- Sex
  - Intradural: M ≤ F
  - Terminal: M < F

Natural History & Prognosis

- Small lipomas may grow dramatically during infancy
  - Spinal lipomas rapidly ↑ in volume before 3 months of age and especially in infants < 1 month old
  - Closely correlates with physiologic growth of normal subcutaneous fat
- Symptomatic patients unlikely to improve spontaneously without intervention

Treatment

- Surgical resection, untethering of cord (if applicable)

DIAGNOSTIC CHECKLIST

Consider

- Follow-up even small lipomas in neonates; these may grow significantly

Image Interpretation Pearls

- Profound hypodensity on CT myelography and T1 hyperintensity distinctively characteristic of lipoma
- Use chemical fat-saturation or inversion recovery MR technique to confirm fat content

SELECTED REFERENCES

1. Aby JL et al: Management of asymptomatic cutaneous lumbosacral findings in newborns: a neurosurgical perspective. J Neurosurg Pediatr. 31(5):484-7, 2023
2. De Vloo P et al: Radical resection of lumbosacral lipomas in children: the Great Ormond Street Hospital experience. Childs Nerv Syst. 38(6):1113-23, 2022
3. Yoshifuji K et al: Physiological rapid growth of spinal lipoma in the early postnatal period. J Neurosurg Pediatr. 1-9, 2022
4. Seki T et al: Surgical outcomes of pediatric patients with asymptomatic tethered cord syndrome. Asian Spine J. 12(3):551-5, 2018
5. Morota N et al: New classification of spinal lipomas based on embryonic stage. J Neurosurg Pediatr. 19(4):428-39, 2017

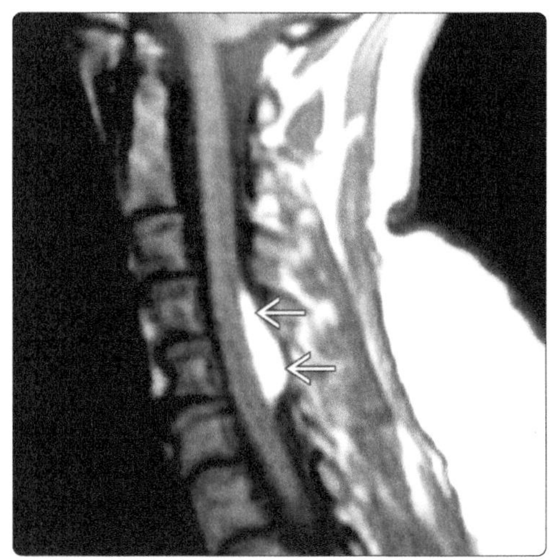

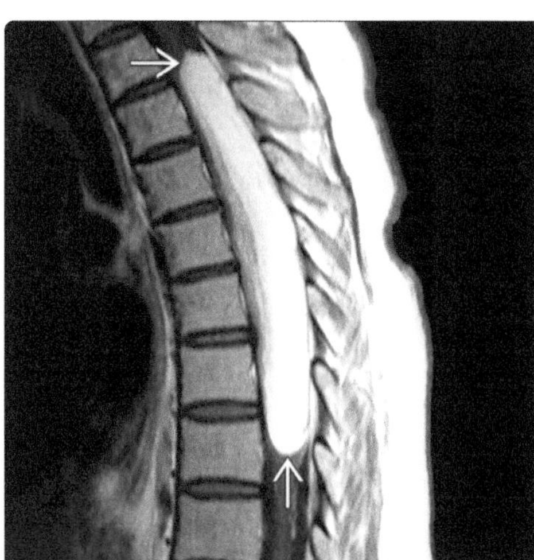

(Left) *Sagittal T1WI MR reveals a classic intradural subpial lipoma ➡ adherent to the dorsal cervical spinal cord. Note that there is very subtle remodeling and enlargement of the osseous spinal canal at the lipoma level.* **(Right)** *Sagittal T1WI MR demonstrates a well-delineated, hyperintense mass ➡ situated along the dorsal surface of the thoracic spinal cord. These findings are classic for a subpial spinal cord lipoma.*

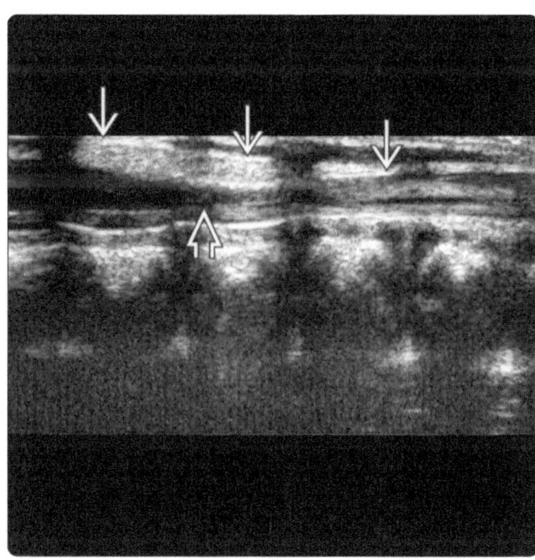

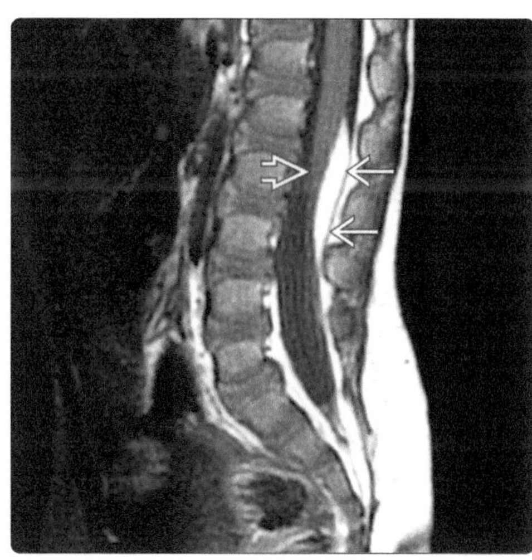

(Left) *Lateral lumbar grayscale real-time ultrasound demonstrates an echogenic dorsal intradural mass ➡ representing a juxtamedullary (subpial) lipoma tethering the low-lying conus tip ➡ at the L3 level.* **(Right)** *Sagittal T1WI MR in the same patient demonstrates a large intradural juxtamedullary (subpial) conus lipoma ➡ intimately associated with the abnormally low-lying conus ➡ at the L3 level.*

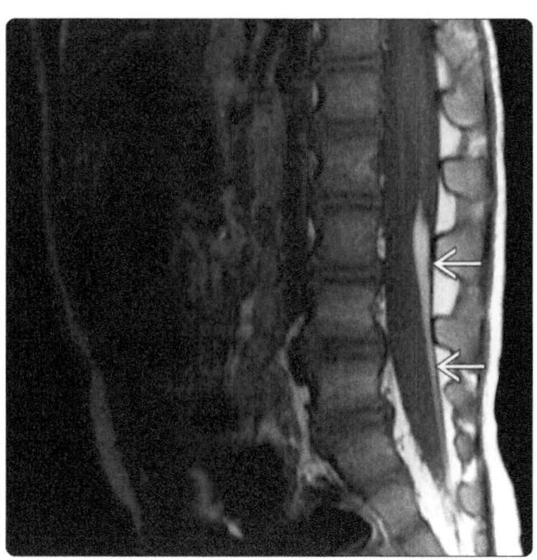

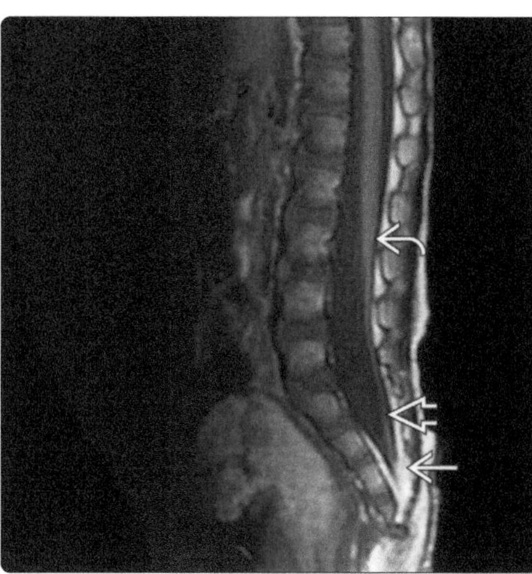

(Left) *Sagittal T1WI MR demonstrates a thick filum lipoma ➡ with low-lying spinal cord terminating at L2/L3.* **(Right)** *Sagittal T1WI MR demonstrates elongation of the low-lying spinal cord conus ➡, terminating at the L4 level. The thickened filum terminale ➡ is fatty infiltrated caudally and inserts into a small terminal lipoma ➡. Note the hypoplastic sacrum reflecting the caudal regression spectrum.*

Epidural Lipomatosis

KEY FACTS

TERMINOLOGY

- Excessive accumulation of intraspinal fat causing cord compression and neurologic deficits

IMAGING

- Over multiple vertebral segments
- Thoracic spine: 58-61%
  - T6-T8, dorsal to spinal cord
  - Epidural fat ≥ 7 mm thick
- Lumbar spine: 39-42%
  - L4-L5, surrounding thecal sac
- Y-shaped configuration to lumbar thecal sac on axial imaging
- Mass effect on thecal sac and nerve roots
- Follows fat signal intensity on all sequences
  - Fat suppression to confirm adipose tissue, exclude blood products

TOP DIFFERENTIAL DIAGNOSES

- Subacute epidural hematoma
- Spinal angiolipoma
- Epidural metastasis
- Epidural abscess

PATHOLOGY

- Exogenous or endogenous steroids
- General obesity
- Idiopathic

CLINICAL ISSUES

- Gradual progression of symptoms
- Weakness: > 85%
- Back pain, sensory loss, polyradiculopathy, altered reflexes, incontinence, ataxia

DIAGNOSTIC CHECKLIST

- Most cases associated with exogenous corticosteroid usage

(Left) *Sagittal graphic illustrates confluent abundant dorsal epidural fat ➡ within the dorsal thoracic canal, producing effacement of the dorsal thecal sac and mild mass effect on the ventrally displaced spinal cord.* **(Right)** *Sagittal T1WI MR in a 31-month-old with autonomic dysfunction on corticosteroids reveals neuromuscular kyphosis and exuberant epidural fat ➡ that narrows the spinal canal.*

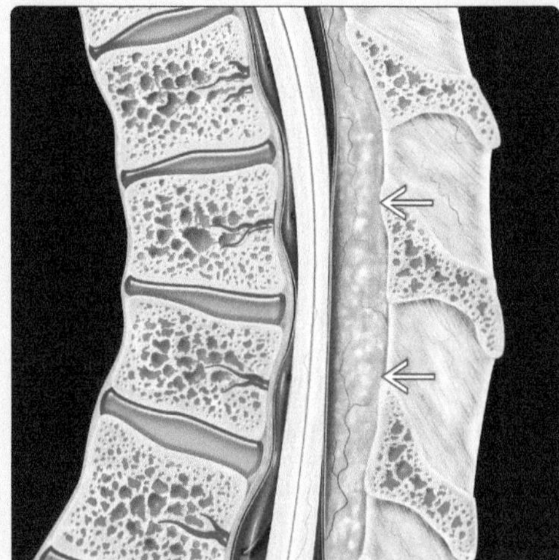

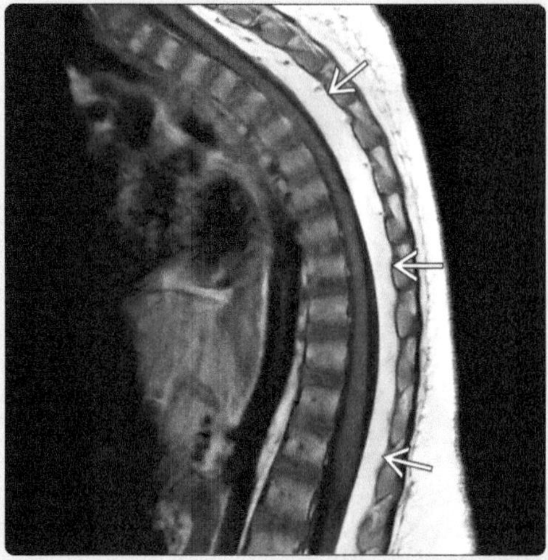

(Left) *Sagittal STIR MR in the same patient reveals signal loss in the epidural fat, compatible with epidural lipomatosis.* **(Right)** *Axial T2WI MR in the same patient confirms dorsal epidural localization of fat ➡ that narrows the central spinal canal and displaces the dura and spinal cord ➡ anteriorly.*

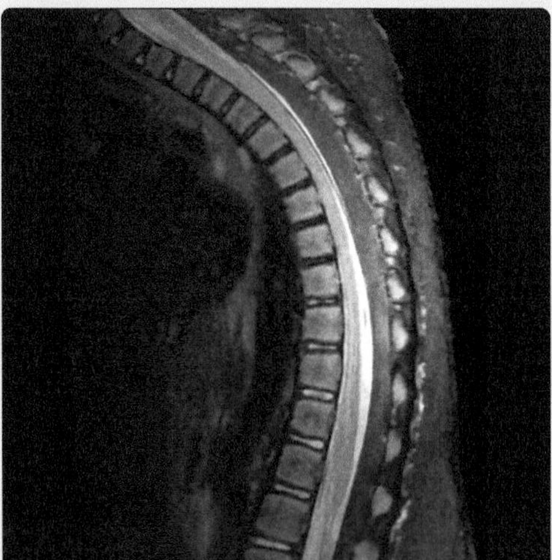

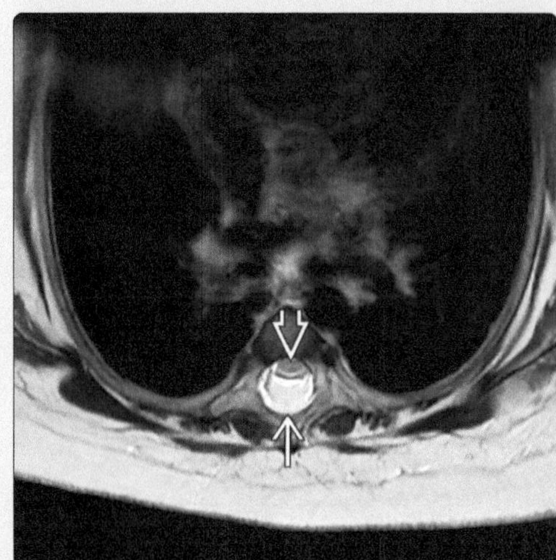

TERMINOLOGY

Definitions

- Excessive accumulation of intraspinal fat causing cord compression and neurologic deficits

IMAGING

General Features

- Best diagnostic clue
  - Abundant epidural fat in midthoracic and distal lumbar spinal canal compressing thecal sac
- Location
  - Thoracic spine: 58-61%
    - T6-T8, dorsal to spinal cord
  - Lumbar spine: 39-42%
    - L4-L5, surrounding thecal sac
- Size
  - Epidural fat ≥ 7 mm thick in thoracic spine
  - Over multiple vertebral segments
- Morphology
  - Y-shaped configuration to lumbar thecal sac on axial imaging

CT Findings

- ↑ fat in spinal canal
- Compression of cord or thecal sac
- No abnormal enhancement
- No osseous erosion

MR Findings

- Mass effect on dural sac, nerve roots
  - Obliterated CSF, cord compression, crowded cauda equina
- Epidural mass follows fat signal intensity on all sequences
- No abnormal enhancement

Imaging Recommendations

- Best imaging tool
  - Sagittal and axial T1 MR
- Protocol advice
  - Use fat suppression to confirm adipose tissue, exclude blood products

DIFFERENTIAL DIAGNOSIS

Subacute Epidural Hematoma

- Acute onset of symptoms
- High signal intensity on T1WI persists on fat-suppressed sequences

Spinal Angiolipoma

- Benign neoplasm with adipose and vascular elements
- Focal, rounded mass
- Infiltrative type invades surrounding bone
- Usually ↓ signal relative to fat on T1 MR, ↑ on STIR MR
  - Attributed to vascular component
- Contrast enhancement of nonlipomatous component

Epidural Metastasis

- Low signal intensity on T1 MR, intermediate to high signal intensity on T2 MR, STIR
- Contrast enhancement of mass

Epidural Abscess

- Hypointense on T1 MR, hyperintense on T2 MR
- Diffuse or peripheral contrast enhancement

PATHOLOGY

General Features

- Etiology
  - Long-term exogenous steroid administration most common
  - Excessive endogenous steroid production
    - Cushing disease
    - Pituitary prolactinoma
  - General obesity
  - Idiopathic
  - Metabolic syndrome association
- Associated abnormalities
  - Vertebral compression fractures
    - Steroid-related osteoporosis

Microscopic Features

- Histologically normal unencapsulated adipose tissue within epidural space

CLINICAL ISSUES

Presentation

- Most common signs/symptoms
  - Weakness: > 85%
- Other signs/symptoms
  - Back pain, sensory loss, polyradiculopathy, altered reflexes, incontinence, ataxia
- Clinical profile
  - Gradual progression of symptoms

Demographics

- Uncommon; most commonly seen in middle-aged patients (M > F)

Natural History & Prognosis

- Presurgical low steroid dose and idiopathic cases have better prognosis
- > 80% with postsurgical symptomatic relief

Treatment

- Correction of underlying endocrinopathies
- Weight reduction in case of general obesity
- Multilevel laminectomy and fusion
  - Indicated when cord compression and radiculopathy present

SELECTED REFERENCES

1. D'Agostino V et al: Could spinal epidural lipomatosis be the hallmark of metabolic syndrome on the spine? A literature review with emphasis on etiology. Diagnostics (Basel). 13(2):322, 2023
2. Alomari S et al: Etiologies and outcomes of spinal epidural lipomatosis: systematic review of the literature and meta-analysis of reported cases. Clin Spine Surg. 35(9):383-7, 2022
3. Walker PB et al: Spinal epidural lipomatosis: a comprehensive review. Orthop Rev (Pavia). 13(2):25571, 2021
4. Ishihara S et al: Spinal epidural lipomatosis is a previously unrecognized manifestation of metabolic syndrome. Spine J. 19(3):493-500, 2018
5. Papastefan ST et al: Management of idiopathic spinal epidural lipomatosis: a case report and review of the literature. Childs Nerv Syst. 34(4):757-63, 2018

Extramedullary Hematopoiesis

KEY FACTS

TERMINOLOGY

- Epidural ± paravertebral proliferation of hematopoietic tissue in response to profound chronic anemia
- Minimally enhancing isointense thoracic intra- or paraspinal masses with associated diffuse marrow hypointensity

IMAGING

- Midthoracic > cervical, lumbar
- Bilateral (a)symmetrically widened paraspinal soft tissues
- ± rib, clavicle medullary expansion
- Look for spinal cord displacement and compression

TOP DIFFERENTIAL DIAGNOSES

- Epidural/paraspinal metastasis
- Spinal epidural lymphoma
- Paravertebral phlegmon/abscess
- Peripheral nerve sheath tumor
- Epidural hematoma

PATHOLOGY

- Ectopic hematopoietic rests stimulated in response to chronic anemic states
  - Intermediate β-thalassemia: Most common
  - Sickle cell anemia
  - Polycythemia vera
  - Myelofibrosis with myeloid metaplasia

CLINICAL ISSUES

- Asymptomatic
- Back ± radicular pain
- Overall, prognosis limited by underlying hemoglobinopathy or myeloproliferative disorder

DIAGNOSTIC CHECKLIST

- Consider spinal extramedullary hematopoiesis (EMH) for thoracic epidural/paraspinal isointense masses in patients with hemoglobinopathies or myeloproliferative disorders

(Left) *Sagittal graphic of extramedullary hematopoiesis (EMH) depicts abundant hematopoietic marrow in lumbar vertebrae, extending into the prevertebral ➡ and dorsal epidural space ⇨.* **(Right)** *Sagittal T2 MR of the spine and paraspinal tissues (thalassemia) demonstrates abnormal marrow signal and intermediate signal deposits of EMH ⇨ breaking through the vertebral bodies into the epidural space.*

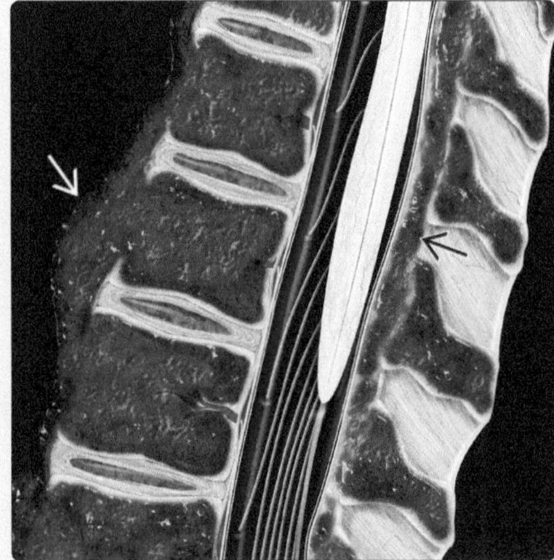

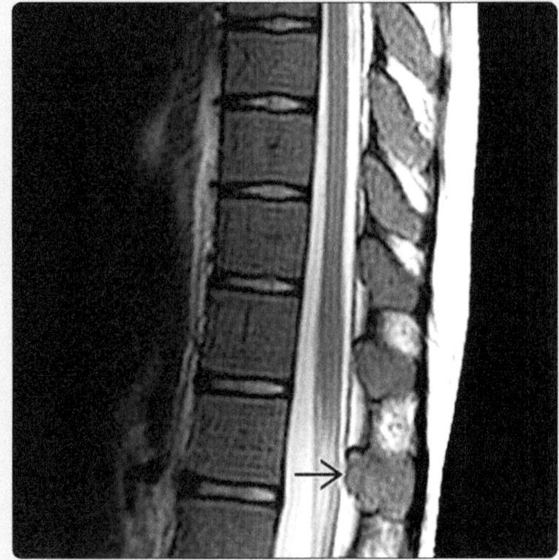

(Left) *Axial T1 MR reveals bilateral paraspinal foci of EMH originating in the ribs ➡, breaking through the vertebral bodies into the neural foramina ➡.* **(Right)** *Coronal T1 C+ FS MR of the thoracic spine and paraspinal tissues in the same patient demonstrates large, symmetric deposits of EMH ➡ extending from the ribs. No extension into the spinal canal is demonstrated on this image.*

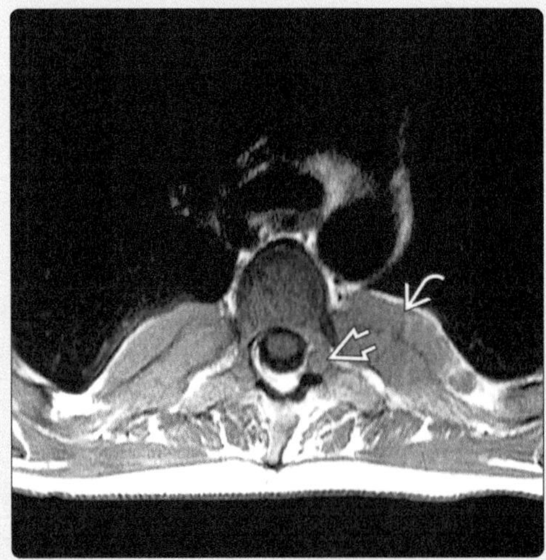

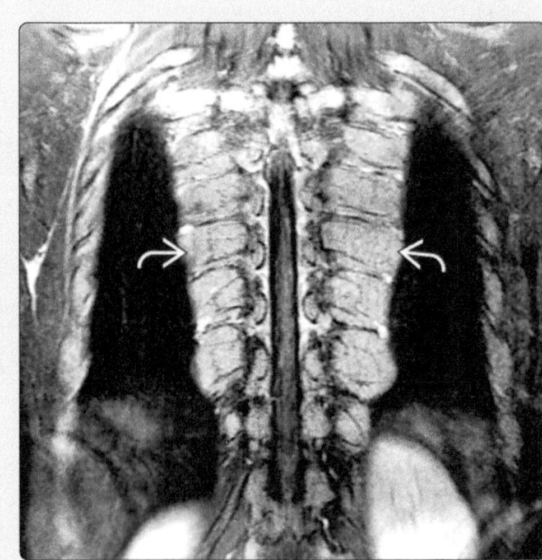

TERMINOLOGY

Abbreviations

- Extramedullary hematopoiesis (EMH)

Definitions

- Epidural ± paravertebral proliferation of hematopoietic tissue in response to profound chronic anemia

IMAGING

General Features

- Best diagnostic clue
  - Minimally enhancing isointense thoracic intra- or paraspinal masses with associated diffuse marrow hypointensity
- Location
  - Midthoracic > cervical, lumbar
    - Epidural, paravertebral
- Size
  - Multisegmental
- Morphology
  - Well circumscribed
  - Homogeneous and lobular soft tissue mass

Radiographic Findings

- Radiography
  - Bilateral (a)symmetrically widened paraspinal stripe on frontal radiograph
  - ± rib, clavicle medullary expansion

CT Findings

- NECT
  - Soft tissue density
  - Central canal narrowing
  - Cord displacement and compression
  - ± rib, clavicle medullary expansion
- CECT
  - Mild enhancement
- Bone CT
  - No bony erosions or calcifications

MR Findings

- T1WI
  - Isointense to cord
- T2WI
  - Isointense to mildly hyperintense to cord
    - Hypointensity may represent ↑ iron content in hematopoietic tissue
- STIR
  - Iso- to hyperintense
- T1WI C+
  - Minimal, mild, or moderate
- Variable mass effect on spinal cord
  - Cord compression most commonly reported with β-thalassemia
  - Intramedullary T2 hyperintensity may be present
    - Edema or myelomalacia
- Nerve root compression
- Diffuse vertebral marrow T1 hypointensity on all sequences

Nonvascular Interventions

- Myelography
  - Nonspecific hypodense epidural mass effacing central canal
  - Vertebrae are enlarged and translucent ~ 86% in one report

Nuclear Medicine Findings

- Technetium sulfur colloid scan
  - Foci of epidural/paraspinal uptake correspond to EMH

Imaging Recommendations

- Best imaging tool
  - Sagittal, axial T2WI, T1WI, T1 C+ MR

DIFFERENTIAL DIAGNOSIS

Epidural/Paraspinal Metastasis

- Extension from adjacent vertebral lesions
  - Posterior cortex typically involved
    - High intensity on STIR
  - Compression fractures
- Isolated epidural/paraspinal disease sparing spinal column rare
- Moderate enhancement invariably present

Spinal Epidural Lymphoma

- Isointense to cord on T1WI
  - Iso- to hyperintense on T2WI
- Intense, homogeneous postgadolinium enhancement
- ± adjacent vertebral involvement
- ± diffuse marrow hypointensity

Paravertebral Phlegmon/Abscess

- Associated with infectious spondylitis
  - Destructive changes in adjacent vertebrae
- Hyperintense on STIR
  - Especially liquefied components
- Diffuse (phlegmon) or peripheral (abscess) enhancement

Peripheral Nerve Sheath Tumor

- Often at single level
- Multiple neurofibromas in neurofibromatosis type 1
- Isointense to cord on T1WI, ↑ signal on T2WI
- Avid postcontrast enhancement
- Widened intervertebral foramina

Epidural Hematoma

- Often hyperintense on T1WI
- Iso- to hypointense on T2WI
- ± postgadolinium enhancement
- Sudden onset of symptoms

PATHOLOGY

General Features

- Etiology
  - Ectopic hematopoietic rests stimulated in response to chronic anemic states
    - Intermediate β-thalassemia: Most common
      - Transfusion independent because of compensatory mechanisms of bone marrow
    - Sickle cell anemia

- Polycythemia vera
- Myelofibrosis with myeloid metaplasia
- Source of extravertebral hematopoiesis controversial
  - Stimulation of embryonic multipleuritant hematopoietic stem cells in epidural space
  - Direct extension of hematopoietic marrow from vertebrae into epidural space
  - Fetal hematopoietic capacity of dura
  - Embolic phenomenon
- Associated abnormalities
  - Marrow expansion in ribs
  - Small infarcted spleen in patients with sickle cell disease
    - Splenomegaly in thalassemia
  - Hemothorax with paraspinal EMH
  - Labs: Chronic microcytosis hemolytic anemia
- Compensatory mechanism when normal marrow insufficient to meet circulatory demands in chronic anemia
- Common sites of EMH: Liver, spleen, lymph nodes
  - Uncommon sites: Retroperitoneal tissue, kidneys, adrenal area, paravertebral region, thymus, breasts, sweat glands, pleura, prostate, broad ligaments
  - Unusual sites: Peripheral nerves and cranial dura matter
  - Sites of fetal hematopoiesis

Gross Pathologic & Surgical Features

- Discrete, flesh-colored mass

Microscopic Features

- Resembles bone marrow on biopsy
  - Trilineage hematopoiesis
    - Erythroid and granulocytic precursors, megakaryocytes

CLINICAL ISSUES

Presentation

- Most common signs/symptoms
  - Asymptomatic
  - Back ± radicular pain
  - Other signs/symptoms
    - Paraparesis
    - Sensory deficit
    - Gait disturbance
    - Bladder, bowel dysfunction
    - Diminished deep tendon reflexes
    - Anemia, pancytopenia
- Clinical profile
  - Cord compression from epidural EMH should be suspected in patients with chronic anemia who present with neurologic complaints

Demographics

- Age
  - More common in adults
    - 3rd-4th decades
- Ethnicity
  - Some hemoglobinopathies more common in certain ethnic groups
    - Sickle cell disease: African Americans
    - Thalassemia: Races along Eastern Mediterranean Sea (Greek, Italian, Persian, etc.)
  - Myeloproliferative disorders: No ethnic predilection
- Epidemiology
  - Spinal involvement most common after hepatosplenic EMH
    - Spinal EMH: 27% of nonhepatosplenic involvement
    - Intraspinal EMH occurs in 11-15% of patients with thalassemia

Natural History & Prognosis

- Excellent prognosis: Resolution of symptoms 3-7 days after radiotherapy
  - Overall, prognosis limited by underlying hemoglobinopathy or myeloproliferative disorder

Treatment

- Intravenous steroids
  - ↓ cord edema
- Radiation therapy
  - Ectopic hematopoietic tissue extremely radiosensitive
  - Alone or in conjunction with surgery
  - Risk of marrow suppression
    - May be stimulus for further EMH
- Decompressive laminectomy with surgical resection
  - Indicated when significant myelopathy present
- Transfusions
  - When radiation or surgery contraindicated
  - Hematopoietic tissues regress as stress of anemia relieved
  - Frequent recurrences
- Hydroxyurea
  - ↑ production of hemoglobin-F
  - Role in myelosuppression
- Fetal hemoglobin-inducing agents that decrease hematopoietic drive

DIAGNOSTIC CHECKLIST

Image Interpretation Pearls

- Consider spinal EMH for thoracic epidural/paraspinal isointense masses in patients with hemoglobinopathies or myeloproliferative disorders

SELECTED REFERENCES

1. Ganapathi SS et al: Extramedullary hematopoiesis in the dura mater during treatment of a CNS embryonal tumor. J Pediatr Hematol Oncol. 43(8):e1217-9, 2021
2. Xue JY et al: Expanding the phenotypic spectrum of TNFRSF11A-associated dysosteosclerosis: a case with intracranial extramedullary hematopoiesis. J Hum Genet. 66(6):607-11, 2021
3. Darole P et al: Unusual presentation of extramedullary haematopoiesis in a young boy. BMJ Case Rep. 12(3), 2019
4. Fareed S et al: Spinal cord compression secondary to extramedullary hematopoiesis: a rareness in a young adult with thalassemia major. Acta Biomed. 88(2):237-42, 2017
5. Hisamud-Din N et al: Incomplete paraplegia caused by extramedullary hematopoiesis in a patient with thalassemia intermedia. Spinal Cord Ser Cases. 3:17020, 2017
6. Soman S et al: A case report of extramedullary haematopoeisis in lumbosacral region presenting as cauda equina syndrome. Int J Spine Surg. 10:25, 2016
7. Ruo Redda MG et al: Complete recovery from paraparesis in spinal cord compression due to extramedullary haemopoiesis in beta-thalassaemia by emergency radiation therapy. Intern Med J. 44(4):409-12, 2014
8. Ghieda U et al: Progressive spinal cord compression due to epidural extramedullary hematopoiesis in thalassemia intermedia. A case report and literature review. Neuroradiol J. 26(1):111-7, 2013

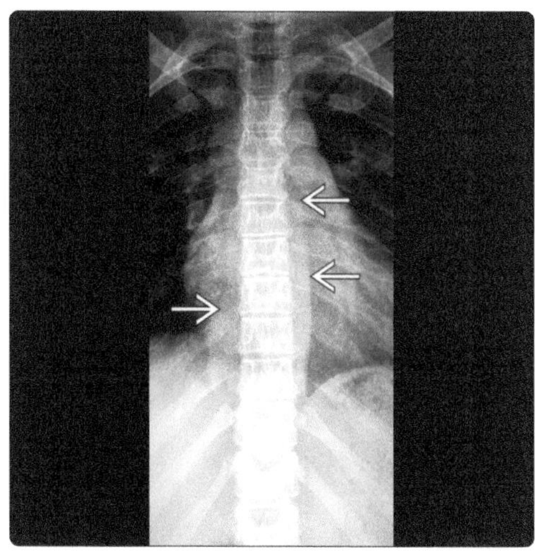

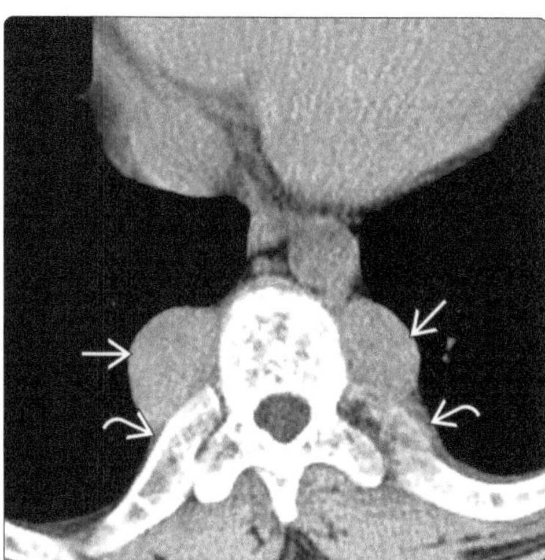

(Left) *Anteroposterior radiograph of the thoracic spine demonstrates the typical appearance of EMH presenting as bilateral, paraspinal, masses with widened bilateral paraspinal stripes* ➡*.* **(Right)** *Axial NECT through the lower thoracic spine in the same patient confirms the presence of large bilateral paraspinal soft tissue masses* ➡ *with medullary expansion of vertebra and ribs* ➡*.*

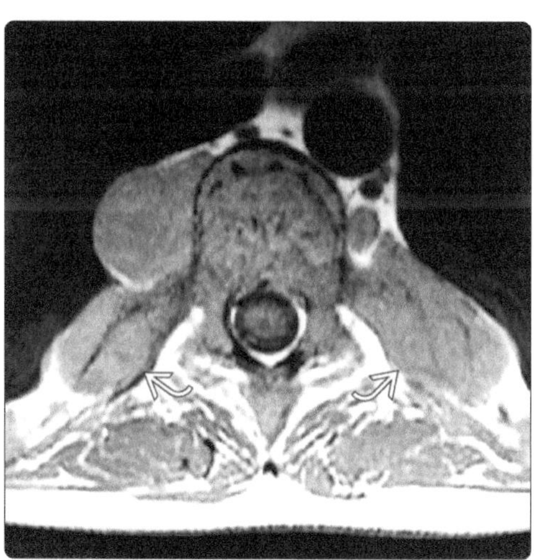

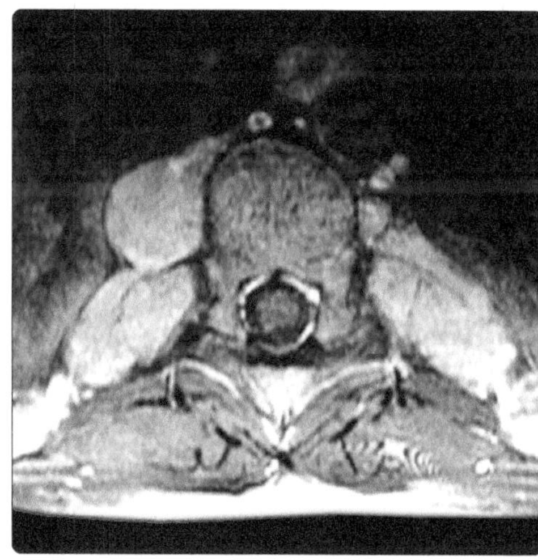

(Left) *Axial T1 MR in a chronically anemic patient with β-thalassemia reveals large, bilateral paraspinal masses that are isointense to the spinal cord. Bilateral rib marrow expansion* ➡ *is also evident.* **(Right)** *Axial T1 C+ MR in the same patient demonstrates moderate enhancement of the bilateral, paraspinal EMH masses.*

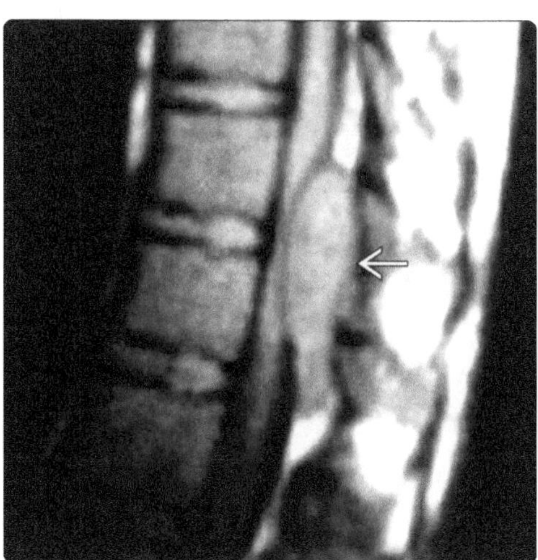

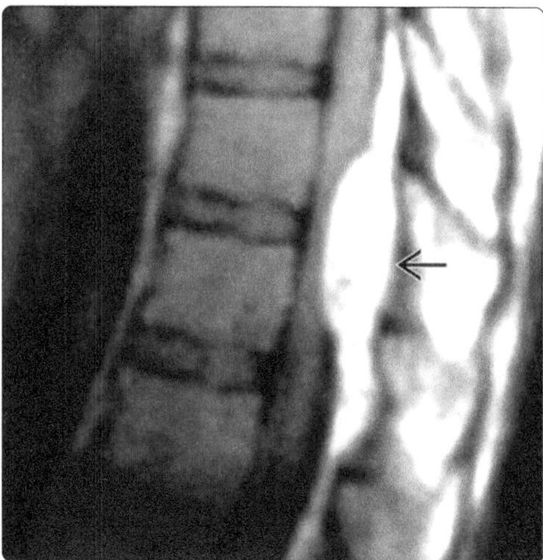

(Left) *Sagittal T1 MR depicts an ovoid, well-circumscribed, isointense epidural soft tissue mass* ➡ *compressing the distal thoracic cord. This is a typical appearance of EMH, presenting as an epidural soft tissue mass with myelopathy.* **(Right)** *Sagittal T1 C+ MR in the same patient confirms diffuse and intense enhancement of the epidural mass* ➡*.*

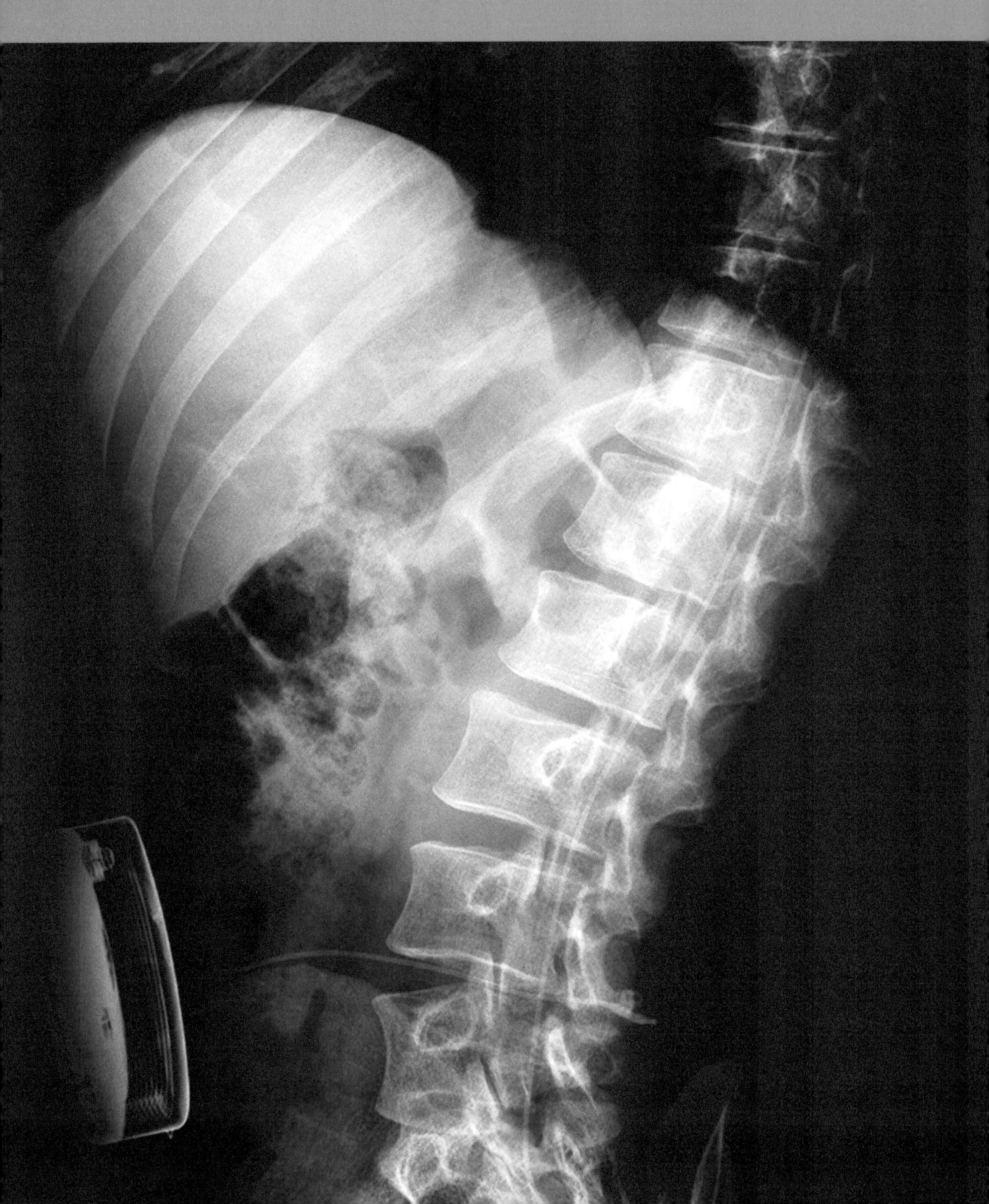

PART III
SECTION 6

Spine Postprocedural Imaging

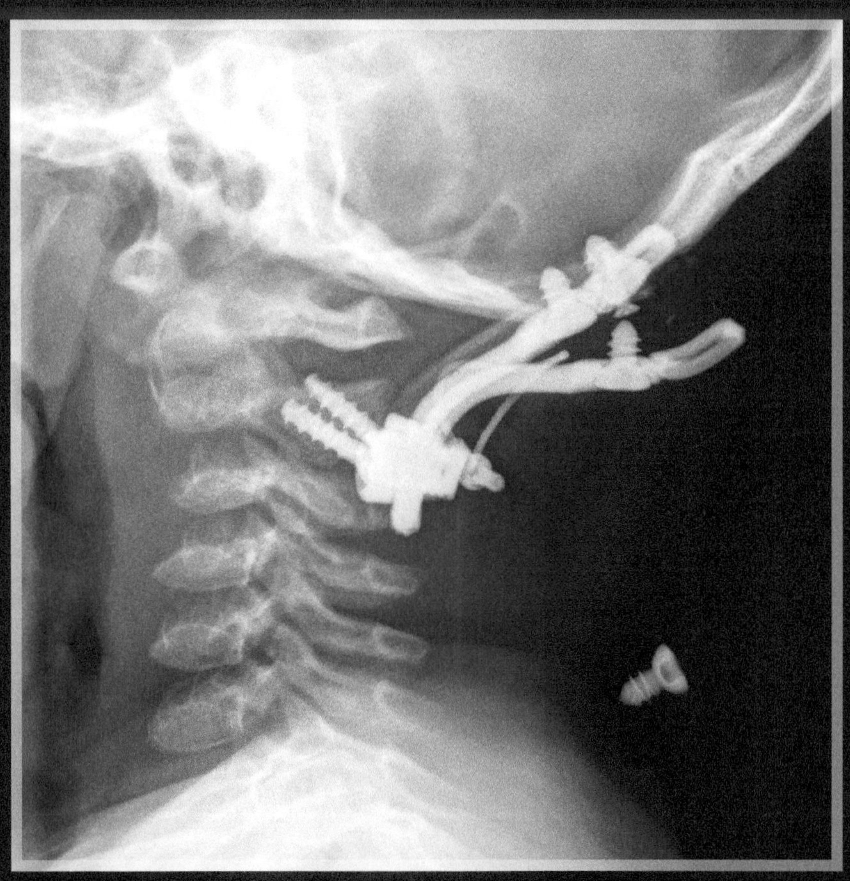

Hardware Failure

KEY FACTS

TERMINOLOGY

- Mechanical breakdown or malfunction of hardware

IMAGING

- Fractured or malpositioned metallic implant
- Lucency ± sclerosis along implant or at vertebral body-graft interface
- Adjacent levels may experience biomechanic stresses with resulting marrow edema and accelerated degenerative changes
- Plain films excellent in evaluating vertebral alignment, hardware integrity, fusion status
- Flexion-extension views if hardware failure present
- CT evaluation if implant breakage suspected but not definitive on radiography
  - Especially with complex constructs &/or in osteopenic patients
  - Enables accurate assessment of degree of osseous fusion; however, surgical exploration remains reference standard for evaluating fusion
- Soft tissue complications, marrow edema (suggesting segmental instability), or spinal cord injury

PATHOLOGY

- Fibrous union may provide satisfactory stability in absence of radiographic osseous fusion

CLINICAL ISSUES

- Pain, tenderness, radiculopathy

DIAGNOSTIC CHECKLIST

- Compare with multiple prior studies to identify subtle progressive changes
- Failed fusion may indicate unsuspected ligamentous injury in trauma or tumor recurrence or progression

(Left) *Lateral radiograph following craniovertebral junction fusion hardware failure (mucopolysaccharidosis type 1) demonstrates failure of 1 of the metal occipital surgical plates ➡, which has pulled out of the occipital bone. One of the fixation screws ➡ has migrated into the surgical wound.* **(Right)** *Sagittal bone CT in the same patient obtained for further clarification confirms that the fixation screws/plate ➡ have pulled away from the occipital bone. The proximal fixation screw in the C2 lateral mass ➡ is in expected position.*

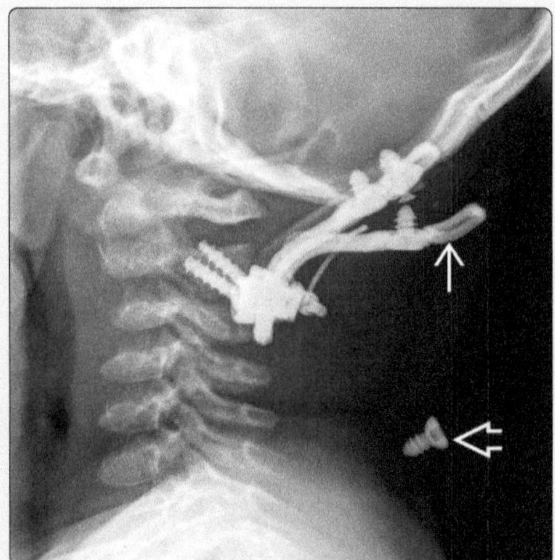

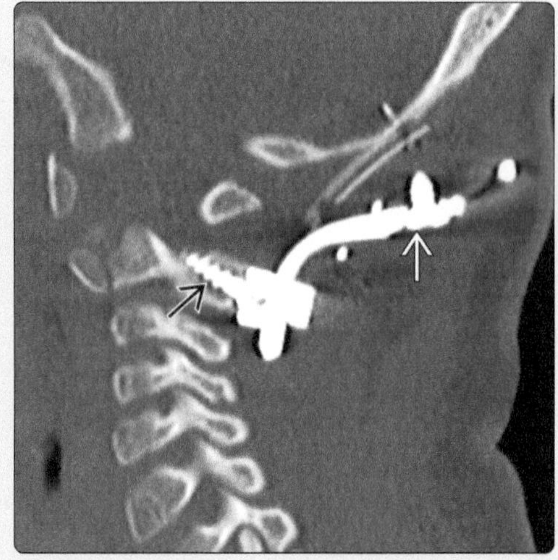

(Left) *Sagittal bone CT in the same patient confirms migration of the fixation screw ➡ in the midline surgical wound. The strut bone graft ➡ is in the proper place.* **(Right)** *Coronal bone CT in the same patient shows that not only has the fixation screws/plate ➡ pulled away from the occipital bone, but the paired strut grafts ➡ remain in the appropriate position.*

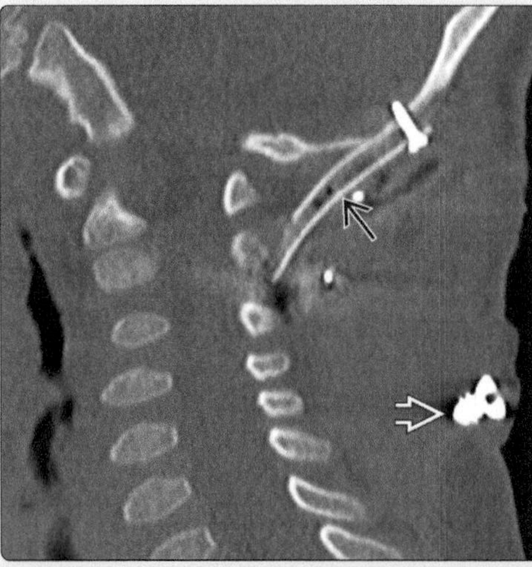

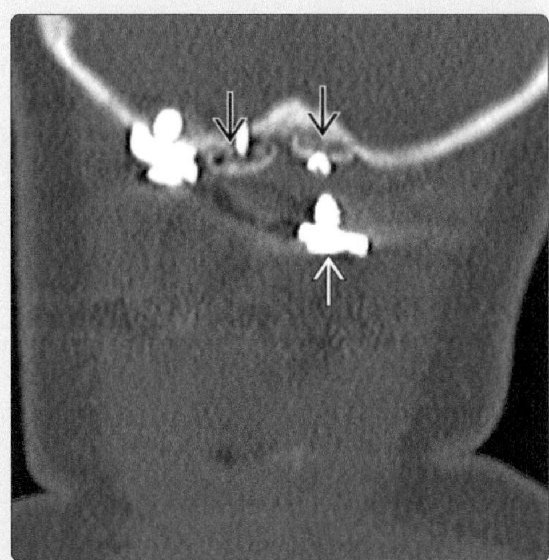

TERMINOLOGY

Synonyms

- Implant or prosthesis failure

Definitions

- Mechanical breakdown or malfunction of hardware
  - Pseudoarthrosis, subsidence

IMAGING

General Features

- Best diagnostic clue
  - Fractured or malpositioned metallic implant
  - Lucency ± sclerosis along implant or at vertebral body-graft interface
- Location
  - Any spinal segment where instrumentations occur
    - Adjacent levels may experience biomechanic stresses with resulting marrow edema and accelerated degenerative changes

Radiographic Findings

- Radiography
  - Cervical spine
    - Lucency along cannulated screw bridging type II odontoid fracture
    - Broken extruded screw
    - Fractured ventrally displaced plate
    - Dislodged allograft
    - Broken detached posterior cervical wire
  - Thoracolumbar and lumbosacral spine
    - Broken sublaminar or subpars wire
    - Bent, loose, or fractured pedicle screw
    - Disengaged hook
    - Broken dislodged rod
    - Intervertebral cage/allograft migration
  - Pseudoarthrosis
    - Lucency between bone graft and adjacent vertebra
    - Sclerosis and rounding of unfused bones
  - Development or progression of vertebral malalignment
  - Progressive graft collapse and increasing kyphosis

Fluoroscopic Findings

- Pseudoarthrosis on flexion/extension views
  - 4 mm of translation or > 10° of angular motion between adjacent vertebrae
    - Up to 3 mm of translation considered normal
  - ≥ 2 mm change in interspinous distance on flexion and extension

CT Findings

- Bone CT
  - Periimplant lucency (suggests loosening)
  - Overextension beyond posterior vertebral cortex by cervical bicortical screws
  - Medial cortex penetration by suboptimally placed lumbar pedicle screw
  - Occult osseous fractures
    - Altered biomechanics with fusion may result in adjacent level stress reaction
  - Osseous nonunion, pseudoarthrosis

MR Findings

- MR generally does not depict hardware location or integrity well
  - Nondiagnostic with extensive artifact from steel hardware
  - Titanium hardware produces less artifact
- MR useful for demonstrating impact on surrounding soft tissue and cord morphology
  - T2/STIR hyperintensity can be seen in adjacent level posterior elements due to stress reaction

Nuclear Medicine Findings

- Bone scan
  - Increased uptake at fusion site suggests nonunion
    - Nonspecific until 1 year after surgery
    - Fused segment should be "cold" after 6-12 months
    - Also useful for detecting infection

Imaging Recommendations

- Best imaging tool
  - Plain films excellent in evaluating vertebral alignment, hardware integrity, fusion status
    - Cost-effective
    - Flexion/extension views
    - Cannot be used to reliably exclude presence of bone metastases or of cauda equina compression
  - CT evaluation if implant breakage suspected but not definitive on radiography
    - Especially with complex constructs &/or in osteopenic patients
    - Enables accurate assessment of degree of osseous fusion; however, surgical exploration remains reference standard for evaluating fusion
  - MR to identify soft tissue complications, marrow edema, suggesting segmental instability, or spinal cord injury
- Protocol advice
  - MR techniques to minimize susceptibility artifact
    - Low magnetic field strength minimizes metal artifact
    - Fast spin-echo technique; avoid gradient-echo sequences
      - Higher receiver bandwidths, short echo time, small voxel
    - SE/FSE susceptibility artifact (signal loss and distortion) projects along frequency encoding direction
      - Frequency encoding direction should be chosen along long axis of hardware
  - Increasing kilovolt peaks/milliamperes to reduce beam hardening on CT

PATHOLOGY

General Features

- Etiology
  - Excessive stress loading on implant
    - Implant malpositioning at surgery
    - Gross spinal instability
    - Failed fusion with pseudoarthrosis
  - Poor bone quality
    - Periimplant bone resorption
    - Osteoporosis

- Osteomyelitis
- Residual or recurrent neoplasm
  - Multisegmental constructs
  - Unconstrained cervical fusion plates: Orozco, Casper
    - Screw not locked to plate with risk of screw extrusion
  - Risks of pseudoarthrosis
    - Comorbidities: Old age, smoking, obesity, diabetes
    - Multiple spine surgeries
    - Multilevel fusions
    - ≥ grade III anterolisthesis
  - Particle disease with disc prostheses
    - Particles resulting from wear debris cause macrophage activation and phagocytosis → joint loosening and implant failure
    - Well-defined, osteolytic, lesion-mimicking tumor
  - Bone morphogenic protein (BMP) in anterior cervical fusion procedures associated with higher complication rate
    - Primary increases seen in wound-related complications and dysphagia or hoarseness
  - BMP, particularly in transforaminal lumbar interbody fusion and posterior lumbar interbody fusion, associated with severe postoperative radiculitis
    - Proinflammatory reaction ± ectopic bone formation
- Associated abnormalities
  - Pseudoarthrosis, instability, fractures
  - Dural laceration, nerve injury
- Hardware intended to stabilize fusion construct while awaiting successful osseous fusion
  - All hardware eventually fails if fusion does not occur in timely fashion
  - Fusion rate improved with direct current electrical stimulation
  - Fusion occurs after 6-9 months, up to 18 months
- Fibrous union may provide satisfactory stability in absence of radiographic osseous fusion
  - Best confirmed with dynamic flexion-extension views

CLINICAL ISSUES

Presentation

- Most common signs/symptoms
  - May be incidental finding
- Other signs/symptoms
  - Pain, weakness, paresthesia, radiculopathy
  - Dysphagia/esophageal perforation due to cervical plate migration
- Clinical profile
  - Hardware failure in early postoperative period
    - Indication of continued gross spinal instability
  - Development or progression of neurologic symptoms
    - Osseous nonunion &/or hardware failure should be suspected

Demographics

- Epidemiology
  - 2-45% reoperation rate for implant failure
  - Hardware failure in scoliosis surgery
    - 31% with anterior approach
    - 1% with posterior approach
  - Unconstrained cervical fusion system
    - 22-46% failure rate vs. 18% in constrained system
  - Lumbar fusion with unconstrained pedicle screw system
    - 22% failure rate
      - 75% due to pseudoarthrosis

Natural History & Prognosis

- Osseous fusion may be expected even if hardware fails
  - Broken hardware need not be removed if spine clinically, radiographically stable
- Fibrous union without radiographic osseous fusion may be satisfactory
  - Best demonstrated on dynamic flexion-extension views
- Repeat surgical fusion may be necessary
  - Especially if hardware failure occurs early

Treatment

- Conservative observation
- Surgical revision to prevent nonunion and instability

DIAGNOSTIC CHECKLIST

Consider

- Consulting references describing expected hardware appearance
- Important to understand hardware commonly used at your institution

Image Interpretation Pearls

- Important not only to evaluate hardware failure but also to look for complicating instability or osseous fracture
- Important to consider original indication for fusion in suspected implant failure
  - Failed fusion for trauma may indicate unsuspected ligamentous injury
  - Failed fusion for neoplasm may indicate tumor recurrence or progression

Reporting Tips

- Important to compare current radiographs with multiple previous studies to identify subtle progressive changes (e.g., in spinal alignment and in position of hardware devices)

SELECTED REFERENCES

1. Ayers R et al: Laser marking of spine rods is strongly associated with risk of clinical rod failure. J Am Acad Orthop Surg. 30(2):e252-63, 2022
2. Luna LP et al: Imaging evaluation of the spinal hardware: what residents and fellows need to know. Curr Probl Diagn Radiol. 50(5):675-86, 2021
3. Song KJ et al: Prognosis of hardware-related problems in anterior cervical discectomy and fusion with cage and plate constructs. World Neurosurg. 134:e249-55, 2020
4. Winegar BA et al: Update on imaging of spinal fixation hardware. Semin Musculoskelet Radiol. 23(2):e56-79, 2019
5. Sellin JN et al: Feasibility and safety of using thoracic and lumbar cortical bone trajectory pedicle screws in spinal constructs in children: technical note. J Neurosurg Pediatr. 21(2):190-6, 2018
6. Singh B et al: Laminar screw fixation of the axis in the pediatric population: a series of eight patients. Spine J. 15(2):e17-25, 2015
7. Mazur MD et al: Avoiding early complications and reoperation during occipitocervical fusion in pediatric patients. J Neurosurg Pediatr. 14(5):465-75, 2014
8. Petscavage-Thomas JM et al: Imaging current spine hardware: part 1, cervical spine and fracture fixation. AJR Am J Roentgenol. 203(2):394-405, 2014
9. Botolin S et al: Aseptic loosening of pedicle screw as a result of metal wear debris in a pediatric patient. Spine (Phila Pa 1976). 38(1):E38-42, 2013
10. Rutherford EE et al: Lumbar spine fusion and stabilization: hardware, techniques, and imaging appearances. Radiographics. 27(6):1737-49, 2007

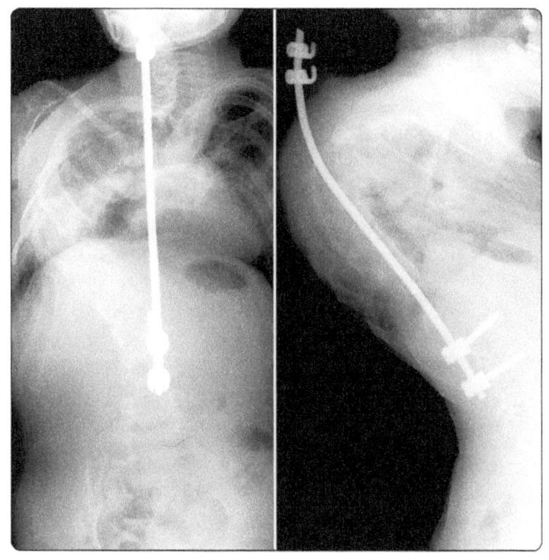

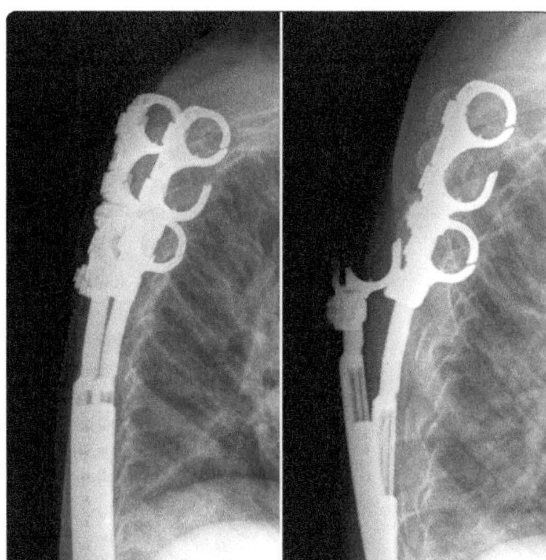

(Left) *AP (left) and lateral (right) radiographs in a patient with neurofibromatosis type 1 who presented with back pain and protrusion of hardware through the back skin are shown. Note that diagnosis is difficult on the frontal radiograph but straightforward on the lateral radiograph.* **(Right)** *Lateral composite radiograph (neuromuscular scoliosis) shows posterior spinal fusion hardware on an asymptomatic clinic visit (left) and after presentation with broken hardware protruding through the skin (right).*

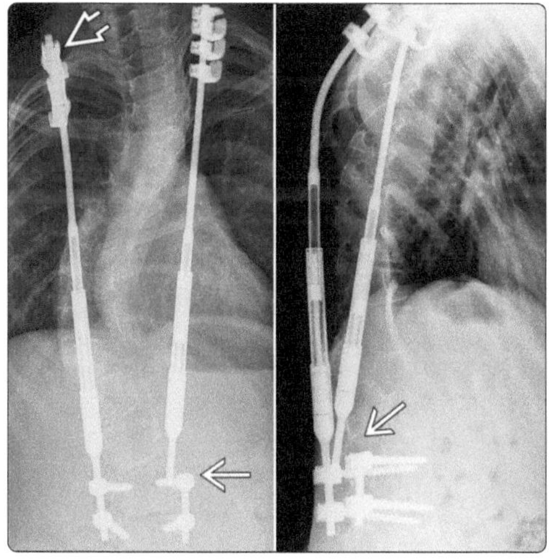

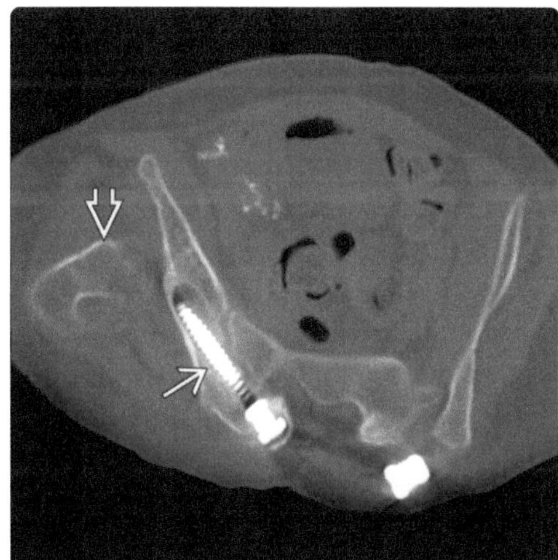

(Left) *AP (left) and lateral (right) radiographs of the thoracic spine show 2 separate areas of hardware failure. The left rod has fractured ➡ with displacement, and the rostral right hook ➡ has dislodged from the ribs.* **(Right)** *Axial bone CT demonstrates lucency surrounding a right sacral fixation screw ➡. Bone loss is greater near the tip, indicating that the screw is toggling back and forth. Incidentally, the right femoral head ➡ is posteriorly and superiorly dislocated and pseudoarticulates with the right iliac wing.*

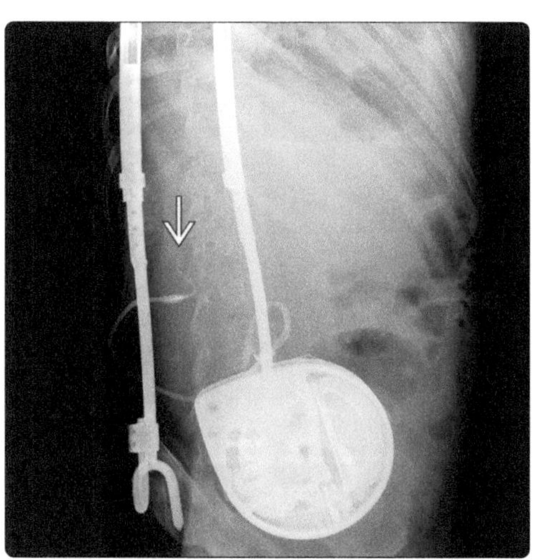

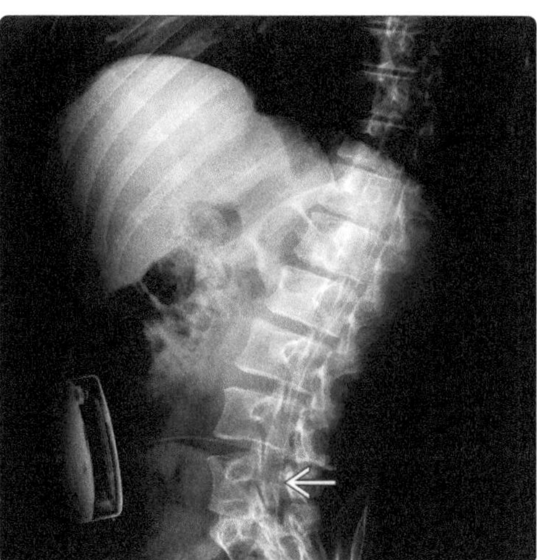

(Left) *Lateral radiograph obtained for Baclofen pump failure shows that the intrathecal catheter ➡ has fractured and resides outside the spinal canal. The remainder of the catheter migrated within the thecal sac (not shown).* **(Right)** *Lateral radiograph obtained for Baclofen pump failure shows that the intrathecal catheter has fractured within the thecal sac with caudal migration of the distal fragment ➡.*

INDEX

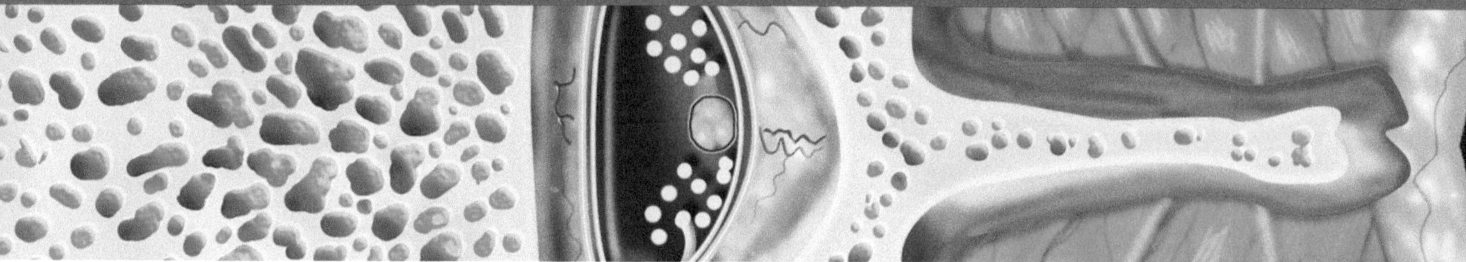

A

INDEX

INDEX

INDEX

INDEX

INDEX

INDEX

INDEX

C

INDEX

INDEX

INDEX

INDEX

D

INDEX

INDEX

E

INDEX

INDEX

F

G

H

INDEX

INDEX

INDEX

I

INDEX

INDEX

INDEX

J

INDEX

K

L

INDEX

M

INDEX

INDEX

INDEX

N

INDEX

O

P

INDEX

Q

R

S

INDEX

INDEX

INDEX

INDEX

T

INDEX

U

V

W

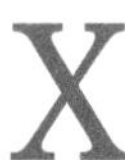

X

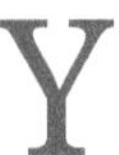

Y

Z